BRIEF CONTENTS

UNIT 1 Children, Their Families, and the Nurse

UNIT 2 Assessment of the Child and Family

UNIT 3 Family-Centered Care of the Newborn

UNIT 4 Family-Centered Care of the Infant

UNIT 5 Family-Centered Care of the Young Child

UNIT 6 Family-Centered Care of the School-Age Child and Adolescent

UNIT 7 Family-Centered Care of the Child With Special Needs

UNIT 8 The Child Who Is Hospitalized

UNIT 9 The Child With Problems Related to the Transfer of Oxygen and Nutrients

UNIT 10 The Child With Problems Related to the Production and Circulation of Blood

UNIT 11 The Child With a Disturbance of Regulatory Mechanisms

UNIT 12 The Child With a Problem That Interferes With Physical Mobility

WONG'S ESSENTIALS OF PEDIATRIC NURSING

ELEVENTH EDITION

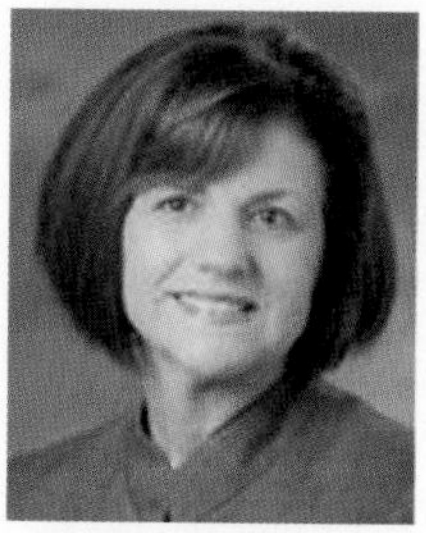

Marilyn J. Hockenberry, PhD, RN, PPCNP-BC, FAAN
Professor of Pediatrics
Baylor College of Medicine
Director, Global HOPE Nursing
Texas Children's Hospital
Houston, Texas
Bessie Baker Professor Emerita of Nursing
Chair, Duke Institutional Review Board
Duke University
Durham, North Carolina

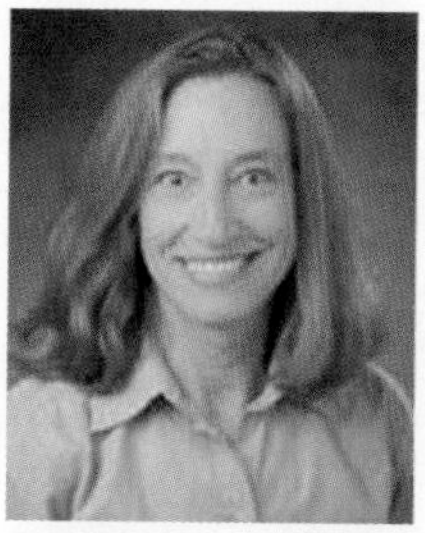

Cheryl C. Rodgers, PhD, RN, CPNP, CPON (deceased)
Associate Professor
Duke University School of Nursing
Durham, North Carolina

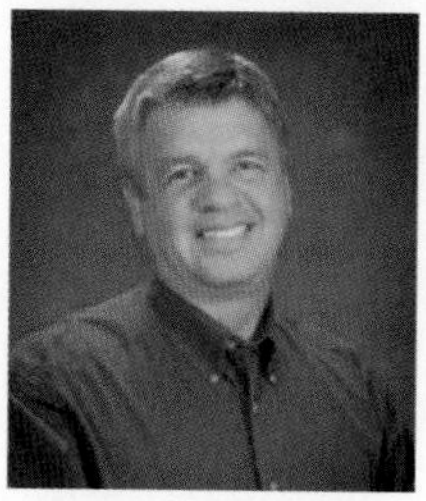

David Wilson, MS, RNC-NIC (deceased)
Staff
Children's Hospital at Saint Francis
Tulsa, Oklahoma

ELSEVIER

Elsevier
3251 Riverport Lane
St. Louis, Missouri 63043

WONG'S ESSENTIALS OF PEDIATRIC NURSING, ELEVENTH EDITION ISBN: 978-0-323-62419-0

Notice

Practitioners and researchers must always rely on their own experience and knowledge in evaluating and using any information, methods, compounds or experiments described herein. Because of rapid advances in the medical sciences, in particular, independent verification of diagnoses and drug dosages should be made. To the fullest extent of the law, no responsibility is assumed by Elsevier, authors, editors or contributors for any injury and/or damage to persons or property as a matter of products liability, negligence or otherwise, or from any use or operation of any methods, products, instructions, or ideas contained in the material herein.

Previous editions copyrighted 2017, 2013, 2009, 2005, 2001, 1997, 1993, 1989, 1985, 1982.

Library of Congress Control Number: 2020952261

Content Strategist: Sandra Clark
Senior Content Development Specialist: Heather Bays-Petrovic
Publishing Services Manager: Julie Eddy
Senior Project Managers: Tracey Schriefer and Rachel E. McMullen
Design Direction: Maggie Reid
Chapter Opener Art: © iStockphoto.com

Printed in Canada

Last digit is the print number: 9 8 7 6 5 4 3 2 1

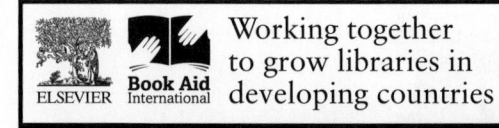

CONTRIBUTORS

Caroline E. Anderson, MSN, RN, CPHON
Clinical Practice & Advanced Education Specialist
Organizational & Professional Development
Cook Children's Health Care System
Fort Worth, Texas

Annette L. Baker, RN, BSN, MSN, CPNP
Nurse Practitioner
Cardiovascular Program/Kawasaki Team
Boston Children's Hospital
Boston, Massachusetts

Rose Ann U. Baker, PhD, PMHCNS-BC
Assistant Lecturer
School of Nursing
College of Health Professions
University of Akron
Akron, Ohio

Amy Barry, RN, MSN, CPNP
Pediatric Nurse Practitioner
Cancer Immunotherapy Program
Children's Hospital of Philadelphia
Philadelphia, Pennsylvania

Heather Bastardi, RN, MSN, CPNP, CCTC
Nurse Practitioner
Advanced Cardiac Therapies
Boston Children's Hospital
Boston, Massachusetts

Rosalind Bryant, PhD, RN, PPCNP-BC
Clinical Instructor
Baylor College of Medicine
Houston, Texas

Alice M. Burch, DNP, MSN-Ed, BSN
Assistant Professor
Nursing
Adams State University
Alamosa, Colorado

Lisa M. Cleveland, PhD, RN, CPNP, IBCLC, FAAN
Associate Professor
School of Nursing
UT Health San Antonio
San Antonio, Texas;, Adjunct Associate Professor
Institute for Interdisciplinary Salivary Bioscience Research
University of California at Irvine
Irvine, California

Erin Connelly, BBA, BSN, MSN
Pediatric Nurse Practitioner
Hematology/Oncology
Children's Healthcare of Atlanta
Atlanta, Georgia

Elizabeth A. Duffy, DNP, RN, CPNP
Clinical Assistant Professor
Health Behavior and Biological Sciences
The University of Michigan School of Nursing
Ann Arbor, Michigan

Kimberley Ann Fisher, PhD
Director, Neonatal Perinatal Research Unit
Pediatrics;
Clinical Associate Faculty
School of Medicine;
Clinical Associate Faculty
School of Nursing
Duke University
Durham, North Carolina;, Director, Neonatal Perinatal Research Unit
School of Medicine
Duke University
Durham, North Carolina

R. Elizabeth Fisher, DNP, APRN, CPNP AC/PC, CPON
Lecturer/Clinical Faculty
School of Nursing
Clemson University
Clemson, South Carolina;, Nurse Practitioner
Pediatric Hematology/Oncology
Greenville Health Systems
Greenville, South Carolina;, Nurse Practitioner
Pediatric Hematology/Oncology
Children's Healthcare of Atlanta
Atlanta, Georgia

Jan M. Foote, DNP, ARNP, CPNP, FAANP
Pediatric Nurse Practitioner
Pediatric Endocrinology
Blank Children's Hospital
Des Moines, Iowa;
Clinical Associate Professor
College of Nursing
The University of Iowa
Iowa City, Iowa

Melody Hellsten, DNP, MSN, MS
Associate Director
Pediatric Hematology Oncology Palliative Care Program
Pediatrics
Texas Children's Hospital
Houston, Texas

Ruth Anne Herring, MSN, RN, CPNP-AC/PC, CPHON
Pediatric Nurse Practitioner
Center for Cancer & Blood Disorders
Children's Health
Dallas, Texas

Joy Hesselgrave, MSN, RN, CPON, CHPPN
Assistant Clinical Director
Palliative Care
Texas Children's Hospital
Houston, Texas

Maryellen S. Kelly, DNP, CPNP
Clinical Associate
School of Nursing;
Pediatric Nurse Practitioner
Division of Urology
Department of Surgery
Duke University
Durham, North Carolina

Patricia McElfresh, PNP-BC
PNP Manager of Advanced Practice Providers
Pediatric Hematology Oncology
Children's Healthcare of Atlanta
Atlanta, Georgia

Tara Taneski Merck, RN, MS, CPNP, APNP
Director, Advanced Practice Providers
Children's Specialty Group
Medical College of Wisconsin
Milwaukee, Wisconsin

Kristina Miller, DNP, RN, PCNS-BC, CNE
Assistant Professor
Maternal Child Nursing
University of South Alabama
Mobile, Alabama

Mary Mondozzi, MSN, BSN, WCC
Burn Center Education/Outreach Coordinator
The Paul and Carol David Foundation Burn Institute
Akron Children's Hospital
Akron, Ohio

Rebecca A. Monroe, MSN, APRN, CPNP
Pediatric Nurse Practitioner
Frisco, Texas

Tadala Mulemba, BSN
Global HOPE Nursing
Baylor College of Medicine–Global HOPE Malawi
Lilongwe, Malawi

Patricia O'Brien, MSN, CPNP-AC, FAHA
Nurse Practitioner
Department of Nursing/Patient Services, Cardiovascular Program
Boston Children's Hospital
Boston, Massachusetts

Kathie Prihoda, RN, MSN, DNP
Assistant Professor
Nursing
Rutgers University
Camden, New Jersey

Cynthia A. Prows, BSN, MSN, APRN
Clinical Nurse Specialist
Human Genetics and Patient Services
Children's Hospital Medical Center
Cincinnati, Ohio

Mpho Raletshegwana, BSN, RN
Global HOPE Nursing
Baylor College of Medicine–Global HOPE Malawi
Lilongwe, Malawi

Kathleen S. Ruccione, PhD, MPH, RN, CPON, FAAN
Department Chair of Doctoral Programs and Associate Professor
Azusa Pacific University
Azusa, California

Gina Santucci, MSN, FNP, APN-BC
Nurse Practitioner
Palliative Care
Texas Children's Hospital
Houston, Texas

Margaret L. Schroeder, MSN, BSN, BA, RN, PPCNP-BC
Pediatric Nurse Practitioner
Cardiac Surgery
Boston Children's Hospital
Boston, Massachusetts

Micah Skeens, PhD, RN, CPNP
Nurse Scientist
Research
Nationwide Children's Hospital
Columbus, Ohio

Laura Tillman, DNP, APRN, CPNP
Pediatric Orthopedic Nurse Practitioner
Orthopedics
Gillette Children's Specialty Healthcare
Saint Paul, Minnesota

Caroline C. Weeks, BS, BA, RDN, LD
Registered Dietitian
Division of Endocrinology
Mayo Clinic Children's Center
Rochester, Minnesota

REVIEWERS

Joy Hesselgrave, MSN, RN, CPON, CHPPN
Assistant Clinical Director of Palliative Care
Texas Children's Hospital
Houston, Texas

Christine B. Kavanagh, RN, DNP, PPCNP-BC
Assistant Professor
School of Nursing and Health Sciences
Pennsylvania College of Technology
Williamsport, Pennsylvania

Jill M. Krell, DNP, MSN, BSN, RN
Assistant Professor
Traditional Undergraduate Program
Concordia University, Wisconsin
Mequon, Wisconsin

Carmella Mikol, PhD, RN-BC, CNE, CPNP-PC, ANEF
Professor and Department Chair
Nursing
College of Lake County
Grayslake, Illinois

Gina Santucci, MSN, FNP
Palliative Care
Texas Children's Hospital
Houston, Texas

Katherine M. Schafer, MSN, APRN, PCNS-BC, CCRN
Instructor Clinical Nurse Specialist
Women, Children, and Family Nursing
Rush University College of Nursing
Rush University Medical Center
Chicago, Illinois

Felisa Smith, RN, BSN, MSA, MSN/Ed, CNE
Acting Accelerated BSN Program Coordinator
Nursing and Allied Health
Norfolk State University
Norfolk, Virginia

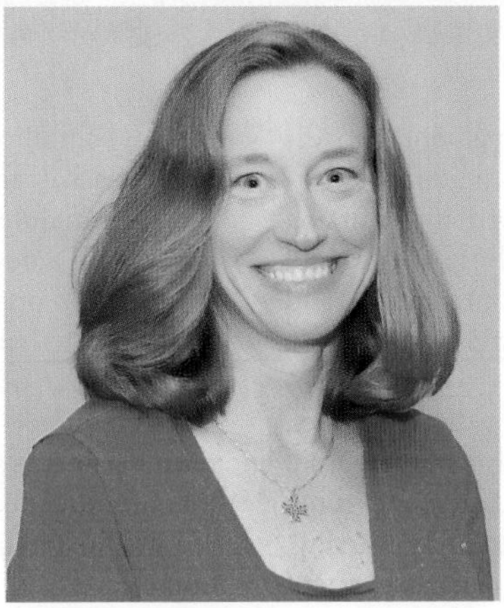

It is with great sadness that we announce the passing of Dr. Cheryl Rodgers on July 7, 2018, following a tragic accident. Cheryl was an exemplary nurse practitioner, educator, and leader in the field of pediatric nursing. Cheryl was an Associate Professor at the Duke University School of Nursing, and she held national leadership positions in the Children's Oncology Group Nursing Discipline and the Association of Pediatric Hematology Nurses. She served on the *Journal of Pediatric Oncology Nursing* Editorial Board, led several funded research studies, authored numerous impactful publications, and had just been selected for induction as a Fellow in the American Academy of Nursing, the profession's highest honor. Her devotion to pediatric nursing education served her well as a Wong textbook editor, and she will be greatly missed. Most important, Cheryl was an outstanding role model and a treasured mentor to so many pediatric nurses; her loss will be felt broadly and deeply throughout the profession.

PREFACE

Wong's Essentials of Pediatric Nursing has been a leading book in pediatric nursing since it was first published. This 11th edition continues its tradition of being an essential resource for pediatric nursing and continues the legacy of Donna Wong, David Wilson, and Cheryl Rodgers, our beloved colleagues. We hold dear their contributions and our memories of their pursuit of excellence in all they did for the Wong textbooks.

To accomplish this, Marilyn J. Hockenberry, as editor-in-chief, and many expert nurses and multidisciplinary specialists have revised, rewritten, or authored portions of the text on areas that are undergoing rapid and complex change. These areas include community nursing, development, immunizations, genetics, home care, pain assessment and management, high-risk newborn care, adolescent health issues, end-of-life care, and numerous pediatric diseases. We have carefully preserved aspects of the book that have met with universal acceptance: its state-of-the-art, research-based information; its strong, integrated focus on the family and community; its logical and user-friendly organization; and its easy-to-read style.

We have tried to meet the increasing demands of faculty and students to teach and to learn in an environment characterized by rapid change, enormous amounts of information, fewer traditional clinical facilities, and less time.

This text encourages students to *think critically.* We have added more case studies that discuss clinical scenarios, allowing the student to visualize how the care plan develops as a clinical situation evolves over time. The Critical Thinking Case Studies are revised and begin with a short case that provides enough details for the student to understand the clinical problem. Questions specific to the initial assessment are asked, and clinical reasoning is emphasized by asking what nursing interventions are important. Teaching points are included with each case study to summarize why specific nursing actions are warranted. Pediatric quality indicators from the 2019 Core Set of Children's Health Care Quality Measures are updated and added throughout the book.

Revised evidence-based practice boxes include the latest knowledge crucial for nurses to practice using quality and safety competencies. Competencies included in the evidence-based practice boxes are designed specifically for prelicensed nurses and are from the Quality and Safety Education for Nurses website.

This text also serves as a reference manual for practicing nurses. The latest recommendations have been included from authoritative organizations such as the American Academy of Pediatrics, the Centers for Disease Control and Prevention, the Institute of Medicine, the Agency for Healthcare Research and Quality, the American Pain Society, the American Nurses Association, and the National Association of Pediatric Nurse Associates and Practitioners. To expand the universe of available information, websites and email addresses have been included for hundreds of organizations and other educational resources.

ORGANIZATION OF THE BOOK

The same general approach to the presentation of content has been preserved from the first edition, although some content has been added, condensed, and rearranged within this framework to improve the flow; minimize duplication; and emphasize health care trends, such as home and community care. The book is divided into two broad parts. The first part of the book, Chapters 1 through 16, follow what is sometimes called the "age and stage" approach, considering infancy, childhood, and adolescence from a developmental context. It emphasizes the importance of the nurse's role in health promotion and maintenance and in considering the family as the focus of care. From a developmental perspective, the care of common health problems is presented, giving readers a sense of the normal problems expected in otherwise healthy children and demonstrating when in the course of childhood these problems are most likely to occur. The remainder of the book, Chapters 17 through 31, presents the more serious health problems of infancy, childhood, and adolescence that are not specific to any particular age-group and that frequently require hospitalization, major medical and nursing intervention, and home care.

UNIT ONE (Chapters 1 through 3) provides a longitudinal view of the child as an individual on a continuum of developmental changes from birth through adolescence and as a member of a family unit maturing within a culture and a community. The latest discussion of morbidity and mortality in infancy and childhood is presented, and child health care is examined from a historical perspective. Because unintentional injury is one of the leading causes of death in children, an overview of this topic is included. In this edition, the critical components of evidence-based practice are presented to provide the template for exploring the latest pediatric nursing research or practice guidelines throughout the book. Quality nursing care is also emphasized, and this sets the stage for quality outcome measures that are included for specific problems in many of the chapters. This book is about families with children, and the philosophy of family-centered care is emphasized. This book is also about providing atraumatic care—care that minimizes the psychologic and physical stress that health promotion and illness treatment can inflict.

In this Unit, the philosophy of delivering nursing care is addressed. We believe strongly that children and families need consistent caregivers. Establishing the therapeutic relationship with the child and family is explored as the essential foundation for providing quality nursing care. Important information is presented on the family, social and cultural, and religious influences on child health promotion. The content clearly describes the role of the nurse, with emphasis on cultural and religious sensitivity and competent care.

Unit One includes discussion of the developmental and genetic influences on child health, continues to provide the latest information on genetics, and also focuses on a theoretic approach to personality development and learning.

UNIT TWO (Chapters 4 to 6) contains guidelines for communicating with children, adolescents, and their families, as well as a detailed description of a health assessment, including discussion of family assessment, nutritional assessment, and sexual history. Content on communication techniques is outlined to provide a concise format for reference. A comprehensive approach to physical examination and developmental assessment is included, with updated material on temperature measurement and body mass index–for-age guidelines. Critical aspects of assessment and management of pain in children is found in this Unit. Although the literature on pain assessment and management in children has grown considerably, this knowledge has not been widely applied in practice. Common infectious diseases occur in children, and the importance of infection control is emphasized with a review of the various bacterial and viral infections encountered in childhood. Hospital-acquired infections, childhood communicable disease, and immunizations are also discussed. Coronavirus disease (COVID 19) is added to the infectious diseases chapter.

UNIT THREE (Chapters 7 and 8) stresses the importance of the neonatal period in relation to child survival during the first few months and the impact on health in later life. Several topics in this Unit have been revised to reflect current issues, especially regarding the educational needs of the family during the infant's transition to extrauterine life as well as the recognition of newborn problems in the first few weeks of life. The nurse's role in caring for the high-risk newborn is stressed, as is the importance of astute observations to the survival of this vulnerable group of infants. Modern advances in neonatal care have mandated extensive revision with a greater sensitivity to the diverse needs of infants, from those with extremely low birth weights, to those born late-preterm, to those of normal gestational age who have difficulty making an effective transition to extrauterine life.

UNITS FOUR through SIX (Chapters 9 through 16) present the major developmental stages outlined in Unit One, which are expanded to provide a broader concept of these stages and the health problems most often associated with each age-group. Special emphasis is placed on preventive aspects of care. The chapters on health promotion follow a standard approach that is used consistently for each age-group. The influence of nutrition in preschool-age and school-age children (especially decreasing fat intake) in relation to later chronic diseases such as obesity and hypertension has been revised. The importance of safety promotion and injury prevention in relation to each age-group is included in these chapters as well.

The chapters on health problems in these units primarily reflect more typical and age-related concerns. The information on many disorders has been revised to reflect recent changes. Examples include sudden infant death syndrome, lead poisoning, severe acute malnutrition, burns, attention-deficit/hyperactivity disorder, contraception, teenage pregnancy, and sexually transmitted infections. The chapters on adolescence include the latest information on substance abuse, adolescent immunizations, and the impact of adolescent nutrition on cardiovascular health.

UNIT SEVEN (Chapters 17 and 18) deals with children who have the same developmental needs as growing children but who, because of congenital or acquired physical, cognitive, or sensory impairment, require alternative interventions to facilitate development. Current trends in the care of families and children with chronic illness or disability, such as providing home care, normalizing children's lives, focusing on developmental needs, enabling and empowering families, and promoting early intervention, are included. This Unit highlights common fears experienced by the child and family and includes discussion of symptom management and nurses' reactions to caring for dying children.

The content on cognitive or sensory impairment includes important updates on the definition and classification of cognitive impairment. Autism spectrum disorders are discussed to provide a cohesive overview of cognitive and sensory impairments.

UNIT EIGHT (Chapters 19 and 20) is concerned with the impact of hospitalization on the child and family and presents a comprehensive overview of the stressors imposed by hospitalization and discusses nursing interventions to prevent or eliminate them. New research on short-stay or outpatient admissions addresses preparing children for these experiences. The effects of illness and hospitalization on children at specific ages and the effects on their development are updated. Revised Evidence-Based Practice boxes that include Quality and Safety Education for Nurses competencies are designed to provide rationales for the interventions discussed. A major focus is the evidence related to preparation of the child for procedures commonly performed by nurses.

UNITS NINE through TWELVE (Chapters 21 through 31) consider serious health problems of infants and children primarily from the biologic systems orientation, which has the practical organizational value of permitting health problems and nursing considerations to relate to specific pathophysiologic disturbances. The most common serious diseases in children are reviewed in these chapters. A section on the multisystem inflammatory syndrome (MIS-C) that is seen in children exposed to COVID-19 has been added.

UNIFYING PRINCIPLES

Several unifying principles have guided the organizational structure of this book since its inception. These principles continue to strengthen the book with each revision to produce a text that is consistent in approach throughout each chapter.

The Family as the Unit of Care

The child is an essential member of the family unit. We refer to parents in this book as a mother and/or father but recognize that parents include of a variety of individuals and do not undervalue the importance of any parent role or family structure.

Nursing care is most effective when it is delivered with the belief that *the family is the patient.* This belief permeates the book. When a child is healthy, the child's health is enhanced when the family is a fully functioning, health-promoting system. The family unit can be manifested in a myriad of structures; each has the potential to provide a caring, supportive environment in which the child can grow, mature, and maximize his or her human potential. In addition to integrating family-centered care in every chapter, an entire chapter is devoted to understanding the family as the focus in children's lives, including the social, cultural, and religious influences that affect family beliefs. Separate sections in another chapter deal in depth with family communication and family assessment. The impact of illness and hospitalization, home care, community care, and the death of a child are covered extensively in additional chapters. The needs of the family are emphasized throughout the text under Nursing Care Management in a separate section on family support. Numerous Family-Centered Care boxes are included to assist nurses in understanding and providing helpful information to families.

An Integrated Approach to Development

Children are not small adults but special individuals with unique minds, bodies, and needs. No book on pediatric nursing is complete without extensive coverage of communication, nutrition, play, safety, dental care, sexuality, sleep, self-esteem, and, of course, parenting. Nurses promote the healthy expression of all of these dimensions of personhood and need to understand how these functions are expressed by different children at different developmental ages and stages. Effective parenting depends on knowledge of development, and it is often the nurse's responsibility to provide parents with a developmental awareness of their children's needs. For these reasons, coverage of the many dimensions of childhood is integrated within the growth and development chapters rather than being presented in separate chapters. For example, safety concerns for a toddler are much different from those for an adolescent. Sleep needs change with age, as do nutritional needs. As a result, the units on each stage of childhood contain complete information on all of these functions as they relate to the specific age. In the unit on school-age children, for instance, information is presented on nutritional needs, age-appropriate play and its significance, safety concerns characteristic of the age-group, appropriate dental care, sleep characteristics, and means of promoting self-esteem—a particularly significant concern for school-age children. The challenges of being the parent of a school-age child are presented, and interventions that nurses can use to promote healthy parenting are suggested. Using the integrated approach, students gain an appreciation for the unique characteristics and needs of children at every age and stage of development.

Focus on Wellness and Illness: Child, Family, and Community

In a pediatric nursing text, a focus on illness is expected. Children become ill, and nurses typically are involved in helping children get well. However, it is not sufficient to prepare nursing students to care primarily for sick children. First, health is more than the absence of disease. Being healthy is being whole in mind, body, and spirit. Therefore most of the first half of the book is devoted to discussions that promote physical, emotional, psychosocial, mental, and spiritual wellness. Much emphasis is placed on anticipatory guidance of parents to prevent injury or illness in their children. Second, health care is more than ever prevention focused. The objectives set forth in the *Healthy People 2030* report clearly establish a health care agenda in which solutions to medical and social problems lie in preventive strategies. Third, health care is moving from acute care settings to the community, the home, short-stay centers, and clinics. Nurses must be prepared to function in all settings. To be successful, they must understand the pathophysiology, diagnosis, and treatment of health conditions. Competent nursing care flows from this knowledge and is enhanced by an awareness of childhood development, family dynamics, and communication skills.

Nursing Care

Although the information in this text incorporates information from numerous disciplines (medicine, pathophysiology, pharmacology, nutrition, psychology, sociology), its primary purpose is to provide information on the nursing care of children and families. Discussions of all disorders conclude with a section on Nursing Care Management. In addition, 14 care plans are included. Taken together, they cover the nursing care for many childhood diseases, disorders, and conditions. The purposes of the care plans, like every other feature of the book, are to teach and to convey information. The care plans are designed to stimulate critical thinking and to encourage the student to individualize outcomes and interventions for the child rather than to provide an extensive picture of all nursing diagnoses, outcomes, and interventions for every given disease or condition.

Culturally Competent Care

Increasing cultural diversity in the United States requires nurses caring for children and their families to develop expertise in the care of children from numerous backgrounds. Culturally competent nursing care requires more than acquiring knowledge about ethnic and cultural groups. It encompasses not only awareness of the influence of culture on the child and family but also the ability to intervene appropriately and effectively. The nurse must learn objective skills to focus on the child's, family's, and community's cultural characteristics. The nurse's self-awareness of unique personal cultural backgrounds must be acknowledged in order to understand how they contribute to cross-cultural communication. The importance of the environment of a cross-cultural care setting must be considered when providing clinical nursing care to culturally diverse families. This edition provides numerous learning experiences that examine cross-cultural communication, cultural assessment, cultural interpretation, and appropriate nursing interventions.

The Critical Role of Research and Evidence-Based Practice

This 11th edition is the product of an extensive review of the literature published since the book was last revised. Many readers and researchers have come to rely on the copious references that reflect significant contributions from a broad audience of professionals. To ensure that information is accurate and current, most citations are less than 5 years old, and almost every chapter has entries dated within 1 year of publication. This book reflects the art and science of pediatric nursing. A central goal in every revision is to base care on research rather than on tradition. Evidence-based practice produces measurable outcomes that nurses can use to validate their unique role in the health care system. Throughout the book, Evidence-Based Practice boxes reflect the importance of the science of nursing care.

SPECIAL FEATURES

Much effort has been directed toward making this book easy to teach from and, more important, easy to learn from. In this edition, the following features have been included to benefit educators, students, and practitioners.

APPLYING EVIDENCE TO PRACTICE boxes are new specialty boxes throughout the text outlining up-to-date procedures to show best practice and focus on applying evidence.

ATRAUMATIC CARE boxes emphasize the importance of providing competent care without creating undue physical and psychologic distress. Although many of the boxes provide suggestions for managing pain, atraumatic care also considers approaches to promoting self-esteem and preventing embarrassment.

CONCEPTS have been added to the beginning of each chapter to focus student attention on unique principles found in each chapter as well as to aid students who are using concept-based curriculum, system-focused curriculum, or a hybrid approach.

COMMUNITY FOCUS boxes address issues that expand to the community, such as increasing immunization rates, preventing lead poisoning, and decreasing smoking among teens.

CRITICAL THINKING CASE STUDIES ask the nurse to examine the evidence, consider the assumptions, establish priorities, and evaluate alternative perspectives regarding each patient situation. Answers to the Case Studies are provided within the box.

CULTURAL CONSIDERATIONS boxes integrate concepts of culturally sensitive care throughout the text. The emphasis is on the clinical application of the information, whether it focuses on toilet training or on male or female circumcision.

DRUG ALERTS highlight critical drug safety concerns for better therapeutic management.

EMERGENCY TREATMENT boxes are flagged by colored thumb tabs, enabling the reader to quickly locate interventions for crisis situations.

FAMILY-CENTERED CARE boxes present issues of special significance to families that have a child with a particular disorder. This feature is another method of highlighting the needs or concerns of families that should be addressed when family-centered care is provided.

NURSING ALERT features call the reader's attention to considerations that, if ignored, could lead to a deteriorating or emergency situation. Key assessment data, risk factors, and danger signs are among the kinds of information included.

NURSING CARE GUIDELINES summarize important nursing interventions for a variety of situations and conditions.

NURSING CARE PLANS are revised to allow students to experience an "unfolding case" written in the format of the next-generation NCLEX-RN examination. These include expected patient outcomes and rationales for the included nursing interventions that may not be immediately evident to the student. The care plans include an unfolding case study that represents a "real" patient and family to demonstrate the principles of clinical judgment.

NURSING TIPS present handy information of a nonemergency nature that makes patients more comfortable and the nurse's job easier.

QUALITY PATIENT INDICATORS are added throughout the text to provide a framework for measuring nursing care performance. Nursing-sensitive outcome measures are integrated into the outcome indicators used throughout the book.

RESEARCH FOCUS boxes review new evidence on important topics in a concise way.

TRANSLATING EVIDENCE INTO PRACTICE boxes have been updated in this edition to focus the reader's attention on application of both research and critical thought processes to support and guide the outcomes of nursing care. These boxes include Quality and Safety Education for Nurses competencies and provide measurable outcomes that nurses can use to validate their unique role in the health care system.

NEXT-GENERATION REVIEW QUESTIONS are found at the end of each chapter that are designed to promote clinical judgment. Using the new format for the Next-Generation NCLEX® examination, questions allow the nurse to process through a case study using clinical reasoning to make appropriate judgments about the patient's plan of care.

Numerous pedagogic devices that enhance student learning have been retained from previous editions:

- A functional and attractive **FULL-COLOR DESIGN** visually enhances the organization of each chapter, as well as the special features.
- A detailed, cross-referenced **INDEX** allows readers to quickly access discussions.
- **KEY TERMS** are highlighted throughout each chapter to reinforce student learning.
- Hundreds of **TABLES** and **BOXES** highlight key concepts and nursing interventions.
- Many of the **COLOR PHOTOGRAPHS** are new, and anatomic drawings are easy to follow, with color appropriately used to illustrate important aspects, such as saturated and desaturated blood. As an example, the full-color heart illustrations in Chapter 23 clearly depict congenital cardiac defects and associated hemodynamic changes.

ACKNOWLEDGMENTS

We are grateful to our mentor and colleague, **Donna Wong,** whose support made us better pediatric nurses. We are fortunate to have worked for many years with David Wilson and Cheryl Rodgers, who served as coeditors on numerous editions. We miss them greatly with this edition. We are also grateful to the many nursing faculty members, practitioners, and students who have offered their comments, recommendations, and suggestions. We are especially grateful to the contributors and the many reviewers who brought constructive criticism, suggestions, and clinical expertise to this edition. This edition could not have been completed without the dedication of these special people.

No book ever becomes a reality without the dedication and perseverance of the editorial staff. Although it is impossible to list every individual at Elsevier who has made exceptional efforts to produce this text, we are especially grateful to **Sandra Clark** and **Heather Bays** for their support and commitment to excellence. We want to say a very special thanks to Heather Bays, who has served the Wong textbooks for many editions with a commitment to excellence that is so appreciated. Her dedication to this book is reflected in every chapter.

Finally, we thank our families and children—for their unselfish love and endless patience that allows us to devote such a large part of our lives to our careers. Our children have given us the opportunity to directly observe the wonders of childhood.

Marilyn J. Hockenberry

CONTENTS

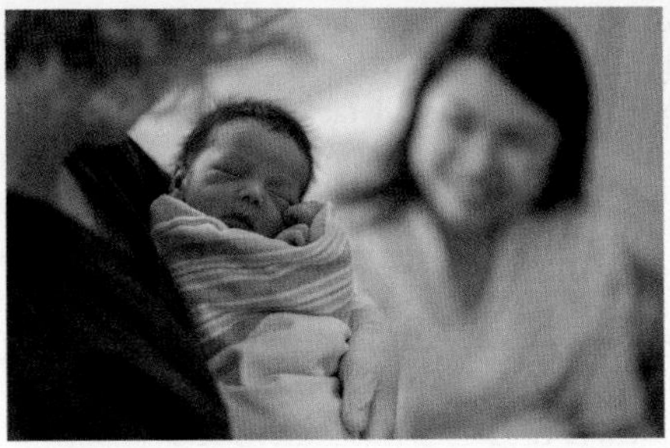

1

Perspectives of Pediatric Nursing

Marilyn J. Hockenberry

http://evolve.elsevier.com/wong/essentials

CONCEPTS

- Family-Centered Care
- Atraumatic Care
- Clinical Reasoning
- Nursing Process
- Research and Evidence-Based Practice
- Quality Outcome Measures

HEALTH CARE FOR CHILDREN

The major goal for pediatric nursing is to improve the quality of health care for children and their families. In 2018 almost 74 million children 0 to 17 years old lived in the United States, making up 22% of the population (Federal Interagency Forum on Child and Family Statistics, 2019). The health status of children in the United States has improved in a number of areas, including increased immunization rates for all children, decreased adolescent birth rate, and improved child health outcomes. The 2019 America's Children in Brief—Indicators of Well-Being reveals that preterm births increased slightly in 2016, after a continuous decline since 2007. Average mathematics scores for fourth- and eighth-grade students has remained stable since 2015, and the violent crime victimization rate among youth decreased during the last 20 years. Although the number of children living in poverty decreased slightly in 2017, overall the rate remains high at 18%. The percentage of children with at least one parent employed full time year round increased to 78% in 2017 (Federal Interagency Forum on Child and Family Statistics, 2019).

Millions of children and their families have no health insurance, which results in a lack of access to care and health promotion services. In addition, disparities in pediatric health care are related to race, ethnicity, socioeconomic status, and geographic factors (Flores & Lesley, 2014). Patterns of child health are shaped by medical progress and societal trends. Urgent priorities for health and health care of children in the United States are the focus for action toward new policy priorities (Box 1.1).

HEALTH PROMOTION

Child health promotion provides opportunities to reduce differences in current health status among members of different groups and to ensure equal opportunities and resources to enable all children to achieve their fullest health potential. The Healthy People 2030 Leading Health Indicators (Box 1.2) provide a framework for identifying essential components for child health promotion programs designed to prevent future health problems in our nation's children. Bright Futures is a national health promotion initiative with a goal to improve the health of our nation's children (Bright Futures, 2018). Major themes of the Bright Futures guideline are promoting family support, child development, mental health, and healthy nutrition that leads to healthy weight, physical activity, oral health, healthy sexual development and sexuality, safety and injury prevention, and the importance of community relationships and resources.[a] Throughout this book, developmentally appropriate health promotion strategies are discussed. Key examples of child health promotion themes essential for all age-groups include promoting development, nutrition, and oral health. Bright Futures recommendations for preventive health care during infancy, early childhood, and adolescence are found throughout the book.

Development

Health promotion integrates surveillance of the physical, psychologic, and emotional changes that occur in human beings between birth and the end of adolescence. Developmental processes are unique to each stage of development, and continuous screening and assessment are essential for early intervention when problems are found. The most dramatic time of physical, motor, cognitive, emotional, and social development occurs during infancy. Interactions between the parent and infant are central to promoting optimal developmental outcomes and are a key component of infant assessment. During early childhood, early identification of developmental delays is critical for establishing early interventions. Anticipatory guidance strategies ensure that parents are aware of the specific developmental needs of each developmental stage. Ongoing surveillance during middle childhood provides opportunities

[a]Bright Futures is supported by the American Academy of Pediatrics (see http://brightfutures.aap.org/about.html).

BOX 1.1 Health and Health Care Priorities for American Children

Poverty
Lack of health insurance
Environmental health
Nutrition
Firearm deaths and injuries
Mental health
Racial and ethnic disparities
Immigration

Adapted from American Academy of Pediatrics. (n.d.). *Federal advocacy*. Retrieved February 8, 2018, from https://www.aap.org/en-us/advocacy-and-policy/federal-advocacy

BOX 1.2 Healthy People 2030

Overarching Goals

- Attain healthy, thriving lives and well-being, free of preventable disease, disability, injury and premature death.
- Eliminate health disparities, achieve health equity, and attain health literacy to improve the health and well-being of all.
- Create social, physical, and economic environments that promote attaining full potential for health and well-being for all.
- Promote healthy development, healthy behaviors and well-being across all life stages.
- Engage leadership, key constituents, and the public across multiple sectors to take action and design policies that improve the health and well-being of all.

From US Department of Health and Human Services, Office of Disease Prevention and Health Promotion. (2019). *Healthy People 2030*. Retrieved from http://www.healthypeople.gov/

to strengthen cognitive and emotional attributes, communication skills, self-esteem, and independence. Recognition that adolescents differ greatly in their physical, social, and emotional maturity is important for surveillance throughout this developmental period.

An important example for health promotion during early child development is to be aware of changing recommendations that address the fast-changing world of technology in our society. An important example is the changes in the latest (American Academy of Pediatrics, 2016) policy statement on screen viewing by infants and children. New guidelines for screen viewing (laptop or phone) shift the importance from what is on the screen to who is viewing the information with the young child (American Academy of Pediatrics, 2016). For infants less than 18 months of age, no screen time is recommended except for video calling with a grandparent or loved one. Parents should be advised to use technology sparingly before 5 years of age and to always participate during screen-time viewing.

Nutrition

Nutrition is an essential component for healthy growth and development. Human milk is the preferred form of nutrition for all infants. Breastfeeding provides the infant with micronutrients, immunologic properties, and several enzymes that enhance digestion and absorption of these nutrients. A recent resurgence in breastfeeding has occurred as a result of the education of mothers and fathers regarding its benefits and increased social support.

Children establish lifelong eating habits during the first 3 years of life, and the nurse is instrumental in educating parents on the importance of nutrition. Most eating preferences and attitudes related to food are established by family influences and culture. During adolescence, parental influence diminishes and the adolescent makes food choices related to peer acceptability and sociability. Occasionally these choices are detrimental to adolescents with chronic illnesses such as diabetes, obesity, chronic lung disease, hypertension, cardiovascular risk factors, and renal disease.

Families that struggle with lower incomes, homelessness, and migrant status generally lack the resources to provide their children with adequate food intake, nutritious foods such as fresh fruits and vegetables, and appropriate protein intake (Flores & Lesley, 2014). The result is nutritional deficiencies with subsequent growth and developmental delays, depression, and behavior problems.

Oral Health

Oral health is an essential component of health promotion throughout infancy, childhood, and adolescence. Preventing dental caries and developing healthy oral hygiene habits must occur early in childhood. Dental caries has been recommended for decades as a significant yet preventable health problem for children. By 3 years of age, 28% of children will have one or more cavities (American Academy of Pediatrics, 2018). Children in racial or cultural minority groups experience disparities in oral health care and are much more likely to have dental disease.

Preschoolers of low-income families are twice as likely to develop tooth decay and only half as likely to visit the dentist as other children. Early childhood caries is a preventable disease, and nurses play an essential role in educating children and parents about practicing dental hygiene, beginning with the first tooth eruption; drinking fluoridated water, including bottled water; and instituting early dental preventive care. Oral health care practices established during the early years of development prevent destructive periodontal disease and dental decay.

CHILDHOOD HEALTH PROBLEMS

Changes in modern society, including advancing medical knowledge and technology, the proliferation of information systems, struggles with insurance disparities, economically troubled times, and various changes and disruptive influences on the family, are leading to significant medical problems that affect the health of children. Problems that can negatively affect a child's development include poverty, violence, aggression, noncompliance, school failure, and adjustment to parental separation and divorce. In addition, mental health issues cause challenges in childhood and adolescence. Emergence of the COVID-19 pandemic impacts children both physically and mentally. Recent concern has focused on groups of children who are at highest risk, such as children born preterm or with very low birth weight (VLBW) or low birth weight (LBW), children attending child care centers, children who live in poverty or are homeless, children of immigrant families, and children with chronic medical and psychiatric illness and disabilities. In addition, these children and their families face multiple barriers to adequate health, dental, and psychiatric care. A perspective of several health problems facing children and the major challenges for pediatric nurses is discussed in the following sections.

Obesity and Type 2 Diabetes

Childhood obesity, the most common nutritional problem among American children, is increasing in epidemic proportions. *Obesity* in children and adolescents is defined as a body mass index (BMI) at or greater than the 95th percentile for youth of the same age and gender. *Overweight* is defined as a BMI at or above the 85th percentile and below the 95th percentile for children and teens of the same age and sex. The prevalence of obesity during childhood was 18.5%, and obesity affects more than 13.7 million children and adolescents in 2016 (Centers for Disease Control and Prevention, 2018; Flores & Lesley, 2014).

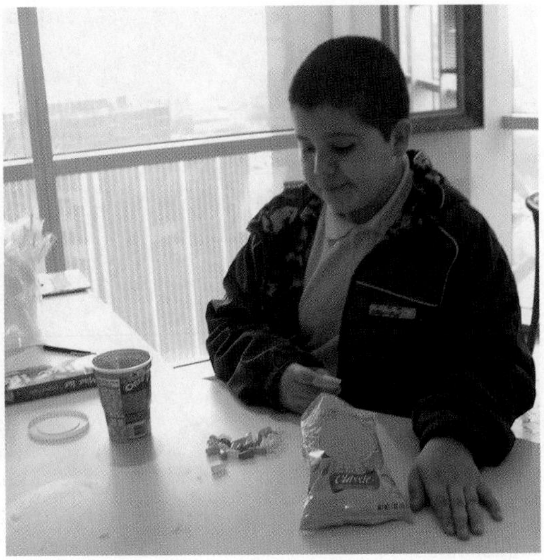

Fig. 1.1 The American culture's intake of high-caloric, fatty food contributes to obesity in children.

Increasing evidence indicates that maternal obesity is a major influence on offspring health during childhood and in adult life (Godfrey, Reynolds, Prescott, et al., 2016). An optimal nutritional and microbial environment during pregnancy may reduce the risk of infants being obese or overweight during early life (Garcia-Mantrana & Collado, 2016). Obesity and overweight research now recommends that education and preventative strategies be implemented beginning in infancy, and some researchers even feel that the prenatal period is best. Emphasis is on preventive strategies that start in infancy and in the prenatal period.

Lack of physical activity and a sedentary lifestyle related to limited resources, unsafe environments, and inconvenient play and exercise facilities, combined with easy access to television and video games, increases the incidence of obesity among low-income, minority children. Overweight youth have increased risk for cardiometabolic changes (a cluster of cardiovascular factors that include hypertension, altered glucose metabolism, dyslipidemia, and abdominal obesity) in the future (Weiss, Bremer, & Lustig, 2013) (Fig. 1.1). The US Department of Health and Human Services (2013) suggests that nurses focus on prevention strategies to reduce the incidence of overweight children from the current 20% in all ethnic groups to less than 6%. Lifestyle interventions show promise in preventing obesity and decreasing occurrence if targeted at children 6 to 12 years old.

Childhood Injuries

Injuries are the most common cause of death and disability among children in the United States (Centers for Disease Control and Prevention, 2017b) (Table 1.1). Mortality rates for suicide, poisoning, and falls rose substantially over the past decade. Other unintentional injuries (head injuries, drowning, burns, and firearm accidents) take the lives of children every day. Implementing programs of accident prevention and health promotion could prevent many childhood injuries and fatalities.

The type of injury and the circumstances surrounding it are closely related to normal growth and development (Box 1.3). As children develop, their innate curiosity compels them to investigate the environment and to mimic the behavior of others. This is essential to acquire competency as an adult, but it can also predispose children to numerous hazards.

The child's developmental stage partially determines the types of injuries that are most likely to occur at a specific age and helps provide clues to preventive measures. For example, small infants are helpless in any environment. When they begin to roll over or propel themselves, they can fall from unprotected surfaces. The crawling infant, who has a natural tendency to place objects in the mouth, is at risk for aspiration or poisoning. The mobile toddler, with the instinct to explore and investigate and the ability to run and climb, may experience falls, burns, and collisions with objects. As children grow older, their absorption with play makes them oblivious to environmental hazards such as street traffic or water. The need to conform and gain acceptance compels older children and adolescents to accept challenges and dares. Although the rate of injuries is high in children younger than 9 years old, most fatal injuries occur in later childhood and adolescence.

The pattern of deaths caused by unintentional injuries, especially from motor vehicle accidents (MVAs), drowning, and burns, is remarkably consistent in most Western societies. The leading causes of death from injuries for each age-group according to sex are presented in Table 1.1. The majority of deaths from injuries occur in boys. It is important to note that accidents continue to account for more than three times as many teen deaths as any other cause (Annie E. Casey Foundation, 2019). Fortunately, prevention strategies such as the use of car restraints, bicycle helmets, and smoke detectors have significantly decreased fatalities for children. Nevertheless,

BOX 1.3 Childhood Injuries: Risk Factors

- *Sex*—Preponderance of males; difference mainly the result of behavioral characteristics, especially aggression
- *Temperament*—Children with difficult temperament profile, especially persistence, high activity level, and negative reactions to new situations
- *Stress*—Predisposes children to increased risk taking and self-destructive behavior; general lack of self-protection
- *Alcohol and drug use*—Associated with higher incidence of motor vehicle injuries, drownings, homicides, and suicides
- *History of previous injury*—Associated with increased likelihood of another injury, especially if initial injury required hospitalization
- *Developmental characteristics*
  - Mismatch between child's developmental level and skill required for activity (e.g., all-terrain vehicles)
  - Natural curiosity to explore environment
  - Desire to assert self and challenge rules
  - In older child, desire for peer approval and acceptance
- *Cognitive characteristics* (age specific)
  - *Infant*—Sensorimotor: explores environment through taste and touch
  - *Young child*—Object permanence: actively searches for attractive object; cause and effect: lacks awareness of consequential dangers; transductive reasoning: may fail to learn from experiences (e.g., perceives falling from a step as a different type of danger from climbing a tree); magical and egocentric thinking: is unable to comprehend danger to self or others
  - *School-age child*—Transitional cognitive processes: is unable to fully comprehend causal relationships; attempts dangerous acts without detailed planning regarding consequences
  - *Adolescent*—Formal operations: is preoccupied with abstract thinking and loses sight of reality; may lead to feeling of invulnerability
- *Anatomic characteristics* (especially in young children)
  - *Large head*—Predisposes to cranial injury
  - *Large spleen and liver with wide costal arch*—Predisposes to direct trauma to these organs
  - *Small and light body*—May be thrown easily, especially inside a moving vehicle
- *Other factors*—Poverty, family stress (e.g., maternal illness, recent environmental change), substandard alternative child care, young maternal age, low maternal education, multiple siblings

TABLE 1.1 Preventable, Unintentional Injury-Related Deaths, United States, 2017 (Rate per 100,000 Population in Each Age-Group)

	AGE (YEARS)		
Type of Accident	**0-4**	**5-14**	**15-24**
Males			
Motor vehicle	2.8 (3)	2.4 (1)	22.0 (1)
Drowning	3.0 (2)	0.8 (2)	1.8 (3)
Fires and burns	0.5 (5)	0.4 (3)	0.2 (5)
Choking	0.6 (4)	—	—
Falls	—	—	0.8 (4)
Mechanical suffocation	6.4 (1)	0.2 (4)	—
Poisoning	—	—	16.2 (2)
Other causes	0.8	0.5	2.2
Females			
Motor vehicle	2.6 (2)	1.7 (1)	9.4 (1)
Drowning	1.6 (3)	0.3 (3)	0.3 (3)
Fires and burns	0.5 (4)	0.3 (2)	0.2 (4)
Choking	0.3 (5)	—	—
Falls	—	0.1 (5)	0.1 (5)
Mechanical suffocation	4.8 (1)	—	—
Poisoning	—	0.1 (4)	6.8 (2)
Other causes	0.4	0.3	0.5

Data Source: National Safety Council, *Injury Facts,* Online database, available at https://injuryfacts.nsc.org.

the overwhelming causes of death in children are MVAs, including occupant, pedestrian, bicycle, and motorcycle deaths; these account for more than half of all injury deaths (Kids Count Data Center, 2016) (Fig. 1.2).

Pedestrian accidents involving children account for significant numbers of motor vehicle–related deaths. Most of these accidents occur at midblock, at intersections, in driveways, and in parking lots. Driveway injuries typically involve small children and large vehicles backing up.

Bicycle-associated injuries also cause a number of childhood deaths. Children ages 5 to 9 years are at greatest risk of bicycling fatalities. The majority of bicycling deaths are from traumatic head injuries (Centers for Disease Control and Prevention, 2017a). Helmets greatly reduce the risk of head injury, but few children wear helmets. Community-wide bicycle helmet campaigns and mandatory-use laws have resulted in significant increases in helmet use. Still, issues such as stylishness, comfort, and social acceptability remain important factors in noncompliance. Nurses can educate children and families about pedestrian and bicycle safety. In particular, school nurses can promote helmet wearing and encourage peer leaders to act as role models.

Drowning and burns are among the leading causes of deaths for males and females throughout childhood (Fig. 1.3). In addition, improper use of firearms is a major cause of death among males (Fig. 1.4). During early childhood, more boys die of aspiration or suffocation than do girls (Fig. 1.5). Each year, more than 500,000 children ages 5 years and younger experience a potential poisoning related to medications (Ferguson, Osterthaler, Kaminski,

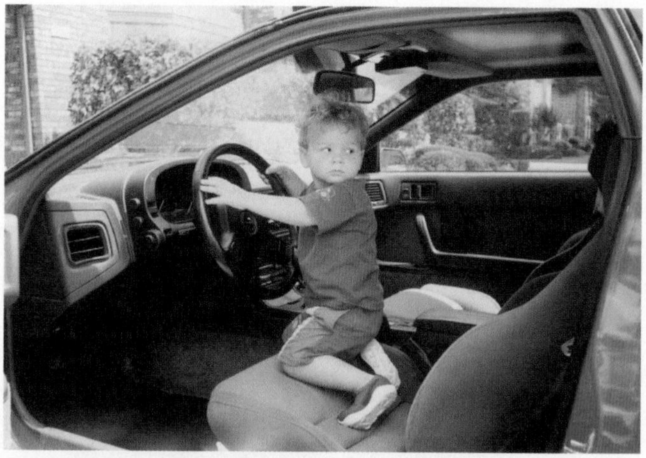

Fig. 1.2 Motor vehicle injuries are the leading cause of death in children older than 1 year of age. The majority of fatalities involve occupants who are unrestrained.

et al., 2015). Currently, more children are brought to emergency departments (EDs) for unintentional medication overdoses. Approximately 95% of medication-related ED visits in children younger than 5 years are due to ingesting medication while unsupervised (Fig. 1.6). Intentional poisoning, associated with drug and alcohol abuse and suicide attempt, is the second leading cause of death in adolescent females and the third leading cause in adolescent males.

Violence

Youth violence is a high-visibility, high-priority concern in every sector of American society (David-Ferdon & Simon, 2014). Strikingly higher homicide rates are found among minority populations, especially African American children. The causes of violence against children and self-inflicted violence are not fully understood. Violence seems to permeate American households through television programs, commercials, video games, and movies, all of which tend to desensitize the child toward violence. Violence also permeates the schools with the availability of guns, illicit drugs, and gangs. The problem of child homicide is extremely complex and involves numerous social, economic, and other influences. Prevention lies in a better understanding of the social and psychologic factors that lead to the high rates of homicide and suicide. Nurses need to be especially aware of young people who harm animals or start fires, are depressed, are repeatedly in trouble with the criminal justice system, or are associated with groups known to be violent. Prevention requires early identification and rapid therapeutic intervention by qualified professionals.

Pediatric nurses can assess children and adolescents for risk factors related to violence. Families that own firearms must be educated about their safe use and storage. The presence of a gun in a household increases the risk of suicide by about fivefold and the risk of homicide by about threefold. Technologic changes such as childproof safety devices and loading indicators could improve the safety of firearms (see Community and Home Health Considerations box).

ADOLESCENT VAPING EPIDEMIC

The use of e-cigarettes has become a national epidemic (Farzal, Perry, Yarbrough, et al., 2019). The rise in vaping (using e-cigarettes), reported in 2018, had increased by 78% in high school

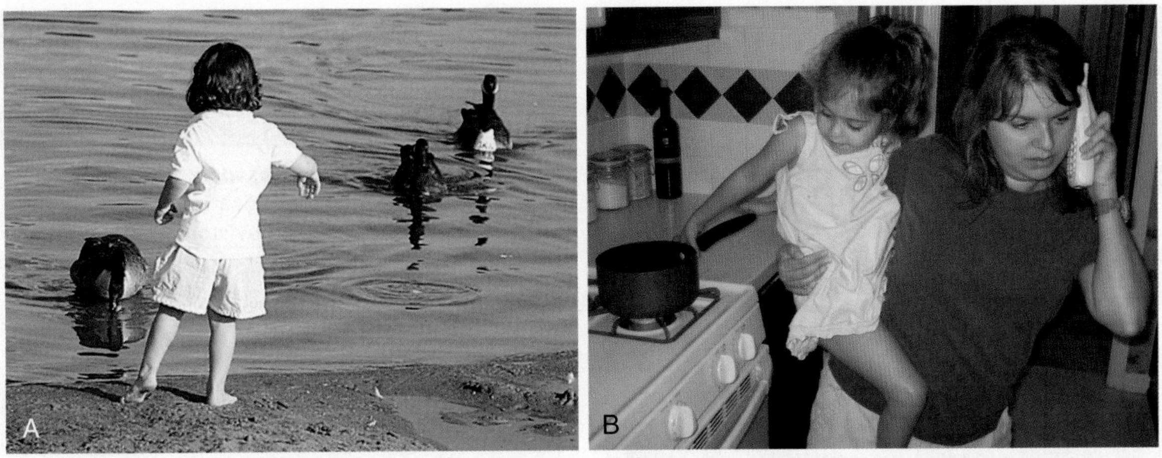

Fig. 1.3 A, Drowning is one of the leading causes of death in children. Children left unattended are unsafe even in shallow water. B, Burns are among the three leading causes of death from injury in children 1 to 14 years old.

COMMUNITY AND HOME HEALTH CONSIDERATIONS

Violence in Children

Community violence has reached epidemic proportions in the United States. The serious problem of community violence affects the lives of many children and expands throughout the family, schools, and the workplace. Nurses working with children, adolescents, and families have a critical role in reducing violence through early identification and symptom recognition of the mental-emotional stress that can result from these experiences.

Violent crimes continue to be a significant health issue for children, with homicide being the second leading cause of death in 15- to 19-year-olds (Annie E. Casey Foundation, 2019). The multifaceted origins of violence include developmental factors, gang involvement, access to firearms, drugs, the media, poverty, and family conflict. Often the silent and underrecognized victims are the children who witness acts of community violence. Studies suggest that chronic exposure to violence has a negative effect on a child's cognitive, social, psychologic, and moral development. Also, multiple exposures to episodes of violence do not inoculate children against the negative effects; continued exposure can result in lasting symptoms of stress.

National concern about the increasing prevalence of violent crimes has prompted nurses to actively participate in ensuring that children grow up in safe environments. Pediatric nurses are positioned to assess children and adolescents for signs of exposure to violence and well-known risk factors; nurses also can provide nonviolent problem-solving strategies, counseling, and referrals. These activities affect community practice and expand the nurse's role in the future health environment. Professional resources include the following:

National Domestic Violence Hotline
PO Box 161810
Austin, TX 78716
800-799-SAFE
https://www.ndvh.org

Child Trends
Child Trends Databank. (2016). *Teen homicide, suicide, and firearm deaths.* Retrieved from http://www.childtrends.org/?indicators=teen-homicide-suicide-and-firearm-deaths

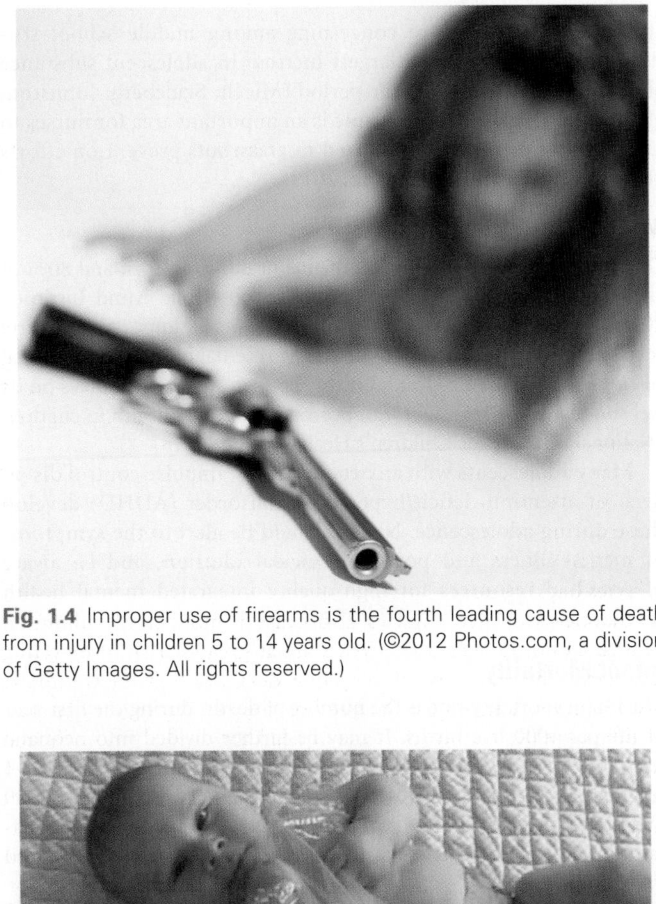

Fig. 1.4 Improper use of firearms is the fourth leading cause of death from injury in children 5 to 14 years old. (©2012 Photos.com, a division of Getty Images. All rights reserved.)

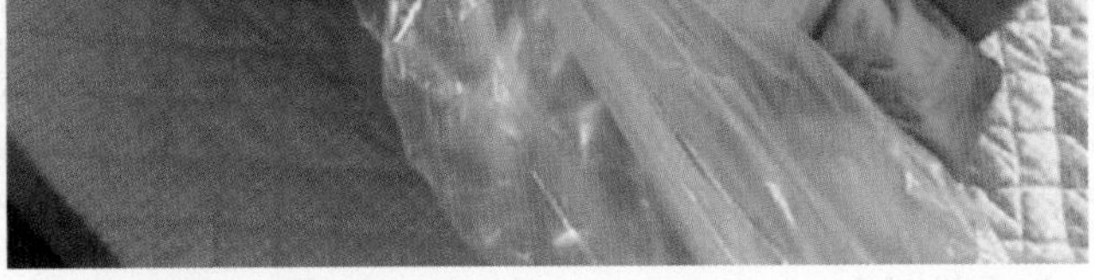

Fig. 1.5 Mechanical suffocation is the leading cause of death from injury in infants.

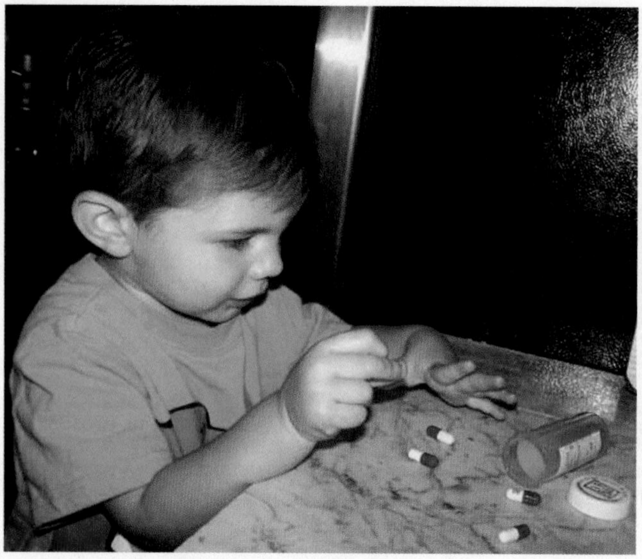

Fig. 1.6 Poisoning causes a considerable number of injuries in children younger than 4 years old. Medications should never be left where young children can reach them.

students and even more concerning among middle school students by 48%. This is the largest increase in adolescent substance abuse recorded over a 1-year period (Miech, Sculeberg, Johnston, et al., 2018). This rising epidemic is an important area for nurses to take action by becoming involved in grassroots prevention efforts (Farzal, Perry, Yarbrough, et al., 2019).

Mental Health Problems

One in five children experiences mental health problems, and 80% of chronic mental disorders begin in childhood (Child Mind Institute, 2016). There is significant research that highlights the importance of early social-emotional support to foster positive mental health. The National Institute for Children's Health Quality hosts numerous resources on its website that provide insight into promoting optimal health in children (National Institute for Children's Health Quality, 2018).

Many adolescents with anxiety disorders, impulse control disorders, or attention-deficit/hyperactivity disorder (ADHD) develop these during adolescence. Nurses should be alert to the symptoms of mental illness and potential suicidal ideation, and be aware of potential resources for high-quality integrated mental health services.

Infant Mortality

The infant mortality rate is the number of deaths during the first year of life per 1000 live births. It may be further divided into neonatal mortality (<28 days of life) and postneonatal mortality (28 days to 11 months). In the United States the infant mortality rate was 5.8 per 1000 live births, the neonatal mortality rate was 3.84, and the postneonatal mortality rate was 1.95 in 2017 (Centers for Disease Control and Prevention, 2017a).

Birth weight is considered the major determinant of neonatal death in technologically developed countries. The relatively high incidence of LBW (<2500 g [5.5 pounds]) in the United States is considered a key factor in its higher neonatal mortality rate compared with other countries. Access to and the use of high-quality prenatal care are promising preventive strategies to decrease early delivery and infant mortality.

As Table 1.2 demonstrates, many of the leading causes of death during infancy continue to occur during the perinatal period. The first four causes—congenital anomalies, disorders relating to short gestation and unspecified LBW, newborn affected by maternal complications of pregnancy, and sudden infant death syndrome—accounted for about half (49.8%) of all deaths of infants younger than 1 year old (Kochanek, Murphy, Xu, et al., 2019). Many birth defects are associated with LBW, and reducing the incidence of LBW will help prevent congenital anomalies. Infant mortality resulting from human immunodeficiency virus (HIV) infection decreased significantly during the 1990s.

When infant death rates are categorized according to race, a disturbing difference is seen. Infant mortality for whites is considerably lower than for all other races in the United States, with African Americans having twice the rate of whites. The LBW rate is also much higher for African American infants than for any other group. One encouraging note is that the gap in mortality rates between white and nonwhite races (other than African Americans) has narrowed in recent years. Infant mortality rates for Hispanics and Asian–Pacific Islanders have decreased dramatically during the past two decades.

TABLE 1.2 Infant Mortality Rate and Percentage of Total Deaths for 10 Leading Causes of Infant Death in 2017 (Rate per 1000 Live Births)

Rank	Cause of Death (Based on International Classification of Diseases, 10th Revision)	Percent	Rate
	All races, all causes	100.0	579.3
1	Congenital anomalies	20.5	118.8
2	Disorders relating to short gestation and unspecified low birth weight	16.8	97.2
3	Newborn affected by maternal complications of pregnancy	6.4	37.1
4	Sudden infant death syndrome	6.1	35.4
5	Accidents (unintentional injuries)	5.9	34.2
6	Newborn affected by complications of placenta, cord, and membranes	3.8	21.9
7	Bacterial sepsis of newborn	2.7	15.4
8	Diseases of the circulatory system	2.0	11.6
9	Respiratory distress of newborn	2.0	11.4
10	Neonatal hemorrhage	1.7	9.8

Kochanek K.D, Murphy, S.L. Xu, J. et al. (2019). Deaths: Final Data for 2017. *National Vital Statistics Reports,* 68(9), 1–77.

Childhood Mortality

Death rates for children older than 1 year of age have always been lower than those for infants. Children ages 5 to 14 years have the lowest rate of death. However, a sharp rise occurs during later adolescence, primarily from injuries, homicide, and suicide (Table 1.3). In 2014 accidental injuries accounted for 34.4% of all deaths. The second leading cause of death was suicide, accounting for 12.1% of all deaths. The trend in racial differences that occurs in infant mortality is also apparent in childhood deaths for all ages and for both sexes. Whites have fewer deaths for all ages, and male deaths outnumber female deaths.

After 1 year of age, the cause of death changes dramatically, with unintentional injuries (accidents) being the leading cause from the

TABLE 1.3 Five Leading Causes of Death in Children in the United States: Selected Age Intervals, 2014[a]

	1–4 YEARS OF AGE		5–9 YEARS OF AGE		10–14 YEARS OF AGE		15–19 YEARS OF AGE	
Rank	Cause	Rate	Cause	Rate	Cause	Rate	Cause	Rate
	All causes	24.0	All causes	11.5	All causes	14.0	All causes	45.5
1	Injuries	7.6	Injuries	3.6	Injuries	3.6	Injuries	17.7
2	Congenital anomalies	2.5	Cancer	2.1	Suicide	2.1	Suicide	8.7
3	Homicide	2.3	Congenital anomalies	0.9	Cancer	2.0	Homicide	6.7
4	Cancer	2.0	Homicide	0.6	Congenital anomalies	0.8	Cancer	2.9
5	Heart disease	0.9	Heart disease	0.3	Homicide	0.8	Heart disease	1.4

[a]Rate per 100,000 population.
Modifi ed from Murphy, S. L., Mathews, T. J., Martin, J. A., et al. (2017). Annual summary of vital statistics: 2013-2014V. *Pediatrics, 139*(6), e20163239.

youngest ages to the adolescent years. Violent deaths have been steadily increasing among young people ages 10 through 25 years, especially among African Americans and males. Homicide is the third leading cause of death in the 15- to 19-year age-group (see Table 1.3). Children 12 years of age and older tend to be killed by non–family members (acquaintances and gangs, typically of the same race) and most frequently by firearms. Suicide, a form of self-violence, is the third leading cause of death among children and adolescents 10 to 19 years old.

Childhood Morbidity

Acute illness is defined as an illness with symptoms severe enough to limit activity or require medical attention. Respiratory illness accounts for approximately 50% of all acute conditions, 11% are caused by infections and parasitic disease, and 15% are caused by injuries. The chief illness of childhood is the common cold.

The types of diseases that children contract during childhood vary according to age. For example, upper respiratory tract infections and diarrhea decrease in frequency with age, whereas other disorders, such as acne and headaches, increase. Children who have had a particular type of problem are more likely to have that problem again. Morbidity is not distributed randomly in children. Recent concern has focused on groups of children who have increased morbidity: homeless children, children living in poverty, LBW children, children with chronic illnesses, foreign-born adopted children, and children in daycare centers. A number of factors place these groups at risk for poor health. A major cause is barriers to health care, especially for the homeless, the poverty stricken, and those with chronic health problems. Other factors include improved survival of children with chronic health problems, particularly infants of VLBW.

THE ART OF PEDIATRIC NURSING

Philosophy of Care

Nursing of infants, children, and adolescents involves the protection, promotion, and optimization of health and abilities, prevention of illness and injury, alleviation of suffering through the diagnosis and treatment of human response, and advocacy in the care of individuals, families, and populations.

Family-Centered Care

The philosophy of family-centered care recognizes the family as the constant in a child's life. Family-centered care is an approach to the planning, delivery, and evaluation of health care that is grounded in mutually beneficial partnerships among health care providers, patients, and families (Institute for Patient- and Family-Centered Care, 2018).

BOX 1.4 Key Elements of Family-Centered Care

- Incorporating into policy and practice the recognition that the family is the constant in a child's life, whereas the service systems and support personnel within those systems fluctuate
- Facilitating family-professional collaboration at all levels of hospital, home, and community care:
  - Care of an individual child
  - Program development, implementation, and evaluation
  - Policy formation
- Exchanging complete and unbiased information between family members and professionals in a supportive manner at all times
- Incorporating into policy and practice the recognition and honoring of cultural diversity, strengths, and individuality within and across all families, including ethnic, racial, spiritual, social, economic, educational, and geographic diversity
- Recognizing and respecting different methods of coping and implementing comprehensive policies and programs that provide developmental, educational, emotional, environmental, and financial support to meet the diverse needs of families
- Encouraging and facilitating family-to-family support and networking
- Ensuring that home, hospital, and community service and support systems for children needing specialized health and developmental care and their families are flexible, accessible, and comprehensive in responding to diverse family-identified needs
- Appreciating families as families and children as children, recognizing that they possess a wide range of strengths, concerns, emotions, and aspirations beyond their need for specialized health and developmental services and support

From Shelton, T. L., & Stepanek, J. S. (2014). *Family-centered care for children needing specialized health and developmental services.* Bethesda, MD: Association for the Care of Children's Health.

Nurses support families in their natural caregiving and decision-making roles by building on their unique strengths and acknowledging their expertise in caring for their child both within and outside the hospital setting. The nurse considers the needs of all family members in relation to the care of the child (Box 1.4). The philosophy acknowledges diversity among family structures and backgrounds; family goals, dreams, strategies, and actions; and family support, service, and information needs.

Two basic concepts in family-centered care are enabling and empowerment. Professionals enable families by creating opportunities and means for all family members to display their current abilities and competencies and to acquire new ones to meet the needs of the child and family. *Empowerment* describes the interaction of professionals with families in such a way that families maintain or acquire a sense of control over their family lives and acknowledge positive changes that result from helping behaviors that foster their own strengths, abilities, and actions.

Although caring for the family is strongly emphasized throughout this text, it is highlighted in features such as Cultural Considerations and Family-Centered Care boxes.

Atraumatic Care

Atraumatic care is the provision of therapeutic care in settings, by personnel, and through the use of interventions that eliminate or minimize the psychologic and physical distress experienced by children and their families in the health care system. Therapeutic care encompasses the prevention, diagnosis, treatment, or palliation of acute or chronic conditions. Setting refers to the place in which that care is given—the home, the hospital, or any other health care setting. Personnel include anyone directly involved in providing therapeutic care. Interventions range from psychologic approaches, such as preparing children for procedures, to physical interventions, such as providing space for a parent to room in with a child. Psychologic distress may include anxiety, fear, anger, disappointment, sadness, shame, or guilt. Physical distress may range from sleeplessness and immobilization to disturbances from sensory stimuli, such as pain, temperature extremes, loud noises, bright lights, or darkness. Thus atraumatic care is concerned with the where, who, why, and how of any procedure performed on a child for the purpose of preventing or minimizing psychologic and physical stress (Wong, 1989).

The overriding goal in providing atraumatic care is as follows: First, do no harm. Three principles provide the framework for achieving this goal: (1) prevent or minimize the child's separation from the family, (2) promote a sense of control, and (3) prevent or minimize bodily injury and pain. Examples of providing atraumatic care include fostering the parent-child relationship during hospitalization, preparing the child before any unfamiliar treatment or procedure, controlling pain, allowing the child privacy, providing play activities for expression of fear and aggression, providing choices to children, and respecting cultural differences.

Role of the Pediatric Nurse

The pediatric nurse is responsible for promoting the health and well-being of the child and family. Nursing functions vary according to regional job structures, individual education and experience, and personal career goals. Just as patients (children and their families) have unique backgrounds, each nurse brings an individual set of variables that affect the nurse-patient relationship. No matter where pediatric nurses practice, their primary concern is the welfare of the child and family.

There are many different roles for nurses specializing in the care of children and their families. For example, a pediatric nurse can pursue an advanced degree and become a Pediatric Nurse Practitioner (PNP) or Clinical Nurse Specialist (CNS) in pediatrics. Many advanced pediatric nurses go on to pursue the Doctorate of Nursing Practice (DNP) degree. PNPs work in a variety of settings and are able to diagnose illnesses and prescribe medication. They provide a spectrum of care from children needing routine examinations and wellness care to caring for children with serious or chronic conditions. CNSs function in a variety of settings in both the direct and the indirect roles. They model expert direct family-centered patient care.

Therapeutic Relationship

The establishment of a therapeutic relationship is the essential foundation for providing high-quality nursing care. Pediatric nurses need to have meaningful relationships with children and their families yet remain separate enough to distinguish their own feelings and needs. In a therapeutic relationship, caring, well-defined boundaries separate the nurse from the child and family. These boundaries are positive and professional and promote the family's control over the child's health care. Both the nurse and the family are empowered and maintain open communication. In a nontherapeutic relationship, these boundaries are blurred, and many of the nurse's actions may serve personal needs, such as a need to feel wanted and involved, rather than the family's needs. Exploring whether relationships with patients are therapeutic or nontherapeutic helps nurses identify problem areas early in their interactions with children and families (see Nursing Care Guidelines box).

Family Advocacy and Caring

Although nurses are responsible to themselves, the profession, and the institution of employment, their primary responsibility is to the consumer of nursing services: the child and family. The nurse must work with family members, identify their goals and needs, and plan interventions that best address the defined problems. As an advocate, the nurse assists the child and family in making informed choices and acting in the child's best interest. Advocacy involves ensuring that families

NURSING CARE GUIDELINES

Exploring Your Relationships With Children and Families

To foster therapeutic relationships with children and families, you must first become aware of your caregiving style, including how effectively you take care of yourself. The following questions should help you understand the therapeutic quality of your professional relationships.

Negative Actions

- Are you overinvolved with children and their families?
- Do you work overtime to care for the family?
- Do you spend off-duty time with children's families, either in or out of the hospital?
- Do you call frequently (either the hospital or home) to see how the family is doing?
- Do you show favoritism toward certain patients?
- Do you buy clothes, toys, food, or other items for the child and family?
- Do you compete with other staff members for the affection of certain patients and families?
- Do other staff members comment to you about your closeness to the family?
- Do you attempt to influence families' decisions rather than facilitate their informed decision making?
- Are you underinvolved with children and families?
- Do you restrict parent or visitor access to children, using excuses such as that the unit is too busy?
- Do you focus on the technical aspects of care and lose sight of the person who is the patient?
- Are you overinvolved with children and underinvolved with their parents?
- Do you become critical when parents do not visit their children?
- Do you compete with parents for their children's affection?

Positive Actions

- Do you strive to empower families?
- Do you explore families' strengths and needs in an effort to increase family involvement?

NURSING CARE GUIDELINES—cont'd

Exploring Your Relationships With Children and Families

- Have you developed teaching skills to instruct families rather than doing everything for them?
- Do you work with families to find ways to decrease their dependence on health care providers?
- Can you separate families' needs from your own needs?
- Do you strive to empower yourself?
- Are you aware of your emotional responses to different people and situations?
- Do you seek to understand how your own family experiences influence reactions to patients and families, especially as they affect tendencies toward overinvolvement or underinvolvement?
- Do you have a calming influence, not one that will amplify emotionality?
- Have you developed interpersonal skills in addition to technical skills?
- Have you learned about ethnic and religious family patterns?
- Do you communicate directly with persons with whom you are upset or take issue?
- Are you able to "step back" and withdraw emotionally, if not physically, when emotional overload occurs, yet remain committed?
- Do you take care of yourself and your needs?
- Do you periodically interview family members to determine their current issues (e.g., feelings, attitudes, responses, wishes), communicate these findings to peers, and update records?
- Do you avoid relying on initial interview data, assumptions, or gossip regarding families?
- Do you ask questions if families are not participating in care?
- Do you assess families for feelings of anxiety, fear, intimidation, worry about making a mistake, a perceived lack of competence to care for their child, or fear of health care professionals overstepping their boundaries into family territory, or vice versa?
- Do you explore these issues with family members and provide encouragement and support to enable families to help themselves?
- Do you keep communication channels open among self, family, physicians, and other care providers?
- Do you resolve conflicts and misunderstandings directly with those who are involved?
- Do you clarify information for families or seek the appropriate person to do so?
- Do you recognize that from time to time a therapeutic relationship can change to a social relationship or an intimate friendship?
- Are you able to acknowledge the fact when it occurs and understand why it happened?
- Can you ensure that there is someone else who is more objective who can take your place in the therapeutic relationship?

are aware of all available health services, adequately informed of treatments and procedures, involved in the child's care, and encouraged to change or support existing health care practices.

As nurses care for children and families, they must demonstrate caring, compassion, and empathy for others. Aspects of caring embody the concept of atraumatic care and the development of a therapeutic relationship with patients. Parents perceive caring as a sign of quality in nursing care, which is often focused on the nontechnical needs of the child and family. Parents describe "personable" care as actions by the nurse that include acknowledging the parent's presence, listening, making the parent feel comfortable in the hospital environment, involving the parent and child in the nursing care, showing interest in and concern for their welfare, showing affection and sensitivity to the parent and child, communicating with them, and individualizing the nursing care. Parents perceive personable nursing care as being integral to establishing a positive relationship.

Disease Prevention and Health Promotion

Every nurse involved in caring for children must understand the importance of disease prevention and health promotion. A nursing care plan must include a thorough assessment of all aspects of child growth and development, including nutrition, immunizations, safety, dental care, socialization, discipline, and education. If problems are identified, the nurse intervenes directly or refers the family to other health care providers or agencies.

The best approach to prevention is education and anticipatory guidance. In this text, each chapter on health promotion includes sections on anticipatory guidance. An appreciation of the hazards or conflicts of each developmental period enables the nurse to guide parents regarding childrearing practices aimed at preventing potential problems. One significant example is safety. Because each age-group is at risk for special types of injuries, preventive teaching can significantly reduce injuries, lowering permanent disability and mortality rates.

Prevention also involves less obvious aspects of caring for children. The nurse is responsible for providing care that promotes mental well-being (e.g., enlisting the help of a child life specialist during a painful procedure, such as an immunization).

Health Teaching

Health teaching is inseparable from family advocacy and prevention. Health teaching may be the nurse's direct goal, such as during parenting classes, or may be indirect, such as helping parents and children understand a diagnosis or medical treatment, encouraging children to ask questions about their bodies, referring families to health-related professional or lay groups, supplying patients with appropriate literature, and providing anticipatory guidance. The importance of carefully assessing health literacy in families and culturally sensitive approaches to teaching should be emphasized.

Health teaching is one area in which nurses often need preparation and practice with competent role models, because it involves transmitting information at the child's and family's level of understanding and desire for information. As an effective educator, the nurse focuses on providing the appropriate health teaching with generous feedback and evaluation to promote learning.

Injury Prevention

Each year, injuries kill or disable more children older than 1 year of age than all childhood diseases combined. The nurse plays an important role in preventing injuries by using a developmental approach to safety counseling for parents of children of all ages. Realizing that safety concerns for a young infant are completely different than injury risks of adolescents, the nurse discusses appropriate injury prevention tips to parents and children as part of routine patient care.

Support and Counseling

Attention to emotional needs requires support and sometimes counseling. The role of child advocate or health teacher is supportive by virtue of the individualized approach. The nurse can offer support by listening, touching, and being physically present. Touching and physical presence are most helpful with children, because they facilitate nonverbal communication. Counseling involves a mutual exchange of ideas and opinions that provides the basis for mutual problem solving. It involves support, teaching, techniques to foster the expression of feelings or thoughts, and approaches to help the family cope with stress. Optimally, counseling not only helps resolve a crisis or problem but also enables the family to attain a higher level of functioning, greater self-esteem, and closer relationships. Although counseling is often the role of nurses in specialized areas, counseling techniques are discussed in various sections of this text to help students and nurses cope with immediate crises and refer families for additional professional assistance.

Coordination and Collaboration

The nurse, as a member of the health care team, collaborates and coordinates nursing care with the care activities of other professionals. A nurse working in isolation rarely serves the child's best interests. The concept of holistic care can be realized through a unified, interdisciplinary approach by being aware of individual contributions and limitations and collaborating with other specialists to provide high-quality health services. Failure to recognize limitations can be nontherapeutic at best and destructive at worst. For example, the nurse who feels competent in counseling but who is really inadequate in this area may not only prevent the child from dealing with a crisis but also impede future success with a qualified professional. Nursing should be seen as a major contributor to ensuring that the health care team focuses on high-quality, safe care.

Ethical Decision Making

Ethical dilemmas arise when competing moral considerations underlie various alternatives. Parents, nurses, physicians, and other health care team members may reach different but morally defensible decisions by assigning different weights to competing moral values. These competing moral values may include autonomy, the patient's right to be self-governing; nonmaleficence, the obligation to minimize or prevent harm; beneficence, the obligation to promote the patient's well-being; and justice, the concept of fairness. Nurses must determine the most beneficial or least harmful action within the framework of societal mores, professional practice standards, the law, institutional rules, the family's value system and religious traditions, and the nurse's personal values.

Nurses must prepare themselves systematically for collaborative ethical decision making. They can accomplish this through formal course work, continuing education, and contemporary literature, and work to establish an environment conducive to ethical discourse.

The nurse also uses the professional code of ethics for guidance and as a means for professional self-regulation. Nurses may face ethical issues regarding patient care, such as the use of life-saving measures for VLBW newborns or the terminally ill child's right to refuse treatment. They may struggle with questions regarding truthfulness, balancing their rights and responsibilities in caring for children with acquired immune deficiency syndrome (AIDS), whistle blowing, or allocating resources. Ethical arguments are presented to help nurses clarify their value judgments when confronted with sensitive issues.

Research and Evidence-Based Practice

Nurses should contribute to research because they are the individuals observing human responses to health and illness. The current emphasis on measurable outcomes to determine the efficacy of interventions (often in relation to the cost) demands that nurses know whether clinical interventions result in positive outcomes for their patients. This demand has influenced the current trend toward evidence-based practice (EBP), which implies questioning why something is effective and whether a better approach exists. The concept of EBP also involves analyzing and translating published clinical research into the everyday practice of nursing. When nurses base their clinical practice on science and research and document their clinical outcomes, they will be able to validate their contributions to health, wellness, and cure, not only to their patients, third-party payers, and institutions but also to the nursing profession. Evaluation is essential to the nursing process, and research is one of the best ways to accomplish this.

EBP is the collection, interpretation, and integration of valid, important, and applicable patient-reported, nurse-observed, and research-derived information. Using the population/patient problem, intervention, comparison, outcome, and time (PICOT) question to clearly define the problem of interest, nurses are able to obtain the best evidence to improve care. Evidence-based nursing practice combines knowledge with clinical experience and intuition. It provides a rational approach to decision making that facilitates best practice (Melnyk & Fineout-Overholt, 2014). EBP is an important tool that complements the nursing process by using critical thinking skills to make decisions based on existing knowledge. The traditional nursing process approach to patient care can be used to conceptualize the essential components of EBP in nursing. During the assessment and diagnostic phases of the nursing process, the nurse establishes important clinical questions and completes a critical review of existing knowledge. EBP also begins with identification of the problem. The nurse asks clinical questions in a concise, organized way that allows for clear answers. Once the specific questions are identified, extensive searching for the best information to answer the question begins. The nurse evaluates clinically relevant research, analyzes findings from the history and physical examination, and reviews the specific pathophysiology of the defined problem. The third step in the nursing process is to develop a care plan. In evidence-based nursing practice, the care plan is established on completion of a critical appraisal of what is known and not known about the defined problem. Next, in the traditional nursing process, the nurse implements the care plan. By integrating evidence with clinical expertise, the nurse focuses care on the patient's unique needs. The final step in EBP is consistent with the final phase of the nursing process—to evaluate the effectiveness of the care plan.

Searching for evidence in this modern era of technology can be overwhelming. For nurses to implement EBP, they must have access to appropriate, recent resources such as online search engines and journals. In many institutions, computer terminals are available on patient care units, with the Internet and online journals easily accessible. Another important resource for the implementation of EBP is time. The nursing shortage and ongoing changes in many institutions have compounded the issue of nursing time allocation for patient care, education, and training. In some institutions, nurses are given paid time away from performing patient care to participate in activities that promote EBP. This requires an organizational environment that values EBP and its potential impact on patient care. As knowledge is generated regarding the significant impact of EBP on patient care outcomes, it is hoped that the organizational culture will change to support the staff nurse's participation in EBP. As the amount of available evidence increases, so does our need to critically evaluate the evidence.

Throughout this book, Translating Evidence into Practice boxes summarize the existing evidence that promotes excellence in clinical care. The GRADE (Grading of Recommendations Assessment, Development and Evaluation) criteria are used to evaluate the quality of research articles used to develop practice guidelines (Guyatt, Oxman, Akl, et al., 2011). Table 1.4 defines how the nurse rates the quality of the evidence using the GRADE criteria and establishes a

TABLE 1.4 The GRADE Criteria to Evaluate the Quality of the Evidence

Quality	Type of Evidence
High	Consistent evidence from well-performed RCTs or exceptionally strong evidence from unbiased observational studies
Moderate	Evidence from RCTs with important limitations (inconsistent results, flaws in methodology, indirect evidence, or imprecise results) or unusually strong evidence from unbiased observational studies
Low	Evidence for at least one critical outcome from observational studies, from RCTs with serious flaws, or from indirect evidence
Very low	Evidence for at least one of the critical outcomes from unsystematic clinical observations or very indirect evidence
Quality	**Recommendation**
Strong	Desirable effects clearly outweigh undesirable effects, or vice versa
Weak	Desirable effects closely balanced with undesirable effects

RCT, Randomized clinical trial.
Adapted from Guyatt, G. H., Oxman, A. D., Akl, E. A., et al. (2011). GRADE guidelines: 1. Introduction—GRADE evidence profiles and summary of findings tables. *Journal of Clinical Epidemiology, 64*(4), 383–394.

strong versus weak recommendation. Each Translating Evidence into Practice box rates the quality of existing evidence and the strength of the recommendation for practice change.

CLINICAL JUDGMENT AND REASONING WHEN PROVIDING NURSING CARE TO CHILDREN AND FAMILIES

Clinical Judgment and Reasoning

A systematic thought process is essential to a profession. It assists the professional in meeting the patient's needs.

The National Council of State Boards of Nursing (NCSBN) definition of clinical judgment is "the observed outcome of critical thinking and decision-making. It is an iterative process that uses nursing knowledge to observe and assess presenting situations, identify a prioritized client concern, and generate the best possible evidence-based solutions in order to deliver safe client care" (NCSBN, 2018a, p. 12). This definition builds on and expands the nursing process, and indicates that clinical judgment skills are not linear steps that are followed in a particular sequence.

Clinical reasoning is a complex developmental process based on rational and deliberate thought. Clinical reasoning provides a common denominator for knowledge that exemplifies disciplined and self-directed thinking. The knowledge is acquired, assessed, and organized by thinking through the clinical situation and developing an outcome focused on optimum patient care. Clinical reasoning transforms the way in which individuals view themselves, understand the world, and make decisions.

The NCSBN developed a Clinical Judgment Measurement and Action Model. Six cognitive (thinking) skills, called cognitive processes, were identified as essential for nurses to make appropriate clinical judgment. Clinical judgment skills are compared to the nursing process in Table 1.5. Judgment skills help nurses identify changes in a client's clinical condition, and know what actions to take and why. The six essential cognitive skills of clinical judgment are described below (NCSBN, 2019).

TABLE 1.5 Comparison of Nursing Process Steps with Clinical Judgment Cognitive Skills

Steps of the Nursing Process	Cognitive Skills for Clinical Judgment
Assessment	Recognize Cues
Analysis	Analyze Cues
Analysis	Prioritize Hypotheses
Planning	Generate Solutions
Implementation	Take Action
Evaluation	Evaluate Outcomes

Six Essential Cognitive Skills of Clinical Judgment

- Recognize Cues
  Cues are elements of assessment data that provide important information for the nurse as a basis for making client decisions. In a clinical situation, the nurse determines which data are relevant (directly related to client outcomes or the priority of care) and of immediate concern to the nurse, or irrelevant (unrelated to client outcomes or priority of care).
- Analyze Cues
  When using this skill, the nurse considers the context of the client's history and situation, and interprets how the identified relevant cues relate to the client's condition. Data that support or contradict a particular cue in the client situation are determined, and potential complications are identified.
- Prioritize Hypotheses
  For this skill, the nurse needs to examine all possibilities about what is occurring in the client situation. The urgency and risk for the client is considered for each possible health condition. The nurse determines which client conditions are the most likely and most serious, and why.
- Generate Solutions
  To generate solutions, the nurse first identifies expected client outcomes. Using the prioritized hypotheses, the nurse then plans specific actions that may achieve the desirable outcomes. Actual or potential evidence-based actions that should be avoided or are contraindicated are also considered because some actions could be harmful for the client in the given situation.
- Take Action
  Using this skill, the nurse decides which nursing actions will address the highest priorities of care and determines in what priority these actions will be implemented. Actions can include, but are not limited to, additional assessment, health teaching, documentation, requested primary healthcare provider orders, performance of nursing skills, and consultation with health care team members.
- Evaluate Outcomes
  After implementing the best evidence-based nursing action, the nurse evaluates the actual client outcomes in the situation and compares them to expected outcomes. The nurse then decides if the selected nursing actions were effective, ineffective, or made no difference in how the client is progressing.

TABLE 1.6 Examples of Core Pediatric Clinical Care Quality Measures[a]

Clinical Care Quality Measure	How the Quality Measure Is Evaluated
Childhood immunization status	Percentage of children 2 years of age who had four diphtheria, tetanus, and acellular pertussis (DTaP); three polio (IPV); one measles, mumps, and rubella (MMR); three *Haemophilus influenzae* type B (HiB); three hepatitis B (Hep B); one chickenpox (VZV); four pneumococcal conjugate (PCV); one hepatitis A (Hep A); two or three rotavirus (RV); and two influenza (flu) vaccines by their second birthday.
Pediatric central line–associated bloodstream infections (CLABSI-CH)	A laboratory confirmed bloodstream infection (LCBI) found in pediatric patients with a central line that is not secondary to an infection at another body site found during hospitalization.
ADHD: follow-up care for children prescribed attention-deficit/hyperactivity disorder (ADHD) medication	Percentage of children 6-12 years of age and newly dispensed a medication for ADHD who had appropriate follow-up care. Two rates are reported.
Appropriate testing for children with pharyngitis	Percentage of children 2-18 years of age who were diagnosed with pharyngitis, ordered an antibiotic, and received a group A streptococcus (strep) test for the episode.

[a]Endorsed by the Centers for Medicaid and Medicare Services. (2019). *Children's health care quality measures.* Retrieved from https://www.medicaid.gov/medicaid/quality-of-care/downloads/performance-measurement/2019-child-core-set.pdf

In recognition of the importance of clinical judgment, case studies throughout the book present the importance of clinical judgment of nursing care. Nursing Care Plans are revised to integrate clinical judgment into nursing decisions. Clinical judgment allows the nurse to gather information and evaluate the relevance of the evidence to the specific clinical problem and patient. This promotes the application of knowledge to real clinical situations (Victor-Chmil, 2013).

The documentation of nursing care is an essential nursing responsibility and essential documentation components are summarized in the Nursing Care Guidelines box.

Quality Outcome Measures

Quality of care refers to the degree to which health services for individuals and populations increase the likelihood of desired health outcomes and are consistent with current professional knowledge (Institute of Medicine, 2000). The progress report to Congress on the National Strategy for Quality Improvement in Health Care focuses on six national quality priorities for health care quality improvement (National Strategy for Quality Improvement in Health Care, 2015)[b]:

NURSING CARE GUIDELINES

Documentation of Nursing Care

- Initial assessments and reassessments
- Nursing problem and/or patient care needs
- Interventions identified to meet the patient's nursing care needs
- Nursing care provided
- Patient's response to and the outcomes of the care provided
- Abilities of patient and/or, as appropriate, significant other(s) to manage continuing care needs after discharge

1. Making care safer by reducing harm caused in the delivery of care.
2. Ensuring that each person and family is engaged as partners in their care.
3. Promoting effective communication and coordination of care.
4. Promoting the most effective prevention and treatment practices for the leading causes of mortality, starting with cardiovascular disease.
5. Working with communities to promote wide use of best practices to enable healthy living.
6. Making quality care more affordable for individuals, families, employers, and governments by developing and spreading new health care delivery models.

[b]National Quality Strategy information can be found at http://www.ahrq.gov/workingforquality/about.htm#priorities.

The Centers for Medicare and Medicaid Services (2019) proposed a core of pediatric clinical care quality measures that align with these high-priority health care improvement goals. These indicators are endorsed by the National Quality Forum and designed to guide the effectiveness of pediatric health care programs. Table 1.6 presents examples of quality indicators from the core set of the Centers for Medicare and Medicaid Services measures. Throughout the chapters, examples of quality indicators endorsed by the Centers for Medicare and Medicaid Services and the National Quality Forum are presented and include a description of how the indicators will be measured. In each of these boxes the measurement name is provided along with the numerator and denominator for the measure to reflect how the indicator is defined. States across the country now use these indicators, usually over 1 year, to determine their success in meeting the quality measures. We also have developed examples of specific patient-centered quality outcome measures for certain diseases throughout the book. These quality outcome measures promote interdisciplinary teamwork, and the boxes throughout this book exemplify measures of effective collaboration to improve care. Pediatric Quality Indicators and Quality Patient Outcomes boxes throughout this book assist nurses in identifying appropriate measures that evaluate the quality of patient care.

Children's Hospitals' Solutions for Patient Safety is an excellent resource for intervention prevention bundles specific to pediatric care. Its website[c] has materials related to national initiatives that are implemented across more than 130 children's hospitals throughout the country. These activities are dedicated to creating safe and healing environments for all children and their families.

The Quality and Safety Education for Nurses Institute has defined quality and safety competencies for nursing. The Quality and Safety Education for Nurses Institute is now being hosted by faculty at the Case Western Reserve University and provides a comprehensive overview for the development of knowledge, skills, and attitudes related to quality and safety in health care.[d] In this book, each Translating Evidence into Practice box includes the Quality and Safety Education for Nurses Institute competencies related to knowledge, skills, and attitudes for evidence-based nursing practice.

[c]Children's Hospitals' Solutions for Patient Safety: https://www.solutionsforpatientsafety.org/

[d]Quality and Safety Education for Nurses Institute, Frances Payne Bolton School of Nursing, Case Western Reserve University: qsen.org

CLINICAL JUDGMENT AND NEXT-GENERATION NCLEX® EXAMINATION-STYLE QUESTIONS

1. Because injuries are the most common cause of death and disability in children in the United States, the stage of development can determine the type of injury that is most likely to occur. A nurse caring for a 2 ½ year old would focus on which of the following areas when discussing safety concerns for the home? **Select all that apply.**
   A. A newborn may roll over and fall off an elevated surface.
   B. The need to conform and gain acceptance from his peers may make a school-age child accept a dare.
   C. Toddlers who can run and climb may be susceptible to burns, falls, and collisions with objects.
   D. A toddler may ride her two-wheel bike in a reckless manner.
   E. A crawling infant may aspirate due to the tendency to place objects on the floor in his mouth.

2. The newest nurse on the pediatric unit is concerned about promoting family-centered care for the patients she cares for. She is working on an inpatient cancer unit and caring for a 7 year old with leukemia. Which of the following are important actions for the nurse to consider that will promote family-centered care for this child and family on her unit? **Select all that apply.**
   A. Striving to empower the family
   B. Purchase toys and clothes for the child
   C. Explore the family's strengths that will support the child
   D. Call the child frequently after discharge to offer support
   E. Assess the family's concerns and anxiety
   F. Restrict visitor access to the child
   G. Have a calming influence

3. The Clinical Judgment Measurement Model (CJMM) presents complex situations to promote nurse decision-making. **Match the Nursing Process skill in Column1 with the cognitive process/skill below found in the CJMM. Answers can be used more than once.**

CJMM Skill	Nursing Process	Match the Nursing Process Skill With CJMM Skill
1. Recognize Cues	Analysis	
2. Analyze Cues	Planning	
3. Prioritize Hypotheses	Implementation	
4. Generate Solutions	Evaluation	
5. Take Action	Assessment	
6. Evaluate Outcomes		

4. A family you are caring for on the pediatric unit asks you about nutrition for their 6-month old baby. What facts will you want to include in this nutritional information at this point in time? **Use an X for the nursing actions listed below that are Indicated (appropriate or necessary), Contraindicated (could be harmful), or Non-Essential (makes no difference or not necessary) for the child's care at this time.**

Nursing Action	Indicated	Contraindicated	Non-Essential
Eating preferences and attitudes related to food are established by family influences and culture.			
Breastfeeding provides micronutrients and immunologic properties.			
Most children establish lifelong eating habits by 18 months old.			
Because of the stress of returning to work, most mothers use this as a time to stop breastfeeding.			
During adolescence, parental influence diminishes, and adolescents make food choices related to peer acceptability and sociability.			
Chronic illness can cause a young child to not want to eat.			

REFERENCES

American Academy of Pediatrics. (2016). *American Academy of Pediatrics Announces New Recommendations for Children's Media Use.* https://www.aap.org.

American Academy of Pediatrics. Federal Advocacy, accessed 2/8/2019 https://www.aap.org/en-us/advocacy-and-policy/federal-advocacy.

American Academy of Pediatrics. (2018). *Dental Health & Hygiene for Young Children.* healthychildren.org. https://www.healthychildren.org/English/healthy-living/oral-health/Pages/Teething-and-Dental-Hygiene.aspx.

Annie, E. Casey Foundation (2019): *2019 Kids count data book: State trends in child well-being.* Baltimore, MD: The Foundation. http://www.aecf.org/databook.

Bright Futures. (2018). *Prevention and health promotion for infants, children, adolescents, and their families.* http://brightfutures.aap.org.

Centers for Disease Control and Prevention. (2017a). *Infant Mortality.* https://www.cdc.gov/reproductivehealth/MaternalInfantHealth/InfantMortality.htm.

Centers for Disease Control and Prevention. (2017b). *Injury and violence prevention and control.* http://www.cdc.gov/injury.

Centers for Disease Control and Prevention. (2018). *Childhood Obesity Facts.* https://www.cdc.gov/obesity/data/childhood.html.

Center for Medicaid and Medicare Services. (2019). *Children's Health Care Quality Measures.* https://www.medicaid.gov/medicaid/quality-of-care/downloads/performance-measurement/2019-child-core-set.pdf.

Child Mind Institute. (2016). *2016 Children's Mental Health Report.* https://www.childmind.org/report/2016-childrens-mental-health-report/.

David-Ferdon, C., & Simon, T. R. (2014). *Preventing youth violence: Opportunities for action.* Atlanta, GA: National Center for Injury Prevention and Control, Centers for Disease Control and Prevention.

Farzal, Z., Perry, M. F., Yarbrough, W. G., et al. (2019). The adolescent vaping epidemic in the United States-how it happened and where we go from here. *JAMA Otolaryngology.* Published online. [Accessed 22 August 2019].

Federal Interagency Forum on Child and Family Statistics. (2019). *America's Children: Key national indicators of well-being.* Washington, DC: U.S. Government Printing Office. http://www.childstats.gov/americaschildren/index.asp.

Ferguson, R. W., Osterthaler, K., Kaminski, S., et al. (2015). *Medicine safety for children: An in-depth look at poison center calls.* Washington, D.C: Safe Kids Worldwide, March.

Flores, G., & Lesley, B. (2014). Children and US federal policy on health and health care. *JAMA Pediatrics, 168*(12), 1155–1163.

Garcia-Mantrana, I., & Collado, M. C. (2016). Obesity and overweight: Impact on maternal and milk microbiome and their role for infant health and nutrition. *Molecular Nutrition & Food Research, 60*(8), 1865–1875.

Godfrey, K. M., Reynolds, R. M., Prescott, S. L., et al. (2016). Influence of maternal obesity on the long-term health of offspring. *Lancet Diabetes Endocrinol,* S2213–8587.

Guyatt, G. H., Oxman, A. D., Akl, E. A., et al. (2011). GRADE guidelines: 1. Introduction—GRADE evidence profiles and summary of findings tables. *Journal of Clinical Epidemiology, 64*(4), 383–394.

Institute of Medicine. (2000). *Crossing the quality chasm.* Washington, DC: The Institute.

Institute for Patient- and Family-Centered Care. (2018). *Patient- and family-centered care.* http://www.ipfcc.org/about/pfcc.html.

Kids Count Data Center. (2016). *Child and teen death rate.* http://datacenter.kidscount.org.

Kochanek, K.D., Murphy, S.L. Xu, J., et. al. (2019). Deaths: final data for 2017. *National vital statistics report,* 68(9), 1–77.

Melnyk, B. M., & Fineout-Overholt, E. (2014). *Evidence-based practice in nursing and healthcare: A guide to best practice.* Philadelphia: Lippincott Williams & Wilkins.

Miech, R.A., Schulenberg, J.E., Johnston, L.D., et al. (2018). National adolescent drug trends in 2018. Monitoring the Future: Ann Arbor, Mi. Retrieved Jan 10, 2019. http://www.monotroingthe.future.org.

National Council of State Boards of Nursing. (Winter, 2018a). Measuring the right things: NCSBN's next generation NCLEX® endeavors to go beyond the leading edge. *In Focus.* Chicago, IL: Author.

National Council of State Boards of Nursing (NCSBN). (2019). The clinical judgment model. *Next generation NCLEX News. (Winter).* 1-6.

National Institute for Children's Health Quality. Promoting optimal child development, accessed 12/5/2018. https://www.nichq.org/project/promoting-optimal-child-development.

National Safety Council. (2000). *Injury facts.* Itasca, IL: The Council.

National Strategy for Quality Improvement in Health Care. (2015). *Annual progress report to congress.* Washington, DC: US Department of Health and Human Services.

US Department of Health and Human Services. (2013). *Healthy people 2020.* http://www.healthypeople.gov/.

US Department of Health and Human Services. (2019). *Office of Disease Prevention and Health Promotion. Healthy People 2030.* Retrieved from http://www.healthypeople.gov/.

Victor-Chmil, J. (2013). Critical thinking versus clinical reasoning versus clinical judgment: differential diagnosis. *Nurse Educator, 38*(1), 34–36.

Weiss, R., Bremer, A. A., & Lustig, R. H. (2013). What is metabolic syndrome, and why are children getting it? *Annals of the New York Academy of Sciences, 1281,* 123–140.

Wong, D. (1989). Principles of atraumatic care. In V. Feeg (Ed.), *Pediatric nursing: forum on the future: Looking toward the 21st century.* Pitman, NJ: Anthony J Jannetti.

2

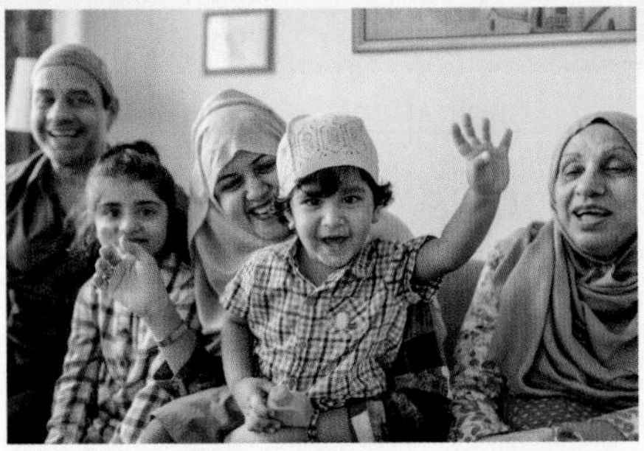

Social, Cultural, Religious, and Family Influences on Child Health Promotion*

Marilyn J. Hockenberry

http://evolve.elsevier.com/wong/essentials

CONCEPTS

- Family Dynamics
- Culture

GENERAL CONCEPTS

DEFINITION OF FAMILY

The term **family** has been defined in many ways according to the individual's own frame of reference, values, or discipline. There is no universal definition of family; a family is what an individual considers it to be. Biology describes the family as fulfilling the biologic function of perpetuation of the species. Psychology emphasizes the interpersonal aspects of the family and its responsibility for personality development. Economics views the family as a productive unit that provides for material needs. Sociology depicts the family as a social unit that interacts with the larger society, creating the context within which cultural values and identity are formed. Others define family in terms of the relationships of the persons who make up the family unit. The most common types of relationships are **consanguineous** (blood relationships), **affinal** (marital relationships), and **family of origin** (family unit a person is born into).

Considerable controversy has surrounded the newer concepts of family, such as communal families, single-parent families, and homosexual families. To accommodate these and other varieties of family styles, the descriptive term *household* is frequently used.

> **! NURSING ALERT**
>
> The nurse's knowledge and the sensitivity with which he or she assesses a household will determine the types of interventions that are appropriate to support family members.

Nursing care of infants and children is intimately involved with care of the child and the family. Family structure and dynamics can have an enduring influence on a child, affecting the child's health and well-being (American Academy of Pediatrics, 2003). Consequently, nurses must be aware of the functions of the family, various types of family structures, and theories that provide a foundation for understanding the changes within a family and for directing family-oriented interventions.

FAMILY THEORIES

A **family theory** can be used to describe families and how the family unit responds to events both within and outside the family. Each family theory makes assumptions about the family and has inherent strengths and limitations (Kaakinen & Coehlo, 2015). Most nurses use a combination of theories in their work with children and families. Commonly used theories are family systems theory, family stress theory, and developmental theory (Table 2.1).

Family Systems Theory

Family systems theory is derived from general systems theory, a science of "wholeness" that is characterized by interaction among the components of the system and between the system and the environment (Bomar, 2004; Papero, 1990). **General systems theory** expanded scientific thought from a simplistic view of direct cause and effect (*A* causes *B*) to a more complex and interrelated theory (*A* influences *B*, but *B* also affects *A*). In family systems theory, the family is viewed as a system that continually interacts with its members and the environment. The emphasis is on the interaction between the members; a change in one family member creates a change in other members, which in turn results in a new change in the original member. Consequently, a problem or dysfunction does not lie in any one member but rather in the type of interactions used by the family. Because the interactions, not the individual members, are viewed as the source of the problem, the family becomes the patient and the focus of care. Examples of the application of family systems theory to clinical problems are nonorganic failure to thrive and child abuse. According to family systems theory, the problem does not rest solely with the parent or child but with the type of interactions between the parent and the child and the factors that affect their relationship.

The family is viewed as a whole that is different from the sum of the individual members. For example, a household of parents and one child consists of not only three individuals but also four interactive units. These units include three dyads (the marital relationship, the mother-child relationship, and the father-child relationship) and a triangle (the mother-father-child relationship). In this ecologic model, the family system functions within a larger system, with the family dyads in the center of a circle surrounded by the extended family, the subculture, and the culture, with the larger society at the periphery.

*This chapter was originally updated by Quinn Franklin and Kim Mooney-Doyle.

TABLE 2.1 Summary of Family Theories and Application

Assumptions	Strengths	Limitations	Applications
Family Systems Theory			
A change in any one part of a family system affects all other parts of the family system (circular causality). Family systems are characterized by periods of rapid growth and change and periods of relative stability. Both too little change and too much change are dysfunctional for the family system; therefore a balance between morphogenesis (change) and morphostasis (no change) is necessary. Family systems can initiate change as well as react to it.	Applicable for family in normal everyday life as well as for family dysfunction and pathology. Useful for families of varying structure and various stages of life cycle.	More difficult to determine cause-and-effect relationships because of circular causality.	Mate selection, courtship processes, family communication, boundary maintenance, power and control within family, parent-child relationships, adolescent pregnancy and parenthood.
Family Stress Theory			
Stress is an inevitable part of family life, and any event, even if positive, can be stressful for family. Family encounters both normative expected stressors and unexpected situational stressors over the life cycle. Stress has a cumulative effect on family. Families cope with and respond to stressors with a wide range of responses and effectiveness.	Potential to explain and predict family behavior in response to stressors and to develop effective interventions to promote family adaptation. Focuses on positive contribution of resources, coping, and social support to adaptive outcomes. Can be used by many disciplines in health care field.	Relationships between all variables in framework not yet adequately described. Not yet known if certain combinations of resources and coping strategies are applicable to all stressful events.	Transition to parenthood and other normative transitions, single-parent families, families experiencing work-related stressors (dual-earner family, unemployment), acute or chronic childhood illness or disability, infertility, death of a child, divorce, adolescent pregnancy and parenthood.
Developmental Theory			
Families develop and change over time in similar and consistent ways. Family and its members must perform certain time-specific tasks set by themselves and by persons in the broader society. Family role performance at one stage of family life cycle influences family's behavioral options at next stage. Family tends to be in stage of disequilibrium when entering a new life cycle stage and strives toward homeostasis within stages.	Provides a dynamic, rather than static, view of family. Addresses both changes within family and changes in family as a social system over its life history. Anticipates potential stressors that normally accompany transitions to various stages and when problems may peak because of lack of resources.	Traditional model more easily applied to two-parent families with children. Use of age of oldest child and marital duration as marker of stage transition sometimes problematic (e.g., in stepfamilies, single-parent families).	Anticipatory guidance, educational strategies, and developing or strengthening family resources for management of transition to parenthood; family adjustment to children entering school, becoming adolescents, leaving home; management of "empty nest" years and retirement.

Bowen's family systems theory (Kaakinen & Coehlo, 2015; Papero, 1990) emphasizes that the key to healthy family function is the members' ability to distinguish themselves from one another both emotionally and intellectually. The family unit has a high level of **adaptability**. When problems arise within the family, change occurs by altering the interaction or feedback messages that perpetuate disruptive behavior. **Feedback** refers to processes in the family that help identify strengths and needs and determine how well goals are accomplished. Positive feedback initiates change; negative feedback resists change (Goldenberg & Goldenberg, 2012). When the family system is disrupted, change can occur at any point in the system.

A major factor that influences a family's adaptability is its **boundary**, an imaginary line that exists between the family and its environment (Kaakinen & Coehlo, 2015). Families have varying degrees of openness and closure in these boundaries. For example, one family has the capacity to reach out for help, whereas another considers help threatening. Knowledge of boundaries is critical when teaching or counseling families. Families with open boundaries may demonstrate a greater receptivity to interventions, whereas families with closed boundaries often require increased sensitivity and skill on the part of the nurse to gain their trust and acceptance. The nurse who uses family systems theory should assess the family's ability to accept new ideas, information, resources, and opportunities, and to plan strategies.

Family Stress Theory

Family stress theory explains how families react to stressful events and suggests factors that promote adaptation to stress (Kaakinen & Coehlo, 2015). Families encounter **stressors** (events that cause stress and have the potential to effect a change in the family social system), including those that are predictable (e.g., parenthood) and those that are unpredictable (e.g., illness, unemployment). These stressors are cumulative, involving simultaneous demands from work, family, and community life. Too many stressful events occurring within a relatively short period (usually 1 year) can overwhelm the family's ability

BOX 2.1 Duvall's Developmental Stages of the Family

Stage I—Marriage and an Independent Home: The Joining of Families
Reestablish couple identity.
Realign relationships with extended family.
Make decisions regarding parenthood.

Stage II—Families With Infants
Integrate infants into the family unit.
Accommodate to new parenting and grandparenting roles.
Maintain marital bond.

Stage III—Families With Preschoolers
Socialize children.
Parents and children adjust to separation.

Stage IV—Families With Schoolchildren
Children develop peer relations.
Parents adjust to their children's peer and school influences.

Stage V—Families With Teenagers
Adolescents develop increasing autonomy.
Parents refocus on midlife marital and career issues.
Parents begin a shift toward concern for the older generation.

Stage VI—Families as Launching Centers
Parents and young adults establish independent identities.
Parents renegotiate marital relationship.

Stage VII—Middle-Aged Families
Reinvest in couple identity with concurrent development of independent interests.
Realign relationships to include in-laws and grandchildren.
Deal with disabilities and death of older generation.

Stage VIII—Aging Families
Shift from work role to leisure and semiretirement or full retirement.
Maintain couple and individual functioning while adapting to the aging process.
Prepare for own death and dealing with the loss of spouse and/or siblings and other peers.

Modified from Wright, L. M., & Leahey, M (1984). *Nurses and families: A guide to family assessment and intervention.* Philadelphia, PA: Davis.

to cope and place it at risk for breakdown or physical and emotional health problems among its members. When the family experiences too many stressors for it to cope adequately, a state of crisis ensues. For adaptation to occur, a change in family structure or interaction is necessary.

The **resiliency model of family stress, adjustment, and adaptation** emphasizes that the stressful situation is not necessarily pathologic or detrimental to the family but demonstrates that the family needs to make fundamental structural or systemic changes to adapt to the situation (McCubbin & McCubbin, 1994).

Developmental Theory

Developmental theory is an outgrowth of several theories of development. Duvall (1977) described eight developmental tasks of the family throughout its life span (Box 2.1). The family is described as a small group, a semiclosed system of personalities that interacts with the larger cultural social system. As an interrelated system, the family does not have changes in one part without a series of changes in other parts.

Developmental theory addresses family change over time, using Duvall's family life cycle stages. This theory is based on the predictable changes in the family's structure, function, and roles, with the age of the oldest child as the marker for stage transition. The arrival of the first child marks the transition from stage I to stage II. As the first child grows and develops, the family enters subsequent stages. In every stage the family faces certain developmental tasks. At the same time, each family member must achieve individual developmental tasks as part of each family life cycle stage.

Developmental theory can be applied to nursing practice. For example, the nurse can assess how well new parents are accomplishing the individual and family developmental tasks associated with transition to parenthood. New applications should emerge as more is learned about developmental stages for nonnuclear and nontraditional families.

BOX 2.2 Family Nursing Intervention

- Behavior modification
- Case management and coordination
- Collaborative strategies
- Contracting
- Counseling, including support, cognitive reappraisal, and reframing
- Empowering families through active participation
- Environmental modification
- Family advocacy
- Family crisis intervention
- Networking, including use of self-help groups and social support
- Providing information and technical expertise
- Role modeling
- Role supplementation
- Teaching strategies, including stress management, lifestyle modifications, and anticipatory guidance

From Friedman, M. M., Bowden, V. R., & Jones, E. G. (2003). *Family nursing: Research theory and practice* (5th ed.). Upper Saddle River, NJ: Prentice Hall.

FAMILY NURSING INTERVENTIONS

In working with children, the nurse must include family members in their care plan. Research confirms parents' desire and expectation to participate in their child's care (Power & Franck, 2008). To discover family dynamics, strengths, and weaknesses, a thorough family assessment is necessary (see Chapter 4). The nurse's choice of interventions depends on the theoretic family model that is used (Box 2.2). For example, in family systems theory, the focus is on the interaction of family members within the larger environment (Goldenberg & Goldenberg, 2012). In this case using group dynamics to involve all members in the intervention process and being a skillful communicator are essential. Systems theory also presents excellent opportunities for anticipatory guidance. Because each family member reacts to every stress experienced by that system, nurses can intervene to help the family prepare for and cope with changes. In family stress theory the nurse uses crisis intervention strategies to help family members cope with the challenging event. In developmental theory the nurse provides anticipatory guidance to prepare members for transition to the next family stage. Nurses who think family involvement plays a key role in the care of a child are more likely to include families in the child's daily care (Fisher, Lindhorst, Matthews, et al., 2008).

FAMILY STRUCTURE AND FUNCTION

FAMILY STRUCTURE

The family structure, or family composition, consists of individuals, each with a socially recognized status and position, who interact with one another on a regular, recurring basis in socially sanctioned ways (Kaakinen & Coehlo, 2015). When members are gained or lost through events such as marriage, divorce, birth, death, abandonment, or incarceration, the family composition is altered and roles must be redefined or redistributed.

Traditionally, the family structure was either a nuclear or an extended family. In recent years family composition has assumed new configurations, with the single-parent family and blended family becoming prominent forms. The predominant structural pattern in any society depends on the mobility of families as they pursue economic goals and as relationships change. It is not uncommon for children to belong to several different family groups during their lifetime.

Nurses must be able to meet the needs of children from many diverse family structures and home situations. A family's structure affects the direction of nursing care. The US Census Bureau uses four definitions for families: (1) the traditional nuclear family, (2) the nuclear family, (3) the blended family or household, and (4) the extended family or household. In addition, numerous other types of families have been defined, such as single-parent; binuclear; polygamous; communal; and lesbian, gay, bisexual, and transgender (LGBT) families.

Traditional Nuclear Family

A traditional nuclear family consists of a married couple and their biologic children. Children in this type of family live with both biologic parents and, if siblings are present, only full brothers and sisters (i.e., siblings who share the same two biologic parents). No other persons are present in the household (i.e., no steprelatives, foster or adopted children, half-siblings, other relatives, or nonrelatives).

Nuclear Family

The nuclear family is composed of two parents and their children. The parent-child relationship may be biologic, step, adoptive, or foster. Sibling ties may be biologic, step, half, or adoptive. The parents are not necessarily married. No other relatives or nonrelatives are present in the household.

Blended Family

A blended family or household, also called a reconstituted family, includes at least one stepparent, stepsibling, or half-sibling. A stepparent is the spouse of a child's biologic parent but is not the child's biologic parent. Stepsiblings do not share a common biologic parent; the biologic parent of one child is the stepparent of the other. Half-siblings share only one biologic parent.

Extended Family

An extended family or household includes at least one parent, one or more children, and one or more members (related or unrelated) other than a parent or sibling. Parent-child and sibling relationships may be biologic, step, adoptive, or foster.

In many nations and among many ethnic and cultural groups, households with extended families are common. Within the extended family, grandparents often find themselves rearing their grandchildren (Fig. 2.1). Young parents are often considered too young or too inexperienced to make decisions independently. Often the older relative holds the authority and makes decisions in consultation with the young parents. Sharing residence with relatives also assists with the management of scarce resources and provides child care for working families.

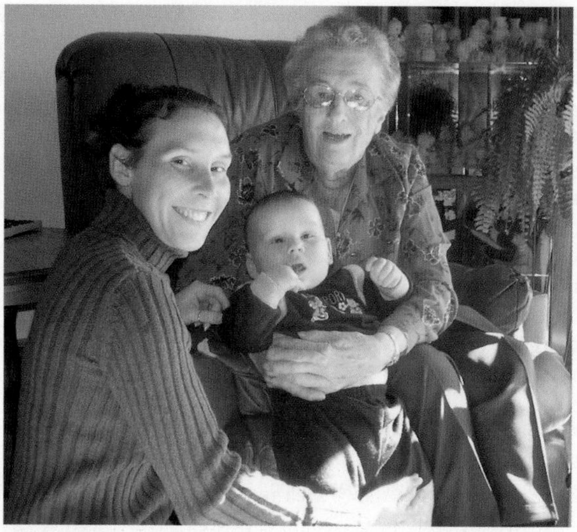

Fig. 2.1 Children benefit from interaction with grandparents, who sometimes assume the parenting role.

Single-Parent Family

In the United States an estimated 24.4 million or 35% of children live in single-parent families (Annie E. Casey Foundation, 2018). The contemporary single-parent family has emerged partially as a consequence of the women's rights movement and also as a result of more women (and men) establishing separate households because of divorce, death, desertion, or single parenthood. In addition, a more liberal attitude in the courts has made it possible for single people, both male and female, to adopt children. Although mothers usually head single-parent families, it is becoming more common for fathers to be awarded custody of dependent children in divorce settlements. With women's increased psychologic and financial independence and the increased acceptability of single parents in society, more unmarried women are deliberately choosing mother-child families. Frequently, these mothers and children are absorbed into the extended family. The challenges of single-parent families are discussed later in the chapter.

Binuclear Family

The term binuclear family refers to parents continuing the parenting role while terminating the spousal unit. The degree of cooperation between households and the time the child spends with each can vary. In joint custody the court assigns divorcing parents equal rights and responsibilities concerning the minor child or children. These alternate family forms are efforts to view divorce as a process of reorganization and redefinition of a family rather than as a family dissolution. Joint custody and coparenting are discussed further later in the chapter.

Polygamous Family

Although it is not legally sanctioned in the United States, the conjugal unit is sometimes extended by the addition of spouses in polygamous matings. Polygamy refers to either multiple wives (polygyny) or, rarely, multiple husbands (polyandry). Many societies practice polygyny that is further designated as sororal, in which the wives are sisters, or nonsororal, in which the wives are unrelated. Sororal polygyny is widespread throughout the world. Most often, mothers and their children share a husband and father, with each mother and her children living in the same or separate household.

Communal Family

The **communal family** emerged from disenchantment with most contemporary life choices. Although communal families may have divergent beliefs, practices, and organization, the basic impetus for formation is often dissatisfaction with the nuclear family structure, social systems, and goals of the larger community. Relatively uncommon today, communal groups share common ownership of property. In cooperatives, property ownership is private, but certain goods and services are shared and exchanged without monetary consideration. There is strong reliance on group members and material interdependence. Both provide collective security for nonproductive members, share homemaking and childrearing functions, and help overcome the problem of interpersonal isolation or loneliness.

Lesbian, Gay, Bisexual, and Transgender Families

A **same-sex**, **homosexual**, or **lesbian/gay/bisexual/transgender (LGBT) family** is one in which there is a legal or common-law tie between two persons of the same sex who have children. There are a growing number of families with same-sex parents in the United States, with an estimated 16.4% of all same-sex couples raising children (US Census Bureau, 2017). Although some children in LGBT households are biologic from a former marriage relationship, children may be present in other circumstances. They may be foster or adoptive parents, lesbian mothers may conceive through artificial fertilization, or a gay male couple may become parents through use of a surrogate mother.

When children are brought up in LGBT families, the relationships seem as natural to them as heterosexual parents do to their offspring. In other cases, however, disclosure of parental homosexuality ("coming out") to children can be a concern for families. There are a number of factors to consider before disclosing this information to children. Parents should be comfortable with their own sexual orientation and should discuss this with the children as they become old enough to understand relationships. Discussions should be planned and take place in a quiet setting where interruptions are unlikely.

Nurses need to be nonjudgmental and to learn to accept differences rather than demonstrate prejudice that can have a detrimental effect on the nurse-child-family relationship. Moreover, the more nurses know about the child's family and lifestyle, the more they can help the parents and the child.

FAMILY STRENGTHS AND FUNCTIONING STYLE

Family function refers to the interactions of family members, especially the quality of those relationships and interactions (Bomar, 2004). Researchers are interested in family characteristics that help families to function effectively. Knowledge of these factors guides the nurse throughout the nursing process and helps the nurse to predict ways that families may cope and respond to a stressful event, to provide individualized support that builds on family strengths and unique functioning style, and to assist family members in obtaining resources.

Family strengths and unique functioning styles (Box 2.3) are significant resources that nurses can use to meet family needs. Building on qualities that make a family work well and strengthening family resources make the family unit even stronger. All families have strengths as well as vulnerabilities.

FAMILY ROLES AND RELATIONSHIPS

Each individual has a position, or status, in the family structure and plays culturally and socially defined roles in interactions within the family. Each family also has its own traditions and values and sets its own standards for interaction within and outside the group. Each determines the experiences the children should have, those they are to be shielded from, and how each of these experiences meets the needs of family members. When family ties are strong, social control is highly effective, and most members conform to their roles willingly and with commitment. Conflicts arise when people do not fulfill their roles in ways that meet other family members' expectations, either because they are unaware of the expectations or because they choose not to meet them.

BOX 2.3 Qualities of Strong Families

- A belief and sense of **commitment** toward promoting the well-being and growth of individual family members, as well as the family unit
- **Appreciation** for the small and large things that individual family members do well and **encouragement** to do better
- Concentrated effort to spend **time** and do things together, no matter how formal or informal the activity or event
- A sense of **purpose** that permeates the reasons and basis for "going on" in both bad and good times
- A sense of **congruence** among family members regarding the value and importance of assigning time and energy to meet needs
- The ability to **communicate** with one another in a way that emphasizes positive interactions
- A clear set of **family rules, values,** and **beliefs** that establishes expectations about acceptable and desired behavior
- A varied repertoire of **coping strategies** that promote positive functioning in dealing with both normative and nonnormative life events
- The ability to engage in **problem-solving** activities designed to evaluate options for meeting needs and procuring resources
- The ability to be **positive** and see the positive in almost all aspects of their lives, including the ability to see crisis and problems as an opportunity to learn and grow
- **Flexibility** and **adaptability** in the roles necessary to procure resources to meet needs
- A **balance** between the use of internal and external family resources for coping and adapting to life events and planning for the future

From Dunst, C., Trivette, C., & Deal, A. (1988). *Enabling and empowering families: Principles and guidelines for practice.* Cambridge, MA: Brookline Books.

PARENTAL ROLES

In all family groups, the socially recognized statuses of father and mother exist with socially sanctioned roles that prescribe appropriate sexual behavior and childrearing responsibilities. The guides for behavior in these roles serve to control sexual conflict in society and provide for prolonged care of children. The degree to which parents are committed and the way they play their roles are influenced by a number of variables and by the parents' unique socialization experience.

Parental role definitions have changed as a result of the changing economy and increased opportunities for women (Bomar, 2004). As the woman's role has changed, the complementary role of the man has also changed. Many fathers are more active in childrearing and household tasks. As the redefinition of sex roles continues in American families, role conflicts may arise in many families because of a cultural lag of the persisting traditional role definitions.

ROLE LEARNING

Roles are learned through the socialization process. During all stages of development, children learn and practice, through interaction with others and in their play, a set of social roles and the characteristics of other roles. They behave in patterned and more or less predictable ways because they learn roles that define mutual expectations in typical social relationships. Although role definitions are changing, the basic determinants of parenting remain the same. Determinants of parenting infants and young children include parental personality and mental well-being, systems of support, and child characteristics. These determinants have been used as consistent measurements to determine a person's success in fulfilling the parental role.

In some cultures the role behavior expected of children conflicts with desirable adult behavior. One of the family's responsibilities is to develop culturally appropriate role behavior in children. Children learn to perform in expected ways consistent with their position in the family and culture. The observed behavior of each child is a single manifestation—a combination of social influences and individual psychologic processes. In this way the uniting of the child's intrapersonal system (the self) with the interpersonal system (the family) is simultaneously understood as the child's conduct.

Role structuring initially takes place within the family unit, in which the children fulfill a set of roles and respond to the roles of their parents and other family members (Kaakinen & Coehlo, 2015). Children's roles are shaped primarily by the parents, who apply direct or indirect pressures to induce or force children into the desired patterns of behavior or direct their efforts toward modification of the role responses of the child on a mutually acceptable basis. Parents have their own techniques and determine the course of the socialization process.

Children respond to life situations according to behaviors learned in reciprocal transactions. As they acquire important role-taking skills, their relationships with others change. For instance, when a teenager is also the mother but lives in a household with the grandmother, the teenager may be viewed more as an adolescent than as a mother. Children become proficient at understanding others as they acquire the ability to discriminate their own perspectives from those of others. Children who get along well with others and attain status in the peer group have well-developed role-taking skills.

Family Size and Configuration

Parenting practices differ between small and large families. Small families place more emphasis on the individual development of the children. Parenting is intensive rather than extensive, and there is constant pressure to measure up to family expectations. Children's development and achievement are measured against those of other children in the neighborhood and social class. In small families, children have more democratic participation than they do in larger families. Adolescents in small families identify more strongly with their parents and rely more on them for advice. They have well-developed, autonomous inner controls as contrasted with adolescents from larger families, who rely more on adult authority.

Children in a large family are able to adjust to a variety of changes and crises. There is more emphasis on the group and less emphasis on the individual (Fig. 2.2). Cooperation is essential, often because of economic necessity. The large number of people sharing a limited amount of space requires a greater degree of organization, administration, and authoritarian control. A dominant family member (a parent or older child) wields control. The number of children reduces the intimate, one-to-one contact between the parent and any individual child. Consequently, children turn to each other for what they cannot get from their parents. The reduced parent-child contact encourages individual children to adopt specialized roles to gain recognition in the family.

Older siblings in large families often administer discipline (Fig. 2.3). Siblings are usually attuned to what constitutes misbehavior. Sibling disapproval or ostracism is frequently a more meaningful disciplinary measure than parental interventions. In situations such as death or illness of a parent, an older sibling often assumes responsibility for the family at considerable personal sacrifice. Large families generate a sense of security in the children that is fostered by sibling support and cooperation. However, adolescents from a large family are more peer oriented than family oriented.

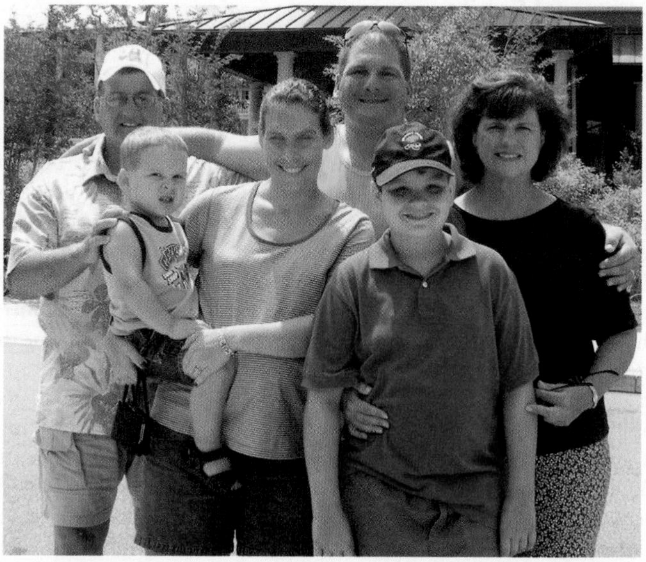

Fig. 2.2 Family structure and function promote strong relationships among its members.

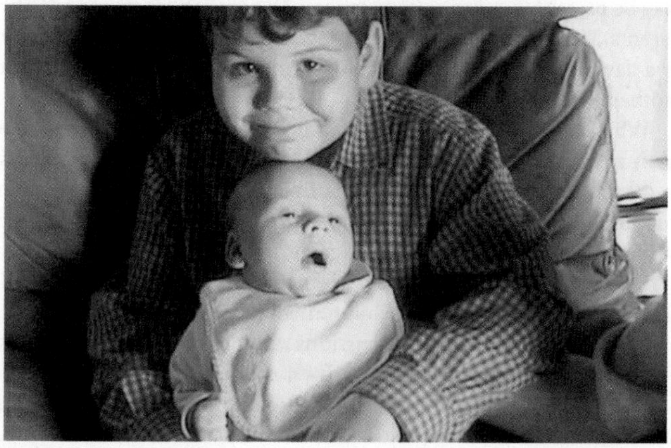

Fig. 2.3 Older school-age children often enjoy taking responsibility for the care of a younger sibling.

PARENTING

PARENTING STYLES

Children respond to their environment in a variety of ways. A child's temperament heavily influences his or her response (see Chapter 10), but styles of parenting have also been show to affect a child and lead to particular behavioral responses. Parenting styles are often classified as authoritarian, permissive, or authoritative (Baumrind, 1971, 1996). **Authoritarian** parents try to control their children's behavior and attitudes through unquestioned mandates. They establish rules and regulations or standards of conduct that they expect to be followed rigidly and unquestioningly. The message is: "Do it because I say so." Punishment need not be corporal but may be stern withdrawal of love and approval. Careful training often results in rigidly conforming behavior in the children, who tend to be sensitive, shy, self-conscious, retiring, and submissive. They are more likely to be courteous, loyal, honest, and dependable, but docile. These behaviors are more typically observed when close supervision and affection accompany parental authority. If not, this style of parenting may be associated with both defiant and antisocial behaviors.

Permissive parents exert little or no control over their children's actions. They avoid imposing their own standards of conduct and allow their children to regulate their own activity as much as possible. These parents consider themselves to be resources for the children, not role models. If rules do exist, the parents explain the underlying reason, elicit the children's opinions, and consult them in decision-making processes. They employ lax, inconsistent discipline; do not set sensible limits; and do not prevent the children from upsetting the home routine. These parents rarely punish the children.

Authoritative parents combine practices from both of the other parenting styles. They direct their children's behavior and attitudes by emphasizing the reason for rules and negatively reinforcing deviations. They respect the individuality of each child and allow the child to voice objections to family standards or regulations. Parental control is firm and consistent but tempered with encouragement, understanding, and security. Control is focused on the issue, not on withdrawal of love or the fear of punishment. These parents foster "inner-directedness," a conscience that regulates behavior based on feelings of guilt or shame for wrongdoing, not on fear of being caught or punished. Parents' realistic standards and reasonable expectations produce children with high self-esteem who are self-reliant, assertive, inquisitive, content, and highly interactive with other children.

There are differing philosophies in regard to parenting. Childrearing is a culturally bound phenomenon, and children are socialized to behave in ways that are important to their family. In the authoritative style, authority is shared and children are included in discussions, fostering an independent and assertive style of participation in family life. When working with individual families, nurses should give these differing styles equal respect.

LIMIT SETTING AND DISCIPLINE

In its broadest sense, **discipline** means "to teach" or refers to a set of rules governing conduct. In a narrower sense, it refers to the action taken to enforce the rules after noncompliance. **Limit setting** refers to establishing the rules or guidelines for behavior. For example, parents can place limits on the amount of time children spend watching television or chatting online. The clearer the limits that are set and the more consistently they are enforced, the less need there is for disciplinary action.

Nurses can help parents establish realistic and concrete "rules." Limit setting and discipline are positive, necessary components of childrearing and serve several useful functions as they help children to:

- Test their limits of control
- Achieve in areas appropriate for mastery at their level
- Channel undesirable feelings into constructive activity
- Protect themselves from danger
- Learn socially acceptable behavior

Children want and need limits. Unrestricted freedom is a threat to their security and safety. By testing the limits imposed on them, children learn the extent to which they can manipulate their environment and gain reassurance from knowing that others are there to protect them from potential harm.

Minimizing Misbehavior

The reasons for misbehavior may include attention, power, defiance, and a display of inadequacy (e.g., the child misses classes because of a fear that he or she is unable to do the work). Children may also misbehave because the rules are not clear or consistently applied. Acting-out behavior, such as a temper tantrum, may represent uncontrolled frustration, anger, depression, or pain. The best approach is to structure interactions with children to prevent or minimize unacceptable behavior (see Family-Centered Care box).

General Guidelines for Implementing Discipline

Regardless of the type of discipline used, certain principles are essential to ensure the efficacy of the approach (see Family-Centered Care box). Many strategies, such as behavior modification, can only be implemented effectively when principles of consistency and timing are followed. A pattern of intermittent or occasional enforcement of limits actually prolongs the undesired behavior because children learn that if they are persistent, the behavior is permitted eventually. Delaying punishment weakens its intent, and practices such as telling the child "Wait until your father comes home" not only are ineffectual but also convey negative messages about the other parent.

FAMILY-CENTERED CARE

Minimizing Misbehavior

- Set realistic goals for acceptable behavior and expected achievements.
- Structure opportunities for small successes to lessen feelings of inadequacy.
- Praise children for desirable behavior with attention and verbal approval.
- Structure the environment to prevent unnecessary difficulties (e.g., place fragile objects in an inaccessible area).
- Set clear and reasonable rules; expect the same behavior regardless of the circumstances; if exceptions are made, clarify that the change is for one time only.
- Teach desirable behavior through own example, such as using a quiet, calm voice rather than screaming.
- Review expected behavior before special or unusual events, such as visiting a relative or having dinner in a restaurant.
- Phrase requests for appropriate behavior positively, such as "Put the book down" rather than "Don't touch the book."
- Call attention to unacceptable behavior as soon as it begins; use distraction to change the behavior or offer alternatives to annoying actions, such as exchanging a quiet toy for one that is too noisy.
- Give advance notice or "friendly reminders," such as "When the TV program is over, it is time for dinner" or "I'll give you to the count of three, and then we have to go."
- Be attentive to situations that increase the likelihood of misbehaving, such as overexcitement or fatigue, or to decreased personal tolerance to minor infractions.
- Offer sympathetic explanations for not granting a request, such as "I am sorry I can't read you a story now, but I have to finish dinner. Then we can spend time together."
- Keep any promises made to children.
- Avoid outright conflicts; temper discussions with statements such as "Let's talk about it and see what we can decide together" or "I have to think about it first."
- Provide children with opportunities for power and control.

Types of Discipline

To deal with misbehavior, parents need to implement appropriate disciplinary action. Many approaches are available. **Reasoning** involves explaining why an act is wrong and is usually appropriate for older children, especially when moral issues are involved. However, young children cannot be expected to "see the other side" because of their egocentrism. Children in the preoperative stage of cognitive development (toddlers and preschoolers) have a limited ability to distinguish between their point of view and that of others. Sometimes children use "reasoning" as a way of gaining attention. For example, they may misbehave, thinking the parents will give them a lengthy explanation of the wrongdoing and knowing that negative attention is better than no attention. When children use this technique, parents should end the explanation by stating, "This is the rule, and this is how I expect you to behave. I won't explain it any further."

FAMILY-CENTERED CARE

Implementing Discipline

- **Consistency**—Implement disciplinary action exactly as agreed on and for each infraction.
- **Timing**—Initiate discipline as soon as child misbehaves; if delays are necessary, such as to avoid embarrassment, verbally disapprove of the behavior and state that disciplinary action will be implemented.
- **Commitment**—Follow through with the details of the discipline, such as timing of minutes; avoid distractions that may interfere with the plan, such as telephone calls.
- **Unity**—Make certain that all caregivers agree on the plan and are familiar with the details to prevent confusion and alliances between child and one parent.
- **Flexibility**—Choose disciplinary strategies that are appropriate to child's age and temperament and the severity of the misbehavior.
- **Planning**—Plan disciplinary strategies in advance and prepare child if feasible (e.g., explain use of time-out); for unexpected misbehavior, try to discipline when you are calm.
- **Behavior orientation**—Always disapprove of the behavior, not the child, with statements such as "That was a wrong thing to do. I am unhappy when I see behavior like that."
- **Privacy**—Administer discipline in private, especially with older children, who may feel ashamed in front of others.
- **Termination**—After the discipline is administered, consider child as having a "clean slate," and avoid bringing up the incident or lecturing.

Unfortunately, reasoning is often combined with **scolding**, which sometimes takes the form of shame or criticism. For example, the parent may state, "You are a bad boy for hitting your brother." Children take such remarks seriously and personally, believing that they are bad.

Positive and negative reinforcement is the basis of **behavior modification theory**—behavior that is rewarded will be repeated; behavior that is not rewarded will be extinguished. Using **rewards** is a positive approach. By encouraging children to behave in specified ways, the parents can decrease the tendency to misbehave. With young children, using paper stars is an effective method. With older children, the "token system" is appropriate, especially if a certain number of stars or tokens yields a special reward, such as a trip to the movies or a new book. In planning a reward system, the parents must explain expected behaviors to the child and establish rewards that are reinforcing. They should use a chart to record the stars or tokens and always give an earned reward promptly. Verbal approval should always accompany extrinsic rewards.

! NURSING ALERT

When reprimanding children, focus only on the misbehavior, not on the child. Use of "I" messages rather than "you" messages expresses personal feelings without accusation or ridicule. For example, an "I" message attacks the behavior—"I am upset when Johnny is punched; I don't like to see him hurt"—not the child.

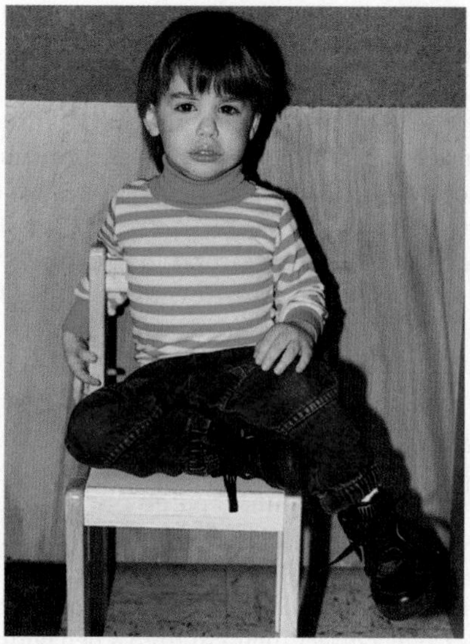

Fig. 2.4 Time-out is an excellent disciplinary strategy for young children.

Consistently **ignoring** behavior will eventually extinguish or minimize the act. Although this approach sounds simple, it is difficult to implement consistently. Parents frequently "give in" and resort to previous patterns of discipline. Consequently, the behavior is actually reinforced because the child learns that persistence gains parental attention. For ignoring to be effective, parents should (1) understand the process, (2) record the undesired behavior before using ignoring to determine whether a problem exists and to compare results after ignoring is begun, (3) determine whether parental attention acts as a reinforcer, and (4) be aware of "response burst." Response burst is a phenomenon that occurs when the undesired behavior increases after ignoring is initiated because the child is "testing" the parents to see if they are serious about the plan.

The strategy of consequences involves allowing children to experience the results of their misbehavior. It includes three types:

1. Natural—Those that occur without any intervention, such as being late and having to clean up the dinner table
2. Logical—Those that are directly related to the rule, such as not being allowed to play with another toy until the used ones are put away
3. Unrelated—Those that are imposed deliberately, such as no playing until homework is completed or the use of time-out

Natural or logical consequences are preferred and effective if they are meaningful to children. For example, the natural consequence of living in a messy room may do little to encourage cleaning up, but allowing no friends over until the room is neat can be motivating. Withdrawing privileges is often an unrelated consequence. After the child experiences the consequence, the parent should refrain from any comment, because the usual tendency is for the child to try to place blame for imposing the rule.

Time-out is a refinement of the common practice of sending the child to his or her room and is a type of unrelated consequence. It is based on the premise of removing the reinforcer (i.e., the satisfaction or attention the child is receiving from the activity). When placed in an unstimulating and isolated place, children become bored and consequently agree to behave in order to reenter the family group (Fig. 2.4). Time-out avoids many of the problems of other disciplinary approaches. No physical punishment is involved; no reasoning or scolding is given; and the parent does not need to be present for all of the time-out, thus facilitating consistent application of this type of discipline. Time-out offers both the child and the parent a "cooling-off" time. To be effective, however, time-out must be planned (see Family-Centered Care box). Implement time-out in a public place by selecting a suitable area, or explain to children that time-out will be spent immediately on returning home.

Corporal or **physical punishment** most often takes the form of spanking (Mendez, Durtschi, Neppl, et al., 2016). Based on the principles of aversive therapy, inflicting pain through spanking causes a dramatic short-term decrease in the behavior. However, this approach has serious flaws: (1) it teaches children that violence is acceptable; (2) it may physically harm the child if it is the result of parental rage; and (3) children become "accustomed" to spanking, requiring more severe corporal punishment over time. Spanking can result in severe physical and psychologic injury, and it interferes with effective parent-child interaction (Gershoff, 2008). In addition, when the parents are not around, children are likely to misbehave, because they have not learned to behave well for their own sake. Parental use of corporal punishment may also interfere with the child's development of moral reasoning.

FAMILY-CENTERED CARE

Using Time-Out

- Select an area for time-out that is safe, convenient, and unstimulating but where the child can be monitored, such as the bathroom, hallway, or laundry room.
- Determine what behaviors warrant a time-out.
- Make certain children understand the "rules" and how they are expected to behave.
- Explain to children the process of time-out:
  - When they misbehave, they will be given one warning. If they do not obey, they will be sent to the place designated for time-out.
  - They are to sit there for a specified period.
  - If they cry, refuse, or display any disruptive behavior, the time-out period will begin after they quiet down.
  - When they are quiet for the duration of the time, they can then leave the designated place.
- A rule for the length of time-out is 1 minute per year of age; use a kitchen timer with an audible bell rather than a watch to record the time.

SPECIAL PARENTING SITUATIONS

Parenting is a demanding task under ideal circumstances, but when parents and children face situations that deviate from "the norm," the potential for family disruption is increased. Situations that are encountered frequently are divorce, single parenthood, blended families, adoption, and dual-career families. In addition, as cultural diversity increases in our communities, many immigrants are making the transition to parenthood and a new country, culture, and language simultaneously. Other situations that create unique parenting challenges are parental alcoholism, homelessness, and incarceration. Although these topics are not addressed here, the reader may wish to investigate them further.

PARENTING THE ADOPTED CHILD

Adoption establishes a legal relationship between a child and parents who are not related by birth but who have the same rights and obligations that exist between children and their biologic parents. In the past the biologic mother alone made the decision to relinquish the rights to her child. In recent years the courts have acknowledged the legal rights of the biologic father regarding this decision. Concerned child advocates have questioned whether decisions that honor the father's rights are in the best interests of the child. As the child's rights have become recognized, older children have successfully dissolved their legal bond with their biologic parents to pursue adoption by adults of their choice. Furthermore, there is a growing interest and demand within the LGBT community to adopt.

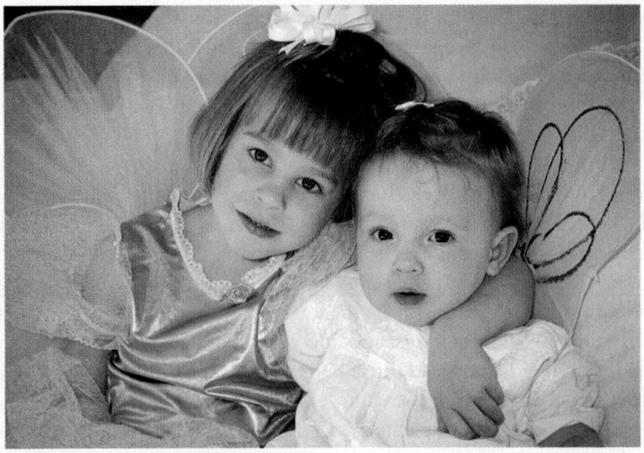

Fig. 2.5 An older sister lovingly embraces her adopted sister.

Unlike biologic parents, who prepare for their child's birth with prenatal classes and the support of friends and relatives, adoptive parents have fewer sources of support and preparation for the new addition to their family. Nurses can provide the information, support, and reassurance needed to reduce parental anxiety regarding the adoptive process and refer adoptive parents to state parental support groups. Such sources can be contacted through a state or county welfare office.

The sooner infants enter their adoptive home, the better the chances of parent-infant attachment. However, the more caregivers the infant had before adoption, the greater the risk for attachment problems. The infant must break the bond with the previous caregiver and form a new bond with the adoptive parents. Difficulties in forming an attachment depend on the amount of time he or she has spent with caregivers early in life, as well as the number of caregivers (e.g., the birth mother, nurse, adoption agency personnel).

Siblings, adopted or biologic, who are old enough to understand should be included in decisions regarding the commitment to adopt, with reassurance that they are not being replaced. Ways that the siblings can interact with the adopted child should be stressed (Fig. 2.5).

Issues of Origin

The task of telling children that they are adopted can be a cause of deep concern and anxiety. There are no clear-cut guidelines for parents to follow in determining when and at what age children are ready for the information. Parents are naturally reluctant to present such potentially unsettling news. However, it is important that parents not withhold the adoption from the child, because it is an essential component of the child's identity.

The timing arises naturally as parents become aware of the child's readiness. Most authorities believe that children should be informed at an age young enough so that, as they grow older, they do not remember a time when they did not know they were adopted. The time is highly individual, but it must be right for both the parents and the child. It may be when children ask where babies come from, at which time children can also be told the facts of their adoption. If they are told in a way that conveys the idea that they were active participants in the selection process, they will be less likely to feel that they were abandoned victims in a helpless situation. For example, parents can tell children that their personal qualities drew the parents to them. It is wise for parents who have not previously discussed adoption to tell children that they are adopted before the children enter school to avoid having them learn it from third parties. Complete honesty between parents and children strengthens the relationship.

Parents should anticipate behavior changes after the disclosure, especially in older children. Children who are struggling with the revelation that they are adopted may benefit from individual and family counseling. Children may use the fact of their adoption as a weapon to manipulate and threaten parents. Statements such as "My real mother would not treat me like this" or "You don't love me as much because I'm adopted" hurt parents and increase their feelings of insecurity. Such statements may also cause parents to become overly permissive. Adopted children need the same undemanding love, combined with firm discipline and limit setting, as any other child.

Adolescence

Adolescence may be an especially trying time for parents of adopted children. The normal confrontations of adolescents and parents assume more painful aspects in adoptive families. Adolescents may use their adoption to defy parental authority or as a justification for aberrant behavior. As they attempt to master the task of identity formation, they may begin to have feelings of abandonment by their biologic parents. Gender differences in reacting to adoption may surface.

Adopted children fantasize about their biologic parents and may feel the need to discover their parents' identity to define themselves and their own identity. It is important for parents to keep the lines of communication open and to reassure their child that they understand the need to search for his or her identity. In some states, birth certificates are made legally available to adopted children when they come of age. Parents should be honest with questioning adolescents and tell them of this possibility (the parents themselves are unable to obtain the birth certificate; it is the children's responsibility if they desire it).

Cross-Racial and International Adoption

Adoption of children from racial backgrounds different from that of the family is commonplace. In addition to the problems faced by adopted children in general, children of a cross-racial adoption must deal with physical and sometimes cultural differences. It is advised that parents who adopt children with a different ethnic background do everything to preserve the adopted children's racial heritage.

Although the children are full-fledged members of an adopting family and citizens of the adopted country, if they have a strikingly different appearance from other family members or exhibit distinct racial or ethnic characteristics, challenges may be encountered outside the family. Bigotry may appear among relatives and friends. Strangers may make thoughtless comments and talk about the children as though they were not members of the family. It is vital that family members declare to others that this is their child and a cherished member of the family.

> **! NURSING ALERT**
>
> As a health care provider, it is important not to ask the wrong questions, such as "Is she yours, or is she adopted?" "What do you know about the 'real' mother?" "Do they have the same father?" or "How much did it cost to adopt him?"

In international adoptions the medical information the parents receive may be incomplete or sketchy; weight, height, and head circumference are often the only objective information present in the child's medical record. Many internationally adopted children were born prematurely, and common health problems such as infant diarrhea and malnutrition delay growth and development. Some children have serious or multiple health problems that can be stressful for the parents.

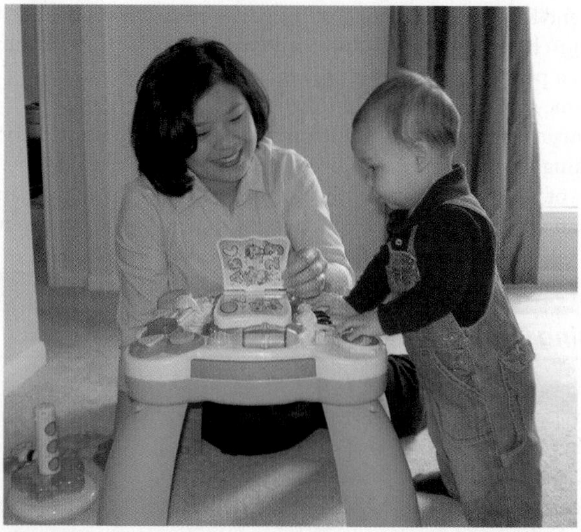

Fig. 2.6 Quality time spent with a child during a divorce is essential to a family's health and well-being.

PARENTING AND DIVORCE

Since the mid-1960s, a marked change in the stability of families has been reflected in increased rates of divorce, single parenthood, and remarriage. In 2017 the divorce rate in the United States was 2.9 per 1000 total population (Centers for Disease Control and Prevention, 2018). The divorce rate has changed little since 1987. In the decade before that, the rate increased yearly, with a peak in 1979. Although almost half of all divorcing couples are childless, it is estimated that more than 1 million children experience divorce each year.

The process of divorce begins with a period of marital conflict of varying length and intensity, followed by a separation, the actual legal divorce, and the reestablishment of different living arrangements. Because a function of parenthood is to provide for the security and emotional welfare of children, disruption of the family structure often engenders strong feelings of guilt in the divorcing parents (Fig. 2.6).

During a divorce, parents' coping abilities may be compromised. The parents may be preoccupied with their own feelings, needs, and life changes and be unavailable to support their children. Newly employed parents, usually mothers, are likely to leave children with new caregivers, in strange settings, or alone after school. The parent may also spend more time away from home, searching for or establishing new relationships. Sometimes, however, the adult feels frightened and alone and begins to depend on the child as a substitute for the absent parent. This dependence places an enormous burden on the child.

Telling the Children

Parents are understandably hesitant to tell children about their decision to divorce. Most parents neglect to discuss either the divorce or its inevitable changes with their preschool child. Without preparation, even children who remain in the family home are confused by the parental separation. Frequently, children are already experiencing vague, uneasy feelings that are more difficult to cope with than being told the truth about the situation.

If possible, the initial disclosure should include both parents and siblings, followed by individual discussions with each child. Sufficient

BOX 2.4 Feelings and Behaviors of Children Related to Divorce

Infancy
- Effects of reduced mothering or lack of mothering
- Increased irritability
- Disturbance in eating, sleeping, and elimination
- Interference with attachment process

Early Preschool Children (Ages 2 to 3 Years)
- Frightened and confused
- Blame themselves for the divorce
- Fear of abandonment
- Increased irritability, whining, tantrums
- Regressive behaviors (e.g., thumb sucking, loss of elimination control)
- Separation anxiety

Later Preschool Children (Ages 3 to 5 Years)
- Fear of abandonment
- Blame themselves for the divorce; decreased self-esteem
- Bewilderment regarding all human relationships
- Become more aggressive in relationships with others (e.g., siblings, peers)
- Engage in fantasy to seek understanding of the divorce

Early School-Age Children (Ages 5 to 6 Years)
- Depression and immature behavior
- Loss of appetite and sleep disorders
- May be able to verbalize some feelings and understand some divorce-related changes
- Increased anxiety and aggression
- Feelings of abandonment by departing parent

Middle School-Age Children (Ages 6 to 8 Years)
- Panic reactions
- Feelings of deprivation—loss of parent, attention, money, and secure future
- Profound sadness, depression, fear, and insecurity
- Feelings of abandonment and rejection
- Fear regarding the future
- Difficulty expressing anger at parents
- Intense desire for reconciliation of parents
- Impaired capacity to play and enjoy outside activities
- Decline in school performance
- Altered peer relationships—become bossy, irritable, demanding, and manipulative
- Frequent crying, loss of appetite, sleep disorders
- Disturbed routine, forgetfulness

Later School-Age Children (Ages 9 to 12 Years)
- More realistic understanding of divorce
- Intense anger directed at one or both parents
- Divided loyalties
- Ability to express feelings of anger
- Ashamed of parental behavior
- Desire for revenge; may wish to punish the parent they hold responsible
- Feelings of loneliness, rejection, and abandonment
- Altered peer relationships
- Decline in school performance
- May develop somatic complaints
- May engage in aberrant behavior such as lying, stealing
- Temper tantrums
- Dictatorial attitude

Adolescents (Ages 12 to 18 Years)
- Able to disengage themselves from parental conflict
- Feelings of a profound sense of loss—of family, childhood
- Feelings of anxiety
- Worry about themselves, parents, siblings
- Expression of anger, sadness, shame, embarrassment
- May withdraw from family and friends
- Disturbed concept of sexuality
- May engage in acting-out behaviors

time should be set aside for these discussions, and they should take place during a period of calm, not after an argument. Parents who physically hold or touch their children provide them with a feeling of warmth and reassurance. The discussions should include the reason for the divorce, if age appropriate, and reassurance that the divorce is not the fault of the children.

Parents should not fear crying in front of the children, because their crying gives the children permission to cry also. Children need to ventilate their feelings. Children may feel guilt, a sense of failure, or that they are being punished for misbehavior. They normally feel anger and resentment and should be allowed to communicate these feelings without punishment. They also have feelings of terror and abandonment (Box 2.4). They need consistency and order in their lives. They want to know where they will live, who will take care of them, if they will be with their siblings, and if there will be enough money to live on. Children may also wonder what will happen on special days such as birthdays and holidays, whether both parents will come to school events, and whether they will still have the same friends. Children fear that if their parents stopped loving each other, they could stop loving them. Their need for love and reassurance is tremendous at this time.

Custody and Parenting Partnerships

In the past, when parents separated, the mother was given custody of the children with visitation agreements for the father. Now both parents and the courts are seeking alternatives. Current belief is that neither fathers nor mothers should be awarded custody automatically. Custody should be awarded to the parent who is best able to provide for the children's welfare. In some cases, children experience severe stress when living or spending time with a parent. Many fathers have demonstrated both their competence and their commitment to care for their children.

Often overlooked are the changes that may occur in the children's relationships with other relatives, especially grandparents. Grandparents are increasingly involved in the care of young children (Pulgaron, Marchante, Agosto, et al., 2016). Grandparents on the noncustodial side are often kept from their grandchildren, whereas those on the custodial side may be overwhelmed by their adult child's return to the household with grandchildren.

Two other types of custody arrangements are divided custody and joint custody. **Divided custody**, or **split custody**, means that each parent is awarded custody of one or more of the children, thereby separating siblings. For example, sons might live with the father and daughters with the mother.

Joint custody takes one of two forms. In **joint physical custody**, the parents alternate the physical care and control of the children on an agreed-upon basis while maintaining shared parenting responsibilities legally. This custody arrangement works well for families who live close to each other and whose occupations permit an active role in the care and rearing of the children. In **joint legal custody**, the children reside with one parent, but both parents are the children's legal guardians, and both participate in childrearing.

Coparenting offers substantial benefits for the family: children can be close to both parents, and life with each parent can be more normal (as opposed to having a disciplinarian mother and a recreational father). To be successful, parents in these arrangements must be highly committed to provide normal parenting and to separate their marital conflicts from their parenting roles. No matter what type of custody arrangement is awarded, the primary consideration is the welfare of the children.

SINGLE PARENTING

An individual may acquire single-parent status as a result of divorce, separation, death of a spouse, or birth or adoption of a child. Although divorce rates have stabilized, the number of single-parent households continues to rise. In 2016, 32% of single-parent families had incomes below the poverty line (Annie E. Casey Foundation, 2018). In addition, 35% of children younger than 18 years of age lived in single-parent families, and the majority of single parents were women (Annie E. Casey Foundation, 2018). Unfortunately, children raised in female-headed households are more likely to drop out of school, be a teen parent, and experience divorce in adulthood. Although some women are single parents by choice, most never planned on being single parents, and many feel pressure to marry or remarry.

Managing shortages of money, time, and energy is often a concern for single parents. Studies repeatedly confirm the financial difficulties of single-parent families, particularly single mothers. In fact, the stigma of poverty may be more keenly felt than the discrimination associated with being a single parent. These families are often forced by their financial status to live in communities with inadequate housing and personal safety concerns. Single parents often feel guilty about the time spent away from their children. Divorced mothers, from marriages in which the father assumed the role of breadwinner and the mother the household maintenance and parenting roles, have considerable difficulty adjusting to their new role of breadwinner. Many single parents have trouble arranging for adequate child care, particularly for a sick child.

Social supports and community resources needed by single-parent families include health care services that are open on evenings and weekends; high-quality child care; respite child care to relieve parental exhaustion and prevent burnout; and parent enhancement centers for advancing education and job skills, providing recreational activities, and offering parenting education. Single parents need social contacts separate from their children for their own emotional growth and that of their children. Parents Without Partners[a] is an organization designed to meet the needs of single parents.

Single Fathers

Fathers who have custody of their children have many of the same problems as divorced mothers. They feel overburdened by the responsibility; depressed; and concerned about their ability to cope with the emotional needs of the children, especially girls. Some fathers lack homemaking skills. They may find it difficult at first to coordinate household tasks, school visits, and other activities associated with managing a household alone (Fig. 2.7).

[a]1650 South Dixie Hwy, Suite 402, Boca Raton, FL 33432; 800-637-7974; http://parentswithoutpartners.org.

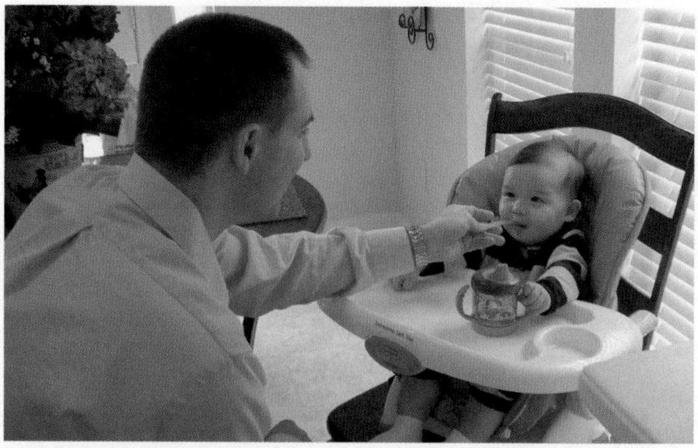

Fig. 2.7 Fathers who assume care of their children may feel more comfortable and successful in their parenting role.

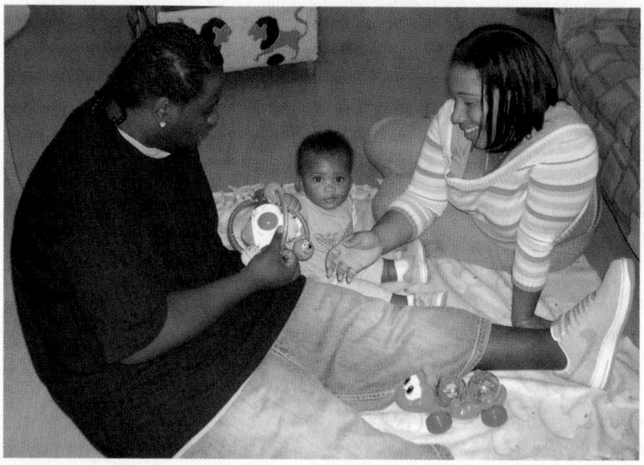

Fig. 2.8 Learning new roles in reconstituted families as a mother and father can enhance parenting relationships.

PARENTING IN RECONSTITUTED FAMILIES

In the United States, many children living in homes where parents have divorced will experience another major change in their lives, such as the addition of a stepparent or new siblings (Kaakinen & Coehlo, 2015). The entry of a stepparent into a ready-made family requires adjustments for all family members. Some obstacles to the role adjustments and family problem solving include disruption of previous lifestyles and interaction patterns, complexity in the formation of new ones, and lack of social supports. Despite these problems, most children from divorced families want to live in a two-parent home.

Cooperative parenting relationships can allow more time for each set of parents to be alone to establish their own relationship with the children. Under ideal circumstances, power conflicts between the two households can be reduced, and tension and anxiety can be lessened for all family members. In addition, the children's self-esteem can be increased, and there is a greater likelihood of continued contact with grandparents. Flexibility, mutual support, and open communication are critical in successful relationships in stepfamilies and stepparenting situations (Fig. 2.8).

PARENTING IN DUAL-EARNER FAMILIES

No change in family lifestyle has had more impact than the large numbers of women moving away from the traditional homemaker role and entering the workplace (Kaakinen & Coehlo, 2015). The trend toward increased numbers of dual-earner families is unlikely to diminish significantly. As a result, the family is subject to considerable stress as members attempt to meet often competing demands of occupational needs and those regarded as necessary for a rich family life.

Working Mothers

Working mothers have become the norm in the United States. Maternal employment may have variable effects on preschool children's health (Lucas-Thompson, Goldberg, & Prause, 2010). The quality of child care is a persistent concern for all working parents. Determinants of child care quality are based on health and safety requirements, responsive and warm interaction between staff and children, developmentally appropriate activities, trained staff, limited group size, age-appropriate caregivers, adequate staff-to-child ratios, and adequate indoor and outdoor space. Nurses play an important role in helping families to find suitable sources of child care and to prepare children for this experience.

Kinship Care

Since the 1980s, the proportion of children in out-of-home care placed with relatives has increased rapidly. More than 2.7 million US children are raised by grandparents or other kin at some time in their lives (Annie E. Casey Foundation, 2012). According to US Census Bureau data, kinship caregivers are more likely to be poor, single, older, less educated, and unemployed than families in which at least one parent is present.

FOSTER PARENTING

The term **foster care** is defined as placement in an approved living situation away from the family of origin (American Academy of Pediatrics, 2000; Annie E. Casey Foundation, 2012). The living situation may be an approved foster home, possibly with other children, or a preadoptive home. Each state provides a standard for the role of foster parent and a process by which to become one. These "parents" contract with the state to provide a home for children for a limited duration. Most states require about 27 hours of training before being on contract and at least 12 hours of continuing education a year. Foster parents may be required to attend a foster parent support group that is often separate from a state agency. Each state has guidelines regarding the relative health of the prospective foster parents and their families, background checks regarding legal issues for the adults, personal interviews, and a safety inspection of the residence and surroundings (Chamberlain, Price, Leve, et al., 2008).

Foster homes include both kinship and nonrelative placements. Since the 1980s, the proportion of children in out-of-home care placed with relatives has increased rapidly and been accompanied by a decrease in the number of foster families. As with their nonfoster counterparts, much of the child's adjustment depends on the family's stability and available resources. Even though foster homes are designed to provide short-term care, it is not unusual for children to stay for many years.

Nurses should be aware that nearly 700,000 children spend time living in foster care in a given year, many of them facing developmental concerns (American Academy of Pediatrics, 2000; Annie E. Casey Foundation, 2015). Children from lower-income, single-mother, and mother-partner families are considerably more likely to be living in foster care (Berger & Waldfogel, 2004). Children in foster care tend to have a higher than normal incidence of acute and chronic health problems and may experience feelings of isolation or confusion (Annie E. Casey Foundation, 2015). Foster children are often at risk because of their previous caretaking environment. Nurses should strive to implement strategies to improve the health care for this group of children. In particular, assessment and case management skills are required to involve other disciplines in meeting their needs.

SOCIOCULTURAL INFLUENCES ON CHILDREN AND FAMILIES

A child and his or her immediate family are nested within a local community of school, peers, and extended family; within a larger community that may be bound by common geography, background, and traditions; and within an even broader community that incorporates the social, political, and economic elements that influence many aspects of family life. These layers of influence are often multifactorial: parents, extended family, and community exert influence most directly when thinking about the religious or ethnic background of the family. These elements come into play when we think about children moving into the wider world, such as their interface with other children at school or potential biases a child or adolescent may face because of religious or ethnic and racial identity. Thus the sociopolitical context, though an outer layer of a social ecologic model, can exert enormous influence on a child's daily life, opportunities, and outcomes. Equally important to child and family health outcomes, the sociopolitical context draws our attention to factors and health policies at the local, regional, state, and federal levels that can serve as barriers to health equity. This is also made evident through research on the social determinants of health. The next section of the chapter will delve into a deeper discussion of such factors.

The social ecologic model (Kazak, 2001; Kazak, Rourke, & Navasaria, 2010), rooted in Bronfenbrenner's ecologic model (Bronfenbrenner, 1979, 2005), offers a perspective of viewing children and their families within the context of various circles of influence, called an ecologic framework. This framework posits that individuals adapt in response to changes in their surrounding environments, whether that be the environment of the immediate family, the school, the neighborhood in which the family lives, or the socioeconomic forces that may shape job availability in their geographic area. In addition, Kazak argues that a person's behavior results from the interaction of his or her traits and abilities with the environment. No single factor can explain the totality of a child and his or her family's health behaviors. Children possess their own factors that influence their behavior (i.e., personal history or biologic factors). In turn, they are surrounded by relationships with family, friends, and peers who influence their behavior. Children and their families are then situated within a community that establishes the context in which social relationships develop. Finally, wider sociocultural factors influence whether a behavior is encouraged or prohibited (e.g., social policy on smoking, cultural norms of mothers as primary caregivers of young children, media that can influence how a teenager thinks he or she should look) (Fig. 2.9).

Promoting the health of children requires a nurse to understand social, cultural, and religious influences on children and their families. The US population is constantly evolving. Patients experience negative health outcomes when social, cultural, and religious factors are not considered as influencing their health care (Chavez, 2012; Williams, 2012). Educating health care providers is one way to reduce disparities in health care.

INFLUENCES IN THE SURROUNDING ENVIRONMENT

SCHOOL COMMUNITIES: SCHOOL HEALTH AND SCHOOL CONNECTEDNESS

Environments differentially support learning through the kinds of opportunities and support provided. Learning and development are cumulative and synergistic; one supports the other. High-quality early

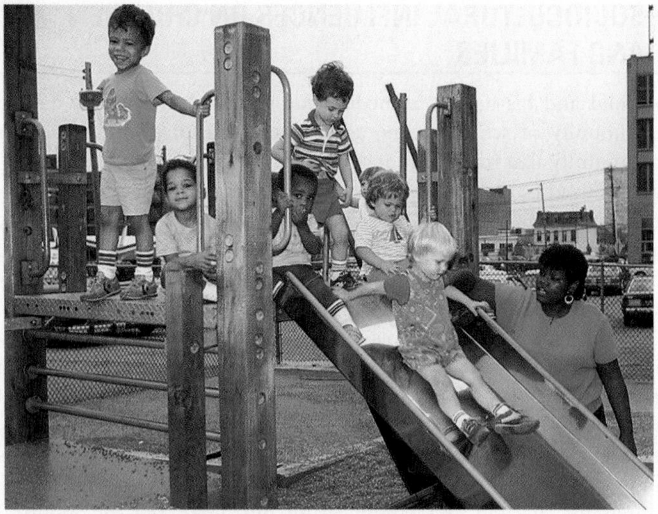

Fig. 2.9 Youngsters from different cultural backgrounds interact within the larger culture.

childhood education is especially beneficial to set children up for success in early grades. This is especially true for children from disadvantaged backgrounds. Access to this high-quality education is key yet also occurs along a socioeconomic gradient, with more highly resourced children attending higher-quality preschool programs.

Within communities, schools are important sites for health promotion. Initiatives such as the Centers for Disease Control and Prevention–sponsored Whole School, Whole Community, Whole Child model emphasize and build on this critical connection between youth academic performance and health by addressing important elements of children's and adolescents' lives that cut across domains. Examples of such elements include physical education and activity, nutritional environment, counseling, psychologic and social services, social and emotional climate, physical environment, family engagement, and community involvement (Michael, Merlo, Basch, et al., 2015). This approach acknowledges the need for multifaceted strategies to improve academic and health outcomes. It situates school not only as a place to learn, but also as a place to practice positive health behaviors and health promotion skills. For example, a nutritional health environment constructed in a way to promote child and adolescent health gives youth a chance to live out these skills by making healthy food choices available, by weaving nutrition education into the health curriculum, and by including supportive messaging about healthy nutrition in the school environment (Lewallen, Hunt, Potts-Datema, et al., 2015).

The Centers for Disease Control and Prevention and the World Health Organization identified place-based settings that contribute to individual, family, and population health, including educational settings. Thus schools and early childhood centers can contribute to the health of children by teaching about health and healthy behaviors and also by offering ways to enact healthy behaviors (e.g., physical education, coordinated psychosocial or mental health services, healthy snacks). This position addresses potential gaps in care or assessment for children and adolescents, because place-based care can improve access for many children, and emphasizes coordination among services in a given neighborhood.

An important concept when considering schools as a site of health promotion is connectedness (Centers for Disease Control and Prevention, 2009). *School connectedness* is defined as students' perception that they and their learning matter to the adults at their school and to their peers. It occurs when youth believe that their teachers, staff, and peers care about them academically and personally. The growth and implementation of this concept into educational practice stems from research indicating greater impact on youth health through bolstering protective factors that help children and adolescents avoid risky or unhealthy behaviors. This focus on strengths and promoting positive choices may also help buffer the impact of negative events on children and their health.

Feeling connected at school has important health benefits. Children and youth who feel more connected are more likely to engage in healthy behaviors and do well academically. School connectedness has been found to be particularly protective against substance abuse, early sexual debut, and violence in both boys and girls. In addition, school connectedness was second only to family connectedness in protection against emotional distress, disordered eating, and suicidal ideation and attempts. Finally, in addition to health outcomes it promotes academic outcomes, including improved grades, decreased absence, and delayed dropout.

Recommended strategies for achieving school connectedness include effective training for teachers and staff to create positive learning environments; opportunities for families to become involved in the process and associated training; and provision of important academic, emotional, and social skills to students (and addressing barriers to achieving these skills) so that students can feel engaged and have a stake in their education (Centers for Disease Control and Prevention, 2009).

SCHOOLS

When children enter school, their radius of relationships extends to include a wider variety of peers and a new source of authority. Although parents continue to exert the major influence on children, in the school environment teachers have the most significant psychologic impact on children's development and socialization. In addition to academic and cognitive progress, teachers are concerned with the emotional and social development of the children in their care. Both parents and teachers act to model, shape, and promote positive behavior; constrain negative behavior; and enforce standards of conduct. Ideally, parents and teachers work together for the benefit of the children in their care.

Schools serve as a major source of socialization for children. Next to the family, schools exert a major force in providing continuity and passing down culture from one generation to the next. This in turn prepares children to carry out the social roles they are expected to assume as they develop into adults. School is the center of **cultural diffusion,** wherein the cultural standards of the larger group are disseminated into the community. It governs what is taught and, to a great extent, how it is taught. School rules and regulations regarding attendance, authority relationships, and the system of rewards and penalties based on achievement transmit to children the expectations of the adult world of employment and relationships. School is an important institution in which children systematically learn about the negative consequences of behavior that departs from social expectations. School also serves as an avenue for children to participate in the larger society in rewarding ways, to promote social mobility, and to connect the family with new knowledge and services. Like parents, teachers are responsible for transmitting knowledge and culture (i.e., values on which there is a broad consensus) to the children in their care. Teachers are also expected to stimulate and guide children's intellectual development and creative problem solving.

PEER CULTURES

Peer groups also have an impact on the socialization of children. Peer relationships become increasingly important and influential as children

TABLE 2.2 Media Effects on Children and Adolescents

Media Effect	Potential Consequences
Violence	Government, medical, and public health data show that exposure to media violence is one factor in violent and aggressive behavior. Both adults and children become desensitized by violence witnessed through various media, including television (including children's programming), movies (including G rated), music, and video games. In addition, cyber-bullying and harassment via text messages are a growing concern among middle school and high school students.
Sex	A significant body of research shows that sexual content in the media can contribute to beliefs and attitudes about sex, sexual behavior, and initiation of intercourse. Teens access sexual content through a variety of media: television, movies, music, magazines, Internet, social media, and mobile devices. Current issues receiving attention for the role they play in teen sexual behavior include sending sexual images via mobile devices (i.e., sexting), the impact of violent media on youth views of women and forced sex or rape, and cyber-bullying LGBT youth. Media can also serve as a positive source of sexual information (i.e., information, apps, social media about sexually transmitted infections, teen pregnancy, and promoting acceptance and support of LGBT youth).
Substance use and abuse	Although the causes of teen substance use and abuse are numerous, media play a significant role. Alcohol and tobacco, including the use of e-cigarettes (vaping), are still heavily marketed to adolescents and young adults. Television and movies featuring the use of these substances can influence initiation of use. Media also show substance use to be pervasive and without consequences. Finally, content shared over social networking sites can serve as a form of peer pressure and can influence likelihood of use.
Obesity	Obesity is a highly prevalent public health issue among children of all ages and in increasing rates around the world. A number of studies have demonstrated a link between the amount of screen time and obesity. Advertising of unhealthy food to children is a long-standing marketing practice, which may increase snacking in the face of decreased activity. In addition, both increased screen time and unhealthy eating may also be related to unhealthy sleep.
Body image	Media may play a significant role in the development of body image awareness, expectations, and body dissatisfaction among young and older adolescent girls. Their beliefs may be influenced by images on television, movies, and magazines. New media also contribute to this through Internet images, social network sites, and websites that encourage disordered eating (Strasburger, Jordan, & Donnerstein, 2012).

proceed through school. In school, children have what can be regarded as a culture of their own. This is even more apparent in unsupervised playgroups because the culture in school is partly produced by adults.

During their lives, children are subjected to many influential factors, such as family, religious community, and social class. In peer-group interactions, they confront a variety of these sets of values. The values imposed by the peer group are especially compelling because children must accept and conform to them to be accepted as members of the group. When the peer values are not too different from those of family and teachers, the mild conflict created by these small differences serves to separate children from the adults in their lives and to strengthen the feeling of belonging to the peer group.

Although the peer group has neither the traditional authority of the parents nor the legal authority of the schools to teach information, it manages to convey a substantial amount of information to its members, especially on taboo subjects such as sex and drugs. Children's need for the friendship of their peers brings them into an increasingly complex social system. Through peer relationships, children learn to deal with dominance and hostility and to relate with persons in positions of leadership and authority. Other functions of the peer subculture are to relieve boredom and to provide recognition that individual members do not receive from teachers and other authority figures.

COMMUNITY

Families and communities are often interwoven in their impact on child health. Although both are essential to socioemotional growth and improved learning outcomes in children, their influence on children is synergistic. When families live in areas of concentrated poverty, residents experience risk at population and individual levels. Children and families living in areas of concentrated poverty are at risk for negative health outcomes and experience higher rates of crime and violence. In addition, affected neighborhoods are more likely to have low-performing schools, limited access to high-quality preschool and diminished school readiness, and poorer overall education outcomes. If parents have grown up in the area or a similar area, they have also experienced untoward effects on their health or educational outcomes. As a result, they may not be able to secure employment that provides greater resources for them to invest in their child or that provides economic stability for the family. Financial stressors in parents contribute to their stress and depression, which can inhibit effective parenting. Thus we see an important need for two-generation programs or strategies to both build on family and community strengths and diminish their stressors.

Community-level factors are especially important as we consider the life, safety, and causes of death in older adolescents. For example, 75% of teen deaths are attributed to accidents, homicide, and suicide, and community-level factors, such as violence, drug use, and alcohol use, influence this number (Annie E. Casey Foundation, 2018).

BROADER INFLUENCES ON CHILD HEALTH

SOCIAL MEDIA AND MASS MEDIA

Digital technologies that serve as an avenue to mass and social media are pervasive in most parts of American society. Technology has a role in the lives of children more than ever before. The American Academy of Pediatrics (2016a) found that children younger than 5 years of age, across socioeconomic levels, use digital technology daily and are frequently targeted by advertisers. This frequent use carries risks for increased rates of obesity; disrupted sleep; and delays in cognitive, social, and language development, potentially related to diminished parent-child interaction in preschoolers (Table 2.2). Research has demonstrated that there is limited benefit of digital technology for children younger than 2 years of age, also likely related to diminished parent-child interaction. Benefits of digital technology use are related to the type of content viewed and used. For example, high-quality programming, such as *Sesame Street,* can bolster cognitive and social outcomes in preschool-age children, and applications from similar organizations (e.g., PBS or Sesame Workshop) can promote literacy skills. Unfortunately, many programs and applications targeted to children and their parents or caregivers are not created under the direction of educators or developmental experts and may not prove as beneficial to child social and cognitive outcomes. In addition, less than 30% of children from lower-income homes view high-quality digital media, perpetuating potential risks posed by the technology and associated disparities. Despite technologic advances, play, social interactions with peers, and parent-child interactions remain vital to young children's development of the skills needed to succeed in school, including persistence, emotional regulation, and creative thinking (American Academy of Pediatrics, 2016b).

The digital landscape for older children and adolescents seems to change and grow on a daily basis and is woven into daily life for many youth. Indeed, recent research indicates that nearly 75% of adolescents have a smart phone or mobile technology device and approximately half report feeling addicted to their phone (American Academy of Pediatrics, 2016b). While using these mobile devices, most adolescents are engaging in social media, with nearly three-fourths engaging in multiple social media sites and cultivating a portfolio (American Academy of Pediatrics, 2016b). This immersion poses both benefits and risks to these youth. In terms of the benefits, youth have an unprecedented chance to learn and gather information and consider new perspectives; to connect with other youth, which is especially important for youth who may feel marginalized or isolated; and to maintain connections with family and friends who live at a distance.

On the other hand, navigating this landscape includes potential risks to physical and mental health, such as obesity, disrupted sleep, addictive behavior, negative impact on academics, bullying and sexual exploitation, and normalization of maladaptive behavior (e.g., sites that promote disordered eating or self-harm). Similar to traditional forms of media (e.g., television), research has demonstrated that social media postings can influence perceptions of alcohol and drug use and younger age of initiating sexual activity as normal in the eyes of adolescents (American Academy of Pediatrics, 2016b). Traditional forms of mass media, such as television and movies, can reify gender and racial stereotypes, thus perpetuating negative mental and emotional health outcomes (American Academy of Pediatrics, 2016b). Finally, communication among adolescents has shifted and become more pervasive through texting, messaging through gaming systems, and messaging on social media sites. This continual access and inlet to the lives of peers can serve as both a source of support and a source of derision and stress. Thus it is essential for nurses and other health care providers to talk with older children and adolescents about the frequency, content, and nature of their digital and social media use and how they maintain their privacy and safety. Equally important, nurses can help families devise strategies and personalized plans for safe and healthy technology use (American Academy of Pediatrics, 2016b) (Box 2.5).

BOX 2.5 Actions to Promote Positive Media Use

Parents

- Follow American Academy of Pediatrics recommendations for 2 total hours of screen time daily for children ages 2 years and older.
- Establish clear guidelines for Internet use and provide direct supervision. Have frank discussions of what youth may encounter in viewing media. Be mindful of own media use in the home.
- Encourage unstructured play in the home and plan to help children readjust to this change in family dynamic. Consider planned, deliberate use of media to experience the benefits (e.g., watching a television show together to bond or start a sensitive discussion).

Nurses and Health Care Providers

- Dedicate a few minutes of each visit to provide media screening and counseling.
- Discourage presence of electronic devices in children's rooms.
- Be sensitive to the challenges that parents face in carrying this out.

Schools

- Offer timely, accurate sexuality and drug education.
- Promote resilience.
- Develop programs to educate youth on wise use of technology.
- Develop and implement policies on dealing with cyber-bullying and sexting.

RACE AND ETHNICITY

Race and ethnicity are socially constructed terms used to group together people who share similar characteristics, traditions, or historical experience. **Race** is a term that groups together people by their outward, physical appearance. **Ethnicity** is a classification aimed at grouping individuals who share common characteristics unique in comparison to others in a society, resulting in a distinctive, cultural behavior (Scott & Marshall, 2009). Ethnicities may be differentiated from one another by customs and language, and may influence family structure, food preferences, and expressions of emotion. The composition and definition of ethnic groups can be fluid in response to changes in geography (i.e., moving from one country to another). Race and ethnicity influence a family's health when they are used as criteria by which a child or family is discriminated against. There is a significant body of work that describes this. In fact, 100 years of research describe racial gaps in health (Williams, 2012).

Racism remains an important social determinant of health. According to Williams (2012), for minority or other groups who experience stigmatization, "inequalities in health are created by larger inequalities in society," meaning that prevailing social conditions and obstacles to equal opportunities for all influences the health of all individuals. For example, from birth forward, African American and American Indian children have a higher mortality rate than white children in general. There is also a higher death rate for babies of African American and Hispanic women versus white women. Even when controlling for maternal levels of education, the infant mortality rate for college-educated African American women is 2.5 times higher than for Hispanic and white women of similar education level (Williams, 2012). These numbers demonstrate that children and families ultimately feel the effects of such health disparities.

Children and families may also experience perceived racism, which also has negative consequences. For example, in a study of more than 5000 fifth-graders, 15% of Hispanic youth and 20% of African American youth reported that they had experienced racial discrimination. Such experiences were then associated with a higher risk of mental health symptoms (Coker, Elliot, Kanouse, et al., 2009). Teens also report racial discrimination through online communities, social networking sites, and texting, which is related to increased anxiety and depression (Tynes, Giang, Williams, et al., 2008).

POVERTY

Opportunities to promote health or risks to health often begin in our families, schools, neighborhoods, and places of employment. Thus to fully promote child health and diminish risks to it, we need to understand how the surrounding context and environments are influential. Children are nested within layers of family, peers, school, and community; we can consider the direct impact of these outside systems interacting with the child and family. Equally important, however, is the influence of factors within the sociopolitical landscape at local, state, regional, national, and international levels. These factors affect the creation of health and social policies that may perpetuate health disparities or make health equity possible.

The circumstances into which a child is born can determine the child's exposure to factors that promote or compromise healthy development. For example, adverse events can have long-lasting impacts into adulthood. Layers of the child's surrounding environment that contribute to health inequity fall into socioeconomic, political, and cultural contexts, including local, state, and federal policies; daily living conditions; and the circumstances in which people live, work, and play.

Child health disparities are discrepancies that are based in avoidable differences and are concerning because of the immense and foundational development that occurs in early childhood. Health inequities, in a similar vein, are defined as differences in health states between populations that are socially produced and systemic in unequal distribution across populations that are avoidable and unfair. Health follows a social gradient; there are better health outcomes with increased socioeconomic status and further improvements with movements upward in socioeconomic status. Similarly, compromised health outcomes are associated with lower economic status. Inequitable access to services maintains or perpetuates health inequities in early childhood because the children most in need of services are most likely to not receive them. Multilevel, multifactorial responses to address these issues include policies that improve access to high-quality services and connect parents to secure, stable, flexible workplaces; service systems that deliver inclusive programs rooted in research and evidence; and timely assistance for parents so that they can feel successful in their parenting role.

Economy and Poverty

A major factor that affects child and family health in the United States is poverty. Nearly one-fifth of all American children live in families with annual incomes below 100% of the federal poverty level for a family of 4 (approximately $24,600), and almost one-half of children live 200% below this federal poverty guideline (Fierman, Beck, Chung, et al., 2016). Poverty affects children and their families across all geographic areas, including urban, suburban, and rural. Several social factors associated with poverty that can negatively affect child health are family disruption, parental depression, substance use, other mental illnesses, unsafe homes or neighborhoods, housing instability, homelessness, decreased educational opportunities, and low parent educational levels and health literacy (Fierman, Beck, Chung, et al., 2016).

Poverty influences these social determinants of health, the circumstances and environments in which people are born, live, work, learn, and play. In turn, these social determinants shape child health in major and lasting ways. Poverty itself is a major cause of acute and chronic stress for adults and children. The daily stressors associated with poverty are overwhelming, and other circumstances, such as trauma or violence, can add to the stress experienced by parents and children. This overwhelming stress can undermine skills in dealing with challenging situations. The stressors associated with poverty can be psychologically and emotionally depleting, yet supports to deal with this depletion, such as adequate mental health services, high-quality and affordable child care, or social supports, may not be available (Center on the Developing Child at Harvard University, 2016).

Infants and toddlers are more likely to live in poverty than older children. Thus some of the most profound effects of poverty are demonstrated in young children, such as increased prevalence of low birth weight and infant mortality and delayed language development. These risks can perpetuate other lifetime hazards, such as diminished health status due to chronic illness or compromised academic performance.

Underinsurance imposes financial difficulties on families. This reminds us that having insurance does not automatically negate financial distress or impact on families. High out-of-pocket costs (e.g., copays, medications, supplies) and associated costs for transportation to appointments, parking at hospitals, meals while a child is hospitalized, and child care for siblings contribute to this distress (Mooney-Doyle, dos Santos, Bousso, et al., 2017).

Parental Education

Parental level of education is another important factor when we consider economic influences on child health. Child economic status is directly tied to parental earnings. Parental earnings from employment in turn are affected by parental level of education. Income inequality is pervasive and has become worse in recent history. Although some families are catching up on what was lost in the Great Recession of 2008, many of the jobs that could help decrease income inequality require a college degree, and only one-third of adults in the United States have such degrees. Thus many children in the United States are living in families in which parents face employment dissatisfaction and barriers, contributing to stress or negative parental or family outcomes (Annie E. Casey Foundation, 2018). Although this issue affects children across races, ethnicities, and geographic settings, children of color disproportionately live in homes without sufficient finances (12% white children versus 36% African American children versus 31% Hispanic children). Gaps in income undermine a family's ability to access social mobility and move permanently out of poverty (American Academy of Pediatrics, 2016c).

The American Academy of Pediatrics recommends that screening be done at each well visit by asking about ability to meet basic needs, such as heat, shelter, and food. To address the issue, the American Academy of Pediatrics recommends that pediatric health care providers build on family strengths such as cohesion, humor, support, and spiritual beliefs, and advocate for creation of programs to address the multiple facets of childhood poverty that are rooted in research (American Academy of Pediatrics, 2016c). Barriers to screening exist, however, and derail providers with the best of intentions. Barriers include not recognizing the impact of poverty or the measurable outcomes associated with it; lack of time; limited and insufficient training in assessment and limited familiarity with assessment tools; and limited knowledge of available community resources. Pediatric nurses and health care providers can initiate surveillance and screening to elicit and address parent concerns; identify risk and protective factors; screen for specific issues; and refer the child and family to the right place with the right services. To address the social determinants of health, screening can be tailored to the most sensitive or sustained issues in the community, to parent sources of concern, and to child developmental stage.

Economic barriers impede parents' ability to provide for their children. Thus pediatric nurses and other health care providers must imbue their practice with an understanding of the challenges that families face, integrate care to minimize the strain of interacting with health and social services (informed by the knowledge that emotional care of the family is within the scope of pediatrics), and minimize the effects of toxic stress through supportive care services that build on family strengths (American Academy of Pediatrics, 2013, 2016c).

LAND OF ORIGIN AND IMMIGRATION STATUS

Cultural factors are woven into social, economic, and political influences on child health, including the misconception that children are oblivious to or not deeply affected by the world around them. This perception of children can color governments' and policy-making bodies' work on behalf of children and families. In addition, young childhood is often perceived to be in the domain of the home; thus calls for universal preschool are not heeded.

The demographics of the United States are changing, yet race and ethnicity remain important social determinants of health for many children. Children of color are disproportionately represented in impoverished communities and schools, yet they will comprise the majority of children in 13 states by 2020. This demonstrates one way in which a child's chances for thriving depend not only on child, family, and community characteristics, but also on the state in which the child lives because of variations in health and social services available. State policy choices and investments can have a tremendous impact on child health (Annie E. Casey Foundation, 2014, 2018).

Considering the broader context of where children and families live, work, and play is complex when we care for children and families who are considered refugees or undocumented immigrants. For these children and families, we must consider not only where they are within the United States and in our particular site for care, but also where they have been and where they have left. Nearly half of the world's displaced people are children (Murray, 2015), amounting to more than 20 million children. Within this group are both children and families who have fled their home countries and those who are internally displaced within their home country. Nonetheless, these children and their families often experience mental and physical trauma; they may have experienced danger and violence in both staying in their homes and fleeing. For children and families who journey to a new destination, there are dangers along the journey, including inclement weather, discrimination in destination countries, potential loss of loved ones along the journey, further threats to safety in refugee camps, and lack of food and water. Children and adolescents who journey alone face heightened threats of abduction, trafficking, sexual violence and exploitation, or abuse.

For nurses caring for children who have arrived in the United States for resettlement, it is important to know that children and families will have already fled one country, arrived in a second country, and could be resettling in yet another country. Thus trauma and psychologic distress may come not only from extraordinary threats of violence, but also from constant disruption to family life. In fact, psychologic distress and mental illness are the major causes of disability among refugee children, as they frequently experience posttraumatic stress, grief, anxiety, and depression (Murray, 2015). In terms of physical health, the greatest risks stem from infectious diseases and malnutrition. The leading causes of infectious disease–related death among refugees are tuberculosis, malaria, and intestinal parasites, often due to overcrowding, poor sanitation, or inability to institute standing transmission-prevention measures in campsites. Nurses caring for these children and families must keep in mind that their assessment and treatment procedures may need to be accommodated because of trauma and stress that children have already experienced. Nurses must also be aware of signs of exploitation or abuse, indicating that a child or adolescent may be a victim of trafficking, such as elevated fear or unexplained injuries. The process of disentangling the child and family's story may unfold over time after trust has been established.

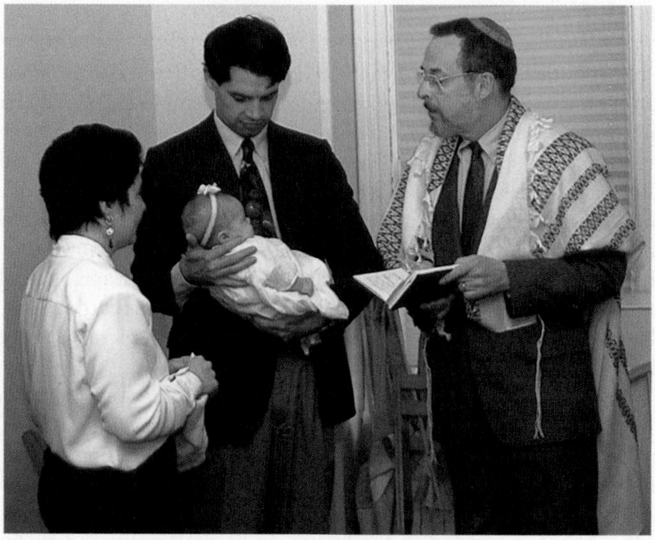

Fig. 2.10 Soon after an infant is born, many families have special religious ceremonies.

Undocumented immigrants are another group of children and families that may have untoward health outcomes and for whom nurses will provide care. Because of their own or their parents' undocumented status, children may be particularly vulnerable to limited access to health care. Negative health effects are often associated with being an undocumented immigrant and are related to poverty, poor living and working conditions, food insecurity, chronic stress, and ongoing fear of deportation and arrest. Despite the negative health effects, research demonstrates that undocumented immigrants seek health care at lower rates than other groups. Although programs such as the Migrant Health Program exist to provide access to low-cost primary care, barriers that families face in accessing this care include language barriers, lack of transportation, difficulty arranging for time off from work, and limited ability to pay.

The health care system is an important layer of influence in the health of children. Although this can be a site of health promotion, health maintenance, and illness management, it may also erect barriers for families to enact the care prescribed. Although child and family factors accounted for some influence (child care, transportation, inadequate insurance), health care system factors had a major impact on completion of referrals. These factors included the ability to get an appointment quickly, the communication style of front-desk staff, and interpreter services.

RELIGION AND SPIRITUAL IDENTITY

Religion and spirituality are powerful forces in the lives of individuals, families, and communities (Fig. 2.10). Spirituality and religion are important principles around which families organize their responses to illness experiences and life transitions. Indeed, nearly 80% of people report that religion is fairly important to them. The terms, however, are often conflated. Religion and spirituality, although frequently grouped together, denote different entities. Religion is a specific set of beliefs enacted through a practice (religiosity) (Taylor, Petersen, Oyedele, et al., 2015). Spirituality is described as a unique awareness, belief, practice, and experience starting in childhood and is rooted over time. Religion and spirituality are important avenues through which children participate in making meaning of important life events, such as

BOX 2.6 Guidelines for Integrating Spiritual Care Into Pediatric Nursing Practice

- Respect the child's and family's religious beliefs and practices.
- Consider the child's development when talking about spiritual concerns.
- Contact the institution's chaplaincy department for patients and families who have symptoms of spiritual distress or ask for specific religious rituals.
- Become knowledgeable about the religious worldviews of cultural groups found in the patients you care for.
- Encourage visitation with family members, members of the patient's spiritual community, and spiritual leaders.
- Allow children and families to teach you about the specifics of their religious beliefs.
- Develop awareness of your own spiritual perspective.
- Listen for understanding rather than agreement or disagreement.

Data from Brooks, B. (2004). Spirituality. In N. Kline (Ed.), *Essentials of pediatric oncology nursing: A core curriculum* (2nd ed.). Glenview, IL: Association of Pediatric Oncology Nurses; Barnes, L. L., Plotnikoff, G. A., Fox, K., et al. (2000). Spirituality, religion, and pediatrics: Intersecting worlds of healing. *Pediatrics, 106*(Suppl. 4), 899–908.

illness in themselves or loved ones, and are shaped by the developmental stage of the child (Taylor, Petersen, Oyedele, et al., 2015). Further, spiritual assessment is necessary to provide family-centered care that is aligned with spiritual and religious needs. Finally, many regulatory bodies that guide practice, including the American Nurses Association, the International Council of Nurses, and The Joint Commission, call for assessment of, and intervention for, spiritual concerns.

Individual, family, and community experiences of religion and spirituality are interrelated, and children experience them from their own, individualized experience as people situated within a community; they also experience what the community as a whole experiences. For example, children whose families practice the Islamic faith experience the religion within the home and what their own relationship to Allah means. They also experience the religion from the perspective of being part of a community when attending mosque or participating in collective prayer. They also might experience being part of a faith community that may face stigma or bias or whose tenets are misunderstood. In many instances, religion and spirituality propel people toward virtuous actions and behaviors. Most of the world's religions share a common thread of "upholding humility, charity, and honesty" (Holden & Williamson, 2014).

When individuals become parents, they may connect to their religion as a guide in raising their children, to enhance their well-being, and to provide a moral and social context for their childrearing. Although parents may use an approach to parenting that is informed by their religion and spirituality, how this is enacted or operationalized varies dramatically because of variability in beliefs about parenting goals and roles, the parent-child relationship, and child discipline and punishment (Holden & Williamson, 2014).

In addition, parents' spirituality, religious practices, and beliefs are a guiding force on their children. Thus with respect to "family-based spirituality care," comprehensive, collaborative, spiritual care is important in addressing the spiritual needs of children who are ill and acknowledges the interrelationships of child, parent, and family spirituality (Box 2.6). In the context of pediatric illness, this is also important because children and families are often isolated from their faith communities and experience crises for which they have no prior experience to draw on or that cause existential questioning and meaning-seeking. Children and families receiving a new or life-threatening diagnosis often experience fear and anxiety and may benefit from health care providers helping them connect to those spiritual and religious practices that are important to them. For example, nurses can help families find a suitable place to pray and ask families which of their health care practices may be most helpful in addressing their spiritual needs.

Children who experience major life transitions, such as being diagnosed with a life-threatening illness or the death of a loved one, often experience spirituality as a source of hope and comfort that promotes their resilience and helps them discern the meaning of the life transition for them. Yet there is a paucity of research on children's spiritual development in a contemporary context (Taylor, Petersen, Oyedele, et al., 2015). Children, adolescents, and young adults have unique spiritual needs related to their developmental stage. For example, adolescents and young adults may be at greater risk for spiritual distress because of their more sophisticated understanding of the impact and risk of illness; diagnosis of a life-threatening illness can cause an internal spiritual struggle and questioning of beliefs. They may engage less with institutionalized religion but still use spirituality as a means of finding meaning and connecting with family and loved ones (Taylor, Petersen, Oyedele, et al., 2015). By asking about and facilitating access to spiritual care, nurses can help build on child and family strengths as they deal with a critical juncture in their lives. Other key practices include avoiding assumptions about spiritual beliefs and practices; asking how the child and family understand the illness's or life event's spiritual impact on the affected individual, other family members, and the family unit; taking time to explore one's own spiritual and religious perspective so that one's values can be clarified and judgments evaluated; active listening that is compassionate and keeps the child's spiritual needs at the center, without false reassurances; and incorporating arts or storytelling into spiritual assessment and intervention. Providing space in the physical environment for children to participate in their spirituality in ways that bring them comfort and provide for meaning-making opportunities is essential, as it can provide a glimpse into their spiritual distress and sources of hope. For example, the provider can elicit an adolescent's narrative of his or her illness situation or life event and invite parents or caregivers to listen and share their reactions to promote family connection and communication.

Nurses can also develop skills and access training to help them feel prepared for when children ask spiritually oriented questions. For example, Ferrell, Wittenberg, Battista, and colleagues (2016) queried children's palliative care nurses and found that children facing life-threatening illnesses most often ask questions about the time-limited nature of their illness, why this has happened to them, and why their deity would allow this to happen to them. They found that children often described the afterlife without fear, sadness, or pain and with angels or predeceased loved ones caring for them there. The authors called for nurses to recognize their ideal position to facilitate spiritual care and communication between child and parents, and child, family, and chaplain or some other spiritual care provider. Ill children, in particular, have spiritual care needs that must be acknowledged. Key components of spiritual care that all nurses can provide are supportive, caring presence to the child and family and taking time to reflect on one's own spirituality or beliefs in order to meet the needs of others. Nurses need not share the belief system of a child or family to sit with and support them in times of spiritual questioning or reflection. Nurses do need skills in supportive, therapeutic listening, answering children's questions about death and the afterlife, facilitating discussion between parents and children, and preserving mindfulness and family relationships (Ferrell, Wittenberg, Battista, et al., 2016).

Regarding physical health, religion has demonstrated mixed effects, with positive effects resulting from the emphasis on healthy behaviors and respect for others. Religiosity and spirituality have been associated with adolescent substance use and older age at sexual debut (Holden & Williamson, 2014). Conversely, deleterious effects may be associated with some religions that are more authoritarian and prohibit health care interventions, such as cases of religiously motivated medical neglect, when a child suffers injury or dies because parents did not seek treatment for a particular ailment, or when immunizations or screenings are declined. In addition, adolescents who identified as highly religious were less likely to use contraception at sexual debut, despite being older than nonreligious adolescents, putting them at risk for unplanned pregnancy or sexually transmitted infections. With respect to mental and emotional health, connection to religion or spirituality has been associated with less adolescent depression, anxiety, and suicidality, as well as lower rates of criminal or delinquent behavior. However, religion or spirituality can contribute to psychologic distress if youth are subjected to negative relationships or experiences that are imbued with demands and criticism. Thus the social context in which the religion is practiced may be more important than the religion itself (Holden & Williamson, 2014).

However, conflicts can arise between religion and health care, and parental religious objections have been a major focus of literature on family spirituality versus other forms of engagement. For example, the American Academy of Pediatrics (2013) cites the intersection of religion, spirituality, and health care as potentially harmful to children based on situations in which parents refuse medical care for their children and there are religious exemptions to child abuse and neglect laws. Although parents' refusal of medical care for their children falls under the scope of parental authority, the child's best interest is the priority. Failure to provide essential health care is increasingly viewed as a form of neglect. Religions and spiritual traditions vary in the depth and nature of treatment they refuse, from refusal of all treatment to refusal of select interventions or therapeutics, such as blood products. Pediatric health care organizations, such as the American Academy of Pediatrics (2013), argue that free exercise of religion should be balanced against protecting children from harm. For example, in a case where parents and health care providers differ on the proposed benefit or burden of a treatment and the primary benefit is spiritual or religious, children's future ability to decide the issue for themselves should be protected and privileged. In addition, the Supreme Court has argued that the free exercise of religion does not include the liberty to subject communities or children to disease or children, in particular, to diminished health or death. These arguments and considerations become murky when the conditions are not life threatening or when the proposed treatment has significant adverse effects or the limited efficacy. Negative psychologic effects must also be considered (American Academy of Pediatrics, 2013).

Complicating this debate is variation in religious exemption laws across states, creating additional uncertainty among families, health care providers, and child protection agencies about when and why to intervene and potential penalties. Thus many health care providers may perceive religion and spirituality as a negative influence in children's lives and believe that such statutes should be abolished, as children may be at greater risk and receive differential care across state lines. These arguments are compelling, and the welfare of children should be prioritized. However, we must walk this line carefully, as health care providers are often in positions of power and families may feel vulnerable, limit their sharing with providers, and ultimately withdraw from care. This hampers spiritual assessment and diminishes communication between child, parent, and health care providers. Overall, pediatric health care providers engage in a limited manner with parents around their spirituality, even if the child is engaged spiritually.

Although many health care providers support the value of religion or spirituality, there is limited discussion in clinical practice, limited assessment and inquiry into families' spiritual beliefs and needs, and limited training in nursing and medical schools on how to conduct such assessment. These limitations create an environment in which limited spiritual and religious interventions that may diminish sorrow and provide comfort and solace can be provided. For example, evaluation and intervention around spiritual beliefs could be helpful for a child who has lost a sibling. Care must be taken, though, to ensure that the right person is available to conduct spiritual care interventions—for example, a trained spiritual counselor or chaplain with expertise in children's spirituality and experience of religion who can skillfully disentangle spiritual from psychologic or emotional issues or parents' spiritual perspectives from those of the child (Holden & Williamson, 2014). Indeed, assessing and addressing child and family spirituality have been incorporated into the standards of various pediatric nursing organizations (e.g., Association of Pediatric Hematology/Oncology Nurses) and other health care organizations (e.g., American Academy of Pediatrics). Spiritual care acknowledges the "transcendent dimensions of life and reflects the reality of the patient" (Taylor, Petersen, Oyedele, et al., 2015). A focused and tiered screening, as proposed by Taylor, Petersen, Oyedele, and colleagues (2015), allows for all children to be screened for spiritual distress and identify immediate needs for support to conducting in-depth spiritual assessment or accessing someone who can. The mnemonic BELIEF also allows for a guided assessment (Taylor, Petersen, Oyedele, et al., 2015):

- Belief system
- Ethics or values
- Lifestyle
- Involvement
- Education
- Future

Religion can influence community standards and norms, although context is key when we consider how religion exerts an effect on children and families. For example, the effect of religion or spirituality may be more pronounced in an isolated rural area versus a major metropolitan area with a more heterogeneous population.

CULTURAL HUMILITY AND HEALTH CARE PROVIDERS' CONTRIBUTION

Health care providers and the wider health care community must reassert the significance of equity, fairness, and caring as the instrumental building blocks of a strong, high-quality, and transformed health care system. One way to get to this point is through teaching and coaching trainees across health care disciplines to be more engaged in understanding the social determinants of health, their impact and roots, and how to counteract their negative effects. Betancourt, Corbett, and Bondaryk (2017) argue that although the concept and practice have limitations, the goal of cultural competence is to "improve the ability of health care providers and health care systems to communicate effectively with and provide quality health care to patients from diverse social backgrounds" (p. 144). Effective communication with patients and families is critical to positive health outcomes, yet many trainees do not feel prepared to engage with patients and families whose backgrounds are different than their own (Betancourt, Corbett, & Bondaryk, 2017; Green, Chun, Cervantes, et al., 2017; Marshall, Cooper, Green, et al., 2017).

It also recognizes the dynamic nature of culture and the influence of context, place, and time. We must also recognize that "culture" is not only race and ethnicity, but also social class, age, sexual orientation, sexuality, gender, ability, and professional discipline, among other things. Thus all of us will be on the receiving and giving ends of care from and for people who do not inhabit the same space as us, yet we can connect on the desire to help and be helped and to minimize suffering.

Foronda, Baptiste, Reinholdt, and colleagues (2016) describe the attributes or characteristics of cultural humility as "openness, self-awareness, egolessness, supportive interactions, self-reflection and critique." They found that the consequences of practicing cultural humility, as published in studies or practice guides, were "mutual empowerment, partnership, respect, optimal care, [and] lifelong learning" (Foronda, Baptiste, Reinholdt, et al., 2016) in clinical encounters. Thus transformational learning environments that can shape students' perspectives and make them aware of power imbalances and inequity in health care can promote humility in future health care encounters.

Although it is imperative to have tools to develop one's presence of mind and to assess one's own values, it is also helpful to have concrete questions and methods with which to elicit a patient's or family's health beliefs or customs. As we have seen, it is not helpful to demonstrate competence by lumping a group of people together and applying an assumed set of beliefs to them, such as "Hispanics have strong family support," as these generalizations can become stereotypical and not illuminate what is important for a particular child and family in a particular context. Thus it is helpful to have a broad understanding of what health beliefs are and how to elicit them.

Religion and culture can influence the ways in which children, youth, and their families interact with health care providers and engage with the health care system. Various avenues for this influence include health beliefs (e.g., children should not know the severity of their illness); health customs (e.g., care of the dead); ethnic customs (e.g., gender roles and division of labor); religious beliefs (e.g., use of blood products); dietary customs (e.g., maintaining a kosher diet); and interpersonal customs (e.g., how children address parents or how touch is used in communication) (Agency for Healthcare Research and Quality, 2015). Questions to begin this conversation can start with the following: "Is there anything you would like for me to know about your child or your family so that I can take the best possible care of you all?" "Can you tell me about your condition (your child's condition)?" or "Do you have any special beliefs or things you do or people you talk to when it comes to your (your child's) health?" These example questions are open-ended and can be adapted to anyone the nurse is caring for at any time in any given location or context. See Box 2.7 for additional questions for exploring a family's culture.

BOX 2.7 Exploring a Family's Culture, Illness, and Care

- What do you think caused your child's health problem?
- Why do you think it started when it did?
- How severe is your child's sickness? Will it have a short or long course?
- How do you think your child's sickness affects your family?
- What are the chief problems your child's sickness has caused?
- What kind of treatment do you think your child should receive?
- What are the most important results you hope to receive from your child's treatment?
- What do you fear most about your child's sickness?

CLINICAL JUDGMENT AND NEXT-GENERATION NCLEX® EXAMINATION-STYLE QUESTIONS

1. The nurse is caring for a 15-year-old girl with diabetes. Parents are concerned about her lack of focus on her diet and glucose testing. What does Duvall's development theory tell you about the focus for this family? In Duvall's Developmental Stage ___1___, the adolescent develops increasing ___2___ and parents focus on ___3___ and ___4___ issues.

Options for 1	Options for 2	Options for 3 and 4
Stage 1	autonomy	marital
Stage II	trust	sibling
Stage III	identity	career
Stage IV	fear	home
Stage V	growth	retirement
Stage VI	height	insurance

2. The nurse caring for a 7-year-old hospitalized because of sickle cell pain finds it difficult to communicate the plan for discharge to the mother who is often absent from the hospital room. Using concepts related to family strengths and functioning style, what are the most appropriate actions for the nurse to take?
Use an X for the nursing actions listed below that are Indicated (appropriate or necessary), Contraindicated (could be harmful), or Non-Essential (makes no difference or not necessary) for the client's care at this time.

Nursing Action: Quality Patient Outcomes	Indicated	Contraindicated	Non-Essential
Realize that parenting roles are learned behaviors and the mother is not prepared to take the child home.			
The family strengths and unique functional style can be a resource for the nurse.			
Parenting styles are all the same and the mother should be forced to listen to the discharge plan.			
Despite difficulty trying to meet with the mother, a sense of purpose to care for this child at home can promote a successful discharge.			
This must be a single family and counseling should be contacted to work with the mother.			

3. The nurse is explaining the importance of limit setting and discipline to a parent of a toddler. In what ways does limit setting and discipline specifically help children? **Select all that apply.**
   A. Protect themselves from danger.
   B. Learn socially acceptable behavior.
   C. Test the limits of their control.
   D. Channel undesirable feelings into constructive activity.
   E. Achieve appropriate mastery at their development level.

4. The nurse is caring for a child and family that has recently moved from China. It is important for the nurse to understand the importance of culture and the impact it has on the child and family. Which of the statements should be used to explore a family's culture? **Select all that apply.**
   A. What do you fear most about your child's illness?
   B. Why did you wait until now to seek treatment?
   C. What do you think caused your child's health problem?
   D. What did you do to cause the child to become ill?
   E. How does your child's sickness affect your family?

REFERENCES

Agency for Healthcare Research and Quality. (2015). *Consider culture, customs, and beliefs (tool 10). AHRQ health literacy universal precautions toolkit* (2nd ed.). Retrieved from. https://www.ahrq.gov/sites/default/files/wysiwyg/professionals/quality-patient-safety/quality-resources/tools/literacy-toolkit/healthlittoolkit2_tool10.pdf.

American Academy of Pediatrics Council on Communications and Media. (2016a). Media use in school-aged children and adolescents. *Pediatrics, 138*(5), e20162592.

American Academy of Pediatrics Council on Communications and Media. (2016b). Media and young minds. *Pediatrics, 138*(5), e20162591.

American Academy Council on Community Pediatrics. (2016c). Poverty and child health in the United States. *Pediatrics, 137*(4), e20160339.

American Academy of Pediatrics Section on Hospice and Palliative Medicine and Hospital Care. (2013). Pediatric palliative care commitments, guidelines, and recommendations. *Pediatrics, 132*, 966–972.

American Academy of Pediatrics, Committee on Early Childhood, Adoption, and Dependent Care. (2000). Development issues for young children in foster care (RE0012). *Pediatrics, 106*(5), 1145–1150.

American Academy of Pediatrics. (2003). Family pediatrics: Report of the task force on the family. *Pediatrics, 111*(6), 1541–1571.

Annie, E. Casey Foundation (2012). *Stepping up for kids: What government and communities should do to support kinship families.* https://www.aecf.org/resources/ stepping-up-for-kids/.

Annie, E. Casey Foundation (2014). *African American, American Indian, and Latino Children have the most barriers.* http://www.aecf.org/blog/african-american-american-indian-and-latino-children-have-the-most-barriers. Retrieved June 20, 2107.

Annie, E. Casey Foundation (2015). *Every kid needs a family.* https://www.aecf.org/m/ resourcedoc/aecf-EveryKidNeedsAFamily-2015.pdf.

Annie, E. Casey Foundation (2018). 2018 kids count data book: State profiles of child well-being. http://www.aecf.org/resources/2018-kids-count-data-bookBetBron.

Baumrind, D. (1971). Harmonious parents and their preschool children. *Developmental Psychology, 41*, 92–102.

Baumrind, D. (1996). The discipline controversy revisited. *Family Relations, 45*, 405–414.

Berger, L., & Waldfogel, J. (2004). Out-of-home placement of children and economic factors: An empirical analysis. *Review of Economics of the Household, 2*(4), 387–411.

Betancourt, J. R., Corbett, J., & Bondaryk, M. R. (2017). Addressing disparities and achieving equity: Cultural competence, ethics, and health-care transformation. *Chest, 145*(1), 145–148.

Bomar, P. J. (2004). *Promoting health in families* (3rd ed.). Philadelphia: Saunders.

Bronfenbrenner, U. (1979). *The ecology of human development: Experiments by nature and design.* Cambridge, Mass: Harvard University Press.

Bronfenbrenner, U. (2005). *Making human beings human: Bioecological perspectives on human development.* Thousand Oaks, Calif: Sage Publications.

Center on the Developing Child at Harvard University. (2016). *Building Core Capabilities for life: The science behind the skills adults need to succeed in parenting and in the workplace.* http://www.developingchild.harvard.edu.

Centers for Disease Control and Prevention. (2009). *School connectedness: Strategies for increasing protective factors among youth.* Atlanta, GA: U.S. Department of Health and Human Services.

Centers for Disease Control and Prevention. (2018). *National marriage and divorce rate trends, 2018.* https://www.cdc.gov/nchs/nvss/marriage-divorce.htm. Retrieved on February 18, 2019.

Chamberlain, P., Price, J., Leve, L. D., et al. (2008). Prevention of behavior problems for children in foster care: Outcomes and mediation effects. *Prevention Science, 9*(1), 17–27.

Chavez, V. (2012). Cultural humility: People, principles, and practices (documentary film). www.youtube.com/watch?v_SaSH<bslv4w. Retrieved March 20, 2013.

Coker, T. R., Elliot, M. N., Kanouse, D. K., et al. (2009). Perceived racial/ethnic discrimination among fifth-grade students and its association with mental health. *American Journal of Public Health, 99*(5), 878–884.

Duvall, E. R. (1977). *Family development* (5th ed.). Philadelphia: Lippincott.

Ferrell, B., Wittenberg, E., Battista, V., et al. (2016). Nurses' experiences of spiritual communication with seriously ill children. *Journal of Palliative Medicine, 19*(11), 1166–1170.

Fierman, A. H., Beck, A. F., Chung, E. K., et al. (2016). Redesigning health-care practices to address childhood poverty. *Academic Pediatrics, 16*, S136–S146.

Fisher, C., Lindhorst, H., Matthews, T., et al. (2008). Nursing staff attitudes and behaviors regarding family presence in the hospital setting. *Journal of Advanced Nursing, 64*(6), 615–624.

Foronda, C., Baptiste, D. L., Reinholdt, M. M., et al. (2016). Cultural humility: A concept analysis. *Journal of Transcultural Nursing, 27*(3), 210–217.

Gershoff, E. T. (2008). *Report on physical punishment in the United States: What research tell us about its effects on children.* Colombus, OH: Center for Effective Discipline.

Goldenberg, I., & Goldenberg, H. (2012). *Family therapy: An overview* (8th ed.). Pacific Grove, Calif: Brooks-Cole Cengage Learning.

Green, A. R., Chun, M. B. J., Cervantes, M., et al. (2017). Measuring medical students' preparedness and skills to provide cross-cultural care. *Health Equity, 1*(1), 15–22.

Holden, G. W., & Williamson, P. A. (2014). Religion and child well-being in B-A. In F. Asher, I. Casas, Frones, & J. E. Corbin (Eds.), *Handbook of child well-being.* Dordrecht: Springer.

Kaakinen, J. R., & Coehlo, D. P. (2015). *Family health care nursing* (5th ed.). Philadelphia: Davis.

Kazak, A. E. (2001). Comprehensive care for children with cancer and their families: A social ecological framework guiding research, practice, and policy. *Children's Services: Social Policy, Research, and Practice, 4*(4), 217–233.

Kazak, A. E., Rourke, M. T., & Navasaria, N. (2010). Families and other systems in pediatric psychology. In Michael C. Roberts, & Ric G. Steele (Eds.), *Handbook of pediatric psychology.* Guilford Press.

Lewallen, T. C., Hunt, H., Potts-Datema, W., et al. (2015). The whole school, whole community, whole child model: A new approach for improving educational attainment and healthy development for students. *The Journal of School Health, 85*, 729–739.

Lucas-Thompson, R. G., Goldberg, W. A., & Prause, J. (2010). Maternal work early in the lives of children and its distal associations with achievement and behavior problems: A meta-analysis. *Psychological Bulletin, 136*(6), 915–942.

Marshall, J. K., Cooper, L. A., Green, A. R., et al. (2017). Residents' attitude, knowledge, and perceived preparedness toward caring for patients from diverse sociocultural backgrounds. *Health Equity*, *1*(1), 43–49. https://doi.org/10.1089/heq.2016.0010.

McCubbin, M. A., & McCubbin, H. I. (1994). Families coping with illness: The resiliency model of family stress, adjustment, and adaptation. In C. B. Danielson, B. H. Bissel, & P. Winstead-Fry (Eds.), *Families, health, and illness*. St. Louis: Mosby.

Mendez, M., Durtschi, J., Neppl, T., et al. (2016). Corporal punishment and externalizing behaviors in toddlers: The moderating role of positive and harsh parenting. *Journal of Family Psychology*, *30*(8), 887–895.

Michael, S. L., Merlo, C. L., Basch, C. E., et al. (2015). Critical connections: Health and academics. *Journal of School Health*, *85*, 740–775.

Mooney-Doyle, dos Santos, M., Bousso, R., & Deatrick, J. A. (2017). Parental expectations for support from healthcare providers: A qualitative secondary analysis. *Journal of Pediatric Nursing*, *36*, 163–172.

Murray, J. S. (2015). Displaced and forgotten child refugees: A humanitarian crisis. *Journal for Specialists in Pediatric Nursing*, *21*, 29–36.

Papero, D. V. (1990). *Bowen family systems theory*. Boston, MA: Pearson.

Power, N., & Franck, L. (2008). Parent participation in the care of hospitalized children: A systematic review. *Journal of Advanced Nursing*, *62*(6), 622–641.

Pulgaron, E. R., Marchante, A. N., Agosto, Y., et al. (2016). Grandparent involvement and children's health outcomes: The current state of the literature. *Family Systems Health Journal*, *34*(3), 260–269.

Scott, J., & Marshall, G. (2009). *Ethnicity, oxford dictionary of sociology, 2009*. Oxford University Press.

Strasburger, V., Jordan, A., & Donnerstein, E. (2012). Children, adolescents, and the media: Health effects. *Pediatric Clinics of North America*, *59*, 533–587.

Taylor, E. J., Petersen, C., Oyedele, O., & Haase, J. (2015). Spirituality and spiritual care of adolescents and young adults with cancer. *Seminars in Oncology Nursing*, *3*, 227–241.

Tynes, B. M., Giang, M. T., Williams, D. R., et al. (2008). Online racial discrimination and psychological adjustment among adolescents. *Journal of Adolescent Health*, *43*(6), 565–569.

US Census Bureau. (2017). *Same sex couple households*. American Community Survey Briefs.

Williams, D. R. (2012). Miles to go before we sleep: Racial inequities in health. *Journal of Health and Social Behavior*, *53*, 279–296.

3

Developmental and Genetic Influences on Child Health Promotion

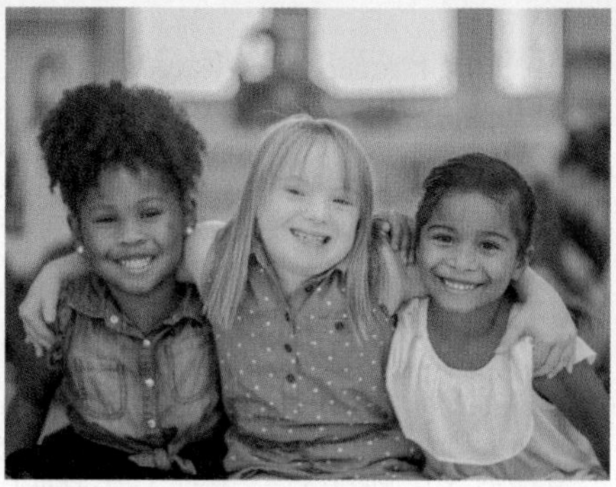

Cynthia A. Prows, Marilyn J. Hockenberry

http://evolve.elsevier.com/wong/essentials

CONCEPTS

- Genetic Influences

GROWTH AND DEVELOPMENT

FOUNDATIONS OF GROWTH AND DEVELOPMENT

Growth and development, usually referred to as a unit, express the sum of the numerous changes that take place during the lifetime of an individual. The entire course is a dynamic process that encompasses several interrelated dimensions:

Growth—an increase in number and size of cells as they divide and synthesize new proteins; results in increased size and weight of the whole or any of its parts

Development—a gradual change and expansion; advancement from lower to more advanced stages of complexity; the emerging and expanding of the individual's capacities through growth, maturation, and learning

Maturation—an increase in competence and adaptability; aging; usually used to describe a qualitative change; a change in the complexity of a structure that makes it possible for that structure to begin functioning; to function at a higher level

Differentiation—processes by which early cells and structures are systematically modified and altered to achieve specific and characteristic physical and chemical properties; sometimes used to describe the trend of mass to specific; development from simple to more complex activities and functions

All of these processes are interrelated, simultaneous, and ongoing; none occurs apart from the others. The processes depend on a sequence of endocrine, genetic, constitutional, environmental, and nutritional influences (Ball, Dains, Flynn, et al., 2019). The child's body becomes larger and more complex; the personality simultaneously expands in scope and complexity. Very simply, growth can be viewed as a **quantitative** change and development as a **qualitative** change.

Stages of Development

Most authorities in the field of child development categorize child growth and behavior into approximate age stages or in terms that describe the features of a developmental age period. The age ranges of these stages are arbitrary, because they do not take into account individual differences and cannot be applied to all children with any degree of precision. Categorization does provide a convenient means to describe the characteristics associated with the majority of children at periods when distinctive developmental changes appear and specific developmental tasks must be accomplished. (A **developmental task** is a set of skills and competencies specific to each developmental stage that children must accomplish or master to function effectively within their environment.) It is also significant for nurses to know that there are characteristic health problems related to each major phase of development. The sequence of descriptive age periods and subperiods that is used here and elaborated in subsequent chapters is listed in Box 3.1.

Patterns of Growth and Development

There are definite and predictable patterns in growth and development that are continuous, orderly, and progressive. These patterns, or trends, are universal and basic to all human beings, but each human being accomplishes these in a manner and time unique to that individual.

Directional Trends

Growth and development proceed in regular, related directions or gradients and reflect the physical development and maturation of neuromuscular functions (Fig. 3.1). The first pattern is the **cephalocaudal**, or **head-to-tail**, direction. The head end of the organism develops first and is large and complex, whereas the lower end is small and simple and takes shape at a later period. The physical evidence of this trend is most apparent during the period before birth, but it also applies to postnatal behavior development. Infants achieve control of the heads before they have control of their trunks and extremities, hold their backs erect before they stand, use their eyes before their hands, and gain control of their hands before they have control of their feet.

Second, the **proximodistal**, or **near-to-far**, trend applies to the midline-to-peripheral concept. A conspicuous illustration is the early embryonic development of limb buds, which is followed by rudimentary fingers and toes. In infants, shoulder control precedes mastery of the hands, the whole hand is used as a unit before the fingers can be manipulated, and the central nervous system develops more rapidly than the peripheral nervous system.

These trends or patterns are bilateral and appear symmetric—each side develops in the same direction and at the same rate as the other. For some of the neurologic functions, this symmetry is only external because of unilateral differentiation of function at an early stage of postnatal development. For example, by the age of approximately 5 years, children have demonstrated a decided preference for the use of one hand over the other, although previously either one had been used.

BOX 3.1 Developmental Age Periods

Prenatal Period—Conception to Birth

Germinal: Conception to approximately 2 weeks old
Embryonic: 2 to 8 weeks old
Fetal: 8 to 40 weeks old (birth)

A rapid growth rate and total dependency make this one of the most crucial periods in the developmental process. The relationship between maternal health and certain manifestations in the newborn emphasizes the importance of adequate prenatal care to the health and well-being of the infant.

Infancy Period—Birth to 12 Months Old

Neonatal: Birth to 27 or 28 days old
Infancy: 1 to approximately 12 months old

The infancy period is one of rapid motor, cognitive, and social development. Through mutuality with the caregiver (parent), the infant establishes a basic trust in the world and the foundation for future interpersonal relationships. The critical first month of life, although part of the infancy period, is often differentiated from the remainder because of the major physical adjustments to extrauterine existence and the psychologic adjustment of the parent.

Early Childhood—1 to 6 Years Old

Toddler: 1 to 3 years old
Preschool: 3 to 6 years old

This period, which extends from the time children attain upright locomotion until they enter school, is characterized by intense activity and discovery. It is a time of marked physical and personality development. Motor development advances steadily. Children at this age acquire language and wider social relationships, learn role standards, gain self-control and mastery, develop increasing awareness of dependence and independence, and begin to develop a self-concept.

Middle Childhood—6 to 11 or 12 Years Old

Frequently referred to as the *school age,* this period of development is one in which the child is directed away from the family group and centered around the wider world of peer relationships. There is steady advancement in physical, mental, and social development with emphasis on developing skill competencies. Social cooperation and early moral development take on more importance with relevance for later life stages. This is a critical period in the development of a self-concept.

Later Childhood—11 to 19 Years Old

Prepubertal: 10 to 13 years old
Adolescence: 13 to approximately 18 years old

The tumultuous period of rapid maturation and change known as *adolescence* is considered to be a transitional period that begins at the onset of puberty and extends to the point of entry into the adult world—usually high school graduation. Biologic and personality maturation are accompanied by physical and emotional turmoil, and there is redefining of the self-concept. In the late adolescent period, the young person begins to internalize all previously learned values and to focus on an individual, rather than a group, identity.

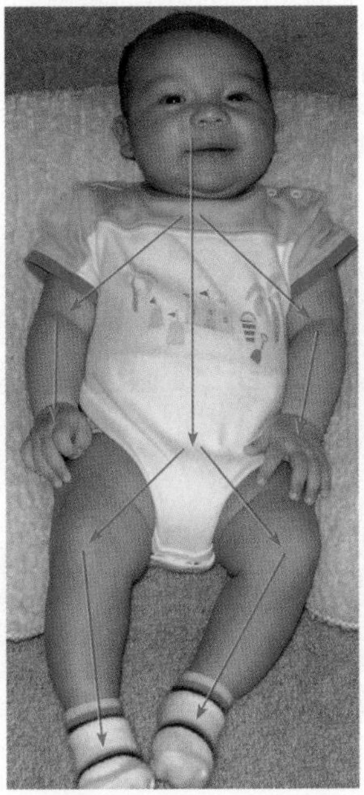

Fig. 3.1 Directional trends in growth.

The third trend, **differentiation**, describes development from simple operations to more complex activities and functions, from broad, global patterns of behavior to more specific, refined patterns. All areas of development (physical, cognitive, social, and emotional) proceed in this direction. Through the process of development and differentiation, early embryonal cells with vague, undifferentiated functions progress to an immensely complex organism composed of highly specialized and diversified cells, tissues, and organs. Generalized development precedes specific or specialized development; gross, random muscle movements take place before fine muscle control.

Sequential Trends

In all dimensions of growth and development, there is a definite, predictable sequence, with each child passing through every stage. For example, children crawl before they creep, creep before they stand, and stand before they walk. Later facets of the personality are built on the early foundation of trust. The child babbles, then forms words and finally sentences; writing emerges from scribbling.

Developmental Pace

Although development has a fixed, precise order, it does not progress at the same rate or pace. There are periods of accelerated growth and periods of decelerated growth in both total body growth and the growth of subsystems. Not all areas of development progress at the same pace. When a spurt occurs in one area (such as gross motor), minimal advances may take place in language, fine motor, or social skills. After the gross motor skill has been achieved, the focus will shift to another area of development. The rapid growth before and after birth gradually levels off throughout early childhood. Growth is relatively slow during middle childhood, markedly increases at the beginning of adolescence, and levels off in early adulthood. Each child grows at his or her own pace. Distinct differences are observed among children as they reach developmental milestones.

NURSING TIP Research suggests that normal growth, particularly height in infants, may occur in brief (possibly even 24-hour) bursts that punctuate long periods in which no measurable growth takes place. The researchers noted sex differences, with girls growing in length during the week they gained weight and boys growing in the week after a significant weight gain. Sex-specific growth hormone pulse patterns may coordinate body composition, weight gain, and linear growth (Lampl, Johnson, & Frongillo, 2001; Lampl, Thompson, & Frongillo, 2005). Furthermore, findings indicate a stuttering or saltatory pattern of growth that follows no regular cycle and can occur after "quiet" periods that last as long as 4 weeks.

Sensitive Periods

There are limited times during the process of growth when the organism interacts with a particular environment in a specific manner. Periods termed **critical**, **sensitive**, **vulnerable**, and **optimal** are the times in the lifetime of an organism when it is more susceptible to positive or negative influences.

The quality of interactions during these sensitive periods determines whether the effects on the organism will be beneficial or harmful. For example, physiologic maturation of the central nervous system is influenced by the adequacy and timing of contributions from the environment, such as stimulation and nutrition. The first 3 months of prenatal life is a sensitive period in the physical growth of fetuses.

Psychosocial development also appears to have sensitive periods when an environmental event has maximal influence on the developing personality. For example, primary socialization occurs during the first year when the infant makes the initial social attachments and establishes a basic trust in the world. A warm and consistently responsive relationship with a parent figure is fundamental to a healthy personality. The same concept might be applied to readiness for learning skills, such as toilet training or reading. In these instances, there appears to be an opportune time when the skill is best learned.

Individual Differences

Each child grows in his or her own unique and personal way. The sequence of events is predictable; the exact timing is not. Rates of growth vary, and measurements are defined in terms of ranges to allow for individual differences. Periods of fast growth, such as the pubescent growth spurt, may begin earlier or later in some children than in others. Children may grow quickly or slowly during the spurt and may finish sooner or later than other children. Gender is an influential factor because girls seem to be more advanced in physiologic growth at all ages.

BIOLOGIC GROWTH AND PHYSICAL DEVELOPMENT

As children grow, their external dimensions change. These changes are accompanied by corresponding alterations in structure and function of internal organs and tissues that reflect the gradual acquisition of physiologic competence. Each part has its own rate of growth, which may be directly related to alterations in the size of the child (e.g., the heart rate). Skeletal muscle growth approximates whole body growth; brain, lymphoid, adrenal, and reproductive tissues follow distinct and individual patterns (Fig. 3.2). When growth deficiency has a secondary cause, such as severe illness or acute malnutrition, recovery from the illness or the establishment of an adequate diet will produce a dramatic acceleration of the growth rate that usually continues until the child's individual growth pattern is resumed.

External Proportions

Variations in the growth rate of different tissues and organ systems produce significant changes in body proportions during childhood. The cephalocaudal trend of development is most evident in total body growth as indicated by these changes. During fetal development, the head is the fastest growing body part, and at 2 months of gestation, the head constitutes 50% of total body length. During infancy, growth of the trunk predominates; the legs are the most rapidly growing part during childhood; in adolescence, the trunk again elongates. In newborn infants, the lower limbs are one-third the total body length but only 15% of the total body weight; in adults, the lower limbs constitute half of the total body height and 30% or more of the total body weight. As growth proceeds, the midpoint in head-to-toe measurements gradually descends from a level even with the umbilicus at birth to the level of the symphysis pubis at maturity.

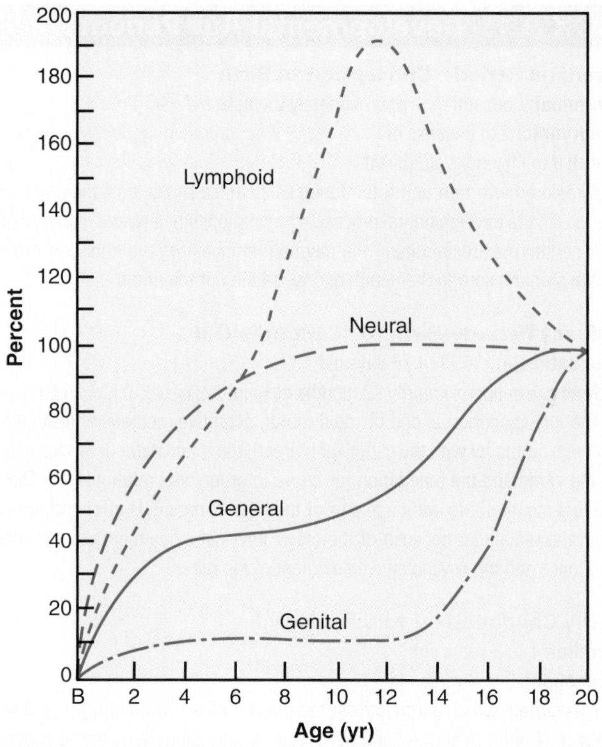

Fig. 3.2 Growth rates for the body as a whole and three types of tissues. *General*—body as a whole; external dimension; and respiratory, digestive, renal, circulatory, and musculoskeletal systems. *Lymphoid*—thymus, lymph nodes, and intestinal lymph masses. *Neural*—brain, dura, spinal cord, optic apparatus, and head dimensions. (Data from Jackson, J. A., Patterson, D. G., & Harris, R. E. [1930]. *The measurement of man.* Minneapolis, MN: University of Minnesota Press.)

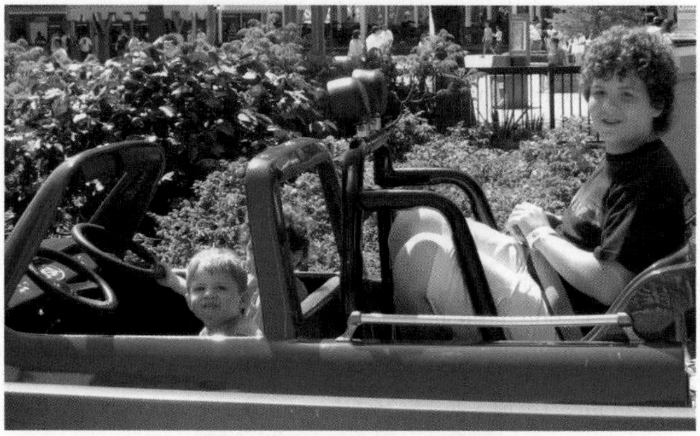

Fig. 3.3 Changes in body proportions occur dramatically during childhood.

Biologic Determinants of Growth and Development

The most prominent feature of childhood and adolescence is physical growth (Fig. 3.3). Throughout development, various tissues in the body undergo changes in growth, composition, and structure. In some tissues, the changes are continuous (e.g., bone growth and dentition); in others, significant alterations occur at specific stages (e.g., appearance of secondary sex characteristics). When these measurements are compared with standardized norms, a child's developmental progress can be determined with a high degree of confidence (Table 3.1). Growth in children with Down syndrome differs from that in other children. Children with Down syndrome have slower growth velocity between 6 months and 3 years of age and then again in adolescence.

TABLE 3.1 General Trends in Height and Weight Gain During Childhood

Age-Group	Weight[a]	Height[a]
Birth to 6 months old	Weekly gain: 140-200 g (5-7 oz) Birth weight doubles by end of first 4-7 months[b]	Monthly gain: 2.5 cm (1 inch)
6 to 12 months old	Weight gain: 85-140 g (3-5 oz) Birth weight triples by end of first year	Monthly gain: 1.25 cm (0.5 inch) Birth length increases by ≈50% by end of first year
Toddlers	Birth weight quadruples by age 2½ years	Height at age 2 years is ≈50% of eventual adult height Gain during second year: about 12 cm (4.7 inches) Gain during third year: about 6-8 cm (2.4-3.1 inches)
Preschoolers	Yearly gain: 2-3 kg (4.5-6.5 pounds)	Birth length doubles by 4 years old Yearly gain: 5-7.5 cm (2-3 inches)
School-age children	Yearly gain: 2-3 kg (4.5-6.5 pounds)	Yearly gain after age 7 years: 5 cm (2 inches) Birth length triples by about 13 years old
Pubertal Growth Spurt		
Females: 10 to 14 years	Weight gain: 7-25 kg (15.5-55 pounds) Mean: 17.5 kg (38.5 pounds)	Height gain: 5-25 cm (2-10 inches); ≈95% of mature height achieved by onset of menarche or skeletal age of 13 years old Mean: 20.5 cm (8 inches)
Males: 11 to 16 years	Weight gain: 7-30 kg (15.5-66 pounds) Mean: 23.7 kg (52.2 pounds)	Height gain: 10-30 cm (4-12 inches); ≈95% of mature height achieved by skeletal age of 15 years old Mean: 27.5 cm (11 inches)

[a]Yearly height and weight gains for each age-group represent averaged estimates from a variety of sources.
[b]Jung, F. E., & Czajka-Narins, D. M. (1985). Birth weight doubling and tripling times: an updated look at the effects of birth weight, sex, race, and type of feeding. *American Journal of Clinical Nutrition, 42*(2), 182–189.

Puberty occurs earlier, and they achieve shorter stature. These patients are frequent users of the health care system, often with multiple providers, and benefit from the use of the Down syndrome growth chart to monitor their growth (Zemel, Pipan, Stallings, et al., 2015).

Linear growth, or **height**, occurs almost entirely as a result of skeletal growth and is considered a stable measurement of general growth. Growth in height is not uniform throughout life but ceases when maturation of the skeleton is complete. The maximum rate of growth in length occurs before birth, but newborns continue to grow at a rapid, although slower, rate.

> **NURSING TIP** Double the child's height at the age of 2 years to estimate how tall he or she may be as an adult.

At birth, **weight** is more variable than height and is, to a greater extent, a reflection of the intrauterine environment. The average newborn weighs 3175 to 3400 g (7 to 7.5 pounds). In general, the birth weight doubles by 4 to 7 months old and triples by the end of the first year. By 2 to 2½ years old, the birth weight usually quadruples. After this point, the "normal" rate of weight gain, just as the growth in height, assumes a steady annual increase of approximately 2 to 2.75 kg (4.4 to 6 pounds) per year until the adolescent growth spurt.

Both **bone age** determinants and state of **dentition** are used as indicators of development. Because both are discussed elsewhere, neither is elaborated here (see the next section for bone age; see Chapters 11 and 12 for dentition).

Skeletal Growth and Maturation

The most accurate measure of general development is **skeletal** or **bone age**, the radiologic determination of osseous maturation. Skeletal age appears to correlate more closely with other measures of physiologic maturity (e.g., onset of menarche) than with chronologic age or height. Bone age is determined by comparing the mineralization of ossification centers and advancing bony form to age-related standards.

Bone formation begins during the second month of fetal life when calcium salts are deposited in the intercellular substance (matrix) to form calcified cartilage first and then true bone. Bone formation exhibits some differences. In small bones, the bone continues to form in the center, and cartilage continues to be laid down on the surfaces. In long bones, the ossification begins in the **diaphysis** (the long central portion of the bone) and continues in the **epiphysis** (the end portions of the bone). Between the diaphysis and the epiphysis, an **epiphyseal cartilage plate** (or **growth plate**) unites with the diaphysis by columns of spongy tissue, the **metaphysis**. Active growth in length takes place in the epiphyseal growth plate. Interference with this growth site by trauma or infection can result in deformity.

The first centers of ossification appear in 2-month-old embryos; at birth, the number is approximately 400, about half the number at maturity. New centers appear at regular intervals during the growth period and provide the basis for assessment of bone age. Postnatally, the earliest centers to appear (at 5 to 6 months old) are those of the capitate and hamate bones in the wrist. Therefore radiographs of the hand and wrist provide the most useful areas for screening to determine skeletal age, especially before 6 years old. These centers appear earlier in girls than in boys.

Nurses must understand that the growing bones of children possess many unique characteristics. Bone fractures occurring at the growth plate may be difficult to discover and may significantly affect subsequent growth and development. Factors that may influence skeletal muscle injury rates and types in children and adolescents include the following (Caine, DiFiori, & Maffulli, 2006):

- Less protective sports equipment for children
- Less emphasis on conditioning, especially flexibility
- In adolescents, fractures that are more common than ligamentous ruptures because of the rapid growth rate of the physeal (segment of tubular bone that is concerned mainly with growth) zone of hypertrophy

Neurologic Maturation

In contrast to other body tissues, which grow rapidly after birth, the nervous system grows proportionately more rapidly before birth. Two periods of rapid brain cell growth occur during fetal life: a dramatic increase in the number of neurons between 15 and 20 weeks of gestation and another increase at 30 weeks, which extends to 1 year of age. The rapid growth of infancy continues during early childhood and then slows to a more gradual rate during later childhood and adolescence.

Postnatal growth consists of increasing the amount of cytoplasm around the nuclei of existing cells, increasing the number and intricacy of communications with other cells, and advancing their peripheral axons to keep pace with expanding body dimensions. This allows for increasingly complex movement and behavior. Neurophysiologic changes also provide the foundation for language, learning, and behavior development. Neurologic or electroencephalographic development is sometimes used as an indicator of maturational age in the early weeks of life.

Lymphoid Tissues

Lymphoid tissues contained in the lymph nodes, thymus, spleen, tonsils, adenoids, and blood lymphocytes follow a growth pattern unlike that of other body tissues. These tissues are small in relation to total body size, but they are well developed at birth. They increase rapidly to reach adult dimensions by 6 years old and continue to grow. At about 10 to 12 years old, they reach a maximum development that is approximately twice their adult size. This is followed by a rapid decline to stable adult dimensions by the end of adolescence.

Development of Organ Systems

All tissues and organ systems undergo changes during development. Some are striking; others are subtle. Many have implications for assessment and care. Because the major importance of these changes relates to their dysfunction, the developmental characteristics of various systems and organs are discussed throughout the book as they relate to these areas. Physical characteristics and physiologic changes that vary with age are included in age-group descriptions.

PHYSIOLOGIC CHANGES

Physiologic changes that take place in all organs and systems are discussed as they relate to dysfunction. Other changes, such as pulse, respiratory rates, and blood pressure, are an integral part of physical assessment (see Chapter 4). In addition, there are changes in basic functions, including metabolism, temperature, and patterns of sleep and rest.

Metabolism

The rate of metabolism when the body is at rest (**basal metabolic rate**, or **BMR**) demonstrates a distinctive change throughout childhood. Highest in newborn infants, the BMR closely relates to the proportion of surface area to body mass, which changes as the body increases in size. In both sexes, the proportion decreases progressively to maturity. The BMR is slightly higher in boys at all ages and further increases during pubescence over that in girls.

The rate of metabolism determines the caloric requirements of the child. The basal energy requirement of infants is about 108 kcal/kg of body weight and decreases to 40 to 45 kcal/kg at maturity. Water requirements throughout life remain at approximately 1.5 ml/calorie of energy expended. Children's energy needs vary considerably at different ages and with changing circumstances. The energy requirement to build tissue steadily decreases with age following the general growth curve; however, energy needs vary with the individual child and may be considerably higher. For short periods (e.g., during strenuous exercise) and more prolonged periods (e.g., illness) the needs can be very high.

! NURSING ALERT

Each degree of fever increases the basal metabolism 10%, with a corresponding increase in fluid requirement.

Temperature

Body temperature, reflecting metabolism, decreases over the course of development. Thermoregulation is one of the most important adaptation responses of infants during the transition from intrauterine to extrauterine life. In healthy neonates, hypothermia can result in several negative metabolic consequences, such as hypoglycemia, elevated bilirubin levels, and metabolic acidosis. Skin-to-skin care, also referred to as *kangaroo care,* is an effective way to prevent neonatal hypothermia in infants. Unclothed, diapered infants are placed on the parent's bare chest after birth, promoting thermoregulation and attachment. After the unstable regulatory ability in the neonatal period, heat production steadily declines as the infant grows into childhood. Individual differences of 0.5°F to 1°F are normal, and occasionally a child normally displays an unusually high or low temperature. Beginning at approximately 12 years old, girls display a temperature that remains relatively stable, but the temperature in boys continues to fall for a few more years. Females maintain a temperature slightly above that of males throughout life.

Even with improved temperature regulation, infants and young children are highly susceptible to temperature fluctuations. Body temperature responds to changes in environmental temperature and is increased with active exercise, crying, and emotional stress. Infections can cause a higher and more rapid temperature increase in infants and young children than in older children. In relation to body weight, an infant produces more heat per unit than adolescents. Consequently, during active play or when heavily clothed, an infant or small child is likely to become overheated.

Sleep and Rest

Sleep, a protective function in all organisms, allows for repair and recovery of tissues after activity. As in most aspects of development, there is wide variation among individual children in the amount and distribution of sleep at various ages. As children mature, there is a change in the total time they spend in sleep and the amount of time they spend in deep sleep.

Newborn infants sleep much of the time that is not occupied with feeding and other aspects of their care. As infants grow older, the total time spent sleeping gradually decreases, they remain awake for longer periods, and they sleep longer at night. For example, the length of a sleep cycle increases from approximately 50 to 60 minutes in newborn infants to approximately 90 minutes in adolescents (National Sleep Foundation, 2019). During the latter part of the first year, most children sleep through the night and take one or two naps during the day. By the time they are 12 to 18 months old, most children have eliminated the second nap. After age 3 years, children have usually given up daytime naps except in cultures in which an afternoon nap or siesta is customary. Sleep time declines slightly from 4 to 10 years old and then increases somewhat during the pubertal growth spurt.

The quality of sleep changes as children mature. As children develop through adolescence, their need for sleep does not decline, but their opportunity for sleep may be affected by social, activity, and academic schedules.

NUTRITION

Nutrition is probably the single most important influence on growth. Dietary factors regulate growth at all stages of development, and their effects are exerted in numerous and complex ways. During the rapid prenatal growth period, poor nutrition may influence development from the time of implantation of the ovum until birth. During infancy and childhood, the demand for calories is relatively great, as evidenced by the rapid increase in both height and weight. At this time, protein and caloric requirements are higher than at almost any period of postnatal development. As the growth rate slows, with its concomitant decrease in metabolism, there is a corresponding reduction in caloric and protein requirements.

Growth is uneven during the periods of childhood between infancy and adolescence, when there are plateaus and small growth spurts. Children's appetites fluctuate in response to these variations until the turbulent growth spurt of adolescence, when adequate nutrition is extremely important but may be subjected to numerous emotional influences. Adequate nutrition is closely related to good health throughout life, and an overall improvement in nourishment is evidenced by the gradual increase in size and early maturation of children in this century.

TEMPERAMENT

Temperament is defined as "the manner of thinking, behaving, or reacting characteristic of an individual" (Chess & Thomas, 1999) and refers to the way in which a person deals with life. From the time of birth, children exhibit marked individual differences in the way they respond to their environment and the way others, particularly the parents, respond to them and their needs. A genetic basis has been suggested for some differences in temperament. Nine characteristics of temperament have been identified through interviews with parents (Box 3.2). Temperament refers to behavioral tendencies, not to discrete behavioral acts. There are no implications of good or bad. Most children can be placed into one of three common categories based on their overall pattern of temperamental attributes:

The easy child: Easygoing children are even tempered, are regular and predictable in their habits, and have a positive approach to new stimuli. They are open and adaptable to change and display a mild to moderately intense mood that is typically positive. Approximately 40% of children fall into this category.

The difficult child: Difficult children are highly active, irritable, and irregular in their habits. Negative withdrawal responses are typical, and they require a more structured environment. These children adapt slowly to new routines, people, and situations. Mood expressions are usually intense and primarily negative. They exhibit frequent periods of crying, and frustration often produces violent tantrums. This group represents about 10% of children.

The slow-to-warm-up child: Slow-to-warm-up children typically react negatively and with mild intensity to new stimuli and, unless pressured, adapt slowly with repeated contact. They respond with only mild but passive resistance to novelty or changes in routine. They are inactive and moody but show only moderate irregularity in functions. Fifteen percent of children demonstrate this temperament pattern.

Thirty-five percent of children either have some, but not all, of the characteristics of one of the categories or are inconsistent in their behavioral responses. Many normal children demonstrate this wide range of behavioral patterns.

BOX 3.2 Attributes of Temperament

Activity: Level of physical motion during activity, such as sleep, eating, play, dressing, and bathing

Rhythmicity: Regularity in the timing of physiologic functions, such as hunger, sleep, and elimination

Approach-withdrawal: Nature of initial responses to a new stimulus, such as people, situations, places, foods, toys, and procedures (**Approach** responses are positive and are displayed by activity or expression; **withdrawal** responses are negative expressions or behaviors.)

Adaptability: Ease or difficulty with which the child adapts or adjusts to new or altered situations

Threshold of responsiveness (sensory threshold): Amount of stimulation, such as sounds or light, required to evoke a response in the child

Intensity of reaction: Energy level of the child's reactions regardless of quality or direction

Mood: Amount of pleasant, happy, friendly behavior compared with unpleasant, unhappy, crying, unfriendly behavior exhibited by the child in various situations

Distractibility: Ease with which a child's attention or direction of behavior can be diverted by external stimuli

Attention span and persistence: Length of time a child pursues a given activity (**attention**) and the continuation of an activity despite obstacles (**persistence**)

Significance of Temperament

Observations indicate that children who display the difficult or slow-to-warm-up patterns of behavior are more vulnerable to the development of behavior problems in early and middle childhood. Any child can develop behavior problems if there is dissonance between the child's temperament and the environment. Demands for change and adaptation that are in conflict with the child's capacities can become excessively stressful. However, authorities emphasize that it is not the temperament patterns of children that place them at risk; rather, it is the **degree of fit** between children and their environment, specifically their parents, that determines the degree of vulnerability. The potential for optimum development exists when environmental expectations and demands fit with the individual's style of behavior and the parents' ability to navigate this period (Chess & Thomas, 1999) (see Chapter 10, Failure to Thrive).

DEVELOPMENT OF PERSONALITY AND COGNITIVE FUNCTION

Personality and cognitive skills develop in much the same manner as biologic growth—new accomplishments build on previously mastered skills. Many aspects depend on physical growth and maturation. This is not a comprehensive account of the multiple facets of personality and behavior development. Many aspects are integrated with the child's social and emotional development in later discussion of various age-groups. Table 3.2 summarizes some of the developmental theories.

THEORETICAL FOUNDATIONS OF PERSONALITY DEVELOPMENT

Psychosexual Development (Freud)

According to Freud (1933), all human behavior is energized by psychodynamic forces, and this psychic energy is divided among three components of personality: the id, ego, and superego. The **id**, the **unconscious mind**, is the inborn component that is driven by instincts.

TABLE 3.2 Summary of Personality, Cognitive, and Moral Development Theories

Psychosexual (Freud)	Psychosocial (Erikson)	Cognitive (Piaget)	Moral Judgment (Kohlberg)
Oral	Trust vs. mistrust	Sensorimotor (birth to 2 years old)	
Anal	Autonomy vs. shame and doubt	Preoperational thought, preconceptual phase (transductive reasoning [e.g., specific to specific]) (2-4 years old)	Preconventional (premoral) level Punishment and obedience orientation
Phallic	Initiative vs. guilt	Preoperational thought, intuitive phase (transductive reasoning) (4-7 years old)	Preconventional (premoral) level Naive instrumental orientation
Latency	Industry vs. inferiority	Concrete operations (inductive reasoning and beginning logic) (7-11 years old)	Conventional level Good-boy, nice-girl orientation Law-and-order orientation
Genital	Identity vs. role confusion	Formal operations (deductive and abstract reasoning) (11-15 years old)	Postconventional or principled level Social-contract orientation

The id obeys the pleasure principle of immediate gratification of needs, regardless of whether the object or action can actually do so. The **ego**, the **conscious mind**, serves the reality principle. It functions as the conscious or controlling self that is able to find realistic means for gratifying the instincts while blocking the irrational thinking of the id. The **superego**, the **conscience**, functions as the moral arbitrator and represents the ideal. It is the mechanism that prevents individuals from expressing undesirable instincts that might threaten the social order.

Freud (1964) considered the sexual instincts to be significant in the development of the personality. However, he used the term *psychosexual* to describe any sensual pleasure. During childhood, certain regions of the body assume a prominent psychologic significance as the source of new pleasures and new conflicts gradually shifts from one part of the body to another at particular stages of development:

Oral stage (birth to 1 year old): During infancy, the major source of pleasure seeking is centered on oral activities, such as sucking, biting, chewing, and vocalizing. Children may prefer one of these over the others, and the preferred method of oral gratification can provide some indication of the personality they develop.

Anal stage (1 to 3 years old): Interest during the second year of life centers in the anal region as sphincter muscles develop and children are able to withhold or expel fecal material at will. At this stage, the climate surrounding toilet training can have lasting effects on children's personalities.

Phallic stage (3 to 6 years old): During the phallic stage, the genitalia become an interesting and sensitive area of the body. Children recognize differences between the sexes and become curious about the dissimilarities. This is the period around which the controversial issues of the Oedipus and Electra complexes, penis envy, and castration anxiety are centered.

Latency period (6 to 12 years old): During the latency period, children elaborate on previously acquired traits and skills. Physical and psychic energy are channeled into acquisition of knowledge and vigorous play.

Genital stage (12 years old and older): The last significant stage begins at puberty with maturation of the reproductive system and production of sex hormones. The genital organs become the major source of sexual tensions and pleasures, but energies are also invested in forming friendships and preparing for marriage.

Psychosocial Development (Erikson)

The most widely accepted theory of personality development is that advanced by Erikson (1963). Although built on Freudian theory, it is known as **psychosocial** development and emphasizes a healthy personality as opposed to a pathologic approach. Erikson also uses the biologic concepts of critical periods and epigenesis, describing key conflicts or core problems that the individual strives to master during critical periods in personality development. Successful completion or mastery of each of these core conflicts is built on the satisfactory completion or mastery of the previous stage.

Each psychosocial stage has two components—the favorable and the unfavorable aspects of the core conflict—and progress to the next stage depends on resolution of this conflict. No core conflict is ever mastered completely but remains a recurrent problem throughout life. No life situation is ever secure. Each new situation presents the conflict in a new form. For example, when children who have satisfactorily achieved a sense of trust encounter a new experience (e.g., hospitalization), they must again develop a sense of trust in those responsible for their care in order to master the situation. Erikson's life span approach to personality development consists of eight stages; however, only the first five relating to childhood are included here:

Trust versus mistrust (birth to 1 year old): The first and most important attribute to develop for a healthy personality is basic **trust**. Establishment of basic trust dominates the first year of life and describes all of the child's satisfying experiences at this age. Corresponding to Freud's oral stage, it is a time of "getting" and "taking in" through all the senses. It exists only in relation to something or someone; therefore consistent, loving care by a mothering person is essential for development of trust. **Mistrust** develops when trust-promoting experiences are deficient or lacking, or when basic needs are inconsistently or inadequately met. Although shreds of mistrust are sprinkled throughout the personality, from a basic trust in parents stems trust in the world, other people, and oneself. The result is **faith** and **optimism**.

Autonomy versus shame and doubt (1 to 3 years old): Corresponding to Freud's anal stage, the problem of autonomy can be symbolized by the holding on and letting go of the sphincter muscles. The development of autonomy during the toddler period is centered on children's increasing ability to control their bodies, themselves, and their environment. They want to do things for themselves using their newly acquired motor skills of walking, climbing, and manipulating, and their mental powers of selecting and decision making. Much of their learning is acquired by imitating the activities and behavior of others. Negative feelings of doubt and shame arise when children are made to feel small and self-conscious, when their choices are disastrous, when others shame them, or when they are forced to be dependent in areas in which they are capable of assuming control. The favorable outcomes are self-control and willpower.

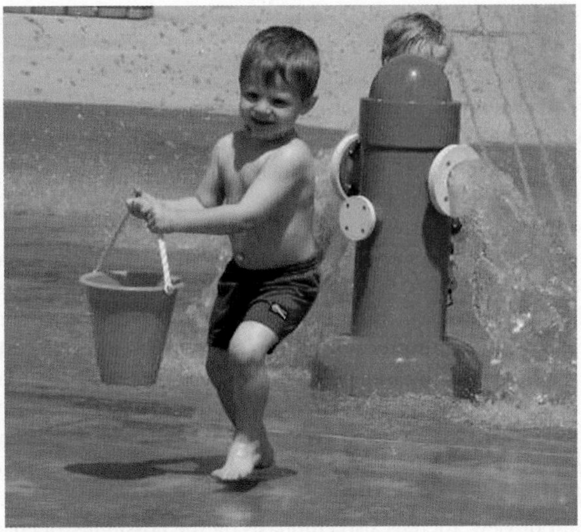

Fig. 3.4 The stage of initiative is characterized by physical activity and imagination while children explore the physical world around them.

Initiative versus guilt (3 to 6 years old): The stage of initiative corresponds to Freud's phallic stage and is characterized by vigorous, intrusive behavior; enterprise; and a strong imagination. Children explore the physical world with all their senses and powers (Fig. 3.4). They develop a conscience. No longer guided only by outsiders, they have an inner voice that warns and threatens. Children sometimes undertake goals or activities that are in conflict with those of parents or others, and being made to feel that their activities or imaginings are bad produces a sense of guilt. Children must learn to retain a sense of initiative without impinging on the rights and privileges of others. The lasting outcomes are direction and purpose.

Industry versus inferiority (6 to 12 years old): The stage of industry is the latency period of Freud. Having achieved the more crucial stages in personality development, children are ready to be workers and producers. They want to engage in tasks and activities that they can carry through to completion; they need and want real achievement. Children learn to compete and cooperate with others, and they learn the rules. It is a decisive period in their social relationships with others. Feelings of inadequacy and inferiority may develop if too much is expected of them or if they believe that they cannot measure up to the standards set for them by others. The ego quality developed from a sense of industry is competence.

Identity versus role confusion (12 to 18 years old): Corresponding to Freud's genital period, the development of identity is characterized by rapid and marked physical changes. Previous trust in their bodies is shaken, and children become overly preoccupied with the way they appear in the eyes of others compared with their own self-concept. Adolescents struggle to fit the roles they have played and those they hope to play with the current roles and fashions adopted by their peers, to integrate their concepts and values with those of society, and to come to a decision regarding an occupation. An inability to solve the core conflict results in role confusion. The outcome of successful mastery is devotion and fidelity to others and to values and ideologies.

THEORETICAL FOUNDATIONS OF COGNITIVE DEVELOPMENT

The term **cognition** refers to the process by which developing individuals become acquainted with the world and the objects it contains. Children are born with inherited potentials for intellectual growth, but they must develop that potential through interaction with the environment. By assimilating information through the senses, processing it, and acting on it, they come to understand relationships between objects and between themselves and their world. With cognitive development, children acquire the ability to reason abstractly, to think in a logical manner, and to organize intellectual functions or performances into higher order structures. Language, morals, and spiritual development emerge as cognitive abilities advance.

Cognitive Development (Piaget)

Jean Piaget (1969), a Swiss psychologist, developed a stage theory to better understand the way a child thinks. According to Piaget, intelligence enables individuals to make adaptations to the environment that increase the probability of survival, and through their behavior individuals establish and maintain equilibrium with the environment. Each stage of cognitive development is derived from and builds on the accomplishments of the previous stage in a continuous, orderly process. This course of development is both maturational and invariant and is divided into four stages (ages are approximate):

Sensorimotor (birth to 2 years old): The sensorimotor stage of intellectual development consists of six substages that are governed by sensations in which simple learning takes place (see Chapters 9 and 11). Children progress from reflex activity through simple repetitive behaviors to imitative behavior. They develop a sense of cause and effect as they direct behavior toward objects. Problem solving is primarily by trial and error. They display a high level of curiosity, experimentation, and enjoyment of novelty and begin to develop a sense of self as they are able to differentiate themselves from their environment. They become aware that objects have **permanence**—that an object exists even though it is no longer visible. Toward the end of the sensorimotor period, children begin to use language and representational thought.

Preoperational (2 to 7 years old): The predominant characteristic of the preoperational stage of intellectual development is **egocentrism**, which in this sense does not mean selfishness or self-centeredness but the inability to put oneself in the place of another. Children interpret objects and events not in terms of general properties but in terms of their relationships or their use to them. They are unable to see things from any perspective other than their own; they cannot see another's point of view, nor can they see any reason to do so (see Chapter 12, Cognitive Development). Preoperational thinking is concrete and tangible. Children cannot reason beyond the observable, and they lack the ability to make deductions or generalizations. Thought is dominated by what they see, hear, or otherwise experience. However, they are increasingly able to use language and symbols to represent objects in their environment. Through imaginative play, questioning, and other interactions, they begin to elaborate concepts and to make simple associations between ideas. In the latter stage of this period, their reasoning is **intuitive** (e.g., the stars have to go to bed just as they do), and they are only beginning to deal with problems of weight, length, size, and time. Reasoning is also **transductive**—because two events occur together, they cause each other, or knowledge of one characteristic is transferred to another (e.g., all women with big bellies have babies).

Concrete operations (7 to 11 years old): At this age, thought becomes increasingly logical and coherent. Children are able to classify, sort, order, and otherwise organize facts about the world to use in problem solving. They develop a new concept of permanence—**conservation** (see Chapter 14, Cognitive Development [Piaget]); that is, they realize that physical factors (such as volume, weight, and number) remain the same even though outward appearances are changed. They are able to deal with a number of different aspects of a situation simultaneously. They do not have the capacity to deal in abstraction; they solve problems in a concrete, systematic fashion based on what they can perceive. Reasoning is **inductive**. Through progressive changes in thought processes and relationships with others, thought becomes less self-centered. They can consider points of view other than their own. Thinking has become socialized.

Formal operations (11 to 15 years old): Formal operational thought is characterized by adaptability and flexibility. Adolescents can think in abstract terms, use abstract symbols, and draw logical conclusions from a set of observations. For example, they can solve the following question: If *A* is larger than *B* and *B* is larger than *C*, which symbol is the largest? (The answer is *A*.) They can make hypotheses and test them; they can consider abstract, theoretic, and philosophic matters. Although they may confuse the ideal with the practical, most contradictions in the world can be dealt with and resolved.

Language Development

Children are born with the mechanism and capacity to develop speech and language skills. However, they do not speak spontaneously. The environment must provide a means for them to acquire these skills. Speech requires intact physiologic structure and function (including respiratory, auditory, and cerebral) plus intelligence, a need to communicate, and stimulation.

The rate of speech development varies from child to child and is directly related to neurologic competence and cognitive development. Gesture precedes speech. As speech develops, gesture recedes but never disappears entirely. Research suggests that infants can learn sign language before vocal language and that it may enhance the development of vocal language (Thompson, Cotner-Bichelman, McKerchar, et al., 2007). At all stages of language development, children's comprehension vocabulary (what they understand) is greater than their expressed vocabulary (what they can say), and this development reflects a continuing process of modification that involves both the acquisition of new words and the expanding and refining of word meanings previously learned. By the time they begin to walk, children are able to attach names to objects and persons.

The first parts of speech used are nouns, sometimes verbs (e.g., "go"), and combination words (e.g., "bye-bye"). Responses are usually structurally incomplete during the toddler period, although the meaning is clear. Next, they begin to use adjectives and adverbs to qualify nouns followed by adverbs to qualify nouns and verbs. Later, pronouns and gender words are added (e.g., "he" and "she"). By the time children enter school, they are able to use simple, structurally complete sentences that average five to seven words.

Moral Development (Kohlberg)

Children also acquire moral reasoning in a developmental sequence. Moral development, as described by Kohlberg (1968), is based on cognitive developmental theory and consists of three major levels, each of which has two stages:

Preconventional level: The preconventional level of moral development parallels the preoperational level of cognitive development and intuitive thought. Culturally oriented to the labels of good/bad and right/wrong, children integrate these in terms of the physical or pleasurable consequences of their actions. At first, children determine the goodness or badness of an action in terms of its consequences. They avoid punishment and obey without question those who have the power to determine and enforce the rules and labels. They have no concept of the basic moral order that supports these consequences. Later, children determine that the right behavior consists of that which satisfies their own needs (and sometimes the needs of others). Although elements of fairness, give and take, and equal sharing are evident, they are interpreted in a practical, concrete manner without loyalty, gratitude, or justice.

Conventional level: At the conventional stage, children are concerned with conformity and loyalty. They value the maintenance of family, group, or national expectations regardless of consequences. Behavior that meets with approval and pleases or helps others is considered good. One earns approval by being "nice." Obeying the rules, doing one's duty, showing respect for authority, and maintaining the social order are the correct behaviors. This level is correlated with the stage of concrete operations in cognitive development.

Postconventional, autonomous, or **principled level:** At the postconventional level, the individual has reached the cognitive stage of formal operations. Correct behavior tends to be defined in terms of general individual rights and standards that have been examined and agreed on by the entire society. Although procedural rules for reaching consensus become important, with emphasis on the legal point of view, there is also emphasis on the possibility of changing law in terms of societal needs and rational considerations.

The most advanced level of moral development is one in which self-chosen ethical principles guide decisions of conscience. These are abstract and ethical but universal principles of justice and human rights with respect for the dignity of persons as individuals. It is believed that few persons reach this stage of moral reasoning.

DEVELOPMENT OF SELF-CONCEPT

Self-concept is how an individual describes him- or herself. The term **self-concept** includes all the notions, beliefs, and convictions that constitute an individual's self-knowledge and that influence that individual's relationships with others. It is not present at birth but develops gradually as a result of unique experiences within the self, significant others, and the realities of the world. However, an individual's self-concept may or may not reflect reality.

In infancy, the self-concept is primarily an awareness of one's independent existence learned in part as a result of social contacts and experiences with others. The process becomes more active during toddlerhood as children explore the limits of their capacities and the nature of their impact on others. School-age children are more aware of differences among people, are more sensitive to social pressures, and become more preoccupied with issues of self-criticism and self-evaluation. During early adolescence, children focus more on physical and emotional changes taking place and on peer acceptance. Self-concept is crystallized during later adolescence as young people organize their self-concept around a set of values, goals, and competencies acquired throughout childhood.

Body Image

A vital component of self-concept, **body image** refers to the subjective concepts and attitudes that individuals have toward their own bodies. It consists of the physiologic (the perception of one's physical characteristics), psychologic (values and attitudes toward the body, abilities, and ideals), and social nature of one's image of self (the self in relation to others). All three of the components interrelate with one another. Body image is a complex phenomenon that evolves and changes during the process of growth and development. Any actual or perceived deviation from the "norm" (no matter how this is interpreted) is cause for concern. The extent to which a characteristic, defect, or disease affects children's body image is influenced by the attitudes and behavior of those around them.

The significant others in their lives exert the most important and meaningful impact on children's body image. Labels that are attached to them (e.g., "skinny," "pretty," or "fat") or their body parts (e.g., "ugly mole," "bug eyes," or "yucky skin") are incorporated into the body image. Because they lack the understanding of deviations from the physical standard or norm, children notice prominent differences in others and unwittingly make rude or cruel remarks about such minor deviations as large or widely spaced front teeth, large or small eyes, moles, or extreme variations in height.

Infants receive input about their bodies through self-exploration and sensory stimulation from others. As they begin to manipulate their environment, they become aware of their bodies as separate from others. Toddlers learn to identify the various parts of their bodies and are able to use symbols to represent objects. Preschoolers become aware of the wholeness of their bodies and discover the genitalia. Exploration of the genitalia and the discovery of differences between the sexes become important.

School-age children begin to learn about internal body structure and function and become aware of differences in body size and configuration. They are highly influenced by the cultural norms of society and current fads. Children whose bodies deviate from the norm are often criticized or ridiculed. Adolescence is the age when children become most concerned about the physical self. The unfamiliar body changes and the new physical self must be integrated into the self-concept. Adolescents face conflicts over what they see and what they visualize as the ideal body structure. Body image formation during adolescence is a crucial element in the shaping of identity, the psychosocial crisis of adolescence.

Self-Esteem

Self-esteem is the value an individual places on oneself and refers to an overall evaluation of oneself (Willoughby, King, & Polatajko, 1996). Whereas self-esteem is described as the affective component of the self, self-concept is the cognitive component; however, the two terms are almost indistinguishable and are often used interchangeably.

The term self-esteem refers to a personal, subjective judgment of one's worthiness derived from and influenced by the social groups in the immediate environment and individuals' perceptions of how they are valued by others. Self-esteem changes with development. Highly egocentric toddlers are unaware of any difference between competence and social approval. On the other hand, preschoolers and early school-age children are increasingly aware of the discrepancy between their competencies and the abilities of more advanced children. Being accepted by adults and peers outside the family group becomes more important to them. Positive feedback enhances their self-esteem; they are vulnerable to feelings of worthlessness and are anxious about failure.

As children's competencies increase and they develop meaningful relationships, their self-esteem rises. Their self-esteem is again at risk during early adolescence when they are defining an identity and sense of self in the context of their peer group. Unless children are continually made to feel incompetent and of little worth, a decrease in self-esteem during vulnerable times is only temporary.

ROLE OF PLAY IN DEVELOPMENT

Through the universal medium of play, children learn what no one can teach them. They learn about their world and how to deal with this environment of objects, time, space, structure, and people. They learn about themselves operating within that environment—what they can do, how to relate to things and situations, and how to adapt themselves to the demands society makes on them. Play is the work of children. In play, children continually practice the complicated, stressful processes of living, communicating, and achieving satisfactory relationships with other people.

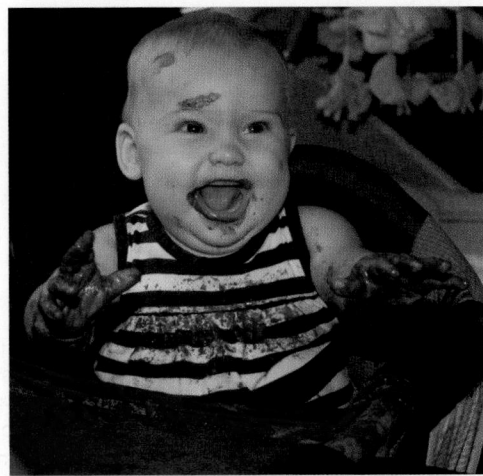

Fig. 3.5 Children derive pleasure from handling raw materials. (Paints in this picture are nontoxic.)

CLASSIFICATION OF PLAY

From a developmental point of view, patterns of children's play can be categorized according to content and social character. In both, there is an additive effect; each builds on past accomplishments, and some element of each is maintained throughout life. At each stage in development, the new predominates.

Content of Play

The content of play involves primarily the physical aspects of play, although social relationships cannot be ignored. The content of play follows the directional trend of the simple to the complex:

Social-affective play: Play begins with social-affective play, wherein infants take pleasure in relationships with people. As adults talk, touch, nuzzle, and in various ways elicit responses from an infant, the infant soon learns to provoke parental emotions and responses with such behaviors as smiling, cooing, or initiating games and activities. The type and intensity of the adult behavior with children vary among cultures.

Sense-pleasure play: Sense-pleasure play is a nonsocial stimulating experience that originates from without. Objects in the environment—light and color, tastes and odors, textures and consistencies—attract children's attention, stimulate their senses, and give pleasure. Pleasurable experiences are derived from handling raw materials (water, sand, food), body motion (swinging, bouncing, rocking), and other uses of senses and abilities (smelling, humming) (Fig. 3.5).

Skill play: After infants have developed the ability to grasp and manipulate, they persistently demonstrate and exercise their newly acquired abilities through skill play, repeating an action again and again. The element of sense-pleasure play is often evident in the practicing of a new ability, but all too frequently the determination to conquer the elusive skill produces pain and frustration (e.g., putting paper in and taking it out of a toy car) (Fig. 3.6).

Unoccupied behavior: In unoccupied behavior, children are not playful but focusing their attention momentarily on anything that strikes their interest. Children daydream, fiddle with clothes or other objects, or walk aimlessly. This role differs from that of onlookers, who actively observe the activity of others.

Dramatic, or pretend, play: One of the vital elements in children's process of identification is dramatic play, also known as *symbolic* or *pretend play*. It begins in late infancy (11 to 13 months) and is the predominant form of play among preschool children. After

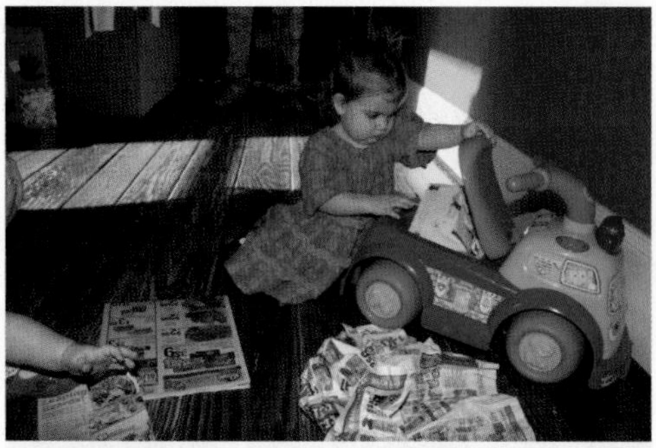

Fig. 3.6 After infants develop new skills to grasp and manipulate, they begin to conquer new abilities, such as putting paper in a toy car and taking it out.

children begin to invest situations and people with meanings and to attribute affective significance to the world, they can pretend and fantasize almost anything. By acting out events of daily life, children learn and practice the roles and identities modeled by the members of their family and society. Children's toys, replicas of the tools of society, provide a medium for learning about adult roles and activities that may be puzzling and frustrating to them. Interacting with the world is one way in which children get to know it. The simple, imitative, dramatic play of toddlers, such as using a telephone, driving a car, or rocking a doll, evolves into the more complex, sustained dramas of preschoolers, which extend beyond common domestic matters to the wider aspects of the world and the society, such as playing police officer, storekeeper, teacher, or nurse. Older children work out elaborate themes, act out stories, and compose plays.

Games: Children in all cultures engage in games alone and with others. Solitary activity involving games begins as very small children participate in repetitive activities and progress to more complicated games that challenge their independent skills, such as puzzles, solitaire, and computer or video games. Very young children participate in simple, **imitative games** such as pat-a-cake and peek-a-boo. Preschool children learn and enjoy **formal games**, beginning with ritualistic, self-sustaining games, such as ring-around-a-rosy and London Bridge. Except for some simple board games, preschool children do not engage in **competitive games**. Preschoolers hate to lose and try to cheat, want to change rules, or demand exceptions and opportunities to change their moves. School-age children and adolescents enjoy competitive games, including cards, checkers, and chess, and physically active games, such as baseball.

SOCIAL CHARACTER OF PLAY

The play interactions of infancy are between the child and an adult. Children continue to enjoy the company of adults but are increasingly able to play alone. As age advances, interaction with age-mates increases in importance and becomes an essential part of the socialization process. Through interaction, highly egocentric infants, unable to tolerate delay or interference, ultimately acquire concern for others and the ability to delay gratification or even to reject gratification at the expense of another. A pair of toddlers will engage in considerable combat because their personal needs cannot tolerate delay or compromise. By the time they reach 5 or 6 years old, children can arrive at compromises or make use of arbitration, usually after they have attempted but failed to gain their own way. Through continued interaction with peers and the growth of conceptual abilities and social skills, children can increase participation with others in the following types of play:

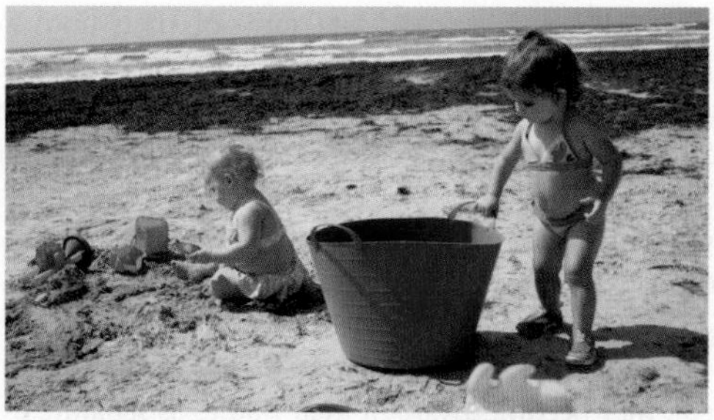

Fig. 3.7 Parallel play at the beach.

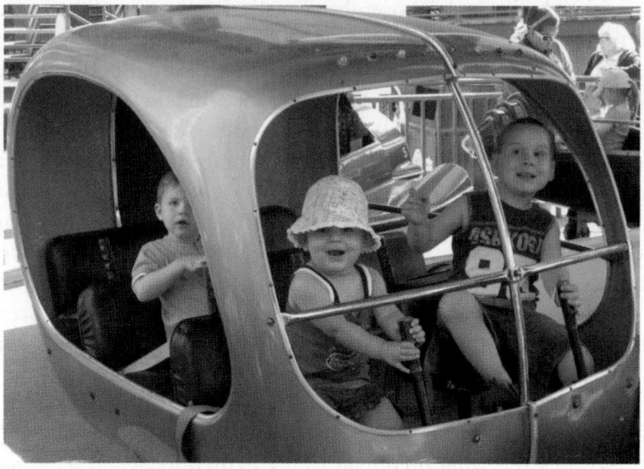

Fig. 3.8 Associative play.

Onlooker play: During onlooker play, children watch what other children are doing but make no attempt to enter the play activity. There is an active interest in observing the interaction of others but no movement toward participating. Watching an older sibling bounce a ball is a common example of the onlooker role.

Solitary play: During solitary play, children play alone with toys different from those used by other children in the same area. They enjoy the presence of other children but make no effort to get close to or speak to them. Their interest is centered on their own activity, which they pursue with no reference to the activities of the others.

Parallel play: During parallel activities, children play independently but among other children. They play with toys similar to those the children around them are using but as each child sees fit, neither influencing nor being influenced by the other children. Each child plays beside, but not with, other children (Fig. 3.7). There is no group association. Parallel play is the characteristic play of toddlers, but it may also occur in other groups of any age. Individuals who are involved in a creative craft with each person separately working on an individual project are engaged in parallel play.

Associative play: In associative play, children play together and are engaged in a similar or even identical activity, but there is no organization, division of labor, leadership assignment, or mutual goal. Children borrow and lend play materials, follow each other with wagons and tricycles, and sometimes attempt to control who may or may not play in the group. Each child acts according to his or her own wishes; there is no group goal (Fig. 3.8). For example, two children play with dolls, borrowing articles of clothing from each other and engaging in similar conversation, but neither directs the other's actions or establishes rules regarding the limits of the play session. There is a great deal of behavioral contagion: When one child initiates an activity, the entire group follows the example.

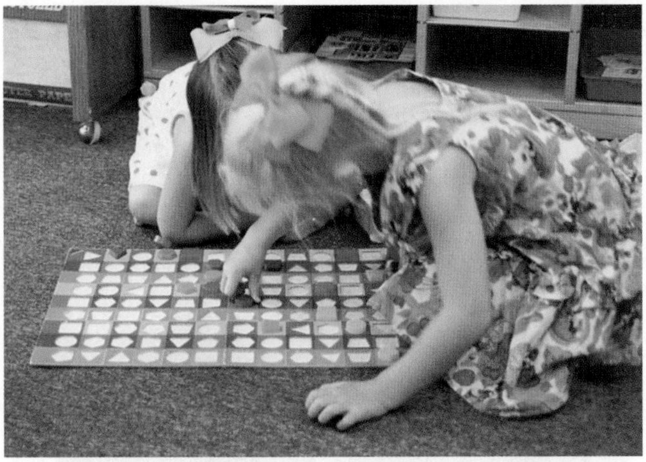

Fig. 3.9 Cooperative play.

Cooperative play: Cooperative play is organized, and children play in a group with other children (Fig. 3.9). They discuss and plan activities for the purposes of accomplishing an end—to make something, attain a competitive goal, dramatize situations of adult or group life, or play formal games. The group is loosely formed, but there is a marked sense of belonging or not belonging. The goal and its attainment require organization of activities, division of labor, and role playing. The leader-follower relationship is clearly established, and the activity is controlled by one or two members who assign roles and direct the activity of the others. The activity is organized to allow one child to supplement another's function to complete the goal.

FUNCTIONS OF PLAY

Sensorimotor Development

Sensorimotor activity is a major component of play at all ages and is the predominant form of play in infancy. Active play is essential for muscle development and serves a useful purpose as a release for surplus energy. Through sensorimotor play, children explore the nature of the physical world. Infants gain impressions of themselves and their world through tactile, auditory, visual, and kinesthetic stimulation. Toddlers and preschoolers revel in body movement and exploration of objects in space. With increasing maturity, sensorimotor play becomes more differentiated and involved. Whereas very young children run for the sheer joy of body movement, older children incorporate or modify the motions into increasingly complex and coordinated activities, such as races, games, roller skating, and bicycle riding.

Intellectual Development

Through exploration and manipulation, children learn colors, shapes, sizes, textures, and the significance of objects. They learn the significance of numbers and how to use them; they learn to associate words with objects; and they develop an understanding of abstract concepts and spatial relationships, such as *up, down, under,* and *over*. Activities such as puzzles and games help them develop problem-solving skills. Books, stories, films, and collections expand knowledge and provide enjoyment as well. Play provides a means to practice and expand language skills. Through play, children continually rehearse past experiences to assimilate them into new perceptions and relationships. Play helps children comprehend the world in which they live and distinguish between fantasy and reality.

Socialization

From very early infancy, children show interest and pleasure in the company of others. Their initial social contact is with the mothering person, but through play with other children they learn to establish social relationships and solve the problems associated with these relationships. They learn to give and take, which is more readily learned from critical peers than from more tolerant adults. They learn the sex role that society expects them to fulfill, as well as approved patterns of behavior and deportment. Closely associated with socialization is development of moral values and ethics. Children learn right from wrong, the standards of the society, and to assume responsibility for their actions.

Creativity

In no other situation is there more opportunity to be creative than in play. Children can experiment and try out their ideas in play through every medium at their disposal, including raw materials, fantasy, and exploration. Creativity is stifled by pressure toward conformity; therefore striving for peer approval may inhibit creative endeavors in school-age or adolescent children. Creativity is primarily a product of solitary activity, yet creative thinking is often enhanced in group settings where listening to others' ideas stimulates further exploration of one's own ideas. After children feel the satisfaction of creating something new and different, they transfer this creative interest to situations outside the world of play.

Self-Awareness

Beginning with active explorations of their bodies and awareness of themselves as separate from their mothers, the process of developing a self-identity is facilitated through play activities. Children learn who they are and their place in the world. They become increasingly able to regulate their own behavior, to learn what their abilities are, and to compare their abilities with those of others. Through play, children can test their abilities, assume and try out various roles, and learn the effects that their behavior has on others. They learn the sex role that society expects them to fulfill, as well as approved patterns of behavior and deportment.

Therapeutic Value

Play is therapeutic at any age (Fig. 3.10). In play, children can express emotions and release unacceptable impulses in a socially acceptable fashion. Children can experiment and test fearful situations and can assume and vicariously master the roles and positions that they are unable to perform in the world of reality. Children reveal much about themselves in play. Through play, children can communicate to the alert observer the needs, fears, and desires that they are unable to express with their limited language skills. Throughout their play, children need the acceptance of adults and their presence to help them control aggression and to channel their destructive tendencies.

Morality

Although children learn at home and at school those behaviors considered right and wrong in the culture, their interaction with peers during play contributes significantly to their moral training. Nowhere is the enforcement of moral standards as rigid as in the play situation. If they are to be acceptable members of the group, children must adhere to the accepted codes of behavior of the culture (e.g., fairness, honesty, self-control, consideration for others). Children soon learn that their peers are less tolerant of violations than are adults and that to maintain a place in the play group, they must conform to the standards of the group (Fig. 3.11).

TOYS

The types of toys chosen by or provided for children can support and enhance children's development in the areas just described. Although no scientific evidence shows that any toy is necessary for optimal

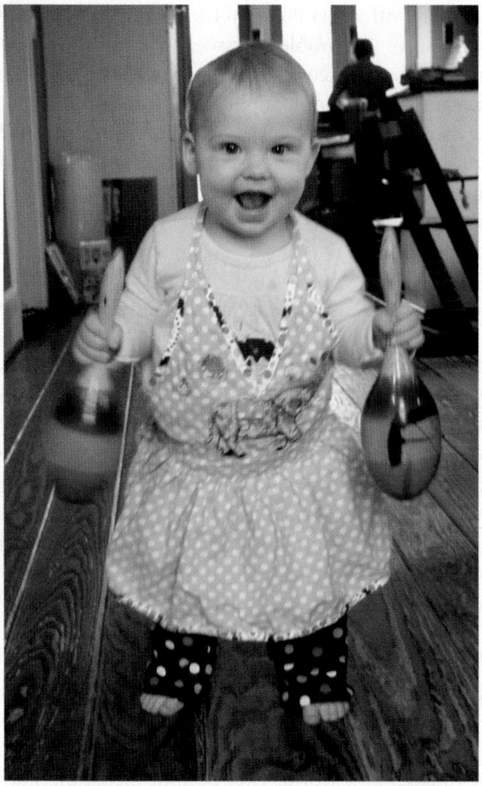

Fig. 3.10 Play is therapeutic at any age and provides a means for release of tension and stress.

learning, toys offer an opportunity to bring children and parents together. Research has indicated that a positive parent-child interaction can enhance early childhood brain development. Toys that are small replicas of the culture and its tools help children assimilate into their culture. Toys that require pushing, pulling, rolling, and manipulating teach them about physical properties of the items and help develop muscles and coordination. Rules and the basic elements of cooperation and organization are learned through board games.

Because they can be used in a variety of ways, raw materials with which children can exercise their own creativity and imaginations are sometimes superior to ready-made items. For example, building blocks can be used to construct a variety of structures, count, and learn shapes and sizes.

DEVELOPMENTAL ASSESSMENT

One of the most essential components of a complete health appraisal is assessment of developmental function. Screening procedures are designed to identify quickly and reliably children whose developmental level is below normal for their age and who therefore require further investigation. They also provide a means of recording objective measurements of present developmental function for future reference. Since the passage of Public Law 99-457, the Education of the Handicapped Act Amendments of 1986, much greater emphasis is placed on developmental assessment of children with disabilities, and nurses can play a vital role in providing this service. There are numerous developmental screening tools, and each uses a different approach.

In the past, the most widely used developmental screening tests for young children were the series of tests known as the Denver Developmental Screening Test (DDST) and its revision, the DDST-R, that have been revised, restandardized, and renamed the Denver II. The American Academy of Neurology and the Child Neurology Society state that research has found that the Denver II is insensitive and lacks specificity, and neither organization recommends use of the Denver II for primary care developmental screening (Filipek, Accardo, Ashwal, et al., 2000). The pediatric health promotion chapters include detailed information on developmental assessment that is unique to the age and each developmental stage of the child.

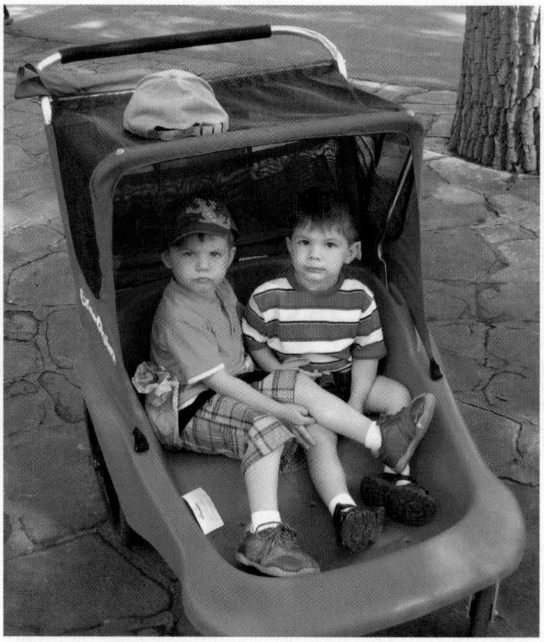

Fig. 3.11 Peers become increasingly important as children develop friendships outside the family group.

BOX 3.3 Ages & Stages Questionnaires[a]

- Type of screening: Developmental (ASQ-3) and social-emotional (ASQ:SE)
- Age range: 1 to 66 months old for ASQ-3, 3 to 66 months old for ASQ:SE
- Number of questionnaires: 21 for ASQ-3, 8 for ASQ:SE
- Number of items: About 30 per questionnaire
- Online components: Data management and questionnaire completion
- Reading level of items: fourth to sixth grade
- Who completes it: Parents
- Time to complete: 10 to 15 minutes
- Who scores it: Professionals
- Time to score: 2 to 3 minutes
- Languages: English and Spanish (for other languages, visit https://agesandstages.com)

[a] Information on the Ages & Stages Questionnaires (ASQ) can be found at https://agesandstages.com.

AGES AND STAGES

Ages and stages is a term used to broadly outline key periods in the human development timeline. During each stage, growth and development occur in the primary developmental domains, including physical, intellectual, language, and social-emotional. The Ages & Stages Questionnaires (ASQ)[a] are high-quality screening tools that include 19 age-specific surveys that ask parents about developmental skills common in daily life for children 1 month to 5½ years old (Box 3.3). Parents or other caregivers answer questions about their child's abilities (e.g.,

[a]The ASQ can be found at https://agesandstages.com.

"Does your child climb on an object such as a chair to reach something he wants?" "When your child wants something, does she tell you by pointing at it?"). Children whose development appears to fall significantly below the results of other children their age are flagged for further evaluation. The ASQ can be used as a universal screening tool in pediatric clinics to identify children at risk for social-emotional developmental delays (Briggs, Stettler, Silver, et al., 2012).

Throughout this book, each of the health promotion chapters includes detailed information on development unique to the age and stage of the child.

GENETIC FACTORS THAT INFLUENCE DEVELOPMENT

OVERVIEW OF GENETICS AND GENOMICS

Nurses and other health care providers are increasingly faced with incorporating genetic and genomic information into their practice. In response to this need, the Consensus Panel on Genetic/Genomic Nursing Competencies was established in 2006. This independent panel of nurse leaders from clinical, research, and academic settings established essential minimal competencies necessary for nurses to deliver competent genetic- and genomic-focused nursing care (Consensus Panel on Genetic/Genomic Nursing Competencies, 2009). In a similar manner, genetic and genomic competencies were created and published for nurses with graduate degrees (Greco, Tinley, & Seibert, 2012). This brief overview identifies key terms and concepts and highlights essential genetics and genomics competencies for all nurses.

Genes, Genetics, and Genomics

Genes are segments of deoxyribonucleic acid (DNA) that contain genetic information necessary to control a certain physiologic function or characteristic. These segments are often referred to as *sites* or *loci,* indicating a physical or "geographic" location on a chromosome. Variant forms of a gene commonly occur within a population. When referring to a particular form of a gene, the term *allele* is used. Variant forms of a gene (variant alleles) may lead to no measurable or observable differences, may cause the person to be susceptible to clinically recognizable pathology within specific environmental contexts, may cause a clinically recognized disease or disorder, or may prove advantageous within a particular environmental context.

In earlier times, human diseases were thought to be either clearly genetic or typically environmental. However, the observation that some genetic disorders are congenital (present at birth) but others are expressed later in life has led scientists to conclude that many, if not most, diseases are caused by a genetic predisposition that can be activated by an environmental trigger. Examples of such interactions are found in single-gene disorders, such as phenylketonuria (PKU) and sickle cell disease, and **multifactorial conditions**, such as cancer and neural tube defects (NTDs). PKU is a disorder resulting from the (genetically determined) absence of an enzyme that metabolizes the amino acid phenylalanine. However, the deleterious effects in the infant are expressed only after sufficient ingestion of phenylalanine-containing substances, such as milk (environmental trigger). Even in the case of a "classic" genetic condition, such as sickle cell disease, its acute symptoms are precipitated by certain conditions, such as lowered oxygen tension, infection, or dehydration.

Congenital Anomalies

Embryogenesis and fetal development are an intricate and precisely timed series of events in which all parts must be properly integrated to ensure a coordinated whole. Insults during development or abnormalities in differentiation or in the proper timing of organogenesis may result in a variety of congenital anomalies. **Congenital anomalies**, or birth defects, occur in 2% to 4% of all live-born children and are often classified as deformations, disruptions, dysplasias, or malformations. **Deformations** are often caused by extrinsic mechanical forces on normally developing tissue. Club foot is an example of a deformation often caused by uterine constraint. **Disruptions** result from the breakdown of previously normal tissue. Congenital amputations caused by amniotic bands (fibrous strands of amnion that wrap around different body parts during development) are examples of disruption anomalies. **Dysplasias** result from abnormal organization of cells into a particular tissue type. Congenital abnormalities of the teeth, hair, nails, or sweat glands may be manifestations of one of the more than 100 different ectodermal dysplasia syndromes (National Foundation for Ectodermal Dysplasias, 2015). **Malformations** are abnormal formations of organs or body parts resulting from an abnormal developmental process. Most malformations occur before 12 weeks of gestation. Cleft lip, an example of a malformation, occurs at approximately 5 weeks of gestation when the developing embryo naturally has two clefts in the area. Normally, between 5 and 7 weeks of gestation, cells rapidly divide and migrate to fill in those clefts. If there is an abnormality in this developmental process, the embryo is left with either a unilateral or a bilateral cleft lip that may also involve the palate.

The types of anomalies that can result from genetic or prenatal environmental causes can be major structural abnormalities with serious medical, surgical, or quality-of-life consequences, or they can be minor anomalies or normal variants with no serious consequences, such as a sacral dimple, an extra nipple, or a café-au-lait spot. Congenital anomalies can occur in isolation, such as congenital heart defect, or multiple anomalies may be present. A recognized pattern of anomalies resulting from a single specific cause is called a **syndrome** (e.g., Down syndrome, fetal alcohol syndrome). A nonrandom pattern of malformations for which a cause has not been determined is called an **association** (e.g., VACTERL [vertebral defects, anal atresia, cardiac defect, tracheoesophageal fistula, and renal and limb defects] association). When a single anomaly leads to a cascade of additional anomalies, the pattern of defects is referred to as a **sequence**. Pierre Robin sequence begins with the abnormal development of the mandible, resulting in abnormal placement of the tongue during development. The normal developmental process for the palate is prevented because the tongue obstructs the migration of the palatal shelves toward the midline, and a cleft palate remains. Consequently, infants born with Pierre Robin sequence have a recessed mandible and an abnormally placed tongue and are at risk for obstructive apnea. NTDs, cleft lip and palate, deafness, congenital heart defects, and cognitive impairment are examples of congenital malformations that can occur in isolation or as part of a syndrome, association, or sequence, and can have different causes, such as single-gene or chromosome abnormalities, prenatal exposures, or multifactorial causes.

Disorders of the Intrauterine Environment

The intrauterine environment can have a profound and permanent effect on developing fetuses with or without chromosome or single-gene abnormalities. Intrauterine growth restriction, for example, can occur with many genetic syndromes, such as Down, Russell-Silver, Prader-Willi, and Turner syndromes (Rimoin, Pyeritz, & Korf, 2013), or it can be caused by nongenetic factors, such as maternal alcohol ingestion. Placental abnormalities are increasingly being found to be the etiologic factor in neurodevelopmental disorders (e.g., cerebral palsy and cognitive impairment) that were previously attributed to asphyxia during delivery (McIntyre, Taitz, Keogh, et al., 2013).

Teratogens, agents that cause birth defects when present in the prenatal environment, account for most adverse intrauterine effects not attributable to genetic factors. Types of teratogens include drugs (phenytoin [Dilantin], warfarin [Coumadin], isotretinoin [Accutane]), chemicals (ethyl alcohol, cocaine, lead), infectious agents (rubella, cytomegalovirus), physical agents (maternal ionizing radiation, hyperthermia), and metabolic agents (maternal PKU). Many of these teratogenic exposures and the resulting effects are completely preventable. For example, pregnant women can avoid having a child with one of the fetal alcohol spectrum disorders by not ingesting alcohol during pregnancy.

Genetic Disorders

Genetic disorders can be caused by chromosome abnormalities as seen in Turner syndrome, Down syndrome, or velocardiofacial syndrome (VCFS); single-gene mutations as seen in sickle cell anemia, neurofibromatosis, or Duchenne muscular dystrophy; a combination of genetic and environmental factors as seen in NTDs or maturity-onset diabetes in the young; and mitochondrial deoxyribonucleic acid (mtDNA) mutations as seen in nonsyndromic deafness susceptibility caused by aminoglycoside sensitivity.

Both numeric and large structural abnormalities of **autosomes** (all chromosomes except the X and Y chromosomes) account for a variety of syndromes usually characterized by cognitive deficiencies. Nurses often note dysmorphic facial features, behavioral characteristics such as an unusual cry and poor feeding behavior, and other neurologic manifestations such as hypotonia or abnormal reflex responses, which may alert them to these and other chromosome abnormalities.

Somatic cells contain 44 autosomes (the 22 pairs of chromosomes that do not greatly influence sex determination at conception) and two sex chromosomes, XX in females and XY in males. In the past, the first-line chromosome test was karyotyping. A karyotype is a laboratory-made arrangement of specially prepared chromosomes that are displayed according to their size, centromere position, and band pattern. Karyotypes can detect too many or too few of one or more chromosomes. Down syndrome is an example of a condition caused by having an extra autosome, chromosome 21. Turner syndrome is the only example of a condition compatible with life that is caused by the absence of a chromosome. Children with Turner syndrome have one X chromosome. Chromosomes are subject to structural alterations resulting from breakage and rearrangement. Some structural chromosome abnormalities are too small to reliably detect with a karyotype but are still clinically relevant. The specific small deletion in chromosome 22 that causes VCFS is often not detectable with karyotype but is reliably detected with a test called chromosome microarray (CMA). Because CMA can detect extra or missing copies of an entire chromosome, large segments of chromosomes, and submicroscopic segments of chromosomes, it has replaced the karyotype as the first-line test for children with developmental delay, intellectual disability, and autism spectrum disorder (Martin & Ledbetter, 2017).

Chromosome anomalies typically affect large numbers of genes; however, a **single-gene disorder** is caused by an abnormality within a gene or in a gene's regulatory region. Single-gene disorders can affect all body systems and may have mild to severe expressions. Single-gene disorders display a Mendelian pattern of dominant or recessive inheritance that was first delineated in the mid-19th century by Gregor Mendel's experiments with plants.

Mendelian inheritance laws allow for risk prediction in single-gene disorders; however, phenotypic expression may be altered by incomplete penetrance or variable expressivity. A phenotype is said to have **reduced** or **incomplete penetrance** in a population when a proportion of persons who possess an allele or pair of alleles associated with the phenotype do not have any signs or symptoms of the phenotype. A phenotype exhibits **variable expressivity** when different individuals possessing the same genotype have different features of the phenotype, the severity of features differs between affected individuals, the onset of features varies, or any combination of these three factors exists. If a person expresses even the mildest possible phenotype, the phenotype associated with the allele or pair of alleles is penetrant in that individual.

BOX 3.4 Pediatric Indications for Genetic Consultation

Family History
- Family history of hereditary diseases, birth defects, or developmental problems
- Family history of sudden cardiac death or early-onset cancer
- Family history of mental illness

Medical History
- Abnormal newborn screen
- Abnormal genetic test result ordered by a nongenetics professional who lacks the knowledge and experience to discuss the implications of results
- Excessive bleeding or excessive clotting
- Progressive neurologic condition
- Recurrent infection or immunodeficiency

Developmental History
- Behavioral disorders
- Cognitive impairment or autism
- Development and speech delays or loss of developmental milestones

Physical Assessment
- Major congenital anomaly
- Minor anomalies and dysmorphic features
- Growth abnormalities
- Skeletal abnormalities
- Visual or hearing problems
- Metabolic disorder (unusual odor of breath, urine, or stool)
- Sexual development abnormalities or delayed puberty
- Skin disorders or abnormalities

Parental Requests
- Parent requests that child be evaluated by a genetics professional

Adapted from Pletcher, B. A., Toriello, H. V., Noblin, S. J., et al. (2007). Indications for genetic referral: a guide for healthcare providers. *Genetics in Medicine, 9*(6), 385–389.

Role of Nurses in Genetics

All nurses need to be prepared to use genetic and genomic information and technology when providing care. The professional practice domains of the essential genetic and genomic competencies include applying and integrating genetic knowledge into nursing assessment; identifying and referring clients who may benefit from genetic information or services; identifying genetics resources and services to meet clients' needs; and providing care and support before, during, and after providing genetic information and services (Consensus Panel on Genetic/Genomic Nursing Competencies, 2009). Often a nurse is the first one to recognize the need for genetic evaluation by identifying an inherited disorder in a family history or by noting physical, cognitive, or behavioral abnormalities when performing a nursing assessment (Box 3.4).

Nursing Assessment: Applying and Integrating Genetic and Genomic Knowledge

Family health history is an important tool to identify individuals and families at increased risk for disease, risk factors for disease (e.g., obesity), and inheritance patterns of diseases. Because of its importance, all nurses need to be able to elicit family history information and, when feasible, document the collected information in pedigree format.

When eliciting a family health history, nurses should collect information about all family members within a minimum of three generations. This process usually takes 20 to 30 minutes. When possible, it is best to include both parents in the interview to elicit information about relatives on both sides of the family. Medical records, birth and death records, family Bibles, and photograph albums are helpful resources, and persons being interviewed should be instructed to bring such items if they are available. It may be necessary to consult other members of the family. The level of education and the degree of understanding vary widely among informants and influence their reliability. The informants may be reticent, particularly if they view the disorder as something to be ashamed of or in some way threatening. Sometimes true relationships may be concealed, such as adoption or misattributed paternity.

In addition to family history, nurses caring for children and families need to collect pregnancy, labor and delivery, perinatal, medical, and developmental histories. Although it is common for genetics nurses to obtain all of these histories before or during an initial genetics consultation, not all nurses are expected to obtain all of these assessment data from each patient during a pediatric encounter. Electronic health records are making it more practical to construct a comprehensive set of histories even when many health care professionals contribute only a portion of the total history.

All nurses are taught to perform physical assessments, but they are seldom taught to recognize minor anomalies and dysmorphology that may suggest a genetic disorder. Yet nurses are keen in recognizing delays in development, behavior differences, and global appearances that raise concern that a newborn, infant, child, or adolescent needs further evaluation (Prows, Hopkin, Barnoy, et al., 2013). Although dysmorphology is beyond the scope of this chapter, readers are encouraged to review the January 2009 issue of *American Journal of Medical Genetics* (Carey, Cohen, Curry, et al., 2009). Drawings and photographs of normal and abnormal morphologic characteristics are provided for the head, face, and extremities together with accepted dysmorphology terminology. Nurses knowledgeable in dysmorphology can articulate specific concerns about a child's appearance rather than relying on the outdated and offensive phrase "funny-looking kid." When a major anomaly is identified, nurses should raise suspicion that the child could have additional congenital anomalies. When three or more minor anomalies are identified, nurses should suspect the possibility of an underlying syndrome. However, it is important to consider the biologic parents' physical appearance, development, and behavior when considering the relevance of the child's combination of minor anomalies.

Identification and Referral

It is nurses' responsibility to learn basic genetic principles, to be alert to situations in which families could benefit from genetic evaluation and counseling, to know about special services that can help manage and support affected children, and to be familiar with facilities in their areas where these services are available. In this way, nurses can direct individuals and families to needed services and be active participants in the genetic evaluation and counseling process. A regularly updated resource for locating genetics professionals can be found at https://ghr.nlm.nih.gov/primer/consult/findingprofessional. In addition, state health departments either offer services or can help identify health professionals with specialty training in genetics.

Early identification of a genetic disorder allows anticipation of associated conditions and implementation of available preventive measures and therapy to avoid potential complications and to enhance the child's health. It may also prevent the unexpected birth of another affected child in the immediate or extended family. Nurses have an important role in identifying patients and families who have or are at risk for developing or transmitting a genetic condition (see Box 3.4). When facilitating genetics consultations, nurses should share with the genetics professional the findings in the histories they collected that triggered the consultation. Nurses can also help the referral process by determining and communicating the family's initial concerns, their state of knowledge about the reason for referral, and their attitudes and beliefs concerning genetics.

Genetic evaluation for diagnostic purposes may occur at any point in the life span. In the newborn period, birth defects and abnormal newborn screen results are obvious reasons for referral. Beyond the newborn period, indicators for referral include metabolic disorders, developmental delays, growth delays, behavioral problems, cognitive delays, abnormal or delayed sexual development, and medical problems known to be associated with genetic diseases. For example, a preschooler with hyperactivity and autistic-like behaviors may need evaluation for fragile X syndrome, and a 17-year-old girl with primary amenorrhea and short stature should be evaluated for Turner syndrome.

With so many recent advances in genetic testing, it is not unusual for a child or adult with long-standing medical problems, including cognitive impairment, to be referred for reevaluation of his or her condition. Expanding testing options are leading to diagnoses that were not possible in the past (Splinter, Adams, Bacino, et al., 2018). After a genetic diagnosis is made, the patient may be referred to relevant specialists, is typically followed by genetics every 6 months to 1 year, and may be referred back to the primary care physician with recommendations for routine management based on the natural history (if known) of the diagnosed genetic disorder.

Providing Education, Care, and Support

Maintaining contact with the family or making a referral to a health care practice or an agency that can provide a sustained relationship is critical. It is becoming more common for genetics health care professionals to provide regular follow-up and management, particularly for children with rare genetic disorders. However, some families choose not to have follow-up visits with genetic experts.

Regardless of whether families choose to receive continued care with a genetics center, clinic, or professional, nurses can help patients and families process and clarify the information they receive during a genetics visit. Misunderstanding of this information can have many causes, including cultural differences, the disparity of knowledge between the counselor and the family, and the heightened emotion surrounding genetic counseling. Family members have difficulty absorbing all of the information presented during a genetics evaluation and counseling session. Knowing this, genetics professionals write and send clinic summary letters to families. The nurse may need to help the family understand terminology in the letter, help them identify and articulate remaining questions or areas of clarification, and coach them through the process of accessing genetics health professionals to get remaining questions and concerns answered. Information often needs to be repeated several times before the family understands the content and its implications.

Nurses must assess for and address parents' feelings of guilt about carrying "bad genes" or having "made my child sick." Families often try to reason that some unrelated event caused the abnormality (e.g., a fall, a urinary tract infection, or "one glass of wine") before the mother was aware that she was pregnant. These misconceptions need to be assessed and dispelled. Depending on the type of cytogenetic disorder, the nurse may be able to absolve the parents of guilt by explaining the random nature of segregation during both gamete formation and fertilization. If the condition is a Mendelian-inherited or mitochondrial disorder, it is important to assess parents' understanding of recurrence risk, help them understand the chances that a subsequent pregnancy will be affected or will not be affected, and ensure they have been given comprehensive and balanced information about available options for future children (such as adoption, use of donor egg or sperm, or prenatal diagnosis to prepare for birth of affected child or to terminate pregnancy).

After a genetics visit, and sometimes before the visit, parents often use the Internet to find answers to their questions. During the initial genetics evaluation, a diagnosis may not be possible. Instead, findings in medical, developmental, and family histories lead the professional to order genetic tests and other diagnostic procedures. Diagnoses under consideration are discussed briefly with the parents. Some parents are satisfied with the brief information and do not care to find out more until the actual diagnosis is established. Other parents go home and seek as much information as they can about the diagnoses under consideration. The information they find can be terrifying and overwhelming and inaccurate or misleading. Nurses can play an important role in helping parents identify reliable, accurate resources for information at whatever time they desire it. It is also important to stress that everything that is described for a genetic condition may not be relevant to their child. Before the follow-up genetics visit when test and procedure results are discussed, nurses can help parents identify and write down the questions and concerns they need addressed before leaving the clinic.

After a genetic diagnosis is made or a genetic predisposition to a delayed-onset disorder is identified, nurses need to have frequent contact with patients and families as they attempt to incorporate recommended therapies or disease prevention strategies into their daily lives. For example, a disorder such as PKU requires conscientious diet management; therefore it is important to make certain that the family understands and follows instructions and is able to navigate the health care system to access the essential formula and low-phenylalanine food products. An infant evaluated for cleft palate and cardiac defect and subsequently found to have VCFS requires surgical intervention for the congenital malformations. Such an infant also benefits from early intervention services and eventually from an individualized education plan in school because developmental delays and eventual learning problems are common.

Initial and ongoing assessment of the family's coping abilities, resources, and support systems is vital to determine their need for additional assistance and support. As with any family who has a child with chronic health care needs, nurses must teach the family to become the child's advocate. Nurses can help families locate agencies and clinics specializing in a specific disorder or its consequences that can provide services (e.g., equipment, medication, and rehabilitation), educational programs, and parent support groups. Referral to local and national support groups or contact with a local family that has a child with the same condition can be helpful for new parents. Privacy and confidentiality are imperative, and both families must give permission before their contact information is given. Nurses can also be instrumental in helping parents start a support group when none is available.

Parental attachment and adjustment to the baby can be supported and facilitated by nursing interventions. Assessing the parents' understanding of the child's disorder and providing simple and truthful explanations can help them begin to understand their child's health issues. Guiding the parents in recognizing their child's cues, responses, and strengths can be helpful even for experienced parents. A caring attitude conveys the value of their child and, by extension, their value as parents. The nurse can help the parents identify their strengths as a family and identify support that is available to them.

Giving birth to and raising a child with a genetic disorder is not necessarily a lifetime burden. It is important for nurses to ask parents to describe their experience raising their child with a genetic condition. What has been the impact on their family? Although parents may initially experience negative outcomes, such as shock, emotional distress, and grief, families can adapt and thrive. Resources for managing stress and restoring balance in the lives of families affected by a genetic condition can help. Van Riper's (2007) research has identified nursing interventions that can promote resilience and adaptation in families of children with Down syndrome. Van Riper's recommendations are useful for families of children with any type of genetic disorder:

- Recognize multiple stressors, strains, and transitions in their lives (e.g., unmet family needs).
- Discuss and implement strategies for reducing family demands (e.g., setting priorities and reducing the number of outside activities family members are involved in).
- Identify and use individual, family, and community resources (e.g., humor, family flexibility, supportive extended family, respite care, local support groups, and Internet resources).
- Expand the range and efficacy of their coping strategies (e.g., increase the use of active strategies such as reframing, mobilize their ability to acquire and accept help, and decrease the use of passive appraisal).
- Encourage the use of an affirming style of family problem-solving communication (e.g., one that conveys support and caring and exerts a calming influence).

Some families do struggle after learning that their child has a genetic disorder. Families may feel ashamed of a hereditary disorder and seek to blame their partner for transmitting a faulty gene or chromosome. Intrafamilial strife, hostility, and marital or couple disharmony, sometimes to the point of family disintegration, can occur. Nurses should be alert for evidence of risk factors that indicate poor adjustment (e.g., child abuse, divorce, or other maladaptive behaviors). Referral to psychosocial professionals for crisis intervention may be necessary.

CLINICAL JUDGMENT AND NEXT-GENERATION NCLEX® EXAMINATION-STYLE QUESTIONS

1. A mother brings her 2 ½-year-old daughter to the well-child clinic and expresses concern that the child's behavior is worrisome and possibly requires therapy or medication. The mother explains that the child constantly responds to the mother's simple requests with a "no" answer, even though the activity has been a favorite in the recent past. Furthermore, the child has had an increase in the number of temper tantrums at bedtime and refuses to go to bed. The mother is afraid her daughter will hurt herself during a temper tantrum because she holds her breath until the mother picks her up and gives in to her request. What responses are most appropriate for the nurse to have based on the mother's concerns. **Select all the apply.**
   - **A.** The child probably would benefit from some counseling with a trained therapist.
   - **B.** The mother and father should evaluate their childrearing practices.
   - **C.** The child's behavior is normal for a toddler and may represent frustration with control of her emotions; further exploration of events surrounding temper tantrums and possible interventions should be explored.
   - **D.** The child's behavior is typical of toddlers, and the parents should do nothing and simply wait for the child to finish this phase because it will end soon.
   - **E.** This is a stage of autonomy versus shame and doubt and can easily result in a young child's frustration and acting out.

2. The nurse is caring for a 9-year-old boy who is hospitalized for sickle cell pain. He is refusing to cooperate and will not talk. The nurse should consider the following regarding the child's stage of development when providing care and communicating with the boy. **Select all that apply.**
   - **A.** Trust versus mistrust is important at this stage.
   - **B.** Concrete operational thought processes are used at this stage.
   - **C.** Engaging in tasks and activities is important at this stage.
   - **D.** Feelings of inadequacy and inferiority can develop at this stage.
   - **E.** Doubt and shame can easily develop at this stage.

3. The nurse is caring for a 2-month-old female infant that parents are concerned may have a genetic disorder. There is a family history of birth defects and the family thinks the infant "looks funny". What are important aspects of the nursing history and assessment listed below that should be integrated into the history and examination of this infant? **Use an X for the nursing assessments listed below that are Indicated (appropriate or necessary), Contraindicated (could be harmful), or Non-Essential (makes no difference or not necessary).**

History and Assessment	Indicated	Contraindicated	Non-Essential
Family history should include information going back at least three generations.			
Family history should include environmental assessment including neighbors and friends.			
Assessment should focus only on the infant's ability to move the arms and legs.			
Assessment should evaluate for Turner Syndrome since girls have a prepubertal growth spurt and then mostly stop growing.			
Awareness of parents' feelings of guilt about causing the disorder is important for the nurse to consider.			

4. When parents consider genetic testing, especially after having a child born with an anomaly, which information is helpful for the nurse to understand when performing a genetic assessment? **Choose the most likely options for the information missing from the statements below by selecting from the lists of options provided.**

   ____1____ is an important tool to identify individuals at increased risk for disease, ____2____ for disease and ____3____ of diseases.

Options for 1	Options for 2	Options for 3
Chromosome analysis	risk factors	etiology
Family health history	medical records	inheritance patterns
Ultrasound	severity	rate of occurrence
Metabolic screening	birth defects	
Anorexia	platelets	
Fever	weight	

REFERENCES

Ball, J. W., Dains, J. E., Flynn, J. A., et al. (2019). *Seidel's guide to physical examination-e book, an interprofessional approach* (9th ed.). St. Louis: Elsevier.

Briggs, R. D., Stettler, E. M., Silver, E. J., et al. (2012). Social-emotional screening for infants and toddlers in primary care. *Pediatrics, 129*(2), e377–e384.

Caine, D., DiFiori, J., & Maffulli, N. (2006). Physeal injuries in children's and youth sports: Reasons for concern? *British Journal of Sports Medicine, 40*(9), 749–760.

Carey, J. C., Cohen, M. M., Curry, C. J., et al. (2009). Elements of morphology: Standard terminology for the lips, mouth, and oral region. *American Journal of Medical Genetics. Part A, 149A*(1), 77–92.

Chess, S., & Thomas, A. (1999). *Goodness of fit: Clinical applications from infancy through adult life*. London: Routledge.

Consensus Panel on Genetic/Genomic Nursing Competencies. (2009). *Essentials of genetic and genomic nursing: Competencies, curricula guidelines, and outcome indicators* (2nd ed.). Silver Spring, MD: American Nurses Association.

Erikson, E. H. (1963). *Childhood and society* (2nd ed.). New York: Norton.

Filipek, P. A., Accardo, P. J., Ashwal, S., et al. (2000). Practice parameter: Screening and diagnosis of autism: Report of the quality standards subcommittee of the american academy of neurology and the child neurology society. *Neurology, 55*(4), 468–479.

Freud, S. (1933). *New introductory lectures in psychoanalysis*. New York: Norton.

Freud, S. (1964). An outline of psychoanalysis. In J. Strachey, & translator (Eds.), *The standard edition of the complete psychological works of Sigmund Freud* (Vol. 23). London: Hogarth Press.

Greco, K. E., Tinley, S., & Seibert, D. (2012). *Essential genetic and genomic competencies for nurses with graduate degrees*. Silver Spring, MD: American Nurses Association and International Society of Nurses in Genetics.

Jackson, J. A., Patterson, D. G., & Harris, R. E. (1930). *The measurement of man*. Minneapolis: University of Minnesota Press.

Kohlberg, L. (1968). Moral development. In D. L. Sills (Ed.), *International encyclopedia of the social sciences*. New York: Macmillan.

Lampl, M., Johnson, M. L., & Frongillo, E. A. (2001). Mixed distribution analysis identifies saltation and stasis growth. *Annals of human biology, 28*(4), 403–411.

Lampl, M., Thompson, A., & Frongillo, E. A. (2005). Sex differences in the relationships among weight gain, subcutaneous skinfold tissue and salutatory length growth spurts in infancy. *Pediatric Research, 58*(6), 1238–1242.

Martin, C. L., & Ledbetter, D. H. (2017). Chromosomal microarray testing for children with unexplained neurodevelopmental disorders. *JAMA, 317*(24), 2545–2546.

Mcintyre, S., Taitz, D., Keogh, J., et al. (2013). A systematic review of risk factors for cerebral palsy in children born at term in developed countries. *Developmental Medicine and Child Neurology, 55*(6), 499–508.

National Foundation for Ectodermal Dysplasias. (2015). *About ectodermal dysplasias*. http://nfed.org/index.php/about_ed/about-ectodermal-dysplasias.

National Sleep Foundation. (2019). How your babie's sleep differs from your own. http:// sleepfoundation.org.

Piaget, J. (1969). *The theory of stages in cognitive development*. New York: McGraw-Hill.

Prows, C. A., Hopkin, R. J., Barnoy, S., et al. (2013). An update of childhood genetic disorders. *The Journal of Nursing Scholarship, 45*(1), 34–42.

Rimoin, D. L., Pyeritz, R. E., & Korf, B. (Eds.). (2013). *Principles and practice of medical genetics* (6th ed.) New York: Elsevier Science.

Splinter, K., Adams, D. R., Bacino, C. A., et al. (2018). Effect of genetic diagnosis on patients with previously undiagnosed disease. *New England Journal of Medicine, 379*(22), 2131–2139. https://doi.org/10.1056/NEJMoa1714458.

Thompson, R., Cotner-Bichelman, N., McKerchar, P., et al. (2007). Enhancing early communication through infant sign training. *Journal of Applied Behavior Analysis, 40*(1), 15–23.

Van Riper, M. (2007). Families of children with Down syndrome: Responding to "a change in plans" with resilience. *Journal of Pediatric Nursing, 22*(2), 116–128.

Willoughby, C., King, G., & Polatajko, H. (1996). A therapist's guide to children's self-esteem. *The American Journal of Occupational Therapy, 50*(2), 124–132.

Zemel, B. S., Pipan, M., Stallings, V. A., Hall, W., Schadt, K., Freedman, D. S., & Thorpe, P. (2015). Growth charts for children with Down syndrome in the United States. *Pediatrics, 136*(5), e1204–1211.

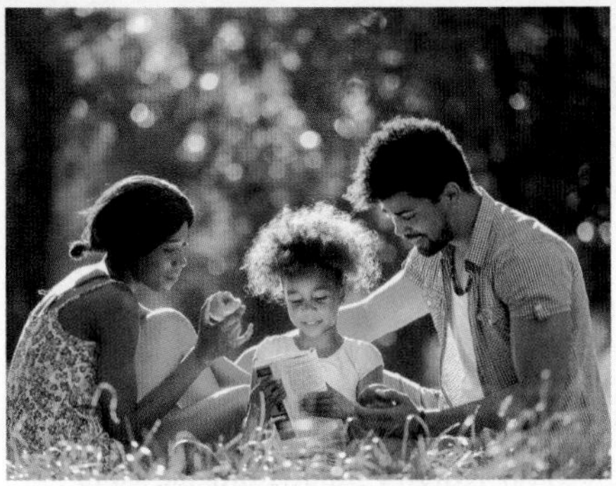

4

Communication and Physical Assessment of the Child and Family

Jan M. Foote

http://evolve.elsevier.com/wong/essentials

CONCEPTS

- Communication
- Assessment

GUIDELINES FOR COMMUNICATION AND INTERVIEWING

The most widely used method of communicating with parents on a professional basis is the interview process. Unlike social conversation, **interviewing** is a specific form of goal-directed communication. As nurses converse with children and adults, they focus on the individuals to determine the kind of persons they are, their usual mode of handling problems, whether they need help, and the way they react to counseling. Developing interviewing skills requires time and practice but following some guiding principles can facilitate this process. An organized approach is most effective when using interviewing skills in patient assessment and patient teaching.

ESTABLISHING A SETTING FOR COMMUNICATION

Appropriate Introduction

Introduce yourself and ask the name of each family member who is present and how they would like to be addressed. Address parents or other adults by their appropriate titles, such as "Mr." and "Mrs.," unless they specify a preferred name. Record the preferred name in the medical record. Using formal address or their preferred names conveys respect and regard for the parents or other caregivers (Ball, Dains, Flynn, et al., 2018).

At the beginning of the visit, include children in the interaction by asking them their name, preferred name, age, and other information. Nurses often direct all questions to adults even when children are old enough to speak for themselves. This only terminates one extremely valuable source of information—the patient. When including children, follow the general rules for communicating with children outlined in Nursing Care Guidelines: Communicating With Children later in the chapter.

Assurance of Privacy and Confidentiality

The place where the nurse conducts the interview is almost as important as the interview itself. The physical environment should allow for as much privacy as possible with distractions (e.g., interruptions, noise, or other visible activity) kept to a minimum. At times it will be necessary to turn off a television, radio, or mobile phone. The environment should also have some play provision for young children to keep them occupied during the parent-nurse interview (Fig. 4.1). Parents who are constantly interrupted by their children are unable to concentrate fully and tend to give brief answers to finish the interview as quickly as possible.

Confidentiality is another essential component of the initial phase of the interview. Because the interview is usually shared with other members of the health care team or the teacher (in the case of students), be certain to inform the family of the limits regarding confidentiality. If confidentiality is a concern in a situation, such as when talking to a parent suspected of child abuse or a teenager contemplating suicide, deal with this directly and inform the person that in such instances confidentiality cannot be ensured. However, the nurse judiciously protects information of a confidential nature.

COMPUTER PRIVACY AND APPLICATIONS IN NURSING

The use of computer technology to store and retrieve health information has become widespread; most institutions now maintain electronic health records for patients. The health care community is increasingly concerned about the privacy and security of this health information, and all nurses are engaged in protecting confidentiality of health care records. Any person accessing confidential health information is charged with managing safeguards for disclosure, including password protection to prevent violation of patient privacy and confidentiality.

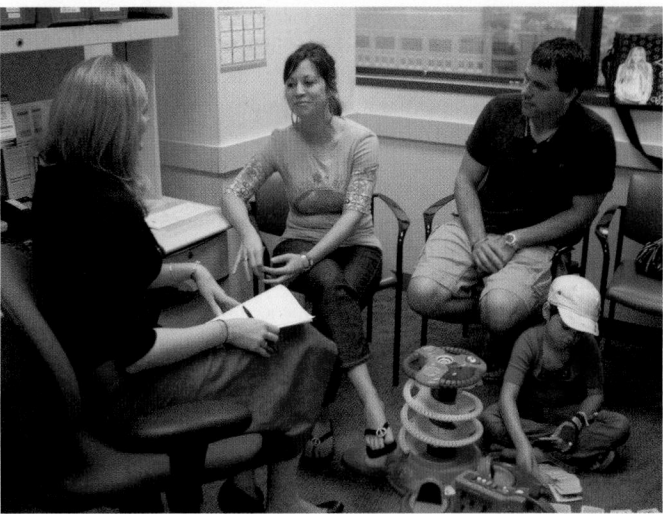

Fig. 4.1 A child plays while the nurse interviews parents.

BOX 4.1 Telephone Triage Guidelines

Date and time
Background
- Name, age, sex, contact information
- Chronic illness
- Allergies, current medications, treatments, or recent immunizations

Chief complaint
General symptoms
- Severity
- Duration
- Other symptoms
- Pain

Systems review
Steps taken
- Advised to call emergency medical services (911)
- Advised to go to emergency department
- Advised to see practitioner (today, tomorrow, or later appointment)
- Advised regarding home care
- Advised to call back if symptoms worsen or fail to improve

Resources for Telephone Triage Protocols

- Beaulieu, R., & Jumphreys, J. (2008). Evaluation of a telephone advice nurse in a nursing faculty managed pediatric community clinic. *Journal of Pediatric Health Care, 22*(3), 175–181.
- Marklund, B., Ström, M., Månsson, J., et al. (2007). Computer-supported telephone nurse triage: An evaluation of medical quality and costs. *Journal of Nursing Management, 15,* 180–187.
- Schmitt, B. D. (2012). *Pediatric telephone protocols: Office version (14th ed.).* Elk Grove Village, IL: American Academy of Pediatrics.
- Simonsen, S. M. (2001). *Telephone assessment: Guidelines for practice* (2nd ed.). St Louis, MO: Mosby.

TELEPHONE TRIAGE AND COUNSELING

Telephone triage care management has increased access to high-quality health care services and empowered parents to participate in their child's health care. Consequently, patient satisfaction has improved significantly. Unnecessary emergency department and clinic visits have decreased, saving health care costs and time (with less absence from work) for families in need of health care.

Telephone triage is more than "just a phone call" because a child's life is a high price to pay for poorly managed or incompetent telephone assessment skills. Typically, guidelines for telephone triage include asking screening questions; determining when to immediately refer to emergency medical services (dial 911) or the emergency department; and determining when to refer to same-day appointments, appointments in 24 to 72 hours, appointments in 4 days or more, or home care (Box 4.1). Successful outcomes are based on the consistency and accuracy of the information provided. A systematic review of 49 studies where nurses triaged calls found that the appropriateness of a decision and subsequent compliance often varied (Blank, Coster, O'Cathain, et al., 2012). A meta-analysis of 13 studies provided further insight and found that patient compliance with triage recommendations were influenced by the quality of provider communication (Purc-Stephenson & Thrasher, 2012). The importance of nurse-patient communication is reinforced as an essential aspect of telephone triage training. Training of communication skills that are patient and family-centered and specifically address active listening and advising skills offers the greatest opportunity for success. Assessment skills used in direct nurse-patient interactions are not directly transferable to the telephone and provide further support for training in decision-making skills for phone triage (Purc-Stephenson & Thrasher, 2010). Evidence-based clinical protocols for telephone triage can provide a structured method for assessment (Stacey, Macartney, Carley, et al., 2013).

COMMUNICATING WITH FAMILIES

COMMUNICATING WITH PARENTS

Although the parent and the child are separate and distinct individuals, the nurse's relationship with the child is frequently mediated by the parent, particularly with younger children. For the most part, nurses acquire information about the child by direct observation and through communication with the parents. Usually it can be assumed that because of the close contact with the child, the parent gives reliable information. Assessing the child requires input from the child (verbal and nonverbal), information from the parent, and the nurse's own observations of the child and interpretation of the relationship between the child and the parent. When children are old enough to be active participants in their own health care, the parent becomes a collaborator.

Encouraging Parents to Talk

Interviewing parents offers the opportunity to determine not only the child's health and developmental status but also information about factors that influence the child's life. Whatever the parent sees as a problem should be a concern of the nurse. These problems are not always easy to identify. Nurses need to be alert for clues and signals by which a parent communicates worries and anxieties. Careful phrasing with broad, open-ended questions (e.g., "What is Andy eating now?") provides more information than several single-answer questions (e.g., "Is Andy eating what the rest of the family eats?").

Sometimes the parent will take the lead without prompting. At other times it may be necessary to direct another question based on an observation, such as "Joseph seems unhappy today." or "How do you feel when Joseph cries?" If the parent appears to be tired or distraught, consider asking, "What do you do to relax?" or "What help do you have with the children?" A comment such as "You handle Jamey very well. What kind of experience have you had with babies?" to new parents who appear comfortable with their first child gives positive reinforcement and provides an opening for questions they might have on the infant's care. Often all that is required to keep parents talking is a nod or saying "yes" or "uh-huh."

Directing the Focus

Directing the focus of the interview while allowing maximum freedom of expression is one of the most difficult goals in effective communication. One approach is the use of open-ended or broad questions followed by guiding statements. For example, if the parent proceeds to list the other children by name, say, "Tell me their ages, too." If the parent continues to describe each child in depth, which is not the purpose of the interview, redirect the focus by stating, "Let's talk about the other children later. You were beginning to tell me about Rachel's activities at school." This approach conveys interest in the other children but focuses the assessment on the patient.

Listening and Cultural Awareness

Listening is the most important component of effective communication. When the purpose of listening is to understand the person being interviewed, it is an active process that requires concentration and attention to all aspects of the conversation—verbal, nonverbal, and abstract. Major blocks to listening are environmental distraction and premature judgment.

Although it is necessary to make some preliminary judgments, listen with as much objectivity as possible by clarifying meanings and attempting to see the situation from the parent's point of view. Effective interviewers consciously control their reactions and responses and the techniques they use (see Cultural Considerations box).

CULTURAL CONSIDERATIONS

Interviewing Without Judgment

It is easy to inject one's own attitudes and feelings into an interview. Often nurses' own prejudices and assumptions, which may include racial, religious, and cultural stereotypes, influence their perceptions of a parent's behavior. What the nurse may interpret as a parent's passive hostility or lack of interest may be shyness or an expression of anxiety. For example, in Western cultures, eye contact and directness are signs of paying attention. However, in many non-Western cultures, including that of American Indians, directness (e.g., looking someone in the eye) is considered rude. Children are sometimes taught to avert their gaze and to look down when being addressed by an adult, especially one with authority. Nurses must make judgments about "listening," as well as verbal interactions, with an appreciation of cultural differences. Nurses must phrase questions in a neutral mode and avoid assumptions about culture without first validating with a parent (Ball, Dains, Flynn, et al., 2018).

Careful listening relies on the use of clues, verbal leads, or signals from the interviewee to move the interview along. Frequent references to an area of concern, repetition of certain key words, or a special emphasis on something or someone serve as cues to the interviewer for the direction of inquiry. Concerns and anxieties are often mentioned in a casual, offhand manner. Even though they are casual, they are important and deserve scrutiny to identify problem areas. For example, a parent who is concerned about a child's habit of bedwetting may casually mention that the child's bed was "wet this morning."

Using Silence

Silence as a response is often one of the most difficult interviewing techniques to learn. The interviewer requires a sense of confidence and comfort to allow the interviewee space in which to think without interruptions. Silence permits the interviewee to sort out thoughts and feelings and search for responses to questions. Silence can also be a cue for the interviewer to go more slowly, reexamine the approach, and not push too hard (Ball, Dains, Flynn, et al., 2018).

Sometimes it is necessary to break the silence and reopen communication. Do this in a way that encourages the person to continue talking about what is considered important. Breaking a silence by introducing a new topic or by prolonged talking essentially terminates the interviewee's opportunity to use the silence. Suggestions for breaking the silence include statements such as the following:

- "Is there anything else you wish to say?"
- "I see you find it difficult to continue; how may I help?"
- "I don't know what this silence means. Perhaps there is something you would like to put into words but find difficult to say."

Being Empathic

Empathy is the capacity to understand what another person is experiencing from within that person's frame of reference; it is often described as the ability to put oneself in another's shoes. The essence of empathic interaction is accurate understanding of another's feelings. Empathy differs from **sympathy**, which is having feelings or emotions similar to those of another person rather than understanding those feelings.

Providing Anticipatory Guidance

The ideal way to handle a situation is to deal with it before it becomes a problem. The best preventive measure is anticipatory guidance. Traditionally, **anticipatory guidance** focused on providing families with information on normal growth and development and nurturing childrearing practices. For example, one of the most significant areas in pediatrics is injury prevention. Beginning prenatally, parents need specific instructions on home safety. Because of the child's maturing developmental skills, parents must implement home safety changes early to minimize risks to the child.

Unprepared parents can be disturbed by many normal developmental changes, such as a toddler's diminished appetite, negativism, altered sleeping patterns, and anxiety toward strangers. The chapters on health promotion provide nurses with information for counseling parents. However, anticipatory guidance should extend beyond giving general information to empowering families to use the information as a means of building competence in their parenting abilities (Dosman & Andrews, 2012). To achieve this level of anticipatory guidance, the nurse should do the following:

- Base interventions on needs identified by the family, not by the professional.
- View the family as competent or as having the ability to be competent.
- Provide opportunities for the family to achieve competence.

Avoiding Blocks to Communication

A number of blocks to communication can adversely affect the quality of the helping relationship. The interviewer introduces many of these blocks, such as giving unrestricted advice or forming prejudged conclusions. Another type of block occurs primarily with the interviewees and concerns **information overload**. When individuals receive too much information or information that is overwhelming, they often demonstrate signs of increasing anxiety or decreasing attention. Such signals should alert the interviewer to give less information or to clarify what has been said. Box 4.2 lists some of the more common blocks to communication, including signs of information overload.

Communicating With Families Through an Interpreter

Sometimes communication is impossible because two people speak different languages. In this case, it is necessary to obtain information through a third party: an interpreter. When using an interpreter, the nurse follows the same interviewing guidelines. Specific guidelines for using an interpreter are given in the Nursing Care Guidelines box.

NURSING CARE GUIDELINES

Using an Interpreter

- Explain to the interpreter the reason for the interview and the type of questions that will be asked.
- Clarify whether a detailed or brief answer is required and whether the translated response can be general or literal.
- Introduce the interpreter to the family and allow some time before the interview for them to become acquainted.
- Communicate directly with family members when asking questions to reinforce interest in them and to observe nonverbal expressions, but do not ignore the interpreter.

Continued

NURSING CARE GUIDELINES—cont'd

Using an Interpreter

- Pose questions to elicit only one answer at a time, such as "Do you have pain?" rather than "Do you have any pain, tiredness, or loss of appetite?"
- Refrain from interrupting family members and the interpreter while they are conversing.
- Avoid commenting to the interpreter about family members, because they may understand some English.
- Be aware that some medical words, such as *allergy,* may have no similar word in another language; avoid medical jargon whenever possible.
- Be aware that cultural differences may exist regarding views on puberty, sex, marriage, or pregnancy.
- Allow time after the interview for the interpreter to share something that he or she thought could not be said earlier; ask about the interpreter's impression of nonverbal clues to communication and family members' reliability or ease in revealing information.
- Arrange for the family to speak with the same interpreter on subsequent visits whenever possible.

BOX 4.2 Blocks to Communication

Communication Barriers (Nurse)

Socializing
Giving unrestricted and sometimes unsought advice
Offering premature or false reassurance
Giving overencouragement
Defending a situation or opinion
Using stereotyped comments or clichés
Using complex medical language
Limiting expression of emotion by asking directed, closed-ended questions
Asking leading questions that suggest only "correct" answers
Interrupting and finishing the person's sentence
Talking more than the interviewee
Forming prejudged conclusions
Deliberately changing the focus

Signs of Information Overload (Patient)

Long periods of silence
Wide eyes and fixed facial expression
Constant fidgeting or attempting to move away
Nervous habits (e.g., tapping, playing with hair)
Sudden interruptions (e.g., asking to go to the bathroom)
Looking around
Yawning, eyes drooping
Frequently looking at a watch or clock
Attempting to change the topic of discussion

Communicating with families through an interpreter requires sensitivity to cultural, legal, and ethical considerations (see Cultural Considerations box). In some cultures, class differences between the interpreter and the family may cause the family to feel intimidated and less inclined to offer information. Therefore it is important to choose the interpreter carefully and provide time for the interpreter and family to establish rapport.

CULTURAL CONSIDERATIONS

Using Children as Interpreters

When no one else is readily available to interpret, there may be temptation to use a bilingual child within the family as an interpreter. However, the use of children in health care interpreting is strongly discouraged because they are often not mature enough to understand health care questions, answers, or messages (American Academy of Pediatrics, 2019). Children may inadvertently commit interpretive errors, such as inaccuracies, omissions, or substitutions. In addition, children can be adversely affected by serious or sensitive information that may be discussed. In some cultures, using a child as an interpreter is considered an insult to an adult because children are expected to show respect by not questioning their elders. Note that some institutions prohibit the use of children as interpreters; check institutional policy for compliance. If a trained on-site or community-based interpreter is not available, a *language line* using a telephonic interpreter may be an option.

In obtaining informed consent through an interpreter, the nurse should fully inform the family of all aspects of the procedure to which they are consenting. Issues of confidentiality may arise when family members related to another patient are asked to interpret for the family, thus revealing sensitive information that may be shared with other families on the unit. With increased sensitivity toward patient rights and confidentiality, many institutions now require consent forms translated in the patient's primary language.

! NURSING ALERT

When using translated materials, such as a health history form, be certain the informant is literate in the foreign language.

COMMUNICATING WITH CHILDREN

Although the greatest amount of verbal communication is usually carried out with the parent, do not exclude the child during the interview. Pay attention to infants and younger children through play or by occasionally directing questions or remarks to them. Include older children as active participants so that they can share their own experiences and perspectives.

In communication with children of all ages, the nonverbal components of the communication process convey the most significant messages. It is difficult to disguise feelings, attitudes, and anxiety when relating to children. They are alert to surroundings and attach meaning to every gesture and move that is made; this is particularly true of very young children.

Active attempts to make friends with children before they have had an opportunity to evaluate an unfamiliar person tend to increase their anxiety. Continue to talk to the child and parent but go about activities that do not involve the child directly, thus allowing the child to observe from a safe position. If the child has a special toy or doll, "talk" to the doll first. Ask simple questions, such as "Does your teddy bear have a name?" to ease the child into conversation. Other guidelines for communicating with children are provided in the Nursing Care Guidelines box. Specific guidelines for preparing children for procedures are provided in Chapter 20.

NURSING CARE GUIDELINES

Communicating With Children

- Allow children time to feel comfortable.
- Avoid sudden or rapid advances, broad smiles, extended eye contact, and other gestures that may be seen as threatening.
- Talk to the parent if the child is initially shy.
- Communicate through transition objects (e.g., dolls, puppets, stuffed animals) before questioning a young child directly.
- Give older children the opportunity to talk without the parents present.
- Assume a position that is at eye level with the child (Fig. 4.2).
- Speak in a quiet, unhurried, and confident voice.
- Speak clearly, be specific, and use simple words and short sentences.
- State directions and suggestions positively.
- Offer a choice only when one exists.
- Be honest with children.
- Allow children to express their concerns and fears.
- Use a variety of communication techniques.

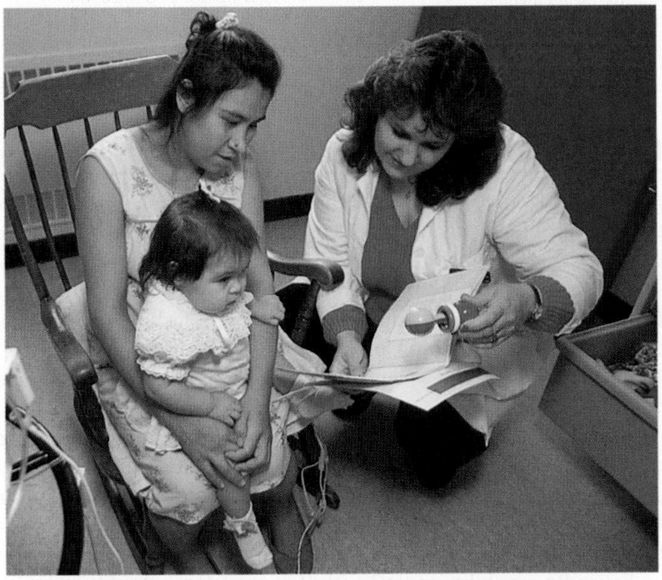
Fig. 4.2 The nurse assumes position at the child's level.

Communication Related to Development of Thought Processes

The normal development of language and thought offers a frame of reference for communicating with children. Thought processes progress from sensorimotor to perceptual to concrete and finally to abstract, formal operations. An understanding of the typical characteristics of these stages provides the nurse with a framework to facilitate social communication.

Infancy

Because they are unable to use words, infants primarily use and understand nonverbal communication. Infants communicate their needs and feelings through nonverbal behaviors and vocalizations that can be interpreted by someone who is around them for a sufficient time. Infants smile and coo when content and cry when distressed. Crying is provoked by unpleasant stimuli from inside or outside, such as hunger, pain, body restraint, or loneliness. Adults interpret this to mean that an infant needs something and consequently try to alleviate the discomfort by meeting their physical needs, speaking softly, and communicating through touch.

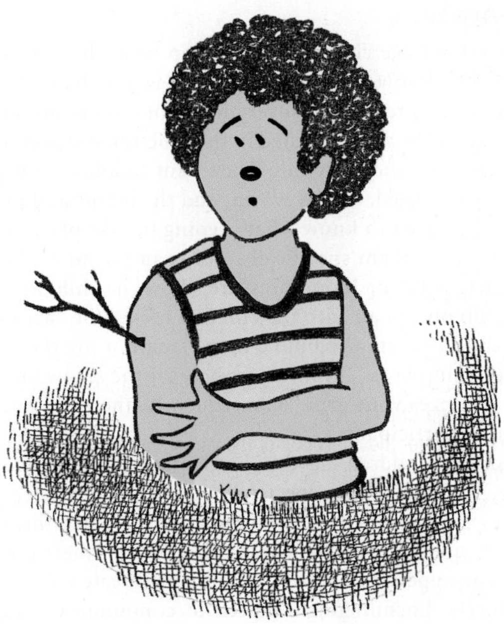
Fig. 4.3 A young child may take the expression "a little stick in the arm" literally.

Infants respond to adults' nonverbal behaviors. They become quiet when they are cuddled, rocked, or receive other forms of gentle physical contact. They receive comfort from the sound of a soft voice even though they do not understand the words that are spoken. Until infants reach the age at which they experience stranger anxiety, they readily respond to any firm, gentle handling and quiet, calm speech. Loud, harsh sounds and sudden movements are frightening.

Early Childhood

Children younger than 5 years old are **egocentric**. They see things only in relation to themselves and from their point of view. Therefore focus communication on them. Tell them what they can do or how they will feel. Experiences of others are of no interest to them. It is futile to use another child's experience in an attempt to gain the cooperation of small children. Allow them to touch and examine articles with which they will come in contact. A stethoscope bell will feel cold; palpating a neck might tickle. Although they have not yet acquired sufficient language skills to express their feelings and wants, toddlers can effectively use their hands to communicate ideas without words. They push an unwanted object away, pull another person to show them something, point, and cover the mouth that is saying something they do not wish to hear.

Everything is direct and concrete to small children. They are unable to work with abstractions and interpret words literally. Analogies escape them because they are unable to separate reality from fantasy. For example, they attach literal meaning to such common phrases as "two-faced," "sticky fingers," and "coughing your head off." Children who are told they will get "a little stick in the arm" may not be able to envision an injection (Fig. 4.3). Therefore use simple, direct language rather than phrases that might be misinterpreted by a small child.

School-Age Years

Younger school-age children rely less on what they see and more on what they know when faced with new problems. They want explanations and reasons for everything but require no verification beyond that. They are interested in the functional aspect of all procedures, objects, and activities. They want to know why an object exists, why it is used, how it works, and the intent and purpose of its user. They need to know what is going to take place and why it is being done to them specifically. For example, to explain a procedure such as taking blood pressure, show the child how squeezing the bulb pushes air into the cuff and makes the "arrow" move. Let the child operate the bulb. An explanation for the procedure might be as simple as "I want to see how far the arrow moves when the cuff squeezes your arm." Consequently, the child becomes an enthusiastic participant.

School-age children have a heightened concern about body integrity. Because of the special importance they place on their body, they are sensitive to anything that constitutes a threat or suggestion of injury to it. This concern extends to their possessions, so they may appear to overreact to loss or threatened loss of treasured objects. Encouraging children to communicate their needs and voice their concerns enables the nurse to provide reassurance, to dispel myths and fears, and to implement activities that reduce their anxiety. For example, if a shy child dislikes being the center of attention, ignore that child by talking and relating to other children in the family or group. When children feel more comfortable, they will usually interject personal ideas, feelings, and interpretations of events.

Adolescence

As children move into adolescence, they fluctuate between child and adult thinking and behavior. They are riding a current that is moving them rapidly toward a maturity that may be beyond their coping ability. Therefore when tensions rise, they may seek the security of the more familiar and comfortable expectations of childhood. Anticipating these shifts in identity allows the nurse to adjust the course of interaction to meet the needs of the moment. No single approach can be relied on consistently, and encountering cooperation, hostility, anger, bravado, and a variety of other behaviors and attitudes is common. It is as much a mistake to regard an adolescent as an adult with an adult's wisdom and control as it is to assume that a teenager has the concerns and expectations of a child.

Interviewing an adolescent presents some special issues. The first may be whether to talk with the adolescent alone or with the adolescent and parents together. If the parents and teenager are together, talking with the adolescent first has the advantage of immediately identifying with the young person, thus fostering the interpersonal relationship. However, talking with the parents initially may provide insight into the family relationship. In either case, give both parties an opportunity to be included in the interview. If time is limited (e.g., during history taking), clarify this at the onset to avoid appearing to "take sides" by talking more with one person than with the other.

Another dilemma in interviewing adolescents is that two views of a problem frequently exist: the teenager's and the parents'. Clarification of the problem is a major task. However, providing both parties an opportunity to discuss their perceptions in an open and unbiased atmosphere can, by itself, be therapeutic. Demonstrating positive communication skills can help families with adolescents to communicate more effectively (see Nursing Care Guidelines box).

NURSING CARE GUIDELINES

Communicating With Adolescents

Build a Foundation

Spend time together.
Encourage expression of ideas and feelings.
Respect their views.
Tolerate differences.
Praise good points.
Respect their privacy.
Set a good example.

Communicate Effectively

Give undivided attention.
Listen, listen, listen.
Be courteous, calm, honest, and open minded.
Try not to overreact. If you do, take a break.
Avoid judging or criticizing.
Avoid the "third degree" of continuous questioning.
Choose important issues when taking a stand.
After taking a stand:

- Think through all options.
- Make expectations clear.

COMMUNICATION TECHNIQUES

Nurses use a variety of verbal techniques to encourage communication. Some of these techniques are useful to pose questions or explore concerns in a less threatening manner. Others can be presented as word games, which are often well received by children. However, for many children and adults, talking about feelings is difficult, and verbal communication may be more stressful than supportive. In such instances, use several nonverbal techniques to encourage communication.

Box 4.3 describes both verbal and nonverbal techniques. Because of the importance of play in communicating with children, play is discussed more extensively in the next section. Any of the verbal or nonverbal techniques can give rise to strong feelings that surface unexpectedly. Be prepared to handle them or to recognize when issues go beyond your ability to deal with them. At that point, consider an appropriate referral.

Play

Play is a universal language of children. It is one of the most important forms of communication and can be an effective technique in relating to them. The nurse can often pick up on clues about physical, intellectual, and social developmental progress from the form and complexity of a child's play behaviors. Play requires minimum equipment or none at all. Many providers use therapeutic play to reduce the trauma of illness and hospitalization (see Chapter 19) and to prepare children for therapeutic procedures (see Chapter 20).

Because their ability to perceive precedes their ability to transmit, infants respond to activities that register with their physical senses. Patting, stroking, and other skin play convey messages. Repetitive actions, such as stretching infants' arms out to the side while they are lying on their back and then folding the arms across the chest or raising and revolving the legs in a bicycling motion, will elicit pleasurable sounds. Colorful items to catch the eye or interesting sounds, such as a ticking clock, chimes, bells, or singing, can be used to attract infants' attention.

BOX 4.3 Creative Communication Techniques With Children

Verbal Techniques

"I" Messages

Relate a feeling about a behavior in terms of "I."

Describe effect behavior had on the person.

Avoid use of "you."

"You" messages are judgmental and provoke defensiveness.

Example: "You" message: "You are being uncooperative about doing your treatments."

Example: "I" message: "I am concerned about how the treatments are going because I want to see you get better."

Third-Person Technique

Express a feeling in terms of a third person ("he," "she," "they"). This is less threatening than directly asking children how they feel because it gives them an opportunity to agree or disagree without being defensive.

Example: "Sometimes when a person is sick a lot, he feels angry and sad because he cannot do what others can." Either wait silently for a response or encourage a reply with a statement, such as "Did you ever feel that way?"

This approach allows children three choices: (1) to agree and, one hopes, express how they feel; (2) to disagree; or (3) to remain silent, which means they probably have such feelings but are unable to express them at that time.

Facilitative Response

Listen carefully and reflect back to patients the feelings and intent of their statements.

Responses are empathic and nonjudgmental and legitimize the person's feelings.

Formula for facilitative responses: "You feel ________ because ________."

Example: If child states, "I hate coming to the hospital and getting needles," a facilitative response is "You feel unhappy because of all the things that are done to you."

Storytelling

Use the language of children to probe areas of their thinking while bypassing conscious inhibitions or fears.

The simplest technique is asking children to relate a story about an event, such as "being in the hospital."

Other approaches:

- Show children a picture of a particular event, such as a child in a hospital with other people in the room, and ask them to describe the scene.
- Cut out comic strips, remove words, and have child add statements for scenes.

Mutual Storytelling

Reveal the child's thinking and attempt to change his or her perceptions or fears by retelling a somewhat different story (more therapeutic approach than storytelling).

Begin by asking the child to tell a story about something; then tell another story that is similar to the child's tale but with differences that help the child in problem areas.

Example: Child's story is about going to the hospital and never seeing his or her parents again. Nurse's story is also about a child (using different names but similar circumstances) in a hospital whose parents visit every day, but in the evening after work, until the child is better and goes home with them.

Bibliotherapy

Use books in a therapeutic and supportive process.

Provide children with an opportunity to explore an event that is similar to their own but sufficiently different to allow them to distance themselves from it and remain in control.

General guidelines for using bibliotherapy are:

1. Assess the child's emotional and cognitive development in terms of readiness to understand the book's message.
2. Be familiar with the book's content (intended message or purpose) and the age for which it is written.
3. Read the book to the child if the child is unable to read.
4. Explore the meaning of the book with the child by having the child:
   - Retell the story.
   - Read a special section with the nurse or parent.
   - Draw a picture related to the story and discuss the drawing.
   - Talk about the characters.
   - Summarize the moral or meaning of the story.

Dreams

Dreams often reveal unconscious and repressed thoughts and feelings.

Ask the child to talk about a dream or nightmare.

Explore with the child what meaning the dream could have.

"What If" Questions

Encourage child to explore potential situations and to consider different problem-solving options.

Example: "What if you got sick and had to go the hospital?" Children's responses reveal what they know already and what they are curious about, providing an opportunity for them to learn coping skills, especially in potentially dangerous situations.

Three Wishes

Ask, "If you could have any three things in the world, what would they be?"

If the child answers, "That all my wishes come true," ask the child for specific wishes.

Rating Game

Use some type of rating scale (numbers, sad to happy faces) to have the child rate an event or feeling.

Example: Instead of asking youngsters how they feel, ask how their day has been "on a scale of 1 to 10, with 10 being the best."

Word Association Game

State key words and ask children to say the first word they think of when they hear the word.

Start with neutral words and then introduce more anxiety-producing words, such as "illness," "needles," "hospitals," and "operation."

Select key words that relate to some relevant event in the child's life.

Sentence Completion

Present a partial statement and have the child complete it. Some sample statements are:

- The thing I like best (least) about school is ________.
- The best (worst) age to be is ________.
- The most (least) fun thing I ever did was ________.
- The thing I like most (least) about my parents is ________.
- The one thing I would change about my family is ________.
- If I could be anything I wanted, I would be ________.
- The thing I like most (least) about myself is ________.

Pros and Cons

Select a topic, such as "being in the hospital," and have the child list "five good things and five bad things" about it.

This is an exceptionally valuable technique when applied to relationships, such as things family members like and dislike about each other.

Continued

BOX 4.3 Creative Communication Techniques With Children—cont'd

Nonverbal Techniques

Writing

Writing is an alternative communication approach for older children and adults.

Specific suggestions include:

- Keep a journal or diary.
- Write down feelings or thoughts that are difficult to express.
- Write "letters" that are never mailed (a variation is making up a "pen pal" to write to).

Keep an account of the child's progress from both a physical and an emotional viewpoint.

Drawing

Drawing is one of the most valuable forms of communication—both nonverbal (from looking at the drawing) and verbal (from the child's story of the picture).

Children's drawings tell a great deal about them because they are projections of their inner selves.

Spontaneous drawing involves giving the child a variety of art supplies and providing the opportunity to draw.

Directed drawing involves a more specific direction, such as "draw a person" or the "three themes" approach (state three things about the child and ask the child to choose one and draw a picture).

Guidelines for Evaluating Drawings

Use spontaneous drawings and evaluate more than one drawing whenever possible.

Interpret the drawings by considering other available information about the child and family, including the child's age and stage of development.

Interpret the drawings as a whole rather than focusing on specific details of the drawings.

Consider individual elements of the drawings that may be significant:

- Sex of figure drawn first: Usually relates to the child's perception of his or her own sex role
- Size of individual figures: Expresses importance, power, or authority
- Order in which figures are drawn: Expresses priority in terms of importance
- Child's position in relation to other family members: Expresses feelings of status or alliance
- Exclusion of a member: May denote feeling of not belonging or desire to eliminate
- Accentuated parts: Usually express concern for areas of special importance (e.g., large hands may be a sign of aggression)
- Absence of or rudimentary arms and hands: Suggest timidity, passivity, or intellectual immaturity; tiny, unstable feet may express insecurity; hidden hands may mean guilt feelings
- Placement of drawing on the page and type of stroke: Free use of paper and firm, continuous strokes express security, whereas drawings restricted to a small area and lightly drawn in broken or wavering lines may be signs of insecurity
- Erasures, shading, or crosshatching: Expresses ambivalence, concern, or anxiety with a particular area

Magic

Use simple magic tricks to help establish rapport with child, encourage compliance with health interventions, and provide effective distraction during painful procedures.

Although the "magician" talks, no verbal response from the child is required.

Play

Play is the universal language and "work" of children.

It tells a great deal about children because they project their inner selves through the activity.

Spontaneous play involves giving child a variety of play materials and providing the opportunity to play.

Directed play involves a more specific direction, such as providing medical equipment or a dollhouse for focused reasons, such as exploring the child's fear of injections or exploring family relationships.

Older infants respond to simple games. The old game of peek-a-boo is an excellent means of initiating communication with infants while maintaining a "safe," nonthreatening distance. After this intermittent eye contact, the nurse is no longer viewed as a stranger but as a friend. This can be followed by touch games. Clapping an infant's hands together for pat-a-cake or wiggling the toes for "this little piggy" delights an infant or small child. Talking to a foot or other part of the child's body is another effective tactic. Much of the nursing assessment can be carried out with the use of games and simple play equipment while the infant remains in the safety of the parent's arms or lap.

The nurse can capitalize on the natural curiosity of small children by playing games, such as "Which hand do you take?" and "Guess what I have in my hand," or by manipulating items such as a flashlight or stethoscope. Finger games are useful. More elaborate materials, such as puppets and replicas of familiar or unfamiliar items, serve as excellent means of communicating with small children. The variety and extent are limited only by the nurse's imagination.

HISTORY TAKING

PERFORMING A HEALTH HISTORY

The format used for history taking may be (1) **direct**, in which the nurse asks for information via direct interview with the informant; or (2) **indirect**, in which the informant supplies the information by completing some type of questionnaire. The direct method is superior to the indirect approach or a combination of both. However, because time is limited, the direct approach is not always practical. If the nurse cannot use the direct approach, he or she should review the parents' written responses and question them regarding any unusual answers. The categories listed in Box 4.4 encompass children's current and past health status and information about their psychosocial environment.

Identifying Information

Much of the identifying information may already be available from other recorded sources. However, if the parent and child seem anxious, use this opportunity to ask about such information to help them feel more comfortable.

Informant

One of the important elements of identifying information is the **informant**, the person or persons who furnish the information. Record (1) who the person is (child, parent, or other), (2) an impression of reliability and willingness to communicate, and (3) any special circumstances such as the use of an interpreter or conflicting answers by more than one person.

Chief Complaint

The **chief complaint** is the specific reason for the child's visit to the clinic, office, or hospital. It may be the theme, with the present illness

BOX 4.4 Outline of a Pediatric Health History

Identifying information
1. Name
2. Address
3. Telephone
4. Birth date and place
5. Race or ethnic group
6. Sex
7. Religion
8. Date of interview
9. Informant

Chief complaint (CC): To establish the major specific reason for the child's and parents' seeking of health care

History of present illness (HPI): To obtain all details related to the chief complaint

Past medical history (PMH): To elicit a profile of the child's previous illnesses, injuries, or surgeries
1. Birth history (pregnancy, labor and delivery, perinatal history)
2. Previous illnesses, injuries, or surgeries
3. Allergies
4. Current medications
5. Immunizations
6. Growth and development
7. Habits

Review of systems (ROS): To elicit information concerning any potential health problem
1. Constitutional
2. Integument
3. Eyes
4. Ears
5. Nose
6. Mouth
7. Throat
8. Neck
9. Chest
10. Respiratory
11. Cardiovascular
12. Gastrointestinal
13. Genitourinary
14. Gynecologic
15. Musculoskeletal
16. Neurologic
17. Endocrine
18. Hematologic/lymphatic
19. Allergic/immunologic
20. Psychiatric

Family medical history: To identify genetic traits or diseases that have familial tendencies and to assess exposure to a communicable disease in a family member and family habits that may affect the child's health, such as smoking and chemical use

Psychosocial history: To elicit information about the child's self-concept

Sexual history: To elicit information concerning the child's sexual concerns or activities and any pertinent data regarding adults' sexual activity that influences the child

Family history: To develop an understanding of the child as an individual and as a member of a family and a community
1. Family composition
2. Home and community environment
3. Occupation and education of family members
4. Cultural and religious traditions
5. Family function and relationships

Nutritional assessment: To elicit information on the adequacy of the child's nutritional intake and needs
1. Dietary intake
2. Clinical examination

viewed as the description of the problem. Elicit the chief complaint by asking open-ended, neutral questions (e.g., "What seems to be the matter?" "How may I help you?" or "Why did you come here today?"). Avoid labeling-type questions (e.g., "How are you sick?" or "What is the problem?"). It is possible that the reason for the visit is not an illness or problem.

History of Present Illness

The history of the present illness[a] is a narrative of the chief complaint from its onset through its progression to the present. Its four major components are the details of onset, a complete interval history, the present status, and the reason for seeking help now. The focus of the present illness is on all factors relevant to the main problem, even if they have disappeared or changed during the onset, interval, and present.

Analyzing a Symptom

Because pain is often the most characteristic symptom denoting the onset of a physical problem, it is used as an example for analysis of a symptom. Assessment includes type, location, severity, duration, and influencing factors (see Nursing Care Guidelines box; see also Chapter 5, Pain Assessment).

[a]The term *illness* is used in its broadest sense to denote any problem of a physical, emotional, or psychosocial nature. Actually, it is a history of the chief complaint.

NURSING CARE GUIDELINES

Analyzing the Symptom: Pain

Type

Be as specific as possible. With young children, asking the parents how they know the child is in pain may help describe its type, location, and severity. For example, a parent may state, "My child must have a severe earache because she pulls at her ears, rolls her head on the floor, and screams. Nothing seems to help." Help older children describe the "hurt" by asking them if it is sharp, throbbing, dull, or stabbing. Record whatever words they use in quotes.

Location

Be specific. "Stomach pain" is too general a description. Children can better localize the pain if they are asked to "point with one finger to where it hurts" or to "point to where mommy or daddy would put a Band-Aid." Determine if the pain radiates by asking, "Does the pain stay there or move? Show me with your finger where the pain goes."

Continued

NURSING CARE GUIDELINES—cont'd

Analyzing the Symptom: Pain

Severity

Severity is best determined by finding out how it affects the child's usual behavior. Pain that prevents a child from playing, interacting with others, sleeping, and eating is most often severe. Assess pain intensity using a rating scale, such as a numeric or Wong-Baker FACES Pain Rating Scale (see Chapter 5).

Duration

Include the duration, onset, and frequency. Describe these in terms of activity and behavior, such as "pain reported to last all night; child refused to sleep and cried intermittently."

Influencing Factors

Include anything that causes a change in the type, location, severity, or duration of the pain: (1) precipitating events (those that cause or increase the pain), (2) relieving events (those that lessen the pain, such as medications), (3) temporal events (times when the pain is relieved or increased), (4) positional events (standing, sitting, lying down), and (5) associated events (meals, stress, coughing).

Past Medical History

The history contains information relating to all previous aspects of the child's health status and concentrates on several areas that are ordinarily passed over in the history of an adult, such as birth history, detailed feeding history, immunizations, and growth and development. Because this section includes a great deal of information, use a combination of open-ended and fact-finding questions. For example, begin interviewing for each section with an open-ended statement (e.g., "Tell me about your child's birth") to provide the informants the opportunity to relate what they think is most important. Ask fact-finding questions related to specific details whenever necessary to focus the interview on certain topics.

Birth History

The **birth history** includes all data concerning (1) the mother's health during pregnancy, (2) the labor and delivery, and (3) the infant's condition immediately after birth. Because prenatal influences have significant effects on a child's physical and emotional development, a thorough investigation of the birth history is essential. Because parents may question what relevance pregnancy and birth have on the child's present condition, particularly if the child is past infancy, explain why such questions are included. An appropriate statement may be, "I will be asking you some questions about your pregnancy and ____'s [refer to child by name] birth. Your answers will give me a more complete picture of his [or her] overall health."

Previous Illnesses, Injuries, and Surgeries

When inquiring about past illnesses, begin with a general question (e.g., "What other illnesses has your child had?"). Because parents are most likely to recall serious health problems, ask specifically about colds, earaches, and childhood diseases, such as measles, rubella (German measles), chickenpox, mumps, pertussis (whooping cough), diphtheria, tuberculosis, scarlet fever, strep throat, recurrent ear infections, influenza, gastroesophageal reflux, tonsillitis, or allergic manifestations.

In addition to illnesses, ask about injuries that required medical intervention, surgeries, procedures, and hospitalizations, including the dates and diagnoses of each incident. Focus on injuries (e.g., accidental falls, poisoning, choking, concussion, fractures, or burns) because these may be potential areas for parental guidance.

Allergies

Ask about commonly known allergic disorders, such as hay fever and asthma; unusual reactions to drugs, food, or latex products; and reactions to other contact agents, such as poisonous plants, animals, household products, or fabrics. If asked appropriate questions, most people can give reliable information about drug reactions (see Nursing Care Guidelines box).

NURSING CARE GUIDELINES

Taking an Allergy History

- Has your child ever taken any prescription or over-the-counter medications that have disagreed with him or her or caused an allergic reaction? If yes, can you remember the name(s) of this medication(s)?
- Can you describe the reaction?
- Was the medication taken by mouth (as a tablet or syrup), or was it an injection?
- How soon after starting the medication did the reaction happen?
- How long ago did this happen?
- Did anyone tell you it was an allergic reaction, or did you decide for yourself?
- Has your child ever taken this medication, or a similar one, again? If yes, did your child experience the same problems?
- Have you told the physicians or nurses about your child's reaction or allergy?

! NURSING ALERT

Information about allergic reactions to drugs or other products is essential. Failure to document a serious reaction places the child at risk if the agent is given.

Current Medications

Inquire about current medications, including vitamins, antipyretics (especially aspirin), antibiotics, antihistamines, decongestants, nutritional supplements, or herbs, essential oils, and homeopathic medications. List all medications, including name, dose, schedule, duration, and reasons for use. Often parents are unaware of a medication's actual name. Whenever possible, ask the parents to bring the containers with them to the next visit, or ask for the name of the pharmacy and call for a list of all the child's recent prescription medications. However, this list will not include over-the-counter medications, which are important to know.

Immunizations

A record of all immunizations is essential. Because many parents are unaware of the exact name and date of each immunization, sources of information include the child's health care provider, the child's school record, and the state's centralized immunization registry. All immunizations and "boosters" are listed, stating (1) the name of the specific disease, (2) the number of injections, (3) the dosage (sometimes lesser amounts are given if a reaction is anticipated), (4) the date administered, and (5) the occurrence of any reaction following immunization. Children should be screened for contraindications and precautions before every vaccine is administered (see Chapter 6, Immunizations).

Dietary History

Because parental concerns are common and nursing interventions are important in ensuring optimum nutrition, the dietary history is discussed in detail in the Nutritional Assessment section later in this chapter.

BOX 4.5 Habits to Explore During a Health Interview

- Behavior patterns, such as nail biting, thumb sucking, pica (habitual ingestion of nonfood substances), rituals ("security" blanket or toy), and unusual movements (head banging, rocking, overt masturbation, walking on toes)
- Activities of daily living, such as hours of sleep and arising, duration of nighttime sleep and naps, type and duration of exercise, regularity of stools and urination, age of toilet training, and daytime or nighttime bedwetting
- Unusual disposition; response to frustration
- Use or abuse of alcohol, drugs, coffee, or tobacco

Growth and Development

Review the child's growth, including:

- Measurements of weight, length, and head circumference at birth
- Patterns of growth on the growth chart and any significant deviations from previous percentiles
- Concerns about growth from the family or child

Developmental milestones include:

- Age of holding up head steadily
- Age of sitting alone without support
- Age of walking without assistance
- Age of saying first words with meaning
- Age of achieving bladder and bowel control
- Present grade in school
- School performance
- If the child has a best friend
- Interactions with other children, peers, and adults

Use specific and detailed questions when inquiring about each developmental milestone. For example, "sitting up" can mean many different activities, such as sitting propped up, sitting in someone's lap, sitting with support, sitting up alone but in a hyperflexed position for assisted balance, or sitting up unsupported with the back slightly rounded. A clue to misunderstanding the requested activity may be an unusually early age of achievement (see Chapter 3, Developmental Assessment).

Habits

Habits are an important area to explore (Box 4.5). Parents frequently express concerns during this part of the history. Encourage their input by saying, "Please tell me any concerns you have about your child's habits, behavior, activities, or development." Investigate further any concerns that parents express.

One of the most common concerns relates to sleep. Many children develop a normal sleep pattern, and all that is required during the assessment is a general overview of nighttime sleep and nap schedules. However, some children develop sleep problems (see Chapters 10 and 13, Sleep Problems). When sleep problems occur, the nurse needs a more detailed sleep history to guide appropriate interventions.

Habits related to use of chemicals apply primarily to older children and adolescents. If a youngster admits to smoking, drinking, or using drugs, ask about the quantity and frequency. Questions such as "Many kids your age are experimenting with drugs and alcohol; have you ever had any drugs or alcohol?" may give more reliable data than questions such as "How much do you drink?" or "How often do you drink or take drugs?" Clarify that "drinking" includes all types of alcohol, including beer and wine. When quantities such as a "glass" of wine or a "can" of beer are given, ask about the size of the container.

If older children deny use of chemical substances, inquire about past experimentation. Asking, "You mean you never tried to smoke or drink?" implies that the nurse expects some such activity, and the youngster may be more inclined to answer truthfully. Be aware of the confidential nature of such questioning, the adverse effect that the parents' presence may have on the adolescent's willingness to answer, and the fact that self-reporting may not be an accurate account of chemical abuse.

BOX 4.6 Anticipatory Guidance: Sexuality

12 to 14 Years Old

Have the adolescent identify a supportive adult with whom to discuss sexuality issues and concerns.
Discuss the advantages of delaying sexual activity.
Discuss making responsible decisions regarding normal sexual feelings.
Discuss the roles of gender, peer pressure, and the media in sexual decision making.
Discuss contraceptive options (advantages and disadvantages).
Provide education regarding sexually transmitted infections (STIs), including human immunodeficiency virus (HIV) infection; clarify risks and discuss condoms.
Discuss abuse prevention, including avoiding dangerous situations, the role of drugs and alcohol, and the use of self-defense.
Have the adolescent clarify his or her values, needs, and ability to be assertive.
If the adolescent is sexually active, discuss limiting partners, use of condoms, and contraceptive options.
Have a confidential interview with the adolescent (including a sexual history).
Discuss the evolution of sexual identity and expression.
Discuss breast examination or testicular examination.

15 to 18 Years Old

Support delaying sexual activity.
Discuss alternatives to intercourse.
Discuss "When are you ready for sex?"
Clarify values; encourage responsible decision making.
Discuss consequences of unprotected sex: early pregnancy and STIs, including HIV infection.
Discuss negotiating with partner and barriers to safer sex.
If the adolescent is sexually active, discuss limiting partners, use of condoms, and contraceptive options.
Emphasize that sex should be safe and pleasurable for both partners.
Have a confidential interview with the adolescent.
Discuss concerns about sexual expression and identity.

Data from Wright, K. (1997). Anticipatory guidance: Developing a healthy sexuality. *Pediatric Annals, 26*(Suppl. 2), S142–S144, C3; Fonseca, H., & Greydanus, D. (2007). Sexuality in the child, teen and young adult: Concepts for the clinician. *Primary Care: Clinics in Office Practice, 34*, 275–292.

Sexual History

The sexual history is an essential component of adolescents' health assessment. The history uncovers areas of concern related to sexual activity, alerts the nurse to circumstances that may indicate the need for screening for sexually transmitted infections or testing for pregnancy, and provides information related to the need for sexual health counseling, such as safer sex practices. Box 4.6 gives guidelines for anticipatory guidance topics for parents and adolescents.

One approach to initiating a conversation about sexual concerns is to begin with a history of peer interactions. Open-ended statements (e.g., "Tell me about your social life" or "Who are your closest friends?") generally lead to a discussion of dating and sexual issues. To probe further, include questions about the adolescent's attitudes on such topics as sex education, "going steady," "living together," and premarital sex. Phrase questions to reflect concern rather than judgment or criticism of sexual practices.

In any conversation regarding sexual history, be aware of the language used in either eliciting or conveying sexual information. For example, avoid asking whether the adolescent is "sexually active," because this term is broadly defined. "Are you having sex with anyone?" is probably the most direct and best understood question. Because same-sex experimentation may occur, refer to all sexual contacts in nongender terms, such as "partners," rather than "girlfriends" or "boyfriends."

Family Health History

The family health history is used primarily to discover any genetic or chronic diseases affecting the child's family members. Assess for the presence or absence of consanguinity (if anyone in the family is related to their spouse's or partner's family). Family health history is generally confined to first-degree relatives (parents, siblings, grandparents, and immediate aunts and uncles). Information includes age, marital status, health status, cause of death if deceased, and any evidence of conditions, such as early heart disease, stroke, sudden death from unknown cause, hypercholesterolemia, hypertension, cancer, diabetes mellitus, obesity, congenital anomalies, inherited diseases, allergies, asthma, seizures, tuberculosis, abnormal bleeding, sickle cell disease, cognitive impairment, hearing or visual deficits, and psychiatric disorders (e.g., depression, psychosis, emotional problems). Confirm the accuracy of the reported disorders by inquiring about the symptoms, course, treatment, and sequelae of each diagnosis.

Geographic Location

One of the important areas to explore when assessing the family health history is geographic location, including the birthplace and travel to different areas in or outside of the country, for identification of possible exposure to endemic diseases. Include current and past housing, whether the family rents or owns, whether the family resides in an urban or rural location, the age of the home, and whether there are significant threats such as molds or pests within the housing structure. Although the primary interest is the child's temporary residence in various localities, also inquire about close family members' travel, especially during tours of military service or business trips.

Family Structure

Assessment of the family, both its structure and its function, is an important component of the history-taking process. Because the quality of the functional relationship between the child and family members is a major factor in emotional and physical health, family assessment is discussed separately and in greater detail apart from the more traditional health history.

Family assessment is the collection of data about the composition of the family and the relationships among its members. In its broadest sense, **family** refers to all those individuals who are considered by the family member to be significant to the nuclear unit, including relatives, friends, and social groups (e.g., daycare, school, church). Although family assessment is not family therapy, it can and frequently is therapeutic. Involving family members in discussing family characteristics and activities can provide insight into family dynamics and relationships.

Because of the time involved in performing an in-depth family assessment as presented here, be selective in deciding when knowledge of family function may facilitate nursing care (see Nursing Care Guidelines box). During brief contacts with families, a full assessment is not appropriate, and screening with one or two questions from each category may reflect the health of the family system or the need for additional assessment.

NURSING CARE GUIDELINES

Initiating a Comprehensive Family Assessment

Perform a comprehensive assessment on:

- Children receiving comprehensive well-child care
- Children experiencing major stressful life events (e.g., chronic illness, disability, parental divorce, family separation, death of a family member)
- Children requiring extensive home care
- Children with developmental delays
- Children with repeated accidental injuries and those with suspected child abuse
- Children with behavioral or physical problems that could be caused by family dysfunction

The most common method of eliciting information on the family structure is to interview family members. The principal areas of concern are family composition, home and community environment, occupation and education of family members, and cultural and religious traditions (Box 4.7).

Psychosocial History

The traditional medical history includes a personal and social section that concentrates on children's personal status, such as school adjustment and any unusual habits, and the family and home environment. Because several personal aspects are covered under development and habits, only those issues related to children's ability to cope and their self-concept are presented here.

Through observation, obtain a general idea of how children handle themselves in terms of confidence in dealing with others, answering questions, and coping with new situations. Observe the parent-child relationship for the types of messages sent to children about their coping skills and self-worth. Do the parents treat the child with respect, focusing on strengths, or is the interaction one of constant reprimands with emphasis on weaknesses and faults? Do the parents help the child learn new coping strategies or support the ones the child uses?

Parent-child interactions also convey messages about body image. Do the parents label the child and body parts (e.g., "bad boy," "skinny legs," or "ugly scar")? Do the parents handle the child gently, using soothing touch to calm an anxious child, or do they treat the child roughly, using force or restraint to make the child obey? If the child touches certain parts of the body, such as the genitalia, do the parents make comments that suggest a negative connotation?

With older children, many of the communication strategies discussed earlier in this chapter are useful in eliciting more definitive information about their coping and self-concept. Children can name or write down five things they like and dislike about themselves. The nurse can use sentence completion statements, such as "The thing I like best (or worst) about myself is ________"; "If I could change one thing about myself, it would be ________"; or "When I am scared, I ________."

Review of Systems

The review of systems is a specific review of each body system, following an order similar to that used in a physical examination (see Nursing Care Guidelines box). Often the history of the present illness provides a complete review of the system involved in the chief complaint. Because asking questions about other body systems may appear irrelevant to the parents or child, precede the questioning with an explanation of why the data are necessary (similar to the explanation concerning the relevance of the birth history) and reassure the parents that the child's main problem has not been forgotten.

BOX 4.7 Family Assessment Interview

General Guidelines

Schedule the interview with the family at a time that is most convenient for all parties; include as many family members as possible; clearly state the purpose of the interview.

Begin the interview by asking each person's name and their relationships to one another.

Restate the purpose of the interview and the objective.

Keep the initial conversation general to put members at ease and to learn the "big picture" of the family.

Identify major concerns and reflect these back to the family to be certain that all parties receive the same message.

Terminate the interview with a summary of what was discussed and a plan for additional sessions, if needed.

Structural Assessment Areas

Family Composition

Immediate members of the household (names, ages, and relationships)
Significant extended family members
Previous marriages, separations, death of spouses, or divorces

Home and Community Environment

Type of dwelling, number of rooms, occupants
Sleeping arrangements
Number of floors, accessibility of stairs and elevators
Adequacy of utilities
Safety features (fire escape, smoke and carbon monoxide detectors, guardrails on windows, use of car restraint)
Environmental hazards (e.g., chipped paint, poor sanitation, pollution, heavy street traffic)
Availability and location of health care facilities, schools, play areas
Relationship with neighbors
Recent crises or changes in home
Child's reaction and adjustment to recent stresses

Occupation and Education of Family Members

Types of employment
Work schedules
Work satisfaction
Exposure to environmental or industrial hazards
Sources of income and adequacy
Effect of illness on financial status
Highest degree or grade level attained

Cultural and Religious Traditions

Religious beliefs and practices
Cultural and ethnic beliefs and practices
Language spoken in home
Assessment questions include the following:

- Does the family identify with a religious or ethnic group? Are both parents from that group?
- How is religious or ethnic background part of family life?
- What special religious or cultural traditions are practiced in the home (e.g., food choices and preparation)?
- Where were family members born, and how long have they lived in this country?
- What language does the family speak most frequently?
- Do they speak and understand English?
- What do they believe causes health or illness?
- What religious or ethnic beliefs influence the family's perception of illness and its treatment?
- What methods are used to prevent or treat illness?
- How does the family know when a health problem needs medical attention?
- Who does the family contact when a member is ill?
- Does the family rely on cultural or religious healers or remedies? If so, ask them to describe the type of healer or remedy.
- Who does the family go to for support (clergy, medical healer, relatives)?
- Does the family experience discrimination because of their race, beliefs, or practices? Ask them to describe.

Functional Assessment Areas

Family Interactions and Roles

Interactions refer to ways in which family members relate to each other. The chief concern is the amount of intimacy and closeness among the members, especially spouses.

Roles refer to behaviors of people as they assume a different status or position.

Observations include the following:

- Family members' responses to each other (cordial, hostile, cool, loving, patient, short tempered)
- Obvious roles of leadership versus submission
- Support and attention shown to various members

Assessment questions include the following:

- What activities does the family perform together?
- Who do family members talk to when something is bothering them?
- What are family members' household chores?
- Who usually oversees what is happening with the children, such as at school or health care?
- How easy or difficult is it for the family to change or accept new responsibilities for household tasks?

Power, Decision Making, and Problem Solving

Power refers to individual member's control over others in family; it is manifested through family decision making and problem solving.

Chief concern is clarity of boundaries of power between parents and children.

One method of assessment involves offering a hypothetical conflict or problem, such as a child failing school, and asking family how they would handle this situation.

Assessment questions include the following:

- Who usually makes the decisions in the family?
- If one parent makes a decision, can the child appeal to the other parent to change it?
- What input do children have in making decisions or discussing rules?
- Who makes and enforces the rules?
- What happens when a rule is broken?

Communication

Communication is concerned with clarity and directness of communication patterns.

Further assessment includes periodically asking family members if they understood what was just said and to repeat the message.

Observations include the following:

- Who speaks to whom
- If one person speaks for another or interrupts
- If members appear uninterested when certain individuals speak
- If there is agreement between verbal and nonverbal messages

Assessment questions include the following:

Continued

BOX 4.7 Family Assessment Interview—cont'd

- How often do family members wait until others are through talking before "having their say?"
- Do parents or older siblings tend to lecture and preach?
- Do parents tend to "talk down" to the children?

Expression of Feelings and Individuality

Expressions are concerned with personal space and freedom to grow, with limits and structure needed for guidance.

Observing patterns of communication offers clues to how freely feelings are expressed.

Assessment questions include the following:

- Is it okay for family members to get angry or sad?
- Who gets angry most of the time? What do they do?
- If someone is upset, how do other family members try to comfort this person?
- Who comforts specific family members?
- When someone wants to do something, such as try out for a new sport or get a job, what is the family's response (offer assistance, discouragement, or no advice)?

NURSING CARE GUIDELINES

Review of Systems

Constitutional: Overall state of health, fatigue, recent or unexplained weight gain or loss (period of time for either), contributing factors (change of diet, illness, altered appetite), exercise tolerance, fevers (time of day), chills, night sweats (unrelated to weather conditions), general ability to carry out activities of daily living

Integument: Pruritus, pigment or other color changes (including birthmarks), acne, eruptions, rashes (location), bruises, petechiae, excessive dryness, general texture, tattoos or piercings, disorders or deformities of nails, hair growth or loss, excess body hair, hair color change (for adolescents, use of hair dyes or other potentially toxic substances, such as hair straighteners)

Eyes: No eye contact in an infant after 8 weeks of age, head tilt or face turn, visual problems (behaviors indicative of poor vision, such as bumping into objects, clumsiness, sitting close to television, holding a book close to face, writing with head near desk, squinting, rubbing the eyes, bending head in an awkward position), crossed eyes or lazy eye (strabismus), eye infections, edema of lids, excessive tearing, photophobia, use of glasses or contact lenses, date of last vision examination

Ears: Earaches, ear discharge, evidence of hearing loss (ask about behaviors, such as the need to repeat requests, loud speech, lack of response to noises, inattentive behavior), results of any previous auditory testing

Nose: Nosebleeds (epistaxis), constant or frequent runny or stuffy nose, nasal obstruction (difficulty breathing through nose), alteration or loss of sense of smell

Mouth: Mouth breathing, gum bleeding, number of teeth and pattern of eruption and loss, toothaches, tooth brushing, use of fluoride, difficulty with teething (symptoms), last visit to dentist (especially if temporary dentition is complete)

Throat: Sore throats, difficulty swallowing, choking, hoarseness or other voice irregularities

Neck: Pain, limitation of movement, stiffness, difficulty holding head straight (torticollis), thyroid enlargement, enlarged nodes or other masses

Chest: Breast enlargement, discharge, masses; for adolescent girls, ask about breast self-examination

Respiratory: Chronic cough, wheezing, shortness of breath at rest or on exertion, difficulty breathing, snoring, sputum production, infections (pneumonia, tuberculosis), skin reaction from tuberculin testing

Cardiovascular: Cyanosis or fatigue on exertion, history of heart murmur or rheumatic fever, tachycardia, syncope, edema

Gastrointestinal: Appetite, nausea, vomiting (not associated with eating; may be indicative of brain tumor or increased intracranial pressure), abdominal pain, jaundice or yellowing skin or sclera, belching, flatulence, distention, diarrhea, constipation, recent change in bowel habits, blood in stools

Genitourinary: Pain on urination, frequency, hesitancy, urgency, hematuria, nocturia, polyuria, enuresis, unpleasant odor to urine, force of stream, discharge, change in size of scrotum, date and result of last urinalysis; for adolescents, sexually transmitted infection and type of treatment; for adolescent boys, ask about testicular self-examination

Gynecologic: Menarche (date of and age at the first occurrence of menstruation), date of last menstrual period, regularity or problems with menstruation, vaginal discharge, pruritus; if sexually active, type of contraception, sexually transmitted infection and type of treatment; if sexually active with weakened immune system or if 21 years old and older, date and result of last Papanicolaou (Pap) smear; obstetric history (as discussed under birth history, when applicable)

Musculoskeletal: Weakness, clumsiness, lack of coordination, unusual movements, scoliosis, back pain, joint pain or swelling, muscle pains or cramps, abnormal gait, deformity, fractures, serious sprains, activity level

Neurologic: Headaches, seizures, tremors, tics, dizziness, head injury (specific details), loss of consciousness episodes, loss of memory, developmental delays or concerns

Endocrine: Intolerance to heat or cold, excessive thirst or urination, excessive sweating, salt craving, rapid or slow growth, signs of early or late puberty (regardless of age)

Hematologic/lymphatic: Easy bruising or bleeding, anemia, date and result of last blood count, blood transfusions, swollen or painful lymph nodes (cervical, axillary, inguinal)

Allergic/immunologic: Allergic responses, anaphylaxis, eczema, rhinitis, unusual sneezing, autoimmunity, recurrent infections, infections associated with unusual complications

Psychiatric: General affect, anxiety, depression, mood changes, hallucinations, attention span, tantrums, behavior problems, suicidal ideation, substance abuse

Begin the review of a specific system with a broad statement (e.g., "How has your child's general health been?" or "Has your child had any problems with his eyes?"). If the parent states that the child has had problems with some body function, pursue this with an encouraging statement, such as "Tell me more about that." If the parent denies any problems, query for specific symptoms (e.g., "Any headaches, bumping into objects, or squinting?"). If the parent confirms the absence of such symptoms, record positive statements in the history, such as "Mother denies headaches, bumping into objects, and squinting." In this way, anyone who reviews the health history is aware of exactly what symptoms were investigated.

NUTRITIONAL ASSESSMENT[b]

DIETARY INTAKE

To best understand a child's health and growth pattern, the nurse needs to assess the child's nutritional status. Obtaining a dietary intake history is an essential component of a nutritional assessment, but it can be one of the most difficult factors to assess due to variance in both types and portions of food consumed. A diet recall of children and adolescents is prone to error, with underreporting being commonplace. Difficulties also lie in cross-cultural communication where people of different ethnic origin may have difficulty adequately describing foods unique to their culture's cuisine. Despite these obstacles, a dietary evaluation is a vital element of the child's health assessment and should be approached in a neutral, judgment-free way for most accurate results.

The Dietary Reference Intakes (DRIs) are a set of four evidence-based nutrient reference values that provide quantitative estimates of nutrient intake for use in assessing and planning dietary intake (US Department of Agriculture, National Agricultural Library, 2014). The specific DRIs are:

Estimated Average Requirement (EAR): Estimated to meet the nutrient requirement of half of healthy individuals for a specific age and gender group

Recommended Dietary Allowance (RDA): Sufficient to meet the nutrient requirement of nearly all healthy individuals for a specific age and gender group

Adequate Intake (AI): Based on estimates of nutrient intake by healthy individuals

Tolerable Upper Intake Level (UL): Highest nutrient intake level likely to pose no risk of adverse health effects

The US Department of Agriculture has an online interactive DRI tool that health care professionals can use to calculate nutrient requirements based on age, gender, height, weight, and activity, although it is important to note that individual requirements may vary (available at http://fnic.nal.usda.gov/fnic/interactiveDRI/).

Fig. 4.4 illustrates ChooseMyPlate.gov, which describes the five food groups that form the foundation for a healthy diet. MyPlate Kids' Place provides resources that promote healthy meal planning and physical activity. Specific questions used to conduct a nutritional assessment are given in Box 4.8. Every nutritional assessment should begin with a dietary history. The questions used by the nurse for a child's dietary history during periods of rapid growth and development should elicit a response that is detailed and specific, and questions may be adapted as the child grows in age. The overview elicited from the dietary history can be helpful in evaluating food frequency records. The history is also concerned with financial and cultural factors that influence food selection and preparation (see Cultural Considerations box).

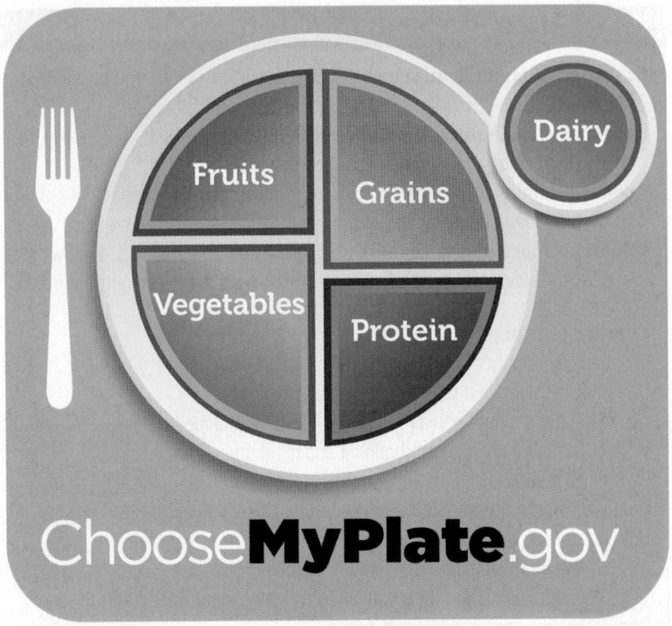

Fig. 4.4 MyPlate advocates building a healthy plate by making half of one's plate fruits and vegetables and the other half grains and lean protein. Avoiding oversized portions, making half of grains whole grains and drinking fat-free or low-fat (1%) milk are among the recommendations for a healthy diet. (From US Department of Agriculture, Center for Nutrition Policy and Promotion. [2015]. *MyPlate.*http://www.ChooseMyPlate.gov.)

CULTURAL CONSIDERATIONS

Food Practices

Because cultural practices are prevalent in food preparation, consider carefully the questions that are asked and the judgments made during counseling. For example, some cultures, such as Hispanic, African American, and American Indian, include many vegetables, legumes, and starches in their diet that together provide sufficient essential amino acids even though the actual amount of meat or dairy protein is low.

The simplest method of assessing daily intake is the 24-hour recall. This involves the child or parent recalling the approximate portion of all foods and liquids consumed in the most recent 24-hour period. This method is most beneficial when history represents a typical day's intake. To increase accuracy of a patient or family's report of portion sizes consumed, it is helpful to use three-dimensional (3D) food models or pictures. In general, this method is most useful in providing *qualitative* information about the child's diet.

To further improve the reliability of the daily recall, the family can complete a food diary by recording every food and liquid consumed for a certain number of days in some sort of chart or log. A 3-day record consisting of 2 weekdays and 1 weekend day is representative for most people. Providing specific charts to record intake can improve overall patient compliance and follow-up.

CLINICAL EXAMINATION OF NUTRITION

A significant amount of information regarding nutritional deficiencies comes from a clinical examination, especially from assessing the child's growth, skeletal development, skin, hair, nails, eyes, mouth, and teeth. Hair, skin, and mouth are vulnerable because of the rapid turnover of epithelial and mucosal tissue. Table 4.1 summarizes some clinical signs of possible nutritional deficiencies. If suspicious signs are found, they must be confirmed with both dietary and biochemical data. Failure to thrive is discussed in Chapter 10. Obesity and eating disorders are discussed in Chapter 16.

Anthropometry, an essential parameter of nutritional status, is the measurement of height (length), weight, head circumference, proportions, skinfold thickness, and arm circumference in children. Height and head circumference reflect quality of nutrition over longer periods of time, whereas weight, skinfold thickness, arm circumference, muscle, and fat stores reflect present nutritional status and are prone to rapid change depending on overall dietary intake. Skinfold thickness is a measurement of the body's fat content, as approximately half of the body's total fat stores are directly beneath the skin. The mid-upper arm circumference is correlated with measurements of total muscle mass. Because muscle serves as the body's major protein reserve, this measurement is considered an index of the body's protein stores and therefore is one objective factor to

[b]Caroline C. Weeks, BS, BA, RDN, LD, updated this section.

BOX 4.8 Assessment of Nutritional Intake

Estimated Average Requirement (EAR): Used to examine the possibility of inadequacy.

Recommended Dietary Allowance (RDA): Dietary intake at or above this level usually has a low probability of inadequacy.

Adequate Intake (AI): Dietary intake at or above this level usually has a low probability of inadequacy.

Tolerable Upper Intake Level (UL): Dietary intake above this level usually places an individual at risk of adverse effects from excessive nutrient intake.

Dietary History

What are the family's usual mealtimes?
Do family members eat together or at separate times?
Are there distractions such as TV or electronics during mealtimes?
Who does the family grocery shopping and meal preparation?
How much money is spent to buy food each week?
How are most foods prepared—baked, broiled, fried, other?
How often does the family or your child eat out?

- What kinds of restaurants do you go to?
- What kinds of food does your child typically eat at restaurants?

Does your child eat breakfast regularly?
Where does your child eat lunch?
What are your child's favorite foods, beverages, and snacks?

- What are the average amounts eaten per day?
- What foods are artificially sweetened?
- What are your child's snacking habits?
- When are sweet foods usually eaten?
- What are your child's tooth brushing habits?

Do you notice your child waking during the night to eat?
What special cultural practices are followed? What ethnic foods are eaten?
What foods and beverages does your child dislike?
How would you describe your child's usual appetite (hearty eater, picky eater)?
What are your child's feeding habits (breast, bottle, cup, spoon, eats by self, needs assistance, any special devices)?
Does your child take vitamins or other supplements? Do they contain iron or fluoride?
Does your child have any known or suspected food allergies? Is your child on a special diet?
Has your child lost or gained weight recently? How much?
Are there any feeding problems (excessive fussiness, spitting up, colic, difficulty sucking or swallowing)?
Are there any dental problems or appliances, such as braces, that affect eating?
What types of exercise does your child do regularly?
Is there a family history of cancer, diabetes, heart disease, high blood pressure, gastrointestinal disease, eating disorders, or obesity?

Additional Questions for Infants

What was the infant's birth weight? When did it double? Triple?
Was the infant premature?
Are you breastfeeding or have you breastfed your infant? How long?

- How long does a typical breastfeeding session last?
- Does the infant nurse from both breasts?

If you use a formula, what is the brand?

- How are you preparing the formula?
- How many ounces does the infant drink at a time? How often?

Have you introduced cow's milk? If so, what kind (whole, low fat, skim)?

- At what age did you start?
- How many ounces does the infant drink a day?

Do you give your infant extra fluids (water, juice)?
If the infant takes a bottle to bed at nap or nighttime, what is in the bottle?
At what age did the child start cereal, vegetables, meat or other protein sources, fruit or juice, finger food, and table food?
Do you make your own baby food or use commercial foods, such as infant cereal?
Has the infant had an allergic reaction to any food(s)? If so, list the foods and describe the reaction.
Does the infant spit up frequently; have unusually loose stools; or have hard, dry stools? If so, how often?
How often do you feed your infant?
Does your infant show eagerness to eat?
Does the infant take a vitamin or mineral supplement? If so, what type?

Modified from Murphy, S. P., & Poos, M. I. (2002). Dietary reference intakes: Summary of applications in dietary assessment. *Public Health Nutrition, 5*(Suppl. 6A), 843–849.

TABLE 4.1 Nutrition-Focused Clinical Findings

Normal Findings	Abnormal Findings	Possible Nutrient Deficiencies
Physical Growth		
Normal weight gain and linear growth for age and gender	Weight loss, poor weight gain, linear growth failure	Protein, fat, calories, zinc, iodine, sodium, other essential nutrients
Normal skeletal development without obvious deformity	Kyphosis, genu varum (bowing of extremities) or genu valgum (knock knees), rickets, history of nontraumatic fractures	Calcium, vitamin D, phosphorus
Skin		
Smooth, slightly dry to touch, elastic and firm, absence of lesions, uniform color appropriate to genetic background	Dry, rough, scaly	Vitamin A, essential fatty acids
	Dermatitis	Essential fatty acids, zinc, niacin, riboflavin, tryptophan
	Petechiae	Riboflavin, vitamin C
	Delayed wound healing	Vitamin C, zinc
	Scaly dermatitis on exposed surfaces	Riboflavin, vitamin C, zinc, niacin, tryptophan
	Wrinkled, flabby	Niacin
	Crusted lesions around orifices, especially nares	Protein, calories, zinc
	Poor turgor	Water, sodium
	Depigmentation	Protein, calories
	Pallor (anemia)	Iron, folic acid; vitamins B_{12}, C, and E (in premature infants); pyridoxine

TABLE 4.1 Nutrition-Focused Clinical Findings—cont'd

Normal Findings	Abnormal Findings	Possible Nutrient Deficiencies
Hair		
Lustrous, silky smooth, strong, elastic, distributed symmetrically	Stringy, friable, dull, dry, thin	Protein, calories, zinc, biotin, essential fatty acids
	Alopecia	Protein, calories, zinc, biotin, essential fatty acids, selenium
	Depigmentation	Protein, calories, copper
	Raised areas around hair follicles	Vitamin C
Nails		
Symmetric and smooth	Transverse lines	Protein
	Flaky	Magnesium
	Poorly blanched	Vitamins A and D
	Brittle nails, spooning	Iron
Eyes		
Clear, bright, moist	Dull, dry with Bitot spots (buildup of keratin superficially in the conjunctiva)	Vitamin A
Good night vision	Night blindness	Vitamin A
Conjunctiva—pink, glossy, tolerates light exposure	Burning, itching, photophobia	Riboflavin
Mouth		
Lips—smooth, moist, darker color than skin, absence of lesions	Fissures and inflammation at corners	Riboflavin
	Dry, swollen	Vitamins B_6 and B_{12}, iron, folate, riboflavin, niacin
Gums—firm, pink, stippled	Spongy, friable, inflamed, bluish red or black, bleed easily	Vitamin C
Mucous membranes—bright pink, smooth, moist	Stomatitis	Niacin
	Dry mucous membranes	Water, zinc
Tongue—moist pink with slightly rough texture, no lesions, normal taste sensation	Glossitis (swollen, inflamed, smooth, and dark red)	Niacin, riboflavin, folate, vitamins B_6 and B_{12}, iron
	Diminished taste sensation	Zinc
Teeth—uniform white color, smooth, intact; normal eruption begins at 4-12 months	Defective enamel	Vitamins A, C, and D; calcium; phosphorus
	Caries	Fluoride, vitamin D
	Delayed dentition	Malnutrition

Adapted from Green Corkins, K., & Teague, E. E. (2017). Pediatric nutrition assessment: Anthropometrics to zinc. *Nutrition in Clinical Practice, 32*(1), 40–51; National Institutes of Health, Office of Dietary Supplements. (n.d.). Vitamin and mineral fact sheets. Retrieved from https://ods.od.nih.gov/factsheets/list-VitaminsMinerals/

consider when diagnosing pediatric malnutrition. Ideally, growth measurements are recorded over time, and comparisons are made regarding the velocity of growth and weight gain based on previous and present values.

Numerous **biochemical tests** may be used, when needed, to complement a clinical nutritional assessment. The most common laboratory studies to assess children for undernutrition are hemoglobin, red blood cell indices, ferritin, albumin, and prealbumin. When albumin or prealbumin is low, inflammatory markers such as C-reactive protein can help determine if levels are reduced due to an inflammatory process or infection, or due to inadequate substrate. Other labs may be needed based on history and physical findings. For obese children, fasting serum glucose, lipids, and liver function studies may be performed to assess for complications.

EVALUATION OF NUTRITIONAL ASSESSMENT

After collecting the data needed for a thorough nutritional assessment, evaluate the findings to plan appropriate counseling. From the data, assess whether the child is malnourished, at risk for becoming malnourished, well-nourished with adequate reserves, or overweight or obese.

Analyze the daily food diary for the variety and amounts of foods suggested in MyPlate (see Fig. 4.4). For example, if the list includes no vegetables, inquire about this rather than assuming that the child dislikes vegetables, because it is possible that none were served that day. Also, evaluate the information in terms of the family's ethnic practices and financial resources. Encouraging increased protein intake with additional meat is not always feasible for families on a limited budget and may conflict with food practices that use meat sparingly, such as in Asian meal preparation.

GENERAL APPROACHES TO EXAMINING THE CHILD

SEQUENCE OF THE EXAMINATION

Ordinarily, the sequence for examining patients follows a head-to-toe direction. The main function of such a systematic approach is to provide a general guideline for assessment of each body area to avoid omitting segments of the examination. The standard recording of data also facilitates exchange of information among different professionals. In examining children, this orderly sequence is frequently altered to accommodate the child's developmental needs, although the examination is recorded following the head-to-toe model. Using developmental and chronologic age as the main criteria for assessing each body system accomplishes several goals:

- Minimizes stress and anxiety associated with assessment of various body parts
- Fosters a trusting nurse-child-parent relationship
- Allows for maximum preparation of the child
- Preserves the essential security of the parent-child relationship, especially with young children
- Maximizes the accuracy and reliability of assessment findings

PREPARATION OF THE CHILD

Although the physical examination consists of painless procedures, for some children the use of a tight arm cuff, probes in the ears and mouth, pressure on the abdomen, and a cold piece of metal to listen to the chest are stressful. Therefore the nurse should use the same considerations discussed in Chapter 20 for preparing children for procedures. In addition to that discussion, general guidelines related to the examining process are given in the Nursing Care Guidelines box.

NURSING CARE GUIDELINES

Performing Pediatric Physical Examination

Perform the examination in an appropriate, nonthreatening area:

- Have room well lit and decorated with neutral colors.
- Have room temperature comfortably warm.
- Place all strange and potentially frightening equipment out of sight.
- Have some toys and games available for child.
- If possible, have rooms decorated and equipped for children of different ages.
- Provide privacy, especially for school-age children and adolescents.
- Provide time for play and becoming acquainted.

Observe behaviors that signal child's readiness to cooperate:

- Talking to the nurse
- Making eye contact
- Accepting the offered equipment
- Allowing physical touching
- Choosing to sit on the examining table rather than parent's lap

If signs of readiness are not observed, use the following techniques:

- Talk to parent while essentially "ignoring" child; gradually focus on child or a favorite object, such as a doll.
- Make complimentary remarks about child, such as about his or her appearance, dress, or a favorite object.
- Tell a funny story or play a simple magic trick.
- Have a nonthreatening "friend" available, such as a hand puppet to "talk" to child for the nurse (see Fig. 4.26A).

If child refuses to cooperate, use the following techniques:

- Assess reason for uncooperative behavior; consider that a child who is unduly afraid may have had a traumatic experience.
- Try to involve child and parent in process.
- Avoid prolonged explanations about examining procedure.
- Use a firm, direct approach regarding expected behavior.
- Perform examination as quickly as possible.
- Have attendant gently restrain child.
- Minimize any disruptions or stimulation.
- Limit number of people in room.
- Use isolated room.
- Use quiet, calm, confident voice.

Begin the examination in a nonthreatening manner for young children or children who are fearful:

- Use activities that can be presented as games, such as test for cranial nerves (see Table 4.11) or parts of developmental screening tests (see Chapter 3).
- Use approaches such as Simon Says to encourage child to make a face, squeeze a hand, stand on one foot, and so on.
- Use paper-doll technique:
  1. Lay child supine on an examining table or floor that is covered with a large sheet of paper.
  2. Trace around child's body outline.
  3. Use body outline to demonstrate what will be examined, such as drawing a heart and listening with a stethoscope before performing activity on the child.

If several children in the family will be examined, begin with the most cooperative child to model desired behavior.

Involve the child in examination process:

- Provide choices, such as sitting on table or in parent's lap.
- Allow child to handle or hold equipment.
- Encourage child to use equipment on a doll, family member, or examiner.
- Explain each step of the procedure in simple language.

Examine child in a comfortable and secure position:

- Sitting on parent's lap
- Sitting upright if in respiratory distress

Proceed to examine the body in an organized sequence (usually head to toe) with the following exceptions:

- Alter sequence to accommodate needs of children of different ages (Table 4.2).
- Examine painful areas last.
- In an emergency, examine vital functions (airway, breathing, and circulation) and injured area first.

Reassure child throughout the examination, especially about bodily concerns that arise during puberty.

Discuss findings with family at the end of the examination.

Praise child for cooperation during the examination; give a reward such as a small toy or sticker.

The physical examination should be as pleasant as possible, as well as educational. The paper-doll technique is a useful approach to teaching children about the body part that is being examined (Fig. 4.5). At the conclusion of the visit, the child can bring home the paper doll as a memento.

Table 4.2 summarizes guidelines for positioning, preparing, and examining children at various ages. Because the child may not fit precisely into one age category, it may be necessary to vary the approach after a preliminary assessment of the child's developmental achievements and needs. Even with the best approach, many toddlers are uncooperative and inconsolable for much of the physical examination. However, some seem intrigued by the new surroundings and unusual equipment and respond more like preschoolers than toddlers. Likewise, some early preschoolers may require more of the "security

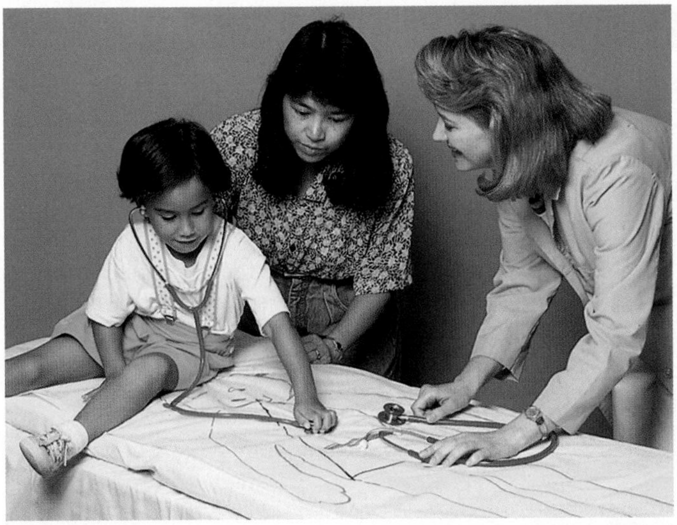

Fig. 4.5 Using the paper-doll technique to prepare a child for physical examination.

measures" used with younger children, such as continued parent-child contact, and fewer of the preparatory measures used with preschoolers, such as playing with the equipment before and during the actual examination (Fig. 4.6).

PHYSICAL EXAMINATION

Although the approach to and sequence of the physical examination differ according to the child's age and development, the following discussion outlines the traditional model for physical assessment. The focus includes all pediatric age-groups (see Chapter 7 for a detailed discussion of a newborn assessment). Because the physical examination is a vital part of preventive pediatric care, Fig. 4.7 gives a schedule for periodic health visits.

GROWTH MEASUREMENTS

Measurement of physical growth in children is a key element in evaluating their health status. Physical growth parameters include weight, height (length), skinfold thickness, arm circumference, and head

TABLE 4.2 Age-Specific Approaches to Physical Examination During Childhood

Position	Sequence	Preparation
Infant		
Before able to sit alone: supine or prone, preferably in parent's lap; before 4-6 months, can place on examining table After able to sit alone: sitting in parent's lap whenever possible; if on table, place with parent in full view	If quiet, auscultate heart, lungs, and abdomen. Record heart and respiratory rates. Palpate and percuss same areas. Proceed in usual head-to-toe direction. Perform traumatic procedures last (eyes, ears, mouth [while crying]). Elicit reflexes as body part is examined. Elicit Moro reflex last.	Completely undress if room temperature permits. Leave diaper on male infant. Gain cooperation with distraction, bright objects, rattles, talking. Smile at infant; use soft, gentle voice. Use pacifier (if used) or bottle with feeding (if bottle feeding). Enlist parent's aid for restraining to examine ears, mouth. Avoid abrupt, jerky movements.
Toddler		
Sitting on parent's lap or standing by parent Prone or supine in parent's lap	Inspect body area through play: "Count fingers," "tickle toes." Use minimum physical contact initially. Introduce equipment slowly. Auscultate, percuss, palpate whenever quiet. Perform traumatic procedures last (same as for infant).	Have parent remove outer clothing. Remove underwear as body part is examined. Allow toddler to inspect equipment; demonstrating use of equipment is usually ineffective. If uncooperative, perform procedures quickly. Use restraint when appropriate; request parent's assistance. Talk about examination if cooperative; use short phrases. Praise for cooperative behavior.
Preschool Child		
Prefer standing or sitting Usually cooperative prone or supine Prefer parent's closeness	If cooperative, proceed in head-to-toe direction. If uncooperative, proceed as with toddler.	Request self-undressing. Allow to wear underwear if shy. Offer equipment for inspection; briefly demonstrate use. Make up story about procedure (e.g., "I'm seeing how strong your muscles are" [blood pressure]). Use paper-doll technique. Give choices when possible. Expect cooperation; use positive statements (e.g., "Open your mouth.").

Continued

TABLE 4.2 Age-Specific Approaches to Physical Examination During Childhood—cont'd

Position	Sequence	Preparation
School-Age Child		
Prefer sitting Cooperative in most positions Younger child prefers parent's presence Older child may prefer privacy	Proceed in head-to-toe direction. May examine genitalia last in older child.	Respect need for privacy. Request self-undressing. Allow to wear underwear. Give gown to wear. Explain purpose of equipment and significance of procedure, such as otoscope to see tympanic membrane, which is necessary for hearing. Teach about body function and care.
Adolescent		
Same as for school-age child Offer option of parent's presence	Same as older school-age child. May examine genitalia last.	Allow to undress in private. Give gown. Expose only area to be examined. Respect need for privacy. Explain findings during examination (e.g., "Your muscles are firm and strong."). Matter-of-factly comment about sexual development (e.g., "Your breasts are developing as they should be."). Emphasize normalcy of development. Examine genitalia as any other body part; may leave to end.

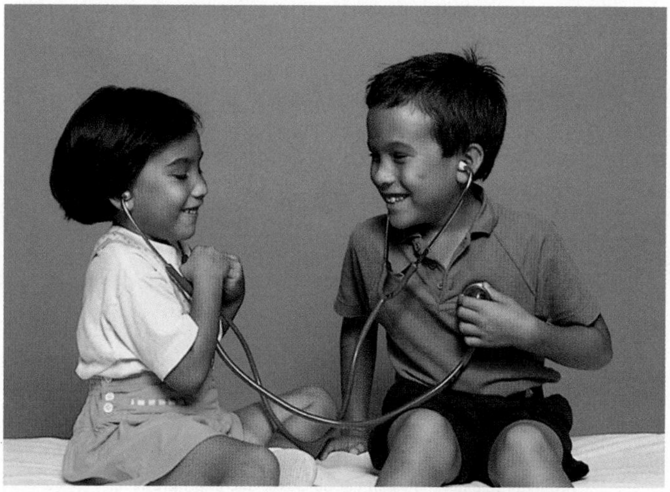

Fig. 4.6 Preparing children for physical examination.

circumference. Values for these growth parameters are plotted on percentile charts, and the child's measurements in percentiles are compared with those of the general population.

Growth Charts

Growth charts use a series of percentile curves to demonstrate the distribution of body measurements in children. The Centers for Disease Control and Prevention recommend that the World Health Organization growth standards be used to monitor growth for infants and children between the ages of 0 and 2 years. Because breastfeeding is the recommended standard for infant feeding, the World Health Organization growth charts are used; they reflect growth patterns among children who were predominately breastfed for at least 4 months and are still breastfeeding at 12 months old. The Centers for Disease Control and Prevention growth charts (http://www.cdc.gov/growthcharts) are used for children 2 years old and older.

Children whose growth may be questionable include:

- Children whose height and weight percentiles are widely disparate (e.g., height in the 10th percentile and weight in the 90th percentile, especially with above-average skinfold thickness)
- Children who fail to follow the expected growth velocity in height and weight
- Children who show a sudden increase or decrease in a previously steady growth pattern (i.e., crossing two major percentile lines, especially after 3 years old)
- Children who are short in the absence of short parents

Because growth is a continuous but uneven process, the most reliable evaluation lies in comparing growth measurements over time because they reflect change. It is important to remember that same-age, same-gender children (whether short, average, or tall in stature) should grow at similar rates (Fig. 4.8).

Length

The term **length** refers to measurements taken when children are supine (also referred to as **recumbent length**). Until children are 24 months old and able to stand alone (or 36 months old if using a chart for birth to 36 months), measure recumbent length using a length board and two measurers (Fig. 4.9A; see Translating Evidence Into Practice box). Because of the normally flexed position during infancy, fully extend the body by (1) holding the head in midline, (2) grasping the knees together gently, and (3) pushing down on the knees until the legs are fully extended and flat against the table. Place the head touching the headboard and the footboard firmly against the heels of both feet. A tape measure should not be used to measure the length of infants and children due to inaccuracy and unreliability (Foote, 2014; Foote, Brady, Burke, et al., 2011). Measure length to the last completed millimeter or 1/16 inch. Measure more than once and record the average length.

	INFANCY								EARLY CHILDHOOD						
AGE	Prenatal	Newborn	3-5 d	By 1 mo	2 mo	4 mo	6 mo	9 mo	12 mo	15 mo	18 mo	24 mo	30 mo	3 y	4 y
HISTORY Initial/Interval	●	●	●	●	●	●	●	●	●	●	●	●	●	●	●
MEASUREMENTS															
Length/Height and Weight		●	●	●	●	●	●	●	●	●	●	●	●	●	●
Head Circumference		●	●	●	●	●	●	●	●	●	●	●			
Weight for Length		●	●	●	●	●	●	●	●	●	●				
Body Mass Index												●	●	●	●
Blood Pressure		★	★	★	★	★	★	★	★	★	★	★	★	●	●
SENSORY SCREENING															
Vision		★	★	★	★	★	★	★	★	★	★	★	★	●	●
Hearing		●	● →	→	→	★	★	★	★	★	★	★	★	★	●
DEVELOPMENTAL/BEHAVIORAL HEALTH															
Developmental Screening								●			●		●		
Autism Spectrum Disorder Screening											●	●			
Developmental Surveillance		●	●	●	●	●	●		●	●		●		●	●
Psychosocial/Behavioral Assessment		●	●	●	●	●	●	●	●	●	●	●	●	●	●
Tobacco, Alcohol, or Drug Use Assessment															
Depression Screening															
Maternal Depression Screening				●	●	●	●								
PHYSICAL EXAMINATION		●	●	●	●	●	●	●	●	●	●	●	●	●	●
PROCEDURES															
Newborn Blood		●	● →	→	→										
Newborn Bilirubin		●													
Critical Congenital Heart Defect		●													
Immunization		●	●	●	●	●	●	●	●	●	●	●	●	●	●
Anemia						★			●	★	★	★	★	★	★
Lead							★	★	● ★		★	● ★		★	★
Tuberculosis				★			★		★			★		★	★
Dyslipidemia												★			★
Sexually Transmitted Infections															
HIV															
Cervical Dysplasia															
ORAL HEALTH							●	●	★		★	★	★	★	★
Fluoride Varnish							←	—	—	—	●	—	—	—	—
Fluoride Supplementation							★	★	★		★	★	★	★	★
ANTICIPATORY GUIDANCE	●	●	●	●	●	●	●	●	●	●	●	●	●	●	●

	MIDDLE CHILDHOOD						ADOLESCENCE							
AGE	5 y	6 y	7 y	8 y	9 y	10 y	11 y	12 y	13 y	14 y	15 y	16 y	17 y	18 y
HISTORY Initial/Interval	●	●	●	●	●	●	●	●	●	●	●	●	●	●
MEASUREMENTS														
Length/Height and Weight	●	●	●	●	●	●	●	●	●	●	●	●	●	●
Head Circumference														
Weight for Length														
Body Mass Index	●	●	●	●	●	●	●	●	●	●	●	●	●	●
Blood Pressure	●	●	●	●	●	●	●	●	●	●	●	●	●	●
SENSORY SCREENING														
Vision	●	●	★	●	★	●	★	●	★	★	●	★	★	★
Hearing	●	●	★	●	★	●	←	—	●	→	←	●	→	
DEVELOPMENTAL/BEHAVIORAL HEALTH														
Developmental Screening														
Autism Spectrum Disorder Screening														
Developmental Surveillance	●	●	●	●	●	●	●	●	●	●	●	●	●	●
Psychosocial/Behavioral Assessment	●	●	●	●	●	●	●	●	●	●	●	●	●	●
Tobacco, Alcohol, or Drug Use Assessment							★	★	★	★	★	★	★	★
Depression Screening								●	●	●	●	●	●	●
Maternal Depression Screening														
PHYSICAL EXAMINATION	●	●	●	●	●	●	●	●	●	●	●	●	●	●
PROCEDURES														
Newborn Blood														
Newborn Bilirubin														
Critical Congenital Heart Defect														
Immunization	●	●	●	●	●	●	●	●	●	●	●	●	●	●
Anemia	★	★	★	★	★	★	★	★	★	★	★	★	★	★
Lead	★	★												
Tuberculosis	★	★	★	★	★	★	★	★	★	★	★	★	★	★
Dyslipidemia		★		★	←	●	→	★	★	★	★	★		
Sexually Transmitted Infections							★	★	★	★	★	★	★	★
HIV							★	★	★	★	←	—	●	→
Cervical Dysplasia														
ORAL HEALTH	★	★												
Fluoride Varnish	→													
Fluoride Supplementation	★	★	★	★	★	★	★	★	★	★	★	★		
ANTICIPATORY GUIDANCE	●	●	●	●	●	●	●	●	●	●	●	●	●	●

KEY: ● = to be performed ★ = risk assessment to be performed with appropriate action to follow, if positive ←●→ = range during which a service may be provided

BFNC 2019.PSMAR 3-351/0319

Fig. 4.7 Preventive pediatric health care chart. (Adapted from American Academy of Pediatrics Committee on Practice and Ambulatory Medicine, Bright Futures Periodicity Schedule Workgroup. [2015]. *2015 Recommendations for pediatric preventive pediatric health care*. Retrieved from https://www.aap.org/en-us/professional-resources/practice-support/Periodicity/Periodicity%20Schedule_FINAL.pdf)

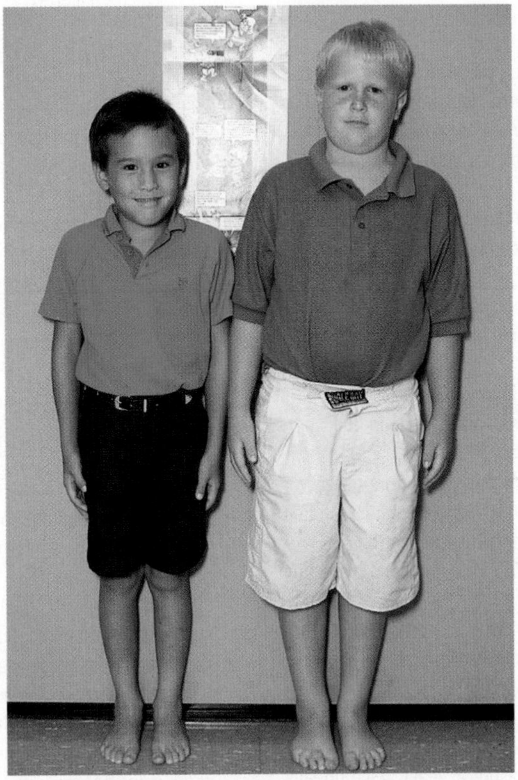

Fig. 4.8 These children of identical age (8 years) are markedly different in size. The child on the left, of Asian descent, is at the 5th percentile for height and weight. The child on the right is above the 95th percentile for height and weight. However, both children demonstrate normal growth patterns.

TRANSLATING EVIDENCE INTO PRACTICE

Linear Growth Measurement in Pediatrics

Ask the Question

PICOT Question

In children, what are the best instruments and techniques to measure linear growth (length and height)?

Search for the Evidence

Search Strategies

Search selection criteria: English language, research-based and review articles and expert opinion from databases, anthropometric and endocrinology textbooks, contact with experts in the field, and informal discovery

Key terms: Length, height, stature, infant, child, adolescent, measurement, instrument, length board, stadiometer, calibration, technique, accuracy, reliability, diurnal variation

Exclusion criteria: Other types of anthropometric measurements, adults

Databases Used

MEDLINE, CINAHL, COCHRANE, EMBASE, OCLC, ERIC, National Guideline Clearinghouse (AHRQ)

Critical Appraisal of the Evidence

An interdisciplinary team systematically and critically appraised the evidence to develop these clinical practice recommendations using an evidence-based practice rating scheme (Foote, Brady, Burke, et al., 2009; Foote, Brady, Burke, et al., 2011; US Preventive Services Task Force, 1996).

Measure recumbent length in children younger than 24 to 36 months old and in children who cannot stand alone (Foote, 2014; Foote, Brady, Burke, et al., 2011) (see Fig. 4.9A).

- Use a length board with these components: Flat, horizontal surface with stationary headboard and smoothly movable footboard, both at 90-degree angles to the horizontal surface, and attached ruler marked in millimeter and/or ¹⁄₁₆-inch increments. Tape measures alone, which are inaccurate and unreliable, should never be used.
- Cover length board with clean, soft, thin cloth or paper.
- Remove all clothing and shoes. Remove or loosen diaper. Remove hair ornaments on crown of head.
- Two measurers are required to accomplish correct positioning; one measurer (assistant) can be a parent or other caregiver when procedures are explained and understood.
- Place child supine on length board. Never leave unattended.
- Assistant holds head in midline with crown of head against headboard, compressing the hair.
- Position head in the Frankfort vertical plane (imaginary line from the lower border of the orbit through the highest point of the auditory meatus; the line is parallel to the headboard and perpendicular to the length board).
- Lead measurer positions the body on length board with one hand placed on both legs to fully extend the body.
- Ensure that head remains against headboard, shoulders and hips are not rotated, back is not arched, and legs are not bent. Reposition as necessary.
- Using the other hand, lead measurer moves footboard against heels of both feet with toes pointing upward.
- Read measurement to the last completed millimeter or ¹⁄₁₆ inch.
- Reposition the child and repeat procedure. Measure at least twice (ideally three times). Average the measurements for the final value. Record immediately.

Measure height in children 24 to 36 months old and older who can stand alone well (Foote, 2014; Foote, Brady, Burke, et al., 2011) (see Fig. 4.9B).

- Use a stadiometer with these components: Vertical surface to stand against, footboard or firm surface to stand on, movable horizontal headboard at 90-degree angle to the vertical surface, and attached ruler marked in millimeter and/or ¹⁄₁₆-inch increments. Wall charts and flip-up horizontal bars (floppy-arm devices) mounted to weighing scales, which are inaccurate and unreliable, should never be used.
- Remove shoes and heavy outer clothing. Remove hair ornaments and undo hairstyles (e.g., braids or buns) on crown of head.
- Stand child on flat surface with back against vertical surface of stadiometer.
- Weight is evenly distributed on both feet with heels together.
- Occiput, scapulae, buttocks, and heels are in contact with vertical surface.
- Encourage child to maintain fully erect position with positional lordosis minimized, knees fully extended, and heels flat. Reposition as necessary.
- Child continues normal breathing with shoulders relaxed and arms hanging down freely.
- Position head in the horizontal Frankfort plane (imaginary line from the lower border of the orbit through the highest point of the auditory meatus; the line is parallel to the headboard and perpendicular to the vertical surface).
- Move headboard down to crown of head, compressing the hair.
- Read measurement at eye level (to avoid parallax error) to the last completed millimeter or ¹⁄₁₆ inch.
- Reposition the child and repeat procedure. Measure at least twice (ideally three times). Average the measurements for the final value. Record immediately.

Special considerations (Foote, 2014; Foote, Brady, Burke, et al., 2009; Lohman, Roche, & Martorell, 1988).

- Some children, such as those who are obese, may not be able to place their occiput, scapulae, buttocks, and heels all in one vertical plane while maintaining their balance, so use at least two of the four contact points.
- If a child has a leg length discrepancy, place a block or wedge of suitable height under the shortest leg until the pelvis is level and both knees are fully extended before measuring height. To measure length, keep the legs together and measure to the heel of the longest leg.
- Children with special health care needs may require alternative measurements, such as arm span, crown-to-rump length, sitting height, knee height, or other segmental lengths. In general, when recumbent length is measured in a child with spasticity or contractures, measure the side of the body that is unaffected or less affected.
- Always document the presence of any condition that may interfere with an accurate and reliable measurement.

Quality control measures (Foote, 2014; Foote, Brady, Burke, et al., 2009; Foote, Brady, Burke, et al., 2011; Foote, Kirouac, & Lipman, 2015).

- Personnel who measure the growth of infants, children, and adolescents need proper education. Competency should be demonstrated. Refresher sessions should occur when a lack of standardization occurs.
- Length boards and stadiometers must be assembled and installed properly and calibrated at regular intervals (ideally daily, at least monthly, and every time they are moved) due to frequent inaccuracy and the variability between different instruments. Calibration can be performed by measuring a rod of known length and adjusting the instrument accordingly.
- All children should be measured at least twice (ideally three times) during each encounter. The measurements should agree within 0.5 cm (ideally 0.3 cm). Use the mean value. If the variation exceeds the limit of agreement, measure again and use the mean of the measures in closest agreement. If none of the measures are within the limit of agreement, then (1) have another measurer assist, (2) check technique, and (3) consider another education session.
- Children between 24 and 36 months of age may have length and/or height measured. Standing height is less than recumbent length due to gravity and compression of the spine. Plot length measurements on a length curve and height measurements on a height curve to avoid misinterpreting the growth pattern.

TRANSLATING EVIDENCE INTO PRACTICE—cont'd

Linear Growth Measurement in Pediatrics

Apply the Evidence: Nursing Implications

Growth is well established as an important and sensitive indicator of health in children. Abnormal growth is a common consequence of many conditions; therefore its measurement can be a useful warning of possible pathology. In a study of 55 primary care practices within 8 geographic areas in the United States, only 30% of children were measured accurately due to faulty instruments and casual techniques; an educational intervention increased measurement accuracy to 70% (Lipman, Hench, Benyi, et al., 2004). Measurement error influences growth assessment and can result in delayed evaluation and treatment of some children, as well as apparent growth deviation in others who are growing normally (Foote, 2014; Foote, Kirouac, & Lipman, 2015). There is good evidence with strong recommendations for using length boards and stadiometers, the described measurement techniques, and the quality control measures. There is fair evidence to recommend procedures for children with special needs (Foote, Brady, Burke, et al., 2009; Lohman, Roche, & Martorell, 1988).

Quality and Safety Competencies: Evidence-Based Practice[a]

Knowledge

Differentiate clinical opinion from research and evidence-based summaries.

Describe the appropriate instruments and techniques to obtain accurate and reliable linear growth measurements of children.

Skills

Base individualized care plan on patient values, clinical expertise, and evidence.

Integrate evidence into practice by using the instruments and techniques for linear growth measurement in clinical care.

Attitudes

Value the concept of evidence-based practice as integral to determining best clinical practice.

Appreciate strengths and weaknesses of evidence for measuring the linear growth of children.

References

Foote, J. M. (2014). Optimizing linear growth measurement in children. *Journal of Pediatric Health Care, 28(5),* 413–419.

Foote, J. M., Brady, L. H., Burke, A. L., Cook, J. S., Dutcher, M. E., Gradoville, K. M., & Walker, B. S. (2009). *Evidence-based clinical practice guideline on linear growth measurement of children.* Retrieved from https://www.unitypoint.org/blankchildrens/education-resources.aspx (to access full-text guideline and implementation tools).

Foote, J. M., Brady, L. H., Burke, A. L., Cook, J. S., Dutcher, M. E., Gradoville, K. M., & Phillips, K. T. (2011). Development of an evidence-based clinical practice guideline on linear growth measurement of children. *Journal of Pediatric Nursing, 26(4),* 312–324.

Foote, J. M., Kirouac, N., & Lipman, T. H. (2015). PENS position statement on linear growth measurement of children. *Journal of Pediatric Nursing, 30(2),* 425–426.

Lipman, T. H., Hench, K. D., Benyi, T., Delaune, J., Johnson, L., Johnson, M. G., & Weber, C. (2004). A multicentre randomised controlled trial of an intervention to improve the accuracy of linear growth measurement. *Archives of Disease in Childhood, 89,* 342–346.

Lohman, T. J., Roche, A. F., & Martorell, R. (1988). *Anthropometric standardization reference manual.* Champaign, IL: Human Kinetics Books.

US Preventive Services Task Force. (1996). *Guide to clinical preventive services: Report of the US Preventive Services Task Force* (2nd ed.). Philadelphia, PA: Lippincott, Williams, & Wilkins.

[a] Adapted from the Quality and Safety Education for Nurses Institute.

Height

The term **height** (or **stature**) refers to the measurement taken when a child is standing upright. Wall charts and flip-up horizontal bars (floppy-arm devices) mounted to weighing scales should not be used to measure the height of children (Foote, 2014; Foote, Brady, Burke, et al., 2011). These devices are not steady and do not maintain a right angle to the vertical ruler, preventing an accurate and reliable height. Measure height by having the child, with the shoes removed, stand as tall and straight as possible with the head in midline and the line of vision parallel to the ceiling and floor (see discussion of the *Frankfort plane* in the Translating Evidence into Practice box). Be certain the child's back is to the wall or other vertical flat surface, with the occiput, scapulae, buttocks, and heels touching the vertical surface and the medial malleoli touching if possible (see Fig. 4.9B). Check for and correct slumping of the shoulders, positional lordosis, bending of the knees, or raising of the heels.

! NURSING ALERT

Normally, height is less if measured in the afternoon than in the morning due to diurnal variation (related to gravity and compression of the spine). The time of day when measurements are taken should be recorded (Foote, Brady, Burke, et al., 2009). For children in whom there are concerns about growth, serial measurements should be taken at the same time of day, when possible, to establish an accurate growth velocity.

For the most accurate measurement, use a wall-mounted unit (**stadiometer**; see Fig. 4.9B). To improvise a flat, vertical surface for measuring height, attach a paper or metal tape or yardstick to the wall, position the child adjacent to the tape, and place a 3D object, such as a thick book or empty box, on top of the head. Rest the side of the object firmly against the wall to form a right angle. Measure height to the last completed millimeter or $\frac{1}{16}$ inch. Measure more than once and record the average height.

Weight

Weight is measured with an appropriately sized electronic or balance beam scale, which measures weight to the nearest 10 g (0.35 oz) for infants and 100 g (0.22 pound) for children. Before weighing the child, balance the scale by setting it at 0 and noting if the balance registers at exactly 0 or in the middle of the mark. If the end of the balance beam rises to the top or bottom of the mark, more or less weight, respectively, is needed. Some scales are designed to self-correct, but others need to be recalibrated according to the manufacturer instructions. Scales vary in their accuracy; infant scales tend to be more accurate than adult platform scales, and newer scales tend to be more accurate than older ones, especially at the upper levels of weight measurement. Weighing more than once and recording the average weight is preferred. Another option is for two nurses to take the weight independently; if there is a discrepancy, take a third reading and use the mean of the measurements in closest agreement.

Take measurements in a comfortably warm room. When the birth-to-2-year or birth-to-36-month growth charts are used, children should be weighed nude. Older children are usually weighed while wearing their underwear, a gown, or light clothing, depending on the setting. However, always respect the privacy of children. If the child must be weighed wearing some type of special device, such as a prosthesis or an armboard for an intravenous device, note this when recording the weight. Children who are measured for recumbent length are usually weighed on an infant scale and placed in a lying or sitting position. Children should be weighed while lying, sitting, or standing in the center of the scale bed. When weighing a young child, place your hand slightly above the infant or young child to prevent him or her from accidentally falling off the scale (Fig. 4.10A) or stand close

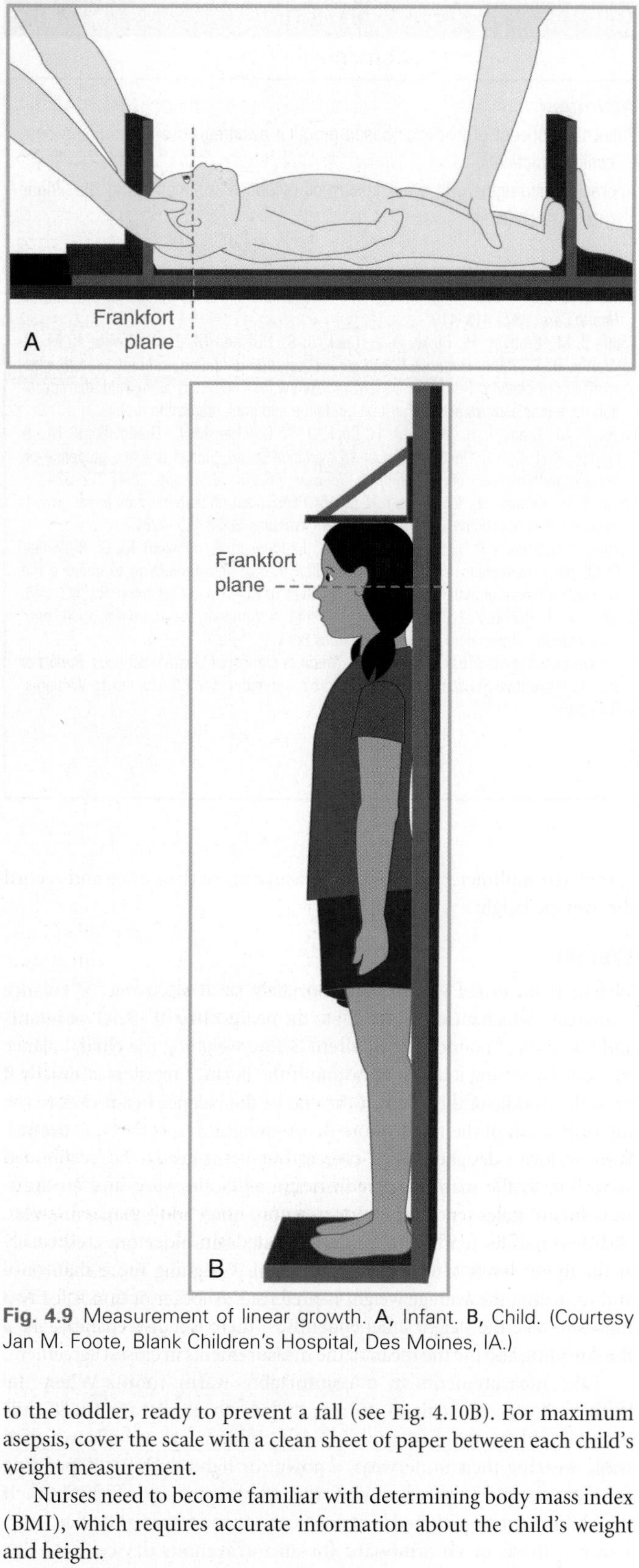

Fig. 4.9 Measurement of linear growth. A, Infant. B, Child. (Courtesy Jan M. Foote, Blank Children's Hospital, Des Moines, IA.)

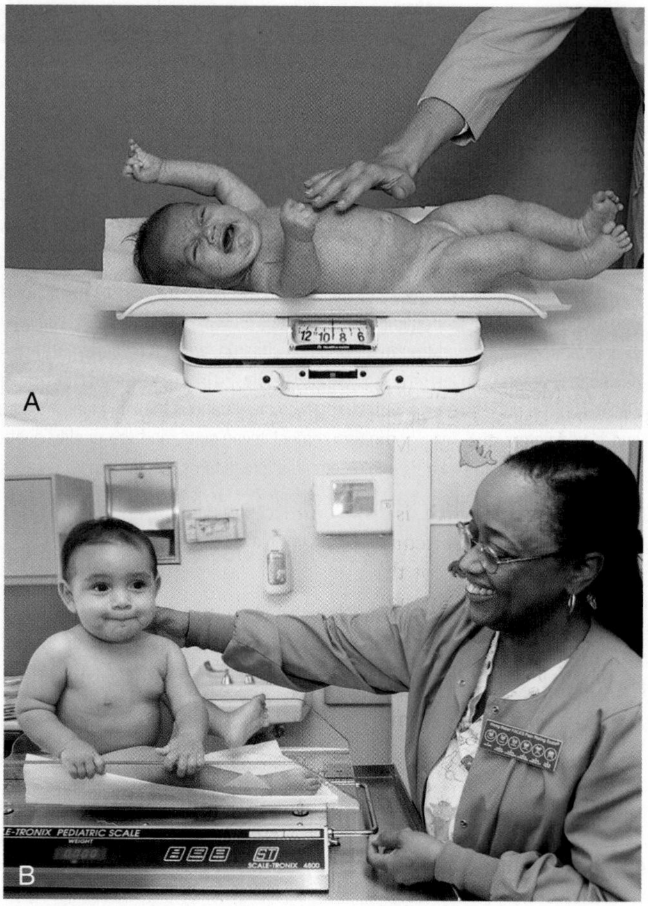

Fig. 4.10 A, Infant on scale. B, Toddler on scale. Note the presence of the nurse to prevent falls. (**B,** Courtesy Paul Vincent Kuntz, Texas Children's Hospital, Houston, TX.)

to the toddler, ready to prevent a fall (see Fig. 4.10B). For maximum asepsis, cover the scale with a clean sheet of paper between each child's weight measurement.

Nurses need to become familiar with determining body mass index (BMI), which requires accurate information about the child's weight and height.

$$\text{BMI} = \text{Weight in kilograms} \div [\text{Height in meters}]^2$$

Or

$$\text{BMI} = [\text{Weight in pounds} \div (\text{Height in inches} \times \text{Height in inches})] \times 703$$

With the increasing number of overweight and obese children in the United States, the BMI charts are a critical component of children's physical assessment.

! NURSING ALERT

BMI for sex and age may be used to identify children and adolescents who are either underweight (<5th percentile), healthy weight (5th percentile to <85th percentile), overweight (≥85th percentile and <95th percentile), or obese (≥95th percentile). Weight per length may be used to identify concerns in infants and other young children whose length (rather than height) is measured.

Skinfold Thickness and Arm Circumference

Measures of relative weight and stature cannot distinguish between adipose (fat) tissue and muscle. One convenient measure of body fat is **skinfold thickness**, which is increasingly recommended as a routine measurement. Measure skinfold thickness with special calipers, such as the Lange calipers. The most common sites for measuring skinfold thickness are the triceps (most practical for routine clinical use), subscapular, suprailiac, abdomen, and upper thigh. For greatest reliability, follow the exact procedure for measurement and record the average of at least two measurements of one site.

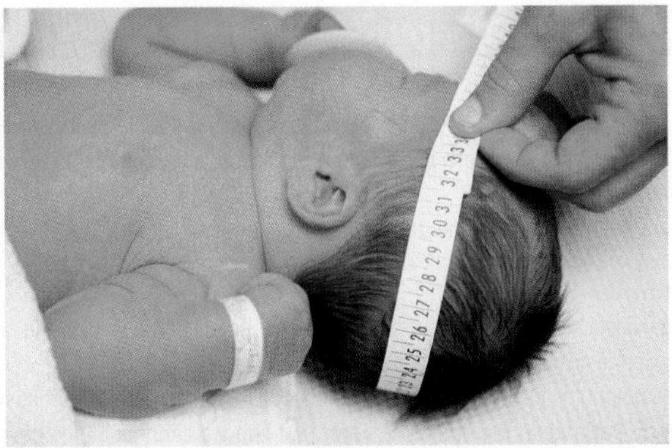

Fig. 4.11 Measurement of head circumference. (From Seidel, H. M., Ball, J. W., Dains, J. E., et al. [1999]. *Mosby's guide to physical examination* [4th ed.]. St Louis, MO: Mosby.)

Arm circumference is an indirect measure of muscle mass. Measurement of arm circumference follows the same procedure as for skinfold thickness except the midpoint is measured with a paper or steel tape. Place the tape vertically along the posterior aspect of the upper arm from the acromial process and to the olecranon process; half of the measured length is the midpoint used to measure the arm circumference. World Health Organization growth curves are available for triceps skinfold and arm circumference measurements.

Head Circumference

Head circumference reflects brain growth. Measure head circumference in children up to 36 months old and in any child whose head size is questionable. Measure the head at its greatest frontooccipital circumference, usually slightly above the eyebrows and pinna of the ears and around the occipital prominence at the back of the skull (Fig. 4.11). Use a paper or nonstretchable tape, or insert-a-tape, marked in millimeter or 1/16-inch increments because a cloth tape can stretch and give a falsely small measurement. Because head shape can affect the location of the maximum circumference and movement of the infant or child can interfere with the measurement, more than one measurement is necessary to obtain the most accurate measure. Measure head circumference to the last completed millimeter or 1/16-inch.

Plot the head size on the appropriate growth chart under head circumference. Generally, head circumference is larger than chest circumference in most newborns. The head and chest circumferences approximate each other around 12 months of age. Later in childhood, chest circumference exceeds head size by about 5 to 7 cm (2 to 2.75 inches). For newborns, see Chapter 7, Physical Assessment.

PHYSIOLOGIC MEASUREMENTS

Physiologic measurements, key elements in evaluating physical status of vital functions, include temperature, pulse, respiration, and blood pressure. Compare each physiologic recording with normal values for that age-group. In addition, compare the values taken on preceding health visits with present recordings. For example, a falsely elevated blood pressure (BP) reading may not indicate hypertension if previous recent readings have been within normal limits. The isolated recording may indicate some stressful event in the child's life.

As in most procedures carried out with children, treat older children and adolescents much the same as adults. However, give special consideration to preschool children (see Atraumatic Care box). For best results in taking vital signs of infants, count respirations first (before the infant is disturbed), take the pulse next, and then measure temperature. If vital signs cannot be taken without disturbing the child, record the child's behavior (e.g., crying) along with the measurement.

ATRAUMATIC CARE

Reducing Young Children's Fears

Young children, especially preschoolers, fear intrusive procedures because of their poorly defined body boundaries. Therefore avoid invasive procedures, such as measuring rectal temperature, whenever possible. Also avoid using the word "take" when measuring vital signs, because young children interpret words literally and may think that their temperature or other function will be taken away. Instead, say, "I want to know how warm you are."

BOX 4.9 Recommended Temperature Screening Routes in Infants and Children

Birth to 2 Years Old

Axillary

Rectal—if definitive temperature reading is needed for infants older than 1 month of age

2 to 5 Years Old

Axillary

Tympanic

Oral—when child can hold thermometer under tongue

Rectal—if definitive temperature reading is needed

Older Than 5 Years Old

Oral

Axillary

Tympanic

Temporal artery

Temperature

Temperature is the measure of heat content within an individual's body. The **core temperature** most closely reflects the temperature of the blood flow through the carotid arteries to the hypothalamus. Core temperature is relatively constant despite wide fluctuations in the external environment. When a child's temperature is altered, receptors in the skin, spinal cord, and brain respond in an attempt to achieve **normothermia**, a normal temperature state. In pediatrics, there is a lack of consensus regarding what temperature constitutes normothermia for every child. For rectal temperatures in children, 37°C to 37.5°C (98.6°F to 99.5°F) is an acceptable range, where heat loss and heat production are balanced. For neonates, a core body temperature between 36.5°C and 37.6°C (97.7°F and 99.7° F) is a desirable range. In the neonate, obtain temperature measurements for monitoring adequacy of thermoregulation, not just for fever; therefore temperature measurements in each infant should be carefully considered in the context of the purpose and the environment.

The nurse can measure temperature in healthy children at several body sites via oral, rectal, axillary, ear canal (tympanic membrane), temporal artery, or skin route (Box 4.9). For the ill child, other sites for temperature measurement have been investigated. Skin temperature sensors are most often used for neonates and infants placed in radiant heat warmers or incubators. The pulmonary artery is the closest to the hypothalamus and best reflects the core temperature (Batra, Saha, & Faridi, 2012). Other sites used are the distal esophagus, urinary bladder, and nasopharynx (Box 4.10). All of these methods are invasive and difficult to use in clinical practice.

Temperature measured by rectal thermometry is considered closest to core temperature, but it has some drawbacks. Tympanic membrane thermometry for children older than 2 years of age and temporal artery thermometry in all age-groups are taking precedence over

BOX 4.10 Alternative Temperature Measurement Sites for Ill Children

Skin

A probe is placed on the skin to determine heat output in response to changes in the patient's skin temperature.

Skin temperature sensors are most often used for neonates and infants placed in radiant heat warmers or isolettes (using servo control feature of the apparatus). In turn, the heater unit warms to a set point to maintain the infant's temperature within a specified range.

ThermoSpot is an example of a device allowing continuous thermal monitoring in neonates.

Urinary Bladder

A thermistor or thermocouple is placed within the indwelling bladder catheter. The catheter tip immersed in the bladder provides a continuous temperature read-out on the bedside monitor.

This is not a true measure of core temperature but responds better than rectal and skin temperatures to core body changes.

Because of thermistor sizes, this method is unusable with neonates and small infants.

Pulmonary Artery

A catheter is placed into the heart to obtain a reading in the pulmonary artery.

It is used in critical care settings or operating rooms only in patients requiring aggressive monitoring.

Catheters are not available in sizes for neonates or small infants.

Esophageal Site

A probe is inserted into the lower third of the esophagus at the level of the heart.

This is used in critical care settings or operating rooms.

Several companies have esophageal stethoscopes with temperature probe monitors for patients in the operating room that show a continuous temperature reading.

Nasopharyngeal Site

A probe is inserted into the nasopharynx, posterior to the soft palate, and provides an estimate of hypothalamic temperature.

This is used in critical care settings or operating rooms.

Data from Kumar, P. R., Nisarga, R., & Gowda, B. (2004). Temperature monitoring in newborns using ThermoSpot. *Indian Journal of Pediatrics, 71*(9), 795–796; Martin, S. A., & Kline, A. M. (2004). Can there be a standard for temperature measurement in the pediatric intensive care unit? *AACN Clinical Issues, 15*(2), 254–266; Maxton, F. J. C., Justin, L., & Gilles, D. (2004). Estimating core temperature in infants and children after cardiac surgery: A comparison of six methods. *Journal of Advanced Nursing, 45*(2), 214–222.

other methods (Batra & Goyal, 2013; Batra, Saha, & Faridi, 2012). One of the most important influences on the accuracy of temperature is improper temperature-taking technique. Detailed discussion of temperature-taking methods and visual examples of proper techniques are given in Table 4.3. For a critical review of the evidence on temperature-taking methods, see the Translating Evidence into Practice box.

TRANSLATING EVIDENCE INTO PRACTICE

Temperature Measurement in Pediatrics

Ask the Question

PICOT Question

In infants and children, what is the most accurate method for measuring temperature in febrile children?

Search for the Evidence

Search Strategies

Clinical research studies related to this issue were identified by searching for English publications with preference for studies in the past 15 years for infant and child populations; comparisons with gold standard: rectal thermometry.

Databases Used

PubMed, Cochrane Collaboration, MD Consult, Joanna Briggs Institute, National Guideline Clearinghouse (AHRQ), TRIP Database Plus, PedsCCM, BestBETs

Critical Appraisal of the Evidence

- **Rectal temperature:** Rectal measurement remains the clinical gold standard for the precise diagnosis of fever in infants and children compared with other methods (Fortuna, Carney, Macy, et al., 2010; Holzhauer, Reith, Sawin, et al., 2009). However, this procedure is more invasive and is contraindicated for infants younger than 1 month old due to risk of rectal perforation (Batra, Saha, & Faridi, 2012). Children with neutropenia, recent rectal surgery, diarrhea, or anorectal lesions or those who are receiving chemotherapy (cancer treatment usually affects the mucosa and causes neutropenia) should not undergo rectal thermometry.
- **Oral temperature (OT):** OT indicates rapid changes in core body temperature, but accuracy may be an issue compared with the rectal site (Batra, Saha, & Faridi, 2012). OTs are considered the standard for temperature measurement, but they are contraindicated in children who have an altered level of consciousness, are receiving oxygen, are mouth breathing, are experiencing mucositis, had recent oral surgery or trauma, or are younger than 5 years old (El-Radhi & Barry, 2006). Limitations of OTs include the effects of ambient room temperature and recent oral intake (Martin & Kline, 2004).
- **Axillary temperature:** This is inconsistent and insensitive in infants and children older than 1 month of age (Falzon, Grech, Caruana, et al., 2003; Stine, Flook, & Vincze, 2012). A systematic review of 20 studies concluded that axillary thermometers showed variation in findings and are not a good method for accurate temperature assessment (Craig, Lancaster, Williamson, et al., 2000). In neonates with fever, the axillary temperature should not be used interchangeably with rectal measurement (Hissink Muller, van Berkel, & de Beaufort, 2008). It can be used as a screening tool for fever in young infants (Batra, Saha, & Faridi, 2012).
- **Ear (aural) temperature:** A meta-analysis of 101 studies comparing tympanic membrane temperatures with rectal temperatures in children concluded that the tympanic method demonstrated a wide range of variability (Craig, Lancaster, Taylor, et al., 2002). Other published reviews found poor sensitivity using infrared ear thermometry (Devrim, Kara, Ceyhan, et al., 2007; Dodd, Lancaster, Craig, et al., 2006). Diagnosis of fever without a focus should not be made based on tympanic thermometry (Batra, Saha, & Faridi, 2012; Devrim, Kara, Ceyhan, et al., 2007; Dodd, Lancaster, Craig, et al., 2006). However, a recent systematic review and meta-analysis of 31 studies found the accuracy of tympanic thermometry in diagnosing fever was high and cautiously recommended its use (Zhen, Xia, Ya Jun, et al., 2015).
- **Temporal artery temperature (TAT):** TAT is not predictable for fever in young children but can be used as a screening tool for detecting fever lower than 38°C (100.4°F) in children 3 months to 4 years old (Al-Mukhaizeem, Allen, Komar,

Temperature Measurement in Pediatrics

et al., 2004; Callanan, 2003; Forrest, Juliano, Conley, et al., 2017; Fortuna, Carney, Macy, et al., 2010; Hebbar, Fortenberry, Rogers, et al., 2005; Hoffman, Etwaru, Dreisinger, et al., 2013; Holzhauer, Reith, Sawin, et al., 2009; Hudson Moore, Dagenhart Carrigan, Solomon, et al., 2015; Odinaka, Edelu, Nwolisa, et al., 2014; Schuh, Komar, Stephens, et al., 2004; Titus, Hulsey, Heckman, et al., 2009). However, a study by Batra and Goyal (2013) found that TAT correlated better with rectal temperature than axillary and tympanic measures in a group of 50 afebrile children between the ages of 2 and 12 years.

Apply the Evidence: Nursing Implications

- No single site used for temperature assessment provides unequivocal estimates of core body temperature.
- Studies show that the axillary and tympanic measures demonstrate poor agreement when these modes are compared with more accurate core temperature methods. The differences are more evident as temperature increases, regardless of age.
- TAT is not predictable for fever and should be used only as a screening tool in young children.
- When an accurate method for obtaining a correct reflection of core temperature is needed, the rectal temperature is recommended in younger children, and the oral route is recommended in older children.

For infants younger than 1 month of age, axillary temperatures are recommended for screening.

Quality and Safety Competencies: Evidence-Based Practice[a]

Knowledge

Differentiate clinical opinion from research and evidence-based summaries.

Demonstrate understanding of thermometry selection based on the developmental age of the child.

Skills

Base individualized care plan on patient values, clinical expertise, and evidence.

Integrate evidence into practice by using the correct type of thermometry to screen for fever compared with measures used for accurate determination of the degree of fever.

Attitudes

Value the concept of evidence-based practice as integral to determining best clinical practice.

Recognize strengths and weaknesses of evidence for the most accurate method for measuring temperature and fever in infants and children.

References

Al-Mukhaizeem, F., Allen, U., Komar, L., Naser, B., Roy, L., Stephens, D., ... Schuh, S. (2004). Comparison of temporal artery, rectal and esophageal core temperatures in children: Results of a pilot study. *Paediatrics & Child Health, 9*(7), 461–465.

Batra, P., & Goyal, S. (2013). Comparison of rectal, axillary, tympanic, and temporal artery thermometry in the pediatric emergency room. *Pediatric Emergency Care, 29*(1), 63–66.

Batra, P., Saha, A., & Faridi, M. M. (2012). Thermometry in children. *Journal of Emergencies, Trauma, and Shock, 5*(3), 246–249.

Callanan, D. (2003). Detecting fever in young infants: Reliability of perceived, pacifier, and temporal artery temperatures in infants younger than 3 months of age. *Pediatric Emergency Care, 19*(4), 240–243.

Craig, J. V., Lancaster, G. A., Taylor, S., Williamson, P. R., & Smyth, R. L. (2002). Infrared ear thermometry compared with rectal thermometry in children: A systemic review. *Lancet, 360*, 603–609.

Craig, J. V., Lancaster, G. A., Williamson, P. R., & Smyth, R. L. (2000). Temperature measured at the axilla compared with rectum in children and young people: Systematic review. *British Medical Journal, 320*, 1174–1178.

Devrim, I., Kara, A., Ceyhan, M., Tezer, H., Uludag, A. K., Cengiz, A. B., ... Secmeer, G. (2007). Measurement accuracy of fever by tympanic and axillary thermometry. *Pediatric Emergency Care, 23*(1), 16–19.

Dodd, S. R., Lancaster, G. A., Craig, J. V., Smyth, R. L., & Williamson, P. R. (2006). In a systematic review, infrared ear thermometry for fever diagnosis in children finds poor sensitivity. *Journal of Clinical Epidemiology, 59*, 354–357.

El-Radhi, A. S., & Barry, W. (2006). Thermometry in paediatric practice. *Archives of Disease in Childhood, 91*(4), 351–356.

Falzon, A., Grech, V., Caruana, B., Magro, A., & Attard-Montalto, S. (2003). How reliable is axillary temperature measurement? *Acta Paediatrica, 92*(3), 309–313.

Forrest, A. J., Juliano, M. L., Conley, S. P., Cronyn, P. D., McGlynn, A., & Auten, J. D. (2017). Temporal artery and axillary thermometry comparison with rectal thermometry in children presenting to the ED. *American Journal of Emergency Medicine, 35*, 1855–1858.

Fortuna, E. L., Carney, M. M., Macy, M., Stanley, R. M., Younger, J. G., & Bradin, S. A. (2010). Accuracy of non-contact infrared thermometry versus rectal thermometry in young children evaluated in the emergency department for fever. *Journal of Emergency Nursing, 36*(2), 101–104.

Hebbar, K., Fortenberry, J. D., Rogers, K., Merritt, R., & Easley, K. (2005). Comparison of temporal artery thermometer to standard temperature measurement in pediatric intensive care unit patients. *Pediatric Critical Care Medicine, 6*(5), 557–561.

Hissink Muller, P. C., van Berkel, L. H., & de Beaufort, A. J. (2008). Axillary and rectal temperature measurements poorly agree in newborn infants. *Neonatology, 94*(1), 31–34.

Hoffman, R. J., Etwaru, K., Dreisinger, N., Khokhar, A., & Husk, G. (2013). Comparison of temporal artery thermometry and rectal thermometry in febrile pediatric emergency department patients. *Pediatric Emergency Care, 29*(3), 301–304.

Holzhauer, J. K., Reith, V., Sawin, K. J., & Yen, K. (2009). Evaluation of temporal artery thermometry in children 3–36 months old. *Journal of Specialty Pediatric Nursing, 14*(4), 239–244.

Hudson Moore, A., Dagenhart Carrigan, J., Solomon, D. M., & Creech Tart, R. (2015). Temporal artery thermometry to detect pediatric fever. *Clinical Nursing Research, 24*(5), 556–563.

Martin, S. A., & Kline, A. M. (2004). Can there be a standard for temperature measurement in the pediatric intensive care unit? *AACN Clinical Issues, 15*(2), 254–266.

Odinaka, K. K., Edelu, B. O., Nwolisa, C. E., Amamilo, I. B., & Okolo, S. N. (2014). Temporal artery thermometry in children younger than 5 years: A comparison with rectal thermometry. *Pediatric Emergency Care, 30*(12), 867–970.

Schuh, S., Komar, L., Stephens, D., Read, S., & Allen, U. (2004). Comparison of the temporal artery and rectal thermometry in children in the emergency department. *Pediatric Emergency Care, 20*(11), 736–741.

Stine, C. A., Flook, D. M., & Vincze, D. L. (2012). Rectal versus axillary temperatures: Is there a significant difference in infants less than 1 years of age? *Journal of Pediatric Nursing, 27*, 265–270.

Titus, M. O., Hulsey, T., Heckman, J., & Losek, J. D. (2009). Temporal artery thermometry utilization in pediatric emergency care. *Clinical Pediatrics, 48*(2), 190–193.

Zhen, C., Xia, Z., Ya Jun, Z., Long, L., Jian, S., Gui Ju, C., & Long, L. (2015). Accuracy of infrared tympanic thermometry used in the diagnosis of fever in children: A systematic review and meta-analysis. *Clinical Pediatrics, 54*(2), 114–126.

[a] Adapted from the Quality and Safety Education for Nurses Institute.

TABLE 4.3 Temperature Measurement Locations for Infants and Children

Temperature Site
Oral Place tip under tongue in right or left posterior sublingual pocket, not in front of tongue. Have child keep mouth closed without biting on thermometer. Pacifier thermometers measure intraoral or supralingual temperature and are available but lack support in the literature. Several factors affect mouth temperature: Eating and mastication, hot or cold beverages, mouth breathing, and ambient temperature. 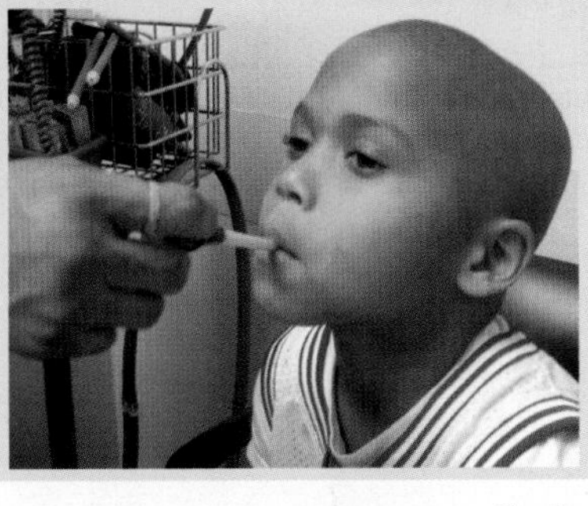

Continued

TABLE 4.3 Temperature Measurement Locations for Infants and Children—cont'd

Temperature Site

Axillary

Place tip under arm in center of axilla and keep close to skin, not clothing. Hold child's arm firmly against side. Temperature may be affected by poor peripheral perfusion (results in lower value), clothing or swaddling, use of radiant warmer, or amount of brown fat in cold-stressed neonate (results in higher value).

Advantages: Avoids intrusive procedure and eliminates risk of rectal perforation.

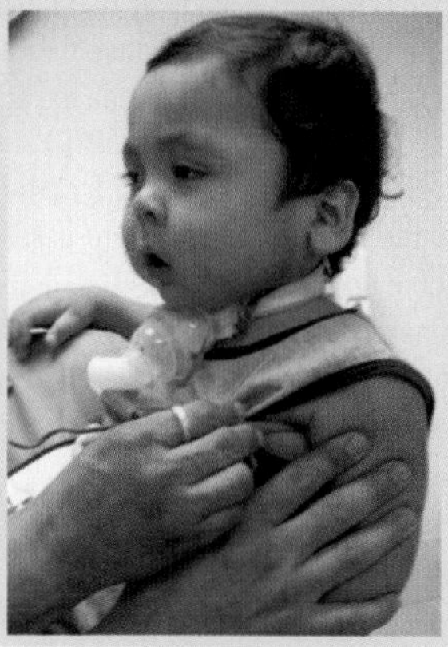

Ear Based (Aural)

Insert small infrared probe deeply into ear canal to allow sensor to obtain measurement from tympanic membrane.

Size of probe (most are 8 mm) may influence accuracy of result. In young children this may be a problem because of small diameter of ear canal.

Proper placement of ear is controversial related to whether the pinna should be pulled in manner similar to that used during otoscopy.

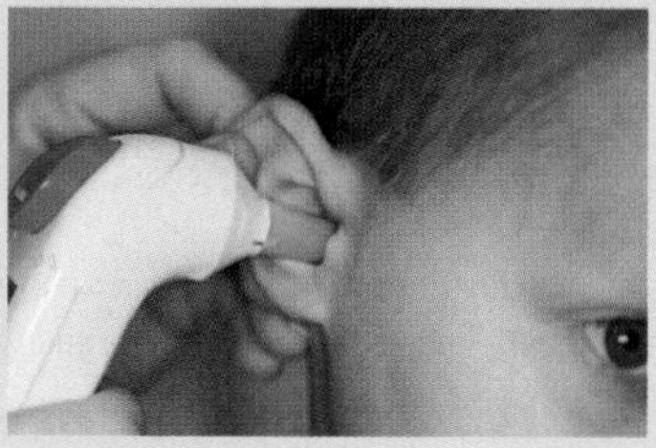

Rectal

Place well-lubricated tip at maximum 2.5 cm (1 inch) into rectum for children and 1.5 cm (0.6 inch) for infants; securely hold thermometer close to anus.

Child may be placed in side-lying, supine, or prone position (i.e., supine with knees flexed toward abdomen); cover penis because procedure may stimulate urination. A small child may be placed prone across parent's lap.

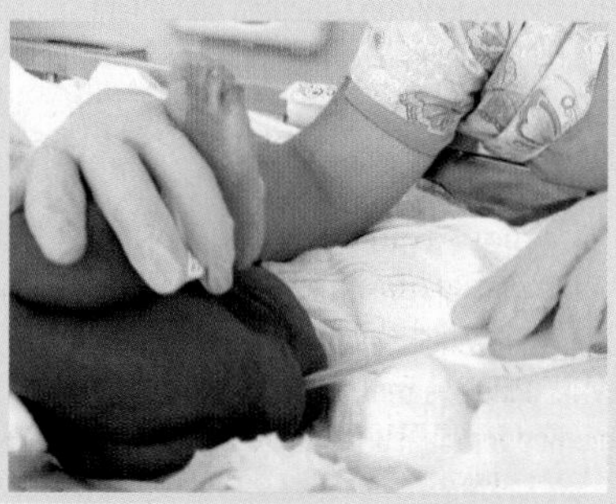

Temporal Artery

An infrared sensor probe scans across forehead, capturing heat from arterial blood flow.

Temporal artery is only artery close enough to skin's surface to provide access for accurate temperature measurement.

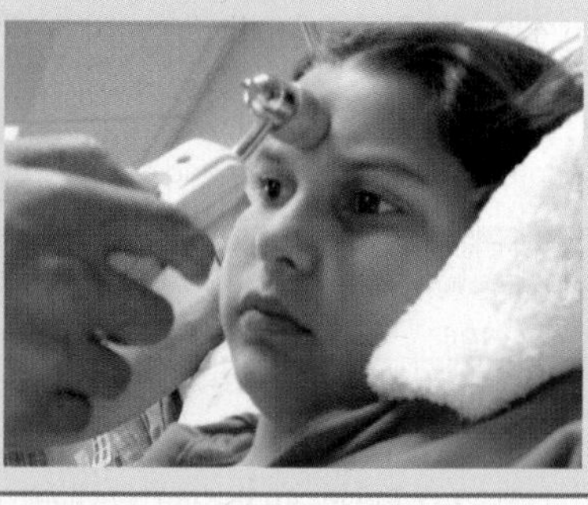

Data from Martin, S. A., & Kline, A. M. (2004). Can there be a standard for temperature measurement in the pediatric intensive care unit? *AACN Clinical Issues, 15*(2), 254–266; Falzon, A., Grech, V., Caruana, B., et al. (2003). How reliable is axillary temperature measurement? *Acta Paediatrica, 92*(3), 309–313. Oral, axillary, rectal, and temporal artery images courtesy Paul Vincent Kuntz, Texas Children's Hospital, Houston, TX.

BOX 4.11 Types of Thermometers Used to Measure Temperature in Infants and Children

Electronic Thermometer

Temperature is sensed with an electronic component called thermistor mounted at the tip of a plastic and stainless steel probe, which is connected to an electronic recorder. A disposable plastic cover is used for infection control.

Temperature measurement appears on digital display within 60 seconds.

The probe can be placed in the mouth, axilla, or rectum.

Infrared Thermometer

Thermal radiation is measured from the axilla, ear canal, or tympanic membrane.

Temperature measurement appears on the digital display in approximately 1 second.

Three types are available for ear-based use: tympanic, ear canal, and arterial heat balance via the ear canal (AHBE).

Often these devices are all inappropriately referred to as *tympanic thermometers.*

Temperatures measured in this way reflect arterial (bloodstream) temperature.

Ear-Based Temperature Sensor

Although this is frequently used in pediatric settings (especially ambulatory clinics), debate on the reliability of ear-based thermometry in screening febrile children continues.

Most models use "offsets" for internal calculations that transform ear temperature into supposedly equivalent oral or rectal temperatures.

Ear Sensor (LighTouch LTX)

This measures the infrared heat energy radiating from ear canal opening, scans ear canal for highest temperature reading, and then calculates arterial temperature (correlates highly with core or internal body temperature).

It is available in two sizes; the smaller size of LighTouch Pedi-Q is for infants and toddlers.

Axillary Sensor (LighTouch LTN)

This measures the infrared heat energy radiating from the axilla.

It can be used on wet skin; in incubators; or under radiant heaters, warming pads, or other heat sources.

Digital Thermometer

A probe is connected to a microprocessor chip, which translates signals into degrees and sends temperature measurement to digital display.

It is used like an oral electronic thermometer and can be used for measuring oral, rectal, and axillary temperature.

It is more accurate and easier to read but somewhat more expensive than a plastic strip thermometer.

Liquid Crystal Skin Contact Thermometer (Chemical Dot Thermometer)

This single-use, disposable, flexible thermometer has a specific chemical mixture in each circle that changes color to measure temperature increments of $\frac{2}{10}$ degree.

There are two types:

1. Kept in mouth (1 minute), axilla (3 minutes), or rectum (3 minutes); color change is read 10 to 15 seconds after removing the thermometer
2. Wearable, continuous-use thermometer, which is placed under axilla; may be read within 2 to 3 minutes after placement and continuously thereafter; discard and replace every 48 hours

The most frequently used temperature measurement devices in infants and children include the following:

Electronic intermittent thermometers measure the patient's temperature at oral, rectal, and axillary sites and are used as primary diagnostic indicators

Infrared thermometers measure the patient's temperature by collecting emitted thermal radiation from a particular site (e.g., ear canal [tympanic membrane])

Electronic continuous thermometers measure the patient's temperature during the administration of general anesthesia, treatment of hypothermia or hyperthermia, and other situations that require continuous monitoring

Box 4.11 provides a detailed description of these devices.

! NURSING ALERT

The belief that oral temperature can be estimated by adding 1°C to the temperature taken in the axilla is incorrect. Axillary temperature is lower than oral temperature, but the difference varies too widely for a standard conversion. Do not add a degree to the finding obtained by taking a temperature by the axillary route.

Pulse

A satisfactory pulse can be taken radially in children older than 2 years of age. However, in infants and young children, the apical impulse (heard through a stethoscope held to the chest at the apex of the heart) is more reliable (see Fig. 4.33 for location of pulses). Count the pulse for 1 full minute in infants and young children because of possible irregularities in rhythm. However, when frequent apical rates are necessary, use shorter counting times (e.g., 15- or 30-second intervals). For greater accuracy, measure the apical rate while the child is asleep; record the child's behavior along with the rate. Grade pulses according to the criteria in Table 4.4. Compare radial and femoral pulses at least once during infancy to detect the presence of circulatory impairment, such as coarctation of the aorta.

TABLE 4.4 Grading of Pulses

Grade	Description
0	Not palpable
+1	Difficult to palpate, thready, weak, easily obliterated with pressure
+2	Difficult to palpate, may be obliterated with pressure
+3	Easy to palpate, not easily obliterated with pressure (normal)
+4	Strong, bounding, not obliterated with pressure

Respiration

Count the respiratory rate in children in the same manner as for adult patients. However, in infants, observe abdominal movements, because respirations are primarily diaphragmatic. Because the movements are irregular, count them for 1 full minute for accuracy (see also the Chest section later in this chapter).

Blood Pressure

BP should be measured annually in children 3 years old through adolescence and in children with underlying renal, adrenal, or cardiovascular disease; children with risk factors for hypertension; children in emergency departments and intensive care units; and high-risk infants (National High Blood Pressure Education Program Working Group on High Blood Pressure in Children and Adolescents, 2004).

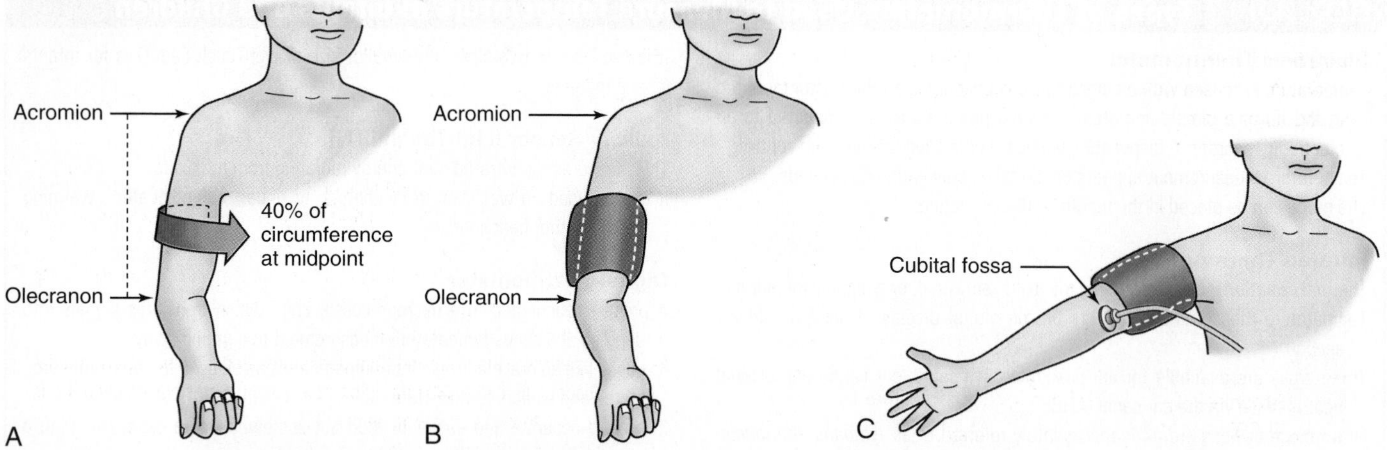

Fig. 4.12 Determination of proper cuff size. **A,** Cuff bladder width should be approximately 40% of circumference of arm measured at a point midway between olecranon and acromion. **B,** Cuff bladder length should cover 80% to 100% of arm circumference. **C,** Blood pressure (BP) should be measured with the cubital fossa at the heart level. The arm should be supported. The stethoscope bell is placed over the brachial artery pulse proximal and medial to the cubital fossa and below the bottom edge of the cuff. (From National Institutes of Health, National Heart, Lung, and Blood Institute. [1996]. *Update on the Task Force Report [1987] on high blood pressure in children and adolescents: A working group report from the National High Blood Pressure Education Program.* NIH Pub No 96-3790. Bethesda, MD: Author.)

Auscultation remains the gold standard method of BP measurement in children under most circumstances. Use of the automated devices is acceptable for BP measurement in newborns and young infants, in whom auscultation is difficult, and in the intensive care setting where frequent BP measurement is needed.

Oscillometric devices measure mean arterial BP and then calculate systolic and diastolic values. The algorithms used by companies are proprietary and differ from company to company and device to device. These devices can yield results that vary widely when one is compared with another, and they do not always closely match BP values obtained by auscultation. An elevated BP reading obtained with an automated or oscillometric device should be repeated using auscultation.

BP readings using oscillometry, such as Dinamap, are generally higher (10 mm Hg higher) than measurements using auscultation (Park, Menard, & Schoolfield, 2005). Differences between Dinamap and auscultatory readings prevent the interchange of the readings by the two methods.

Selection of Cuff

No matter what type of noninvasive technique is used, the most important factor in accurately measuring BP is the use of an appropriately sized cuff (**cuff size** refers only to the inner inflatable bladder, not the cloth covering). A technique to establish an appropriate cuff size is to choose a cuff with a bladder width that is at least 40% of the arm circumference midway between the olecranon and the acromion. This will usually be a cuff bladder that covers 80% to 100% of the circumference of the arm (Fig. 4.12). Cuffs that are either too narrow or too wide affect the accuracy of BP measurements. If the cuff size is too small, the reading on the device is falsely high. If the cuff size is too large, the reading is falsely low.

Using limb circumference for selecting cuff width more accurately reflects direct arterial blood pressure (BP) than using limb length because this method considers variations in arm thickness and the amount of pressure required to compress the artery. For measurement on sites other than the upper arms, use the limb circumference, although the shape of the limb (e.g., conical shape of the thigh) may prevent appropriate placement of the cuff and inaccurately reflect intra-arterial BP (Table 4.5).

When using a site other than the arm, BP measurements using noninvasive techniques may differ. Generally, systolic BP in the lower extremities (thigh or calf) is greater than pressure in the upper extremities, and systolic BP in the calf is higher than that in the thigh (Schell, Briening, Lebet, et al., 2011) (Fig. 4.13).

TABLE 4.5 Recommended Dimensions for Blood Pressure Cuff Bladders

Age	Width (cm)	Length (cm)	Maximum Arm Circumference (cm)[a]
Newborn	4	8	10
Infant	6	12	15
Child	9	18	22
Small adult	10	24	26
Adult	13	30	34
Large adult	16	38	44
Thigh	20	42	52

[a]Calculated so that largest arm would still allow bladder to encircle arm by at least 80%.

From National High Blood Pressure Education Program Working Group on High Blood Pressure in Children and Adolescents. (2004). The fourth report on the diagnosis, evaluation, and treatment of high blood pressure in children and adolescents. *Pediatrics, 114*(Suppl. 2, 4th report), 555–576.

! NURSING ALERT

When taking blood pressure (BP), use an appropriately sized cuff. When the correct size is not available, use an oversized cuff rather than an undersized one or use another site that more appropriately fits the cuff size. Do not choose a cuff based on the name of the cuff (e.g., an "infant" cuff may be too small for some infants).

! NURSING ALERT

Compare BP in the upper and lower extremities to detect abnormalities, such as coarctation of the aorta, in which the lower extremity pressure is less than the upper extremity pressure.

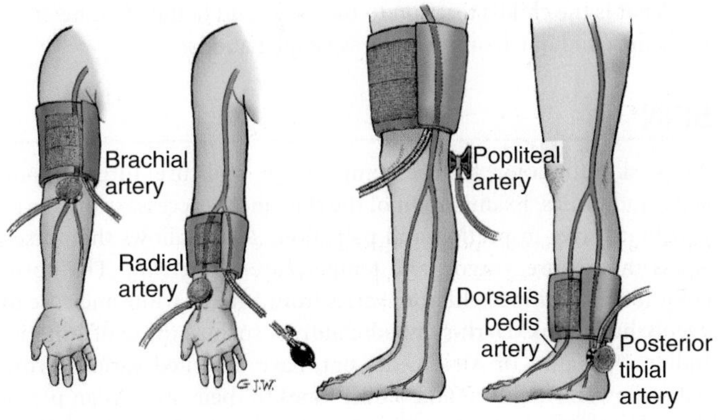

Fig. 4.13 Sites for measuring blood pressure. **A**, Upper arm. **B**, Lower arm or forearm. **C**, Thigh. **D**, Calf or ankle.

Measurement and Interpretation

Measuring and interpreting BP in infants and children requires attention to correct procedure because (1) limb sizes vary and cuff selection must accommodate the circumference; (2) excessive pressure on the antecubital fossa affects the Korotkoff sounds; (3) children easily become anxious, which can elevate BP; and (4) BP values change with age and growth. In children and adolescents, determine the normal range of BP. BP standards that are based on gender, age, and height provide a more precise classification of BP according to body size. This approach avoids misclassifying children who are very tall or very short. The BP tables (http://www.nhlbi.nih.gov/files/docs/guidelines/child_tbl.pdf) include the 50th, 90th, 95th, and 99th percentiles (with standard deviations) by gender, age, and height.

To use the tables in a clinical setting, determine the height percentile by using the Centers for Disease Control and Prevention growth charts (http://www.cdc.gov/growthcharts). The child's measured systolic BP and diastolic BP are compared with the numbers provided in the table (boys or girls) according to the child's age and height percentile. The child is **normotensive** if the BP is below the 90th percentile. If the BP is at or above the 90th percentile, repeat the BP measurement to verify an elevated BP. BP measurements between the 90th and 95th percentiles indicate prehypertension and necessitate reassessment and consideration of other risk factors. In addition, if an adolescent's BP is more than 120/80 mm Hg, consider the patient prehypertensive, even if this value is below the 90th percentile. This BP level typically occurs for systolic BP at 12 years old and for diastolic BP at 16 years old. If the child's BP (systolic or diastolic) is at or above the 95th percentile, the child may be hypertensive, and the measurement must be repeated on at least two occasions to confirm diagnosis (National High Blood Pressure Education Program Working Group on High Blood Pressure in Children and Adolescents, 2004) (see Nursing Care Guidelines box).

NURSING CARE GUIDELINES

Using the Blood Pressure Tables

1. Use the standard height charts to determine the height percentile.
2. Measure and record the child's systolic BP and diastolic BP.
3. Use the correct gender table for systolic BP and diastolic BP.
4. Find the child's age on the left side of the table. Follow the age row horizontally across the table to the intersection of the line for the height percentile (vertical column).
5. Then, find the 50th, 90th, 95th, and 99th percentiles for systolic BP in the left columns and for diastolic BP in the right columns.
   - BP less than 90th percentile is normal.
   - BP between the 90th and 95th percentiles is prehypertension. In adolescents, BP of 120/80 mm Hg or greater is prehypertension even if this figure is less than the 90th percentile.
   - BP over the 95th percentile may be hypertension.
6. If the BP is over the 90th percentile, the BP should be repeated twice, and an average systolic BP and diastolic BP should be used.
7. If the BP is over the 95th percentile, BP should be staged. If BP is stage 1 (95th to 99th percentile plus 5 mm Hg), BP measurements should be repeated on two more occasions. If hypertension is confirmed, evaluation should proceed. If BP is stage 2 (>99th percentile plus 5 mm Hg), prompt referral should be made for evaluation and therapy. If the patient is symptomatic, immediate referral and treatment are indicated.

BP, Blood pressure.
From National High Blood Pressure Education Program Working Group on High Blood Pressure in Children and Adolescents (2004). The fourth report on the diagnosis, evaluation, and treatment of high blood pressure in children and adolescents. *Pediatrics, 114*(Suppl. 2, 4th report), 555–576.

Orthostatic Hypotension

Orthostatic hypotension (OH), also called *postural hypotension* or *orthostatic intolerance*, often manifests as **syncope** (fainting), **vertigo** (dizziness), or lightheadedness and is caused by decreased blood flow to the brain (**cerebral hypoperfusion**). Normally blood flow to the brain is maintained at a constant level by compensating mechanisms that regulate systemic BP. When one assumes a sitting or standing position from a supine or recumbent position, peripheral capillary vasoconstriction occurs, and blood that was pooling in the lower vasculature is returned to the heart for redistribution to the head and remainder of the body. When this mechanism fails or is slow to respond, the person may experience vertigo or syncope. One of the most common causes of OH is hypovolemia, which may be induced by medications such as diuretics, vasodilator medications, and prolonged immobility or bed rest. Other causes of OH include dehydration, diarrhea, emesis, fluid loss from sweating and exertion, alcohol intake, dysrhythmias, diabetes mellitus, sepsis, and hemorrhage.

BP measurements taken with the child first supine and then standing (at least 2 minutes in each position) may demonstrate variability and assist in the diagnosis of OH. The child with a sustained drop in systolic BP of more than 20 mm Hg or in diastolic BP of more than 10 mm Hg after standing for 2 minutes without an increase in heart rate of more than 15 beats/min most likely has an autonomic deficit. Nonneurogenic causes of OH have a compensatory increase in pulse of more than 15 beats/min, as well as a drop in BP, as noted previously. For children and adolescents with vertigo, lightheadedness, nausea, syncope, diaphoresis, and pallor, it is important to monitor BP and heart rate to determine the original cause. BP is an important diagnostic measurement in children and adolescents and must be a part of the routine monitoring of vital signs.

> **! NURSING ALERT**
>
> Published norms for blood pressure (BP) are valid only if you use the same method of measurement (auscultation and cuff size determination) in clinical practice.

GENERAL APPEARANCE

The child's general appearance is a cumulative, subjective impression of the child's physical appearance, state of nutrition, behavior, personality, interactions with parents and nurse (also siblings if present), posture, development, and speech. Although the nurse records general appearance at the beginning of the physical examination, it encompasses all the observations of the child during the interview and physical assessment.

Note the **facies**, the child's facial expression and appearance. For example, the facies may give clues to children who are in pain; have difficulty breathing; feel frightened, discontented, or unhappy; are mentally delayed; or are acutely ill.

Observe the posture, position, and types of body movement. A child with hearing or vision loss may characteristically tilt the head in an awkward position to hear or see better. A child in pain may favor a body part. The child with low self-esteem or a feeling of rejection may assume a slumped, careless, and apathetic pose. Likewise, a child with confidence, a feeling of self-worth, and a sense of security usually demonstrates a tall, straight, well-balanced posture. While observing such body language, do not interpret too freely but rather record objectively.

Note the child's hygiene in terms of cleanliness; unusual body odor; the condition of the hair, neck, nails, teeth, and feet; and the condition of the clothing. Such observations are excellent clues to possible instances of neglect, inadequate financial resources, housing difficulties (e.g., no running water), or lack of knowledge concerning children's needs.

Behavior includes the child's personality, activity level, reaction to stress, requests, frustration, interactions with others (primarily the parent and nurse), degree of alertness, and response to stimuli. Some mental questions that serve as reminders for observing behavior include the following:

- What is the child's overall personality?
- Does the child have a long attention span, or is he or she easily distracted?
- Can the child follow two or three commands in succession without the need for repetition?
- What is the child's response to delayed gratification or frustration?
- Does the child use eye contact during conversation?
- What is the child's reaction to the nurse and family members?
- Is the child quick or slow to grasp explanations?

SKIN

Assess skin for color, texture, temperature, moisture, turgor, lesions, acne, and rashes. Examination of the skin and its accessory organs primarily involves inspection and palpation. Touch allows the nurse to assess the texture, turgor, and temperature of the skin. The normal color in light-skinned children varies from a milky white and rose to a deeply hued pink. Dark-skinned children, such as those of American Indian, Hispanic, or African descent, have inherited various brown, red, yellow, olive green, and bluish tones in their skin. Asian persons have skin that is normally of a yellow tone. Several variations in skin color can occur, some of which warrant further investigation. The types of color change and their appearance in children with light or dark skin are summarized in Table 4.6.

Normally, the skin texture of young children is smooth, slightly dry, and not oily or clammy. Evaluate skin temperature by symmetrically feeling each part of the body and comparing upper areas with lower ones. Note any difference in temperature.

Determine **tissue turgor**, or elasticity in the skin, by grasping the skin on the abdomen between the thumb and index finger, pulling it taut, and quickly releasing it. Elastic tissue immediately resumes its normal position without residual marks or creases. In children with poor skin turgor, the skin remains suspended or tented for a few seconds before slowly falling back on the abdomen. Skin turgor is one of the best estimates of adequate hydration and nutrition.

TABLE 4.6 Differences in Color Changes of Racial Groups

Description	Appearance in Light Skin	Appearance in Dark Skin
Cyanosis—bluish tone through skin; reflects reduced (deoxygenated) hemoglobin	Bluish tinge, especially in palpebral conjunctiva (lower eyelid), nail beds, earlobes, lips, oral membranes, soles, and palms	Ashen gray lips and tongue
Pallor—paleness; may be sign of anemia, chronic disease, edema, or shock	Loss of rosy glow in skin, especially face	Ashen gray appearance in black skin More yellowish-brown color in brown skin
Erythema—redness; may be result of increased blood flow from climatic conditions, local inflammation, infection, skin irritation, allergy, or other dermatoses, or may be caused by increased numbers of red blood cells as compensatory response to chronic hypoxia	Redness easily seen anywhere on body	Much more difficult to assess; rely on palpation for warmth or edema
Ecchymosis—large, diffuse areas, usually black and blue, caused by hemorrhage of blood into skin; typically result of injuries	Purplish to yellow-green areas; may be seen anywhere on skin	Very difficult to see unless in mouth or conjunctiva
Petechiae—same as ecchymosis except for size: small, distinct, pinpoint hemorrhages ≤2 mm in size; can denote some type of blood disorder, such as leukemia	Purplish pinpoints most easily seen on buttocks, abdomen, and inner surfaces of arms or legs	Usually invisible except in oral mucosa, conjunctiva of eyelids, and conjunctiva covering eyeball
Jaundice—yellow staining of skin usually caused by bile pigments	Yellow staining seen in sclerae of eyes, skin, fingernails, soles, palms, and oral mucosa	Most reliably assessed in sclerae, hard palate, palms, and soles

Accessory Structures

Inspection of the accessory structures of the skin may be performed while examining the skin, scalp, or extremities. Inspect the hair for color, texture, quality, distribution, and elasticity. Children's scalp hair is usually lustrous, silky, strong, and elastic. Genetic factors affect the appearance of hair. For example, the hair of African American children is usually curlier and coarser than that of white children. Hair that is stringy, dull, brittle, dry, friable, and depigmented may suggest poor nutrition. Record any bald or thinning spots. Loss of hair in infants may indicate lying in the same position and may be a cue to counsel parents concerning the child's stimulation needs.

Inspect the hair and scalp for general cleanliness. Persons in some ethnic groups condition their hair with oils or lubricants that, if not thoroughly washed from the scalp, clog the sebaceous glands, causing scalp infections. Examine the scalp for lesions, scaliness, evidence of infestation (e.g., lice or ticks), and signs of trauma (e.g., ecchymosis, masses, or scars).

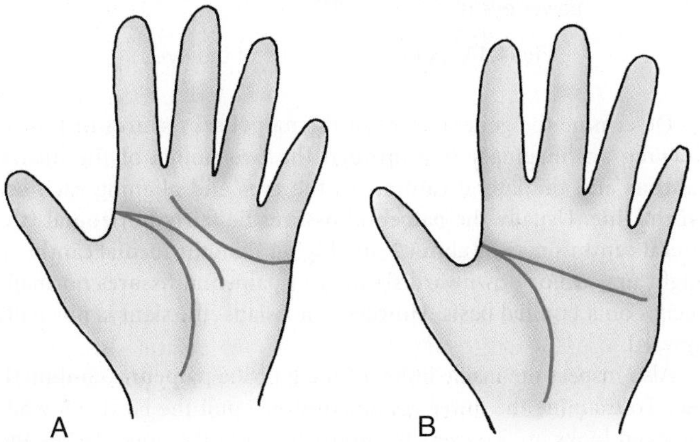

Fig. 4.14 Examples of flexion creases on palm. **A,** Normal. **B,** Transpalmar crease.

In children who are approaching puberty, look for growth of secondary hair as a sign of normally progressing pubertal changes. Note premature or delayed appearance of hair growth because although not always suggestive of hormonal dysfunction, it may be of great concern to the early-maturing child or late-maturing adolescent.

Inspect the nails for color, shape, texture, and quality. Normally, the nails are pink, convex, smooth, and hard but flexible (not brittle). The edges, which are usually white, should extend over the fingers. Dark-skinned individuals may have more deeply pigmented nail beds. Short, ragged nails are typical of habitual biting. Uncut, dirty nails are a sign of poor hygiene.

The palm normally shows three flexion creases (Fig. 4.14A). In some conditions such as Down syndrome, the two distal horizontal creases may be fused to form a single horizontal crease (the single palmar crease, or transpalmar crease) (see Fig. 4.14B). If grossly abnormal lines or folds are observed, sketch a picture to describe them and refer the finding to a specialist for further investigation.

LYMPH NODES

Lymph nodes are usually assessed during examination of the part of the body in which they are located. The body's lymphatic drainage system is extensive. Fig. 4.15 shows the usual sites for palpating accessible lymph nodes.

Palpate nodes using the distal portion of the fingers and gently but firmly pressing in a circular motion along the regions where nodes are normally present. During assessment of the nodes in the head and neck, tilt the child's head upward slightly but without tensing the sternocleidomastoid or trapezius muscles. This position facilitates palpation of the **submental**, **submandibular**, **tonsillar**, and **cervical nodes**. Palpate the **axillary nodes** with the child's arms relaxed at the sides

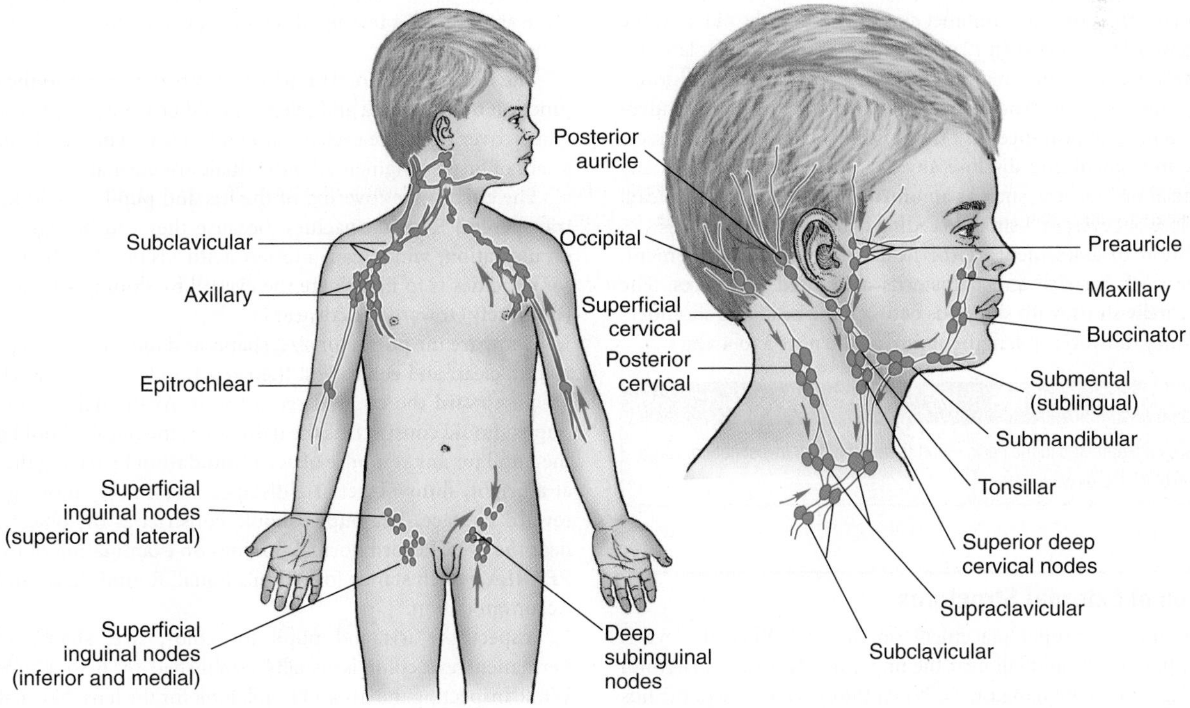

Fig. 4.15 Location of superficial lymph nodes. *Arrows* indicate directional flow of lymph.

but slightly abducted. Palpate the **inguinal nodes** with the child in the supine position. Note size, mobility, temperature, and tenderness, as well as reports by the parents regarding any visible change of enlarged nodes. In children, small, nontender, movable nodes are usually normal. Tender, enlarged, warm, erythematous lymph nodes generally indicate infection or inflammation close to their location. Report such findings for further investigation.

HEAD AND NECK

Observe the head for general shape and symmetry. A flattening of one part of the head, such as the occiput, may indicate that the child continually lies in this position. Marked asymmetry is usually abnormal and may indicate premature closure of the sutures (**craniosynostosis**).

> **! NURSING ALERT**
>
> After 6 months old, significant head lag strongly indicates cerebral injury and is referred for further evaluation.

Note head control in infants and head posture in older children. By 4 months old, most infants should be able to hold the head erect and in midline when in a vertical position.

Evaluate range of motion by asking the older child to look in each direction (to either side, up and down) or by manually putting the younger child through each position. Limited range of motion may indicate **torticollis**, in which the child holds the head to one side with the chin pointing toward the opposite side as a result of a congenital disorder or injury to the sternocleidomastoid muscle.

> **! NURSING ALERT**
>
> Hyperextension of the head (**opisthotonos**) with pain on flexion is a serious indication of meningeal irritation and is referred for immediate medical evaluation.

Palpate the skull for patent sutures, fontanels, fractures, and swellings. Normally the posterior fontanel closes by 2 months old, and the anterior fontanel fuses between 12 and 18 months old. Early or late closure is noted, because either may be a sign of a pathologic condition.

While examining the head, observe the face for symmetry, movement, and general appearance. Ask the child to "make a face" to assess symmetric movement and disclose any degree of paralysis. Note any unusual facial proportion, such as an unusually high or low forehead; wide- or close-set eyes; or a small, receding chin.

In addition to assessment of the head and neck for movement, inspect the neck for size and palpate its associated structures. The neck is normally short, with skinfolds between the head and shoulders during infancy; however, it lengthens during the next 3 to 4 years.

> **! NURSING ALERT**
>
> If any masses are detected in the neck, report them for further investigation. Large masses can block the airway.

EYES

Inspection of External Structures

Inspect the lids for proper placement on the eye. When the eye is open, the upper lid should fall near the upper iris. Note any structural anomaly (e.g., ptosis, hemangioma). When the eyes are closed, the lids should completely cover the cornea and sclera (Fig. 4.16).

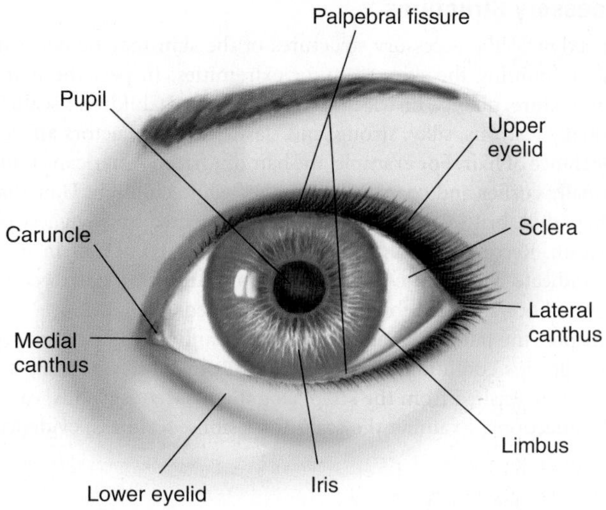

Fig. 4.16 External structures of the eye.

Determine the general slant of the **palpebral fissures** or lids by drawing an imaginary line through the two points of the medial canthus and the lateral canthus of the eyes and aligning each eye on the line. Usually the palpebral fissures lie fairly horizontal (the lateral canthus may lie about 1 mm higher than the medial canthus). Slight upward or downward slanting of palpebral fissures normally occurs on a familial basis. However, in Asians, the slant is normally upward.

Also inspect the inside lining of the lids, the **palpebral conjunctivae**. To examine the lower conjunctival sac, pull the lid down while the child looks up. To evert the upper lid, hold the upper lashes and gently pull down and forward as the child looks down. Normally the conjunctiva appears pink and glossy. Vertical yellow striations along the edge are the **meibomian glands**, or **sebaceous glands**, near the hair follicle. Located in the medial canthus and situated on the inner edge of the upper and lower lids is a tiny opening, the **lacrimal punctum**. Note any excessive tearing, discharge, or inflammation of the lacrimal apparatus.

The **bulbar conjunctiva**, which covers the eye up to the limbus, or junction of the cornea and sclera, should be transparent. The sclera, or white covering of the eyeball, should be clear. Tiny black marks in the sclera of heavily pigmented individuals are normal.

The **cornea**, or covering of the iris and pupil, should be clear and transparent. Record opacities, because they can be signs of scarring or ulceration, which can interfere with vision. The best way to test for opacities is to illuminate the eyeball by shining a light at an angle (**obliquely**) toward the cornea.

Compare the pupils for size, shape, and movement. They should be round, clear, and equal. Test their reaction to light by quickly shining a light toward the eye and removing it. As the light approaches, the pupils should constrict; as the light fades, the pupils should dilate. Test the pupil for any response of **accommodation** by having the child look at a bright, shiny object at a distance and quickly moving the object toward the face. The pupils should constrict as the object is brought near the eyes. Record normal findings on examination of the pupils as **PERRLA**, which stands for "Pupils Equal, Round, React to Light, and Accommodation."

Inspect the iris and pupil for color, size, shape, and clarity. Permanent eye color is usually established by 6 to 12 months old. While inspecting the iris and pupil, look for the lens. Normally the lens is not visible through the pupil.

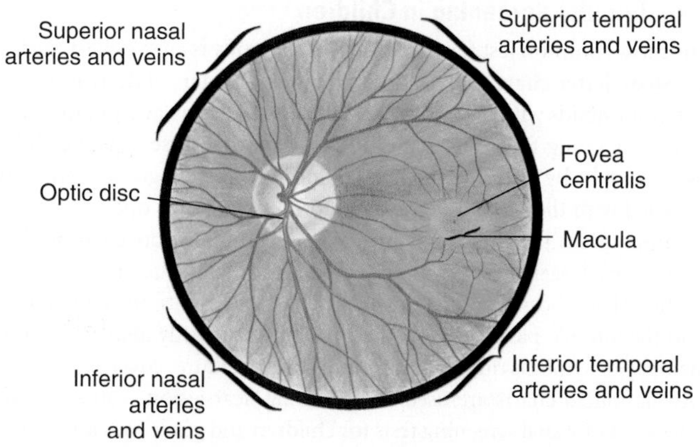

Fig. 4.17 Structures of fundus. (From Ball, J. W., Dains, J. E., Flynn, J. A., et al. [2014]. *Seidel's guide to physical examination* [8th ed.]. St Louis, MO: Elsevier.)

Inspection of Internal Structures

The ophthalmoscope permits visualization of the interior of the eyeball with a system of lenses and a high-intensity light. The lenses permit clear visualization of eye structures at different distances from the nurse's eye and correct visual acuity differences in the examiner and child. A dark room, with a dim light source, facilitates the examination because the pupils will enlarge. Use of the ophthalmoscope requires practice to know which lens setting produces the clearest image.

The ophthalmic and otic heads are often interchangeable on one "body" or handle, which encloses the power source—either disposable or rechargeable batteries. The nurse should practice changing the heads, which snap on and are secured with a quarter turn, and replacing the batteries and light bulbs. Nurses who may not be directly involved in this aspect of physical assessment in some settings are often responsible for ensuring that the instruments function properly.

Preparing the Child

The nurse can prepare the child for the ophthalmoscopic examination by showing the child the instrument, demonstrating the light source and how it shines in the eye, and explaining the reason for darkening the room. For infants and young children who do not respond to such explanations, it is best to use distraction to encourage them to keep their eyes open. Forcibly parting the eyelids results in an uncooperative, watery-eyed child and a frustrated nurse. Usually, with some practice, the nurse can elicit a red reflex almost instantly while approaching the child and may also gain a momentary inspection of the blood vessels, macula, or optic disc.

Funduscopic Examination

Fig. 4.17 shows the structures of the back of the eyeball, or the **fundus**. The fundus is immediately apparent as the **red reflex**. The intensity of the color increases in darkly pigmented individuals.

> **! NURSING ALERT**
>
> A brilliant, uniform red reflex is an important sign because it rules out many serious defects of the cornea, aqueous chamber, lens, and vitreous chamber. Absent, white, dull, or asymmetric red reflexes warrant further investigation.

As the ophthalmoscope is brought closer to the eye, the most conspicuous feature of the fundus is the **optic disc**, the area where the blood vessels and optic nerve fibers enter and exit the eye. The disc is orange to creamy pink with a pale center and lighter in color than the surrounding fundus. Normally, it is round or vertically oval.

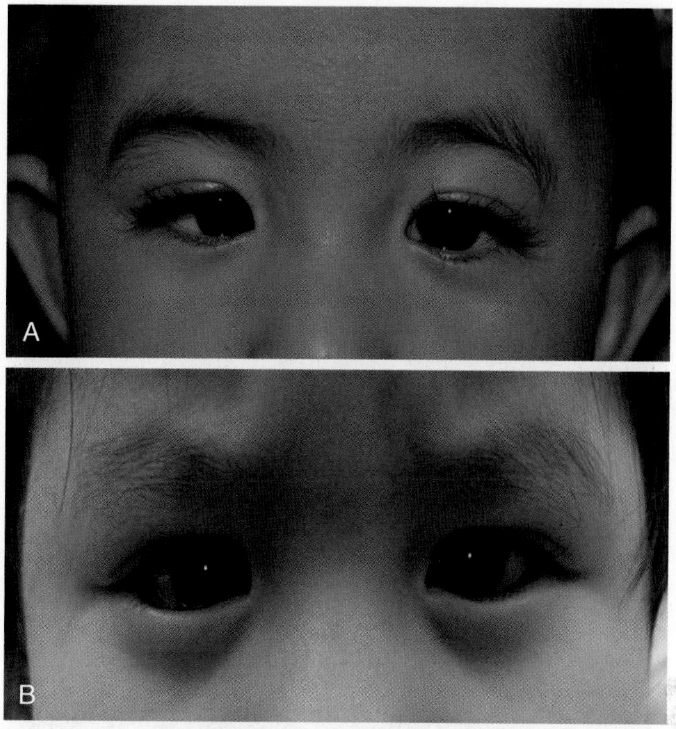

Fig. 4.18 A, Corneal light reflex test demonstrating orthophoric eyes. **B,** Pseudostrabismus. Inner epicanthal folds cause the eyes to appear misaligned; however, the corneal light reflexes fall perfectly symmetrically. (From Gleason, C. A. & Juul, S. E. [2018]. Avery's diseases of the newborn [10th ed.]. Philadelphia, PA: Elsevier.)

After locating the optic disc, inspect the area for blood vessels. The central retinal artery and vein appear in the depths of the disc and emanate outward with visible branching. The veins are darker and about one-fourth larger than the arteries. Normally, the branches of the arteries and veins cross one another.

Other structures include the **macula**, the area of the fundus with the greatest concentration of visual receptors, and in the center of the macula, a minute glistening spot of reflected light called the **fovea centralis**; this is the area of most perfect vision.

Vision Screening

The US Preventive Services Task Force (2017) recommends vision screening for the presence of amblyopia and its risk factors for all children 3 to 5 years old. Several tests are available for assessing vision. This discussion focuses on ocular alignment, visual acuity, peripheral vision, and color vision. Chapter 18 discusses behavioral and physical signs of visual impairment. Nurses can provide accurate vision screening with appropriate training (Mathers, Keyes, & Wright, 2010).

Ocular Alignment

Normally, by 3 to 4 months old, children can fixate on one visual field with both eyes simultaneously (binocularity). In **strabismus**, or cross-eye, one eye deviates from the point of fixation. If the misalignment is constant, the weak eye becomes "lazy," and the brain eventually suppresses the image produced by that eye. If strabismus is not detected and corrected by 4 to 6 years old, blindness from disuse, known as **amblyopia**, may result.

Tests commonly used to detect misalignment are the corneal light reflex and the cover tests. To perform the **corneal light reflex test**, or **Hirschberg test**, shine a penlight or the light of the ophthalmoscope directly into the patient's eyes, while he or she is looking straight ahead, from a distance of about 40.5 cm (16 inches). If the eyes are **orthophoric**, or normal, the light falls symmetrically within each pupil (Fig. 4.18A). If the light falls

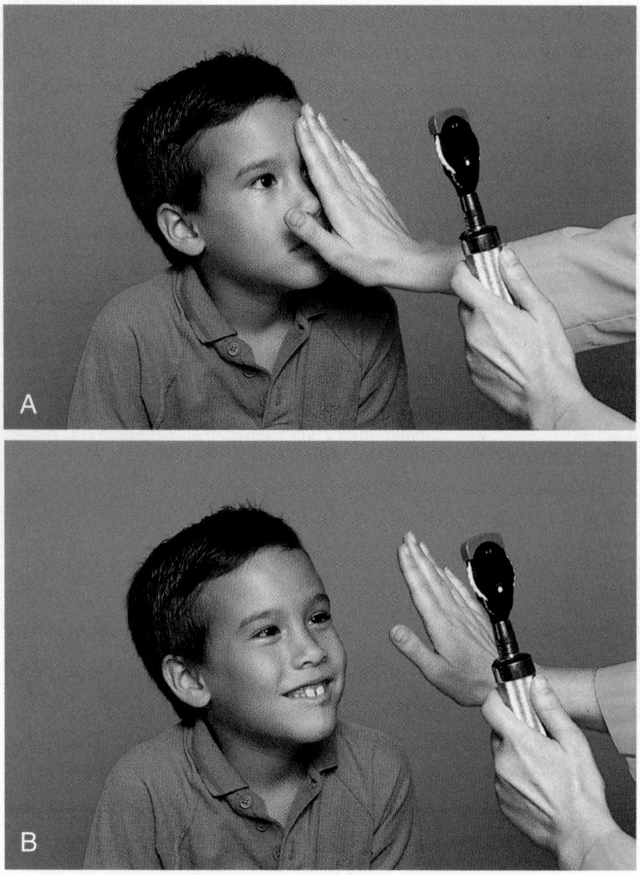

Fig. 4.19 Alternate cover test to detect amblyopia in a patient with strabismus. **A,** The eye is occluded, and the child is fixating on the light source. **B,** If the eye does not move when uncovered, the eyes are aligned.

off-center in one eye, the eyes are misaligned. **Epicanthal folds**, excess folds of skin that extend from the roof of the nose to the inner termination of the eyebrow and that partially or completely overlap the inner canthus of the eye, may give a false impression of misalignment (**pseudostrabismus**) (see Fig. 4.18B). Epicanthal folds are often found in Asian children.

In the **cover test**, one eye is covered, and the movement of the uncovered eye is observed while the child looks at a near (33 cm [13 inches]) or distant (6 m [20 feet]) object. If the uncovered eye does not move, it is aligned. If the uncovered eye moves, a misalignment is present because when the stronger eye is temporarily covered, the misaligned eye attempts to fixate on the object.

In the **alternate cover test**, occlusion shifts back and forth from one eye to the other, and movement of the eye that was covered is observed as soon as the occluder is removed while the child focuses on a point in front of him or her (Fig. 4.19). If normal alignment is present, shifting the cover from one eye to the other will not cause the eye to move. If misalignment is present, eye movement will occur when the cover is moved. This test takes more practice than the other cover test because the occluder must be moved back and forth quickly and accurately to see the eye move. Because deviations can occur at different ranges, it is important to perform the cover tests at both close and far distances.

> **! NURSING ALERT**
>
> The cover test is usually easier to perform if the examiner uses his or her hand rather than a card-type occluder (see Fig. 4.19). Attractive occluders fashioned like an ice cream cone or happy-face lollipop cut from cardboard are also well received by young children.

Visual Acuity Screening in Children

The most common test for measuring visual acuity is an eye chart, such as the **Sloan letter chart**, which consists of lines of letters of decreasing size. The child stands with his or her heels at a line 10 feet away from the chart. When screening for visual acuity in children, the nurse tests the child's right eye first by covering the left. Children who wear glasses should be screened with them on. Tell the child to keep both eyes open during the examination. If the child fails to read the current line, move up the chart to the next larger line. Continue up the chart until the child can read the line. Then begin moving down the chart again until the child fails to read the line. To pass each line, the child must correctly identify a simple majority of symbols on the line. Repeat the procedure, covering the right eye. Handheld charts are used for screening near vision. Table 4.7 provides a list of visual screening tests for children and guidelines for referral.

For children unable to read letters and numbers, optotypes (figures or letters of different sizes) are used. The LEA Symbols consist of four figures, and the child calls them what he or she wants to call them. The HOTV test consists of a wall chart composed of the letters H, O, T, and V. The child is given a board containing a large H, O, T, and V. The examiner points to a letter on the wall chart, and the child matches the correct letter on the board held in his or her hand. The LEA Symbols and HOTV are preferred screening tests for preliterate children.

Visual Acuity Screening in Infants and Difficult-to-Test Children

In newborns, vision is tested mainly by checking for **light perception** by shining a light into the eyes and noting responses, such as pupillary constriction, blinking, following the light to midline, increased alertness, or refusal to open the eyes after exposure to the light. Although the simple maneuver of checking light perception and eliciting the pupillary light reflex indicates that the anterior half of the visual apparatus is intact, it does not confirm that the infant can see. In other words, this test does not assess whether the brain receives the visual message and interprets the signals.

Another test of visual acuity is the infant's ability to fix on and follow a target. Although any brightly colored or patterned object can be used, the human face is excellent. Hold the infant upright while moving your face slowly from side to side. Other signs that may indicate visual loss or other serious eye problems include fixed pupils, strabismus, constant nystagmus, the setting-sun sign, and slow lateral movements. Unfortunately, it is difficult to test each eye separately; the presence of such signs in one eye could indicate unilateral blindness.

Special tests are available for testing infants and other difficult-to-test children to assess visual acuity or confirm blindness. For example, in **visually evoked potentials**, the eyes are stimulated with a bright light or pattern, and electrical activity to the visual cortex is recorded through scalp electrodes.

Evidence supports the use of elective instrument-based vision screening, primarily photoscreening and autorefraction, in children 12 months old until the child can reliably read an eye chart (Donahue, Baker, Committee on Practice and Ambulatory Medicine, et al., 2016; Miller, Lessin, American Academy of Pediatrics Section on Ophthalmology, et al., 2012). Neither instrument measures visual acuity itself but rather measures risk factors for vision problems. Photoscreening uses optical images of the eye's red reflex to estimate refractive error, media opacity, ocular alignment, and other factors putting a child at risk for amblyopia. Handheld autorefraction is used to evaluate the refractive error of each eye.

> **! NURSING ALERT**
>
> If visual fixation and following are not present by 3 months old, further ophthalmologic evaluation is necessary.

TABLE 4.7 Pediatric Vision Assessment

Assessment	Ages: Newborn-6 mos	6-12 mos	1-3 yrs	3-4 yrs	4-5 yrs	Every 1-2 yrs after 5 yrs	When to be Concerned
Assess for red light reflex	•	•	•	•	•	•	No reflex, dull, white, looks opaque, unequal
Exam outside of eye	•	•	•	•	•	•	Structure abnormality (e.g., swelling, drooping)
Examine pupils	•	•	•	•	•	•	Irregular shape, unequal size, slow reaction to light
Assess for corneal light reflex		•	•	•	•	•	Unequal when looking at both eyes
Perform cover test				•	•	•	One eye is covered, and uncovered eye is observed for shift in fixation
Assess ability to focus and follow	infant ≥3 mos	•	•	•	•	•	Unable to fix and follow
Evaluate visual acuity				•	•	•	20/50 or worse in either eye or 2 lines of differences between the eyes
					•	•	20/40 or worse in either eye

Adapted From Hagan, J. F., Shaw, J. S. (Eds.). (2017). *Bright futures: Guidelines for health supervision of infants, children and adolescents* (4th ed.). Elk Grove Village, IL: American Academy of Pediatrics.

Peripheral Vision

In children who are old enough to cooperate, estimate peripheral vision, or the visual field of each eye, by having the children fixate on a specific point directly in front of them while an object, such as a finger or a pencil, is moved from beyond the field of vision into the range of peripheral vision. As soon as children see the object, have them say, "Stop." At that point, measure the angle from the anteroposterior axis of the eye (straight line of vision) to the peripheral axis (point at which the object is first seen). Check each eye separately and for each quadrant of vision. Normally children see about 50 degrees upward, 70 degrees downward, 60 degrees nasalward, and 90 degrees temporally. Limitations in peripheral vision may indicate blindness from damage to structures within the eye or to any of the visual pathways.

Color Vision

The tests available for color vision include the Ishihara test and the Hardy-Rand-Rittler test. Each consists of a series of cards (pseudoisochromatic) containing a color field composed of spots of a certain "confusion" color. Against the field is a number or symbol similarly printed in dots but of a color likely to be confused with the field color by a person with a color vision deficit. As a result, the figure or letter is invisible to an affected individual but is clearly seen by a person with normal vision.

EARS

Inspection of External Structures

The entire external ear is called the pinna, or auricle; one is located on each side of the head. Measure the height alignment of the pinna by drawing an imaginary line from the outer orbit of the eye to the occiput, or most prominent protuberance of the skull. The top of the pinna should meet or cross this line. Low-set ears are commonly associated with renal anomalies or genetic syndromes. Measure the angle of the pinna by drawing a perpendicular line from the imaginary horizontal line and aligning the pinna next to this mark. Normally the pinna lies within a 10-degree angle of the vertical line (Fig. 4.20). If it falls outside this area, record the deviation and look for other anomalies.

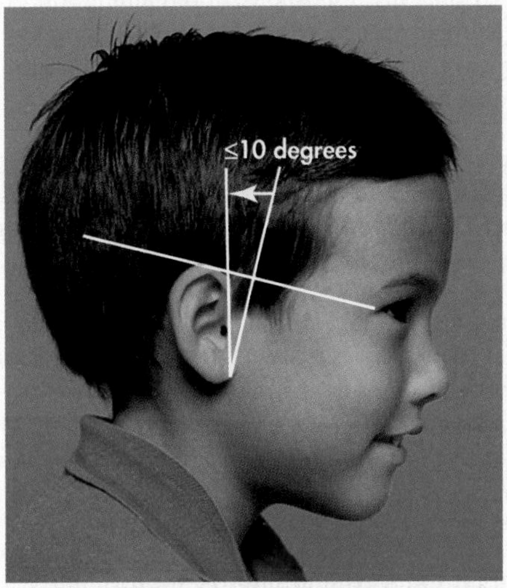

Fig. 4.20 Ear alignment.

Normally the pinna extends slightly outward from the skull. Except in newborn infants, ears that are flat against the head or protruding away from the scalp may indicate problems. Flattened ears in an infant may suggest a frequent side-lying position and, just as with isolated areas of hair loss, may be a clue to investigate parents' understanding of the child's stimulation needs.

Inspect the skin surface around the ear for small openings, extra tags of skin, sinuses, or earlobe creases. If a sinus is found, note this because it may represent a fistula that drains into some area of the neck or ear. Note an earlobe crease, if found, because it may be associated with a rare syndrome. However, having one small abnormality is not uncommon and is often not associated with a serious condition. Cutaneous tags represent no pathologic process but may cause parents concern in terms of the child's appearance.

Also assess the ears for hygiene. An otoscope is not necessary for looking into the external ear canal to note the presence of cerumen, a waxy substance produced by the ceruminous glands in the outer portion of the ear canal. Cerumen is usually yellow-brown and soft. If an otoscope is used and any discharge is visible, note its color and odor. Avoid transmitting potentially infectious material to the other ear or to another child by hand washing and using disposable specula or sterilizing reusable specula between each examination.

Inspection of Internal Structures

The head of the otoscope permits visualization of the tympanic membrane by use of a bright light, a magnifying glass, and a speculum. Some otoscopes have an attachment for a pneumonic device to insert air into the ear canal to determine membrane compliance (movement). The speculum, which is inserted into the external ear canal, comes in a variety of sizes to accommodate different ear canal widths. The largest speculum that fits comfortably into the ear is used to achieve the greatest area of visualization. The lens, or magnifying glass, is movable, allowing the examiner to insert an object, such as a curette, into the ear canal through the speculum while still viewing the structures through the lens.

Positioning the Child

Before beginning the otoscopic examination, position the child properly and gently restrain (child sits on parent's lap, and parent holds child's body and head) if necessary. Older children usually cooperate and do not need restraint. However, prepare them for the procedure by allowing them to play with the instrument, demonstrating how it works, and stressing the importance of remaining still. A helpful suggestion is to let them observe you examining the parent's ear. Restraint is needed for younger children because the ear examination often upsets them (see Atraumatic Care box).

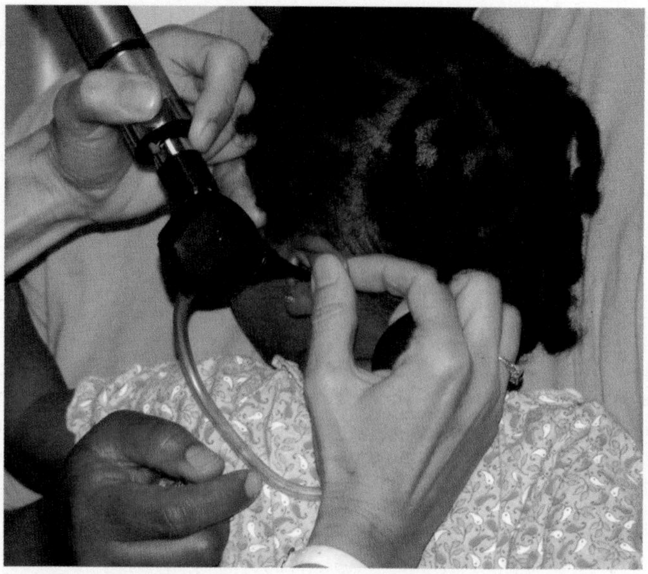

Fig. 4.21 Position for a young child for a pneumatic otoscopic examination where a puff of air is introduced into the ear canal.

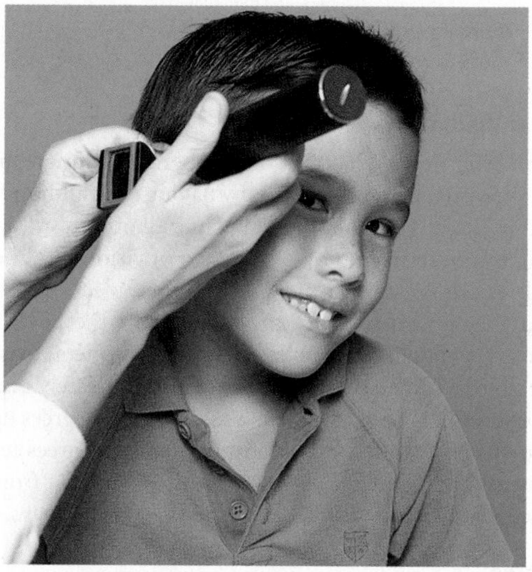

Fig. 4.22 Positioning the head by tilting it toward the opposite shoulder for full view of the tympanic membrane.

ATRAUMATIC CARE

Reducing Distress From Otoscopy in Young Children

Make examining the ear a game by explaining that you are looking for a "bunny" in the ear. This kind of make-believe is an absorbing distraction and usually elicits cooperation. After examining the ear, clarify that "looking for a bunny" was only pretend and thank the child for letting you look in his or her ear. Another great distraction technique is asking the child to put a finger on the opposite ear to keep the light from getting out.

As you insert the speculum into the meatus, move it around the outer rim to accustom the child to the feel of something entering the ear. If examining a painful ear, examine the unaffected ear first, then return to the painful ear and touch a nonpainful part of the affected ear first. By this time, the child is usually less fearful of anything causing discomfort to the ear and will cooperate more.

For their protection and safety, restrain infants and toddlers for the otoscopic examination. There are two general positions of restraint. In one, the child is seated sideways in the parent's lap with one arm hugging the parent and the other arm at the side. The ear to be examined is toward the nurse. With one hand the parent holds the child's head firmly against his or her chest and hugs the child with the other arm, thereby securing the child's free arm (Fig. 4.21). Examine the ear using the same procedure for holding the otoscope as described later.

The other position involves placing the child on the side, back, or abdomen with the arms at the side and the head turned so that the ear to be examined points toward the ceiling. Lean over the child, use the upper part of the body to restrain the arms and upper trunk movements, and use the examining hand to stabilize the head. This position is practical for young infants and for older children who need minimum restraint, but it may not be feasible for other children who protest vigorously. For safety, enlist the parent's or an assistant's help in immobilizing the head by firmly placing one hand above the ear and the other on the child's side, abdomen, or back.

With cooperative children, examine the ear with the child in a side-lying, sitting, or standing position. One disadvantage to standing is that the child may "walk away" as the otoscope enters the ear canal. If the child is standing or sitting, tilt the head slightly toward the child's opposite shoulder to achieve a better view of the tympanic membrane (eardrum) (Fig. 4.22).

With the thumb and forefinger of the free hand, grasp the auricle. For the two positions of restraint, hold the otoscope upside down at the junction of its head and handle with the thumb and index finger. Place the other fingers against the skull to allow the otoscope to move with the child in case of sudden movement. In examining a cooperative child, hold the handle with the otic head upright or upside down. Use the dominant hand to examine both ears or reverse hands for each ear, whichever is more comfortable.

Before using the otoscope, visualize the external ear and the tympanic membrane as being superimposed on a clock (Fig. 4.23). The numbers are important geographic landmarks. Introduce the speculum into the meatus between the 3 and 9 o'clock positions in a downward and forward position. Because the ear canal is curved, the speculum does not permit a panoramic view of the tympanic membrane unless the ear canal is straightened. In infants, the ear canal curves upward. Therefore pull the pinna down and back (toward the 6 to 9 o'clock range for the right ear and toward the 3 to 6 o'clock range for the left ear) to straighten the ear canal (Fig. 4.24A). With older children, usually those older than 3 years of age, the ear canal curves downward and forward. Therefore pull the pinna up and back (toward a 2 o'clock position for the left ear and toward a 10 o'clock position for the right ear) (see Fig. 4.24B). If you have difficulty visualizing the tympanic membrane, try repositioning the head, introducing the speculum at a different angle, and pulling the pinna in a slightly different direction. Do not insert the speculum past the cartilaginous (outermost) portion of the ear canal, usually a distance of 0.60 to 1.25 cm (0.23 to 0.5 inch) in older children. Insertion of the speculum into the posterior or bony portion of the ear canal causes pain.

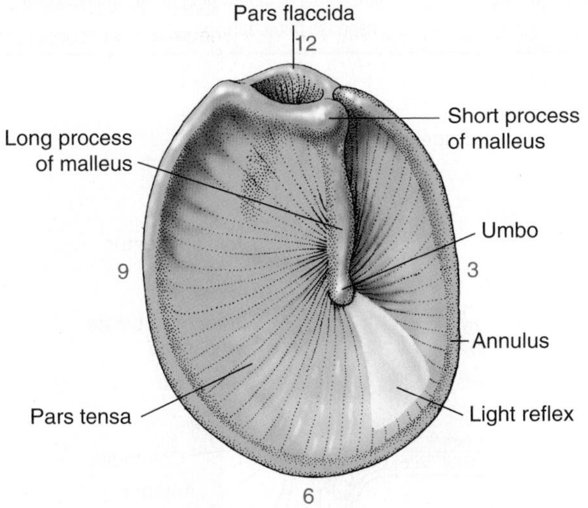

Fig. 4.23 Landmarks of the right tympanic membrane. (From Ignatavicius, D. D., & Workman, M. L. [2013]. *Medical-surgical nursing: Patient-centered collaborative care* [7th ed.]. St Louis, MO: Saunders.)

In neonates and young infants, the walls of the ear canal are pliable and floppy because of the underdeveloped cartilaginous and bony structures. Therefore the very small 2-mm speculum usually needs to be inserted deeper into the ear canal than in older children. Exercise great care not to damage the walls or tympanic membrane. For this reason, only an experienced examiner should insert an otoscope into the ears of very young infants.

Otoscopic Examination

As you introduce the speculum into the external ear canal, inspect the walls of the ear canal, the color of the tympanic membrane, the light reflex, and the usual landmarks of the bony prominences of the middle ear. The walls of the external auditory ear canal are pink, although they are more pigmented in dark-skinned children. Minute hairs are evident in the outermost portion, where cerumen is produced. Note signs of irritation, foreign bodies, or infection.

Foreign bodies in the ear are common in children and range from erasers to beans. Symptoms may include pain, discharge, and affected hearing. Remove soft objects, such as paper or insects, with forceps. Remove small, hard objects, such as pebbles, with a suction tip, a hook, or irrigation. However, irrigation is contraindicated if the object is vegetative matter, such as beans or pasta, which swells when in contact with fluid.

> **! NURSING ALERT**
>
> If there is any doubt about the type of object in the ear and the appropriate method to remove it, refer the child to the appropriate practitioner.

The **tympanic membrane** is a translucent, light pearly pink or gray. Note marked erythema (which may indicate suppurative otitis media); a dull, nontransparent grayish color (sometimes suggestive of serous otitis media); or ashen gray or white areas (signs of scarring from a previous perforation). A black area usually suggests a perforation of the membrane that has not healed.

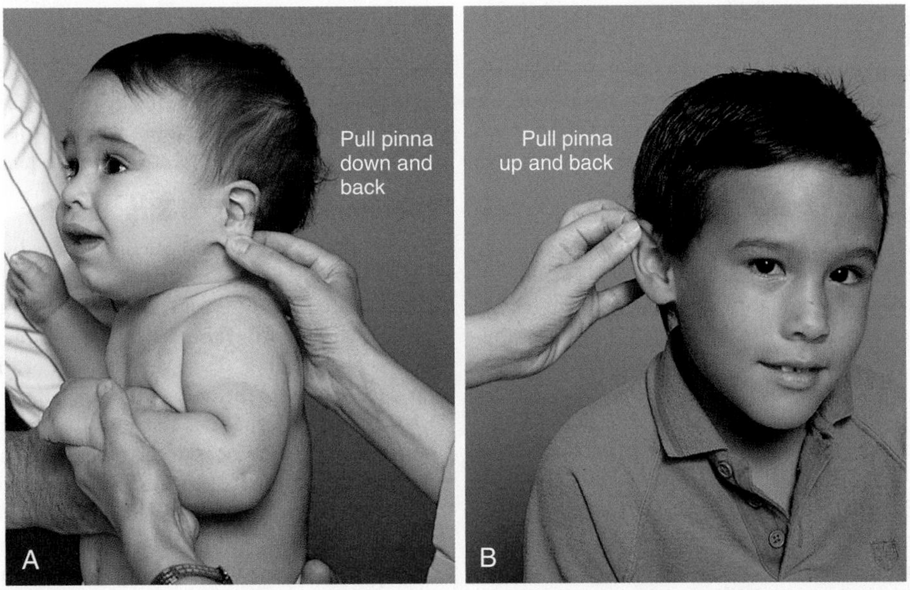

Fig. 4.24 Positioning for visualizing the tympanic membrane (A) in an infant and (B) in a child older than 3 years of age.

TABLE 4.8 Auditory Tests for Infants and Children

Age	Auditory Test	Type of Measurement	Procedure
Newborns	Auditory brainstem response (ABR)	Electrophysiologic measurement of activity in auditory nerve and brainstem pathways	Placement of electrodes on child's head detects auditory stimuli presented though earphones one ear at a time.
Infants	Behavioral audiometry	Used to observe behavior in response to certain sounds heard through speakers or earphones	The child's responses to the sounds heard are observed.
Toddlers	Play audiometry	Uses an audiometer to transmit sounds at different volumes and pitches	The toddler is asked to do something with a toy (e.g., touch a toy, move a toy) every time the sound is heard.
Children and adolescents	Pure tone audiometry	Uses an audiometer that produces sounds at different volumes and pitches in the child's ears	The child is asked to respond in some way when the tone is heard in the earphone.
	Tympanometry (also called *impedance* or *admittance*)	Determines how the middle ear is functioning and detects any changes in pressure in the middle ear	A soft plastic tip is placed over the ear canal, and the tympanometer measures tympanic membrane movement when the pressure changes.
All ages	Evoked optoacoustic emissions (EOAE)	Physiologic test specifically measuring cochlear (outer hair cell) response to presentation of stimulus	Small probe containing sensitive microphone is placed in ear canal for stimulus delivery and response detection.

The characteristic tenseness and slope of the tympanic membrane cause the light of the otoscope to reflect at about the 5 o'clock position (in the right ear) or the 7 o'clock position (in the left ear). The **light reflex** is a fairly well-defined, cone-shaped reflection, which normally points away from the face.

The **bony landmarks** of the tympanic membrane are formed by the **umbo**, or tip of the malleus. It appears as a small, round, opaque, concave spot near the center of the tympanic membrane. The **manubrium** (long process or handle) of the malleus appears to be a whitish line extending from the umbo upward to the margin of the membrane. At the upper end of the long process near the 1 o'clock position (in the right ear) or 11 o'clock position (in the left ear) is a sharp, knoblike protuberance, representing the **short process** of the malleus. Note the absence or distortion of the light reflex, or loss or abnormal prominence of any of these landmarks.

Auditory Testing

Several types of hearing tests are available and recommended for screening in infants and children (Table 4.8). The American Academy of Pediatrics recommends pure tone audiometry testing at 500, 1000, 2000, and 4000 Hz, with children failing if they cannot hear the tones at 20 dB (Harlor, Bower, & Committee on Practice and Ambulatory Medicine, Section on Otolaryngology—Head and Neck Surgery, 2009). Universal newborn hearing screening is available in all US states. The nurse must operate under a high index of suspicion for those children who may have conditions associated with hearing loss, whose parents are concerned about hearing loss, and who may have developed behaviors that indicate auditory impairment. Chapter 18 discusses types of hearing loss, causes, clinical manifestations, and appropriate treatment.

NOSE

Inspection of External Structures

Compare the placement and alignment of the nose by drawing an imaginary vertical line from the center point between the eyes down to the notch of the upper lip. The nose should lie in the middle of the face, with each side exactly symmetric on both sides of the imaginary line. Note its location, any deviation to one side, and asymmetry in overall size and in diameter of the nares (nostrils). The bridge of the nose is sometimes flat in Asian and African American children. Observe the **alae nasi** for any sign of flaring, which indicates respiratory difficulty. Always report any flaring of the alae nasi. Fig. 4.25 illustrates the external landmarks and internal structures of the nose.

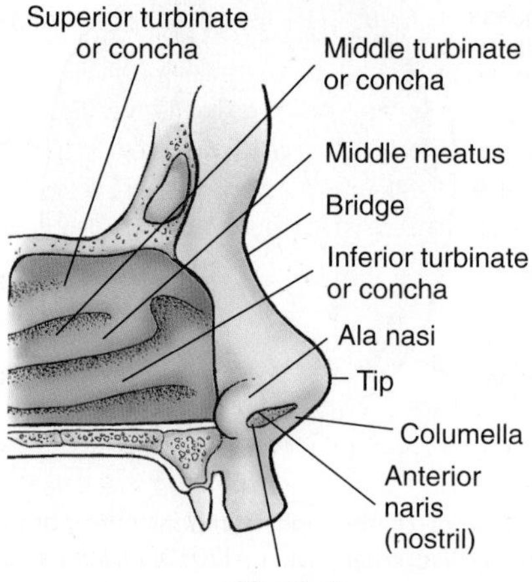

Fig. 4.25 External landmarks and internal structures of the nose.

Inspection of Internal Structures

Inspect the **anterior vestibule** of the nose by pushing the tip upward, tilting the head backward, and illuminating the cavity with a flashlight or otoscope without the attached ear speculum. Note the color of the **mucosal lining**, which is normally redder than the oral membranes, as well as any swelling, discharge, dryness, or bleeding. There should be no discharge from the nose.

On looking deeper into the nose, inspect the **turbinates**, or **concha**, plates of bone that jut into the nasal cavity and are enveloped by the mucous membranes. The turbinates greatly increase the surface area of the nasal cavity as air is inhaled. The spaces or channels between the turbinates are called the **meatus** and correspond to each of the three turbinates. Normally, the front end of the inferior and middle turbinate and the middle meatus are seen. They should be the same color as the lining of the vestibule.

Inspect the **septum**, which should divide the vestibules equally. Note any deviation, especially if it causes an occlusion of one side of the nose. A perforation may be evident within the septum. If this is suspected, shine the light of the otoscope into one naris and look for admittance of light to the other. Because olfaction is an important function of the nose, testing for smell may be done at this point or as part of cranial nerve assessment (see Table 4.11).

MOUTH AND THROAT

With a cooperative child, the nurse can accomplish almost the entire examination of the mouth and throat without the use of a tongue blade. Ask the child to open the mouth wide; to move the tongue in different directions for full visualization; and to say "ahh," which depresses the tongue for full view of the back of the mouth (tonsils, uvula, and oropharynx). For a closer look at the **buccal mucosa**, or lining of the cheeks, ask children to use their fingers to move the outer lip and cheek to one side (see Atraumatic Care box).

ATRAUMATIC CARE

Encouraging Opening the Mouth for Examination

- Perform the examination in front of a mirror.
- Let the child first examine someone else's mouth, such as the parent's, the nurse's, or a puppet's (Fig. 4.26A), and then examine child's mouth.
- Instruct the child to tilt the head back slightly, breathe deeply through the mouth, and hold the breath; this action lowers the tongue to the floor of the mouth without the use of a tongue blade.
- Lightly brushing the palate with a cotton swab also may open the mouth for assessment.

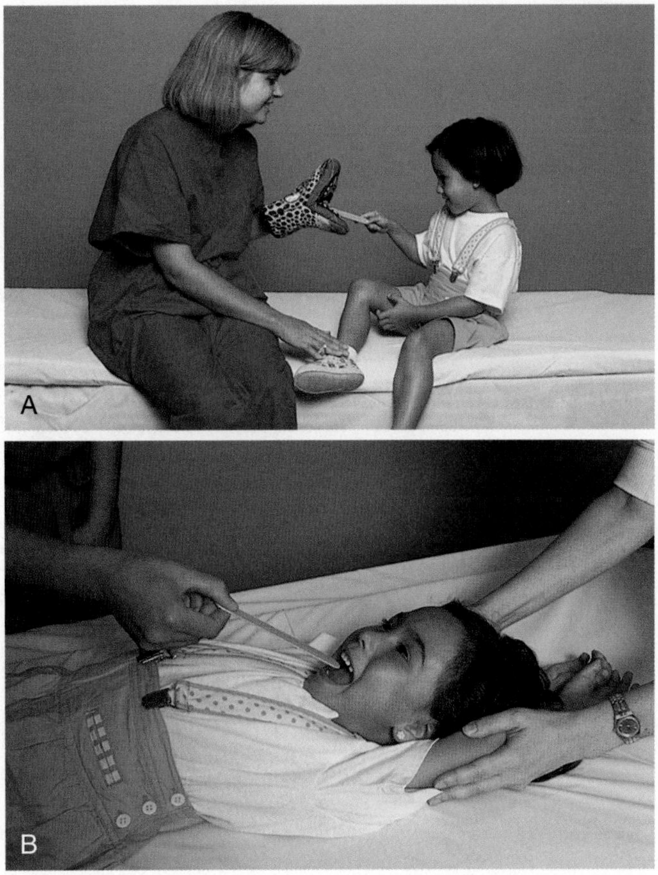

Fig. 4.26 **A,** Encouraging a child to cooperate. **B,** Positioning a child for examination of the mouth.

Infants and toddlers usually resist attempts to keep the mouth open. Because inspecting the mouth is upsetting, leave it for the end of the physical examination (along with examination of the ears) or do it during episodes of crying. However, the use of a tongue blade (preferably flavored) to depress the tongue may be needed. Place the tongue blade along the side of the tongue, not in the center back area where the gag reflex is elicited. Fig. 4.26B illustrates proper positioning of the child for the oral examination.

The major structure of the exterior of the mouth is the lips. The lips should be moist, soft, smooth, and pink, or a deeper hue than the surrounding skin. The lips should be symmetric when relaxed or tensed. Assess symmetry when the child talks or cries.

Inspection of Internal Structures

The major structures that are visible within the oral cavity and oropharynx are the mucosal lining of the lips and cheeks, gums (or gingiva), teeth, tongue, palate, uvula, tonsils, and posterior oropharynx (Fig. 4.27). Inspect all areas lined with **mucous membranes** (inside the lips and cheeks, gingiva, underside of the tongue, palate, and back of the pharynx) for color, any areas of white patches or ulceration, petechiae, bleeding, sensitivity, and moisture. The membranes should be bright pink, smooth, glistening, uniform, and moist.

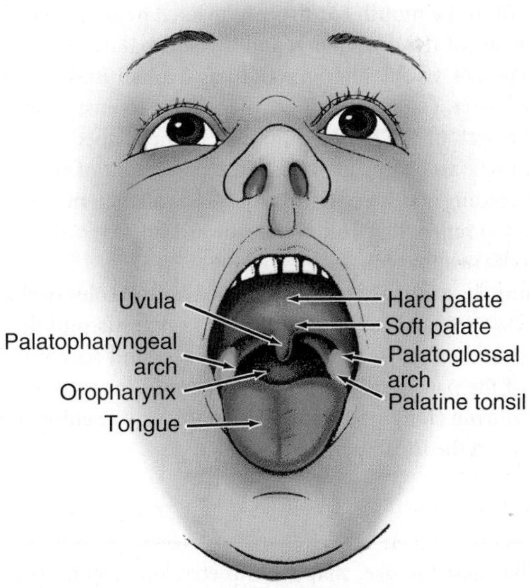

Fig. 4.27 Interior structures of the mouth.

Inspect the teeth for number (deciduous, permanent, or mixed dentition) in each dental arch, for hygiene, and for occlusion or bite (see also Chapter 9, Teething). Discoloration of tooth enamel with obvious **plaque** (whitish coating on the surface of the teeth) is a sign of poor dental hygiene and indicates a need for counseling. Brown spots in the crevices of the crown of the tooth or between the teeth may be **caries** (cavities). Chalky white to yellow or brown areas on the enamel may indicate **fluorosis** (excessive fluoride ingestion). Teeth that appear greenish black may be stained temporarily from ingestion of supplemental iron.

Examine the gums (**gingiva**) surrounding the teeth. The color is normally coral pink, and the surface texture is stippled, similar to that of an orange peel. In dark-skinned children, the gums are more deeply colored, and a brownish area is often observed along the gum line.

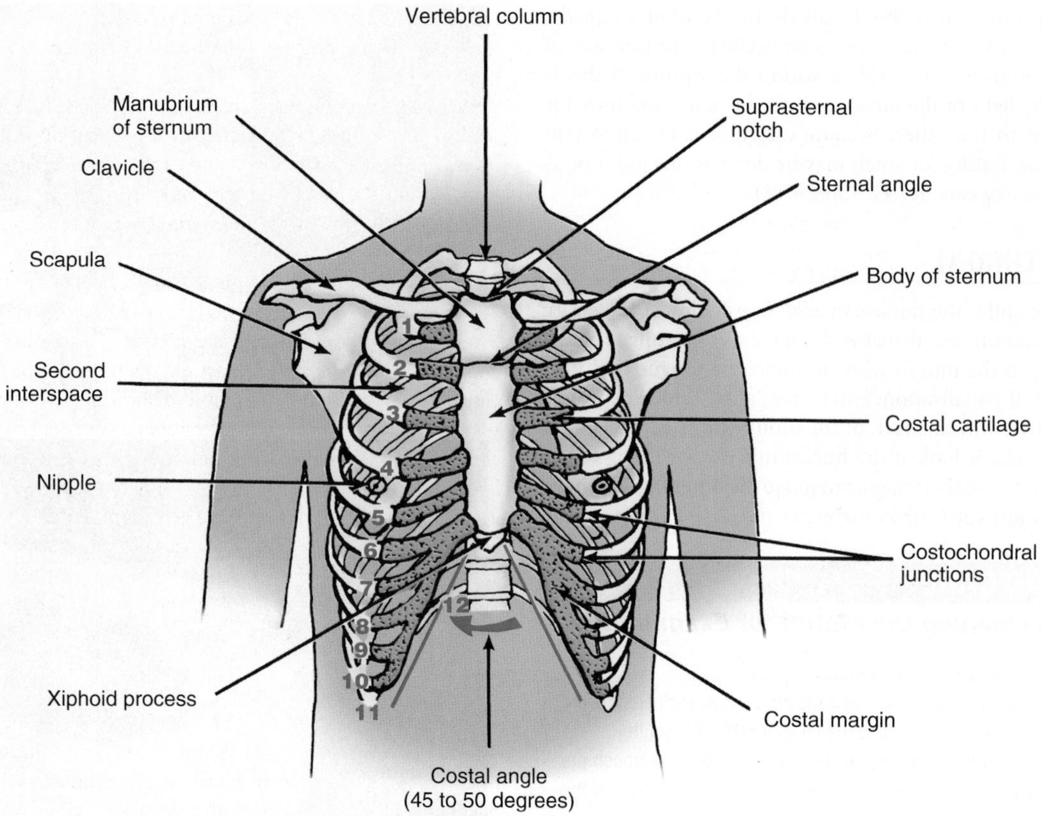

Fig. 4.28 The rib cage.

Inspect the tongue for papillae, small projections that contain several taste buds and give the tongue its characteristic rough appearance. Note the size and mobility of the tongue. Normally the tip of the tongue should extend to the lips or beyond.

The roof of the mouth consists of the **hard palate**, which is located near the front of the oral cavity, and the **soft palate**, which is located toward the back of the pharynx and has a small midline protrusion called the **uvula**. Carefully inspect the palates to ensure that they are intact. The arch of the palate should be dome shaped. A narrow, flat roof or a high, arched palate affects the placement of the tongue and can cause feeding and speech problems. Test movement of the uvula by eliciting a gag reflex. It should move upward to close off the nasopharynx from the oropharynx.

Examine the oropharynx and note the size and color of the **palatine tonsils**. They are normally the same color as the surrounding mucosa, glandular rather than smooth in appearance, and barely visible over the edge of the palatoglossal arches. The size of the tonsils varies considerably during childhood. However, report any swelling, redness, or white areas on the tonsils.

CHEST

Inspect the chest for size, shape, symmetry, movement, breast development, and the bony landmarks formed by the ribs and sternum. The **rib cage** consists of 12 ribs on each side and the sternum, or breastbone, located in the midline of the trunk (Fig. 4.28). The **sternum** is composed of three main parts. The **manubrium**, the uppermost portion, can be felt at the base of the neck at the **suprasternal notch**. The largest segment of the sternum is the body, which forms the **sternal angle (angle of Louis)** as it articulates with the manubrium. At the end of the body is a small, movable process called the **xiphoid**. The angle of the costal margin as it attaches to the sternum is called the **costal angle** and is normally about 45 to 50 degrees. These bony structures are important landmarks in the location of ribs and **intercostal spaces (ICSs)**, which are the spaces between the ribs. They are numbered according to the rib directly above the space. For example, the space immediately below the second rib is the second ICS.

The **thoracic cavity** is also divided into segments by drawing imaginary lines on the chest and back. Fig. 4.29 illustrates the anterior, lateral, and posterior divisions.

Measure the size of the chest by placing the measuring tape around the rib cage at the nipple line. For greatest accuracy, take two measurements—one during inspiration and the other during expiration—and record the average. Chest size is important mainly in relation to head circumference (see Head Circumference earlier in this chapter). Always report marked disproportions because most are caused by abnormal head growth, although some may be a result of altered chest shape, such as **barrel chest** (chest is round), **pectus excavatum** (sternum is depressed), or **pectus carinatum** (sternum protrudes outward).

During infancy the chest's shape is almost circular, with the anteroposterior (front-to-back) diameter equaling the transverse, or lateral (side-to-side), diameter. As the child grows, the chest normally increases in the transverse direction, causing the anteroposterior diameter to be less than the lateral diameter. Note the angle made by the lower costal margin and the sternum and palpate the junction of the ribs with the costal cartilage (costochondral junction) and sternum, which should be fairly smooth.

Movement of the chest wall should be symmetric bilaterally and coordinated with breathing. During inspiration, the chest rises and expands, the diaphragm descends, and the costal angle increases. During expiration, the chest falls and decreases in size, the diaphragm rises, and the costal angle narrows (Fig. 4.30). In children younger than 6 or 7 years old, respiratory movement is principally abdominal or diaphragmatic. In older children, particularly girls,

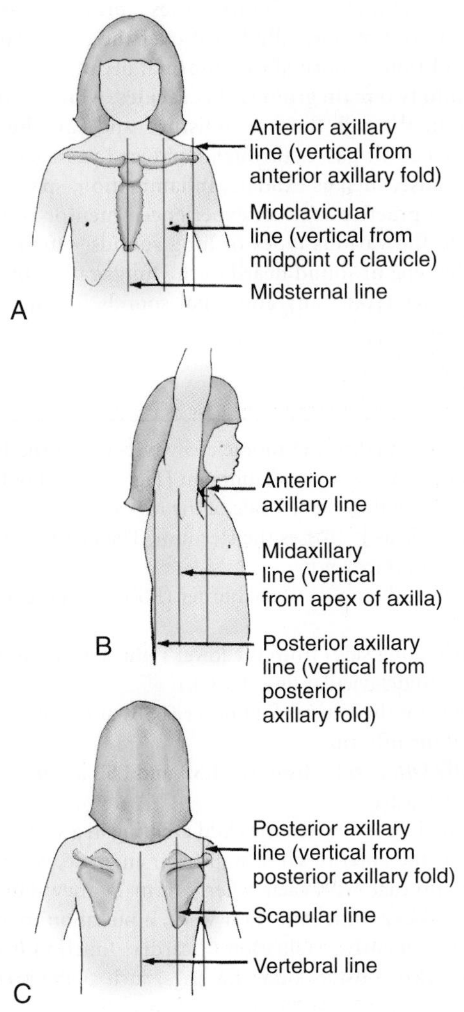

Fig. 4.29 Imaginary landmarks of the chest. **A,** Anterior. **B,** Right lateral. **C,** Posterior.

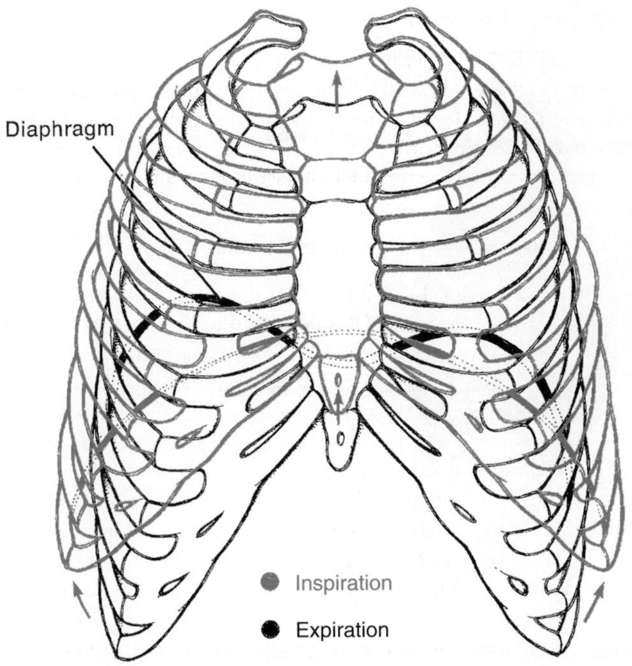

Fig. 4.30 Movement of the chest during respiration.

respirations are chiefly thoracic. In either case, the chest and abdomen should rise and fall together. Always report any asymmetry of movement.

While inspecting the skin surface of the chest, observe the position of the nipples and any evidence of breast development. Normally the nipples are located slightly lateral to the midclavicular line between the fourth and fifth ribs. Note symmetry of nipple placement and normal configuration of a darker pigmented areola surrounding a flat nipple in prepubertal children.

Pubertal breast development usually begins in girls between 8 and 12 years of age (see Chapter 15). Record early (precocious) or delayed breast development, as well as evidence of any other secondary sexual characteristics. In males, breast enlargement (**gynecomastia**) may be caused by hormonal or systemic disorders but more commonly is a result of adipose tissue from obesity or a transient body change during early puberty. In either situation, investigate the child's feelings about breast enlargement.

In adolescent girls who have achieved sexual maturity, palpate the breasts for evidence of any masses or hard nodules. Use this opportunity to discuss the importance of routine breast self-examination. Emphasize that most palpable masses are benign to decrease any fear or concern that results when a mass is felt.

LUNGS

The lungs are situated inside the thoracic cavity, with one lung on each side of the sternum. Each lung is divided into an **apex**, which is slightly pointed and rises above the first rib; a **base**, which is wide and concave and rides on the dome-shaped diaphragm; and a **body**, which is divided into lobes. The right lung has three lobes: the right superior (upper) lobe, right middle lobe, and right inferior (lower) lobe. The left lung has only two lobes, the left superior (upper) and left inferior (lower) lobes, because of the space occupied by the heart (Fig. 4.31).

Inspection of the lungs primarily involves observation of respiratory movements. Evaluate respirations for (1) rate (number per minute), (2) rhythm (regular, irregular, or periodic), (3) depth (deep or shallow), and (4) quality (effortless, automatic, difficult, or labored). Note the character of breath sounds, such as noisy, grunting, snoring, or heavy.

Evaluate respiratory movements by placing each hand flat against the back or chest with the thumbs in midline along the lower costal margin of the lungs. The child should be sitting during this procedure and, if cooperative, should take several deep breaths. During respiration, your hands will move with the chest wall. Assess the amount and speed of respiratory excursion and note any asymmetry of movement.

Experienced examiners may percuss the lungs. Percuss the anterior lung from apex to base, usually with the child in the supine or sitting position. Percuss each side of the chest in sequence to compare the sounds. When percussing the posterior lung, the procedure and sequence are the same, although the child should be sitting. Resonance is heard over all the lobes of the lungs that are not adjacent to other organs. Record and report any deviation from the expected sound.

Auscultation

Auscultation involves using the stethoscope to evaluate breath sounds (see Nursing Care Guidelines box). Breath sounds are best heard if the child inspires deeply (see Atraumatic Care box). In the lungs, breath sounds are classified as vesicular, bronchovesicular, or bronchial (Box 4.12).

NURSING CARE GUIDELINES

Effective Auscultation

- Make certain child is relaxed and not crying, talking, or laughing. Record if child is crying.
- Check that room is comfortable and quiet.
- Warm stethoscope before placing it against skin.
- Apply firm pressure on chest piece but not enough to prevent vibrations and transmission of sound.
- Avoid placing stethoscope over hair or clothing, moving it against the skin, breathing on tubing, or sliding fingers over chest piece, which may cause sounds that falsely resemble pathologic findings.
- Use a symmetric and orderly approach to compare sounds on each side.

ATRAUMATIC CARE

Encouraging Deep Breaths

- Ask child to "blow out" the light on an otoscope or pocket flashlight; discreetly turn off the light on the last try so that child feels successful.
- Place a cotton ball in child's palm; ask child to blow the ball into the air and have parent catch it.
- Hold a tissue in front of child and ask child to blow the tissue in the air.
- Have child blow a pinwheel, a party horn, or bubbles.

Absent or diminished breath sounds are always an abnormal finding warranting investigation. Fluid, air, or solid masses in the pleural space interfere with the conduction of breath sounds. Diminished breath sounds in certain segments of the lung can alert the nurse to pulmonary areas that may benefit from chest physiotherapy. Increased breath sounds after pulmonary therapy indicate improved passage of air through the respiratory tract. Box 4.13 lists terms used to describe various respiration patterns.

Various pulmonary abnormalities produce **adventitious sounds** that are not normally heard over the chest. These sounds occur in addition to normal or abnormal breath sounds. They are classified into two main groups: (1) **crackles**, which result from the passage of air through fluid or moisture, and (2) **wheezes**, which are produced as air passes through narrowed passageways, regardless of the cause, such as exudate, inflammation, spasm, or tumor. Considerable practice with an experienced mentor is necessary to differentiate the various types of lung sounds. Often it is best to describe the type of sound heard in the lungs rather than trying to label it. Always report any abnormal sounds for further medical evaluation.

HEART

The heart is situated in the thoracic cavity between the lungs in the mediastinum and above the diaphragm (Fig. 4.32). About two-thirds of the heart lies within the left side of the rib cage, with the other third on the right side as it crosses the sternum. The heart is positioned in the thorax like a trapezoid:

Vertically along the right sternal border (RSB) from the second to the fifth rib

Horizontally (long side) from the lower right sternum to the fifth rib at the left midclavicular line (LMCL)

Diagonally from the left sternal border (LSB) at the second rib to the LMCL at the fifth rib

Horizontally (short side) from the RSB and LSB at the second ICS—base of the heart

Inspection is easiest when the child is sitting in a semi-Fowler position. Look at the anterior chest wall from an angle, comparing both sides of the rib cage with each other. Normally they should be symmetric. In children with thin chest walls, a pulsation may be visible. Because comprehensive evaluation of cardiac function is not limited to the heart, also consider other findings, such as the presence of all

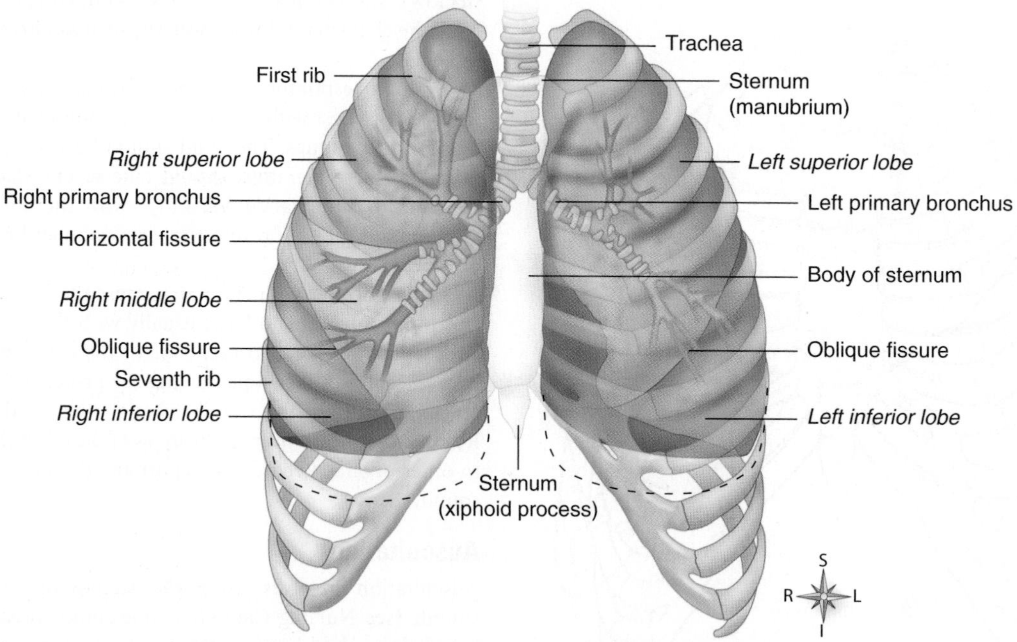

Fig. 4.31 Location of the lobes of the lungs within the thoracic cavity. (From Patton, K. T., & Thibodeau, G. A. [2013]. *Anatomy and physiology* [8th ed.]. St Louis, MO: Mosby.)

BOX 4.12 Classification of Normal Breath Sounds

Vesicular Breath Sounds

Heard over the entire surface of the lungs, except for the upper intrascapular area and the area beneath the manubrium.

Inspiration is louder, longer, and higher pitched than expiration.

The sound is a soft, swishing noise.

Bronchovesicular Breath Sounds

Heard over the manubrium and in the upper intrascapular regions where the trachea and bronchi bifurcate.

Inspiration is louder and higher pitched than in vesicular breathing.

Bronchial Breath Sounds

Heard only over the trachea near the suprasternal notch.

The inspiratory phase is short, and the expiratory phase is long.

BOX 4.13 Various Patterns of Respiration

Tachypnea: Increased rate

Bradypnea: Decreased rate

Dyspnea: Distress during breathing

Apnea: Cessation of breathing

Hyperpnea: Increased depth

Hypoventilation: Decreased depth (shallow) and irregular rhythm

Hyperventilation: Increased rate and depth

Kussmaul respiration: Hyperventilation, gasping and labored respiration; usually seen in diabetic coma or other states of respiratory acidosis

Cheyne-Stokes respiration: Gradually increasing rate and depth with periods of apnea

Biot respiration: Periods of hyperpnea alternating with apnea (similar to Cheyne-Stokes except that depth remains constant)

Seesaw (paradoxic) respirations: Chest falls on inspiration and rises on expiration

Agonal: Last gasping breaths before death

pulses (especially the femoral pulses) (Fig. 4.33), distended neck veins, clubbing of the fingers, peripheral cyanosis, edema, blood pressure, and respiratory status.

Use palpation to determine the location of the **apical pulse (AP)**, the most lateral cardiac impulse that may correspond to the apex. The AP is found:

- At the fifth ICS and LMCL in children older than 7 years of age
- At the fourth ICS and just lateral to the LMCL in children younger than 7 years of age

Although the AP gives a general idea of the size of the heart (with enlargement, the apex is lower and more lateral), its normal location is variable, making it an unreliable indicator of heart size.

The **point of maximum intensity (PMI)**, as the name implies, is the area of most intense pulsation. Usually the PMI is located at the same site as the AP, but it can occur elsewhere. For this reason, the two terms should not be used synonymously.

Assess the **capillary refill time**, an important test for circulation, by pressing the pad of a fingertip between the nurse's thumb and forefinger for 5 seconds at moderate pressure at an ambient temperature of 68°F to 77°F (Fleming, Gill, Van den Bruel, et al., 2016). The time it takes for the blanched area to return to its original color is the capillary refill time.

! NURSING ALERT

Capillary refill should be brisk—2 seconds or less. Prolonged refill of 3 seconds or more is an important warning sign.

Auscultation

Origin of Heart Sounds

The heart sounds are produced by the opening and closing of the valves and the vibration of blood against the walls of the heart and vessels. Normally, two sounds—S_1 and S_2—are heard, which correspond, respectively, to the familiar "lub dub" often used to describe the sounds. S_1 is caused by closure of the **tricuspid** and **mitral valves** (sometimes called the **atrioventricular valves**). S_2 is the result of closure of the **pulmonic** and **aortic valves** (sometimes called **semilunar**

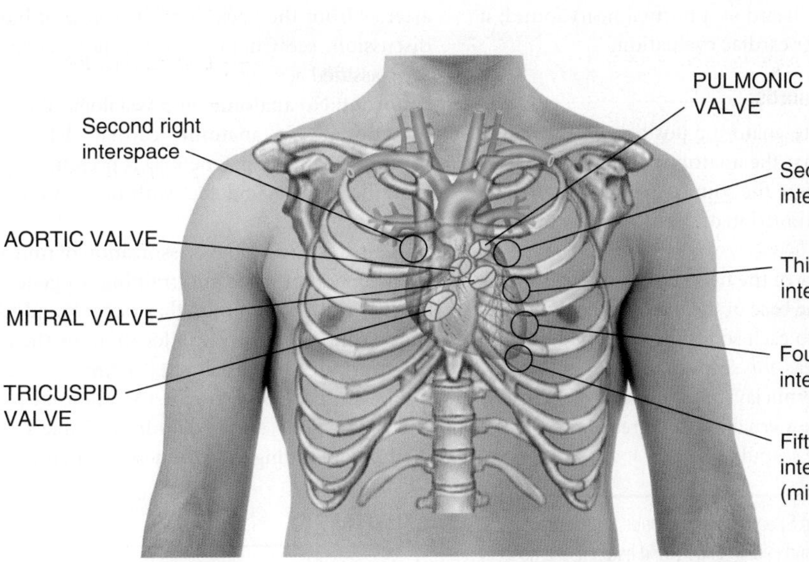

Fig. 4.32 Position of the heart within the thorax. (From Ball, J. W., Dains, J. E., Flynn, J. A., et al. [2014]. *Seidel's guide to physical examination* [8th ed.]. St Louis, MO: Elsevier.)

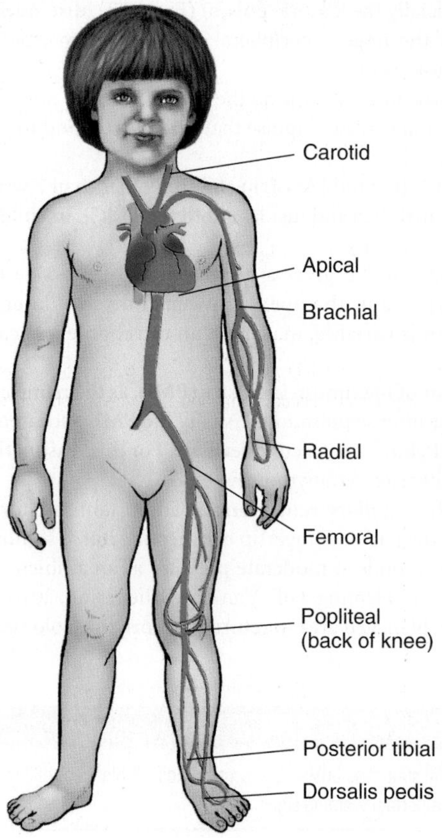

Fig. 4.33 Location of pulses.

valves). Normally the split of the two sounds in S_2 is distinguishable and widens during inspiration. **Physiologic splitting** is a significant normal finding.

> **! NURSING ALERT**
>
> Fixed splitting, in which the split in S_2 does not change during inspiration, is an important diagnostic sign of atrial septal defect.

Two other heart sounds, S_3 and S_4, may be produced. S_3 is normally heard in some children; S_4 is rarely heard as a normal heart sound; it usually indicates the need for further cardiac evaluation.

Differentiating Normal Heart Sounds

Fig. 4.34 illustrates the approximate anatomic position of the valves within the heart chambers. Note that the anatomic location of valves does not correspond to the area where the sounds are heard best. The auscultatory sites are located in the direction of the blood flow through the valves.

Normally S_1 is louder at the apex of the heart in the mitral and tricuspid area, and S_2 is louder near the base of the heart in the pulmonic and aortic area (Table 4.9). Listen to each sound by inching down the chest. Auscultate the following areas for sounds, such as murmurs, which may radiate to these sites: sternoclavicular area above the clavicles and manubrium, area along the sternal border, area along the left midaxillary line, and area below the scapulae.

> **NURSING TIP** To distinguish between S_1 and S_2 heart sounds, simultaneously palpate the carotid pulse with the index and middle fingers and listen to the heart sounds; S_1 is synchronous with the carotid pulse.

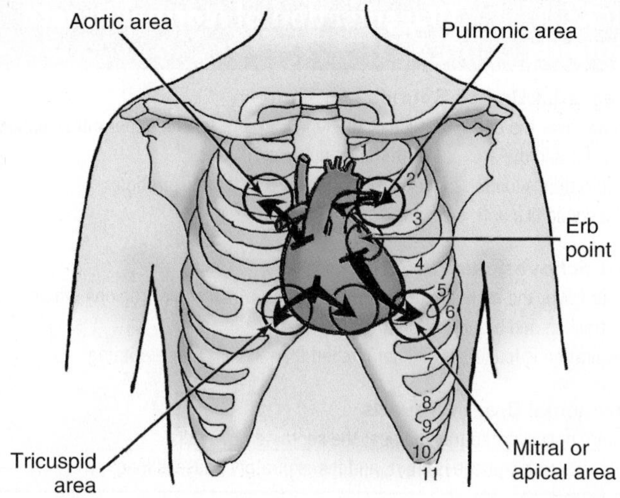

Fig. 4.34 Direction of heart sounds for anatomic valve sites and areas *(circled)* for auscultation.

Auscultate the heart with the child in at least two positions: sitting and reclining. If adventitious sounds are detected, further evaluate them with the child standing, sitting and leaning forward, and lying on the left side. For example, atrial sounds such as S_4 are heard best with the person in a recumbent position and usually fade if the person sits or stands.

Evaluate heart sounds for (1) quality (they should be clear and distinct, not muffled, diffuse, or distant); (2) intensity, especially in relation to the location or auscultatory site (they should not be weak or pounding); (3) rate (they should have the same rate as the radial pulse); and (4) **rhythm** (they should be regular and even). An arrhythmia that occurs normally in many children is **sinus arrhythmia**, in which the heart rate increases with inspiration and decreases with expiration. Differentiate this rhythm from a truly abnormal arrhythmia by having children hold their breath. In sinus arrhythmia, cessation of breathing causes the heart rate to remain steady.

Heart Murmurs

Another important category of the heart sounds is **murmurs**, which are produced by vibrations within the heart chambers or in the major arteries from the back-and-forth flow of blood. (For a more detailed discussion, see Chapter 23, Cardiovascular Dysfunction). Murmurs are classified as:

Innocent: No anatomic or physiologic abnormality exists.

Functional: No anatomic cardiac defect exists, but a physiologic abnormality (e.g., anemia) is present.

Organic: A cardiac defect with or without a physiologic abnormality exists.

The description and classification of murmurs are skills that require considerable practice and training. In general, recognize murmurs as distinct swishing sounds that occur in addition to the normal heart sounds and record the (1) location, or the area of the heart in which the murmur is heard best; (2) time of the occurrence of the murmur within the S_1–S_2 cycle; (3) intensity (evaluate in relation to the child's position); and (4) loudness. Table 4.10 lists the usual subjective method of grading the loudness or intensity of a murmur.

ABDOMEN

Examination of the abdomen involves inspection followed by auscultation and then palpation. Experienced examiners may also percuss the

TABLE 4.9 Sequence of Auscultating Heart Sounds[a]

Auscultatory Site	Chest Location	Characteristics of Heart Sounds
Aortic area	Second right ICS close to sternum	S_2 heard louder than S_1; aortic closure heard loudest
Pulmonic area	Second left ICS close to sternum	Splitting of S_2 heard best, normally widens on inspiration; pulmonic closure heard best
Erb point	Third left ICS close to sternum	Frequent site of innocent murmurs and those of aortic or pulmonic origin
Tricuspid area	Fourth right and left ICSs close to sternum	S_1 heard as louder sound preceding S_2 (S_1 synchronous with carotid pulse)
Mitral or apical area	Fifth ICS, LMCL (fourth ICS and lateral to LMCL in infants)	S_1 heard loudest; splitting of S_1 may be audible because mitral closure is louder than tricuspid closure S_1 heard best at beginning of expiration with child in recumbent or left side-lying position; occurs immediately after S_2; sounds like word S_1 S_2 S_3: "Ken-tuc-ky" S_4 heard best during expiration with child in recumbent position (left side-lying position decreases sound); occurs immediately before S_1; sounds like word S_4 S_1 S_2: "Ten-nes-see"

[a]Use both diaphragm and bell chest pieces when auscultating heart sounds. Bell chest piece is necessary for low-pitched sounds of murmurs, S_3, and S_4.
ICS, Intercostal space; *LMCL,* left midclavicular line.

TABLE 4.10 Grading the Intensity of Heart Murmurs

Grade	Description
I	Very faint; barely heard in a quiet room; often not heard if child sits up
II	Quiet but clearly heard; slightly louder than grade I; audible in all positions
III	Moderately loud; no thrill palpated
IV	Loud; accompanied by a thrill
V	Very loud; heard with the stethoscope barely touching the chest; accompanied by a thrill
VI	Heard without the stethoscope in direct contact with the chest wall; often heard with the human ear close to the chest; accompanied by a thrill

! NURSING ALERT

A tense, board-like abdomen is a serious sign of paralytic ileus and intestinal obstruction.

abdomen to assess for organomegaly, masses, fluid, and flatus. Perform palpation last because it may distort the abdominal sounds. Knowledge of the anatomic placement of the abdominal organs is essential to differentiate normal, expected findings from abnormal ones (Fig. 4.35).

For descriptive purposes, the abdominal cavity is divided into four quadrants by drawing a vertical line midway from the sternum to the symphysis pubis and a horizontal line across the abdomen through the umbilicus. The sections are named:

- Left upper quadrant
- Left lower quadrant
- Right upper quadrant
- Right lower quadrant

Inspection

Inspect the contour of the abdomen with the child erect and supine. Normally the abdomen of infants and young children is cylindric and, in the erect position, fairly prominent because of the physiologic lordosis of the spine. In the supine position, the abdomen appears flat. A midline protrusion from the xiphoid to the umbilicus or symphysis pubis is usually **diastasis recti**, or failure of the rectus abdominis muscles to join in utero. In a healthy child, a midline protrusion is usually a variation of normal muscular development.

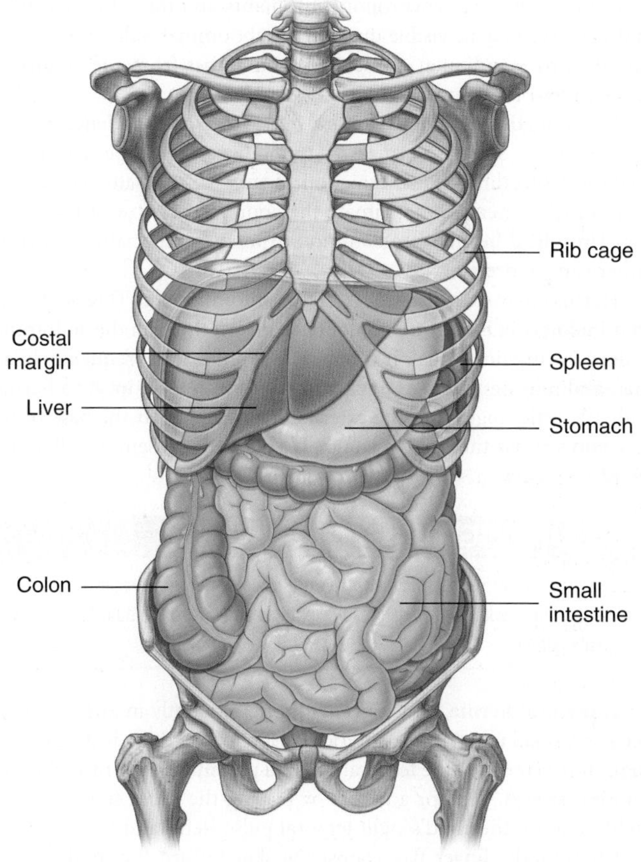

Fig. 4.35 Location of structures in the abdomen. (From Drake, R. L., Vogl, W., & Mitchell, A. W. M. [2015]. *Gray's anatomy for students* [3rd ed.]. New York, NY: Churchill Livingstone.)

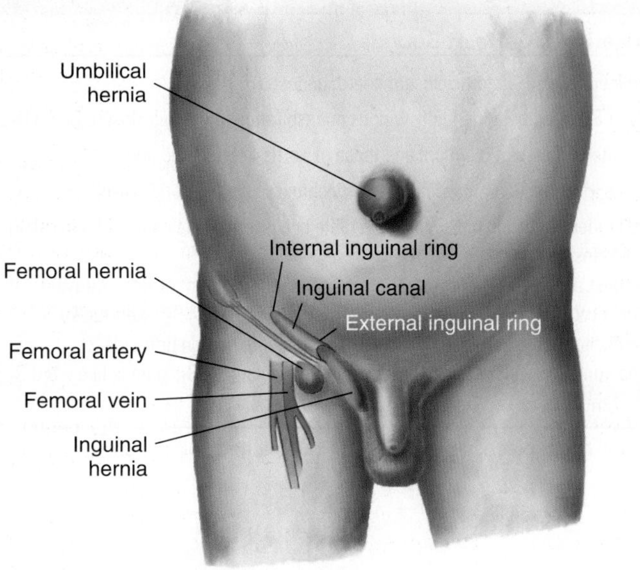

Fig. 4.36 Location of hernias.

The skin covering the abdomen should be uniformly taut, without wrinkles or creases. Sometimes silvery, whitish striae (stretch marks) are seen, especially if the skin has been stretched as in obesity. Superficial veins are usually visible in light-skinned, thin infants, but distended veins are an abnormal finding.

Observe movement of the abdomen. Normally chest and abdominal movements are synchronous. In infants and thin children, **peristaltic waves** may be visible through the abdominal wall; they are best observed by standing at eye level to and across from the abdomen. Always report this finding.

Examine the umbilicus for size, hygiene, and evidence of any abnormalities, such as hernias. The umbilicus should be flat or only slightly protruding. If a herniation is present, palpate the sac for abdominal contents and estimate the approximate size of the opening. **Umbilical hernias** are common in infants, especially in African American children.

Hernias may exist elsewhere on the abdominal wall (Fig. 4.36). An **inguinal hernia** is a protrusion of peritoneum through the abdominal wall in the inguinal canal. It occurs mostly in boys, is frequently bilateral, and may be visible as a mass in the scrotum. To locate a hernia, slide the little finger into the external inguinal ring at the base of the scrotum and ask the child to cough. If a hernia is present, it will hit the tip of the finger.

! NURSING TIP

If the child is too young to cough, have the child blow on a tissue or laugh to raise the intra-abdominal pressure sufficiently to demonstrate the presence of an inguinal hernia.

A **femoral hernia**, which occurs more frequently in girls, is felt or seen as a small mass on the anterior surface of the thigh just below the inguinal ligament in the femoral canal (a potential space medial to the femoral artery). Feel for a hernia by placing the index finger of your right hand on the child's right femoral pulse (left hand for left pulse) and the middle finger flat against the skin toward the midline. The ring finger lies over the femoral canal, where the herniation occurs. Palpation of hernias in the pelvic region is often part of the genital examination.

Auscultation

The most important finding to listen for is **peristalsis**, or **bowel sounds**, which sound like short metallic clicks and gurgles. Record their frequency per minute (e.g., 5 sounds/min). Listen for up to 5 minutes before determining that bowel sounds are absent. Stimulate bowel sounds by stroking the abdominal surface with a fingernail. Report absence of bowel sounds or hyperperistalsis, because either usually denotes a gastrointestinal disorder.

Palpation

There are two types of palpation: superficial and deep. For **superficial palpation**, lightly place your hand against the skin and feel each quadrant, noting any areas of tenderness, muscle tone, and superficial lesions, such as cysts. Because superficial palpation is often perceived as tickling, use several techniques to minimize this sensation and relax the child (see Atraumatic Care box). Admonishing the child to stop laughing only draws attention to the sensation and decreases cooperation.

ATRAUMATIC CARE

Promoting Relaxation During Abdominal Palpation

- Position child comfortably, such as in a semireclining position in the parent's lap, with knees flexed.
- Warm your hands before touching the skin.
- Use distraction, such as telling stories or talking to child.
- Teach child to use deep breathing and to concentrate on an object.
- Give infant a bottle or pacifier.
- Begin with light, superficial palpation and gradually progress to deeper palpation.
- Palpate any tender or painful areas last.
- Have child hold the parent's hand and squeeze it if palpation is uncomfortable.
- Use the nonpalpating hand to comfort the child, such as placing the free hand on child's shoulder while palpating abdomen.
- To minimize sensation of tickling during palpation:
  - Have children "help" with palpation by placing one of their hands over the palpating hand.
  - Have them place a hand on the abdomen with the fingers spread wide apart and palpate between their fingers.

Deep palpation is for palpating organs and large blood vessels and for detecting masses and tenderness that were not discovered during superficial palpation. Palpation usually begins in the lower quadrants and proceeds upward to avoid missing the edge of an enlarged liver or spleen. Except for palpating the liver, successful identification of other organs (e.g., the spleen, kidney, and part of the colon) requires considerable practice with mentored supervision. Report any questionable mass. The lower edge of the liver is sometimes felt in infants and young children as a superficial mass 1 to 2 cm (0.4 to 0.8 inch) below the right costal margin (the distance is sometimes measured in fingerbreadths). Normally the liver descends during inspiration as the diaphragm moves downward. Do not mistake this downward displacement as a sign of liver enlargement.

! NURSING ALERT

If the liver is palpable 3 cm (1.2 inch) below the right costal margin or the spleen is palpable more than 2 cm (0.8 inch) below the left costal margin, these organs are enlarged—a finding that is always reported for further medical investigation.

Palpate the **femoral pulses** by placing the tips of two or three fingers (index, middle, or ring) along the inguinal ligament about midway between the iliac crest and symphysis pubis. Feel both pulses simultaneously to make certain they are equal and strong (Fig. 4.37).

> **! NURSING ALERT**
>
> Absence of femoral pulses is a significant sign of coarctation of the aorta and is referred for evaluation.

GENITALIA

Examination of genitalia conveniently follows assessment of the abdomen while the child is still supine. In examining the genitalia, wear gloves when touching the child and adolescent. The examination should be performed in the presence of a parent, guardian, or another health care professional. The best approach is to examine the genitalia matter-of-factly, placing no more emphasis on this part of the assessment than on any other segment. It helps relieve children's and parents' anxiety by telling them the results of the findings; for example, the nurse might say, "Everything looks fine here." In adolescents, inspection of the genitalia may be left to the end of the examination.

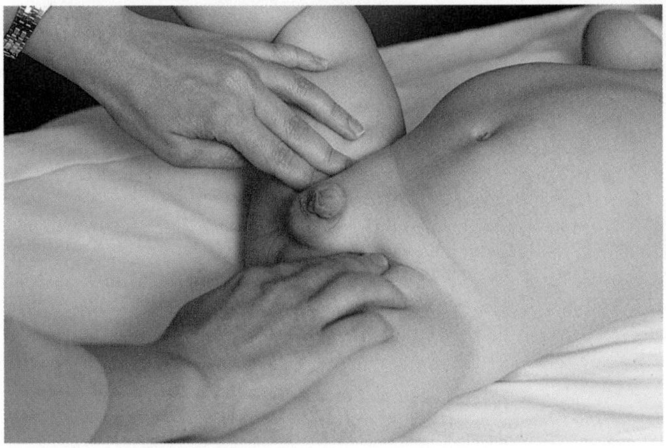

Fig. 4.37 Palpating for femoral pulses.

If it is necessary to ask questions, such as about discharge or difficulty urinating, respect the child's privacy by covering the lower abdomen with the gown or underpants. To prevent embarrassing interruptions, keep the door or curtain closed and post a "do not disturb" sign. Have a drape ready to cover the genitalia if someone enters the room.

The genital examination is an excellent time for eliciting questions or concern about body function or sexual activity. Also use this opportunity to increase or reinforce the child's knowledge of reproductive anatomy by naming each body part and explaining its function. This part of the health assessment is an opportune time to teach about appropriate and inappropriate touch and, in adolescent boys, testicular self-examination.

Male Genitalia

Note the external appearance of the **glans** (head of the penis), the **prepuce** (foreskin), the **shaft** (portion between the perineum and prepuce), the urethral meatus, and the scrotum (Fig. 4.38). The **penis** is generally small in infants and young boys until puberty, when it begins to increase in both length and width. In an obese child, the penis often looks abnormally small because of the folds of adipose tissue partially covering it at the base. Be familiar with normal pubertal growth of the external male genitalia to compare the findings with the expected sequence of maturation (see Chapter 15).

Examine the glans and shaft of the penis for signs of swelling, skin lesions, inflammation, or other irregularities. Any of these signs may indicate underlying disorders, especially sexually transmitted infections.

Carefully inspect the **urethral meatus** for location and evidence of discharge. Normally it is centered at the tip of the glans. Also note pubic hair distribution. Normally, before puberty, no pubic hair is present. Soft, downy hair at the base of the penis is an early sign of pubertal maturation. In older adolescents, hair distribution is diamond shaped from the umbilicus to the anus.

Note the location and size of the **scrotum**. The scrotum hangs freely from the perineum behind the penis, and the left scrotum normally hangs lower than the right. In infants, the scrotum appears large in relation to the rest of the genitalia. The skin of the scrotum is loose and highly rugated (wrinkled). During early adolescence, the skin normally becomes redder and thinner. In dark-skinned boys, the scrotum is usually more deeply pigmented.

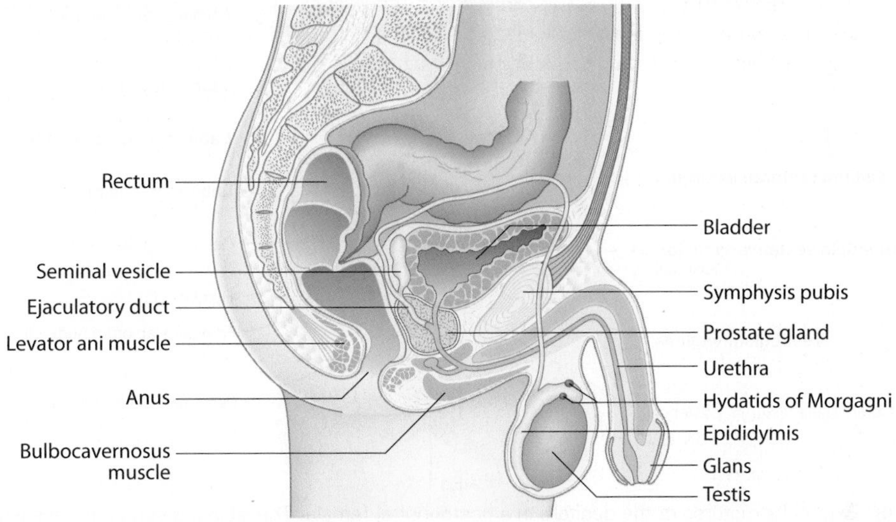

Fig. 4.38 Major structures of genitalia in an uncircumcised postpubertal male. (From Douglas, G., Nicol, F., & Robertson, C. [2013]. *Macleod's clinical examination* [13th ed.]. Philadelphia, PA: Elsevier.)

Palpation of the scrotum includes identification of the testes, epididymis, and, if present, inguinal hernias. Before puberty, the two testes are felt as small, ovoid bodies less than 2.5 cm (1 inch) in length and less than 4 ml in volume—one in each scrotal sac. They do not enlarge until puberty (see Chapter 15). Pubertal testicular development normally begins in boys between 9 and 13 years old. Record early (precocious) or delayed pubertal development, as well as evidence of any other secondary sexual characteristics.

When palpating for the presence of the testes, avoid stimulating the **cremasteric reflex**, which is stimulated by cold, touch, emotional excitement, or exercise. This reflex pulls the testes higher into the pelvic cavity. Several measures are useful in preventing the cremasteric reflex during palpation of the scrotum. First, warm the hands. Second, if the child is old enough, examine him in a tailor or "Indian" position, which stretches the muscle, preventing its contraction (Fig. 4.39A). Third, block the normal pathway of ascent of the testes by placing the thumb and index finger over the upper part of the scrotal sac along the inguinal canal (see Fig. 4.39B). If there is any question concerning the existence of two testes, place the index and middle fingers in a scissors fashion to separate the right and left scrota. If, after using these techniques, you have not palpated the testes, feel along the inguinal canal and perineum to locate masses that may be undescended testes. Report any failure to palpate the testes for further evaluation.

Female Genitalia

The examination of female genitalia is limited to inspection and palpation of external structures. If a vaginal examination is required, the nurse should make an appropriate referral unless he or she is qualified to perform the procedure.

A convenient position for examination of the genitalia involves placing the young child supine on the examining table or in a semireclining position on the parent's lap with the feet supported on your knees as you sit facing the child. Divert the child's attention from the examination by instructing her to try to keep the soles of her feet pressed against each other. Separate the labia majora with the thumb and index finger and retract outward to expose the labia minora, urethral meatus, and vaginal orifice.

Examine the female genitalia for size and location of the structures of the **vulva**, or **pudendum** (Fig. 4.40). The **mons pubis** is a pad of

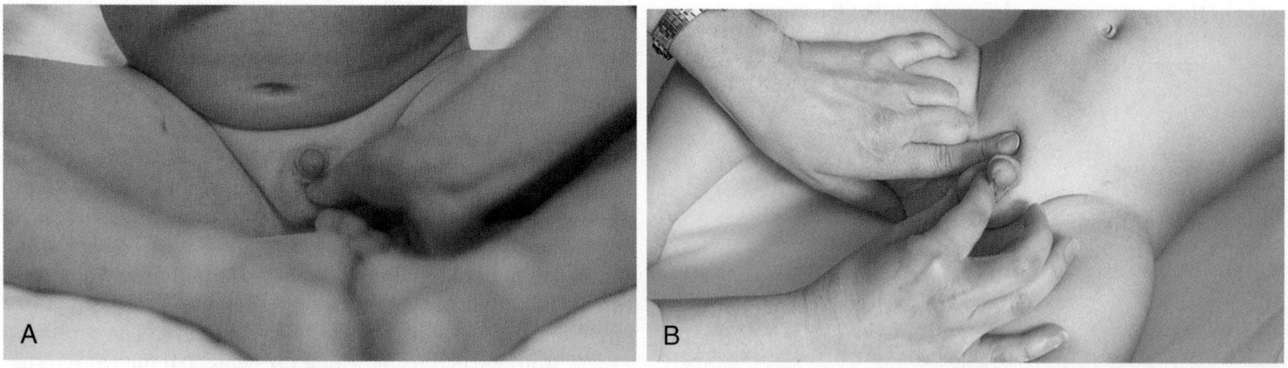

Fig. 4.39 **A,** Preventing the cremasteric reflex by having the child sit in the tailor position. **B,** Blocking the inguinal canal during palpation of the scrotum for descended testes.

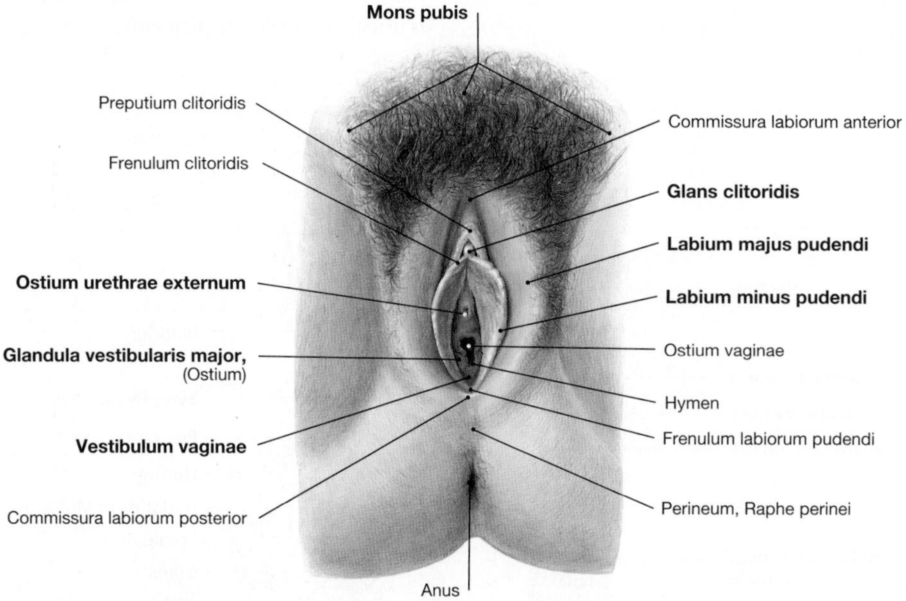

Fig. 4.40 External structures of the genitalia in a postpubertal female. The labia are spread to reveal deeper structures. (From Paulsen, F., & Waschke, J. [2014]. *Sobotta atlas of human anatomy* [Vol. 2, 15th ed.]. Munich, Germany: Elsevier.)

adipose tissue over the symphysis pubis. At puberty, the mons is covered with hair, which extends along the labia. The usual pattern of female hair distribution is an inverted triangle. The appearance of soft, downy hair along the labia majora is an early sign of sexual maturation. Note the size and location of the **clitoris**, a small, erectile organ located at the anterior end of the labia minora. It is covered by a small flap of skin, the **prepuce**.

The **labia majora** are two thick folds of skin running posteriorly from the mons to the posterior commissure of the vagina. Internal to the labia majora are two folds of skin called the **labia minora**. Although the labia minora are usually prominent in newborns, they gradually atrophy, which makes them almost invisible until their enlargement during puberty. The inner surface of the labia should be pink and moist. Note the size of the labia and any evidence of fusion, which may suggest labial adhesion or male scrota. Normally, no masses are palpable within the labia.

The **urethral meatus** is located posterior to the clitoris and is surrounded by the Skene glands and ducts. Although not a prominent structure, the meatus appears as a small V-shaped slit. Note its location, especially if it opens from the clitoris or inside the vagina. Gently palpate the glands, which are common sites of cysts and sexually transmitted lesions.

The **vaginal orifice** is located posterior to the urethral meatus. Its appearance varies depending on individual anatomy and sexual activity. Ordinarily, examination of the vagina is limited to inspection. In virgins, a thin crescent-shaped or circular membrane, called the **hymen**, may cover part of the vaginal opening. In some instances, it completely occludes the orifice. After rupture, small rounded pieces of tissue called **caruncles** remain. Although an imperforate hymen denotes lack of penile intercourse, a perforate one does not necessarily indicate sexual activity.

> **! NURSING ALERT**
>
> In girls who have been circumcised, the genitalia will appear different. Do not show surprise or disgust but note the appearance and discuss the procedure with the child and/or parent (see also Chapter 2, Cultural Considerations "Circumcision").

Surrounding the vaginal opening are **Bartholin glands**, which secrete a clear, mucoid fluid into the vagina for lubrication during intercourse. Palpate the ducts for cysts. Also note the discharge from the vagina, which is usually clear, white, or slightly yellow with odor.

ANUS

After examination of the genitalia, it is easy to identify the anal area, although the child should be placed on the abdomen or side. Note the general firmness of the **buttocks** and symmetry of the **gluteal folds**. Assess the tone of the anal sphincter by eliciting the **anal reflex (anal wink)**. Gently scratching the anal area results in an obvious quick contraction of the external anal sphincter.

BACK AND EXTREMITIES

Spine

Note the general **curvature** of the spine. Normally the back of a newborn is rounded or C-shaped from the thoracic and pelvic curves. The development of the cervical and lumbar curves approximates development of various motor skills, such as cervical curvature with head control, and gives older children the typical double S curve.

Marked curvatures in posture are abnormal. **Scoliosis**, lateral curvature of the spine, is an important childhood problem, and more common in girls. Although scoliosis may be identified by observing and palpating the spine and noting a sideways displacement, more objective tests include:

- With the child (clothed in a gown that is open in the back, with underwear that exposes the iliac crests and posterior and anterior superior iliac spines) bending forward from the waist so that the back is parallel to the floor with knees straight and arms hanging freely, observe from the back, noting thoracic and/or lumbar asymmetry.
- With the child standing erect, observe from behind, noting asymmetry of the shoulders, scapulae, waistline, and hips or distance that the arms hang from the trunk.

Inspect the back, especially along the spine, for any tufts of hair, dimples, or discoloration. Mobility of the vertebral column is easy to assess in most children because of their tendency to be in constant motion during the examination. However, you can test mobility by asking the child to sit up from a prone position or to do a modified sit-up exercise.

Movement of the cervical spine is an important diagnostic sign of neurologic problems, such as meningitis. Normally movement of the head in all directions is effortless.

> **! NURSING ALERT**
>
> Hyperextension of the neck and spine, or *opisthotonos,* which is accompanied by pain when the head is flexed, is always referred for immediate evaluation.

Extremities

Inspect each extremity for symmetry of length and size; refer any deviation for orthopedic evaluation. Count the fingers and toes to be certain of the normal number. This is so often taken for granted that an extra digit (**polydactyly**) or fusion of digits (**syndactyly**) may go unnoticed.

Inspect the arms and legs for temperature and color, which should be equal in each extremity, although the feet may normally be colder than the hands.

Assess the shape of bones. There are several variations of bone shape in children. Although many of them cause parents concern, most are benign and require no treatment. **Bowleg**, or **genu varum**, is lateral bowing of the tibia. It is clinically present when the child stands with an outward bowing of the legs, giving the appearance of a bow. Usually, there is an outward curvature of both femur and tibia (Fig. 4.41A). Toddlers are usually bowlegged after beginning to walk until

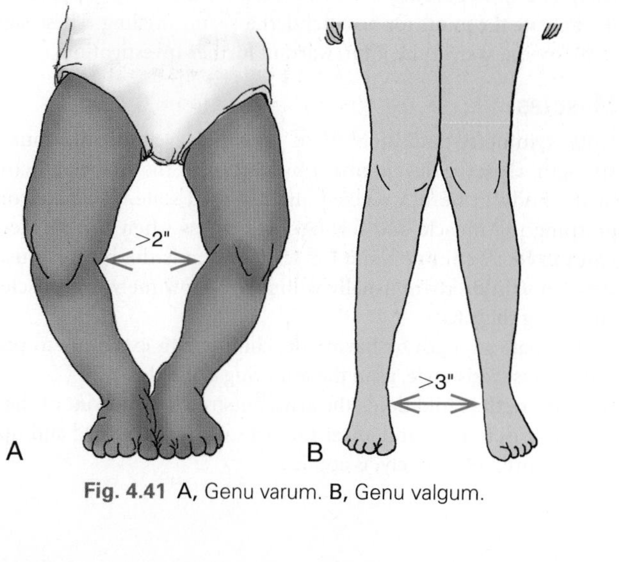

Fig. 4.41 **A,** Genu varum. **B,** Genu valgum.

all of their lower back and leg muscles are well developed. Unilateral or asymmetric bowlegs that are present beyond 2 to 3 years old, particularly in African American children, may represent pathologic conditions requiring further investigation.

Knock-knee, or genu valgum, appears as the opposite of bowleg, in that the knees are close together but the feet are spread apart. It is determined clinically by using the same method as for genu varum but by measuring the distance between the medial malleoli, which normally should be less than 7.5 cm (3 inches) (see Fig. 4.41B). Knock-knee is normally present in children from about 2 to 7 years old. Knock-knee that is excessive, asymmetric, accompanied by short stature, or evident in a child nearing puberty requires further evaluation.

Next inspect the feet. Infants' and toddlers' feet appear flat because the foot is normally wide and the arch is covered by a fat pad. Development of the arch occurs naturally from the action of walking. Normally at birth the feet are held in a valgus (outward) or varus (inward) position. To determine whether a foot deformity at birth is a result of intrauterine position or development, scratch the outer, then inner, side of the sole. If the foot position is self-correctable, it will assume a right angle to the leg. As the child begins to walk, the feet turn outward less than 30 degrees and inward less than 10 degrees.

Toddlers have a "toddling" or broad-based gait, which facilitates walking by lowering the center of gravity. As the child reaches preschool age, the legs are brought closer together. By school age, the walking posture is much more graceful and balanced.

The most common gait problem in young children is pigeon toe, or toeing in, which usually results from torsional deformities, such as internal tibial torsion (abnormal rotation or bowing of the tibia). Tests for tibial torsion include measuring the thigh–foot angle, which requires considerable practice for accuracy.

Elicit the plantar or grasp reflex by exerting firm but gentle pressure with the tip of the thumb against the lateral sole of the foot from the heel upward to the little toe and then across to the big toe. The normal response in children who are walking is flexion of the toes. Babinski sign, dorsiflexion of the big toe and fanning of the other toes, is normal during infancy but abnormal after about 1 year old or when locomotion begins (see Fig. 7.8).

Joints

Evaluate the joints for range of motion. Normally this requires no specific testing if you have observed the child's movements during the examination. However, routinely investigate the hips in infants for congenital dislocation by checking for subluxation of the hip (see Chapter 29). Report any evidence of joint immobility or hyperflexibility. Palpate the joints for heat, tenderness, and swelling. These signs, as well as redness over the joint, warrant further investigation.

Muscles

Note symmetry and quality of muscle development, tone, and strength. Observe development by looking at the shape and contour of the body in both a relaxed and a tensed state. Estimate tone by grasping the muscle and feeling its firmness when it is relaxed and contracted. A common site for testing tone is the biceps muscle of the arm. Children are usually willing to "show me your muscles" by clenching their fists.

Estimate strength by having the child use an extremity to push or pull against resistance, as in the following examples:

Arm strength: Child holds the arms outstretched in front of the body and tries to raise and lower the arms while downward and upward pressure, respectively, is applied.

Hand strength: Child shakes hands with nurse and squeezes one or two fingers of the nurse's hand.

Leg strength: Child sits on a table or chair with the legs dangling and tries to raise and lower the legs while downward and upward pressure, respectively, is applied.

Note symmetry of strength in the extremities, hands, and fingers, and report evidence of paresis, or weakness.

> **BOX 4.14 Tests for Cerebellar Function**
>
> **Finger-to-nose test:** With the child's arm extended, ask the child to touch the nose with the index finger with the eyes open and then closed.
>
> **Heel-to-shin test:** Have the child stand and run the heel of one foot down the shin or anterior aspect of the tibia of the other leg, both with the eyes open and then closed.
>
> **Romberg test:** Have the child stand with the eyes closed and heels together; falling or leaning to one side is abnormal and is called the Romberg sign.

NEUROLOGIC ASSESSMENT

The assessment of the nervous system is the broadest and most diverse part of the examination process because every human function, both physical and emotional, is controlled by neurologic impulses. Much of the neurologic examination has already been discussed, such as assessment of behavior, sensory testing, and motor function. The following focuses on a general appraisal of cerebellar function, deep tendon reflexes, and the cranial nerves.

Cerebellar Function

The cerebellum controls balance and coordination. Much of the assessment of cerebellar function is included in observing the child's posture, body movements, gait, and development of fine and gross motor skills. Tests (e.g., balancing on one foot and the heel-to-toe walk) assess balance. Test coordination by asking the child to reach for a toy, button clothes, tie shoes, or draw a straight line on a piece of paper (provided the child is old enough to do these activities). Coordination can also be tested by any sequence of rapid, successive movements, such as quickly touching each finger with the thumb of the same hand.

Several tests for cerebellar function can be performed as games (Box 4.14). When a Romberg test is done, stay beside the child if there is a possibility that he or she might fall. School-age children should be able to perform these tests, although in the finger-to-nose test, preschoolers normally can bring the finger only within 5 to 7.5 cm (2 to 3 inches) of the nose. Difficulty in performing these exercises indicates a poor sense of position (especially with the eyes closed) and incoordination (especially with the eyes open).

Reflexes

Testing reflexes is an important part of the neurologic examination. Persistence of primitive reflexes (see Chapter 7), loss of reflexes, or hyperactivity of deep tendon reflexes is usually a result of a cerebral insult.

Elicit reflexes by using the rubber head of the reflex hammer, edge of the stethoscope diaphragm, flat of the finger, or side of the hand. If the child is easily frightened by equipment, use your hand or finger. Although testing reflexes is a simple procedure, the child may inhibit the reflex by unconsciously tensing the muscle. To avoid tensing, distract younger children with toys or talk to them. Older children can concentrate on the exercise of grasping their two

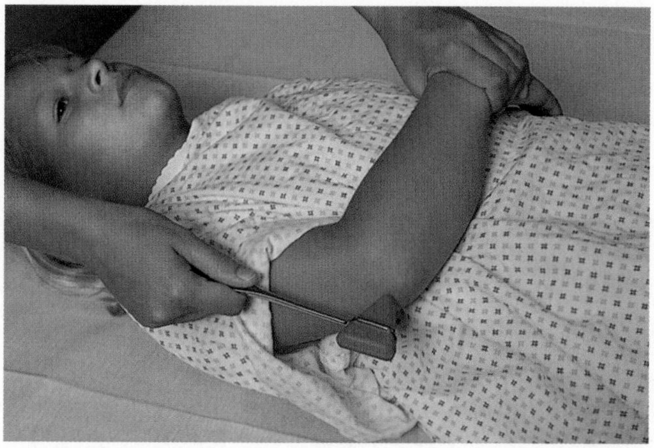

Fig. 4.42 Testing for the triceps reflex. The child is placed supine, with the forearm resting over the chest, and the triceps tendon is struck. *Alternate procedure:* The child's arm is abducted with the upper arm supported and the forearm allowed to hang freely. The triceps tendon is struck. Normal response is partial extension of the forearm.

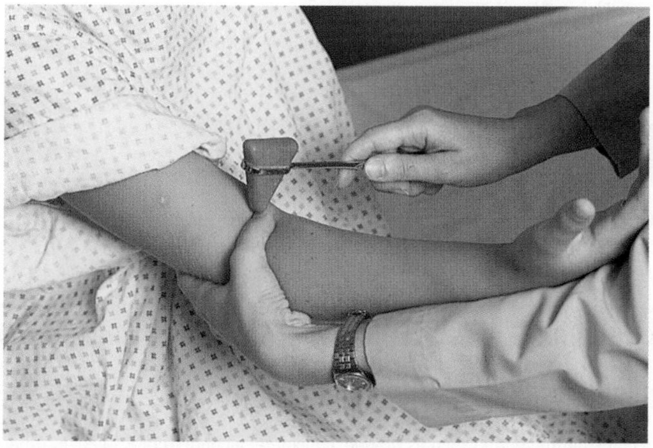

Fig. 4.43 Testing for the biceps reflex. The child's arm is held by placing the partially flexed elbow in the examiner's hand with the thumb over the antecubital space. The examiner's thumbnail is struck with a hammer. Normal response is partial flexion of the forearm.

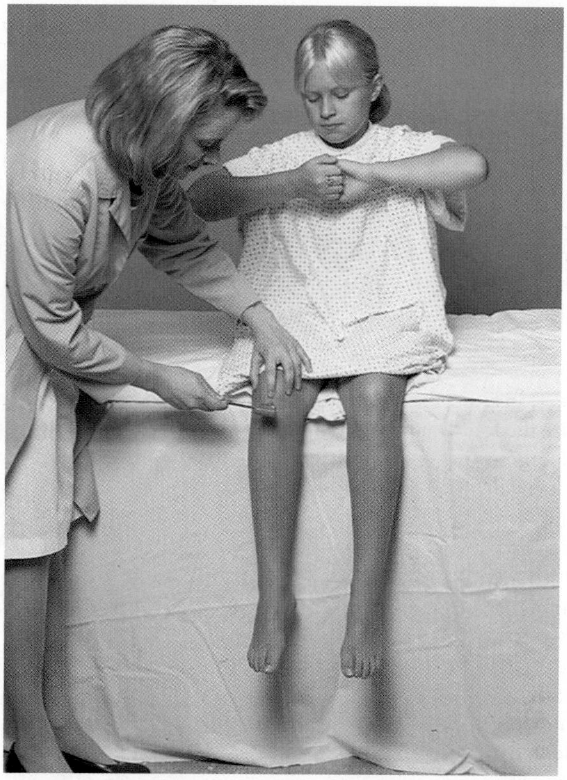

Fig. 4.44 Testing for the patellar, or knee-jerk, reflex using distraction. The child sits on the edge of the examining table (or on the parent's lap) with the lower legs flexed at the knee and dangling freely. The patellar tendon is tapped just below the kneecap. Normal response is partial extension of the lower leg.

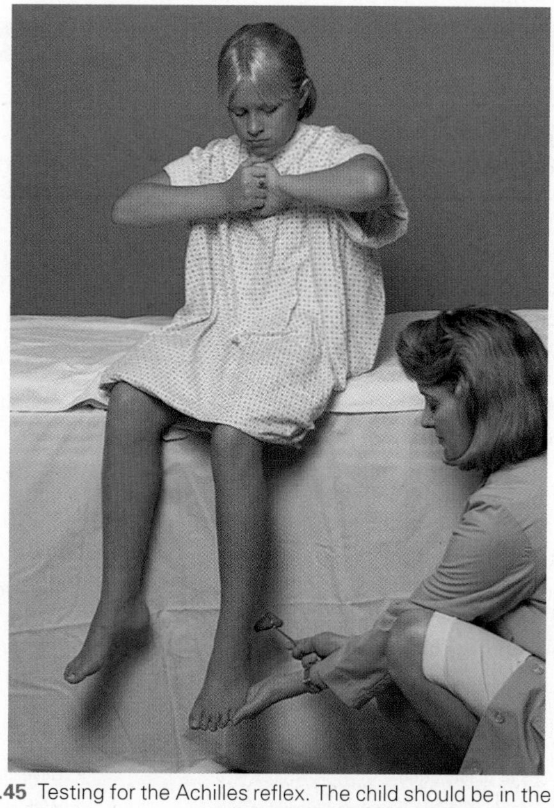

Fig. 4.45 Testing for the Achilles reflex. The child should be in the same position as for the knee-jerk reflex. The foot is supported lightly in the examiner's hand, and the Achilles tendon is struck. Normal response is plantar flexion of the foot (the foot pointing downward).

hands in front of them and trying to pull them apart. This diverts their attention from the testing and causes involuntary relaxation of the muscles.

Deep tendon reflexes are stretch reflexes of a muscle. The most common deep tendon reflex is the **knee jerk reflex**, or **patellar reflex** (sometimes called the **quadriceps reflex**). Figs. 4.42 to 4.45 illustrate the reflexes normally elicited. Report any diminished or hyper-reflexive response for further evaluation.

Cranial Nerves

Assessment of the cranial nerves is an important area of neurologic assessment (Fig. 4.46; Table 4.11). With young children, present the tests as games to foster trust and security at the beginning of the examination. Include the cranial nerve test when examining each system, such as cardinal positions (extraocular movements) of gaze (Fig. 4.47) during examination of the eyes and tongue movement and strength, gag reflex, swallowing, and position of the uvula during examination of the mouth.

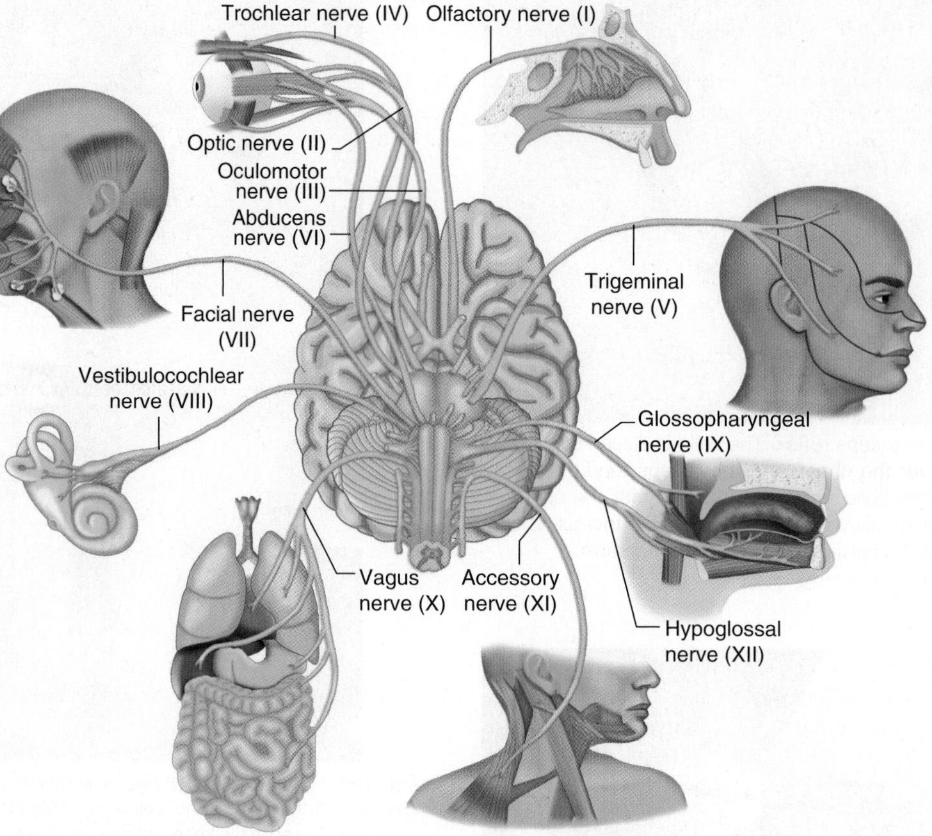

Fig. 4.46 Cranial nerves. (From Patton, K. T., & Thibodeau, G. A. [2013]. *Anatomy and physiology* [8th ed.]. St Louis, MO: Mosby.)

TABLE 4.11 Assessment of Cranial Nerves

Description and Function	Tests
I—Olfactory Nerve	
Olfactory mucosa of nasal cavity Smell	With eyes closed, have child identify odors, such as orange, chocolate, alcohol from a swab, or other smells; test each nostril separately.
II—Optic Nerve	
Rods and cones of retina, optic nerve Vision	Check for perception of light, visual acuity, peripheral vision, color vision, and normal optic discs.
III—Oculomotor Nerve	
Extraocular muscles of eye: • Superior rectus—moves eyeball up and in • Inferior rectus—moves eyeball down and in • Medial rectus—moves eyeball nasally • Inferior oblique—moves eyeball up and out	Have child follow an object (toy) or light in six cardinal positions of gaze (see Fig. 4.47).
Pupil constriction and accommodation	Assess for PERRLA (Pupils Equal, Round, React to Light, and Accommodation).
Eyelid closing	Check for proper placement of eyelid.
IV—Trochlear Nerve	
Superior oblique (SO) muscle—moves eye down and out	Have child look down and in (see Fig. 4.47).
V—Trigeminal Nerve	
Muscles of mastication	Have child bite down hard and open jaw; test symmetry and strength.
Sensory—face, scalp, nasal and buccal mucosa	With child's eyes closed, see if child can detect light touch in mandibular and maxillary regions. Test corneal and blink reflex by touching cornea lightly with a whisk of cotton ball twisted into a point (approach from side so that the child does not blink before cornea is touched).

TABLE 4.11 Assessment of Cranial Nerves—cont'd

Description and Function	Tests
VI—Abducens Nerve	
Lateral rectus (LR) muscle—moves eye temporally	Have child look toward temporal side (see Fig. 4.47).
VII—Facial Nerve	
Muscles for facial expression	Have child smile, frown, make funny face, or show teeth to see symmetry of expression.
Anterior two-thirds of tongue (sensory)	Have child identify sweet or salty solution; place each taste on anterior section and sides of protruding tongue; if child retracts tongue, solution will dissolve toward posterior part of tongue.
VIII—Auditory, Acoustic, or Vestibulocochlear Nerve	
Internal ear Hearing and balance	Test hearing; whisper words in each ear to be repeated; note any loss of equilibrium or presence of vertigo.
IX—Glossopharyngeal Nerve	
Pharynx, tongue	Stimulate posterior pharynx with a tongue blade; child should gag.
Posterior third of tongue Sensory	Test sense of sour or bitter taste on posterior segment of tongue.
X—Vagus Nerve	
Muscles of larynx, pharynx, some organs of gastrointestinal system, sensory fibers of root of tongue, heart, and lung	Note hoarseness of voice, gag reflex, and ability to swallow.Check that uvula is in midline; when stimulated with tongue blade, it should deviate upward and to stimulated side.
XI—Accessory Nerve	
Sternocleidomastoid and trapezius muscles of shoulder	Have child shrug shoulders while applying mild pressure; with examiner's palms placed laterally on child's cheeks, have child turn head against opposing pressure on either side; note symmetry and strength.
XII—Hypoglossal Nerve	
Muscles of tongue	Have child move tongue in all directions; have child protrude tongue as far as possible; note any midline deviation. Test strength by placing tongue blade on one side of tongue and having child move it away.

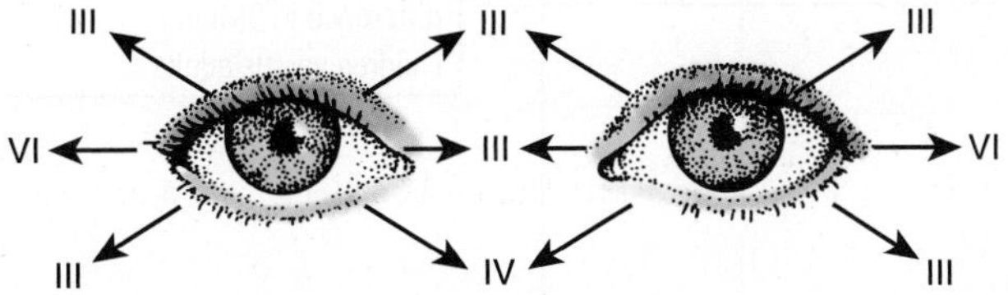

Fig. 4.47 Checking extraocular movements in the six cardinal positions indicates the functioning of cranial nerves III, IV, and VI. (From Ignatavicius, D. D., & Workman, L. M. [2016]. *Medical-surgical nursing: Patient-centered collaborative care* [8th ed.]. St Louis, MO: Elsevier.)

CLINICAL JUDGMENT AND NEXT-GENERATION NCLEX® EXAMINATION-STYLE QUESTIONS

1. The parents of a young infant have arrived for a well child visit. The nurse begins the interview and notices that the mother becomes extremely anxious with the interview questions. Since blocks to communication can adversely affect the child's care, the nurse must look for and recognize clues that indicate communication may be less than optimal. The possible blocks to communication that may interfere with a successful interview during the well child visit are shown below. **Select all that apply.**
   A. Long periods of silence before answering a question.
   B. Sudden, frequent interruptions during the interview.
   C. Concern is raised about the child's feeding schedule.
   D. Nervous habits that distract from the interview.
   E. Questions are asked by both the mother and father.

2. The nurse is communicating with a 6-year-old girl hospitalized for pneumonia. She needs to take the child's blood pressure and is selecting the blood pressure cuff for the assessment. **Choose the *most likely* options for the information missing from the statements below by selecting from the list of options provided.** The nurse recognizes that when measuring blood pressure in the upper arm, a blood pressure cuff with a bladder width equal to ___1___ of the upper arm circumference most accurately reflects ___2___ pressure.

OPTIONS for 1	OPTIONS for 2
20%	radial arterial
30%	radial venous
40%	dorsal arterial
50%	popliteal venous
60%	brachial arterial

3. Organized approaches to performing a physical examination on a child is important. The orderly sequence may be altered to accommodate the child's developmental needs. **For each physical examination assessment approach below, use an X to indicate whether the approach is Effective, Ineffective, or Unrelated.**

Nursing Action: Approach to Physical Examination	Effective	Ineffective	Unrelated
With toddlers, restraints help keep the child still and requesting a parent's assistance is inappropriate.			
An infant's physical examination is always done head to toe, similarly to the adult.			
When examining a preschooler, giving a choice of which body parts to examine first may be helpful in gaining the child's cooperation.			
Giving explanations about body systems can make adolescents nervous due to their egocentricities.			
With an adolescent it is best to have a parent present during the examination.			
The parent's knowledge of stethoscopes can help with cooperation during the examination			

4. Growth measurement is a key element to assess the health status in children. One measurement is linear growth measurement. What is essential in the nursing actions listed below, for the nurse to understand to appropriately perform this technique? **Use an X for the nursing actions listed below that are Indicated (appropriate or necessary), Contraindicated (could be harmful), or Non-Essential (makes no difference or not necessary).**

Nursing Action	Indicated	Contraindicated	Non-Essential
Understand the difference in measurement for children who can stand alone and for those who must lie recumbent.			
Use a stadiometer to measure infant length.			
Two measurers are required for a recumbent child.			
Reposition the child and repeat the procedure. Measure at least twice (ideally three times). Average the measurements for the final value.			
Demonstrate competency when measuring the growth of infants, children, and adolescents. Refresher sessions should be taken when a lack of standardization occurs.			
Understand the difference in BMI in children versus adults.			

REFERENCES

American Academy of Pediatrics. (2019). *Providing culturally effective care.* Retrieved from https://www.aap.org/en-us/professional-resources/practice-transformation/managing-patients/Pages/effective-care.aspx.

Ball, J. W., Dains, J. E., Flynn, J. A., Solomon, B. S., & Stewart, R. W. (2018). *Seidel's guide to physical examination* (9th ed.). St. Louis, MO: Elsevier.

Batra, P., & Goyal, S. (2013). Comparison of rectal, axillary, tympanic, and temporal artery thermometry in the pediatric emergency room. *Pediatric Emergency Care, 29*(1), 63–66.

Batra, P., Saha, A., & Faridi, M. M. (2012). Thermometry in children. *Journal of Emergencies, Trauma, and Shock, 5*(3), 246–249.

Blank, L., Coster, J., O'Cathain, A., Knowles, E., Tosh, J., Turner, J., & Nicholl, J. (2012). The appropriateness of, and compliance with, telephone triage decisions: A systematic review and narrative synthesis. *Journal of Advanced Nursing, 68*(12), 2610–2621.

Clark, J. A., Lieh-Lai, M. W., Sarnaik, A., & Mattoo, T. K. (2002). Discrepancies between direct and indirect blood pressure measurements using various recommendations for arm cuff selection. *Pediatrics, 110*(5), 920–923.

Donahue, S. P., Baker, C. N., Committee on Practice and Ambulatory Medicine, Section on Ophthalmology, American Association of Certified Orthoptists, American Association for Pediatric Ophthalmology and Strabismus, American Academy of Ophthalmology. (2016). Procedure for evaluation of the visual system by pediatricians. *Pediatrics, 137*(1), 1–9.

Dosman, C., & Andrews, D. (2012). Anticipatory guidance for cognitive and social-emotional development: Birth to five years. *Paediatrics & Child Health, 17*(2), 75–80.

Fleming, S., Gill, P. J., Van den Bruel, A., & Thompson, M. (2016). Capillary refill time in sick children: A clinical guide for practice. *British Journal of General Practice, 66*(652), 587–588.

Foote, J. M. (2014). Optimizing linear growth measurement in children. *Journal of Pediatric Health Care, 28*(5), 413–419.

Foote, J. M., Brady, L. H., Burke, A. L., Cook, J. S., Dutcher, M. E., Gradoville, K. M., & Walker, B. S. (2009). *Evidence-based clinical practice guideline on linear growth measurement of children.* Retrieved from http://www.unitypoint.org/blankchildrens/education-resources.aspx (to access full-text guideline and implementation tools).

Foote, J. M., Brady, L. H., Burke, A. L., Cook, J. S., Dutcher, M. E., Gradoville, K. M., & Phillips, K. T. (2011). Development of an evidence-based clinical practice guideline on linear growth measurement of children. *Journal of Pediatric Nursing, 26*(4), 312–324.

Hagan, J. F., & Shaw, J. S. (Eds.). (2017). *Bright futures: guidelines for health supervision of infants, children and adolescents* (4th ed.) Elk Grove Village, IL: American Academy of Pediatrics.

Harlor, A. D., Jr., Bower, C., & Committee on Practice and Ambulatory Medicine, Section on Otolaryngology—Head and Neck Surgery. (2009). Hearing assessment in infants and children: Recommendations beyond neonatal screening. *Pediatrics, 124*(4), 1252–1263.

Mathers, M., Keyes, M., & Wright, M. (2010). A review of the evidence on the effectiveness of children's vision screening. *Child: Care, Health and Development, 36*(6), 754–780.

Miller, J. M., Lessin, H. R., American Academy of Pediatrics Section on Ophthalmology; Committee on Practice and Ambulatory Medicine; American Academy of Ophthalmology and Strabismus; & American Association of Certified Orthoptists. (2012). Instrument-based pediatric vision screening policy statement. *Pediatrics, 130*(5), 983–986.

National High Blood Pressure Education Program Working Group on High Blood Pressure in Children and Adolescents. (2004). The fourth report on the diagnosis, evaluation, and treatment of high blood pressure in children and adolescents. *Pediatrics, 114*(suppl. 2), 555–576.

Park, M. K., Menard, S. W., & Schoolfield, J. (2005). Oscillometric blood pressure standards for children. *Pediatric Cardiology, 26*(5), 601–607.

Purc-Stephenson, R. J., & Thrasher, C. (2010). Nurses' experiences with telephone triage and advice: A meta-ethnography. *Journal of Advanced Nursing, 66*(3), 482–494.

Purc-Stephenson, R. J., & Thrasher, C. (2012). Patient compliance with telephone triage recommendations: A meta-analytic review. *Patient Education and Counseling, 87*(2), 135–142.

Schell, K., Briening, E., Lebet, R., Pruden, K., Rawheiser, S., & Jackson, B. (2011). Comparison of arm and calf automatic noninvasive blood pressures in pediatric intensive care patients. *Journal of Pediatric Nursing, 26*(1), 3–12.

Stacey, D., Macartney, G., Carley, M., Harrison, M. B., & The Pan-Canadian Oncology Symptom Triage and Remote Support Group. (2013). Development and evaluation of evidence-informed clinical nursing protocols for remote assessment, triage and support of cancer treatment-induced symptoms. *Nursing Research and Practice,* article ID:171872. Retrieved from https://www.hindawi.com/journals/nrp/2013/171872/

U.S. Department of Agriculture, National Agricultural Library. (2014). *Food and nutrition information center: Interactive DRI for healthcare professionals.* Retrieved from http://fnic.nal.usda.gov/fnic/interactiveDRI/.

U.S. Preventive Services Task Force. (2017). Vision screening in children aged 6 months to 5 years: US Preventive Task Force Recommendation statement. *Journal of the American Medical Association, 318*(9), 836–844.

5

Pain Assessment and Management in Children

Melody Hellsten

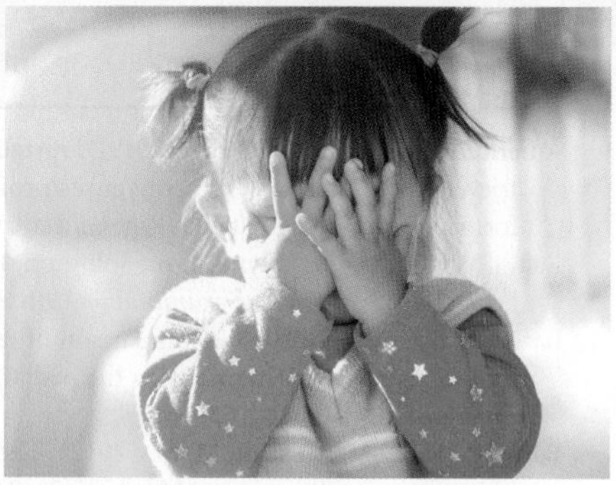

http://evolve.elsevier.com/wong/essentials

CONCEPTS

- Pain
- Sensory Perception

The evidence-based literature on pediatric pain assessment and management grows considerably each year. Treatment options for pediatric acute and chronic pain are continually being evaluated, and new technologies and administration options become available every day (Arane, Behboudi, & Goldman, 2017; Ria, Edmund Allen, & Darren, 2017; Tobias, 2014a; Wiegele, Marhofer, & Lönnqvist, 2019). Unfortunately, despite advances in acute and chronic pediatric pain management, many children and adolescents continue to suffer from inadequately treated pain of all types. Pain is a frequent occurrence in children, with more than 25% of children experiencing pain during hospitalization (Friedrichsdorf, 2015; Harrison, Joly, Chretien, et al., 2014; Kozlowski, Kost-Byerly, Colantuoni, et al., 2014). Effective management of pain in children requires a comprehensive approach of assessment, pain intervention, and reassessment (Habich, Wilson, Thielk, et al., 2012).

PAIN ASSESSMENT

The purpose of a pediatric pain assessment is to determine the pain experience of children receiving medical care. The Pediatric Initiative on Methods, Measurement, and Pain Assessment in Clinical Trials (PedIMMPACT) recommends specific core domains to assess pain in children that include pain intensity, global judgment of satisfaction with treatment, symptoms and adverse events, physical recovery, and emotional response (Dosenovic, Jelicic Kadic, Jeric, et al., 2018; McGrath, Walco, Turk, et al., 2008; Stahlschmidt, Zernikow, & Wager, 2018). Assessing the severity of pain using a number-based pain scale is the first step in understanding the individual child's pain experience. A thorough pain assessment is essential for effective pain management and includes understanding the child's previous experience of pain, pain quality (e.g., sharp, achy, burning), what makes pain better or worse, and how pain interferes with the child's ability to do activities necessary to return to his or her usual state of health. Numerous pediatric pain scales exist and are most commonly identified as behavioral pain measures, self-report pain rating scales, and multidimensional pain assessment tools.

BEHAVIORAL PAIN MEASURES

Behavioral or observational measures of pain are generally used for children from neonate to 4 years old (Table 5.1) or for children of any age who are unable to report pain due to neurocognitive or communication challenges. Behavioral pain assessment may provide a more complete picture of the total pain experience when administered in conjunction with a subjective self-report measure. Distress behaviors—such as moaning, crying, or protestation; changes in facial expression; and unexpected or unusual body movements—have been associated with pain (Figs. 5.1 and 5.2). Understanding that these behaviors are associated with pain makes assessing pain in infants and children with no or limited communication skills a little easier. However, discriminating between pain behaviors and reactions to other sources of distress, such as hunger, anxiety, or other types of discomfort, is not always easy. Behavioral pain measures are most reliable when used to measure short, sharp procedural pain, such as during injections or lumbar punctures, or when assessing pain in infants and young children. They are less reliable when measuring recurrent or chronic pain and when assessing pain in older children, where pain scores on behavioral measures do not always correlate with the children's own reports of pain intensity. Box 5.1 describes pain responses by infants and children of various ages.

The FLACC Pain Assessment Tool is an interval scale that includes the five categories of behavior: **F**acial expression, **L**eg movement, **A**ctivity, **C**ry, and **C**onsolability (Babl, Crellin, Cheng, et al., 2012; Merkel, Voepel-Lewis, Shayevitz, et al., 1997). It measures each behavior on a 0 to 10 scale, with total scores ranging from 0 (no pain behaviors) to 10 (most possible pain behaviors).

The only behavior pain measurement tool recommended for use with children in critical care settings is the COMFORT scale (Ambuel, Hamlett, Marx, et al., 1992). The COMFORT scale is a behavioral, unobtrusive method of measuring distress in unconscious and ventilated infants, children, and adolescents. This scale has eight indicators: alertness, calmness/agitation, respiratory response, physical movement, blood pressure, heart rate, muscle tone, and facial tension. Each indicator is scored between 1 and 5 based on the behaviors exhibited by the patient. The provider observes the patient unobtrusively for 2 minutes and derives the total score by adding the scores of each indicator. The total scores can range between 8 and 40. A score of 17 to 26 generally indicates adequate sedation and pain control. The COMFORT behavior (COMFORT-B) scale is able to detect specific changes in pain or distress intensity in critically ill children and in young children with burns (Boerlage, Ista, Duivenvoorden, et al., 2015; de Jong, Tuinebreijer, Bremer, et al., 2012). The COMFORT scale performed best when compared to other validated observational scales such as the Children's and Infants' Postoperative Pain Scale (CHIPPS), CRIES neonatal pain assessment scale, and the Premature Infant Pain Profile (PIPP) in assessing behavioral and physiologic components of pain in newborns following cardiac surgery (Franck, Ridout, Howard, et al., 2011).

TABLE 5.1 Summary of Selected Behavioral Pain Assessment Scales for Young Children

Ages of Use	Reliability and Validity	Variables	Scoring Range
FLACC Postoperative Pain Tool			
2 months old to 7 years old	Validity using analysis of variance for repeated measures to compare FLACC scores before and after analgesia; preanalgesia FLACC scores significantly higher than postanalgesia scores at 10, 30, and 60 minutes ($p < 0.001$ for each time) Correlation coefficients used to compare FLACC pain scores and OPS; significant positive correlation between FLACC and OPS ($r = 0.80$; $p < 0.001$); positive correlation also found between FLACC scores and nurses' global ratings of pain ($r[47] = 0.41$; $p < 0.005$)	Face (0-2) Legs (0-2) Activity (0-2) Cry (0-2) Consolability (0-2)	0 = no pain; 10 = worst pain

FLACC SCALE

FLACC	0	1	2
Face	No particular expression or smile	Occasional grimace or frown, withdrawn, disinterested	Frequent to constant frown, clenched jaw, quivering chin
Legs	Normal position or relaxed	Uneasy, restless, tense	Kicking, or legs drawn up
Activity	Lying quietly, normal position, moves easily	Squirming, shifting back and forth, tense	Arched, rigid, or jerking
Cry	No cry (awake or asleep)	Moans or whimpers, occasional complaint	Crying steadily, screams or sobs, frequent complaints
Consolability	Content, relaxed	Reassured by occasional touching, hugging, or talking to; distractible	Difficult to console or comfort

From Merkel, S. I., Voepel-Lewis, T., Shayevitz, J. R., et al. (1997). The FLACC: A behavioral scale for scoring postoperative pain in young children. *Pediatric Nursing, 23*(3), 293–297. Used with permission of Jannetti Publications, Inc., and the University of Michigan Health System. Can be reproduced for clinical and research use.

FLACC, Face, Legs, Activity, Cry, Consolability; OPS, observational pain scores.

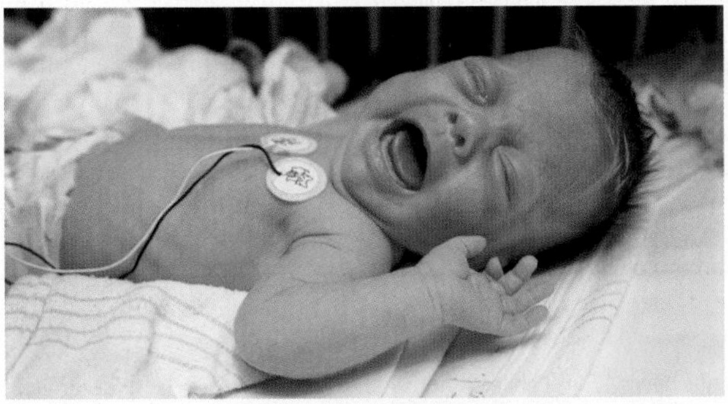

Fig. 5.1 Full, robust crying of preterm infant after heel stick. (Courtesy Halbouty Premature Nursery, Texas Children's Hospital, Houston, TX; photo by Paul Vincent Kuntz.)

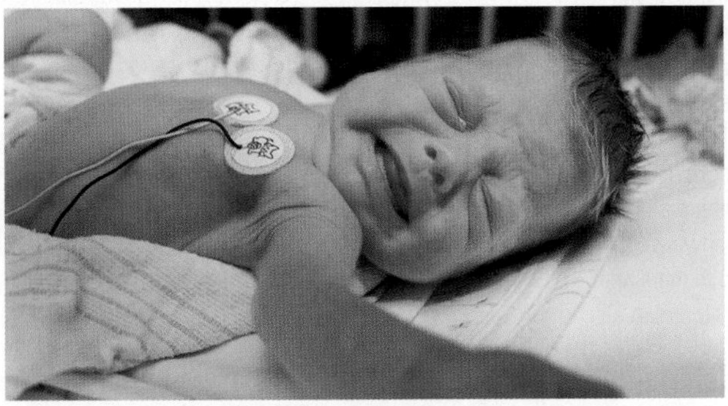

Fig. 5.2 The face of pain after heel stick. Note eye squeeze, brow bulge, nasolabial furrow, and wide-spread mouth. (Courtesy Halbouty Premature Nursery, Texas Children's Hospital, Houston, TX; photo by Paul Vincent Kuntz.)

BOX 5.1 Children's Responses to Pain at Various Ages

Newborn and Young Infant
- Uses crying
- Reveals facial appearance of pain (brows lowered and drawn together, eyes tightly closed, and mouth open and squarish)
- Exhibits generalized body response of rigidity or thrashing, possibly with local reflex withdrawal from what is causing the pain
- Shows no relationship between what is causing the pain and subsequent response

Older Infant
- Uses crying
- Shows a localized body response with deliberate withdrawal from what is causing the pain
- Reveals expression of pain or anger
- Demonstrates a physical struggle, especially pushing away from what is causing the pain

Young Child
- Uses crying and screaming
- Uses verbal expressions, such as "Ow," "Ouch," or "It hurts"
- Uses thrashing of arms and legs to combat pain
- Attempts to push what is causing the pain away before it is applied
- Displays lack of cooperation; need for physical restraint
- Begs for the procedure to end
- Clings to parent, nurse, or other significant person
- Requests physical comfort, such as hugs or other forms of emotional support
- Becomes restless and irritable with ongoing pain
- Worries about the anticipation of the actual painful procedure

BOX 5.1 Children's Responses to Pain at Various Ages—cont'd

School-Age Child

- Demonstrates behaviors of the young child, especially during actual painful procedure, but less before the procedure
- Exhibits time-wasting behavior, such as "Wait a minute" or "I'm not ready"
- Displays muscular rigidity, such as clenched fists, white knuckles, gritted teeth, contracted limbs, body stiffness, closed eyes, wrinkled forehead

Adolescent

- Less vocal with less physical resistance
- More verbal in expressions, such as "It hurts" or "You're hurting me"
- Displays increased muscle tension and body control

SELF-REPORT PAIN RATING SCALES

The number of self-report pain measures available for use in young children and adolescents has increased dramatically and adds a layer of complexity to the assessment of pain in children (Birnie, Chambers, Chorney, et al., 2016). Self-report measures are most often used for children older than 4 years of age (Table 5.2) and generally provide a report of the severity of the child's pain on a scale of 0 to 10, with 0 representing absence of pain and 10 representing the highest severity of pain.

There are many different "faces" scales for the measurement of pain intensity. Faces scales provide a series of facial expressions depicting gradations of pain. The faces are appealing because children can simply point to the face that represents how they feel.

TABLE 5.2 Pain Rating Scales for Children

Pain Scale, Description	Instructions	Recommended Age, Comments
Wong-Baker FACES Pain Rating Scale[a]		
Consists of six cartoon faces ranging from smiling face for "no pain" to tearful face for "worst pain"	*Brief word instructions:* Point to each face using the words to describe the pain intensity. Ask child to choose face that best describes own pain and record appropriate number.	For children as young as 3 years old. Using original instructions without affect words, such as happy or sad, or brief words resulted in same range of pain rating, probably reflecting child's rating of pain intensity. For coding purposes, numbers 0, 2, 4, 6, 8, and 10 can be substituted for 0 to 5 system to accommodate 0 to 10 system.The Wong-Baker FACES Pain Rating Scale provides three scales in one: facial expressions, numbers, and words. Research supports cultural sensitivity of FACES for Caucasian, African-American, Hispanic, Thai, Chinese, and Japanese children.

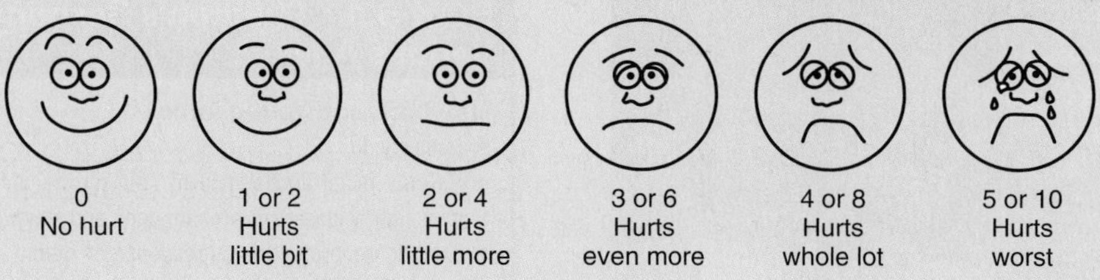

Pain Scale, Description	Instructions	Recommended Age, Comments
Word-Graphic Rating Scale[b] (Tesler, Savedra, Holzemer, et al., 1991)		
Uses descriptive words (may vary in other scales) to denote varying intensities of pain	Explain to child, "This is a line with words to describe how much pain you may have. This side of the line means no pain, and over here the line means worst possible pain." (Point with your finger where "no pain" is, and run your finger along the line to "worst possible pain," as you say it.) "If you have no pain, you would mark like this." (Show example.) "If you have some pain, you would mark somewhere along the line, depending on how much pain you have." (Show example.) "The more pain you have, the closer to worst pain you would mark. The worst pain possible is marked like this." (Show example.) "Show me how much pain you have right now by marking with a straight, up-and-down line anywhere along the line to show how much pain you have right now." With millimeter rule, measure from the "no pain" end to mark and record this measurement as pain score.	For children from 4 to 17 years old.

No pain — Little pain — Medium pain — Large pain — Worst possible pain

Continued

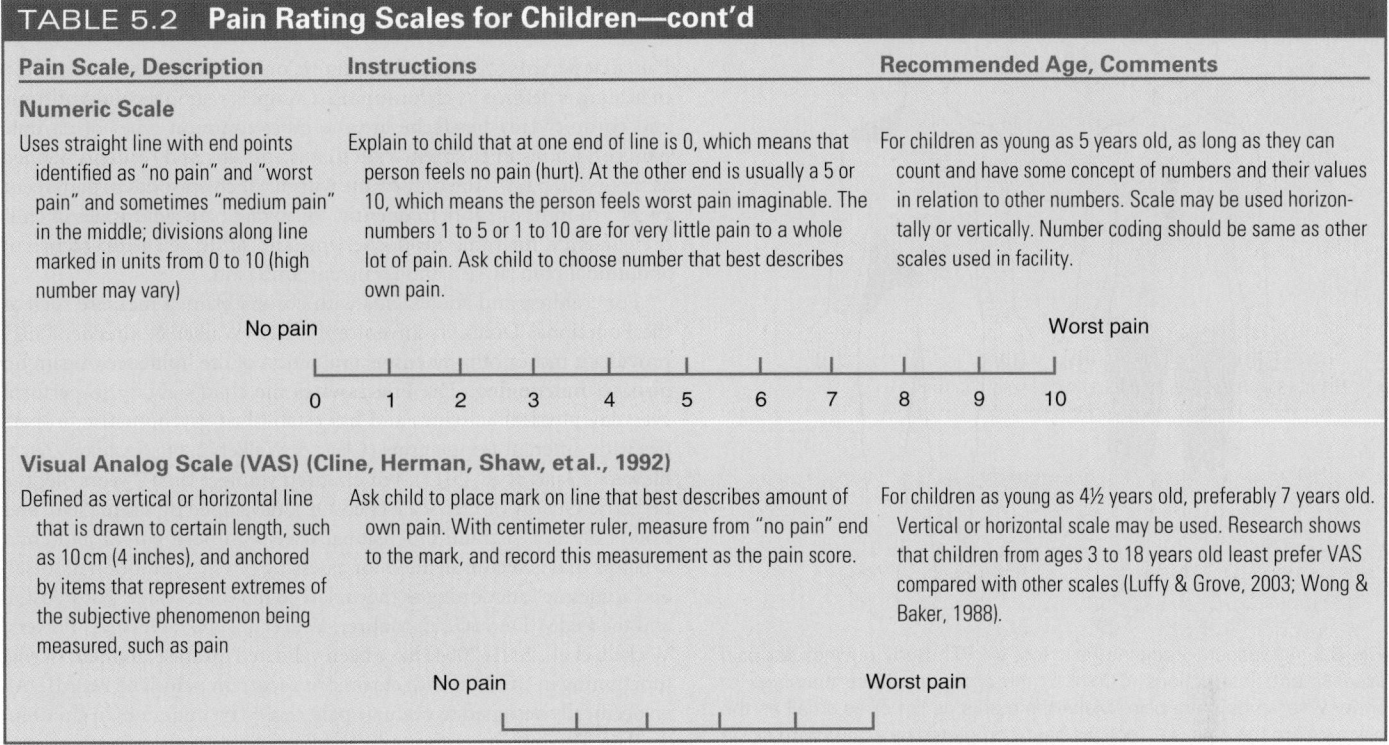

TABLE 5.2 Pain Rating Scales for Children—cont'd

Pain Scale, Description	Instructions	Recommended Age, Comments
Numeric Scale		
Uses straight line with end points identified as "no pain" and "worst pain" and sometimes "medium pain" in the middle; divisions along line marked in units from 0 to 10 (high number may vary)	Explain to child that at one end of line is 0, which means that person feels no pain (hurt). At the other end is usually a 5 or 10, which means the person feels worst pain imaginable. The numbers 1 to 5 or 1 to 10 are for very little pain to a whole lot of pain. Ask child to choose number that best describes own pain.	For children as young as 5 years old, as long as they can count and have some concept of numbers and their values in relation to other numbers. Scale may be used horizontally or vertically. Number coding should be same as other scales used in facility.
No pain 0 1 2 3 4 5 6 7 8 9 10 Worst pain		
Visual Analog Scale (VAS) (Cline, Herman, Shaw, et al., 1992)		
Defined as vertical or horizontal line that is drawn to certain length, such as 10 cm (4 inches), and anchored by items that represent extremes of the subjective phenomenon being measured, such as pain	Ask child to place mark on line that best describes amount of own pain. With centimeter ruler, measure from "no pain" end to the mark, and record this measurement as the pain score.	For children as young as 4½ years old, preferably 7 years old. Vertical or horizontal scale may be used. Research shows that children from ages 3 to 18 years old least prefer VAS compared with other scales (Luffy & Grove, 2003; Wong & Baker, 1988).
No pain — Worst pain		

[a] *Wong-Baker FACES Foundation. (2020). Wong-Baker FACES® Pain Rating Scale. Published with permission from http://www.WongBakerFACES.org. Originally published in Whaley & Wong's Nursing Care of Infants and Children. © Elsevier Inc.*

[b] *Instructions for Word-Graphic Rating Scale from Acute Pain Management Guideline Panel. (1992). Acute pain management in infants, children, and adolescents: Operative and medical procedures; Quick reference guide for clinicians. ACHPR Pub. No. 92-0020. Rockville, MD: Agency for Health Care Research and Quality, US Department of Health and Human Services. Word-Graphic Rating Scale is part of the Adolescent Pediatric Pain Tool and is available from Pediatric Pain Study, University of California, School of Nursing, Department of Family Health Care Nursing, San Francisco, CA 94143-0606; 415-476-4040.*

Although children at 4 or 5 years old are able to use self-report measures, cognitive characteristics of the preoperational stage influence their ability to separate feelings of pain and mood. Smiling faces on pain assessment scales can result in inadequacies of the pain rating (Quinn, Sheldon, & Cooley, 2014). Simple, concrete anchor words, such as "no hurt" to "biggest hurt," are more appropriate than "least pain sensation to worst intense pain imaginable." The ability to discriminate degrees of pain in facial expressions appears to be reasonably established by 3 years old (see Table 5.2).

The Faces Pain Scale–Revised (FPS-R) (Hicks, von Baeyer, Spafford, et al., 2001) and the Wong-Baker FACES Pain Rating Scale (Wong & Baker, 1988) are the most widely used faces pain measurement tools. The FPS-R scale consists of six faces depicting increasing gradation of pain severity from 0 = "no pain" on the left face to 5 = "most pain possible" on the right face. In developing this scale, the authors did not include a smiling face at the "no pain" end or tears at the "most pain" end and validated it so that it is equivalent to a 0 to 10 metric system. The Wong-Baker FACES Pain Rating Scale consists of six cartoon faces ranging from a smiling face for "no pain" to a tearful face for "worst pain." The child is asked to choose a face that describes his or her pain. The Wong-Baker FACES Pain Rating Scale can differentiate pain from fear in school-age children (Garra, Singer, Domingo, et al., 2013). The Wong-Baker FACES Pain Rating Scale is the most preferred and widely used in children's hospitals across the United States and has been translated into many languages (Oakes, 2011).

For children age 8 years and older, the Numeric Rating Scale (NRS), specifically the 0 to 10 scale, is most widely used in clinical practice because it is easy to use. The Visual Analogue Scale (VAS) uses descriptors along a line that provides a highly subjective evaluation of a pain or other symptom. VASs are often used with older children and adults. Although the VAS requires a higher degree of abstraction than the NRS, the PedIMMPACT group recommends the VAS because of the lack of supportive evidence through psychometric studies with the NRS in children and adolescents.

MULTIDIMENSIONAL MEASURES

Several cognitive skills, such as measurement, classification, and seriation (the ability to accurately place in ascending or descending order), become apparent between 7 and 10 years old. Older children are able to use a 0 to 10 NRS used by adolescents and adults. Other dimensions (such as pain quality, pain location, and spatial distribution of pain) may change without a change in pain intensity.

Pain charts or pain drawings are used to obtain information about the location of pain and have been well validated for children age 8 years and older (von Baeyer, Lin, Seidman, et al., 2011). The Adolescent Pediatric Pain Tool (APPT), modeled after the McGill Pain Questionnaire (Melzack, 1975), is a multidimensional pain measurement instrument used with children and adolescents to assess pain location, intensity, and quality (Fernandes, De Campos, Batalha, et al., 2014) (Fig. 5.3). The APPT is an instrument with an anterior and posterior body outline on one side and a 100-mm word-graphing rating scale with a pain descriptor on the other side (Savedra, Holzemer, Tesler, et al., 1993; Savedra, Tesler, Holzemer, et al., 1989; Tesler, Savedra, Holzemer, et al.,

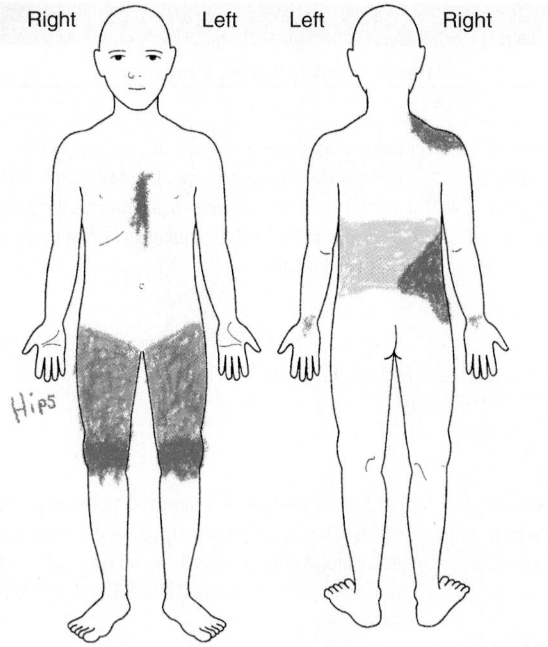

Fig. 5.3 Adolescent Pediatric Pain Tool (APPT): Body outlines for pain assessment. Instructions: "Color in the areas on these drawings to show where you have pain. Make the marks as big or as small as the place where the pain is." Tool has been completed by a child with sickle cell disease. (Redrawn from Savedra, M. C., Tesler, M. D., Holzemer, W. L., & Ward, J. A. [1989]. *Adolescent Pediatric Pain Tool [APPT]: Preliminary user's manual.* San Francisco, CA: University of California.)

1991). Each of the three components of the APPT is scored separately. The body outline is scored by placing a clear plastic template overlay with 43 body areas on the body outline diagram. An estimate of the pervasiveness of the pain is made by counting the number of body areas marked. A ruler or micrometer preprinted on the APPT is used to score the word-graphic rating scale. The number of millimeters from the left side of the scale to the point marked by the child is measured, and the numeric value provides an overall evaluation of the amount of pain the child is experiencing. The total number of words on the descriptor list is counted, and scores range from 0 to 56. The clinician then counts the number of words selected in each of three categories—evaluative (0–8), sensory (0–37), and affective (0–11)—and calculates a percentage score for each one (Savedra, Holzemer, Tesler, et al., 1993). The APPT was identified as the preferred pain assessment tool by hospitalized adolescents when compared to the NRS, Oucher, and FPS-R (Becker, Wilson, Chen-Lim, et al., 2019). A systematic review of the APPT found that it can be helpful in customizing pain management interventions for adolescents (Fernandes, De Campos, Batalha, et al., 2014).

The Pediatric Pain Questionnaire (PPQ) is a multidimensional pain instrument to assess patient and parental perceptions of the pain experience in a manner appropriate for the cognitive-developmental level of children and adolescents (Lootens & Rapoff, 2011). The PPQ consists of eight areas of inquiry: pain history, pain language, the colors children associate with pain, emotions children experience, the worst pain experiences, the ways in which children cope with pain, the positive aspects of pain, and the location of their current pain. The three components of the PPQ include (1) VASs; (2) color-coded rating scales; and (3) verbal descriptors to provide information about the sensory, affective, and evaluative dimensions of chronic pain. There is also information about the child and family's pain history, symptoms, pain relief interventions, and socioenvironmental situations that may influence pain. The child, parent, and physician each complete the form separately.

CHRONIC AND RECURRENT PAIN ASSESSMENT

Pain that persists for 3 months or more, or beyond the expected period of healing is defined as **chronic pain**. Complex regional pain syndrome and chronic daily headache are the most common types of chronic pain conditions in children. Pain that is episodic and recurs is defined as **recurrent pain**—the time frame within which episodes of pain recur every 3 months or more frequently. Recurrent pain syndromes in children include migraine headache, episodic sickle cell pain, recurrent abdominal pain (RAP), and recurrent limb pain.

For children and adolescents with chronic pain, a measure such as the Functional Disability Inventory (FDI) (Walker & Greene, 1991) provides a more comprehensive evaluation of the influence of pain on physical functioning. The FDI assesses the child's ability to perform everyday physical activities and has established psychometric properties with different populations (Claar & Walker, 2006; Kashikar-Zuck, Flowers, Claar, et al., 2011). For children younger than 7 years old, the Pediatric Quality of Life Scale (PedsQL), developed by Varni, Seid, and Rode (1999), is a multidimensional scale with both parent and child versions that is recommended for assessing physical, emotional, social, and academic functioning as they relate to the child's pain. The PedsQL and the PedMIDAS (Gold, Mahrer, Yee, et al., 2009; Hershey, Powers, Vockell, et al., 2001, 2004) have been validated for measurement of role functioning in children with chronic or recurrent pain. The PedMIDAS is specifically designed to evaluate pain caused by migraines in children.

Pain diaries are commonly used to assess pain symptoms and response to treatment in children and adolescents with recurrent or chronic pain (Fortier, Wahi, Bruce, et al., 2014; Stinson, Stevens, Feldman, et al., 2008). Diary studies have included children as young as 6 years old. Conventional paper-and-pencil measures have been associated with several limitations, such as poor compliance, missing data, hoarding of responses, and back and forward filling. An electronic diary to assess pediatric chronic pain is a developing area that holds promise for the future (see Research Focus box).

RESEARCH FOCUS

The Use of Pain Diaries in Pediatric Chronic Pain Research

Pain diaries have been used in a wide variety of pediatric pain research studies to gain insight into the pain experience of children. A study evaluating the relationship between pain recall and momentary pain assessment used the e-Ouch electronic diary to capture momentary pain assessment in addition to a weekly pain recall questionnaire in children with chronic arthritis pain. The findings demonstrated that recalled pain reports did not equate with "in the moment" pain reports, suggesting the need to use electronic momentary reports when collecting pain data (Stinson, Jibb, Lalloo, et al., 2014). Another pain diary study evaluated the role of anxiety and somatization in children with pain-related functional gastrointestinal disorders (painFGIDs) (Williams, Czyzewski, Self, et al., 2015). Children completed anxiety and somatization questionnaires and documented abdominal pain frequency and severity for 2 weeks using a pain diary. Findings demonstrated that somatization was more strongly associated with pain compared to anxiety. Lastly, parent diaries were used to collect parent report of pain episodes experienced by children with profound cognitive impairment and the parent's response to such episodes in addition to two face-to-face interviews (Carter, Arnott, Simons, et al., 2017). Diary data and interviews were reviewed and coded, yielding a metatheme of "developing a sense of knowing" and three core themes of learning to know, learning to be a convincing advocate, and learning to endure and find balance. The findings provide insight into how parents of children with profound cognitive impairment engage in experiential learning to assess and manage their child's pain. In each of these examples, patient- and parent-reported diaries added depth of knowledge to the pain experience of children.

BOX 5.2 Manifestations of Acute Pain in the Neonate

Physiologic Responses

Vital signs: Observe for variations
- Increased heart rate
- Increased blood pressure
- Rapid, shallow respirations

Oxygenation
- Decreased transcutaneous oxygen pressure ($TcPO_2$)
- Decreased arterial oxygen saturation (SaO_2)

Skin: Observe color and character
- Pallor or flushing
- Diaphoresis
- Palmar sweating

Other observations
- Increased muscle tone
- Dilated pupils
- Decreased vagal nerve tone
- Increased intracranial pressure
- Laboratory evidence of metabolic or endocrine changes: Hyperglycemia, lowered pH, elevated corticosteroids

Behavioral Responses

Vocalizations: Observe quality, timing, and duration
- Crying
- Whimpering
- Groaning

Facial expression: Observe characteristics, timing, orientation of eyes and mouth
- Grimaces
- Brow furrowed
- Chin quivering
- Eyes tightly closed
- Mouth open and squarish

Body movements and posture: Observe type, quality, and amount of movement or lack of movement; relationship to other factors
- Limb withdrawal
- Thrashing
- Rigidity
- Flaccidity
- Fist clenching

Changes in state: Observe sleep, appetite, activity level
- Changes in sleep-wake cycles
- Changes in feeding behavior
- Changes in activity level
- Fussiness, irritability
- Listlessness

Sleep disruption is also common in those with chronic or recurrent pain (Fisher, Laikin, Sharp, et al., 2018; Rabbitts, Zhou, Narayanan, et al., 2017; Valrie, Bromberg, Palermo, et al., 2013). A sleep diary can be useful in keeping a record of activities surrounding sleep, including bedtime, time to fall asleep, number of night awakenings, waking in the morning, and especially any pain or other circumstance that interferes with sleeping. The Children's Sleep Habits Questionnaire (Owens, Spirito, & McGuinn, 2000), which is useful for assessing sleep behaviors in school-age children with chronic or recurrent pain, has also been evaluated for use in infants, toddlers, and preschoolers using parent proxy (Sneddon, Peacock, & Crowley, 2013).

ASSESSMENT OF PAIN IN SPECIFIC POPULATIONS

PAIN IN NEONATES

The impact of early pain exposure greatly affects the developing nervous system, with persistent long-term effects. This makes neonatal assessment extremely important, although difficult because the most reliable indicator of pain, self-report, is not possible. Evaluation must be based on physiologic changes and behavioral observations with validated instruments (Hatfield & Ely, 2015) (Box 5.2). Although behaviors (such as vocalizations, facial expressions, body movements, and general relaxation state) are common to all infants, they vary with different situations. Crying associated with pain is more intense and sustained (see Fig. 5.1). Facial expression is the most consistent and specific characteristic; scales to systematically evaluate facial features, such as eye squeeze, brow bulge, open mouth, and taut tongue, are available (see Fig. 5.2). Most infants respond with increased body movements, but the infant may be experiencing pain even when lying quietly with eyes closed. The preterm infant's response to pain may be behaviorally blunted or absent; however, there is ample evidence that such infants are neurologically capable of feeling pain. In addition, infants in awake or alert states demonstrate a more robust reaction to painful stimuli than infants in sleep states. Also, an infant receiving a muscle-paralyzing agent (vecuronium) is incapable of a behavioral or visible pain response.

Several pain assessment tools for infants have been developed (Table 5.3). One tool used by nurses who work with premature and full-term infants in the neonatal intensive care setting is called *CRIES*, which is an acronym for the tool's physiologic and behavioral indicators of pain: **C**rying, **R**equiring increased oxygen, **I**ncreased vital signs, **E**xpression, and **S**leeplessness. Each indicator is scored from 0 to 2, with a total possible pain score, representing the worst pain, of 10. A pain score greater than 4 is considered significant. This tool has been tested for reliability and validity for postoperative pain in infants between the ages of 32 weeks of gestation and 20 weeks postterm (60 weeks) (Sweet & McGrath, 1998).

The Premature Infant Pain Profile (PIPP) was developed specifically for preterm infants (Stevens, Gibbons, Yamada, et al., 2014; Sweet & McGrath, 1998). The category "gestational age at time of observation" gives a higher pain score to infants with lower gestational age, to account for inability to mount emotional response. Infants who are asleep 15 seconds before the painful procedure also receive additional points for their blunted behavioral responses to painful stimuli.

The Neonatal Pain, Agitation, and Sedation Scale (NPASS) was originally developed to measure pain or sedation in preterm infants after surgery (Hillman, Tabrizi, Gauda, et al., 2015). It measures five criteria (see Table 5.3) in two dimensions (pain and sedation) and is used in neonates as young as 23 weeks of gestation up to infants 100 days old. Extra points are added in the pain scale dimension for preterm infants based on gestational age.

CHILDREN WITH COMMUNICATION AND COGNITIVE IMPAIRMENT

The assessment of pain in children with communication and cognitive impairment can be challenging (Cascella, Bimonte, Saettini, et al., 2019; Crosta, Ward, Walker, et al., 2014). Children who have significant difficulties in communicating with others about their pain include

TABLE 5.3 Summary of Pain Assessment Scales for Infants

	PIPP-revised (Stevens, Gibbins, Yamada, et al., 2014)	NIPS (Lawrence, Alcock, McGrath, et al., 1993)	NPASS (Hummel, Puchalski, Creech, et al., 2008)	COMFORT-neo (van Dijk, Roofthooft, Anand, et al., 2009)	CRIES (Krechel & Bildner, 1995)
Age range	25-40 weeks	26-40 weeks	23-40 weeks	24-42 weeks	32-40 weeks
Type of pain	Procedural and postoperative		Procedural and prolonged	Prolonged pain	Postoperative pain
Variables assessed	Scored at (0-3) each Heart rate Oxygen saturation Brow bulge Eye squeeze Nasolabial furrow Behavioral state	Breathing (0-1) Face (0-1) Arms (0-1) Legs (0-1) Cry (0-2) Arousal (0-1)	Scored at (0-2) each Vital signs Crying/ irritability Facial expressions Behavioral state Extremities/tone	Scored at (1-5) each Alertness Calmness/agitation Respiratory response or crying Body movement Muscle tone Facial tension	Scored at (0-2) each Crying Oxygen requirement Changes to vital signs Facial expressions Sleeplessness
Score range	0-21	0-7	Pain: 0-10	6-30	0-10
Adjusted for gestational age	Yes Scored at (0-3)	No	Yes	No	No

Table 5.3 depicts various neonatal assessment scales with variables assessed and score ranges.
Adapted from Harris, J., Ramelet, A., van Dijk, M., et al. (2016). Clinical recommendations for pain, sedation, withdrawal and delirium assessment in critically ill infants and children: An ESPNIC position statement for healthcare professionals. *Intensive Care Medicine, 42,* 972–986.

those who have significant neurologic impairments (e.g., cerebral palsy), cognitive impairment, metabolic disorders, autism, severe brain injury, and communication barriers (e.g., critically ill children who are on ventilators or heavily sedated or have neuromuscular disorders, loss of hearing, or loss of vision) and consequently are at greater risk for undertreatment of pain. Children with communication and cognitive deficits often experience spasticity, contractures, injury, infection, and orthopedic surgical treatment that may be painful. Behaviors include moaning, inconsistent patterns of play and sleep, changes in facial expression, and other physical problems that may mask expression of pain and be difficult to interpret (see Research Focus box).

RESEARCH FOCUS

Pain Reporting in Children with Cognitive Impairment

Children, adolescents, and young adults with cerebral palsy (CP) experience pain from a variety of causes. In a population-based study, Poirot and colleagues (2017) reviewed data from a longitudinal cohort of 240 nonambulatory children ages 3 to 10 years with CP in France. Orthopedic pain was reported in all 65 children with pain (27% prevalence), and 45% of children experienced pain from another origin such as joint movement (58%), scoliosis (43%), and hips (43%) and spasticity treatment (32%). Pain is a frequent experience for children with CP, necessitating regular pain assessment and interventions aimed at preventing scoliosis, hip luxation, reducing scoliosis, and providing analgesics prior to physical therapies or range-of-motion activities.

The revised FLACC observational pain scale uses a behavioral approach that observes the child's face, legs, activity, cry, and consolability and is supported for use in clinical practice for children with cognitive impairment (Voepel-Lewis, Malviya, Tait, et al., 2008). Nurses can assist parents to individualize the scale with their child's unique pain behaviors.

The Non-Communicating Children's Pain Checklist–Revised (NCCPC) is a pain measurement tool specifically designed for children with cognitive impairments (Breau, McGrath, Camfield, et al., 2002). The scale discriminates between periods of pain and calm, and can predict behavior during subsequent episodes of pain. The scale consists of six subscales (vocal, social, facial, activity, body and limbs, physiologic signs), which are scored based on the number of times the items are observed over a 10-minute period (0 = not at all; 1 = just a little; 2 = fairly often; 3 = very often). The NCCPC has been used during the postoperative period and was effective in measuring pain in the clinical setting (Massaro, Ronfani, Ferrara, et al., 2014).

CULTURAL DIFFERENCES

Expression of pain can be greatly affected by communication barriers (Azize, Humphreys, & Cattani, 2011; Jenkins & Fortier, 2014). A major challenge in the assessment and management of pain in children is the cultural appropriateness of pain assessment tools that have been validated only in white and English-speaking children (see Cultural Considerations and Research Focus boxes). Cultural background may influence the validity and reliability of pain assessment tools developed in a single cultural context. However, there is a growing trend toward translating and validating established pediatric pain assessment instruments in different languages (Bueno, Moreno-Ramos, Forni, et al., 2019; Dionysakopoulou, Giannakopoulou, Lianou, et al., 2018; Matsuishi, Hoshino, Shimojo, et al., 2018; Özalp Gerçeker, Bilsin, Binay, et al., 2018).

CULTURAL CONSIDERATIONS

Pain Scales

Observational scales and interview questionnaires for pain may not be as reliable for pain assessment as self-report scales in children of Hispanic origin. Children of Asian descent, who may learn to read Chinese characters vertically downward and from right to left, may have difficulty using horizontally oriented scales.

RESEARCH FOCUS

Pain Reporting in Non–English-Speaking Families

There is a growing body of knowledge demonstrating that ethnic and racial disparities can have a negative effect on pain assessment and management in children in non–English-speaking families. Hispanic children have been shown to receive less analgesia at home after tonsillectomy, with caregivers stating that their child was not in pain or refused to take the medication (Brown, Fortier, Zolghadr, et al., 2016). In a study of the influence of primary language use on reporting musculoskeletal pain, adolescents of Spanish-speaking Hispanic and English-speaking Hispanic parents were less likely to report musculoskeletal pain than adolescents of English-speaking white parents. Parental education and employment was also found to influence children's report of pain. Children of parents with a college degree or who were currently employed reported more pain than did children of parents with a high school degree or who were currently unemployed (Zamora-Kapoor, Omidpanah, Monico, et al., 2015)

CHILDREN WITH CHRONIC ILLNESS AND COMPLEX PAIN

Questionnaires and pain assessment scales do not always provide the most meaningful means of assessing pain in children, particularly for those with complex pain. Some children cannot relate to a face or a number that describes their pain. Other children, such as those with cancer, are experiencing multiple symptoms and may find it difficult to isolate the pain from other symptoms. Rating the pain is only one aspect of assessment and does not always accurately convey to others how they experience and cope with pain (Yetwin, Mahrer, John, et al., 2018).

Important components of assessment include the onset of pain; pain duration or pattern; the effectiveness of the current treatment; factors that aggravate or relieve the pain; other symptoms and complications concurrently felt; and interference with the child's mood, function, and interactions with family (Pasero & McCaffrey, 2011). In addition to asking the child or parent when the pain started and how long the pain lasts, the nurse can assess variations and rhythms by asking whether the pain is better or worse at certain times of the day or night. If the child has had pain for a while, the child or parent may know which medications and doses are helpful. They may also have found some nonpharmacologic methods that have helped. The nurse may ask the child or parent to keep a diary of activities, positions, and other events that may increase or decrease the pain. Pain may be accompanied by other symptoms (such as nausea and poor appetite), and it may interfere with sleep and other activities. A diary can help families identify triggers that may cause pain and interventions that work.

Other aspects warranting careful assessment that may pose barriers to effective management include family issues and relationships, fears and concerns about addictions, the clinician's and family's lack of knowledge about pain, inappropriate use of pain medications, ineffective management of adverse effects from medications, and the use of different pain management modalities.

PAIN MANAGEMENT

Children may experience pain as a result of surgery, injuries, acute and chronic illnesses, and medical or surgical procedures. Unrelieved pain may lead to potential long-term physiologic, psychosocial, and behavioral consequences. Improving pain management requires a multifactorial approach encompassing education, institutional support, attitude shifts, and change leaders (Twycross, 2010). Nonpharmacologic interventions and adequate pain medications are both essential to providing optimal pain management (Ria et al., 2017).

NONPHARMACOLOGIC MANAGEMENT

Pain is often associated with fear, anxiety, and stress. A number of nonpharmacologic techniques, such as distraction, relaxation, guided imagery, and cutaneous stimulation, can help with pain control (see Nursing Care Guidelines box). It is also important to provide coping strategies that help reduce pain perception, make pain more tolerable, decrease anxiety, and enhance the effectiveness of analgesics or reduce the dosage required. Recent changes in The Joint Commission requirements for pain assessment and management (Baker, 2017) have focused on the importance of nonpharmacologic pain management modalities as a means of minimizing opioid exposure in children and adolescents. Nurses play a vital role in providing effective nonpharmacologic pain management interventions tailored to the individual child and family.

NURSING CARE GUIDELINES

Nonpharmacologic Strategies for Pain Management

General Strategies

Consult child life specialist.

Use nonpharmacologic interventions to supplement, not replace, pharmacologic interventions and for mild pain and pain that is reasonably well controlled with analgesics.

Form a trusting relationship with child and family.

Express concern regarding their reports of pain and intervene appropriately.

Take an active role in seeking effective pain management strategies.

Use general guidelines to prepare child for procedure.

Prepare child before potentially painful procedures but avoid "planting" the idea of pain.

- For example, instead of saying, "This is going to (or may) hurt," say, "Sometimes this feels like pushing, sticking, or pinching, and sometimes it doesn't bother people. Tell me what it feels like to you."
- Use "nonpain" descriptors when possible (e.g., "It feels like heat" rather than "It's a burning pain"). This allows for variation in sensory perception, avoids suggesting pain, and gives the child control in describing reactions.
- Avoid evaluative statements or descriptions (e.g., "This is a terrible procedure" or "It really will hurt a lot").

Stay with child during a painful procedure.

Allow parents to stay with child if child and parent desire; encourage parent to talk softly to child and to remain near child's head.

Involve parents in learning specific nonpharmacologic strategies and in assisting child with their use.

Educate child about the pain, especially when explanation may lessen anxiety (e.g., that pain may occur after surgery and does not indicate that something is wrong); reassure child that he or she is not responsible for the pain.

For long-term pain control, offer the child a doll, which represents "the patient," and allow child to do everything to the doll that is done to him or her; emphasize pain control through the doll by stating, "Dolly feels better after the medicine."

Teach procedures to child and family for later use.

NURSING CARE GUIDELINES—cont'd

Nonpharmacologic Strategies for Pain Management

Specific Strategies

Distraction

Involve parent and child in identifying strong distractors.

Involve child in play; use radio, tape recorder, CD player, or computer game; have child sing or use rhythmic breathing.

Have child take a deep breath and blow it out until told to stop.

Have child blow bubbles to "blow the hurt away."

Have child concentrate on yelling or saying "ouch," with instructions to "yell as loud or soft as you feel it hurt; that way I know what's happening."

Have child look through kaleidoscope (type with glitter suspended in fluid-filled tube) and encourage him or her to concentrate by asking, "Do you see the different designs?"

Use humor, such as watching cartoons, telling jokes or funny stories, or acting silly with child.

Have child read, play games, or visit with friends.

Relaxation

With an infant or young child:

- Hold in a comfortable, well-supported position, such as vertically against the chest and shoulder.
- Rock in a wide, rhythmic arc in a rocking chair or sway back and forth, rather than bouncing child.
- Repeat one or two words softly, such as "Mommy's here."

With a slightly older child:

- Ask child to take a deep breath and "go limp as a rag doll" while exhaling slowly; then ask child to yawn (demonstrate if needed).
- Help child assume a comfortable position (e.g., pillow under neck and knees).
- Begin progressive relaxation: starting with the toes, systematically instruct child to let each body part "go limp" or "feel heavy." If child has difficulty relaxing, instruct child to tense or tighten each body part and then relax it.
- Allow child to keep eyes open, since children may respond better if eyes are open rather than closed during relaxation.

Guided Imagery

Have child identify some highly pleasurable real or imaginary experience.

Have child describe details of the event, including as many senses as possible (e.g., "feel the cool breezes," "see the beautiful colors," "hear the pleasant music").

Have child write down or tape record script.

Encourage child to concentrate only on the pleasurable event during the painful time; enhance the image by recalling specific details by reading the script or playing the tape.

Combine with relaxation and rhythmic breathing.

Positive Self-Talk

Teach child positive statements to say when in pain (e.g., "I will be feeling better soon," or "When I go home, I will feel better, and we will eat ice cream").

Thought Stopping

Identify positive facts about the painful event (e.g., "It does not last long").

Identify reassuring information (e.g., "If I think about something else, it does not hurt as much").

Condense positive and reassuring facts into a set of brief statements and have child memorize them (e.g., "Short procedure, good veins, little hurt, nice nurse, go home").

Have child repeat the memorized statements whenever thinking about or experiencing the painful event.

Behavioral Contracting

Informal: May be used with children as young as 4 or 5 years old:

- Use stars, tokens, or cartoon character stickers as rewards.
- Give a child who is uncooperative or procrastinating during a procedure a limited time (measured by a visible timer) to complete the procedure.
- Proceed as needed if child is unable to comply.
- Reinforce cooperation with a reward if the procedure is accomplished within specified time.

Formal: Use written contract, which includes:

- Realistic (seems possible) goal or desired behavior
- Measurable behavior (e.g., agrees not to hit anyone during procedures)
- Contract written, dated, and signed by all persons involved in any of the agreements
- Identified rewards or consequences that are reinforcing
- Goals that can be evaluated
- Commitment and compromise requirements for both parties (e.g., while timer is used, nurse will not nag or prod child to complete procedure)

There is growing evidence that nonpharmacologic approaches such as distraction, hypnosis, cognitive-behavioral therapy (CBT), and breathing-focused interventions are effective in managing needle-related pain and distress in children and adolescents (Bembich, Cont, Causin, et al., 2018; Birnie, Chambers, Chorney, et al., 2016). CBT is an evidence-based psychologic approach for managing pediatric pain (Logan, Coakley, & Garcia, 2014). CBT uses strategies that focus on thoughts and behaviors that modify negative beliefs and enhance the child's ability to solve pain-related problems that result in better pain management.

Nutritive (breast or formula feeding) and nonnutritive sucking (pacifier) (Fig. 5.4), kangaroo care (Fig. 5.5), and swaddling or facilitated tucking interventions reduce behavioral, physiologic, and hormonal responses to pain from procedures, such as heel punctures, in preterm and newborn infants (Bembich et al., 2018; Bos-Veneman, Otter, & Reijneveld, 2018; Meek & Huertas, 2012; Pillai Riddell, Racine, Gennis, et al., 2015) (see Research Focus box).

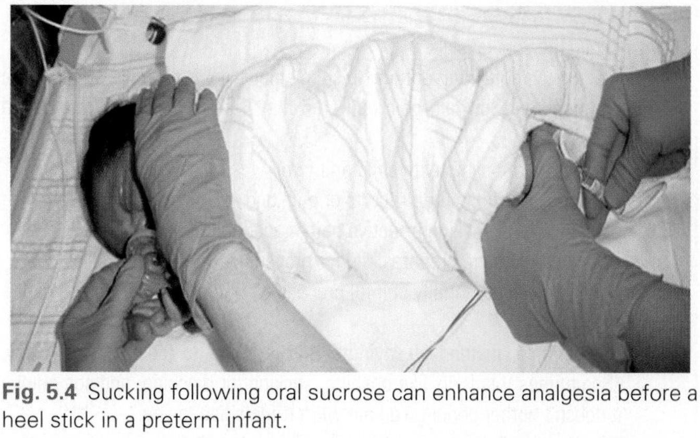

Fig. 5.4 Sucking following oral sucrose can enhance analgesia before a heel stick in a preterm infant.

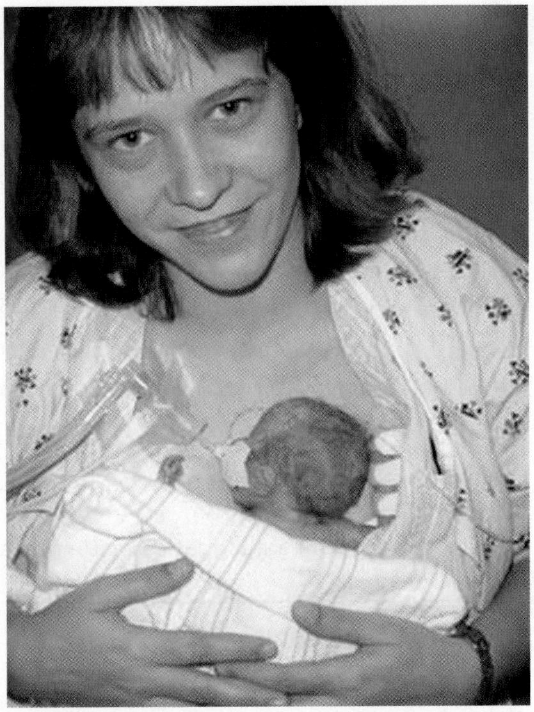

Fig. 5.5 Mother using kangaroo hold with her newborn infant. Note placement of the infant directly on the mother's skin.

RESEARCH FOCUS

Nonpharmacologic Methods of Pain Management: Preterm and Newborn Infants

A Cochrane review of sucrose for analgesia in preterm and newborn infants demonstrated efficacy in reducing procedural pain experienced during single episodes such as heel lance, venipuncture, and intramuscular injections (Stevens, Yamada, Ohlsson, et al., 2016). A multicenter randomized controlled trial of 245 neonates was conducted to ascertain the minimally effective dose of 24% sucrose during heel lance. Neonates were prospectively randomized to three different sucrose volumes (0.1 ml, 0.5 ml, and 1 ml) followed by measurement of pain at 30 and 60 seconds after the procedure using the Premature Infant Pain Profile–Revised. Findings indicated that the 0.1-ml volume of 24% sucrose was a sufficiently effective dose for management of heel lance–related pain in neonates (Stevens, Yamada, Campbell-Yeo, et al., 2018).

A study of 109 preterm infants comparing nonnutritive sucking, oral breast milk, and facilitated tucking during heel stick procedures found that the combined use of sucking, breast milk, and tucking significantly reduced moderate to severe pain, with the addition of facilitated tucking aiding in postprocedure recovery (Peng, Yin, Yang, et al., 2018). Gao and colleagues (2015) found that infants who received kangaroo mother care had significantly lower heart rates and shorter crying and facial grimacing than infants in incubators.

Lastly, data from several individual studies evaluated in a large systematic review found that sucrose significantly reduced pain during needle-related procedures in infants 1 month to 1 year of age (Kassab, Foster, Foureur, et al., 2012). Other randomized controlled trials have also found sucrose effective in reducing distress in older infants during immunizations (Despriee & Langeland, 2016; Yilmaz, Caylan, Oguz, et al., 2014).

If the child cannot identify a familiar coping technique, the nurse can describe several strategies (e.g., distraction, breathing, guided imagery) and let the child select the most appealing one. Experimentation with several strategies that are suitable to the child's age, pain intensity, and abilities is often necessary to determine the most effective approach. Parents should be involved in the selection process; they may be familiar with the child's usual coping skills and can help identify potentially successful strategies. Involving parents also encourages their participation in learning the skill with the child and acting as coach. If the parent cannot assist the child, other appropriate persons may include a grandparent, older sibling, nurse, or child life specialist.

Children should learn to use a specific strategy before pain occurs or before it becomes severe. To reduce the child's effort, instructions for a strategy, such as distraction or relaxation, can be audiotaped and played during a period of comfort. However, even after they have learned an intervention, children often need help using it during a painful procedure. The intervention can also be used after the procedure. This gives the child a chance to recover, feel mastery, and cope more effectively.

COMPLEMENTARY AND INTEGRATIVE HEALTH APPROACHES TO PAIN MANAGEMENT

Complementary therapies are evidence-based health care interventions used in conjunction with conventional Western medicine, while integrative health promotes patient-centered evidence-based care by blending complementary and conventional therapies. Alternative therapies are unconventional interventions used in place of conventional care and are not considered to be evidence based (National Center for Complementary and Integrative Health, 2019). Pediatric integrative medicine is an emerging field that promotes the use of complementary therapies such as natural products and/or mind and body practices alone or in combination with conventional medical interventions with the goal of maximizing patient outcomes (McClafferty, Vohra, Bailey, et al., 2017). The therapies that are increasingly used include herbal medicine, massage, megavitamins, self-help groups, folk remedies, energy healing, and homeopathy (Groenewald, Beals-Erickson, Ralston-Wilson, et al., 2017).

Classification of Complementary and Integrative Medicine (McClafferty et al., 2017)

Natural products

- Biologically based—foods, special diets, herbal or plant preparations, traditional medicines, folk medicines, homeopathic remedies, probiotics, vitamins, other supplements

Mind and body practices

- Manipulative treatments—chiropractic, osteopathy, massage
- Energy based—Reiki, bioelectric or magnetic treatments, pulsed fields, alternating and direct currents
- Mind-body techniques—mental healing, expressive treatments, spiritual healing, hypnosis, relaxation

Creative arts therapies—music therapy, art therapy, animal-assisted therapy

- Alternative medical systems—homeopathy; naturopathy; ayurvedic; traditional Chinese medicine, including acupuncture and moxibustion

Integrative medicine options are used frequently with children at the end of life and are found by their caregivers to be beneficial (Heath, Oh, Clarke, et al., 2012; Schütze, Längler, Zuzak, et al., 2016).

PHARMACOLOGIC MANAGEMENT

The World Health Organization (2012) states that the principles for pharmacologic pain management should include:

- Using a two-step strategy
- Dosing at regular intervals
- Using the appropriate route of administration
- Adapting treatment to the individual child

TABLE 5.4 Nonsteroidal Antiinflammatory Drugs for Children

Drug	Dosage	Comments
Acetaminophen (Tylenol)	10-15 mg/kg/dose q4-6h PO not to exceed five doses in 24 h or 75 mg/kg/day, or 4000 mg/day	Available in numerous preparations Nonprescription Higher dosage range may provide increased analgesia
Choline magnesium trisalicylate (Trilisate)	10-15 mg/kg q8-12h PO Maximum dose 3000 mg/day	Available in suspension, 500 mg/5 ml Prescription
Ibuprofen (children's Motrin, children's Advil)	Children >6 months old: 5-10 mg/kg/dose q6-8h Maximum dose 30 mg/kg/day or 3200 mg/day	Available in numerous preparations Available in suspension, 100 mg/5 ml, and drops, 100 mg/2.5 ml Nonprescription
Naproxen (Naprosyn)	Children >2 years old: 5-7 mg/kg/dose every 12 h Maximum 20 mg/kg/day or 1250 mg/day	Available in suspension, 125 mg/5 ml, and several different dosages for tablets Prescription
Indomethacin	1-2 mg/kg q6-12h Maximum 4g/kg/day or 200 mg/day	Available in 25-mg and 50-mg capsules and suspension 25 mg/5 ml Prescription
Diclofenac	0.5-0.75 mg/kg q6-12h PO Maximum 3 mg/kg/day or 200 mg/day	Available in 50-mg tablet and extended release 100-mg tablets Prescription

PO, By mouth.
Data from McAuley, D. F. (2013). *GlobalRPh: NSAIDs*. Retrieved from http://globalrph.com/nsaids.htm

The traditional World Health Organization stepladder has been replaced with a two-step approach for use with children. This two-step strategy consists of a choice of category of analgesic medications, according to the child's level of pain severity. For children older than 3 months with mild pain, the first step is to administer a nonopioid; nonsteroidal antiinflammatory drugs (NSAIDs) are frequently used for mild pain. A strong opioid is usually administered to children with moderate or severe pain. Morphine is the medicine of choice for the second step, although other opioids may be considered (World Health Organization, 2012). The following sections discuss the most common pain medications used in children in the nonopioid and opioid categories (see Safety Alert).

Nonopioids

Nonopioids, including acetaminophen (Tylenol, paracetamol) and NSAIDs are suitable for mild to moderate pain (Table 5.4). These agents are known for their antipyretic, antiinflammatory, and/or analgesic actions (Tobias, 2014a). Nonopioids are usually the first analgesics for pain related to tissue injury, also known as *nociceptive pain.* NSAIDs can provide safe and effective pain relief when dosed at appropriate levels with adequate frequency. Most NSAIDs take about 1 hour for effect, so timing is crucial.

Opioids

Opioids are needed for moderate to severe pain (Table 5.5). Morphine remains the standard agent used for comparison to other opioid agents. When morphine is not a suitable opioid, drugs such as hydromorphone hydrochloride (Dilaudid) and fentanyl citrate (Sublimaze) are used. Dilaudid has a longer duration of action than morphine (4 to 6 hours) and is less associated with nausea and pruritus than morphine. Sublimaze is a synthetic product that is 100 times more potent than morphine (Tobias, 2014b).

Codeine, a once commonly used oral opiate analgesic, is a weak opioid and has well-known safety and efficacy problems related to genetic variability in biotransformation (Racoosin, Roberson, Pacanowski, et al., 2013; World Health Organization, 2012; Yellon, Kenna, Cladis, et al., 2014). Codeine is a prodrug, requiring the medication to be metabolized to its active form (morphine) via the cytochrome P450 family 2 subfamily D type 6 (CYP2D6) pathway. Children with mutations of particular CYP2D6 alleles can fall into one of four categories: (1) poor metabolizer, (2) intermediate metabolizer, (3) extensive metabolizer, or (4) ultrarapid metabolizer. Patients who are poor metabolizers receive minimal to no analgesic effect from morphine, whereas patients who are extensive or ultrarapid metabolizers are at higher risk of excessive morphine levels, leading to respiratory depression (Andrzejowski & Carroll, 2016; Chidambaran, Sadhasivam, & Mahmoud, 2017). For this reason, codeine is excluded as a recommendation for treatment of moderate pain in the *WHO Guidelines on the Pharmacological Treatment of Persisting Pain in Children With Medical Illnesses.*

SAFETY ALERT

The optimum dosage of an analgesic is one that controls pain without causing undesirable side effects. This usually requires titration, the gradual adjustment of drug dosage (usually by increasing the dose) until optimum pain relief without excessive sedation is achieved. Dosage recommendations are only safe initial dosages (see Tables 5.5 to 5.7), not optimum dosages.

Coanalgesic Drugs

Several drugs, known as **coanalgesic drugs** or **adjuvant analgesics**, may be used alone or with opioids to control pain symptoms and opioid side effects (Table 5.6). Drugs frequently used to relieve anxiety, cause sedation, and provide amnesia are diazepam (Valium) and midazolam (Versed); however, these drugs are not analgesics and should be used to enhance the effects of analgesics, not as a substitute for them. Other adjuvants include tricyclic antidepressants (e.g., amitriptyline, imipramine) and antiepileptics (e.g., gabapentin, carbamazepine, clonazepam) for neuropathic pain (Rastogi & Campbell, 2014; Rodrigues & Kang, 2016). Other medications commonly prescribed include stool softeners and laxatives for constipation, antiemetics for nausea and vomiting, diphenhydramine for itching, steroids for inflammation and bone pain, and dextroamphetamine and caffeine for possible increased pain and sedation (Table 5.7).

TABLE 5.5 Starting Dosages for Opioid Analgesics in Opioid-Naive Children (for Infants Start at 25% to 33% of Dose and Titrate Analgesia and Sedation)

Medicine	Route of Administration	Starting Dosage
Morphine	Oral (immediate release)	0.3 mg/kg q3-4h PO
	Oral (prolonged release)	0.3-0.9 mg/kg q8-12h PO
	IV injection[a]	0.1 mg/kg q1-2h IV or SC
	SC injection	
	IV infusion	0.02 mg/kg/h
	SC infusion	
Fentanyl	IV injection	0.5-1 mcg/kg,[a] repeated q30-60min
	IV infusion	0.5-1 mcg/kg[a]
Hydromorphone[c]	Oral (immediate release)	60 mcg/kg q3-4h (maximum: 2-4 mg/dose)
	IV injection[a] or SC injection	15 mcg/kg q2-3h
Methadone	Oral (immediate release)	0.1 mg/kg
	IV injection[b] or SC injection	Every 4 h for the first two to three doses, then as analgesia duration increases, wean to q6-8h; intervals of analgesia beyond q8h are rare, but it may be dosed q12-24h to treat withdrawal[d]
Oxycodone	Oral (immediate release)	0.2 mg/kg q3-4h (maximum: 10 mg/dose)
	Oral (prolonged release)	0.2-0.6 mg/dose or 10 mg q12h

[a]*Administer IV opioids over 3 to 5 minutes.*

[b]*Due to the complex nature and wide interindividual variation in the pharmacokinetics of methadone, methadone should be commenced only by practitioners experienced with its use.*

[c]*Hydromorphone is a potent opioid, and significant differences exist between oral and IV dosing. Use extreme caution when converting from one route to another.*

[d]*Methadone initially should be titrated like other strong opioids. The dosage may need to be reduced by 50% 2 to 3 days after the effective dose has been found to prevent adverse effects due to methadone accumulation. From then on, dosage increases should be performed at intervals of 1 week or longer and with a maximum increase of 50%.*

IV, Intravenous; PO, by mouth; SC, subcutaneous.

Data from American Pain Society. (2016). *Principles of analgesic use* (7th ed.). Chicago, IL: Author.

TABLE 5.6 Coanalgesic Adjuvant Drugs

Drug	Dosage	Indications	Comments
Antidepressants			
Amitriptyline	0.2-0.5 mg/kg PO hs Titrate upward by 0.25 mg/kg q5-7days prn Available in 10- and 25-mg tablets Usual starting dose: 10-25 mg	Continuous neuropathic pain with burning, aching, dysesthesia with insomnia	Provides analgesia by blocking reuptake of serotonin and norepinephrine, possibly slowing transmission of pain signals Helps with pain related to insomnia and depression (use nortriptyline if patient is oversedated) Analgesic effects seen earlier than antidepressant effects
Nortriptyline	0.2-1.0 mg/kg PO AM or bid Titrate up by 0.5 mg q5-7days Maximum: 25 mg/dose	Neuropathic pain as above without insomnia	Side effects include dry mouth, constipation, urinary retention
Anticonvulsants			
Gabapentin	5 mg/kg PO hs Increase to bid on day 2, tid on day 3 Maximum: 300 mg/day	Neuropathic pain	Mechanism of action unknown Side effects include sedation, ataxia, nystagmus, dizziness
Carbamazepine	<6 years old: 2.5-5 mg/kg PO bid initially Increase 20 mg/kg/24 h, divide bid every week prn Maximum: 100 mg bid 6-12 years old: 5 mg/kg PO bid initially Increase 10 mg/kg/24 h, divide bid every week prn to usual Maximum: 100 mg/dose bid >12 years old: 200 mg PO bid initially Increase 200 mg/24 h, divide bid every week prn to maximum: 1.6-2.4 g/24 h	Sharp, lancinating neuropathic pain Peripheral neuropathies Phantom limb pain	Similar analgesic effect to amitriptyline Monitor blood levels for toxicity only Side effects include decreased blood counts, ataxia, gastrointestinal irritation

TABLE 5.6 Coanalgesic Adjuvant Drugs—cont'd

Drug	Dosage	Indications	Comments
Anxiolytics			
Lorazepam	0.03-0.1 mg/kg q4-6h PO or IV Maximum: 2 mg/dose	Muscle spasm Anxiety	May increase sedation in combination with opioids Can cause depression with prolonged use
Diazepam	0.1-0.3 mg/kg q4-6h PO or IV Maximum: 10 mg/dose		
Corticosteroids			
Dexamethasone	Dose dependent on clinical situation; higher bolus doses in cord compression, then lower daily dose Try to wean to NSAIDs if pain allows Cerebral edema: 1-2 mg/kg load, then 1-1.5 mg/kg/day divided q6h Maximum: 4 mg/dose Antiinflammatory: 0.08-0.3 mg/kg/day divided q6-12h	Pain from increased intracranial pressure Bony metastasis Spinal or nerve compression	Side effects include edema, gastrointestinal irritation, increased weight, acne Use gastro protectants such as H_2-blockers (ranitidine) or proton pump inhibitors, such as omeprazole for long-term administration of steroids or NSAIDs in end-stage cancer with bony pain
Others			
Clonidine	2-4 mcg/kg PO q4-6h May also use a 100-mcg transdermal patch q7days for patients >40 kg (88 pounds)	Neuropathic pain Lancinating, sharp, electrical, shooting pain Phantom limb pain	α_2-Adenoreceptor agonist modulates ascending pain sensations Routes of administration: oral, transdermal, and spinal Management of withdrawal symptoms Monitor for orthostatic hypertension, decreased heart rate Sedation common
Mexiletine	2-3 mg/kg/dose PO tid, may titrate 0.5 mg/kg q2-3wk prn Maximum: 300 mg/dose		Similar to lidocaine, longer acting Stabilizes sodium conduction in nerve cells, reduces neuronal firing Can enhance action of opioids, antidepressants, anticonvulsants Side effects include dizziness, ataxia, nausea, vomiting May measure blood levels for toxicity

bid, Twice a day; hs, at bedtime; IV, intravenous; NSAID, nonsteroidal antiinflammatory drug; PO, by mouth; prn, as needed; q, every; tid, three times a day.

Choosing the Pain Medication Dose

Children (except infants younger than 3 to 6 months old) metabolize drugs more rapidly than adults and show great variability in drug elimination and side effects (Oakes, 2011; Samardzic, Allegaert, & Bajcetic, 2015). Younger children may require higher doses of opioids to achieve the same analgesic effect. Therefore the therapeutic effect and duration of analgesia vary. Children's dosages are usually calculated according to body weight, except in children with a weight greater than 50 kg (110 pounds), where the weight formula may exceed the average adult dose. In this case, the adult dose is used.

A reasonable starting dose of an opioid for infants younger than 6 months old who are not mechanically ventilated is one-fourth to one-third of the recommended starting dose for older children. The infant is monitored closely for signs of pain relief and respiratory depression. The dose is titrated to effect. Because tolerance can develop rapidly, large doses may be needed for continued severe pain. If pain relief is inadequate, the initial dose is increased (usually by 25% to 50% if pain is moderate or by 50% to 100% if pain is severe) to provide greater analgesic effectiveness. Decreasing the interval between doses may also provide more continuous pain relief.

A major difference between opioids and nonopioids is that nonopioids have a **ceiling effect**, which means that doses higher than the recommended dose will not produce greater pain relief. Opioids do not have a ceiling effect other than that imposed by side effects; therefore larger dosages can be safely given for increasing severity of pain.

Parenteral and oral dosages of opioids are not the same. Because of the first-pass effect, an oral opioid is rapidly absorbed from the gastrointestinal tract and is partially metabolized in the liver before reaching the central circulation. Therefore oral dosages must be larger to compensate for the partial loss of analgesic potency to achieve an equal analgesic effect. Conversion factors (Table 5.8) for selected opioids must be used when a change is made from intravenous (IV) (preferred) or intramuscular (IM) to oral. Immediate conversion from IM or IV to the suggested equianalgesic oral dose may result in a substantial error. For example, the dose may be significantly more or less than what the child requires. Small changes ensure small errors.

Choosing the Timing of Analgesia

The right timing for administering analgesics depends on the type of pain. For continuous pain control, such as for postoperative or cancer pain, a preventive schedule of medication around the clock (ATC)

TABLE 5.7 Management of Opioid Side Effects

Side Effect	Adjuvant Drugs	Nonpharmacologic Techniques
Constipation	Senna and docusate sodium *Tablet:* 2-6 years old: Start with ½ tablet once a day; maximum: 1 tablet twice a day 6-12 years old: Start with 1 tablet once a day; maximum: 2 tablets twice a day >12 years old: Start with 2 tablets once a day; maximum: 4 tablets twice a day *Liquid:* 1 month–1 year old: 1.25-5 ml q hs 1-5 years old: 2.5-5 ml q hs 5-15 years old: 5-10 ml q hs >15 years old: 10-25 ml q hs Casanthranol and docusate sodium *Liquid:* 5-15 ml q hs *Capsules:* 1 cap PO q hs Bisacodyl: PO or PR 3-12 years old: 5 mg/dose/day >12 years old: 10-15 mg/dose/day Lactulose 7.5 ml/day after breakfast Adult: 15-30 ml/day PO Mineral oil: 1-2 tsp/day PO Magnesium citrate <6 years old: 2-4 ml/kg PO once 6-12 years old: 100-150 ml PO once >12 years old: 150-300 ml PO once Milk of magnesia <2 years old: 0.5 ml/kg/dose PO once 2-5 years old: 5-15 ml/day PO 6-12 years old: 15-30 ml PO once >12 years old: 30-60 ml PO once	Increase water intake Prune juice, bran cereal, vegetables Exercise
Sedation	Caffeine: Single dose of 1-1.5 mg PO Dextroamphetamine: 2.5-5 mg PO in AM and early afternoon Methylphenidate: 2.5-5 mg PO in AM and early afternoon Consider opioid switch if sedation persists	Caffeinated drinks (e.g., Mountain Dew, cola drinks)
Nausea, vomiting	Promethazine: 0.5 mg/kg q4-6h; maximum: 25 mg/dose Ondansetron: 0.1-0.15 mg/kg IV or PO q4h; maximum: 8 mg/dose Granisetron: 10-40 mcg/kg q2-4h; maximum: 1 mg/dose Droperidol: 0.05-0.06 mg/kg IV q4-6h; can be very sedating	Imagery, relaxation Deep, slow breathing
Pruritus	Diphenhydramine: 1 mg/kg IV or PO q4-6h prn; maximum: 25 mg/dose Hydroxyzine: 0.6 mg/kg/dose PO q6h; maximum: 50 mg/dose Naloxone: 0.5 mcg/kg q2min until pruritus improves (diluted in solution of 0.1 mg naloxone per 10 ml saline) Butorphanol: 0.3-0.5 mg/kg IV (use cautiously in opioid-tolerant children; may cause withdrawal symptoms); maximum: 2 mg/dose because mixed agonist-antagonist	Oatmeal baths, good hygiene Exclude other causes of itching Change opioids
Respiratory depression—mild to moderate	Hold dose of opioid Reduce subsequent doses by 25%	Arouse gently, give oxygen, encourage to deep breathe
Respiratory depression—severe	Naloxone During disease pain management: 0.5 mcg/kg in 2-min increments until breathing improves (Pasero & McCaffrey, 2011) Reduce opioid dose if possible Consider opioid switch During sedation for procedures: 5-10 mcg/kg until breathing improves Reduce opioid dose if possible Consider opioid switch	Oxygen, bag and mask if indicated
Dysphoria, confusion, hallucinations	Evaluate medications, eliminate adjuvant medications with central nervous system effects as symptoms allow Consider opioid switch if possible Haloperidol (Haldol): 0.05-0.15 mg/kg/day divided in two to three doses; maximum: 2-4 mg/day	Rule out other physiologic causes

TABLE 5.7 Management of Opioid Side Effects—cont'd

Side Effect	Adjuvant Drugs	Nonpharmacologic Techniques
Urinary retention	Evaluate medications, eliminate adjuvant medications with anticholinergic effects (e.g., antihistamines, tricyclic antidepressants) Occurs more frequently with spinal analgesia than with systemic opioid use Oxybutynin 1 year old: 1 mg tid 1-2 years old: 2 mg tid 2-3 years old: 3 mg tid 4-5 years old: 4 mg tid >5 years old: 5 mg tid	Rule out other physiologic causes In/out or indwelling urinary catheter

hs, At bedtime; IV, intravenous; PO, by mouth; PR, by rectum; prn, as needed; q, every; tid, three times a day.

TABLE 5.8 Approximate Equianalgesia Ratios for Switching Between Parenteral and Oral Dosage Forms

Medicine	Dosage Ratio Parenteral	Dosage Ratio Oral
Morphine	1	3
Hydromorphone	0.15	0.6
Fentanyl	0.01	—
Hydrocodone	—	3
Oxycodone	—	2

Data from American Pain Society. (2016). *Principles of analgesic use* (7th ed.). Chicago, IL: Author.

is effective. The ATC schedule avoids the low plasma concentrations that permit breakthrough pain. If analgesics are administered only when pain returns (a typical use of the prn, or "as needed," order), pain relief may take several hours. This may require higher doses, leading to a cycle of undermedication of pain alternating with periods of overmedication and drug toxicity. This cycle of erratic pain control also promotes "clock watching," which may be erroneously equated with addiction. Nurses can effectively use prn orders by giving the drug at regular intervals because "as needed" should be interpreted as "as needed to prevent pain," not "as little as possible."

Choosing the Method of Administration

Several routes of analgesic administration can be used (Box 5.3), and the most effective and least traumatic route of administration should be selected. Continuous analgesia is not always appropriate because not all pain is continuous. Frequently, temporary pain control or conscious sedation is needed to provide analgesia before a scheduled procedure. When pain can be predicted, the drug's peak effect should be timed to coincide with the painful event. For example, with opioids the peak effect is approximately a half-hour for the IV route; with nonopioids the peak effect occurs about 2 hours after oral administration. For rapid onset and peak of action, opioids that quickly penetrate the blood-brain barrier (e.g., IV fentanyl) provide excellent pain control.

Severe pain that is uncontrolled by large variations in plasma concentrations of opioids is best controlled through continuous IV infusion rather than intermittent boluses. If intermittent boluses are given, make certain the intervals between doses do not exceed the drug's expected duration of effectiveness. For extended pain control with fewer administration times, drugs that provide longer duration of action (e.g., some NSAIDs, time-released morphine or oxycodone, methadone) can be used.

Patient-Controlled Analgesia

A significant advance in the administration of IV, epidural, or subcutaneous analgesics is the use of patient-controlled analgesia (PCA). As the name implies, the patient controls the amount and frequency of the analgesic, which is typically delivered through a special infusion device. Children who are physically able to "push a button" (i.e., 5 to 6 years old) and who can understand the concept of pushing a button to obtain pain relief can use PCA. Although it is controversial, parents and nurses have used the IV PCA system for children. Nurses can efficiently use the infusion device on a child of any age to administer analgesics to avoid signing for and preparing opioid injections every time one is needed (Fig. 5.6). When PCA is used as "nurse- or parent-controlled" analgesia, the concept of patient control is negated, and the inherent safety of PCA needs to be monitored. Research has reported safe and effective analgesia in children when the patient, parent, or nurse controlled the PCA (Anghelescu, Faughnan, Oakes, et al., 2012; Donado, Solodiuk, Rangel, et al., 2019; Oakes, 2011; Walia, Tumin, Wrona, et al., 2016).

PCA infusion devices typically allow for three methods or modes of drug administration to be used alone or in combination:

1. Patient-administered boluses that can be infused only according to the preset amount and lockout interval (time between doses). More frequent attempts at self-administration may mean the patient needs the dose and time adjusted for better pain control.
2. Nurse-administered boluses that are typically used to give an initial loading dose to increase blood levels rapidly and to relieve breakthrough pain (pain not relieved with the usual programmed dose).
3. Continuous basal rate infusion that delivers a constant amount of analgesic and prevents pain from returning during those times, such as sleep, when the patient cannot control the infusion.

As with any type of analgesic management plan, continued assessment of the child's pain relief is essential for the greatest benefit from PCA. Typical uses of PCA are for controlling pain from surgery, sickle cell crisis, trauma, and cancer. Morphine is the drug of choice for PCA and usually comes in a concentration of 1 mg/ml. Other options are hydromorphone (0.2 mg/ml) and fentanyl (0.01 mg/ml). Hydromorphone is often used when patients are not able to tolerate side effects, such as pruritus and nausea from the morphine PCA. Table 5.9 provides initial PCA settings for opioid-naive children.

Epidural Analgesia

Epidural analgesia is used to manage pain in selected cases. Although an epidural catheter can be inserted at any vertebral level, it is usually placed into the epidural space of the spinal column at the lumbar or caudal level (Suresh, Birmingham, & Kozlowski, 2012; Wiegele et al., 2019). The thoracic level is usually reserved for older children

BOX 5.3 Routes and Methods of Analgesic Drug Administration

Oral

Oral route preferred because of convenience, cost, and relatively steady blood levels

Higher dosages of oral form of opioids required for equivalent parenteral analgesia

Peak drug effect occurring after 1 to 2 hours for most analgesics

Delay in onset a disadvantage when rapid control of severe or fluctuating pain is desired

Sublingual, Buccal, or Transmucosal

Tablet or liquid placed between cheek and gum (buccal) or under tongue (sublingual)

Highly desirable because more rapid onset than oral route

- Produces less first-pass effect through liver than oral route, which normally reduces analgesia from oral opioids (unless sublingual or buccal form is swallowed, which occurs often in children)

Few drugs commercially available in this form

Many drugs can be compounded into sublingual troche or lozenge.[a]

- Actiq: Oral transmucosal fentanyl citrate in hard confection base on a plastic holder; indicated only for management of breakthrough cancer pain in patients with malignancies who are already receiving and are tolerant to opioid therapy, but can be used for preoperative or preprocedural sedation and analgesia

Intravenous (Bolus)

Preferred for rapid control of severe pain

Provides most rapid onset of effect, usually in about 5 minutes

Advantage for acute pain, procedural pain, and breakthrough pain

Needs to be repeated hourly for continuous pain control

Drugs with short half-life (morphine, fentanyl, hydromorphone) preferable to avoid toxic accumulation of drug

Intravenous (Continuous)

Preferred over bolus and intramuscular (IM) injection for maintaining control of pain

Provides steady blood levels

Easy to titrate dosage

Subcutaneous (Continuous)

Used when oral and intravenous (IV) routes not available

Provides equivalent blood levels to continuous IV infusion

Suggested initial bolus dose to equal 2-hour IV dose; total 24-hour dose usually requires concentrated opioid solution to minimize infused volume; use smallest gauge needle that accommodates infusion rate

Patient-Controlled Analgesia

Generally refers to self-administration of drugs, regardless of route

Typically uses programmable infusion pump (IV, epidural, subcutaneous [SC]) that permits self-administration of boluses of medication at preset dose and time interval (lockout interval is time between doses)

Patient-controlled analgesia (PCA) bolus administration often combined with initial bolus and continuous (basal or background) infusion of opioid

Optimum lockout interval not known but must be at least as long as time needed for onset of drug

- Should effectively control pain during movement or procedures
- Longer lockout provides larger dose

Family-Controlled Analgesia

One family member (usually a parent) or other caregiver designated as child's primary pain manager with responsibility for pressing PCA button

Guidelines for selecting a primary pain manager for family-controlled analgesia:

- Spends a significant amount of time with the patient
- Is willing to assume responsibility of being primary pain manager
- Is willing to accept and respect patient's reports of pain (if able to provide) as best indicator of how much pain the patient is experiencing; knows how to use and interpret a pain rating scale
- Understands the purpose and goals of patient's pain management plan
- Understands concept of maintaining a steady analgesic blood level
- Recognizes signs of pain and side effects and adverse reactions to opioid

Nurse-Activated Analgesia

Child's primary nurse designated as primary pain manager and is only person who presses PCA button during that nurse's shift

Guidelines for selecting primary pain manager for family-controlled analgesia also applicable to nurse-activated analgesia

May be used in addition to basal rate to treat breakthrough pain with bolus doses; patient assessed every 30 minutes for need for bolus dose

May be used without a basal rate as a means of maintaining analgesia with around-the-clock bolus doses

Intramuscular

Note: Not recommended for pain control; not current standard of care

Painful administration (hated by children)

Tissue and nerve damage caused by some drugs

Wide fluctuation in absorption of drug from muscle

Faster absorption from deltoid than from gluteal sites

Shorter duration and more expensive than oral drugs

Time consuming for staff and unnecessary delay for child

Intranasal

Available commercially as butorphanol (Stadol NS); approved for those older than 18 years

Should not be used in patient receiving morphine-like drugs because butorphanol is partial antagonist that will reduce analgesia and may cause withdrawal

Intradermal

Used primarily for skin anesthesia (e.g., before lumbar puncture, bone marrow aspiration, arterial puncture, skin biopsy)

Local anesthetics (e.g., lidocaine) cause stinging, burning sensation

Duration of stinging dependent on type of "caine" used

To avoid stinging sensation associated with lidocaine:

- Buffer the solution by adding 1 part sodium bicarbonate (1 mEq/ml) to 9 to 10 parts 1% or 2% lidocaine with or without epinephrine

Normal saline with preservative, benzyl alcohol, anesthetizes venipuncture site

Same dose used as for buffered lidocaine

Topical or Transdermal

EMLA (eutectic mixture of local anesthetics [lidocaine and prilocaine]) cream and anesthetic disk or LMX4 (4% liposomal lidocaine cream)

- Eliminates or reduces pain from most procedures involving skin puncture
- Must be placed on intact skin over puncture site and covered by occlusive dressing or applied as anesthetic disc for 1 hour or more before procedure

Lidocaine-tetracaine (Synera, S-Caine)

- Apply for 20 to 30 minutes
- Do not apply to broken skin

LAT (lidocaine-adrenaline-tetracaine), tetracaine-phenylephrine (tetraphen)

- Provides skin anesthesia about 15 minutes after application on nonintact skin
- Gel (preferable) or liquid placed on wounds for suturing
- Adrenaline not for use on end arterioles (fingers, toes, tip of nose, penis, earlobes) because of vasoconstriction

BOX 5.3 Routes and Methods of Analgesic Drug Administration—cont'd

Transdermal fentanyl (Duragesic)

- Available as patch for continuous pain control
- Safety and efficacy not established in children younger than 12 years old
- Not appropriate for initial relief of acute pain because of long interval to peak effect (12 to 24 hours); for rapid onset of pain relief, give an immediate-release opioid
- Orders for "rescue doses" of an immediate-release opioid recommended for breakthrough pain, a flare of severe pain that breaks through the medication being administered at regular intervals for persistent pain
- Has duration of up to 72 hours for prolonged pain relief
- If respiratory depression occurs, possible need for several doses of naloxone

Vapo-coolant

- Use of prescription spray coolant, such as Fluori-Methane or ethyl chloride (Pain Ease); applied to the skin for 10 to 15 seconds immediately before the needle puncture; anesthesia lasts about 15 seconds
- Some children dislike cold; may be more comfortable to spray coolant on a cotton ball and then apply this to the skin
- Application of ice to the skin for 30 seconds found to be ineffective

Rectal

Alternative to oral or parenteral routes
Variable absorption rate
Generally disliked by children
Many drugs able to be compounded into rectal suppositories[a]

Regional Nerve Block

Use of long-acting local anesthetic (bupivacaine or ropivacaine) injected into nerves to block pain at site
Provides prolonged analgesia postoperatively, such as after inguinal herniorrhaphy
May be used to provide local anesthesia for surgery, such as dorsal penile nerve block for circumcision or for reduction of fractures

Inhalation

Use of anesthetics, such as nitrous oxide, to produce partial or complete analgesia for painful procedures
Side effects (e.g., headache) possible from occupational exposure to high levels of nitrous oxide

Epidural or Intrathecal

Involves catheter placed into epidural, caudal, or intrathecal space for continuous infusion or single or intermittent administration of opioid with or without a long-acting local anesthetic (e.g., bupivacaine, ropivacaine)
Analgesia primarily from drug's direct effect on opioid receptors in spinal cord
Respiratory depression rare but may have slow and delayed onset; can be prevented by checking level of sedation and respiratory rate and depth hourly for initial 24 hours and decreasing dose when excessive sedation is detected
Nausea, itching, and urinary retention common dose-related side effects from the epidural opioid
Mild hypotension, urinary retention, and temporary motor or sensory deficits common unwanted effects of epidural local anesthetic
Catheter for urinary retention inserted during surgery to decrease trauma to child; if inserted when child is awake, anesthetize urethra with lidocaine

[a]For further information about compounding drugs in troche or suppository form, contact Professional Compounding Centers of America (PCCA), 9901 S. Wilcrest Drive, Houston, TX 77009; 800-331-2498; https://www.pccarx.com.
Data from Pasero, C., & McCaffrey, M. (2011). *Pain assessment and pharmacologic management.* St Louis, MO: Elsevier.

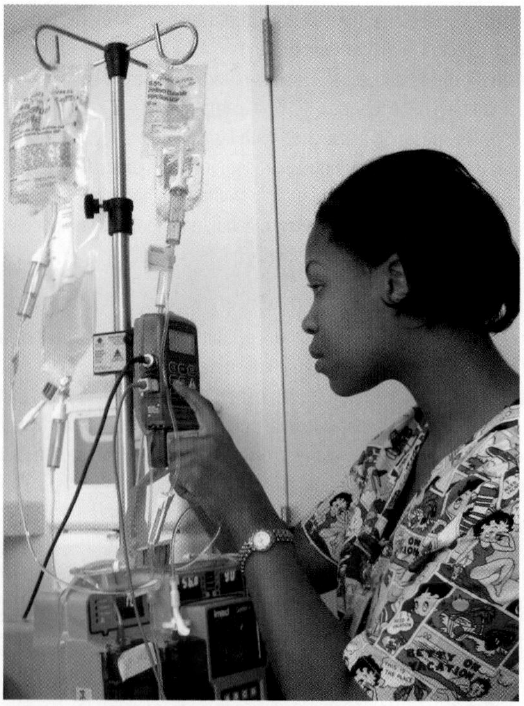

Fig. 5.6 Nurse programming a patient-controlled analgesia (PCA) pump to administer analgesia.

TABLE 5.9 Initial Patient-Controlled Analgesia Settings for Opioid-Naive Children

Drug	Continuous Infusion Dosage	Bolus Dosage/ Frequency
Morphine	0-0.02 mg/kg/h	0.02 mg/kg q15-30min
Hydromorphone	0-0.004 mg/kg/h	0.004 mg/kg q15-30min
Fentanyl	0-0.5 to 1 mcg/kg/h	0.5-1 mcg/kg q10-15min

or adolescents who have had an upper abdominal or thoracic procedure, such as a lung transplant. An opioid (usually fentanyl, hydromorphone, or preservative-free morphine, which is often combined with a long-acting local anesthetic, such as bupivacaine or ropivacaine) is instilled via single or intermittent bolus, continuous infusion, or patient-controlled epidural analgesia. Analgesia results from the drug's effect on opiate receptors in the dorsal horn of the spinal cord, rather than the brain. As a result, respiratory depression is rare, but if it occurs, it develops slowly, typically 6 to 8 hours after administration. Careful monitoring of sedation level and respiratory status is critical to prevent opioid-induced respiratory depression. Assessment of pain and the skin condition around the catheter site are important aspects of nursing care.

Transmucosal and Transdermal Analgesia

Oral transmucosal fentanyl (Oralet) and intranasal fentanyl (Mudd, 2011; Setlur & Friedland, 2018) provide nontraumatic preoperative and preprocedural analgesia and sedation. Fentanyl is also available as a transdermal patch (Duragesic). Duragesic is contraindicated for acute pain management, but it may be used for older children and adolescents who have chronic cancer pain or sickle cell pain or for patients who are opioid tolerant.

One of the most significant improvements in the ability to provide atraumatic care to children undergoing procedures is the anesthetic cream (Chua, Firaza, Ming, et al., 2017; Oakes, 2011; Sansone, Passavanti, Fiorelli, et al., 2017; Zempsky, 2014). LMX4 (a 4% liposomal lidocaine cream) and EMLA (a eutectic mixture of local anesthetics) are the most well-studied topical anesthetics found to be effective in children. (Fig. 5.7). Transdermal patches, such as Synera (lidocaine and tetracaine), are effective methods to administer topical analgesia before painful procedures (Table 5.10). See Box 5.6 for pain prevention resources online.

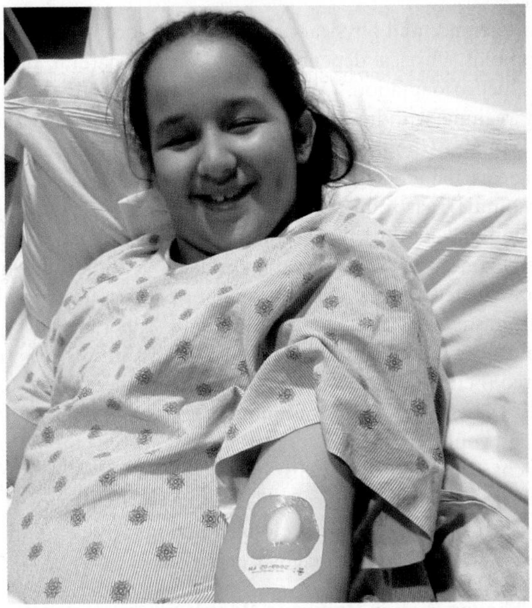

Fig. 5.7 LMX4 (liposomal lidocaine cream) is an effective analgesic before intravenous (IV) insertion or blood draw.

In emergency situations, there is not enough time for topical preparations like LMX4 or EMLA to take effect, and refrigerant sprays, such as ethyl chloride and fluoromethane, can be used. When sprayed on the skin, these sprays vaporize, rapidly cool the area, and provide superficial anesthesia. Hospital formularies may have other products with lidocaine, prilocaine, or amethocaine topical preparations that require less time for application.

The intradermal route is sometimes used to inject a local anesthetic, typically lidocaine, into the skin to reduce the pain from a lumbar puncture, bone marrow aspiration, or venous or arterial access. One problem with the use of lidocaine is the stinging and burning that initially occur. However, the use of buffered lidocaine with sodium bicarbonate reduces the stinging sensation.

Monitoring Side Effects

Both NSAIDs and opioids have side effects, although the major concern is those from opioids (Box 5.4). Respiratory depression is the most serious complication and is most likely to occur in sedated patients. The respiratory rate may decrease gradually, or respirations may cease abruptly; lower limits of normal are not established for children, but any significant change from a previous rate calls for increased vigilance. A slower respiratory rate does not necessarily reflect decreased arterial oxygenation; an increased depth of ventilation may compensate for the altered rate. If respiratory depression or arrest occurs, be prepared to intervene quickly (see Nursing Care Guidelines box).

TABLE 5.10 Needlestick Pain Prevention Products

Product	Onset	Duration	Appropriate Age/Weight	Potential Adverse Effects; Contraindications
EMLA	1 hour	4 hours	Approved by FDA for use in neonates over 27 weeks of gestation Has been used in preterm infants <37 weeks; safety of repeated dosages in preterm infants not established (Biran, Gourrier, Cimerman, et al., 2011)	Blanching, erythema Methemoglobinemia
LMX4	30 min	1 hour	Not recommended for use < 1 month of age	Redness, irritation at the site of the cream Swelling, abnormal sensation at the site of the cream
Needle-free jet injection with buffered lidocaine	10-30 seconds	1-4 hours	Theoretic safety for ≥37 weeks of gestation but no published research Safety established for use in children ≥1 year of age (Lunoe, Drendel, Levas, et al., 2015)	Blanching, erythema, bleeding with improper placement; do not use in children with bleeding disorders or especially fragile skin
Sucrose pacifier	2 minutes	10 minutes	Newborn to 6 months	
Cold vibration device	15 seconds	Limit use to 3 minutes	≥1 year of age; assess cold tolerance before use	Blanching, erythema

FDA, US Food and Drug Administration.

NURSING CARE GUIDELINES

Managing Opioid-Induced Respiratory Depression

If Respirations Are Depressed

Assess sedation level.
Reduce infusion by 25% when possible.
Stimulate patient (shake shoulder gently, call by name, ask to breathe).
Administer oxygen.

If Patient Cannot Be Aroused or Is Apneic

Initiate resuscitation efforts as appropriate.
Administer naloxone (Narcan):

- For children weighing less than 40 kg (88 pounds), dilute 0.1 mg naloxone in 10 ml sterile saline to make 10 mcg/ml solution and give 0.5 mcg/kg.
- For children weighing more than 40 kg (88 pounds), dilute 0.4-mg ampule in 10 ml sterile saline and give 0.5 ml.

Administer bolus by slow intravenous (IV) push every 2 minutes until effect is obtained.
Closely monitor patient. Naloxone's duration of antagonist action may be shorter than that of the opioid, requiring repeated doses of naloxone.

Note: Respiratory depression caused by benzodiazepines (e.g., diazepam [Valium] or midazolam [Versed]) can be reversed with flumazenil (Romazicon). Pediatric dosing experience suggests 0.01 mg/kg (0.1 ml/kg); if no (or inadequate) response after 1 to 2 minutes, administer same dose and repeat as needed at 60-second intervals for maximum dose of 1 mg (10 ml).

BOX 5.4 Side Effects of Opioids

General

Constipation (possibly severe)
Respiratory depression
Sedation
Nausea and vomiting
Agitation, euphoria
Mental clouding
Hallucinations
Orthostatic hypotension
Pruritus
Urticaria
Sweating
Miosis (may be sign of toxicity)
Anaphylaxis (rare)

Signs of Tolerance

Decreasing pain relief
Decreasing duration of pain relief

Signs of Withdrawal Syndrome in Patients With Physical Dependence

Initial Signs of Withdrawal

Lacrimation
Rhinorrhea
Yawning
Sweating

Later Signs of Withdrawal

Restlessness
Irritability
Tremors
Anorexia
Dilated pupils
Gooseflesh
Nausea, vomiting

Although respiratory depression is the most dangerous side effect, constipation is a common and sometimes serious side effect of opioids, which decrease peristalsis and increase anal sphincter tone. Prevention with stool softeners and laxatives is more effective than treatment once constipation occurs. Dietary treatment, such as increased fiber, is usually not sufficient to promote regular bowel evacuation. However, dietary measures, such as increased fluid and fruit intake, and physical activity are encouraged. Pruritus from epidural or IV infusion is treated with low doses of IV naloxone, nalbuphine, or diphenhydramine. Nausea, vomiting, and sedation usually subside after 2 days of opioid administration, although oral or rectal antiemetics are sometimes necessary.

Both tolerance and physical dependence can occur with prolonged use of opioids. Physical dependence is a normal, natural, physiologic state of "neuroadaptation." When opioids are abruptly discontinued without weaning, withdrawal symptoms occur 24 hours later and reach a peak within 72 hours. Symptoms of withdrawal include signs of neurologic excitability (irritability, tremors, seizures, increased motor tone, insomnia), gastrointestinal dysfunction (nausea, vomiting, diarrhea, abdominal cramps), and autonomic dysfunction (sweating, fever, chills, tachypnea, nasal congestion, rhinitis). Withdrawal symptoms can be anticipated and prevented by weaning patients from opioids that were administered for more than 5 to 10 days. Adherence to a weaning protocol to prevent or minimize withdrawal symptoms from opioids is required (Fenn & Plake, 2017). A weaning flowsheet (Fig. 5.8A) may be used to assess the efficacy of opioid weaning in neonates. In older infants and young children (7 months to 10 years old) the Withdrawal Assessment Tool–1 (see Fig. 5.8B) may be used to assess and monitor withdrawal symptoms in critically ill children who are exposed to opioids and benzodiazepines for prolonged periods (Best, Wypij, Asaro, et al., 2017; Franck, Harris, Soetenga, et al., 2008).

Opioid Misuse Risk in Pediatric Populations

It has been standard teaching to both health care providers and patients and families that the risk of developing addiction related to the medical use of opioids is low, and there has been very little effort to date to measure the risk of addiction after opioid exposure (Pinkerton & Hardy, 2017). Several recent studies have documented the level of opioid exposure in pediatric populations. A retrospective review of children receiving opioids while hospitalized found that 43% of patients received some opioid therapy, with 75% receiving opioids for up to 5 days and less than 5% receiving opioids for more than 20 days. Those receiving longer term opioids were primarily children with cancer and other complex medical conditions as well as children in pediatric intensive care units (PICUs) and neonatal intensive care units (NICUs) (Walco, Gove, Phillips, et al., 2017).

A review of national data of children with newly diagnosed acute myeloid leukemia (AML) found that nearly 80% were exposed to opioids over the course of their care, with morphine, fentanyl, and oxycodone most frequently prescribed (Getz, Miller, Seif, et al., 2018). Similarly, a study of childhood cancer survivors found that in the first 3 years after therapy, survivors had a 1.5 to 4.5 times greater risk for filling opioid prescriptions compared to noncancer peers (Smitherman, Mohabir, Wilkins, et al., 2018).

Children undergoing various surgical procedures and discharged with opioid prescriptions who reported prior presurgical opioid or marijuana use or had higher discharge pain scores consumed more opioids after discharge (Whiteside, Russo, Wang, et al., 2016). Two studies reported on postoperative opioid prescription and found that outpatient opioid consumption was influenced by age of the patient (younger children take fewer opioids after discharge than do adolescents) and type of surgical procedure (Nuss orthopedic surgical patients consumed more opioids compared to those who had other types of surgery) (Monitto, Hsu, Gao, et al., 2017). Lastly, three studies reported that pediatric providers generally prescribed more opioids than were needed after discharge, citing concern about having unconsumed opioids at home creating the potential for diversion or misuse (Harbaugh & Gadepalli, 2019; Monitto et al., 2017; Nelson, Adams, Buczek, et al., 2019).

Lastly, data from the National Poison Data System between 2000 and 2015 were analyzed to evaluate the prevalence of opioid exposure in children and adolescents (Allen, Casavant, Spiller, et al., 2017). During that period, the National Poison Data System received reports of nearly 190,000 children under 20 years of age, with hydrocodone the most frequently reported opioid exposure. Adolescents were more likely to be admitted to a health care facility and had higher odds of serious medical outcomes related to opioid exposure than children under 12 years of age. Tragically, the rate of prescription opioid–related suspected suicides by teens rose by 53% over the 15-year study period.

Opioid Stewardship and Risk Screening

Opioid stewardship essentially refers to a structured interprofessional approach by health care providers and institutions to improve, monitor, and evaluate the safe use of opioids in health care settings as well as to develop strategies for identifying and caring for patients who are at high risk for opioid dependence (Phelps, Achey, Mieure, et al., 2018). Components of opioid stewardship recommended by The Joint Commission include the use of state-based prescription monitoring programs that allow prescribers to view a patient's prescription history; expert pharmacy consultation and monitoring of opioid use; patient risk screening; education of patients and families on safe use,

Children's Hospital Oakland Opioid Weaning Flowsheet and Guidelines for Use of the Form
Analgesia/sedation orders (drug/dose/frequency)

Date		
Drug		
Administration time		
Dose ↑ or ↓ or freq change		

		Time:	
Choose one: Crying/agitated 25%-50% of interval Crying/agitated >50% of interval	2 3		
Choose one: Sleeps ≤25% of interval Sleeps 26%-75% of interval Sleeps >75% of interval	3 2 1		
Choose one: Hyperactive Moro Markedly hyperactive Moro	2 3		
Choose one: Mild tremors, disturbed Moderate/severe tremors, disturbed	1 2		
Increased muscle tone	2		
Temperature 37.2°-38.4°C	1		
Temperature >38.4°C	2		
Respiratory rate >60 (extubated)	2		
Suction >twice/interval (intubated)	2		
Sweating	1		
Frequent yawning (>3-4/interval)	1		
Sneezing (>3-4/interval)	1		
Nasal stuffiness	1		
Emesis	2		
Projectile vomiting	3		
Loose stools	2		
Watery stools	3		
TOTAL SCORE			
ADJUSTED SCORE			
INITIALS OF PERSON SCORING			

Directions: Score every 2-4 hours per guideline
Score greater than 8-12 may indicate withdrawal

Guidelines for use of the flow sheet

Use of form

Use the flowsheet for all infants who have received continuous or around-the-clock opioid medication for 3 days or more, or more than 3 doses per day for more than 5 days. This patient population will most often include postoperative patients, agitated intubated infants, and all post-ECMO patients.

Instructions

1. Write drug, dose, and frequency of analgesics and sedatives ordered.
2. Enter date, name of drug (abbreviated MS=morphine sulfate or FENT=fentanyl), and administration time of drugs given in the appropriate boxes; indicate if dose frequency given is an increase or decrease from the ordered dose.
3. Scoring must be performed every 4 hours during weaning of opioids, every 2 hours if score is 8 or greater. The score for each item indicates the presence of the sign during the previous 2-4 hours (depending on the scoring interval). Every 4-hour scoring should continue until the patient is off all opioids for 48-72 hours. Place a "0" in the column after the sign if it is not seen during the scoring period.

Central nervous system

Crying behavior: Score 2 points if patient exhibits crying or cry behavior for a duration of ≤50% of the scoring interval. Score 3 points if cumulative crying behavior totals >50% of the scoring interval.
NOTE: Crying behavior is accompanied by the facial expressions associated with crying, but without audible sounds because of endotracheal intubation.
Sleeping: Score 3 points if patient sleeps for ≤25% of the scoring interval. Score 2 points if patient sleeps for 26%-75% of the scoring interval. Score 1 point if patient sleeps for >75% of the scoring interval.
Moro (startle) reflex: Score 2 points if patient has some arm and/or leg extension when touched or when disturbed by loud noises. Score 3 points if patient has marked arm and/or leg extension that is accompanied by crying behavior, hyperalert state, or continued arm and/or leg tremors after being startled.
Tremors—disturbed: Score 1 point if patient has mild tremors when disturbed. Score 2 points if patient has moderate to severe tremors when disturbed. NOTE: Tremors are alternating movements that are rhythmic, of equal rate and amplitude, and can usually be stopped by flexion of the limb.
Increased muscle tone: Score 2 points if patient exhibits fisting or tight flexion of extremities that are difficult to extend.

Metabolic

Temperature: Score 1 point if patient's temperature is 37.2°-38.4°C. Score 2 points if patient's temperature is >38.4°C.
Respiratory rate: Score 1 point if patient's spontaneous respiratory rate is >60/minute. Score 2 points if patient's spontaneous respiratory rate is >60/minute and accompanied by retractions.
Suction: Score 2 points if patient is suctioned more than twice during a 4-hour period.
Sweating: Score 1 point if patient exhibits any type of sweating, including beads of sweat, or if skin is moist to touch.
Yawning: Score 1 point if patient yawns >3-4 times in succession or yawns 1-2 times often during a 4-hour period.
Sneezing: Score 1 point if patient sneezes >3-4 times in succession or sneezes 1-2 times during a 4-hour period.
Nasal stuffiness: Score 1 point for nasal stuffiness.

Gastrointestinal

Emesis of formula/stomach contents: Score 2 points if patient has 1 or more episodes of emesis during a 4-hour period.
Projectile vomiting: Score 3 points if patient has 1 or more episodes of projectile vomiting.
Loose stools: Score 2 points if patient has loose stools characterized by a water ring around some solid stool. The stools will often be frequent. NOTE: Do not score for "breast milk" stools: frequent, small, seedy, yellow stools.
Watery stools: Score 3 points if patient has stools that consist of only liquid. The stools will often be frequent.

Total score: Add up all the scores in the column and place the total score in this box. Clinical signs that appear continuously, such as respiratory rate >60 or regular poor feeding, should be included in the total score.
Adjusted score: The adjusted score is used when a sign is detected that is expected to occur independently of withdrawal, due to a preexisting condition (high respiratory rate in infant with bronchopulmonary dysplasia). The decision to adjust the score should be made after discussion with the healthcare team during rounds, and the rationale should be recorded in a problem-oriented note. Circle the signs to be excluded and deduct the points from the total score to obtain the adjusted score.
Initials of person scoring: The person scoring should write his/her initials in this space.

A

Fig. 5.8 A, Weaning flowsheet to monitor opioid weaning in neonates.

WITHDRAWAL ASSESSMENT TOOL – 1 (WAT – 1)

Patient Identifier														
	Date:													
	Time:													
Information from patient record, previous 12 hours														
Any loose /watery stools	No = 0 Yes = 1													
Any vomiting/wretching/gagging	No = 0 Yes = 1													
Temperature > 37.8°C	No = 0 Yes = 1													
2 minute pre-stimulus observation														
State	SBS* ≤ 0 or asleep/awake/calm = 0 SBS* ≥ +1 or awake/distressed = 1													
Tremor	None/mild = 0 Moderate/severe = 1													
Any sweating	No = 0 Yes = 1													
Uncoordinated/repetitive movement	None/mild = 0 Moderate/severe = 1													
Yawning or sneezing	None or 1 = 0 ≥2 = 1													
1 minute stimulus observation														
Startle to touch	None/mild = 0 Moderate/severe = 1													
Muscle tone	Normal = 0 Increased = 1													
Post-stimulus recovery														
Time to gain calm state (SBS* ≤ 0)	< 2min = 0 2 - 5min = 1 > 5 min = 2													
Total Score (0-12)														

WITHDRAWAL ASSESSMENT TOOL (WAT – 1) INSTRUCTIONS

- Start WAT-1 scoring from the **first day of weaning** in patients who have received opioids +/or benzodiazepines by infusion or regular dosing for prolonged periods (e.g., > 5 days). Continue twice daily scoring until 72 hours after the last dose.
- The Withdrawal Assessment Tool (WAT-1) should be completed along with the SBS[1] at least once per 12 hour shift (e.g., at 08:00 and 20:00 ± 2 hours). The progressive stimulus used in the SBS[1] assessment provides a standard stimulus for observing signs of withdrawal.

Obtain information from patient record (this can be done before or after the stimulus):

✓ **Loose/watery stools**: Score 1 if any loose or watery stools were documented in the past 12 hours; score 0 if none were noted.
✓ **Vomiting/wretching/gagging**: Score 1 if any vomiting or spontaneous wretching or gagging were documented in the past 12 hours; score 0 if none were noted
✓ **Temperature > 37.8°C**: Score 1 if the modal (most frequently occurring) temperature documented was greater than 37.8 °C in the past 12 hours; score 0 if this was not the case.

2 minute pre-stimulus observation:

✓ **State**: Score 1 if awake and distress (SBS[1]: ≥ +1) observed during the 2 minutes prior to the stimulus; score 0 if asleep or awake and calm/cooperative (SBS[1] ≤ 0).
✓ **Tremor**: Score 1 if moderate to severe tremor observed during the 2 minutes prior to the stimulus; score 0 if no tremor (or only minor, intermittent tremor).
✓ **Sweating**: Score 1 if any sweating during the 2 minutes prior to the stimulus; score 0 if no sweating noted.
✓ **Uncoordinated/repetitive movements**: Score 1 if moderate to severe uncoordinated or repetitive movements such as head turning, leg or arm flailing or torso arching observed during the 2 minutes prior to the stimulus; score 0 if no (or only mild) uncoordinated or repetitive movements.
✓ **Yawning or sneezing** > 1: Score 1 if more than 1 yawn or sneeze observed during the 2 minutes prior to the stimulus; score 0 if 0 to 1 yawn or sneeze.

1 minute stimulus observation:

✓ **Startle to touch**: Score 1 if moderate to severe startle occurs when touched during the stimulus; score 0 if none (or mild).
✓ **Muscle tone**: Score 1 if tone increased during the stimulus; score 0 if normal.

Post-stimulus recovery:

✓ **Time to gain calm state** (SBS[1] ≤ 0): Score 2 if it takes greater than 5 minutes following stimulus; score 1 if achieved within 2 to 5 minutes; score 0 if achieved in less than 2 minutes.

Sum the 11 numbers in the column for the total WAT-1 score (0-12).

B

Fig. 5.8, cont'd B, Withdrawal assessment tool for infants and children. *SBS*, State behavioral scale. (A, Modified from Franck, L., & Vilardi, J. [1995]. Assessment and management of opioid withdrawal in ill neonates. *Neonatal Network, 14*[2], 39–48; B, ©2007 LS Franck and MAQ Curley. All rights reserved. Reprinted in Franck, L. S., Harris, S. K., Soetenga, D. J., et al. [2008]. The Withdrawal Assessment Tool–1 [WAT–1]: An assessment instrument for monitoring opioid and benzodiazepine withdrawal symptoms in pediatric patients. *Pediatric Critical Care Medicine, 9*[6], 577.)
*From Curley, M. Q., Harris, S. K., Fraser, K. A., et al. (2008). State behavioral scale: A sedation assessment instrument for infants and young children supported on mechanical ventilation. *Pediatric Critical Care Medicine, 7*(2), 107–114.

storage, and disposal of opioids; and multimodal integrative health approaches to pain management to maximize comfort and minimize opioid exposure.

In pediatrics, there are many children who live with complex chronic and life-threatening conditions that place them at high risk for opioid misuse behaviors. Children with cancer and hematology disorders are at risk for chronic pain conditions and, as such, at risk for opioid misuse. Risk screening should take a "universal precautions" approach and should be done at the initiation of opioid therapy (Passik, 2009). Risk screening processes were reported in two children's cancer centers, and in both settings approximately 35% of adolescents receiving opioid therapy were found to have high risk of opioid misuse. Mental health factors and concurrent use of two or more opioids were significantly associated with one or more risk behaviors (Anghelescu, Ehrentraut, & Faughnan, 2013; Ehrentraut, Kern, Long, et al., 2014; Thienprayoon, Porter, Tate, et al., 2017).

Tolerance occurs when the dose of an opioid needs to be increased to achieve the same analgesic effects that were previously achieved at a lower dose. Tolerance may develop after 10 to 21 days of morphine administration. Treatment of tolerance involves increasing the dose or decreasing the duration between doses.

Parents and older children may fear addiction when opioids are prescribed. Nurses should provide appropriate reassurance that opioids are effective analgesics for acute pain and discuss other integrative techniques that can be used to reduce the overall dose and length of opioid therapy. Reassuring parents and children that just as the effects of other medications are monitored, the child's response to opioids will be closely monitored and adjusted to minimize any risks or adverse events. Nurses should also explain to parents the differences between physical dependence, tolerance, and addiction, and allow them to express concerns about the use and duration of use of opioids. Lastly, if opioids are included in the discharge medications for home, nurses should provide guidance about safe use, storage, and disposal (Manworren & Gilson, 2015).

Weaning opioids requires a systematic approach. For children on opioids for less than 5 days, decrease the opioid dose by 20% to 30% every 1 to 2 days (Oakes, 2011). For children who have been on opioids for longer than 5 to 7 days, a slower weaning is recommended: Wean by 20% on the first day, then follow that with reductions of 5% to 10% on each day as tolerated, until a total daily dose of morphine (or its equivalent) of 30 mg for an adolescent or a dose of 0.6 mg/kg/day is reached (Oakes, 2011).

CONSEQUENCES OF UNTREATED PAIN IN INFANTS

Despite current research on the neonate's experience of pain, infant pain often remains inadequately managed. The mismanagement of infant pain is partially the result of misconceptions about the effects of pain on the neonate and the lack of knowledge of immediate and long-term consequences of untreated pain. Infants respond to noxious stimuli through physiologic indicators (increased heart rate and blood pressure, variability in heart rate and intracranial pressure, and decreases in arterial oxygen saturation [SaO_2] and skin blood flow) and behavioral indicators (muscle rigidity, facial expression, crying, withdrawal, and sleeplessness) (Clark, 2011; Oakes, 2011). The physiologic and behavioral changes, as well as a variety of neurophysiologic responses to noxious stimulation, are responsible for acute and long-term consequences of pain (Kesavan, 2015).

Several harmful effects occur with unrelieved pain, particularly when pain is prolonged. Pain triggers a number of physiologic stress responses in the body, and they lead to negative consequences that involve multiple systems. Unrelieved pain may prolong the stress response and adversely affect an infant's or child's recovery, whether it is from trauma, surgery, or disease.

Poorly controlled acute pain can predispose patients to chronic pain syndromes. Box 5.5 provides a list of numerous complications of untreated pain in infants. A guiding principle in pain management is that prevention of pain is always better than treatment. Pain that is established and severe is often more difficult to control. When pain is unrelieved, sensory input from injured tissues reaches spinal cord neurons and may enhance subsequent responses. Long-lasting changes in cells within spinal cord pain pathways may occur after a brief painful stimulus and may lead to the development of chronic pain conditions.

An experience known as the *windup phenomenon*, or hyperalgesia, has been attributed to a decreased pain threshold and chronic pain. Central and peripheral mechanisms that occur in response to noxious tissue injury have been studied in an attempt to explain a prolonged neonatal response to pain characteristic of the windup phenomenon. After exposure to noxious stimuli, multiple levels of the spinal cord experience an altered excitability. This altered excitability may cause nonnoxious stimuli, such as routine nursing care and handling, to be perceived as noxious stimuli. Nurses who care for infants and children should consider the potential acute and long-term effects of pain on their young patients and be advocates in treating and preventing pain.

BOX 5.5 Consequences of Untreated Pain in Infants

Acute Consequences

Periventricular-intraventricular hemorrhage
Increased chemical and hormone release
Breakdown of fat and carbohydrate stores
Prolonged hyperglycemia
Higher morbidity for neonatal intensive care unit patients
Memory of painful events
Hypersensitivity to pain
Prolonged response to pain
Inappropriate innervation of the spinal cord
Inappropriate response to nonnoxious stimuli
Lower pain threshold

Potential Long-Term Consequences

Higher somatic complaints of unknown origin
Greater physiologic and behavioral responses to pain
Increased prevalence of neurologic deficits
Psychosocial problems
Neurobehavioral disorders
Cognitive deficits
Learning disorders
Poor motor performance
Behavioral problems
Attention deficits
Poor adaptive behavior
Inability to cope with novel situations
Problems with impulsivity and social control
Learning deficits
Emotional temperament changes in infancy or childhood
Accentuated hormonal stress responses in adult life

BOX 5.6 Needlestick Pain Prevention Resources

Online at the Centers for Disease Control and Prevention website at https://www.cdc.gov/vaccines/pubs/pinkbook/vac-admin.html and https://www.cdc.gov/vaccines/parents/downloads/parent-ver-sch-0-6yrs.pdf.

In addition, handouts with tips for clinical staff and parents are available at https://www.pediatricnursing.net/ce/2018/article4206267274.pdf.

Clinical practice guidelines for reducing pain during immunization) are found online at http://www.apsoc.org.au/PDF/SIG-Pain_in_Childhood/20150824_CMAJ_Reducing_pain_during_vaccine_injections_full.pdf

COMMON PAIN STATES IN CHILDREN

PAINFUL AND INVASIVE PROCEDURES

Procedures that infants and children must experience as part of routine medical care often cause pain and distress. For example, infants and children experience a substantial amount of pain due to routine immunizations. Translating Evidence Into Practice: Reducing Injection Pain During Childhood Immunizations provides interventions that can minimize pain during these procedures. Resources for pain interventions for injections can be found in Box 5.6.

TRANSLATING EVIDENCE INTO PRACTICE

Reducing Injection Pain During Childhood Immunizations

Introduction

Infants and children experience a substantial amount of pain due to routine immunizations. Recent evidence shows that infant and childhood pain not only is immediately distressing to both the infant and the caregiver, but also can have lifelong consequences. Recent evidence has shown that infants who exhibit vaccine-related pain early in life are more likely to do so at subsequent injections (McMurtry, Pillai Riddell, Taddio, et al., 2015). There exist many simple, scientifically grounded strategies that reduce injection pain in infants (Shah, Taddio, McMurty, et al., 2015). This box examines the line of evidence supporting strategies to reduce vaccine-related pain among healthy infants and children (birth to 18 months old) receiving routine immunizations.

Ask the Question

What measures are effective in reducing pain experienced during routine childhood immunizations for infants and children 0 to 18 months old?

Search for the Evidence

Search Strategies

Search selection criteria included English publications within the past 10 years, research-based articles (level 1 or lower) on infants and children (0 to 18 months old) receiving routine childhood immunizations.

Databases Used

PubMed, Cochrane Collaboration, MD Consult, Joanna Briggs Institute, National Guideline Clearinghouse (AHQR), TRIP Database Plus, PedsCCM, BestBETs

Critically Analyze the Evidence

Injection Techniques

What needle length to use? (longer versus shorter needle)

- A Cochrane review conducted by Beirne and colleagues (2018) found that a 25-mm (23- or 25-gauge) needle likely reduces occurrence of local reactions while maintaining immune response compared to a 16-mm needle when used during routine childhood immunizations.

Does tactile stimulation help reduce injection pain in infants?

- A randomized controlled trial conducted by Hogan and colleagues (2014) evaluated whether parent-led tactile stimulation would reduce injection pain in 124 four- to six-month-old infants scheduled to receive a routine immunization. The trial demonstrated no reduction in modified behavioral pain score (MBPS) for infants receiving tactile stimulation in the presence of other pain-reducing strategies, compared to infants receiving no tactile stimulation.

Does aspiration increase injection pain?

- Rapid intramuscular (IM) injection without aspiration reduces injection pain by shortening the time of the procedure and avoiding displacement of the needle (Taddio, Ilersich, Ipp, et al., 2009).
- In a randomized controlled trial conducted by Ipp and colleagues (2007), 113 four- to six-month-old infants were randomized to either the slow injection–aspiration–slow withdrawal (standard) immunization technique or the rapid immunization without aspiration (intervention) immunization technique. Infants in the intervention group ($n = 56$) had lower MBPSs, were less likely to cry, cried for a shorter time, and had lower pain scores when scored by both parents and physicians using a Visual Analogue Scale (VAS).

Positioning

Vertical versus lying down

- Supine positioning is associated with increased fear in children who experience a greater feeling of lost control, confusion, anxiety, and anger (Gaskell, Binns, Heyhoe, et al., 2005).
- In a trial conducted by Sparks, Setlik, and Luhman (2007), 118 nine-month-old to four-year-old children were randomized to either upright or supine positioning for intravenous (IV) insertion. The upright group had lower Procedural Behavior Rating Scale–Revised (PBRS-R) scores, indicating less anxiety, fear, and pain compared to the supine group.
- In a trial of 106 two- to six-month-old infants, there was no difference in pain score or duration of cry between infants placed supine and upright (Ipp, Taddio, Goldbach, et al., 2004).

Breastfeeding

- In a systematic review of 11 randomized and quasi-randomized controlled trials examining the use of breastfeeding to reduce vaccine-related pain, the breastfed infants cried for shorter periods and had less increased heart rates than swaddled infants or infants offered a pacifier (Shah, Aliwalis, & Shah, 2007). There was no difference in crying time or pain scores for infants offered high doses of sucrose (2 ml of 12% sucrose in sterile water) compared to breastfeeding infants. Breastfeeding, where feasible and appropriate, is recommended over sucrose because breastfeeding is a no-cost intervention, promotes mother-infant bonding, and provides comfort to the infant.
- Sixty-six infants between 2 and 4 months old were randomized to receive a routine diphtheria, tetanus, and acellular pertussis (DTaP) vaccine while breastfeeding or receiving standard care (swaddled and placed in bassinet) (Efe & Ozer, 2007). Pain was measured using change in heart rates, oxygen saturation levels, and duration of cry. Crying time was shorter in the breastfed group compared to the control group, but heart rate and oxygen saturation were unaffected by breastfeeding.
- One hundred and twenty infants younger than 1 year old were randomized to either standard care or breastfeeding during administration of a routine pediatric immunization (Abdel Razek & Az El-Dein, 2009). The breastfeeding group experienced lower pain by all measures used, including change in heart rate. Care was taken in this study to ensure that infants had a secure latch prior to injection and were encouraged to continue breastfeeding if there was a pause.
- One hundred and fifty-eight infants between 0 and 6 months old were randomized to either no intervention or breastfeeding during routine vaccine administration (Dilli, Küçük, & Dallar, 2009). Breastfed infants cried on average for 20 seconds, and nonbreastfed infants cried on average for 150 seconds ($p < 0.001$). Neonatal Infant Pain Scale (NIPS) scores were significantly lower for breastfed infants (NIPS average = 3) compared to nonbreastfed infants (NIPS average = 6, $p < 0.001$).

Skin-to-Skin or Kangaroo Care

- Kostandy, Anderson, and Good (2013) conducted an in-hospital randomized controlled trial among healthy, full-term newborns examining the impact of skin-to-skin infant cry time and consolability among infants receiving a hepatitis B vaccine within the first hour of life. Thirty-six mother-infant dyads were randomized to either routine (infant placed supine in bassinet) or skin-to-skin (prone on mother's chest) vaccine administration. Skin-to-skin infants had shorter cry times and calmed more quickly after vaccine administration.
- Saeidi and colleagues (2011) conducted a randomized controlled trial of 60 healthy, full-term newborns randomized to either swaddling and placed next to mother or skin-to-skin positioning for in-hospital hepatitis B vaccine administration. Infants placed skin-to-skin had lower pain intensity scores, cried for a shorter time, and returned to preprocedure behavior more quickly compared to the swaddled infants.
- Chermont and colleagues (2009) conducted a trial in which 640 infants between 12 and 72 hours old were randomized to standard care (no analgesia), skin-to-skin initiated 2 minutes prior to injection, 25% sucrose administered

Continued

TRANSLATING EVIDENCE INTO PRACTICE—cont'd

Reducing Injection Pain During Childhood Immunizations

2 minutes prior to injection, or a combination of skin-to-skin and 25% sucrose for routine hepatitis B vaccination. Infants in the skin-to-skin branch of the trial had lower pain scores (NIPS, Premature Infant Pain Profile [PIPP], and Neonatal Facial Coding System [NFCS]) and experienced procedural pain for a shorter time than the other infants. Infants receiving 25% dextrose had decreased pain duration but not decreased pain scores compared to the skin-to-skin group. The combination of 25% dextrose and skin-to-skin had stronger analgesic effects than either intervention alone.

Verbal Reassurance and Soothing

- Racine and colleagues (2012) conducted a cross-sectional analysis of infant distress and parent soothing (combination of verbal reassurance and rocking or picking up the infant) among 606 infants between 2 and 12 months old. At 2 months old, caregiver soothing did not affect infant distress. However, among infants 4, 6, and 12 months old, infant distress increased caregiver soothing and produced further increases in infant distress.
- Campbell and colleagues (2013) conducted a cross-sectional study examining the relationship between caregiver soothing and infant distress among 760 infants between 2 and 12 months old. Infants who were soothed did not have lower observer-rated distress scores compared to infants who were not soothed. Caregiver soothing did not affect infant distress, but physical soothing (e.g., picking up the infant or rocking) is encouraged because it promotes infant-caregiver bonding and trust elements that have long-term implications for infant development.
- In a naturalistic observation study of 49 infants conducted by Blount and colleagues (2008), verbal reassurance, empathy, and apology were shown to increase anxiety and crying in participating infants (Child-Adult Medical Procedure Interaction Scale–Infant Version IV [CAMPIS-IV]). This same study showed that skin-to-skin contact between caregiver and infant decreased CAMPIS-IV scores, as did rocking or physically soothing the infant.

Pharmacologic and Additional Techniques

Topical numbing agents

- O'Brien and colleagues (2004) conducted a randomized controlled trial examining the effect of topical 4% amethocaine gel in reducing pain associated with routine, subcutaneous measles, mumps, and rubella (MMR) administration among 120 twelve-month-old children. Change from baseline MBPS postinjection was used to measure pain. Children in the nonintervention branch ($n = 59$) had a much greater increase in MBPS score compared to the intervention group (change in MBPS = 2.3 versus 1.5, respectively, $p = 0.029$).
- In a double-blind, placebo-controlled, randomized trial, 110 full-term newborns received 1 g of amethocaine gel 4% or placebo 30 minutes prior to IM injection of 0.5 ml of vitamin K (Shah, Taddio, Hancock, et al., 2008). Pain was measured using VAS to assess for percent facial grimacing score, percent cry duration, and time to cry. There was no statistically significant difference for percent facial grimacing or percent cry duration between the two groups ($p = 0.41$ and $p = 0.34$, respectively). Time to cry was longer for the amethocaine group (4.7 versus 2.7 seconds, $p = 0.01$) compared to the placebo group.
- Twenty-seven 6- to 12-month-old infants were randomized to topical lidocaine-prilocaine ($n = 7$), 12% oral sucrose ($n = 7$), or no intervention ($n = 13$) for routine immunization administration (Dilli et al., 2009). Pain was measured using NIPS and duration of cry. Both intervention groups cried for an average of 35 seconds compared to the nonintervention group cry time average of 150 seconds ($p < 0.001$). NIPS scores were similarly reduced for the intervention infants (average of 3.5 compared to 6, $p < 0.001$). There was no measurable difference in pain reduction between the sucrose and lidocaine-prilocaine group, and both interventions were effective in reducing vaccine-associated pain in this study.

Oral sucrose to diminish vaccine-pain

- Hatfield and colleagues (2008) conducted a randomized controlled trial comparing 24% oral sucrose to placebo for pain control in infants receiving 2- or 4-month routine immunizations. Eighty-three infants received either sucrose ($n = 38$) or placebo ($n = 45$) 2 minutes prior to injection of combined DTaP, inactivated poliovirus (IPV), and hepatitis B virus (HepB) vaccines, followed 1 minute later by a *Haemophilus influenzae* type B (Hib) vaccine and 3 minutes later by a pneumococcal conjugate vaccine (PCV). The University of Wisconsin Children's Hospital Pain Scale was used to measure pain response at baseline and 2, 5, 7, and 9 minutes after administration of sucrose or placebo. The oral sucrose infants had lowered pain scores at minutes 5, 7, and 9. Pain scores peaked in both groups of infants at 7 minutes, with an average pain score of 3.8 for sucrose infants and 4.8 for placebo infants. By minute 9, pain scores for infants in the sucrose group had returned to baseline, whereas infants in the placebo group had an average pain score of 2.91.
- A double-blind randomized controlled trial was conducted by Kassab and colleagues (2012) to examine the effectiveness of 25% oral glucose in relieving pain for 120 infants receiving 2-month routine vaccinations. Infants received either 2 ml of glucose ($n = 60$) or sterile water ($n = 60$) 2 minutes prior to consecutive administration of DTaP-HepB-IPV (right thigh) or Hib (left thigh) vaccines. Pain was measured with the MBPS, crying time, and duration of full-lung cry. Infants in the intervention group spent an average of 38 seconds crying compared to 77.9 seconds in the placebo group. MBPS during immunization and after immunization was statistically lower in the intervention group ($p = 0.005$ and $p < 0.001$, respectively). Average full-lung crying time was 7.38 seconds in the sucrose infants compared to 13.84 seconds in the placebo infants ($p < 0.001$).
- One hundred and ten 3-month-old infants were randomized to receive either 2 ml 30% glucose ($n = 55$) or water ($n = 55$) prior to routine immunization (Thyr, Sundholm, Teeland, et al., 2007). Infants were enrolled in the study and remained in their respective study branch for 3-, 5-, and 12-month vaccines. Pain was evaluated by measuring crying time in both groups. At 3 months old, infants in the glucose group cried for an average of 18 seconds compared to 23 seconds in the placebo group ($p = 0.664$). At 5 and 12 months old, the intervention infants cried for an average of 6 seconds and 14 seconds compared to 16 seconds ($p = 0.017$) and 29 seconds ($p = 0.031$), respectively. In the water group, there was a significant correlation between infants who cried at 3 months old and subsequently cried at 5 and 12 months old ($r = 0.515$, $p < 0.001$ and $r = 0.332$, $p = 0.199$, respectively). However, this correlation was not repeated in the glucose group, suggesting that glucose is an effective intervention for reducing vaccine-related pain in very young infants.
- One hundred and thirteen infants were randomized to receive 2 ml 50% sucrose, 75% sucrose, or water by mouth prior to administration of 2-, 4-, and 6-month vaccines (Curry, Brown, & Wrona, 2012). Pain was measured by the FLACC Pain Assessment Tool (Facial expression, Leg movement, Activity, Cry, and Consolability) score and crying time. There was no significant difference between the intervention groups and control group in terms of FLACC scores or crying time ($p = 0.646$ and $p = 0.24$, respectively). Parents were not instructed to withhold comfort measures, and infants who were rocked, held, or patted had significantly lower FLACC scores ($p = 0.029$).

Apply the Evidence: Nursing Implications

There is moderate evidence with strong recommendations using the GRADE (Grading of Recommendations, Assessment, Development and Evaluations) criteria (Balshem, Helfand, Schunemann, et al., 2011) that the following interventions reduce pain during routine immunizations for infants and children between 0 and 18 months old:

- Skin-to-skin or breastfeeding where appropriate and agreeable to the caregiver and infant
- Upright positioning of child (sitting or held by caregiver)
- Sucrose administration prior to injection
- Use of topical anesthetics prior to injection (see Table 5.10)
- Use of the proper vaccine site and needle length for age and size of child
- Rapid injection without aspiration

TRANSLATING EVIDENCE INTO PRACTICE—cont'd

Reducing Injection Pain During Childhood Immunizations

There is low evidence and strong recommendation for implementation supporting the following interventions to reduce pain during routine immunizations for infants and children between 0 and 18 months old:

- Administering the least painful vaccine first when administering multiple vaccines in one visit
- Parent-led or clinician-led distraction or redirection
- Caregivers and nurses should *avoid* verbal reassurance, empathy, and apology

Quality and Safety Competencies: Evidence-Based Practice[a]

Knowledge

Differentiate clinical opinion from research and evidence-based summaries. Describe the most reliable methods to reduce pain during routine immunizations for infants and children between 0 and 18 months old.

Skills

Base the individualized care plan on patient values, clinical expertise, and evidence. Integrate evidence into practice by using the most reliable methods to reduce pain when administering routine vaccinations to infants and children between 0 and 18 months old.

Attitudes

Value the concept of evidence-based practice as integral in determining the best clinical practice. Appreciate strength and weakness of the evidence for the interventions listed in this box.

References

Abdel Razek A, Az El-Dein N: Effect of breast-feeding on pain relief during infant immunization injections, *International Journal of Nursing Practice* 15(2):99–104, 2009.

Balshem H, Helfand M, Schunemann HJ, et al.: GRADE guidelines: 3. Rating the quality of evidence, *Journal of Clinical Epidemiology* 64(4):401–406, 2011.

Beirne PV, Hennessy S, Cadogan SL, Shiely F, Fitzgerald T, MacLeod F: Needle size for vaccination procedures in children and adolescents, *Cochrane Database of Systematic Reviews* 8, 2018, CD010720.

Blount RL, Devine KA, Cheng PS, et al.: The impact of adult behaviors and vocalizations on infant distress during immunizations, *Journal of Pediatric Psychology* 33(10):1163–1174, 2008.

Campbell L, Pillai Riddell R, Garfield H, et al.: A cross-sectional examination of the relationship between caregiver proximal soothing and infant pain over the first year of life, *Pain* 154(6):813–823, 2013.

Chermont AG, Falcão LF, de Souza Silva EH, et al.: Skin-to-skin contact and/or oral 25% dextrose for procedural pain relief for term newborn infants, *Pediatrics* 124(6):e1101–e1107, 2009.

Curry DM, Brown C, Wrona S: Effectiveness of oral sucrose for pain management in infants during immunizations, *Pain Management Nursing* 13(3):139–149, 2012.

Dilli D, Küçük IG, Dallar Y: Interventions to reduce pain during vaccination in infancy, *Journal of Pediatrics* 154(3):385–390, 2009.

Efe E, Ozer ZC: The use of breast-feeding for pain relief during neonatal immunization injections, *Applied Nursing Research* 20(1):10–16, 2007.

Gaskell S, Binns F, Heyhoe MB, et al.: Taking the sting out of needles: Education for staff in primary care, *Paediatric Nursing* 17(4):24–28, 2005.

Hatfield LA, Gusic ME, Dyer AM, et al.: Analgesic properties of oral sucrose during routine immunizations at 2 and 4 months of age, *Pediatrics* 121(2):e327–e334, 2008.

Hogan ME, Probst J, Wong K, et al.: A randomized-controlled trial of parent-led tactile stimulation to reduce pain during infant immunization injections, *Clinical Journal of Pain* 30(3):259–265, 2014.

Ipp M, Taddio A, Goldbach M, et al.: Effects of age, gender and holding on pain response during infant immunization, *Canadian Journal of Clinical Pharmacology* 11(1):e2–e7, 2004.

Ipp M, Taddio A, Sam J, et al.: Vaccine-related pain: Randomised controlled trial of two injection techniques, *Archives of Disease in Childhood* 92(12):1105–1108, 2007.

Kassab M, Sheehy A, King M, et al.: A double-blind randomised controlled trial 25% oral glucose for pain relief in 2-month old infants undergoing immunization, *International Journal for Nursing Studies* 49(3):249–256, 2012.

Kostandy R, Anderson GC, Good M: Skin-to-skin contact diminishes pain from hepatitis B vaccine injection in healthy full-term neonates, *Neonatal Network* 32(4):274–280, 2013.

McMurtry CM, Pillai Riddell R, Taddio A, Racine N, Asmundson GJG, Noel M, Adults T: Far from "just a poke": Common painful needle procedures and the development of needle fear, *Clinical Journal of Pain* 31(Suppl. 10):S3–S11, 2015.

O'Brien L, Taddio A, Ipp M, et al.: Topical 4% amethocaine gel reduces the pain of subcutaneous measles-mumps-rubella vaccination, *Pediatrics* 114(6):e720–e724, 2004.

Racine NM, Pillai Riddell RR, Flora D, et al.: A longitudinal examination of verbal reassurance during infant immunization: Occurrence and examination of emotional availability as a potential moderator, *Journal of Pediatric Psychology* 37(8):935–944, 2012.

Saeidi R, Asnaashari Z, Amirnejad M, et al.: Use of "kangaroo care" to alleviate the intensity of vaccination pain in newborns, *Iranian Journal of Pediatrics* 21(1):99–102, 2011.

Shah PS, Aliwalas L, Shah V: Breastfeeding or breastmilk to alleviate procedural pain in neonates: A systematic review, *Breastfeeding Medicine* 2(2):74–84, 2007.

Shah VS, Taddio A, Hancock R, et al.: Topical amethocaine gel 4% for intramuscular injection in term neonates: A double-blind, placebo-controlled, randomized trial, *Clinical Therapeutics* 30(1):166–174, 2008.

Shah V, Taddio A, McMurtry CM, Halperin SA, Noel M, Pillai Riddell R, Team HE: Pharmacological and combined interventions to reduce vaccine injection pain in children and adults: Systematic review and meta-analysis, *Clinical Journal of Pain* 31(Suppl. 10):S38–S63, 2015.

Sparks LA, Setlik J, Luhman J: Parental holding and positioning to decrease IV distress in young children: A randomized controlled trial, *Journal of Pediatric Nursing* 22(6):440–447, 2007.

Taddio A, Ilersich AL, Ipp M, et al.: Physical interventions and injection techniques for reducing injection pain during routine childhood immunizations: Systematic review of randomized controlled trials and quasi-randomized controlled trials, *Clinical Therapeutics* 31(Suppl. 2):S48–S76, 2009.

Thyr M, Sundholm A, Teeland L, et al.: Oral glucose as an analgesic to reduce infant distress following immunization at the age of 3, 5 and 12 months, *Acta Paediatrica* 96(2):233–236, 2007.

Originally prepared by Rebecca Njord

[a]Adapted from the Quality and Safety Education for Nurses Institute.

Combining pharmacologic and nonpharmacologic interventions provides the best approach for reducing pain. Local anesthetic administration is crucial to minimize pain from the procedure and is discussed in the Transmucosal and Transdermal Analgesia section earlier in the chapter. Common systems that do not require needles for providing local analgesics are found in Table 5.10.

Procedural Sedation and Analgesia

Severe pain associated with invasive procedures and anxiety associated with diagnostic imaging can be managed with sedation and analgesia. Sedation involves a wide range of levels of consciousness (Box 5.7). A thorough patient assessment including the child's history is essential before procedural sedation.

Key components to include in the patient history are:

- Past medical history: Major illnesses, such as asthma, psychiatric disorders, cardiac disease, hepatic or renal impairment; previous hospitalizations or surgeries; history of previous anesthesia or sedation
- Allergies: Opiates, benzodiazepines, barbiturates, local anesthetics, others
- Current medications: Cardiovascular medications, central nervous system depressants; use caution with chronic benzodiazepine and opiate users; administration of reversal agents may induce withdrawal or seizures
- Drug use: Narcotics, benzodiazepines, barbiturates, cocaine, alcohol
- Last oral intake: For nonemergent cases, some guidelines recommend more than 6 hours for solid food and more than 2 hours for clear liquid

BOX 5.7 Levels of Sedation

Minimal Sedation (Anxiolysis)
Patient responds to verbal commands.
Cognitive function may be impaired.
Respiratory and cardiovascular systems are unaffected.

Moderate Sedation (Previously Conscious Sedation)
Patient responds to verbal commands but may not respond to light tactile stimulation.
Cognitive function is impaired.
Respiratory function is adequate; cardiovascular system is unaffected.

Deep Sedation
Patient cannot be easily aroused except with repeated or painful stimuli.
Ability to maintain airway may be impaired.
Spontaneous ventilation may be impaired; cardiovascular function is maintained.

General Anesthesia
Loss of consciousness, patient cannot be aroused with painful stimuli.
Airway cannot be maintained adequately and ventilation is impaired.
Cardiovascular function may be impaired.

From Meredith, J. R., O'Keefe, K. P., & Galwankar, S. (2008). Pediatric procedural sedation and analgesia. *Journal of Emergencies, Trauma, and Shock, 1*(2), 88–96.

BOX 5.8 Procedural Sedation and Analgesia Equipment Needs

- High-flow oxygen and delivery method
- Airway management materials: Endotracheal tubes, bag valve masks, and laryngoscopes
- Pulse oximetry, blood pressure monitor, electrocardiography,[a] capnography[a]
- Suction and large-bore catheters
- Vascular access supplies
- Resuscitation drugs, intravenous (IV) fluids
- Reversal agents, including flumazenil and naloxone

[a]May be optional devices.

- Volume status: Vomiting, diarrhea, fluid restriction, urinary output, making tears

A physical status evaluation using the American Society of Anesthesiologists Physical Status Classification (Leahy, Berry, Johnson, et al., 2018; Meredith, O'Keefe, & Galwankar, 2008) is documented before administering analgesia and sedation:

- Class I: A normally healthy patient
- Class II: A patient with mild systemic disease
- Class III: A patient with severe systemic disease
- Class IV: A patient with severe systemic disease that is a constant threat to life
- Class V: A moribund patient who is not expected to survive without the operation

To provide a safe environment for procedural sedation and analgesia (PSA), equipment should be readily available to prevent or manage adverse events and complications (Box 5.8). The patient should have an IV access for titration of sedation and analgesic medications and for administration of possible antagonists and fluids. Trained personnel (physician, registered nurse, respiratory therapist) whose sole responsibility is to monitor the patient (rather than performing or assisting with the procedure) should be present to monitor for adverse events and complications.

POSTOPERATIVE PAIN

Surgery and traumatic injuries (fractures, dislocations, strains, sprains, lacerations, burns) generate a catabolic state as a result of increased secretion of catabolic hormones; lead to alterations in blood flow, coagulation, fibrinolysis, substrate metabolism, and water and electrolyte balance; and increase the demands on the cardiovascular and respiratory systems. The major endocrine and metabolic changes occur during the first 48 hours after surgery or trauma. Local anesthetics and opioid neural blockade may effectively mitigate the physiologic responses to surgical injury.

Pain associated with surgery to the chest (e.g., repair of congenital heart defects, chest trauma) or abdominal regions (e.g., appendectomy, cholecystectomy, splenectomy) may result in pulmonary complications. Pain leads to decreased muscle movement in the thorax and abdominal area and to decreased tidal volume, vital capacity, functional residual capacity, and alveolar ventilation. The patient is unable to cough and clear secretions, and the risk for complications (such as pneumonia and atelectasis) is high. Severe postoperative pain also results in sympathetic overactivity that leads to increases in heart rate, peripheral resistance, blood pressure, and cardiac output. The patient eventually experiences an increase in cardiac demand and myocardial oxygen consumption and a decrease in oxygen delivery to the tissues.

The basis for good postoperative pain control in children is preemptive analgesia (Cicvaric, Divkovic, Tot, et al., 2018; Michelet, Andreu-Gallien, Bensalah, et al., 2012). Preemptive analgesia involves administration of medications (e.g., local and regional anesthetics, analgesics) before the child experiences the pain or before surgery is performed so that the sensory activation and changes in the pain pathways of the peripheral and central nervous system can be controlled. Preemptive analgesia lowers postoperative pain, lowers analgesic requirement, lowers hospital stay, lowers complications after surgery, and minimizes the risks for peripheral and central nervous system sensitization that can lead to persistent pain.

A combination of medications (multimodal or balanced analgesia) is used for postoperative pain and may include NSAIDs, local anesthetics, nonopioids, and opioid analgesics to achieve optimum relief and minimize side effects. Opioids (see Table 5.5) administered ATC during the first 48 hours or administered via PCA are commonly prescribed. Perioperative NSAID administration is shown to reduce opioid consumption and postoperative nausea and vomiting in children (Cicvaric et al., 2018; Michelet et al., 2012). Scheduled acetaminophen is supported as the preferred medication in children after tonsillectomy; codeine is not recommended due to the risk of children experiencing ultrarapid metabolizers caused by abnormal function of the CYP2D6 enzyme (Yellon et al., 2014).

The combination of the IV NSAID ketorolac and morphine using a PCA device is frequently prescribed after thoracic surgery. Morphine delivered by PCA leads to a lower total dosage of opioid analgesia when compared with the administration of intermittent doses of analgesia as required. After bowel surgery, a mixture of a local anesthetic (bupivacaine) and a low-dose opioid (fentanyl) delivered by epidural route improves the rate of recovery and minimizes the gastrointestinal effects (e.g., bowel stasis, nausea, vomiting). Once bowel function has been restored, oral opioids (such as immediate-release and controlled-release preparations) are preferred in older children. Controlled-release opioids facilitate ATC dosing and improve sleep. They are also associated with a lower incidence of nausea, sedation, and breakthrough pain.

BURN PAIN

Because burn pain has multiple components, involves repeated manipulations over the injured painful sites, and has changing patterns over time, it is difficult and challenging to control. Burn pain includes a constant background pain that is felt at the wound sites and surrounding areas. Burn pain is exacerbated (breakthrough pain) by movements, such as changing position, turning in bed, walking, or even breathing. Areas of normal skin that have been harvested for skin grafts (donor sites) also are painful. Pain is commonly experienced with intense tingling or itching sensations when skin grafting is required. During the healing process, when the tissue and nerve regenerate, the necrotic tissue (eschar) is excised until viable tissue is reached. The healing process may last for months to years. Pain or paresthetic sensations (itching, tingling, cold sensations, and so on) may persist. In addition, discomfort may be associated with immobilization of limbs in splints or garments, as well as multiple surgical interventions such as skin grafting and reconstructive surgery.

Multiple therapeutic procedures are carried out during treatment. These procedures (dressing changes, wound debridement and cleansing, physical therapy sessions) occur daily or even several times a day (see Chapter 31). Providing proper analgesia without interfering with the patient's awareness during and after the procedure is the biggest challenge in the management of burn pain. Fentanyl or alfentanil has a major advantage over morphine because of the short duration. Fentanyl can prevent oversedation after the procedure. For less painful procedures, premedication with oral morphine, oral ketamine, or milder opioids 15 minutes before the procedure may be sufficient. Depending on the patient's anxiety level, a benzodiazepine (e.g., lorazepam) before the procedure may be beneficial. For longer procedures, morphine is the mainstay of treatment. Some patients may require moderate to deep sedation and analgesia. Oral oxycodone with midazolam and acetaminophen, in addition to nitrous oxide, may be needed. IV ketamine administered at subtherapeutic doses has been one of the most extensively used anesthetics for burn patients. The dysphoria and unpleasant reactions associated with ketamine administration may be minimized by premedication with a benzodiazepine. If ketamine is used with either morphine or fentanyl, the regimen could have opioid-sparing actions and reduce the opioid-related side effects.

RECURRENT HEADACHES IN CHILDREN

Recurrent headaches in children can be caused by several factors, including tension, dental braces, imbalance or weakness of eye muscles causing deviation in alignment and refractive errors, sequelae to accidents, sinusitis and other cranial infection or inflammation, increased intracranial pressure, epileptic attacks, drugs, obstructive sleep apnea, and, rarely, hypertension (Connelly & Sekhon, 2019) (see Chapter 27). Other causes may include arteriovenous malformations, disturbances in cerebrospinal fluid flow or absorption, intracranial hemorrhages, ocular and dental diseases, bacterial infections, and brain tumors.

Severe pain is the most disturbing symptom in migraine. Tension-type headache is usually mild or moderate, often producing a pressing feeling in the temples, like a "tight band around the head." Continuous, daily, or near-daily headache with no specific cause occurs in a small subgroup of children. In epilepsy, headaches commonly occur immediately before, during, or after a seizure attack.

Headache management involves two main behavioral approaches: (1) teaching patients self-control skills to prevent headache (biofeedback techniques and relaxation training), and (2) modifying behavior patterns that increase the risk of headache occurrence or reinforce headache activity (cognitive-behavioral stress management techniques). Families may be able to identify factors that trigger the headache and avoid the triggers in the future. Biofeedback is a technology-based form of relaxation therapy and can be useful in assessing and reinforcing learning of relaxation skills, such as progressive muscle relaxation, deep breathing, and imagery. Children as young as 7 years old can learn these skills and with 2 to 3 weeks of practice are able to decrease the time needed to achieve relaxation.

To modify behavior patterns that increase the risk of headache or reinforce headache activity, the nurse instructs parents to avoid giving excessive attention to their child's headache and to respond matter-of-factly to pain behavior and requests for special attention. Parents learn to assess whether the child is avoiding school or social performance demands because of headache. Parents are taught to focus attention on adaptive coping, such as the use of relaxation techniques and maintenance of normal activity patterns. When using cognitive-behavioral stress management techniques, the parents identify negative thoughts and situations that may be associated with increased risk for headache. The parent teaches the child to activate positive thoughts and engage in adaptive behavior appropriate to the situation.

RECURRENT ABDOMINAL PAIN IN CHILDREN

RAP or functional abdominal pain is defined as pain that occurs at least once per month for 3 consecutive months, accompanied by pain-free periods, and is severe enough that it interferes with a child's normal activities (Hyman, 2016) (see Chapter 16). Management of RAP is highly individualized to reflect the causes of the pain and the psychosocial needs of the child and family. A clear understanding of the child's characteristics (anxiety, physical health, temperament, coping skills, experience, learned response, depression), the child's disability (school attendance, activities with family, social interactions, pain behaviors), environmental factors (family attitudes and behavioral patterns, school environment, community, friendships), and the pain stimulus (disease, injury, stress) is important in planning management strategies (Oakes, 2011).

Before any workup of the pain, the nurse informs the family that RAP is common in children and only 10% of children with RAP have an identifiable organic cause for their pain symptom. Medical workup is dictated by the child's symptoms and signs in combination with knowledge about common organic causes of RAP. If an organic cause is found, it will be treated appropriately. Even if no organic cause is found, the nurse needs to communicate to the child and family a belief that the pain is real. Usually the abdominal pain goes away, but even if problems are identified, they may not be the actual cause, and pain may persist, may be replaced by another symptom, or may go away on its own. The management plan includes regular follow-up at 3- to 4-month intervals, a list of symptoms that call for earlier contact, and biobehavioral pain management techniques. The goal is to minimize the impact of the pain on the child's activities and the family's life.

The use of CBT has been documented to reduce or eliminate pain in children with RAP and highlights the involvement of parents in supporting their child's self-management behavior. Case reports have demonstrated the effectiveness of implementing a time-out procedure, token systems, and positive reinforcement based on operant theory treatment modalities. Stress management and cognitive-behavioral strategies have also been successful. Parent training in how to avoid positive reinforcement of sick behaviors and focus on rewarding healthy behaviors is important. Over the course of several sessions, parents are educated about RAP, how to distinguish between sick and well behaviors, a reward system for well behaviors, and the importance of reinforcing relaxation and coping skills taught to children for pain management. Treatment may consist of a varying number of sessions over 1 to 6 months and may include various components, such as monitoring symptoms, limiting parent attention, relaxation training, increasing dietary fiber, and requiring school attendance. No negative side effects of symptom substitution occurred with the interventions.

PAIN IN CHILDREN WITH SICKLE CELL DISEASE

A painful episode is the most frequent cause for emergency department visits and hospital admissions among children with sickle cell disease (see Chapter 24). The acute painful episode in sickle cell disease is the only pain syndrome in which opioids are considered the major therapy and are started in early childhood and continued throughout adult life. A source of frustration for patients and clinicians is that most current analgesic regimens are inadequate in controlling some of the most severe painful episodes. A multidisciplinary approach that involves both pharmacologic and nonpharmacologic modalities (cognitive-behavioral intervention, heat, massage, physical therapy) is needed but not often implemented. The goals of treatment of the acute episode may not be to take all of the pain away, which is usually impossible, but to make the pain tolerable to the patient until the episode resolves and to increase function and patient participation in activities of daily living (Oakes, 2011; Telfer & Kaya, 2017).

Patients coming to an emergency department for acute painful episodes usually have exhausted all home care options or outpatient therapy. The nurse should ask patients what the usual medication, dosage, and side effects were in the past; the usual medication taken at home; and medication taken since the onset of present pain. The patient may be on long-term opioid therapy at home and therefore may have developed some degree of tolerance. A different potent opioid or a larger dose of the same medication may be indicated. Because mixed opioid-agonist-antagonists may precipitate withdrawal syndromes, avoid these if patients were taking long-term opioids at home. A "passport" card with patient information about the diagnosis, previous complications, suggested pain management regimen, and name and contact information of the primary hematologist is helpful for parents and facilitates patient-centered management of pain in the emergency department.

The patient is admitted for inpatient management of severe pain if adequate relief is not achieved in the emergency department. For severe pain, IV administration with bolus dosing and continuous infusion using a PCA device may be necessary. Patients requiring more than 5 to 7 days of opioids should have tapering doses to avoid the physiologic symptoms of withdrawal (dysphoria, nasal congestion, diarrhea, nausea and vomiting, sweating, and seizures). Appropriate weaning of the PCA schedules start with reduction of the continuous infusion rate before discontinuation while the patient continues to use demand doses for analgesia. Morphine-equivalent equianalgesic conversions may be used to convert continuous infusion rates to equivalent oral analgesics. Doses of long-acting oral analgesics, such as sustained-release oral morphine, may also be used to replace continuous infusion dosing. The demand doses can be subsequently reduced if analgesia remains adequate.

Patients who are administered doses of opioids that are inadequate to relieve their pain or whose doses are not tapered after a course of treatment may develop iatrogenic pseudoaddiction (Greene & Chambers, 2015; Passik, 2009). Pseudoaddiction is a phenomenon that suggests that undertreatment of pain leads to patient behaviors that "mimic" addiction, such as asking for specific medications by name and preferred dose, asking for pain medicines on schedule (clock watching), and reporting high pain scores on a frequent basis. Such a scenario can be experienced by patients with sickle cell disease, cancer, and other chronic pain conditions when presenting in busy emergency departments where they encounter a different provider each time. Although there are few data regarding the role of pseudoaddiction in chronic pain, at its core it can be seen as a fundamental issue of miscommunication and mistrust between a patient and a caregiver. Communicating with patients to ensure accurate pain history and assessment and participating in shared decision making about safe and effective pain management can provide both patients and providers with a satisfactory encounter and outcome.

CANCER PAIN IN CHILDREN

Pain in children with cancer is present before diagnosis and treatment and may resolve after initiation of anticancer therapy. However, treatment-related pain is common (Table 5.11). Pain may be related to surgery, mucositis, a phantom limb, or infection. Pain can also be related to chemotherapy and procedures, such as bone marrow aspiration, needle puncture, and lumbar puncture. Tumor-related pain frequently occurs when the child relapses or when tumors become resistant to treatment. Intractable pain may occur in patients with bulky solid tumors that occupy space in the lungs, limbs, abdomen, pelvis, or brain. In young adult survivors of childhood cancer, chronic pain conditions may develop, including complex regional pain syndrome of the lower extremity, phantom limb pain, avascular necrosis, mechanical pain related to leg lengthening procedures, and postherpetic neuralgia.

Oral mucositis (ulceration of the oral cavity and throat) frequently occurs in patients undergoing chemotherapy or radiotherapy and in patients undergoing bone marrow transplant. Treatment includes single agents (saline, opioids, sodium bicarbonate, hydrogen peroxide, sucralfate suspension, clotrimazole, nystatin, viscous lidocaine, amphotericin B, dyclonine) or mouthwash mixtures using a combination of agents (lidocaine, diphenhydramine, Maalox or Mylanta, nystatin). Mucositis after bone marrow transplantation may be prolonged, continuously intense, exacerbated by mouth care and swallowing, or worse during waking hours. The patient may be unable to eat or swallow. Morphine administered as a continuous infusion or delivered by PCA device may be required until mucositis is resolved (Bennett, 2016; Hickman, Varadarajan, & Weisman, 2014; Sung, Robinson, Treister, et al., 2017).

Other treatment-related pain includes (1) abdominal pain after allogeneic bone marrow transplantation, which may be associated with acute graft-versus-host disease; (2) abdominal pain associated with typhlitis (infection of the cecum), which occurs when the patient is immunocompromised; (3) phantom sensations and phantom limb pain after an amputation; (4) peripheral neuropathy after administration of vincristine and other chemotherapy agents with neurotoxic effects; and (5) medullary bone pain, which may be associated with administration of granulocyte colony–stimulating factor or disease burden in the medullary bone spaces.

Survivors of childhood cancer describe vivid memories of their experience with repeated painful procedures during treatment. These procedures include needle puncture for IM chemotherapy (L-asparaginase), IV lines, port access and blood draws, lumbar puncture, bone marrow aspiration and biopsy, removal of central venous catheters, and other invasive diagnostic procedures. Fear and anxiety related to these procedures may be minimized with parent and child preparation. The preparation starts with obtaining information from the parent about the child's coping styles, explaining the procedure, and enlisting their support, followed by an age-appropriate explanation to the child. CBT (guided imagery, relaxation, music therapy, hypnosis), conscious sedation, and general anesthesia have been effective in decreasing pain and distress during the procedure. Topical analgesics (cold sprays, EMLA, amethocaine gels), as discussed earlier in the chapter, are effective in providing analgesia before needle procedures.

If the patient is neutropenic (absolute neutrophil count $<500/mm^3$), the antipyretic action of acetaminophen may mask a fever. In patients with thrombocytopenia (platelet count $<50,000/mm^3$), who may be at

TABLE 5.11 Cancer Pain in Children

Type	Clinical Presentation	Causes
Bone		
Skull Vertebrae Pelvis and femur	Aching to sharp, severe pain generally more pronounced with movement; point tenderness common Skull—headaches, blurred vision Spine—tenderness over spinous process Extremities—pain associated with movement or lifting Pelvis and femur—pain associated with movement; pain with weight bearing and walking	Infiltration of bone Skeletal metastases—irritation and stretching of pain receptors in periosteum and endosteum Prostaglandins released from bone destruction
Neuropathic		
Peripheral Plexus Epidural Cord compression	Complaints of pain without any detectable tissue damage Abnormal or unpleasant sensations, generally described as tingling, burning, or stabbing Often a delay in onset Brief, shooting pain Increased intensity of pain with receptive stimuli	Nerve injury caused by tumor infiltration; can also be caused by injury from treatment (e.g., vincristine toxicity) Infiltration or compression of peripheral nerves Surgical interruption of nerves (phantom pain after amputation)
Visceral		
Soft tissue Tumors of bowel Retroperitoneum	Poorly localized Varies in intensity Pressure, deep or aching	Obstruction—bowel, urinary tract, biliary tract Mucosal ulceration Metabolic alteration Nociceptor activation, generally from distention or inflammation of visceral organs
Treatment Related		
Mucositis Infection Post–lumbar puncture headaches Radiation dermatitis Postsurgical	Difficulty swallowing, pain from lesions in oropharynx; may extend throughout entire gastrointestinal tract Infection may be localized pain from focused infection or generalized (i.e., tissue infection versus septicemia) Severe headache after lumbar puncture Skin inflammation causing redness and breakdown Pain related to tissue trauma secondary to surgery	Direct side effects of treatment for cancer: Chemotherapy Radiation Surgery

risk for bleeding, NSAIDs are contraindicated. Morphine is the most widely used opioid for moderate to severe pain and may be administered via the oral (including sustained-release formulations, such as MS Contin), IV, subcutaneous, epidural, and intrathecal routes.

The most common clinical syndrome of neuropathic pain is painful peripheral neuropathy caused by chemotherapeutic agents, particularly vincristine and cisplatin and rarely cytarabine (Hickman et al., 2014). After withdrawal of the chemotherapy, the neuropathy may resolve over weeks to months, or it may persist even after withdrawal. Neuropathic pain is associated with at least one of the following: (1) pain that is described as electric or shocklike, stabbing, or burning; (2) signs of neurologic involvement (paralysis, neuralgia, pain hypersensitivity) other than those associated with the progression of the tumor; and (3) the location of the solid organ cancer consistent with neurologic damage that could give rise to neuropathic pain. An epidural or subarachnoid infusion may be initiated if the patient experiences dose-limiting side effects of opioids or if pain is resistant to opioids. Tricyclic antidepressants (amitriptyline, desipramine) and anticonvulsants (gabapentin, carbamazepine) have demonstrated effectiveness in neuropathic cancer pain (Anghelescu, Faughnan, Popenhagen, et al., 2014).

PAIN AND SEDATION IN END-OF-LIFE CARE

Children living with terminal illnesses or conditions experience pain at various points on their disease trajectory. The cumulative effects of treatments, procedures, medications, and symptoms can lead to increased suffering as they near the end of life. Palliative care and hospice professionals are skilled at managing the pain and complex symptoms that accompany complex medical illness and end of life, allowing children to remain in the comfort of their homes as they reach the end of life (Kaye, Gattas, Kiefer, et al., 2019). In most cases, pain and symptoms can be adequately managed, and the child can remain comfortable throughout the dying process. However, there are some children for whom pain and other symptoms are difficult to control, leading to suffering for both the child and the family. Palliative sedation can be considered when a child is imminently dying and intolerable symptoms are causing distress and suffering during the dying process. Palliative sedation should not be considered unless all other means of achieving comfort have been exhausted (Bodnar, 2017).

Initiating conversations about palliative sedation should be focused on clarifying the goal of sedation. In some circumstances, palliative sedation may be a time-limited process to allow rest and the opportunity to adjust symptom management, with the hope of improved comfort and the possibility of returning to a more awake state. In more intractable situations, the goal may be to initiate a deep sedation aimed at creating a restful state until death. In either case, the interdisciplinary palliative or hospice team should meet with the family to discuss their perception of the child's suffering and preferences for palliative sedation and to determine clinical outcomes that would indicate when to titrate or discontinue sedation (Anghelescu, 2012).

The use of palliative sedation at end of life is rooted in ethical principles of beneficence (to act in the best interest of the patient, to be merciful) and nonmaleficence (to do no harm). The intent of palliative sedation is to reduce suffering by inducing a sedated state of rest, not to hasten death, and it is not considered euthanasia or assisted suicide (Anghelescu, 2012).

Euthanasia involves a person other than the patient determining that the patient is suffering and then acting with the intent to end the person's life (Saad, 2017). Euthanasia is illegal at any age in the United States. Physician-assisted suicide involves terminally ill individuals requesting that their doctor provide the means to end their life at the time of their choosing, and then these individuals acting with the intent to end their life. Several states allow physician-assisted suicide for adults only (Campbell & Black, 2014; Orentlicher, Pope, & Rich, 2016).

CLINICAL JUDGMENT AND NEXT-GENERATION NCLEX® EXAMINATION-STYLE QUESTIONS

1. When caring for a 6-month infant hospitalized for bronchiolitis, a parent asks the nurse, "Is she in pain? How would you know since she can't tell you?" On the previous nursing assessment the infant has a temperature of 99°F (37°C), respirations of 32, pulse-100 beats/min and blood pressure- 98/50 mm/Hg. The infant is sleeping. **Use an X for the nursing response to the mother who is concerned about pain listed below that is Indicated (appropriate or necessary), Contraindicated (could be harmful), or Non-Essential (makes no difference or not necessary) regarding whether the child is experiencing pain and how the nurses will know.**

Nursing Action	Indicated	Contraindicated	Non-Essential
"Infants don't feel pain as adults do because their pain receptors are not fully developed yet."			
"Although we try to give the baby medicine before pain is felt, we watch very closely and use different techniques to help relieve the pain."			
"The nurses give pain medication before the infant really feels pain to all hospitalized patients when needed."			
"We assess pain using a pain assessment tool for children of all ages and give the medicine as needed."			
"We wait until the infant cries or is fussy, and then we know that pain is being experienced"			

2. A 9-year-old boy who is experiencing pain following surgery for appendicitis. Which of . He was operated on this morning and had no complications from surgery. The nurse performs an assessment 30 minutes after giving him pain medication and notes assessment finding warrants. Which of these indicators warrant further nursing action? He currently rates his pain as a "5" on a scale of 0-5. **Select all that apply.**
   - **A.** Pain rating is a 4 on a 0-5 scale obtained 30 minutes after IV pain medication
   - **B.** Respiration rate is 20 breaths/min- 2 hours after IV pain medication
   - **C.** Respiration rate of 20 breaths/min
   - **D.** Pain score changed from 4/5 to 2/5- 30 minutes after IV pain medication
   - **E.** Blood pressure rate of 112/74 mm/Hg
   - **F.** Pulse rate of 85 beats/min
   - **G.** Vomiting immediately after administration of oral pain medication
   - **H.** Sitting in bed talking with parent 45 minutes after pain medication given
   - **I.** Reports pain as 5 on scale of 0-5 while asking for ice cream – needs follow-up because behavior is incongruent with what is being reported
   - **J.** The wound is warm to touch and red

3. The nurse is caring for four pediatric patients who could be experiencing pain for different reasons. **Indicate which pain scale listed in the far-left column is appropriate for the child experiencing pain listed in the middle column. Place the number of the pain scale that should be used for the patient described in the middle column in the far-right column. Note that NOT all pain scales will be used.**

Pain Assessment Scale	Patient and Type of Pain Experienced	Correct Pain Scale
1. CRIES: Crying, Requiring increased oxygen, Inability to console, Expression, and Sleeplessness	2-year-old with Down Syndrome in recovery from morning surgery	
2. FLACC Pain Assessment Tool: Facial expression, Leg movement, Activity, Cry, and Consolability	Newborn in intensive care for low birth weight and born to an addicted mother	
3. Non-Communicating Children's Pain Checklist (NCCPC): Parent and health care giver questionnaire assessing acute and chronic pain	17-year-old admitted for sickle cell crisis	
4. Neonatal Pain, Agitation, and Sedation Scale (NPASS): For infants from 3 to 6 months old	5-year-old with leukemia undergoing a lumbar puncture	
5. Wong-Baker FACES Scale		
6. Premature Infant Pain Profile (PIPP)		
7. Visual Analogue Numeric Scale		

4. A 5-year-old girl with sickle cell disease is admitted for an acute painful episode and was placed on opioids in the emergency room. On admission her pain score was 5/5 using the Wong-Baker Pain Scale. Two hours later she is feeling better and rates her pain as a 2/5 using the Wong-Baker Pain Scale. **Choose the most likely options for the information missing from the statements below by selecting from the lists of options provided.**

The best option for her at this time is to maintain a ____1____ infusion of pain medication with ____2____ dosing as needed. If she continues opioids for more than 5-7 days, ____3____ doses over time is needed to avoid withdrawal symptoms.

Options for 1	Options for 2	Options for 3
intermittent	bolus	increasing
continuous	triple	changing
as needed	half	stopping
prn	full	tapering
one-time	continuous	adjusting
daily	daily	holding

REFERENCES

Allen, J. D., Casavant, M. J., Spiller, H. A., Chounthirath, T., Hodges, N. L., & Smith, G. A. (2017). Prescription opioid exposures among children and adolescents in the United States: 2000–2015. *Pediatrics, 139*(4), e20163382.

Ambuel, B., Hamlett, K. W., Marx, C. M., et al. (1992). Assessing distress in pediatric intensive care environments: The COMFORT scale. *Journal of Pediatric Psychology, 17*(1), 95–109.

Andrzejowski, P., & Carroll, W. (2016). Codeine in paediatrics: Pharmacology, prescribing and controversies. Archives of disease in childhood. *Education & Practice edition, 101*(3), 148–151.

Anghelescu, D. L. (2012). Pediatric palliative sedation therapy with propofol: Recommendations based on experience in children with terminal cancer. *Journal of Palliative Medicine, 15*(10), 1082–1090.

Anghelescu, D. L., Ehrentraut, J. H., & Faughnan, L. G. (2013). Opioid misuse and abuse: Risk assessment and management in patients with cancer pain. *Journal of the National Comprehensive Cancer Network, 11*(8), 1023–1031.

Anghelescu, D. L., Faughnan, L. G., Oakes, L. L., Windsor, K. B., Pei, D., & Burgoyne, L. L. (2012). Parent-controlled PCA for pain management in pediatric oncology: Is it safe? *Journal of Pediatric Hematology Oncology, 34*(6), 416–420.

Anghelescu, D. L., Faughnan, L. G., Popenhagen, M. P., Oakes, L. L., Pei, D., & Burgoyne, L. L. (2014). Neuropathic pain referrals to a multidisciplinary pediatric cancer pain service. *Pain Management Nursing, 15*(1), 126–131.

Anghelescu, D. L., Patel, R. M., Mahoney, D. P., Trujillo, L., Faughnan, L. G., Steen, B. D., et al. (2016). Methadone prolongs cardiac conduction in young patients with cancer-related pain. *Journal of Opioid Management, 12*(2), 131–138.

Arane, K., Behboudi, A., & Goldman, R. D. (2017). Virtual reality for pain and anxiety management in children. *Canadian Family Physician Medecin de famille canadien, 63*(12), 932–934.

Azize, P. M., Humphreys, A., & Cattani, A. (2011). The impact of language on the expression and assessment of pain in children. *Intensive and Critical Care Nursing, 27*(5), 235–243.

Babl, F. E., Crellin, D., Cheng, J., et al. (2012). The use of faces, legs, activity, cry and consolability scale to assess procedural pain and distress in young children. *Pediatric Emergency Care, 28*(12), 1281–1296.

von Baeyer, C. L., Lin, V., Seidman, L. C., et al. (2011). Pain charts (body maps or manikins) in assessment of the location of pediatric pain. *Pain Management, 1*(1), 61–68.

Baker, D. W. (2017). History of the joint commission's pain standards: Lessons for today's prescription opioid epidemic. The joint commission's pain standards and the prescription opioid epidemic. *The Journal of the American Medical Association, 317*(11), 1117–1118.

Becker, E. M., Wilson, B., Chen-Lim, M. L., & Ely, E. (2019). The experience of pain and pain tool preferences of hospitalized youth. *Pain Management Nursing.*

Bembich, S., Cont, G., Causin, E., Paviotti, G., Marzari, P., & Demarini, S. (2018). Infant analgesia with a combination of breast milk, glucose, or maternal holding. *Pediatrics, 142*(3), e20173416.

Bennett, M. (2016). Pain management for chemotherapy-induced oral mucositis. *Nursing Child Young People, 28*(10), 25–29.

Best, K. M., Wypij, D., Asaro, L. A., & Curley, M. A. (2017). Patient, process, and system predictors of iatrogenic withdrawal syndrome in critically ill children. *Critical Care Medicine, 45*(1), e7–e15.

Biran, V., Gourrier, E., Cimerman, P., et al. (2011). Analgesic effects of EMLA cream and oral sucrose during venipuncture in preterm infants. *Pediatrics, 128*(1), e63–e70.

Birnie, K. A., Chambers, C. T., Chorney, J., Fernandez, C. V., & McGrath, P. J. (2016). A multi-informant multi-method investigation of family functioning and parent–child coping during children's acute pain. *Journal of Pediatric Psychology*.

Bodnar, J. (2017). A review of agents for palliative sedation/continuous deep sedation: Pharmacology and practical applications. *Journal of Pain & Palliative Care Pharmacotherapy, 31*(1), 16–37.

Boerlage, A. A., Ista, E., Duivenvoorden, H. J., et al. (2015). The COMFORT behavior scale detects clinically meaningful effects of analgesic and sedative treatment. *European Journal of Pain, 19*(4), 473–479.

Bos-Veneman, N. G. P., Otter, M., & Reijneveld, S. A. (2018). Using feeding to reduce pain during vaccination of formula-fed infants: A randomised controlled trial. *Archives of Disease in Childhood, 103*(12), 1132.

Breau, L. M., McGrath, P. J., Camfield, C. S., et al. (2002). Psychometric properties of the non-communicating children's pain checklist—revised. *Pain, 99*(1–2), 349–357.

Brown, R., Fortier, M. A., Zolghadr, S., Gulur, P., Jenkins, B. N., & Kain, Z. N. (2016). Postoperative pain management in children of hispanic origin: A descriptive cohort study. *Anesthesia & Analgesia, 122*(2), 497–502.

Bueno, M., Moreno-Ramos, M. C., Forni, E., & Kimura, A. F. (2019). Adaptation and initial validation of the premature infant pain profile–revised (PIPP-R) in Brazil. *Pain Management Nursing*.

Campbell, C. S., & Black, M. A. (2014). Dignity, death, and dilemmas: A study of Washington hospices and physician-assisted death. *Journal of Pain and Symptom Management, 47*(1), 137–153.

Carter, B., Arnott, J., Simons, J., & Bray, L. (2017). Developing a sense of knowing and acquiring the skills to manage pain in children with profound cognitive impairments: Mothers' perspectives. *Pain Research & Management*, 2514920–2514920.

Cascella, M., Bimonte, S., Saettini, F., & Muzio, M. R. (2019). The challenge of pain assessment in children with cognitive disabilities: Features and clinical applicability of different observational tools. *Journal of Paediatrics and Child Health, 55*(2), 129–135.

Chidambaran, V., Sadhasivam, S., & Mahmoud, M. (2017). Codeine and opioid metabolism: Implications and alternatives for pediatric pain management. *Current Opinion in Anaesthesiology, 30*(3), 349–356.

Chua, M. E., Firaza, P. N. B., Ming, J. M., Silangcruz, J. M. A., Braga, L. H., & Lorenzo, A. J. (2017). Lidocaine gel for urethral catheterization in children: A meta-analysis. *The Journal of Pediatrics, 190*, 207–214 e201.

Cicvaric, A., Divkovic, D., Tot, O. K., & Kvolik, S. (2018). Effect of pre-emptive paracetamol infusion on postoperative analgesic consumption in children undergoing elective herniorrhaphy. *Turkish Journal of Anaesthesiology and Reanimation, 46*(3), 197–200.

Claar, R. L., & Walker, L. S. (2006). Functional assessment of pediatric pain patients: Psychometric properties of the functional disability inventory. *Pain, 121*(1–2), 77–84.

Clark, L. (2011). Pain management in the pediatric population. *Critical Care Nursing Clinics of North, 23*(2), 291–301.

Cline, M. E., Herman, J., Shaw, E. R., et al. (1992). Standardization of the visual analogue scale. *Nursing Research, 41*(6), 378–380.

Connelly, M., & Sekhon, S. (2019). Current perspectives on the development and treatment of chronic daily headache in children and adolescents. *Pain Management, 9*(2), 175–189.

Crosta, Q. R., Ward, T. M., Walker, A. J., et al. (2014). A review of pain measures for hospitalized children with cognitive impairment. *Journal for Specialists in Pediatric Nursing, 19*(2), 109–118.

De Jong, A. E., Tuinebreijer, W. E., Bremer, M., et al. (2012). Construct validity of two pain behavior observation measurement instruments for young children with burns by Rasch analysis. *Pain, 153*(11), 2260–2266.

Despriee, Å. W., & Langeland, E. (2016). The effect of sucrose as pain relief/comfort during immunisation of 15-month-old children in health care centres: A randomised controlled trial. *Journal of Clinical Nursing, 25*(3–4), 372–380.

van Dijk, M., Roofthooft, D. W., Anand, K. J., et al. (2009). Taking up the challenge of measuring prolonged pain in (premature) neonates: The COMFORTneo scale seems promising. *The Clinical Journal of Pain, 25*(7), 607–616.

Dionysakopoulou, C., Giannakopoulou, M., Lianou, L., Bozas, E., Zannikos, K., & Matziou, V. (2018). Validation of Greek versions of the neonatal infant pain scale and premature infant pain profile in neonatal intensive care unit. *Pain Management Nursing, 19*(3), 313–319.

Donado, C., Solodiuk, J., Rangel, S. J., Nelson, C. P., Heeney, M. M., Mahan, S. T., et al. (2019). Patient- and nurse-controlled analgesia: 22-Year experience in a pediatric hospital. *Hospital Pediatrics, 9*(2), 129.

Dosenovic, S., Jelicic Kadic, A., Jeric, M., Boric, M., Markovic, D., Vucic, K., et al. (2018). Efficacy and safety outcome domains and outcome measures in systematic reviews of neuropathic pain conditions. *The Clinical Journal of Pain, 34*(7), 674–684.

Ehrentraut, J. H., Kern, K. D., Long, S. A., An, A. Q., Faughnan, L. G., & Anghelescu, D. L. (2014). Opioid misuse behaviors in adolescents and young adults in a hematology/oncology setting. *Journal of Pediatric Psychology, 39*(10), 1149–1160.

Fenn, N. E., & Plake, K. S. (2017). Opioid and benzodiazepine weaning in pediatric patients: Review of current literature. *Pharmacotherapy: The Journal of Human Pharmacology and Drug Therapy, 37*(11), 1458–1468.

Fernandes, A. M., De Campos, C., Batalha, L., et al. (2014). Pain assessment using the adolescent pediatric pain tool: A systematic review. *Pain Research and Management, 19*(4), 212–218.

Fisher, K., Laikin, A. M., Sharp, K. M. H., Criddle, C. A., Palermo, T. M., & Karlson, C. W. (2018). Temporal relationship between daily pain and actigraphy sleep patterns in pediatric sickle cell disease. *Journal of Behavioral Medicine, 41*(3), 416–422.

Fortier, M. A., Wahi, A., Bruce, C., et al. (2014). Pain management at home in children with cancer: A daily diary study. *Pediatric Blood and Cancer, 61*(6), 1029–1033.

Franck, L. S., Harris, S. K., Soetenga, D. J., et al. (2008). The withdrawal assessment tool–1 (WAT-1): An assessment instrument for monitoring opioid and benzodiazepine withdrawal symptoms in pediatric patients. *Pediatric Critical Care Medicine, 9*(6), 573–580.

Franck, L. S., Ridout, D., Howard, R., et al. (2011). A comparison of pain measures in newborn infants after cardiac surgery. *Pain, 152*(8), 1758–1765.

Friedrichsdorf, S. J. (2015). Pain outcomes in a US children's hospital: A prospective cross-sectional survey. *Hospital Pediatrics, 5*(1), 18–26.

Gao, H., Xu, G., Gao, H., Dong, R., Fu, H., Wang, D., et al. (2015). Effect of repeated kangaroo mother care on repeated procedural pain in preterm infants: A randomized controlled trial. *International Journal of Nursing Studies, 52*(7), 1157–1165.

Garra, F., Singer, A. J., Domingo, A., et al. (2013). The Wong-Baker pain FACES scale measures pain, not fear. *Pediatric Emergency Care, 29*(1), 17–20.

Getz, K. D., Miller, T. P., Seif, A. E., Li, Y., Huang, Y.-S. V., Fisher, B. T., et al. (2018). Opioid utilization among pediatric patients treated for newly diagnosed acute myeloid leukemia. *PLoS One, 13*(2), 1–15.

Gold, J. I., Mahrer, N. E., Yee, J., et al. (2009). Pain, fatigue and health-related quality of life in children and adolescents with chronic pain. *The Clinical Journal of Pain, 25*(5), 407–412.

Greene, M. S., & Chambers, R. A. (2015). Pseudoaddiction: Fact or fiction? an investigation of the medical literature. *Current Addiction Reports, 2*(4), 310–317.

Groenewald, C. B., Beals-Erickson, S. E., Ralston-Wilson, J., Rabbitts, J. A., & Palermo, T. M. (2017). Complementary and alternative medicine use by children with pain in the United States. *Academic Pediatrics, 17*(7), 785–793.

Habich, M., Wilson, D., Thielk, D., et al. (2012). Evaluating the effectiveness of pediatric pain management guidelines. *Journal of Pediatric Nursing, 27*(4), 336–345.

Harbaugh, C. M., & Gadepalli, S. K. (2019). Pediatric postoperative opioid prescribing and the opioid crisis. *Current Opinion in Pediatrics, 31*(3), 378–385.

Harrison, D., Joly, C., Chretien, C., Cochrane, S., Ellis, J., Lamontagne, C., et al. (2014). Pain prevalence in a pediatric hospital: Raising awareness during pain awareness week. *Pain Research and Management : The Journal of the Canadian Pain Society, 19*(1), e24–e30.

Hatfield, L. A., & Ely, E. A. (2015). Measurement of acute pain in infants: A review of behavioural and physiological variables. *Biological Research For Nursing, 17*(1), 100–111.

Heath, J. A., Oh, L. J., Clarke, N. E., et al. (2012). Complementary and alternative medicine use in children with cancer at the end of life. *Journal of Palliative Medicine, 15*(11), 1218–1221.

Hershey, A. D., Powers, S. W., Vockell, A. L., et al. (2001). PedMIDAS: Development of a questionnaire to assess disability of migraines in children. *Neurology*, *57*(11), 2034–2039.

Hershey, A. D., Powers, S. W., Vockell, A. L., et al. (2004). Development of a patient-based grading scale for PedMIDAS. *Cephalalgia*, *24*(10), 844–849.

Hickman, J., Varadarajan, J., & Weisman, S. J. (2014). Paediatric cancer pain. In P. C. McGrath, B. J. Stevens, S. M. Walker, et al. (Eds.), *Oxford textbook of paediatric pain*. Oxford UK: Oxford University Press.

Hicks, C. L., von Baeyer, C. L., Spafford, P. A., et al. (2001). The faces pain scale–revised: Toward a common metric in pediatric pain measurement. *Pain*, *93*(2), 173–183.

Hillman, B. A., Tabrizi, M. N., Gauda, E. B., et al. (2015). The neonatal pain, agitation and sedation scale and the bedside nurse's assessment of neonates. *Journal of Perinatology*, *35*(2), 128–131.

Hummel, P., Puchalski, M., & Creech, S. D. (2008). Clinical reliability and validity of the N-PASS: Neonatal pain, agitation and sedation scale with prolonged pain. *Journal of Perinatology*, *28*(1), 55–60.

Hyman, P. E. (2016). Chronic and recurrent abdominal pain. *Pediatrics in Review*, *37*(9), 377.

Jenkins, B. N., & Fortier, M. A. (2014). Developmental and cultural perspectives on children's postoperative pain management at home. *Pain Management*, *4*(6), 407–412.

Kashikar-Zuck, S., Flowers, S. R., Claar, R. L., et al. (2011). Clinical utility and validity of the Functional Disability Inventory among a multicenter sample of youth with chronic pain. *Pain*, *152*(7), 1600–1607.

Kassab, M., Foster, J. P., Foureur, M., et al. (2012). Sweet-tasting solutions for needle-related procedural pain in infants one month to one year of age. *Cochrane Database of Systematic Reviews*.

Kaye, E. C., Gattas, M., Kiefer, A., Reynolds, J., Zalud, K., Li, C., et al. (2019). Provision of palliative and hospice care to children in the community: A population study of hospice nurses. *Journal of Pain and Symptom Management*, *57*(2), 241–250.

Kesavan, K. (2015). Neurodevelopmental implications of neonatal pain and morphine exposure. *Pediatric Annals*, *44*(11), e260–264. https://doi.org/10.3928/00904481-20151112-08.

Kozlowski, L. J., Kost-Byerly, S., Colantuoni, E., et al. (2014). Pain prevalence, intensity, assessment and management in a hospitalized pediatric population. *Pain Management Nursing*, *15*(1), 22–35.

Krechel, S. W., & Bildner, J. (1995). Cries: A new neonatal postoperative pain measurement score: Initial testing of validity and reliability. *Paediatric Anaesthesia*, *5*(1), 53–61.

Lawrence, J., Alcock, D., McGrath, P., et al. (1993). The development of a tool to assess neonatal pain. *Neonatal Network*, *12*(6), 59–66.

Leahy, I., Berry, J. G., Johnson, C. J., Crofton, C., Staffa, S. J., & Ferrari, L. (2018). Does the current American Society of Anesthesiologists physical status classification represent the chronic disease burden in children undergoing general anesthesia? Anesthesia & Analgesia. Publish Ahead of Print.

Logan, D. E., Coakley, R. M., & Garcia, B. N. B. (2014). Cognitive-behavioural interventions. In P. C. McGrath, B. J. Stevens, S. M. Walker, et al. (Eds.), *Oxford textbook of paediatric pain*. Oxford UK: Oxford University Press.

Lootens, C. C., & Rapoff, M. A. (2011). Measures of pediatric pain: 21-numbered circle visual analog scale (VAS), E-Ouch electronic pain diary, oucher, pain behavior observation method, pediatric pain assessment yool (PPAT), and pediatric pain questionnaire (PPQ). *Arthritis Care & Research*, *63*(Suppl. 11), S253–S262.

Luffy, R., & Grove, S. K. (2003). Examining the validity, reliability, and preference of three pediatric pain measurement tools in African-American children. *Pediatric Nursing*, *29*(1), 54–60.

Lunoe, M. M., Drendel, A. L., Levas, M. N., et al. (2015). A randomized clinical trial of jet-injected lidocaine to reduce venipuncture pain for young children. *Annals of Emergency Medicine*, *66*(5), 466–474.

Manworren, R. C. B., & Gilson, A. M. (2015). CE: Nurses' role in preventing prescription opioid diversion. *AJN: American Journal of Nursing*, *115*(8), 34–40.

Massaro, M., Ronfani, L., Ferrara, G., et al. (2014). A comparison of three scales for measuring pain in children with cognitive impairment. *Acta Paediatrica*, *103*(11), e495–e500.

Matsuishi, Y., Hoshino, H., Shimojo, N., Enomoto, Y., Kido, T., Hoshino, T., et al. (2018). Verifying the validity and reliability of the Japanese version of the face, legs, activity, cry, consolability (FLACC) behavioral scale. *PLoS One*, *13*(3), e0194094-e0194094.

McClafferty, H., Vohra, S., Bailey, M., Brown, M., Esparham, A., Gerstbacher, D., et al. (2017). Pediatric integrative medicine. *Pediatrics*, *140*(3), e20171961.

McGrath, P. J., Walco, G. A., Turk, D. C., et al. (2008). Core outcome domains and measures for pediatric acute and chronic/recurrent pain clinical trials: PedIMMPACT recommendations. *The Journal of Pain*, *9*(9), 771–783.

Meek, J., & Huertas, A. (2012). Cochrane review: Non-nutritive sucking, kangaroo care and swaddling/facilitated tucking are observed to reduce procedural pain in infants and young children. *Evidence-Based Nursing*, *15*(3), 84–85.

Melzack, R. (1975). The McGill pain questionnaire: Major properties and scoring methods. *Pain*, *1*(3), 277–299.

Meredith, J. R., O'Keefe, K. P., & Galwankar, S. (2008). Pediatric procedural sedation and analgesia. *Journal of Emergencies, Trauma, and Shock*, *1*(2), 88–96.

Merkel, S. I., Voepel-Lewis, T., Shayevitz, J. R., et al. (1997). The FLACC: A behavioral scale for scoring postoperative pain in young children. *Pediatric Nursing*, *23*(3), 293–297.

Michelet, D., Andreu-Gallien, J., Bensalah, T., et al. (2012). A meta-analysis of the use of nonsteroidal antiinflammatory drugs for pediatric postoperative pain. *Anesthesia & Analgesia*, *114*(2), 393–406.

Monitto, C. L., Hsu, A., Gao, S., Vozzo, P. T., Park, P. S., Roter, D., et al. (2017). Opioid prescribing for the treatment of acute pain in children on hospital discharge. *Anesthesia & Analgesia*, *125*(6), 2113–2122.

Mudd, S. (2011). Intranasal fentanyl for pain management in children: A systematic review of the literature. *Journal of Pediatric Health Care*, *25*(5), 316–322.

National Center for Complementary and Integrative Health. (2019). Complementary, alternative or integrative health: what's in a name? Available at: https://nccih.nih.gov/health/integrative-health. Accessed May 4th 2019

Nelson, S. E., Adams, A. J., Buczek, M. J., Anthony, C. A., & Shah, A. S. (2019). Postoperative pain and opioid use in children with supracondylar humeral fractures: Balancing analgesia and opioid stewardship. *The Journal of Bone & Joint Surgery*, *101*(2), 119–126.

Oakes, L. L. (2011). *Infant and child pain management*. New York: Springer Publishing.

Orentlicher, D., Pope, T. M., & Rich, B. A. (2016). Clinical criteria for physician aid in dying. *Journal of Palliative Medicine*, *19*(3), 259–262.

Owens, J. A., Spirito, A., & McGuinn, M. (2000). The children's sleep habits questionnaire (CSHQ): Psychometric properties of a survey instrument for school-aged children. *Sleep*, *23*(8), 1043–1051.

Özalp Gerçeker, G., Bilsin, E., Binay, Ş., Bal Yılmaz, H., & Jacob, E. (2018). Cultural adaptation of the adolescent pediatric pain tool in Turkish children with cancer. *European Journal of Oncology Nursing*, *34*, 28–34.

Pasero, C., & McCaffrey, M. (2011). *Pain assessment and pharmacologic management*. St Louis: Elsevier.

Passik, S. D. (2009). Issues in long-term opioid therapy: Unmet needs, risks, and solutions. *Mayo Clinic Proceedings*, *84*(7), 593–601.

Peng, H. F., Yin, T., Yang, L., Wang, C., Chang, Y. C., Jeng, M. J., et al. (2018). Non-nutritive sucking, oral breast milk, and facilitated tucking relieve preterm infant pain during heel-stick procedures: A prospective, randomized controlled trial. *International Journal of Nursing*, *77*, 162–170.

Phelps, P., Achey, T. S., Mieure, K. D., Cuellar, L., MacMaster, H., Pecho, R., et al. (2018). A survey of opioid medication stewardship practices at academic medical centers. *Hospital Pharmacy*, *54*(1), 57–62.

Pillai Riddell, R. R., Racine, N. M., Gennis, H. G., Turcotte, K., Uman, L. S., Horton, R. E., et al. (2015). Non-pharmacological management of infant and young child procedural pain. *Cochrane Database of Systematic Reviews*, (12), CD006275-CD006275.

Pinkerton, R., & Hardy, J. R. (2017). Opioid addiction and misuse in adult and adolescent patients with cancer. *Internal Medicine Journal*, *47*(6), 632–636.

Poirot, I., Laudy, V., Rabilloud, M., Roche, S., Ginhoux, T., Kassaï, B., et al. (2017). Prevalence of pain in 240 non-ambulatory children with severe cerebral palsy. *Annals of Physical and Rehabilitation Medicine*, *60*(6), 371–375.

Quinn, B. L., Sheldon, L. K., & Cooley, M. E. (2014). Pediatric pain assessment by drawn faces scales: A review. *Pain Management Nursing*, *15*(4), 909–918.

Rabbitts, J. A., Zhou, C., Narayanan, A., & Palermo, T. M. (2017). Longitudinal and temporal associations between daily pain and sleep patterns after major pediatric surgery. *The Journal of Pain : Official Journal of the American Pain Society*, 18(6), 656–663.

Racoosin, J. A., Roberson, D. W., Pacanowski, M. A., et al. (2013). New evidence about an old drug—risk with codeine after adenotonsillectomy. *New England Journal of Medicine, 368*(23), 2155–2157.

Rastogi, S., & Campbell, F. (2014). Drugs for neuropathic pain. In P. C. McGrath, B. J. Stevens, S. M. Walker, et al. (Eds.), *Oxford textbook of paediatric pain*. Oxford UK: Oxford University Press.

Ria, D., Edmund Allen, L., & Darren, F. (2017). Acute pain management in hospitalized children. *Reviews on Recent Clinical Trials, 12*(4), 277–283.

Rodrigues, A. C., & Kang, P. B. (2016). Neuropathic and myopathic pain. *Seminars in Pediatric Neurology, 23*(3), 242–247.

Saad, T. C. (2017). Euthanasia in Belgium: Legal, historical and political review. *Issues in Law & Medicine, 32*(2), 183–204.

Samardzic, J., Allegaert, K., & Bajcetic, M. (2015). Developmental pharmacology: A moving target. *International Journal of Pharmaceutics, 492*(1), 335–337.

Sansone, P., Passavanti, M. B., Fiorelli, A., Aurilio, C., Colella, U., De Nardis, L., et al. (2017). Efficacy of the topical 5% lidocaine medicated plaster in the treatment of chronic post-thoracotomy neuropathic pain. *Pain Management, 7*(3), 189–196.

Savedra, M. C., Holzemer, W. L., Tesler, M. D., et al. (1993). Assessment of postoperation pain in children and adolescents using the adolescent pediatric pain tool. *Nursing Research, 42*(1), 5–9.

Savedra, M. C., Tesler, M. D., Holzemer, W. L., et al. (1989). Pain location: Validity and reliability of body outline markings by hospitalized children and adolescents. *Research in Nursing & Health, 12*(5), 307–314.

Schütze, T., Längler, A., Zuzak, T. J., Schmidt, P., & Zernikow, B. (2016). Use of complementary and alternative medicine by pediatric oncology patients during palliative care. *Supportive Care in Cancer, 24*(7), 2869–2875.

Setlur, A., & Friedland, H. (2018). Treatment of pain with intranasal fentanyl in pediatric patients in an acute care setting: A systematic review. *Pain Management, 8*(5), 341–352.

Smitherman, A. B., Mohabir, D., Wilkins, T. M., Blatt, J., Nichols, H. B., & Dusetzina, S. B. (2018). Early post-therapy prescription drug usage among childhood and adolescent cancer survivors. *The Journal of Pediatrics, 195*, 161–168.e167.

Sneddon, P., Peacock, G. G., & Crowley, S. L. (2013). Assessment of sleep problems in preschool aged children: An adaptation of the children's sleep habits questionnaire. *Behavioral Sleep Medicine, 11*(4), 283–296.

Stahlschmidt, L., Zernikow, B., & Wager, J. (2018). Satisfaction with an intensive interdisciplinary pain treatment for children and adolescents: An independent outcome measure? *The Clinical Journal of Pain, 34*(9), 795–803.

Stevens, B. J., Gibbins, S., Yamada, J., et al. (2014). The premature infant pain profile-revised (PIPP-R): Initial validation and feasibility. *The Clinical Journal of Pain, 30*(3), 238–243.

Stevens, B., Yamada, J., Campbell-Yeo, M., Gibbins, S., Harrison, D., Dionne, K., et al. (2018). The minimally effective dose of sucrose for procedural pain relief in neonates: A randomized controlled trial. *BioMed Central Pediatrics, 18*(1), 85–85.

Stevens, B., Yamada, J., Ohlsson, A., Haliburton, S., & Shorkey, A. (2016). Sucrose for analgesia in newborn infants undergoing painful procedures. *Cochrane Database of Systematic Reviews, 7*(7), CD001069-CD001069.

Stinson, J. N., Jibb, L. A., Lalloo, C., Feldman, B. M., McGrath, P. J., Petroz, G. C., et al. (2014). Comparison of average weekly pain using recalled paper and momentary assessment electronic diary reports in children with arthritis. *The Clinical Journal of Pain, 30*(12), 1044–1050.

Stinson, J. N., Stevens, B. J., Feldman, B. M., et al. (2008). Construct validity of a multidimensional electronic pain diary for adolescents with arthritis. *Pain, 136*(3), 281–292.

Sung, L., Robinson, P., Treister, N., Baggott, T., Gibson, P., Tissing, W., et al. (2017). Guideline for the prevention of oral and oropharyngeal mucositis in children receiving treatment for cancer or undergoing haematopoietic stem cell transplantation. *BMJ Supportive & Palliative Care, 7*(1), 7–16.

Suresh, S., Birmingham, P. K., & Kozlowski, R. J. (2012). Pediatric pain management. *Anesthesiology Clinics, 30*(1), 101–117.

Sweet, S., & McGrath, P. (1998). Physiological measures of pain. In G. A. Finley, & P. J. McGrath (Eds.), *Measurement of pain in infants and children*. Seattle: IASP Press.

Telfer, P., & Kaya, B. (2017). Optimizing the care model for an uncomplicated acute pain episode in sickle cell disease. *Hematology. American Society of Hematology. Education Program, 2017*(1), 525–533.

Tesler, M. D., Savedra, M. C., Holzemer, W. L., et al. (1991). The word-graphic rating scale as a measure of children's and adolescents' pain intensity. *Research in Nursing & Health, 14*(5), 361–371.

Thienprayoon, R., Porter, K., Tate, M., Ashby, M., & Meyer, M. (2017). Risk stratification for opioid misuse in children, adolescents, and young adults: A quality improvement project. *Pediatrics, 139*(1).

Tobias, J. D. (2014a). Acute pain management in infants and children-Part 1: Pain pathways, pain assessment, and outpatient pain management. *Pediatric Annals, 43*(7), e163–e168.

Tobias, J. D. (2014b). Acute pain management in infants and children-Part 2: Intravenous opioids, intravenous nonsteroidal anti-inflammatory drugs, and managing adverse effects. *Pediatric Annals, 43*(7), e169–e175.

Twycross, A. (2010). Managing pain in children: Where to from here? *Journal of Clinical Nursing, 19*(15–16), 2090–2099.

Valrie, C. R., Bromberg, M. H., Palermo, T., et al. (2013). A systematic review of sleep in pediatric pain populations. *Journal of Developmental and Behavioral Pediatrics, 34*(2), 120–128.

Varni, J. W., Seid, M., & Rode, C. A. (1999). The PedsQL: Measurement model for the pediatric quality of life inventory. *Medical Care, 37*(2), 126–139.

Voepel-Lewis, T., Malviya, S., Tait, A. R., et al. (2008). A comparison of the clinical utility of pain assessment tools for children with cognitive impairment. *Anesthesia & Analgesia, 106*(1), 72–78.

Walco, G. A., Gove, N., Phillips, J., & Weisman, S. J. (2017). Opioid analgesics administered for pain in the inpatient pediatric setting. *The Journal of Pain, 18*(10), 1270–1276.

Walia, H., Tumin, D., Wrona, S., Martin, D., Bhalla, T., & Tobias, J. D. (2016). Safety and efficacy of nurse-controlled analgesia in patients less than 1 year of age. *Journal of Pain Research, 9*, 385–390.

Walker, L. S., & Greene, J. W. (1991). The functional disability inventory: Measuring a neglected dimension of child health status. *Journal of Pediatric Psychology, 16*(1), 39–58.

Whiteside, L. K., Russo, J., Wang, J., Ranney, M. L., Neam, V., & Zatzick, D. F. (2016). Predictors of sustained prescription opioid use after admission for Trauma in adolescents. *The Journal of Adolescent Health : Official Publication of the Society for Adolescent Medicine, 58*(1), 92–97.

Wiegele, M., Marhofer, P., & Lönnqvist, P. A. (2019). Caudal epidural blocks in paediatric patients: A review and practical considerations. *British Journal of Anaesthesia, 122*(4), 509–517.

Williams, A. E., Czyzewski, D. I., Self, M. M., & Shulman, R. J. (2015). Are child anxiety and somatization associated with pain in pain-related functional gastrointestinal disorders? *Journal of Health Psychology, 20*(4), 369–379.

Wong, D. L., & Baker, C. M. (1988). Pain in children: Comparison of assessment scales. *Pediatric Nursing, 14*(1), 9–17.

World Health Organization. (2012). *WHO guidelines on the pharmacological treatment of persisting pain in children with medical illnesses*. Geneva: World Health Organization.

Yellon, R. F., Kenna, M. A., Cladis, F. P., et al. (2014). What is the best non-codeine post adenotonsilectomy pain management for children? *The Laryngoscope, 124*(8), 1737–1738.

Yetwin, A. K., Mahrer, N. E., John, C., & Gold, J. I. (2018). Does pain intensity matter? the relation between coping and quality of life in pediatric patients with chronic pain. *Journal of Pediatric Nursing, 40*, 7–13.

Yilmaz, G., Caylan, N., Oguz, M., et al. (2014). Oral sucrose administration to reduce pain response during immunization in 16-19-month infants: A randomized, placebo-controlled trial. *European Journal of Pediatrics, 173*(11), 1527–1532.

Zamora-Kapoor, A., Omidpanah, A., Monico, E., Buchwald, D., Harris, R., & Jimenez, N. (2015). The role of language use in reports of musculoskeletal pain among hispanic and non-hispanic white adolescents. *Journal of Transcultural Nursing, 28*(2), 144–151.

Zempsky, W. T. (2014). Topical anesthetics and analgesics. In P. C. McGrath, B. J. Stevens, S. M. Walker, et al. (Eds.), *Oxford textbook of paediatric pain*. Oxford UK: Oxford University Press.

6

Childhood Communicable and Infectious Diseases

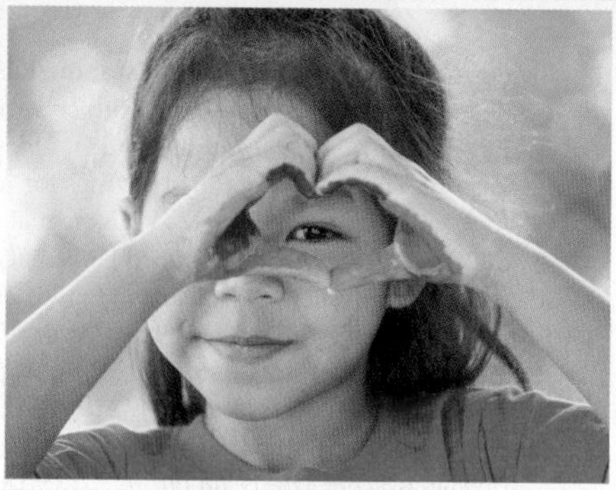

Marilyn J. Hockenberry

http://evolve.elsevier.com/wong/essentials

CONCEPTS

- Immunity
- Infection
- Safety

INFECTION CONTROL

According to the Centers for Disease Control and Prevention, although progress has been made on hospital-acquired infections (HAIs), each day about 1 in 31 patients will acquire at least one HAI (Centers for Disease Control and Prevention, 2018). These infections occur when there is interaction among patients, health care personnel, equipment, and bacteria. HAIs are preventable if caregivers practice meticulous hand washing, cleaning, and disposal techniques.

Standard Precautions synthesize the major features of universal (i.e., blood and body fluid) precautions (designed to reduce the risk of transmission of bloodborne pathogens) and body substance isolation (designed to reduce the risk of transmission of pathogens from moist body substances). Standard Precautions involve the use of barrier protection (personal protective equipment [PPE]), such as gloves, goggles, gowns, and masks, to prevent contamination from blood; all body fluids, secretions, and excretions, except sweat, regardless of whether they contain visible blood; nonintact skin; and mucous membranes. Standard Precautions are designed for the care of all patients to reduce the risk of transmission of microorganisms from both recognized and unrecognized sources of infection.

Several years ago, the Centers for Disease Control and Prevention recommended adding Respiratory Hygiene/Cough Etiquette and safe injection practices to Standard Precautions. Respiratory Hygiene/Cough Etiquette stresses the importance of source control measures to contain respiratory secretions to prevent droplet and fomite transmission of viral respiratory tract infections such as respiratory syncytial virus, influenza, and adenovirus. Safe injection practices involve the use of safety-engineered sharps devices to prevent sharps injury as a component of Standard Precautions.

Hand hygiene continues to be the single most important practice to reduce the transmission of infectious diseases in health care settings (Bolon, 2016). Hand hygiene includes hand washing with soap and water, as well as the use of alcohol-based products for hand disinfection.

Transmission-Based Precautions are designed for patients with documented or suspected infection or colonization (i.e., presence of microorganisms in or on patient but without clinical signs and symptoms of infection) with highly transmissible or epidemiologically important pathogens for which additional precautions beyond Standard Precautions are needed to interrupt transmission in hospitals. The three types of Transmission-Based Precautions are (1) Airborne Precautions, (2) Droplet Precautions, and (3) Contact Precautions. They may be combined for diseases that have multiple routes of transmission (Box 6.1). They are to be used in addition to Standard Precautions.

Airborne Precautions reduce the risk of airborne transmission of infectious agents. Airborne transmission occurs by dissemination of either airborne droplet nuclei (i.e., small-particle residue [≤5 mm] of evaporated droplets that may remain suspended in the air for long periods) or dust particles containing the infectious agent. Microorganisms carried in this manner can be dispersed widely by air currents and may become inhaled by or deposited on a susceptible host within the same room or over a longer distance from the source patient, depending on environmental factors. Special air handling and ventilation are required to prevent airborne transmission. The term *airborne infection isolation room* (AIIR) has replaced *negative pressure isolation room;* this room is used to isolate persons with a suspected or confirmed airborne infectious disease transmitted by the airborne route such as measles, varicella, and tuberculosis.

Droplet Precautions reduce the risk of droplet transmission of infectious agents. Droplet transmission involves contact of the conjunctivae or the mucous membranes of the nose or mouth of a susceptible person with large-particle droplets (>5 mm) containing microorganisms generated from a person who has a clinical disease or who is a carrier of the microorganism. Droplets are generated from the source person primarily during coughing, sneezing, or talking, and during procedures such as suctioning and bronchoscopy. Transmission requires close contact between source and recipient persons because droplets do not remain suspended in the air and generally travel only short distances, usually 3 feet or less, through the air. Because droplets do not remain suspended in the air, special air handling and ventilation are not required to prevent droplet transmission. Droplet Precautions apply to any patient with known or suspected infection with pathogens that can be transmitted by infectious droplets (see Box 6.1).

Contact Precautions reduce the risk of transmission of microorganisms by direct or indirect contact. Direct-contact transmission involves skin-to-skin contact and physical transfer of microorganisms to a susceptible host from an infected or colonized person, such as occurs when turning or bathing patients. Direct-contact transmission also can occur between two patients (e.g., by hand contact). Indirect contact transmission involves contact of a susceptible host with a

BOX 6.1 Types of Precautions and Patients Requiring Them

Standard Precautions for Prevention of Transmission of Pathogens

Use Standard Precautions for the care of all patients. Hand hygiene should be emphasized as part of Standard Precautions.

Respiratory Hygiene/Cough Etiquette

In addition to Standard Precautions, the Centers for Disease Control and Prevention suggest a combination of measures designed to minimize the transmission of respiratory pathogens via droplet or airborne routes in the health care environment. Measures include covering the mouth and nose during coughing and sneezing; offering a surgical mask to persons who are coughing; using tissues to contain respiratory secretions; and turning the head away from others and keeping a space of 3 feet or more when coughing. These measures should be used on entry to the health care institution for patients and visitors or family members who have symptoms of respiratory infection.

Airborne Precautions

In addition to Standard Precautions, use Airborne Precautions and an airborne infection isolation room (AIIR) for patients known or suspected to have serious illnesses transmitted by airborne droplet nuclei. Examples of such illnesses include measles, varicella (including disseminated zoster), and tuberculosis.

Droplet Precautions

In addition to Standard Precautions, use Droplet Precautions for patients known or suspected to have serious illnesses transmitted by large particle droplets. Examples of such illnesses include the following:

- Invasive *Haemophilus influenzae* type b disease, including meningitis, pneumonia, epiglottitis, and sepsis
- Invasive *Neisseria meningitidis* disease, including meningitis, pneumonia, and sepsis
- Other serious bacterial respiratory tract infections spread by droplet transmission, including diphtheria (pharyngeal), mycoplasmal pneumonia, pertussis, pneumonic plague, streptococcal pharyngitis, pneumonia, or scarlet fever in infants and young children
- Serious viral infections spread by droplet transmission, including adenovirus, influenza, mumps, human parvovirus B19, and rubella

Contact Precautions

In addition to Standard Precautions, use Contact Precautions for patients known or suspected to have serious illnesses easily transmitted by direct patient contact or by contact with items in the patient's environment. Examples of such illnesses include the following:

- Gastrointestinal, respiratory, skin, or wound infections or colonization with multidrug-resistant bacteria judged by the infection control program, based on current state, regional, or national recommendations, to be of special clinical and epidemiologic significance
- Enteric infections with a low infectious dose or prolonged environmental survival, including *Clostridium difficile;* for diapered or incontinent patients: enterohemorrhagic *Escherichia coli* 0157:H7, *Shigella* organisms, hepatitis A, or rotavirus
- Respiratory syncytial virus, parainfluenza virus, or enteroviral infections in infants and young children
- Skin infections that are highly contagious or that may occur on dry skin, including diphtheria (cutaneous), herpes simplex virus (neonatal or mucocutaneous), impetigo, major (noncontained) abscesses, cellulitis or decubitus, pediculosis, scabies, staphylococcal furunculosis in infants and young children, zoster (disseminated or in the immunocompromised host)
- Viral or hemorrhagic conjunctivitis
- Viral hemorrhagic infections (Ebola, Lassa, or Marburg)

Modified from Siegel, J. D., Rhinehart, E., Jackson, M., et al. (2007). *2007 Guideline for isolation precautions: Preventing transmission of infectious agents in healthcare settings.* Retrieved from https://www.cdc.gov/hicpac/pdf/isolation/Isolation2007.pdf

contaminated intermediate object, usually inanimate, in the patient's environment (see Nursing Alert box). Contact Precautions apply to specified patients known or suspected to be infected or colonized with microorganisms that can be transmitted by direct or indirect contact.

! NURSING ALERT

The most common piece of medical equipment, the stethoscope, can be a potent source of harmful microorganisms and nosocomial infections. Consider also the keyboard and desktop as potential sources.

Nurses caring for young children are frequently in contact with body substances, especially urine, feces, and vomitus. Nurses need to exercise judgment concerning those situations when gloves, gowns, or masks are necessary. For example, wear gloves and possibly gowns for changing diapers when there are loose or explosive stools. Otherwise, the plastic lining of disposable diapers provides a sufficient barrier between the hands and body substances, and therefore gloves are adequate.

Antimicrobial-resistant organisms are causing increasing numbers of HAIs. In hospitals, patients are the most significant sources of methicillin-resistant *Staphylococcus aureus* (MRSA), and the main mode of transmission is patient-to-patient transmission via the hands of a health care provider. Hand washing is the most critical infection control practice.

During feedings, wear gowns if the child is likely to vomit or spit up, which often occurs during burping. When wearing gloves, wash the hands thoroughly after removing them because gloves fail to provide complete protection. The absence of visible leaks does not indicate that gloves are intact.

Another essential practice of infection control is that all needles (uncapped and unbroken) are disposed of in a rigid, puncture-resistant container located near the site of use. Consequently, these containers are installed in each patient's room. Because children are naturally curious, extra attention is needed in selecting a suitable type of container and a location that prevents access to the discarded needles (Fig. 6.1). The use of needleless systems allows secure syringe or intravenous (IV) tubing attachment to vascular access devices without the risk of needlestick injury to the child or nurse.

IMMUNIZATIONS

One of the most dramatic advances in pediatrics has been the decline of infectious diseases during the 20th century because of the widespread use of immunization for preventable diseases. This trend has continued into the 21st century with the development of newer vaccines. Although many of the immunizations can be given to individuals of any age, the recommended primary schedule begins during infancy and, with the exception of boosters, is completed during early childhood. This section includes a discussion of childhood immunizations for diphtheria, tetanus, and acellular pertussis (DTaP); poliovirus; measles, mumps, and rubella (MMR); *Haemophilus influenzae* type B (Hib); hepatitis B virus (HBV); hepatitis A virus (HAV); meningococcal disease; pneumococcal conjugate vaccine (PCV); influenza (and H1N1); varicella-zoster virus (VZV; chickenpox); rotavirus; and human papillomaviruses. Selected vaccines generally reserved for children considered at high risk for the disease are discussed here and as appropriate throughout the text.

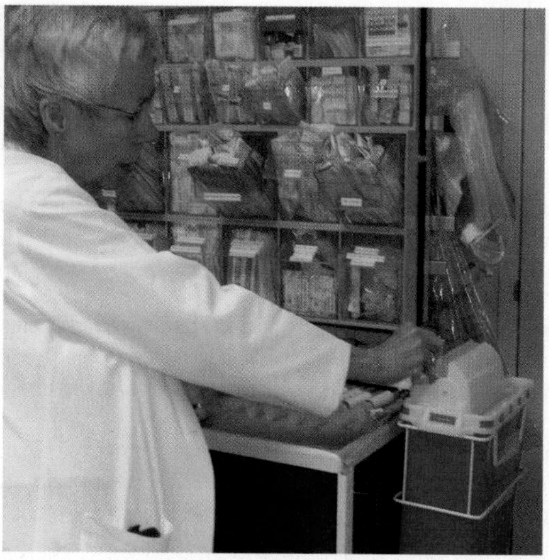

Fig. 6.1 To prevent needlestick injuries, used needles (and other sharp instruments) are not capped or broken and are disposed of in a rigid, puncture-resistant container located near site of use. Note placement of container to prevent children's access to contents.

To facilitate an understanding of immunizations, key terms are listed in Box 6.2. Although in this discussion the terms *vaccination* and *immunization* are used interchangeably in reference to active immunization, they are not synonymous because the administration of an immunobiologic such as a vaccine cannot automatically be equated with the development of adequate immunity.

Schedule for Immunizations

In the United States, two organizations, the Advisory Committee on Immunization Practices of the Centers for Disease Control and Prevention and the Committee on Infectious Diseases of the American Academy of Pediatrics, govern the recommendations for immunization policies and procedures. In Canada, recommendations are from the National Advisory Committee on Immunization under the authority of the Minister of Health and Public Health Agency of Canada. The policies of each committee are recommendations, not rules, and they change as a result of advances in the field of immunology. Nurses need to be knowledgeable about the purpose of each organization, view immunization practices in light of the needs of each child and the community, and keep informed of the latest advances and changes in policy.

The recommended age for beginning primary immunizations of infants is at birth or within 2 weeks of birth. Children born preterm

BOX 6.2 Key Immunization Terms

Immunization—Inclusive term denoting the process of inducing or providing active or passive immunity artificially by administering an immunobiologic

Immunity—An inherited or acquired state in which an individual is resistant to the occurrence or the effects of a specific disease, particularly an infectious agent

Natural immunity—Innate immunity or resistance to infection or toxicity

Acquired immunity—Immunity from exposure to the invading agent, either bacteria, virus, or toxin

Active immunity—A state in which immune bodies are actively formed against specific antigens, either naturally by having had the disease clinically or subclinically, or artificially by introducing the antigen into the individual

Passive immunity—Temporary immunity obtained by transfusing immunoglobulins or antitoxins either artificially from another human or an animal that has been actively immunized against an antigen or naturally from the mother to the fetus via the placenta

Antibody—A protein, found mostly in serum, that is formed in response to exposure to a specific antigen

Antigen—A variety of foreign substances, including bacteria, viruses, toxins, and foreign proteins, that stimulate the formation of antibodies

Attenuate—Reduce the virulence (infectiousness) of a pathogenic microorganism by such measures as treating it with heat or chemicals or cultivating it on a certain medium

Immunobiologic—Antigenic substances (e.g., vaccines and toxoids) or antibody-containing preparations (e.g., globulins and antitoxins) from human or animal donors, used for active or passive immunization or therapy

Vaccine—A suspension of live (usually attenuated) or inactivated microorganisms (e.g., bacteria, viruses, rickettsiae) or fractions of the microorganism administered to induce immunity and prevent infectious disease or its sequelae

Toxoid—A modified bacterial toxin that has been made nontoxic but retains the ability to stimulate the formation of antitoxin

Antitoxin—A solution of antibodies (e.g., diphtheria antitoxin, botulinum antitoxin) derived from the serum of animals immunized with specific antigens and used to confer passive immunity and for treatment

Immunoglobulin (Ig) or intravenous immunoglobulin (IVIG)—A sterile solution containing antibodies from large pools of human blood plasma; primarily indicated for routine maintenance of immunity of certain immunodeficient persons and for passive immunization against measles and hepatitis A

Specific immunoglobulins—Special preparations obtained from blood plasma from donor pools preselected for a high antibody content against a specific antigen (e.g., hepatitis B immunoglobulin, varicella-zoster immunoglobulin, rabies immunoglobulin, tetanus immunoglobulin, and cytomegalovirus immunoglobulin); as with Ig and IVIG, do not transmit hepatitis B virus, human immunodeficiency virus, or other infectious diseases

Vaccination—Originally referred to inoculation with vaccinia smallpox virus to make a person immune to smallpox; currently denotes physical act of administering any vaccine or toxoid

Herd immunity—A condition in which the majority of the population community is vaccinated and the spread of certain diseases is stopped because the population that has been vaccinated protects those in the same population who are unvaccinated

Monovalent vaccine—Vaccine designed to vaccinate against a single antigen or organism

Conjugate vaccine—A carrier protein with proven immunologic potential combined with a less antigenic polysaccharide antigen to enhance the type and magnitude of the immune response (e.g., *Haemophilus influenzae* type b [Hib])

Combination vaccine—Combination of multiple vaccines into one parenteral form

Polyvalent vaccine—Vaccine designed to vaccinate against two or more antigens or organisms (e.g., inactivated poliovirus vaccine [IPV])

Cocooning—Strategy of protecting infants from pertussis by vaccinating all persons who come in close contact with the infant, including the mother, grandparents, and health care workers.

TABLE 6.1 Pediatric Quality Indicator[a]

Immunizations for Adolescents	
Measure	The percentage of adolescents 13 years of age who had the recommended immunizations by their 13th birthday.
Numerator	Adolescents who had one dose of meningococcal vaccine on or between the patient's 11th and 13th birthdays Adolescents who had one tetanus, diphtheria toxoids, and acellular pertussis vaccine (Tdap) on or between the patient's 10th and 13th birthdays Adolescents who had at least three human papillomavirus (HPV) vaccines on or between the patient's 9th and 13th birthdays.
Denominator	Adolescents who turn 13 years of age during the measurement period.

[a]Endorsed by the National Quality Forum NQF #0394 and 2019 Core Set of Children's Health Care Quality Measures for Medicaid and CHIP. https://www.medicaid.gov/federal-policy-guidance/downloads/cib112018.pdf.

should receive the full dose of each vaccine at the appropriate chronologic age. A recommended catch-up schedule for children not immunized during infancy is available at the Centers for Disease Control and Prevention website (https://www.cdc.gov/vaccines/schedules/downloads/child/0-18yrs-child-combined-schedule.pdf). Immunization recommendation schedules for Canadian children are available at http://www.phac-aspc.gc.ca/im/is-cv/index-eng.php.

Children who began primary immunization at the recommended age but fail to receive all doses do not need to begin the series again but instead receive only the missed doses. Table 6.1 reports the quality indicators for immunizations for adolescents. For situations in which there is doubt that the child will return for immunization according to the optimum schedule, HBV vaccine (HepB), DTaP, IPV, MMR, varicella, and Hib vaccines can be administered simultaneously at separate injection sites. Parenteral vaccines are given in separate syringes in different injection sites (Kimberlin, Brady, Jackson, et al., 2018).

Recommendations for Routine Immunizations[a]

Hepatitis B Virus

HBV is a significant pediatric disease because HBV infections that occur during childhood and adolescence can lead to fatal consequences from cirrhosis or liver cancer during adulthood. Up to 90% of infants infected perinatally and 25% to 50% of children infected before age 5 years become chronically infected (Kimberlin et al., 2018). It is recommended that newborns receive HepB before hospital discharge if the mother is hepatitis B surface antigen (HBsAg) negative. Monovalent HepB should be given as the birth dose, whereas combination vaccine containing HepB may be given for subsequent doses in the series. Both full-term and preterm infants born to mothers whose HBsAg status is positive or unknown should receive HepB and hepatitis B immune globulin (HBIG), 0.5 ml, within 12 hours of birth at two different injection sites. Because the immune response to HepB is not optimum in newborns weighing less than 2000 grams (4.4 pounds), the first HepB dose should be given to such infants at a chronologic age of 1 month, as long as the mother's HBsAg status is negative (Kimberlin et al., 2018). If a preterm infant is given a dose at birth, the current recommendation is that the infant be given the full series (three additional doses) at 1, 2, and 6 months of age. The American Academy of Pediatrics (2018) also encourages immunization of all children by age 11 years (Kimberlin et al., 2018).

The vaccine is given intramuscularly in the vastus lateralis in newborns or in the deltoid for older infants and children. Regardless of age, avoid the dorsogluteal site because it has been associated with low antibody seroconversion rates, indicating a reduced immune response. No data exist regarding the seroconversion when the ventrogluteal site is used. The vaccine can be safely administered simultaneously at a separate site with DTaP, MMR, and Hib vaccines.

Hepatitis A Virus

Hepatitis A has been recognized as a significant child health problem, particularly in communities with unusually high infection rates. HAV is spread by the fecal-oral route and from person-to-person contact, by ingestion of contaminated food or water, and, rarely, by blood transfusion. The illness has an abrupt onset, with fever, malaise, anorexia, nausea, abdominal discomfort, dark urine, and jaundice being the most common clinical signs of infection. In children under 6 years of age, who represent approximately one-third of all cases of hepatitis A, the disease may be asymptomatic, and jaundice is rarely evident.

HAV vaccine (HepA) is now recommended for all children beginning at age 1 year (i.e., 12 months to 23 months). The second dose in the two-dose series may be administered no sooner than 6 months after the first dose. Since the implementation of widespread childhood HepA vaccination, infection rates among children ages 5 to 14 years have declined significantly.

Diphtheria

Although cases of diphtheria are rare in the United States, the disease can result in significant morbidity. Respiratory manifestations include respiratory nasopharyngitis or obstructive laryngotracheitis with upper airway obstruction. The cutaneous manifestations of the disease include vaginal, otic, conjunctival, or cutaneous lesions, which are primarily seen in urban homeless persons and in the tropics (Kimberlin et al., 2018). Administer a single dose of equine antitoxin intravenously to the child with clinical symptoms because of the often fulminant progression of the disease (Kimberlin et al., 2018). Diphtheria vaccine is commonly administered (1) in combination with tetanus and pertussis vaccines (DTaP) or DTaP and Hib vaccines for children younger than 7 years of age, (2) in combination with a conjugate Hib vaccine, (3) in a combined vaccine with tetanus (DT) for children younger than 7 years of age who have some contraindication to receiving pertussis vaccine, (4) in combination with tetanus and acellular pertussis (Tdap) for children 11 years and older, or (5) as a single antigen when combined antigen preparations are not indicated. Although the diphtheria vaccine does not produce absolute immunity, protective antitoxin persists for 10 years or more when given according to the recommended schedule, and boosters are given every 10 years for life (see following section for adolescent diphtheria and acellular pertussis and tetanus toxoid recommendation). Several vaccines contain diphtheria toxoid (e.g., Hib, meningococcal, pneumococcal), but this does not confer immunity to the disease.

Tetanus

Three forms of tetanus vaccine—tetanus toxoid, tetanus immunoglobulin (TIG) (human), and tetanus antitoxin (equine antitoxin)—are available; however, tetanus antitoxin is no longer available in the United States. Tetanus toxoid is used for routine primary immunization, usually in one of the combinations listed for diphtheria, and provides protective antitoxin levels for approximately 10 years.

[a]Because of constant changes in the pharmaceutical industry, trade names of single and combination vaccines in this section may differ from those currently available. The reader is encouraged to access the vaccine page of the Center for Biologics Evaluation and Research of the US Food and Drug Administration for the latest licensed vaccine trade names: http://www.fda.gov/BiologicsBloodVaccines/Vaccines/ApprovedProducts/ucm093833.htm.

Tetanus and diphtheria toxoids along with acellular pertussis vaccine (Tdap) are now recommended for persons ages 11 to 12 years who have completed the recommended DTaP/DTP vaccine series but have not received the tetanus (Td) booster dose. Adolescents 13 to 18 years of age who have not received the Td/Tdap booster should receive a single Tdap booster, provided that the routine DTaP/DTP childhood immunization series has been previously received. In addition, children ages 7 to 10 years who are not fully vaccinated for pertussis (i.e., did not receive five doses of DTaP or four doses of DTaP with the fourth dose being administered on or after the fourth birthday) should receive a dose of Tdap (Kimberlin et al., 2018). It is recommended that children receive subsequent Td boosters every 10 years (Kimberlin et al., 2018). Boostrix (Tdap) is currently licensed for persons 10 years of age (including those ≥65 years of age) and older, whereas Adacel (Tdap) is licensed for individuals 10 to 64 years of age.

For wound management, passive immunity is available with TIG. Persons with a history of two previous doses of tetanus toxoid can receive a booster dose of the toxoid. Separate syringes and different sites are used when tetanus toxoid and TIG are given concurrently.

For children older than 7 years of age who require wound prophylaxis, tetanus immunization may be accomplished by administering Td (adult-type diphtheria and tetanus toxoids). If TIG is not available, the equine antitoxin (not available in the United States) may be administered after appropriate testing for sensitivity. The antitoxin is administered in a separate syringe and at a separate intramuscular site if given concurrently with tetanus toxoid.

Pertussis

Pertussis vaccine is recommended for all children 6 weeks through 6 years of age (up to the seventh birthday) who have no neurologic contraindications to its use. Concerns over outbreaks of the disease in the past decade have prompted discussion about vaccinating infants and adults. Many cases of pertussis have occurred in children younger than 6 months or persons older than 7 years, both groups falling in the category for which pertussis immunization previously was not recommended. The Tdap is now recommended at ages 11 to 12 years for persons who have completed the DTaP/DTP childhood series. The Tdap is also recommended for adolescents 13 to 18 years old who have not received a tetanus booster (Td) or Tdap dose and have completed the childhood DTaP/DTP series. When the Tdap is used as a booster dose, it may be administered regardless of the interval from the previous tetanus, diphtheria, and pertussis–containing vaccine. Children ages 7 through 10 years who are not fully vaccinated for pertussis (i.e., did not receive five doses of DTaP or four doses of DTaP with the fourth dose being administered on or after the fourth birthday) should receive a dose of Tdap (Kimberlin et al., 2018) (see discussion in the Tetanus section earlier).

The Advisory Committee on Immunization Practices and the American College of Obstetricians and Gynecologists have recommended that pregnant adolescents and women who are not protected against pertussis receive the Tdap vaccine optimally between 27 and 36 weeks of gestation or postpartum before discharge from the hospital; breastfeeding is not a contraindication to Tdap vaccination (Centers for Disease Control and Prevention, 2013a). The concept of cocooning has been promoted since 2006 to reduce the spread of pertussis to vulnerable infants. Cocooning involves the strategy of vaccinating pregnant women during or after pregnancy, as well as all persons who will have close contact with the infants (including health care workers, fathers, and adults [especially those ages 65 years and older]) (Blain, Lewis, Banerjee, et al., 2016). Cocooning can prevent pertussis in vulnerable infants; however, actual implantation of the cocooning strategy among all family members is difficult (Blain, Lewis, Banerjee, et al., 2016).

Currently, two forms of pertussis vaccine are available in the United States. The whole-cell pertussis vaccine is prepared from inactivated cells of *Bordetella pertussis* and contains multiple antigens. In contrast, the acellular pertussis vaccine contains one or more immunogens derived from the *B. pertussis* organism. The highly purified acellular vaccine is associated with fewer local and systemic reactions than those occurring with the whole-cell vaccine in children of similar age. The acellular pertussis vaccine is recommended by the American Academy of Pediatrics (2018) for the first three immunizations and is usually given at 2, 4, and 6 months of age with diphtheria and tetanus (DTaP) (Kimberlin et al., 2018). Several forms of acellular pertussis vaccine are currently licensed for use in infants: Daptacel, Pediarix, Kinrix (DTaP and IPV), and Infanrix (diphtheria, tetanus toxoid, and acellular pertussis conjugate). Pentacel is licensed for use in infants 4 weeks of age and older; in addition to acellular pertussis, diphtheria, and tetanus, this vaccine contains inactivated poliovirus (IPV) and Hib conjugate. Either the acellular or the whole-cell vaccine may be given for the fourth and fifth doses, but the acellular vaccine is preferred. It is also recommended that the first three DTaP vaccinations be from the same manufacturer. The fourth dose may be from a different manufacturer. The child who has received one or more whole-cell vaccines may complete the series of five with the acellular vaccine.

Health care workers who may be susceptible to pertussis as a result of waning immunity and who have potential exposure to children or adults with pertussis should receive a single dose of Tdap (if not previously vaccinated with same) and take the necessary protective precautions against droplet contamination (i.e., wear procedural or surgical masks and practice hand washing). The diagnosis of pertussis may be missed or delayed in unvaccinated infants, who often are seen with respiratory distress and apnea without the typical cough.

Additional guidelines for prevention and treatment of pertussis among health care workers and close contacts can be found on the Centers for Disease Control and Prevention website at http://www.cdc.gov/vaccines/.

Polio

An all-IPV (inactivated poliovirus vaccine) schedule for routine childhood polio vaccination is now recommended for children in the United States. All children should receive four doses of IPV at 2 months, 4 months, 6 to 18 months, and 4 to 6 years of age (Kimberlin et al., 2018).

The change from the exclusive use of oral polio vaccine (OPV) to the exclusive use of IPV is related to the rare risk of vaccine-associated polio paralysis (VAPP) from OPV. The exclusive use of IPV eliminates the risk of VAPP but is associated with an increased number of injections and increased cost. Since IPV usage was instituted in the United States in 2000, no new indigenously acquired cases of VAPP have occurred. Pediarix is a combination vaccine containing DTaP, HepB, and IPV; this may be used as the primary immunization beginning at 2 months of age (Kimberlin et al., 2018). Kinrix contains DTaP and IPV, and it may be used as the fifth dose in the DTaP series and as the fourth dose in the IPV series in children ages 4 to 6 years whose previous vaccine doses have been with Infanrix and/or Pediarix for the first three doses and Infanrix for the fourth dose. As noted earlier, Pentacel is also licensed for use in infants 4 weeks of age and older and contains DTaP, Hib, and inactivated poliovirus. Pediarix has been licensed for use in children as young as 6 weeks and contains DTaP, Hep B, and IPV.

Measles

The measles (rubeola) vaccine is given at 12 to 15 months of age. During measles outbreaks, the vaccine can be given at 6 to 11 months of age, followed by a second inoculation after age 12 months. The second measles immunization is recommended at 4 to 6 years of age (at school entry) but may be given earlier provided that 4 weeks have elapsed since the administration of the previous dose. Revaccination should occur by 11 to 12 years of age if the measles vaccine was not administered at school entry (4 to 6 years). Any child who is vaccinated before 12 months of age should receive two additional doses beginning at 12 to 15 months and separated by at least 4 weeks (Kimberlin et al., 2018). Revaccination should include all individuals born after 1956 who have not received two doses of measles vaccine after 12 months of age. Individuals born before this date are thought to be immune from exposure to natural measles virus. Because of the continuing occurrence of measles in older children and young adults, identify potentially susceptible adolescents and young adults and immunize them if two doses of measles vaccine have not been administered previously or the person had a confirmed case of the illness. For postexposure prophylaxis, one dose of MMR may be administered within 72 hours of exposure in vaccine-eligible individuals 12 months of age or older and is preferable to immunoglobulin (Centers for Disease Control and Prevention, 2013b).

The measles, mumps, rubella, and varicella (MMRV) vaccine is an attenuated live virus vaccine and may be given to children 12 to 15 months of age or at 4 through 6 years of age concurrent with other vaccines. Children with human immunodeficiency virus (HIV) should not receive the MMRV vaccine because of a lack of evidence of its safety in this population. The risks and benefits of administering the MMRV vaccine should be fully explained to the parent or caregiver; the risk for a febrile seizure at 5 to 12 days in children 12 to 23 months of age remains relatively low and should be weighed against the benefit of one fewer intramuscular injection (Kimberlin et al., 2018). The American Academy of Pediatrics (2018) recommends that either the MMR or the MMRV vaccine be given as the first dose at ages 12 through 47 months; for children 48 months and older, the first dose with MMRV is recommended to decrease the number of injections; for the second dose at any age (15 months through 12 years), MMRV is also recommended for the same reason (Kimberlin et al., 2018).

Vitamin A supplementation has been effective in decreasing the morbidity and mortality risks associated with measles in developing countries.

Mumps

Mumps virus vaccine is recommended for children at 12 to 15 months of age and is typically given in combination with measles and rubella. It should not be administered to infants younger than 12 months of age because persisting maternal antibodies can interfere with the immune response. Because of continued occurrence of the disease, especially in children 10 to 19 years of age, mumps immunization is recommended for all individuals born after 1957 who may be susceptible to mumps (i.e., those who have no history of having had the disease or vaccine and who have no laboratory evidence of immunity).

Rubella

Rubella is a relatively mild infection in children, but in a pregnant woman the actual infection presents serious risks to the developing fetus. The aim of rubella immunization is protection of the unborn child rather than the recipient of the immunization.

Rubella immunization is recommended for all children at 12 to 15 months of age and at age of school entry or 4 to 6 years of age or sooner, according to the routine recommendations for the MMRV vaccine (Kimberlin et al., 2018). Increased emphasis should also be placed on vaccinating all unimmunized prepubertal children and susceptible adolescents and adult women in the childbearing age-group. Postpubertal females without evidence of rubella immunity should be immunized unless they are pregnant; they should be counseled not to become pregnant for 28 days after receiving the rubella-containing vaccine (Kimberlin et al., 2018). Because the live attenuated virus may cross the placenta and theoretically present a risk to the developing fetus, rubella vaccine is currently not given to any pregnant woman. Although this is standard practice, current evidence from women who received the vaccine while pregnant and delivered unaffected offspring indicates that the risk to the fetus is negligible (de Martino, 2016). In addition, there is no reported danger of administering rubella vaccine to a child if the mother is pregnant.

Haemophilus influenzae Type B

Hib conjugate vaccines protect against a number of serious infections caused by *H. influenzae* type B, especially bacterial meningitis, epiglottitis, bacterial pneumonia, septic arthritis, and sepsis (Hib is not associated with the viruses that cause influenza, or "flu"). Hib vaccines that are currently available include PedvaxHIB and Pentacel, which are combination vaccines, and Hiberix and ActHib. Pentacel is described in the Pertussis section earlier in the chapter. These conjugate vaccines connect Hib to a nontoxic form of another organism, such as meningococcal protein, tetanus toxoid, or diphtheria protein. There is no antibody response to these nontoxic proteins, but they significantly improve the antibody response to Hib, especially in infants. The use of combination vaccines provides equivalent immunogenicity and decreases the number of injections an infant receives. However, it is important that they be given to the appropriate-age child. The American Academy of Pediatrics (2018) clarified that only one dose of Hib should be given to children 15 months of age or older who have not been previously vaccinated(Kimberlin et al., 2018).

When possible, the Hib conjugate vaccine used at the first vaccination should be used for all subsequent vaccinations in the primary series. All Hib vaccines are administered by intramuscular injection using a separate syringe and at a site separate from any concurrent vaccinations.

> **! NURSING ALERT**
>
> The use of meningococcal and diphtheria proteins in combination vaccines does not mean that the child has received adequate immunization for meningococcal or diphtheria illnesses; the child must be given the appropriate vaccine for each specific disease.

Varicella

Administration of the cell-free live attenuated varicella vaccine is recommended for any susceptible child (i.e., one who lacks proof of varicella vaccination or has a reliable history of varicella infection). A single dose of 0.5 ml should be given by subcutaneous injection. The first dose of varicella vaccine is recommended for children ages 12 to 15 months, and to ensure adequate protection, a second varicella vaccine is recommended for children at 4 to 6 years of age. The second varicella vaccine may be administered before 4 years of age as long as a period of 3 months occurs between the first and second doses. Children 13 years of age or older who are susceptible should receive two doses administered at least 4 weeks apart. Children in the same age-group (13 to 18 years) who have received only one previous varicella vaccine should receive a second varicella vaccine. The two-dose regimen was adopted to protect children who did not have adequate protection with one dose, not because of waning immunity to the vaccine (Kimberlin et al., 2018). The combination vaccine MMRV (ProQuad) is licensed for use in children ages 12 months to 12 years (see discussion in the Measles section earlier in the chapter.)

According to the American Academy of Pediatrics (2018), children who have received two doses of the varicella vaccine are one-third less likely to have breakthrough illness in the first 10 years of immunization in comparison with those who have received one dose (Kimberlin et al., 2018). Children who do contract varicella after immunization reportedly have milder cases with fewer vesicles, lower degree of fever, and faster recovery. Antibodies persist for at least 8 years.

Keep the vaccine frozen in the lyophilic form (i.e., stable particles that readily go into solution) and use it within 30 minutes of being reconstituted to ensure viral potency.

Varicella vaccine may be administered simultaneously with MMR. However, separate syringes and injection sites should be used. If these vaccines are not administered simultaneously, the interval between administration of varicella vaccine and MMR should be at least 1 month. Varicella vaccine may also be given simultaneously with DTaP, IPV, HepB, or Hib (Kimberlin et al., 2018). The vaccine is administered subcutaneously.

Pneumococcal Disease

Streptococcus pneumoniae bacteria are responsible for a number of infections in children under 2 years of age that may cause serious morbidity and mortality. Among these are generalized infections, such as septicemia and meningitis, and localized infections, such as otitis media, sinusitis, and pneumonia. These illnesses are particularly problematic in children who attend daycare facilities (the incidence in children attending daycare is two to three times higher than in those not attending out-of-home daycare) and in those who are immunocompromised. A 13-valent pneumococcal vaccine (PCV13 [Prevnar 13]) has been licensed for use and is currently recommended as the standard pneumococcal vaccine for children ages 6 weeks to 24 months. Children who have started the PCV series with PCV7 may complete the vaccine series with PCV13 (Kimberlin et al., 2018).

The PCV13 vaccine is administered at 2, 4, and 6 months of age, with a fourth dose at 12 to 15 months of age. A single supplemental dose of PCV13 is recommended for children ages 14 through 59 months who have received an age-appropriate series of PCV7. PCV13 is also recommended for all children younger than 24 months of age and for children 24 to 71 months of age with sickle cell disease; functional or anatomic asplenia; nephrotic syndrome or chronic renal failure; conditions associated with immunosuppression, such as solid organ transplantation, drug therapy, or cytoreduction therapy (including long-term systemic corticosteroid therapy); diabetes mellitus; cochlear implants; congenital immunodeficiency; HIV infection; cerebrospinal fluid leaks; chronic cardiovascular disease (e.g., congestive heart failure or cardiomyopathy); chronic pulmonary disease (e.g., emphysema or cystic fibrosis but not asthma); chronic liver disease (e.g., cirrhosis); or exposure to living environments or social settings in which the risk of invasive pneumococcal disease or its complications is very high (e.g., Alaskan Native, African American, and certain American Indian populations). The PCV13 vaccine may be administered in conjunction with all other immunizations in a separate syringe and at a separate intramuscular site.

The PPSV23 (pneumococcal polysaccharide [23-valent] vaccine) is not recommended for children younger than 24 months of age who do not have one of the high-risk conditions described previously. One dose of PPSV23 is recommended in children older than 23 months of age who have one of the high-risk conditions after primary immunization with PCV13.

Influenza

The influenza vaccine is recommended annually for children ages 6 months to 18 years. Influenza vaccine (inactivated influenza vaccine [IIV]) may be given to any healthy children 6 months of age and older. The trivalent inactivated influenza vaccine (TIV) was changed to inactivated influenza vaccine (IIV) (Kimberlin et al., 2018). It is administered in early fall before the flu season begins and is repeated yearly for ongoing protection. The intramuscular vaccine is administered as two separate doses 4 weeks apart in first-time recipients younger than 9 years old. The dose is 0.25 ml of Fluzone or 0.5 ml of FluLaval or Fluarix for children 6 to 35 months old and 0.5 ml for children 3 years of age and older. An intradermal form of IIV has been licensed for persons 18 to 64 years of age. The vaccine may be given simultaneously with other vaccines but in a separate syringe and at a separate site. The vaccine is administered yearly because different strains of influenza are used each year in the manufacture of the vaccine. According to the American Academy of Pediatrics (2018), recent data have shown that IIV administered in a single, age- appropriate dose is tolerated by those with egg allergy of any severity, suggesting that special precautions for egg-allergic recipients of IIV are not warranted (Kimberlin et al., 2018). An age-appropriate recombinant or cell-cultured product may be used for patients who refuse to receive an egg-based vaccine. Several options for administering the influenza vaccine are described in the literature, and individuals should discuss the risks and benefits with a knowledgeable health care practitioner.

During the 2016–17 influenza season, the live attenuated influenza vaccine (LAIV) was determined not to be an acceptable alternative for the influenza vaccine due to concerns about its effectiveness (Belongia, Karron, Reingold, et al., 2017). The US Advisory Committee on Immunization Practices is monitoring ongoing research to determine recommendations for future influenza seasons.

The H1N1 virus (swine flu) is a subtype of influenza type A. The pandemic of H1N1 in 2009–10 caused significant morbidity and mortality worldwide (Kimberlin et al., 2018). The signs and symptoms of H1N1 flu are the same as those mentioned for influenza. The most updated information on the status of this disease may be found at the Centers for Disease Control and Prevention website (http://www.cdc.gov/flu/about/season/index.html).

Meningococcal Disease

Invasive meningococcal disease continues to be the cause of high morbidity in children in the United States. Infants younger than 1 year of age are particularly susceptible, yet the highest fatalities occur in adolescents and young adults, with 50 to 60 cases and 5 to 10 deaths reported annually (Centers for Disease Control and Prevention, 2015). There is also evidence that the risk of meningococcal infections is high in college freshmen living in dormitories. Meningococcal infections are also responsible for significant morbidities, including limb or digit amputation, skin scarring, hearing loss, and neurologic disabilities.

Neisseria meningitidis is the leading cause of bacterial meningitis in the United States. It is not recommended that children 9 months to 10 years old routinely receive the meningococcal conjugate vaccines (MCVs) because the infection rate is low in this age-group. Children at increased risk for meningococcal infection should receive a two-dose series of either MenACWY-D (Menactra) or MenACWY-CRM (Menveo), both of which are MCV4 vaccines, or the infant series of Menveo (MenACWY-CRM) given at least 2 months apart. These include children with terminal complement component deficiency, anatomic or functional asplenia, or HIV. Children ages 2 to 18 years who travel to or reside in countries where *N. meningitidis* is hyperendemic or epidemic or who are at risk during a community outbreak should receive one dose of MCV4 (either Menveo or Menactra). Menactra is licensed for administration in children as young as 9 months of age, and Menveo is licensed for children 2 months of age and older.

Children and adolescents 11 to 12 years of age should receive a single immunization of MCV4 (either Menactra or Menveo) and a booster of the same at age 16 to 18 years. Others at high risk who should receive MCV4 include college freshmen living in dormitories and military recruits. Children ages 2 to 23 months with high-risk conditions can be administered a four-dose series of Menveo at 2, 4, 6, and 12 months. Persons who are at high risk for the disease and received meningococcal polysaccharide vaccine (MPSV4) 3 or more years earlier should be reimmunized with MCV4. MCV4 (Menveo or Menactra) is administered as an intramuscular injection (0.5 mL) and may be administered in conjunction with other vaccines in a separate syringe and at a separate site. Immunization with MCV4 is contraindicated in persons with hypersensitivity to any components of the vaccine, including diphtheria toxoid, and to rubber latex (part of the vial stopper).

Rotavirus

Rotavirus is one of the leading causes of severe diarrhea in infants and young children and is transmitted by the fecal-oral route. The incidence of rotavirus has decreased dramatically since rotavirus vaccines became available in 2006. Two rotavirus vaccines, RotaTeq (RV5) and Rotarix (RV1), have received a license from the US Food and Drug Administration for distribution in the United States. Infants in the United States are routinely immunized with three doses of RotaTeq at 2, 4, and 6 months of age or two doses of Rotarix at 2 and 4 months of age. RotaTeq is licensed for administration to infants at 6 to 14 weeks of age, with two additional doses administered at 4- to 10-week intervals but not after 32 weeks of age (Kimberlin et al., 2018). Rotarix (1 ml) may be administered beginning at 6 weeks of age, with a second dose at least 4 weeks after the first dose but before 32 weeks of age (Kimberlin et al., 2018). Both vaccines are administered orally. Infants who contract rotavirus infection before completing the vaccine series should complete the vaccinations following the standard intervals (Kimberlin et al., 2018).

Human Papillomavirus

Human papillomaviruses (HPVs) are a large family of viruses that consist of cutaneous (i.e., skin warts) and genital (i.e., mucosal) types. Genital HPVs can be classified as low risk and high risk according to their association with cancers. Three HPV vaccines have been licensed for use in adolescents, but Gardasil 9 is the only available HPV vaccine in the United States (Centers for Disease Control and Prevention, 2016a). The vaccine is administered intramuscularly, preferably in the deltoid muscle, in three separate doses; the first dose in the series is commonly administered at 11 to 12 years of age, and the second dose is given 1 to 2 months after the first, with the third dose given 6 months after the first dose (Kimberlin et al., 2018). The vaccine is recommended for both boys and girls at a minimum age of 9 years and a maximum age of 26 years (Centers for Disease Control and Prevention, 2016a). Women who receive the HPV vaccine must continue to have regular Papanicolaou (Pap) tests (Kimberlin et al., 2018).

Reactions

Vaccines for routine immunizations are among the safest and most reliable drugs available. However, minor side effects do occur after many of the immunizations and, rarely, a serious reaction may result from the vaccine. A number of inactive components are incorporated in vaccines to enhance their effectiveness and safety. Some of these components include preservatives, stabilizers, adjuvants, antibiotics (e.g., neomycin), and purified culture medium proteins (e.g., egg) to enhance effectiveness. A child may react to the preservative in the vaccine rather than the vaccine component; an example of this is the hepatitis B vaccine, which is prepared from yeast cultures. Yeast hypersensitivity therefore would preclude an individual from receiving that vaccine without consulting an allergist. Trace amounts of neomycin are used to decrease bacterial growth within certain vaccine preparations, and persons with documented anaphylactic reactions to neomycin should avoid those vaccines.

Most vaccine preparations now contain vial stoppers with a synthetic rubber to prevent latex allergy reactions, but health care personnel administering vaccines should make sure that the package insert specifies that there is no latex in the stopper. If an individual has a severe reaction to a vaccine and subsequent immunizations are required, an allergist should be consulted to determine the best course of action. Although influenza vaccines contain small amounts of egg protein, recent evidence shows no risk of an anaphylactic reaction with the inactivated influenza vaccine among children with an egg allergy, and these children should receive the influenza vaccine (American Academy of Pediatrics, Committee on Infectious Diseases, 2016). Some vaccines contain a preservative, thimerosal, which contains ethyl mercury. Concerns regarding possible mercury poisoning in the 1990s prompted many to put off vaccination of infants and small children for fear of childhood developmental problems, such as autism. A number of manufacturers have since stopped producing vaccines containing thimerosal. No local hypersensitivity reactions to thimerosal have been recorded, and studies on thimerosal and the potential link to autism or any other pervasive developmental disorder failed to establish a causal relationship between the two (DeStefano, Price, & Weintraub, 2013; Yoshimasu, Kiyohara, Takemura, et al., 2014). The Institute of Medicine (2004), following an in-depth 3-year study, concluded that there was no link between autism and the MMR vaccine or vaccines containing the preservative thimerosal.

With inactivated antigens, such as DTaP, side effects are most likely to occur within a few hours or days of administration and are usually limited to local tenderness, erythema, and swelling at the injection site; low-grade fever; and behavioral changes (e.g., drowsiness, eating less, prolonged or unusual cry). Local reactions tend to be less severe when a needle of sufficient length to deposit the vaccine in the muscle is used (see Atraumatic Care box). Rarely, more severe reactions may occur (see Drug Alert box). If epinephrine is administered, observe for adverse reactions such as tachycardia, hypertension, irritability, headaches, nausea, and tremors.

ATRAUMATIC CARE

Immunizations

Needle length and injection techniques are important factors and must be considered for each child. Fewer reactions to immunizations are observed when the vaccine is given deep into the muscle rather than into subcutaneous tissue. The dorsogluteal site is not recommended as an injection site for children because of the potential for sciatic nerve damage (Rishovd, 2014). In addition, aspiration for blood is no longer recommended for an intramuscular injection because large blood vessels are not present at recommended injection sites and slow aspiration causes more pain than injection without aspiration (Rishovd, 2014).

To ensure appropriate needle size for vaccine administration (Rishovd, 2014):

- Newborns (0 to 28 days old): recommended needle size is 5/8 inch, 22 to 25 gauge; recommended injection site: vastus lateralis.
- Infant/toddler (1 month to 2 years old): recommended needle size and site is 1 inch, 22 to 25 gauge in vastus lateralis or 5/8 to 1 inch, 22 to 25 gauge in the deltoid only if muscle mass is adequately developed.
- Child/adolescent (3 to 18 years old): less than 60 kg: 5/8 to 1 inch, 22 to 25 gauge in the deltoid; greater than 60 kg: 1 to 1½ inch, 22 to 25 gauge in the deltoid.

Use one or more of the following techniques to minimize pain (Rishovd, 2014; World Health Organization, 2015):

- Apply the topical anesthetic EMLA (lidocaine-prilocaine) to the injection site and cover with an occlusive dressing for at least 1 hour[a] or apply the topical anesthetic LMX4 (4% lidocaine) to the injection site and cover with an occlusive dressing for 30 minutes before the injection.
- Apply a vapocoolant spray (e.g., ethyl chloride or Fluori-Methane) directly to the skin; however, some children may report pain associated with the cooling sensation.
- Ensure beneficial positioning of the patient: being held by a parent or caregiver for infants and young children and sitting upright for older children and adolescents.
- Encourage breastfeeding during or before the immunizations.
- For children younger than 6 years old, use distraction, such as asking the child to blow bubbles or telling the child to "take a deep breath and blow and blow and blow until I tell you to stop." Evidence does not show any benefit to using distraction during injections with adolescents.
- Nurses administering the injections should remain calm and use neutral words such as "here I go" instead of "here comes the sting."
- Do not manually stimulate (i.e., rub or apply pressure to) the injection site.

[a] The use of an EMLA patch before administration of diphtheria-tetanus–acellular pertussis–inactivated poliovirus–*Haemophilus influenzae* type b (DTaP-IPV-Hib) and hepatitis B vaccine.

DRUG ALERT

Emergency Management of Anaphylaxis

EpiPen Jr (0.15 mg; 0.3 ml of 1:2000) intramuscularly (IM) for child weighing 15 to 30 kg (33 to 66 pounds)
EpiPen (0.3 mg; 0.3 ml of 1:1000) IM for child weighing 30 kg (66 pounds) or more

Contraindications and Precautions

Nurses need to be aware of the reasons for withholding immunizations—both for the child's safety in terms of avoiding reactions and for the child's maximum benefit from receiving the vaccine. Unfounded fears and lack of knowledge regarding contraindications can needlessly prevent a child from having protection from life-threatening diseases. Issues that have surfaced regarding vaccines include the misconception that administering combination vaccines may overload the child's immune system; the combined vaccines have undergone rigorous study in relation to side effects and immunogenicity rates following administration. Others may express concern that vaccines are not a part of the individual's natural immunity and that administering too many vaccines may decrease the child's immunity to such diseases. A recent evaluation of parents' vaccination concerns identified through posts on social media found that parents were concerned about adverse reactions, such as autism, pain, compromised immunity, and death associated with vaccinations (Tangherlini, Roychowdhury, Glenn, et al., 2016).

A *contraindication* is a condition in an individual that increases the risk for a serious adverse reaction (e.g., not administering a live virus vaccine to a severely immunocompromised child). Thus one would not administer a vaccine when a contraindication is present. A *precaution* is a condition in a recipient that might increase the risk for a serious adverse reaction or that might compromise the ability of the vaccine to produce immunity. If conditions are such that the benefit of receiving the vaccine would outweigh the risk of an adverse event or incomplete response, a precaution would not prevent vaccine administration (Kimberlin et al., 2018).

The general contraindication for all immunizations is a severe febrile illness. This precaution avoids adding the risk of adverse side effects from the vaccine to an already ill child or mistakenly identifying a symptom of the disease as having been caused by the vaccine. The presence of minor illnesses, such as the common cold, is not a contraindication. Live virus vaccines are generally not administered to anyone with an altered immune system because multiplication of the virus may be enhanced, causing a severe vaccine-induced illness.

In general, live virus vaccines should not be administered to persons who are severely immunocompromised or among persons whose immune function is not known (Kimberlin et al., 2018). Another contraindication to live virus vaccines (e.g., MMR, varicella, and rotavirus) is the presence of recently acquired passive immunity through blood transfusions, immunoglobulin, or maternal antibodies. Administration of MMR and varicella should be postponed for a minimum of 3 months after passive immunization with immunoglobulins and blood transfusions (except washed red blood cells, which do not interfere with the immune response). Suggested intervals between administration of immunoglobulin preparations and MMR and varicella depend on the type of immune product and dosage. If the vaccine and immunoglobulin are given simultaneously because of imminent exposure to disease, the two preparations are injected at sites far from each other. Vaccination should be repeated after the suggested intervals unless there is serologic evidence of antibody production.

A final contraindication is a known allergic response to a previously administered vaccine or a substance in the vaccine. An anaphylactic reaction to a vaccine or its component is a true contraindication. MMR vaccines contain minute amounts of neomycin; measles and mumps vaccines, which are grown on chick embryo tissue cultures, are not believed to contain significant amounts of egg cross-reacting proteins. Therefore only a history of anaphylactic reaction to neomycin, gelatin, or the vaccine itself is considered a contraindication to their use.

Pregnancy is a contraindication to MMR vaccines, although the risk of fetal damage is primarily theoretic. Breastfeeding is not a contraindication for any vaccine. The only vaccine virus that has been isolated in human milk is rubella, and there is no indication that this is harmful to infants; rubella infection in an infant as a result of exposure to rubella virus in human milk would likely be well tolerated because the vaccine is attenuated (Kimberlin et al., 2018).

To identify the rare child who may not be able to receive the vaccines, take a careful allergy history. If the child has a history of anaphylaxis, report this to the practitioner before administering the vaccine. Contact dermatitis in reaction to neomycin is not considered a contraindication to immunization. Evidence indicates that children who are egg sensitive are not at increased risk for untoward reactions to MMR vaccine. Furthermore, skin testing of egg-allergic children with vaccine has failed to predict immediate hypersensitivity reactions (Kimberlin et al., 2018). A family history of seizures or adverse event following vaccination, penicillin allergy, allergies to duck meat or duck feathers, and a family history of sudden infant death syndrome (SIDS) are not considered contraindications to receiving childhood vaccines (Kimberlin et al., 2018).

Nurses are at the forefront in providing parents with appropriate information about childhood immunization benefits, contraindications, and side effects and the effects of nonvaccination on the child's health. Some suggestions for communicating with parents about the benefits of immunizations in childhood include the following (portions adapted from Coyer, 2002; Fredrickson, Davis, Arnold, et al., 2004; Rosenthal, 2004):

- Provide accurate and user-friendly information on vaccines (the need for each one, the disease each prevents, potential adverse effects).
- Realize that the parent is expressing concern for the child's health.
- Acknowledge the parent's concerns in a genuine, empathetic manner.
- Tailor the discussion to the needs of the parent; avoid judgmental or threatening language.
- Be knowledgeable about the benefits of individual vaccines, the common adverse effects, and how to minimize those effects.
- Give the parent the **vaccine information statement (VIS)** before vaccination and be prepared to answer any questions that may arise.
- Help the parent make an informed decision regarding the administration of each vaccine.
- Be flexible and provide parents with options regarding the administration of multiple vaccines, especially in infants, who must receive multiple injections at 2, 4, and 6 months of age (i.e., allow parents to space the vaccinations at different visits to decrease the total number of injections at each visit; make provisions for office visits for immunization purposes only [does not incur a practitioner fee except for administration of vaccine], provided the child is healthy).
- Involve the parent in minimizing the potential adverse effects of the vaccine (e.g., administering an appropriate dose of acetaminophen 45 minutes before administering the vaccine [as warranted]; applying eutectic mixture of local anesthetics [EMLA; lidocaine-prilocaine] or 4% lidocaine [LMX4] to the injection sites before administration [see Atraumatic Care box earlier in the chapter]; following up to check on the child if untoward reactions have occurred in the past or the parent is especially anxious about the child's well-being).
- Respect the parent's ultimate wishes.

Administration

The principal precautions in administering immunizations include proper storage of the vaccine to protect its potency and institution of recommended procedures for injection. The nurse must be familiar with the manufacturer's directions for storage and reconstitution of the vaccine. For example, if the vaccine is to be refrigerated, it should be stored on a center shelf, not in the door, where frequent temperature increases from opening the refrigerator can alter the vaccine's potency. For protection against light, the vial can be wrapped in aluminum foil. Periodic checks are established to ensure that no vaccine is used after its expiration date.

The DTP (or DTaP) vaccines contain an adjuvant to retain the antigen at the injection site and prolong the stimulatory effect. Because subcutaneous or intracutaneous injection of the adjuvant can cause local irritation, inflammation, or abscess formation, excellent intramuscular injection technique must be used (see Atraumatic Care box earlier in the chapter).

The total series requires several injections, and every attempt is made to rotate the sites and administer the injections as painlessly as possible. (See Chapter 20, Intramuscular Administration.) When two or more injections are given at separate sites, the order of injections is arbitrary. Some practitioners suggest injecting the less painful one first. Some believe this is DTP (or DTaP), whereas others suggest the MMR or Hib vaccine. Still others advocate injecting at two sites simultaneously (requires two operators) (see Research Focus box).

RESEARCH FOCUS

Order of Injections

Ipp and colleagues (2009) evaluated the administration order of the vaccines diphtheria-tetanus–acellular pertussis–*Haemophilus influenzae* type B (DTaP-Hib) and pneumococcal conjugate vaccine (PCV) and pain perception in 120 infants 2 to 6 months of age. The infants who were given the primary DTaP-Hib vaccine before the PCV had significantly lower pain scores than those who received the PCV first. Fallah and colleagues (2016) evaluated the best order for immunizations: intramuscular injection (diphtheria, pertussis, and tetanus) versus subcutaneous injection (measles, mumps, and rubella) among 70 children. Pain was significantly lower when the subcutaneous injection was administered before the intramuscular injection.

One of the most important features of injecting vaccines is adequate penetration of the muscle for deposition of the drug intramuscularly and not subcutaneously (depending on the manufacturer's recommendation for administration). The use of appropriate needle length is an essential component of administering vaccines. A recent systematic review reported the appropriate needle size to be ⅝ inch for infants less than 28 days old, 1 inch for infants 1 month to 2 years old, and ⅝ inch if the skin is stretched tightly and not bunched to 1 inch for children 3 to 18 years old (Beirne, Hennessy, Cadogan, et al., 2015). In two studies, the use of longer needles significantly decreased the incidence of localized edema and tenderness when vaccines were administered to a group of infants (Diggle & Deeks, 2000; Diggle, Deeks, & Pollard, 2006). Similar findings have been recorded for children 4 to 6 years of age receiving the fifth DTaP vaccine (Jackson, Yu, Nelson, et al., 2011).

Nurses often administer vaccines, and thus they may have the responsibility for adequately informing parents of the nature, prevalence, and risks of the disease; the type of immunization product to be used; the expected benefits and risks of side effects of the vaccine; and the need for accurate immunization records. Referring to immunizations as "baby shots" and limiting the discussion to vague statements about the vaccines are unacceptable practices.

Although immunization rates have increased significantly, health professionals should use every opportunity to encourage complete immunization of all children (see Community Focus box). Table 6.2 reports the quality indicator for childhood immunization status.

COMMUNITY FOCUS

Keeping Current on Vaccine Recommendations

It is much easier to keep current if you know where to look for the official recommendations of the American Academy of Pediatrics and the Centers for Disease Control and Prevention's Advisory Committee on Immunization Practices. The primary sources are publications and the Internet. You can also contact each organization to request information:

American Academy of Pediatrics
141 Northwest Point Blvd.
Elk Grove Village, IL 60007
847-434-4000
Fax: 847-434-8000
http://www.aap.org

Centers for Disease Control and Prevention
1600 Clifton Road
Atlanta, GA 30333
404-639-3311
Information: 800-232-4636
https://www.cdc.gov
Vaccine and immunization information: https://www.cdc.gov/vaccines

Another important nursing responsibility is accurate documentation. Each child should have an immunization record for parents to keep, especially for families who move frequently. Blank immunization records may be downloaded from a number of websites, including the Immunization Action Coalition (http://www.immunize.org), which has vaccine information and records in a number of languages.

Document the following information on the medical record: day, month, and year of administration; manufacturer and lot number of vaccine; and name, address, and title of the person administering the vaccine. Additional data to record are the site and route of administration and evidence that the parent or legal guardian gave informed consent before the immunization was administered. Report any adverse reactions after the administration of a vaccine to the Vaccine Adverse Event Reporting System (http://www.vaers.hhs.gov; 1-800-822-7967).

Many states and territories participate in the immunization information system (IIS), which provides immunization information for parents and health professionals, as well as a local or regional registry of immunizations that children have received. In addition, the IIS can provide parents with information about missed scheduled immunizations. This information is also useful for schools and health clinics.

An additional source of vaccine information that must be given to parents (as required by the National Childhood Vaccine Injury Act of 1986) before the administration of vaccines is the VIS for the particular vaccine being administered. Practitioners are required by law to fully inform families of the risks and benefits of the vaccines. VISs are designed to provide updated information to the adult vaccinee or parents or legal guardians of children being vaccinated regarding the risks and benefits of each vaccine. The practitioner should answer questions regarding the information in the VIS. VISs are available for the following vaccines: adenovirus, anthrax, tetanus, diphtheria, pertussis, MMR, MMRV, IPV, HPV, varicella, Hib, influenza, meningococcal, pneumococcal (13 and 23), rabies, rotavirus, shingles, smallpox, yellow fever, Japanese encephalitis, typhoid, and hepatitis A and B. An updated VIS should be provided, and documentation in the patient's chart should state that the VIS was given and include its publication date; this represents **informed consent** once the parent or caregiver gives permission to administer the vaccines. VISs are available from state or local health departments or from the Immunization Action Coalition (http://www.immunize.org/vis) and Centers for Disease Control and Prevention (https://www.cdc.gov/vaccines/hcp/vis/index.html).

TABLE 6.2 Pediatric Quality Indicator[a]

Childhood Immunization Status	
Measure	Children 2 years of age who had four diphtheria, tetanus, and acellular pertussis (DTaP); three inactivated polio vaccine (IPV); one measles, mumps, and rubella (MMR); three *Haemophilus influenzae* type B (Hib); three hepatitis B vaccine (HepB); one varicella-zoster virus (VZV); four pneumococcal conjugate vaccine (PCV); two hepatitis A vaccine (HepA); two or three rotavirus (RV); and two influenza (flu) vaccines by their second birthday.
Numerator	Number of children who have evidence showing they received recommended vaccines during the measurement time.
Denominator	Number of children who turn 2 years of age during the measurement year are eligible for inclusion.

[a]Endorsed by the National Quality Forum NQF #0038 and 2019 Core Set of Children's Health Care Quality Measures for Medicaid and CHIP. https://www.medicaid.gov/federal-policy-guidance/downloads/cib112018.pdf.

In response to the concerns of manufacturers, practitioners, and parents of children with serious vaccine-associated injuries, the National Childhood Vaccine Injury Act of 1986 and the Vaccine Compensation Amendments of 1987 were passed. These laws are designed to provide fair compensation for children who are inadvertently injured and provide greater protection from liability for vaccine manufacturers and providers. (See *2018 Red Book: Report of the Committee on Infectious Diseases* [Kimberlin et al., 2018] for further details of this program.)

The American Academy of Pediatrics' Report of the Committee on Infectious Diseases, known as the *Red Book*, is an authoritative source of information on vaccines and other important pediatric infectious diseases. However, it lacks an in-depth review and reference list of controversial issues. The recommendations in the *Red Book* first appear in the journal *Pediatrics* and/or the *AAP News*. Typically, the most recent immunization schedule appears in the January issue of the journal.

The Centers for Disease Control and Prevention now offers a valuable online resource tool for parents and clinicians. The tool prints out an individualized vaccination schedule with dates associated with each vaccination based on the child's date of birth. Clinicians can use this tool for children under 5 years of age to serve as a reminder for parents. Nurses should note that the personalized tool is based on the current immunization schedule and may need to be adjusted with the yearly updates from the American Academy of Pediatrics and the Advisory Committee on Immunization Practices. The tool is available at https://www2a.cdc.gov/vaccines/childquiz/.

A publication of the Centers for Disease Control and Prevention, *Morbidity and Mortality Weekly Report* (MMWR) contains comprehensive reviews of the literature and important background data regarding vaccine efficacy and side effects. To subscribe to this free publication, visit https://www.cdc.gov/mmwr/mmwrsubscribe.html. An electronic copy also is available from the Centers for Disease Control and Prevention's website at https://www.cdc.gov.

COMMUNICABLE DISEASES

The incidence of childhood communicable diseases has declined significantly since the advent of immunizations. The use of antibiotics and antitoxins has further reduced serious complications resulting from such infections. However, infectious diseases do occur, and nurses must be familiar with the infectious agent to recognize the disease and to institute appropriate preventive and supportive interventions (Table 6.3 and Figs. 6.2 to 6.7).

NURSING CARE MANAGEMENT

Table 6.3 describes the more common communicable diseases of childhood, their therapeutic management, and specific nursing care. The following is a general discussion of nursing care management for communicable diseases.

Identification of the infectious agent is of primary importance to prevent exposure to susceptible individuals. Nurses in ambulatory care settings, child care centers, and schools are often the first persons to see signs of a communicable disease, such as a rash or sore throat. The nurse must operate under a high index of suspicion for common childhood diseases to identify potentially infectious cases and to recognize diseases that require medical intervention. An example is the common complaint of sore throat. Although most often a symptom of a minor viral infection, it can signal diphtheria or a streptococcal infection, such as scarlet fever. Each of these bacterial conditions requires appropriate medical treatment to prevent serious complications.

When the nurse suspects a communicable disease, it is important to assess the following:

- Recent exposure to a known case
- **Prodromal symptoms** (symptoms that occur between early manifestations of the disease and its overt clinical syndrome) or evidence of constitutional symptoms, such as a fever or rash (see Table 6.3)
- Immunization history
- History of having the disease

Immunizations are available for many diseases, and infection usually confers lifelong immunity; therefore the possibility of many infectious agents can be eliminated based on these two criteria.

Prevent Spread

Prevention consists of two components: prevention of the disease and control of its spread to others. **Primary prevention** rests almost exclusively on immunization.

Control measures to prevent spread of disease should include techniques to reduce risk of cross-transmission of infectious organisms between patients and to protect health care workers from organisms harbored by patients. If the child is hospitalized, follow the facility's policies for infection control. The most important procedure is hand washing. Persons directly caring for the child or handling contaminated articles must wash their hands and practice effective Standard Precautions in care of their patients.

Instruct the child to practice good hand-washing technique after toileting and before eating. For those diseases spread by droplets, instruct the parents in measures to reduce airborne transmission. The child who is old enough should use a tissue to cover the face during coughing or sneezing; otherwise the parent should cover the child's mouth with a tissue and then discard it (see Respiratory Hygiene/Cough Etiquette in the Infection Control section discussed earlier in the chapter and in Box 6.1). Stress the usual hygiene measures of not sharing eating and drinking utensils to the family.

! NURSING ALERT

If a child is admitted to the hospital with an undiagnosed exanthema, institute strict Transmission-Based Precautions (Contact, Airborne, and Droplet) and Standard Precautions until a diagnosis is confirmed. Childhood communicable diseases requiring these precautions include diphtheria, varicella-zoster virus (VZV; chickenpox), measles, tuberculosis, adenovirus, *Haemophilus influenzae* type b (Hib), influenza, mumps, *Neisseria meningitides, Mycoplasma pneumoniae* infection, pertussis, plague, rhinovirus, group A streptococcal pharyngitis, severe acute respiratory syndrome, pneumonia, or scarlet fever (Kimberlin et al., 2018).

TABLE 6.3 Communicable Diseases of Childhood

Disease	Clinical Manifestations	Therapeutic Management and Complications	Nursing Care Management
Chickenpox (Varicella) (Fig. 6.2)			
Agents—Varicella-zoster virus (VZV) **Source**—Primary secretions of respiratory tract of infected persons; to a lesser degree, skin lesions (scabs not infectious) **Transmissions**—Direct contact, droplet (airborne) spread, and contaminated objects **Incubation period**—2-3 wk, usually 14-16 days **Period of communicability**—Probably 1 day before eruption of lesions (prodromal period) to 6 days after first crop of vesicles when crusts have formed	**Prodromal stage**—Slight fever, malaise, and anorexia for first 24 h; rash highly pruritic; begins as macule, rapidly progresses to papule and then vesicle (surrounded by erythematous base; becomes umbilicated and cloudy; breaks easily and forms crusts); all three stages (papule, vesicle, crust) present in varying degrees at one time **Distribution**—Centripetal, spreading to face and proximal extremities but sparse on distal limbs and less on areas not exposed to heat (i.e., from clothing or sun) **Constitutional signs and symptoms**—Elevated temperature from lymphadenopathy, irritability from pruritus	**Specific**—Antiviral agent acyclovir (Zovirax); varicella-zoster immune globulin or intravenous immunoglobulin (IVIG) after exposure in high-risk children **Supportive**—Diphenhydramine hydrochloride or antihistamines to relieve itching; skin care to prevent secondary bacterial infection **Complications**—Secondary bacterial infections (abscesses, cellulitis, necrotizing fasciitis, pneumonia, sepsis) Encephalitis Varicella pneumonia (rare in healthy children) Hemorrhagic varicella (tiny hemorrhages in vesicles and numerous petechiae in skin) Chronic or transient thrombocytopenia **Preventive**—Childhood immunization	Maintain Standard, Airborne, and Contact Precautions if hospitalized until all lesions are crusted; for immunized child with mild breakthrough varicella, isolate until no new lesions are seen. Keep child in home away from susceptible individuals until vesicles have dried (usually 1 wk after onset of disease) and isolate high-risk children from infected children. Administer skin care: give bath and change clothes and linens daily; administer topical calamine lotion; keep child's fingernails short and clean; apply mittens if child scratches. Keep child cool (may decrease number of lesions). Lessen pruritus; keep child occupied. Remove loose crusts that rub and irritate skin. Teach child to apply pressure to pruritic area rather than scratching it. Avoid use of aspirin (possible association with Reye syndrome).
Diphtheria			
Agent—*Corynebacterium diphtheriae* **Source**—Discharges from mucous membranes of nose and nasopharynx, skin, and other lesions of infected person **Transmission**—Direct contact with infected person, a carrier, or contaminated articles **Incubation period**—Usually 2-5 days, possibly longer **Period of communicability**—Variable; until virulent bacilli are no longer present (identified by three negative cultures); usually 2 wk but as long as 4 wk	Vary according to anatomic location of pseudomembrane **Nasal**—Resembles common cold, serosanguineous mucopurulent nasal discharge without constitutional symptoms; may have frank epistaxis **Tonsillar-pharyngeal**—Malaise; anorexia; sore throat; low-grade fever; pulse increased above expected for temperature within 24 h; smooth, adherent, white or gray membrane; lymphadenitis possibly pronounced ("bull's neck"); in severe cases, toxemia, septic shock, and death within 6-10 days **Laryngeal**—Fever, hoarseness, cough, with or without previous signs listed; potential airway obstruction; apprehensive; dyspneic retractions; cyanosis	Equine antitoxin (usually intravenously); preceded by skin or conjunctival test to rule out sensitivity to horse serum Antibiotics (penicillin G procaine or erythromycin) in addition to equine antitoxin Complete bed rest (prevention of myocarditis) Tracheostomy for airway obstruction Treatment of infected contacts and carriers **Complications**—Toxic cardiomyopathy (wk 2 to 3) Toxic neuropathy **Preventive**—Childhood immunization	Follow Standard and Droplet Precautions until two cultures are negative for *C. diphtheriae;* use Contact Precautions with cutaneous manifestations. Administer antibiotics in timely manner. Participate in sensitivity testing; have epinephrine available. Administer complete care to maintain bed rest. Use suctioning as needed. Observe respiration for signs of obstruction. Administer humidified oxygen as prescribed.

TABLE 6.3 Communicable Diseases of Childhood—cont'd

Disease	Clinical Manifestations	Therapeutic Management and Complications	Nursing Care Management
Erythema Infectiosum (Fifth Disease) (Fig. 6.3)			
Agent—Human parvovirus B19 **Source**—Infected persons, mainly school-age children **Transmission**—Respiratory secretions and blood, blood products **Incubation period**—4-14 days; may be as long as 21 days **Period of communicability**—Uncertain but before onset of symptoms in children with aplastic crisis	Rash appears in three stages: I—Erythema on face, chiefly on cheeks ("slapped face" appearance); disappears by 1-4 days II—About 1 day after rash appears on face, maculopapular red spots appear, symmetrically distributed on upper and lower extremities; rash progresses from proximal to distal surfaces and may last ≥1 wk III—Rash subsides but reappears if skin is irritated or traumatized (sun, heat, cold, friction) In children with aplastic crisis, rash usually absent and prodromal illness includes fever, myalgia, lethargy, nausea, vomiting, and abdominal pain Child with sickle cell disease may have concurrent vasoocclusive crisis	**Symptomatic and supportive**—Antipyretics, analgesics, antiinflammatory drugs Possible blood transfusion for transient aplastic anemia **Complications**—Self-limited arthritis and arthralgia (arthritis may become chronic); more common in adult women May result in serious complications (anemia, hydrops) or fetal death if mother infected during pregnancy (primarily second trimester) Aplastic crisis in children with hemolytic disease or immunodeficiency Myocarditis (rare)	Isolation of child is not necessary, except hospitalized child (immunosuppressed or with aplastic crises) suspected of parvovirus infection is placed on Droplet Precautions and Standard Precautions. Pregnant women need not be excluded from workplace where parvovirus infection is present; they should not care for patients with aplastic crises. Explain low risk of fetal death to those in contact with affected children; assist with routine fetal ultrasound for detection of fetal hydrops.
Exanthem Subitum (Roseola Infantum) (Fig. 6.4)			
Agent—Human herpesvirus 6 (HHV-6; rarely HHV-7) **Source**—Possibly acquired from saliva of healthy adult person; entry via nasal, buccal, or conjunctival mucosa **Transmission**—Year round; no reported contact with infected individual in most cases (virtually limited to children <3 years but peak age is 6-15 months) **Incubation period**—Usually 5-15 days **Period of communicability**—Unknown	Persistent high fever >39.5°C (103°F) for 3-7 days in child who appears well Precipitous drop in fever to normal with appearance of rash Bulging fontanel **Rash**—Discrete rose-pink macules or maculopapules appearing first on trunk, then spreading to neck, face, and extremities; nonpruritic; fades on pressure; lasts 1-2 days **Associated signs and symptoms**—Cervical and postauricular lymphadenopathy, inflamed pharynx, cough, coryza	Nonspecific Antipyretics to control fever **Complications**—Recurrent febrile seizures (possibly from latent infection of central nervous system that is reactivated by fever) Encephalitis Hepatitis (rare)	Use Standard Precautions. Teach parents measures for lowering temperature (antipyretic drugs); ensure adequate parental understanding of specific antipyretic dosage to prevent accidental overdose. If child is prone to seizures, discuss appropriate precautions and possibility of recurrent febrile seizures.
Mumps			
Agent—Paramyxovirus **Source**—Saliva of infected persons **Transmission**—Direct contact with or droplet spread from an infected person **Incubation period**—14-21 days **Period of communicability**—Most communicable immediately before and after swelling begins	**Prodromal stage**—Fever, headache, malaise, and anorexia for 24 h, followed by "earache" that is aggravated by chewing **Parotitis**—By third day, parotid gland(s) (either unilateral or bilateral) enlarges and reaches maximum size in 1-3 days; accompanied by pain and tenderness; other exocrine glands (submandibular) may also be swollen	**Preventive**—Childhood immunization **Symptomatic and supportive**—Analgesics for pain and antipyretics for fever Intravenous fluid if needed for child who refuses to drink or vomits because of meningoencephalitis **Complications**—Sensorineural deafness Postinfectious encephalitis Myocarditis Arthritis Hepatitis Epididymo-orchitis Oophoritis Pancreatitis Sterility (extremely rare in adult men) Meningitis	Maintain isolation during period of communicability; institute Droplet and Contact Precautions during hospitalization. Encourage rest and decreased activity during prodromal phase until swelling subsides. Give analgesics for pain; if child is unwilling to swallow pills or tablets medication, use elixir form. Encourage fluids and soft, bland foods; avoid foods requiring chewing. Apply hot or cold compresses to neck, whichever is more comforting. To relieve orchitis, provide hot or cold packs for analgesia and scrotal elevation.

Continued

TABLE 6.3 Communicable Diseases of Childhood—cont'd

Disease	Clinical Manifestations	Therapeutic Management and Complications	Nursing Care Management
Measles (Rubeola) (Fig. 6.5)			
Agent—Virus Source—Respiratory tract secretions, blood, and urine of infected person Transmission—Usually by direct contact with droplets of infected person; primarily in the winter Incubation period—10-20 days Period of communicability—From 4 days before to 5 days after rash appears but mainly during prodromal (catarrhal) stage	Prodromal (catarrhal) stage— Fever and malaise, followed in 24h by coryza, cough, conjunctivitis, Koplik spots (small, irregular red spots with a minute, bluish-white center first seen on buccal mucosa opposite molars 2 days before rash); symptoms gradually increasing in severity until second day after rash appears, when they begin to subside Rash—Appears 3-4 days after onset of prodromal stage; begins as erythematous maculopapular eruption on face and gradually spreads downward; more severe in earlier sites (appears confluent) and less intense in later sites (appears discrete); after 3-4 days assumes brownish appearance, and fine desquamation occurs over area of extensive involvement Constitutional signs and symptoms—Anorexia, abdominal pain, malaise, generalized lymphadenopathy	Preventive—Childhood immunization Supportive—Bed rest during febrile period; antipyretics Antibiotics to prevent secondary bacterial infection in high-risk children Complications—Otitis media Pneumonia (bacterial) Obstructive laryngitis and laryngotracheitis Encephalitis (rare but has high mortality) Treatment—Administer vitamin A (World Health Organization recommendation) for children with acute illness: 200,000 IU for children ≥12 months old;100,000 IU for children 6-11 months old; 50,000 IU for infants <6 months old (Kimberlin et al., 2018)	Maintain isolation until fifth day of rash; if child is hospitalized, institute Airborne Precautions.Encourage rest during prodromal stage; provide quiet activity. Fever—Instruct parents to administer antipyretics; avoid chilling; if child is prone to seizures, institute appropriate precautions. Eye care—Dim lights if photophobia present; clean eyelids with warm saline solution to remove secretions or crusts; keep child from rubbing eyes. Coryza, cough—Use cool-mist vaporizer; protect skin around nares with layer of petrolatum; encourage fluids and soft, bland foods. Skin care—Keep skin clean; use tepid baths as necessary.
Pertussis (Whooping Cough)			
Agent—*Bordetella pertussis* Source—Discharge from respiratory tract of infected persons Transmission—Direct contact or droplet spread from infected person; indirect contact with freshly contaminated articles Incubation period—6-20 days; usually 7-10 days Period of communicability—Greatest during catarrhal stage before onset of paroxysms	Catarrhal stage—Begins with symptoms of upper respiratory tract infection, such as coryza, sneezing, lacrimation, cough, and low-grade fever; symptoms continue for 1-2wk, when dry, hacking cough becomes more severe Paroxysmal stage—Cough most common at night, consists of short, rapid coughs followed by sudden inspiration associated with a high-pitched crowing sound or "whoop"; during paroxysms, cheeks become flushed or cyanotic, eyes bulge, and tongue protrudes; paroxysm may continue until thick mucus plug is dislodged; vomiting frequently follows attack; stage generally lasts 4-6 wk, followed by convalescent stage Infants <6 months old may not have characteristic whoop cough but have difficulty maintaining adequate oxygenation with amount of secretions, frequent vomiting of mucus and formula or breast milk Pertussis may occur in adolescents and adults with varying manifestations; cough and whoop may be absent, but as many as 50% of adolescents may have a cough for up to 10 wk (Kimberlin et al., 2018) Additional symptoms in adolescents include difficulty breathing and posttussive vomiting (*See also* the Pertussis section earlier in the chapter for discussion of pertussis immunization schedule.)	Preventive—Immunization; current belief is that childhood immunizations for pertussis do not confer lifelong immunity to adolescents and adults, so a pertussis booster is recommended for adolescents (see the Pertussis section earlier in the chapter) Antimicrobial therapy (e.g., erythromycin, clarithromycin, azithromycin) Supportive—Hospitalization sometimes required for infants, children who are dehydrated, or those who have complications Increased oxygen intake and humidity Adequate fluids Intensive care and mechanical ventilation if needed for infants <6 months old Complications—Pneumonia (usual cause of death in younger children) Atelectasis Otitis media Seizures Hemorrhage (scleral, conjunctival, epistaxis; pulmonary hemorrhage in neonate) Weight loss and dehydration Hernias (umbilical and inguinal) Prolapsed rectum Complications reported among adolescents include syncope, sleep disturbance, rib fractures, incontinence, and pneumonia (Kimberlin et al., 2018)	Maintain isolation during catarrhal stage; if child is hospitalized, institute Standard and Droplet Precautions. Obtain nasopharyngeal culture for diagnosis. Encourage oral fluids; offer small amount of fluids frequently. Ensure adequate oxygenation during paroxysms; position infant on side to decrease chance of aspiration with vomiting. Provide humidified oxygen; suction as needed to prevent choking on secretions. Observe for signs of airway obstruction (e.g., increased restlessness, apprehension, retractions, cyanosis). Encourage compliance with antibiotic therapy for household contacts. Encourage adolescents to obtain pertussis booster (Tdap) (see Pertussis section earlier in the chapter). Use Standard and Droplet Precautions in health care workers exposed to children with persistent cough and high suspicion of pertussis.

TABLE 6.3 Communicable Diseases of Childhood—cont'd

Disease	Clinical Manifestations	Therapeutic Management and Complications	Nursing Care Management
Poliomyelitis			
Agent—Enteroviruses, three types: type 1, most frequent cause of paralysis, both epidemic and endemic; type 2, least frequently associated with paralysis; type 3, second most frequently associated with paralysis Source—Feces and oropharyngeal secretions of infected persons, especially young children Transmission—Direct contact with persons with apparent or inapparent active infection; spread via fecal-oral and pharyngeal-oropharyngeal routes; vaccine-acquired paralytic polio may occur as a result of the live oral polio vaccination (no longer available in the United States) Incubation period—Usually 7-14 days, with range of 5-35 days Period of communicability—Not exactly known; virus present in throat and feces shortly after infection and persists for about 1 wk in throat and 4-6 wk in feces	May be manifested in three different forms: Abortive or inapparent—Fever, uneasiness, sore throat, headache, anorexia, vomiting, abdominal pain; lasts a few hours to a few days Nonparalytic—Same manifestations as abortive but more severe, with pain and stiffness in neck, back, and legs Paralytic—Initial course similar to nonparalytic type, followed by recovery and then signs of central nervous system paralysis	Preventive—Childhood immunization Supportive—Complete bed rest during acute phase Mechanical or assisted ventilation in case of respiratory paralysis Physical therapy for muscles after acute stage Complications—Permanent paralysis Respiratory arrest Hypertension Kidney stones from demineralization of bone during prolonged immobility	Institute Contact Precautions. Administer mild sedatives as necessary to relieve anxiety and promote rest. Participate in physical therapy procedures (use of moist hot packs and range-of-motion exercises). Position child to maintain body alignment and prevent contractures or skin breakdown; use footboard or appropriate orthoses to prevent foot drop; use pressure mattress for prolonged immobility. Encourage child to perform activities of daily living to capability; promote early ambulation with assistive devices; administer analgesics for maximum comfort during physical activity; give high-protein diet and bowel management for prolonged immobility. Observe for respiratory paralysis (e.g., difficulty talking, ineffective cough, inability to hold breath, shallow and rapid respirations); report such signs and symptoms to practitioner.
Rubella (German Measles) (Fig. 6.6)			
Agent—Rubella virus Source—Primarily nasopharyngeal secretions of person with apparent or inapparent infection; virus also present in blood, stool, and urine Incubation period—14-21 days Period of communicability—7 days before to about 5 days after appearance of rash Constitutional signs and symptoms—Occasionally low-grade fever, headache, malaise, and lymphadenopathy	Prodromal stage—Absent in children, present in adults and adolescents; consists of low-grade fever, headache, malaise, anorexia, mild conjunctivitis, coryza, sore throat, cough, and lymphadenopathy; lasts 1-5 days, subsides 1 day after appearance of rash Rash—First appears on face and rapidly spreads downward to neck, arms, trunk, and legs; by end of first day, body is covered with discrete, pinkish-red maculopapular exanthema; disappears in same order as it began and is usually gone by third day	Preventive—Childhood immunization No treatment necessary other than antipyretics for low-grade fever and analgesics for discomfort Complications—Rare (arthritis, encephalitis, or purpura); most benign of all childhood communicable diseases; greatest danger is teratogenic effect on fetus	Institute Droplet Precautions. Reassure parents of benign nature of illness in affected child. Use comfort measures as necessary. Avoid contact with pregnant women. Monitor rubella titer in pregnant adolescent.

Continued

TABLE 6.3 Communicable Diseases of Childhood—cont'd

Disease	Clinical Manifestations	Therapeutic Management and Complications	Nursing Care Management
Scarlet Fever (Fig. 6.7)			
Agent—Group A beta-hemolytic streptococci **Source**—Usually from nasopharyngeal secretions of infected persons and carriers **Transmission**—Direct contact with infected person or droplet spread; indirectly by contact with contaminated articles or ingestion of contaminated milk or other food **Incubation period**—2-5 days, with range of 1-7 days **Period of communicability**—During incubation period and clinical illness, approximately 10 days; during first 2 wk of carrier phase, although may persist for months	**Prodromal stage**—Abrupt high fever, pulse increased out of proportion to fever, vomiting, headache, chills, malaise, abdominal pain, halitosis **Enanthema**—Tonsils enlarged, edematous, reddened, and covered with patches of exudates; in severe cases appearance resembles membrane seen in diphtheria; pharynx is edematous and beefy red; during first 1-2 days tongue is coated and papillae become red and swollen (white strawberry tongue); by fourth or fifth day white coat sloughs off, leaving prominent papillae (red strawberry tongue); palate is covered with erythematous punctate lesions **Exanthema**—Rash appears within 12 h after prodromal signs; red pinhead-sized punctate lesions rapidly become generalized but are absent on face, which becomes flushed with striking circumoral pallor; rash more intense in folds of joints; by end of first week desquamation begins (fine, sandpaper-like on torso; sheetlike sloughing on palms and soles), which may be complete by 3 wk or longer	Full course of penicillin (or erythromycin in penicillin-sensitive children) or oral cephalosporin Antibiotic therapy for newly diagnosed carriers (nose or throat cultures positive for streptococci) **Supportive**—Rest during febrile phase, analgesics for sore throat; antipruritics for rash if bothersome **Complications**—Peritonsillar and retropharyngeal abscess Sinusitis Otitis media Acute glomerulonephritis Acute rheumatic fever Polyarthritis (uncommon)	Institute Standard and Droplet Precautions until 24 h after initiation of treatment. Ensure compliance with oral antibiotic therapy; intramuscular benzathine penicillin G [Bicillin] may be given. Encourage rest during febrile phase; provide quiet activity during convalescent period. Relieve discomfort of sore throat with analgesics, gargles, lozenges, antiseptic throat sprays, and inhalation of cool mist. Encourage fluids during febrile phase; avoid irritating liquids (e.g., citrus juices) or rough foods (e.g., chips); when child can eat, begin with soft diet. Advise parents to consult practitioner if fever persists after beginning therapy. Discuss procedures for preventing spread of infection—discard toothbrush; avoid sharing drinking and eating utensils.

Tdap, Tetanus, diphtheria toxoids, and acellular pertussis vaccine.

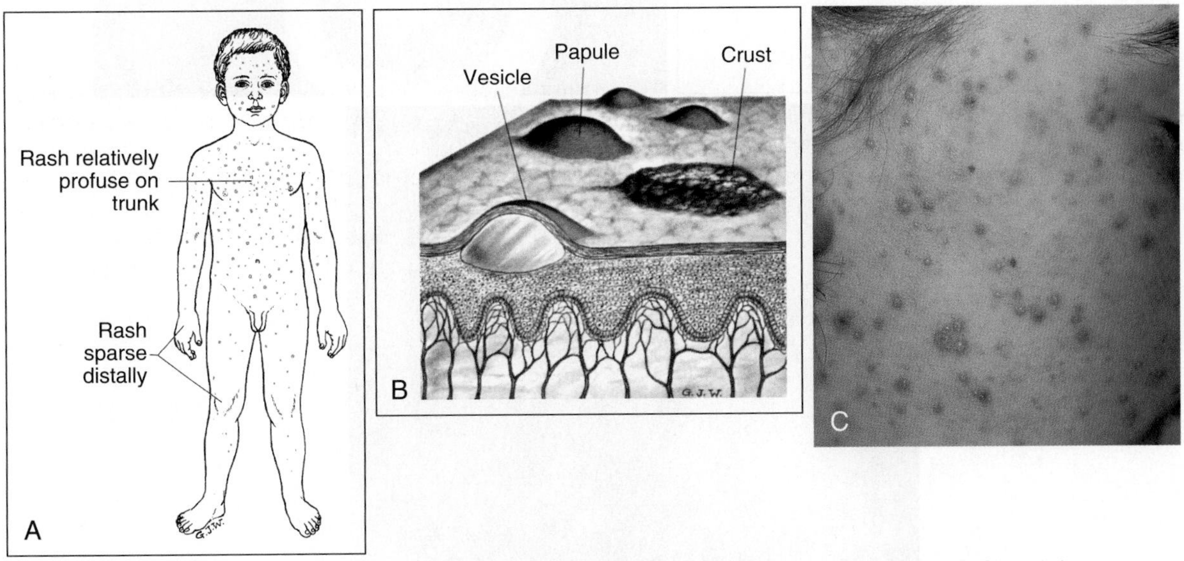

Fig. 6.2 Chickenpox (varicella). **A,** Progression of disease. **B,** Simultaneous stages of lesions. **C,** Clinical view. (**C,** From Habif, T. P. [2016]. *Clinical dermatology: A color guide to diagnosis and therapy* [6th ed.]. St. Louis, MO: Mosby.)

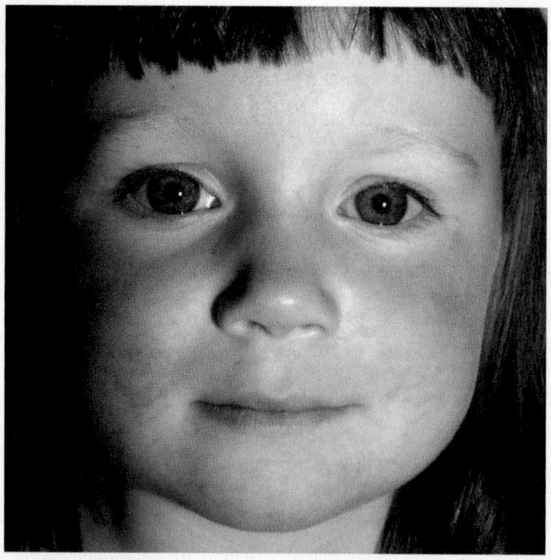

Fig. 6.3 Erythema infectiosum (fifth disease). (From Habif, T. P. [2016]. *Clinical dermatology: A color guide to diagnosis and therapy* [6th ed.]. St. Louis, MO: Mosby.)

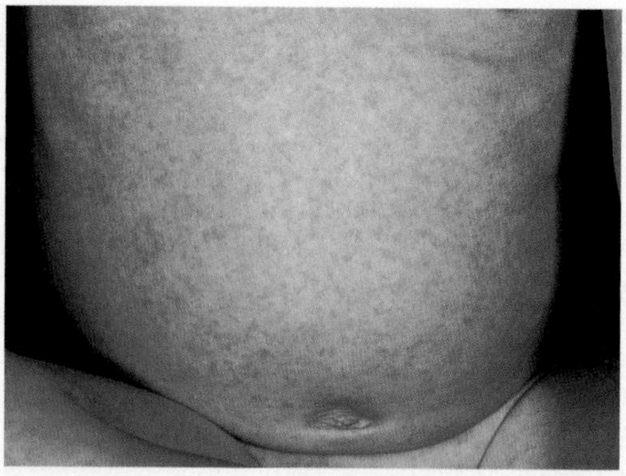

Fig. 6.4 Exanthem subitum (roseola infantum). (From Habif, T. P. [2016]. *Clinical dermatology: A color guide to diagnosis and therapy* [6th ed.]. St. Louis, MO: Mosby.)

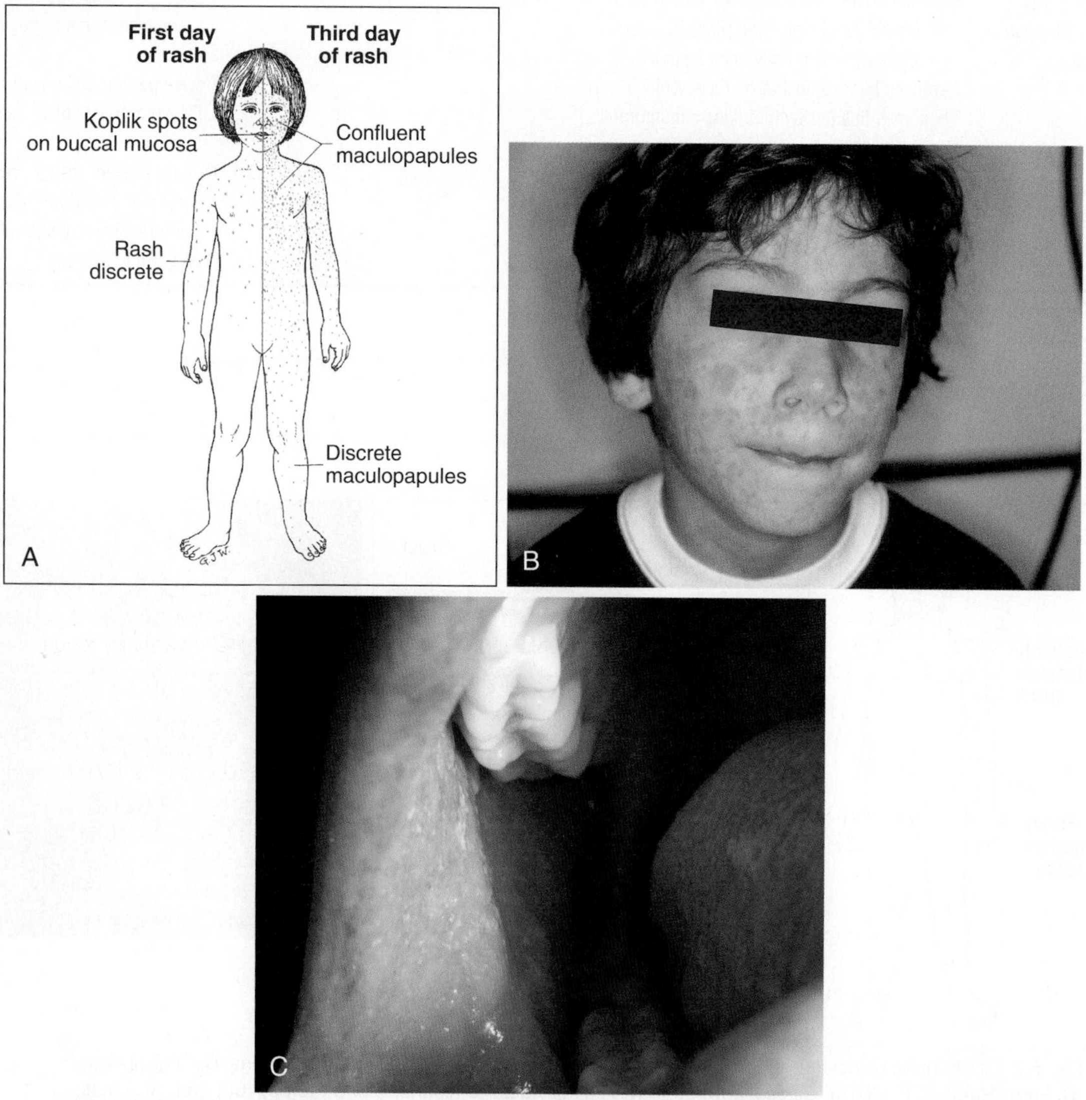

Fig. 6.5 Measles (rubeola). **A,** Progression of disease. **B,** Clinical view. **C,** Koplik spots. (**B,** From Paller, S. A., & Mancini, A. J. [2011]. *Hurwitz clinical pediatric dermatology* [4th ed.]. St. Louis, MO: Saunders; **C,** From Habif, T. P. [2016]. *Clinical dermatology: A color guide to diagnosis and therapy* [6th ed.]. St. Louis, MO: Mosby.)

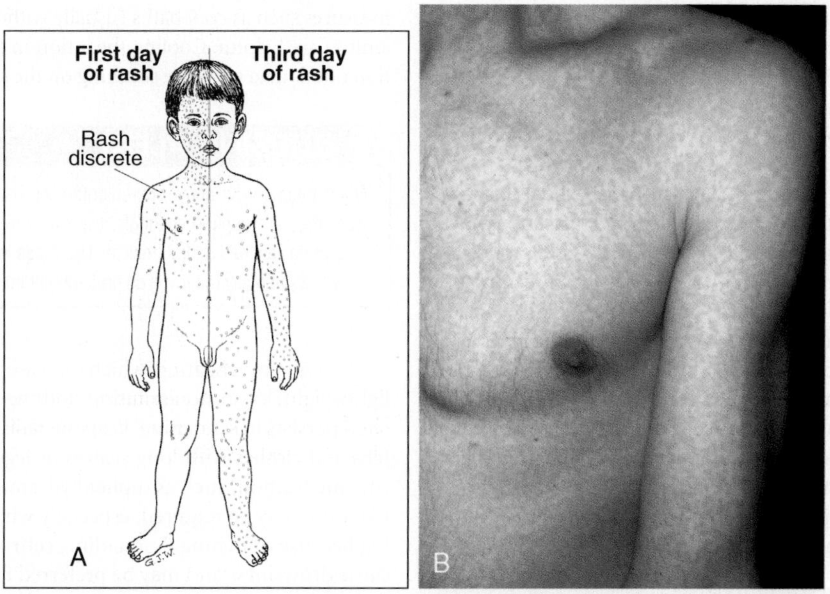

Fig. 6.6 Rubella (German measles). A, Progression of rash. B, Clinical view. (B, From Zitelli, B. J., & Davis, H. W. [2007]. *Atlas of pediatric physical diagnosis* [5th ed.]. St. Louis, MO: Mosby; courtesy Dr. Michael Sherlock, Lutherville, MD.)

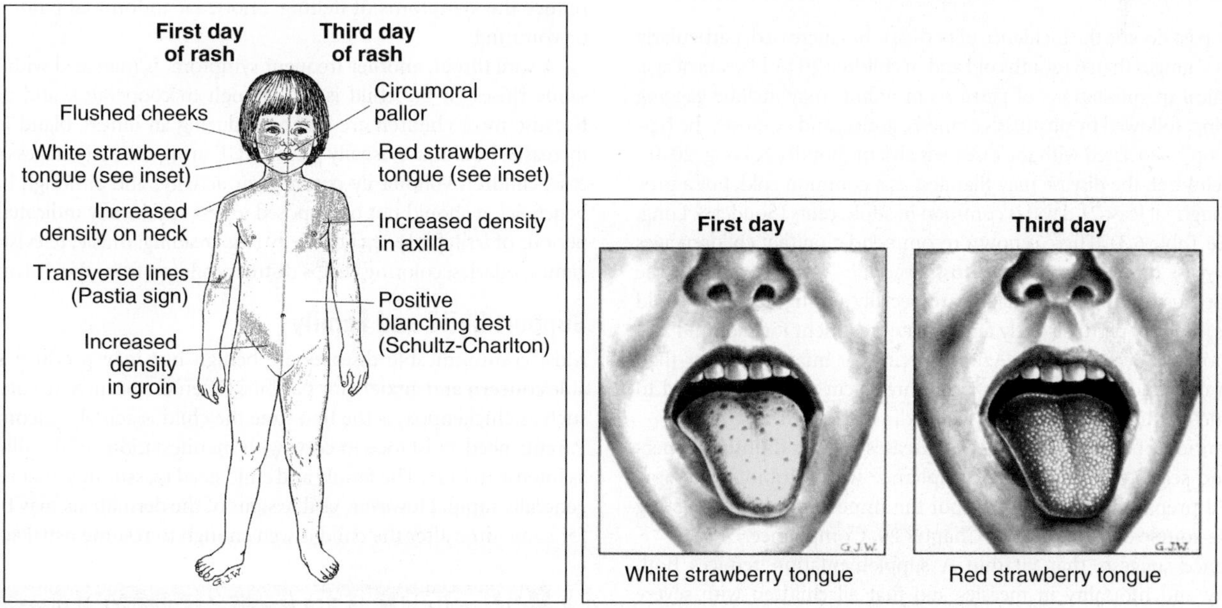

Fig. 6.7 Scarlet fever.

Prevent Complications

Although most children recover without difficulty, certain groups are at risk for serious, even fatal, complications from communicable diseases, especially the viral diseases chickenpox and erythema infectiosum (fifth disease) caused by **human parvovirus B19**.

Children with immunodeficiency—those receiving steroid or other immunosuppressive therapy, those with a generalized malignancy such as leukemia or lymphoma, or those with an immunologic disorder—are at risk for viremia from replication of the **varicella-zoster virus (VZV)**[b] in the blood. VZV is so named because it causes two distinct diseases: **varicella (chickenpox)** and **zoster (herpes zoster** or **shingles)**. Varicella occurs primarily in children younger than 15 years of age. However, it leaves the threat of herpes zoster, an intensely painful varicella that is localized to a single **dermatome** (body area innervated by a particular segment of the spinal cord). Immunocompromised patients and healthy infants younger than 1 year of age (who also have reduced immunity) are at a higher risk for reactivation of VZV causing herpes zoster, probably as a result of a deficiency in cellular immunity (Kimberlin et al., 2018). Complications of herpes zoster virus in children include secondary bacterial infection, depigmentation, and scarring. Postherpetic neuralgia in children is uncommon (Kimberlin et al., 2018).

The use of varicella-zoster immune globulin (VariZIG) or intravenous immunoglobulin (IVIG) is recommended for children who are immunocompromised, who have no previous history of varicella, and who are likely to contract the disease and have complications as a result (Kimberlin et al., 2018). The antiviral agent acyclovir (Zovirax) or valacyclovir may be used to treat varicella infections in susceptible immunocompromised

[b]Educational materials may be obtained from the National Shingles Foundation, 590 Madison Ave., 21st Floor, New York, NY 10022; 212-222-3390; http://www.vzvfoundation.org.

persons. It is effective in decreasing the number of lesions; shortening the duration of fever; and decreasing itching, lethargy, and anorexia. Consider oral valacyclovir for immunocompromised children without a history of varicella disease, newborns whose mother had varicella within 5 days before delivery or within 48 hours after delivery, and hospitalized preterm infants with significant varicella exposure (Kimberlin et al., 2018).

Children with hemolytic disease, such as sickle cell disease, are at risk for aplastic anemia from erythema infectiosum. Human parvovirus B19 infects and lyses red blood cell precursors, thus interrupting the production of red blood cells. Therefore the virus may precipitate a severe aplastic crisis in patients who need increased red blood cell production to maintain normal red blood cell volumes. Thrombocytopenia and neutropenia may also occur as a result of human parvovirus B19 infection. The fetus has a relatively high rate of red blood cell production and an immature immune system; it may develop severe anemia and hydrops as a result of maternal human parvovirus infection. Fetal death rates as a result of human parvovirus B19 have been estimated to be between 2% and 6%, with the greatest risk appearing to be in the first 20 weeks (Kimberlin et al., 2018; Koch, 2020).

! NURSING ALERT

Refer children at risk for contracting these communicable diseases to the practitioner immediately in case of known exposure or outbreaks.

In the past decade the incidence of pertussis has increased, particularly in infants younger than 6 months old and in children 10 to 14 years of age. Early clinical manifestations of pertussis in infants may include gagging and gasping, followed by posttussive emesis, apnea, and cyanosis; the typical "whoop" associated with the disease is absent (Souder & Long, 2020). In older children the disease may manifest as a common cold, but a prolonged cough (at least 21 days) is common in adolescents (Souder & Long, 2020) (see Table 6.3). There is now a recommendation that children ages 11 to 12 years receive a booster pertussis vaccine (Tdap) to prevent the disease. Because pertussis is contagious, especially among close household members, identify pertussis early and initiate treatment for the child and those who have been exposed. Azithromycin (for infants younger than 1 month old) and erythromycin or clarithromycin are administered to infants and children with pertussis (Kimberlin et al., 2018).

Prevention of complications from diseases such as diphtheria, pertussis, and scarlet fever requires compliance with antibiotic therapy. With oral preparations, educate about the importance of completing the entire course of therapy. (See Chapter 20, Compliance.)

Evidence suggests that vitamin A supplementation reduces both morbidity and mortality in measles and that all children with severe measles should receive vitamin A supplements. A single oral dose of 200,000 IU for children at least 1 year old is recommended (use half that dose for children 6 to 12 months of age) (see Table 6.3). The higher dose may be associated with vomiting and headache for a few hours. The dose should be repeated on the next day and at 4 weeks for children with ophthalmologic evidence of vitamin A deficiency (Kimberlin et al., 2018).

! NURSING ALERT

Although the risk of vitamin A toxicity from these doses (they are 100 to 200 times the recommended dietary allowance) is relatively low, nurses should instruct parents on safe storage of the drug. Ideally, vitamin A should be dispensed in the age-appropriate unit dose to prevent excessive administration and possible toxicity.

Provide Comfort

Many communicable diseases cause skin manifestations that are bothersome to the child. The chief discomfort from most rashes is itching, and measures such as cool baths (usually without soap) and lotions (e.g., calamine) are helpful. Cooling the lotion in the refrigerator before application often makes it more soothing on the skin than at room temperature.

! NURSING ALERT

When lotions with active ingredients such as diphenhydramine in Caladryl are used, they are applied sparingly, especially over open lesions, where excessive absorption can lead to drug toxicity. Use these lotions with caution in children who are simultaneously receiving an oral antihistamine.

To avoid overheating, which increases itching, children should wear lightweight, loose, nonirritating clothing and keep out of the sun. If the child persists in scratching, keep the nails short and smooth or use mittens and clothes with long sleeves or legs. For severe itching, antipruritic medication, such as diphenhydramine (Benadryl) or hydroxyzine (Atarax), may be required, especially when the child has trouble sleeping because of itching. Loratadine, cetirizine, and fexofenadine do not cause drowsiness and may be preferred for urticaria during the day.

An elevated temperature is common, and both antipyretic medicine (acetaminophen or ibuprofen) and environmental manipulation are implemented. (See Chapter 20, Controlling Elevated Temperatures.) Acetaminophen is effective in lowering fever but does not significantly reduce the symptoms of itching, anorexia, abdominal pain, fussiness, or vomiting.

A sore throat, another frequent symptom, is managed with lozenges, saline rinses (if the child is old enough to cooperate), and analgesics. Because most children are anorectic during an illness, bland foods and increased liquids are usually preferred. During the early stages of the disease, children voluntarily curtail their activity, and although bed rest is beneficial, it should not be imposed unless specifically indicated. During periods of irritability, quiet activity (e.g., reading, music, television, video games, puzzles, coloring) helps distract children from the discomfort.

Support Child and Family

Most communicable diseases are benign but may produce considerable concern and anxiety for parents. Often the occurrence of a disease, such as chickenpox, is the first time the child is acutely uncomfortable. Parents need assistance to cope with manifestations of the illness, such as intense itching. The family and child need reassurance that recovery is generally rapid. However, visible signs of the dermatosis may be present for some time after the child is well enough to resume usual activities.

! NURSING ALERT

The occurrence of a communicable disease provides the opportunity to ask parents about the child's immunization status and reinforce the benefits of vaccines for children.

CONJUNCTIVITIS

Acute **conjunctivitis** (inflammation of the conjunctiva) occurs from a variety of causes that are typically age related. In newborns, conjunctivitis can occur from infection during birth, most often from *Chlamydia trachomatis* (inclusion conjunctivitis) or *Neisseria gonorrhoeae.* Conjunctivitis in a neonate is a serious condition and can potentially lead to blindness; all signs of conjunctivitis require prompt reporting and a comprehensive evaluation (Olitsky & Marsh, 2020). The clinical signs of conjunctivitis are similar regardless of the cause: redness and swelling of the conjunctiva, eyelid edema, and discharge (Olitsky & Marsh, 2020). In infants, recurrent conjunctivitis may be a sign of nasolacrimal (tear) duct obstruction or dacryocystitis, an infection of the lacrimal sac. Timing of the infection may provide signs of the cause. A chemical conjunctivitis may occur within 24 hours of instillation of neonatal ophthalmic prophylaxis; *N. gonorrhoeae* usually occurs within 2 to 5 days after birth, and *C. trachomatis* occurs 5 to 14 days after birth (Olitsky & Marsh, 2020). In children, the usual causes of conjunctivitis are viral, bacterial, allergic, or related to a foreign body. Bacterial infection accounts for most instances of acute conjunctivitis in children. Diagnosis is made primarily from the clinical manifestations (Box 6.3), although cultures of purulent drainage may be needed to identify the specific cause.

Therapeutic Management

Treatment of conjunctivitis depends on the cause. Viral conjunctivitis is self-limiting, and treatment is limited to removal of the accumulated secretions. Bacterial conjunctivitis has traditionally been treated with topical antibacterial agents such as polymyxin and bacitracin (Polysporin), sodium sulfacetamide (Sulamyd), or trimethoprim and polymyxin (Polytrim). Infants with bacterial conjunctivitis may require systemic antibiotics (Olitsky & Marsh, 2020). For children age 1 year and older, fluoroquinolones and aminoglycosides are commonly used ophthalmic antimicrobial agents. Fourth-generation fluoroquinolones such as moxifloxacin, gatifloxacin, and besifloxacin provide broad-spectrum coverage, are bactericidal, and are generally well tolerated (Alter, Vidwan, Sobande, et al., 2011). Drops may be used during the day and an ointment used at bedtime because the ointment preparation remains in the eye longer but blurs the vision. Corticosteroids are avoided because they reduce ocular resistance to bacteria.

Nursing Care Management

Nursing care includes keeping the eye clean and properly administering ophthalmic medication. Remove accumulated secretions by wiping from the inner canthus downward and outward, away from the opposite eye. Warm, moist compresses, such as a clean washcloth wrung out with hot tap water, are helpful in removing the crusts. Compresses are *not* kept on the eye because an occlusive covering promotes bacterial growth. Instill medication immediately after the eyes have been cleaned and according to correct procedure (see Chapter 20).

Prevention of infection in other family members is an important consideration with bacterial conjunctivitis. Keep the child's washcloth and towel separate from those used by others. Discard tissues used to clean the eye. Instruct the child to refrain from rubbing the eye and to use good hand-washing technique.

STOMATITIS

Stomatitis is inflammation of the oral mucosa, which may include the buccal (cheek) and labial (lip) mucosa, tongue, gingiva, palate, and floor of the mouth. It may be infectious or noninfectious and may be caused by local or systemic factors. In children, aphthous stomatitis and herpetic stomatitis are typically seen. Children with immunosuppression and those receiving chemotherapy or head and neck radiotherapy are at high risk for developing mucosal ulceration and herpetic stomatitis.

Aphthous stomatitis (aphthous ulcer, canker sore) is a benign but painful condition whose cause is unknown. Its onset is usually associated with mild traumatic injury (e.g., biting the cheek, hitting the mucosa with a toothbrush, a mouth appliance rubbing on the mucosa), allergy, or emotional stress. The lesions are painful, small, whitish ulcerations surrounded by a red border. They are distinguished from other types of stomatitis by healthy adjacent tissues, absence of vesicles, and no systemic illness. The ulcers persist for 4 to 12 days and heal uneventfully.

Herpetic gingivostomatitis (HGS) is caused by herpes simplex virus (HSV), most often type 1, and may occur as a primary infection or recur in a less severe form known as **recurrent herpes labialis** (commonly called *cold sores* or *fever blisters*). The primary infection usually begins with a fever; the pharynx becomes edematous and erythematous; and vesicles erupt on the mucosa, causing severe pain (Fig. 6.8). Cervical lymphadenitis often occurs, and the breath has a distinctly foul odor. In the recurrent form, the vesicles appear on the lips, usually singly or in groups. The precipitating factors for the cold sores include emotional stress, trauma (often related to dental procedures), immunosuppression, or exposure to excessive sunlight. The disease can last 5 to 14 days, with varying degrees of severity.

Stomatitis may occur as a manifestation of hand-foot-and-mouth disease (HFMD) and herpangina; both manifest with scattered vesicles on the buccal mucosa and are commonly caused by the nonpolio enteroviruses (primarily coxsackieviruses). Children with either HFMD or herpangina often have poor intake as a result of the mouth sores; infants may refuse to nurse or take a bottle or may pull away and cry after a few seconds of nursing.

Therapeutic Management

Treatment for all types of stomatitis is aimed at relief of symptoms, primarily pain. Acetaminophen and ibuprofen are usually sufficient for mild cases, but with more severe HGS, stronger analgesics such as codeine may be needed. Topical anesthetics are helpful and include over-the-counter preparations such as Orabase, Anbesol, and Kank-A. Lidocaine (Xylocaine Viscous) can be prescribed for the child who can keep 1 tsp of the solution in the mouth for 2 to 3 minutes and then expectorate the drug. A mixture of equal parts

BOX 6.3 Clinical Manifestations of Conjunctivitis

Bacterial Conjunctivitis ("Pink Eye")
Purulent drainage
Crusting of eyelids, especially on awakening
Inflamed conjunctiva
Swollen eyelids

Viral Conjunctivitis
Usually occurs with upper respiratory tract infection
Serous (watery) drainage
Inflamed conjunctiva
Swollen eyelids

Allergic Conjunctivitis
Itching
Watery to thick, stringy discharge
Inflamed conjunctiva
Swollen eyelids

Conjunctivitis Caused by Foreign Body
Tearing
Pain
Inflamed conjunctiva
Usually only one eye affected

! NURSING ALERT

Signs of serious conjunctivitis include reduction or loss of vision, ocular pain, photophobia, exophthalmos (bulging eyeball), decreased ocular mobility, corneal ulceration, and unusual patterns of inflammation (e.g., the perilimbal flush associated with iritis or localized inflammation associated with scleritis). If a patient has any of these signs, refer him or her immediately to an ophthalmologist.

of diphenhydramine elixir and Maalox (aluminum and magnesium hydroxide) provides mild analgesia, antiinflammatory properties, and a protective coating for the lesions. Sucralfate can also be used as a coating agent for oral mucous membranes. Treatment for children with severe cases of HGS includes the use of antiviral agents such as acyclovir (Dhar, 2020).

Nursing Care Management

The chief nursing goals for children with stomatitis are relief of pain and prevention of spread of the herpes virus. Analgesics and topical anesthetics are used as needed to provide relief, especially before meals to encourage food and fluid intake. For younger infants and toddlers who cannot swish and swallow, apply the diphenhydramine and Maalox solution with a cotton-tipped applicator before feedings to minimize pain. Educating parents about the use of these medications is important to maintain adequate hydration in the child whose mouth is too sore to take liquids. Drinking bland fluids through a straw is helpful in avoiding the painful lesions. Encourage mouth care; the use of a very soft–bristle toothbrush or disposable foam-tipped toothbrush provides gentle cleaning near ulcerated areas.

Careful hand washing is essential when caring for children with HGS. Because the infection is autoinoculable, children should keep their fingers out of the mouth; contaminated hands can infect other body parts. Very young children may require elbow restraints to ensure compliance. Articles placed in the mouth are cleaned thoroughly. Newborns and individuals with immunosuppression should not be exposed to infected children.

! NURSING ALERT

When examining herpetic lesions, wear gloves. The virus easily enters any breaks in the skin and can cause herpetic whitlow of the fingers.

Because herpes infection is often associated with sexual transmission, explain to parents and older children that HGS is usually caused by type 1 HSV, the type not associated with sexual activity.

ZIKA VIRUS

The Zika virus (ZIKV) was initially discovered almost 70 years ago in the Zika Forest in Uganda with sporadic outbreaks, but in 2013 occurrences of the virus in Polynesia then spread to various areas of South America, leading to a major epidemic by 2016. ZIKV is transmitted to humans primarily via an infected *Aedes* species mosquito bite; however, the virus can also be transferred from mother to child during pregnancy (transplacental) and to others by contact with urine, blood, semen, or vaginal fluid (Centers for Disease Control and Prevention, 2016b). There is no current evidence that the Zika virus is in breast milk, and mothers are encouraged to continue breastfeeding (Centers for Disease Control and Prevention, 2016b).

Most infected individuals are asymptomatic, but approximately 18% will develop fever, arthralgia, maculopapular rash, or conjunctivitis 3 to 12 days after being infected, with symptoms lasting up to 7 days (Murray, 2016). The most serious manifestations of ZIKV are fetal brain defects, including microcephaly, that occur in the developing fetus when a pregnant woman contracts the virus (Murray, 2016). Preliminary diagnosis is based on the patient's symptoms and recent travel (Centers for Disease Control and Prevention, 2016b). Confirmation of the diagnosis can be made through molecular diagnostic techniques of blood or urine from the individual.

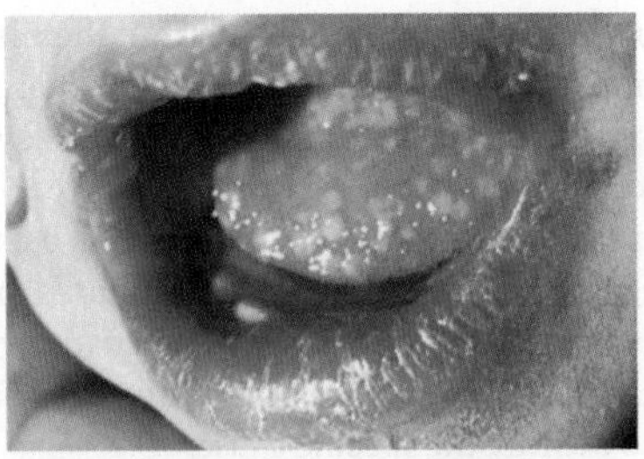

Fig. 6.8 Primary gingivostomatitis. (From Thompson, J. M., McFarland, G. M., Hirsch, J. E., et al. [2002]. *Mosby's clinical nursing* [5th ed.]. St. Louis, MO: Mosby.)

Therapeutic Management

There is no current therapy available to treat ZIKV (Murray, 2016). Provide the patient with supportive care measures, including rest, adequate hydration, analgesics, and antipyretics as needed. As with any other viral illness, aspirin and other salicylates should not be administered to children to avoid Reye syndrome (Murray, 2016). Avoiding mosquito bites is the best method to prevent the disease.

Nursing Care Management

Nurses must remain informed about emerging ZIKV developments and educate patients, parents, and caretakers with accurate information. The Centers for Disease Control and Prevention provides thorough and updated information on ZIKV on its website (https://www.cdc.gov/zika). Resources such as fact sheets, posters, and communication toolkits in several different languages are also available on the website.

Preventing mosquito bites is one of the most effective ways to prevent ZIKV infection. When traveling to areas known to have ZIKV, preventive measures include wearing appropriate clothing to have as little skin exposed as possible, using insect repellent, and using screens on windows and doors or insecticide-treated nets if windows and doors are not available (Murray, 2016).

INTESTINAL PARASITIC DISEASES

Intestinal parasitic diseases, including helminths (worms) and protozoa, constitute the most frequent infections in the world. In the United States, the incidence of intestinal parasitic disease, especially giardiasis, has increased among young children who attend daycare centers. Young children are especially at risk because of typical hand-to-mouth activity and uncontrolled fecal activity.

Various infecting organisms cause intestinal parasitic diseases in humans. This discussion is limited to three common parasitic infections among children in the United States: giardiasis, pinworms, and bed bugs. Table 6.4 describes the outstanding features of selected helminths that belong to the family of nematodes.

GENERAL NURSING CARE MANAGEMENT

Nursing responsibilities related to intestinal parasitic infections involve assistance with identification of the parasite, treatment of the infection, and prevention of initial infection or reinfection. Laboratory examination of substances containing the worm, its larvae, or its ova can identify the organism. Most are identified by examining fecal smears from the stools of persons suspected of harboring the parasite. Fresh specimens are best for revealing parasites or larvae; therefore take collected specimens directly to the laboratory for examination. If this is not possible, place the specimen in a container with a preservative. Parents need clear instructions on obtaining an adequate sample and the number of samples required (see Chapter 20, Stool Specimens). In most parasitic infections, other family members, especially children, may be examined to identify those who are similarly affected.

After the diagnosis is confirmed and appropriate treatment is planned, parents need further explanation and reinforcement. Compliance in terms of drug therapy and other measures, such as thorough hand washing, is essential for eradication of the parasite. The family needs to understand the nature of transmission and that in some cases the medication must be repeated in 2 weeks to 1 month to kill organisms hatched since initial treatment.

The nurse's most important function is preventive education of children and families regarding hygiene and health habits. Thorough hand washing before eating or handling food and after using the toilet is the most important precautionary method. The Family-Centered Care box lists other preventive practices.

GIARDIASIS

Giardiasis is caused by the protozoan *Giardia intestinalis* (formerly called *Giardia lamblia* and *Giardia duodenalis*). It is the most common intestinal parasitic pathogen in the United States, with an estimated 1.2 million people affected annually (Painter, Gargano, Collier, et al., 2015). Child care centers and institutions providing care for persons with developmental disabilities are common sites for urban giardiasis, and the children may pass cysts for months. Also consider giardiasis in those with a history of recent travel to an endemic area or drinking untreated water.

The potential for transmission is great because the cysts—the nonmotile stage of the protozoa—can survive in the environment for months. Chief modes of transmission are person to person, food, and animals. Contaminated water, especially in lakes and streams, and swimming or wading pools frequented by diapered infants are common sources of transmission (Painter et al., 2015). In children, person-to-person transmission is the most likely cause. Although individuals infected with giardiasis may be asymptomatic, common symptoms include abdominal cramps, bloating, and diarrhea (Box 6.4).

Diagnosis of giardiasis may be made by microscopic examination of stool specimens or duodenal fluid or by identification of *G. intestinalis* antigens in these specimens by techniques such as enzyme immunoassay (EIA) and direct fluorescence antibody (DFA) assays. Because the *Giardia* organisms live in the upper intestine and are excreted in a highly variable pattern, repeated microscopic examination of stool specimens may be required to identify trophozoites (active parasites) or cysts. Duodenal specimens are obtained by direct aspiration, biopsy, or the string test. In the string test, the child swallows a gelatin capsule with a nylon string attached. Several hours later, the string is withdrawn, and the contents are sent for laboratory analysis. With the availability of EIA techniques to identify *Giardia* antigens in stool specimens, other tests are being used less often.

Therapeutic Management

The drugs of choice for treatment of giardiasis are metronidazole (Flagyl), tinidazole (Tindamax), and nitazoxanide (Alinia). Tinidazole is said to have an 80% to 100% cure rate after a single dose (Kimberlin et al., 2018). Metronidazole and tinidazole have a metallic taste and gastrointestinal side effects, including nausea and vomiting. Nitazoxanide does not have a bitter taste and should be taken with food to avoid gastrointestinal symptoms; it reportedly has very few adverse effects and is available in suspension form. Alternative drug therapy includes albendazole, furazolidone, and quinacrine (John, 2020). Quinacrine is only available from a compounding pharmacy.

FAMILY-CENTERED CARE

Preventing Intestinal Parasitic Disease

- Always wash hands and fingernails with soap and water before eating and handling food and after toileting.
- Avoid placing fingers in mouth and biting nails.
- Discourage children from scratching bare anal area.
- Use superabsorbent disposable diapers to prevent leakage.
- Change diapers as soon as soiled and dispose of diapers in closed receptacle out of children's reach.
- Do not rinse cloth or disposable diapers in toilet.
- Disinfect toilet seats and diaper-changing areas; use dilute household bleach (10% solution) or ammonia (Lysol) and wipe clean with paper towels.
- Drink only treated water or bottled water, especially if camping.
- Wash all raw fruits and vegetables and food that have fallen on the floor.
- Avoid growing foods in soil fertilized with human or untreated animal excreta.
- Teach children to defecate only in a toilet, not on the ground.
- Keep dogs and cats away from playgrounds and sandboxes.
- Avoid swimming in pools frequented by diapered children.
- Wear shoes outside.

The most important nursing consideration is prevention of giardiasis and education of parents, child care center staff, and others who assume the daily care of small children. Attention to meticulous sanitary practices, especially during diaper changes, is essential (see Family-Centered Care box and Fig. 6.9). Nurses can play an important role in educating parents of small children and daycare staff regarding appropriate sanitation practices. In addition, discourage young children who are infected or who have diarrhea from swimming in community or private pools until they have been infection-free for 2 weeks (Kimberlin et al., 2018). Lakes and streams may contain high numbers of *Giardia* spore cysts, which can be swallowed in the water. Discourage children from swimming in stagnant bodies of water and in water where there are known infected children swimming when there is a high chance of swallowing water. *Giardia* organisms are resistant to chlorine (Painter et al., 2015). Encourage parents to take small children to the restroom frequently when swimming, to avoid letting children in diapers in swimming areas, and to change diapers away from the water source. (See also Centers for Disease Control and Prevention information on recreational water illnesses, http://www.cdc.gov/healthywater/swimming.) After children are infected, family education regarding drug administration is essential.

ENTEROBIASIS (PINWORMS)

Enterobiasis, or pinworms, caused by the nematode *Enterobius vermicularis,* is the most common helminthic infection in the United States. It is universally present in temperate climatic zones and may infect more than 30% of all children at any one time. Transmission is favored in crowded conditions, such as in classrooms and daycare centers. Infection begins when the eggs are ingested or inhaled (the eggs float in the air). The eggs hatch in the upper intestine and then mature and migrate through the intestine. After mating, adult females migrate out the anus and lay eggs (Kimberlin et al., 2018).

TABLE 6.4 Selected Intestinal Parasites

Clinical Manifestations	Comments
Ascariasis—*Ascaris lumbricoides* (Common Roundworm)	
Light infections or asymptomatic: Parent may find roundworm in child's diaper with or without stool or see roundworms in the toilet Heavy infections: Anorexia, irritability, nervousness, enlarged abdomen, weight loss, fever, intestinal colic Severe infections: Intestinal obstruction, appendicitis, perforation of intestine with peritonitis, obstructive jaundice, lung involvement (pneumonitis)	Transferred to mouth via contaminated food, fingers, or toys (*Ascaris* lays eggs in soil, which children play in) No person-to-person transmission Largest of the intestinal helminths Affects principally young children 1-4 years of age Prevalent in warm climates Treatment with albendazole (single dose) OR mebendazole for 3 days OR oral ivermectin (children >15 kg) as a single dose OR nitazoxanide for 3 days Reexamine stool specimen in 2 wk to establish need for further pharmacologic therapy (Kimberlin et al., 2018).
Hookworm—*Necator americanus* and *Ancylostoma duodenale*	
Light infections in well-nourished individuals: No problems Heavier infections: Mild to severe hypochromia, microcytic anemia, malnutrition, hypoproteinemia and edema May be itching and burning followed by erythema and a papular eruption in areas to which the organism migrates	Transmitted by discharging eggs on the soil, which are picked up by human host, commonly in the feet, causing infection from direct skin contact with contaminated soil Recommend wearing shoes, although children playing in contaminated soil expose many skin surfaces Diagnosis established by presence of hookworm eggs in stool (humans are the only host of hookworms) Treat with albendazole, mebendazole, and pyrantel pamoate
Strongyloidiasis—*Strongyloides stercoralis* (Threadworm)	
Light infection: Asymptomatic Heavy infection: Respiratory signs and symptoms; abdominal pain, distention; nausea and vomiting; diarrhea (large, pale stools, often with mucus) Larva migration manifests as pruritic skin lesions in the perianal area, buttocks, and upper thighs, creating serpiginous, erythematous tracks called *larva currens* (Kimberlin et al., 2018) Life threatening in children with weakened immunologic defenses	Transmission is same as for hookworm except autoinfection common; humans are hosts, but cats, dogs, and other animals may also be hosts for the threadworm Older children and adults affected more often than young children Severe infections may lead to severe nutritional deficiency Diagnosis: Often difficult; several stool specimens may be required Treat with oral ivermectin (preferred) OR thiabendazole and albendazole (both less effective than oral ivermectin)
Visceral Larva Migrans—*Toxocara canis* (Dogs) (Roundworm) **Intestinal Toxocariasis—*Toxocara cati* (Cats) (Roundworm)**	
Depends on reactivity of infected individual May be asymptomatic except for eosinophilia or pulmonary wheezing Specific diagnosis difficult Visceral toxocariasis: Fever, leukocytosis, eosinophilia, hepatomegaly, hypogammaglobulinemia, malaise, anemia, cough (Kimberlin et al., 2018) Ocular invasion may occur Rarely pneumonia, myocarditis, encephalitis	Transmitted by direct contamination of hands from contact with soil or contaminated objects; less commonly by direct contact with dog or cat More common in children or adults with pica Keep dogs and cats away from areas where children play; sandboxes especially important transmission areas; more common in hot, humid regions Hand washing is imperative in children playing in soil or around domestic animals such as cats and dogs Periodic deworming of diagnosed dogs and cats Control of dog and cat population Diagnosis: Hypergammaglobulinemia and hypereosinophilia; increased titers of anti-A or anti-B blood group antigens; liver biopsy in some cases Treatment: Albendazole; specific symptoms may require additional treatment
Trichuriasis—*Trichuris trichiura* (Whipworm or Human Whipworm)	
Light infections: Asymptomatic Heavy infections: Abdominal pain and distention, diarrhea; failure to thrive, impaired cognitive development; stools may have mucus, water, and blood	Transmitted from contaminated soil, fruit, vegetables, toys, and other objects Most frequent in warm, moist climates Occurs most often in undernourished children living in unsanitary conditions where human feces is not disposed of properly. Diagnosis by microscopic examination of stool specimen Treat with albendazole, mebendazole, or oral ivermectin

The movement of the worms on skin and mucous membrane surfaces causes intense itching. As the child scratches, eggs are deposited on the hands and underneath the fingernails. The typical hand-to-mouth activity of young children makes them especially prone to reinfection. Pinworm eggs persist in the indoor environment for 2 to 3 weeks, contaminating anything they contact, such as toilet seats, doorknobs, bed linens, underwear, and food. Except for the intense rectal itching associated with pinworms, the clinical manifestations are nonspecific (Box 6.5).

Diagnostic Evaluation

Diagnosis is most commonly made from the tape test (see Nursing Care Management section that follows). Repeated tests to collect eggs may be necessary (3 consecutive days in the early morning before the child washes are recommended for testing [Kimberlin et al., 2018]), and if there is a possibility that other family members may be infected, a tape test should be performed on them as well.

Therapeutic Management

The drugs available for treatment of pinworms include pyrantel pamoate (Pin-Rid, Antiminth) and albendazole. Mebendazole is not recommended for children younger than 2 years of age. Because pinworms are easily transmitted, all household members should be treated. The dose of antiparasitic medication should be repeated in 2 weeks to completely eradicate the parasite and prevent reinfection.

Nursing Care Management

Direct nursing care at identifying the parasite, eradicating the organism, and preventing reinfection. Parents need clear, detailed instructions for the tape test. A loop of transparent (not "frosted" or "magic") tape, sticky side out, is placed around the end of a tongue depressor, which is then firmly pressed against the child's perianal area. A convenient, commercially prepared tape is also available for this purpose. Pinworm specimens are collected in the morning as soon as the child awakens and *before* the child has a bowel movement or bathes. The procedure may need to be performed on 3 or more consecutive days before eggs are collected. Parents are instructed to place the tongue blade in a glass jar or loosely in a plastic bag so it can be brought in for microscopic examination. For specimens collected in the hospital, practitioner's office, or clinic, place the tape smoothly on a glass slide, sticky side down, for examination.

Adherence to the drug regimen is usually excellent because only one or two doses are needed. The family should be reminded of the need to take a second dose in 2 weeks to ensure eradication of the eggs.

To prevent reinfection, washing all clothes and bed linens in hot water and vacuuming the house may be recommended. However, there is little documentation of the effectiveness of these measures because pinworms survive on many surfaces. Helpful suggestions include hand washing after toileting and before eating, keeping the child's fingernails short to minimize the chance of ova collecting under the nails, dressing children in one-piece sleeping outfits, and daily showering rather than tub bathing. Inform families that recurrence is common. Treat repeated infections in the same manner as the first one.

BED BUGS

Bed bugs are classified as insects, and the most common types seen are *Cimex lectularius* (common bed bug) and *Cimex hemipterus* (tropical bed bug). Although once considered to be practically nonexistent in the United States, these parasites have reemerged and are increasing by 100% to 500% annually (Lai, Ho, Glick, et al., 2016). Bed bugs are troublesome because they are difficult to diagnose and among the most challenging pests to eradicate. They are mentioned here primarily because of the secondary health problems that may occur as a result of their bites: infection, cellulitis, folliculitis, intense urticaria, impetigo, anaphylactic reaction, and sleep loss. However, in some cases a person may be asymptomatic (McMenaman & Gausche-Hill, 2016).

Bed bugs undergo various life stages, but the small ones are approximately 5 mm in length and light yellow; once the bed bugs "feed" on blood, they enlarge and become reddish-brown. They tend to inhabit warm, dark areas such as bed mattresses, sofas, and other

BOX 6.4 Clinical Manifestations of Giardiasis

Infants and young children:
- Diarrhea
- Vomiting
- Anorexia
- Failure to thrive—if chronic exposure

Children older than 5 years of age:
- Abdominal cramps
- Intermittent loose stools
- Constipation
- Stools that are malodorous, watery, pale, and greasy
- Spontaneous resolution of most infections in 4 to 6 weeks

Rare, chronic form:
- Intermittent loose, foul-smelling stools
- Possibility of abdominal bloating, flatulence, sulfur-tasting belches, epigastric pain, vomiting, headache, and weight loss

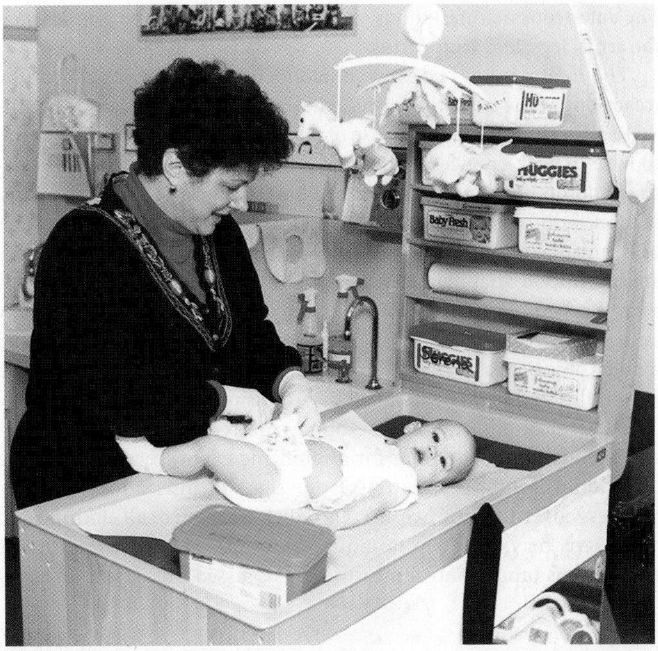

Fig. 6.9 Prevention of giardiasis, especially in daycare centers, requires sanitary practices during diaper changes, such as discarding paper diapers in a covered receptacle, changing paper covers on the diaper-changing surface, and having facilities for hand washing nearby. Note: Soiled cloth diapers and clothing should be stored in a plastic bag for transport home.

BOX 6.5 Clinical Manifestations of Pinworms

Intense perianal itching is the principal symptom. Evidence of itching in young children includes the following:

- General irritability
- Restlessness
- Poor sleep
- Bedwetting
- Distractibility
- Short attention span
- Perianal dermatitis and excoriation secondary to itching
- If worms migrate, possible vaginal (vulvovaginitis) and urethral infection

furniture and emerge at night to feed. Although there is speculation of bed bugs being vectors to transmit other diseases, there is currently no evidence that bed bugs are associated with disease transmission (Lai et al., 2016).

The clinical manifestations of bed bug bites are outlined in Box 6.6. The cutaneous manifestations of bed bug bites tend to be primarily on the arms, legs, and trunk areas.

The treatment of bed bugs should focus on proper identification, treatment of the symptoms, and eradication. Bed bugs can be identified on bedding at night because of their nighttime activity. They tend to hide in dark crevices (e.g., floor, walls, furniture) during the daytime and do not stay on the human host. Contrary to several myths, bed bugs do not fly or jump. It is not uncommon for bed bug bites to be misdiagnosed as scabies, chickenpox, spider or mosquito bites, and even food anaphylaxis in some cases. There is no specific treatment for bed bugs; topical steroids and systemic antihistamines may be used to treat the urticaria. Secondary skin infections are treated with antibiotics as described in this chapter. Eradication of bed bugs is complex and must be handled by professional exterminators; multiple chemical applications are often required to completely eradicate the insects. Suggestions for minimizing exposure when traveling include inspecting the mattresses for signs of infestation; encasing mattress covers may be helpful. Thorough washing of all clothing and bed linens may also help minimize exposure. The use of pesticides and various other control measures is discussed in Bennett and colleagues (2016).

CORONAVIRUS DISEASE (COVID-19)

COVID-19 is a new disease, caused by a novel human coronavirus that has not been previously seen in humans. There are many types of human coronaviruses including some that commonly cause mild upper-respiratory tract illnesses (Centers for Disease Control, 2020). Signs and symptoms of COVID-19 in children may be similar to those for common viral respiratory infections or other childhood illnesses. Many children have no symptoms at all (MMWR, 2020; Shekerdemian, Mahmood, Wolfe, et al., 2020). The largest study of pediatric patients (>2,000) with COVID-19 from China reported that symptoms ranged from asymptomatic to critical (Don, Mo, Hu, et al., 2020).

- Asymptomatic (no clinical signs or symptoms with normal chest imaging): 4%
- Mild (mild symptoms, including fever, fatigue, myalgia, cough): 51%

BOX 6.6 Clinical Manifestations of Bed Bugs

Cutaneous Reactions

- Erythematous papule
- Linear papules
- Red macular lesion
- Rash
- Wheal
- Vesicles
- Bullae
- Urticaria

Secondary

- Impetiginous lesions with scratching
- Folliculitis
- Cellulitis
- Eczematoid dermatitis

Systemic Reactions

- Asthma exacerbation
- Anaphylaxis
- Fever and malaise (chronic exposure)

Data from Doggett, S. L., Dwyer, D., Peñas, P. F., et al. (2012). Bed bugs: Clinical relevance and control options. *Clinical Microbiology Reviews, 25*(1), 164–192; Haisley-Royster, C. (2011). Cutaneous infestations and infections. *Adolescent Medicine: State of the Art Reviews, 22*(1), 129–145.

- Moderate (pneumonia with symptoms or subclinical disease with abnormal chest imaging): 39%
- Severe (dyspnea, central cyanosis, hypoxia): 5%
- Critical (acute respiratory distress syndrome [ARDS], respiratory failure, shock, or multi-organ dysfunction): 0.6%

In 2020, there is considerable uncertainty among infectious disease epidemiology experts in forecasting the timing and extent of the COVID-19 pandemic in the United States. The first reports describe the burden of COVID-19 infection in North American PICUs and confirms that severe illness in children is significant but far less frequent than in adults (MMWR, 2020; Patel, 2020).

Therapeutic Management

There is no approved therapy to treat COVID-19 in children and insufficient data to recommend for or against the use of specific antivirals or immunomodulatory agents for the treatment of COVID-19 in pediatric patients (National Institutes of Health, 2020). The emergence of a life-threatening multisystem inflammatory syndrome across the United States is seen in children and causes damage to multiple organ systems. This syndrome has symptoms similar to Kawasaki's Disease and is discussed in Chapter 23.

Nursing Care Management

For children who have no underlying health conditions, supportive care measures similar to those for the common cold or flu are recommended including rest, adequate hydration, analgesics, and antipyretics as needed. Children with underlying conditions such as chronic lung disease (including asthma), heart disease, and conditions that weaken the immune system may have to be hospitalized because they may be at risk for more severe illness.

CLINICAL JUDGMENT AND NEXT-GENERATION NCLEX® EXAMINATION-STYLE QUESTIONS

1. Use of standard precautions for the prevention of transmission of pathogens is crucial to the spread of disease. Nursing caring for children must be knowledgeable of the types of precautions and when to use them. The nurse is triaging individuals that have presented to the emergency department (ED) for various needs. **Indicate which type of precautions listed in the far-left column the nurse will place the client from the middle column into, upon arrival to the ED in order to prevent transmission of various pathogens that children listed in the middle column may be exposed to.**

Standard Precautions	History and Assessment Findings	Type of Precaution to Implement
1. Transfusion-Based Precautions	15-year-old returning from summer in India who presents with symptoms of tuberculosis	
2. Airborne Precautions	3-year-old who has a respiratory illness with cough	
3. Standard Precautions	5-year-old admitted with fever and productive cough; bacterial pneumonia confirmed by lab and xray	
4. Droplet Precautions	7-year-old admitted tonsillectomy	
5. Respiratory Hygiene / Cough Etiquette		
6. No precautions needed		

2. A 14-year old client is preparing to travel outside of the United States on a mission trip. When the client meets with the pediatric nurse to review immunizations, the nurse determines that the client needs an immunization to remain safe while traveling. **Choose the most likely options for the information missing from the statements below by selecting from the lists of options provided.** Based upon this information, the nurse will administer hepatitis ___1___ vaccine ___2___ in the ___3___ muscle.

Options for 1	Options for 2	Options for 3
A Virus	subcutaneously	dorsogluteal
B Virus	intravenously	vastus lateralis
Tetanus	intramuscularly	pectoral
Infection	intrathecally	subclavicular

3. A 6-year-old girl is brought to the clinic by a foster parent who assumed care of her a week ago. The foster parent reports that the girl has "not been acting right for a couple of days" after developing a fever and cough 2 days ago. The foster parents also states, "she had a rash on her face and some small red spots in her mouth 2 days ago, but they are gone now." When asked about an outbreak of measles she states the teacher called her last night about another child in the school who had measles. The foster parent reports that no immunizations records exist, so it is unknown whether the child has ever been immunized. Which assessment findings require follow-up? **Select all that apply.**
   - **A.** Temperature of 101.5 F (38.6 C)
   - **B.** Pulse 95 beats/min
   - **C.** Respirations 20 breaths/min
   - **D.** Cough for 2 days
   - **E.** Small spots on the buccal mucosa 3 days ago that disappeared, described as white with a red ring
   - **F.** Weight in the 25th% for age
   - **G.** Rash on the face, chest and arms
   - **H.** Abdominal pain
   - **I.** Generalized lymphadenopathy

4. A 7-year-old child is brought by a parent to the clinic due to an outbreak of pediculosis capitis at the school. Assessment confirms that the child is scratching her scalp and there are nits on the hair. Which intervention will the nurse implement at this time? **Select all that apply.**
   - **A.** Teach parent to soak combs, brushes and hair accessories in lice-killing products for 1 hour or in boiling water for 10 minutes.
   - **B.** Shave the child's head and cleanse the scalp with rubbing alcohol.
   - **C.** Tell parent to machine wash clothing, towels and bed linens in hot water and dry in hot dryer for at least 20 minutes.
   - **D.** Dispose of the child's clothing in a plastic garbage bag at the clinic.
   - **E.** Recommend that parent vacuum carpets, car seats, pillows, stuffed animals, rugs, mattresses and upholstered furniture.
   - **F.** Explain to child that she can only share hats, scarves, combs and brushes with family members.
   - **G.** Administer intramuscular antibiotics to limit the spread of infection.
   - **H.** Use a natura l remedy such a mayonnaise on the hair to suffocate nits.

REFERENCES

Alter, S. J., Vidwan, N. K., Sobande, P. O., et al. (2011). Common childhood bacterial infections. *Current Problems in Pediatric and Adolescent Health Care, 41*(10), 256–283.

American Academy of Pediatrics, Committee on Infectious Diseases. (2016). Recommendations for prevention and control of influenza in children, 2016-2017. *Pediatrics, 138*, 1–20.

Beirne, P. V., Hennessy, S., Cadogan, S. L., et al. (2015). Needle size for vaccination procedures in children and adolescents. *Cochrane Database of Systematic Reviews* (6), CD010720.

Belongia, E. A., Karron, R. A., Reingold, A., et al. (2017). The Advisory Committee on Immunization Practices recommendation regarding the use of live influenza vaccine: A rejoinder. *Vaccine*, epub ahead of print.

Bennett, G. W., Gondhalekar, A. D., Wang, C., et al. (2016). Using research and education to implement practical bed bug control programs in multifamily housing. *Pest Management Science, 72*, 8–14.

Blain, A. E., Lewis, M., Banerjee, E., et al. (2016). An assessment of the cocooning strategy for preventing infant pertussis – United States, 2011. *Clinical Infectious Diseases, 63*(suppl. 4), S221–S226.

Bolon, M. K. (2016). Hand hygiene: An update. *Infectious Disease Clinics of North America, 30*, 591–607.

CDC COVID-19 Response Team. (2020). Coronavirus Disease 2019 in Children — United States, February 12–April 2, 2020. *MMWR. Morbidity and Mortality Weekly Report*, *69*(14), 422–426.

Centers for Disease Control and Prevention. (2013a). Updated recommendations for use of tetanus toxoid, reduced diphtheria toxoid and acellular pertussis vaccine (Tdap) in pregnant women—Advisory Committee on Immunization Practices (ACIP), 2012. *MMWR. Morbidity and Mortality Weekly Report*, *62*(7), 131–135.

Centers for Disease Control and Prevention. (2013b). Prevention of measles, rubella, congenital rubella syndrome, and mumps, 2013: Summary recommendations of the Advisory Committee on Immunization Practices (ACIP). *Morbidity and Mortality Weekly Report. Recommendations and Reports*, *62*(4), 1–25.

Centers for Disease Control and Prevention. (2015). Use of serogroup B meningococcal vaccines in adolescents and young adults: Recommendations of the Advisory Committee on Immunization Practices, 2015. *Morbidity and Mortality Weekly Report*, *64*(41), 1171–1176.

Centers for Disease Control and Prevention. (2016a). *Human papillomavirus (HPV)*. Obtained from https://www.cdc.gov/hpv/.

Centers for Disease Control and Prevention. (2016b). *Zika virus*. Retrieved from https://www.cdc.gov/zika/.

Centers for Disease Control and Prevention. (2018). Health care associated infections. Obtained from https://www.cdc.gov.

Centers for Disease Control and Prevention. (2020, June 17). *Coronavirus Disease 2019 Covid-19*. Retrieved June 24, 2020, from https://www.cdc.gov-/ncird/dvd.html.

Coyer, S. M. (2002). Understanding parental concerns about immunizations. *Journal of Pediatric Health Care*, *16*(4), 193–196.

de Martino, M. (2016). Dismantling the taboo against vaccines in pregnancy. *International Journal of Molecular Sciences*, *17*, 1–8.

DeStefano, F., Price, C. S., & Weintraub, E. S. (2013). Increasing exposure to antibody- stimulating proteins and polysaccharides in vaccines is not associated with risk of autism. *The Journal of Pediatrics*, *163*(2), 561–567.

Dhar, V. (2020). Common lesions of the oral soft tissues. In R. M. Kliegman, J. W. St. Geme, N. J. Blum, et al. (Eds.), *Nelson textbook of pediatrics* (21st ed.). Philadelphia: Saunders/Elsevier.

Diggle, L., & Deeks, J. (2000). Effect of needle length on incidence of local reactions to routine immunizations in infants aged 4 months: Randomized controlled trial. *BMJ (Clinical Research Ed.)*, *321*(7266), 931–993.

Diggle, L., Deeks, J. J., & Pollard, A. J. (2006). Effect of needle size and immunogenecity and reactogenecity of vaccines in infants: A randomized controlled trial. *BMJ (Clinical Research Ed.)*, *333*(7568), 571.

Dong, Y., Mo, X., Hu, Y., et al. (2020). Epidemiological characteristics of 2,143 pediatric patients with 2019 coronavirus disease in China. *Pediatrics*, *145*(6), e20200702.

Fallah, R., Gholami, H., Ferdosian, F., et al. (2016). Evaluation of vaccines injection order on pain score of intramuscular injection of diphtheria, whole cell pertussis and tetanus vaccine. *Indian Journal of Pediatrics*, *83*, 1405–1409.

Fredrickson, D. D., Davis, T. C., Arnold, C. L., et al. (2004). Childhood immunization refusal: Provider and parent perceptions. *Family Medicine*, *36*(6), 431–438.

Institute of Medicine. (2004). *Immunization safety review: Vaccines and autism*. Washington, DC: National Academies Press.

Ipp, M., Parkin, P. C., Lear, N., et al. (2009). Order of vaccine injection and infant pain response. *Archives of Pediatrics and Adolescent Medicine*, *163*(5), 469–472.

Jackson, L. A., Yu, O., Nelson, J. C., et al. (2011). Injection site and risk of medically attended local reactions to acellular pertussis vaccine. *Pediatrics*, *127*(3), e681–e687.

John, C. C. (2020). Giardiasis and Balantidiasis. In R. M. Kliegman, J. W. St. Geme, N. J. Blum, et al. (Eds.), *Nelson textbook of pediatrics* (21st ed.). Philadelphia: Saunders/Elsevier.

Kimberlin, D. W., Brady, M. T., Jackson, M. A., et al. (Eds.). (2018). *Red Book: Report of the committee on infectious diseases* (31st ed.) Elk Grove Village, Ill: The Academy.

Koch, W. C. (2020). Parvoviruses. In R. M. Kliegman, J. W. St. Geme, N. J. Blum, et al. (Eds.), *Nelson textbook of pediatrics* (21st ed.). Philadelphia: Saunders/Elsevier.

Lai, O., Ho, D., Glick, S., et al. (2016). Bed bugs and possible transmission of human pathogens: A systematic review. *Archives of Dermatological Research*, *308*, 531–538.

McMenaman, K. S., & Gausche-Hill, M. (2016). Cimex lectularius ("Bed Bugs") recognition, management, and eradication. *Pediatric Emergency Care*, *32*, 801–806.

Murray, J. S. (2016). Understanding zika virus. *Journal for Specialists in Pediatric Nursing*, *22*(1), e12164.

National Childhood Vaccine Injury Act. (1986). *42 U.S.C. Sec 300aa-1 to 300aa-34*. Rockville, Md: Public Health Service.

National Institutes of Health. (n. d.). (Special considerations in Children. Retrieved June 11. 2020, from https://www.covid19treatmentguidelines.nih.gov/overview/children/.Olitsky, S. E., & Marsh, J. D. (2020). Disorders of the conjunctiva. In R. M. Kliegman, J. W. St. Geme, N. J. Blum, et al. (Eds.), *Nelson textbook of pediatrics* (21st ed.). Philadelphia: Saunders/Elsevier.

Painter, J. E., Gargano, J. W., Collier, S. A., et al. (2015). Giardiasis surveillance – United States, 2011-2012. *MMWR Supplements*, *64*(3), 15–25.

Patel, N. A. (2020). Pediatric COVID-19: Systematic review of the literature. *American Journal of Otolaryngology*, *41*(5), 102573.

Rishovd, A. (2014). Pediatric intramuscular injections: Guidelines for best practice. *MCN: The American Journal of Maternal Child Nursing*, *39*, 107–112.

Rosenthal, M. (2004). Bacterial colonization, hyperresponsive immune systems conspire in eczema: Diagnosing dermatological disorders. *Infectious Diseases in Children*, *17*(3), 47–48.

Shekerdemian, L. S., Mahmood, N. R., Wolfe, K. K., et al. (2020). Characteristics and outcomes of children with Coronavirus Disease 2019 (COVID-19) infection admitted to US and Canadian Pediatric Intensive Care Units. *JAMA Pediatrics*. https://doi.org/10.1001/jamapediatrics.2020.1948. Advance online publication.

Souder, E., & Long, S. S. (2020). Pertussis. In R. M. Kliegman, J. W. St. Geme, N. J. Blum, et al. (Eds.), *Nelson textbook of pediatrics* (21st ed.). Philadelphia: Saunders/Elsevier.

Tangherlini, T. R., Roychowdhury, V., Glenn, B., et al. (2016). "Mommy blogs" and the vaccination exemption narrative: Results from a machine-learning approach for story aggregation on parenting social media sites. *JMIR Public Health and Surveillance*, *2*, 1–15.

World Health Organization. (2015). Reducing pain at the time of vaccination: WHO position paper – September 2015. *World Health Organization Weekly Epidemiological Record*, *39*, 505–516.

Yoshimasu, K., Kiyohara, C., Takemura, S., et al. (2014). A meta-analysis of the evidence on the impact of prenatal and early infancy exposures to mercury on autism and attention deficit/hyperactivity disorder in the childhood. *Neurotoxicology*, *44*, 121–131.

7

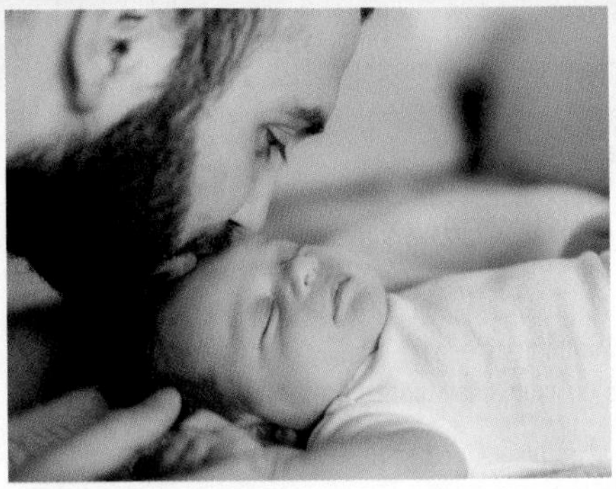

Health Promotion of the Newborn and Family

Lisa M. Cleveland

http://evolve.elsevier.com/wong/essentials

CONCEPTS

- Perfusion
- Thermoregulation

ADJUSTMENT TO EXTRAUTERINE LIFE

The most profound physiologic change required of neonates is transition from fetal or placental circulation to independent respiration. The loss of the placental connection means the loss of complete metabolic support, especially the supply of oxygen and the removal of carbon dioxide. The normal stresses of labor and delivery produce alterations of placental gas exchange patterns, acid-base balance in the blood, and cardiovascular activity in the infant. Factors that interfere with this normal transition or that interfere with fetal **oxygenation** (including conditions such as hypoxemia, hypercapnia, and acidosis) affect the fetus's adjustment to extrauterine life.

IMMEDIATE ADJUSTMENTS

Respiratory System

The most critical and immediate physiologic change required of newborns is the onset of breathing. The stimuli that help initiate the first breath are primarily chemical and thermal. **Chemical factors** in the blood (low oxygen, high carbon dioxide, and low pH) initiate impulses that excite the respiratory center in the medulla. The primary **thermal stimulus** is the sudden chilling of the infant, who leaves a warm environment and enters a relatively cooler atmosphere. This abrupt change in temperature excites sensory impulses in the skin that are transmitted to the respiratory center.

Tactile stimulation may assist in initiating respiration. Descent through the birth canal and normal handling during delivery help stimulate respiration in uncompromised infants. Acceptable methods of tactile stimulation include tapping or flicking the soles of the feet or gently rubbing the newborn's back, trunk, or extremities. Slapping the newborn's buttocks or back is a harmful technique and should not be used. Prolonged tactile stimulation, beyond one or two taps or flicks to the soles of the feet or rubbing the back once or twice, can waste precious time in the event of respiratory difficulty and can cause additional damage in infants who have become hypoxemic before or during the birth process (Kimberlin, Brady, Jackson, et. al., 2018).

The initial entry of air into the lungs is opposed by the surface tension of the fluid that filled the fetal lungs and the alveoli. Some lung fluid is removed during the normal forces of labor and delivery. As the chest emerges from the birth canal, fluid is squeezed from the lungs through the nose and mouth. After complete delivery of the chest, brisk recoil of the thorax occurs, and air enters the upper airway to replace the lost fluid. Remaining lung fluid is absorbed by the pulmonary capillaries and lymphatic vessels.

In the alveoli, the surface tension of the fluid is reduced by **surfactant**, a substance produced by the alveolar epithelium that coats the alveolar surface. The effect of surfactant in facilitating breathing is discussed in relation to respiratory distress syndrome (see Chapter 8).

Circulatory System

As important as the initiation of respiration is the circulatory changes that allow blood to flow through the lungs. These changes, which occur more gradually, are the result of pressure changes in the lungs, heart, and major vessels. The transition from fetal to postnatal circulation involves the functional closure of the **fetal shunts**: the foramen ovale, the ductus arteriosus, and eventually the ductus venosus. (For a review of fetal circulation, see Chapter 23.) Increased blood flow dilates the pulmonary vessels, pulmonary vascular resistance decreases, and systemic resistance increases, thus maintaining blood pressure (BP). As the pulmonary vessels receive blood, the pressure in the right atrium, right ventricle, and pulmonary arteries decreases. Left atrial pressure increases above right atrial pressure, with subsequent foramen ovale closure. With the increase in pulmonary blood flow and dramatic reduction of pulmonary vascular resistance, the ductus arteriosus begins to close.

The most important factors controlling ductal closure are the increased oxygen concentration of the blood and the fall in endogenous prostaglandins. The foramen ovale closes functionally at or soon after birth. The ductus arteriosus is closed functionally by the fourth day. Anatomic closure takes considerably longer. Failure of the ductus arteriosus or foramen ovale to close results in persistence of fetal shunting of blood away from the lungs (see Chapter 23).

Because of the reversible flow of blood through the ductus during the early neonatal period, a functional murmur occasionally may be heard. In conditions such as crying or straining, the increased pressure shunts deoxygenated blood from the right side of the heart across the ductal opening, which may cause **transient cyanosis**.

PHYSIOLOGIC STATUS OF OTHER SYSTEMS

Thermoregulation

Next to establishing respiration, heat regulation is most critical to the newborn's survival. Although the newborn's capacity for heat production is adequate, three factors predispose newborns to excessive heat loss:

- The newborn's large surface area facilitates heat loss to the environment, although this is partially compensated for by the newborn's usual position of flexion, which decreases the amount of surface area exposed to the environment.
- The newborn's thin layer of subcutaneous fat provides poor insulation for conservation of heat.
- The newborn's mechanism for producing heat is different from that of the adult, who can increase heat production through shivering. A chilled neonate cannot shiver but produces heat through **nonshivering thermogenesis (NST)**, which involves increased metabolism and oxygen consumption.

The principal thermogenic sources are the heart, liver, and brain. An additional source, once believed to be unique to newborns, is known as **brown adipose tissue**, or **brown fat** (Symonds, Aldiss, Pope, et al., 2018). Brown fat, which owes its name to its larger content of mitochondrial cytochromes, has a greater capacity for heat production through intensified metabolic activity than ordinary adipose tissue. Heat generated in brown fat is distributed to other parts of the body by the blood, which is warmed as it flows through the layers of this tissue. Superficial deposits of brown fat are located between the scapulae, around the neck, in the axillae, and behind the sternum. Deeper layers surround the kidneys, trachea, esophagus, some major arteries, and adrenals. The location of brown fat may explain why the nape of the neck often feels warmer than the rest of the infant's body. Due to factors that predispose newborns to heat loss, they must be quickly dried and ideally placed skin-to-skin with their mothers or provided with warm, dry blankets after delivery. Although the newborn's ability to conserve heat is usually of greatest concern, they may also have difficulty dissipating heat in an overheated environment, which increases their risk of hyperthermia.

Hematopoietic System

The blood volume of the newborn depends on the amount of placental transfer of blood. The blood volume of a full-term infant is about 80 to 85 ml/kg of body weight. Immediately after birth, the total blood volume averages 300 ml, but depending on how long umbilical cord clamping is delayed or if the umbilical cord is milked, as much as 100 ml can be added to the blood volume (American College of Obstetrics & Gynecology, 2017).

Fluid and Electrolyte Balance

Changes occur in the total body water volume, extracellular fluid volume, and intracellular fluid volume during the transition from fetal to postnatal life. At birth, the total weight of an infant is 73% fluid compared with 58% in an adult. Infants have a proportionately higher ratio of extracellular fluid than adults. An important aspect of fluid balance is its relationship to other systems. An infant's rate of metabolism is twice that of an adult in relation to body weight. As a result, twice as much acid is formed, leading to more rapid development of acidosis. In addition, immature kidneys cannot sufficiently concentrate urine to conserve body water. These three factors make infants more prone to dehydration, acidosis, and possible overhydration or water intoxication.

BOX 7.1 Change in Stooling Patterns of Newborns

Meconium

Infant's first stool; composed of amniotic fluid and its constituents, intestinal secretions, shed mucosal cells, and possibly blood (ingested maternal blood or minor bleeding of alimentary tract vessels).

Passage of meconium should occur within the first 24 to 48 hours, although it may be delayed up to 7 days in very low birth weight infants.

Transitional Stools

Usually appear by third day after initiation of feeding; greenish brown to yellowish brown, thin, and less sticky than meconium; may contain some milk curds.

Milk Stool

Usually appears by fourth day.

In **breastfed infants,** stools are yellow to golden, are pasty in consistency, and have an odor similar to that of sour milk.

In **formula-fed infants,** stools are pale yellow to light brown, are firmer in consistency, and have a more offensive odor.

Gastrointestinal System

The ability of newborns to digest, absorb, and metabolize food is sufficient but limited in certain functions. Enzymes are adequate to handle proteins and simple carbohydrates (monosaccharides and disaccharides), but deficient production of pancreatic amylase impairs use of complex carbohydrates (polysaccharides). Deficiency of pancreatic lipase limits absorption of fats, especially with ingestion of foods with high saturated fatty acid content, such as cow's milk. Human milk, despite its high fat content, is easily digested because the milk itself contains enzymes (such as lipase), which assist in digestion.

The liver is the most immature of the gastrointestinal organs. The activity of the enzyme **glucuronyl transferase** is reduced, which affects the conjugation of bilirubin with glucuronic acid and contributes to physiologic jaundice of newborns. The liver is also deficient in forming plasma proteins. The decreased plasma protein concentration probably plays a role in the edema usually seen at birth. Prothrombin and other coagulation factors are also low. The liver stores less glycogen at birth than later in life. Consequently, newborns are prone to hypoglycemia, which may be prevented by early and effective feeding, ideally breastfeeding.

Some salivary glands are functioning at birth, but the majority do not begin to secrete saliva until about age 2 to 3 months, when drooling is frequent. Newborn stomach capacity is difficult to determine; however, small quantities of early breast milk (called *colostrum*) ideally meet or exceed the newborn's needs (Academy of Breastfeeding Medicine, 2017). The newborn colon has a small volume, thus newborns may have a bowel movement after each feeding. Newborns who breastfeed usually have more frequent feedings, resulting in more frequent stools than infants who receive commercially prepared infant formula.

An infant's intestines are longer in relation to their body size when compared to that of an adult. Therefore they have a larger number of secretory glands and a larger surface area for absorption in comparison. Infants have rapid peristaltic waves and simultaneous nonperistaltic waves along the entire esophagus, which propel nutrients forward. The relative immaturity of the peristaltic waves combined with decreased lower esophageal sphincter (LES) pressure, inappropriate relaxation of the LES, and delayed gastric emptying make regurgitation a common occurrence. Progressive changes in the stooling pattern indicate a properly functioning gastrointestinal tract (Box 7.1).

The neonatal gastrointestinal mucosa performs an important function as a barrier to foreign antigens. Both immune and nonimmune factors may play a vital role in decreasing the absorption of antigens capable of causing serious neonatal illness; however, the functional capacity of this system may be immature or altered. Feeding an infant human milk increases the effectiveness of this defense mechanism (Molès, Tuaillon, Kankasa, et al., 2018).

Renal System

All structural components are present in the renal system, but there is a functional deficiency in the kidneys' ability to concentrate urine and to cope with conditions of fluid and electrolyte stress, such as dehydration or a concentrated solute load. Total volume of urine per 24 hours is about 200 to 300 ml by the end of the first week. However, the bladder voluntarily empties when stretched by a volume of 15 ml, resulting in as many as 20 voidings per day. The first voiding should occur within 24 hours. The urine is colorless and odorless and has a specific gravity of about 1.020.

Integumentary System

At birth, all structures within the skin are present, but many functions of the integument are immature. The outer two layers of the skin, the epidermis and dermis, are loosely bound to each other and very thin. **Rete pegs**, which later in life anchor the epidermis to the dermis, are not developed. Slight friction across the epidermis, such as from rapid removal of adhesive tape, can cause separation of these layers and blister formation. The transitional zone between the cornified and living layers of the epidermis is effective in preventing fluid from reaching the skin surface.

The **sebaceous glands** are active late in fetal life and in early infancy because of the high levels of maternal androgens. They are most densely located on the scalp, face, and genitalia and produce the greasy vernix caseosa that covers infants at birth. Plugging of the sebaceous glands causes **milia**.

The **eccrine glands**, which produce sweat in response to heat or emotional stimuli, are functional at birth, and by 3 weeks of age palmar sweating on crying reaches levels equivalent to those of anxious adults. The eccrine glands produce sweat in response to higher temperatures than those required in adults, and the retention of sweat may result in milia. The **apocrine glands** remain small and nonfunctional until puberty.

The growth phases of hair follicles usually occur simultaneously at birth. During the first few months, the synchrony between hair loss and regrowth is disrupted, and there may be overgrowth of hair or temporary alopecia.

Because the amount of melanin is low at birth, newborns are lighter skinned than they will be as children. Consequently, they are more susceptible to the harmful effects of the sun.

Musculoskeletal System

At birth, the skeletal system contains more cartilage than ossified bone, although the process of ossification is rapid during the first year. The nose, for example, is predominantly cartilage at birth and may be temporarily flattened or asymmetric because of the force of delivery. The six skull bones are relatively soft and are separated only by membranous seams. The sinuses are incompletely formed in newborns.

Unlike the skeletal system, the muscular system is almost completely formed at birth. Growth in size of muscular tissue is caused by hypertrophy, rather than hyperplasia, of cells.

Defenses Against Infection

Infants are born with several defenses against infection. The first line of defense is the skin and mucous membranes, which protect the body from invading organisms. The mature neonatal intestinal mucosal (gut) barrier also plays a vital role as an important defense mechanism against antigens. The second line of defense is the macrophage system, which produces several types of cells capable of attacking a pathogen. The **neutrophils** and **monocytes** are phagocytes, which means they can engulf, ingest, and destroy foreign agents. **Eosinophils** also probably have a phagocytic property because they increase in number in the presence of foreign protein. The **lymphocytes** (T cells and B cells) are capable of being converted to other cell types, such as monocytes and antibodies. Although the phagocytic properties of the blood are present in infants, the inflammatory response of the tissues to localize an infection is immature.

The third line of defense is the formation of specific antibodies to an antigen. Exposure to various foreign agents is necessary for antibody production to occur. Infants are generally not capable of producing their own immunoglobulin until the beginning of the second month of life, but they receive considerable passive immunity in the form of immunoglobulin G (IgG) from the maternal circulation and from human milk (see the Human Milk section later in the chapter). They are protected against most major childhood diseases, including diphtheria, measles, poliomyelitis, and rubella, for about 3 months, provided the mother has developed antibodies to these illnesses.

Endocrine System

Ordinarily, the endocrine system of newborns is adequately developed, but its functions are immature. For example, the posterior lobe of the pituitary gland produces limited quantities of **antidiuretic hormone**, or **vasopressin**, which inhibits diuresis. This renders young infants highly susceptible to dehydration.

The effect of maternal sex hormones is particularly evident in newborns. The labia are hypertrophied, and the breasts of both genders may be engorged and secrete milk from the first few days of life up to 2 months of age. Female newborns may have **pseudomenstruation** (more often seen as a milky secretion than actual blood) from a sudden drop in progesterone and estrogen levels.

Neurologic System

At birth, the nervous system is incompletely integrated but sufficiently developed to sustain extrauterine life. Most neurologic functions are primitive reflexes. The autonomic nervous system is crucial during transition because it stimulates initial respirations, helps maintain acid-base balance, and partially regulates temperature control.

Myelination of the nervous system follows cephalocaudal and proximodistal (head-to-toe and center-to-periphery) laws of development and is closely related to observed mastery of fine and gross motor skills. Myelin is necessary for rapid and efficient transmission of some, but not all, nerve impulses along the neural pathway. The tracts that develop myelin earliest are the sensory, cerebellar, and extrapyramidal tracts. This accounts for the acute senses of taste, smell, and hearing in newborns, as well as the perception of pain. All cranial nerves are present and myelinated except for the optic and olfactory nerves.

Sensory Functions

Newborns' sensory functions are remarkably well developed and have a significant effect on growth and development, including the attachment process.

Vision

At birth, the eye is structurally incomplete. The fovea centralis is not yet completely differentiated from the macula. The ciliary muscles are also immature, limiting the eyes' ability to accommodate and focus on an object for any length of time. The infant can track and follow objects. The pupils react to light, the blink reflex is responsive to minimal stimulus, and the corneal reflex is activated by a light touch. Tear glands usually do not begin to function until 2 to 4 weeks of age.

Newborns can focus momentarily on a bright or moving object that is within 20 cm (8 inches) and in the midline of the visual field. In fact, infants' ability to fixate on coordinated movement is greater during the first hour of life than during the succeeding several days. Visual acuity is reported to be between 20/100 and 20/400, depending on the vision measurement techniques.

Infants also demonstrate visual preferences: medium colors (yellow, green, pink) over bright (red, orange, blue) or dim colors; black-and-white contrasting patterns, especially geometric shapes and checkerboards; large objects with medium complexity rather than small, complex objects; and reflecting objects over dull ones.

Hearing

After the amniotic fluid has drained from the ears, infants probably have **auditory acuity** like that of adults. Neonates react to loud sounds of about 90 decibels with a startle (Moro) reflex. The newborn's response to sounds of low and high frequency differs; the former, such as a heartbeat, metronome, or lullaby, tends to decrease an infant's motor activity and crying, whereas the latter elicits an alerting reaction. There is an early sensitivity to the sound of human voices. For example, infants younger than 3 days old can discriminate the mother's voice from that of other women. As early as 5 days old, newborns can differentiate between stories repeated to them during the last trimester of pregnancy by their mother and the same stories read after birth by a different woman.

The internal and middle ear is large at birth, but the external canal is small. The mastoid process and the bony part of the external canal have not yet developed. Consequently, the tympanic membrane and facial nerve are very close to the surface and can be easily damaged.

Smell

Newborns react to strong odors such as alcohol and vinegar by turning their heads away. Breastfed infants can smell breast milk and will cry for their mothers when they smell leaking milk. Infants are also able to differentiate the breast milk of their mothers from the breast milk of other women by scent alone. Maternal odors are believed to influence the attachment process and successful breastfeeding. Unnecessary routine washing of the breast may interfere with establishment of early breastfeeding.

Taste

The newborn can distinguish among tastes, and various types of solutions elicit differing facial reflexes. A tasteless solution elicits no facial expression; a sweet solution elicits an eager suck and a look of satisfaction; a sour solution causes puckering of the lips; and a bitter liquid produces an angry, upset expression.

Touch

At birth, infants can perceive tactile sensation in any part of their body, although the face (especially the mouth), hands, and soles of the feet seem to be the most sensitive. Evidence shows that touch and motion are essential to normal growth and development. Gentle patting of the back or rubbing of the abdomen usually elicits a calming response from infants. In turn, painful stimuli, such as a pinprick, elicit an upset response.

NURSING CARE OF THE NEWBORN AND FAMILY

Assessment

Newborns require thorough, skilled observation to ensure a satisfactory adjustment to extrauterine life. Physical assessment after delivery can be divided into four phases:

1. The initial assessment, which includes the Apgar scoring system
2. Transitional assessment during the periods of reactivity
3. Assessment of gestational age
4. Systematic physical examination

In addition, the nurse must be aware of behaviors that signal successful reciprocal attachment between the infant and parents. Awareness of the expected normal findings during each assessment process helps the nurse recognize any deviation that may prevent the infant from progressing uneventfully through the early postnatal period. With shorter hospitalizations, the accomplishment of thorough newborn assessment and parent teaching may be a challenge.

Initial Assessment: Apgar Scoring

The most frequently used method to assess newborns' immediate adjustment to extrauterine life is the **Apgar** scoring system, which is based on newborn heart rate, respiratory effort, muscle tone, reflex irritability, and color (Table 7.1). Each item is given a score of 0, 1, or 2. Evaluations of all five categories are made at 1 and 5 minutes after birth and repeated until the infant's condition stabilizes. Total scores of 0 to 3 represent severe distress, scores of 4 to 6 signify moderate difficulty, and scores of 7 to 10 indicate absence of difficulty in adjusting to extrauterine life. The Apgar score is affected by the degree of physiologic immaturity, infection, congenital malformations, maternal sedation or analgesia, and neuromuscular disorders.

The Apgar score reflects the general condition of the infant at 1 and 5 minutes based on the five parameters described earlier. However, the Apgar score is not a tool that stands on its own to interpret past events, determine need for newborn resuscitation, or predict future events linked to the infant's eventual neurologic or physical status. Considerable discussion and controversy have centered on Apgar scoring because of its misuse as an indicator for the presence or absence of perinatal asphyxia in the medicolegal field (American Academy of Pediatrics, Committee on Fetus and Newborn & American College of Obstetricians and Gynecologists, Committee on Obstetric Practice, 2015a).

Clinical Assessment of Gestational Age

Assessment of gestational age is an important criterion because perinatal morbidity and mortality are related to gestational age and birth weight. A frequently used method of determining gestational age is the **New Ballard Scale (NBS)** by Ballard and colleagues (1991) (Fig. 7.1A). This scale, an abbreviated version of the **Dubowitz scale**, assesses six external physical and six neuromuscular signs. Each sign has a number score, and the cumulative score correlates with a maturity rating of 20 to 44 weeks of gestation.

The NBS includes scores that reflect signs of extremely preterm infants, such as fused eyelids; imperceptible breast tissue; sticky, friable, transparent skin; no lanugo; and square-window (flexion

TABLE 7.1 Infant Evaluation at Birth: Apgar Scoring System

Sign	0	1	2
Heart rate	Absent	Slow, <100 beats/min	>100 beats/min
Respiratory effort	Absent	Irregular, slow, weak cry	Good, strong cry
Muscle tone	Limp	Some flexion of extremities	Well flexed
Reflex irritability	No response	Grimace	Cry, sneeze
Color	Blue, pale	Body pink, extremities blue	Completely pink

of wrist) angle greater than 90 degrees (see Fig. 7.1A and the description of the tests in Box 7.2). For infants with a gestational age of at least 26 weeks, the examination may be performed up to 96 hours after birth; however, it is recommended that the initial examination be performed within the first 48 hours of life. In a study of preterm infants ranging from 29 to 35 weeks at birth, NBS scores completed more than 7 days following birth were found to either overestimate or underestimate gestational age by up to 2 weeks (Sasidharan, Dutta, & Narang, 2009). Further, in a study published in 2017, researchers found that the NBS overestimated the physical component scores of small for gestational age (SGA) infants. However, reanalysis after reducing skin and plantar crease physical parameter scores showed that NBS scores were more consistent with infants' gestational age (Singhal, Jain, Chawla, et al., 2017).

Weight Related to Gestational Age

Birth weight is correlated with perinatal morbidity and mortality. However, birth weight alone is a poor indicator of gestational age and fetal maturity. Maturity implies **functional capacity**—the degree to which the neonate's organ systems can adapt to the requirements of extrauterine life. Therefore gestational age is more closely related to fetal maturity than birth weight. Because heredity influences a newborn's size, noting the size of other family members is part of the assessment process.

Intrauterine growth curves are used to classify infants according to birth weight and gestational age. The primary intrauterine growth charts that provide national reference data include the work of Alexander and colleagues (1996), which is representative of more than 3.1 million live births in the United States, and Thomas and colleagues (2000). In 2010 new intrauterine growth curves based on more than

ESTIMATION OF GESTATIONAL AGE BY MATURITY RATING

NEUROMUSCULAR MATURITY

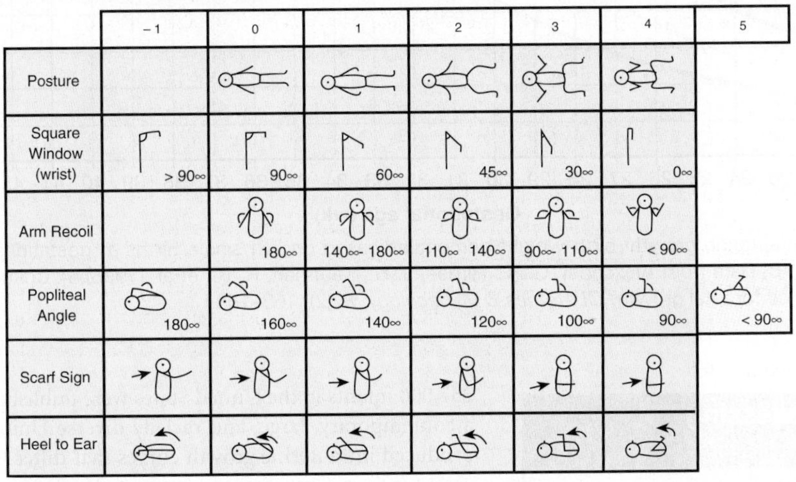

PHYSICAL MATURITY

	−1	0	1	2	3	4	5
Skin	sticky friable transparent	gelatinous red, translucent	smooth pink, visible veins	superficial peeling &/or rash, few veins	cracking pale areas rare veins	parchment deep cracking no vessels	leathery cracked wrinkled
Lanugo	none	sparse	abundant	thinning	bald areas	mostly bald	
Plantar Surface	heel-toe 40-50 mm: –1 <40 mm: –2	>50 mm no crease	faint red marks	anterior transverse crease only	creases ant. 2/3	creases over entire sole	
Breast	imperceptible	barely perceptible	flat areola no bud	stippled areola 1-2 mm bud	raised areola 3-4 mm bud	full areola 5-10 mm bud	
Eye/Ear	lids fused loosely: –1 tightly: –2	lids open pinna flat stays folded	slightly curved pinna; soft; slow recoil	well-curved pinna; soft but ready recoil	formed & firm instant recoil	thick cartilage ear stiff	
Genitals (male)	scrotum flat, smooth	scrotum empty faint rugae	testes in upper canal rare rugae	testes descending few rugae	testes down good rugae	testes pendulous deep rugae	
Genitals (female)	clitoris prominent labia flat	prominent clitoris small labia minora	prominent clitoris enlarging minora	majora & minora equally prominent	majora large minora small	majora cover clitoris & minora	

MATURITY RATING

score	weeks
−10	20
−5	22
0	24
5	26
10	28
15	30
20	32
25	34
30	36
35	38
40	40
45	42
50	44

A

Fig. 7.1 **A,** Ballard scale for newborn maturity rating. Expanded scale includes extremely premature infants and has been refined to improve accuracy in more mature infants. (**A,** From Ballard, J. L., Khoury, J. C., Wedig, K., et al. [1991].New Ballard score expanded to include extremely premature infants. *Journal of Pediatrics, 119,* 417.)

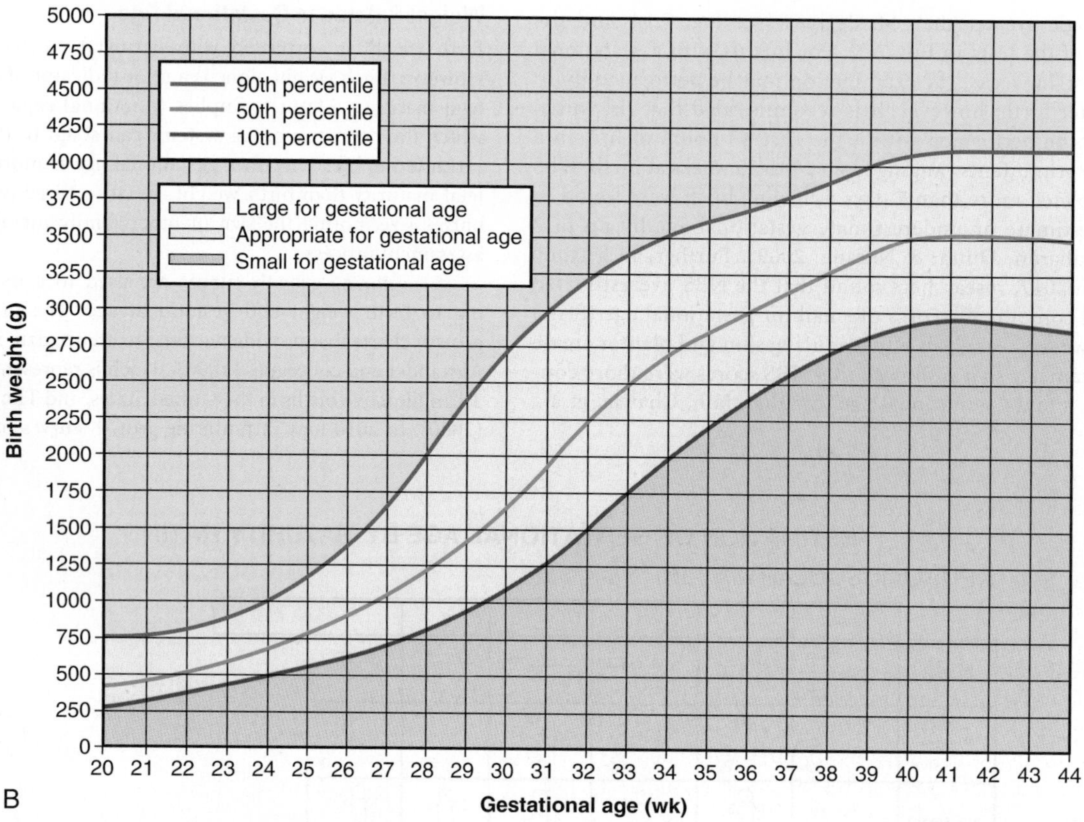

Fig. 7.1, cont'd B, Intrauterine growth: birth weight percentiles based on live single births at gestational ages 20 to 44 weeks. (**B,** Data from Alexander, G. R., Himes, J. H., Kaufman, R. B., et al. [1996]. A United States national reference for fetal growth. *Obstetrics & Gynecology, 87*(2), 163–168.)

BOX 7.2 Tests Used in Assessing Gestational Age

Posture: With infant quiet and in a supine position, observe degree of flexion in arms and legs. Muscle tone and degree of flexion increase with maturity.
Full flexion of the arms and legs—4[a]

Square window: With thumb supporting back of arm below wrist, apply gentle pressure with index and third fingers on dorsum of hand without rotating infant's wrist. Measure angle between base of thumb and forearm.
Full flexion (hand lies flat on ventral surface of forearm)—4

Arm recoil: With infant supine, fully flex both forearms on upper arms, hold for 5 seconds; pull down on hands to fully extend and rapidly release arms. Observe rapidity and intensity of recoil to a state of flexion.
A brisk return to full flexion—4

Popliteal angle: With infant supine and pelvis flat on a firm surface, flex lower leg on thigh and then flex thigh on abdomen. While holding knee with thumb and index finger, extend lower leg with index finger of other hand. Measure degree of angle behind knee (popliteal angle).
An angle of less than 90 degrees—5

Scarf sign: With infant supine, support head in midline with one hand; use other hand to pull infant's arm across the shoulder so that infant's hand touches shoulder. Determine location of elbow in relation to midline.
Elbow does not reach midline—4

Heel to ear: With infant supine and pelvis flat on a firm surface, pull foot as far as possible up toward ear on same side. Measure degree of knee flexion (same as popliteal angle).
Knees flexed with a popliteal angle of less than 90 degrees—4

[a]Numeric ratings correspond to Fig. 7.1A.

257,000 infants in the United States were published, noting that use of a contemporary, large, and racially diverse United States sample has produced intrauterine growth curves that differ from those produced earlier (Olsen, Groveman, Lawson, et al., 2010).

Until recently, commonly used reference ranges have been based solely on single populations largely from industrialized countries. Therefore, in 2018, the World Health Organization made the establishment of fetal growth charts for international use a priority and included countries where perinatal morbidity and mortality are high. As a result, it developed new fetal growth charts for common fetal measurements and estimated fetal weight based on a longitudinal study of 1387 low-risk pregnant women from 10 countries (Argentina, Brazil, Democratic Republic of Congo, Denmark, Egypt, France, Germany, India, Norway, and Thailand) that provided 8203 ultrasound measurements. It discovered that fetal growth may not be uniform even under ideal maternal conditions. Thus, it recommends the use of carefully adjusted growth charts that reflect optimal local growth when public health issues are being addressed (Kiserud, Benachi, Kecher, et al., 2018).

Classification of infants at birth by both weight and gestational age provides a more accurate method for predicting morbidity and mortality risks and providing guidelines for management of the neonate than estimating gestational age or birth weight alone. The infant's birth weight, length, and head circumference are plotted on standardized graphs with normal values for gestational age (for birth weight, see Fig. 7.1B). Infants whose weight is **appropriate for gestational age (AGA)** (between the 10th and 90th percentiles) are classified as having grown at a normal rate regardless of the time of birth—preterm, term, or postterm. Infants who are **large for gestational age (LGA)** (above

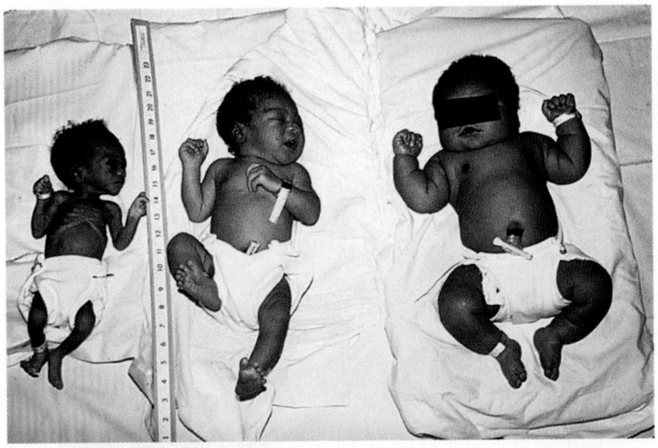

Fig. 7.2 Three infants of the same gestational age, weight 600 g, 1400 g, and 2750 g, respectively, from left to right. (From Perinatal assessment of maturation, National Audiovisual Center, Washington, DC.)

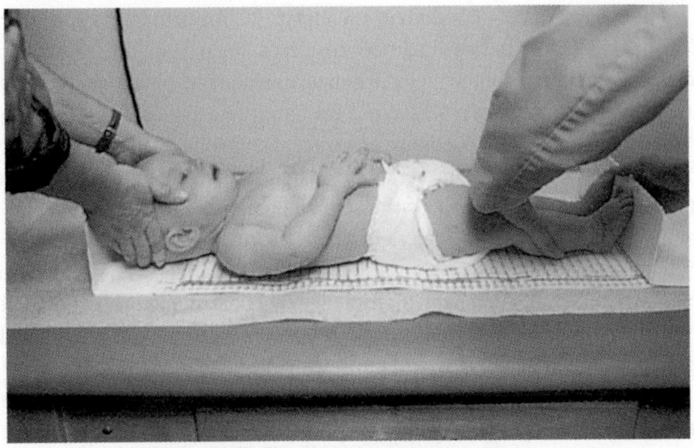

Fig. 7.3 Measurement of infant length.

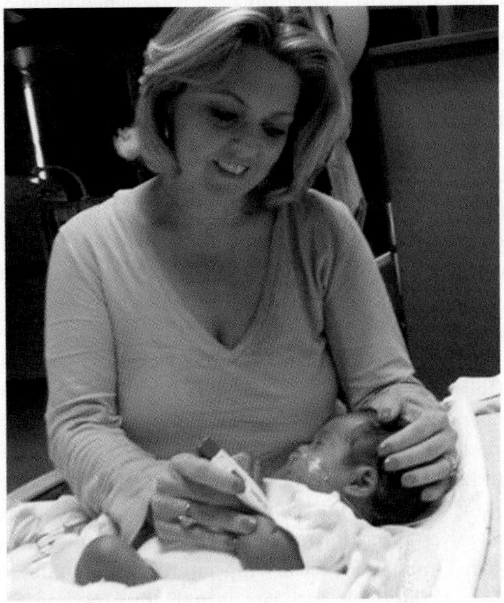

Fig. 7.4 Mother taking axillary temperature with digital thermometer.

the 90th percentile) are considered to have grown at an accelerated rate during fetal life; **small for gestational age (SGA)** infants (below the 10th percentile) are classified as having experienced intrauterine growth restriction or delay.

When gestational age is determined according to a standardized gestational age scale such as the NBS, the newborn will fall into one of the following nine possible categories for birth weight and gestational age: AGA—term, preterm, postterm; SGA—term, preterm, postterm; LGA—term, preterm, postterm. Fig. 7.2 illustrates the disparity between birth weights of three preterm infants of the same gestational age, 32 weeks. Birth weight and gestational age both influence morbidity and mortality; the lower the birth weight and gestational age, the higher the rate of morbidity and mortality.

General Measurements

Several important newborn measurements are significant when compared and recorded over time on a graph. For full-term infants, average head circumference is between 33 and 35.5 cm (13 and 14 inches). Head circumference may be somewhat smaller and inaccurate immediately following birth due to the molding process that occurs with vaginal deliveries. However, usually by the second or third day after birth, the skull is normal in size and contour.

Head circumference may be compared with crown-to-rump length or sitting height. Crown-to-rump measurements are usually 31 to 35 cm (12.2 to 13.8 inches), thus head circumference is generally equal to or up to 2 cm more than crown-to-rump length. Comparing neonatal head circumference with crown-to-rump length may provide a means for identifying infants at risk for microcephaly, hydrocephalus, cephalohematoma, subgaleal hemorrhage, and subdural hematoma. Prematurity and intrauterine malnutrition may also disrupt the relationship between head circumference and crown-to-rump length.

Abdominal circumference is not routinely monitored in full-term newborns but should be done in the event of abdominal distention to determine changes in girth over time. Since the umbilical cord is still intact, abdominal circumference is measured just above the level of the umbilicus. Measuring the abdominal circumference below the umbilical region may be inaccurate since bladder fullness may affect the reading.

Head-to-heel length is also measured, and since the usual position of the newborn is flexed, it will be necessary to extend the legs completely when measuring total body length. The average length of newborns is 48 to 53 cm (19 to 21 inches) (Fig. 7.3).

Body weight should be measured soon after birth since weight loss may occur rapidly. Normally, neonates lose about 10% of their birth weight by day 3 or 4 because of loss of extracellular fluid and passing of meconium, as well as limited food intake, particularly in breastfed infants. Newborns are expected to return to their birth weight by no later than 10 to 14 days of life. Most newborns weigh 2700 to 4000 g (6 to 9 pounds), with the average weight being about 3400 g (7.5 pounds). Accurate birth weight and length are important since these measurements provide a baseline for assessing future growth.

A newborn's vital signs are another important measurement of well-being. Axillary temperatures rather than rectal temperatures are assessed because an incorrectly inserted thermometer in the rectum can potentially cause perforation of the mucosa (Fig. 7.4). Core body temperature varies according to the periods of reactivity but is usually 36.5° to 37.6°C (97.7° to 99.7°F). Skin temperature is slightly lower than core body temperature. The single best method for determining a newborn's temperature remains elusive when considering the available studies. Despite their usefulness in older children and adults, the accuracy of tympanic membrane sensors is problematic in infants. A comprehensive review of the literature exploring methods and devices for temperature measurement in the newborn resulted in the authors concluding that the accuracy of the tympanic route in the neonate is controversial (Smith, 2014; Smith, Alcock, & Usher, 2013).

The Canadian Paediatric Society, Community Paediatrics Committee (2017a) has outlined concerns regarding the safety and accuracy of tympanic temperature measurement in newborns because of the size of a newborn's external ear canal relative to the size of the thermometer probe. To ensure accuracy, the probe, which may be up to 8 mm (0.3 inch) in diameter, must be inserted deeply into the ear canal to allow orientation of the sensor near or against the tympanic membrane. At birth, the average diameter of the canal is just 4 mm (0.16 inch); at 2 years old, it is just 5 mm (0.2 inch). The Canadian Paediatric Society (2017a) concluded that current infrared tympanic thermometry lacks sufficient safety and precision to meet clinical needs for use in newborn infants and children younger than 2 years old.

Infrared axillary and digital thermometers are used in many neonatal units because they give rapid readings and are easy to clean; studies demonstrate their usefulness in well, full-term newborns. Smith, Alcock, and Usher (2013) conducted an extensive review of the literature on temperature measurement in term and preterm infants. These researchers concluded that the most commonly used route when using digital and electronic thermometers for temperature measurement is the axillary route. Advantages of digital thermometers in neonatal care include relatively easy readability by parents and caretakers in the home, improvement of discharge planning effectiveness, and decreased risk of breakage and associated complications compared with glass thermometers.

Temporal artery thermometers (TATs), in which a battery-powered instrument is gently slid across the newborn's forehead, are available for use in the general pediatric population. A benefit of this type of temperature measurement is that it is not necessary to undress the newborn. Research findings in the neonatal population suggests that TAT may be a reasonable method for newborn temperature measurement, although no more accurate than the standard axillary method (Syrkin-Nikolau, Johnson, Colaizy, et al., 2017). Further, TAT has been found to accurately detect temperature in febrile and normothermic full-term neonates but not in hypothermic neonates (Goswami, Batra, Khurana, et al., 2017). In most studies regarding newborn temperature, the glass mercury thermometer is the gold standard against which other methods are compared. There is no universal agreement on placement times for glass thermometers, although 3 minutes for rectal temperature and 5 minutes for axillary temperature are considered adequate. In 2009 the American Academy of Pediatrics, Committee on Environmental Health reaffirmed its statement recommending that mercury thermometers no longer be used in clinics and homes to decrease mercury exposure hazard (Wyckoff, 2009).

Nurses must be cognizant of the many variables involved:

Site—axillary, rectal, tympanic, skin

Environment—radiant warmer, open crib, incubator, clothing, or nesting

Purpose—fever, possible sepsis (in which case the temperature may be lower than normal in newborns), and thermoregulation in the transition phase

Instrument—electronic, digital, infrared

Nurses must also make clear clinical decisions based on accurate and objective data. Further research is needed to perfect thermometers that accurately reflect infants' core temperature to effectively plan nursing care and maintain a stable temperature.

Pulse and respirations also vary according to the periods of reactivity and the infant's behaviors but are usually in the range of 120 to 140 beats/min and 30 to 60 breaths/min. Both are counted for a full 60 seconds to detect irregularities in rate or rhythm. The heart rate is taken apically with a stethoscope, and the femoral arteries are palpated for equality of strength or fullness.

Measurement of BP provides baseline data and may indicate cardiovascular problems. BP is most easily and accurately assessed using oscillometry (Dinamap) when the newborn is in a quiet or sleep state using an appropriate cuff width–to-arm ratio of 0.45 to 0.70 (approximately half to three-quarters) (Fig. 7.5). For healthy term infants, the average oscillometric systolic/diastolic BP is 68/38 mm Hg on day 1 of life, changing to 75.5/44 mm Hg by day 4 (Novak & Gill, 2018). Blood pressure should be compared in the upper and lower extremities and should be equal.

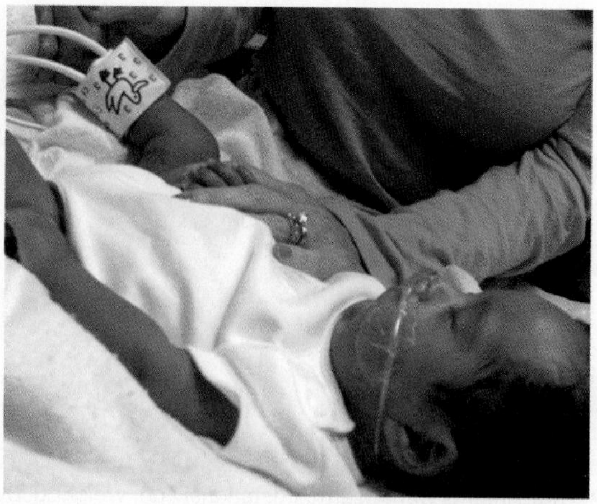

Fig. 7.5 Measurement of blood pressure using oscillometry.

! NURSING ALERT

Although uncommon, the presence of neonatal hypertension may be a sign of a significant underlying problem (such as renal, cardiac, or thromboembolic pathologic condition), or it may be associated with a medication treatment regimen. Neonatal hypertension is brought to the primary practitioner's attention for further evaluation.

The American Academy of Pediatrics, Section on Cardiology and Cardiac Surgery Executive Committee recommends routine pulse oximetry screening for critical congenital heart disease (CCHD) for all newborns (Ewer & Martin, 2016). Delayed diagnosis of CCHD can result in morbidity or mortality to infants. Research has demonstrated that adding pulse oximetry, a noninvasive, painless technology, to newborn assessment can detect CCHD. Practitioners are directed to use motion-tolerant pulse oximeters and to screen infants after 24 hours of age to reduce false-positive results. Oxygen saturation must be measured in the right hand and in one foot; a reading of 95% or greater in either extremity with a 3% or less difference between the upper and lower extremities would be a "pass." Infants with oxygen saturation of less than 90% need immediate evaluation.

A suggested schedule for monitoring heart rate, respiratory rate, and temperature is on admission to the nursery, once every 30 minutes until the newborn has been stable for 2 hours, and then once every 8 hours until discharge. However, this schedule may vary according to institutional policy. Any change in the infant, such as color, breathing, muscle tone, or behavior, necessitates more frequent monitoring.

General Appearance

Before each body system is assessed, it is important to describe the general posture and behavior of the newborn. The overall appearance yields valuable clues to the infant's physical status. In full-term neonates, the posture is one of complete flexion as a result of in utero position. Most infants are born in a vertex presentation with the head flexed and the chin resting on the upper chest, the arms flexed with the

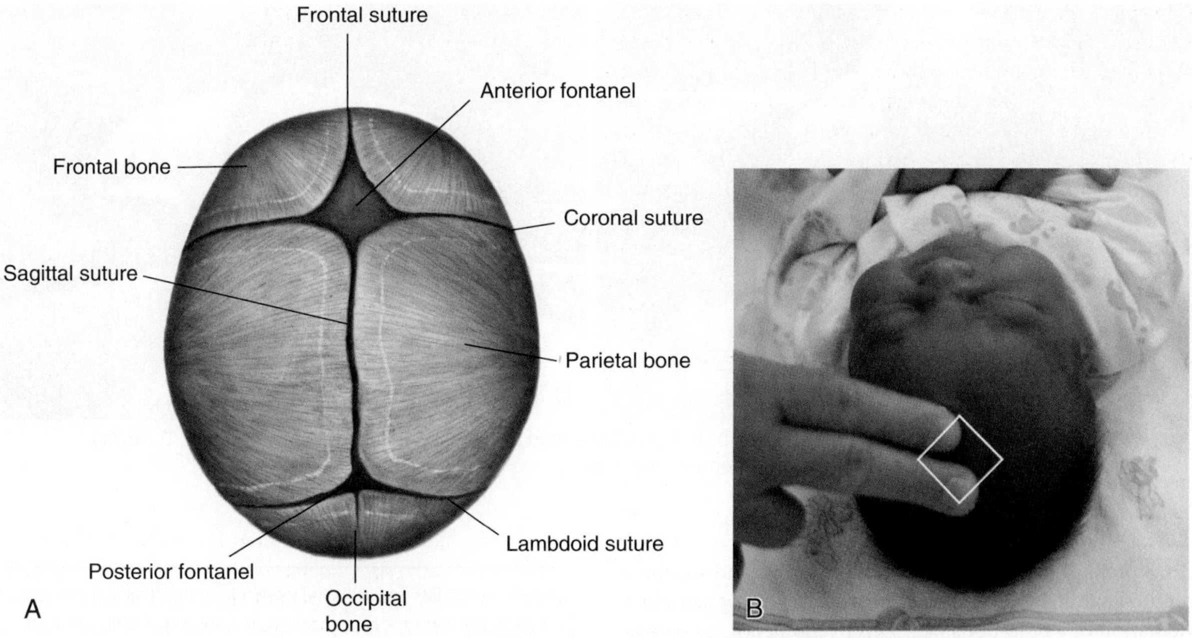

Fig. 7.6 A, Location of sutures and fontanels. B, Palpating the anterior fontanel.

hands clenched, the legs flexed at the knees and hips, and the feet dorsiflexed. The vertebral column is also flexed. It is important to recognize any deviation from this characteristic fetal position.

The infant's behavior is carefully noted, especially the degree of alertness, drowsiness, and irritability; the latter two factors may reflect common signs of neurologic problems. Some questions to mentally ask when assessing behavior are:

- Is the infant awakened easily by a loud noise?
- Is the infant comforted by rocking, sucking, or cuddling?
- Do there seem to be periods of deep and light sleep?
- When awake, does the infant seem satisfied after a feeding?
- What stimuli elicit responses from the infant?
- When disturbed, how much does the infant protest?

Skin

The texture of the newborn's skin is velvety smooth and puffy, especially about the eyes, the legs, the dorsal aspect of the hands and the feet, and the scrotum or labia. Skin color depends on racial and familial background and varies greatly among newborns. In general, white infants are usually pink to red. African American newborns may appear a pinkish or yellowish brown. Infants of Hispanic descent may have an olive tint or a slight yellow cast to the skin. Infants of Asian descent may be a rosy or yellowish tan. The color of American Indian newborns varies from a light pink to a dark reddish brown. By the second or third day of life, the skin turns to its more natural tone and is drier and flakier. Several other color changes that may be noted on the skin are described later in this chapter (see Table 7.4).

At birth, the skin may be partially covered with a grayish white, cheese-like substance called **vernix caseosa**, a mixture of sebum and desquamating cells. It is absorbed by 24 to 28 hours. A fine, downy hair called **lanugo** may be present on the skin, especially on the forehead, cheeks, shoulders, and back.

Head

General observation of the contour of the head is important because molding occurs in almost all vaginal deliveries. In a vertex delivery, the head is usually flattened at the forehead, with the apex rising and forming a point at the end of the parietal bones and the posterior skull or occiput dropping abruptly. The usual, more oval contour of the head is apparent by 1 to 2 days after birth. The change in shape occurs because the bones of the cranium are not fused, allowing for overlapping of the edges of these bones to accommodate to the size of the birth canal during delivery. Such molding usually does not occur in infants born by elective cesarean section.

Six bones—the frontal, occipital, two parietals, and two temporals—make up the cranium. Between the junction of these bones are bands of connective tissue called **sutures**. At the junction of the sutures are wider spaces of unossified membranous tissue called **fontanels**. The two most prominent fontanels in infants are the anterior fontanel formed by the junction of the sagittal, coronal, and frontal sutures and the posterior fontanel formed by the junction of the sagittal and lambdoid sutures (Fig. 7.6A).

> **NURSING TIP** The location of the sutures is easily remembered because the coronal suture "crowns" the head, and the sagittal suture "separates" the head.

The skull is palpated for all patent sutures and fontanels, noting size, shape, molding, or abnormal closure. The sutures feel like cracks between the skull bones, and the fontanels feel like wider soft spots at the junction of the sutures. These are palpated by using the tip of the index finger and running it along the ends of the bones (see Fig. 7.6B).

The anterior fontanel is diamond shaped and measures anywhere from barely palpable to 4 to 5 cm (≈2 inches) at its widest point (from bone to bone rather than from suture to suture). The posterior fontanel is easily located by following the sagittal suture toward the occiput. The posterior fontanel is triangular, usually measuring between 0.5 and 1 cm (<0.5 inch) at its widest part. The fontanels should feel flat, firm, and well demarcated against the bony edges of the skull. Frequently, pulsations are visible at the anterior fontanel. Coughing, crying, or lying down may temporarily cause the fontanels to bulge and become taut.

Palpate the skull for any unusual masses or prominences, particularly those resulting from birth trauma, such as caput succedaneum or cephalohematoma (see Chapter 8). Because of the pliability of the

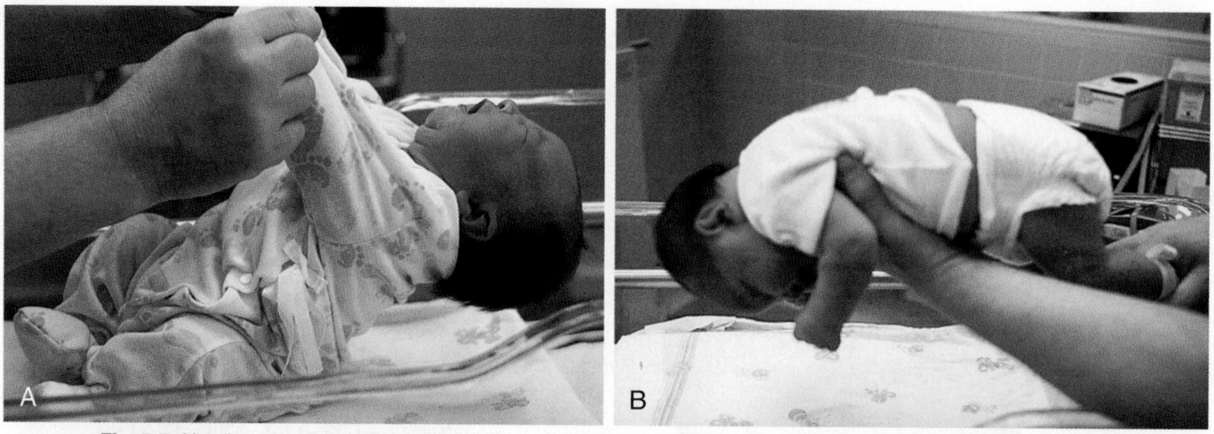

Fig. 7.7 Head control in an infant. **A**, Inability to hold the head erect when pulled to sitting position. **B**, Ability to hold the head erect when placed in ventral suspension.

skull, exerting pressure at the margin of the parietal and occipital bones along the lambdoid suture may produce a snapping sensation like the indentation of a ping-pong ball. This phenomenon, known as **physiologic craniotabes**, may be found normally, especially in newborns of breech birth, but also may indicate hydrocephalus, congenital syphilis, or rickets.

Assess the degree of head control. Although head lag is normal in newborns, the degree of ability to control the head in certain positions should be recognized. If a supine infant is pulled by the arms into a semi-Fowler position, marked head lag and hyperextension are noted (Fig. 7.7A). However, as the infant is brought forward into a sitting position, the infant will attempt to control the head in an upright position. As the head falls forward onto the chest, many infants will attempt to right it into the erect position. Also, if the infant is held in ventral suspension (i.e., held prone above and parallel to the examining surface), the infant will hold the head in a straight line with the spinal column (see Fig. 7.7B). When lying on the abdomen, newborns have the ability to lift the head slightly, turning it from side to side. Marked head lag is seen in neonates with Down syndrome, prematurity, hypoxia, and neuromuscular compromise.

Eyes

Because newborns tend to have their eyes tightly closed, it is best to begin the examination of the eyes by observing the eyelids for edema, which is normally present for the first 2 days after delivery. The eyes are observed for symmetry. Tears may be present at birth, but purulent discharge from the eyes shortly after birth is abnormal. To visualize the surface structures of the eyes, the infant is held supine, and the head is gently lowered. The eyes will usually open, like the mechanism of a doll's eyes. The sclera should be white and clear.

The cornea is examined for the presence of any opacities or haziness. The corneal reflex is normally present at birth but may not be elicited unless neurologic or eye damage is suspected. The pupil will usually respond to light by constricting. The pupils are normally malaligned. A searching nystagmus is common. Strabismus is a normal finding because of the lack of binocularity. The color of the iris is noted. Most light-skinned newborns have slate gray or dark blue eyes, and dark-skinned infants have brown eyes.

A funduscopic examination may be difficult to perform because of the infant's tendency to keep the eyes tightly closed. However, a red reflex should be elicited. The absence of a red reflex in a newborn may indicate a cataract, glaucoma, retinal abnormalities, or retinoblastoma (see Chapter 4).

> **NURSING TIP** To elicit a red reflex, place the infant in a dark room. In an alert state, many newborns open their eyes in a supported sitting position.

Ears

The ears are examined for position, structure, and auditory function. The top of the pinna should lie in a horizontal plane to the outer canthus of the eye. The pinna is often flattened against the side of the head from pressure in utero. An otoscopic examination may be difficult to perform if the canals are filled with vernix caseosa and amniotic fluid, making visualization of the tympanic membrane difficult.

Auditory ability is tested by a number of objective hearing tests. Making a loud noise close to the infant's head may or may not elicit a response; the lack of a response, however, is not a definite indication of hearing loss. The startle reflex (Table 7.2) may be observed when there is a sudden loud noise near the infant or the bassinet is accidentally bumped, but this often depends on the infant's state at the time.

Nose

The nose is usually flattened after birth, and bruises are common. Patency of the nasal canals can be assessed by holding a hand over the infant's mouth and one canal and noting the passage of air through the unobstructed opening. If nasal patency is questionable, report it because most newborns are obligatory nose breathers and are unable to breathe orally in response to nasal occlusion. Sneezing and thin white mucus are common up to several hours after birth.

Mouth and Throat

An external defect of the mouth (such as cleft lip) is obvious; however, the internal structures require careful inspection. The palate is normally highly arched and somewhat narrow. Rarely, teeth may be present. A common finding is **Epstein pearls**, small, white, epithelial cysts along both sides of the midline of the hard palate. They are insignificant and disappear in several weeks.

The **frenulum** of the upper lip is a band of thick pink tissue that lies under the inner surface of the upper lip and extends to the maxillary alveolar ridge. It is particularly evident when the infant yawns or smiles. It disappears as the maxilla grows. The lingual frenulum attaches the underside of the tongue to the lower palate midway between the ventral surface of the tongue and the tip. In some cases, a tight lingual frenulum, formerly referred to as *tongue-tie*, may restrict adequate sucking (Brookes & Bowley, 2014). Further evaluation may

TABLE 7.2 Assessment of Reflexes in the Newborn

Reflexes	Expected Behavioral Responses
Localized	
Eyes	
Blinking or corneal	Infant blinks at sudden appearance of a bright light or at approach of an object toward cornea; persists throughout life.
Pupillary	Pupil constricts when a bright light shines toward it; persists throughout life.
Doll's eye	As head is moved slowly to right or left, eyes lag behind and do not immediately adjust to new position of head; disappears as fixation develops; if persists, indicates neurologic damage.
Nose	
Sneeze	Sneezing is a spontaneous response of nasal passages to irritation or obstruction; persists throughout life.
Glabellar	Tapping briskly on glabella (bridge of nose) causes eyes to close tightly.
Mouth and Throat	
Sucking	Infant begins strong sucking movements of circumoral area in response to stimulation; persists throughout infancy even without stimulation, such as during sleep.
Gag	Stimulation of posterior pharynx by food, suction, or passage of a tube causes infant to gag; persists throughout life.
Rooting	Touching or stroking the cheek alongside the mouth causes infant to turn head toward that side and begin to suck; should disappear at about 3 to 4 months old but may persist for up to 12 months.
Extrusion	When tongue is touched or depressed, infant responds by forcing it outward; disappears by 4 months old.
Yawn	Yawning is a spontaneous response to decreased oxygen by increasing amount of inspired air; persists throughout life.
Cough	Irritation of mucous membranes of larynx or tracheobronchial tree causes coughing; persists throughout life; usually present after first day of birth.
Extremities	
Grasp	Touching palms of hands or soles of feet near base of digits causes flexion of fingers and toes (Fig. 7.8A); palmar grasp lessens after 3 months old to be replaced by voluntary movement; plantar grasp lessens by 8 months old.
Babinski	Stroking outer sole of foot upward from heel and across ball of foot causes toes to hyperextend and hallux to dorsiflex (see Fig. 7.8B); disappears after 1 year old.
Ankle clonus	Briskly dorsiflexing foot while supporting knee in partially flexed position results in one or two oscillating movements ("beats"); eventually no beats should be felt.
Mass	
Moro	Sudden jarring or change in equilibrium causes sudden extension and abduction of extremities and fanning of fingers, with index finger and thumb forming a C shape followed by flexion and adduction of extremities; legs may weakly flex; infant may cry (Fig. 7.9A); disappears after 3 to 4 months old, usually strongest during first 2 months.
Startle	A sudden loud noise causes abduction of the arms with flexion of elbows; hands remain clenched; disappears by 4 months old.
Perez	While infant is prone on a firm surface, thumb is pressed along spine from sacrum to neck; infant responds by crying, flexing extremities, and elevating pelvis and head; lordosis of the spine, as well as defecation and urination, may occur; disappears by 4 to 6 months old.
Tonic neck	When infant's head is turned to one side, arm and leg extend on that side, and opposite arm and leg flex (see Fig. 7.9B); disappears by 3 to 4 months old to be replaced by symmetric positioning of both sides of body.
Trunk incurvation (Galant)	Stroking infant's back alongside the spine causes hips to move toward stimulated side; disappears by 4 weeks old.
Dance or step	If infant is held so that sole of foot touches a hard surface, there is a reciprocal flexion and extension of the leg, simulating walking (see Fig. 7.9C); disappears after 3 to 4 weeks old to be replaced by deliberate movement.
Crawl	When placed on abdomen, infant makes crawling movements with arms and legs (see Fig. 7.9D); disappears at about 6 weeks old.
Placing	When infant is held upright under arms and dorsal side of foot is briskly placed against hard object, such as a table, leg lifts as if foot is stepping on table; age of disappearance varies.

be required to ascertain adequate sucking, particularly in breastfed infants. The treatment for a tight lingual frenulum is frenotomy, which is a safe and effective surgical procedure to improve comfort, effectiveness, and ease of breastfeeding for mother and infant. A recent Cochrane review of five published studies concluded, however, that although a reduction in maternal pain was generally reported, breastfeeding was not consistently improved postprocedure (O'Shea, Foster, O'Donnell, et al., 2017). Research continues to determine how best to select which infants may benefit from the procedure and when to perform it (Emond, Ingram, Johnson, et al., 2014; Power & Murphy, 2015).

Elicit the sucking reflex by placing a nipple or nonlatex gloved finger in the infant's mouth. The infant should exhibit a strong, vigorous suck. The rooting reflex is elicited by stroking the cheek and noting the infant's response of turning toward the stimulated side and sucking.

The uvula can be inspected while the infant is crying, and the chin is depressed. However, it may be retracted upward and backward during crying. Tonsillar tissue is generally not seen in newborns. **Natal teeth**, teeth present at birth, as opposed to **neonatal teeth**, which erupt during the first month of life, are seen infrequently and erupt chiefly at the position of the lower incisors. Teeth are reported because they are

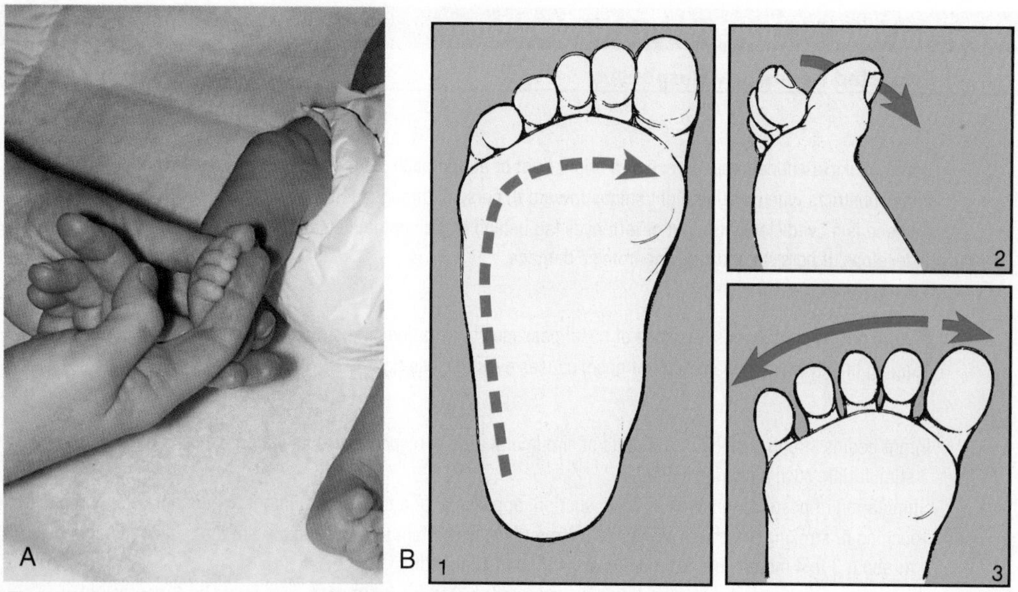

Fig. 7.8 A, Plantar or grasp reflex. B, Babinski reflex. *1,* Direction of stroke. *2,* Dorsiflexion of big toe. *3,* Fanning of toes. (**A,** From Zitelli, B. J., McIntire, S. C., & Nowalk, A. J. [2012]. *Zitelli and Davis' atlas of pediatric physical diagnosis* [16th ed.]. St Louis, MO: Saunders/Elsevier.)

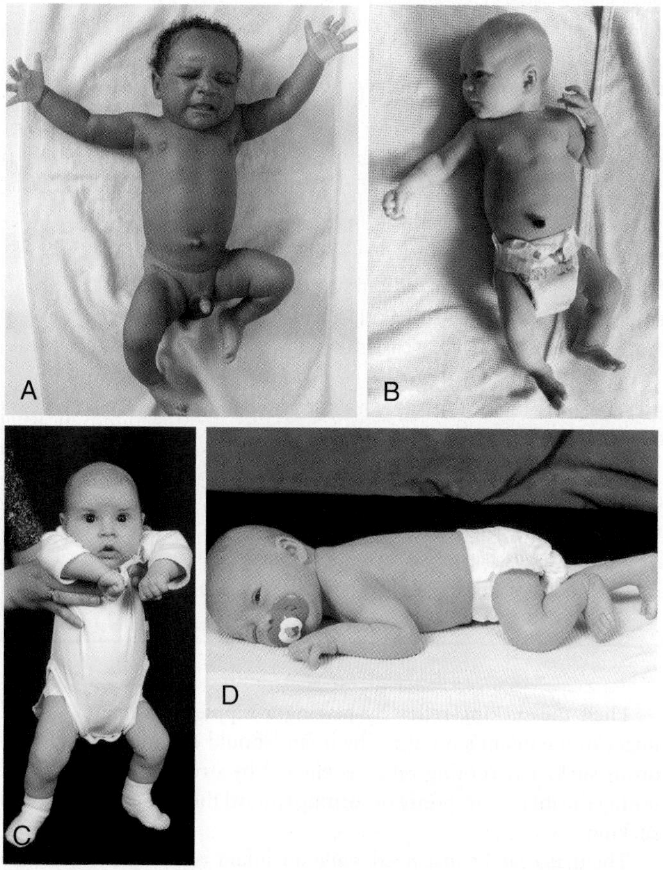

Fig. 7.9 A, Moro reflex. B, Tonic neck reflex. C, Dance reflex. D, Crawl reflex. (Courtesy Paul Vincent Kuntz, Texas Children's Hospital, Houston, TX.)

frequently found with developmental abnormalities and syndromes, including cleft lip and palate. Most natal teeth are loosely attached. However, current thinking suggests preserving them until they exfoliate naturally (Maheswari, Kumar, Karunakaran, et al., 2012) unless the teeth are attached loosely or breastfeeding is impaired by the neonate's biting the breast.

Neck

Because the newborn's neck is short and covered with folds of tissue, adequate assessment of the neck requires allowing the head to fall gently backward in hyperextension while the back is supported in a slightly raised position. Observe for range of motion, shape, and any abnormal masses and palpate each clavicle for possible fractures.

Chest

The shape of the newborn's chest is almost circular because the anteroposterior and lateral diameters are equal. The ribs are flexible, and slight intercostal retractions are normally seen on inspiration. The xiphoid process is commonly visible as a small protrusion at the end of the sternum. The sternum is generally raised and slightly curved.

Inspect the breasts for size, shape and nipple formation, location, and number. Breast enlargement appears in many newborns of both genders by the second or third day and is caused by maternal hormones. Occasionally, a milky substance is secreted by the infant's breasts. Supernumerary nipples may be found on the chest, on the abdomen, or in the axilla.

Lungs

The normal respirations of newborns are irregular and abdominal, and the rate is between 30 and 60 breaths/min. Pauses in respiration of less than 20 seconds' duration are considered normal. After the initial forceful breaths required to initiate respiration, subsequent breaths should be nonlabored and fairly regular in rhythm. Periodic breathing is commonly seen in full-term newborns and consists of rapid nonlabored respirations followed by pauses of less than 20 seconds; periodic breathing may be more prominent during sleep and is not accompanied by status changes, such as cyanosis or bradycardia. Occasional irregularities occur in relation to crying, sleeping, stooling, and feeding.

Perform auscultation when the infant is quiet. Bronchial breath sounds should be equal bilaterally. Any differences in auscultatory findings between symmetric sites are reported. Crackles soon after birth indicate the presence of fluid, which represents the normal transition of the lungs to extrauterine life. However, wheezes, persistence of medium or coarse crackles after the first few hours of life, and stridor should be reported for further investigation.

Heart

Heart rate is auscultated and may range from 100 to 180 beats/min shortly after birth and, when the infant's condition has stabilized, from 120 to 140 beats/min. The point of maximum intensity (PMI) may be palpated and is usually found at the fourth to fifth intercostal space, medial to the left midclavicular line. The PMI gives some indication of the location of the heart, which may be displaced in conditions such as congenital diaphragmatic hernia or pneumothorax. **Dextrocardia**, an anomaly wherein the heart is on the right side of the body, is reported because the abdominal organs may also be reversed, with associated circulatory abnormalities.

Auscultation of the specific components of the heart sounds is difficult because of the rapid rate and effective transmission of respiratory sounds. However, the first (S_1) and second (S_2) sounds should be clear and well defined; the second sound is somewhat higher in pitch and sharper than the first. A murmur is frequently heard in newborns, especially over the base of the heart or at the left sternal border at the third or fourth interspace. In newborns, a murmur is not necessarily associated with specific cardiac defects but frequently represents the incomplete functional closure of fetal shunts (see Chapter 4 for other characteristics of murmurs). However, always record and report all murmurs and other unusual heart sounds.

Abdomen

The normal contour of the abdomen is cylindric and usually prominent with few visible veins. Bowel sounds are heard within the first 15 to 20 minutes after birth. Visible peristaltic waves may be observed in some newborns.

Inspect the umbilical cord to determine the presence of two arteries, which look like papular structures, and one vein, which has a larger lumen than the arteries and a thinner vessel wall. At birth, the umbilical cord appears bluish white and moist. After clamping, it begins to dry and appears a dull, yellowish brown. It progressively shrivels in size and turns greenish black.

If the umbilical cord appears unusually large in diameter at the base, inspect for the presence of a hematoma or small omphalocele. If the cord is clamped over an existing omphalocele, part of the intestine will be clamped, causing tissue necrosis. One practical rule of thumb is to cut the cord distally 4 to 5 inches from a questionable enlargement until further examination is carried out by a practitioner. The extra length can later be cut if no pathologic condition has been identified.

! NURSING ALERT

An umbilical cord that is draining and erythematous at the base should be investigated by the primary practitioner. The cord undergoes a process of dry gangrene decay, which has an odor; therefore odor alone may not be a reliable index of suspicion for omphalitis.

Palpate after inspecting the abdomen. The liver is normally palpable 1 to 3 cm (≈0.5 to 1 inch) below the right costal margin. The tip of the spleen can sometimes be felt, but a palpable spleen more than 1 cm below the left costal margin suggests enlargement and warrants further investigation. Although both kidneys should be palpated, this maneuver requires considerable practice. When felt, the lower half of the right kidney and the tip of the left kidney are 1 to 2 cm above the umbilicus. During examination of the lower abdomen, palpate for femoral pulses, which should be strong and equal bilaterally.

Female Genitalia

Normally, the labia minora, labia majora, and clitoris are edematous, especially after a breech delivery. However, the labia and clitoris must be carefully inspected to identify any evidence of ambiguous genitalia or other abnormalities. Normally, in a girl, the urethral opening is located behind and below the clitoris.

A **hymenal tag** is occasionally visible from the posterior opening of the vagina. It is composed of tissue from the hymen and the labia minora. It usually disappears in several weeks. Generally, the vaginal vault is not inspected.

Vaginal discharge may be noted during the first week of life. This pseudomenstruation is a manifestation of the abrupt decrease of maternal hormones and usually disappears by 2 to 4 weeks of age. Fecal discharge from the vaginal opening indicates a rectovaginal fistula and is always reported. Vernix caseosa may be present in large amounts between the labia; it will disappear after several days with routine bathing and care.

Male Genitalia

The penis is inspected for the urethral opening, which is located at the tip. However, the opening may be totally covered by the **prepuce**, or foreskin, which covers the glans penis. A tight prepuce is a common finding in newborns. It should not be forcefully retracted; locating the urinary meatus is usually possible without retracting the foreskin. **Smegma**, a white cheesy substance, is commonly found around the glans penis under the foreskin. Small, white, firm lesions called *epithelial pearls* may be seen at the tip of the prepuce. An erection is common in newborns.

The scrotum may be large, edematous, and pendulous in full-term neonates, especially in infants born in breech position. It is more deeply pigmented in dark-skinned infants. A noncommunicating hydrocele commonly occurs unilaterally and disappears within a few months. Always palpate the scrotum for the presence of testes (see Chapter 4). In small newborns, particularly preterm infants, the undescended testes may be palpable within the inguinal canal. Absence of the testes may also be a sign of ambiguous genitalia (disorders of sex development), especially when accompanied by a small scrotum and penis. Inguinal hernias may or may not be manifested immediately after birth. A hernia is more easily detected when the infant is crying. Palpable lymph nodes are most commonly found in the inguinal area.

Back and Rectum

Inspect the spine with the infant prone. The shape of the spine is gently rounded, with none of the characteristic S-shaped curves seen later in life. Any abnormal openings, masses, dimples, or soft areas are noted. A protruding sac anywhere along the spine, but most commonly in the sacral area, indicates some type of spina bifida. A small sinus, which may or may not be communicating with the spine, is a pilonidal sinus. It is frequently covered with a tuft of hair. Although it may have no pathologic significance, a pilonidal cyst may indicate the existence of spina bifida occulta or be a portal of entry into the spinal column.

With the infant still prone, note symmetry of the gluteal folds. Report any evidence of asymmetry. Skilled examiners test for developmental dysplasia of the hip (see Chapter 29).

The presence of an anal orifice and passage of meconium from the anal orifice during the first 24 to 48 hours of life indicates anal patency. If an imperforate anus is suspected, report this to the primary practitioner for further evaluation.

! NURSING ALERT

The presence of meconium or stool in the rectal area is not an indication of rectal patency; a fistula may exist wherein stool is evacuated via the vagina, scrotum, or raphe. Therefore it is imperative that anal patency be checked with a small rubber catheter if doubt regarding patency exists.

Extremities

Examine the extremities for symmetry, range of motion, and signs of malformation. Count the fingers and toes and note any supernumerary digits (**polydactyly**) or fusion of digits (**syndactyly**). A partial syndactyly between the second and third toes is a common variation seen in otherwise normal infants. The nail beds should be pink, although slight blueness is evident in acrocyanosis.

The palms of the hands should have the usual creases. Full-term newborns usually have creases covering the entire sole of the foot. The soles of the feet are flat with prominent fat pads.

Observe range of motion of the extremities throughout the entire examination. The absence of arm movement signals a potential birth injury paralysis, such as Klumpke or Erb-Duchenne palsy. An asymmetric or partial Moro reflex should alert the practitioner to further evaluate upper extremity mobility. Examine the lower extremities for limb length, symmetry, and hip abduction and flexion. Newborns demonstrate full range of motion in the elbow, hip, shoulder, and knee joints. Movements should be symmetric, smooth, and unrestricted.

Also assess muscle tone. By attempting to extend a flexed extremity, determine if tone is equal bilaterally. Extension of any extremity is usually met with resistance, and when released, the extremity returns to its previous flexed position. Hypotonia suggests some degree of hypoxia or neurologic disorder and is common in an infant with Down syndrome. Asymmetry of muscle tone may indicate a degree of paralysis from brain damage or nerve damage. Failure to move the lower limbs suggests a spinal cord lesion or injury. Sustained rhythmic tremors, twitches, and myoclonic jerks characterize neonatal seizures or may indicate neonatal abstinence syndrome (see Chapter 8, Neonatal Seizures and Drug-Exposed Infants). Sudden asynchronous jerking movements, quivering, or momentary tremors are usually normal.

Neurologic System

Assessing neurologic status is a critical part of the physical examination of newborns. Much of the neurologic testing takes place during evaluation of body systems, such as eliciting localized reflexes and observing posture, muscle tone, head control, and movement. However, several important mass (total body) reflexes also need to be elicited. These should be tested at the end of the examination because they may disturb the infant and interfere with auscultation. Two common newborn reflexes are elicited. The first is the grasp reflex. Touching the palms of the hands or soles of the feet near the base of the digits causes flexion or grasping (see Fig. 7.8A). The other is the Babinski reflex. Stroking the outer sole of the foot upward from the heel across the ball of the foot causes the big toe to dorsiflex and the other toes to hyperextend (see Fig. 7.8B).

These reflexes, as well as several local reflexes, are described in Table 7.2. Record and report the absence, asymmetry, persistence, or weakness of a reflex.

Transitional Assessment: Periods of Reactivity

Newborns exhibit behavioral and physiologic characteristics that may at first appear to be signs of stress. However, during the initial 24 hours, changes in heart rate, respiration, motor activity, color, mucus production, and bowel activity occur in an orderly, predictable sequence that is normal and indicates lack of stress.

For 6 to 8 hours after birth, the newborn is in the first period of reactivity. During the first 30 minutes, the infant is very alert, cries vigorously, may suck his or her fingers or fist, and appears very interested in the environment. At this time, the newborn's eyes are usually open, making this an excellent opportunity for the mother, father, and child to see each other. Because the healthy newborn has a vigorous suck, this is also an opportune time to begin breastfeeding. The infant will usually grasp the nipple quickly, satisfying both the mother and the infant. This is particularly important to point out to the parents because after this initially highly active state, the infant may be sleepy and uninterested in sucking. Physiologically, the respiratory rate during this period is as high as 80 breaths/min, crackles may be heard, heart rate reaches 180 beats/min, bowel sounds are active, mucus secretions are increased, and temperature may decrease. Maintaining appropriate temperature for newborns is best accomplished by practicing skin-to-skin care, whereby only a diaper is worn to allow majority of skin surface to be in contact with the mother's skin. A light blanket is used to cover the mother and newborn. Research has shown that skin-to-skin mother-infant holding is effective in ensuring that the newborn does not become hypothermic (Cleveland, Hill, Pulse, et al., 2017).

After this initial stage of alertness and activity, the infant enters the second stage of the first reactive period, which generally lasts 2 to 4 hours. Heart and respiratory rates decrease, temperature continues to fall, mucus production decreases, and urine and stool are usually not passed. The infant is in a state of sleep and relative calm. Any attempt at stimulation usually elicits minimal response. Because of the continued decline in body temperature, undressing or bathing is avoided during this time.

The second period of reactivity begins when the infant awakens from this deep sleep; it lasts about 2 to 5 hours and provides another excellent opportunity for child and parents to interact. The infant is again alert and responsive, heart and respiratory rates increase, the gag reflex is active, gastric and respiratory secretions are increased, and passage of meconium frequently occurs. This period is usually over when the amount of respiratory mucus has decreased. After this stage is a period of stabilization of physiologic systems and a vacillating pattern of sleep and activity.

Behavioral Assessment

An important area of assessment is observation of behavior. Infants' behavior helps shape their environment, and their ability to react to various stimuli affects how others relate to them. The principal areas of behavior for newborns are sleep, wakefulness, and activity such as crying.

One method of systematically assessing the infant's behavior is use of the Brazelton Neonatal Behavioral Assessment Scale (BNBAS) (Brazelton & Nugent, 1996). The BNBAS is an interactive examination that assesses the infant's response to 28 items organized in clusters

BOX 7.3 Clusters of Neonatal Behaviors in Brazelton Neonatal Behavioral Assessment Scale

Habituation: Ability to respond to and then inhibit response to discrete stimulus (light, rattle, bell, pinprick) while asleep
Orientation: Quality of alert states and ability to attend to visual and auditory stimuli while alert
Motor performance: Quality of movement and tone
Range of state: Measure of general arousal level or arousability of infant
Regulation of state: How infant responds when aroused
Autonomic stability: Signs of stress (tremors, startles, skin color) related to homeostatic (self-regulating) adjustment of the nervous system
Reflexes: Assessment of several neonatal reflexes

(Box 7.3). It is generally used as a research or diagnostic tool and requires special training.

The scale may be used to assess and support parent-child relationships, guiding parents to focus on their infant's individuality and develop a deeper attachment. Studies have demonstrated that exposure to the BNBAS results in increased maternal confidence and in improved parent-infant interaction and developmental outcome (Nugent, Bartlett, Von Ende, et al., 2017).

The Newborn Behavioral Observations (NBO) system, inspired by the BNBAS, is an interactive relationship-building instrument that highlights the baby's capacities and individuality (Nugent et al., 2017). It is much shorter than the BNBAS, consisting of 18 neurobehavioral observations, which are easily integrated into routine care (Sanders & Buckner, 2006). There has been renewed interest in the NBO recently, and it is now being used by nurses, doctors, home visitors, and others to optimize parent-infant relationships (Holland & Watkins, 2015). However, in a recent Cochrane review it was discovered that currently there is only very low-quality evidence for the effectiveness of the BNBAS and NBO in improving parent-infant interaction. Further, this evidence only applies to mostly low-risk, first-time caregivers and their infants. Additional research is underway to better explore the effectiveness of the NBO and is necessary to corroborate the findings of this review (Barlow, Herath, Bartram, et al., 2018).

Patterns of Sleep and Activity

Newborns begin life with a systematic schedule of sleep and wakefulness that is initially evident during the periods of reactivity. After this initial period, it is not unusual for the infant to sleep almost constantly for the next 2 to 3 days to recover from the exhausting birth process.

Infants have six distinct sleep–wake states, which represent a particular form of neural control (Table 7.3). As maturity increases, each state becomes more precisely defined according to the behaviors observed. **State** is defined as a "group of characteristics that regularly occur together" (Leigh, 2016) and includes body activity, eye and facial movements, respiratory pattern, and response to internal and external stimuli. The six sleep–wake states are quiet (deep) sleep, active (light) sleep, drowsy, quiet alert, active alert, and crying. Infants respond to internal and external environmental factors by controlling sensory input and regulating the sleep–wake states; the ability to make smooth transitions between states is called **state modulation**. The ability to regulate sleep–wake states is essential in infants' neurobehavioral development. The more immature the infant, the less he or she can cope with external and internal factors that affect the sleep–wake patterns.

TABLE 7.3 States of Sleep and Activity

State and Behavior	Implications for Parenting
Deep Sleep (Quiet) Closed eyes Regular breathing No movement except for occasional sudden bodily twitch No eye movement	Continue usual house noises because external stimuli do not arouse infant. Leave infant alone if sudden loud noise awakens infant and he or she cries. Do not attempt to feed.
Light Sleep (Active) Closed eyes Irregular breathing Slight muscular twitching of body Rapid eye movement (REM) under closed eyelids May smile	External stimuli that did not arouse infant during deep sleep may minimally arouse child. Periodic groaning or crying is usual; do not interpret as an indication of pain or discomfort.
Drowsy Eyes may be open Irregular breathing Active body movement variable with occasional mild startles	Most stimuli arouse infant but may return to sleep state. Pick up infant during this time rather than leaving in crib. Provide mild stimulus to awaken. Infant may enjoy nonnutritive sucking.
Quiet Alert Eyes wide open and bright Responds to environment by active body movement and staring at close-range objects Minimal body activity Regular breathing Focuses attention on stimuli	Satisfy infant's needs such as hunger or nonnutritive sucking. Place infant in area of home where activity is continuous. Place a toy in crib or play yard. Place objects within 17.5 to 20 cm (7 to 8 inches) of infant's view. Intervene to console.
Active Alert May begin with whimpering and slight body movement Eyes open Irregular breathing	Remove intense internal or external stimuli because infant has increased sensitivity to stimuli.
Crying Progresses to strong, angry crying and uncoordinated thrashing of extremities Eyes open or tightly closed Grimaces Irregular breathing	Comforting measures that were effective during alert state are usually ineffective. Rock and swaddle to decrease crying. Intervene to reduce fatigue, hunger, or discomfort.

Portions adapted from Blackburn, S., & Loper, D. L. (1992). *Maternal, fetal, and neonatal physiology: A clinical perspective.* Philadelphia, PA: Saunders.

Recognition and knowledge of sleep–wake states are important in the planning of nursing care. It is also important for nurses to help parents and caregivers understand the significance of the infant's behavioral responses to daily caregiving and how these states can be altered. A classic example is a newborn who feeds vigorously in the active alert state but poorly when he or she progresses to the crying state.

The neurologic assessment of a newborn in the active alert state will differ significantly from that performed during the deep sleep state.

Newborns typically spend as much as 16 to 18 hours sleeping and do not necessarily follow a pattern of light–dark diurnal rhythm. With increasing age, sleep–wake states change, with increasing amounts of time spent in awake alert states and decreasing amounts of sleep time. Approximately 50% of total sleep time is spent in irregular or rapid eye movement sleep.

Cry

Newborns should begin extrauterine life with a strong, lusty cry. The duration of crying is as variable in each infant as the duration of sleep patterns. Newborns may cry for as little as 5 minutes or as much as 2 hours or more per day. Feeding usually terminates the state of crying when hunger is the cause. Holding the infant skin-to-skin, swaddling, or wrapping an infant snugly in a blanket (while ensuring that the hands remain free to allow for self-calming and avoid overheating) calms infants, promotes sleep, and maintains body temperature. Rocking the infant may reduce crying and induce quiet alertness or sleep.

Variations in the initial cry can indicate abnormalities. A weak, groaning cry or grunting during expiration usually indicates respiratory disturbance. Absent, weak, or constant crying requires further investigation for possible drug withdrawal or a neurologic problem.

Assessment of Attachment Behaviors

One of the most important areas of assessment is careful observation of behaviors that are thought to indicate the formation of emotional bonds between the newborn and family, especially the mother. Such behaviors include the en face position; undressing and touching the infant; smiling, kissing, and talking to the infant; and holding, rocking, and cradling the child close to the body (see Nursing Care Guidelines box). Because assessment is closely related to interventions that promote attachment (e.g., encouraging these behaviors in parents), assessing attachment behaviors is discussed further later in the chapter.

NURSING CARE GUIDELINES

Assessing Attachment Behaviors

- When the infant is brought to the parents, do they reach out for the child and call the child by name?
- Do the parents speak about the child in terms of identification—who the infant looks like; what appears special about their child compared with other infants?
- When parents are holding the infant, what kind of body contact is there? Do they feel at ease in changing the infant's position? Are fingertips or whole hands used? Are there parts of the body they avoid touching or parts of the body they investigate and scrutinize?
- When the infant is awake, what kinds of stimulation do the parents provide? Do they talk to the infant, to each other, or to no one? How do they look at the infant—direct visual contact, avoidance of eye contact, or looking at other people or objects?
- How comfortable do the parents appear in terms of caring for the infant? Do they express any concern regarding their ability or disgust for certain activities, such as changing diapers?
- What type of affection do they demonstrate to the newborn, such as smiling, stroking, kissing, or rocking?
- If the infant is fussy, what kinds of comforting techniques do the parents use, such as rocking, swaddling, talking, or stroking?

Physical Assessment

An essential aspect of the care of the newborn is a thorough physical assessment that includes estimation of gestational age and physical examination to identify normal characteristics and existing abnormalities. These initial and ongoing assessments are critical to establishing baseline data for planning, implementing, and evaluating care and are a nursing priority in caring for the newborn. The discussion of physical examination focuses on normal findings and variations from the norm that require little or no intervention. Readers are encouraged to review Chapter 4 for further discussion of examination techniques. General guidelines for conducting a physical examination are presented in the Nursing Care Guidelines box. Table 7.4 summarizes physical examination of newborns.

NURSING CARE GUIDELINES

Physical Examination of the Newborn

1. Provide a normothermic and nonstimulating examination area.
2. Check that equipment and supplies are working properly and are accessible.
3. Undress only the body area examined to prevent heat loss.
4. Proceed in an orderly sequence (usually head to toe) with the following exceptions:
   - Observe the infant's attitude and position of flexion first to avoid disturbing him or her.
   - Perform all procedures that require quiet next, such as auscultating the lungs, heart, and abdomen.
   - Perform disturbing procedures, such as testing reflexes, last.
   - Measure head and length at the same time to compare results.
5. Proceed quickly to avoid stressing the infant.
6. Comfort the infant during and after the examination.
   - Talk softly.
   - Hold the infant's hands against his or her chest.
   - Swaddle and hold the infant.
   - Offer a nonlatex gloved finger to suck.
   - Use containment and positioning to maximize developmental state regulation.

The nursing care of newborns is discussed on the following pages.

MAINTAIN A PATENT AIRWAY

Establishing a patent airway is a primary objective in the delivery room. When the newborn is supine, a neutral neck position (i.e., avoiding neck flexion or hyperextension) is critical to achieving and maintaining a patent airway.

The American Academy of Pediatrics (2016b) recommends the supine position during sleep for healthy newborns. This recommendation is based on the association between sleeping prone and sudden infant death syndrome (see Chapter 10). Since the initial recommendation in 1992 that all infants be placed in the supine position to sleep, there has been no evidence of an increased number of complications, such as choking or vomiting, when infants are placed in this position. However, there has been an increase in the number of infants with cranial asymmetry, particularly unilateral flattening of the occiput, and the American Academy of Pediatrics (2016c) has endorsed guidelines for the management of positional plagiocephaly. Health care professionals must educate parents on prevention of positional plagiocephaly by encouraging alternate positions when infants are awake (see also Chapter 10, Positional Plagiocephaly).

TABLE 7.4 **Physical Assessment of the Newborn**

Usual Findings	Common Variations or Minor Abnormalities	Potential Signs of Distress or Major Abnormalities
General Appearance		
Posture: Flexion of head and extremities, which rest on chest and abdomen	**Frank breech:** Extended legs, abducted and fully rotated thighs, flattened occiput, extended neck	Limp posture, extension of extremities
Skin		
At birth, bright red, puffy, smooth Second to third day, pink, flaky, dry Vernix caseosa Lanugo Edema around eyes, face, legs, dorsa of hands, feet, and scrotum or labia **Acrocyanosis:** Cyanosis of hands and feet **Cutis marmorata:** Transient mottling when infant is exposed to decreased temperature	Neonatal jaundice after first 24 hours Ecchymoses or petechiae caused by birth trauma **Milia:** Distended sebaceous glands that appear as tiny white papules on cheeks, chin, and nose **Miliaria** or **sudamina:** Distended sweat (eccrine) glands that appear as minute vesicles, especially on face **Erythema toxicum:** Pink papular rash with vesicles superimposed on thorax, back, buttocks, and abdomen; may appear in 24 to 48 hours and resolve after several days **Harlequin color change:** Clearly outlined color change as infant lies on side; lower half of body becomes pink, and upper half is pale **Mongolian spots:** Irregular areas of deep blue pigmentation, usually in sacral and gluteal regions; seen predominantly in newborns of African, American Indian, Asian, or Hispanic descent **Telangiectatic nevi ("stork bites"):** Flat, deep pink localized areas usually seen on back of neck	Jaundice appearing in first 24 hours Generalized cyanosis Pallor Mottling Grayness Plethora Hemorrhage, ecchymoses, or petechiae that persist **Sclerema:** Hard and stiff skin Poor skin turgor Rashes, pustules, or blisters **Café-au-lait spots:** Light brown spots **Nevus flammeus:** Port-wine stain
Head		
Fontanels flat, soft, and firm Widest part of fontanel measured from bone to bone, not suture to suture	Molding after vaginal delivery Third sagittal (parietal) fontanel Bulging fontanel because of crying or coughing **Caput succedaneum:** Edema of soft scalp tissue **Cephalohematoma** (uncomplicated): Hematoma between periosteum and skull bone	Fused sutures Bulging or depressed fontanels when quiet Widened sutures and fontanels **Craniotabes:** Snapping sensation along lambdoid suture that resembles indentation of ping-pong ball
Eyes		
Eyelids usually edematous **Color:** Slate gray, dark blue, brown Absence of tears Presence of red retinal reflex Corneal reflex in response to touch Pupillary reflex in response to light Blink reflex in response to light or touch Rudimentary fixation on objects and ability to follow to midline	Epicanthal folds in Asian infants Searching nystagmus or strabismus **Subconjunctival (scleral) hemorrhages:** Ruptured capillaries, usually at limbus	Pink color of iris Purulent discharge Upward slant in non-Asians Hypertelorism (3 cm) Hypotelorism Congenital cataract(s) Constricted or dilated fixed pupil Absence of red retinal reflex White reflex (leukocoria) Absence of pupillary or corneal reflex Inability to follow object or bright light to midline Yellow sclera
Ears		
Position: Top of pinna on horizontal line with outer canthus of eye Startle reflex elicited by a loud, sudden noise Pinna flexible, cartilage present	Inability to visualize tympanic membrane because of filled aural canals Pinna flat against head Irregular shape or size Pits or skin tags Preauricular sinus	Low placement of ears Absence of startle reflex in response to loud noise should be evaluated but is not diagnostic Minor abnormalities may be signs of various syndromes, especially renal

TABLE 7.4 Physical Assessment of the Newborn—cont'd

Usual Findings	Common Variations or Minor Abnormalities	Potential Signs of Distress or Major Abnormalities
Nose		
Nasal patency **Nasal discharge:** Thin white mucus (transient) Sneezing	Flattened and bruised	Nonpatent canals Thick, bloody nasal discharge Flaring of nares (alae nasi) Copious nasal secretions or stuffiness (may be minor)
Mouth and Throat		
Intact, high-arched palate Uvula in midline Frenulum of tongue Frenulum of upper lip **Sucking reflex:** Strong and coordinated Rooting reflex Gag reflex Extrusion reflex Absent or minimal salivation Vigorous cry	**Natal teeth:** Teeth present at birth; benign but may be associated with congenital defects **Epstein pearls:** Small, white epithelial cysts along midline of hard palate	Cleft lip Cleft palate Large, protruding tongue or posterior displacement of tongue Receding chin (lower jaw): Micrognathia Profuse salivation or drooling **Candidiasis (thrush):** White, adherent patches on tongue, palate, and buccal surfaces Inability to pass nasogastric tube Hoarse, high-pitched, weak, absent, or other abnormal cry
Neck		
Short, thick, usually surrounded by skinfolds Tonic neck reflex	**Torticollis (wry neck):** Head held to one side with chin pointing to opposite side	Excessive skinfolds Resistance to flexion Absence of tonic neck reflex Fractured clavicle; crepitus
Chest		
Anteroposterior and lateral diameters equal Slight sternal retractions evident during inspiration Xiphoid process evident Breast enlargement	Funnel chest (pectus excavatum) Pigeon chest (pectus carinatum) Supernumerary nipples Secretion of milky substance from breasts	Depressed sternum Marked retractions of chest and intercostal spaces during respiration Asymmetric chest expansion Redness and firmness around nipples Wide-spaced nipples
Lungs		
Respirations chiefly abdominal Cough reflex absent at birth; may be present by 1 to 2 wk Bilateral equal bronchial breath sounds	Irregular rate and depth of respirations, periodic breathing Crackles shortly after birth	Inspiratory stridor Expiratory grunt Intercostal, substernal, or suprasternal retractions Persistent irregular breathing Periodic breathing with repeated apneic spells lasting >20 seconds Seesaw respirations (paradoxic) Unequal breath sounds Persistent fine, medium, or coarse crackles Wheezing Cough Diminished breath sounds Peristaltic bowel sounds on one side with diminished breath sounds on same side
Heart		
Apex: Fourth to fifth intercostal space, lateral to left sternal border S_2 slightly sharper and higher in pitch than S_1	**Sinus arrhythmia:** Heart rate increasing with inspiration and decreasing with expiration Transient cyanosis on crying or straining	**Dextrocardia:** Heart on right side Displacement of apex, muffled or distant Cardiomegaly Abdominal bruit Murmur Thrill Persistent central cyanosis Hyperactive precordium

TABLE 7.4 Physical Assessment of the Newborn—cont'd

Usual Findings	Common Variations or Minor Abnormalities	Potential Signs of Distress or Major Abnormalities
Abdomen		
Cylindric **Liver:** Palpable 2 to 3 cm below right costal margin **Spleen:** Tip palpable at end of first week of age **Kidneys:** Palpable 1 to 2 cm above umbilicus **Umbilical cord:** Bluish white at birth with two arteries and one vein **Femoral pulses:** Equal bilaterally	Umbilical hernia **Diastasis recti:** Midline gap between recti muscles **Wharton jelly:** Unusually thick umbilical cord	Abdominal distention Localized bulging Distended veins Absent bowel sounds Enlarged liver and spleen Ascites Visible peristaltic waves Scaphoid or concave abdomen Moist umbilical cord Presence of only one artery in umbilical cord Urine, stool, or pus leaking from umbilical cord or cord insertion site Periumbilical erythema Palpable bladder distention after scanty voiding Absent femoral pulses Cord bleeding or hematoma **Omphalocele** or **gastroschisis:** Protrusion of abdominal contents through abdominal wall or cord
Female Genitalia		
Labia and clitoris usually edematous Urethral meatus behind clitoris Vernix caseosa between labia Urination within 24 h	**Pseudomenstruation:** Blood-tinged or mucoid discharge Hymenal tag	Enlarged clitoris with urethral meatus at tip Fused labia Absence of vaginal opening Meconium from vaginal opening No urination within 24 h Mass in labia Ambiguous genitalia Bladder exstrophy
Male Genitalia		
Urethral opening at tip of glans penis Testes palpable in each scrotum Scrotum usually large, edematous, pendulous, and covered with rugae; usually deeply pigmented in dark-skinned ethnic groups Smegma Urination within 24 h	Urethral opening covered by prepuce Inability to retract foreskin **Epithelial pearls:** Small, firm, white lesions at tip of prepuce Erection or priapism Testes palpable in inguinal canal Scrotum small	**Hypospadias:** Urethral opening on ventral surface of penis **Epispadias:** Urethral opening on dorsal surface of penis **Chordee:** Ventral curvature of penis Testes not palpable in scrotum or inguinal canal No urination within 24 h Inguinal hernia Hypoplastic scrotum **Hydrocele:** Fluid in scrotum Masses in scrotum Meconium from scrotum Discoloration of testes Ambiguous genitalia Bladder exstrophy
Back and Rectum		
Spine intact; no openings, masses, or prominent curves Trunk incurvation reflex Anal reflex Patent anal opening Passage of meconium within 48 h	Green liquid stools in infant under phototherapy Delayed passage of meconium in very low birth weight neonates	Anal fissures or fistulas Imperforate anus Absence of anal reflex No meconium within 36-48 h Missing vertebrae Pilonidal cyst or sinus Tuft of hair along spine Spina bifida cystica

Continued

TABLE 7.4 Physical Assessment of the Newborn—cont'd

Usual Findings	Common Variations or Minor Abnormalities	Potential Signs of Distress or Major Abnormalities
Extremities		
Ten fingers and toes Full range of motion Nail beds pink with transient cyanosis immediately after birth Creases on anterior two-thirds of sole Sole usually flat Symmetry of extremities Equal muscle tone bilaterally, especially resistance to opposing flexion Equal bilateral brachial pulses	Partial syndactyly between second and third toes Second toe overlapping third toe Wide gap between first (hallux) and second toes Deep crease on plantar surface of foot between first and second toes Asymmetric length of toes Dorsiflexion and shortness of hallux	**Polydactyly:** Extra digits **Syndactyly:** Fused or webbed digits **Phocomelia:** Hands or feet attached close to trunk **Hemimelia:** Absence of distal part of extremity Hyperflexibility of joints Persistent cyanosis of nail beds Yellowing of nail beds Sole covered with creases Transverse palmar (simian) crease Fractures Decreased or absent range of motion Dislocated or subluxated hip Limitation in hip abduction Unequal gluteal or leg folds Unequal knee height Audible clunk on abduction of hip Asymmetry of extremities Unequal muscle tone or range of motion
Neuromuscular System		
Extremities usually in some degree of flexion Extension of an extremity followed by previous position of flexion Head lag while sitting but momentary ability to hold head erect Ability to turn head from side to side when prone Ability to hold head in horizontal line with back when held prone	Quivering or momentary tremors	**Hypotonia:** Floppy, poor head control, extremities limp **Hypertonia:** Jittery, arms and hands tightly flexed, legs stiffly extended, startles easily Asymmetric posturing (except tonic neck reflex) Opisthotonic posturing: Arched back Signs of paralysis Tremors, twitches, and myoclonic jerks Marked head lag in all positions

A bulb syringe is kept near the infant and is used if suctioning is required. If more forceful removal of secretions is required, mechanical suction is used. The use of a properly sized catheter and correct suctioning technique is essential to prevent mucosal damage and edema. Gentle suctioning is necessary to prevent reflex bradycardia, laryngospasm, and cardiac arrhythmias from vagal stimulation. Oropharyngeal suctioning is performed for up to 5 seconds, leaving sufficient time between each attempt to allow the infant to reoxygenate.

! NURSING ALERT

To avoid aspiration of amniotic fluid or mucus, clear the pharynx first and then the nasal passages using a bulb syringe; remember, **m**outh before **n**ose. Vital signs are closely monitored, and any indication of respiratory distress is reported immediately.

! NURSING ALERT

The cardinal signs of respiratory distress in a newborn include tachypnea, nasal flaring, grunting, intercostal retractions, and cyanosis.

MAINTAIN A STABLE BODY TEMPERATURE

Conserving the newborn's body heat is an essential nursing goal. At birth, a major cause of heat loss is **evaporation**, the loss of heat through moisture. The amniotic fluid that bathes the infant's skin favors evaporation, especially when combined with the cool atmosphere of the delivery room. Heat loss through evaporation is minimized by rapidly drying the skin and hair with a warmed towel and placing the infant in skin-to-skin contact with the mother, covered by a blanket.

Another major cause of heat loss is **radiation**, the loss of heat to cooler solid objects in the environment that are not in direct contact with the infant. Loss of heat through radiation increases as these solid objects become colder and closer to the infant. The temperature of ambient or surrounding air has no effect on loss of heat through radiation. This is a critical point to remember when attempting to maintain a constant temperature for the infant because even though the temperature of the ambient air is optimal, the infant can become hypothermic.

An example of radiant heat loss is the placement of the crib close to a cold window or air-conditioning unit. The cold from either source will cool the crib walls and, subsequently, the body of the neonate. To prevent this, place cribs as far away as possible from exterior walls, windows, and ventilating units. Heat loss can also occur through conduction and convection. **Conduction** involves loss of heat from the body because of direct contact of skin with a cooler solid object. Placing the infant on a padded, covered surface and providing insulation through clothes and blankets rather than directly on a cool hard table can minimize heat loss. Placing the newborn skin-to-skin with the mother on her chest or abdomen immediately after delivery is physically beneficial in terms of conserving heat as well as fostering maternal attachment and breastfeeding.

Convection is like conduction except that heat loss is aided by surrounding air currents. For example, placing the infant in the direct flow of air from a fan or air conditioning vent will cause rapid heat loss through convection. Transporting the neonate in a crib with solid sides reduces airflow around the infant.

PROTECT FROM INFECTION AND INJURY

The most important practice for preventing cross-infection is thorough hand washing of all individuals involved in the infant's care. Other procedures to prevent infection include eye care, umbilical care, bathing, and care of the circumcision. Artificial nails are prohibited (World Health Organization, 2009), and long fingernails are discouraged for health care providers because the former have been implicated in the transmission of sepsis. Vitamin K is administered to protect against hemorrhage.

Identification

Proper identification of the newborn is essential. The nurse must verify that identifying bands are securely fastened and verify the information on them (name, gender, mother's admission number, date, and time of birth) against the birth records. Optimally, this identification process should take place in the delivery room. Some institutions use methods of infant identification such as a color photograph kept in the medical record, storage of cord blood for DNA genotyping, and electronic surveillance systems for infant security. The National Center for Missing and Exploited Children recommends the use of footprints as a form of identification in addition to a cord blood sample, which is stored until the day after discharge. Electronic tags that give off a radio frequency may also be used to prevent newborn abductions (Rabun, 2014). A tag is placed on the newborn and removed at the time of discharge by hospital personnel.

A proactive hospital emergency plan should be implemented to prevent infant abduction and to respond promptly and effectively if one happens. A mock newborn abduction drill is an effective method that can be used to evaluate staff competence and response to the incident (Rabun, 2014). All hospital personnel should be educated regarding newborn abduction, preventive aspects, and methods to identify the potential risk of such an occurrence.

The nurse should discuss safety issues with the mother the first time the infant is brought to her. According to the National Center for Missing and Exploited Children,[a] 58% of infant abductions occur in the mother's hospital room (Rabun, 2014). A written copy of the safety instructions should also be given to parents. Parents are instructed to look at the identification badges of nurses and hospital personnel who come to take infants and not to relinquish their infants to anyone without proper identification. Mothers are also advised not to leave infants alone in the crib while they shower or use the bathroom; rather, they should ask to have infants observed by a health care worker if a family member is not present in the room. Parents and staff are encouraged to use a password system when the newborn is taken from the room as a routine security measure. The nurse should document in the chart that these instructions were given and that appropriate identification band checks are routinely made throughout each shift. Nursing staff are also educated about the "typical" abductor profile and to be constantly aware of visitors with unusual behavior. The typical profile of an abductor is a female between the ages of 12 and 55 years (generally in early 20s) who is often overweight and has low self-esteem; she may be emotionally disturbed because of the loss of her own child or an inability to conceive and may have a strained relationship with her husband or partner. The typical abductor may also be seen visiting the newborn nursery or neonatal intensive care unit area before the abduction and may ask questions about the care or health of a specific newborn. The abductor may familiarize herself with the hospital routine and may also impersonate a health care worker. Parents are made aware of the fact that infant safety measures must be implemented in the home as well. Measures to prevent and decrease infant abduction after discharge to the home include avoiding the publication of birth announcements in the local newspaper and avoiding using yard decorations to announce a newborn's arrival (Rabun, 2014).

Eye Care

Prophylactic eye treatment against **ophthalmia neonatorum**, infectious conjunctivitis of the newborn, includes the use of (1) silver nitrate (1%) solution, (2) erythromycin (0.5%) ophthalmic ointment or drops, or (3) tetracycline (1%) ophthalmic ointment or drops (preferably in single-dose ampules or tubes). All three are effective against gonococcal conjunctivitis. *Chlamydia trachomatis* is the major cause of ophthalmia neonatorum in the United States; topical antibiotics (tetracycline and erythromycin) and silver nitrate are not effective in the prevention and treatment of chlamydial conjunctivitis. A 14-day course of oral erythromycin or a 3-day course of azithromycin may be given for chlamydial conjunctivitis (American Academy of Pediatrics, 2018). The administration of oral erythromycin to infants younger than 6 weeks old has been associated with the development of infantile hypertrophic pyloric stenosis; therefore parents should be informed of the potential risks and signs of the illness (American Academy of Pediatrics, 2018).

Although eye prophylaxis is mandatory in the United States, health care facilities are free to choose the specific drugs used. Effective prophylaxis may be better directed toward treating maternal chlamydia infections in areas where the organism is prevalent. Studies on maternal attachment have shown that in the first hour of life a newborn has a greater ability to focus on coordinated movement than at any other time during the next several days. Since eye contact is very important in the development of maternal-infant bonding, the routine administration of silver nitrate or topical ophthalmic antibiotics can be postponed for up to an hour following birth. However, practitioners must ensure that the drug is given by 1 hour of age.

Vitamin K Administration

Shortly after birth, vitamin K is administered to prevent hemorrhagic disease of the newborn. Normally, vitamin K is synthesized by the intestinal flora. However, because infants' intestines are relatively sterile at birth and because breast milk contains low levels of vitamin K, the supply is inadequate for at least the first 3 or 4 days. The major

[a]National Center for Missing and Exploited Children has a variety of resources for parents and health professionals aimed at preventing child abduction. Contact 800-THE-LOST (800-843-5678); http://www.missingkids.com.

function of vitamin K is to catalyze the synthesis of prothrombin in the liver, which is needed for blood clotting. The vastus lateralis muscle is the traditionally recommended injection site, but the ventrogluteal (not the dorsogluteal) muscle can be used.

Several countries have noted resurgence in later onset of vitamin K deficiency bleeding (VKDB) after practicing orally administered prophylaxis (American Academy of Pediatrics, 2014). Current recommendations are that vitamin K be given to all newborns as a single intramuscular dose of 0.5 to 1.0 mg (American Academy of Pediatrics, 2014; Ng & Loewy, 2018). Additional study is needed on the efficacy, safety, and bioavailability of oral preparations and on the most effective dosing regimens to prevent VKDB.

Hepatitis B Vaccine Administration

To decrease the incidence of hepatitis B virus (HBV) in children and its serious consequences (cirrhosis and liver cancer) in adulthood, the first of three doses of hepatitis B vaccine is recommended soon after birth and before hospital discharge for all newborns born to hepatitis B surface antigen (HBsAg)–negative mothers. The injection is given in the vastus lateralis muscle because this site is associated with a better immune response than the dorsogluteal area (American Academy of Pediatrics, 2018). Giving the infant concentrated oral sucrose can reduce the pain of the injection (Stevens, Yamada, Ohlsson, et al., 2016).

Preterm infants born to HBsAg-negative women should be vaccinated as early as 30 days of age, regardless of gestational age or birth weight. Infants born to HBsAg-positive women should be immunized within 12 hours after birth with hepatitis B vaccine and hepatitis B immune globulin (HBIG) at separate sites, regardless of gestational age or birth weight (American Academy of Pediatrics, 2018).

Newborn Screening for Disease

Several genetic disorders can be detected in the newborn period. There is no national policy for newborn screening in the United States; therefore the extent of neonatal screening is determined by state laws and voluntary guidelines. All states require screening for phenylketonuria (PKU) and congenital hypothyroidism; many states also have programs that include screening for sickle cell disease and galactosemia. Because there is concern about inconsistency among states in screening for genetic disorders based on cost, population demographics, resource availability, and political environment, the Task Force on Newborn Screening was formed by the American Academy of Pediatrics and other federal health care agencies to address this issue. Several resolutions and policies have been developed to better address the issue of newborn screening (American Academy of Pediatrics, 2016d).

The nurse's responsibility is to educate parents about the importance of screening and to collect appropriate specimens at the recommended time (after 24 hours of age). With early newborn discharge before 24 hours of age, some authorities recommend a repeat screening for PKU within 2 weeks. Accurate screening depends on high-quality blood spots on approved filter paper forms. The blood should completely saturate the filter paper spot on one side only. The paper should not be handled, placed on wet surfaces, or contaminated with any substance (see Atraumatic Care box).

The American Academy of Pediatrics (2018) recommends routine prenatal and perinatal human immunodeficiency virus (HIV) counseling and testing for all pregnant women. Benefits of early identification of HIV-infected infants include the following:

- Early antiretroviral therapy and aggressive nutritional supplementation
- Appropriate changes in their immunization schedule
- Monitoring and evaluation of immunologic, neurologic, and neuropsychologic functions for possible changes caused by antiretroviral therapy
- Initiation of special educational services
- Evaluation of the need for other therapies, such as immunoglobulin for the prevention of bacterial infections
- Tuberculosis screening and treatment
- Management of communicable disease exposures

ATRAUMATIC CARE

Heel Punctures

Heel lancing is necessary to obtain blood for newborn tests, including newborn metabolic screening. Heel lancing is recognized as a painful procedure, and numerous nonpharmacologic strategies have demonstrated pain relief potential.

The American Academy of Pediatrics (2016e) has written a comprehensive policy statement on prevention and management of pain in the neonate. It outlines the importance of preventing and minimizing pain with interventions such as nonnutritive sucking, skin-to-skin holding, swaddling or facilitated tucking, and breastfeeding or oral sucrose. These strategies can significantly manage pain behaviors associated with painful procedures in neonates. Oral sucrose and nonnutritive sucking have proved effective in decreasing the pain associated with heel punctures and other painful procedures in preterm and full-term infants; however, the exact dosage range that provides optimal effectiveness varies among studies. Evidence indicates that as little as 0.05 to 0.5 ml of a 24% oral sucrose solution is effective in decreasing pain in full-term and preterm infants (Stevens et al., 2016). The best analgesic effect is achieved when sucrose is administered 2 minutes before the painful procedure with a pacifier or syringe and is repeatedly administered in small amounts (i.e., 0.05 to 0.5 ml) at 2-minute intervals throughout the painful procedure. The effect appears to begin at 2 minutes and lasts about 4 minutes, thus analgesic effect may wane if procedures are prolonged (Stevens et al., 2016).

Several commercially available oral sucrose solutions now exist. When these are not available, the pharmacy may mix an oral sucrose solution to ensure a clean product. Strict attention to aseptic technique must be paid with this method to prevent contamination of the solution and subsequent problems. Breastfeeding is correlated with pain relief in full-term newborns undergoing painful procedures, as demonstrated by a reduction in infants' crying time and pain scores (Cleveland et al., 2017), but breast milk given by syringe has not shown the same efficacy as breastfeeding itself (Shah, Herbozo, Aliwalas, et al., 2012). Comparison of sucrose with breastfeeding has produced mixed results, thus it is difficult to determine optimal pain prevention treatment when comparing breastfeeding with sucrose, and more research is needed (Shah et al., 2012).

In a review of eight randomized controlled studies, the use of topical anesthetics, such as the eutectic mixture of local anesthetics (EMLA) cream before venipuncture, in term and preterm infants was explored. The authors concluded that analgesic effects were of uncertain clinical significance and concerns regarding the risk of methemoglobinemia needed to be further evaluated in future studies (Foster, Taylor, & Spence, 2017).

Mother-infant skin-to-skin holding, also known as kangaroo mother care, has been shown to significantly reduce an infant's distress during painful procedures (Cleveland et al., 2017). This has been measured with physiologic indices such as heart rate and behaviors such as crying. Published studies are diverse with respect to outcomes measured, and it is impossible to have observers be blinded to pain prevention treatments. The authors of a comprehensive review of 25 studies concluded that more research is needed to better understand optimal strategies for and the effects of skin-to-skin holding for pain prevention and relief (Johnston, Campbell-Yeo, Disher, et al., 2017).

There are many effective interventions for decreasing the pain associated with heel puncture in newborns. Nurses should use all available resources to advocate for the prevention and management of neonatal pain during painful procedures (see also Atraumatic Care box later in the chapter).

The American Academy of Pediatrics (2018) provides comprehensive direction for care of mothers affected with HIV and their newborns. Cesarean section performed before the rupture of membranes or the onset of labor may prevent mother-to-child transmission of HIV in optimally treated women and is associated with a reduction in the risk of mother-to-child transmission among HIV-infected women who are either not receiving antiretroviral therapy or receiving minimal therapy. For infants whose mother's HIV status is unknown, rapid HIV antibody testing provides information within 12 hours of the infant's birth. Antiretroviral prophylaxis is started as soon as possible, pending completion of confirmatory HIV testing. Breastfeeding is delayed until confirmatory testing is done. If the test is negative, prophylaxis is discontinued, and breastfeeding may start. If the test is positive, infants should be treated with antiretroviral prophylaxis for 6 weeks, and the mother should not breastfeed (American Academy of Pediatrics, 2018).

Universal Newborn Hearing Screening

Assessment of risk factors alone may fail to identify as many as 50% of newborns with hearing loss. Auditory deprivation in early infancy results in structural and functional reorganization at a cortical level, leading to lifelong deficits (Canadian Paediatric Society, 2016). Without early diagnosis and intervention, hearing loss leads to irreversible deficits in communication and psychosocial skills, cognition, and literacy (Canadian Paediatric Society, 2016). For these reasons the American Academy of Pediatrics (2016d) and the Canadian Paediatric Society (2016) recommend universal hearing screening of all newborns before discharge from the birthing hospital.

Infants may be screened for hearing loss by auditory brainstem response or evoked otoacoustic emissions. For infants born by cesarean delivery, it is preferable to delay otoacoustic emission (OAE) testing until after 48 hours of age, since earlier testing is associated with significantly higher rates of failure, possibly because of retained fluid in the middle ear (Smolkin, Mick, Dabbah, et al., 2012). Newborns who fail the initial screening require referral for outpatient retesting and intervention by 1 month of age; newborns who do not receive initial screening before discharge should also be tested within the first month of life (American Academy of Pediatrics, 2016d).

Bathing

Bath time is an opportunity for the nurse to accomplish much more than general hygiene. It is an excellent time for observing the infant's behavior, state of arousal, alertness, and muscular activity. Because of the possibility of transmission of organisms such as HBV and HIV via maternal blood and blood-stained amniotic fluid, as part of Standard Precautions nurses should wear gloves when handling the newborn until blood and amniotic fluid are removed by bathing.

Early bathing (within the first hour of life) interferes with skin-to-skin holding and breastfeeding, thus compromising basic protection against neonatal infection. Recent recommendations from the World Health Organization advise delaying a newborn's first bath for 24 hours (World Health Organization, 2018a). If there are cultural reason for earlier bathing, the World Health Organization recommends delaying the first bath for a minimum of 6 hours following birth. Further, in a recent quality improvement project, nurses discovered that delaying the first bath for at least 12 hours resulted in greater rates of in-hospital exclusive breastfeeding (Condo DiCioccio, Ady, Bena, et al., 2018).

The bath time provides an opportunity for the nurse to involve the parents in the care of their child, to teach correct hygiene procedures, and to help parents learn about their infant's individual characteristics

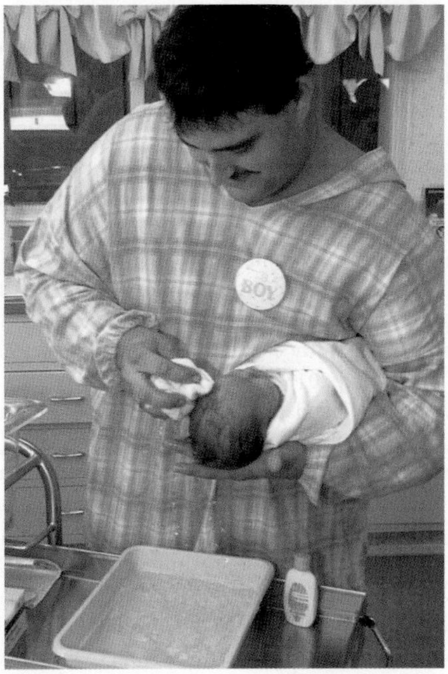

Fig. 7.10 Bath time is an excellent opportunity for parents to learn about their newborn.

(Fig. 7.10). The bath may also be used to help parents learn and better understand their newborn's behavioral characteristics. The nurse stresses appropriate bathing supplies and the need for safety in terms of water temperature and supervision of the infant at all times during the bath.

The infant's skin surface has a pH of about 5 soon after birth, and the bacteriostatic effects of this pH are significant. In addition, newborn skin is covered with vernix caseosa, a chemical and mechanical skin barrier for newborns. Vernix protects newborns from infection and assists in the development of the skin's acid mantle. Vernix should not be removed with bathing; allow it to absorb or wear off with normal care and handling (Lund, 2016). Consequently, plain warm water is appropriate for routine bathing. If a cleanser is needed, it should be mild and have a neutral pH. Alkaline soaps, oils, powder, and lotions are not used because they alter the acid mantle, thus providing a medium for bacterial growth. Talcum or cornstarch powders have the added risk of aspiration if they are applied close to the infant's face (see Chapter 10, Diaper Dermatitis).

Parents should be involved in a discussion of the newborn's bath at home. It is recommended that for the first 2 to 4 weeks the infant be bathed no more than two or three times per week with a plain warm sponge bath. This practice will help maintain the integrity of the newborn's skin and allow time for the umbilical cord to dry completely. Routine daily bathing for newborns is no longer recommended.

Cleansing should proceed in the cephalocaudal (head-to-toe) direction. Remind parents not to vigorously rub infant's skin to remove vernix. A diaper is applied after the bath, and the infant is clothed appropriately to prevent heat loss.

Care of the Umbilicus

Since the umbilical stump is an excellent medium for bacterial growth, various methods of cord care have been practiced for prevention of infection. Some methods popular in the past include the use of an antimicrobial agent such as bacitracin or triple dye or agents such as alcohol or povidone. A Cochrane review of 21 studies (most of which were conducted in developed countries) found no significant difference between cords treated with antiseptics compared with dry cord care or placebo; there were no reported systemic infections or deaths, and a trend toward reduced colonization was found in cords treated with antibiotics (Zupan, Garner, & Omari, 2004). Further, in a clinical review published by the American Academy of Pediatrics in 2016, the authors reported that no benefit occurred from applying antimicrobials to the umbilicus of an infant born in the hospital of a high-resource country (Stewart & Benitz, 2016). Thus current recommendations for cord care for infants in the developed world include cleaning the cord initially with sterile water or a neutral pH cleanser, then subsequently cleaning the cord with water (American Academy of Pediatrics, 2016f).

Nurses working in neonatal care must carefully evaluate the available studies and compare the risks and benefits regarding the method of cord care within their own population of newborns and families. Particularly in the developing world, infants may encounter increased risk of potentially life-threatening sepsis, thus antimicrobial treatment may be appropriate in such settings (American Academy of Pediatrics, 2016f).

Regardless of the method used, nurses must teach parents about the importance of observation and monitoring of the cord, in addition to cord care methods, in discharge planning. The diaper is positioned below the cord to avoid irritation and wetness of the site. Parents are educated about stump deterioration and proper umbilical care. The stump deteriorates through the process of dry gangrene, with an average separation time of 5 to 15 days. Cord separation time is influenced by several factors, including type of cord care, type of delivery, and other perinatal events. It takes a few more weeks for the cord base to heal completely after cord separation. During this time, care consists of keeping the base clean and dry and observing for any signs of infection.

Circumcision

Circumcision, the surgical removal of the foreskin on the glans penis, is not a common practice in most countries. In the United States, however, between 40% and 70% of newborn males are circumcised, depending on the region (Owings, Uddin, & Williams, 2013). The Centers for Disease Control and Prevention reports that the overall rate of newborn circumcision in the United States has fallen from 64.5% in 1979 to 58.3% in 2010 (Owings et al., 2013). Despite the frequency of the procedure in the United States, there is some controversy regarding the benefits and risks (Box 7.4).

Researchers have explored the possible link between circumcision and reduced transmission of communicable illnesses such as human papillomavirus (HPV) and HIV in later life. Current evidence suggests that circumcision reduces the incidence of urinary tract infections, penile and vaginal cancer, and the acquisition of sexually transmitted infections; however, benefits are most significant for high-risk populations in the developing world (Canadian Paediatric Society, 2015; Morris, Krieger, & Klausnerc, 2017). The American Academy of Pediatrics (2012a) states that current evidence indicates that the health benefits of newborn male circumcision outweigh the risks and that the procedure should be made available to families who choose it. Despite encouraging outcome data, the health benefits are not yet great enough to recommend *routine* circumcision for all male newborns (Canadian Paediatric Society, 2015; Jagannath, Fedorowicz, Sud, et al., 2012; Morris et al., 2017).

The American Academy of Pediatrics (2012a) statement emphasizes parental autonomy to determine what is in the best interest of their newborn. The policy encourages the primary care practitioner to ensure that parents have been given accurate and unbiased information about the risks, benefits, and alternatives before making an informed choice and that they understand that circumcision is an elective procedure. In addition to examining the medical benefits of newborn circumcision, the American Academy of Pediatrics recommends that if parents decide to have their male infant circumcised, procedural analgesia should be provided.

Nurses are in a unique position to educate parents on the care of their newborns, and they must ensure that parents have accurate and unbiased information with which to make an informed decision. Parents should discuss the options for pain control, and the possibility of observing the procedure, with the primary practitioner.[b]

The nurse should use nonpharmacologic interventions as an adjunct to reduce the pain of this operative procedure (see Atraumatic Care box). Despite adequate scientific evidence that newborns feel and respond to pain, circumcisions may still be performed with either insufficient analgesia or no analgesia at all. Nurses should use the American Academy of Pediatrics' policy statement to advocate for the use of optimum pain relief during circumcision.

BOX 7.4 Risks and Benefits of Neonatal Circumcision

Risks

Complications:
- Hemorrhage
- Infection
- Meatitis (from loss of protective foreskin)
- Adhesions
- Concealed penis
- Urethral fistula
- Meatal stenosis
- Necrosis or amputation

Pain in unanesthetized infants: Long-term consequences unknown, but short-term stresses include increased heart rate, behavior changes, prolonged crying, increased cortisol levels, and decreased blood oxygenation

Benefits[a]

Prevention of penile cancer and posthitis (inflammation of prepuce)

Decreased incidence of balanitis (inflammation of glans), urinary tract infections in male infants, and some sexually transmitted infections later in life (herpes, syphilis, gonorrhea)

Decreased incidence of human immunodeficiency virus (HIV) infection, human papillomavirus (HPV), and cervical cancer (in female partner)

Prevention of complications associated with later circumcision

Preservation of male's body image that is consistent with peers (only in countries or cultures where procedure is common)

[a]Although there is risk reduction for these conditions with circumcision, the absolute risk of conditions (such as penile cancer and infant urinary tract infections) is so low that neither the American Academy of Pediatrics nor the American Medical Association recommends circumcision for prevention. There is growing evidence regarding circumcision and decreased transmission of sexually transmitted infections (Morris, Krieger, & Klausnerc, 2017). The Centers for Disease Control and Prevention's male circumcision recommendations represent a key public health measure for long-term HIV prevention and are likely to include the provision of neonatal circumcision.

[b]*Should the baby be circumcised?* is available from the American Academy of Pediatrics, 141 Northwest Point Blvd., Elk Grove Village, IL 60009-1098; 847-434-4000; fax: 847-434-8000; http://www.aap.org.

ATRAUMATIC CARE

Guidelines for Pain Management During Neonatal Circumcision[a]

Pharmacologic Interventions

Use of Dorsal Penile Nerve Block or Ring Block With Topical Analgesia

Topical creams such as EMLA are used to numb the operative site and lidocaine, which is administered by injection to perform a nerve block.

Nonpharmacologic Interventions

Comfort measures such as music, sucking on a pacifier, and soothing voices are helpful; however, these strategies have *not* proved to be sufficient in reducing the pain of circumcision when used alone. In addition to the practitioner-ordered pharmacologic interventions:

- If using a circumcision board, pad as needed with blankets or other thick, soft material. A more comfortable, padded, and physiologic restraint that places the infant in a semireclining position may also decrease distress.
- Provide the parents with the option to be present during the circumcision, after ascertaining that this is an option by discussing it with the primary practitioner.
- Swaddle the infant's upper body and legs to provide warmth and containment and to reduce movement.
- If the newborn is not swaddled and is unclothed, use a radiant warmer to prevent hypothermia. Shield the newborn's eyes from overhead lights.
- Prewarm any topical solutions to be used in sterile preparation of the surgical site by placing them in a warm blanket or towel.
- Play infant relaxation music before, during, and after the procedure; allow the parents or other caregiver the option of choosing the music.
- After the procedure, remove restraints and swaddle. Immediately have the parents, other caregiver, or nursing staff hold the infant. Continue to have the infant suck on a pacifier or offer feeding.

[a]There is sufficient evidence and support for the use of pharmacologic and nonpharmacologic interventions to holistically manage neonatal pain. Combined analgesia, including pharmaceuticals and nonpharmacologic interventions (such as swaddling, sucking, and sucrose), are recommended during the procedure to provide holistic pain management (American Academy of Pediatrics, 2016d).

Circumcision is usually performed in the nursery. It should not be performed immediately after delivery because of the neonate's unstable physiologic status and increased susceptibility to stress. Preoperative nursing care includes allowing the infant nothing by mouth before the procedure to prevent aspiration of vomitus (about 1 to 2 hours); however, the necessity of this practice has been challenged. Additional measures include the surgical time-out, checking for a signed consent form, and adequately restraining the infant, usually on a special board (Fig. 7.11) or physiologic circumcision restraint chair. The circumcision chair is padded and allows free movement of the newborn's extremities without compromising the surgical field. In addition, the chair allows the infant to sit at a 30- to 45-degree angle, and it is adjustable to accommodate smaller newborns. All the equipment used for the procedure, such as gloves, instruments, dressings, and draping towels, must be sterile.

The procedure involves freeing the foreskin from the glans penis by using a scalpel, Gomco or Mogen clamp (see Cultural Considerations box), or Plastibell. In the Gomco technique the foreskin is clamped, cut with a scalpel, and removed; the clamp crushes the nerve endings and blood vessels, promoting hemostasis. In the Plastibell procedure

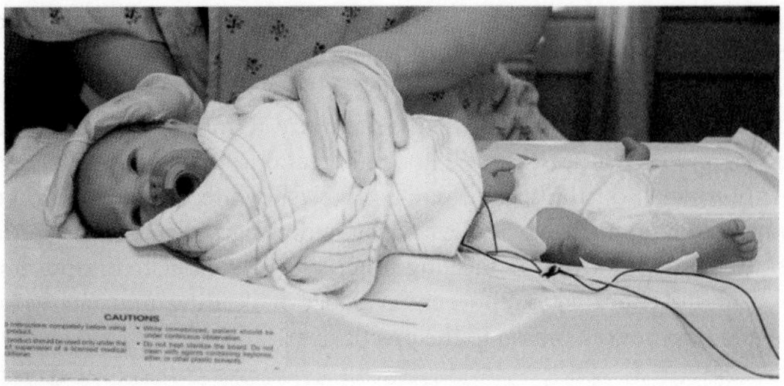

Fig. 7.11 Proper positioning of infant in Circumstraint. (Photo by Paul Vincent Kuntz, Texas Children's Hospital, Houston, TX.)

the foreskin is removed using a plastic ring and a string tied around the foreskin like a tourniquet. The excess foreskin is trimmed. In about 5 to 8 days the plastic ring separates and falls off.

CULTURAL CONSIDERATIONS

Circumcision

In the Jewish culture circumcision is performed during a ceremony called a berith, or bris, which takes place on the eighth day of life. A specially trained professional known as a mohel stretches the prepuce over the glans, pulling it through a slit in a shield (usually a Mogen clamp) and cutting it with a knife. The traditional technique is not sterile, and bleeding is controlled by tight bandaging around the penis. The infant may be given some sweet wine before the procedure. Blankets instead of straps are usually used to restrain the infant to a board, and the parents are present. Although the risk of injury from neonatal circumcision is low, risk is increased when circumcision is done outside of the hospital by nonprofessional practitioners. Suggested techniques for avoiding injury, and for repair of injury, are available (Banihani, Fox, Gander, et al., 2014; Pippi Salle, Jesus, Lorenzo, et al., 2013).

Female circumcision (mutilation) is practiced in some parts of Africa, the Middle East, Southeast Asia, and South America—and in some immigrants from these areas. In the most extensive operations, the vaginal orifice is narrowed with creation of a covering seal by cutting and appositioning the labia minora and/or the labia majora, with or without excision of the clitoris (Bazi, 2017). Sharp objects such as glass, razors, scissors, or sharpened rocks are typically used, often without anesthesia of any type. Hemorrhage, trauma, and sepsis are potential complications. Female genital mutilation may be done on infants or may be delayed until puberty. In some cultures, female circumcision is used to prove virginity and to reduce sexual pleasure, thus promoting fidelity.

The World Health Organization (2018b) condemns all forms of female genital mutilation. It is associated with an increased risk for adverse obstetric outcomes and numerous physical problems, which often may not receive adequate medical care.

Once the procedure is completed, the infant is released from the restraints and comforted. If the parents were not present during the procedure, they are informed of the infant's status and reunited with their son.

Care of the circumcision depends on the type of procedure. If a clamp was used, a petrolatum gauze dressing may be applied loosely to prevent adherence to the diaper. If the Plastibell was applied, no special dressing is required; however, a petrolatum jelly gauze dressing may be used to prevent adherence of the glans to the diaper. Because the area is tender, the diaper is applied loosely to prevent friction against the penis. The circumcision is evaluated for excessive bleeding in the first few hours after the procedure, and the first void is recorded. A recommended standard is to evaluate the site every 30 minutes for at least 2 hours and then at least every 2 hours thereafter.

Normally, on the second day a yellowish white exudate forms as part of the granulation process. This is not a sign of infection and is not forcibly removed. As healing progresses, the exudate disappears. Parents are educated to report any evidence of bleeding, unusual swelling, or absence of voiding to the practitioner.

> **NURSING TIP** To check for the first void in disposable diapers made of absorbent gelling material, pinch the crotch of the diaper for a "clumpy, doughy" feeling because these diapers will feel dry despite voiding.

PROVIDE OPTIMAL NUTRITION

Selection of a feeding method is one of the major decisions that parents face. In general, there are two choices: (1) human milk and (2) commercially prepared whole cow's milk infant formula. These two methods have significant nutritional, economic, and psychologic advantages and differences. Nurses should be at the forefront in providing parents with accurate and unbiased information needed to make a conscientious informed decision regarding the feeding method.

Cultural Influences on Infant Feeding

Cultural beliefs and practices may significantly influence infant feeding methods. Many cultures typically do not give colostrum to newborns and only begin breastfeeding after the milk has "come in" (i.e., milk is produced in larger volumes than those seen with initial colostrum production). These groups include mothers in Asia, Latin America, and sub-Saharan Africa and often mothers who have emigrated from these areas (Agho, Ogeleka, Ogbo, et al, 2016). When breastfeeding is delayed until the mother's milk is available in larger volumes (generally a few days after delivery), babies are given prelacteal liquids such as tea, juice, water, or water sweetened with sugar or honey before the initiation of breastfeeding (Agho et al., 2016). Some rationales for this practice include a concern that because colostrum volume is small, the baby may be at risk for dehydration, or that nonmilk feeds are needed to "cleanse" the gastrointestinal tract for digestion. Although perhaps intuitively logical, neither of these rationales is based on evidence. The use of prelacteal feedings significantly increases the risk of infection, particularly in developing countries where sanitation may be poor. In addition, failure to empty the breasts regularly in the early hours and days after delivery contributes to suboptimal milk supply.

A recent study of Chinese immigrant women in Australia reported that Chinese women were more likely to combine breastfeeding with formula and to introduce solids earlier than the general Australian population (Kuswara, Laws, Kremer, et al., 2016). Chinese mothers shared that although they supported exclusive breastfeeding, grandparents frequently pressured them to use formula, believing that "a fat baby is a healthy baby." Wandel and colleagues (2016) reported similar findings after studying a small group of Somali women who immigrated to Norway. Although family support for breastfeeding is generally reported as strong, early formula supplementation is common, as is the belief in the need to introduce water feedings early. Somali culture apparently favors "chubby" babies, and formula is seen as the best way ensure this weight gain.

Waldrop (2016) describes the practice of *los dos* (which means *the two* or *both*) among Hispanic women living in the United States, which involves supplementing breastfeeding with infant formula. Women in this study stated that reasons for choosing *los dos* were based on previous experience with infant feeding, not wanting the baby to cry from hunger, a desire to improve the infant's health, and wanting to prevent the baby from suffering when the mother had to return to work. Many mothers believed that breast milk alone was inadequate for infants' nutrition and that they did not have an adequate supply of breast milk to keep their infants satisfied. Breastfeeding was also perceived as being somewhat laborious and at times painful and embarrassing in comparison to bottle-feeding. Family and cultural beliefs were also cited as reasons for not exclusively breastfeeding and practicing *los dos.*

In a recent small study of Mexican American women from a midwestern US city, the authors reported that 43% of women exclusively breastfed and only a minority of these mothers used formula in the early days of breastfeeding (Wambach, Domain, Page-Goertz, et al., 2016). This finding illustrates the danger of making assumptions about any cultural group, as education and exposure to different practices may influence change in breastfeeding practice. Traditional cultural ideas and practices may evolve over time, thus cultural background does not always predict behavior and individual assessment is necessary.

Sociocultural values may preclude the mother receiving adequate information regarding breastfeeding. If the family is strongly patriarchal and the father is the only English-speaking person in the family, the necessary information being conveyed to the family by the health care provider may not be translated correctly, thus the need to continually assess mothers' beliefs and practices. Variation in dialect may also contribute to confusion. For example, among Hispanic Spanish-speaking people, terminology used in one country for the act of breastfeeding or describing the breasts may be offensive in another country. Cultural attitudes regarding modesty and breastfeeding are sometimes important considerations (see Cultural Considerations box).

> **CULTURAL CONSIDERATIONS**
>
> ***Acculturation***
>
> Acculturation is a process whereby members of one cultural group adopt the beliefs and behaviors of another group. There may be language or literacy issues that interfere with acquisition of up-to-date breastfeeding information. There may be limited family support for immigrant women, and cultural norms may be at odds with information presented by care providers in their new country.
>
> Jones and colleagues (2015) reported that although some potential barriers to breastfeeding are common to all women, such as pain, embarrassment, employment, or inconvenience, immigrant women often have additional concerns. Strategies to increase the likelihood of breastfeeding success include prenatal breastfeeding education, enhanced breastfeeding support programs in hospitals, and linking mothers with nonprofessional peer supporters (Jones et al., 2015).

With the increasing numbers of immigrants in the United States, it is incumbent on nurses to discuss cultural values related to breastfeeding and the benefits of breastfeeding so that mothers can make an informed decision. Nurses must clarify with mothers what their expectations are regarding infant feeding and assist them in meeting those goals.

Human Milk

Human milk is the best option for infant nutrition up to 1 year old. It contains micronutrients that are **bioavailable**, meaning that these nutrients are available in quantities and qualities that make them easily digestible by the newborn's intestine and absorbed for energy and growth. Human milk offers a variety of immunologic properties not found in commercially prepared infant formula. Further, human milk has been shown to be effective in protecting newborns against respiratory tract infections, gastrointestinal infections, otitis media, numerous allergies, type 2 diabetes, and atopy.

Lysozyme is found in large quantities in human milk with bacteriostatic functions against gram-positive bacteria and Enterobacteriaceae organisms. Human milk also contains numerous other host defense factors such as macrophages, granulocytes, and T and B lymphocytes. Casein in human milk greatly enhances the absorption of iron, thus preventing iron-dependent bacteria from proliferating in the gastrointestinal tract. Secretory immunoglobulin A (IgA) is found in high levels in colostrum, but levels gradually decrease over the first 14 days of life. Secretory IgA is an immunoglobulin that prevents viruses and bacteria from invading the intestinal mucosa in breastfed newborns, thus protecting them from infection. This whey protein is also believed to play an important role in preventing the development of allergies.

The fat content of human milk is composed of lipids, triglycerides, and cholesterol; cholesterol is an essential element for brain growth. The function of these lipids is to allow optimum intestinal absorption of fatty acids and provide essential fatty acids and polyunsaturated fatty acids. Furthermore, lipids contribute approximately 50% of the total calories in human milk. Although the overall fat content in human milk is higher than that of cow's milk–based formula, it is used more efficiently by the infant.

The primary source of carbohydrate in human milk is lactose, which is present in higher concentrations (6.8 g/dl) than in cow's milk–based formula (4.9 g/dl). Other carbohydrates found in human milk include glucose, galactose, and glucosamine. The carbohydrates serve not only as a large percentage of the total calories in human milk but also have a protective function; the oligosaccharides (**prebiotic**) in human milk stimulate the growth of *Lactobacillus bifidus* (a **probiotic**) and prevent bacteria from adhering to epithelial surfaces.

Human milk contains the two proteins whey (lactalbumin) and casein (curd) in a whey-dominant ratio of 70 to 80:20 to 30 in early lactation, decreasing to 50:50 in late lactation. Cow's milk is casein dominant, with a ratio of approximately 20:80 whey to casein. Cow's milk–based formulas vary in their whey-to-casein ratios, as some have added whey to alter their formulation to more closely resemble human milk (Martin, Ling, & Blackburn, 2016). This ratio of whey dominance in human milk makes it more digestible and produces the soft stools seen in breastfed infants. Thus human milk has a laxative effect, and constipation is uncommon. The whey protein lactoferrin in human milk has iron-binding characteristics with bacteriostatic capabilities, particularly against gram-positive and gram-negative aerobes, anaerobes, and yeasts.

Several digestive enzymes, such as amylases, lipases, proteases, and ribonucleases, are present in human milk and enhance digestion and absorption of various nutrients. The amounts of lipid- and water-soluble vitamins, as well as electrolytes, minerals, and trace elements, in human milk are sufficient for infant growth, development, and energy needs during the first 6 months of life. The one possible exception is vitamin D, which is found in varying amounts depending on the mother's intake of vitamin D–fortified food and exposure to ultraviolet light. Therefore, to prevent vitamin D–deficiency rickets, the Centers for Disease Control and Prevention (2018) recommends that unless the lactating mother is taking supplements of approximately 6000 IU/day, breastfed and partially breastfed infants should be supplemented with 400 IU of vitamin D (oral) per day, beginning in the first few days of life. Supplementation should continue until the infant is consuming at least 1 L/day of vitamin D–fortified infant formula or cow's milk (Centers for Disease Control and Prevention, 2018). The Canadian Paediatric Society (2017b) suggests that for infants and children living in Canada's northernmost climates, it may be reasonable to supplement with 800 IU/day, to compensate for extremely limited exposure to sunlight.

Breastfeeding is associated with a decrease in the incidence of type 2 diabetes and obesity, fewer hospital admissions for respiratory tract illnesses in generally healthy infants, and higher intelligence scores compared with formula-fed infants (Horta, Loret de Mola, & Victora, 2015; Wang, Collins, Ratliff, et al., 2017). Breastfeeding has an analgesic effect on newborns during painful procedures such as heel puncture (Shah et al., 2012), and it has also been found to decrease pain scores in full-term and older infants receiving routine childhood immunizations (Modarres, Jazayeri, Rahnama, et al., 2013). Additional beneficial components of human milk include stem cells, prostaglandins, epidermal growth factor, docosahexaenoic acid (DHA), arachidonic acid (AA), taurine, carnitine, cytokine, interleukins, and natural hormones such as thyroid-releasing hormone, gonadotropin-releasing hormone, and prolactin.

Human milk changes over the course of the lactation cycle. **Colostrum**, for example, is rich in immunoglobulins and vitamin K and has a higher protein content than mature milk; however, it has a lower fat content. Transitional milk replaces colostrum when the mother's milk supply starts increasing, and eventually mature milk becomes the primary milk source. There is also diurnal variation in the biochemistry of mature human milk. Human milk also varies with respect to gestational age; preterm human milk differs from mature milk in its biochemical composition. Nonphysiologic advantages of human milk are discussed in the next section.

Breastfeeding

Human milk is the preferred form of nutrition for all infants. Healthy People 2020 has a goal to increase breastfeeding rates in the United States to 81.9% in early postpartum and to 61% for mothers who continue to breastfeed for at least 6 months (United States Breastfeeding Committee, 2019). Rates of breastfeeding vary among different demographic groups, with lower breastfeeding rates at 6 months reported in African American women and higher rates reported in women of Asian descent. Interestingly, enrollment in the Women, Infants, and Children (WIC) program is consistently found to have a negative impact on breastfeeding rates in the United States (Houghtaling, Byker Shanks, & Jenkins, 2017). Several strategies have been identified to mitigate the negative influences, including environmental, social, and individual WIC participant strategies (Houghtaling et al., 2017).

Studies exploring mothers' reasons for early cessation of breastfeeding suggest that several factors may contribute to this decision, such as the perception of insufficient milk, difficulties with lactation such as nipple trauma, and concerns with maternal or newborn health (Newby & Davies, 2016; Odom, Li, Scanlon, et al., 2013). Modifiable factors associated with decreased risk of early cessation of breastfeeding include professional and social support (Newby & Davies, 2016; Odom et al., 2013). These findings have important implications for nurses in education and discussion regarding breastfeeding before, during, and after the pregnancy. Teaching families about the importance of breastfeeding and supporting mothers who are learning this skill will contribute to mothers' success.

The American Academy of Pediatrics (2012b) has reaffirmed its position recommending exclusive breastfeeding until 6 months of age, with continued breastfeeding to at least 1 year of age and beyond if mutually desirable by mother and infant. The American Academy of Pediatrics also supports programs that enable women to continue breastfeeding after returning to work. In its support of breastfeeding practices, the American Academy of Pediatrics further discourages the advertisement of infant formula to breastfeeding mothers and distribution of formula discharge packs without the advice of a health care provider.

BOX 7.5 Ten Steps to Successful Breastfeeding

Every facility providing maternity services and care for newborn infants should:

1. Have a written breastfeeding policy that is routinely communicated to all health care staff.
2. Train all health care staff in skills necessary to implement this policy.
3. Inform all pregnant women about the benefits and management of breastfeeding.
4. Help mothers initiate breastfeeding within ½ hour of birth.
5. Show mothers how to breastfeed and how to maintain lactation even if they should be separated from their infants.
6. Give newborn infants no food or drink other than breast milk unless medically indicated.
7. Practice rooming-in—allowing mothers and infants to remain together—24 hours a day.
8. Encourage breastfeeding on demand.
9. Give no artificial teats or pacifiers (also called *dummies* or *soothers*) to breastfeeding infants.
10. Foster the establishment of breastfeeding support groups and refer mothers to them on discharge from the hospital or clinic.

Data from World Health Organization, United Nations Children's Fund, and Wellstart International. (2012). *The baby-friendly hospital initiative.* Retrieved from https://www.babyfriendlyusa.org/about/

The Baby-Friendly Initiative (BFI) is a joint effort of the World Health Organization and UNICEF to encourage, promote, and support breastfeeding as the model for optimum infant nutrition. BFI developed 10 research-supported practices as guidelines for caregivers worldwide to promote breastfeeding (World Health Organization, United Nations Children's Fund, & Wellstart International, 2009) (Box 7.5). Research indicates that BFI designation is sometimes associated with higher rates of breastfeeding initiation; however, the designation does not appear to affect breastfeeding rates among women with higher educational levels in US populations (Hawkins, Stern, Baum, et al., 2014, 2015). Howe-Heyman and Lutenbacher (2016), after reviewing 25 studies published over 23 years, concluded that although there are more studies that support the BFI as an intervention to increase breastfeeding rates than there are studies that demonstrate no effect, many of the studies are methodologically weak. These authors suggest that peer support, formal prenatal breastfeeding education, and needs-based informal postpartum support may be more effective than the BFI for increasing breastfeeding rates (Howe-Heyman & Lutenbacher, 2016).

In addition to the physiologic qualities of human milk, the most outstanding psychologic benefit of breastfeeding is the close maternal-child relationship. The infant is nestled close to the mother's skin, can hear the rhythm of her heartbeat, can feel the warmth of her body, and has a sense of peaceful security. The mother has a close feeling of union with her child and feels a sense of accomplishment and satisfaction as the infant suckles milk from her.

Human milk is the most economical form of feeding. It is always available, ready to serve at room temperature, and free of contamination. Although human milk is not sterile, healthy full-term infants can tolerate and in fact benefit from varying amounts of nonpathogenic and pathogenic organisms. The protection against infection can provide additional cost savings in terms of fewer medical visits and less time lost from work for the employed mother. Breastfed infants, especially beyond 2 to 3 months of age, tend to grow at a satisfactory but slower rate than bottle-fed infants.

Contraindications to breastfeeding include the following (American Academy of Pediatrics, 2012b):

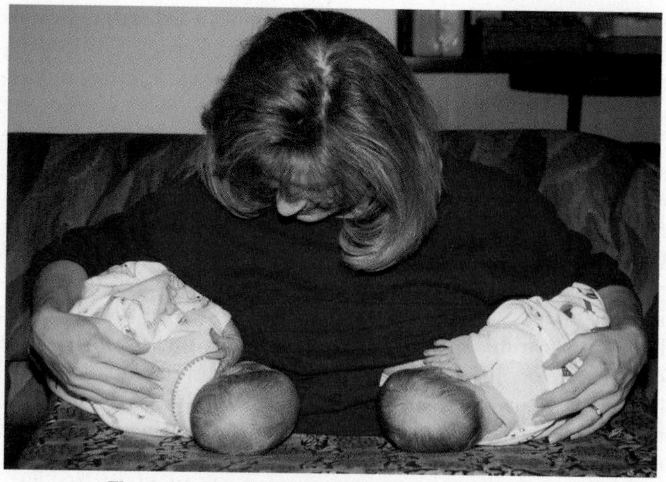

Fig. 7.12 Simultaneous breastfeeding of twins.

- Maternal chemotherapy—antimetabolites and certain antineoplastic drugs
- Active tuberculosis not under treatment in mother
- HIV in mothers *in the developed world;* in the developing world, risks to nonbreastfeeding infants from malnutrition and infectious disease are significant, so the benefits of breastfeeding may outweigh the risk of acquiring HIV from human milk (American Academy of Pediatrics, 2018)
- Galactosemia in infant
- Maternal herpes simplex lesion on a breast
- Cytomegalovirus (CMV): may be a risk to extremely low birth weight preterm infants (<1500 g); not a risk for full-term infants whose mother is seropositive for CMV
- Maternal use of illicit street drugs (e.g., phencyclidine [PCP], cocaine, methamphetamine, heroin); note that women in treatment and receiving medication-assisted treatment (using medications such as methadone or buprenorphine) should be encouraged to breastfeed if they screen negative for HIV and illicit drugs (Cleveland, 2016)
- Human T-cell leukemia virus type I or II
- Mothers receiving diagnostic or radioactive isotopes or who have had exposure to radioactive materials (for as long as there is radioactivity in the milk)

A small number of medications are contraindicated for breastfeeding mothers. Consult a reference such as LactMed, an online source published by the National Library of Medicine/National Institutes of Health (US National Library of Medicine, 2019). Mastitis is usually not a contraindication if the discomfort is tolerable; however, each case should be treated on an individual basis.

Some herbal products are marketed as safe and effective alternatives to prescription medications, and claims about efficacy for which there is no evidence may be made. Certain agents, called galactogogues, are reported to increase breast milk production. Data are insufficient to confirm or deny the assertion of increased milk production using herbal galactogogues, and nurses should caution mothers to seek advice from a practitioner to ensure that the herbal preparations do not have the potential for harm (Bazzano, Hofer, Thibeau, et al., 2016).

Breastfeeding with twins and other multiples requires specialized professional support. If the infants are full term, they can begin feedings immediately after birth (Fig. 7.12); late preterm infants should be evaluated individually but may be put to breast if stable. Simultaneous feeding promotes the rapid production of milk needed for both infants and makes the milk that would normally be lost in the let-down reflex available to one of the twins. When only one infant is hungry, the mother should feed singly. She should also alternate breasts when feeding each infant and avoid favoring one breast for one infant. The sucking patterns of infants vary, and each infant needs the visual stimulation and exercise that alternating breasts provides.

> **! NURSING ALERT**
>
> Do not use microwaves to defrost or warm human milk. High-temperature microwaving (72° to 98°C [162° to 208°F]) significantly destroys the anti-infective factors and vitamin C and may cause hot spots that could burn the baby's mouth (Eglash & Simon, 2017). Human milk may be thawed or warmed in warm tap water (be sure that the milk is not contaminated by the water bath) or by placing it in a commercial bottle warmer. Test the temperature of the milk before feeding.

Bottle-Feeding

Bottle-feeding generally refers to the use of bottles for feeding commercial or evaporated milk formula rather than using the breast, although in some instances human milk may be expressed and fed with a bottle. Bottle-feeding is an acceptable method of feeding. Nurses should not assume that new parents know how to bottle-feed their infant. Parents who choose bottle-feeding also need support and assistance in meeting their infant's needs.

Providing newborns with nutrition is only one aspect of the feeding. Holding them close to the body while rocking or cuddling them helps ensure the emotional component of feeding. Like breastfed infants, bottle-fed infants need to be held on alternate sides of the lap to expose them to different stimuli. The feeding should not be hurried. Even though they may suck vigorously for the first 5 minutes and seem to be satisfied, they should be allowed to continue sucking. Infants need at least 2 hours of sucking a day. If there are six feedings per day, about 20 minutes of sucking at each feeding provides for oral gratification.

Propping the bottle is discouraged for the following reasons:

- It denies the infant the important component of close human contact.
- The infant may aspirate formula into the trachea and lungs.
- It may facilitate the development of middle ear infections. As the infant lies flat and sucks, milk that has pooled in the pharynx becomes a suitable medium for bacterial growth. Bacteria may then enter the eustachian tube, which leads to the middle ear, causing acute otitis media.
- It encourages continuous pooling of formula in the mouth, which can lead to caries when the teeth erupt (see Chapter 12).

> **! NURSING ALERT**
>
> Warming bottles in the microwave oven is not recommended because of the risk of burns from excessively hot temperatures of the milk or from bottles exploding. When milk is warmed in the microwave, it is not warmed evenly and may be too hot in places, causing mouth burns (US Food & Drug Administration, 2018). Milk may be warmed in warm tap water (be sure the milk is not contaminated by the water bath) or in a commercial bottle warmer. Test the temperature of the milk before feeding.

Commercially Prepared Infant Formulas

The analysis of human and whole cow's milk indicates that the latter is unsuitable for infant nutrition. Whole cow's milk has a high protein content and low fat and lipid content, and it may cause intestinal bleeding and lead to iron-deficiency anemia in infants. Questions have also been raised regarding the unmodified protein content of whole cow's milk, which may trigger an undesired immune response and thus increase the incidence of allergies in children at an early age.

Commercially prepared infant formulas are cow's milk based and have been modified to resemble the nutritional content of human milk. These formulas are altered from cow's milk by removing butterfat, decreasing the protein content, and adding vegetable oil and carbohydrate. Some cow's milk–based formulas have demineralized whey added to yield a whey-to-casein ratio of 60:40. The standard cow's milk–based formulas, regardless of the commercial brand, have essentially the same compositions of vitamins, minerals, protein, carbohydrates, and essential amino acids with minor variations, such as the source of carbohydrate; nucleotides to enhance immune function; and long-chain polyunsaturated fatty acids (LCPUFAs), DHA, and AA. DHA and AA are both found in large quantities in human milk but until recently were not present in most infant formulas. Studies suggest that both preterm and full-term infants receiving formula supplemented with DHA and AA have improved brain function and visual acuity when compared with those receiving formula without DHA and AA (Hadley, Ryan, Forsyth, et al., 2016). Sources for LCPUFAs include egg yolk lipid, phospholipids, and triglycerides. The results of recent Cochrane reviews showed no benefit from supplementing full-term or preterm infants with LCPUFAs and that the overall quality of evidence for LCPUFA supplementation was low (Jasani, Simmer, Patole, et al., 2017; Moon, Rao, Schulzke, et al., 2016).

The US Food and Drug Administration regulates the manufacture of infant formula in the United States to ensure product safety. Standard cow's milk–based formulas are sold as low iron and iron fortified; however, the American Academy of Pediatrics (2015b) states that only the iron-fortified formulas meet the requirements of infants.

There are four main categories of commercially prepared infant formulas: (1) **cow's milk–based formulas**, available in 20 kcal/fl oz as liquid (ready to feed), powder (requires reconstitution with water), or concentrated liquid (requires dilution with water); (2) **soy-based formulas**, commercially available in ready-to-feed 20 kcal/fl oz powder and concentrated liquid forms and commonly used for children who are lactose or cow's milk protein intolerant; (3) **casein-** or **whey-hydrolysate formulas**, commercially available in ready-to-feed and powder forms and used primarily for children who cannot tolerate or digest cow's milk– or soy-based formulas; and (4) **amino acid formulas**.

The American Academy of Pediatrics (2015b) states that there are few circumstances in which soy-based formula should be chosen instead of cow's milk–based formula for full-term infants; however, it does recommend the use of soy protein–based formulas for infants with galactosemia and hereditary lactose intolerance and when a vegetarian diet is preferred.

For infants with documented allergies caused by cow's milk, extensively hydrolyzed protein formula should be considered because up to 14% of these infants will also have a soy protein allergy. The casein- or whey-hydrolysate formulas are less antigenic than either cow's milk– or soy-based formulas. The protein hydrolysate formulas (casein and whey) are derived from cow's milk–based formula by a process of heat, filtration, and enzyme treatment designed to break the peptide chains into more digestible proteins. There are also amino acid formulas, designed for infants who are extremely sensitive to cow's milk–based, soy-based, and partially or extensively hydrolyzed casein- and whey-based formulas. Various formulas are manufactured for infants and children with special needs. A formula company representative can provide product books that describe the purpose and content of each formula.

Follow-up formulas are marketed as a transitional formula for infants older than 6 months who are also eating solid foods.

These generally contain a higher percentage of calories from protein and carbohydrate sources, a higher amount of iron and vitamins, and a lower amount of fat than standard cow's milk–based formulas. However, many nutrition experts and the American Academy of Pediatrics Committee on Nutrition (Kleinman & Greer, 2014) discount the necessity of follow-up formulas if the infant is receiving an adequate amount of solid food containing sufficient iron, vitamins, and minerals.

Preparation of Formula

Persons preparing infant formula must wash their hands well and then wash all equipment used to prepare the formula (including the cans of formula) with soap and water. Sterilizing bottles and nipples may be done in a dishwasher or a commercial home sterilizer (electric or microwave steam sterilizer or chemical sterilizer), following the manufacturer's instructions. Equipment may also be sterilized by boiling. Fill a large pan with water and completely submerge all washed equipment, ensuring that there are no trapped air bubbles. Cover the pan with a lid and bring it to a rolling boil, making sure that the pan does not boil dry. Keep the pan covered until the equipment is needed.

Powdered infant formula is not sterile, and it has been associated with severe illness attributable to *Cronobacter* species (Xinjie, Shukula, Lee, et al., 2016) and *Salmonella enterica* (Morlay, Piat, Mercey, et al., 2016). Careful preparation and handling reduce the risk of illness. Recommendations include reconstitution of powdered infant formula with water brought to a rolling boil and mixed when it is at or above 70°C, since this is thought to be hot enough to inactivate *Cronobacter* and other pathogens (World Health Organization, 2007). More recent research shows that temperatures higher that 70°C may be necessary (Losio, Pavoni, Finazzi, et al., 2018). Bottled water is not considered sterile and must also be boiled before use.

Following the manufacturer's instructions for preparing the formula is essential to ensure that the infant receives adequate calories and fluid for adequate growth. Parents are cautioned not to alter the reconstitution or dilution of infant formula except under the specific directions of the primary practitioner. Powdered formula and concentrated formula are prepared and bottled and refrigerated if not used for feeding immediately. Warming the formula is optional, although many parents prefer to warm it before feeding. Any milk remaining in the bottle after the feeding is discarded because it is an excellent medium for bacterial growth. Opened cans of ready-to-feed or concentrated formula are covered and refrigerated immediately until the next feeding. Because of incidents involving contamination of powdered formula with *Cronobacter* species and subsequent infant death in a neonatal unit, it is now recommended that hospital formula preparation for newborns follow separate guidelines.

Laws governing the labeling of infant formulas require that the directions for preparation and use of the formula include pictures and symbols for nonreading individuals. In addition, manufacturers are translating directions into foreign languages, such as Spanish and Vietnamese, to prevent misunderstanding and errors in formula preparation.

! NURSING ALERT

Stress to families that the proportions must not be altered when preparing formula—neither diluted with extra water to extend the amount of formula nor concentrated to provide more calories.

Alternate Milk Products

In the United States, few infants are fed evaporated milk formula, and its use is not recommended by the American Academy of Pediatrics Committee on Nutrition (Kleinman & Greer, 2014). However, it has advantages over whole milk. It is readily available in cans; needs no refrigeration if unopened; is less expensive than commercial formula; provides a softer, more digestible curd; and contains more lactalbumin and a higher calcium-to-phosphorus ratio. Disadvantages of evaporated milk for infant nutrition include low iron and vitamin C concentrations, excessive sodium and phosphorus, decreased vitamin A and D (except in fortified forms), and poorly digested fat. A common rule for preparing evaporated milk formula is diluting the 13-oz can of milk with 19.5 oz of water and adding 3 Tbsp of sugar or commercially processed corn syrup.

Evaporated milk must not be confused with condensed milk, which is a form of evaporated milk with 45% more sugar. Because of its high carbohydrate concentration and disproportionately low fat and protein content, condensed milk is not used for infant feeding. Likewise, skim and low-fat milk must not be used for infant milk, because they are deficient in caloric concentration, significantly increase the renal solute load and water demands, and deprive the body of essential fatty acids.

Goat's milk is a poor source of iron and folic acid. It has an excessively high renal solute load because of its high protein content, making it unsuitable for infant nutrition (Kleinman & Greer, 2014). Some believe that goat's milk is less allergenic than other available milk sources and may feed it to their infants to reduce allergic milk reactions. However, infants allergic to cow's milk are just as likely to be allergic to goat's milk; other complications (such as hypernatremia and metabolic acidosis) may ensue because of the high sodium and protein concentration found in goat's milk compared with human milk (Basnet, Schneider, Gazit, et al., 2010). Raw, unpasteurized milk from any animal source is unacceptable for infant nutrition.

Feeding Schedules

Ideally, feeding schedules should be determined by the infant's hunger. **Demand feedings** involve feeding infants when they signal readiness. **Scheduled feedings** are arranged at predetermined intervals. Although this may be satisfactory for bottle-fed infants, it hinders the breastfeeding process. Breastfed infants tend to be hungry every 2 to 3 hours because of the easy digestibility of the milk; therefore they should be fed on demand.

Supplemental feedings should *not* be offered to breastfed infants before lactation is well established, because they may satiate the infant and may cause nipple preference. Supplemental water is not needed in breastfed infants even in hot climates. Satiated infants suck less vigorously at the breast, and milk production depends on the breast being emptied at each feeding. If milk accumulates in the ducts (causing breast engorgement), ischemia results, suppressing the activity of the acini, or milk-secreting cells. Consequently, milk production is reduced. In addition, the process of sucking from a bottle is different from breast nipple compression. The relatively inflexible rubber nipple prevents the tongue from its usual rhythmic action. Infants learn to put the tongue against the nipple holes to slow down the more rapid flow of fluid. When infants use these same tongue movements during breastfeeding, they may push the human nipple out of the mouth and may not grasp the areola properly.

Usually by 3 weeks of age, lactation is well established. Bottle-fed infants consume about 2 to 3 oz of formula at each feeding and are fed approximately six times a day. The quantity of formula consumed is based on the caloric need of 108 kcal/kg/day; therefore a newborn who weighs 3 kg requires 324 kcal/day. Because commercial formula has 20 kcal/oz, approximately 16 oz (480 ml) provides the daily caloric requirement. Breastfed infants may feed as frequently as 10 to 12 times a day.

Feeding Behavior

Five behavioral stages occur during successful feeding. Recognizing these steps can assist nurses in identifying potential feeding problems caused by improper feeding techniques. **Prefeeding behavior**, such as crying or fussing, demonstrates the infant's level of arousal and degree of hunger. To encourage the infant to grasp the breast properly, it is preferable to begin feeding during the quiet alert state before the infant becomes upset. **Approach behavior** is indicated by sucking movements or the rooting reflex. **Attachment behavior** includes activities that occur from the time the infant receives the nipple and sucks (sometimes more pronounced during initial attempts at breastfeeding). **Consummatory behavior** consists of coordinated sucking and swallowing. Persistent gagging might indicate unsuccessful consummatory behavior. **Satiety behavior** is observed when the infant lets the parent know that he or she satisfied, usually by falling asleep.

PROMOTE PARENT-INFANT BONDING (ATTACHMENT)

The process of parenting is based on a relationship between the parent and infant. Neonates are complex individuals, capable of influencing and shaping their environments, particularly their interaction with significant others. Promoting positive parent-child relationships necessitates an understanding of behavioral steps in attachment, variables that enhance or hinder this process, and methods of teaching parents to develop a stronger relationship with their children, especially by recognizing potential problems (see also the Assessment of Attachment Behaviors section earlier in the chapter).

Infant Behavior

Nurses must appreciate the individuality and uniqueness of each infant. According to their individual temperaments, infants change and shape the environment, which influences their future development (see the Patterns of Sleep and Activity section earlier in the chapter). An infant who sleeps 20 hours a day will be exposed to fewer stimuli than one who sleeps 16 hours a day. In turn, each infant will likely elicit a different response from parents. An infant who is quiet, undemanding, and passive may receive much less attention than one who is responsive, alert, and active. Behavioral characteristics such as irritability and consolability can influence the ease of transition to parenthood and the parents' perception of the infant.

Nurses can positively influence the attachment of the parent and child. The first step is recognizing individual differences and explaining to the parents that such characteristics are normal. For example, some people believe that infants sleep throughout the day except for feedings. For some newborns, this may be true, but for many, it is not. Understanding that the infant's wakefulness is part of a biologic rhythm and not a reflection of inadequate parenting can be crucial in promoting healthy parent-child relationships. Another aspect of helping parents with their concerns includes supplying guidelines on how to enhance the infant's development during awake periods. Placing the child in a crib to stare at the same mobile every day is not exciting, but carrying the infant into each room as one does daily chores can be fascinating.

Infants enjoy human contact and often respond to visual and auditory stimuli in different ways depending on their sleep–wake state and the type of stimuli provided. Infants prefer black and white objects, geometric patterns and shapes, and reflective surfaces such as mirrors and eyeglasses. However, evidence indicates that infants prefer contact with human faces and enjoy interactions with others more than they enjoy objects or television images.

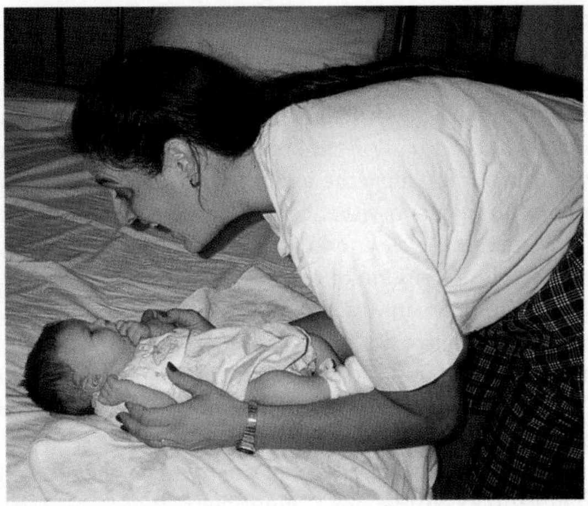

Fig. 7.13 En face position between the parent and infant can be significant in the attachment process.

Maternal Attachment

Mothers may demonstrate a predictable and orderly pattern of behavior during the development of the attachment process. When mothers are presented with their nude infants, they begin to examine the infant with their fingertips, concentrating on touching the extremities, and then proceed to massage and encompass the trunk with their entire hands. Assuming the **en face position**, in which the mother's and infant's eyes meet in visual contact in the same vertical plane, is significant in the formation of affectional ties (Fig. 7.13).

Some authors have reported that mothers experiencing depression, as well as adolescent mothers, may have lower rates of secure attachment with their infants (Flaherty & Sadler, 2011; Riva Crugnola, Ierardi, Ferro, et al., 2016a; 2016b), necessitating that caregivers monitor such mothers closely and model attachment behaviors. Nurses must observe for maternal attachment behaviors and exercise caution in interpreting such behaviors.

The long-term benefits of providing parents with opportunities to bond with their infant during the initial postpartum period are unclear; however, skin-to-skin contact with the mother immediately after delivery enhances the likelihood of success in breastfeeding. The nurse should stress to parents that, although early bonding may be valuable, it does not represent an "all or none" phenomenon. Throughout the child's life there will be multiple opportunities for the development of parent-child attachment. Bonding is a complex process that develops gradually and is influenced by numerous factors, only one of which is the type of initial contact between the newborn and parent.

One component of successful maternal attachment is **reciprocity** (Brazelton, 1974). As the mother responds to the infant, the infant must respond to the mother by some signal, such as sucking, cooing, eye contact, grasping, or molding (conforming to another's body during close physical contact). The first step in this complex process is *initiation,* in which interaction between infant and parent begins. Next is *orientation,* which establishes the partners' expectations of each other during the interaction. Following orientation is *acceleration* of the attention cycle to a peak of excitement. The infant reaches out and coos, both arms jerk forward, the head moves backward, the eyes dilate, and the face brightens. After a short time, *deceleration* of the excitement and *turning away* occur, in which the infant's eyes shift away from the mother's and the child may grasp his or her own shirt.

During this cycle of nonattention, repeated verbal or visual attempts to reinitiate the infant's attention are ineffective. This deceleration and turning away probably prevent the infant from being overwhelmed by excessive stimuli. In a good-quality interaction, both participants have synchronized their attention-nonattention cycles. Parents or other caregivers who do not allow the infant to turn away and who continually attempt to maintain visual contact may encourage the infant to turn off the attention cycle and thus prolong the nonattention phase.

Although this description of reciprocal interacting behavior is usually observed in the infant by 2 to 3 weeks of age, nurses can use this information to teach parents how to interact with their newborn infant. Recognizing the attention versus nonattention cycles and understanding that the latter is not a rejection of the parent helps parents develop competence in parenting.

Paternal Engrossment

Fathers also show specific attachment behaviors to their newborns. This process of **paternal engrossment**, forming a sense of absorption, preoccupation, and interest in the infant, includes (1) visual awareness of the newborn, especially focusing on the child's beauty; (2) tactile awareness, often expressed in a desire to hold the infant; (3) awareness of distinct characteristics with emphasis on those features of the infant that resemble the father; (4) perception of the infant as perfect; (5) development of a strong feeling of attraction to the child that leads to intense focusing of attention on the infant; (6) extreme elation; and (7) a sense of deep self-esteem and satisfaction. These responses are greatest during the early contacts with the infant and are intensified by the neonate's normal reflex activity, especially the grasp reflex and visual alertness. In addition to behavioral reactions, fathers also demonstrate physiologic responses such as increased heart rate and blood pressure during interactions with their newborns.

The process of engrossment has significant implications for nurses. It is imperative to recognize the importance of early father-infant contact in this process. Fathers need to be encouraged to express their positive feelings, especially if such emotions are contrary to any belief that fathers should remain stoic. If this is not clarified, fathers may feel confused and attempt to suppress the natural sensations of absorption, preoccupation, and interest to conform to societal expectations.

Mothers also need to be aware of the responses of the father toward the newborn because one of the consequences of paternal preoccupation with the infant is less overt attention toward the mother. If both parents are able to share their feelings, each can appreciate the process of attachment toward their child and will avoid the unfortunate conflict of being insensitive and unaware of the other's needs. In addition, a father who is encouraged to form a relationship with his newborn is less likely to feel excluded and abandoned once the family returns home and the mother directs her attention toward caring for the infant.

Ideally, the process of engrossment should be discussed with parents before the delivery, such as in prenatal classes, to reinforce the father's awareness of his natural feelings toward the expected child. Focusing on the future experience of seeing, touching, and holding one's newborn may also help expectant fathers become more comfortable in accepting their paternal feelings. This in turn can assist them in being more supportive toward the mother, especially as labor and delivery draw near.

At the infant's birth the nurse can play a vital role in helping the father express engrossment by assessing the neonate in front of the couple; pointing out normal characteristics; encouraging identification through consistent referral to the child by name; encouraging the father to cuddle, hold, and talk to the infant; and demonstrating whenever necessary the soothing powers of caressing, stroking, and rocking the child (Fig. 7.14).

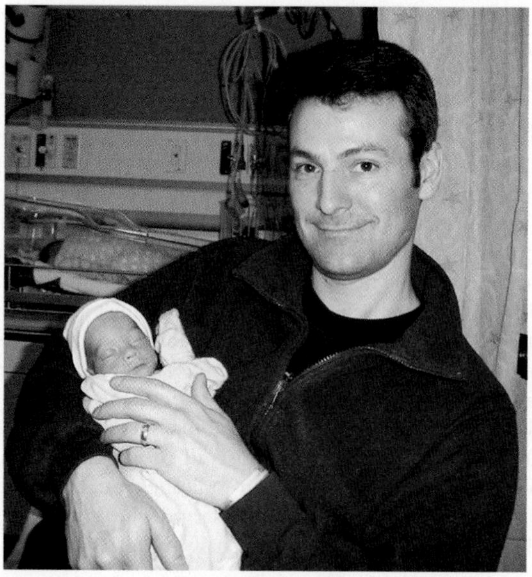

Fig. 7.14 A desire to hold the infant and participate in caregiving activities is an indication of paternal engrossment.

The father's role in supporting the mother during this period cannot be overemphasized. Once the mother has held the newborn skin-to-skin, the father may also be encouraged to hold the newborn skin-to-skin while the mother rests. Fathers are encouraged to be with the mother during labor and delivery, to spend time alone with the mother and newborn after delivery, and to "room-in" with the mother and infant. Education programs should be made available to new fathers and include information on holding the newborn, bathing, assisting the mother with breastfeeding, problems associated with breastfeeding and potential solutions, and care of the newborn at home (including safety). The integration of the father into the existing dyad of mother-newborn to form a new family—a triad—will help solidify his role as parent and partner in the care and support of his family.

The indications of affection from the father are the same as those expected in the mother, such as visual contact in the en face position and embracing the infant close to the body. When present, such behaviors should be reinforced. If such responses are not obvious, the nurse needs to assess the father's feelings regarding this birth, cultural beliefs that may prevent his expression of emotions, and other factors to facilitate his positive attachment during the newborn period.

Siblings

Although the attachment process has been discussed almost exclusively in terms of parents and infants, it is essential that nurses be aware of other family members, such as siblings and members of the extended family, who need preparation for the acceptance of this new child. Young children in particular need sensitive preparation for the birth to minimize sibling jealousy.

In support of family-centered care, siblings are generally encouraged to visit the mother in hospital and to hold the newborn (Fig. 7.15). Another trend has been the presence of siblings at childbirth. Unlike sibling visitation, the evidence supporting this practice has been controversial, yet family-centered care encompasses siblings, grandparents, and other significant persons who comprise the extended family unit. Children exhibit different degrees of involvement in the birth process. Some reported benefits include children's increased knowledge of the birth process, less regressive behavior after the birth, and more mothering and caregiving behavior toward the infant. Some practitioners add facilitated family bonding and assimilation of the

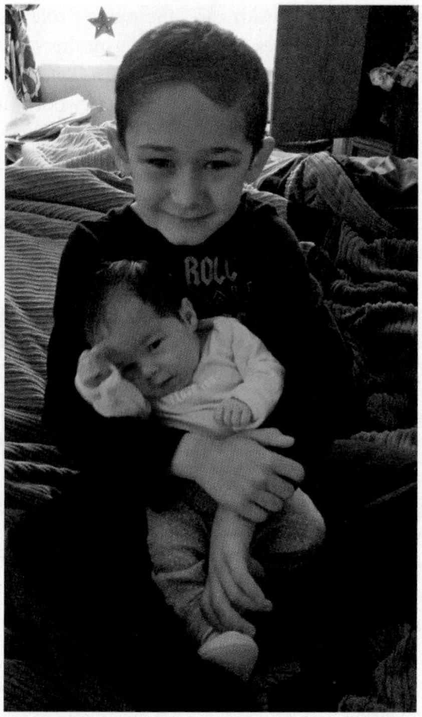

Fig. 7.15 Sibling holds infant sister on the first day home from the hospital.

newborn into the family as positive outcomes. Parents whose children attended the birth have echoed these same benefits and have expressed their desire to repeat the experience should another pregnancy occur. Despite these positive findings, opponents believe that allowing children to observe a delivery could lead to emotional difficulties, although there is no research to support this contention. As research mounts, birthing centers that allow siblings at the birth are developing more definitive guidelines, such as an age requirement of at least 4 to 5 years old, the presence of a supportive person for the sibling only, and an adequate sequence of preparation in which parents explore all options for preparing their other children.

From observations during sibling visitation, there is evidence that sibling attachment occurs. However, the en face position is assumed much less often between the newborn and siblings than between the mother and newborn, and when this position is used, it is brief. Siblings focus more on the head or face than on touching or talking to the infant. The siblings' verbalizations often focus less on attracting the infant's attention and more on addressing the mother about the newborn. Children who have established a prenatal relationship with the fetus have demonstrated more attachment behaviors, supporting the suggestion of encouraging prenatal acquaintance. Additional research is needed to establish theories on sibling bonding as have been constructed for parental bonding.

Multiple Births and Subsequent Children

A component of attachment that has special meaning for families with multiple births, **monotropy** refers to the principle that a person can become optimally attached to only one individual at a time. If a parent can form only one attachment at a time, how can all siblings of a multiple birth receive optimum emotional care? Research on bonding and multiple births is still lacking despite the recent increase in multiple births, and even less is known about paternal engrossment and sibling attachment. Regarding mother-twin bonding, the conclusions of different authors vary. Some report that mothers bond equally to each twin at the time of birth, even if one twin is ill. Others suggest that mothers of twins may take months or years to form individual attachments to each child or even longer if the twins are identical.

Nurses can be instrumental in promoting bonding of multiple births. The most important principle is to assist the parents in recognizing the individuality of the children, especially in monozygotic (identical) twins. The mother should visit with each newborn, including a sick infant, as much as possible after birth. Nonseparation and breastfeeding are encouraged. Any characteristics that are unique to each child are emphasized, and each infant is called by name rather than referring to "the twins." Asking the family questions (such as "How do you tell Ashley and Amy apart?" and "In what ways are Ashley and Amy different and similar?") helps point out the siblings' individual characteristics. Behaviors on the BNBAS can be used to illustrate these differences and to stress effective strategies for dealing with multiple personalities at the same time.

Co-bedding of twins or other multiples in the hospital has at times been suggested to maintain the bond between siblings that was formed in utero. A review of five studies exploring the safety and benefits of the practice of co-bedding stable preterm twins concluded that available evidence is insufficient to recommend this practice (Lai, Foong, Foong, et al., 2016) (see also Chapter 10, Sudden Infant Death Syndrome). The American Academy of Pediatrics (2016b) has also recommended against parents or other family members sleeping in the same bed with infants at home. Because neither the safety nor the benefits of co-bedding for newborns has been documented in the literature, the American Academy of Pediatrics recommends that families be counseled to follow safe sleeping practices, which currently dictate that infants sleep alone for optimal safety.

Another area of attachment that has received minimal attention is maternal bonding of multiparous mothers. Research suggests that "taking on" a second or third child has several additional tasks:

- Promoting acceptance and approval of the second child
- Grieving and resolving the loss of an exclusive dyadic relationship with the first child
- Planning and coordinating family life to include a second child
- Reformulating a relationship with the first child
- Identifying with the second child by comparing this child with the first child in terms of physical and psychologic characteristics
- Assessing one's affective capabilities in providing sufficient emotional support and nurturance simultaneously to two children

PREPARE FOR DISCHARGE AND HOME CARE

With shorter postpartum stays, as well as a trend toward mother-infant care (also called dyad or couplet care), discharge planning and postdischarge follow-up have become important components of comprehensive newborn care. First-time, as well as experienced, parents benefit from guidance and assistance with the infant's care, such as breastfeeding or bottle-feeding, and with the family's integration of a new member, particularly sibling adjustment.

To assess and meet these needs, teaching must begin early, ideally before the birth. Not only is the postpartum stay sometimes very short (as little as 12 to 24 hours), but mothers are also in the taking-in phase, where they may demonstrate passive and dependent behaviors. On the first postpartum day, because of fatigue and excitement about the newborn, mothers may not be able to absorb large amounts of information. This time may need to be spent highlighting essential aspects of care, such as infant safety and feeding. Parents may also be given a list of mother and infant care topics so that they can choose issues they wish to review before going home. Teaching before discharge should focus on newborn feeding patterns, monitoring diapers for stools and voiding, jaundice, and infant crying (see Family-Centered Care box).

FAMILY-CENTERED CARE

Healthy Term Newborn Discharge Criteria[a]

- Infant born between 37 and 41 completed weeks of gestation.
- Clinical course and physical examination at discharge have not revealed abnormalities that require continued hospitalization.
- Vital signs are within normal range and stable for the 12 hours preceding discharge.
- Infant has urinated regularly and passed at least one stool spontaneously.
- Infant has completed at least two successful feedings. For breastfed infants: A caregiver knowledgeable in breastfeeding must observe a feeding and assess latch, swallow, and infant satiety. For bottle-fed infants: Assess ability to coordinate sucking, swallowing, and breathing while feeding. These assessments must be documented in the health record.
- There is no significant bleeding at the circumcision site.
- Clinical risk of development of hyperbilirubinemia has been assessed, and follow-up plans per American Academy of Pediatrics clinical practice guidelines are in place.
- Infant has been adequately evaluated and monitored for sepsis based on maternal risk factors, including group B streptococcal disease.
- Maternal blood test and screening results are available and have been reviewed, including syphilis, hepatitis B, and HIV as per state regulations.
- Infant blood tests are available and have been reviewed, including cord or infant blood type and direct Coombs test results, as clinically indicated.
- Initial hepatitis B vaccine has been administered.
- If a mother has not previously been vaccinated, she should receive tetanus toxoid, reduced diphtheria toxoid, and acellular pertussis vaccine (Tdap) immediately after delivery.
- If a mother who delivers during flu season has not been previously immunized, she should receive the flu vaccine.
- Newborn metabolic, hearing, and congenital heart disease screening has been completed per hospital protocol and state regulations.
- Family, environmental, and social risk factors have been assessed, and proactive management is in place.
- Mother's knowledge, ability, and confidence to provide adequate infant care have been assessed for competency.
- An appropriate car seat is available before hospital discharge, and mother has demonstrated competence in its use.
- Continuing medical care is planned; infants discharged sooner than 48 hours should be examined within 48 hours of discharge from the hospital.
- Barriers to adequate follow-up care (e.g., lack of telephone or transportation) have been assessed, and a plan is in place to manage issues.

[a]See American Academy of Pediatrics (2015c) for comprehensive discussion of each criterion.
Data from American Academy of Pediatrics. (2015c). Policy statement: Hospital stay for healthy term newborn infants. *Pediatrics, 135*(5), 948–953.

Although legislation has been enacted guaranteeing most mothers a minimum of 48 hours' hospitalization, some mothers leave the hospital as early as 8 to 12 hours after vaginal delivery. The American Academy of Pediatrics (2015c) has established guidelines for discharge criteria for healthy term newborns. The American Academy of Pediatrics emphasizes that the primary care practitioner, in consultation with the mother, the midwife or obstetrician, and other health care providers, should make the determination of appropriate discharge time.

Follow-up home care within days (or even hours after discharge when minor problems are anticipated) is important to provide adequate maternal-newborn care with minimal complications. Despite the changing spectrum of well-newborn health care, the nurse's role continues to be that of providing ongoing assessments of each mother-newborn dyad to ensure a safe transition to home and a successful adaptation into the family unit. The ultimate safety and success of early newborn discharge from the hospital are contingent on using clear discharge criteria and having a high-quality early follow-up program (see Community Focus box).

With family structures changing, it is essential that nurses identify the primary caregiver, which may not always be the mother but may be a father, grandparent, or babysitter. Depending on the family composition, the mother's primary support system in caring for the newborn may not always be the traditional husband or male companion.

COMMUNITY FOCUS

Newborn Home Care After Early Discharge[a]

Wet diapers: Minimum of 1 for each day of life (day 2 = 2 wets; day 3 = 3 wets) until fifth or sixth day, at which time 5 or 6 per day to 14 days, then 6 to 10 per day

Breastfeeding: Successful latch-on and feeding every 1.5 to 3 hours daily; audible swallowing

Formula feeding: Successfully taking at least 1 to 2 oz every 3 to 4 hours; voiding as described earlier

Circumcision: Wash with warm water only; yellow exudate forming, with no bleeding; Plastibell intact for 48 hours

Stools: At least one every 48 to 72 hours (bottle feeding), or two or three per day (breastfeeding)

Color: Pink to ruddy when crying; pink centrally when at rest or asleep

Activity: Has four or five wakeful periods per day and alerts to environmental sounds and voices

Jaundice: Physiologic jaundice (i.e., jaundice not appearing in the first 24 hours); feeding, voiding, and stooling as noted earlier or practitioner notification for suspicion of pathologic jaundice (appears within 24 hours of birth; hemolysis and ABO/Rh problem suspected); decreased activity, poor feeding, or dark orange skin color persisting on the fifth day in light-skinned newborn; obtain transcutaneous (or serum) bilirubin before discharge and identify risk with an hour-specific nomogram (see Chapter 8, Hyperbilirubinemia)

Umbilical cord: Kept above diaper line; drying, no drainage; periumbilical area nonerythematous

Vital signs: Heart rate, 120 to 140 beats/min at rest; respiratory rate, 30 to 55 breaths/min at rest without evidence of sternal retractions, grunting, or nasal flaring; temperature, 36.3° to 37°C (97.3° to 98.6°F) axillary

Position of sleep: On back

[a]Any deviation from this list or suspicion of poor newborn adaptation should be reported immediately to the practitioner.

Nurses should not assume that terminology associated with mother-infant care is understood. Words relating to the anatomy (e.g., *meconium, labia, edema,* and *genitalia*) and to breastfeeding (e.g., *areola, colostrum,* and *let-down reflex*) may be unfamiliar to mothers. Mothers with other children do not necessarily understand more words, and younger, less educated mothers may be at risk for not understanding teaching.

An essential area of discharge counseling is the safe transportation of the newborn home from the hospital. Ideally, this information should be provided *before* delivery to allow parents an opportunity to purchase a suitable infant car safety seat. When purchasing a car safety seat, parents should consider cost and convenience. The convertible-type seats are more expensive initially but cost less than two separate systems (infant-only model and infant-toddler convertible model). Convenience is a major factor because a cumbersome restraint may be used less often or used improperly. Before buying a car safety seat, it is best to look carefully at different models. For example, some types are too large for subcompact cars. Asking friends about the advantages and disadvantages of their restraints is helpful, but borrowing a car seat or purchasing a used one can be dangerous. Parents should use only a restraint that has directions for use and a certification label stating that it complies with federal motor vehicle safety standards (both should be on the seat). They should not use a restraint that has been involved in a crash. Some service clubs and hospitals have loan programs for restraints. Information about approved models and other aspects of car safety seat restraints is available from several organizations and sources.[c]

[c]American Academy of Pediatrics, 141 Northwest Point Blvd., Elk Grove Village, IL 60007-1098; 847-434-4000; *Car Seats: Information for Families*, http://www.healthychildren.org.

Parents are cautioned against placing an infant in the front seat of a car with a passenger-side air bag. The American Academy of Pediatrics (2018) provides the following recommendations for children and car seats: (1) rear-facing car safety seats for as long as possible; (2) forward-facing car safety seats from the time a child outgrows a rear-facing seat for most children through at least 4 years of age; (3) belt-positioning booster seats from the time a child outgrows forward-facing seats for most children through at least 8 years of age; and (4) lap and shoulder seat belts for all who have outgrown booster seats. In addition, the American Academy of Pediatrics (2018) recommends that all children younger than 13 years old ride in the rear seats of vehicles.

CLINICAL JUDGMENT AND NEXT-GENERATION NCLEX® EXAMINATION-STYLE QUESTIONS

1. A newborn full-term infant was just born. The 1-minute Apgar Score was 8. Which would the nurse assess when performing an Apgar assessment at 5 minutes? Select the indicators below. **Select all that apply.**
   A. Respiratory effort
   B. Heart rate
   C. Core temperature
   D. Reflex irritability
   E. Muscle tone
   F. Color

2. A mother and her full-term newborn boy are being discharged 24 hours after birth. **Indicate which nursing education action listed in the far-left column is appropriate to teach the mother about specific newborn home care needs in the middle column. Place the number in the far-right column. Note that not all nursing actions will be used.**

Nursing Action: Early Discharge Newborn Care	Topic	Appropriate Nursing Education Action
1. The newborn should be fed every 1.5–3 hours	Wet Diapers	
2. This could occur within 24 hours of birth and hemolysis or ABO/Rh problem suspected	Position of Sleep	
3. The newborn should be fed 1–2oz every 4–6 hours	Umbilical Cord	
4. Wash with warm water, check for bleeding	Stools	
5. Keep it above the diaper line and allow to dry, check for drainage	Breast Feeding	
6. Place the newborn on his back	Pathologic Jaundice	
7. The newborn should have 4-5 wakeful periods a day		
8. The newborn should have 6-10 a day after 14 days of age		
9. The newborn should have 2-3 a day if breastfeeding		

3. A full-term newborn after birth will need to have a number of interventions as part of routine care as well as to prevent infection. **Select all the items below that the nurse is required to administer as part of routine newborn care. Select all that apply.**
   A. Prophylactic eye treatment
   B. Hepatitis C vaccine
   C. PKU and congenital hypothyroidism
   D. Pneumococcal vaccine
   E. Vitamin K Administration

4. A healthy infant is born to a mother with known high-risk behaviors whose HIV status is undetermined. The mother states that she wishes to breastfeed her infant. The nurse's response to the mother's request will be based on which of the following information? **Use an X for the health teaching below that is Indicated (appropriate or necessary), Contraindicated (could be harmful), or Non-Essential (makes no difference or not necessary).**

Health Teaching	Indicated	Contraindicated	Non-Essential
HIV is rarely transmitted to the newborn through maternal milk.			
In such infants, antiretroviral medication will be started within 12 hours of birth.			
Breastfeeding will be avoided completely in mothers with high-risk behaviors.			
Breastfeeding will be withheld until HIV status (maternal) is determined.			

REFERENCES

Academy of Breastfeeding Medicine. (2017). ABM clinical protocol #3: Supplementary feedings in the healthy term breastfed neonate, revised 2017. *Breastfeeding Medicine, 12*(3).

Agho, K. E., Ogeleka, P., Ogbo, F. A., et al. (2016). Trends and predictors of prelacteal feeding practices in Nigeria (2003–2013). *Nutrients, 8*(8), E462.

Alexander, G. R., Himes, J. H., Kaufman, R. B., et al. (1996). A United States national reference for fetal growth. *Obstetrics and Gynecology, 87*(2), 163–168.

American Academy of Pediatrics, Task Force on Circumcision. (2012a). Circumcision policy statement. *Pediatrics, 130*(3), 585–586.

American Academy of Pediatrics. (2012b). Policy statement: Breastfeeding and the use of human milk. *Pediatrics, 129*(3), e827–e841.

American Academy of Pediatrics (2003; reaffirmed 2014). Policy statement: Controversies concerning vitamin K and the newborn, *Pediatrics. 112*(1):191–192.

American Academy of Pediatrics, Committee on Fetus and Newborn, American College of Obstetricians and Gynecologists, Committee on Obstetric Practice. (2015a). The Apgar score. *Pediatrics, 136*(4), 819–822.

American Academy of Pediatrics. (2015b). *Caring for Your Baby and Young child: Birth to age 5* (6th ed.). Retrieved January 27, 2019 from https://www.healthychildren.org/English/ages-stages/baby/formula-feeding/Pages/Choosing-an-Infant-Formula.aspx.

American Academy of Pediatrics, Committee on Fetus & Newborn, Policy statement. (2015c). Hospital stay for healthy term newborn infants. *Pediatrics, 135*(5), 948–953.

American Academy of Pediatrics. (2016a). *Neonatal resuscitation textbook* (7th ed.). Elk Grove Village, IL: American Academy of Pediatrics & American Heart Association.

American Academy of Pediatrics Task Force on Sudden Infant Death Syndrome Policy Statement. (2016b). SIDS and other sleep-related infant deaths. updated 2016 recommendations for a safe infant sleeping environment. *Pediatrics, 138*(5), e20162938.

American Academy of Pediatrics, Statement of Endorsement. (2016c). Systematic review of and evidence-based guidelines for the management of patients with positional plagiocephaly. *Pediatrics, 138*(5), e20162802.

American Academy of Pediatrics, Clinical Report. (2008; reaffirmed 2016d). Newborn screening expands: Recommendations for pediatricians and medical homes – implications for the system. *Pediatrics, 121*(1), 192–217.

American Academy of Pediatrics, Committee on Fetus and Newborn, and Section on Anesthesiology and Pain Medicine, Policy Statement. (2016e). Prevention and management of procedural pain in the neonate: An update. *Pediatrics, 137*(2), e20154217.

American Academy of Pediatrics, Committee on fetus and newborn. (2016f). Umbilical cord care in the newborn infant. *Pediatrics, 138*(3), e201622149.

American College of Obstetrics & Gynecology. (2017). Delayed umbilical cord clamping after birth. committee opinion No. 684. *Obstetrics & Gynecology, 129*, e5–e10.

Ballard, J. L., Khoury, J. C., Wedig, K., et al. (1991). New Ballard score expanded to include extremely premature infants. *The Journal of Pediatrics, 119*(3), 417–423.

Banihani, O. I., Fox, J. A., Gander, B. H., et al. (2014). Complete penile amputation during ritual neonatal circumcision and successful replantation using postoperative leech therapy. *Urology, 84*(2), 472–474.

Barlow, J., Herath, N., Bartram, T. C., et al. (2018). The neonatal behavioral assessment scale (NBAS) and newborn behavioral observations (NBO) system for supporting caregivers and improving outcomes in caregivers and their infants. *Cochrane Database of Systematic Reviews, 3*, CD011754.

Basnet, S., Schneider, M., Gazit, A., et al. (2010). Fresh goat's milk for infants: Myths and realities—a review. *Pediatrics, 125*(4), e973–e977.

Bazi, T. (2017). Female genital mutilation: The role of medical professional organizations. *International Urogynecology Journal, 28*(4), 537–541.

Bazzano, A. N., Hofer, R., Thibeau, S., et al. (2016). A review of herbal and pharmaceutical galactogogues for breast-feeding. *The Ochsner Journal, 16*(4), 511–514.

Brazelton, T. B. (1974). Mother–infant reciprocity. In M. Klaus, T. Leger, & M. A. Trause (Eds.), *Maternal attachment and mothering disorders*. New Brunswick, NJ: Johnson & Johnson Baby Products.

Brazelton, T. B., & Nugent, J. K. (1996). *Neonatal behavioral assessment scale*. London: MacKeith Press.

Brookes, A., & Bowley, D. M. (2014). Tongue tie: The evidence for frenotomy. *Early Human Development, 90*(11), 765–768.

Canadian Paediatric Society, Position Statement. (2015). Newborn male circumcision. *Paediatrics & Child Health, 20*(6), 311–315.

Canadian Paediatric Society, Community Paediatrics Committee. (2011, reaffirmed 2016). Universal newborn hearing screening. *Paediatrics & child Health*, 16(5), 301–305.

Canadian Paediatric Society, Community Paediatrics Committee. (2017a). *Temperature Measurement in Paediatrics*. Retrieved January 21, 2019 from: https://www.cps.ca/en/documents/position/temperature-measurement.

Canadian Paediatric Society, First Nations, Inuit, and Métis Health Committee. (2007, reaffirmed 2017b). Vitamin D supplementation: Recommendations for Canadian mothers and infants, *Paediatric Child Health 12*(7):583–598. Retrieved January 27, 2019 from: https://www.cps.ca/en/documents/position/vitamin-d.

Centers for Disease Control & Prevention. (2018). Vitamin D. Retrieved January 27, 2019 from: https://www.cdc.gov/breastfeeding/breastfeeding-special-circumstances/diet-and-micronutrients/vitamin-d.html.

Cleveland, L. M. (2016). Breastfeeding recommendations for women who receive medication-assisted treatment for opioid use disorders: AWHONN practice brief number 4. *Journal of Obstetrics, Gynecology and Neonatal Nurses, 45*(4), 574–576.

Cleveland, L. M., Hill, C. M., Pulse, W. S., et al. (2017). Systematic review of skin-to-skin care for full-term, healthy newborns. *Journal of Obstetric, Gynecologic & Neonatal Nursing, 46*(6), 857–869.

Condo DiCioccio, H., Ady, C., Bena, J. F., et al. (2018). Initiative to improve exclusive breastfeeding by delaying the newborn bath. *Journal of Obstetric, Gynecologic & Neonatal Nurses, 7*(3), S30–S31.

Eglash, A., & Simon, L. (2017). ABM clinical protocol #8: Human milk storage information for home use for full-term infants. *Breastfeeding Medicine, 12*(7), 390–395.

Emond, A., Ingram, J., Johnson, D., et al. (2014). Randomized controlled trial of early frenotomy in breastfed infants with mild-moderate tongue-tie. archives of disease in childhood. *Fetal and Neonatal Edition, 99*(3), F189–F195.

Ewer, A. K., & Martin, G. R. (2016). Newborn pulse oximetry screening: Which algorithm is best? *Pediatrics, 138*(5). Retrieved January 21, 2019 from: http://pediatrics.aappublications.org/content/138/5/e20161206. .

Flaherty, S. C., & Sadler, L. S. (2011). A review of attachment theory in the context of adolescent parenting. *Journal of Pediatric Health Care, 25*(2), 114–121.

Foster, J. P., Taylor, C., & Spence, K. (2017). Topical anaesthesia for needle-related pain in newborn infants. *Cochrane Database of Systematic Reviews, 2*, CD010331.

Goswami, E., Batra, P., Khurana, R., et al. (2017). Comparison of temporal artery thermometry with axillary and rectal thermometry in full term neonates. *Indian Journal of Pediatrics, 84*(3), 195–199.

Hadley, K. B., Ryan, A. S., Forsyth, S., et al. (2016). The essentiality of arachidonic acid in infant development. *Nutrients, 8*(4), 40–47.

Hawkins, S. S., Stern, A. D., Baum, C. F., et al. (2014). Compliance with the baby-friendly hospital initiative and impact on breastfeeding rates. *Archives of Disease in Childhood. Fetal and Neonatal Edition, 99*(2), F138–F143.

Hawkins, S. S., Stern, A. D., Baum, C. F., et al. (2015). Evaluating the impact of the baby-friendly hospital initiative on breast-feeding rates: A multi-state analysis. *Public Health Nutrition, 18*(2), 179–187.

Holland, A., & Watkins, D. (2015). Flying start health visitors' views of implementing the newborn behavioural observation: Barriers and facilitating factors. *Community Practitioner, 88*(6), 33–36.

Horta, B. L., Loret de Mola, C., & Victora, C. G. (2015). Breastfeeding and intelligence: A systematic review and meta-analysis. *Acta Paediatrica, 104*(467), 14–19.

Houghtaling, B., Byker Shanks, C., & Jenkins, M. (2017). Likelihood of breastfeeding within the USDA's food and nutrition service special supplementation nutrition program for women, infants, and children population. *Journal of Human Lactation, 33*(1), 83–97.

Howe-Heyman, A., & Lutenbacher, M. (2016). The baby-friendly hospital initiative as an intervention to improve breastfeeding rates: A review of the literature. *Journal of Midwifery & Women's Health, 61*(1), 77–102.

Jagannath, V. ,A. „ Fedorowicz, Z., Sud, V., et al. (2012). Routine neonatal circumcision for the prevention of urinary tract infections in infancy. *Cochrane Database Systematic Reviews, 11*, CD009129.

Jasani, B., Simmer, K., Patole, S. K., et al. (2017). Long chain polyunsaturated fatty acid supplementation in infants born at term. *Cochrane Database of Systematic Reviews, 3*, CD000376.

Johnston, C., Campbell-Yeo, M., Disher, T., et al. (2017). Skin-to-skin care for procedural pain in neonates. *Cochrane Database of Systematic Reviews, 2*, CD008435.

Jones, K. M., Power, M. L., Queenan, J. T., et al. (2015). Racial and ethnic disparities in breastfeeding. *Breastfeeding Medicine, 10*(4), 186–196.

Kimberlin, Brady, Jackson, et al. (2018). *American Academy of Pediatrics, Committee on Infectious Diseases. Red Book: 2018 Report of the Committee on Infectious Diseases* (31st ed.). Elk Grove Village, IL: The Academy.

Kiserud, T., Benachi, A., Hecher, K., et al. (2018). The World Health Organization fetal growth charts: concept, findings, interpretation, and application. *American Journal of Obstetrics & Gynecology, 218*(2), S619–S629.

Kleinman, R. E., & Greer, F. R. (Eds.). (2014). *Pediatric nutrition* (7th ed.). Elk Grove Village, IL: American Academy of Pediatrics.

Kuswara, K., Laws, R., Kremer, P., et al. (2016). The infant feeding practices of Chinese immigrant mothers in Australia: A qualitative exploration. *Appetite, 105*, 375–384.

Lai, N. M., Foong, S. C., Foong, W. C., et al. (2016). Co-bedding in neonatal nursery for promoting growth and neurodevelopment in stable preterm twins. *Cochrane Database of Systematic Reviews, 4*, CD008313.

Leigh, B. (2016). *Six States of Alertness for Newborns*. Centre for Perinatal Psychology. Retrieved January 21, 2019 from: https://www.centreforperinatalpsychology.com.au/states-of-alertness/. Retrieved from.

Losio, M. N., Pavoni, E., Finazzi, G., et al. (2018). Preparation of powdered infant formula: Could product's safety be improved? *Journal of Pediatric Gastroenterology & Nutrition, 67*(4), 543–546.

Lund, C. (2016). Bathing and beyond: Current bathing controversies for newborn infants. *Advances in Neonatal Care, 16*(5S), S13–S20.

Maheswari, N. U., Kumar, B. P., Karunakaran, A., et al. (2012). "Early baby teeth": Folklore and facts. *Journal of Pharmacy and Bioallied Sciences*, 4(Suppl 2, part 3), S329–S333.

Martin, C. R., Ling, P. R., & Blackburn, G. L. (2016). Review of infant feeding: Key features of breast milk and infant formula. *Nutrients, 8*(5), 279–290.

Modarres, M., Jazayeri, Q., Rahnama, P., et al. (2013). Breastfeeding and pain relief in full-term neonates during immunization injections: A clinical randomized trial. *BMC Anesthesiology, 13*(1), 22–28.

Molès, J. P., Tuaillon, E., Kankasa, C., et al. (2018). Breastmilk cell trafficking induces microchimerism-mediated immune system maturation in the infant. *Pediatric Allergy & Immunology, 29*(2), 133–143.

Moon, K., Rao, S. C., Schulzke, S. M., et al. (2016). Longchain polyunsaturated fatty acid supplementation in preterm infants. *Cochrane Database of Systematic Reviews, 12*, CD000375.

Morlay, A., Piat, F., Mercey, T., et al. (2016). Immunological detection of cronobacter and salmonella in powdered infant formula by plasmonic label-free assay. *Letters in Applied Microbiology, 62*(2), 459–465.

Morris, B. J., Krieger, J. N., & Klausnerc, J. D. (2017). CDC's male circumcision recommendations represent a key public health measure. *Global Health: Science & Practice, 5*(1), 15–27.

Newby, R. M., & Davies, P. S. (2016). Why do women stop breast-feeding? Results from a contemporary prospective study in a cohort of Australian women. *European Journal of Clinical Nutrition, 70*(12), 1428–1432.

Ng, E., & Loewy, A. D. (2018). *Policy Statement: Guidelines for Vitamin K Prophylaxis in Newborns.* Canadian Paediatric Society. Fetus & Newborn Committee & College of Family Physicians of Canada. Retrieved January 21, 2019 from: https://www.cps.ca/en/documents/position/vitamin-k-prophylaxis-in-newborns.

Novak, C., & Gill, P. (2018). Pediatric Vital Signs Reference Chart. *PedsCases.* Retrieved January 21, 2019 from: http://www.pedscases.com/pediatric-vital-signs-reference-chart.

Nugent, K. J., Bartlett, J. D., Von Ende, A., et al. (2017). The effects of the newborn behavioral observations (NBO) system on sensitivity in mother–infant interactions. *Infants & Young Children, 30*(4), 257–268.

Odom, E. C., Li, R., Scanlon, K. S., Perrine, C. G., et al. (2013). Reasons for earlier than desired cessation of breastfeeding. *Pediatrics, 131*(3), e726–e732.

Olsen, I. E., Groveman, S. A., Lawson, M. L., et al. (2010). New intrauterine growth curves based on United States data. *Pediatrics, 125*(2), e214–e224.

O'Shea, J. E., Foster, J. P., O'Donnell, C. P. F., et al. (2017). Frenotomy for tongue-tie in newborn infants. *The Cochrane Database of Systemic Reviews, 3*, CD011065.

Owings, M., Uddin, S., & Williams, S. (2013). Trends in circumcision for male newborns in US hospitals: 1979-2010.

Pippi Salle, J. L., Jesus, L. E., Lorenzo, A. J., et al. (2013). Glans amputation during routine neonatal circumcision: Mechanisms of injury and strategy for prevention. *Journal of Pediatric Urology, 9*(6 Pt A), 763–768. Epub 2012 Nov 5.

Power, R. F., & Murphy, J. F. (2015). Tongue-tie and frenotomy in infants with breastfeeding difficulties: Achieving a balance. *Archives of Disease in Childhood, 100*(5), 489–494.

Rabun, J. B. (2014). For health care professionals: Guidelines on prevention of and response to infant abductions. *National Center for Missing and Exploited Children* (10th ed.).

Riva Crugnola, C., Ierardi, E., Ferro, V., et al. (2016a). Mother-infant emotion regulation at three months: The role of maternal anxiety, depression and parenting stress. *Psychopathology, 49*, 285–294.

Riva Crugnola, C., Ierardi, E., Ferro, V., et al. (2016b). Post-natal mother-to-infant attachment in sub-clinically depressed mothers: Dyads at risk? *Psychopathology, 49*(4), 269–276.

Sanders, L., & Buckner, E. B. (2006). The newborn behavioral observations (NBO) system as a nursing intervention to enhance engagement in first-time mothers: Feasibility and desirability. *Pediatric Nursing, 32*(5), 455–459.

Sasidharan, K., Dutta, S., & Narang, A. (2009). Validity of new Ballard score until 7th day of postnatal life in moderately preterm neonates. archives of disease in childhood. *Fetal and Neonatal Edition, 94*, F39–F44.

Shah, P. S., Herbozo, C., Aliwalas, L. L., et al. (2012). Breastfeeding or breast milk for procedural pain in neonates. *Cochrane Database of Systematic Reviews, 12*, CD004950.

Singhal, R., Jain, S., Chawla, D., et al. (2017). Accuracy of new Ballard score in small-for-gestational age neonates. *Journal of Tropical Pediatrics, 63*(6), 489–494.

Smith, J. (2014). Methods and devices of temperature measurement in the neonate: A narrative review of practice recommendations. *Newborns and Infant Nursing Reviews, 14*(2), 64–71.

Smith, J., Alcock, G., & Usher, K. (2013). Temperature measurement in the preterm an term neonate: A review of literature. *Neonatal Network, 32*(1), 16–25.

Smolkin, T., Mick, O., Dabbah, M., et al. (2012). Birth by cesarean delivery and failure on first otoacoustic emissions hearing test. *Pediatrics, 130*(1), e95–e100.

Stevens, B., Yamada, J., Ohlsson, A., et al. (2016). Sucrose for analgesia in newborn infants undergoing painful procedures. *The Cochrane Database Systematic Reviews, 7*, CD0010690. CD001069.pub5.

Stewart, D., & Benitz, W. (2016). AAP committee on fetus and newborn: Umbilical cord care in the newborn infant. *Pediatrics, 138*(3), e20162149.

Symonds, M. E., Aldiss, P., Pope, M., et al. (2018). Recent advances in our understanding of brown and beige adipose tissue: The good fat that keeps you healthy, *F1000Res 7*.

Syrkin-Nikolau, M. E., Johnson, K. J., Colaizy, T. T., et al. (2017). Temporal artery temperature measurement in the neonate. *American Journal of Perinatology, 34*(10), 1026–1031.

Thomas, P., Peabody, J., Turnier, V., et al. (2000). A new look at intrauterine growth and the impact of race, altitude, and gender. *Pediatrics, 106*(2), e21.

United States Breastfeeding Committee. (2019). *Healthy people 2020.* Retrieved January 27, 2019 from: http://www.usbreastfeeding.org/p/cm/ld/fid=221.

US Food & Drug Administration. (2018). *Once Baby Arrives From Food Safety for Moms to be.* Retrieved January 27, 2019 from: https://www.fda.gov/Food/ResourcesForYou/HealthEducators/ucm089629.htm.

US National Library of Medicine, Toxicology Data Network, Drugs and Lactation Database. LactMed. Retrieved January 27, 2019 from: http://toxnet.nlm.nih.gov/newtoxnet/lactmed.htm.

Wambach, K., Domain, E. W., Page-Goertz, S., et al. (2016). Exclusive breastfeeding experiences among Mexican-American women. *Journal of Human Lactation, 32*(1), 103–111.

Wandel, M., Terragni, L., Nguyen, C., et al. (2016). Breastfeeding among soMali mothers living in Norway: Attitudes, practices and challenges. *Women and Birth, 29*(6), 487–493.

Wang, L., Collins, C., Ratliff, M., et al. (2017). Breastfeeding reduces childhood obesity risks. *Childhood Obesity, 13*(3).

World Health Organization. (2007). *Safe Preparation, Storage and Handling of Powdered Infant Formula: Guidelines.* Food and Agriculture Organization of the United Nations. Retrieved January 28, 2019 from: https://apps.who.int/iris/bitstream/handle/10665/43659/9789241595414_eng.pdf?sequence=1&isAllowed=y.

World Health Organization. (2009). *WHO Guidelines on Hand Hygiene in Health Care.* Retrieved January 27, 2019 from: https://apps.who.int/iris/bitstream/handle/10665/44102/9789241597906_eng.pdf;jsessionid=2EA5179FC8C081BA7FE1307832E630CF?sequence=1.

World Health Organization, United Nations Children's Fund, and Wellstart International. (2009). Baby-friendly hospital initiative: Revised, updated and expanded for integrated care. https://apps.who.int/iris/bitstream/handle/10665/43593/9789241594981_eng.pdf?sequence

World Health Organization. (2018a). *WHO Recommendation on Bathing and Other Immediate Postnatal Care of the Newborn.* Retrieved January 26, 2019 from: https://extranet.who.int/rhl/topics/newborn-health/care-newborn-infant/who-recommendation-bathing-and-other-immediate-postnatal-care-newborn.

World Health Organization. (2018b). *Female Genital Mutilation.* Retrieved January 27, 2019 from: https://www.who.int/news-room/fact-sheets/detail/female-genital-mutilation.

Wyckoff, A. S. (2009). Thermometer use 101. *AAP News.* Retrieved January 21, 2019 from: http://www.aappublications.org/content/30/11/29.2.

Xinjie, S., Shukla, S., Lee, G., et al. (2016). Detection of *Cronobacter* genus in powdered infant formula by enzyme-linked immunosorbent assay using anti-*Cronobacter* antibody. *Frontiers of Microbiology, 7*(1124), 1–10.

8

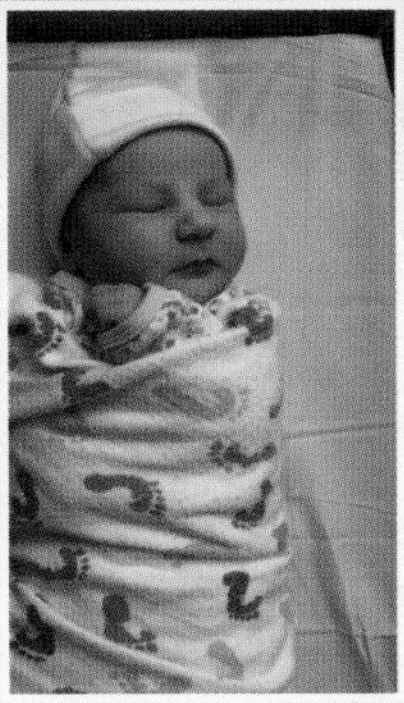

Health Problems of Newborns

Kimberley Ann Fisher

http://evolve.elsevier.com/wong/essentials

CONCEPTS

- Birth Injuries
- Congenital Abnormalities
- Thermoregulation
- Glucose Regulation

BIRTH INJURIES

Several factors predispose an infant to birth injuries (Mangurten, Puppala, & Prazad, 2015; Parsons, Seay, & Jacobson, 2016). Maternal factors include uterine dysfunction that leads to prolonged or precipitous labor, preterm or postterm labor, and cephalopelvic disproportion. Injury may result from dystocia caused by fetal macrosomia, multifetal gestation, abnormal or difficult presentation (not caused by maternal uterine or pelvic conditions), and congenital anomalies. Intrapartum events that can result in scalp injury include the use of intrapartum monitoring of fetal heart rate and collection of fetal scalp blood for acid-base assessment. Obstetric birth techniques can cause injury. Forceps birth, vacuum extraction, version and extraction, and cesarean birth are potential contributory factors. Often more than one factor is present, and multiple predisposing factors may be related to a single maternal condition.

SOFT TISSUE INJURY

Various types of soft tissue injury may be sustained during the process of birth, primarily in the form of bruises or abrasions secondary to dystocia. Soft tissue injury usually occurs when there is some degree of disproportion between the presenting part and the maternal pelvis (**cephalopelvic disproportion**). The use of forceps to facilitate a difficult vertex delivery may produce bruising or abrasion on the sides of the neonate's face. Petechiae or ecchymoses may be observed on the presenting part after a breech or brow delivery. After a difficult or precipitous delivery, the sudden release of pressure on the head can produce scleral hemorrhages or generalized petechiae over the face and head. Petechiae and ecchymoses may also appear on the head, neck, and face of an infant born with a nuchal cord, giving the infant's face a cyanotic appearance. A well-defined circle of petechiae and ecchymoses or abrasions may also be seen on the occipital region of the newborn's head when a vacuum suction cup is applied during delivery. Rarely, lacerations occur during cesarean section.

These traumatic lesions generally fade spontaneously within a few days without treatment. However, petechiae may be a manifestation of an underlying bleeding disorder or a systemic illness (such as an infection) and should be further evaluated as to their origin. Nursing care is primarily directed toward assessing and monitoring the injury and providing an explanation and reassurance to the parents.

HEAD TRAUMA

Trauma to the head and scalp that occurs during the birth process is usually benign but occasionally results in more serious injury. The injuries that produce serious trauma, such as intracranial hemorrhage and subdural hematoma, are discussed in relation to neurologic disorders in the newborn (Table 8.1). Skull fractures are discussed in association with other fractures sustained during the birth process. The three most common types of extracranial hemorrhagic injury are caput succedaneum, cephalhematoma, and subgaleal hemorrhage.

Caput Succedaneum

The most commonly observed scalp lesion is **caput succedaneum**, a vaguely outlined area of edematous tissue situated over the portion of the scalp that presents in a vertex delivery (Fig. 8.1A). The swelling consists of serum, blood, or both accumulated in the tissues above the bone, and it often extends beyond the bone margins. The swelling may be associated with overlying petechiae or ecchymoses. No specific treatment is needed, and the swelling subsides within a few days. Careful observation for signs of infection is needed if the skin over the caput is abraded or broken down.

Cephalhematoma

Infrequently, a cephalhematoma is formed when blood vessels rupture during labor or delivery producing bleeding into the area between the bone and its periosteum. The injury occurs most often with primiparous delivery and is more likely with forceps delivery and vacuum extraction. Unlike caput succedaneum, the boundaries of the cephalhematoma are sharply demarcated and do not extend beyond the limits of the bone (suture lines) (see Fig. 8.1B). The cephalhematoma may involve one or both parietal bones. The occipital bones are less commonly affected, and the frontal bones are rarely affected. The swelling is usually minimal or absent at birth and increases in size on the second or third day. Blood loss is usually not significant.

No treatment is indicated for uncomplicated cephalhematoma. Most lesions are absorbed within 2 weeks to 3 months. Lesions that result in severe blood loss to the area or that involve an underlying fracture require further evaluation. Hyperbilirubinemia may result during resolution of the hematoma. A local infection can develop and is suspected when a sudden increase in swelling occurs. Parents should be counseled that, in some cases, a small area of calcification may develop and persist.

TABLE 8.1 **Neurologic Complications**

Description	Clinical Manifestations	Therapeutic Management	Nursing Care Management
Hypoxic-Ischemic Brain Injury			
Nonprogressive neurologic (brain) impairment caused by intrauterine or postnatal asphyxia resulting in hypoxemia or cerebral ischemia Hypoxic-ischemic encephalopathy—the resultant cellular damage causes the clinical manifestations	Appears within first 6-12 h after hypoxic episode Seizures Abnormal muscle tone (usually hypotonia) Disturbance of sucking and swallowing Apneic episodes Stupor or coma Muscular weakness in hips and shoulders (full term), lower limb weakness (preterm)	Prevent hypoxia. Provide supportive care. Provide adequate ventilation. Maintain cerebral perfusion. Prevent cerebral edema. Treat underlying cause. Administer antiseizure drugs. Initiate therapeutic hypothermia if criteria met.	See Nursing Care of the High-Risk Newborn and Family later in the chapter. Observe for signs that indicate cerebral hypoxia. Monitor ventilatory and IV therapy. Observe for and manage seizures. Support family. Provide guidelines for family management of potential mild to severe neurologic damage.
Germinal Matrix or Intraventricular Hemorrhage			
Hemorrhage into and around ventricles caused by ruptured vessels as a result of an event that increases cerebral blood flow to area	Sudden deterioration in condition if bleed is large Most bleeds initially asymptomatic Tense, bulging anterior fontanel Neurologic signs: • Twitching • Stupor • Apnea • Seizures Evident on cranial ultrasonography or MRI	Supportive care: Maintain oxygenation. Regulate fluid and electrolytes, acid-base balance. Suppress or prevent seizures. Provide ventricular shunting or drainage.	See Nursing Care of the High-Risk Newborn and Family later in the chapter. Prevent increased cerebral BP. Avoid events that may increase or decrease cerebral blood flow (e.g., pain, unnecessary stimulation, ET suctioning, hypoxia, hyperosmolar drugs, rapid volume expansion). Elevate head of bed 20-30 degrees; keep head in midline for the first 72 h after birth. Support family. Monitor for posthemorrhagic hydrocephalus after diagnosis. Provide developmental care and enhancement.
Intracranial Hemorrhage			
Subdural Subarachnoid Intracerebellar	Sudden decrease in hematocrit Change in sensorium Poor feeding See Chapter 27	See Chapter 27.	Same as for germinal matrix or intraventricular hemorrhage.

BP, Blood pressure; *ET*, endotracheal; *IV*, intravenous; *MRI*, magnetic resonance imaging.

Subgaleal Hemorrhage

Subgaleal hemorrhage is bleeding into the subgaleal compartment (see Fig. 8.1C). The **subgaleal compartment** is a potential space that contains loosely arranged connective tissue; it is located beneath the galea aponeurosis, the tendinous sheath that connects the frontal and occipital muscles and forms the inner surface of the scalp. The injury occurs as a result of forces that compress and then drag the head through the pelvic outlet (Parsons et al., 2016). Instrumented delivery, particularly vacuum extraction and forceps delivery, increases the risk of subgaleal hemorrhage. Additional risk factors include prolonged second stage of labor, prolonged rupture of membranes, fetal distress, failed vacuum extraction, malposition of the fetal head and maternal primiparity (Colditz, Lai, Cartwright, et al., 2015). The bleeding extends beyond bone, often posteriorly into the neck, and continues after birth with the potential for serious complications, such as anemia or hypovolemic shock.

Early detection of the hemorrhage is vital; serial head circumference measurements and inspection of the back of the neck for increasing edema and a firm mass are essential. A boggy fluctuant mass over the scalp that crosses the suture line and moves as the baby is repositioned is an early sign of subgaleal hemorrhage (Parsons et al., 2016). Other signs include pallor, hypotonia, and increasing head circumference (Mangurten et al., 2015). Another sign of subgaleal hemorrhage is a forward and lateral positioning of the newborn's ears because the hematoma extends posteriorly (Mangurten et al., 2015). Disseminated intravascular coagulation (DIC) has also been reported in association with subgaleal hemorrhage (Colditz et al., 2015). Computed tomography (CT) or magnetic resonance imaging (MRI) is useful in confirming the diagnosis. Replacement of lost blood and clotting factors is required in acute cases of hemorrhage. Monitoring the infant for changes in level of consciousness and a decrease in the hematocrit are also key to early recognition and management. An increase in serum bilirubin levels may be seen as a result of the degradation of red blood cells (RBCs) within the hematoma.

Nursing Care Management

Nursing care is directed toward assessment and observation of the common scalp injuries and vigilance in observing for possible associated complications (such as infection) or, as in the case of subgaleal hemorrhage, acute blood loss and hypovolemia. Nursing care of a newborn with a subgaleal hemorrhage includes careful monitoring for signs of hemodynamic instability and shock (Parsons et al., 2016).

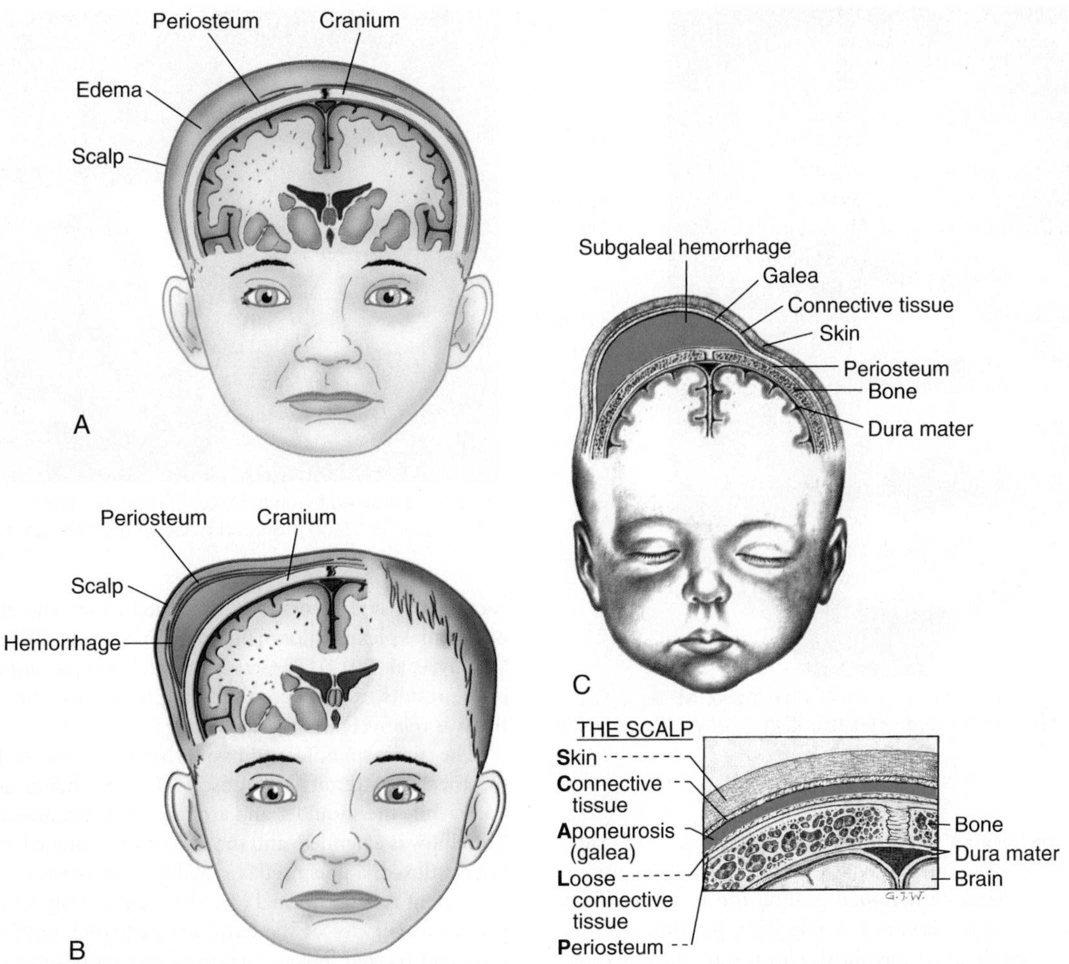

Fig. 8.1 A, Caput succedaneum. B, Cephalhematoma. C, Subgaleal hemorrhage. (**A** and **B**, From Seidel, H. M., Ball, J. M., Davis, J. E., et al. [2006]. *Mosby's guide to physical examination* [6th ed.]. St Louis, MO: Mosby.)

Because caput succedaneum and cephalhematoma usually resolve spontaneously, parents need reassurance of their usual benign nature.

FRACTURES

The clavicle, or collarbone, is the bone most frequently fractured during the birth process. Clavicular fracture is more common with shoulder dystocia, a vertex or breech delivery of infants who are large for gestational age or extended arms in breech deliveries (Mangurten et al., 2015). Crepitus (the coarse crackling sensation produced by the rubbing together of fractured bone fragments) may be felt or heard on examination. A palpable, spongy mass, representing localized edema and hematoma, may also be a sign of a fractured clavicle. The infant may be reluctant to move the arm on the affected side, and the Moro reflex may be asymmetric. Radiographs usually reveal a complete fracture with overriding of the fragments.

Fractures of long bones, such as the femur or the humerus, are sometimes difficult to detect by radiographic examination in infants. Although osteogenesis imperfecta is a rare finding, a newborn infant with a fracture should be assessed for other evidence of this congenital disorder.

Fractures of the neonatal skull are uncommon. The bones, which are less mineralized and more compressible than bones in older infants and children, are separated by membranous seams that allow sufficient alteration in the head contour so that it adjusts to the birth canal during delivery. Skull fractures usually follow a prolonged, difficult delivery or forceps extraction. Most fractures are linear, but some may be visible as depressed indentations that compress or decompress like a ping-pong ball. Management of depressed skull fractures is controversial; many resolve without intervention. Nonsurgical elevation of the indentation using a hand breast pump or vacuum extractor has been reported (Mangurten et al., 2015). Surgery may be required in the presence of bone fragments or signs of significant blood clots (intracranial pressure [ICP]) (Roland & Hill, 2016). A similar finding in neonates is craniotabes, which is usually benign and may be associated with prematurity or uterine compression (Brady, Barnes-Davis, & Poindexter, 2020). In this condition, the cranial bone(s) move freely on palpation; further investigation is needed if the condition persists.

> **! NURSING ALERT**
>
> A newborn with a fractured clavicle may have no symptoms, but suspect a fracture if an infant has limited use of the affected arm, malpositioning of the arm, asymmetric Moro reflex, or focal swelling or tenderness or if he or she cries in pain when the arm is moved.

> **! NURSING ALERT**
>
> Any newborn who is large for gestational age or weighs more than 3855 g (8.5 pounds) and is delivered vaginally should be evaluated for a fractured clavicle.

Nursing Care Management

Often no intervention is needed other than maintaining proper body alignment, careful dressing and undressing of the infant, along with

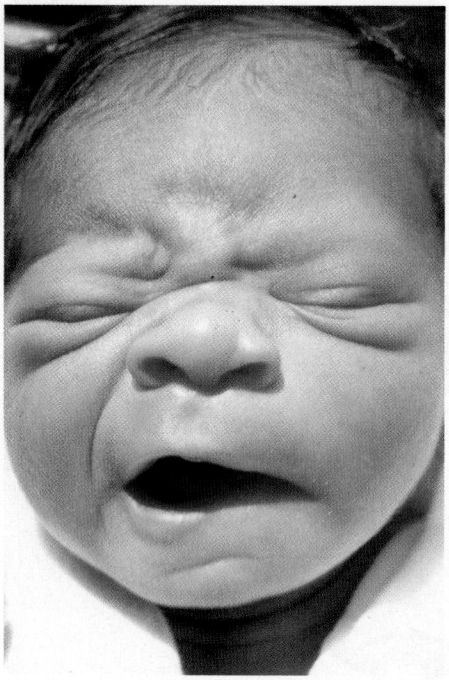

Fig. 8.2 Facial nerve palsy. (From Clark-Gambelunghe, M. B., & Clark, D. [2015]. Sensory development. *Pediatric Clinics of North America, 62*[2], 367–384.)

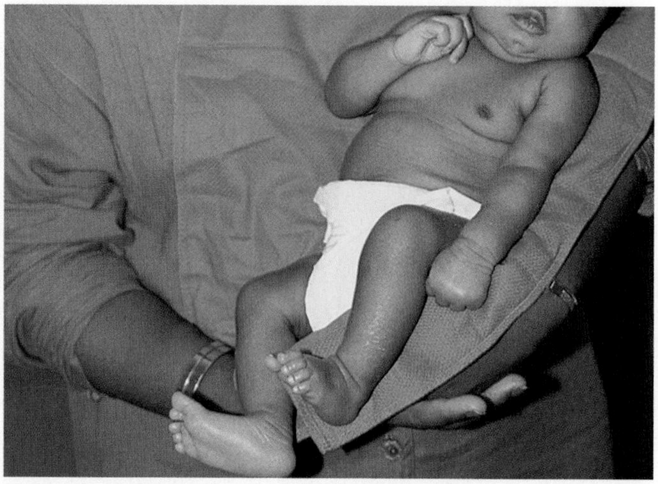

Fig. 8.3 Left-sided brachial plexus (Erb) palsy. Note the extended, internally rotated arm and pronated wrist on the affected side.

handling and carrying that support the affected bone. For example, if the infant has a fractured clavicle, it is important to support the upper and lower back rather than pulling the infant up from under the arms. Placing the infant in a side-lying position with the affected side down should also be avoided. Linear skull fractures usually require no treatment. A ping-pong ball–type skull fracture may require decompression by surgical intervention. The infant is carefully observed for signs of neurologic complications. The parents of infants with a fracture of any bone should be involved in caring for the infant during hospitalization as part of discharge planning for care at home.

PARALYSIS

Facial Paralysis

Pressure on the facial nerve (cranial nerve VII) during delivery may result in injury to that nerve. The primary clinical manifestations are loss of movement on the affected side, such as an inability to completely close the eye, drooping of the corner of the mouth, and absence of wrinkling of the forehead and nasolabial fold (Fig. 8.2). The paralysis is most noticeable when the infant cries. The mouth is drawn to the unaffected side, the wrinkles are deeper on the normal side, and the eye on the involved side remains open.

No medical intervention is necessary. The paralysis usually disappears spontaneously in a few days but may take as long as several months.

Brachial Palsy

Plexus injury results from forces that alter the normal position and relationship of the arm, shoulder, and neck. **Erb palsy (Erb-Duchenne paralysis)** is caused by damage to the upper plexus and usually results from stretching or pulling away of the shoulder from the head, as might occur with shoulder dystocia or with a difficult vertex or breech delivery. Other identified risk factors include an infant with birth weight of more than 4000 g (8.8 pounds), multiparous pregnancy, a vacuum-assisted extraction, prolonged labor, and a previous history of brachial plexus injury (Buterbaugh & Shah, 2016; Lindqvist, Ajne, Cooray, et al., 2014). The less common lower plexus palsy, or **Klumpke palsy**, results from severe stretching of the upper extremity while the trunk is relatively less mobile.

The clinical manifestations of Erb palsy are related to the paralysis of the affected extremity and muscles. The arm hangs limp alongside the body while the shoulder and arm are adducted and internally rotated. The elbow is extended, and the forearm is pronated, with the wrist and fingers flexed; a grasp reflex may be present because finger and wrist movement remain normal (Tappero, 2015) (Fig. 8.3). In lower plexus palsy, the muscles of the hand are paralyzed, with consequent wrist drop and relaxed fingers. In a third and more severe form of brachial palsy, the entire arm is paralyzed and hangs limp and motionless at the side. The Moro reflex is absent on the affected side for all forms of brachial palsy.

Treatment of the affected arm is aimed at preventing contractures of the paralyzed muscles and maintaining correct placement of the humeral head within the glenoid fossa of the scapula. Complete recovery from stretched nerves usually takes 3 to 6 months. Full recovery is expected in 88% to 92% of infants (Parsons et al., 2016). However, avulsion of the nerves (complete disconnection of the ganglia from the spinal cord that involves both anterior and posterior roots) results in permanent damage. For injuries that do not improve spontaneously by 3 to 6 months, surgical intervention may be needed to relieve pressure on the nerves or to repair the nerves with grafting. In some cases, injection of botulinum toxin A into the pectoralis major muscle may be effective in reducing muscle contractures after birth-related brachial plexus injuries (Buterbaugh & Shaw, 2016).

Phrenic Nerve Paralysis

Phrenic nerve paralysis results in diaphragmatic paralysis as demonstrated by ultrasonography, which shows paradoxic chest movement and an elevated diaphragm. Initially, radiography may not demonstrate an elevated diaphragm if the neonate is receiving positive pressure ventilation (Parsons et al., 2016). The injury sometimes occurs in conjunction with brachial palsy. Respiratory distress is the most common and important sign of injury. Because injury to the phrenic nerve is usually unilateral, the lung on the affected side does not expand, and respiratory efforts are ineffectual. Breathing is primarily thoracic, and cyanosis, tachypnea, or complete respiratory failure may be seen. Pneumonia and atelectasis on the affected side may also occur.

Nursing Care Management

Nursing care of an infant with facial nerve paralysis involves aiding the infant in sucking and helping the mother with feeding techniques. A comprehensive evaluation of the infant's oral motor skills by both an infant feeding specialist and a lactation consultant are recommended to develop an effective multidisciplinary feeding regimen. The infant may require gavage feeding and supplemental oral stimulation with a minimum amount of expressed breast milk to prevent aspiration. Breastfeeding is recommended, and the mother will need assistance in helping the infant grasp and compress the areolar area to ensure effective milk transfer from mother to infant (Lawrence & Lawrence, 2016a).

If the eyelid of the eye on the affected side does not close completely, artificial tears can be instilled daily to prevent drying of the conjunctiva, sclera, and cornea. The eyelid is often taped shut to prevent accidental injury. If eye care is needed at home, the parents are taught the procedure for administering eye drops before the infant is discharged from the nursery (see Chapter 20).

Nursing care of the newborn with brachial palsy is concerned primarily with proper positioning of the affected arm. The affected arm should be gently immobilized on the upper abdomen if a fracture is present; passive range-of-motion exercises of the shoulder, wrist, elbow, and fingers are initiated at 7 to 10 days of age (Yang, 2014). Wrist flexion contractures may be prevented with the use of supportive splints. In dressing the infant, preference is given to the affected arm. Undressing begins with the unaffected arm, and redressing begins with the affected arm to prevent unnecessary manipulation and stress on the paralyzed muscles. Teach parents to use the "football" position when holding the infant and to avoid picking up the child from under the axillae or by pulling on the arms.

The infant with phrenic nerve paralysis requires the same nursing care as any infant with respiratory distress. Mechanical ventilation may be required to prevent further respiratory compromise.

The family's emotional needs are also an important part of nursing care; the family will need reassurance regarding the neonate's progress toward an optimal outcome. Follow-up is also essential because of the extended length of recovery.

CRANIAL DEFORMITIES

In a normal newborn, the cranial sutures are separated by membranous seams several millimeters wide. Up to 2 days after birth, the cranial bones are highly mobile, which allows them to mold and slide over one another, adjusting the circumference of the head to accommodate to the changing shape and character of the birth canal. The principal sutures in the infant's skull are the sagittal, coronal, and lambdoidal sutures, and the major soft areas at the juncture of these sutures are the anterior and posterior fontanels.

After birth, growth of the skull bones occurs in a direction **perpendicular** to the line of the suture, and normal closure occurs in a regular and predictable order. Although there are wide variations in the age at which closure takes place in individual children, normally all sutures and fontanels are ossified by the following ages:

Eight weeks: Posterior fontanel closed
Six months: Fibrous union of suture lines and interlocking of serrated edges
Eighteen months: Anterior fontanel closed
After 12 years: Sutures unable to be separated by increased ICP

Solid union of all sutures is not completed until late childhood. Craniostenosis, closure of a suture before the expected time, inhibits the perpendicular growth. Because normal increase in brain volume requires expansion, the skull is forced to grow in a direction *parallel* to the fused suture. This alteration in skull growth always produces a distortion of the head shape when the underlying brain growth is normal. A small head with closed and normal shape is a result of deficient brain growth; the suture closure is secondary to this brain growth failure. Failure of brain growth is not secondary to suture closure.

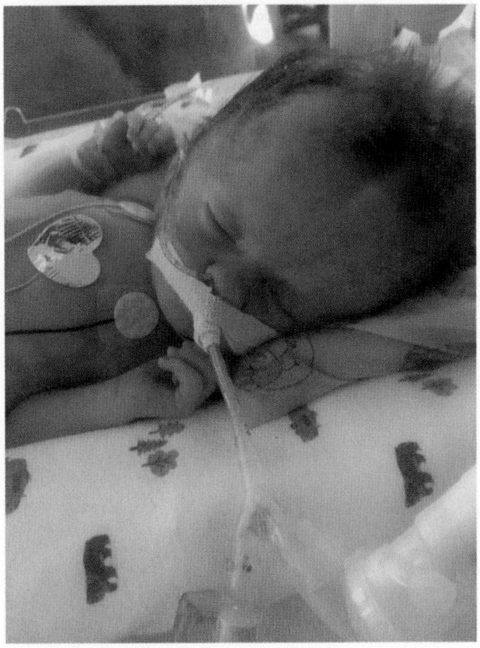

Fig. 8.4 Infant with hydrocephalus. (Courtesy K. Fisher, Duke University Medical Center, Durham, NC.)

Various types of cranial deformities are encountered in early infancy. These include an enlarged head with frontal protrusion (**bossing**; characteristic of hydrocephalus [Fig. 8.4]), parietal bossing that is seen in chronic subdural hematoma, a small head, and a variety of skull deformities. Some occur during prenatal development; in others, head circumference is usually within normal limits at birth, and the deviation from normal development becomes apparent with advancing age.

PROGNOSIS

The majority of infants with craniostenosis have normal brain development. The exceptions are those with genetic disorders that involve brain pathologic conditions.

NURSING CARE MANAGEMENT

Nursing care of families in which there is a child with a cranial defect involves identifying children with deformities and referring them for evaluation. Because no therapy is available for children with microcephaly, nursing care is directed toward helping parents adjust to caring for a child with brain damage (see Chapter 18).

Infants who benefit from surgery require special emphasis on observation for signs of anemia because of the large blood loss during surgery (see Family-Centered Care box). Nursing care includes observation for signs of hemorrhage, infection, pain, and swelling, as well as parental education for suture care and safety (Fig. 8.5). Surgical sutures should remain dry and intact. Parents need to observe for any signs of redness, drainage, or swelling, and report any temperature greater than 38.4°C (101°F).

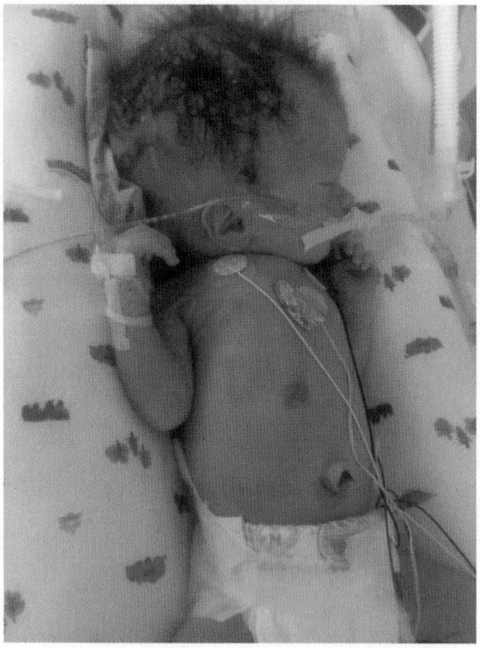

Fig. 8.5 Infant after surgical shunt placement. (Courtesy K. Fisher, Duke University Medical Center, Durham, NC.)

FAMILY-CENTERED CARE

Blood Donation

Parents may wish to provide a compatible blood donor for their infant undergoing a planned surgical correction for craniostenosis. Nurses need to inform and guide parents through the blood bank procedure.

Early surgical management of craniostenosis in children before 1 year of age allows proper expansion of the brain and the creation of an acceptable appearance (Lee, Hwang, Doumit, et al., 2017). Parents require special support and education during this time, especially from the health care team.

STRUCTURAL DEFECTS

Cleft Lip and Cleft Palate

Clefts of the lip (CL) and palate (CP) are facial malformations that occur during embryonic development and are the most common congenital deformities in the United States. They may appear separately or, more often, together.

The palate can be divided into the primary and secondary palates. The primary palate consists of the medial portion of the upper lip and the portion of the alveolar ridge that contains the central and lateral incisors. The secondary palate consists of the remaining portion of the hard palate and all of the soft palate. CL may vary from a small notch in the upper lip to a complete cleft extending into the base of the nose, including the lip and the alveolar ridge (Fig. 8.6). CL can be unilateral or bilateral. Deformed dental structures are associated with CL. Isolated CP occurs in the midline of the secondary palate and may also vary from a bifid uvula (the mildest form of CP) to a complete cleft extending from the soft palate to the hard palate.

Cleft lip and palate (CL/P) is more common than CP alone and varies by ethnicity. The occurrence is 1 in 750 births in whites, 1 in 500 births in Asians, 1 in 300 births in American Indians, and 1 in 2500 births in African Americans (Dhar, 2020). CL/P tends to be more common in males, and isolated CP occurs more frequently in females.

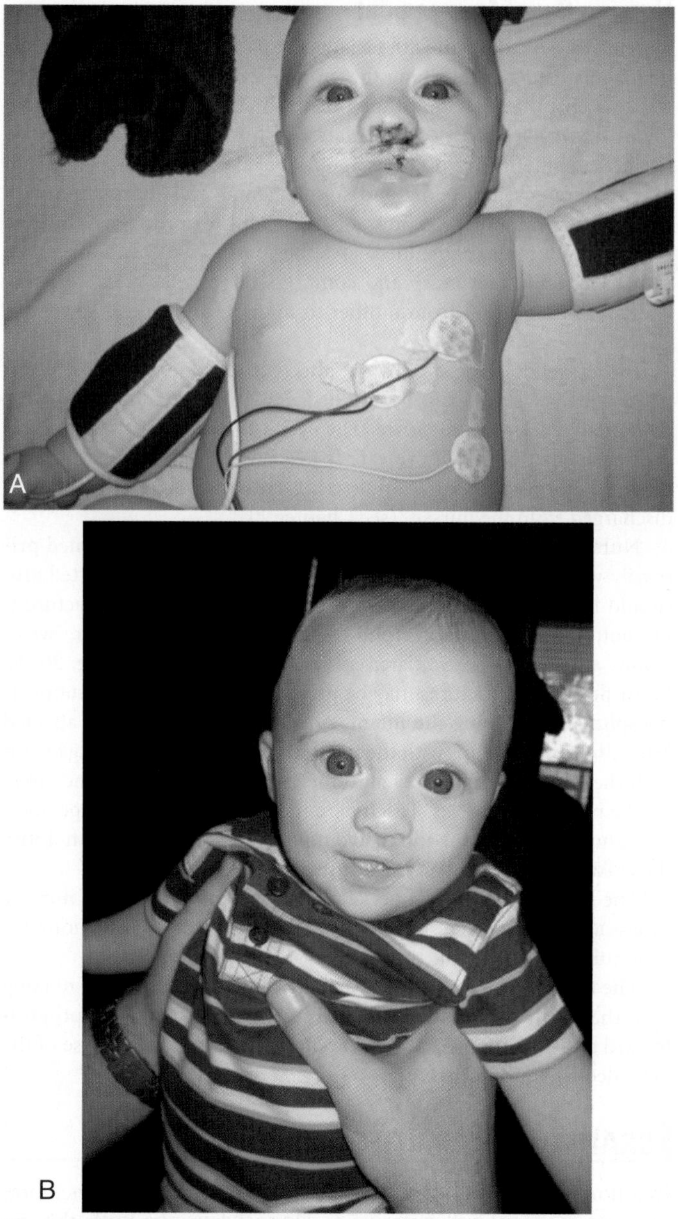

Fig. 8.6 A, Cleft lip (CL) repair at 16 weeks old. Note the elbow restraints. B, CL 3 weeks after surgery repair. (Photo courtesy E. Danks.)

Etiology

Cleft deformities may be an isolated anomaly, or they may occur with a recognized syndrome. CL/P and CP are distinct from isolated CP. Clefts of the secondary palate alone are more likely to be associated with syndromes than are isolated CL or CL/P.

Most cases of CL and CP have multifactorial inheritance, which is generally caused by a combination of genetic and environmental factors. Researchers do not yet know which gene(s) are responsible for clefting or to what extent environmental factors affect the developing structures. Exposure to teratogens such as alcohol, cigarette smoking, anticonvulsants, steroids, and retinoids are associated with higher rates of oral clefting. Folate deficiency is also a risk factor for clefting.

Pathophysiology

Cleft deformities represent a defect in cell migration that results in a failure of the maxillary and premaxillary processes to come together between the fourth and tenth weeks of embryonic development.

Although often appearing together, CL and CP are distinct malformations embryologically, occurring at different times during the developmental process. Merging of the primary palate (upper lip and alveolus bilaterally) is completed by the seventh week of gestation. Fusion of the secondary palate (hard and soft palate) takes place later, between the seventh and tenth weeks of gestation. In the process of migrating to a horizontal position, the palates are separated by the tongue for a short time. If there is delay in this movement or if the tongue fails to descend soon enough, the remaining development proceeds, but the palate never fuses.

Diagnostic Evaluation

CL and CL/P are apparent at birth. CP is less obvious than CL and may not be detected immediately without a thorough assessment of the mouth. CP is identified through visual examination of the oral cavity or when the examiner places a gloved finger directly on the palate. Clefts of the hard and soft palate form a continuous opening between the mouth and the nasal cavity. The severity of the CP has an impact on feeding; the infant is unable to create suction in the oral cavity that is necessary for feeding. However, in most cases, the infant's ability to swallow is normal.

Prenatal diagnosis with fetal ultrasonography is not reliable until the soft tissues of the fetal face can be visualized at 13 to 14 weeks. About 20% to 30% of infants with CL and CL/P are prenatally diagnosed through ultrasonography (Abramson, Peacock, Cohen, et al., 2015), although infants with CP only are rarely diagnosed prenatally.

Therapeutic Management

Treatment of the infant with CL and CP involves the cooperative efforts of a multidisciplinary health care team, including pediatrics, plastic surgery, orthodontics, otolaryngology, lactation consultants, speech/language pathology, audiology, nursing, and social work. Management is directed toward closure of the cleft(s), prevention of complications, and facilitation of normal growth and development in the child.

Surgical Correction of Cleft Lip. CL repair typically occurs at most centers between 2 and 3 months of age. The two most common procedures for repair of CL are the Fisher repair and the Millard rotational advancement technique. Surgeons often use a combination of techniques to address individual differences. Improved surgical techniques and postoperative wound care have minimized scar retraction, and in the absence of infection or trauma, most heal very well (see Fig. 8.6). Nasoalveolar molding may also be used to bring the cleft segments closer together before definitive CL repair, reducing the need for CL revision. Optimal cosmetic results, however, may be difficult to obtain in severe defects. Additional revisions may be necessary at a later age.

Surgical Correction of Cleft Palate. CP repair typically occurs before 12 months of age to enhance normal speech development (Dhar, 2020). The most common techniques to repair CP include the Veau-Wardill-Kilner V-Y pushback procedure and the Furlow double-opposing Z-plasty. Approximately 20% to 30% of children with repaired CP will need a secondary surgery to improve velopharyngeal closure for speech. Secondary procedures may include palatal lengthening, pharyngeal flap, sphincter pharyngoplasty, or posterior pharyngeal wall augmentation. If the child is not a candidate for surgical revision to improve velopharyngeal function, prosthetic management should be considered.

Prognosis

Children with CL may require multiple surgeries to achieve optimal aesthetic outcomes but are not at risk for increased speech problems. Although some children with CP and CL/P do not require speech therapy, many have some degree of speech impairment that requires speech therapy at some point throughout childhood. Articulation errors result from a history of velopharyngeal dysfunction, incorrect articulatory placement, improper tooth alignment, and varying degrees of hearing loss. Improper drainage of the middle ear as a result of inefficient function of the eustachian tube relating to the history of CP contributes to recurrent otitis media, which leads to conductive hearing loss in many children with CP; many children with clefts will have pressure-equalization tubes placed. Extensive orthodontics and prosthodontics may be needed to correct malposition of the teeth and maxillary arches. Academic achievement, social adjustment, and behavior should be monitored, particularly in children with syndromic cleft conditions.

Nursing Care Management

The immediate nursing problems for an infant with CL/P deformities are related to feeding. Parents of newborns with clefts place high priority on learning how to feed their infants and identify when they are sick, but they also express interest in learning about the infant's "normal" features. Whenever possible, they should be referred to a comprehensive CP team.

Feeding. Feeding the infant with a cleft presents a challenge to nurses and parents. Growth failure in infants with CL/P or CP has been attributed to preoperative feeding difficulties. After surgical repair, most infants who have isolated CL, CP, or CL/P with no associated syndromes gain weight or achieve adequate weight and height for age.

CL may interfere with an infant's ability to achieve an adequate anterior lip seal. An infant with an isolated CL typically has no difficulty breastfeeding because the breast tissue is able to conform to the cleft. If bottle-fed, an infant with an isolated CL may have greater success using bottles with a wide base of the nipple, such as a Playtex nurser or a NUK (orthodontic) nipple. Cheek support (squeezing the cheeks together to decrease the width of the cleft) may be useful in improving lip seal during feeding.

Mothers should be encouraged to provide the protective benefits of breast milk. Infants with CP and CL/P should be individually evaluated for breastfeeding and provided knowledgeable support. It is important to assess the following: (1) size and location of the baby's CL/P, (2) mother's desire to provide breast milk, and (3) previous experience with breastfeeding (Reilly, Reid, Skeat, et al., 2013). CP reduces the infant's ability to suck, which interferes with breastfeeding and traditional bottle-feeding. Modifications to positioning, bottle selection, and feeder supportive techniques can help infants with CP feed efficiently. Begin by positioning an infant with CP in an upright position with the head supported by the caregiver's hand or cradled in the arm; this position allows gravity to assist with the flow of the liquid so that it is swallowed instead of lost through the nose.

Suction is almost certainly impaired in infants with CP because the velum is unable to elevate and separate the oral nasal cavities while generating adequate negative intraoral pressure. Several types of bottles work well with infants unable to generate adequate suction, including the SpecialNeeds Feeder (formerly Haberman), the Pigeon bottle, and the Mead Johnson Cleft Palate Nurser. The SpecialNeeds Feeder and the Pigeon bottles use a one-way flow valve that allows the infant to feed successfully by compressing the nipple with either the intact segments of the palate and the mandible or the tongue. With the one-way flow valve in place, the liquid flows into the oral cavity rather than back into the bottle chamber when the nipple is compressed. The SpecialNeeds Feeder also has a large nipple chamber that allows the feeder to provide extra assistance by squeezing the chamber if needed. The tip of the SpecialNeeds Feeder has a slit cut, which allows the feeder to control the flow of liquid by positioning the slit vertically or horizontally within the mouth, which can reduce choking and gagging. The Pigeon bottle comes with two nipple sizes—standard and small—each with a Y-cut nipple that increases the flow of liquid. The third bottle, the Mead Johnson Cleft Palate Nurser, is a squeezable bottle with a long, thin X-cut nipple; this bottle requires the feeder to rhythmically squeeze the bottle throughout the feeding and does not require the infant to actively compress the nipple during the feeding.

Infants with clefts tend to swallow excessive air during feedings, so it is important to pause during feedings and burp the infant. Some CP specialists advocate for the use of feeding obturators to assist with feeding; these devices may increase compression surfaces within the oral cavity but do not improve feeding efficiency or growth within the first year of life (Lawrence & Lawrence, 2016a).

Regardless of the feeding method used, the mother should begin feeding the infant as soon as possible. When maternal feeding is initiated early, the mother can help to determine the method best suited to her and the infant and can become adept in the technique before discharge from the hospital.

Preoperative Care. In preparation for surgical repair, parents may be taught to use alternative feeding systems (e.g., syringes) several days before surgery. For CL, many surgeons allow babies to return to their typical feeding system. However, for CP, some surgeons require that the child be off the bottle and drinking from an open cup or sippy cup.

Postoperative Care. The major efforts in the postoperative period are directed toward protecting the operative site. For CL, parents may be advised to apply petroleum jelly to the operative site for several days after surgery. For CL, CP, or CL/P, elbow immobilizers may be used to prevent the infant from rubbing or disturbing the suture line; they are applied immediately after surgery and may be used for 7 to 10 days. Some centers advocate using a syringe for feeding for 7 to 10 days after CL or CP repair. Adequate analgesia is required to relieve postoperative pain and to prevent restlessness. Feeding is resumed when tolerated. An upright or infant seat position is helpful in the immediate postoperative period (especially for infants who have difficulty handling secretions). Avoid the use of suction or other objects in the mouth, such as tongue depressors, thermometers, pacifiers, spoons, and straws.

The older infant or child may be discharged on a blenderized or soft diet, and parents are instructed to continue the diet until the surgeon directs them otherwise. Parents are cautioned against allowing the child to eat hard items (e.g., toast, hard cookies, and potato chips) that can damage the repaired palate.

Long-Term Care. Children with CL/P often require a variety of services during recovery. Family members need support and encouragement by health professionals and guidance in activities that facilitate a normal outcome for their child. Parents frequently cite financial stress as a difficult issue. With the combined efforts of the family and the health team, most children achieve a satisfactory outcome. Many children with CL/P have surgical correction that creates a near normal–appearing lip and permits good function of the palate for speech and feeding. Parents need to understand the function of speech therapy and the purpose and care of all orthodontic appliances, as well as the importance of establishing good mouth care and proper brushing habits.

Throughout the child's development, an important goal is the development of a healthy personality and self-esteem. Many communities have CP parents' groups that offer help and support to families. Agencies that provide services and information for children with CL/P and their families include the American Cleft Palate–Craniofacial Association (http://www.acpa-cpf.org), the Cleft Palate Foundation (http://www.cleftline.org), Cleft Advocate (http://www.cleftadvocate.org), the March of Dimes (http://www.marchforbabies.org), and various state children's medical services.

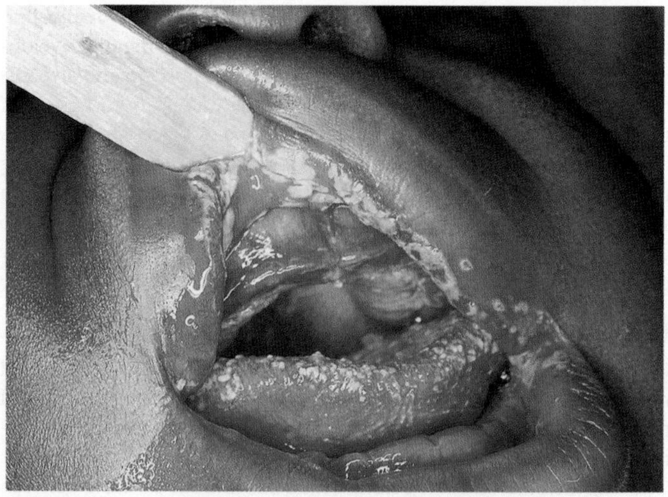

Fig. 8.7 Oral candidiasis (thrush). (From Paller, A. S., & Mancini, A. J. [2016]. *Hurwitz clinical pediatric dermatology* [5th ed.]. St Louis, MO: Elsevier.)

COMMON PROBLEMS IN THE NEWBORN

ERYTHEMA TOXICUM NEONATORUM

Erythema toxicum neonatorum, also known as **flea-bite dermatitis** or **newborn rash**, is a benign, self-limiting eruption of unknown cause that usually appears within the first 2 days of life. The lesions are firm, 1- to 3-mm, pale yellow or white papules or pustules on an erythematous base; they resemble flea bites. The rash appears most commonly on the face, proximal extremities, trunk, and buttocks, but it may be located anywhere on the body except the palms and soles. The rash is more obvious during crying episodes. There are no systemic manifestations, and successive crops of lesions heal without pigmentation changes. The rash usually lasts about 5 to 7 days. The etiology is unknown. However, a smear of the pustule will show numerous eosinophils and a relative absence of neutrophils. When the diagnosis is questionable, bacterial, fungal, or viral cultures should be obtained. Although no treatment is necessary, parents are usually concerned about the rash and need to be reassured of its benign and transient nature.

CANDIDIASIS

Candidiasis, also known as **moniliasis**, is not uncommon in newborns. *Candida albicans*, the usual organism responsible, may cause disease in any organ system. It is a yeastlike fungus (it produces yeast cells and spores) that can be acquired from a maternal vaginal infection during delivery; from person-to-person transmission (especially from poor hand-washing technique); or from contaminated hands, bottles, nipples, or other articles. Mucocutaneous, cutaneous, and disseminated candidal infections are all observed in this age-group. Candidiasis is usually a benign disorder in neonates, often confined to the oral and diaper regions. In extremely preterm infants, there is an increased risk of serious systemic infections caused by *Candida*. **Diaper dermatitis** caused by *Candida* organisms manifests as a moist, erythematous eruption with small white or yellow pebbly pustules. Small areas of skin erosion may also be seen (see Chapter 10, Diaper Dermatitis).

Oral Candidiasis

Oral candidiasis (**thrush**) is characterized by white, adherent patches on the tongue, palate, and inner aspects of the cheeks (Fig. 8.7). It is often difficult to distinguish from coagulated milk. The infant may refuse to suck because of pain in the mouth.

This condition tends to be acute in newborns and chronic in infants and young children. Thrush appears when the oral flora is altered as a result of antibiotic therapy or poor hand washing by the infant's caregiver. Although the disorder is usually self-limiting, spontaneous resolution may take as long as 2 months, during which time lesions may spread to the larynx, trachea, bronchi, and lungs, and along the gastrointestinal tract. The disease is treated with good hygiene, application of a fungicide, and correction of any underlying disturbance. The source of infection should be treated to prevent reinfection.

Topical application of 1 ml nystatin (Mycostatin) over the surfaces of the oral cavity four times a day, or every 6 hours, is usually sufficient to prevent spread of the disease or prolongation of its course. Several other drugs may be used, including amphotericin B (Fungizone), clotrimazole (Lotrimin, Mycelex), fluconazole (Diflucan), or miconazole (Monistat, Micatin) given intravenously, orally, or topically. To prevent relapse, therapy should be continued for at least 2 days after the lesions disappear (Lawrence & Lawrence, 2016a). Gentian violet solution may be used in addition to one of the antifungal drugs in chronic cases of oral thrush; however, the former does not treat gastrointestinal *Candida* infection. Some practitioners avoid its use because it is messy, easily stains clothing, and may be irritating to the oral mucosa.

! NURSING ALERT

Oral candidiasis can be distinguished from coagulated milk when attempts to remove the patches with a tongue blade are unsuccessful. The primary caregiver may also report that the infant does not nurse well or bottle-feed as previously.

Nursing Care Management

Nursing care is directed toward preventing spread of the infection and correctly applying the prescribed topical medication. For candidiasis in the diaper area, the caregiver is taught to keep the diaper area clean and to apply the medication to affected areas as prescribed (see also Chapter 10, Diaper Dermatitis). Older infants with *Candida* diaper dermatitis can introduce the yeast into the mouth from contaminated hands. Placing clothes over the diaper can prevent this cycle of self-infection.

In cases of oral thrush, nystatin is administered after feedings. Distribute the medication over the surface of the oral mucosa and tongue with an applicator or syringe; the remainder of the dose is deposited in the mouth to be swallowed by the infant to treat any gastrointestinal lesions.

In addition to good hygienic care, other measures to control thrush include rinsing the infant's mouth with plain water after each feeding before applying the medication and boiling reusable nipples and bottles for at least 20 minutes after a thorough washing (spores are heat resistant). If used, pacifiers should be boiled for at least 20 minutes once daily. If the mother is breastfeeding, it is recommended that simultaneous treatment of the infant and mother occur if either is infected (Lawrence & Lawrence, 2016a).

HERPES SIMPLEX VIRUS

Neonatal herpes is one of the most serious viral infections in newborns, with a mortality rate of up to 60% in infants with disseminated disease. Approximately 85% of herpes simplex virus (HSV) transmission occurs during passage through the birth canal (James, Sheffield, & Kimberlin, 2014). The risk of infection during vaginal birth in the presence of genital herpes is estimated to be 25% to 60% with active primary infection at term (American Academy of Pediatrics, 2018). Globally, the incidence of neonatal herpes infection continues to warrant vigilance, as genital HSV infections among adolescents and adults are a global health problem estimated to affect more than half a billion people worldwide (Looker, Magaret, May, et al., 2017).

Neonatal herpes manifests in one of three ways: (1) with skin, eye, and mouth (SEM) involvement; (2) as localized central nervous system (CNS) disease; or (3) as disseminated disease involving multiple organs. In skin and eye disease, a rash appears as vesicles or pustules on an erythematous base. Clusters of lesions are common. The lesions ulcerate and crust over rapidly. Ophthalmologic findings include keratoconjunctivitis, chorioretinitis, cataracta, and retinal detachment; neurologic involvement (such as microcephaly and encephalomalacia) may also develop (Baley & Gonzalez, 2015). Disseminated infections may involve virtually every organ system, but the liver, adrenal glands, and lungs are most commonly affected. In HSV meningitis, infants develop multiple lesions with cortical hemorrhagic necrosis. It can occur alone or with oral, eye, or skin lesions. The presenting symptoms, which may occur in the second to fourth weeks of life, include lethargy, poor feeding, irritability, and local or generalized seizures.

Nursing Care Management

Neonates with herpesvirus or suspected infection (as a result of exposure) should be carefully evaluated for clinical manifestations. The absence of skin lesions in the neonate exposed to maternal herpesvirus does not indicate absence of disease. Contact Precautions (in addition to Standard Precautions) should be instituted according to the American Academy of Pediatrics and American College of Obstetricians and Gynecologists (2017) guidelines or hospital protocol. It is recommended that swabs of the mouth, nasopharynx, conjunctivae, rectum, and any skin vesicles be obtained from the exposed neonate; in addition, urine, blood, and cerebrospinal fluid (CSF) specimens should be obtained for culture. Therapy with acyclovir is initiated if the culture results are positive or if there is strong suspicion of herpesvirus infection (Kimberlin, 2018). High-dose acyclovir (60 mg/kg/day) has been shown to decrease mortality rates in infants with disseminated HSV (Ericson, Gostelow, Autmizguine, et al., 2017).

BIRTHMARKS

Discolorations of the skin are common findings in newborn infants (see discussion of skin assessment of newborns in Chapter 7). Most, such as mongolian spots or telangiectatic nevi, involve no therapy other than reassurance to parents of the benign nature of these discolorations. However, some can be a manifestation of a disease that suggests further examination of the child and other family members (e.g., the multiple light brown **café-au-lait spots** that often characterize the autosomal dominant hereditary disorder neurofibromatosis and are common findings in Albright syndrome).

Darker or more extensive lesions demand further scrutiny, and excision of the lesion is recommended when feasible. Such lesions include a reddish brown solitary nodule that appears on the face or upper arm and usually represents a spindle and epithelioid cell nevus (**juvenile melanoma**); a **giant pigmented nevus** (or **bathing trunk nevus**), a dark brown to black, irregular plaque that is at risk of transformation to malignant melanoma; and the dark brown or black macules that become more numerous with age (**junctional** or **compound nevi**).

Vascular birthmarks may be divided into the following categories: vascular malformations, capillary hemangiomas, and mixed hemangiomas. **Vascular stains (malformations)** are permanent lesions that are present at birth and are initially flat and erythematous. Any vascular

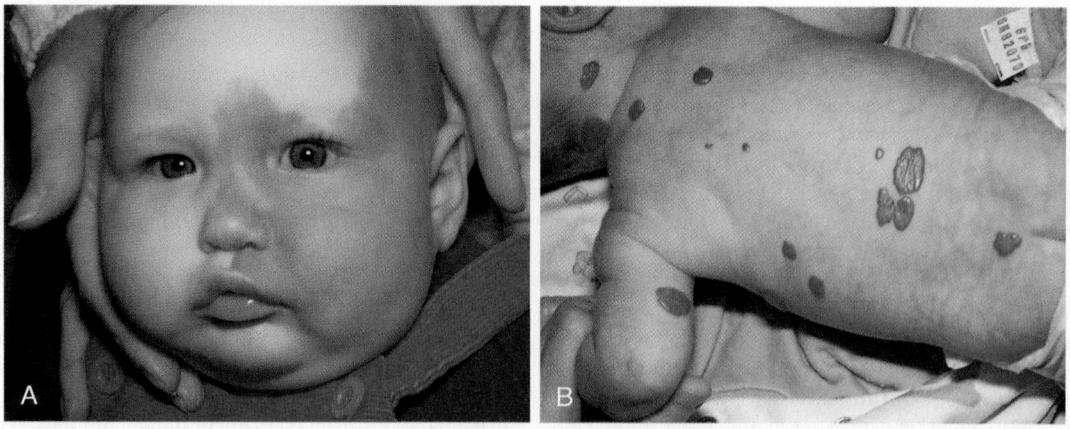

Fig. 8.8 **A,** Port-wine stain. **B,** Strawberry hemangioma. (From Zitelli, B. J., McIntire, S. C., & Nowalk, A. J. *Zitelli and Davis' atlas of pediatric physical diagnosis* [6th ed.]. St Louis, MO: Saunders/Elsevier.)

structure, capillary, vein, artery, or lymphatic may be involved. The two most common vascular stains are the **transient macular stain** (stork bite, salmon patch, or angel kiss) and the **port-wine stain**, or **nevus flammeus**. The port-wine lesions are pink, red, or, rarely, purple stains of the skin that thicken, darken, and proportionately enlarge as the child grows (Fig. 8.8A). The macular stain is most often located on the eyelids, glabella, or nape of the neck and usually fades over several months but may be prominent with crying or environmental temperature changes.

Port-wine stains may also be associated with structural malformations, such as glaucoma or leptomeningeal angiomatosis (tumor of blood or lymph vessels in the pia-arachnoid) (**Sturge-Weber syndrome**) or bony or muscular overgrowth (**Klippel-Trenaunay-Weber syndrome**). Children with port-wine stains on the eyelids, forehead, or cheeks should be monitored for these syndromes with periodic ophthalmologic examination, neurologic imaging, and measurement of extremities.

The treatment of choice for port-wine stains is the use of the pulsed-dye laser. A series of treatments is usually needed. The treatments can significantly lighten or completely clear the lesions with almost no scarring or pigment change.

Capillary hemangiomas, sometimes referred to as **strawberry hemangiomas**, are benign cutaneous tumors that involve only capillaries. These hemangiomas are bright red, rubbery nodules with a rough surface and a well-defined margin (see Fig. 8.8B). Strawberry hemangiomas may not be apparent at birth but may appear within a few weeks and enlarge considerably during the first year of life and then begin to involute spontaneously. It may take 5 to 12 years for complete resolution, and a significant number of patients may be left with residual findings, such as telangiectasia, redundant fatty tissue, or skin atrophy (Ji, Chen, Li, et al., 2014). Topical timolol solution (0.5% gel; maximum dose 0.5 mg/day) is effective for cases that require intervention, and systemic propranolol may be used in severe cases to shrink the lesions (Martin, 2020). **Cavernous venous hemangiomas** involve deeper vessels in the dermis and have a bluish red color and poorly defined margins. These latter forms may be associated with the trapping of platelets (**Kasabach-Merritt syndrome**) and subsequent thrombocytopenia (Martin, 2020; Witt, 2015).

Hemangiomas may also occur as part of the PHACE syndrome (Valdivielso-Ramos, Torrelo, Martin-Santiago, et al., 2018):

Posterior fossa brain malformation
Hemangiomas (segmental cervicofacial)
Arterial anomalies
Cardiac defects, including coarctation of the aorta
Eye anomalies

Although most hemangiomas require no treatment because of their high rate of spontaneous involution, some vision and airway obstruction may necessitate therapy. Systemic propranolol or prednisone may deter further growth. Subcutaneous injections of interferon or vincristine may be required if prednisone therapy and the pulsed-dye laser fail to control a problematic hemangioma; however, the associated side effects may outweigh the benefits of therapy in some cases (Martin, 2020).

Nursing Care Management

Birthmarks, especially those on the face, are upsetting to parents. Families need an explanation of the type of lesion, its significance, and possible treatment.[a] Parents can benefit from seeing photographs of other infants before and after treatment for port-wine stains or after the passage of time for hemangiomas. Pictures taken to follow the involution process may further help parents gain confidence that progress is taking place.

If laser therapy is performed, the lesion will have a purplish black appearance for 7 to 10 days, after which the blackness fades and gives way to redness with an eventual lightening of the treated area. During the treatment phase, parents are cautioned to avoid any trauma to the lesion or picking at the scab. The child's fingernails are trimmed as an added precaution. Washing the area gently with water and dabbing it dry is adequate, although in some cases a topical antibiotic ointment may be used. No salicylates should be taken during the treatment phase because they decrease the effects of the therapy. The child should be kept out of the sun for several weeks and then protected with a sunscreen that has a sun protection factor (SPF) of at least 25. Complications associated with laser treatment include redness and bruising and, less commonly, hyperpigmentation, hypopigmentation, and atrophic scarring (Furuta, Sato, Tsuji, et al., 2016).

NURSING CARE OF THE HIGH-RISK NEWBORN AND FAMILY

IDENTIFICATION OF HIGH-RISK NEWBORNS

A **high-risk neonate** can be defined as a newborn, regardless of gestational age or birth weight, who has a greater than average chance of morbidity or mortality because of conditions or circumstances

[a] Laboratories should verify that these ranges are appropriate for use in their own settings.

associated with birth and adjustment to the extrauterine environment. The high-risk period encompasses human growth and development from the time of viability (the gestational age at which survival outside the uterus is believed to be possible, or as early as 23 weeks of gestation) up to 28 days after birth; thus it includes threats to life and health that occur during the prenatal, perinatal, and postnatal periods.

There has been increased interest in late-preterm infants of 34 to $36^6/_7$ weeks of gestation who may receive the same treatment as term infants. Late-preterm infants often experience similar morbidities to preterm infants, including respiratory distress, hypoglycemia requiring treatment, temperature instability, poor feeding, jaundice, and adverse neurodevelopmental outcomes (Horgan, 2015). Therefore assessment and prompt intervention in life-threatening perinatal emergencies often make the difference between a favorable outcome and a lifetime of disability. It is estimated that late-preterm infants represent 70% of the total preterm infant population and that the mortality rate for this group is up to five times higher than that of term infants (Horgan, 2015). Because late-preterm infants' birth weights often range from 2000 to 2500 g (4.4 to 5.5 pounds) and they appear relatively mature compared with smaller preterm infants, they may be cared for in the same manner as healthy term infants, leaving risk factors for late-preterm infants overlooked. Late-preterm infants are often discharged early from the birth institution and have a significantly higher rate of rehospitalization than term infants (Reedy, 2014). Discussions of high-risk infants in this chapter also refer to late-preterm infants who are experiencing a delayed transition to extrauterine life. Nurses in newborn nurseries should be familiar with the characteristics of neonates and recognize the significance of serious deviations from expected observations. When providers can anticipate the need for specialized care and plan for it, the probability of successful outcome is increased.

The Association of Women's Health, Obstetric and Neonatal Nurses (2017) has published the *Assessment and Care of the Late Preterm Infant* guide for the education of perinatal nurses, regarding the late-preterm infant's risk factors and appropriate care and follow-up care.

Classification of High-Risk Newborns

High-risk infants are most often classified according to birth weight, gestational age, and predominant pathophysiologic problems. The more common problems related to physiologic status are closely associated with the state of maturity of the infant and usually involve chemical disturbances (e.g., hypoglycemia, hypocalcemia) or consequences of immature organs and systems (e.g., hyperbilirubinemia, respiratory distress, hypothermia). Because high-risk factors are common to several specialty areas—particularly obstetrics, pediatrics, and neonatology—specific terminology is needed to describe the developmental status of the newborn (Box 8.1).

Formerly, weight at birth was considered to reflect a reasonably accurate estimation of gestational age; that is, if an infant's birth weight exceeded 2500 g (5.5 pounds), the infant was considered mature. However, accumulated data have shown that intrauterine growth rates are not the same for all infants and that other factors (e.g., heredity, placental insufficiency, maternal disease) influence intrauterine growth and birth weight. From these data, a more definitive and meaningful classification system that encompasses birth weight, gestational age, and neonatal outcome has been developed.

BOX 8.1 Classification of High-Risk Infants

Classification According to Size

Low birth weight (LBW) infant: An infant whose birth weight is less than 2500 g (5.5 pounds) regardless of gestational age

Very low birth weight (VLBW) infant: An infant whose birth weight is less than 1500 g (3.3 pounds)

Extremely low birth weight (ELBW) infant: An infant whose birth weight is less than 1000 g (2.2 pounds)

Appropriate for gestational age (AGA) infant: An infant whose weight falls between the 10th and 90th percentiles on intrauterine growth curves

Small for date (SFD) or small for gestational age (SGA) infant: An infant whose rate of intrauterine growth was slowed and whose birth weight falls below the 10th percentile on intrauterine growth curves

Intrauterine growth restriction (IUGR): Found in infants whose intrauterine growth is restricted (sometimes used as a more descriptive term for SGA infants)

Symmetric IUGR: Growth restriction in which the weight, length, and head circumference are all affected

Asymmetric IUGR: Growth restriction in which the head circumference remains within normal parameters while the birth weight falls below the 10th percentile

Large for gestational age (LGA) infant: An infant whose birth weight falls above the 90th percentile on intrauterine growth charts

Classification According to Gestational Age

Preterm (premature) infant: An infant born before completion of 37 weeks of gestation regardless of birth weight

Full-term infant: An infant born between the beginning of 38 weeks and the completion of 42 weeks of gestation regardless of birth weight

Late-preterm infant: An infant born between 34 0/7 and 36 0/7 weeks of gestation regardless of birth weight

Postterm (postmature) infant: An infant born after 42 weeks of gestational age regardless of birth weight

Classification According to Mortality

Live birth: Birth in which the neonate manifests any heartbeat, breathes, or displays voluntary movement regardless of gestational age

Fetal death: Death of the fetus after 20 weeks of gestation and before delivery with absence of any signs of life after birth

Neonatal death: Death that occurs in the first 27 days of life; early neonatal death occurs in the first week of life; late neonatal death occurs at 7 to 27 days

Perinatal mortality: Total number of fetal and early neonatal deaths per 1000 live births

CARE OF HIGH-RISK NEWBORNS

Systematic Assessment

A thorough systematic physical assessment is an essential component in the care of high-risk infants (see Nursing Care Guidelines box). Subtle changes in feeding behavior, activity, color, oxygen saturation (SaO_2), or vital signs often indicate an underlying problem. Low birth weight (LBW) preterm infants, especially very low birth weight (VLBW) or extremely low birth weight (ELBW) infants, are ill equipped to withstand prolonged physiologic stress and may die within minutes of exhibiting abnormal symptoms if the underlying pathologic process is not corrected. Alert nurses are aware of subtle changes and react promptly to implement interventions that promote optimum functioning in high-risk neonates. Changes in the infant's status are noted through ongoing observations of the infant's adaptation to the extrauterine environment.

Monitoring Physiologic Data

Most neonates needing close observation are placed in a controlled thermal environment and monitored for heart rate, respiratory

NURSING CARE GUIDELINES

Physical Assessment

General Assessment

Using an accurate scale, weigh daily, or more often if indicated.
Measure length and head circumference at birth.
Describe general body shape and size, posture at rest, ease of breathing, presence and location of edema.
Describe any apparent deformities.
Describe any signs of distress—poor color, hypotonia, lethargy, apnea.

Respiratory Assessment

Describe shape of chest (barrel, concave), symmetry, presence of incisions, chest tubes, or other deviations.
Describe use of accessory muscles—nasal flaring or substernal, intercostal, or suprasternal retractions.
Determine respiratory rate and regularity.
Auscultate and describe breath sounds—crackles, wheezing, wet or diminished sounds, grunting, diminished air movement, stridor, equality of breath sounds.
Describe cry if not intubated.
Describe ambient oxygen and method of delivery; if intubated, describe size and position of tube, type of ventilator, and settings.
Determine oxygen saturation by pulse oximetry and partial pressure of oxygen, and describe carbon dioxide by transcutaneous carbon dioxide ($tcPCO_2$).

Cardiovascular Assessment

Determine heart rate and rhythm.
Describe heart sounds, including any murmurs.
Determine the point of maximum impulse (PMI), the point at which the heartbeat sounds and palpates loudest (a change in the PMI may indicate a mediastinal shift).
Describe infant's color—cyanosis (may be of cardiac, respiratory, or hematopoietic origin), pallor, plethora, jaundice, mottling.
Assess color of mucous membranes, lips.
Determine blood pressure (BP) as indicated. Indicate extremity used and cuff size.
Describe femoral pulses, capillary refill, and peripheral perfusion (mottling).
Describe monitors, their parameters, and whether alarms are in the "on" position.

Gastrointestinal Assessment

Determine presence of abdominal distention—increase in circumference, shiny skin, evidence of abdominal wall erythema, visible peristalsis, visible loops of bowel, status of umbilicus.
Determine any signs of regurgitation and time related to feeding; describe character and amount of residual if gavage fed; if nasogastric tube is in place, describe type of suction and drainage (color, consistency, pH).
Describe amount, color, consistency, and odor of any emesis.
Palpate liver margin (1 to 3 cm below right costal margin).
Describe amount, color, and consistency of stools.
Describe bowel sounds—presence or absence (must be present if feeding).

Genitourinary Assessment

Describe any abnormalities of genitalia.
Describe amount (as determined by weight), color, pH, lab stick findings, and specific gravity of urine.
Check weight.

Neurologic–Musculoskeletal Assessment

Describe infant's movements—random, purposeful, jittery, twitching, spontaneous, elicited; describe level of activity with stimulation; evaluate based on gestational age.
Describe infant's position or attitude—flexed, extended.
Describe reflexes observed—Moro, sucking, Babinski, plantar, and other expected reflexes.
Determine level of response and consolability.
Determine changes in head circumference (if indicated), size and tension of fontanels, suture lines.
Determine pupillary responses in infant older than 32 weeks of gestation.
Check hip alignment (only experienced practitioner should perform).

Temperature

Determine axillary temperature.
Determine relationship to environmental temperature.

Skin Assessment

Note any skin lesions or birthmarks.
Describe any discoloration, reddened area, signs of irritation, blisters, abrasions, or denuded areas, especially where monitoring equipment, infusions, or other apparatus come in contact with skin; also check and note any skin preparation used (e.g., skin disinfectants).
Determine texture and turgor of skin—dry, smooth, flaky, peeling, and so on.
Describe any rash, skin lesion, or birthmarks.
Determine whether intravenous (IV) infusion catheter is in place and observe for signs of infiltration.
Describe parenteral infusion lines—location, type (arterial, venous, peripheral, umbilical, central, peripheral central venous), type of infusion (medication, saline, dextrose, electrolyte, lipids, total parenteral nutrition), type of infusion pump and rate of flow, type of catheter, and appearance of insertion site.
Observational assessments of high-risk infants are made according to each infant's acuity; critically ill infants require close observation and assessment of respiratory function, including continuous pulse oximetry, electrolytes, and evaluation of blood gases. Accurate documentation of the infant's status is an integral component of nursing care. With the aid of continuous, sophisticated cardiopulmonary monitoring, nursing assessments and daily care may be coordinated to allow for minimal handling of the infant (especially very low birth weight [VLBW] or extremely low birth weight [ELBW] infants) to decrease the effects of environmental stress.

activity, and temperature. The monitoring devices are equipped with an alarm system that indicates when the vital signs are above or below preset limits. However, it is essential to check the apical heart rate and compare it with the monitor reading.

Blood pressure (BP) is monitored routinely in sick neonates by either internal or external means. Direct recording with arterial catheters may be used but carries the risks inherent in any procedure in which a catheter is introduced into an artery. BP values gradually increase over the first month of life in preterm and term infants. BP norms vary by gestational age and weight, medications (such as corticosteroids), and disease process. One of the primary considerations in the preterm infant is the relationship between systemic BP and the determination of adequate cerebral blood flow. In the neonatal intensive care unit (NICU), frequent laboratory examinations and their interpretation are integral parts of the ongoing assessment of infants' progress. Accurate intake and output records are kept on all acutely ill infants. An accurate output can be obtained by weighing first the dry diaper followed by the soiled diaper and then subtracting the difference; this is the simplest and least traumatic means of measuring urinary output. The preweighed wet diaper is weighed on a gram scale, and the gram weight of the urine is converted directly to milliliters (e.g., 25 g = 25 ml).

Blood examinations are a necessary part of the ongoing assessment and monitoring of the high-risk newborn's progress. The tests most often performed are blood glucose, bilirubin, calcium, hematocrit, serum electrolytes, and blood gases. Samples may be obtained from the heel; by venipuncture; by arterial puncture; or by an indwelling catheter in an umbilical vein, an umbilical artery, or a peripheral artery (see the Atraumatic Care box in Chapter 7 and Chapter 20, Collection of Specimens).

When numerous blood samples must be drawn, it is important to maintain an accurate record of the amount of blood being removed, especially in ELBW and VLBW infants. There is an increased emphasis on drawing as little blood as possible from high-risk neonates to minimize the depletion of blood volume and avoid blood transfusions and associated complications. To avoid the need for repeated arterial punctures, pulse oximetry, which measures the saturation or percentage of oxygen in the hemoglobin, is typically used. The nurse notes changes in oxygenation (or other aspects being monitored) associated with handling and adjusts the infant's care accordingly. The frequency of vital signs is determined by the infant's acuity level (seriousness of condition) and response to handling.

Respiratory Support

The primary objective in the care of high-risk infants is to establish and maintain adequate respiration. Many infants require supplemental oxygen and assisted ventilation. All infants require appropriate positioning to maximize oxygenation and ventilation. Oxygen therapy is provided on the basis of the infant's requirements and illness (see the Respiratory Distress Syndrome section later in this chapter).

Thermoregulation

After or concurrent with the establishment of respiration, the most crucial need of LBW infants is application of external warmth. Prevention of heat loss in distressed infants is essential for survival, and maintaining a neutral thermal environment is a challenging aspect of neonatal intensive nursing care. Heat production is a complicated process that involves the cardiovascular, neurologic, and metabolic systems; and immature neonates have all of the problems related to heat production that are faced by full-term infants (see Chapter 7, Thermoregulation). However, LBW infants are placed at further disadvantage by a number of additional problems. They have an even smaller muscle mass and fewer deposits of brown fat for producing heat, lack insulating subcutaneous fat, and have poor reflex control of skin capillaries.

To reduce the risk of cold stress, at-risk newborns are placed skin-to-skin with their mother if medically stable or in a heated environment immediately after birth, where they remain until they are able to maintain **thermal stability**, which is the capacity to balance heat production and conservation with heat dissipation. Because overheating produces an increase in oxygen and calorie consumption, infants are also jeopardized in a hyperthermic environment. A **neutral thermal environment** is one that permits the infant to maintain a normal core temperature with minimum oxygen consumption and calorie expenditure. Studies indicate that optimum thermoneutrality cannot be predicted for every high-risk infant's needs. In healthy term infants, it is recommended that axillary temperatures be maintained at 36.5° to 37.5°C (97.7° to 99.5°F) (American Academy of Pediatrics, Committee on Fetus and Newborn & American College of Obstetricians and Gynecologists, Committee on Obstetric Practice, 2017); in preterm infants, admission temperatures of 36.5° and 37.2°C (97.7° and 98.9°F) are considered optimal (Lyu, Shah, Ye, et al., 2015).

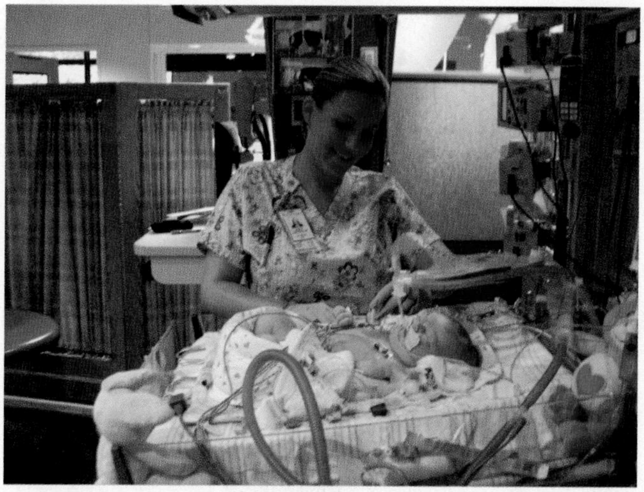

Fig. 8.9 Nurse caring for an infant in a radiant warmer. (Photo courtesy E. Jacobs, Texas Children's Hospital, Houston, TX.)

VLBW and ELBW infants, with thin skin and almost no subcutaneous fat, can control body heat loss or gain only within a limited range of environmental temperatures. In these infants, heat loss from radiation, evaporation, and transepidermal water loss is three to five times greater than in larger infants, and a decrease in body temperature is associated with an increase in mortality. Further research is needed to define a neutral thermal environment for ELBW infants.

The consequences of cold stress that produce additional hazards to neonates are (1) hypoxia, (2) metabolic acidosis, and (3) hypoglycemia. Increased metabolism in response to chilling creates a compensatory increase in oxygen and calorie consumption. If available oxygen is not increased to accommodate this need, arterial oxygen tension is decreased. This is further complicated by a smaller lung volume in relation to the metabolic rate, which creates diminished oxygen in the blood and concurrent pulmonary disorders. A small advantage is gained by the presence of fetal hemoglobin because its increased capacity to carry oxygen allows the infant to exist for longer periods in conditions of lowered oxygen tension.

The three primary methods for maintaining a neutral thermal environment are the use of an incubator, a radiant warmer (Fig. 8.9), and an open bassinet with cotton blankets. A dressed infant under blankets can maintain a certain temperature within a wider range of environmental temperatures; however, the need for closer observation of a high-risk infant may require that the infant remain partially unclothed. The incubator should always be prewarmed before placing an infant in it. The use of **double-walled incubators** significantly improves the infant's ability to maintain a desirable temperature and reduce energy expenditure related to heat regulation. Inside or outside the incubator, head coverings are effective in preventing heat loss. A fabric-insulated or wool cap is more effective than one fashioned from stockinette. The use of a heated gel mattress with radiant heat has been shown to significantly decrease the incidence of radiation heat loss and preserve an adequate neutral thermal environment for the VLBW neonate (Fastman, Howell, Holzman, et al., 2014). An effective means for maintaining the desired range of temperature in the infant is the use of a **manually adjusted** or **automatically controlled (servo-controlled) incubator**. The latter mechanism, when set at the upper and lower limits of the desired circulating air temperature range, adjusts automatically in response to signals from a thermal sensor attached to the abdominal skin. If the infant's temperature drops, the warming device is triggered to increase heat output. The servo control is usually set to a desired skin temperature between 36.5° and 37°C (97.7° and 98.6°F) (Gardner & Hernandez, 2016a).

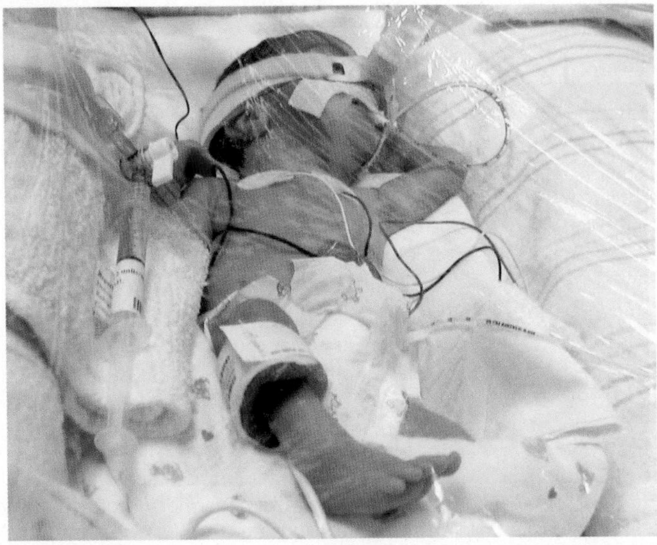

Fig. 8.10 Infant under plastic wrap, which produces a draft-free environment. (Photo courtesy E. Jacobs, Texas Children's Hospital, Houston, TX.)

A high-humidity atmosphere contributes to body temperature maintenance by reducing evaporative heat loss. A number of "microenvironments" may be used with VLBW and ELBW infants to minimize evaporative and insensible water losses. These include items such as food-grade plastic bags or plastic wrap, humidified reservoirs for incubators, and humidified plastic heat shields covered with plastic wrap (Fig. 8.10). When such environments are used, special care must be taken to avoid bacterial contamination of the warm and humid environment by organisms such as *Pseudomonas* and *Serratia,* which have an affinity for moist environments; postnatally acquired pneumonia from such organisms may be fatal, particularly in VLBW infants. A systematic review of practices to decrease hypothermia at birth in LBW infants found that plastic wraps (polyethylene) or bags kept preterm infants warmer, leading to higher temperatures on admission to neonatal units and less hypothermia (McCall, Alderdice, Halliday, et al., 2014; Wilson, Maier, Norman, et al., 2016). This practice is now recommended in the Neonatal Resuscitation Program guidelines published by the American Heart Association (Zaichkin, 2017).

Skin-to-skin (kangaroo) contact between a stable preterm infant and parent is also a viable option for interaction because of the maintenance of appropriate body temperature by the infant. Other benefits of skin-to-skin contact are discussed later in this chapter.

Protection From Infection

Protection from infection is an integral part of all newborn care, but preterm and sick neonates are particularly susceptible. The protective environment of a regularly cleaned and changed incubator provides effective isolation from airborne infective agents. However, thorough, meticulous, and frequent hand washing is the foundation of a preventive program. This includes *all* persons who come in contact with infants and their equipment. After handling another infant or equipment, no one should ever touch an infant without first washing their hands.

Personnel with infectious disorders are either barred from the unit until they are no longer infectious or are required to wear suitable shields, such as masks or gloves, to reduce the likelihood of contamination. An annual influenza vaccination is recommended for NICU personnel. Standard Precautions as a method of infection control are instituted in all nursery areas to protect the infants and staff (see Chapter 20). The benefit of "gowning" by visitors and hospital staff to control infection is not supported by research. Sibling visitation in the NICU has not been shown to increase nosocomial infections (American Academy of Pediatrics & American College of Obstetricians and Gynecologists, 2017); however, appropriate screening for upper respiratory illness in siblings is often recommended.

The sources of infection rise in direct relation to the number of persons and pieces of equipment coming in contact with the infants. Equipment used in the care of infants is cleaned on a regular basis in accordance with the manufacturer's recommendations or institutional protocol; this includes cleaning of cribs, mattresses, incubators, radiant warmers, cardiorespiratory monitors, pulse oximeters, and vital sign–monitoring equipment after usage with one infant and before usage with another. Because organisms thrive best in water, plumbing fixtures and humidifying equipment are particularly hazardous. Disposable equipment used for water-related therapies, such as nebulizers and plastic tubing, is changed regularly.

Hydration

High-risk infants often receive supplemental parenteral fluids to supply additional calories, electrolytes, and water. Adequate hydration is particularly important in preterm infants because their extracellular water content is higher (70% in full-term infants and up to 90% in preterm infants), their body surface is larger, and the capacity for handling fluid shifts is limited in preterm infants' underdeveloped kidneys. Therefore these infants are highly vulnerable to fluid depletion.

Parenteral fluids may be given to the high-risk neonate via several routes depending on the nature of the illness, the duration and type of fluid therapy, and unit preference. Common routes of fluid infusion include peripheral, peripherally inserted central venous (or percutaneous central venous), surgically inserted central venous, and umbilical venous catheters. The preferred sites for peripheral intravenous (IV) infusions in neonates are the peripheral veins on the dorsal surfaces of the hands or feet. Alternative sites are scalp veins and antecubital veins. Special Precautions and frequent observations must accompany the use of peripheral lines. In many neonatal centers, the percutaneous central venous catheter (peripherally inserted central catheter [PICC]) is used for parenteral therapy and medication administration because of less expense and decreased neonatal trauma.

In most facilities, NICU nurses insert peripheral IV catheters and maintain the infusions. IV fluids must always be delivered by continuous infusion pumps that deliver minute volumes at a preset flow rate. The catheter is secured to the skin with a transparent dressing (see the Skin Care section later in this chapter), with care taken not to cause undue pressure from the catheter hub and tubing. Because all infants, especially those who are ELBW and VLBW, are highly vulnerable to any fluid shifts, infusion rates are carefully regulated and checked hourly to prevent tissue damage from extravasation, fluid overload, or dehydration (Nyp, Brunkhorst, Reavey, et al., 2016). Pulmonary edema, congestive heart failure, patent ductus arteriosus, and intraventricular hemorrhage may occur with fluid overload. Dehydration may cause electrolyte disturbances with potentially serious CNS effects.

Infants who are ELBW, tachypneic, receiving phototherapy, or in a radiant warmer have increased insensible water losses that require appropriate fluid adjustments. Nurses must monitor fluid status by daily (or more frequent) weights and accurate intake and output of all fluids, including medications and blood products. Serum electrolytes are monitored per unit protocol, and urine electrolytes are obtained as warranted by the infant's condition. ELBW infants often require more frequent monitoring of these parameters because of their inordinate transepidermal fluid loss, immature renal function, and propensity to dehydration or overhydration. Intolerance of even dextrose 5%

is not uncommon in ELBW infants, with subsequent glycosuria and osmotic diuresis. Alterations in behavior, alertness, or activity level in these infants receiving IV fluids may signal an electrolyte imbalance, hypoglycemia, or hyperglycemia. Nurses should also be observant for tremors or seizures in VLBW or ELBW infants, because these may be a sign of hyponatremia or hypernatremia.

! NURSING ALERT

Nurses should be constantly alert for signs of intravenous (IV) infiltration (e.g., erythema, edema, color change of tissue, blanching at site) and for signs of overhydration (weight gain >30 g [1 oz] in 24 hours, periorbital edema, tachypnea, and crackles on lung auscultation).

A common problem observed in infants who have an umbilical artery catheter in place is vasoconstriction of peripheral vessels, which can seriously impair circulation. The response is triggered by arterial vasospasm caused by the presence of the catheter, the infusion of fluids, or injection of medication. Blanching of the buttocks, genitalia, or legs or feet is an indication of vasospasm. The problem is recognized promptly and reported to the practitioner. The nurse must also observe for signs of thrombi in infants with umbilical venous or arterial lines. The precipitation of microthrombi in the vascular bed with the use of such catheters is commonly manifested by a sudden bluish discoloration seen in the toes, called **catheter toes**. The problem is promptly reported to the practitioner because failure to alleviate the existing pathologic condition may result in the loss of toes or even a foot or leg.

Infants with umbilical venous or arterial catheters should also be observed closely for catheter dislodging and subsequent bleeding or hemorrhage; urinary output, renal function, and gastrointestinal function are also evaluated in these infants. Although the intent of such catheters is to effectively deliver IV fluids (and sometimes medications) and to obtain arterial blood gas samples, they are not without inherent complications.

Nutrition

Optimum nutrition is critical in the management of LBW and preterm infants, but there are difficulties in meeting their nutritional needs. The various mechanisms for ingestion and digestion of foods are not fully developed, and the problem of providing optimal nutrition to the infant is greatest in the more immature infant. In addition, the nutritional requirements for this group of infants are not known with certainty. It is known that all preterm infants are at risk because of poor nutritional stores and several physical and developmental characteristics.

An infant's nutritional needs for rapid growth and daily maintenance must be met in the presence of several anatomic and physiologic disabilities. Although some sucking and swallowing activities are demonstrated before birth and in preterm infants, coordination of these mechanisms does not occur until approximately 32 to 34 weeks of gestation, and they are not fully synchronized until 36 to 37 weeks. Initial sucking is not accompanied by swallowing, and esophageal contractions are uncoordinated. Consequently, infants are highly prone to aspiration and its attendant dangers. As infants mature, the suck–swallow pattern develops but is slow and ineffectual, and these reflexes may also become easily exhausted.

The amount and method of feeding are determined by the infant's size and condition. Nutrition can be provided by either the parenteral or the enteral route or by a combination of the two. Infants who are ELBW, VLBW, or critically ill often obtain the majority of their nutrients by the parenteral route because of their inability to digest and absorb enteral nutrition. Hypoxic insults or illness and major organ immaturity further preclude the use of enteral feeding until the infant's condition has stabilized; necrotizing enterocolitis (NEC) has previously been associated with enteral feedings in acutely ill or distressed infants (see the Necrotizing Enterocolitis section later in this chapter). Total parenteral nutritional support of acutely ill infants may be accomplished successfully with commercially available IV solutions specifically designed to meet the infant's nutritional needs, including protein, amino acids, trace minerals, vitamins, carbohydrates (dextrose), and fat (lipid emulsion).

Studies have shown that there are benefits to the early introduction of small amounts of enteral feedings in metabolically stable preterm infants. These **minimal enteral (trophic gastrointestinal priming) feedings** have been shown to stimulate the infant's gastrointestinal tract, preventing mucosal atrophy and subsequent enteral feeding difficulties. Minimal enteral feedings with as little as 1 ml/kg of breast milk or donor milk may be given by gavage as soon as the infant is medically stable. Parenteral nutrition is continued until the infant is able to tolerate an amount of enteral feeding sufficient to sustain growth. An increased incidence of NEC in VLBW infants receiving minimal enteral nutrition has not been substantiated (Poindexter & Ehrenkranz, 2015. Minimal enteral feedings have been proven to increase mineral absorption, increase gut hormone activity, and substantially decrease the incidence of feeding intolerance in preterm infants (Poindexter & Ehrenkranz, 2015). Minimal enteral feedings are recommended as the standard of care for feeding VLBW infants (Malhotra, Nzegwu, Harrington, et al., 2016).

Although the timing of the first feeding has been a matter of controversy, most authorities now believe that early feeding (provided that the infant is medically stable) reduces the incidence of complicating factors, such as hypoglycemia and dehydration, and the degree of hyperbilirubinemia. The feeding regimen used varies in different units.

Breastfeeding

Human milk is the best source of nutrition for term and preterm infants. Studies indicate that small preterm infants can breastfeed if they have adequate sucking and swallowing reflexes and there are no other contraindications, such as respiratory complications or concurrent illness (Cartwright, Atz, Newman, et al., 2017; Rayfield, Oakley, & Quigley, 2015). Mothers who wish to breastfeed their preterm infants are encouraged to pump their breasts until their infants are sufficiently stable to tolerate breastfeeding. Appropriate guidelines for the storage of **expressed mother's milk** should be followed to decrease the risk of milk contamination and destruction of its beneficial properties (Steele, 2018).

The American Academy of Pediatrics Section on Breastfeeding (2012) recommends human milk for all infants, including sick newborns and preterm infants (with rare exceptions). The American Academy of Pediatrics recognizes that the choice of what to feed is the parents' prerogative but advises that providers give parents complete and accurate information on the benefits and the risks of not providing breast milk to ensure that an informed decision is made. Barriers to initiation and continuation of breastfeeding include physician indifference, misinformation, lack of prenatal education about breastfeeding, distracting hospital policies, lack of follow-up, maternal employment, lack of support from family or society, hospital discharge packs with formula or coupons for formula, and media portrayal of bottle-feeding.

Milk produced by mothers whose infants are born before term contains higher concentrations of protein, sodium, chloride, and immunoglobulin A (IgA). Growth factors, hormones, prolactin, calcitonin, thyroxine (T_4), steroids, and taurine (an essential amino acid) are also present in human milk. Secretory IgA concentration is higher in the milk from mothers of preterm infants than in the milk from mothers of full-term infants. IgA is important in the control of bacteria in the intestinal tract, where it inhibits adherence and proliferation of bacteria on epithelial surfaces. Additional protection from infection is provided by leukocytes, lactoferrin, and lysozyme, all of which are present in human milk. The milk produced by mothers for their infants changes in content over the first 30 days postnatally, at which time it is similar to full-term human milk. Despite its benefits, LBW infants (<1500 g [3.3 pounds]) who are exclusively fed unfortified human milk demonstrate decreased growth rates and nutritional deficiencies even beyond the hospitalization period. These infants often have inadequacies of calcium, phosphorus, protein, sodium, vitamins, and energy. Specially designed supplements for human milk have been developed to address these deficits. Fortifiers containing protein; carbohydrate; calcium; phosphorus; magnesium; sodium; and varied amounts of zinc, copper, and vitamins are used to supplement breast milk. Because fortifiers do not contain sufficient iron, supplemental iron is added, usually when the infant reaches 1 month of age.

A number of studies regarding the effects of long-chain polyunsaturated fatty acids on cognitive development, visual acuity, and physical growth in full-term and preterm infants have prompted formula companies to add docosahexaenoic acid (DHA) and arachidonic acid (AA) to their infant formulas. AA and DHA are present in human milk, and their presence has been reported to lead to an increase in cognitive development in human milk–fed infants compared with infants fed a formula without these fatty acids. However, one meta-analysis demonstrated no clinically significant developmental benefits to supplementation of formula with AA and DHA in term infants up to 24 months of age (Jasani, Simmer, Patole, et al., 2017).

Preterm infants may be able to successfully breastfeed earlier than previously believed (28 to 36 weeks); in addition, preterm infants who are breastfed rather than bottle-fed demonstrate fewer incidences of oxygen desaturation; absence of bradycardia; warmer skin temperature; and better coordination of breathing, sucking, and swallowing (Lawrence & Lawrence, 2016b). Preterm infants should be carefully evaluated for readiness to breastfeed, including assessment of behavioral state, ability to maintain body temperature outside an artificial heat source, respiratory status, and readiness to suckle at the mother's breast. The latter may be accomplished with nonnutritive sucking at the breast during skin-to-skin (kangaroo) contact so that the mother and newborn may become accustomed to each other (Lawrence & Lawrence, 2016b). Nasal cannula oxygen may also be provided during preterm breastfeeding based on the infant's assessed requirements.

Time, patience, and dedication on the part of the mother and the nursing staff are needed to help infants with breastfeeding. The process is begun slowly—beginning with one feeding daily and gradually increasing the feedings as the infant tolerates them. Human milk provides both short-term and long-term advantages in a dose-dependent relationship in that the more breast milk the preterm receives, the more benefits are gained (Gardner & Lawrence, 2016; Johnson, Patra, Greene, et al., 2019). Supplementary bottle feeding is inefficient because the infant expends energy and calories to feed twice. Supplementing by gavage feeding or using a training nipple is more energy and calorie efficient. Breastfeeding preterm infants often requires additional guidance by a lactation consultant; continued support and encouragement by the nursing staff and family members are essential. In addition, postdischarge breastfeeding often requires further guidance, counseling, and support by nursing staff (Dennison, Nguyen, Gregg, et al., 2016).

Because of the anti-infective and growth-promoting properties of human milk, as well as its superior nutrition, donor milk is used in many NICUs for preterm or sick infants when the mother's milk is not available (American Academy of Pediatrics Section on Breastfeeding, 2012). Donor milk is also used therapeutically for medical purposes, such as in transplant recipients who are immunocompromised. Unprocessed human milk from unscreened donors is not recommended because of the risk of transmission of infectious agents (American Academy of Pediatrics Section on Breastfeeding, 2012).

The Human Milk Banking Association of North America[b] has established guidelines for the operation of donor human milk banks (Human Milk Banking Association, 2015). Donor milk banks collect, screen, process (pasteurize), and distribute milk donated by breastfeeding mothers who are feeding their own infants and pumping a few extra ounces each day for the milk bank.

Nipple Feeding

Vigorous infants can be fed from a nipple with little difficulty, but compromised preterm infants require alternative methods. The amount to be fed is determined largely by the infant's weight gain and tolerance of previous feeding and is increased by small increments until a satisfactory caloric intake is ensured.

The rate of increase that is well tolerated varies from one infant to another, and determining this rate is often a nursing responsibility. Preterm infants require more time and patience to feed compared with full-term infants, and the oropharyngeal mechanism may be stressed by an attempt to feed too rapidly. It is important not to tire the infants or overtax their capacity to retain the feedings. When infants require a prolonged time (arbitrarily, more than 30 minutes) to complete a feeding, gavage feeding may be considered for the next time.

Cue-based (also known as infant-driven) feeding is a developmental approach to oral feeding that considers the individual infant's readiness rather than initiating feedings based on weight and age or a predetermined time schedule (Fry, Marfurt, & Wengier, 2018; Gennattasio, Perri, Baranek, et al., 2015; Whetten, 2016). Feeding readiness is determined by each infant's medical status, energy level, ability to sustain a brief quiet alert state, gag reflex, spontaneous rooting and sucking behaviors, and hand-to-mouth behaviors (Fry et al., 2018). A preterm infant may experience difficulty coordinating sucking, swallowing, and breathing with resultant apnea, bradycardia, and decreased oxygen saturation. The infant's ability to suck on a pacifier does not indicate complete readiness for nipple feeding or ability to coordinate the aforementioned activities without some degree of stress; a gradual introduction of nippling in preterm infants is based on careful evaluation of their ability to maintain adequate cardiopulmonary functions while feeding. When infants are unable to tolerate bottle feedings, intermittent feedings by gavage are instituted until they gain enough strength and coordination to use the nipple.

! NURSING ALERT

Poor feeding behaviors such as apnea, bradycardia, cyanosis, pallor, and decreased oxygen saturation in any infant who has previously fed well may indicate an underlying illness.

The nipple used should be relatively firm and stable. Although a high-flow, pliable nipple requires less energy to use, it may provide a flow rate that is too rapid for some preterm infants to manage without a risk of aspiration. A firmer nipple facilitates a more "cupped" tongue configuration and allows for a more controlled, manageable flow rate.

[b]http://www.hmbana.org.

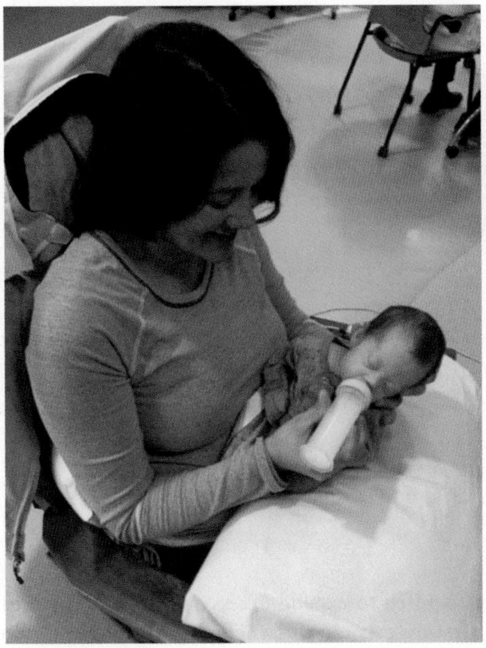

Fig. 8.11 Parent demonstrating nipple feeding of preterm infant using the ESL technique. (Courtesy K. Fisher, Duke University Medical Center, Durham, NC.)

Brown and colleagues (2016) used the semielevated side-lying (ESL) position when introducing bottle feedings to preterm infants between 32 and 36 weeks of age. The ESL position better mimics the breastfeeding position and allows for better coordination of breathing with swallowing. Supported infants had fewer and shorter pauses during feeding and had higher postfeeding oxygen saturations than infants not receiving oral support (Brown et al., 2016). The infant is positioned in the feeder's arms or placed semiupright in the lap (Fig. 8.11) and is held with the back curved slightly to simulate the position assumed naturally by most full-term newborns. The use of gentle cheek and jaw support for preterm infants has been shown to facilitate feedings. Stroking the infant's lips, cheeks, and tongue before feeding helps promote oral sensitivity. Inward and upward support to the infant's cheeks and a slightly upward lift to the chin are provided by the fingers to assist nipple compression during feeding.

Bottle feedings are continued if infants are able to tolerate the feedings and take the required amount. Some preterm infants respond more slowly than full-term infants; therefore the feeding interval and the amount of the feeding are individualized. Preterm infants are often slow feeders and require patience, frequent rest periods, and burping (or bubbling).

Gavage Feeding

Gavage feeding is a safe means of meeting the nutritional requirements of infants who are unable to feed orally. These infants are usually too weak to suck effectively, are unable to coordinate swallowing, and lack a gag reflex. Studies have demonstrated that both bolus and continuous feeding are equally suitable feeding strategies for preterm neonates, with only a slight preference for bolus feeding to allow for more parent-infant bonding (Bozzetti, Paterlini, De Lorenzo, et al., 2016; Rövekamp-Abels, Hogewind-Schoonenboom, de Wijs-Meijller, et al., 2015). The goal for any feeding strategy is to optimize the overall health of the infant and thus reduce the time to reach full feeding.

A size 5-, 6-, or 8-Fr feeding tube is used to instill the feeding, and the usual methods for determining correct placement are used (see Chapter 20 for technique). Although the more relaxed lower esophageal sphincter makes passage of the tube easier, there may be changes in heart rate and BP in response to vagal stimulation. When an indwelling tube is required, consideration should be given to using a product made of Silastic rather than polyvinyl chloride (PVC) because PVC becomes stiff when exposed to body fluids. Compared to the PVC and Silastic tubes, polyurethane (poly) tubes offer another viable option for use. Poly tubes are easier to insert and have a larger inner lumen (Wallace & Steward, 2014).

The stomach is aspirated, the contents are measured, and the aspirate is returned as part of the feeding. However, this practice may vary depending on circumstances and individual unit protocol. The amount of aspirate depends on the time since the previous feeding or concurrent illness.

The milk or formula is allowed to flow by gravity, and the length of time varies. This procedure is not used as a timesaving method for the nurse. Complications of indwelling tubes include aspiration, obstructed nares, mucous plugs, purulent rhinitis, epistaxis, infection, and possible stomach perforation. Current practice dictates a radiograph as the only certain way to determine nasogastric tube placement. Methods such as nose-ear–midway to umbilicus (NEMU), nose-ear-xiphoid (NEX) measurements for insertion depth, and pH measurements are considered imprecise when used as the only method for determining placement (Ellett, Cohen, Croffie, et al., 2014; Parker, Withers, & Talage, 2018; Taylor, Allan, McWilliam, et al., 2014). One study determined that the NEMU method was used most often by the majority of nurses polled (64%) and that it was incorporated in approximately 50% of the NICU policy guidelines (Parker et al., 2018). The NEMU method is also recommended for use in the delivery room by the Neonatal Resuscitation Program (Weiner & Zaichkin, 2015). Research focusing on magnetic resonance–guided nasogastric feeding tube placement for neonates has demonstrated feasibility and benefits (Daniels, Ireland, Kraus, et al., 2016). Further research is needed to determine optimal positioning of feeding tubes in high-risk infants on intermittent bolus or continuous gavage feedings.

! NURSING ALERT

The nurse must observe preterm infants closely for behaviors that indicate readiness for oral feedings. These include:

- A strong, vigorous suck
- Coordination of sucking and swallowing
- A gag reflex
- Sucking on the gavage tube, hands, or a pacifier
- Rooting and wakefulness before and sleeping after feedings

When these behaviors are noted, infants can be challenged with oral feedings that are introduced slowly.

The infant may be held during gavage feedings by the caregiver or parent. If necessary, oxygen may be supplied via nasal cannula to facilitate handling. It is not recommended that the infant be removed from a primary source of oxygen for feedings, because doing so decreases oxygen availability. **Nonnutritive sucking (NNS)** on a pacifier may help bring the infant to a quiet alert state in preparation for feeding. Proposed benefits of NNS include improved weight gain, improved milk intake, more stable heart rate and oxygen saturation, earlier age at full oral feeds, and improved behavioral state. A systematic review of NNS found that infants receiving NNS were discharged significantly earlier than non-NNS infants and that they experienced a more rapid transition from tube to bottle feedings and better bottle-feeding performance (Harding, Frank, Van Someren, et al., 2014). Additional research suggests that NNS may provide relief of mild to moderate pain associated with procedures such as heel sticks (Liu, Huang, Luo, et al., 2017).

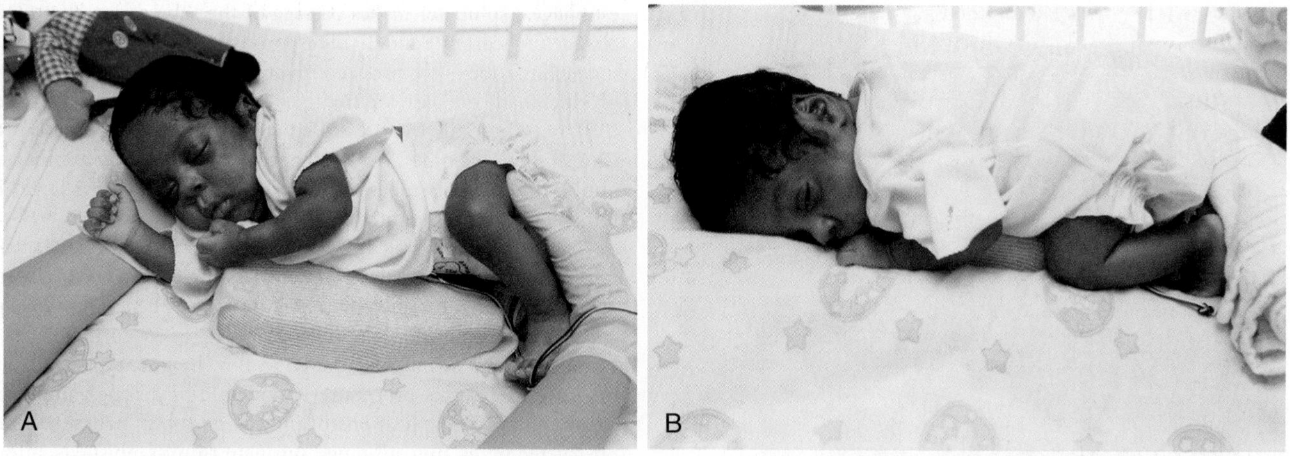

Fig. 8.12 **A,** Preterm infant slowly transitioned to the prone position on a prone roll. **B,** Preterm infant positioned on a prone roll. (Courtesy Halbouty Premature Nursery, Texas Children's Hospital, Houston, TX; photos by Paul Vincent Kuntz.)

> **! NURSING ALERT**
>
> An increase in gastric residuals, abdominal distention, bilious vomiting, temperature instability, apneic episodes, and bradycardia may be indicative of early necrotizing enterocolitis (NEC) and should be reported to the practitioner.

Feeding Resistance

Any feeding technique that bypasses the mouth precludes the opportunity for the infant to practice sucking and swallowing or to experience normal hunger and satiation cycles. Infants may demonstrate aversion to oral feedings by such behaviors as averting the head to the presentation of the nipple, extruding the nipple by tongue thrust, gagging, or even vomiting.

Other observations include disinterest in or active resistance to oral play, diminished spontaneity and motivation, and shallow interpersonal relationships, probably related to the absence of some early incorporative patterns of normal oral experiences. The longer the period of nonoral feeding, the more severe the feeding problems, especially if this period occurs during a time when the infant progresses from reflexive to learned and voluntary feeding actions. Infancy is the period during which the mouth is the primary instrument for reception of stimulation and pleasure.

Infants identified as being at risk for feeding resistance should be provided with regular oral stimulation, such as stroking the oral area from the cheeks to the lips, touching the tongue, placing some of the feeding on the lips and tongue, and associating feeding with pleasurable activities (holding, talking, making eye contact) based on the child's developmental level. Those who exhibit feeding aversion should begin a stimulation program to overcome resistance and acquire the ability to take nourishment by the oral route. Because management requires long-term commitment, successful implementation of a plan for oral stimulation depends on maximum parental involvement and a multidisciplinary team approach.

Energy Conservation

One of the major goals of care for the high-risk infant is conservation of energy. Much of the care described in this section is directed toward this end (e.g., disturbing the infant as little as possible, maintaining a neutral thermal environment, gavage feeding as appropriate, promoting oxygenation, and judiciously implementing any caregiving activities that increase oxygen intake and caloric consumption). An infant who is not required to expend excess energy to breathe, eat, or alter body temperature can use this energy for growth and development. Diminishing environmental noise levels and shading the infant from bright lights also promote rest (see the Developmental Outcome section later in this chapter).

Early in hospitalization, the prone position is best for most preterm infants and results in improved oxygenation, better-tolerated feedings, and more organized sleep–rest patterns. Infants exhibit less physical activity and energy expenditure when placed in the prone position (Fig. 8.12). Prolonged supine positioning for preterm infants is also not desirable because they appear to lose their sense of equilibrium when supine and use vital energy in attempts to recover balance by postural changes. In addition, prolonged supine positioning is associated with long-term problems, such as widely abducted hips (frog-leg position), retracted and abducted shoulders, ankle and foot eversion, and increased neck extension (Gardner, Goldson, & Hernandez, 2016). The American Academy of Pediatrics, Task Force on Sudden Infant Death Syndrome (2016) continues to affirm its position that healthy infants be placed to sleep in a supine position.[c] When medically stable, preterm infants should also be placed in a supine position to sleep unless conditions such as gastroesophageal reflux or upper airway anomalies make this impractical (see also Chapter 10, Sudden Infant Death Syndrome). Prone positioning for play should be provided in the nursery and encouraged after discharge.

Skin Care

The skin of preterm infants is characteristically immature relative to that of full-term infants. In most preterm infants, the skin barrier properties resemble those of the term infant by 2 to 4 weeks' postnatal age, regardless of gestational age at birth. Because of its increased sensitivity and fragility, alkaline-based soap that might destroy the skin's **acid mantle** is avoided. The increased permeability of the skin facilitates absorption of ingredients. All skin products (e.g., alcohol, chlorhexidine, povidone iodine) should be used with caution; the skin is rinsed with water afterward because these substances may cause severe irritation and chemical burns in VLBW and ELBW infants.

---

[c]Information is available from the National Institute of Child Health and Human Development's Safe to Sleep Public Education Campaign, http://www.nichd.nih.gov/sts.

The skin is easily excoriated and denuded; therefore care must be taken to avoid damage to the delicate structure. The total skin is thinner than that of full-term infants and lacks rete pegs, appendages that anchor the epidermis to the dermis. Therefore there is less cohesion between the thinner skin layers. The use of adhesive tape or bandages may excoriate the skin or adhere to the skin surface so well that the epidermis can be separated from the dermis and pulled away with the tape. The use of pectin barriers and hydrocolloid adhesives may be useful, because these products mold well to skin contours and adhere in moist conditions. Recommendations for protecting the integrity of the skin of preterm infants include using minimal adhesive tape, backing the tape with cotton, and delaying adhesive and pectin barrier removal until adherence is reduced (Lund & Kuller, 2014). Emollients, such as Eucerin or Aquaphor, have been used to promote skin integrity and prevent dry, cracking, and peeling skin in infants at risk for skin breakdown; however, the use of such agents has been shown to increase the risk for coagulase-negative infections in preterm infants and therefore should not be routinely used (Lund & Kuller, 2014).

It is unsafe to use scissors to remove dressings or tape from the extremities of very small and immature infants, because it is easy to snip off tiny extremities or nick loosely attached skin. Solvents used to remove tape are avoided, because they tend to dry and burn the delicate skin. Guidelines for skin care are listed in the Nursing Care Guidelines box.

NURSING CARE GUIDELINES

Neonatal Skin Care

General Skin Care

Assessment

Assess skin every day or more often as needed for redness, dryness, flaking, scaling, rashes, lesions, excoriation, and breakdown.

Identify risk factors for skin injury: Gestational age of 32 weeks or less, high-frequency ventilation, extracorporeal membrane oxygenation (ECMO), hypotension requiring vasopressors.

Use a valid assessment tool to provide reliable and objective measurement of skin condition.

Evaluate and report abnormal skin findings and analyze for possible causes.

Intervene according to interpretation of findings or physician order.

Bathing

Initial Bath

Assess to ensure that the infant has a stable temperature for a minimum of 2 to 4 hours before first bath.

Use cleansing agents with neutral pH and minimal dyes or perfume.

Use Standard Precautions; wear gloves.

Do not completely remove vernix; allow vernix to wear off with normal care and handling.

Bathe preterm infant younger than 32 weeks in warm water only for the first week.

Routine

Decrease frequency of baths to every second or third day by daily cleansing of eye, oral, and diaper areas and pressure points.

Use pH-neutral cleanser or soaps no more than two or three times a week.

Avoid rubbing skin during bathing or drying.

Immerse stable infants fully (except head) in an appropriate-size tub.

Use swaddled immersion bathing technique: Slowly unwrap after gently lowering into water for sensitive but stable infants needing assistance with motor system reactivity.

Emollients

Apply sparingly to dry, flaking, fissured areas as needed.

Choose petrolatum-based products that are free of preservatives, dyes, and perfumes.

Observe neonates who weigh 750 g or less and are receiving emollient therapy for increased risk of coagulase-negative *Staphylococcus* (ConS) infections. Consider dispensing emollients from hospital pharmacy, unit dose, or patient-specific container.

Adhesives

Decrease use as much as possible.

Use semipermeable dressings to secure intravenous (IV) lines, nasogastric or orogastric tubes, silicone catheters, and central lines.

Use hydrogel electrodes.

Consider pectin barriers beneath adhesives to protect skin.

Secure pulse oximeter probe or electrodes with elasticized dressing material (carefully avoid restricting blood flow).

Do not use adhesive remover, solvents, or bonding agents.

Avoid removing adhesives for at least 24 hours after application.

Adhesive removal can be facilitated using water, mineral oil, or petrolatum.

Remove adhesives or skin barriers slowly, supporting the skin underneath with one hand and gently peeling away the product from the skin with the other hand.

Antiseptic Agents

Apply before invasive procedures.

Consider the potential for skin breakdown or irritation with disinfectant.

No specific disinfectant is recommended over another for all neonates; remove completely with water or saline after use.

Avoid use of isopropyl alcohol for skin prep or removal of other disinfectants.

Transepidermal Water Loss

Minimize transepidermal water loss (TEWL) and heat loss in small preterm infants at less than 30 weeks of gestation by:

- Maintaining ambient humidity during first weeks of life.
- Applying occlusive polyethylene body bag immediately at delivery and removing after infant is stabilized in the neonatal intensive care unit (NICU).
- Considering increasing humidity to 70% to 90% by using a humidified incubator for first 7 days; decrease to 50% until 28 days of age.
- Using supplemental conductive heat and reduce radiant heat source.

Skin Breakdown

Prevention

Decrease pressure from externally applied forces using water, air, or gel mattresses or cotton bedding.

Provide adequate nutrition, including protein, fat, and zinc.

Apply transparent adhesive dressings to protect arms, elbows, and knees from friction injury.

Use emollient in the diaper area (groin and thighs) to reduce urine irritation.

Treating Skin Breakdown

Irrigate wound every 4 to 8 hours with warm half-strength normal saline.

Culture wound and treat if signs of infection are present (excessive redness, swelling, pain on touch, heat, or resistance to healing).

Use transparent adhesive dressing for uninfected wounds.

Apply hydrogel with or without antibacterial or antifungal ointments (as ordered) for infected wounds (may need to moisten before removal).

NURSING CARE GUIDELINES—CONT'D

Use hydrocolloid for deep, uninfected wounds (leave in place for 5 to 7 days) or as an ostomy barrier and to improve appliance adhesion.
Avoid use of antiseptic solutions for wound cleansing (use for intact skin only).

Treating Diaper Dermatitis

Maintain clean, dry skin; use absorbent diapers and change often.
If mild irritation occurs, use petrolatum barrier.
For developing dermatitis, apply a generous quantity of zinc-oxide barrier.
For severe dermatitis, identify cause and treat (frequent stooling from spina bifida, severe opiate withdrawal, or malabsorption syndrome).
Treat *Candida albicans* with antifungal ointment or cream.
Avoid powders and antibiotic ointments (see Chapter 7, Care of the Umbilicus and Circumcision).

Other Skin Care Concerns

Use of Substances on Skin

Evaluate all substances that come in contact with infant's skin.
Before using any topical agent, analyze components of preparation and:

- Use sparingly and only when necessary.
- Confine use to smallest possible area.
- Whenever possible and appropriate, wash off with water.
- Monitor infant carefully for signs of toxicity and systemic effects.

Use of Thermal Devices

When prewarming heels before phlebotomy, avoid temperatures over 40°C.
Provide warm ambient humidity, directed away from infant; use aerosolized sterile water and maintain ambient temperature so as to not exceed 40°C.
Document use of all heating devices.

Use of Fluid Therapy and Hemodynamic Monitoring

Be certain fingers or toes are visible whenever extremity is used for peripheral IV or arterial line.
Secure catheter or needle with transparent dressing and tape to promote easy visualization of site.
Assess site hourly for signs of infiltration and inadequate perfusion (check capillary refill, pulses, color).
Avoid use of restraints (e.g., armboards); if used, check that they are secured safely and not restricting circulation or movement (check for pressure areas).

Data from Association of Women's Health, Obstetric and Neonatal Nurses. (2018). *Evidence-based clinical practice guideline: Neonatal skin care* (4th ed.). Washington, DC: Author; Edraki, M., Paran, M., Montaseri, S., et al. (2014). Comparing the effects of swaddled and conventional bathing methods on body temperature and crying duration in premature infants. *Journal of Caring Sciences, 3*(2), 83–91; Lund, C. H., & Durand, D. J. (2016). Skin and skin care. In S. L. Gardner, B. S. Carter, M. Enzman-Hines, & J. A. Hernandez (Eds.), *Merenstein & Gardner's handbook of neonatal intensive care* (8th ed.). St Louis, MO: Mosby/Elsevier; Lund, C. H., & Kuller, J. M. (2014). Integumentary system. In C. Kenner & J. Lott (Eds.), *Comprehensive neonatal care: An interdisciplinary approach* (5th ed.). New York, NY: Springer.

During skin assessment of preterm infants, nurses are alert to the subtle signs that indicate **zinc deficiency**, a problem sometimes seen in infants who have inadequate intake or abnormal losses of zinc. Breakdown usually occurs in the areas around the mouth, buttocks, fingers, and toes. In preterm and VLBW infants, it may also occur in the creases of the neck, wrists, ankles, and around wounds. Zinc deficiency is most likely to appear in preterm infants with inadequate zinc intake, an ileostomy, short bowel syndrome, or chronic diarrhea. Suspicious lesions are reported to the practitioner so that zinc supplements can be prescribed. Skin injuries have been reported during the use of phototherapy and hypothermia cooling blankets. Caution is warranted in using these products in ELBW infants and infants who are at risk for skin breakdown.

Administration of Medications

Administration of therapeutic agents (such as drugs, ointments, IV infusions, and oxygen) requires judicious handling and meticulous attention to detail. The computation, preparation, and administration of drugs in minute amounts often require collaboration among members of the health care team to reduce the chance for error. In addition, the immaturity of an infant's detoxification mechanisms and inability to demonstrate symptoms of toxicity (e.g., signs of auditory nerve involvement from ototoxic drugs, such as gentamicin) complicate drug therapy and require that nurses be particularly alert for signs of adverse reaction (see Chapter 20, Administration of Medication).

Nurses should be aware of the hazards of administering bacteriostatic and hyperosmolar solutions to infants. Benzyl alcohol, a common preservative in bacteriostatic water and saline, has been shown to be toxic to newborns, and products containing this preservative should not be used to flush IV catheters, to dilute or reconstitute medications, or as an anesthetic to start IV lines. It is recommended that medications with preservative (such as benzyl alcohol) be avoided whenever possible. *Nurses must read labels carefully to detect the presence of preservatives in any medication to be administered to an infant.*

Hyperosmolar solutions present a potential danger to preterm infants. Hyperosmolar solutions given orally to infants can produce clinical, physiologic, and morphologic alterations, the most serious of which is NEC. Oral and parenteral medications should be sufficiently diluted to prevent complications related to hyperosmolality.

There has been heightened awareness of the impact of medication errors and subsequent poor outcomes for high-risk neonates. Nurses, physicians, and pharmacists must work in cooperation to implement strategies in the NICU environment to eradicate medication errors. Technology alone has not proved to be the solution; therefore nurses must be extremely vigilant when administering medications to preterm and high-risk infants.

Developmental Outcome

Much attention has been focused on the effects of early developmental intervention on both normal and preterm infants. Infants respond to a great variety of stimuli, and the atmosphere and activities of the NICU are overstimulating. Consequently, infants in NICUs are subjected to inappropriate stimulation that can be harmful. For example, the noise level that results from monitoring equipment, alarms, and general unit activity has been correlated with the incidence of intracranial hemorrhage, especially in ELBW and VLBW infants. Personnel should reduce noise-generating activities, such as closing doors (including incubator portholes), listening to loud radios, talking loudly, and handling equipment (e.g., trash containers). Planned noise control training for care providers who work in the NICU environment can be an effective method to address problem areas (Calikusu & Balci, 2017). Nursing care activities (such as taking vital signs, changing the infant's position, weighing, and changing diapers) are associated with frequent periods of hypoxia, oxygen desaturation, and elevated ICP. The more immature the infant, the less able he or she is to habituate to a single procedure, such as taking an oscillometric BP, without becoming overstimulated.

Twenty-four-hour surveillance of sick infants implies maximum visibility and often bright lights. Units should establish a night–day sleep pattern by darkening the room, covering cribs with blankets, or placing eye patches over infants' eyes at night. Infants need scheduled rest periods during which the lights are dimmed, the incubators are covered with blankets, and the infants are not disturbed for handling of any kind (Altimier & White, 2014). Sleep periods should be undisturbed for at least 50 minutes to allow for complete sleep cycles.

Infants' eyes should be shielded from bright procedure lights to prevent potential harm. Many experts suggest that the human face, especially a parent's, is the best visual stimulus and that visual stimuli be kept to a minimum early in development. Developmental care, accentuating the infant's unique ability to achieve behavioral state organization, is tailored to the developmental level and tolerance of each infant based on a comprehensive behavioral assessment. During the early stages of development (especially before 33 weeks of gestation), external stimulation produces uncoordinated, random activity, such as jerky limb extension, hyperflexion, and irregular vital signs. At this stage, infants need to have minimum environmental stimulation. Using the developmental model of supportive care, the nurse closely monitors physiologic and behavioral signs to promote organization and well-being of the high-risk infant during handling. Softly calling the infant by name and then gently placing a hand on the body signal that care is beginning and alleviate the abrupt interruption that precedes caregiving. Infants are handled with slow, controlled movements (some infants are unstable if moved abruptly), and their random movements are controlled with limbs held flexed close to their bodies during turning or other position changes. This containment or facilitated tucking may also be used before invasive procedures, such as heel stick, to alleviate distress. Blanket swaddling and nesting or containment have been shown to decrease physiologic and behavioral stress during routine care procedures, such as bathing, weighing, and heel stick. A nest constructed by placing blanket rolls under the bed sheet helps infants maintain an attitude of flexion when prone or side lying.

Although it must be individually adjusted, skin-to-skin contact (kangaroo care) and short periods of gentle massage can help reduce stress in preterm infants. Regular passive skin-to-skin contact between parents (mother or father) and LBW infants has been shown to alleviate stress. The parent wears a loose-fitting, open-front top, and the undressed (except for diaper) infant is placed in a vertical position on the parent's bare chest, which permits direct eye contact, skin-to-skin sensations, and close proximity (Fig. 8.13). Skin-to-skin contact between the parent and infant, in addition to being a safe and effective method for VLBW infant-parent acquaintance, can have a positive healing effect for the mother with a high-risk pregnancy. Mothers may experience psychologic healing related to preterm delivery and regain the mothering role through early skin-to-skin contact with their VLBW infants. Major neonatal benefits of skin-to-skin care include a reduced risk of mortality, fewer nosocomial infections, decreased length of hospital stay, maintenance of neonatal thermal stability and oxygen saturation, increased feeding vigor, and improved growth (Evereklian & Posmontier, 2017; Gardner & Hernandez, 2016b). In full-term newborns, skin-to-skin contact has a strong analgesic effect during procedures, such as heel lance (Liu, Zhao, & Li, 2015). LBW infants receiving skin-to-skin contact with breastfeeding mothers maintained higher oxygen saturation and were less likely to have desaturations below 90%, and their mothers were more likely to continue breastfeeding both in the hospital and for 1 month after discharge. Kangaroo care of preterm infants fosters appropriate neurobehavioral development by promoting stability of heart and respiratory function, minimizes purposeless movements, offers maternal proximity for attention, improves the infant's behavioral state, and permits self-regulating behaviors (Gardner & Hernandez, 2016b).

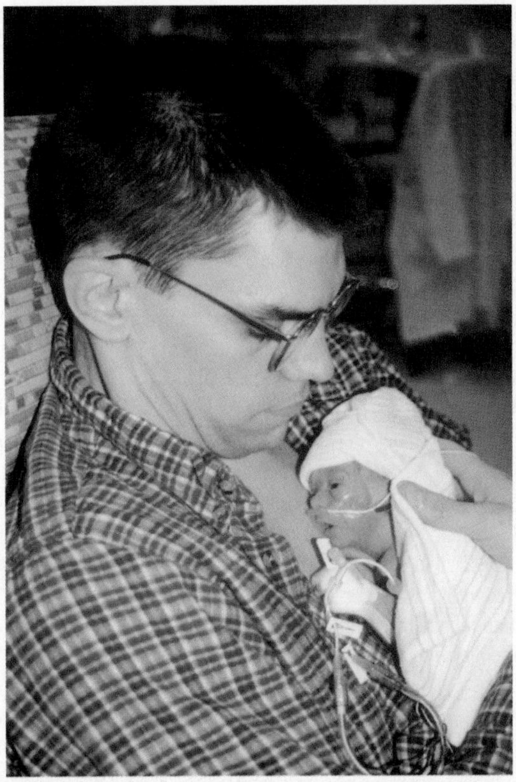

Fig. 8.13 Father providing skin-to-skin (kangaroo) care. (Courtesy Judy Meyr, St Louis, MO.)

Additional research studies have confirmed the beneficial effects of developmental care with preterm infants. In addition to requiring fewer days of mechanical ventilation, preterm infants who received individualized developmental care had shorter hospital stays; a significant decrease in complications, such as nosocomial infection and bronchopulmonary dysplasia; improved neurodevelopmental scores; and increased breastfeeding (Casper, Sarapuk, & Pavlyshyn, 2018; Deng, Li, Wang, et al., 2018; Lorenz, Marulli, Dawson, et al., 2018).

The arena of developmental care for preterm infants has expanded to include a wide variety of interventions, such as infant massage, soothing soft music, recordings of parents reading stories, positioning to enhance self-regulatory abilities, enhancement of hand-to-mouth activities, uninterrupted sleep periods, decreased environmental light and noise, and even the use of stuffed animals to facilitate infant positioning. As a result of such interventions, parents may perceive the NICU environment as less threatening. Active participation in providing such an environment for their special infant also involves the parents in the provision of daily care when the newborn is critically ill and cannot be fed or held.

When infants have reached sufficient developmental organization and stability, interventions are designed and implemented to support their growing abilities. Nurses and parents become adept at learning to read infants' behavioral cues and supplying appropriate interventions (Table 8.2). Cues include both approach and avoidance behaviors. **Approach behaviors** that are supported and enhanced include tongue extension, hand clasp, hand-to-mouth movements, sucking, looking, and cooing. Signs of stress or fatigue that signal the infant's need for "time-out" are described in Table 8.2.

When infants are recovering and are free of support systems, medically stable, and on room air or smaller amounts of oxygen, they are assessed to

TABLE 8.2 Signs of Stress or Fatigue in Neonates

Subsystem	Signs of Stress
Autonomic	Physiologic instability
Respiratory	Tachypnea, pauses, gasping, sighing
Color	Mottled, dusky, pale or gray
Visceral	Hiccups, gagging, choking, spitting up, grunting and straining as if having a bowel movement, coughing, sneezing, yawning
Autonomic	Tremors, startles, twitches
Motor	Fluctuating tone; lack of control over movement, activity, and posture
Flaccidity	Low tone in trunk; limp, floppy upper and lower extremities; limp, drooping jaw (gape face)
Hypertonicity	Arm or leg extensions, arm(s) outstretched with fingers splayed in salute gesture, fingers stiffly outstretched, trunk arching, neck hyperextended
Hyperflexion	Trunk, extremities
Activity	Squirming; frantic, diffuse activity or little or no activity or responsiveness
State	Disorganized quality to state behaviors, including available states, maintenance of state control, and transition from one state to another
Sleep	Whimpering sounds, irregular respirations, fussing, grimacing, restless appearance
Awake	Glazed, unfocused look; staring; worried or pained expression; hyperalert or panicked appearance; eye roving; crying; cry-face; actively averting gaze or closing eyes; irritability; prolonged awake periods; inconsolability
	Abrupt or rapid state changes
Other state-related behaviors and attention interaction	Efforts to attend to and interact with environmental stimulation eliciting signs of stress and disorganized subsystem functioning
Autonomic	Physiologic instability of varying degrees with autonomic, respiratory, color, and visceral responses
Motor	Fluctuating tone, increased motor activity, progressively frantic diffuse activity if stimulation continues
State	Roving eyes; gaze averting; glazed, unfocused look or worried, panicked expression; weak cry; cry-face; irritability
	Closed eyes and sleeplikeww withdrawal
	Abrupt state changes
	Signs of stress when presented with more than one type of stimulus at a time

Data from Bradley, C., & Ritter, R. (2014). Developmental care for the sick and preterm infant. In C. Kenner & J. Lott (Eds.), *Comprehensive neonatal care: An interdisciplinary approach* (5th ed.). New York, NY: Springer; Gardner, S. L., Goldson, E., & Hernandez, J. A. (2016). The neonate and the environment: Impact on development. In S. L. Gardner, B. S. Carter, M. Enzman-Hines, et al. (Eds.), *Merenstein and Gardner's handbook of neonatal intensive care* (8th ed.). St Louis, MO: Mosby/Elsevier; Lin, H.-C., Huang, L.-C., Li, T.-C., et al. (2014). Relationship between energy expenditure and stress behaviors of preterm infants in the neonatal intensive care unit. *Journal for Specialists in Pediatric Nursing, 19*(4), 331–338.

document behavioral state organization and ability to self-regulate. When the infant is stable and mature enough to begin developmental intervention, activities are individualized according to each infant's cues, temperament, state, behavioral organization, and particular needs. Intervention periods are short (e.g., 2 to 3 minutes of voices, 5 minutes of quiet music). Hearing and vestibular interventions are initiated earlier than visual stimulation. One type of intervention at a time is applied to document the infant's tolerance and response (see Nursing Care Guidelines box). An intervention program for convalescing infants includes parents and siblings early in the infant's hospitalization; teaching parents to be responsive to the infant's individual cues is an important function of the NICU nurse. Parents, siblings, and health care providers are encouraged to adhere to the established developmental care plan to avoid disruption in sleep–wake cycles and minimize inappropriate stimuli.

Developmental care of preterm neonates is an ongoing process in the NICU and is incorporated into the daily care given to each infant. The nurse is cognizant of the preterm infant's developmental needs, temperament, and newborn state, as well as environmental conditions that adversely affect the infant; nursing care is planned accordingly to enhance optimum physical, psychosocial, and neurologic development. This task is often difficult to accomplish when invasive treatments or interventions are required to stabilize the critically ill neonate.

Family Support and Involvement

Professional health workers often are so absorbed in the lifesaving physical aspects of care that they ignore the emotional needs of infants and their families. The significance of early parent-child interaction and infant stimulation has been documented by reliable research. Nurses, aware of these infant and family needs, must incorporate activities that facilitate family interaction into the nursing care plan.

The birth of a preterm infant is an unexpected and stressful event for which families are emotionally unprepared. They find themselves simultaneously coping with their own needs, the needs of their infant, and the needs of their family (especially when they have other children). To compound the situation, their infant's precarious condition engenders an atmosphere of apprehension and uncertainty. Parents are faced with multiple crises and overwhelming feelings of responsibility, helplessness, and frustration.

All parents have some anxieties about the outcome of a pregnancy, but after a preterm birth, the concern is heightened regarding both the viability and the normalcy of their infant. Mothers may see their infant only briefly before the newborn is removed to the intensive care unit or even to another hospital, leaving them with just the recollection of the infant's very small size and unusual appearance. They often feel alone or lost on the mother-baby unit, belonging neither with mothers who

NURSING CARE GUIDELINES

Developmental Interventions

General Guidelines

Individualize interventions for each infant.
Offer stimulus only during periods of alertness.
Begin one type of stimulus at a time.
Provide intervention for short periods.
Space periods according to infant's tolerance.
Continually assess infant's response to developmental interventions.
Titrate interventions according to infant's cues.
Terminate stimulation if infant displays evidence of overstimulation (see Table 8.2).
Provide 50-minute uninterrupted sleep periods.
Handle to promote or maintain behavioral organization, providing for flexion, containment, firm pressure, grasp, and nonnutritive sucking (NNS).

Tactile

Stroke skin slowly and gently in head-to-toe direction (assess tolerance first).
Provide alternate textures (e.g., satin, velvet).
Provide firm boundaries: Foot bracing, blankets, "nesting."
Encourage skin-to-skin (kangaroo) holding by parents and siblings as tolerated.
Provide containment holding in cupped palms of hand for nesting and comfort.

Auditory

Reduce noise levels.
Mother's voice is the best.
Maintain 50 dB with maximum 55 dB for only 10 minutes per hour.
Play audio recording of parents' and siblings' voices.
Softly play simple, soothing music[a]; recording of womb sounds; or music box for short periods only.
Call infant by name at each interaction.

Vestibular

Position with limbs and trunk in flexion with hands to face at midline.
Slowly change position during handling; avoid quick position changes.
Side-to-side slow movement is preferred over rocking.
Place in sling (hammock) and rock.
Close infant's fist around cloth toy.
Lift head to upright position, tip to right and then to left, stopping at midline (only with stable, more mature infants).
Avoid rapid horizontal to vertical movements in ill infant to minimize intracranial pressure (ICP) and autonomic consequences (desaturation, apnea, bradycardia).

Olfactory

Pass open container or a cotton gauze dipped in breast milk under nose.
Place cloth doll that has been in close contact with mother's skin in the infant's bed; avoid perfumes, scented soaps, and powders.
Use a pacifier dipped in mother's breast milk during gavage feeding for NNS.

Gustatory

Place infant's hand or a pacifier in mouth when sucking movements are observed or during gavage feeding.
Place one or two drops of milk in infant's mouth with each tube feeding.
Provide NNS at mother's breast.

Visual

Reduce light levels and protect eyes from direct lights, such as examination or procedure lights.
Place photographs of parents and siblings in visual range (19 to 22 cm [7.5 to 8.5 inches]) in en face position (maintain for short periods when awake and alert; constant picture in close proximity may be too much stimulus).
Initiate eye contact; repeat as tolerated once the infant reaches equivalent of 30 weeks of gestation. Monitor carefully for stress responses.

[a]Suggested infant relaxation music: *Heartbeat Lullabies* by Terry Woodford. Available from Baby-Go-To-Sleep Center, Audio Therapy Innovations, Inc., PO Box 550, Colorado Springs, CO 80901; 800-537-7748; http://www.babygotosleep.com.

have lost their infants nor with those who have delivered healthy, full-term infants. The staff and physicians are often guarded in discussing the infant's condition; mothers are continually expecting to hear that their infant has died, and they are sensitive to the anxieties of other mothers and staff members. Going home without their infant only compounds their feelings of disappointment, failure, and deprivation.

When an infant is to be transported from the hospital, the parents need a description of the facility where the infant is going. They need to know the location, reputation, and nature of the facility and the care that the infant is expected to receive. The name of the infant's physician and the telephone number of the nursery should be given to them, and unfamiliar terms (such as *neonatologist, ventilator, infusion,* and *incubator*) should be explained. Explanations should be kept simple, and parents given the opportunity to ask questions. If booklets are available that describe the facility, they are given to the family.

Perhaps most important, the parents should have some contact with the infant before the transport. Being able to see, touch, and (if possible) hold their infant may help decrease the parents' anxiety. Often a photograph or even a videotape of their infant can serve as tangible evidence of the newborn's existence until the parents are able to travel to the regional facility. When possible, it is often advisable to transfer the mother to the same institution as her infant.

Parents need to be informed of their infant's progress and reassured that the infant is receiving proper care. They need to understand the smallest aspects of the infant's condition and treatment. Parents need a realistic, honest, and direct assessment of the situation. Using nonmedical terminology, moving at a pace that is comfortable for parents to assimilate the information, and avoiding lengthy technical explanations facilitate communication with family members. Psychologic tasks that must be accomplished by parents during their infant's care are presented in Box 8.2.

BOX 8.2 Psychologic Tasks of Parents of a High-Risk Infant

- Work through the events surrounding labor and delivery.
- Acknowledge that the infant's life is endangered and begin the anticipatory grieving process.
- Confront and recognize feelings of inadequacy and guilt in not delivering a healthy child.
- Adapt to the neonatal intensive care environment.
- Resume parental relationships with the sick infant and initiate the caregiving role.
- Prepare to take the infant home.

Modified from Gardner, S. L., Voos, K., & Hills, P. (2016). Families in crisis: Theoretical and practical considerations. In S. L. Gardner, B. S. Carter, M. Enzman-Hines, et al. (Eds.), *Merenstein and Gardner's handbook of neonatal intensive care* (8th ed.). St Louis, MO: Mosby/Elsevier.

Facilitating Parent-Infant Relationships

Because of their physiologic instability, infants are separated from their mothers immediately and surrounded by a complex, impenetrable barrier of glass windows, mechanical equipment, and special caregivers. There is some evidence indicating that the emotional separation that accompanies the physical separation of mothers and infants may interfere with the normal mother-infant attachment process discussed in Chapter 7. Maternal attachment is a cumulative process that begins before conception, strengthens by significant events during pregnancy, and matures through mother-infant contact during the neonatal period and infancy.

When an infant is sick, the necessary physical separation appears to be accompanied by an emotional estrangement by the parents, which may seriously damage the capacity for parenting their infant. This detachment is further hampered by the tenuous nature of the infant's condition. When survival is in doubt, parents may be reluctant to establish a relationship with their infant. They prepare themselves for the infant's death while continuing to hope for recovery. This **anticipatory grief** (see Chapter 17) and hesitancy to embark on a relationship are evidenced by behaviors such as delay in giving the infant a name, reluctance in visiting the nursery (or when they do visit, focusing on equipment and treatments rather than on the infant), and hesitancy to touch or handle the infant when given the opportunity.

Family-centered care of high-risk newborns includes encouraging and facilitating parental involvement rather than isolating parents from their infant and associated care. This is particularly important in relation to mothers; to reduce the effects of physical separation, mothers are united with their newborn at the earliest opportunity.

Preparing the parents to see their infant for the first time is an important nursing responsibility. The nurse prepares parents for their infant's appearance, the equipment attached to the child, and the general atmosphere of the unit. The initial encounter with the intensive care unit is a stressful experience, and the frightening array of people, equipment, and activity is likely to be overwhelming. A book of photographs or pamphlets describing the NICU environment (infants in incubators or under radiant warmers, monitors, mechanical ventilators, and IV equipment) provides a useful and nonthreatening introduction to the NICU.

Parents are encouraged to visit their infant as soon as possible. Even if they saw the infant at the time of transport or shortly after birth, the infant may have changed considerably, especially if a number of medical and equipment requirements are associated with the infant's hospitalization. At the bedside, the nurse should explain the function of each piece of equipment and the role it plays in facilitating recovery. Explanations may often need to be patiently repeated because parents' anxiety over the infant's condition and the surroundings may prevent them from really "hearing" what is being said. When possible, some items related to therapy can be removed; for example, phototherapy can be temporarily discontinued and eye patches removed to permit eye-to-eye contact.

Parents appreciate the support of a nurse during the initial visit with their infant, but they may also appreciate some time alone with the infant for a short while. It is important during the early visits to emphasize the positive aspects of their infant's behavior and development so that the parents can focus on their infant as an individual rather than on the equipment that surrounds the child. For example, the nurse may describe the infant's spontaneous behaviors during care, such as the grasp reflex and spontaneous movement, or make comments about the infant's biologic functions. Most institutions have open visiting policies so that parents and siblings may visit their infant as often as they wish.

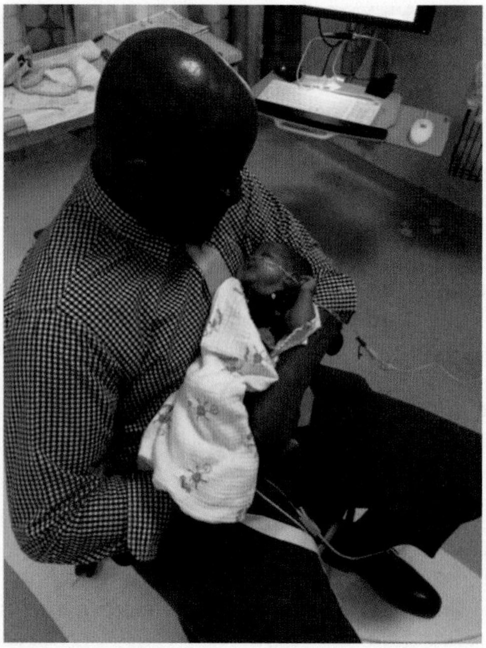

Fig. 8.14 Father interacting with newborn receiving intensive care. (Photo courtesy K. Fisher, Duke University Medical Center, Durham, NC.)

Parents vary greatly in the degree to which they are able to interact with their infant. Some may wish to touch or hold their infant during the first visit, but others may not feel comfortable enough to even enter the nursery. These reactions depend on a variety of prenatal and postnatal factors, such as the parity of the mother and her preparation before birth; the infant's size, condition, and physical appearance; and the type of treatment the infant is receiving. It is essential to recognize that the individualized pacing and quality of the interactions are more important than an early onset of these interactions. Parents may not be receptive to early and extended infant contact because they need time to adjust to the impact of an infant with birth problems and must be helped to grieve before they can accept their infant.

The parents' inability to focus on their infant is a clue for the nurse to assist the parents in expressing feelings of guilt, anxiety, helplessness, inadequacy, anger, and ambivalence. Nurses can help parents deal with these distressing feelings and recognize that they are normal responses shared by other parents. It is important to point out and reinforce the positive aspects of parents' behavior and interactions with their infant.

Most parents feel shaky and insecure about initiating interaction with their infant. Nurses can sense parents' level of readiness and offer encouragement in these initial efforts. Parents of preterm infants follow the same acquaintance process as do parents of term infants. They may quickly proceed through the process or may require several days or even weeks to complete it. Parents begin by touching their infant's extremities with their fingertips and poking the infant tenderly and then proceed to caresses and fondling (Figs. 8.14 and 8.15). Touching is the first act of communication between parents and child. Parents need to be prepared for their infant's exaggerated and generalized startle responses to touch so that they will not interpret these as negative reactions to their overtures. It may be necessary to limit tactile stimuli when the infant is critically ill and labile, but the nurse can offer other options such as speaking softly or sitting at the bedside.

Parents of acutely ill preterm infants may express feelings of helplessness and lack of control. Involving the parent in some type of caregiving activity, no matter how minor it may seem to the nurse, enables the parent to "take on" a more active role. Examples of such

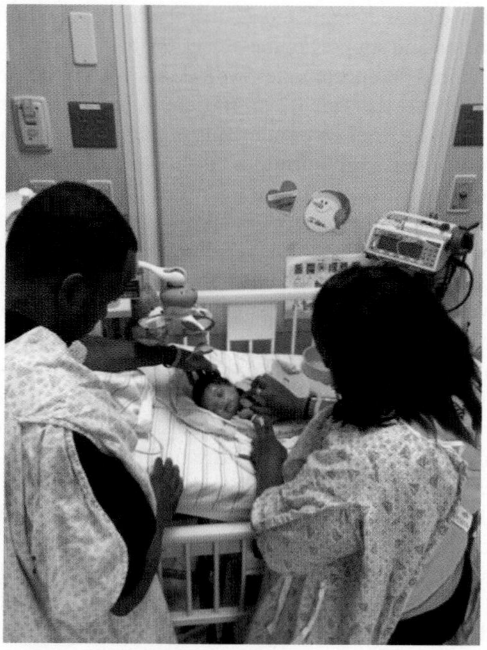

Fig. 8.15 Mother and father interacting with their preterm infant. (Photo courtesy K. Fisher, Duke University Medical Center, Durham, NC.)

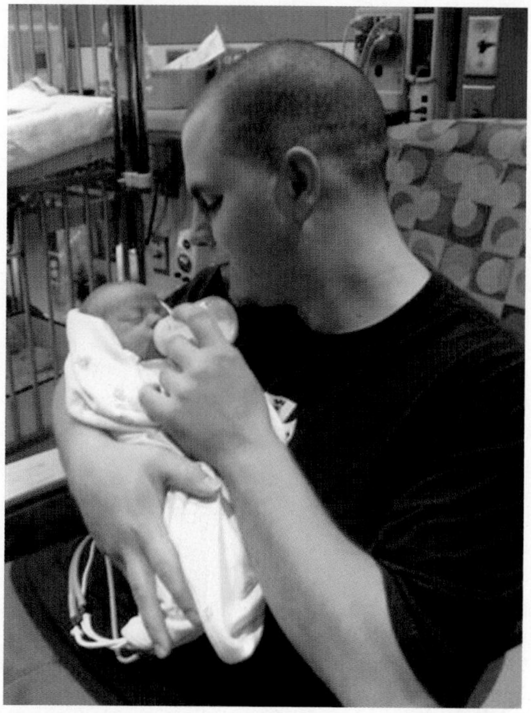

Fig. 8.16 Father feeding preterm infant. (Photo courtesy E. Jacobs, Texas Children's Hospital, Houston, TX.)

caregiving for an acutely ill infant who cannot be held and is seemingly not responding positively include moistening the infant's lips with a small amount of sterile water on a cotton-tipped swab or slipping the diaper from under the infant when it is wet or soiled.

Eventually, parents begin to endow their infant with an identity—as part of the family. When an infant no longer appears as a foreign object and begins to take on aspects of family members, such as the father's chin or the sister's nose, nurses can facilitate this incorporation. Parents are encouraged to bring in clothes, a toy, a stuffed animal, or a family snapshot for their infant, and the nurse can help parents set goals for themselves and for the infant. Parents may become involved by reading a children's storybook or nursery rhymes in a soft, soothing voice. Some families record the parents' voices telling or reading stories and play the audio when the infant is able to cope with such stimuli. Feeding schedules are discussed, and parents are encouraged to visit at times when they can become involved in the care of their infant (Fig. 8.16).

Throughout the parent-infant acquaintance process, the nurse listens carefully to what the parents say to assess their concerns and their progress toward incorporating the infant into their lives. The manner in which parents refer to their infant and the questions they ask reveal their worries and feelings and can serve as valuable clues to future relationships with the infant. The alert nurse is attuned to these subtle indications of parents' needs, which provide guidelines for nursing intervention. Often all that the parents need is reassurance that they will have the support of the nurse during caregiving activities and that the behaviors about which they are concerned are normal reactions and will disappear as the infant matures.

Parents need guidance in their relationships with their infant and assistance in their efforts to meet their infant's physical and developmental needs. The nursing staff must help parents understand that their preterm infant offers few behavioral rewards and show them how to accept small rewards from their infant. The infant's reactions and behaviors are explained to parents, who take their infant's jerky, rejective behavior personally. They need reassurance that these behaviors are not a reflection on their parenting skills. Parents are taught to recognize their infant's cues regarding stimulation, handling, and other interaction, especially aversive behaviors that indicate a need for rest. Nurses need to include parents in planning their infant's care and sensory stimulation materials, such as a music box or recording.

Above all, nurses must encourage and reinforce parents during their caregiving activities and interactions with their infant to promote healthy parent-child relationships. It is also helpful for the parents to have contact and communication with a consistent group of nurses. This decreases the different information given to parents and often instills confidence that although the parents cannot be at their infant's bedside 24 hours a day, there are competent and caring nurses whom they may call to inquire about the infant's status. Periodic parent conferences involving the staff caring for the child serve to clarify misunderstandings or problems related to the infant's condition.

Siblings

In the past, concerns about sibling visitation in the NICU focused on fears of infection and disruption of nursing routines. These fears have not been substantiated, and sibling visits should be a part of the normal operation of NICUs (Fig. 8.17). Clearly defined policies and procedures should be developed to facilitate sibling visitation (American Academy of Pediatrics & American College of Obstetricians and Gynecologists, 2017; Maree & Downes, 2016).

The birth of a preterm infant is a difficult time for siblings, who rely on the support of understanding parents. When the happy anticipation is changed to sadness, worry, and altered routines, siblings are bewildered and deprived of their parents' attention. They know something is wrong, but they have only a dim understanding of what it is. Concern about the negative effects on visiting siblings of seeing the ill newborn has not been confirmed. Children have not hesitated to approach or touch the infant, and children younger than 5 years old have been less reluctant than older children; in addition, there have been no measurable differences between previsit and postvisit behaviors.

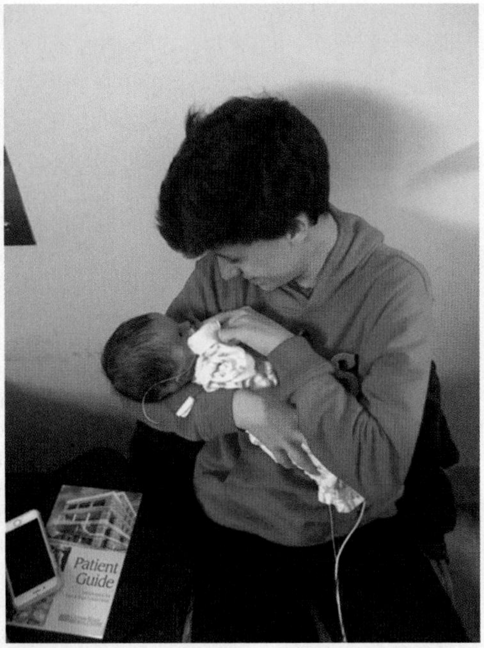

Fig. 8.17 Sibling holding brother in the neonatal intensive care unit (NICU). (Photo courtesy K. Fisher, Duke University Medical Center, Durham, NC.)

The potential benefits of sibling visits must be weighed against exposure of the child to the environment of the NICU. Children must be prepared for the unfamiliar NICU atmosphere, but contact with the infant appears to have a positive effect on siblings by helping them deal with the reality rather than the bizarre fantasies that are characteristic of young children. Such visits also help to bond the family as a unit.

Support Groups

Parents need to feel that they are not alone. Parent support groups have been of immeasurable value to families of infants in the NICU. Some groups consist of parents who have infants in the hospital and share the same anxieties and concerns. Other groups include parents who have had infants in the NICU and who have dealt with the crisis effectively. The groups are usually under the leadership of a staff person and involve physicians, nurses, and social workers, but the parents can offer other parents something that no one else can provide.

An excellent resource for parents of preterm infants is the book *Understanding the NICU: What Parents of Preemies and Other Hospitalized Newborns Need to Know* (Zaichkin, Weiner, & Loren, 2017). This resource, published by the American Academy of Pediatrics, has technical and anecdotal information on different problems facing preterm infants, common treatments and therapies, preparation for home discharge, and home care for the preterm infant.

Discharge Planning and Home Care

Parents become apprehensive and excited as the time for discharge approaches. They have many concerns and insecurities regarding the care of their infant. They fear that the child may still be in danger, that they will be unable to recognize signs of distress or illness in their infant, and that the infant may not yet be ready for discharge. Nurses need to begin early to assist parents in acquiring or increasing their skills in the care of their infant. Appropriate instruction must be provided and sufficient time allowed for the family to assimilate the information and learn the continuing special care requirements. Where rooming-in or other live-in arrangements are available, parents can stay for a few days and nights and assume the care of their infant under the supervision and support of the nursery staff.

There should be appropriate medical and nursing follow-up and referrals to services that can benefit the family, including developmental follow-up. Parents of preterm infants should also be given adequate information about immunizations with other discharge planning information. With the trend toward earlier discharge, many hospital-based home health care agencies become involved in the follow-up and care of NICU "graduates" in the home. For the parents of an infant being discharged with equipment (such as an oxygen tank, apnea monitor, or even a ventilator), discharge planning requires a multidisciplinary collaborative approach to ensure that the family has not only the appropriate resources but also the available assistance for dealing with the infant's needs. Many communities have organized support groups, including those discussed previously, those designed for parents of infants who require special care because of specific defects or disabilities, and those for parents of multiple births.

Since 1991, the American Academy of Pediatrics has recommended a car seat tolerance screen (CSTS) for all preterm infants or infants who are small for gestational age prior to being discharged from the hospital (Davis, 2015). The CSTS is meant to detect possible apnea, bradycardia, and decreased oxygen saturation during the required 90- to 120-minute screening process or the duration of the car ride home, whichever is longer (Bull, Engle, Committee on Injury, Violence, and Poison Prevention and the Committee on Fetus and Newborn, et al., 2009) (see Community Focus box). For adequate support without slumping, the seat back–to–crotch strap distance must be 14 cm (5.5 inches) or less; a small rolled blanket may be placed between the crotch strap and the infant to reduce slouching. The distance from the lower harness strap to the seat bottom should be 25.5 cm (10 inches) or less to decrease the potential for the harness straps to cross the infant's ears. The rear-facing position provides support for the head, neck, and back, thereby reducing the stress to the neck and spinal cord in a vehicle crash. Car seat manufacturers must specify recommended minimum and maximum weights for the occupant; therefore it is important to check the manufacturer's recommendations before purchasing a car seat for a smaller infant. Additional guidelines are available from the American Academy of Pediatrics (Durbin & Committee on Injury, Violence, and Poison Prevention, 2011). See Chapter 9 for a discussion of infant car restraints.

COMMUNITY FOCUS

Preterm and Near-Term Infant Car Seat Evaluation

The American Academy of Pediatrics (Bull et al., 2009) recommends that infants born before 37 weeks of gestation be evaluated for apnea, bradycardia, and oxygen desaturation episodes before hospital discharge.[a] The American Academy of Pediatrics suggests that facilities develop policies for the implementation of a program of evaluation; however, few evidence-based practice recommendations have been published to date delineating specific requirements for such a program. Based on the available literature, suggestions for providing a car seat evaluation of infants born before 37 weeks of gestation include:

- Use the parents' car seat for the evaluation.
- Perform the evaluation 1 to 7 days before the infant's anticipated discharge.
- Set the pulse oximeter low alarm at 88% (or per unit protocol).
- Set the heart rate low alarm limit at 80 beats/min and apnea alarm at 20 seconds (cardiorespiratory monitor).
- Leave the infant undisturbed semiupright in the car seat for a minimum of 90 to 120 minutes or for the time parents state it takes to arrive at their home (whichever is longer).

Continued

COMMUNITY FOCUS—cont'd

- Document the infant's tolerance to the car seat evaluation.
- An episode of desaturation, bradycardia, or apnea (20 seconds or more) constitutes a failure, and evaluation by the practitioner must occur before discharge. If the infant experiences this in a semiupright position, a car bed with the infant supine should be considered, and similar testing should be undertaken in the car bed.
- Repeat the test in 24 hours after modifications have been made to the car seat, car bed, or infant's position in either restraint system.
- It is recommended that a certified car seat technician place the infant in the car seat (or bed) if a failure occurs (see National Highway Traffic Safety Administration website[b] for car seat inspection station).
- If the infant is being discharged on an apnea or cardiorespiratory monitor, this equipment should be used during the trip home.
- The technician will demonstrate appropriate positioning of the infant in the restraint device to the parents and have the parents do a return demonstration.
- Document the interventions, the infant's tolerance, and the parents' return demonstration.

[a]Infants at risk for obstructive apnea (e.g., Pierre Robin sequence or congenital neuromuscular disorders such as spinal muscular atrophy) may also need to be evaluated in a semiupright car seat or car bed before discharge.
[b]http://www.nhtsa.gov
Modified from American Academy of Pediatrics. (2009). Safe transportation of premature and low birth weight infants. *Pediatrics, 123*(5), 1424–1429; O'Neil, J., Yonkman, J., Taltry, J., et al. (2009). Transporting children with special health care needs. *Pediatrics, 124*(2), 596–603; Bull, M. J., Engle, W. A., Committee on Injury, Violence, and Poison Prevention and the Committee on Fetus and Newborn, et al. (2009). Safe transportation of preterm and low birth weight infants at hospital discharge. *Pediatrics, 123*(5), 1424–1429.

An important part of discharge planning and care of preterm infants is nutrition for continued growth; thus the choice of feeding must be carefully addressed. Human milk is the recommended form of infant nutrition. The feeding of human milk to all infants, term and preterm, is supported by the American Academy of Pediatrics.

An enriched postdischarge formula has been used for preterm infants born at less than 36 weeks to meet appropriate growth standards (Poindexter & Ehrenkranz, 2015). However, a Cochrane review of studies examining growth in preterm infants fed an enriched postdischarge formula did not find strong evidence of enhanced growth and development compared with infants fed standard formula (Young, Embleton, & McGuire, 2016). Various products are available to fortify human milk, and these should be used to maintain adequate growth and development for the preterm infant (Radmacher & Adamkin, 2017).

Knowing that staff members are available for telephone or personal contact when the parents take the infant home provides a measure of security to anxious parents. Many NICU facilities maintain a policy of open communication between staff and parents both during the infant's hospitalization and after discharge. It is the responsibility of the NICU staff to make certain that parents are prepared to care for their infant, both emotionally and physically. At the same time, it is important that parents establish a trusting relationship with the infant's primary care provider in the community before discharge from the acute care facility.

Neonatal Loss

The precarious nature of many high-risk infants makes death a real and ever-present possibility. Although infant mortality has been reduced sharply with improved technology, the mortality rate is still greatest during the neonatal period. Nurses in the NICU are the persons who must prepare the parents for an inevitable death, provide end-of-life care for the infant and family, and facilitate a family's grieving process after an expected or unexpected death.

The loss of an infant has special meaning for the grieving parents. It represents a loss of a part of themselves, a loss of the potential for immortality that offspring represent, and the loss of the dream child that has been fantasized about throughout the pregnancy. There is often a sense of emptiness and failure. In addition, when an infant has lived for such a short time, there may be few, if any, pleasant memories to serve as a basis for the identification and idealization that are part of the resolution of a loss.

To help parents understand that the death is a reality, it is important that they be encouraged to hold their infant before death and, if possible, be present at the time of death so that their infant can die in their arms if they choose. Many who deny the need to hold their infant may later regret the decision.

Parents are given the opportunity to actually "parent" the infant in any manner they wish or are able to do before and after the death. This may include seeing, touching, holding, caressing, and talking to their infant privately; the parents may also wish to bathe and dress the infant. If parents are hesitant about seeing their dead infant, it is advisable to keep the body in the unit for a few hours because many parents change their minds after the initial shock of the death.

Parents may need to see and hold the infant more than once—the first time to say "hello" and the last time to say "goodbye." If parents wish to see the infant after the body has been taken to the morgue, the infant should be retrieved, wrapped in a blanket, rewarmed in a radiant warmer, and taken to the mother's room or other private place. The nurse should stay with the parents and provide them with an opportunity for private time alone with their dead infant. Individual grief responses of the mother and father should be recognized and handled appropriately; gender differences and cultural and religious beliefs will affect the parents' grief responses.

A hospice approach for families with infants for whom the decision has been made to not prolong life and who are receiving only palliative care may be implemented in such cases. Another approach is to send the family home with the infant and allow them to spend time together until the eventual death; hospice services may be available, and supportive care is provided in the home setting. Some families find this option less restrictive and more family oriented than being in the hospital setting. See Chapter 17 for further discussion of hospice care.

When available, providers trained in palliative care bring additional expertise in effective acute and chronic pain management for infants and their families (Marc-Aurele & English, 2016). Early integration of palliative care permits involvement of decision support for both the family and the clinicians. A fundamental focus of palliative care is on maximizing quality of life for both the patient and the family throughout the process of illness (Lemmon, Bidegain, & Boss, 2016). Integrating this focus early may help families begin to formulate their goals related to quality of life and thus lessen the burden of decision making on the family.

A photograph of the infant taken before or after death is highly desirable. Parents may wish to have a special family portrait taken with the infant and other family members; this often helps personalize the experience and make it more tangible. The parents may not wish to see the photograph at the time of death, but the chance to refer to it later will help make their infant seem more real, which is a part of the normal grief process. A photograph of their infant being held by the hand or touched by an adult offers a more positive image than a morgue-type photograph. A bereavement or memory packet can be given to the grieving parents and family; it may include the infant's handprints and footprints; a lock of hair; the bedside name card; the ID bracelet or armbands; and as appropriate to the family's religious beliefs, a certificate of baptism.

Naming the deceased infant is an important step in the grieving process. Some parents may hesitate to give the newborn a name that was chosen during the pregnancy for their "special baby." However, having a tangible person for whom to grieve is an important component of the grieving process.

A nurse who is familiar to the family should be present during the discussion about the dead or dying infant. The nurse should talk with parents openly and honestly about funeral arrangements, because few parents have had experience with this aspect of death. Many funeral homes now offer inexpensive arrangements for these special cases. Someone from the NICU should take the responsibility for acquiring this type of information. It is often helpful to parents for the NICU to have a list of local funeral homes, services offered, and prices. Families need to be informed of the options available, but a funeral is preferable because the ritual provides an opportunity for parents to feel the support of friends and relatives. A member of the clergy of the appropriate faith may be notified if the parents wish. Issues regarding an autopsy or organ donation (when appropriate) are approached in a multidisciplinary fashion (primary practitioner and primary nurse) with respect, sensitivity to cultural and religious beliefs, tact, and consideration of the family's wishes.

Before the parents leave the hospital, they are given the telephone number of the unit (if they do not have it) and invited to call any time they have further questions. Many intensive care units make a point to contact the parents several weeks after a neonatal death to assess the parents' coping mechanisms, evaluate the grieving process, and provide support as needed. Several organizations are available to offer support and understanding to families who have lost a newborn; these organization include the Compassionate Friends,[d] Aiding Mothers and Fathers Experiencing Neonatal Death,[e] and Share Pregnancy and Infant Loss Support, Incorporated.[f] See Chapter 17 for further discussion of the family and the grief process.

Nurses who care for critically ill infants also experience grief; NICU nurses may feel helpless and sorrowful. It is important that such grief be allowed and that nurses attend the funeral or memorial service as a part of working through the grief process. Nurses may fear that showing emotion is unprofessional and that the expression of grief indicates "loss of control." These fears are unfounded. Studies have demonstrated that to continue to be effective managers and providers of care, nurses must be allowed to grieve and support each other through the process (Gardner & Carter, 2016).

Baptism

Because many Christian parents wish to have their child baptized if death is anticipated or is a decided possibility, this may become a nursing responsibility. Whenever possible, it is most desirable that a representative of the parents' faith (e.g., Roman Catholic priest, Protestant minister) perform such a ritual. When death is imminent, a nurse or a physician can perform the baptism by simply pouring water on the infant's forehead (a medicine dropper is a convenient means) while repeating the words, "I baptize you in the name of the Father and of the Son and of the Holy Spirit." This includes a birth of any gestational age, particularly when the parents are Roman Catholic.

When the parents' faith is uncertain, a conditional baptism can be carried out by saying, "If you are capable of receiving baptism, I baptize you in the name of the Father and of the Son and of the Holy Spirit." The baptism is recorded in the infant's chart, and a notice is placed on the crib or incubator. Parents are informed at the first opportunity.

HIGH RISK RELATED TO DYSMATURITY

PRETERM INFANTS

Prematurity accounts for the largest number of admissions to NICUs. Immaturity of most organ systems places infants at risk for a variety of neonatal complications (e.g., hyperbilirubinemia, respiratory distress syndrome [RDS], intellectual and motor delays). According to the Centers for Disease Control and Prevention, low birth weight and prematurity were the second leading cause of infant mortality in the United States in 2011 (Kochanek, Murphy, & Xu, 2015). The actual cause of prematurity is not known in most instances. Factors such as poverty, maternal infections, previous preterm delivery, multiple pregnancies, pregnancy-induced hypertension, and placental problems that interrupt the normal course of gestation before completion of fetal development are responsible for a large number of preterm births. Additional factors are listed in Box 8.3.

BOX 8.3 Etiology of Preterm Birth

Maternal Factors

Socioeconomic
- Malnutrition
- Age
- Race

Chronic Medical Conditions
- Heart disease
- Renal disease
- Diabetes
- Hypertension

Behavioral
- Substance abuse
- Smoking
- Poor or absent prenatal care

Factors Related to Pregnancy

Multiple pregnancy
Low body mass index (<19.8 kg/m^2) (Markham & Fanaroff, 2015)
Abruptio placentae or placenta previa
Incompetent cervix
Maternal hypertension
Premature rupture of membranes or chorioamnionitis
Polyhydramnios or oligohydramnios
Infection
Trauma

Fetal Factors

Chromosomal abnormalities
Congenital anomalies
Nonimmune hydrops
Erythroblastosis

Unknown Factors

[d]PO Box 3696, Oakbrook, IL 60522-3696; 630-990-0010, 877-969-0010; http://www.compassionatefriends.org
[e]Contact Maureen Connelly, 4324 Berrywick Terrace, St Louis, MO 63128; 314-487-7582; or Martha Eise, Martha@amendgroup.com; http://www.amendgroup.com
[f]National Share Office, 402 Jackson Street, St Charles, MO 63301; 800-821-6819.

The outlook for preterm infants is largely, but not entirely, related to the state of physiologic and anatomic immaturity of the various organs and systems at the time of birth. Infants at term have advanced to a state of maturity sufficient to allow a successful transition to the extrauterine environment. Preterm infants must make the same adjustments but with functional immaturity proportional to the stage of development reached at the time of birth. However, these adjustments may be limited or even hindered by the external environment to which the preterm infant is exposed. Exposure to excessive stimuli, bacteria, and viruses make the environment less conducive for preterm infants to grow and develop. The degree to which infants are prepared for extrauterine life can be predicted to some extent by birth weight and estimated gestational age (see Chapter 7, Clinical Assessment of Gestational Age).

Within the past decade, increasing attention has been given to **late preterm infants**, that is, infants born between 34 and $36^{6}/_{7}$ weeks' gestation. Such infants have some of the same risk factors as those born before 34 weeks' gestation, but physical characteristics and adaptation to extrauterine life are variable. Late preterm infants have metabolic and physical immaturity that places them at risk for greater mortality and morbidity than term infants (Aliaga, Zhang, Long, et al., 2016). Studies have demonstrated decreased cognitive and motor function in late preterm infants at 24 months compared with term infants (Natarajan & Shankaran, 2016). In the following sections, the discussion of preterm infants continues to apply to all infants who are born before a completed gestational age of 37 weeks. Because prematurity now encompasses a wider age, weight, and physiologic maturity range, physical characteristics described may also vary; such descriptions are generalized for description purposes.

Diagnostic Evaluation

Preterm infants have a number of distinct characteristics at various stages of development. Identification of these characteristics provides valuable clues to the gestational age and hence to the infant's physiologic capabilities. The general, outward physical appearance changes as the infant progresses to maturity. Characteristics of skin, general attitude (or posture) when supine, appearance of hair, and amount of subcutaneous fat provide clues to a newborn's physical development. Observation of spontaneous, active movements and response to stimulation and passive movement contributes to the assessment of neurologic status. The appraisal is made as soon as possible after admission to the nursery because much of the observation and management of infants depends on this information.

On inspection, preterm infants are very small and appear scrawny, because they have only minimal subcutaneous fat deposits (or none, in some cases) and have a proportionately large head in relation to the body, which reflects the cephalocaudal direction of growth. The skin is bright pink (often translucent, depending on the degree of immaturity), smooth, and shiny, with small blood vessels clearly visible underneath the thin epidermis. The fine lanugo hair is abundant over the body (depending on gestational age) but is sparse, fine, and fuzzy on the head. The ear cartilage is soft and pliable, and the soles and palms have minimal creases, resulting in a smooth appearance. The bones of the skull and the ribs feel soft, and the eyes may be closed. Male infants have few scrotal rugae, and the testes are undescended; in girls, the labia and clitoris are prominent. Fig. 8.18 compares the features of full-term and preterm infants.

In contrast to full-term infants' overall attitude of flexion and continuous activity, preterm infants may be inactive and listless. The extremities maintain an attitude of extension and remain in any position in which they are placed. Reflex activity is only partially developed—sucking is absent, weak, or ineffectual; swallow, gag, and cough reflexes are absent or weak; and other neurologic signs are absent or diminished. Physiologically immature, preterm infants are unable to maintain body temperature, have limited ability to excrete solutes in the urine, and have increased susceptibility to infection. A pliable thorax, immature lung tissue, and an immature regulatory center lead to periodic breathing, hypoventilation, and frequent periods of apnea. They are more susceptible to biochemical alterations such as hyperbilirubinemia and hypoglycemia, and they have a higher extracellular water content that renders them more vulnerable to fluid and electrolyte derangements. Preterm infants exchange fully half of their extracellular fluid volume every 24 hours compared with one-seventh of the volume in adults. The soft cranium is subject to characteristic unintentional deformation (dolichocephaly) caused by positioning from one side to the other on a mattress (McCarty, Peat, Malcolm, et al., 2017). The head looks disproportionately longer from front to back, is flattened on both sides, and lacks the usual convexity seen at the temporal and parietal areas. This positional molding is often a concern to parents and may influence the parents' perception of the infant's attractiveness and their responsiveness to the infant. Positioning the infant on a waterbed or gel mattress and the use of a midliner positioning system can reduce or minimize cranial molding (McCarty, O'Donnell, Goldstein, et al., 2018).

Neurologic impairment (e.g., intraventricular hemorrhage) and serious sequelae correlate with the size and gestational age of infants at birth and with the severity of neonatal complications. The greater the degree of immaturity, the greater the degree of potential disability. A greater incidence of cerebral palsy, attention-deficit/hyperactivity disorder (ADHD), visual-motor deficits, and altered intellectual functioning is observed in preterm than in full-term infants. However, behavioral development can be enhanced when families are provided with support and infants are referred to appropriate services for neurologic and developmental interventions. Parental interest and involvement are important variables in the developmental progress of infants.

Therapeutic Management

When delivery of a preterm infant is anticipated, the intensive care nursery is alerted and a team approach implemented. Ideally, a neonatologist, an advanced practice nurse, a staff nurse, and a respiratory therapist are present for the delivery. Infants who do not require resuscitation are immediately transferred in a heated incubator to the NICU, where they are weighed and where IV lines, oxygen therapy, and other therapeutic interventions are initiated as needed. Resuscitation is conducted in the delivery area until infants can be safely transported to the NICU.

Subsequent care is determined by the infant's status. The general care of preterm infants differs from that of full-term infants primarily in the areas of respiratory support, temperature regulation, nutrition, susceptibility to infection, activity intolerance, neurodevelopmental care, and other consequences of physical immaturity.

Nursing Care Management

The nursing care, similar to the therapeutic management, is individualized for each infant. See appropriate discussions in the Nursing Care of the High-Risk Newborn and Family section for additional details of care.

POSTTERM INFANTS

Infants born beyond 42 weeks as calculated from the mother's last menstrual period (or by gestational age assessment) are considered postterm regardless of birth weight. This constitutes 3.5% to 15% of all pregnancies. The cause of delayed birth is unknown. Some infants

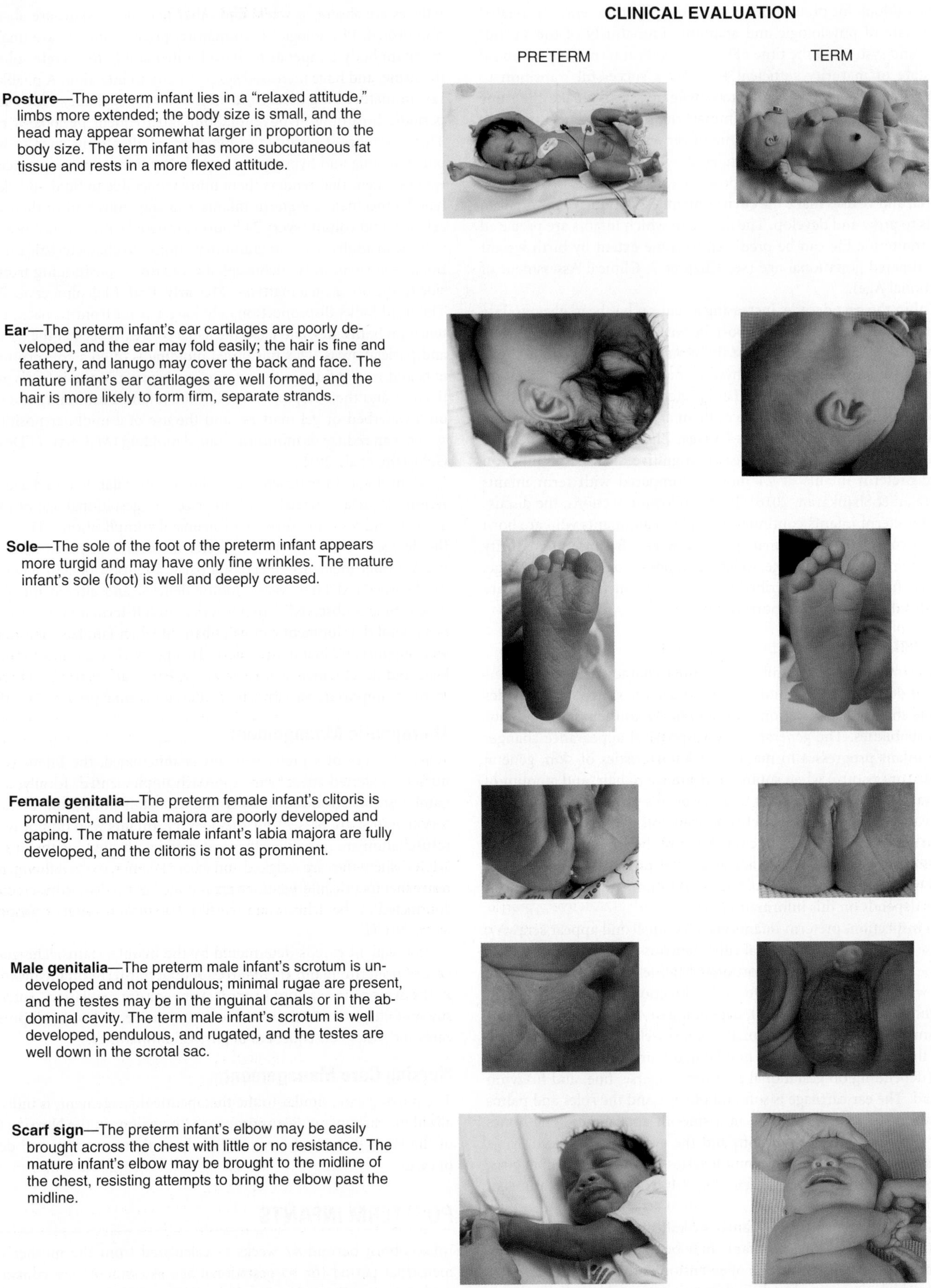
CLINICAL EVALUATION
PRETERM
TERM
Posture—The preterm infant lies in a "relaxed attitude," limbs more extended; the body size is small, and the head may appear somewhat larger in proportion to the body size. The term infant has more subcutaneous fat tissue and rests in a more flexed attitude.
Ear—The preterm infant's ear cartilages are poorly developed, and the ear may fold easily; the hair is fine and feathery, and lanugo may cover the back and face. The mature infant's ear cartilages are well formed, and the hair is more likely to form firm, separate strands.
Sole—The sole of the foot of the preterm infant appears more turgid and may have only fine wrinkles. The mature infant's sole (foot) is well and deeply creased.
Female genitalia—The preterm female infant's clitoris is prominent, and labia majora are poorly developed and gaping. The mature female infant's labia majora are fully developed, and the clitoris is not as prominent.
Male genitalia—The preterm male infant's scrotum is undeveloped and not pendulous; minimal rugae are present, and the testes may be in the inguinal canals or in the abdominal cavity. The term male infant's scrotum is well developed, pendulous, and rugated, and the testes are well down in the scrotal sac.
Scarf sign—The preterm infant's elbow may be easily brought across the chest with little or no resistance. The mature infant's elbow may be brought to the midline of the chest, resisting attempts to bring the elbow past the midline.

Fig. 8.18 Clinical and neurologic examinations comparing preterm and full-term infants. (Data from Pierog, S. H., & Ferrara, A. [1976]. *Medical care of the sick newborn* [2nd ed.]. St Louis, MO: Mosby.)

NEUROLOGIC EVALUATION

PRETERM TERM

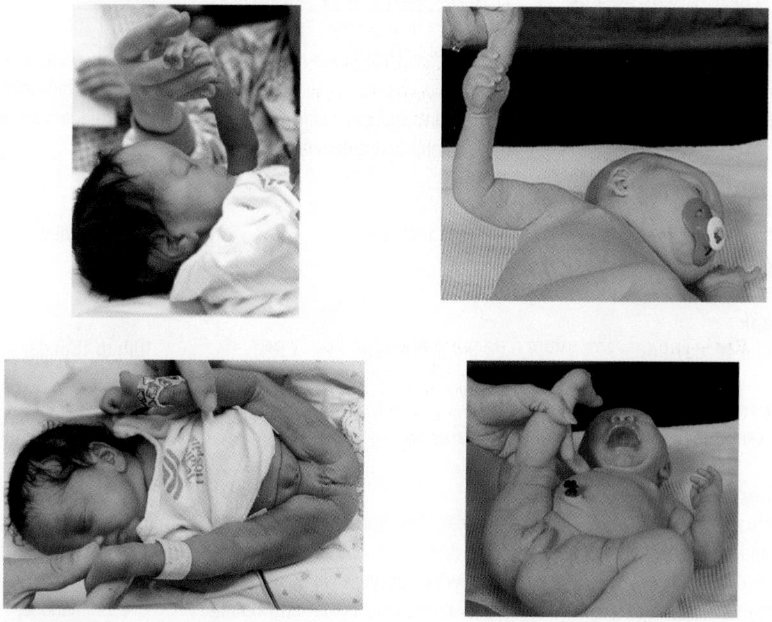

Grasp reflex—The preterm infant's grasp is weak; the term infant's grasp is strong, allowing the infant to be lifted up from the mattress.

Heel-to-ear maneuver—The preterm infant's heel is easily brought to the ear, meeting with no resistance. This maneuver is not possible in the term infant, since there is considerable resistance at the knee.

Fig. 8.18—cont'd

are appropriate for gestational age but show the characteristics of progressive placental dysfunction. These infants display characteristics such as absence of lanugo, little if any vernix caseosa, abundant scalp hair, and long fingernails. The skin is often cracked, parchment-like, and desquamating. A common finding in postterm infants is a wasted physical appearance that reflects intrauterine deprivation. Depletion of subcutaneous fat gives them a thin, elongated appearance. The little vernix caseosa that remains in the skinfolds may be stained a deep yellow or green, which is usually an indication of meconium in the amniotic fluid.

There is a significant increase in fetal and neonatal mortality in postterm infants compared with those born at term. They are especially prone to fetal distress associated with the decreasing efficiency of the placenta, macrosomia, and meconium aspiration syndrome. The greatest risk occurs during the stresses of labor and delivery, particularly in an infant of a **primigravida**, or a woman delivering her first child. Close surveillance with fetal assessment and induction of labor is usually recommended when infants are significantly overdue.

HIGH RISK RELATED TO PHYSIOLOGIC FACTORS

HYPERBILIRUBINEMIA

Hyperbilirubinemia refers to an excessive level of accumulated bilirubin in the blood and is characterized by **jaundice**, or **icterus**, a yellowish discoloration of the skin, sclerae, and nails. Hyperbilirubinemia is a common finding in newborns and in most instances is relatively benign. However, in extreme cases, it can indicate a pathologic state.

Hyperbilirubinemia may result from increased unconjugated or conjugated bilirubin. The unconjugated form or indirect hyperbilirubinemia (Table 8.3) is the type most commonly seen in newborns. The following discussion of hyperbilirubinemia is limited to unconjugated hyperbilirubinemia.

Pathophysiology

Bilirubin is one of the breakdown products of the hemoglobin that results from RBC destruction. When RBCs are destroyed, the breakdown products are released into the circulation, where the hemoglobin splits into two fractions: heme and globin. The globin (protein) portion is used by the body, and the heme portion is converted to **unconjugated bilirubin**, an insoluble substance bound to albumin.

In the liver, the bilirubin is detached from the albumin molecule and, in the presence of the enzyme **glucuronyl transferase**, is conjugated with glucuronic acid to produce a highly soluble substance, **conjugated bilirubin**, which is then excreted into the bile. In the intestine, bacterial action reduces the conjugated bilirubin to urobilinogen, the pigment that gives stool its characteristic color. Most of the reduced bilirubin is excreted through the feces; a small amount is eliminated in the urine.

Normally, the body can maintain a balance between the destruction of RBCs and the use or excretion of byproducts. However, when developmental limitations or a pathologic process interferes with this balance, bilirubin accumulates in the tissues to produce jaundice. Possible causes of hyperbilirubinemia in newborns are:

- Physiologic (developmental) factors (prematurity)
- An association with breastfeeding or breast milk
- Dehydration (limited oral intake)
- Excess production of bilirubin (e.g., hemolytic disease, biochemical defects, bruises)
- Disturbed capacity of the liver to secrete conjugated bilirubin (e.g., enzyme deficiency, bile duct obstruction)
- Combined overproduction and undersecretion (e.g., sepsis)
- Some disease states (e.g., hypothyroidism, galactosemia, infant of diabetic mother [IDM])
- Genetic predisposition to increased production or delayed metabolism (American Indians, Asians, Mediterranean)

TABLE 8.3 Comparison of Major Types of Unconjugated Hyperbilirubinemia[a]

Physiologic Jaundice	Breastfeeding-Associated Jaundice (Early Onset)	Breast Milk Jaundice (Late Onset)	Hemolytic Disease
Cause			
Immature hepatic function plus increased bilirubin load from RBC hemolysis	Decreased milk intake related to fewer calories consumed by infant before mother's milk is well established; enterohepatic shunting	Possible factors in breast milk that prevent bilirubin conjugation Less frequent stooling	Blood antigen incompatibility causing hemolysis of large numbers of RBCs Liver's inability to conjugate and excrete excess bilirubin from hemolysis
Onset			
After 24 h (preterm infants, prolonged)	2nd to 4th day	4th to 8th day	During first 24 h (levels increase >5 mg/dl/day)
Peak			
3rd to 4th day	3rd to 5th day	10th to 15th day	Variable
Duration			
Declines on 5th to 7th day	Variable	May remain jaundiced for 3-12 wk or more	Depends on severity and treatment
Therapy			
Increase frequency of feedings and avoid supplements. Evaluate stooling pattern. Monitor TcB or TSB level. Perform risk assessment (see Fig. 8.19A). Use phototherapy if bilirubin levels increase significantly or significant hemolysis is present.	Breastfeed frequently (10-12 times/day); avoid supplements such as water, dextrose water, and formula. Evaluate stooling pattern; stimulate as needed. Perform risk assessment (see Fig. 8.19A). Use phototherapy if bilirubin levels increase significantly or significant hemolysis is present. If phototherapy is instituted, evaluate benefits and harm of temporarily discontinuing breastfeeding; additional assessments may be required. Assist mother with maintaining milk supply; feed expressed milk as appropriate. After discharge, follow up according to hour of discharge.	Increase frequency of breastfeeding; use no supplementation, such as glucose water; cessation of breastfeeding is not recommended. Perform risk assessment (see Fig. 8.19A). Consider performing additional evaluations: G6PD, direct and indirect serum bilirubin, family history, and others as necessary. May include home phototherapy with a temporary (10-12 h) discontinuation of breastfeeding; a subsequent TSB may be drawn to evaluate a drop in serum levels. Assist mother with maintenance of milk supply and reassurance regarding her milk supply and therapy. Use formula supplements only at practitioner's discretion.	Monitor TcB or TSB level. Perform risk assessment (see Fig. 8.19A). Postnatal: Use phototherapy; administer IV immunoglobulin per protocol; if severe, perform exchange transfusion. Prenatal: Perform transfusion (fetus). Prevent sensitization (Rh incompatibility) of Rh-negative mother with $Rh_o(D)$ immune globulin (RhIg). If mother is breastfeeding, assist with maintenance and storage of milk; may bottle-feed expressed milk as appropriate to therapy. Minimize maternal-infant separation and encourage contact as appropriate.

[a]Table depicts patterns of jaundice in term infants; patterns in preterm infants vary according to factors such as gestational age, birth weight, and illness.

G6PD, Glucose-6-phosphate dehydrogenase; *IV,* intravenous; *RBC,* red blood cell; *RhIg,* Rh immunoglobulin; *TcB,* transcutaneous bilirubin; *TSB,* total serum bilirubin.

The most common cause of hyperbilirubinemia is the relatively mild and self-limited **physiologic jaundice**. Unlike hemolytic disease of the fetus and newborn (HDFN) (see discussion later in the chapter), physiologic jaundice is not associated with any pathologic process. Although almost all newborns experience elevated bilirubin levels, only about 50% to 60% demonstrate observable signs of jaundice (Blackburn, 2018).

Two phases of physiologic jaundice have been identified in full-term infants. In the first phase, bilirubin levels of formula-fed white and African American infants gradually increase to approximately 5 to 6 mg/dl by 3 to 4 days of life and then decrease to a plateau of 2 to 3 mg/dl by the fifth day (Blackburn, 2018). Bilirubin levels maintain a steady plateau state in the second phase without increasing or decreasing until approximately 12 to 14 days, at which time levels decrease to the normal value of 1 mg/dl (Blackburn, 2018). This pattern varies according to racial group, method of feeding (breast vs. bottle), and gestational age. In preterm formula-fed infants, serum bilirubin levels may peak as high as 10 to 12 mg/dl at 5 or 6 days of life and decrease slowly over a period of 2 to 4 weeks (Blackburn, 2018).

As noted earlier, infants of Asian descent (as well as American Indians) have mean bilirubin levels almost twice those seen in whites or African Americans. An increased incidence of hyperbilirubinemia is seen in newborns from certain geographic areas, particularly areas around Greece. These populations may have glucose-6-phosphate dehydrogenase (G6PD) deficiency, which can cause hemolytic anemia.

On average, newborns produce twice as much bilirubin as adults because of higher concentrations of circulating erythrocytes and a shorter life span of RBCs (only 70 to 90 days in contrast to 120 days in older children and adults). In addition, the liver's ability to conjugate bilirubin is reduced because of limited production of glucuronyl transferase. Newborns also have a lower plasma-binding capacity for bilirubin because of reduced albumin concentrations compared with older children. Normal changes in hepatic circulation after birth may contribute to excess demands on liver function.

Normally, conjugated bilirubin is reduced to urobilinogen by the intestinal flora and excreted in feces. However, the relatively sterile and less motile newborn bowel is initially less effective in excreting urobilinogen. In the newborn intestine, the enzyme β-glucuronidase is able to convert conjugated bilirubin into the unconjugated form, which is subsequently reabsorbed by the intestinal mucosa and transported to the liver. This process, known as **enterohepatic circulation**, or **shunting**, is accentuated in newborns and is thought to be a primary mechanism in physiologic jaundice (Blackburn, 2018). Feeding (1) stimulates peristalsis and produces more rapid passage of meconium, thus diminishing the amount of reabsorption of unconjugated bilirubin; and (2) introduces bacteria to aid in the reduction of bilirubin to urobilinogen. Colostrum, a natural cathartic, facilitates meconium evacuation.

Breastfeeding is associated with an increased incidence of jaundice as a result of two distinct processes. **Breastfeeding-associated jaundice (early-onset jaundice)** begins at 2 to 4 days of age and occurs in approximately 12% to 35% of breastfed newborns (Blackburn, 2018). The jaundice is related to the process of breastfeeding and results from decreased caloric and fluid intake by breastfed infants before the milk supply is well established because decreased milk intake is associated with increased enterohepatic circulation of bilirubin (Chantry, Eglash, Labbok, et al., 2015). Reduced fluid intake results in dehydration, which also concentrates the bilirubin in the blood.

Breast milk jaundice (late-onset jaundice) begins at age 5 to 7 days and occurs in 2% to 4% of breastfed infants (Blackburn, 2018). Rising levels of bilirubin peak during the second week and gradually diminish. Despite high levels of bilirubin that may persist for 3 to 12 weeks, these infants are well. The jaundice may be caused by factors in the breast milk (pregnanediol, fatty acids, and β-glucuronidase) that either inhibit the conjugation or decrease the excretion of bilirubin. Less frequent stooling by breastfed infants may allow for an extended time for reabsorption of bilirubin from stools.

Diagnostic Evaluation

The degree of jaundice is determined by serum bilirubin measurements. Normal values of unconjugated bilirubin are 0.2 to 1.4 mg/dl. In newborns, levels must exceed 5 mg/dl before jaundice (icterus) is observable. It is important to note, however, that the evaluation of jaundice is not based solely on serum bilirubin levels but also on the timing of the appearance of clinical jaundice; gestational age at birth; age in days since birth; family history, including maternal Rh factor; evidence of hemolysis; feeding method; infant's physiologic status; and the progression of serial serum bilirubin levels. The following criteria are indicators of pathologic jaundice that, when present, warrant further investigation as to the cause of the jaundice:

- Persistent jaundice over 2 weeks in a full-term formula-fed infant
- Total serum bilirubin levels over 12.9 mg/dl (term infant) or over 15 mg/dl (preterm infant); the upper limit for breastfed infant is 15 mg/dl
- Increase in serum bilirubin by 5 mg/dl/day
- Direct bilirubin exceeding 1.5 to 2 mg/dl
- Total serum bilirubin level over the 95th percentile for age (in hours) on an hour-specific nomogram (Fig. 8.19)

This is not an all-inclusive list; other factors are also evaluated.

Factors placing newborns at higher risk for hyperbilirubinemia include maternal race (e.g., Asian or Asian American), late preterm birth, jaundice observed in the first 24 hours of life, significant bruising, cephalhematoma, exclusive breastfeeding, blood group incompatibility or hemolytic disease (such as G6PD), and history of sibling with hyperbilirubinemia (Muchowski, 2014).

Noninvasive monitoring of bilirubin via cutaneous reflectance measurements (**transcutaneous bilirubinometry [TcB]**) allows for repetitive estimations of bilirubin and, when used correctly, may decrease the need for invasive monitoring. The new TcB monitors provide accurate measurements within 2 mg/dl in most neonatal populations at serum levels below 15 mg/dl (Shabuj, Hossain, & Dey, 2019). TcB monitors must be used according to published guidelines as a screening tool, not as a predictor of need for therapy; multiple readings over time at a consistent site (e.g., sternum or forehead) are of more value than a single reading. After phototherapy has been initiated, TcB is no longer useful as a screening tool.

The use of hour-specific serum bilirubin levels to predict newborns at risk for rapidly rising levels has now become the standard of care as well as an official recommendation by the American Academy of Pediatrics, Subcommittee on Hyperbilirubinemia (2004) for the monitoring of healthy neonates of 35 weeks of gestation or older. The use of a nomogram with three levels (high, intermediate, or low risk) of rising total serum bilirubin values assists in the determination of which newborns might need further evaluation after discharge (Lai, Ahmad, Choo, et al., 2017) (see Fig. 8.19A). The hour-specific bilirubin risk nomogram is used to determine the infant's risk for developing hyperbilirubinemia requiring medical treatment or more frequent screening. Risk factors recognized to place infants in the high-risk category include gestational age of younger than 38 weeks, maternal age, maternal diabetes, breastfeeding, a sibling who had significant jaundice, delayed bowel movement, weight loss, cutaneous bruising and early-appearing jaundice (Shaughnessy & Goyal, 2020a; Kamath-Rayne, Thilo, Deacon, et al., 2016).

It is also recommended that healthy term infants receive follow-up care and bilirubin risk assessment with TcB or the hour-specific nomogram within 3 days of discharge if discharged at less than 24 hours of age. Newborns discharged at 24 to 48 hours should receive follow-up evaluation within 4 days (96 hours), and those discharged between 48 and 72 hours should receive follow-up within 5 days (American Academy of Pediatrics, Subcommittee on Hyperbilirubinemia, 2004; Blackburn, 2018). The serum bilirubin may be obtained at the time of the metabolic screening, thus precluding the need for additional blood sampling. The newest guidelines for monitoring and treating neonatal hyperbilirubinemia are published extensively elsewhere, and readers are referred to "Management of Hyperbilirubinemia in the Newborn Infant 35 or More Weeks of Gestation (Clinical Practice Guideline)" (American Academy of Pediatrics, Subcommittee on Hyperbilirubinemia, 2004) for an in-depth overview of management guidelines.

Complications

Unconjugated bilirubin is highly toxic to neurons; therefore an infant with severe jaundice is at risk of developing **bilirubin encephalopathy**, a syndrome of severe brain damage resulting from the deposition of unconjugated bilirubin in brain cells. **Kernicterus** describes the yellow staining of the brain cells that may result in bilirubin encephalopathy. The damage occurs when the serum concentration reaches toxic levels, regardless of cause. There is evidence that a fraction of unconjugated bilirubin crosses the blood-brain barrier in neonates with physiologic hyperbilirubinemia. When certain pathologic conditions exist in addition to elevated bilirubin levels, there is an increase in the permeability of the blood-brain barrier to unconjugated bilirubin and thus potential irreversible damage. The exact level of serum bilirubin required to cause damage is not yet known.

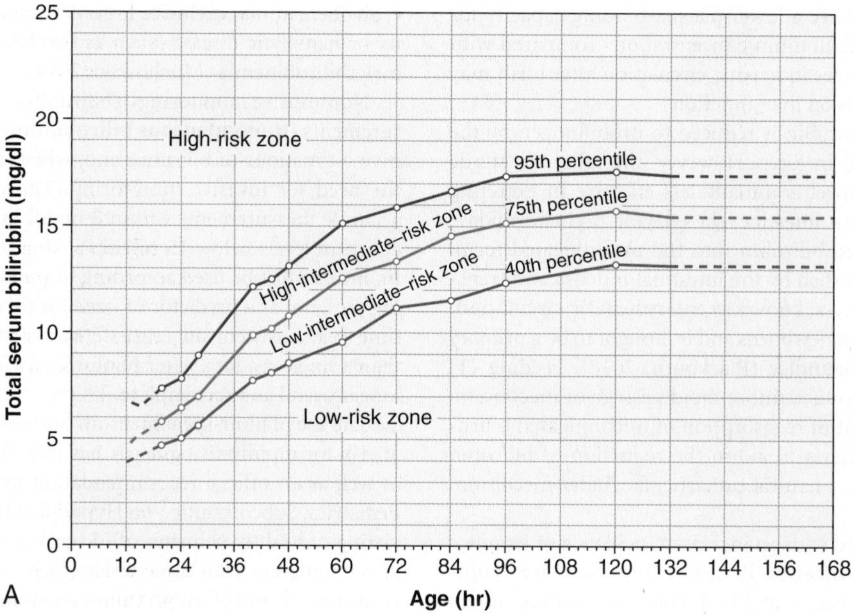

A

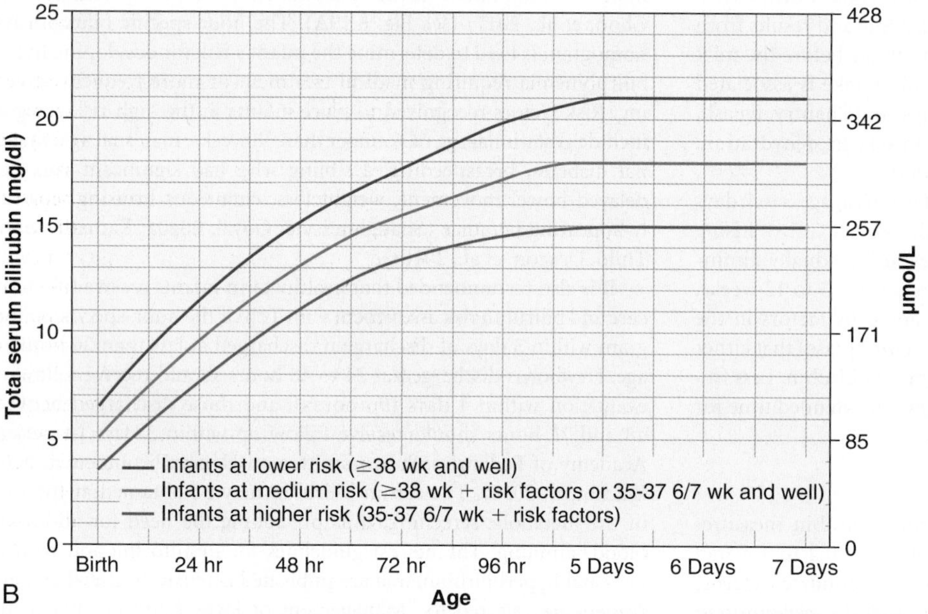

- Use total bilirubin. Do not subtract direct reacting or conjugated bilirubin.
- Risk factors = isoimmune hemolytic disease. G6PD deficiency, asphyxia, significant lethargy, temperature instability, sepsis, acidosis, or albumin <3.0 g/dl (if measured).
- For well infants 35-37 6/7 wk, can adjust total serum bilirubin (TSB) levels for intervention around the medium-risk line. It is an option to intervene at lower TSB levels for infants closer to 35 wk and at higher TSB levels for those closer to 37 6/7 wk.
- It is an option to provide conventional phototherapy in the hospital or at home at TSB levels 2-3 mg/dl (35-50 mmol/L) below those shown, but home phototherapy should not be used in any infant with risk factors.

B

Fig. 8.19 **A,** Nomogram for designation of risk in 2840 well newborns at 36 or more weeks of gestational age with birth weights of 2000 g (4.4 pounds) or more or at 35 or more weeks of gestational age with birth weights of 2500 g (5.5 pounds) or more based on the hour-specific serum bilirubin values. (This nomogram should not be used to represent the natural history of neonatal hyperbilirubinemia.) **B,** Guidelines for phototherapy in hospitalized infants of 35 or more weeks of gestation. *G6PD,* Glucose-6-phosphate dehydrogenase. (**A,** From Bhutani, V. K., Johnson, L., & Sivieri, E. M. [1999]. Predictive ability of a predischarge hour-specific serum bilirubin for subsequent significant hyperbilirubinemia in healthy term and near-term newborns. *Pediatrics, 103*[1], 6–14. **B,** From American Academy of Pediatrics, Subcommittee on Hyperbilirubinemia. [2004]. Management of hyperbilirubinemia in the newborn infant 35 or more weeks of gestation. *Pediatrics, 114*[1], 297–316.)

Multiple factors contribute to bilirubin neurotoxicity; therefore *serum bilirubin levels alone do not predict the risk of brain injury.* Factors that are known to enhance the development of bilirubin encephalopathy include metabolic acidosis, lowered serum albumin levels, intracranial infections (such as meningitis), and abrupt fluctuations in BP. In addition, any condition that increases the metabolic demands for oxygen or glucose (e.g., fetal distress, hypoxia, hypothermia, hypoglycemia) also increases the risk of brain damage at lower serum levels of bilirubin.

The signs of bilirubin encephalopathy are those of CNS depression or excitation. Prodromal symptoms consist of decreased activity, lethargy, irritability, hypotonia, and seizures. Later these subtle findings are followed by development of hypertonia of extensor muscles, opisthotonos, retrocolis, and fever (Shaughnessy & Goyal, 2020b). Motor skills are delayed, and dental enamel hypoplasia may also occur. Those who survive may eventually show evidence of neurologic damage, such as cognitive delay, ADHD, delayed or abnormal motor movement

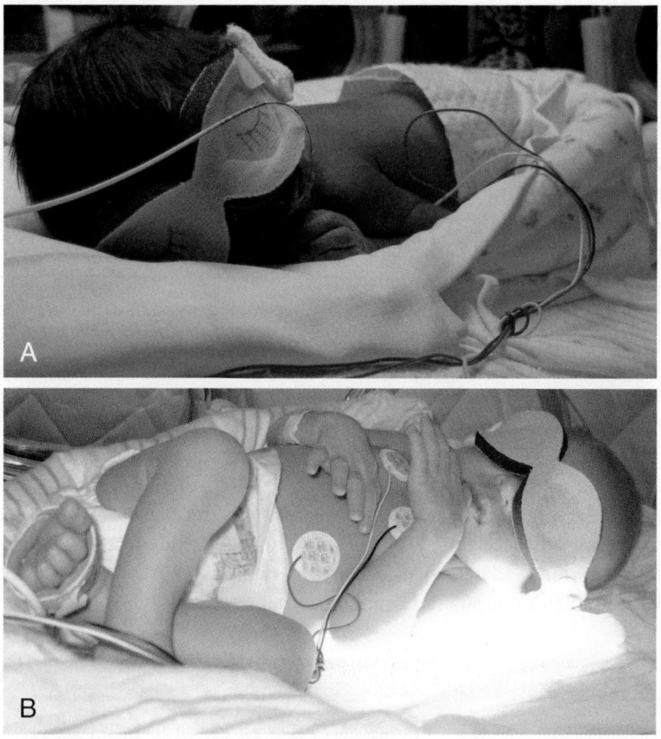

Fig. 8.20 A, An infant receiving phototherapy; note the nested boundaries for comfort and eye protection. B, A newborn laying on a BiliBlanket, which may be used with overhead lights to provide intensive phototherapy. (Courtesy E. Jacobs, Texas Children's Hospital, Houston, TX.)

(especially ataxia or athetosis), behavior disorders, perceptual problems, or sensorineural hearing loss.

Therapeutic Management

The primary goals in the treatment of hyperbilirubinemia are to identify infants at high risk for hyperbilirubinemia; monitor serum bilirubin levels; prevent bilirubin encephalopathy; and, as in any blood group incompatibility, reverse the hemolytic process. The main form of treatment involves the use of phototherapy. Exchange transfusion is generally used for reducing dangerously high bilirubin levels that may occur with hemolytic disease.

Intravenous immunoglobulin (IVIG) is an adjunctive treatment in reducing bilirubin levels in infants with Rh alloimmunization and ABO incompatibility (Shaughnessy & Goyal, 2020b) and is recommended by the American Academy of Pediatrics (American Academy of Pediatrics, Subcommittee on Hyperbilirubinemia, 2004).

Healthy near-term and full-term infants with jaundice may also benefit from early initiation of feedings and frequent breastfeeding. These preventive measures are aimed at promoting increased intestinal motility, decreasing enterohepatic shunting, and establishing normal bacterial flora in the bowel to effectively enhance the excretion of unconjugated bilirubin.

Phototherapy consists of the application of a special source of light (irradiance) to the infant's exposed skin (Fig. 8.20). Light promotes bilirubin excretion by **photoisomerization**, which alters the structure of bilirubin to a soluble form (**lumirubin**) for easier excretion.

Studies indicate that blue fluorescent light is more effective than white fluorescent in reducing bilirubin levels. However, because blue light alters the infant's coloration, the normal light of fluorescent bulbs in the spectrum of 420 to 460 nm is often preferred so that the infant's skin can be better observed for color (jaundice, pallor, cyanosis) or other conditions. Increasing irradiance to the 430 to 490 nm band provides best results. For phototherapy to be effective, the infant's skin must be fully exposed to an adequate amount of the light source. A diaper and boundary materials for postural support may be left in place; periodically turning the neonate under phototherapy has not been shown to accelerate bilirubin clearance. When serum bilirubin levels are rapidly increasing or approximating critical levels, intensive phototherapy is recommended. Intensive phototherapy with a higher irradiance is considered more effective than standard phototherapy for rapid reduction of serum bilirubin levels (Edris, Ghany, Razek, et al., 2014). The color of the infant's skin does not influence the efficacy of phototherapy. Best results occur within the first 4 to 6 hours of treatment (Cai, Qi, Su, et al., 2016). Phototherapy alone is not effective in the management of hyperbilirubinemia when levels are at a critical level or are rising rapidly; it is designed primarily for the treatment of moderate hyperbilirubinemia.

The American Academy of Pediatrics, Subcommittee on Hyperbilirubinemia (2004) practice parameter guidelines provide suggestions for initiating phototherapy (see Fig. 8.19B) and for implementing exchange transfusion in healthy term infants. However, each infant should be carefully evaluated with other illness and risk factors in mind rather than depending on absolute values for all infants in a specific group. Prophylactic phototherapy may be used in preterm infants to prevent a significant increase in serum bilirubin levels (Waite & Taylor, 2016).

Phototherapy has not been found to cause long-term adverse effects. The effectiveness of treatment is determined by a decrease in total serum bilirubin levels. Concurrently, the infant's total physical status is assessed continually because the suppression of jaundice by phototherapy may mask signs of sepsis, hemolytic disease, or hepatitis.

Recommendations for prevention and management of early-onset jaundice in breastfed infants include encouraging frequent breastfeeding, preferably every 1.5 to 2 hours; avoiding glucose water, formula, and water supplementation; and monitoring for early stooling. The infant's weight, voiding, and stooling should be evaluated along with the breastfeeding pattern (Lawrence & Lawrence, 2016a). Parents are taught to evaluate the number of voids and evidence of adequate breastfeeding after the infant is home, and they are encouraged to call the primary care practitioner if the infant is not feeding well, is difficult to arouse for feedings, or is not voiding and stooling adequately.

Phototherapy as a treatment for hyperbilirubinemia is discussed further later in the chapter.

Prognosis

Early recognition and treatment of hyperbilirubinemia prevents unnecessary medical therapies, parent-infant separation, breastfeeding disruption and possibly failure, and neurologic damage (bilirubin encephalopathy). Phototherapy is a safe and effective method of decreasing serum bilirubin levels in newborns with mild to moderate hyperbilirubinemia.

Nursing Care Management

Part of routine nursing care management includes observing for evidence of jaundice at regular intervals. Jaundice is most reliably assessed by observing the infant's skin color from head to toe and the color of the sclerae and mucous membranes. Applying direct pressure to the skin, especially over bony prominences (such as the tip of the nose or the sternum), causes blanching and allows the yellow stain to be more pronounced. For dark-skinned infants, the color of the sclerae, conjunctivae, and oral mucosa is the most reliable indicator. Also, bilirubin (especially at high levels) is not uniformly distributed in the skin. The nurse should observe the infant in natural daylight for a true assessment of color.

The TcB is a useful screening device and is used to detect neonatal jaundice in full-term infants. Because phototherapy reduces the accuracy of the instrument, its value is limited to assessments made before the initiation of phototherapy. Institutions in which the device is used set up their own criteria based on their experience with their particular instrument. Blood samples are also taken for the measurement of bilirubin in the laboratory.

With short hospital stays, jaundice may appear after discharge. A careful history from the parents may reveal significant familial patterns of hyperbilirubinemia (e.g., older siblings who had jaundice). Other considerations in assessment include the ethnic origin of the family (e.g., higher incidence in Asian infants); type of delivery (e.g., induction of labor); and infant characteristics, such as weight loss after birth, gestational age, sex, and the presence of any bruising. The method and frequency of feeding are assessed. Prevention of jaundice may be possible with early introduction of feedings and frequent nursing without supplementation. Every effort is made to provide an optimum thermal environment to reduce metabolic needs.

! NURSING ALERT

While blood is drawn, phototherapy lights are turned off. Blood is transported in a covered tube to avoid a false reading as a result of bilirubin destruction in the test tube.

QUALITY PATIENT OUTCOMES: NEONATAL HYPERBILIRUBINEMIA

Total serum bilirubin level will be maintained below high-risk critical value (as determined on the hour-specific total serum bilirubin nomogram).

! NURSING ALERT

Evidence of jaundice that appears before the infant is 24 hours old is an indication for assessing bilirubin levels.

Phototherapy

The infant who receives phototherapy is placed seminude (diaper may be left in place) under the light source and periodically evaluated to ensure tolerance of the procedure. After phototherapy has been initiated, frequent serum bilirubin levels (every 6 to 24 hours) are necessary because visual assessment of jaundice or transcutaneous bilirubin monitoring is no longer considered valid.

Several precautions are instituted to protect the infant during phototherapy. The infant's eyes are shielded by an opaque mask to prevent exposure to the light (see Fig. 8.20). The eye shield should be properly sized and correctly positioned to cover the eyes completely but prevent any occlusion of the nares. The infant's eyelids are closed before the mask is applied because the corneas may become excoriated if they come in contact with the dressing. On each nursing shift, the eyes are checked for evidence of discharge, excessive pressure on the eyelids, and corneal irritation. Eye shields are removed during feedings, which provide the opportunity for visual and sensory stimulation.

Infants who are in an open crib must have a protective Plexiglas shield between them and the overhead fluorescent lights to minimize the amount of undesirable ultraviolet light reaching their skin and to protect them from accidental bulb breakage. Their temperature is closely monitored to prevent hyperthermia or hypothermia. Maintaining the infant in a flexed position with rolled blankets along the sides of the body helps maintain heat and provides comfort.

Accurate documentation is another important nursing responsibility and includes (1) times that phototherapy is started and stopped, (2) proper shielding of the eyes, (3) type of light source (by manufacturer), (4) use of phototherapy in combination with an incubator or open bassinet, (5) photometer measurement of light intensity according to hospital protocol, (6) feeding and elimination pattern, (7) body temperature, and (8) serum bilirubin levels.

Minor side effects for which the nurse should be alert include loose, greenish stools; transient skin rashes; hyperthermia; increased metabolic rate; dehydration; electrolyte disturbances, such as hypocalcemia; and priapism. To prevent or minimize these effects, the temperature is monitored to detect early signs of hypothermia or hyperthermia, and the skin is observed for evidence of dehydration and drying, which can lead to excoriation and breakdown. Oily lubricants or lotions are not used on the skin while the infant is under phototherapy. Infants receiving phototherapy may require additional fluid volume to compensate for insensible and intestinal fluid loss. Breastfeeding or bottle-feeding by the parent(s) and parental interaction (such as holding) is encouraged once phototherapy is initiated, provided the infant receives adequate exposure to the treatment. Because phototherapy enhances the excretion of unconjugated bilirubin through the bowel, loose stools may indicate accelerated bilirubin removal. Frequent stooling can cause perianal irritation; therefore meticulous skin care, especially keeping the skin clean and dry, is essential.

! NURSING ALERT

Parents may be told by some practitioners to place the infant in the sunlight when the infant has jaundice; however, this practice is not recommended. If performed, the infant should only be placed in indirect sunlight (e.g., in a room where sunlight filters through a glass window), because direct sunlight may cause skin burns in a newborn.

After phototherapy is permanently discontinued, there is often a subsequent increase in the serum bilirubin level, often called the **rebound effect**. This is usually transient and resolves without resuming therapy; however, serum bilirubin level should be checked on follow-up.

Family Support

Parents need reassurance concerning their infant's progress. All procedures are explained to familiarize them with the benefits and risks. Parents need to be reassured that the naked infant under the bilirubin light is warm and comfortable. Eye shields are removed when the parents are visiting to facilitate the attachment process. The parents can be reassured that the neonate is accustomed to darkness after months of intrauterine existence and benefits a great deal from auditory and tactile stimulation (see Family-Centered Care box).

FAMILY-CENTERED CARE

Phototherapy and Parent-Infant Interaction

The traditional use of phototherapy has evoked concerns about a number of psychobehavioral issues, including parent-infant separation, potential social isolation, decreased sensorineural stimulation, altered biologic rhythms, altered feeding patterns, and activity changes. Parental anxiety is greatly increased, particularly at the sight of the newborn blindfolded and under special lights. The interruption of breastfeeding for phototherapy is a potential deterrent to successful mother-infant attachment and interaction. Because research has demonstrated that bilirubin catabolism occurs primarily within the first few hours of the initiation of phototherapy, there is increased support for the periodic removal of the infant from treatment for feeding and holding. The benefits of stopping phototherapy for parental feeding and holding outweigh concerns related to the clearance of bilirubin in healthy full-term newborns with mild hyperbilirubinemia. Home phototherapy offers an additional opportunity to foster parent-infant attachment.

The initiation of any treatment requires **informed consent** by the parents for the therapy prescribed; however, in the case of phototherapy, considerable anxiety may rightfully occur when words such as *kernicterus* and *neurologic damage* are used to describe possible effects of nontreatment. It is imperative that nurses remain sensitive to parents' feelings and information needs during this process; an important nursing intervention is assessment of the parents' understanding of the treatment involved and clarification of the nature of the therapy.

An important nursing intervention is recognition of breastfeeding jaundice. Lack of familiarity among health professionals has caused many newborns prolonged hospitalization, termination of breastfeeding, and unnecessary phototherapy. Care of the new mother may include supporting successful and frequent breastfeeding. Parents also need reassurance of the benign nature of the jaundice in a healthy infant and encouragement to resume breastfeeding if temporary cessation is prescribed. In some situations, jaundice may increase the risk of the parents discontinuing breastfeeding and developing the **vulnerable child syndrome**—a belief that their child has experienced a "close call" and is vulnerable to serious injury (see Critical Thinking Case Study box).

CRITICAL THINKING CASE STUDY

Jaundice

A full-term, 120-hour-old newborn is brought to the urgent care department late in the evening for evaluation of newborn jaundice. A serum bilirubin level was drawn earlier in the day at the birth hospital by heel stick; the results were total bilirubin 13.6 mg/dl and direct bilirubin 0.6 mg/dl. The father is concerned because he saw an online medical report saying that newborns could develop brain damage if the bilirubin levels were to increase to high levels. The mother is breastfeeding every 2 to 3 hours, and the newborn has had five wet diapers and three semiliquid stools over the past 18 hours. The newborn's birth weight was 2834 g (6.2 pounds), and her current weight (nude) is 2722 g (6 pounds). On examination, the infant is active and alert, with visibly jaundiced skin and sclerae, intact neurologic reflexes, and a strong suck reflex. The history reveals no prenatal or delivery complications. Apgar scores at 1 and 5 minutes were 8 and 9, respectively, and the initial assessment did not reveal any problems. The mother's blood type is A positive, and the direct Coombs test result is negative. The newborn was discharged from the birth hospital on the second day of life in apparent good health.

Initial Assessment. What findings in the case study provide evidence for unconjugated hyperbilirubinemia?

Clinical Reasoning. What risks factors are commonly associated with this type of jaundice?

Teaching Points

- Recommend frequent breastfeeding every 2 hours
- Avoid glucose water, supplemental water, and formula
- Monitor for early stooling
- Advise to call if not feeding well, difficult to arouse for feedings, or not voiding and stooling adequately

Critical Thinking Answers

Initial Assessment. Total bilirubin 13.6 mg/dl and direct bilirubin 0.6 mg/dl in a 120-hour-old full-term newborn; visibly jaundiced skin and sclerae. This is newborn jaundice in a healthy full-term infant who is being breastfed every 2 to 3 hours (see Table 8.3 and Fig. 8.19)

Clinical Reasoning. Breastfeeding-associated jaundice begins 2 to 4 days after birth. Jaundice related to decreasing caloric and fluid intake before the milk supply is well established.

Discharge Planning and Home Care

With short hospital stays, mothers and infants may be discharged before evidence of jaundice is present. It is important for the nurse to discuss signs of jaundice with the mother because any clinical symptoms will probably appear at home. Home visits within 2 to 3 days after discharge to evaluate feeding and elimination patterns and jaundice are often routine for some health care organizations. Others may have an outpatient bilirubin clinic or laboratory where the infant can be evaluated by a nurse and weighed and a serum bilirubin can be drawn for evaluation. Assessment of breastfeeding is essential.

If home phototherapy is instituted, the hospital or home health care nurse or medical equipment company representative is usually responsible for teaching the family members and assessing their abilities to implement the treatment safely. General guidelines for home care preparation and education are discussed in Chapter 20. Written instructions and supervision of care—especially the application of eye shields, if needed—are essential. The minor side effects of phototherapy are reviewed, and parents may need instruction in taking axillary temperatures and recording times and amounts of feedings and the number of wet diapers and stools. Regardless of how benign the disorder or the therapy, the parents need support and understanding. Measures should be taken to assist the mother in achieving successful breastfeeding, including consultation with a lactation specialist on an outpatient basis. Infants treated with phototherapy for neonatal jaundice are at greater risk for breastfeeding failure. Research has demonstrated that infants treated with phototherapy for neonatal jaundice experience decreased rates of exclusive breastfeeding in the first 4 months of life (Waite & Taylor, 2016). For breastfeeding infants it is important to emphasize an approach that focuses on modifying any factors that could affect early-onset jaundice in breastfed infants (Lawrence & Lawrence, 2016a).

HEMOLYTIC DISEASE OF THE NEWBORN

Hyperbilirubinemia in the first 24 hours of life is most often the result of HDFN, an abnormally rapid rate of RBC destruction. Anemia caused by this destruction stimulates the production of RBCs, which in turn provides increasing numbers of cells for hemolysis. Major causes of increased erythrocyte destruction are red cell alloimmunization (primarily Rh) and ABO incompatibility.

Blood Incompatibility

The membranes of human blood cells contain a variety of **antigens**, also known as **agglutinogens**, substances capable of producing an immune response if recognized by the body as foreign. The reciprocal relationship between antigens on RBCs and antibodies in the plasma causes **agglutination** (clumping). In other words, antibodies in the plasma of one blood group (except the AB group, which contains no antibodies) produce agglutination when mixed with antigens of a different blood group. In the **ABO blood group system**, the antibodies occur naturally. In the **Rh system**, the person must be exposed to the Rh antigen before significant antibody formation takes place and causes a sensitivity response known as **alloimmunization**.

Rh Incompatibility (Alloimmunization)

The Rh blood group consists of several antigens (with D being the most prevalent). For simplicity, only the terms **Rh positive** (presence of antigen) and **Rh negative** (absence of antigen) are used in this discussion. The presence or absence of the naturally occurring Rh factor determines the blood type.

Ordinarily, no problems are anticipated when the Rh blood types are the same in both the mother and the fetus or when the mother is Rh positive and the infant is Rh negative. Difficulty may arise when

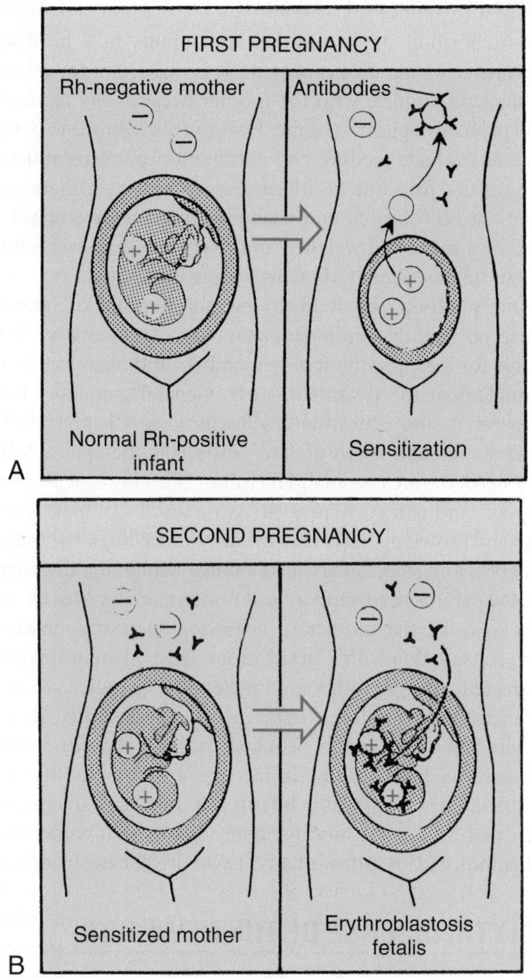

Fig. 8.21 Development of maternal sensitization to Rh antigens. **A**, Fetal Rh-positive erythrocytes enter the maternal system. Maternal anti-Rh antibodies are formed. **B**, Anti-Rh antibodies cross the placenta and attack fetal erythrocytes.

the mother is Rh negative and the infant is Rh positive. Although the maternal and fetal circulations are separate, there is evidence that fetal RBCs and cell-free deoxyribonucleic acid (DNA) can enter the maternal circulation during pregnancy (Moise, 2017). More commonly, however, fetal RBCs enter into the maternal circulation at the time of delivery. The mother's natural defense mechanism responds to these alien cells by producing anti-Rh antibodies.

Under normal circumstances, this process of alloimmunization has no effect during the first pregnancy with an Rh-positive fetus, because the initial sensitization to Rh antigens rarely occurs before the onset of labor. However, with the increased risk of fetal blood being transferred to the maternal circulation during placental separation, maternal antibody production is stimulated. During a subsequent pregnancy with an Rh-positive fetus, these previously formed maternal antibodies to Rh-positive blood cells may enter the fetal circulation, where they attack and destroy fetal erythrocytes (Fig. 8.21). The American College of Obstetricians and Gynecologists recommends antepartum administration of Rh immunoglobulin (RhIG) for the following indications: spontaneous miscarriage, elective abortion, ectopic pregnancy, genetic amniocentesis, chorionic villus sampling, and fetal blood sampling (Moise, 2017).

Because the condition begins in utero, the fetus attempts to compensate for the progressive hemolysis and anemia by accelerating the rate of erythropoiesis. As a result, immature RBCs (**erythroblasts**) appear in the fetal circulation, hence the term **erythroblastosis fetalis**.

TABLE 8.4 Potential Maternal-Fetal ABO Incompatibilities

Maternal Blood Group	Incompatible Fetal Blood Group
O	A or B
B	A or AB
A	B or AB

There is wide variability in the development of maternal sensitization to Rh-positive antigens. Sensitization may occur during the first pregnancy if the woman had previously received an Rh-positive blood transfusion. No sensitization may occur in situations in which a strong placental barrier prevents transfer of fetal blood into the maternal circulation. In approximately 10% to 15% of sensitized mothers, there is no hemolytic reaction in the newborn.

In the most severe form of erythroblastosis fetalis, **hydrops fetalis**, the progressive hemolysis causes fetal hypoxia; cardiac failure; generalized edema (anasarca); and fluid effusions into the pericardial, pleural, and peritoneal spaces (hydrops). The fetus may be delivered stillborn or in severe respiratory distress. Maternal RhIg administration, early intrauterine detection of fetal anemia by ultrasonography (serial Doppler assessment of the peak velocity in the fetal middle cerebral artery), and subsequent treatment by fetal blood transfusions or high-dose IVIG have dramatically improved the outcome of affected fetuses (Niss & Ware, 2020).

ABO Incompatibility

Hemolytic disease can also occur when the major blood group antigens of the fetus are different from those of the mother. The major blood groups are A, B, AB, and O. In the North American white population, 46% have type O blood, 42% have type A blood, 9% have type B blood, and 3% have type AB blood.

The presence or absence of antibodies and antigens determines whether agglutination will occur. Antibodies in the plasma of one blood group (except the AB group, which contains no antibodies) will produce agglutination (clumping) when mixed with antigens of a different blood group. Naturally occurring antibodies in the recipient's blood cause agglutination of a donor's RBCs. The agglutinated donor cells become trapped in peripheral blood vessels, where they hemolyze, releasing large amounts of bilirubin into the circulation.

The most common blood group incompatibility in the neonate is between a mother with O blood group and an infant with A or B blood group (see Table 8.4 for possible ABO incompatibilities). Naturally occurring anti-A or anti-B antibodies already present in the maternal circulation cross the placenta and attack the fetal RBCs, causing hemolysis. Usually the hemolytic reaction is less severe than in Rh incompatibility. Unlike the Rh reaction, ABO incompatibility may occur in the first pregnancy.

Clinical Manifestations

Jaundice may appear shortly after birth (during the first 24 hours) in newborns affected by HDFN, and serum levels of unconjugated bilirubin rise rapidly. Anemia results from the hemolysis of large numbers of erythrocytes, and hyperbilirubinemia and jaundice result from the liver's inability to conjugate and excrete the excess bilirubin. Most newborns with HDFN are not jaundiced at birth. However, hepatosplenomegaly and varying degrees of hydrops may be evident. If the infant is severely affected, signs of anemia (notably, marked pallor) and hypovolemic shock are apparent. Hypoglycemia may occur as a result of pancreatic cell hyperplasia.

Diagnostic Evaluation

Early identification and diagnosis of RhD sensitization are important in the management and prevention of fetal complications. A maternal antibody titer (**indirect Coombs test**) should be drawn at the first prenatal visit. Genetic testing allows early identification of paternal zygosity at the RhD gene locus, thus allowing earlier detection of the potential for alloimmunization and avoiding further maternal or fetal testing (Liao, Gronowski, & Zhao, 2014). Amniocentesis can be used to test the fetal blood type of a woman whose antibody screen result is positive; the use of polymerase chain reaction may determine the fetal blood type and presence of maternal antibodies. The fetal hemoglobin and hematocrit can also be measured (Moise, 2017). Testing for the presence of cell-free fetal DNA in the maternal plasma of RhD-negative women to detect an RhD-positive fetus has been used successfully (Moise, 2017). Such testing negates the need for amniocentesis for fetal blood type.

Ultrasonography is considered an important adjunct in the detection of alloimmunization; alterations in the placenta, umbilical cord, and amniotic fluid volume, as well as the presence of fetal hydrops, can be detected with high-resolution ultrasonography and allow early treatment before the development of erythroblastosis. Doppler ultrasonography of fetal middle cerebral artery peak velocity has been used to detect and measure fetal hemoglobin and, subsequently, fetal anemia (Moise, 2017). Erythroblastosis fetalis caused by Rh incompatibility can also be monitored by evaluating rising anti-Rh antibody titers in the maternal circulation or by testing the optical density of amniotic fluid (ΔOD450 test) (Moise, 2017).

Hemolysis in the newborn is suspected based on the timing and appearance of jaundice (see Table 8.3) and can be confirmed postnatally by detecting antibodies attached to the circulating erythrocytes of affected infants (**direct Coombs test** or **direct antiglobulin test**). The Coombs test may be performed on umbilical cord blood samples from infants born to Rh-negative mothers if there is a history of incompatibility or further investigation is warranted.

Therapeutic Management

The primary aim of therapeutic management of alloimmunization is prevention. Postnatal therapy is usually phototherapy for mild cases of hemolysis and exchange transfusion for more severe forms. Although phototherapy may control bilirubin levels in mild cases, the hemolytic process may continue, causing significant anemia between 7 and 21 days of life. In some institutions, an IVIG is administered to decrease the formation of bilirubin in neonates with ABO incompatibility.

Prevention of Rh Isoimmunization

The administration of RhIg, a human gamma globulin concentrate of anti-D, to all unsensitized Rh-negative mothers at 28 weeks of gestation and after delivery or abortion of an Rh-positive infant or fetus prevents the development of maternal sensitization to the Rh factor. The injected anti-Rh antibodies are thought to destroy (by subsequent phagocytosis and agglutination) fetal RBCs passing into the maternal circulation before they can be recognized by the mother's immune system. Because the immune response is blocked, anti-D antibodies and memory cells (which produce the primary and secondary immune responses, respectively) are not formed (Bagwell, 2014; Blackburn, 2018). The inhibition of memory cell formation is especially important because memory cells provide long-term immunity by initiating a rapid immune response after the antigen is reintroduced.

To be effective, RhIg (e.g., RhoGAM) must be administered to unsensitized mothers within 72 hours (but possibly as long as 3 to 4 weeks) after the first delivery or abortion and repeated after subsequent pregnancies or losses. The administration of RhIg at 26 to 28 weeks of gestation further reduces the risk of Rh alloimmunization. RhIg is not effective against existing Rh-positive antibodies in the maternal circulation.

Studies have demonstrated the effectiveness of IVIG at decreasing the severity of RBC destruction (hemolysis) in HDFN and subsequent development of neonatal jaundice; however, further studies including a blinding intervention by use of a placebo are recommended (Zwiers, Scheffer-Rath, Lopriore, et al., 2018). This therapy, often used in conjunction with phototherapy, may decrease the necessity for exchange transfusion. Maternal administration of high-dose IVIG, alone or in combination with plasmapheresis, decreases the fetal effects of RhD alloimmunization (Bellone & Boctor, 2014).

DRUG ALERT

RhIg is administered intramuscularly, not intravenously, and only to Rh-negative women with a negative Coombs test result—never to the newborn or father.

Intrauterine Transfusion

Infants of mothers already sensitized may be treated by intrauterine transfusion, which consists of infusing blood into the umbilical vein of the fetus. The need for therapy is based on the antenatal diagnosis of alloimmunization by determining the optical density of amniotic fluid (by amniocentesis) as an index of fetal hemolysis or by serial ultrasonography, which may detect the presence of fetal hydrops as early as 16 weeks of gestation. With the advance of ultrasound technology, fetal transfusion may be accomplished directly via the umbilical vein, infusing type O Rh-negative packed RBCs to raise the fetal hematocrit to 40% to 50%. The frequency of intrauterine transfusions may vary according to institution and fetal hydropic status, but they are most often done every 2 to 3 weeks until the fetus reaches pulmonary maturity at approximately 36 weeks of gestation (Sainio, Nupponen, Kuosmanen, et al., 2015). Intraperitoneal blood transfusions are used less commonly for alloimmunization because of higher associated fetal risks; however, they may be used when intravascular access is impossible.

Exchange Transfusion

Exchange transfusion, in which the infant's blood is removed in small amounts (usually 5 to 10 ml at a time) and replaced with compatible blood (e.g., Rh-negative blood), is a standard mode of therapy for treatment of severe hyperbilirubinemia and is the treatment of choice for hyperbilirubinemia and hydrops caused by Rh incompatibility (Fig. 8.22). Exchange transfusion removes the sensitized erythrocytes, lowers the serum bilirubin level to prevent bilirubin encephalopathy, corrects the anemia, and prevents cardiac failure. Indications for exchange transfusion in full-term infants may include a rapidly increasing serum bilirubin level and hemolysis despite intensive phototherapy. The criteria for exchange transfusions in preterm infants vary according to associated illness factors. The American Academy of Pediatrics, Subcommittee on Hyperbilirubinemia (2004) practice parameter guidelines provide recommendations for initiating phototherapy and for exchange transfusion in infants at 35 weeks of gestation or more. An infant born with hydrops fetalis or signs of cardiac failure is a candidate for immediate exchange transfusion with fresh whole blood.

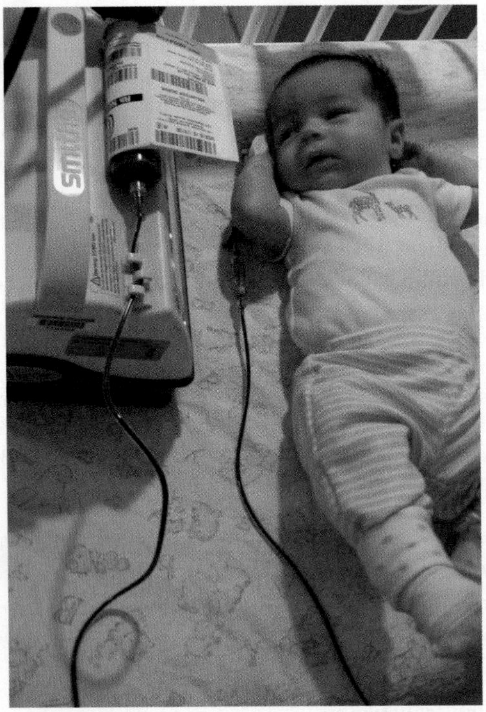

Fig. 8.22 Preterm infant who is Rh positive born to an Rh-negative mother who received intrauterine transfusions and is receiving postnatal transfusions.

For exchange transfusion, fresh whole blood is typed and cross-matched to the mother's serum. The amount of donor blood used is usually double the blood volume of the infant, which is approximately 85 ml/kg body weight but is limited to no more than 500 ml. The two-volume exchange transfusion replaces approximately 85% of the neonate's blood.

An exchange transfusion is a sterile surgical procedure. A catheter is inserted into the umbilical vein and threaded into the inferior vena cava. Depending on the infant's weight, 5 to 10 ml of blood is withdrawn within 15 to 20 seconds, and the same volume of donor blood is infused over 60 to 90 seconds. If the blood has been **citrated** (addition of citrate phosphate dextrose adenine to prevent coagulation), calcium gluconate may be given after the infusion of each 100 ml of donor's blood to prevent hypocalcemia.

Prognosis

The severe anemia of alloimmunization may result in stillbirth, shock, congestive heart failure, or pulmonary or cerebral complications, such as cerebral palsy. As a result of early detection and intrauterine treatment, erythroblastotic newborns are seen less often and exchange transfusions for the condition are less common. Despite the availability of effective preventive measures, Rh HDFN continues to cause significant fetal morbidity and mortality in the United States.

Nursing Care Management

The initial nursing responsibility is recognizing newborn jaundice. The possibility of hemolytic disease can be anticipated from the prenatal and perinatal history. Prenatal evidence of incompatibility and a positive Coombs test result are cause for increased vigilance for early signs of jaundice in an infant. Data indicate that the hour-specific bilirubin nomogram can be used in infants born at 35 weeks or more with ABO incompatibility and a positive Coombs test result to follow the infant's serum bilirubin to determine the need for additional follow-up after hospital discharge (Shaughnessy & Goyal, 2020).

If an exchange transfusion is required, the nurse prepares the infant and the family and assists the practitioner with the procedure. The infant receives nothing by mouth (NPO) during the procedure; therefore a peripheral infusion of dextrose and electrolytes is established. The nurse documents the blood volume exchanged, including the amount of blood withdrawn and infused, the time of each procedure, and the cumulative record of the total volume exchanged. Vital signs, monitored electronically, are evaluated frequently and correlated with the removal and infusion of blood. If signs of cardiac or respiratory problems occur, the procedure is stopped temporarily and resumed after the infant's cardiorespiratory function stabilizes. The nurse also observes for signs of blood transfusion reaction and maintains the infant's blood glucose levels and fluid balance.

Throughout the procedure, attention must be given to the infant's thermoregulation. Hypothermia increases oxygen and glucose consumption, causing metabolic acidosis. These consequences not only hinder the infant's overall physical ability to withstand the long procedure, but also inhibit the binding capacity of albumin and bilirubin and the hepatic enzymatic reactions, thus increasing the risk of kernicterus. Conversely, hyperthermia damages the donor erythrocytes, elevating the free potassium content and predisposing the infant to cardiac arrest.

The exchange transfusion is performed with the infant in a radiant warmer. However, the infant is usually covered with sterile drapes that may prevent the radiant heat from sufficiently warming the skin. The blood may also be warmed (using specially designed blood warming devices) before infusion.

After the procedure is completed, the nurse inspects the umbilical site for evidence of bleeding. The catheter may remain in place in case repeated exchanges are required.

! NURSING ALERT

Signs of blood exchange transfusion reaction include tachycardia or bradycardia, respiratory distress, dramatic change in blood pressure (BP), temperature instability, and generalized rash.

METABOLIC COMPLICATIONS

High-risk infants are subject to a variety of complications related to physiologic function and the transition to extrauterine life. Prominent among these are fluid and electrolyte derangements, hypoglycemia, and hypocalcemia. These complications often occur concurrently with or as a secondary result of other neonatal disorders and may therefore be difficult to differentiate from other conditions. The major characteristics of hypoglycemia and hypocalcemia are outlined in Table 8.5.

DRUG ALERT

Calcium preparations should *never* be administered by bolus rapid infusion in infants.

QUALITY PATIENT OUTCOMES: NEONATAL HYPOGLYCEMIA

- Maintains serum blood glucose level above 45 mg/dl
- No clinical evidence of hypoglycemia or its effects
- Receives adequate carbohydrate intake

TABLE 8.5 Metabolic Complications

	Hypoglycemia	Hypocalcemia
Definition	Blood glucose concentration significantly lower than that in the majority of infants of the same age and weight (usually <45 mg/dl) (see also Adamkin & American Academy of Pediatrics, Committee on Fetus and Newborn, 2011, for parameters for SGA, late preterm, and IDM or LGA infants)	Abnormally low levels of calcium in circulating blood (see values listed below)
Type	**Increased or impaired glucose use:** Large or normal-size infants who appear to have hyperinsulinism; infants born to women with diabetes; infants with increased metabolic demands, such as those with cold stress, sepsis, or after resuscitation; infants with enzymatic or metabolic endocrine defects **Decreased glucose stores:** Small or growth-restricted infants, preterm infants	**Early onset:** Appears in first 48 h; appears in preterm infants who experienced perinatal hypoxia or sometimes in IDM **Late onset:** Cow's milk–induced hypocalcemia (neonatal tetany); apparent after first 3-4 days (high phosphorus-to-calcium ratio of cow's milk depresses parathyroid activity, reducing serum calcium levels); infants with intestinal malabsorption, hypoparathyroidism, or hypomagnesemia
Clinical Manifestations	Vague, often indistinguishable from other newborn conditions **Cerebral signs:** Jitteriness, tremors, twitching, weak or high-pitched cry, lethargy, limpness, apathy, convulsions, and coma **Other:** Cyanosis, apnea, rapid irregular respirations, sweating, eye rolling, poor feeding Signs often transient but recurrent	**Early onset:** Jitteriness, apnea, cyanotic episodes, edema, high-pitched cry, abdominal distention **Late onset:** Twitching, tremors, seizures
Screening	Bedside monitoring or serum blood glucose for all infants at risk	At-risk infants or those who are symptomatic
Laboratory Diagnosis	Plasma glucose concentrations <47-50 mg/dl (2.6-2.8 mmol/L) (see also Adamkin & American Academy of Pediatrics, Committee on Fetus and Newborn, 2011, for parameters for SGA, late preterm, and IDM or LGA infants)	Serum calcium <7.8-8 mg/dl (1.95-2.0 mmol/L) in full-term infant OR Ionized calcium <4.4 mg/dl (1.1 mmol/L)
Treatment	Early feeding (within 1 h) in normoglycemic and asymptomatic infants (preventive); IV glucose administration if breastfeeding or formula feedings not tolerated or glucose level extremely low (<25 mg/dL)	**Early onset:** Increased appropriate infant formula feedings; administration of calcium supplements (sometimes) **Late onset:** Administration of calcium gluconate orally or intravenously (slowly); vitamin D Correct hypoparathyroidism
Nursing	Identify infants at risk or with hypoglycemia (e.g., SGA, IUGR, LGA, IDM, late preterm). Reduce environmental factors that predispose to hypoglycemia (e.g., cold stress, respiratory distress). Administer IV dextrose as prescribed. Initiate early breastfeeding or formula feedings in healthy infant. Ensure adequate intake of carbohydrate (breast milk or formula).	Identify infants at risk or with hypocalcemia. Administer calcium as prescribed.[a] Observe for signs of acute hypercalcemia (e.g., vomiting, bradycardia). Manipulate environment to reduce stimuli that might precipitate a seizure or tremors (e.g., picking up infant suddenly, sudden jarring of crib).

[a]See Drug Alert box.

IDM, Infant of diabetic mother; *IUGR,* intrauterine growth restriction; *IV,* intravenous; *LGA,* large for gestational age; *SGA,* small for gestational age.

RESPIRATORY DISTRESS SYNDROME

Respiratory distress is a name applied to respiratory dysfunction in neonates and is primarily a disease related to developmental delay in lung maturation. The terms **respiratory distress syndrome (RDS)** and **hyaline membrane disease** are most often applied to this severe lung disorder, which not only is responsible for more infant deaths than any other disease but also carries the highest risk in terms of long-term respiratory and neurologic complications (see Chapter 21 for a discussion of acute RDS). It is seen almost exclusively in preterm infants. The disorder is rare in drug-exposed infants and infants who have been subjected to chronic intrauterine stress (e.g., maternal preeclampsia or hypertension). Respiratory distress of a nonpulmonary origin in neonates may also be caused by sepsis, cardiac defects (structural or functional), exposure to cold, airway obstruction (atresia), intraventricular hemorrhage, hypoglycemia, metabolic acidosis, acute blood loss, and drugs. Pneumonia in the neonatal period may result in respiratory distress caused by bacterial or viral agents and may occur alone or as a complication of RDS.

Pathophysiology

Preterm infants are born before the lungs are fully prepared to serve as efficient organs for gas exchange. This appears to be a critical factor in the development of RDS. The effects of lung immaturity are compounded by the presence of more cartilage in the chest wall, leading to increased compliance of the chest wall, which collapses inward in response to less compliant (stiffer) lung tissue.

There is evidence of fetal respiratory activity before birth. The lungs make feeble respiratory movements, and fluid is excreted through the alveoli. Because the final unfolding of the alveolar septa, which increases the surface area of the lungs, occurs during the last trimester of pregnancy, preterm infants are born with numerous underdeveloped and many uninflatable alveoli. Pulmonary blood flow is limited as a result of the collapsed state of the fetal lungs, poor vascular development in general, and an immature capillary network. Because of increased pulmonary vascular resistance (PVR), the major portion of fetal blood is shunted from the lungs by way of the ductus arteriosus and foramen ovale.

At birth, infants must initiate breathing and keep the previously fluid-filled lungs inflated with air. At the same time, the pulmonary capillary blood flow increases by approximately tenfold to provide for adequate lung perfusion and to alter the intracardiac pressure that closes the fetal cardiac shunts. Most full-term infants successfully accomplish these adjustments, but preterm infants with respiratory distress are unable to do so. Although numerous factors are involved, a lack of stable surfactant plays a central role.

Surfactant is a surface-active phospholipid secreted by the alveolar epithelium. Acting much like a detergent, this substance reduces the surface tension of fluids that line the alveoli and respiratory passages, resulting in uniform expansion and maintenance of lung expansion at low intra-alveolar pressure. Deficient surfactant production causes unequal inflation of alveoli on inspiration and the collapse of alveoli on end expiration. Without surfactant, infants are unable to keep their lungs inflated and therefore exert a great deal of effort to reexpand the alveoli with each breath. With increasing exhaustion, infants are able to open fewer and fewer alveoli. This inability to maintain lung expansion produces widespread atelectasis.

Following birth, the oxygen concentration in the blood normally increases, the ductus arteriosus constricts, and the pulmonary vessels dilate to decrease PVR. In the absence of alveolar stability (normal functional residual capacity) and with progressive atelectasis, PVR increases as resistance to blood flow into the lungs increases hypoperfusion to the lung tissue. With the increase in PVR, fetal shunts (ductus arteriosus and foramen ovale) remain open, allowing right-to-left shunting of blood through the persisting fetal shunts.

Inadequate pulmonary perfusion and ventilation produce hypoxemia and hypercapnia. Pulmonary arterioles, with their thick, muscular layer, constrict in response to hypoxia. Thus a decrease in oxygen tension causes vasoconstriction in the pulmonary arterioles that is further enhanced by a decrease in blood pH. This vasoconstriction contributes to a further increase in PVR.

Prolonged hypoxemia activates anaerobic glycolysis, which produces increased amounts of lactic acid. An increase in lactic acid causes metabolic acidosis; an inability of the atelectatic lungs to blow off excess carbon dioxide produces respiratory acidosis. Acidosis causes further vasoconstriction. With deficient pulmonary circulation and alveolar perfusion, partial pressure of oxygen in arterial blood continues to fall, pH falls, and the materials needed for surfactant production are not circulated to the alveoli.

BOX 8.4 Clinical Manifestations of Respiratory Distress Syndrome

Tachypnea (>80 to 120 breaths/min) initially[a]
Dyspnea
Pronounced intercostal or substernal retractions (see Fig. 8.23)
Fine inspiratory crackles
Audible expiratory grunt
Flaring of the external nares
Cyanosis or pallor

[a]Not all infants born with respiratory distress syndrome (RDS) manifest these characteristics; very low birth weight (VLBW) and extremely low birth weight (ELBW) infants may have respiratory failure and shock at birth because of physiologic immaturity.

Diagnostic Evaluation

The diagnosis of RDS is made based on clinical signs (Box 8.4) and chest x-ray studies. Radiographic findings characteristic of RDS include (1) a diffuse granular pattern over both lung fields that closely resembles ground glass and represents alveolar atelectasis and (2) dark streaks, or bronchograms, within the ground glass areas that represent dilated, air-filled bronchioles. It is difficult to distinguish between RDS and pneumonia in infants with respiratory distress. The extent of respiratory compromise and acid-base status is determined by blood gas analysis. Criteria for visually evaluating the degree of respiratory distress are illustrated in Fig. 8.23. Pulse oximetry and carbon dioxide monitoring, as well as pulmonary function studies, assist in differentiating pulmonary and extrapulmonary illness and are used in the management of RDS.

QUALITY PATIENT OUTCOMES: NEONATAL RESPIRATORY DISTRESS SYNDROME

- Room air or oxygen saturation of 88% or higher
- Respiratory rate less than 60 breaths/min
- Blood pH 7.30 or higher

Therapeutic Management

The treatment of RDS involves immediate establishment of adequate oxygenation and ventilation and supportive care and measures required for any preterm infant, as well as those instituted to prevent further complications associated with preterm birth. The supportive measures most crucial to a favorable outcome are to:

- Maintain adequate ventilation and oxygenation
- Maintain acid-base balance
- Maintain a neutral thermal environment
- Maintain adequate tissue perfusion and oxygenation
- Prevent hypotension
- Maintain adequate hydration and electrolyte status

Nipple feedings are contraindicated in any situation that creates a marked increase in respiratory rate because of the greater hazards of aspiration. Nutrition is provided by parenteral therapy during the acute stage of the disease, and minimal enteral feeding is provided to enhance maturation of the neonate's gastrointestinal system.

The administration of **exogenous surfactant** to preterm neonates with RDS has become an accepted therapy in neonatal centers worldwide. Numerous clinical trials involving the administration of exogenous surfactant to infants with or at high risk for RDS demonstrate improvements in blood gas values and ventilator settings, decreased incidence of pulmonary air leaks, intraventricular hemorrhage,

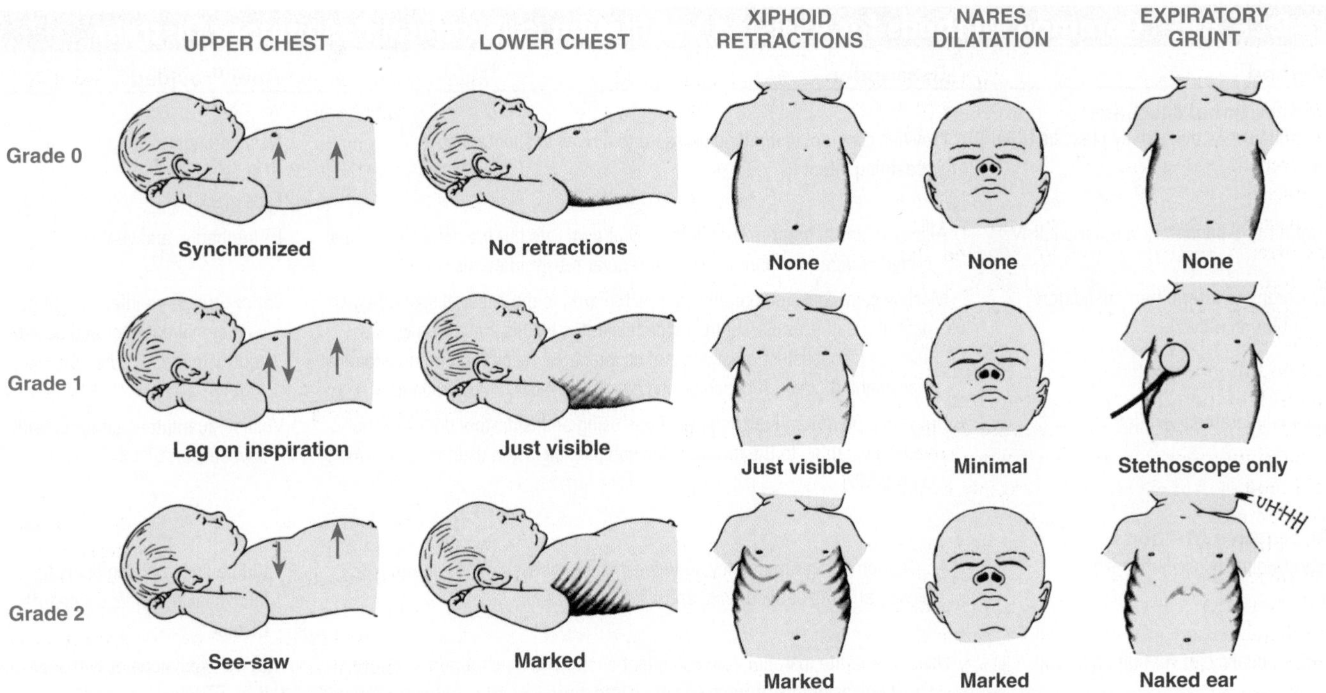

Fig. 8.23 Criteria for evaluating respiratory distress. (Modified from Silvermann, W. A., & Anderson, D. H. [1956]. A controlled clinical trial of effects of water mist on obstructive respiratory signs, death rate, and necropsy findings among premature infants. *Pediatrics, 17,* 1.)

decreased deaths from RDS, and an overall decreased infant mortality rate (Polin, Carlo, & American Academy of Pediatrics, Committee on Fetus and Newborn, 2014). The overall rates of some associated comorbidities (bronchopulmonary dysplasia, NEC, patent ductus arteriosus) have not decreased with surfactant replacement. Currently, exogenous surfactant is derived from a natural source (e.g., porcine, bovine).

Surfactant therapy is also being used in infants with meconium aspiration, infectious pneumonia, sepsis, persistent pulmonary hypertension, and congenital diaphragmatic hernia (Polin et al., 2014). Surfactant may be administered at birth as a preventive or prophylactic treatment of RDS or later on in the course of RDS as a rescue treatment; however, research has demonstrated improved clinical outcomes and fewer adverse effects when surfactant is administered prophylactically to infants at risk for developing RDS (Polin et al., 2014). Use of surfactant in late preterm infants with RDS has demonstrated improvement in respiratory function but did not affect short-term outcomes (Dani, Mosca, Vento, et al., 2018). Surfactant is administered via an endotracheal (ET) tube directly into the infant's trachea. Complications seen with surfactant administration include pulmonary hemorrhage and mucus plugging. Nursing responsibilities with surfactant administration include assistance in the delivery of the product, collection and monitoring of blood gases, scrupulous monitoring of oxygenation with pulse oximetry, and assessment of the infant's tolerance of the procedure. After surfactant is absorbed, there is usually an increase in respiratory compliance that requires adjustment of ventilator settings to decrease mean airway pressure and prevent overinflation or hyperoxemia. Suctioning is usually delayed for an hour or so (depending on the type of surfactant and unit protocol) to allow maximum effects to occur. Studies have shown the benefit of administering surfactant early (prophylactic) in infants at risk for developing RDS, then extubating and placing them on nasal continuous positive airway pressure (CPAP); this decreased the overall incidence of bronchopulmonary dysplasia, need for mechanical ventilation, and fewer air leak syndromes (Gardner, Enzman-Hines, & Nyp, 2016). Research is in progress to investigate the possibility of delivering an aerosolized surfactant (Rey-Santano, Mielgo, Lopez, et al., 2016). This method would decrease the problems associated with current delivery systems (contamination of the airway, interruption of mechanical ventilation, and loss of the drug in the ET tubing from reflux).

The goals of oxygen therapy are to provide adequate oxygen to the tissues, prevent lactic acid accumulation resulting from hypoxia, and at the same time avoid the potentially negative effects of oxygen and barotrauma. Numerous methods have been devised to improve oxygenation (Table 8.6). All require that the gas be warmed and humidified before entering the respiratory tract. If the infant does not require mechanical ventilation, oxygen can be supplied by nasal cannula or via nasal prongs in conjunction with CPAP (see Chapter 20, Oxygen Therapy). If oxygen saturation of the blood cannot be maintained at a satisfactory level and the arterial carbon dioxide ($PaCO_2$) level rises, infants will require ventilatory assistance.

Prevention

The most successful approach to prevention of RDS is prevention of preterm delivery, especially in elective early delivery and cesarean section. Improved methods for assessing the maturity of the fetal lung by amniocentesis, although not a routine procedure, allow a reasonable prediction of adequate surfactant formation. Because estimation of a delivery date can be miscalculated by as much as 1 month, such tests are particularly valuable when scheduling an elective cesarean section. The combination of maternal steroid administration before delivery and surfactant administration postnatally seems to have a synergistic effect on neonatal lungs, with the net result being

TABLE 8.6 Common Methods for Assisted Ventilation in Neonatal Respiratory Distress

Method	Description	How Provided
Conventional Methods		
Continuous positive airway pressure (CPAP)	Provides constant distending pressure to airway in spontaneously breathing infant	Nasal prongs ET tube Face mask
Intermittent mandatory ventilation (IMV)[a]	Allows infant to breathe spontaneously at own rate but provides mechanical cycled respirations and pressure at regular preset intervals	ET intubation and ventilator
Synchronized intermittent mandatory ventilation (SIMV)	Mechanically delivered breaths are synchronized to the onset of spontaneous patient breaths; assist/control mode facilitates full inspiratory synchrony; involves signal detection of onset of spontaneous respiration from abdominal movement, thoracic impedance, and airway pressure or flow changes	Patient-triggered infant ventilator with signal detector and assist/control mode; ET tube
Volume guarantee ventilation	Delivers a predetermined volume of gas using an inspiratory pressure that varies according to the infant's lung compliance (often used in conjunction with SIMV)	Volume guarantee ventilator with flow sensor; ET tube
Alternative Methods		
High-frequency oscillation (HFO)	Application of high-frequency, low-volume, sine-wave flow oscillations to airway at rates between 480 and 1200 breaths/min	Variable-speed piston pump (or loudspeaker, fluidic oscillator); ET tube
High-frequency jet ventilation (HFJV)	Uses a separate, parallel, low-compliant circuit and injector port to deliver small pulses or jets of fresh gas deep into airway at rates between 250 and 900 breaths/min	May be used alone or with low-rate IMV; ET tube

[a]Also referred to as *conventional ventilation* (vs. high-frequency ventilation [HFV]).
ET, Endotracheal.

a decrease in infant mortality, decreased incidence of intraventricular hemorrhage, fewer pulmonary air leaks, and fewer problems with pulmonary interstitial emphysema and RDS (Shaughnessy & Goyal, 2020).

Prognosis

RDS is a self-limiting disease. Before the use of surfactant, infants typically experienced a period of deterioration (≈48 hours) and, in the absence of complications, improved by 72 hours. Often heralded by the onset of diuresis, this improvement was attributed primarily to increased production and greater availability of surfactant. With the administration of surfactant, lung compliance begins to improve almost immediately, resulting in lower oxygen requirements and a decreased need for ventilatory support.

Infants with RDS who survive the first 96 hours have a reasonable chance of recovery. However, complications of RDS include associated respiratory conditions and problems associated with prematurity, including patent ductus arteriosus and congestive heart failure, intraventricular hemorrhage, bronchopulmonary dysplasia, retinopathy of prematurity, pneumonia, air leak syndrome, sepsis, NEC, and neurologic sequelae.

Nursing Care Management

Care of infants with RDS involves all of the observations and interventions previously described for high-risk infants. In addition, the nurse is concerned with the complex problems related to respiratory therapy and the constant threat of hypoxemia and acidosis that complicates the care of patients in respiratory difficulty.

The respiratory therapist, an important member of the NICU team, is often responsible for the maintenance of respiratory equipment. Although it may be the respiratory therapist's responsibility to regulate the apparatus, nurses should understand the equipment and be able to recognize when it is not functioning correctly. The most essential nursing function is to observe and assess the infant's response to therapy. Continuous monitoring and close observation are mandatory because an infant's status can change rapidly and because oxygen concentration and ventilation parameters are prescribed according to the infant's blood gas measurements and pulse oximetry readings.

Changes in oxygen concentration are based on these observations. The amount of oxygen administered, expressed as the fraction of inspired oxygen (FiO_2), is determined on an individual basis according to pulse oximetry or direct or indirect measurement of arterial oxygen concentration. Capillary samples collected from the heel (see Chapter 20 for procedure) are useful for pH and $PaCO_2$ determinations but not for oxygenation status. Continuous transcutaneous or pulse oximetry readings are recorded at least hourly. Blood sampling is performed after ventilator changes for the acutely ill infant and thereafter when clinically indicated.

Mucus may collect in the respiratory tract as a result of the infant's pulmonary condition. Secretions interfere with gas flow and predispose the infant to obstruction of the passages, including the ET tube. Suctioning should be performed only when necessary and should be based on individual infant assessment, which includes auscultation of the chest, evidence of decreased oxygenation, excess moisture in the ET tube, or increased infant irritability. During suctioning, a variety of techniques can be used to minimize complications, including the use of a closed suctioning system (Gardner, Enzman-Hines, & Nyp, 2016).

! NURSING ALERT

Endotracheal (ET) suctioning is not an innocuous procedure (it may cause bronchospasm, bradycardia resulting from vagal nerve stimulation, hypoxia, or increased intracranial pressure [ICP], predisposing the infant to intraventricular hemorrhage) and should never be carried out on a routine basis. Improper suctioning technique can also cause infection, airway damage, or even pneumothoraces.

When nasopharyngeal passages, the trachea, or the ET tube is being suctioned, the catheter should be inserted gently but quickly; intermittent suction is applied as the catheter is withdrawn. Negative airway pressure should be applied for no more than 10 to 15 seconds because continuous suction removes air from the lungs along with the mucus. It is recommended that the "two-person" suctioning procedure be used on infants who are acutely ill and who do not tolerate any procedure without profound decreases in oxygen saturation, BP, and heart rate. The object of suctioning an artificial airway is to maintain patency of that airway, not the bronchi. Suction applied beyond the ET tube can cause traumatic lesions of the trachea. The use of in-line suction catheters may decrease airway contamination and hypoxia. Serious complications associated with ET tube suctioning can be mitigated with proper training and technique (Gardner, Enzman-Hines, & Nyp, 2016).

The most advantageous positions for facilitating an infant's open airway are on the side with the head supported in alignment by a small folded blanket or, when on the back, positioned to keep the neck slightly extended. With the head in the "sniffing" position, the trachea is opened at its maximum; hyperextension reduces the tracheal diameter in neonates.

Inspection of the skin is part of routine infant assessment. Position changes and the use of water pillows are helpful in guarding against skin breakdown.

Mouth care is especially important when infants are receiving respiratory support. Thick oral secretions and dry mucous membranes may result from the drying effect of oxygen therapy. Drying and cracking can be prevented by good oral hygiene using sterile water. Irritation to the nares or mouth that occurs from appliances used to administer oxygen (e.g., nasal CPAP) may be reduced by the use of a water-soluble ointment. Routine oral hygiene care in intubated adults and older children has been shown to decrease the incidence of ventilator-associated pneumonia (see Chapter 21).

The nursing care of an infant with RDS is a demanding role; meticulous attention must be given to subtle changes in the infant's oxygenation status. The importance of attention to detail cannot be overemphasized, particularly in regard to medication administration.

RESPIRATORY COMPLICATIONS

Newborn infants are vulnerable to a variety of pulmonary complications, some requiring oxygen therapy (Table 8.7). For example, the preterm infant is subject to periods of apnea, and in term, late preterm, and post-term infants, intrauterine stress often causes fetuses to pass meconium, which may be aspirated before or during birth. Oxygen therapy, although lifesaving, is not without its hazards. Positive pressure introduced by mechanical apparatus has created an increase in the incidence of ruptured alveoli and subsequent pneumothorax and bronchopulmonary dysplasia (chronic lung disease). The use of nasal CPAP decreases the incidence of adverse effects associated with intubation and positive pressure ventilation in preterm infants with RDS. Retinopathy of prematurity is observed almost exclusively in preterm infants and is related primarily to prematurity and oxygen therapy (see Table 8.7). Evidence supports the resuscitation of asphyxiated newborns with 21% oxygen rather than 100% oxygen; preliminary studies reduced mortality and neurologic morbidities in newborns resuscitated with 21% oxygen (Manley, Owen, Hooper, et al., 2017). Proponents for room air resuscitation suggest that fewer complications are associated with oxidative stress and hyperoxemia when room air is administered (Vento, 2015. The 2015 American Heart Association Neonatal Resuscitation Guidelines recommend the initiation of neonatal resuscitation using room air (no supplemental oxygen); if the neonate does not improve within 60 seconds ("the Golden Minute"), the use of supplemental oxygen is recommended (see Translating Evidence Into Practice box). Pulse oximetry is recommended to monitor the infant's oxygenation status during resuscitation and to prevent excessive use of oxygen in both term and preterm infants (Wyckoff, Aziz, Escobedo, et al., 2015).

TRANSLATING EVIDENCE INTO PRACTICE

Use of Room Air or Low Oxygen for Newborn Stabilization and Resuscitation in the Delivery Room

Ask the Question

Is room air or low oxygen better for newborn stabilization and resuscitation in the delivery room?

Search for Evidence

Search Strategies

Search selection included English publications on room air or low oxygen use for newborn stabilization and resuscitation in delivery room in past 3 years.

Database Used

PubMed

Critically Analyze the Evidence

- In infants younger than 32 weeks' gestation, initial oxygen supplementation of 30% oxygen is as safe as 65% oxygen with no differences in chronic lung disease or oxidative stress markers (Rook, Schierbeek, Vento, et al., 2014).
- Systematic review of 21% oxygen versus 100% oxygen use for stabilization or resuscitation of newborns found a significant reduction in risk for newborn mortality as well as hypoxic ischemic encephalopathy when 21% oxygen was used (Saugstad, Ramji, Soll, et al., 2008).

In moderately asphyxiated term infants, those resuscitated with 100% oxygen had elevated oxidative stress markers in their blood at 28 days of age, whereas those resuscitated with 21% oxygen had levels similar to nonasphyxiated control infants (Vento, Escobar, Cernada, et al., 2012).

- In neonates 24 to 34 weeks' gestational age, a low-oxygen strategy beginning with room air with a 10% increase in oxygen concentration every 30 seconds until satisfactory oxygen saturations were achieved resulted in less oxygen exposure, lower oxidative stress, and decreased respiratory morbidities compared to infants resuscitated with a high-oxygen strategy (100% oxygen to start followed by 10% decreases in oxygen concentration every 30 seconds).
- In neonates 32 weeks' gestational age or younger, initiating resuscitation with 100% oxygen and titrating downward was more effective than initiating resuscitation with 21% oxygen (Rabi, Singhal, & Nettel-Aguirre, 2011).
- Use of heated and humidified air in neonates 32 weeks' gestational age or younger during resuscitation or stabilization in the delivery room minimized postnatal heat loss (te Pas, Lopriore, Dito, et al., 2010).
- Infants receiving 100% oxygen with positive pressure ventilation and healthy infants transitioned in room air had similar increase in oxygen saturation, but a slower increase in oxygen saturation was observed in infants receiving 100% oxygen free flow (Rabi, Chen, Yee, et al., 2009).
- Newborns with spontaneous circulation (heart rate >60 beats/min) should be stabilized or resuscitated with room air, but asphyxiated newborns with depressed circulation (heart rate <60 beats/min) should be stabilized or resuscitated with 100% oxygen (Ten & Matsiukevich, 2009).
- In very preterm infants (<30 weeks' gestational age) stabilized or resuscitated with 100% oxygen, the majority (80%) had SpO_2 95% in the first 10 minutes. Infants stabilized or resuscitated with room air followed a similar course as

TRANSLATING EVIDENCE INTO PRACTICE—cont'd

Use of Room Air or Low Oxygen for Newborn Stabilization and Resuscitation in the Delivery Room

full-term and preterm newborns when 100% oxygen was administered along with titration against SpO_2. Similar changes in heart rate were observed in both groups (Dawson, Kamlin, Wong, et al., 2009).

Apply the Evidence: Nursing Implications

The International Liaison Committee on Resuscitation recommends that "in term infants receiving resuscitation at birth with positive pressure ventilation, it is best to begin with air rather than 100% oxygen" (Perlman, Wyllie, Kattwinkel, et al., 2010). Decisions to increase the oxygen concentration should be based on the oxygen saturation and the infant's clinical response.

When the oxygen saturation is below the recommended levels, increase fraction of inspired oxygen (FiO_2) by 10% every 30 seconds until the saturation level reaches the desired range. Rapid FiO_2 changes may cause constriction of the pulmonary blood vessels (Ramji, Saugstad, & Jain, 2015).

Quality and Safety Competencies: Evidence-Based Practice[a]

Knowledge

Differentiate clinical opinion from research and evidence-based summaries.

Describe the various interventions for newborn stabilization and delivery room resuscitations with room air or low oxygen.

Skills

Base individualized care plan on patient values, clinical expertise, and evidence.

Integrate evidence into practice by using interventions for newborn stabilization and delivery room resuscitations with room air or low oxygen.

Attitudes

Value the concept of evidence-based practice as integral to determining best clinical practice.

Appreciate strengths and weakness of evidence for newborn stabilization and delivery room resuscitations with room air or low oxygen.

References

Dawson, J. A., Kamlin, C. O., Wong, C., et al. (2009). Oxygen saturation and heart rate during delivery room resuscitation of infants <30 weeks' gestation with air or 100% oxygen. *Archives of Disease in Childhood: Fetal and Neonatal Edition, 94*(2), F87–F91.

Perlman, J. M., Wyllie, J., Kattwinkel, J., et al. (2010). Part 11: Neonatal resuscitation: 2010 international consensus on cardiopulmonary resuscitation and emergency cardiovascular care science with treatment recommendations. *Circulation, 122*(16 Suppl. 2), S516–S538.

Rabi, Y., Chen, S. Y., Yee, W. H., et al. (2009). Relationship between oxygen saturation and the mode of oxygen delivery used in newborn resuscitation. *Journal of Perinatology, 29*(2), 101–105.

Rabi, Y., Singhal, N., & Nettel-Aguirre, A. (2011). Room-air versus oxygen administration for resuscitation of preterm infants: The roar study. *Pediatrics, 128*(2), e374–e381.

Ramji, S., Saugstad, O. D., & Jain, A. (2015). Current concepts of oxygen therapy in neonates. *Indian Journal of Pediatrics, 82*(1), 46–52.

Rook, D., Schierbeek, H., Vento, M., et al. (2014). Resuscitation of preterm infants with different inspired oxygen fractions. *Journal of Pediatrics, 164*(6), 1322–1326.

Saugstad, O. D., Ramji, S., Soll, R. F., et al. (2008). Resuscitation of newborn infants with 21% or 100% oxygen: An updated systematic review and meta-analysis. *Neonatology, 94*(3), 176–182.

te Pas, A. B., Lopriore, E., Dito, I., et al. (2010). Humidified and heated air during stabilization at birth improves temperature in preterm infants. *Pediatrics, 125*(6), e1427–e1432.

Ten, V. S., & Matsiukevich, D. (2009). Room air or 100% oxygen for resuscitation of infants with prenatal depression. *Current Opinion in Pediatrics, 21*(2), 188–193.

Vento, M., Escobar, J., Cernada, M., et al. (2012). The use and misuse of oxygen during the neonatal period. *Clinics in Perinatology, 39*(1), 165–176.

Updated by Deb Fraser

[a]Adapted from the Quality and Safety Education for Nurses Institute.

QUALITY PATIENT OUTCOMES: MECONIUM ASPIRATION SYNDROME

- Room air oxygen saturation 90% or greater
- Maintains arterial/venous pH 7.35 or greater

Inhaled nitric oxide (INO) and **extracorporeal membrane oxygenation (ECMO)** are additional therapies used in the treatment of respiratory distress and respiratory failure in neonates. INO is used in term and late preterm infants with conditions such as persistent pulmonary hypertension, meconium aspiration syndrome (see Table 8.7), pneumonia, sepsis, and congenital diaphragmatic hernia to decrease or reverse pulmonary hypertension, pulmonary vasoconstriction, acidosis, and hypoxemia. Nitric oxide is a colorless, highly diffusible gas that can be administered through the ventilator circuit blended with oxygen. INO therapy may be used in conjunction with surfactant replacement therapy, high-frequency ventilation, or ECMO. Although INO is used in preterm infants with respiratory distress and respiratory failure, its use has not proved to be significantly effective in decreasing rates of bronchopulmonary dysplasia or in improving survival rates in preterm infants (Barrington, Finer, & Pennaforte, 2017).

ECMO may be used in the management of term infants with acute severe respiratory failure for the same conditions as those mentioned for INO. This therapy involves a modified heart–lung machine, although in ECMO the heart is not stopped and blood does not entirely bypass the lungs. Blood is shunted from a catheter in the right atrium or right internal jugular vein by gravity to a servo-regulated roller pump, pumped through a membrane lung where it is oxygenated and through a small heat exchanger, and then returned to the systemic circulation via a major artery, such as the carotid artery, to the aortic arch. ECMO provides oxygen to the circulation; allows the lungs to "rest"; and decreases pulmonary hypertension and hypoxemia in such conditions as persistent pulmonary hypertension of the newborn, congenital diaphragmatic hernia, sepsis, meconium aspiration, and severe pneumonia.

Acid-Base Imbalance

Many respiratory and metabolic conditions in infants and children may cause an acid-base imbalance. Disease states such as diarrhea (see Chapter 22), RDS, bronchopulmonary dysplasia, and respiratory failure may interfere with the body's ability to regulate and maintain acid-base balance. Simply stated, **acidosis** (acidemia) results from either accumulation of acid or loss of base, and **alkalosis** (alkalemia) results from either accumulation of base or loss of acid. Several laboratory tests are used to assess the nature and extent of acid-base disturbances; these are outlined in Table 8.8. To determine the acid-base status, three variables—the respiratory component (PCO_2), the metabolic component (arterial bicarbonate or serum carbon dioxide [HCO_3^-]), and the serum pH—must be determined. In addition, the anion gap may be useful in determining the cause and extent of metabolic acidosis; therefore serum chemistry is obtained as well. Measurement of any two variables (PCO_2, pH, HCO_3^-) allows computation of the third using the Henderson-Hasselbalch equation. A summary of the relationships between these and other variables is outlined in Table 8.9.

TABLE 8.7 Respiratory Complications

Description	Clinical Manifestations	Therapeutic Management	Nursing Care Management
Meconium Aspiration Syndrome			
Aspiration of amniotic fluid containing meconium into fetal or newborn trachea in utero or at first breath	Meconium stained at birth Tachypnea Hypoxia Acidemia Hyperventilation (early) Hypoventilation (later)	Suction hypopharynx after delivery. Infants who are vigorous with strong, stable respiratory effort; good muscle tone; and heart rate >100 beats/min should not undergo tracheal suctioning but should be closely monitored. Infants who demonstrate poor respiratory effort, low heart rate, and poor tone should be rapidly intubated, suctioned appropriately, and resuscitated according to clinical status after suctioning. Monitor for respiratory distress; manage with supplemental oxygen. Prevent acidosis and hypoxemia. May use exogenous surfactant, INO, or ECMO.	See Respiratory Distress Syndrome, Nursing Care Management earlier in the chapter.
Apnea of Prematurity			
Lapse of spontaneous breathing for ≥20 seconds, which may or may not be followed by bradycardia, oxygen desaturation, and color change	Persistent apneic spells	Observe for apnea. Check for thermal stability and metabolic problem such as hypoglycemia. Administer caffeine as prescribed. Administer nasal CPAP.	Provide continuous electronic monitoring (respiratory and heart rates). Observe for presence of respirations. Observe color. Provide gentle tactile stimulation. Suction nose and oropharynx if still apneic. Apply positive pressure ventilation with bag valve mask using the minimum pressure needed to gently lift rib cage. Assess for and manage any precipitating factors (e.g., temperature instability, abdominal distention, ambient oxygen). Observe for signs of caffeine toxicity: tachycardia (rate ≥180 beats/min) and (later) vomiting, restlessness, irritability. Assess skin (with use of nasal CPAP) for breakdown, irritation at nasal septum.
Pneumothorax			
Presence of extraneous air in pleural space as a result of alveolar rupture	Tachypnea or apnea Systemic hypotension Sudden or persistent oxygen desaturation Grunting, nasal flaring Retractions Absent or diminished breath sounds Shift in point of maximum impulse of heart sounds Bradycardia, cyanosis	Evacuate trapped air in pleural space through needle aspiration or insertion of chest tube. In otherwise healthy term infants who do not require high oxygen concentration or mechanical ventilation, supplemental oxygen to maintain normal saturation levels and close observation may be the only treatment required.	Maintain close vigilance of infants with respiratory distress and those on assisted ventilation. Provide appropriate care of chest drainage apparatus. Ensure emergency needle aspiration setup is available.

Continued

TABLE 8.7 Respiratory Complications—cont'd

Description	Clinical Manifestations	Therapeutic Management	Nursing Care Management
Bronchopulmonary Dysplasia			
Pathologic process related to alveolar damage from lung disease, prolonged exposure to mechanical ventilation, high peak inspiratory pressures and oxygen, and immature alveoli and respiratory tract	Dyspnea Barrel chest Inability to wean from oxygen or mechanical ventilation after course of RDS (surfactant deficiency) Wheezing	Prevention: Administer maternal steroids; administer exogenous surfactant postnatally. Avoid intubation and mechanical ventilation when the infant's condition allows. Extubate mechanically ventilated infants as soon as medically indicated. Provide early detection with pulmonary function tests. Use synchronized or volume guarantee ventilation, decreased inspiratory pressures, or nasal CPAP. Prevent air leaks. Use high-frequency ventilation. Prevent or control respiratory or systemic infections. Minimize use of high oxygen concentrations in neonatal resuscitation and on mechanical ventilation; monitor oxygen saturation and implement resuscitation according to neonate response to low oxygen administration. Diagnosis established: Support respiratory efforts. Maintain adequate oxygenation and avoid hypoxemia. Administer bronchodilators and, in select cases, postnatal steroids. Provide supplemental oxygen in hospital or home.	Provide individualized developmental care and enhancement. Monitor oxygen saturations closely in preterm infants and avoid hyperoxemia Provide opportunities for additional rest during feedings. Observe for signs of fluid overload or pulmonary edema. Assist with home oxygen therapy as needed. Assess susceptibility to upper respiratory tract infections and need for frequent hospitalization for respiratory dysfunction. Provide increased caloric density (feedings) with human milk fortifier or protein supplements.
Persistent Pulmonary Hypertension of the Newborn			
Severe pulmonary hypertension and large right-to-left shunt through foramen ovale and ductus arteriosus	Hypoxia Marked cyanosis Tachypnea with grunting and retractions Decreased peripheral pulses and prolonged capillary refill (poor perfusion) Shock	Regulate IV fluids. Provide supplemental oxygen and assisted ventilation. Administer systemic vasodilators, such as sildenafil. Maintain acid-base balance. Prevent hypoxemia and hypercarbia. Administer INO or ECMO.	See Nursing Care of the High-Risk Newborn and Family and Respiratory Distress Syndrome earlier in the chapter. Provide nursing care to reduce stress to infant, especially noxious stimuli that cause increased oxygen demands. Decrease physical manipulation and disturbance.
Retinopathy of Prematurity			
Severe vascular constriction in the immature retinal vasculature followed by hypoxemia in the retina, which in turn stimulates abnormal vascular proliferation of retinal capillaries into the hypoxic area; as retinal veins dilate and multiply in the direction of the lens, retinal detachment may occur if untreated Multifactorial etiology: Preterm birth is major risk factor	Progressive vascular growth of retina Eventual blindness if not treated Diagnosed by ophthalmologic examination	Prevent preterm birth. Provide early screening and detection in infants born at <30 wk of gestation and weight <1500 g (3.3 pounds). Decrease exposure to bright, direct lighting; although exposure to bright light has not been proven to contribute to retinopathy of prematurity, such exposure is undesirable from a neurobehavioral developmental perspective. Use supplemental oxygen judiciously and monitor oxygen blood levels carefully; prevent wide fluctuations in oxygen blood levels (hyperoxemia and hypoxemia). Arrest vascular proliferation process—laser photocoagulation; surgical repair of detached retina. Recently there has been increased interest in the administration of an antivascular endothelial growth factor drug bevacizumab, which arrests the proliferation of vessels and prevents retinal detachment commonly seen in retinopathy of prematurity. If successful, this therapy may preclude the use of laser therapy (Hartnett, 2014).	See Nursing Care of the High-Risk Newborn and Family and earlier in the chapter. Provide preventive care by closely monitoring blood oxygen levels, responding promptly to saturation alarms, and preventing fluctuations in blood oxygen levels. Provide postoperative pain management if surgery is performed. Provide parental education and support. Provide nursing care using principles of individualized developmental care.

CPAP, Continuous positive airway pressure; *ECMO,* extracorporeal membrane oxygenation; *INO,* inhaled nitric oxide; *IV,* intravenous; *RDS,* respiratory distress syndrome.

TABLE 8.8 Laboratory Tests Used in Assessment of Acid-Base Status

Abbreviation	Test	Normal Values[a]	Description
pH	Partial pressure of hydrogen	Birth: 7.11-7.36 1 day: 7.29-7.45 Child: 7.35-7.45	Expression of hydrogen ion concentration
PCO_2	Partial pressure of carbon dioxide or carbon dioxide tension	Newborn: 27-40 mm Hg Infant: 27-41 mm Hg	Measure of carbon dioxide tension; reflects carbonic acid (H_2CO_3) concentrations of plasma
HCO_3^- (serum) arterial	Carbon dioxide content or carbon dioxide combining power	Infant: 21-28 mEq/ml Thereafter: 22-26 mEq/ml	Concentration of base bicarbonate
Base excess	Base excess (whole blood)	Newborn: −2 to −10 Infant: −1 to −7 Child: +2 to −4 Thereafter: +3 to −3	Used to express extent of deviation from normal buffer base concentration; indicates quantity of blood buffers remaining after hydrogen ion is buffered
Anion gap	Anion gap; using chemistry profile and serum bicarbonate	10-12[a] (4-11)[b]	Reflects difference between measured cation sodium and anions (also measured) of chloride and bicarbonate

[a]Huether, S. E. (2019). The cellular environment: Fluids and electrolytes, acids and bases. In K. L. McCance and S. E. Huether (Eds.), *Pathophysiology: The biologic basis for disease in adults and children* (8th ed.). St Louis, MO: Elsevier.
[b]Data from Kliegman, R. M., Stanton, B. F., St. Geme, J. W., et al. (Eds.). (2020). *Nelson textbook of pediatrics* (21st ed.). Philadelphia, PA: Elsevier.

TABLE 8.9 Summary of Simple Acid-Base Disturbances (Partially Compensated)

Disturbance	Plasma pH	Plasma PCO_2	Plasma HCO_3^-
Respiratory acidosis	↓	↑	↑
Respiratory alkalosis	↑	↓	↓
Metabolic acidosis	↓	↓	↓
Metabolic alkalosis	↑	↑	↑

The pH represents the concentration of hydrogen (H^+) in solution and indicates only whether the imbalance is more acidic or more alkaline. It does not reflect the nature of the imbalance (i.e., whether it is of metabolic or respiratory origin). Body metabolism affects primarily the base bicarbonate (HCO_3^-); therefore alterations in the concentration of bicarbonate are called *metabolic disturbances of acid-base balance*. Also, because the amount of carbon dioxide (CO_2) exhaled through the lungs affects the carbonic acid (H_2CO_3), changes in carbonic acid concentration are referred to as *respiratory disturbances*. Consequently, the simple disturbances (those with a single primary cause) are categorized as metabolic acidosis or alkalosis and respiratory acidosis or alkalosis.

When the fundamental acid-base ratio is altered for any reason, the body attempts to correct the deviation. In a simple disturbance, a single primary factor affects one component of the acid-base pair and is usually accompanied by a compensatory or secondary change in the component that is not primarily affected. For example, when the concentration of metabolic acids in the body increases, they combine with bicarbonate (a buffer) to form carbonic acid. The lungs immediately attempt to compensate for the imbalance by eliminating the carbonic acid through exhaled carbon dioxide and water (compensation). The imbalance is corrected when the kidneys excrete hydrogen and ammonium ions in exchange for reabsorbed sodium bicarbonate.

When the secondary changes (the hyperventilation and renal excretion of hydrogen ions in the preceding example) succeed in preventing a distortion of the acid-base ratio and the pH is restored to normal, the disturbance is described as **compensated**. The **uncompensated** state exists when there is no compensatory effect and the pH remains uncorrected. The imbalance is said to be corrected when physiologic mechanisms fully correct the primary abnormality. *Mixed* acid-base imbalances may also occur in diseases states, and the patient will manifest two simultaneous acid-base imbalances rather than a single imbalance. It is not within the scope of this text to discuss the many variations of mixed acid-base imbalances; readers are referred to other published sources for such material.

CARDIOVASCULAR COMPLICATIONS

The most serious cardiovascular disorders of newborns are the congenital heart defects. Other conditions that occur in the newborn period are usually related to prematurity (e.g., anemia, patent ductus arteriosus) or other diseases (e.g., respiratory distress). Some of these disorders are outlined in Table 8.10.

NEUROLOGIC COMPLICATIONS

Neurologic injury in newborn infants is common. Newborn infants are particularly vulnerable to ischemic injury caused by variable (both increased and decreased) cerebral blood flow subsequent to asphyxia; and preterm infants, with a fragile cerebrovascular network, are highly prone to periventricular or intraventricular hemorrhage. Fragility and increased permeability of capillaries and prolonged prothrombin time predispose preterm infants to trauma when delicate structures are subjected to the forces of labor. The more common neurologic complications are outlined in Table 8.1.

The highest incidence of abnormal neurologic findings occurs in VLBW infants and those with intracranial hemorrhage. Major neurologic problems, such as cerebral palsy, seizures, and hydrocephalus, are

TABLE 8.10 Cardiovascular and Hematologic Complications

Description	Clinical Manifestations	Therapeutic Management	Nursing Care Management
Patent Ductus Arteriosus			
Failure of ductus arteriosus to close at birth, resulting in shunting of oxygenated blood from aorta through open ductus arteriosus into pulmonary artery, increasing workload on left side of heart and increasing pulmonary vascular congestion (see Chapter 23)	Decreased PaO_2 Increased PCO_2 Recurrent apnea Bounding peripheral pulses Systolic or continuous murmur	Regulate parenteral fluids. Provide respiratory support. Administer course of indomethacin or ibuprofen or perform surgical ductal ligation.	See Nursing Care of the High-Risk Newborn and Family earlier in the chapter.
Anemia			
Hemoglobin (<14 mg/dl) inadequate to carry oxygenated blood to tissues Anemia commonly occurs in ill preterm infants as a result of increased blood sampling and deficient erythropoiesis	Pallor Apnea Tachycardia Diminished activity Poor feeder Poor weight gain Respiratory distress—grunting, nasal flaring, intercostal retractions Respiratory difficulty	Administer volume expanders for acute hypovolemia at birth (e.g., normal saline). Transfuse with packed RBCs or administer recombinant human erythropoietin.	Use microsamples for blood tests. Monitor amount of blood drawn for tests. Administer recombinant human erythropoietin as prescribed. Administer iron supplements as prescribed.
Polycythemia or Hyperviscosity Syndrome			
Venous hematocrit ≥65% results in venous stasis in vital organs and risk for microthrombus development	High incidence of: Cardiovascular symptoms (PPHN, cyanosis, apnea) Seizures Hyperbilirubinemia Gastrointestinal abnormalities	Implement partial exchange transfusion with blood product or appropriate volume expander. Provide appropriate therapy for associated problems.	See Nursing Care of the High-Risk Newborn and Family and Hyperbilirubinemia earlier in the chapter.
Vitamin K Deficiency Bleeding (Formerly Hemorrhagic Disease of the Newborn)			
Bleeding disorder resulting from transient deficiency of vitamin K–dependent blood factors; newborn's sterile gut does not produce adequate amounts of vitamin K	Oozing blood from umbilicus or circumcision Bloody or black stools Hematuria Petechiae	Administer prophylactic vitamin K.	Administer prophylactic vitamin K via intramuscular route. Observe for complications, such as bleeding umbilical cord, prolonged circumcision bleeding, and petechiae.

PPHN, Persistent pulmonary hypertension of the newborn; *RBC,* red blood cell.

usually diagnosed in the first 2 years of life. Less severe deficits, such as learning disorders, ADHD, and fine and gross motor incoordination, may not be diagnosed until preschool or even school age. Cerebral palsy is one of the most common neurologic deficits in survivors of prematurity (see Chapter 30).

NEONATAL SEIZURES

Seizures in the neonatal period are usually the clinical manifestation of a serious underlying disease. The most common cause of seizures for term and preterm neonates is hypoxic ischemic encephalopathy secondary to perinatal asphyxia (Parsons et al., 2016). Although not life threatening as an isolated entity, seizures constitute a medical emergency because they signal a disease process that may produce irreversible cerebral damage. Consequently, it is imperative to recognize a seizure and its significance so that the cause, as well as the seizure, can be treated (Box 8.5).

The features of neonatal seizures are different from those observed in older infants and children. For example, the well-organized, generalized tonic-clonic seizures seen in older children are rare in infants, especially preterm infants. The newborn brain, with its immature anatomic and physiologic status and less cortical organization, is unable to allow ready development and maintenance of a generalized seizure. Instead, signs of seizures in newborns, especially preterm neonates, are subtle and include findings such as lip smacking, tongue thrusting, eye rolling, and swimming movements (Parsons et al., 2016).

Jitteriness or tremulousness in newborns is a repetitive shaking of an extremity or extremities that may be observed with crying, occur with changes in sleeping state, or is elicited with stimulation. Jitteriness is relatively common in newborns and in a mild degree may be considered normal during the first 4 days of life. Jitteriness can be distinguished from seizures by several characteristics:

- Jitteriness is not accompanied by ocular movement as are seizures.
- Whereas the dominant movement in jitteriness is tremor, seizure movement is clonic jerking that cannot be stopped by flexion of the affected limb.
- Jitteriness is highly sensitive to stimulation, but seizures are not.

Jitteriness may be a sign of hypoglycemia, and infants with jitteriness should have their blood glucose level evaluated.

A **tremor** is defined as repetitive movements of both hands (with or without movement of legs or jaws) at a frequency of two to five per second and lasting more than 10 minutes. It is common in newborn infants and has a variety of causes, including neurologic damage,

BOX 8.5 Causes of Neonatal Seizures

Metabolic
Hypoglycemia, hyperglycemia
Hypocalcemia
Hypernatremia, hyponatremia
Hypomagnesemia
Pyridoxine deficiency
Aminoaciduria (e.g., phenylketonuria, maple syrup urine disease)
Hyperammonemia

Toxic
Uremia
Bilirubin encephalopathy (kernicterus)

Prenatal Infections
Toxoplasmosis
Syphilis
Cytomegalovirus
Herpes simplex

Postnatal Infections
Bacterial meningitis
Viral meningoencephalitis
Sepsis
Brain abscess

Trauma at Birth
Hypoxic brain injury
Subarachnoid, subdural hemorrhage
Intraventricular hemorrhage

Malformations
Central nervous system (CNS) agenesis
Hydranencephaly
Tuberous sclerosis

Miscellaneous
Neonatal stroke
Narcotic withdrawal
Degenerative disease
Benign familial neonatal seizures

TABLE 8.11 Classifications of Neonatal Seizures

Type	Characteristics
Clonic	Slow, rhythmic jerking movements Approximately 1-3/second
Focal	Involves face, upper or lower extremities on one side of body May involve neck or trunk Infant is conscious during event
Multifocal	May migrate randomly from one part of the body to another Movements may start at different times
Tonic	Extension, stiffening movements
Generalized	Extension of all four limbs (similar to decerebrate rigidity) Upper limbs maintained in a stiffly flexed position (resembles decorticate rigidity)
Focal	Sustained posturing of a limb Asymmetric posturing of trunk or neck
Subtle	May develop in either full-term or preterm infants but more common in preterm Often overlooked by inexperienced observers Signs: • Horizontal eye deviation • Repetitive blinking or fluttering of the eyelids, staring • Sucking or other oral-buccal-lingual movements • Arm movements that resemble rowing or swimming • Leg movements described as pedaling or bicycling • Apnea (common) Signs may appear alone or in combination
Myoclonic	Rapid jerks that involve flexor muscle groups
Focal	Involves upper extremity flexor muscle group No EEG discharges observed
Multifocal	Asynchronous twitching of several parts of the body No associated EEG discharges observed
Generalized	Bilateral jerks of upper and lower limbs Associated with EEG discharges

EEG, Electroencephalogram.
Adapted from Volpe, J. (2008). Neonatal seizures. In J. Volpe, *Neurology of the newborn* (4th ed.). Philadelphia, PA: Saunders.

hypoglycemia, and hypocalcemia. In most instances, tremors are of no pathologic significance.

Spasms are sudden generalized jerks lasting briefly (1 to 2 seconds) that are distinguished from generalized tonic spells by their short duration and by the fact that spasms are most often associated with a single, brief generalized discharge (Mikati & Tchapjnikov, 2020).

Neonatal seizures can be divided into four major types. These classifications are outlined in order of frequency in Table 8.11 and consist of clonic, tonic, subtle, and myoclonic seizures (Parsons et al., 2016). Clonic, multifocal clonic, and migratory clonic seizures are more common in term infants.

Diagnostic Evaluation

Early evaluation and diagnosis of seizures are urgent. In addition to a careful physical examination, the pregnancy and family histories are investigated for familial and prenatal causes. Blood is drawn for glucose and electrolyte examination, and CSF may be obtained for testing of cell count and differential, protein, glucose, and culture. Electroencephalography (EEG) may help identify subtle seizures but is less helpful in establishing a diagnosis. Other diagnostic procedures, such as CT, MRI, and cerebral ultrasonography, may be indicated. A video EEG may be used to identify seizure activity in some newborns. More extensive metabolic testing may be needed when initial test results do not provide a diagnosis or the history is suggestive of an inherited metabolic disorder.

Therapeutic Management

Treatment is directed toward prevention of neurologic damage and involves correction of metabolic derangements, respiratory and cardiovascular support, and suppression of the seizure activity. The underlying cause is treated (e.g., glucose infusion for hypoglycemia, calcium for hypocalcemia, antibiotics for infection). If needed, respiratory support is provided for hypoxia, and anticonvulsants may be administered, especially when the other measures fail to control the seizures. Lorazepam is the initial drug of choice used to control acute seizures because it is distributed to the brain quickly and exerts its anticonvulsant effect in less than 5 minutes (Mikati & Tchapjnikov,

2020). Phenobarbital, given intravenously or orally, is the first drug of choice for a long-acting drug and is used if seizures are severe and persistent. Other drugs that may be used are phenytoin (Dilantin) and lorazepam.

Fosphenytoin sodium is a water-soluble prodrug and may also be used for seizures. Fosphenytoin metabolizes to form phenytoin in the body yet can easily be diluted or mixed in dextrose and normal saline and may be given via IV or intramuscular routes. In addition, fosphenytoin does not cause pain during IV administration. If EEG done at the time of discharge does not show evidence of epileptiform activity, medications are usually tapered at that time.

Recent research has shown that therapeutic hypothermia provided by cooling either the infant's head or the whole body reduces the severity of the neurologic damage in hypoxic ischemic encephalopathy when it is applied in the early stages of injury (first 6 hours after delivery) in infants with a gestational age of 35 to 36 weeks or more (Azzopardi, Strohm, Marlow, et al., 2014; Parsons et al., 2016). Clinical trials are currently ongoing to evaluate the efficacy and safety of using whole body cooling for infants with hypoxic ischemic encephalopathy (HIE) born at 33 to 35 weeks' gestational age.

A pilot study assessing the safety and feasibility of providing autologous umbilical cord blood (UCB) cells to neonates with HIE has demonstrated feasibility (Cotten, Murtha, Goldberg, et al., 2014). The study hypothesized that early infusion of autologous volume- and RBC-reduced UCB cells in infants with HIE would improve outcomes (Cotten et al., 2014).

Nursing Care Management

The major nursing responsibilities in the care of infants with seizures are to recognize when the infant is having a seizure so that therapy can be instituted, to carry out the therapeutic regimen, and to observe the response to the therapy and any further evidence of seizures or other symptomatology. Assessment and other aspects of care are the same as for all high-risk infants. Parents need to be informed of their infant's status, and the nurse should reinforce and clarify the practitioner's explanations. The infant's behaviors need to be interpreted for the parents, and the infant's responses to the treatment must be assessed and their significance explained. Parents are encouraged to visit their infant and perform the parenting activities consistent with the care plan. Seizures are a frightening phenomenon and generate a great deal of anxiety and fear, which is easily compounded by the justifiable concern of the staff. Providing support and guidance is an important nursing function.

HIGH RISK RELATED TO INFECTIOUS PROCESSES

SEPSIS

Sepsis, or **septicemia**, refers to a generalized bacterial infection in the bloodstream. Neonates are highly susceptible to infection as a result of diminished nonspecific (inflammatory) and specific (humoral) immunity, such as impaired phagocytosis, delayed chemotactic response, minimal or absent IgA and immunoglobulin M (IgM), and decreased complement levels. Because of infants' poor response to pathogenic agents, there is usually no local inflammatory reaction at the portal of entry to signal an infection, and the resulting symptoms tend to be vague and nonspecific. Consequently, diagnosis and treatment may be delayed.

Breastfeeding has a protective benefit against infection and should be promoted for all newborns. It is of particular benefit to high-risk neonates. Colostrum contains immunoglobulins that are effective against gram-negative bacteria.

Sepsis in the neonatal period can be acquired prenatally across the placenta from the maternal bloodstream or during labor from ingestion or aspiration of infected amniotic fluid. Prolonged rupture of the membranes always presents a risk for this type from maternal-fetal transfer of pathogenic organisms. In utero transplacental transfer can occur with organisms and viruses such as cytomegalovirus, toxoplasmosis, and *Treponema pallidum* (syphilis), which cross the placental barrier during the latter half of pregnancy. Intrapartum infection may occur via contact with an infected mother; examples of such infections include herpesvirus and human immunodeficiency virus (HIV).

Early-onset sepsis (less than 3 days after birth) is acquired in the perinatal period; infection can occur from direct contact with organisms from the maternal gastrointestinal and genitourinary tracts. The most common infecting organism in term infants is group B streptococcus (GBS); in preterm infants, it is *Escherichia coli* (Mukhopadhyay & Puopolo, 2017). Despite the development of maternal screening and prophylaxis, infection rates for early-onset GBS infection remain at approximately 0.1 to 0.3 per 1000 live births (Berardi, Rossi, Spada, et al., 2018). GBS is an extremely virulent organism in neonates, it remains the predominant pathogen responsible for neonatal sepsis (Cortese, Scicchitano, Gesualdo, et al., 2016). Other bacteria noted to cause early-onset infection include *E. coli, Haemophilus influenzae, Enterobacter* organisms and coagulase-negative *Staphylococcus* (ConS) (Pammi, Brand, & Weisman, 2016; Resch, Renoldner, & Hofer, 2016). Other pathogens that are harbored in the vagina and may infect the infant include gonococci, *C. albicans,* HSV (type II), and *Chlamydia.*

Late-onset sepsis (1 to 3 weeks after birth) is primarily nosocomial, and the offending organisms are usually staphylococci, *Klebsiella* organisms, enterococci, *E. coli,* and *Pseudomonas* or *Candida* (Pammi, Flores, Versalovic, et al., 2017). ConS, considered to be primarily a contaminant in older children and adults, is the most common cause of late-onset septicemia in ELBW and VLBW infants. Bacterial invasion can occur through sites such as the umbilical stump; the skin; mucous membranes of the eye, nose, pharynx, and ear; and internal systems, such as the respiratory, nervous, urinary, and gastrointestinal systems. Risk factors for ConS include low birth weight and early gestational age, poor hand hygiene, previous antibiotic exposure, and the presence of central IV lines (Nour, Eldegla, Nasef, et al., 2017).

Postnatal infection is acquired by cross-contamination from other infants, personnel, or objects in the environment. Bacteria that are commonly called "water bugs" (because they are able to grow in water) are found in water supplies, humidifying apparatus, sink drains, suction machines, and most respiratory equipment. Organisms such as ConS, which usually colonize the skin, may infect indwelling venous and arterial catheters used for infusions, blood sampling, and monitoring of vital signs. Neonatal sepsis is most common in infants at risk, particularly preterm infants and infants born after a difficult or traumatic labor and delivery, who are least capable of resisting such bacterial invasion. These organisms are often transmitted by personnel from person to person or object to person by poor hand washing, crowded conditions, and inadequate housecleaning.

Diagnostic Evaluation

Diagnosis of sepsis is often based on suspicion of presenting clinical signs and symptoms. Because sepsis is so easily confused with other neonatal disorders, the definitive diagnosis is established by laboratory and radiographic examination. Cultures of blood, urine, and CSF are collected to identify the causative organism. Blood studies may show signs of anemia, leukocytosis, or leukopenia. Leukopenia is usually an ominous sign because of its frequent association with high mortality. An elevated number of immature neutrophils (a **left shift**), decreased or increased total neutrophils, and changes in neutrophil morphology also suggest an infectious process in the neonate. Other diagnostic data may be helpful in the determination of neonatal sepsis and include C-reactive protein and other acute phase reactants, such as serum amyloid A; procalcitonin; and interleukins, specifically interleukin-6 (Pammi et al., 2017).

Prevention

Several measures are important in the prevention of both early- and late-onset infection. Programs to screen pregnant women for GBS colonization (culture-based) and treatment of those women in labor have dramatically reduced the incidence of GBS infection in neonates (Parsons et al., 2016). Screening programs for other maternal infections, including hepatitis B and HIV, are also recommended. In developed countries, breastfeeding by mothers infected with HIV is not recommended because the virus may be transmitted in breast milk.

Nursery procedures aimed at minimizing the risk of nosocomial infections include the practice of good hand-washing techniques, appropriate isolation precautions where indicated, and the adoption of recommended standards for spacing of infant beds. Strategies such as the early introduction of enteral feeding, preferential breastfeeding, and standardized nutrition protocols have been shown to reduce the risk of nosocomial infection (i.e., NEC) (Uberos, Aguilera-Rodríguez, Jerez-Calero, et al., 2017).

Therapeutic Management

In addition to the institution of rigorous therapeutic measures, early recognition (Box 8.6) and diagnosis are essential to increase the infant's chance for survival and reduce the likelihood of permanent neurologic damage. Antibiotic therapy is initiated before laboratory results are available for confirmation and identification of the exact organism. Treatment consists of circulatory support, respiratory support, aggressive administration of antibiotics, and immunotherapy.

Supportive therapy usually involves administration of oxygen (if respiratory distress or hypoxia is evident), careful regulation of fluids, correction of electrolyte or acid-base imbalance, and temporary discontinuation of oral feedings. Blood transfusions may be needed to correct anemia and shock, and electronic monitoring of vital signs and regulation of the thermal environment are mandatory.

Antibiotic therapy, usually administered intravenously, is continued for 7 to 10 days if culture results are positive and discontinued in 48 to 72 hours if culture results are negative and the infant is asymptomatic. Antifungal and antiviral therapies are implemented as appropriate, depending on causative agents.

Prognosis

The prognosis for neonatal sepsis is variable. Severe neurologic and respiratory sequelae may occur in ELBW and VLBW infants with early-onset sepsis. Late-onset sepsis and meningitis may also result in poor outcomes for immunocompromised neonates.

The introduction of new markers for neonatal sepsis such as acute phase reactants, cytokines, cell surface antigens, and bacterial genomes may prove to be particularly helpful in guidance for antibiotic therapy (Gilfillan & Bhandari, 2017). Future experimental methods being explored to combat infection in neonates include monoclonal antibody therapy, fibronectin infusion, and lymphokine enhancement.

Nursing Care Management

Nursing care of infants with sepsis involves observation and assessment as outlined for any high-risk infant. Recognition of the existing problem is of paramount importance; it is usually the nurse who observes and assesses infants and identifies that "something is wrong" with them. Awareness of the potential modes of infection transmission also helps the nurse identify infants at risk for developing sepsis. Much of the care of infants with sepsis involves the medical treatment of the illness. Knowledge of the side effects of the specific antibiotic and proper regulation and administration of the drug are vital.

Prolonged antibiotic therapy poses additional hazards for affected infants. Antibiotics predispose infants to growth of resistant organisms and superinfection from fungal or mycotic agents, such as *C. albicans.* Nurses must be alert for evidence of such complications. Nystatin oral suspension is swabbed on the buccal mucosa for prophylaxis against oral candidiasis.

Part of the total care of infants with sepsis is to decrease any additional physiologic or environmental stress. This includes providing an optimum thermoregulated environment and anticipating potential problems such as dehydration or hypoxia. Precautions are implemented to prevent the spread of infection to other newborns, but to be effective, activities must be carried out by all caregivers. Proper hand washing, the use of disposable equipment (e.g., linens, catheters, feeding supplies, IV equipment), disposal of excretions (e.g., vomitus, stool), and adequate housekeeping of the environment and equipment are essential. Because nurses are the most consistent caregivers involved with sick infants, it is usually their

BOX 8.6 Manifestations of Neonatal Sepsis

General Signs
Infant generally "not doing well"
Poor temperature control—hypothermia, hyperthermia (rare in neonates)

Circulatory System
Pallor, cyanosis, or mottling
Cool, clammy skin
Hypotension
Edema
Irregular heartbeat—bradycardia, tachycardia

Respiratory System
Irregular respirations, apnea, or tachypnea
Cyanosis
Grunting
Dyspnea
Retractions

Central Nervous System
Diminished activity—lethargy, hyporeflexia, coma
Increased activity—irritability, tremors, seizures
Full fontanel
Increased or decreased tone
Abnormal eye movements

Gastrointestinal System
Poor feeding
Vomiting
Diarrhea or decreased stooling
Abdominal distention
Hepatomegaly
Hemoccult-positive stools

Hematopoietic System
Jaundice
Pallor
Petechiae, ecchymosis
Splenomegaly

responsibility to see that Standard Precautions are maintained by everyone.

In recent years, ventilator-associated pneumonia has received considerable attention in adult and pediatric intensive care units. Hand hygiene (staff) and oral hygiene (patient) have been shown to decrease the incidence of ventilator-associated pneumonia in children (see Chapter 21).

Another aspect of caring for infants with sepsis involves observation for signs of complications, including meningitis and septic shock, a severe complication caused by toxins in the bloodstream.

NECROTIZING ENTEROCOLITIS

NEC is an acute inflammatory disease of the bowel with increased incidence in preterm infants. The precise cause of NEC is still uncertain, but it appears to occur in infants whose gastrointestinal tracts have experienced vascular compromise. Intestinal ischemia of unknown etiology, immature gastrointestinal host defenses, bacterial proliferation, and feeding substrate are now believed to have a multifactorial role in the etiology of NEC. Frequent use of antibiotic therapy and anti-acid medications, followed by enteral feeding, are believed to increase the risk of NEC (Chang, Chen, Chang, et al., 2017). Prematurity remains the most prominent risk factor in the development of NEC (Bucher, Pacetti, Lovvorn, et al., 2016).

The damage to mucosal cells lining the bowel wall may be significant. Diminished blood supply to these cells causes their death in large numbers; they stop secreting protective, lubricating mucus; and the thin, unprotected bowel wall is attacked by proteolytic enzymes. Thus the bowel wall continues to swell and break down; it is unable to synthesize protective IgM, and the mucosa is permeable to macromolecules (e.g., exotoxins), which further hampers intestinal defenses. Gas-forming bacteria invade the damaged areas to produce **pneumatosis intestinalis**, a radiologic finding reflecting the presence of gas in the submucosal or subserosal surfaces of the bowel.

A consistent relationship has been observed between the development of NEC and enteric feeding of hypertonic substances (e.g., formula, hyperosmolar medications). It is unclear whether this connection is a result of the formula imposing a stress on an ischemic bowel, serving as a substrate for bacterial growth, or both.

Diagnostic Evaluation

Radiographic studies show a sausage-shaped dilation of the intestine that progresses to marked distention and the characteristic pneumatosis intestinalis—"soapsuds," or the bubbly appearance of thickened bowel wall and ultra lumina. There may be air in the portal circulation or free air observed in the abdomen, indicating perforation. Laboratory findings may include anemia, leukopenia, leukocytosis, metabolic acidosis, and electrolyte imbalance. In severe cases, coagulopathy (DIC) or thrombocytopenia may be evident. Gram-negative organisms are often cultured from blood, although bacteremia or septicemia may not be prominent early in the course of the disease.

Therapeutic Management

Treatment of infants with NEC begins with prevention. Oral feedings may be withheld for at least 24 to 48 hours from infants who are believed to have experienced birth asphyxia. Breast milk is the preferred enteral nutrient because it confers some passive immunity (IgA), macrophages, and lysozymes.

Minimal enteral feedings (trophic feeding, gastrointestinal priming) have gained acceptance with no evidence of increased incidence of NEC. In particular, the use of fresh human milk has been shown to promote intestinal maturation, reduce liver dysfunction, and improve feeding tolerance (Poindexter & Ehrenkranz, 2015). A systematic review of the role of lactoferrin, a normal component of human milk, given as a supplement to enteral feeds decreases the incidence of NEC in preterm infants (Pammi & Suresh, 2017). Many randomized controlled trials have confirmed that oral probiotics effectively prevent NEC when given within the first 7 days and continued for 14 days in preterm infants (<34 weeks' gestation) and/or those with a birth weight less than 1500 g (Aceti, Gori, Barone, et al., 2015; Alfaleh, Anabrees, Bassler, et al., 2014; Athalye-Jape, Rao, & Patole, 2016; Lau & Chamberlain, 2015). The preferred type and optimal dosing of probiotics remain to be determined.

Medical treatment of infants with confirmed NEC consists of discontinuation of all oral feedings; institution of abdominal decompression via nasogastric suction; administration of IV antibiotics; and correction of extravascular volume depletion, electrolyte abnormalities, acid-base imbalances, and hypoxia. Replacing oral feedings with parenteral fluids decreases the need for oxygen and circulation to the bowel. Serial abdominal radiographs (every 6 to 8 hours in the acute phase) are taken to monitor for possible progression of the disease to intestinal perforation.

Prognosis

With early recognition and treatment, medical management is increasingly successful. If there is progressive deterioration under medical management or evidence of perforation, surgical resection and anastomosis are performed. Extensive involvement may necessitate surgical intervention and establishment of an ileostomy, jejunostomy, or colostomy. Sequelae in surviving infants include short bowel syndrome (see Chapter 22), colonic stricture with obstruction, fat malabsorption, and growth failure secondary to intestinal dysfunction. A variety of surgical interventions for NEC is available and depends on the extent of bowel necrosis, associated illness factors, and infant stability. Intestinal transplantation has been successful in some former preterm infants with NEC-associated short bowel syndrome who had already developed life-threatening total parenteral nutrition–related complications. Transplantation may be a lifesaving option for infants who previously faced high morbidity and mortality. Research is now underway to examine the use of tissue-engineered small intestine (Liu, Cromeens, Wang, et al., 2018).

Nursing Care Management

Nursing responsibilities begin with the prompt recognition of the early warning signs of NEC. Because the signs are similar to those observed in many other disorders of newborns, nurses must constantly be aware of the possibility of this disease in infants who are at high risk for developing NEC (Box 8.7).

When the disease is suspected, the nurse assists with diagnostic procedures and implements the therapeutic regimen. Vital signs, including BP, are monitored for changes that might indicate bowel perforation, septicemia, or cardiovascular shock, and measures are instituted to prevent possible transmission to other infants. It is especially important to avoid rectal temperatures because of the increased danger of perforation. To avoid pressure on the distended abdomen and to facilitate continuous observation, infants are often left undiapered and positioned supine or on the side.

Observe for indications of early development of NEC by checking the appearance of the abdomen for distention (measuring abdominal girth, measuring residual gastric contents before feedings, and listening for bowel sounds) and performing all routine assessments for high-risk neonates.

Conscientious attention to nutritional and hydration needs is essential, and antibiotics are administered as prescribed. The time at which oral feedings are reinstituted varies considerably but is usually

BOX 8.7 Clinical Manifestations of Necrotizing Enterocolitis

Nonspecific Clinical Signs
Lethargy
Poor feeding
Hypotension
Vomiting
Apnea
Decreased urinary output
Unstable temperature
Jaundice

Specific Signs
Distended (often shiny) abdomen
Blood in the stools or gastric contents
Gastric retention (undigested formula)
Localized abdominal wall erythema or induration
Bilious vomitus

at least 7 to 10 days after diagnosis and treatment. Feeding is usually reestablished using human milk, if available.

Because NEC is an infectious disease, one of the most important nursing functions is control of infection. Strict hand washing is the primary barrier to spread, and confirmed multiple cases are isolated. Persons with symptoms of a gastrointestinal disorder should not care for these or any other infants.

Infants who require surgery require the same careful attention and observation as any infant with abdominal surgery, including ostomy care (as applicable). This disorder is one of the most common reasons for performing ostomies on newborns. Throughout the medical and surgical management of infants with NEC, the nurse should be continually alert to signs of complications, such as septicemia, DIC, hypoglycemia, and other metabolic derangements.

HIGH RISK RELATED TO MATERNAL CONDITIONS

The health of fetuses and newborns may be affected by a number of maternal conditions; essentially, any condition affecting the mother also has the potential to negatively affect the health of the newborn. Pregnancy-induced hypertension or HELLP (hemolysis, elevated liver enzymes, low platelets) syndrome may cause preterm delivery, intrauterine growth restriction (IUGR), asphyxia, and death if it is not detected early and appropriate interventions implemented. It is not within the scope of this text to elaborate on the pathophysiology and treatment of these conditions; however, readers are referred to any one of the excellent maternity texts available for a detailed discussion of these conditions.

INFANTS OF DIABETIC MOTHERS

Before insulin therapy, few women with diabetes were able to conceive; for those who did, the mortality rate for both the mother and the infant was high. The morbidity and mortality of infants of diabetic mothers (IDMs) have been significantly reduced as a result of effective control of maternal diabetes and an increased understanding of fetal disorders. Because infants born to women with gestational diabetes mellitus are at risk for the same complications as IDMs, the following discussion of IDMs includes infants born to women with gestational diabetes mellitus.

The severity of the maternal diabetes affects infant survival. The severity of maternal diabetes is determined by the duration of the disease before pregnancy; age at onset; extent of vascular complications; and abnormalities of the current pregnancy, such as pyelonephritis, diabetic ketoacidosis, pregnancy-induced hypertension, and noncompliance. The single most important factor influencing fetal well-being is the euglycemic status of the mother. It has been found that reasonable metabolic control that begins before conception and continues during the first weeks of pregnancy can prevent malformation in an IDM. Elevated levels of hemoglobin A1c during the periconceptional period appear to be associated with a higher incidence of congenital malformations. In the case of gestational diabetes, macrosomia is the most common finding; serious complications are rare (Tieu, McPhee, Crowther, et al., 2017).

Hypoglycemia may appear a short time after birth and in IDMs is associated with increased insulin activity in the blood (see also Table 8.5). The serum glucose level that corresponds to clinical hypoglycemia has not been well defined. Because some infants experience metabolic complications at higher levels than previously thought, some researchers recommend that serum glucose levels be maintained above 45 mg/dl (2.5 mmol/L) in infants with abnormal clinical symptoms and as high as 50 mg/dl in other infants (Sperling, 2016). The American Academy of Pediatrics recommends that symptomatic infants receive treatment if their blood glucose is less than 40 mg/dl (Adamkin & American Academy of Pediatrics, Committee on Fetus and Newborn, 2011).

Hypoglycemia in IDMs is related to hypertrophy and hyperplasia of the pancreatic islet cells and thus is a transient state of hyperinsulinism. High maternal blood glucose levels during fetal life provide a continual stimulus to the fetal islet cells for insulin production (glucose easily passes the placental barrier from maternal to fetal side; insulin, however, does not cross the placental barrier). This sustained state of hyperglycemia promotes fetal insulin secretion that ultimately leads to excessive growth and deposition of fat, which probably accounts for the infants who are large for gestational age, or macrosomic (Sheanon & Muglia, 2020). When the neonate's glucose supply is removed abruptly at the time of birth, the continued production of insulin soon depletes the blood of circulating glucose, creating a state of hyperinsulinism and hypoglycemia within 0.5 to 4 hours, especially in infants of mothers with poorly controlled diabetes (formerly class C diabetes or beyond [class D through R]). Precipitous drops in blood glucose levels can cause serious neurologic damage or death.

IDMs have a characteristic appearance (Box 8.8 and Fig. 8.24). IDMs are more likely to have disproportionately large abdominal circumferences and shoulders, leading to an increased risk of shoulder dystocia and birth injury (Sheanon & Muglia, 2020). Infants of mothers with advanced diabetes may be small for gestational age, may have IUGR, or may be the appropriate size for gestational age because of the maternal vascular (placental) involvement. There is an increase in congenital anomalies in IDMs in addition to a high susceptibility to hypoglycemia, hypocalcemia, hypomagnesemia, polycythemia, hyperbilirubinemia, cardiomyopathy, and RDS (Sheanon & Muglia, 2020). Hyperinsulinemia and hyperglycemia in the diabetic mother may be factors in reducing fetal surfactant synthesis, thus contributing to the development of RDS. Although large, these infants may be delivered before term as a result of maternal complications or increased fetal size.

Congenital hyperinsulinism, a condition that causes neonatal macrosomia and profound hypoglycemia, is often present in the neonatal period. However, this condition is usually not associated with maternal diabetes mellitus but appears to have a genetic etiology; the condition is also associated with syndromes, such as Beckwith-Wiedemann syndrome (Sperling, 2016).

BOX 8.8 Clinical Manifestations of Infants of Diabetic Mothers

- Large for gestational age
- Very plump and full faced
- Abundant vernix caseosa
- Plethora (polycythemia)
- Listless and lethargic
- Jitteriness

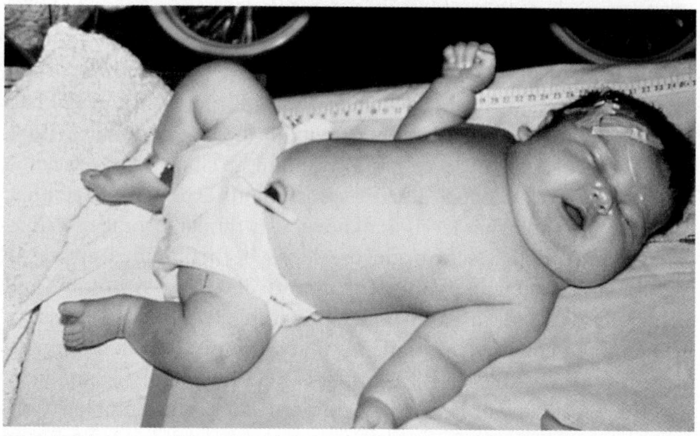

Fig. 8.24 Large for gestational age infant. This infant of a diabetic mother (IDM) weighed 5 kg at birth and exhibits the typical round facies. (From Zitelli, B. J., McIntire, S. C., & Nowalk, A. J. [2012]. *Zitelli and Davis' atlas of pediatric physical diagnosis* [6th ed.]. St Louis, MO: Saunders/Elsevier.)

Therapeutic Management

The most important management of IDMs is careful monitoring of serum glucose levels and observation for accompanying complications such as RDS. The infants are examined for the presence of any anomalies or birth injuries, and blood studies for determination of glucose, calcium, hematocrit, and bilirubin are obtained on a regular basis.

Because the hypertrophied pancreas is so sensitive to blood glucose concentrations, the administration of oral glucose may trigger a massive insulin release, resulting in rebound hypoglycemia. Therefore feedings of breast milk or formula begin within the first hour after birth, provided that the infant's cardiorespiratory condition is stable. Approximately half of these infants do well and adjust without complications. Infants born to mothers with poorly controlled diabetes may require IV dextrose infusions. Treatment with 10% dextrose and water (IV) is initiated with the goal of maintaining serum blood glucose levels above 45 mg/dl (Adamkin & American Academy of Pediatrics, Committee on Fetus and Newborn, 2011). Oral and IV intake may be titrated to maintain adequate blood glucose levels. Frequent blood glucose determinations are needed for the first 2 to 4 days of life to assess the degree of hypoglycemia present at any given time. Testing blood taken from the heel with calibrated portable reflectance meters (e.g., glucometers) is a simple and effective screening evaluation that can then be confirmed by laboratory examination.

Nursing Care Management

The nursing care of IDMs involves early examination for congenital anomalies, signs of possible respiratory or cardiac problems, maintenance of adequate thermoregulation, early introduction of carbohydrate feedings as appropriate, and monitoring of serum blood glucose levels. The latter is of particular importance because many infants with hypoglycemia may remain asymptomatic. IV glucose infusion requires careful monitoring of the site and the neonate's reaction to therapy; high glucose concentrations (≥12.5%) should be infused via a central line instead of a peripheral site.

Because macrosomic infants are at risk for problems associated with a difficult delivery, they are monitored for birth injuries, such as brachial plexus injury and palsy, fractured clavicle, and phrenic nerve palsy. Additional monitoring of the infant for problems associated with this condition (polycythemia, hypocalcemia, poor feeding, and hyperbilirubinemia) is also a vital nursing function.

DRUG-EXPOSED INFANTS[g]

Maternal habits hazardous to the fetus and neonate include drug addiction, smoking, and alcohol abuse. Occasional withdrawal reactions have been reported in neonates of mothers who use excessive amounts of drugs, such as barbiturates, alcohol, amphetamines, or antidepressants. Serious reactions are seen in neonates whose mothers abuse psychoactive drugs or are treated with methadone.

Narcotics, which have a low molecular weight, readily cross the placental membrane and enter the fetal system. Illicit substances may also be transmitted to the newborn through breast milk. When the mother is a habitual user of opiates, especially oxycodone (OxyContin), heroin, or methadone, the unborn child may also become chemically dependent or passively addicted to the drug, which places such infants at risk during the perinatal and early neonatal periods. **Neonatal abstinence syndrome (NAS)** is the term used to describe the set of behaviors exhibited by infants exposed to narcotics in utero.

Clinical Manifestations

The adverse effects of exposure of a fetus to drugs are varied. They include transient behavioral changes such as alterations in fetal breathing movements and irreversible effects such as fetal death, IUGR, structural malformations, or cognitive impairment. Determining the specific effects of individual drugs on an individual fetus is made difficult by polydrug use, which is common; errors or omissions in reporting drug use; and variations in the strength, purity, and types of additives found in street drugs. Maternal conditions such as poverty, malnutrition, and comorbid conditions (such as sexually transmitted infections) further compound the difficulty in identifying the presence and consequences of intrauterine drug exposure. Most infants who are exposed to drugs in utero may demonstrate no immediate untoward effects and appear normal at birth. Infants exposed only to heroin may begin to exhibit signs of drug withdrawal within 12 to 24 hours. If mothers have been taking methadone, the signs appear somewhat later—anywhere from 1 or 2 days to 2 to 3 weeks or more after birth. The clinical manifestations may fall into any one or all of the following categories: CNS, gastrointestinal, respiratory, and autonomic nervous system signs (Weiner & Finnegan, 2016). The manifestations become most pronounced between 48 and 72 hours of age and may last from 6 days to 8 weeks, depending on the severity of the withdrawal (Box 8.9). Although these infants suck avidly ssson

[g]Note that the term *addiction* is often associated with behaviors whereby the person seeks the drug(s) to experience a high or euphoria, escape from reality, or satisfy a personal need. Newborns who have been exposed to drugs in utero are not addicted in a behavioral sense, yet they may experience mild to strong physiologic signs as a result of the exposure. Therefore to say that an infant born to a mother who uses substances is addicted is incorrect; *drug-exposed newborn* is a better term, which implies intrauterine drug exposure.

BOX 8.9 Signs of Withdrawal in Neonates

Neurologic
Irritability
Seizures
Hyperactivity
High-pitched cry
Tremors
Exaggerated Moro reflex
Hypertonicity of muscles

Gastrointestinal
Poor feeding
Diarrhea
Dehydration
Vomiting
Frantic, uncoordinated sucking
Gastric residuals

Autonomic
Diaphoresis
Fever
Mottled skin
Nasal stuffiness

Miscellaneous
Disrupted sleep patterns
Tachypnea (>60 breaths/min)
Excoriations (knees, face, perianal)
Temperature instability

fists and display an exaggerated rooting reflex, they are poor feeders with uncoordinated and ineffectual sucking and swallowing reflexes.

Because of irregular and varying degrees of drug use, quality of drug, and mixed-drug usage by the mother, some infants display mild or variable manifestations. Most manifestations are the vague, nonspecific signs characteristic of all infants in general; therefore it is important to differentiate between drug withdrawal and other disorders before specific therapy is instituted. Other conditions (e.g., hypocalcemia, hypoglycemia, sepsis) often coexist with the drug withdrawal. Additional signs seen in drug-exposed newborns include loose stools; tachycardia; fever; projectile vomiting; crying; nasal stuffiness; and generalized perspiration, which is unusual in newborns.

Diagnostic Evaluation

Newborn urine, hair, or meconium sampling may be required to identify drug exposure and implement appropriate early interventional therapies aimed at minimizing the consequences of intrauterine drug exposure. Meconium sampling for fetal drug exposure is reported to provide more screening accuracy than urine screening because drug metabolites accumulate in meconium (Weiner & Finnegan, 2016). Urine toxicology screening may be less accurate because it reflects only recent substance intake by the mother (Malcolm, 2015). Meconium and hair testing for drug metabolites has the advantages of being noninvasive, more accurate, and easy to collect.

Therapeutic Management

The treatment of drug-exposed infants initially consists of early identification through maternal history, presenting symptoms of NAS, or toxicology screening when substance abuse is strongly suspected. Early identification and intervention are essential to prevent further adverse effects; early discharge from the birth institution should be postponed until further assessment of the maternal situation and establishment of a treatment plan for the mother and infant. Drug therapies to decrease withdrawal effects include parenteral or oral administration of phenobarbital, buprenorphine, clonidine, methadone, and morphine. A combination of these drugs may be necessary to treat infants exposed to multiple drugs in utero, and careful attention should be given to possible adverse effects of the treatment drugs (Malcolm, 2015).

Prognosis

The prognosis for drug-exposed infants depends on the type and amount of drug(s) taken by the mother and the stage(s) of fetal development in which the drug was taken. The overall mortality rate of infants born to narcotic-addicted mothers is increased, but with early recognition, proper treatment, and long-term follow-up, the morbidity and mortality associated with drug exposure are decreased.

Often drug-exposed infants exhibit poor brain and body growth at birth; however, at times infants do not exhibit any signs that indicate exposure to harmful agents, and their condition may therefore be overlooked until symptoms appear later in life. Drug-exposed infants may have chronic feeding problems; irritability; abnormal neurologic responses; abnormal parent-infant interactions; developmental and cognitive delays; learning disabilities in childhood; and behavioral problems, including ADHD.

Nursing Care Management

One of the key factors in the treatment of drug-exposed neonates is early identification of substance abuse in the pregnant woman so that treatment can be initiated and side effects minimized. This is especially problematic from a social and legal standpoint because the pregnant woman is often aware of the consequences of admitting to substance abuse and may therefore be less likely to readily admit to the problem for fear of social and legal repercussions. If the mother has had good prenatal care, the practitioner is aware of the problem and may have instituted therapy before delivery. However, a number of mothers deliver their infants without the benefit of adequate care, and the condition is unknown to health care personnel at the time of delivery.

The degree of withdrawal is closely related to the amount of drug the mother has habitually taken, the length of time she has been taking the drug, and her drug level at the time of delivery. The most severe symptoms are observed in the infants of mothers who have taken large amounts of drugs over a long period. In addition, the nearer to the time of delivery that the mother takes the drug, the longer it takes the child to develop withdrawal and the more severe the manifestations. The infant may not exhibit withdrawal symptoms until 7 to 10 days after delivery, by which time most newborns have been discharged from the birth center and caregivers are less likely to recognize signs of irritability and poor feeding as withdrawal, thus predisposing the newborn to abuse or neglect and growth failure (failure to thrive). The infant may be at further risk for subsequent abuse or neglect because of home conditions that preclude adequate newborn care and follow-up.

After the presence of NAS is identified in an infant, nursing care is directed toward treatment of the presenting signs, decreasing stimuli that may precipitate hyperactivity and irritability (e.g., dimming the lights, decreasing noise levels), providing adequate nutrition and hydration, and promoting the mother-infant relationship. Appropriate individualized developmental care is implemented to facilitate self-consoling and self-regulating behaviors. Irritable and hyperactive infants have been found to respond to physical comforting, movement, and close contact. Wrapping infants snugly and rocking and holding them tightly limit their ability to self-stimulate. Arranging nursing activities to reduce the amount of disturbance helps decrease exogenous stimulation.

Breastfeeding is encouraged in mothers who are not using illicit substances, do not have HIV infection, and are compliant with a methadone program; breastfeeding promotes mother-infant bonding, and small quantities of methadone passed through breast milk have not proven to be harmful.

The Neonatal Abstinence Scoring System was developed to monitor infants in an objective manner and evaluate their response to clinical and pharmacologic interventions (Finnegan, 1985). This system is also designed to assist nurses and other health care workers in evaluating the severity of infants' withdrawal symptoms. Another tool that may be used to evaluate withdrawal behavior and treatment in newborns is the Neonatal Withdrawal Inventory developed by Zahorodny and colleagues (1998).

The Neonatal Intensive Care Unit Network Neurobehavioral Scale (NNNS) is a comprehensive neurologic and behavioral assessment tool that may be used to identify newborns at risk as a result of intrauterine drug exposure. The tool measures stress or abstinence, state, neurologic status, and muscle tone in the context of the newborn's medical condition at the time of examination. The NNNS may be used for medically stable newborns who are at least 30 weeks of gestation and up to 48 weeks of corrected or conceptional age (Lester, Tronick, & Brazelton, 2004).

Loose stools, poor intake, and regurgitation after feeding predispose these infants to malnutrition, dehydration, skin breakdown, and electrolyte imbalance. In addition, these infants burn up energy with continual activity and increased oxygen consumption at the cellular level. Frequent weighing, careful monitoring of intake and output and electrolytes, and additional caloric supplementation may be necessary. Hyperactive infants must be protected from skin abrasions on the knees, toes, and cheeks that are caused by rubbing on bed linens while in a prone position (awake). Monitoring and recording the activity level and its relationship to other activities, such as feeding and preventing complications, are important nursing functions.

A valuable aid to anticipating problems in the newborn is recognizing substance abuse in the mother. Unless the mother is enrolled in a methadone rehabilitation program, she seldom risks calling attention to her habit by seeking prenatal care. Consequently, infants and mothers are exposed to the additional hazards of obstetric and medical complications. Moreover, the nature of substance use and addiction makes the user susceptible to disorders, such as infection (hepatitis B, HIV), foreign body reaction, and the hazards of inadequate nutrition and preterm birth. Methadone treatment does not prevent withdrawal reaction in neonates, but the clinical course may be modified. Also, the intensive psychologic support of mothers is a factor in the treatment and reduction of perinatal mortality. Experience has indicated that these mothers are usually anxious and depressed, lack confidence, have a poor self-image, and have difficulty with interpersonal relationships. They may have a psychologic need for the pregnancy and an infant.

Initial symptoms or the recurrence of withdrawal symptoms may develop after discharge from the hospital; therefore it is important to establish rapport and maintain contact with the family so that they will return for treatment if this occurs. The demands of the drug-exposed infant on the caregiver are enormous and unrewarding in terms of positive feedback. The infants are difficult to comfort, and they cry for long periods, which can be especially trying for the caregiver after the infant's discharge from the hospital. Long-term follow-up to evaluate the status of the infant and family is very important. Sudden infant death syndrome (SIDS) and HIV infection are observed more commonly in infants born to users of methadone and heroin.

Many problems arise in relation to the disposition of infants of drug-dependent mothers. Those who advocate separation of mothers and children argue that the mothers are not capable of assuming responsibility for their infants' care, that child care is frustrating to them, and that their existence is too disorganized and chaotic. Others encourage the mother-infant bond and recommend a protected environment, such as a therapeutic community; a halfway house; or continuous ongoing, supportive services in the home after discharge. Careful evaluation and the cooperative efforts of a variety of health professionals are required whether the choice is foster home placement or supportive follow-up care of mothers who keep their infants.

Alcohol Exposure

Alcohol ingestion during pregnancy is associated with both short- and long-term effects on the fetus and newborn. The quantity of alcohol required to produce fetal effects is unclear, but it is known that infants born to heavy drinkers have twice the risk of congenital abnormalities than those born to moderate drinkers (Weitzman, 2020). Alcohol withdrawal can occur in neonates, particularly when maternal ingestion occurs near the time of delivery. Signs and symptoms include jitteriness, increased tone and reflex responses, and irritability. Seizures are also common. Fetal effects of alcohol exposure vary from subtle learning disabilities to obvious facial features and growth abnormalities. In 2004 the National Organization on Fetal Alcohol Syndrome clarified terminology for fetal alcohol exposure by adopting the term *fetal alcohol spectrum disorder (FASD)* as an umbrella term to describe the range of clinical effects. Fetal alcohol syndrome (FAS) falls within this spectrum but is reserved for individuals who display the triad of characteristic facial features, growth restriction, and neurodevelopmental deficits with a confirmed history of maternal alcohol consumption (Denny, Coles, & Blitz, 2017). Craniofacial features include microcephaly, small eyes or short palpebral fissures, a thin upper lip, a flat midface, and an indistinct philtrum. Neurologic problems in FAS children include some degree of intelligence quotient (IQ) deficit, ADHD, diminished fine motor skills, and poor speech. These children have been shown to lack inhibition, have no stranger anxiety, and lack appropriate judgment skills.

Infants who do not display the signs of FAS but are born to mothers who are also heavy alcohol drinkers have significantly more tremors, hypertonia, restlessness, excessive mouthing movements, crying, and inconsolability than infants of substance-abusive mothers who do not consume alcohol during pregnancy. An added concern regarding substance abuse is that many of the mothers often use several drugs, such as tranquilizers, sedatives, amphetamines, phencyclidine, marijuana, and other psychotropic agents.

Cocaine Exposure

Cocaine is a CNS stimulant and peripheral sympathomimetic. Legally, it is classified as a narcotic, but it is not an opioid. Prenatal cocaine exposure is commonly associated with a number of adverse consequences throughout development (Ross, Graham, Money, et al., 2015). The effects on fetuses are secondary to maternal effects, which include increased BP, decreased uterine blood flow, and increased vascular resistance. Consequently, the fetus experiences decreased blood flow and oxygenation because of placental and fetal vasoconstriction. Researchers have concluded that variables such as the mother's lack of prenatal care; poor nutrition; and use of tobacco, alcohol, and other drugs during pregnancy compound the effects of cocaine exposure in the infant (Parcianello, Mardini, Cereser, et al., 2018).

Infants may appear normal or may show neurologic problems at birth that may continue during the neonatal period. In much of the research literature, these findings were transient, and there has been variable evidence demonstrating permanent sequelae. Either of two types of behavior may emerge as a result of cocaine's effects on fetal development: neurobehavioral depression or excitability. The behaviors of a depressed infant include lethargy, hypotonia, a weak cry, and difficulty in arousing. The behaviors of an excitable neonate may include a high-pitched cry, hypertonicity, jitteriness, irritability, and an inability to be consoled (Hudak, 2015).

Sequelae of prenatal cocaine exposure include preterm birth, a smaller head circumference, decreased birth length, and decreased weight. The areas of the brain that appear to be particularly vulnerable to the effects of prenatal cocaine exposure include those that regulate attention and executive functioning. Early studies of cocaine exposure identified an increased incidence of gastroschisis, genitourinary anomalies, and periventricular and intraventricular hemorrhage; however, meta-analyses have not confirmed these complications (Hudak, 2015). Exposure to cocaine is typified by abnormal arousal and attention regulation. One study demonstrated functional connectivity and behavioral disruptions in the thalamus of neonates exposed to cocaine prenatally (Salzwedel, Grewen, Goldman, et al., 2016).

Follow-up at adolescence of 218 children exposed prenatally to cocaine demonstrated poorer perceptual organization IQ, visual-spatial information processing, attention, language, executive function, and behavior regulation through age 14 years (Singer, Minnes, Min, et al., 2015). Another compounding factor for prenatal drug exposure and later substance abuse risk is that cocaine-exposed adolescents self-reported that they were more likely to use alcohol, tobacco, and/or marijuana by age 15 years compared with non–cocaine-exposed adolescents (Minnes, Singer, Min, et al., 2014).

Therapeutic Management

Treatment of these infants is similar to that for other drug-exposed infants, including reduction of external stimuli; supportive treatment aimed at alleviating symptoms; and, at times, mild sedation.

Nursing Care Management

Nursing care of cocaine-exposed infants is the same as that for other drug-exposed infants. Because they have increased flexor tone, these infants respond to swaddling (Sherman, 2015). Positioning, infant massage, and limited tactile stimulation have been shown to be effective interventions. Significant amounts of cocaine have been found in breast milk (Hale, 2019); therefore mothers should be cautioned about this hazard to their infants.

Referral to early intervention programs, including child health care, parental drug treatment, individualized developmental care, and parenting education, is essential in promoting optimum outcome for these children. Because these children often live in impoverished environments, they are at high risk for cognitive delays, lack of child health care, and inadequate nutrition and benefit from early intervention programs.

Methamphetamine Exposure

The fetal and neonatal effects of maternal use of methamphetamines in pregnancy are not well known, and findings are often confounded by polydrug use and the effects of the newborn or child's environment. LBW, preterm birth, and anomalies such as cleft lip and palate and cardiac defects have been reported in infants exposed to methamphetamines in utero (Sherman, 2015).

Methamphetamine use has increased significantly in the past 10 years in certain regions of the United States. A higher incidence of preterm delivery and placental abruption was associated with methamphetamine use. In addition, fetal growth restriction (small for gestational age) was slightly higher in methamphetamine-exposed offspring; however, 80% of these neonates' mothers also had significant alcohol and tobacco use.

Study reports vary in the time of clinical manifestations of withdrawal from this drug. Continuous methamphetamine use during pregnancy is associated with preterm delivery and low birth weight, both of which contribute to neonatal morbidity and mortality (Wright, Schuetter, Tellei, et al., 2015). Stopping methamphetamine use at any time during pregnancy improves birth outcomes (Wright et al., 2015). After birth, infants may experience abnormal sleep patterns, agitation, poor feeding, and state disorganization (Sherman, 2015).

The long-term effects of methamphetamine exposure on children remain unclear; however, some studies have shown problems with math and language skills. It is postulated that, similar to cocaine, methamphetamine exposure may affect areas of the brain responsible for higher order functioning, with effects more likely to be manifest when the child reaches school age (Hudak, 2015).

Marijuana Exposure

Marijuana has replaced cocaine as the most common illicit drug used by women ages 18 to 44 years (nonpregnant and pregnant) in the United States (Oh, Salas-Wright, Vaughn, et al., 2017). Marijuana crosses the placenta; however, specific effects on the fetus have been difficult to determine. Some studies have reported an association between the chronic use of marijuana and a decrease in infant birth weight and the need for placement in a NICU (Conner, Carter, Tuuli, et al., 2015; Gunn, Rosales, Center, et al., 2016). Compounding the issue of the effects of marijuana is multidrug use, which combines the harmful effects of marijuana, tobacco, alcohol, opiates, and cocaine. Long-term follow-up studies on exposed infants are needed.

Selective Serotonin Reuptake Inhibitors

Studies estimate that about 12.4% of pregnant women experience major depression (Zhao, Liu, Cao, et al., 2018.). For many of these women, selective serotonin reuptake inhibitors (SSRIs) provide an important therapeutic benefit; however, these drugs may result in side effects in their newborns. Signs of withdrawal are present in up to one-third of infants exposed to SSRIs in utero (Zhao et al., 2018). Findings include hypertonia, tremulousness, wakefulness, high-pitched crying, and feeding problems. An increased risk of persistent pulmonary hypertension has been reported in neonates exposed to SSRIs early in pregnancy (Zhao et al., 2018); however, this finding has not been consistently reported (Zullino & Simoncini, 2018). Some SSRIs are transferred into breast milk. Breastfeeding infants whose mothers are taking SSRIs should be monitored for sleep disturbances, irritability, and poor feeding.

MATERNAL INFECTIONS

The range of pathologic conditions produced by infectious agents is large, and the difference between the maternal and fetal effects caused by any one agent is also great. Some maternal infections, especially during early gestation, can result in fetal loss or malformations because the fetus's ability to handle infectious organisms is limited and the fetal immunologic system is unable to prevent the dissemination of infectious organisms to the various tissues.

Not all prenatal infections produce teratogenic effects. Furthermore, the clinical picture of disorders caused by transplacental transfer of infectious agents is not always well defined. Some viral agents can cause remarkably similar manifestations, and it is common to test for all of them when a prenatal infection is suspected. This is the so-called **TORCH complex**, an acronym for:

Toxoplasmosis
Other (e.g., hepatitis B, parvovirus, HIV, West Nile)
Rubella
Cytomegalovirus infection
Herpes simplex

To determine the causative agent in a symptomatic infant, tests are performed to rule out each of these infections. The *O* category may involve testing for several viral infections (e.g., hepatitis B, varicella zoster, measles, mumps, HIV, syphilis, and human parvovirus). Bacterial infections are not included in the TORCH workup because they are usually identified by clinical manifestations and readily available laboratory tests. Gonococcal conjunctivitis (ophthalmia neonatorum) and chlamydial conjunctivitis have been significantly reduced by prophylactic measures at birth (see Chapter 7). The major maternal infections, their possible effects, and specific nursing considerations are outlined in Table 8.12.

Nursing Care Management

One of the major goals in care of infants suspected of having an infectious disease is identification of the causative organism. Standard Precautions are implemented according to institutional policy. In suspected cytomegalovirus and rubella infections, pregnant health care personnel are cautioned to avoid contact with these infants. HSV is easily transmitted from one infant to another; therefore the risk of cross-contamination is reduced or eliminated by wearing gloves for patient contact. The American Academy of Pediatrics' *Red Book: 2018 Report of the Committee on Infectious Diseases* provides guidelines for the type and duration of precautions for most bacterial and viral exposures (Kimberlin, Brady & Jackson, 2018). Careful hand washing is the most important nursing intervention in reducing the spread of any infection.

Specimens need to be obtained for laboratory examinations, and the infant and parents need to be prepared for diagnostic procedures. When possible, long-term disabilities are prevented by early evaluation and implementation of therapy. The family is taught any special handling techniques needed for the care of their infant and signs of complications or possible sequelae. If sequelae are inevitable, the family will need assistance in determining how they can best cope with the problems, such as assistance with home care, referral to appropriate agencies, or placement in an institution for care. The major goal of nursing care is prevention of these disorders with provision of adequate prenatal care for the expectant mother and precautions regarding exposure to teratogenic infections.

DEFECTS CAUSED BY CHEMICAL AGENTS

Prenatal environmental influences from chemicals such as alcohol, medications, or drugs of abuse; infectious disease; or radiation or other environmental influences may be regarded as nongenetic causes of congenital anomalies because these effects can produce congenital structural, functional, or growth defects. An agent that produces congenital malformations or increases their incidence is called a **teratogen**.

The relationship of the fetal and maternal circulations allows for the interchange of chemical substances across the placental membrane. Many drugs have been suspected of producing congenital malformations, and some have been definitely implicated. Some of the most recognized teratogenic drugs include alcohol, tobacco, antiepileptic medications, isotretinoin (Accutane), lithium, cocaine, and diethylstilbestrol (Table 8.13).

The extent to which chemical agents affect the unborn child depends on the interplay of several factors, including the nature of the agent and its accessibility to the fetus, the gestational age at which exposure occurred, the level and duration of the dosage, and the genetic makeup of the fetus. For example, fetal exposure to valproic acid in the first 3 months of pregnancy may result in congenital anomalies such as neural tube defects, congenital heart defects, and distinctive facial features. The limited metabolic capabilities of the fetal liver and its immature enzyme and transport systems render the unborn child ill equipped for maintaining homeostasis when chemical disturbances are imposed by the mother or the environment. This includes both substances produced by the mother in response to a disease state (e.g., diabetes) and exogenous substances ingested or inhaled by the mother.

The teratogenic effect of drugs is not believed to have an effect on developing tissue until day 15 of gestation, when tissue differentiation begins to take place. Before that time, drugs usually have little effect because they are believed to have an insignificant affinity for undifferentiated tissue. Also, until implantation takes place, at approximately 7 days after conception, the embryo is not exposed to maternal blood that contains the drug. However, some drugs may affect the uterine lining, making it unsuitable for implantation. Drugs administered between days 15 and 90 may produce an effect if the tissue for which the drug has an affinity is in the process of differentiation at that time. After 90 days, when differentiation is complete, most fetal tissues are believed to be relatively resistant to teratogenic effects of drugs. However, the impact on ongoing neurologic development is not known.

Nursing Care Management

Expectant mothers are cautioned against ingesting any medication without first consulting a practitioner. To help ensure that fewer women will inadvertently take some chemical that might be harmful to their fetuses, labels on medications are now required to include information on the possible teratogenic effects of each drug. All women of childbearing age should be educated regarding the effects of chemicals, especially alcohol, on unborn fetuses. FAS is an irreversible condition but is completely preventable. The March of Dimes[h] and Centers for Disease Control and Prevention[i] have information about prevention tips, and the Genetic Alliance[j] has information about support groups for families of children with FAS. Genetic counseling is recommended for women who are concerned about a possible teratogen during pregnancy.

> **! NURSING ALERT**
>
> One drug recognized for its carcinogenic effect is diethylstilbestrol. Large doses of this hormone, given to pregnant women in the United States between 1938 and 1971 to prevent abortion, caused adenocarcinoma of the vagina in a significant proportion of the female offspring when they reach adolescence and early adulthood.

CONGENITAL HYPOTHYROIDISM

Congenital hypothyroidism (CH) may have a number of causes and can be either permanent or transient. Transient CH is frequently associated with maternal Graves disease that was treated with antithyroid drugs. The majority of cases are sporadic (nonhereditary), but approximately 15% of all cases are transmitted as an autosomal dominant trait. The most common pathogenesis is thyroid dysgenesis, mostly with unknown causes. Worldwide, the most common cause

[h] 1275 Mamaroneck Ave., White Plains, NY 10605; 914-997-4488; http://www.marchofdimes.com.
[i] http://www.cdc.gov/.
[j] 4301 Connecticut Ave. NW, Suite 404, Washington, DC 20008; http://www.geneticalliance.org.

TABLE 8.12 Infections Acquired From the Mother Before, During, or After Birth[a]

Fetal or Newborn Effect	Transmission	Nursing Considerations[b]
Human Immunodeficiency Virus		
No significant difference between infected and uninfected infants at birth in some instances Embryopathy reported by some observers: • Depressed nasal bridge • Mild upward or downward obliquity of eyes • Long palpebral fissures with blue sclerae • Patulous lips • Ocular hypertelorism • Prominent upper vermilion border (see also Chapter 24)	Transplacental; during vaginal delivery; potentially in breast milk	Administer antiviral prophylaxis to the HIV-positive mother. The time of initiation (if not already on treatment) and the choice of regimens is determined by examining a number of factors, including the mother's current treatment. Detailed recommendations can be obtained from Office of AIDS Research Advisory Council (2014). During labor, *ZDV is recommended for all HIV-infected pregnant women, regardless of the antepartum treatment regimen.* Cesarean section in HIV-positive mothers is recommended to reduce transmission. HIV-exposed neonates should receive a 6-week course of ZDV (consider addition of another antiretroviral drug based on maternal treatment and exposure). Avoid breastfeeding in HIV-positive mother. Documented routine HIV education and routine testing with consent for all pregnant women in United States are recommended.
Chickenpox (Varicella-Zoster Virus)		
Intrauterine exposure—congenital varicella syndrome: limb dysplasia, microcephaly, cortical atrophy, chorioretinitis, cataracts, cutaneous scars, other anomalies, auditory nerve palsy, motor and cognitive delays Severe symptoms (rash, fever) and higher mortality in infant whose mother develops varicella 5 days before to 2 days after delivery	First trimester (fetal varicella syndrome); perinatal period (infection)	Use varicella zoster immunoglobulin (VariZIG) or IVIG to treat infants born to mothers with onset of disease within 5 days before or 2 days after delivery. Institute isolation precautions in newborn born to mother with varicella up to 21 to 28 days (latter time if newborn received VariZIG or IVIG after birth) if hospitalized. Prevention: Universal immunization of all children with varicella vaccine.
Chlamydia Infection *(Chlamydia Trachomatis)*		
Conjunctivitis, pneumonia	Last trimester or perinatal period	Standard ophthalmic prophylaxis for gonococcal ophthalmia neonatorum (topical antibiotics, silver nitrate, or povidone iodine) is not effective in treatment or prevention of chlamydial ophthalmia. Treat with oral erythromycin for 14 days.
Coxsackievirus (Group B Enterovirus–Nonpolio)		
Poor feeding, vomiting, diarrhea, fever; cardiac enlargement, arrhythmias, congestive heart failure; lethargy, seizures, meningeal involvement Mimics bacterial sepsis	Peripartum	Treatment is supportive. Provide IVIG in neonatal infections.
Cytomegalovirus		
Variable manifestation from asymptomatic to severe Microcephaly, cerebral calcifications, chorioretinitis Jaundice, hepatosplenomegaly Petechial or purpuric rash Neurologic sequelae—seizure disorders, sensorimotor deafness, cognitive impairment	Throughout pregnancy	Infection acquired at birth, shortly thereafter, or via human milk is not associated with clinical illness. Affected individuals excrete virus. Virus is detected in urine or tissue by electron microscopy. Pregnant women should avoid close contact with known cases. To treat infection, administer IV antivirals such as ganciclovir to newborn.

Continued

TABLE 8.12 Infections Acquired From the Mother Before, During, or After Birth[a]—cont'd

Fetal or Newborn Effect	Transmission	Nursing Considerations[b]
Parvovirus B19 (Erythema Infectiosum)		
Fetal hydrops and death from anemia and heart failure with early exposure Anemia with later exposure No teratogenic effects established Ordinarily, low risk of adverse effect to fetus	Transplacental	First trimester infection has most serious effects. Pregnant health care workers should not care for patients who might be highly contagious (e.g., child with sickle cell anemia, aplastic crisis). Routine exclusion of pregnant women from workplace where disease is occurring is not recommended.
Gonococcal Disease *(Neisseria Gonorrhoeae)*		
Ophthalmitis Neonatal gonococcal arthritis, septicemia, meningitis	Last trimester or perinatal period	Apply prophylactic medication to eyes at time of birth. Obtain smears for culture. To treat infection, administer penicillin.
Hepatitis B Virus		
May be asymptomatic at birth Acute hepatitis, changes in liver function	Transplacental; contaminated maternal fluids or secretions during delivery	Administer HBIg to all infants of HBsAG-positive mothers within 12 hours of birth; in addition, administer hepatitis B vaccine at separate site. Prevention: Universal immunization of all infants with hepatitis B vaccine (see Chapter 6, Immunizations).
Listeriosis *(Listeria Monocytogenes)*		
Maternal infection associated with abortion, preterm delivery, and fetal death Preterm birth, sepsis, and pneumonia seen in early-onset disease; late-onset disease usually manifests as meningitis	Transplacental by ascending infection or exposure at delivery	Hand washing is essential to prevent nosocomial spread. Treat infected newborn with antibiotics—ampicillin and gentamicin.
Rubella, Congenital (Rubella Virus)		
Eye defects—cataracts (unilateral or bilateral), microphthalmia, retinitis, glaucoma CNS signs—microcephaly, seizures, severe cognitive impairment Congenital heart defects—patent ductus arteriosus Auditory—high incidence of delayed hearing loss IUGR Hyperbilirubinemia, meningitis, thrombocytopenia, hepatomegaly	First trimester; early second trimester	Pregnant women should avoid contact with all affected persons, including infants with rubella syndrome. Emphasize vaccination of all unimmunized prepubertal children, susceptible adolescents, and women of childbearing age (nonpregnant). Caution women against pregnancy for at least 3 months after vaccination.
Syphilis, Congenital *(Treponema Pallidum)*		
Stillbirth, prematurity, hydrops fetalis May be asymptomatic at birth and in first few weeks of life or may have multisystem manifestations: hepatosplenomegaly, lymphadenopathy, hemolytic anemia, and thrombocytopenia Copper-colored maculopapular cutaneous lesions (usually after first few weeks of life), mucous membrane patches, hair loss, nail exfoliation, snuffles (syphilitic rhinitis), profound anemia, poor feeding, pseudoparalysis of one or more limbs, dysmorphic teeth (older child)	Transplacental; can be anytime during pregnancy or at birth	This is most severe form of syphilis. Treatment consists of IV penicillin. Diagnostic evaluation depends on maternal serology testing and infant symptoms (American Academy of Pediatrics, Committee on Infectious Diseases, 2012).

TABLE 8.12 Infections Acquired From the Mother Before, During, or After Birth[a]—cont'd

Fetal or Newborn Effect	Transmission	Nursing Considerations[b]
Toxoplasmosis *(Toxoplasma Gondii)*		
May be asymptomatic at birth (70% to 90% of cases) or have maculopapular rash, lymphadenopathy, hepatosplenomegaly, jaundice, thrombocytopenia Hydrocephaly, cerebral calcifications, chorioretinitis (classic triad) Microcephaly, seizures, cognitive impairment, deafness Encephalitis, myocarditis, hepatosplenomegaly, anemia, jaundice, diarrhea, vomiting, purpura	Throughout pregnancy Predominant host for organism is cats May be transmitted through cat feces or poorly cooked or raw infected meats	Caution pregnant women to avoid contact with cat feces (e.g., emptying cat litter boxes). Administer a combination of sulfadiazine and pyrimethamine (Daraprim) along with supplemental folinic acid.

[a]This table is not an exhaustive representation of all perinatally transmitted infections. For further information regarding specific diseases or treatment not listed here, refer to American Academy of Pediatrics, Committee on Infectious Diseases. (2018). *2018–2021 Red book: Report of the Committee on Infectious Diseases* (31st ed.). Elk Grove Village, IL: American Academy of Pediatrics.
[b]Isolation precautions depend on institutional policy (see Chapter 20, Infection Control).
CNS, Central nervous system; *HBsAG,* hepatitis B surface antigen; *HBIg,* hepatitis B immunoglobulin; *HIV,* human immunodeficiency virus; *IUGR,* intrauterine growth restriction; *IV,* intravenous; *IVIG,* intravenous immunoglobulin; *ZDV,* zidovudine.
From Nussbaum, R. L., McInnes, R. R., & Willard, H. F. (2007). *Thompson and Thompson genetics in medicine* (6th ed., rev reprint). Philadelphia, PA: Saunders/Elsevier.

of CH resulting in hypothyroidism is iodine deficiency. However, no matter what the cause, the manifestations and management are similar. In some conditions, the thyroid deficiency is severe, and manifestations develop early; in others, the symptoms may be delayed for months or years. Early detection and prompt initiation of treatment are essential because their delay will result in various degrees of cognitive impairment, in which the IQ loss has a direct relationship to the time at which treatment is initiated. If treatment is implemented from 0 to 3 months of age, the mean IQ attained is 89 (range, 64 to 107); if treatment begins at 3 to 6 months, mean IQ will reach 71 (range, 36 to 96); treatment initiated after 6 months of age will result in a mean IQ of 54 (range, 25 to 80).

Results of screening tests indicate that CH occurs in approximately 1 in 4000 to 1 in 3000 newborns (Sheanon & Muglia, 2020). It affects all races and ethnicities but is more prevalent among Hispanic and American Indian or Alaskan Native people (1 in 2000 to 1 in 700 newborns) and less prevalent among African Americans (1 in 3200 to 1 in 17,000 newborns). Also, a higher incidence of other congenital abnormalities has been observed in infants with CH. Many preterm infants have transient hypothyroidism (hypothyroxinemia) at birth as a result of hypothalamic and pituitary immaturity. Infants born before 28 weeks of gestation may require temporary thyroid hormone replacement. Some screening programs target both primary (thyroid-based) and secondary (pituitary-based) hypothyroidism.

Diagnostic Evaluation

Because CH is one of the most common preventable causes of cognitive impairment, early diagnosis and treatment of this disease are essential interventions. Neonatal screening consists of an initial filter paper blood spot T_4 measurement followed by measurement of thyroid-stimulating hormone (TSH) in specimens with low T_4 values.

Tests are mandatory in all US states and territories. Although a blood sample obtained by heel stick for the spot test is best obtained between 2 and 6 days of age, specimens are usually taken within the first 24 to 48 hours or before discharge as part of a concurrent screen for other metabolic defects. Early screening can result in overdiagnosis (false positives) but is preferable to missing the diagnosis.

For screening results that show a low level of T_4 (<10%), obtain TSH levels, and if these are elevated (>40 mU/L), further tests to determine the cause of the disease should be carried out (Stokowski, 2014). Additional tests include serum measurement of T_4, triiodothyronine (T_3), resin uptake, free T_4, and thyroid-bound globulin. Tests of thyroid gland function (thyroid scan and uptake) usually involve oral administration of a radioactive isotope of iodine (^{131}I) and measurement of iodine uptake by the thyroid, usually within 24 hours. In CH, protein-bound iodine, T_4, T_3, and free T_4 levels are low, and thyroid uptake of ^{131}I is decreased. Skeletal radiography is used to assess age.

In newborns, thyroid function studies are elevated in comparison with values in older children; therefore it is important to document the timing of the tests. In preterm and sick full-term infants, thyroid function tests are usually lower than in healthy full-term infants; a repeat T_4 and TSH may be evaluated after 30 weeks (corrected age) in newborns born before that time and after resolution of the acute illness in sick full-term infants.

Therapeutic Management

Treatment involves lifelong thyroid hormone replacement therapy as soon as possible after diagnosis to abolish all signs of hypothyroidism and reestablish normal physical and mental development. The drug of choice is synthetic levothyroxine sodium (Synthroid, Levothroid). Optimum dosage of L-thyroxine should be able to maintain blood TSH concentration between 0.5 and 4.0 mU/L during the first 3 years of life (Stokowski, 2014). Regular measurement of T_4 levels is important in ensuring optimum treatment. Bone age surveys are also performed to ensure optimum growth.

Prognosis

If treatment is started shortly after birth, normal physical growth and intelligence are possible. The most significant factor adversely affecting eventual intellectual development appears to be inadequate treatment, which may be related to noncompliance. An appropriate approach to treatment remains a subject of debate. Some studies have shown that delay in diagnosis and late or no treatment of CH may lead to irreversible brain damage or cretinism (Chuang, Gutmark-Little, & Rose, 2015).

TABLE 8.13 Congenital Effects of Maternal Alcohol Ingestion and Tobacco Smoking

Fetal or Newborn Effects	Comments and Nursing Care Management
Alcohol (Fetal Alcohol Spectrum Disorder)	
Features vary—infant may not display physical features; involves three main categories: • Growth failure in utero and after birth, including microcephaly • Midfacial dysmorphic features • CNS involvement, including cognitive impairment, irritability, hyperactivity, hypertonia, and behavioral problems Facial features include hypoplastic maxilla; micrognathia; short palpebral fissures; thinned upper lip; hypoplastic philtrum; short, upturned nose. One or a combination of these features present in infancy or later (may not appear until later in life). Children or adults who demonstrate cognitive, behavioral, and psychosocial problems without physical features and growth delay are referred to as having ARND. Affected infants may display nonspecific signs, such as irritability, lethargy, difficulty establishing respirations, seizures, tremors, poor suck reflex, and abdominal distention. Birth defects may occur but are less common. Diagnosis is made more difficult by a lack of a single biologic marker and may be made based on maternal history of alcohol ingestion. A number of terms (including ARND and FASD) have been proposed to describe the combination of findings.	Quantity of alcohol consumed is not the determinant; rather, it is the amount consumed in excess of the liver's ability to detoxify the alcohol. Free alcohol has an affinity for brain tissue, hence the CNS symptoms. Ethanol byproducts also contribute to toxicity, as do other substances consumed in addition to alcohol and poor maternal self-care. The effects of alcohol on the fetus occur across a continuum ranging from subtle neurologic deficits to full-blown FAS. The term *FASD* is used to describe the range of clinical presentations ascribed to fetal alcohol exposure. Early gestation is considered the most vulnerable period; however, exposure at any period may cause subtle damage to the developing fetus. Effects of alcohol on CNS are not reversible. FASD is the leading cause of preventable cognitive impairment in the United States. Early intervention with mothers is aimed at minimizing fetal effects, education, and involvement in prevention and treatment counseling. Early intervention with newborns focuses on reducing the effects of alcohol exposure on growing child, especially in relation to cognitive deficits and learning disabilities. Treatment in the neonatal period is similar to that of drug-exposed infants and should involve extensive assessment and individualized developmental care. Provide resources to help decrease or eliminate alcohol intake. *During Your Pregnancy: Alcohol During Pregnancy* is available at the March of Dimes website.[a] Further information is available from the National Organization on Fetal Alcohol Syndrome[b] and Centers for Disease Control and Prevention.
Maternal Tobacco Smoking	
Smoking is associated with significant birth weight deficits; positive dose-response relationship is related to size of fetus. Two active substances—nicotine and cotinine—are higher in newborns of mothers who smoke than in mothers who do not. Postnatal growth deficits occur, as do deficits in emotional and behavioral development in the growing child. Maternal smoking is associated with an increased risk of SIDS, respiratory tract illnesses in childhood, and childhood learning deficits. There is evidence that even secondhand smoke can be deleterious to unborn fetuses and growing children.	Counseling regarding fetal and postnatal effects should be made available to all pregnant women, and they are encouraged to stop smoking. Smoking cessation during pregnancy decreases the chance of fetal complications. Encourage pregnant women to enroll in smoking cessation programs. Evaluate polydrug use in conjunction with smoking. An increased incidence of perinatal complications leading to preterm birth includes abruptio placentae, placenta previa, and premature rupture of membranes. Provide resources to help eliminate smoking. *During Your Pregnancy: Smoking During Pregnancy* is available from the March of Dimes.[a]

[a]http://www.marchofdimes.com.
[b]1200 Eton Court NW, Third Floor, Washington, DC 20007; 202-785-4585; 800 66 NOFAS; http://www.nofas.org.
ARND, Alcohol-related neurodevelopmental disorder; *CNS,* central nervous system; *FAS,* fetal alcohol syndrome; *FASD,* fetal alcohol spectrum disorder; *SIDS,* sudden infant death syndrome.

Nursing Care Management

The most important nursing objective is early identification of the disorder. Nurses caring for neonates must be certain that screening is performed, especially in infants who are preterm, discharged early, or born at home. Approximately 10% of cases are detected only by a second screening at 2 to 6 weeks old. Nurses in community health need to be aware of the earliest signs of the disorder. Parental remarks about an unusually "quiet and good" baby and demonstrated symptoms (such as prolonged jaundice, constipation, and umbilical hernia) should lead to a suspicion of hypothyroidism, which requires a referral for specific tests.

After the diagnosis is confirmed, parents need an explanation of the disorder and the necessity of lifelong treatment. The child should be referred to a pediatric endocrinologist for care. The importance of compliance with the drug regimen for the child to achieve normal growth and development must be stressed (Chuang et al., 2015). Because the drug is tasteless, it can be crushed and added to formula, water, or food. If a dose is missed, twice the dose should be given the next day. Unless there are maternal contraindicative factors, breastfeeding is acceptable and encouraged in infants with hypothyroidism (Lawrence & Lawrence, 2016a). Parents also need to be aware of signs indicating overdose, such as a rapid pulse, dyspnea, irritability, insomnia, fever, sweating, and weight loss. Ideally, they should know how to count the pulse and be instructed to withhold a dose and consult their practitioner if the pulse rate is above a certain value. Signs of inadequate treatment are fatigue, sleepiness, decreased appetite, and constipation.

If the diagnosis was delayed past early infancy, the chance of permanent cognitive impairment is great. Parents need the same guidance in caring for their child as others who have an offspring with cognitive impairment (see Chapter 18). They need an opportunity to discuss their feelings regarding late recognition of the disorder. Although treatment will not reverse the intellectual deficit, it may prevent further damage. Genetic counseling is important for the rare families in which the etiology of CH is thyroid dyshormonogenesis, which is inherited in an autosomal recessive manner (see the Genetic Evaluation and Counseling section later in this chapter).

PHENYLKETONURIA

Phenylketonuria (PKU), an inborn error of metabolism inherited as an autosomal recessive trait (the *PAH* gene is located on chromosome 12q24), is caused by a deficiency or absence of the enzyme needed to metabolize the essential amino acid phenylalanine. Classic PKU is at one end of a spectrum of conditions known as **hyperphenylalaninemia**. Within the spectrum of hyperphenylalaninemia are conditions with varying degrees of severity depending on the degree of enzyme deficiency. Because rarer forms are a result of a deficiency in other enzymes and are diagnosed and treated differently, the following discussion of PKU is limited to the severe, classic form.

In PKU, the hepatic enzyme phenylalanine hydroxylase, which normally controls the conversion of phenylalanine to tyrosine, is deficient. This results in the accumulation of phenylalanine in the bloodstream and urinary excretion of abnormal amounts of its metabolites, the phenyl acids. One of these phenylketones, phenylacetic acid, gives urine the characteristic musty odor associated with the disease. Another is phenylpyruvic acid, which is responsible for the term *phenylketonuria*.

Tyrosine, the amino acid produced by the metabolism of phenylalanine, is absent in PKU. Tyrosine is needed to form the pigment melanin and the hormones epinephrine and T_4. Decreased melanin production results in similar phenotypes of most individuals with PKU, which is blond hair, blue eyes, and fair skin that is particularly susceptible to eczema and other dermatologic problems. Children with a genetically darker skin color may be red haired or brunette.

The prevalence of PKU varies widely in the United States because different states have different definition criteria for what constitutes hyperphenylalaninemia and PKU. The reported figure for PKU in the United States is 1 case per 10,000 live births. The disease has a wide variation of incidence by ethnic groups. Asian populations report rates of 1 case per 17,000 births in China to 1 case per 125,000 births in Japan, whereas European populations report Ireland with a prevalence rate of 1 case per 4500 births and Finland with a rate of 1 case in 200,00 births. However, in Turkey a PKU prevalence rate of 1 case per 2600 births was identified. The wide variation in prevalence demonstrates the need for research to investigate the true prevalence of PKU using comprehensive population screening tests (El-Metwally, Yousef, Ayman, et al., 2018).

Clinical manifestations in untreated PKU include failure to thrive (growth failure); frequent vomiting; irritability; hyperactivity; and unpredictable, erratic behavior. Cognitive impairment is thought to be caused by the accumulation of phenylalanine and presumably by decreased levels of the neurotransmitters dopamine and tryptophan, which affect the normal development of the brain and CNS, resulting in defective myelinization, cystic degeneration of the gray and white matter, and disturbances in cortical lamination. Older children commonly display bizarre or schizoid behavior patterns such as fright reactions, screaming episodes, head banging, arm biting, disorientation, failure to respond to strong stimuli, and catatonia-like positions.

Diagnostic Evaluation[k]

The objective in diagnosing and treating the disorder is to prevent cognitive impairment. Every newborn should be screened for PKU. The most commonly used test for screening newborns is the **Guthrie blood test**, a bacterial inhibition assay for phenylalanine in the blood. *Bacillus subtilis,* present in the culture medium, grows if the blood contains an excessive amount of phenylalanine. If performed properly, this test detects serum phenylalanine levels greater than 4 mg/dl (normal value, 1.6 mg/dl), but it will not quantify the results. Other methods for testing include quantitative fluorometric assay and tandem mass spectrometry, which will give an absolute value. Only fresh heel blood, not cord blood, can be used for the test.

Avoid "layering" the blood specimen on the special Guthrie paper. Layering is placing one drop of blood on top of the other or overlapping the specimen. This practice results in a falsely high reading, or false positive, which will lead the newborn screening department to call the family and physician to arrange for a diagnostic blood phenylalanine test to determine whether the newborn truly has PKU. Best results are obtained by collecting the specimen with a pipette from the heel stick and spreading the blood uniformly over the blot paper.

Because of the possibility of variant forms of hyperphenylalaninemia, PKU cofactor variant screen should be performed in all children diagnosed with PKU. A major concern is that a significant number of infants are not rescreened for PKU after early discharge and are at risk for a missed or delayed diagnosis. Give special consideration to screening infants born at home who have no hospital contact and infants adopted internationally.

Therapeutic Management[l]

Treatment of PKU involves restricting phenylalanine in the diet. Because the genetic enzyme is intracellular, systemic administration of phenylalanine hydroxylase is of no value. Phenylalanine cannot be eliminated because it is an essential amino acid in tissue growth. Therefore dietary management must meet two criteria: (1) meet the child's nutritional need for optimum growth and (2) maintain phenylalanine levels within a safe range (2 to 6 mg/dl in neonates and children up to 12 years old and 2 to 10 mg/dl through adolescence) (Soltanizadeh & Mirmoghtadaie, 2014).

Professionals agree that infants with PKU who have blood phenylalanine levels higher than 10 mg/dl should be started on treatment to establish metabolic control as soon as possible, ideally by 7 to 10 days of age (Shchelochkov & Venditti, 2020). The daily amounts of phenylalanine are individualized for each child and require frequent changes on the basis of appetite, growth and development, and blood phenylalanine and tyrosine levels.

Because all natural food proteins contain phenylalanine and will be limited, the diet must be supplemented with a specially prepared phenylalanine-free formula (e.g., Phenex-1 for infants or Phenex-2 for children and adults).[m] The phenylalanine-free formula is an amino acid–modified formula essential in the low-phenylalanine diet to provide the appropriate protein, vitamins, minerals, and calories for optimal growth and development. Because tyrosine becomes an essential amino acid, the phenylalanine-free formula supplies an adequate amount, but in some cases additional supplementation may be needed. The phenylalanine-free amino acid–modified formula for infants has all of the nutrients necessary for adequate infant growth. Because of the low phenylalanine content of breast milk, total or partial

[k]Always refer patient to a genetic metabolic specialist. For a reference list, visit the American Society of Human Genetics website, http://www.ashg.org.

[l]For more information, contact American Society of Human Genetics, 9650 Rockville Pike, Bethesda, MD 20814; 301-634-7300, 866-HUM-GENE; http://www.ashg.org.

[m]A resource for dietary management is Acosta, P. B., & Yannicelli, S. (2001). *The Ross metabolic formula system nutrition support protocols* (4th ed.). Columbus, OH: Abbott Nutrition; 800-227-5767; http://abbottnutrition.com.

breastfeeding may be possible with close monitoring of phenylalanine levels (Lawrence & Lawrence, 2016a).

When treatment for PKU was first instituted, it was believed that phenylalanine withdrawal during only the first 3 years of age would suffice to avoid cognitive impairment and other deleterious manifestations of PKU. However, most clinicians now agree that to achieve optimal metabolic control and outcome, a restricted phenylalanine diet, including medical foods and low-protein products, most likely will be medically required for virtually all individuals with classic PKU for their entire lives (Soltanizadeh & Mirmoghtadaie, 2014). Such lifetime reduction of phenylalanine intake is necessary to prevent neuropsychologic and cognitive deficits because even mild hyperphenylalaninemia (20 mg/dl) would produce such effects. To evaluate the effectiveness of dietary treatment, frequent monitoring of blood phenylalanine and tyrosine levels is necessary.

Phenylalanine levels greater than 6 mg/dl in mothers with PKU affect the normal embryologic development of the fetus, including cognitive impairment, cardiac defects, and LBW. It is recommended that phenylalanine levels below 5 mg/dl be achieved during pregnancy in women with PKU (Grange, Hillman, Burton, et al., 2014).

Prognosis

Although many individuals with treated PKU manifest no cognitive and behavioral deficits, many comparisons of individuals with PKU with control participants show lower performance on IQ tests, with larger differences in other cognitive domains; however, their performance is still in the average range. Evidence for differences in behavioral adjustment is inconsistent despite anecdotal reports suggesting greater risk for internalizing psychopathology and attention disorders. In addition, insufficient data are available on the effects of phenylalanine restriction over many decades of life (Shchelochkov & Venditti, 2020). Recent data suggest that treatment with tetrahydrobiopterin in addition to the phenylalanine-restricted diet may be beneficial to PKU patients (Kor, Yilmaz, Bulut, et al., 2017). Total bone mineral density is considerably lower in children who are on a low-phenylalanine diet even though calcium, phosphorus, and magnesium intakes are higher than normal.

Nursing Care Management

The principal nursing considerations involve teaching the family regarding the dietary restrictions. Although the treatment may sound simple, the task of maintaining such a strict dietary regimen is demanding, especially for older children and adolescents. In addition, mothers of children with PKU may have to spend many hours preparing special foods, such as low-phenylalanine snacks. Foods with low phenylalanine levels (e.g., vegetables, fruits, juices, and some cereals, breads, and starches) must be measured to provide the prescribed amount of phenylalanine. High-protein foods, such as meat and dairy products, are eliminated from the diet. The sweetener aspartame (NutraSweet) should be avoided because it is composed of two amino acids, aspartic acid and phenylalanine, and if used will decrease the amount of natural phenylalanine that is prescribed for the day. However, medications that use aspartame as the sweetener may be used if no other nonaspartame medications are available because the content of the artificial sweetener is minimal or can be counted in the total daily phenylalanine allowance.

Maintaining the diet during infancy presents few problems. Solid foods such as cereal, fruits, and vegetables are introduced as usual to the infant. Difficulties arise as the child gets older. Long-term management of patients with PKU is best accomplished with a team of experienced professionals (Shchelochkov & Venditti, 2020).

A decreased appetite and refusal to eat may reduce intake of the calculated phenylalanine requirement. The child's increasing independence may also inhibit absolute control of what he or she eats. Either factor can result in decreased or increased phenylalanine levels. During the school years, peer pressure becomes a major force in deterring the child from eating the prescribed foods or abstaining from high-protein foods, such as milkshakes and ice cream. Limitations of this diet are best illustrated by an example: a quarter-pound hamburger may provide a 2-day phenylalanine allowance for a school-age child.

The assistance of a registered dietitian is essential. Parents need a basic understanding of the disorder and practical suggestions regarding food selection and preparation.[n] Meal planning is based on weighing the food on a gram scale; a less accurate method is the exchange list. As soon as children are old enough, usually by early preschool, they should be involved in the daily calculation, menu planning, and formula preparation. Using a computer, voice-activated calculator, cards, or colored beads can help children keep track of the daily allowance of phenylalanine foods. A system of goal setting, self-monitoring, contracts, and rewards can promote compliance in adolescents.

Preparation of the phenylalanine-free formula can present some challenges. The formula tends to be lumpy; mixing the powder with a small amount of water to make a paste and then adding the rest of the required liquid helps alleviate this problem. A blender or mixer dissolves the powder more easily; a rechargeable hand mixer can be used when traveling. Although the taste is virtually impossible to camouflage, many new products are on the market today. Some of the complete formulas are chocolate, vanilla, strawberry, and orange flavored. Incomplete formulas that do not contain the vitamins and minerals and are plain tasting are also available; these can be added to cold foods instead of mixing them as a formula. Formula bars are convenient for active adolescents. Formula capsules are also available, but the patient would need to take 20 or more capsules per day.

Family Support[o]

In addition to the problems related to a child with a chronic disorder (see Chapter 17), parents have the burden of knowing that they are carriers of the defect. Genetic counseling is especially important to inform the parents that prenatal testing is now available to detect the presence of the defective gene in heterozygotes. Counseling is also important for adults with PKU to inform them that all of their offspring will be carriers for PKU (see the Genetic Evaluation and Counseling section later in the chapter).

GALACTOSEMIA

Galactosemia is a rare autosomal recessive disorder that results from various gene mutations leading to three distinct enzymatic deficiencies. The most common type of galactosemia (classic galactosemia) results from a deficiency of a hepatic enzyme, galactose 1-phosphate uridyltransferase (GALT), and affects approximately 1 in 50,000 births. The other two varieties of galactosemia involve deficiencies in the enzymes galactokinase (GALK) and galactose 4′-epimerase (GALE); these are extremely rare disorders. All three enzymes (GALT, GALK, and GALE) are involved in the conversion of galactose into glucose.

[n]A helpful resource is Schuett, V. (Ed.). (1997). *Low protein cookery for phenylketonuria* (3rd ed.). Madison, WI: University of Wisconsin Press.

[o]National support groups include the Children's PKU Network, which offers a variety of support services; contact 3790 Via de la Valle, Suite 120, Del Mar, CA 92014; 800-377-6677; email: PKUnetwork@aol.com; http://www.pkunetwork.org, and the National PKU Alliance, contact Christine Brown, Executive Director, PO Box 501, Tomahawk, WI 54487; 715-437-0477; http://www.npkua.org.

As galactose accumulates in the blood, several organs are affected. Hepatic dysfunction leads to cirrhosis, resulting in jaundice in the infant by the second week of life. The spleen subsequently becomes enlarged as a result of portal hypertension. Cataracts are usually recognizable by 1 or 2 months of age; cerebral damage, manifested by the symptoms of lethargy and hypotonia, is evident soon afterward. Infants with galactosemia appear normal at birth, but within a few days of ingesting milk (which has a high lactose content), they begin to experience vomiting and diarrhea, leading to weight loss. *E. coli* sepsis is also a common presenting clinical sign. Death during the first month of life is frequent in untreated infants. Occasionally classic galactosemia is seen with milder, chronic manifestations, such as growth failure, feeding difficulty, and developmental delay. This presentation is more frequent among African American children with galactosemia (Kishnani & Chen, 2020).

Diagnostic Evaluation

Diagnosis is made on the basis of the infant's history, physical examination, galactosuria, increased levels of galactose in the blood, and decreased levels of GALT activity in erythrocytes. The infant may display characteristics of malnutrition: hypoglycemia, jaundice, hepatosplenomegaly, sepsis, cataracts, and decreased muscle tone (Kishnani & Chen, 2020). Newborn screening for this disease is required in most states. Heterozygotes can also be identified because heterozygotic individuals have significantly lower levels of the essential enzyme.

Therapeutic Management

During infancy, treatment consists of eliminating all milk and lactose-containing formula, including breast milk. Traditionally, lactose-free formulas are used, with soy protein formula being the feeding of choice; however, some research suggests that elemental formula (galactose-free) may be more beneficial than soy formulas (Kishnani & Chen, 2020). However, the American Academy of Pediatrics recommends the use of soy protein–based formula for infants with galactosemia, and it is considerably less expensive than elemental formula (Bhatia, Greer, & Committee on Nutrition, 2008). As the infant progresses to solids, only foods low in galactose should be consumed. Certain fruits are high in galactose, and some dietitians recommend that they be avoided. Food lists should be given to the family to ensure that appropriate foods are chosen.

If galactosemia is suspected, supportive treatment and care are implemented, including monitoring for hypoglycemia, liver failure, bleeding disorders, and *E. coli* sepsis.

Prognosis

Follow-up studies of children treated from birth or within the first 2 months of life after symptoms appear have found long-term complications, such as hypogonadism, cognitive impairment, growth restriction, and verbal and motor delays (Kishnani & Chen, 2020). These findings have revealed that eliminating sources of galactose does not significantly improve the outcome. New therapeutic strategies, such as enhancing residual transferase activity, replacing depleted metabolites, and using gene replacement therapy, are needed to improve the prognosis for these children.

Nursing Care Management[p]

Nursing interventions are similar to those for PKU except that dietary restrictions are easier to maintain because many more foods are allowed. However, reading food labels carefully for the presence of any form of lactose, especially dairy products, is mandatory. Many drugs, such as some of the penicillin preparations, contain lactose as filler and also must be avoided. Unfortunately, lactose is an unlabeled ingredient in many pharmaceuticals. Therefore instruct parents to ask their local pharmacist about galactose content of any over-the-counter or prescription medication.

GENETIC EVALUATION AND COUNSELING

Genetic counseling is a communication process concerned with the human problems associated with the occurrence, or risk of occurrence, of a genetic disorder in a family. It involves relaying information about the diagnosis, treatment options, recurrence risk, and availability of prenatal diagnosis. With the completion of the Human Genome Project, the international project to determine the total genetic information in humans, a new era of human genetics is unfolding (International Human Genome Sequencing Consortium, 2004), and it will lead to a better understanding of specifically how genetic variation contributes to health and disease. It is essential that nurses master the basic principles of heredity, understand how heredity contributes to disorders, and be aware of the types of genetic testing available.

Nurses frequently encounter children with genetic diseases and families in which there is a risk that a disorder may be transmitted to or occur in an offspring. It is a responsibility of nurses to be alert to situations in which persons could benefit from a genetic evaluation and counseling (see Nursing Care Guidelines box), to be aware of the local genetic resources, to aid families in finding services, and to offer support and care for children and families affected by genetic conditions. Local genetic clinics can be located through several sites; for example, GeneTests,[q] a publicly funded medical genetics information resource developed for physicians and other health care providers, is available at no cost to all interested persons. Another resource is the National Society of Genetic Counselors,[r] which lists genetic counselors by state in the United States.

NURSING CARE GUIDELINES

Common Indications for Referral

- Previous child with multiple congenital anomalies; cognitive impairment; or an isolated birth defect, such as neural tube defect, cleft lip, or cleft palate
- Family history of a hereditary condition, such as cystic fibrosis, fragile X syndrome, or diabetes
- Prenatal diagnosis of advanced maternal age or other indication
- Consanguinity
- Teratogen exposure, such as to occupational chemicals, medications, or alcohol
- Repeated pregnancy loss or infertility
- Newly diagnosed abnormality or genetic condition
- Before undertaking genetic testing and after receiving results, particularly when testing for susceptibility to late-onset disorders, such as cancer or neurologic disease
- As follow-up for a positive newborn test, as with phenylketonuria, or a heterozygote screening test, such as Tay-Sachs disease

From Nussbaum, R., McInnes, R., & Willard, H. (2007). *Thompson and Thompson genetics in medicine* (6th ed.). Philadelphia, PA: Saunders/Elsevier.

[p]Information and support for parents can be found at the American Liver Foundation, http://www.liverfoundation.org, and at Parents of Galactosemic Children, Inc., PO Box 2401, Mandeville, LA 70470-2401; 866-900-PGC1; http://www.galactosemia.org.

[q]http://www.ncbi.nlm.nih.gov/sites/GeneTests.

[r]http://www.nsgc.org.

Maintaining contact with the family or referring the family to an agency that can provide a sustained relationship, usually the public health agency in their locality, is one of the most important aspects in the care of the patient and family. In a disorder that requires conscientious diet management, such as PKU or galactosemia, it is important to make certain that the family understands and follows the advice. A vital role for nurses is to advocate for the child and family as they make their way through the various specialty clinics. This is especially important for families that are more vulnerable because of cognitive, hearing, language, or financial issues, and those who otherwise may have difficulty accessing health services. Nurses can reinforce the genetic information or arrange for additional genetic counseling if a family has additional questions or misunderstandings.

One of the current ethical concerns is the testing of healthy children for carrier status of a genetic condition that either will not have adverse consequences until adulthood or has only reproductive implications. The American Academy of Pediatrics, Committee on Bioethics (2001, reaffirmed 2008) policy statement does not support the broad use of carrier testing or screening in children or adolescents. When there is no clear medical benefit to testing in childhood, the child should be permitted to wait until adulthood to choose whether to be tested. Genetic counseling is recommended to help the family weigh all of the issues.

PSYCHOLOGICAL ASPECTS OF GENETIC DISEASE

The diagnosis of a genetic disorder in a child can be a life-altering experience for families. They may have to reassess their perception of "self" and the loss of the dream of the perfect infant. Parents may change educational, employment, and reproductive plans after the diagnosis of a genetic disorder in their child.

Families may need to have the genetic information repeated several times. Families may also encounter ethical or moral dilemmas regarding genetic evaluation and testing options, as well as potential involvement of other family members. Nurses are pivotal caregivers in assessing the family's understanding of the genetic disorder, psychological responses, and coping mechanisms. Nurses may help families by providing support and attempting to alleviate possible feelings of guilt and by helping the family make the best possible adjustment to the disorder.

It is important to stress that there is nothing shameful about an inherited or congenital defect and to emphasize any appropriate remedy. The thought of a hereditary disorder often creates intrafamily strife, hostility, and marital disharmony, sometimes to the point of family disintegration. Relatives may change their reproductive plans after the diagnosis of a genetic disorder in a member, or the decision to reproduce may be postponed indefinitely on the basis of a disorder in a relative, even a remote one. Although people may understand the information on an intellectual level, they may still harbor fears on an emotional level. Nurses can help the family identify their personal strengths and offer them information about local and national support groups. (The Genetic Alliance[s] is a nonprofit organization that has a database of support groups for genetic conditions.) Finally, it is important to keep in mind that the infant or child has the same basic needs after the diagnosis of a genetic disorder as he or she had before the diagnosis.

[s]http://www.geneticalliance.org.

CLINICAL JUDGMENT AND NEXT-GENERATION NCLEX® EXAMINATION-STYLE QUESTIONS

1. **Choose the most likely options for the information missing from the statements below by selecting from the lists of options provided.**
When assessing temperature in a newborn, ______1______ temperatures are taken because insertion of a thermometer in the ______2______ may cause perforation if done incorrectly.

Options for 1	Options for 2
oral	mouth
rectal	ear
axillary	rectum
temporal	nose

2. The nurse is developing a plan of care for a 4-day old full-term newborn boy who is being seen in the pediatrician's office. At discharge 2 days ago, the serum total bilirubin level was 12 mg/dl and direct bilirubin as 0.6 mg.dl. Today he returns for a bilirubin follow-up and his serum total bilirubin level is 14mg/dl and direct bilirubin is 0.7 mg.dl. The newborn is being breast fed for 10 minutes every 3-4 hours on each side. The mother reports no changes in wet diapers or stools since being home. **Use an X for the health teaching below that is Indicated (appropriate or necessary), Contraindicated (could be harmful), or Non-Essential (makes no difference or not necessary).**

Nursing Action	Indicated	Contraindicated	Non-Essential
Review the medical history to assess what laboratory studies were performed after birth.			
Encourage frequent breastfeeding			
Switch to formula feeding for 72 hours			
Teach mother how to swaddle the newborn			
Administer IV immunoglobulin			

3. A late pre-term infant (6 weeks of gestation) who was just born has experienced meconium aspiration. The newborn has stable respiratory effort and good muscle tone. Heart rate is 120 beats/minute. When planning care for this pre-term newborn, which nursing interventions would the nurse consider at this time? **Select all that apply.**
   A. Tracheal suctioning should be done immediately
   B. Suction the hypopharynx after delivery
   C. Monitory for respiratory distress
   D. Prevent acidosis
   E. Prevent hypoxemia
   F. Administer nasal CPAP
   G. Place child in strict isolation

4. A newborn born yesterday has a possible viral infection thought to be obtained from the mother. The nurse caring for the newborn is to obtain specimens for the TORCH workup. **Select all of the viral infections that are assessed in the TORCH workup. Select all that apply.**
   A. Tetanus
   B. Toxoplasmosis
   C. HIV
   D. Gonorrhea
   E. Cytomegalovirus
   F. Rubella
   G. Herpes Simplex
   H. Klebsiella

REFERENCES

Abramson, A. R., Peacock, Z. S., Cohen, H. L., & Choudhri, A. F. (2015). Radiology of cleft lip and palate: Imaging for the prenatal period and throughout life. *Radiographics, 35*(7), 2053–2063.

Aceti, A., Gori, D., Barone, G., et al. (2015). Probiotics for prevention of necrotizing enterocolitis in preterm infants: Systematic review and meta-analysis. *Italian Journal of Pediatrics, 41*, 1–20.

Adamkin, D. H., & American Academy of Pediatrics, Committee on Fetus and Newborn (2011). Postnatal glucose homeostasis in late-preterm and term infants. *Pediatrics, 127*(3), 575–579.

Alfaleh, K., Anabrees, J., Bassler, D., et al. (2014). Probiotics for prevention of necrotizing enterocolitis in preterm infants. *The Cochrane Database of Systematic Reviews* (4), CD005496.

Aliaga, S., Zhang, J., Long, D. L., et al. (2016). Center variation in the delivery of indicated late preterm births. *American Journal of Perinatology, 33*(10), 1008–1016.

Athalye-Jape, G., Rao, S., & Patole, S. (2016). Lactobacillus reuteri DSM 17938 as a probiotic for preterm neonates: A strain-specific systematic review. *Journal of Parenteral and Enteral Nutrition, 40*, 783–794.

Altimier, L., & White, R. D. (2014). The neonatal intensive care unit (NICU) environment. In C. Kenner, & J. Lott (Eds.), *Comprehensive neonatal care: An interdisciplinary approach* (5th ed.). New York: Springer.

American Academy of Pediatrics & American College of Obstetricians and Gynecologists. (2017). In S. Kilpatrick, L. Papile, (Associate eds) & G. A. Macones, K. L. Watterberg, (Eds.), *Guidelines for perinatal care.* (8th ed.). Elk Grove Village, IL: American Academy of Pediatrics.

American Academy of Pediatrics, Committee on Bioethics. (2001). Ethical issues with genetic testing in pediatrics. *Pediatrics, 107*(6), 1451–1455, Reaffirmed 2008.

American Academy of Pediatrics Section on Breastfeeding. (2012). Breastfeeding and the use of human milk. *Pediatrics, 129*(3), e827–e841.

American Academy of Pediatrics, Subcommittee on Hyperbilirubinemia. (2004). Management of hyperbilirubinemia in the newborn infant 35 or more weeks of gestation (clinical practice guideline). *Pediatrics, 114*(1), 297–316.

American Academy of Pediatrics, Task Force on Sudden Infant Death Syndrome. (2016). SIDS and other sleep-related infant death: Expansion of recommendations for a safe infant sleeping environment. *Pediatrics, 138*(5), e1341–e1367.

Association of Women's Health, Obstetric and Neonatal Nurses. (2017). *Assessment and care of the late preterm infant.* Washington, DC: Association of Women's Health, Obstetric and Neonatal Nurses.

Azzopardi, D., Strohm, B., Marlow, N., et al. (2014). Effects of hypothermia for perinatal asphyxia on childhood outcomes. *The New England Journal of Medicine, 371*(2), 140–149.

Bagwell, G. A. (2014). Hematologic system. In C. Kenner, & J. Lott (Eds.), *Comprehensive neonatal care: An interdisciplinary approach* (5th ed.). St Louis: Saunders/Elsevier.

Baley, J. E., & Gonzalez, B. E. (2015). Perinatal viral infants. In R. J. Martin, A. A. Fanaroff, & M. C. Walsh (Eds.), *Fanaroff and Martin's neonatal-perinatal medicine: Diseases of the fetus and infant* (10th ed.). St Louis: Elsevier.

Barrington, K. J., Finer, N., & Pennaforte, T. (2017). Inhaled nitric oxide for respiratory failure in preterm infants. *Cochrane Database Systematic Reviews, 3*(1), CD000509.

Bellone, M., & Boctor, F. N. (2014). Therapeutic plasma exchange and intravenous immunoglobulin as primary therapy for D alloimmunization in pregnancy precludes the need for intrauterine transfusion. *Transfusion, 54*(8), 2118–2121.

Berardi, A., Rossi, C., Spada, C., et al. (2018). GBS prevention working group of emilia-romagna: strategies for preventing early-onset sepsis and for managing neonates at-risk: Wide variability across six Western countries. *The Journal of Maternal-Fetal and Neonatal Medicine, 1*, 1–7.

Bhatia, J., Greer, F., & Committee on Nutrition. (2008). Use of soy protein-based formulas in infant feeding. *Pediatrics, 121*(5), 1062–1068.

Blackburn, S. T. (2018). *Maternal, fetal, and neonatal physiology: A clinical perspective* (5th ed.). Philadelphia: Saunders/Elsevier.

Bozzetti, V., Paterlini, G., De Lorenzo, P., et al. (2016). Impact of continuous vs bolus feeding on splanchnic perfusion in very low birth weight infants: A randomized trial. *The Journal of Pediatrics, 9*, 86–92.

Brown, L. D., Hendrickson, K., Evans, R., et al. (2016). Enteral nurtition. In S. L. Gardner, B. S. Carter, M. Enzman-Hines, et al. (Eds.), *Merenstein & Gardner's handbook of neonatal intensive care* (8th ed.). St. Louis: Mosby.

Bucher, B. T., Pacetti, A., Lovvorn, III., et al. (2016). Neonatal surgery. In S. L. Gardner, B. S. Carter, M. Enzman-Hines, et al. (Eds.), *Merenstein and Gardner's handbook of neonatal intensive care* (8th ed.). St Louis: Mosby/Elsevier.

Bull, M. J., Engle, W. A., Committee on Injury, Violence and Poison Prevention and the Committee on Fetus and Newborn, et al. (2009). Safe transportation of preterm and low birth weight infants at hospital discharge. *Pediatrics, 123*(5), 1424–1429.

Buterbaugh, K. L., & Shah, A. S. (2016). The natural history and management of brachial plexus birth palsy. *Pediatric Orthopedics, 9*(4), 418–426.

Cai, A., Qi, S., Su, Z., et al. (2016). A pilot metabolic profiling study of patients with neonatal jaundice and response to phototherapy. *Clinical and Translational Science, 9*(4), 216–220.

Calikusu, M., & Balci, S. (2017). The effect of training on noise reduction in neonatal intensive care units. *Journal for Specialists in Pediatric Nursing, 22*(3), 1–8.

Cartwright, J., Atz, T., Newman, S., et al. (2017). Integrative review of interventions to promote breastfeeding in the late preterm infant. *The Journal of Obstetric, Gynecologic, & Neonatal Nursing, 46*(3), 347–356.

Casper, C., Sarapuk, I., & Pavlyshyn, H. (2018). Regular and prolonged skin-to-skin contact improves short-term outcomes for very preterm infants: A dose-dependent intervention. *Archives of Pediatric, 25*(8), 469–475.

Chang, H., Chen, J., Chang, J., et al. (2017). Multiple strains probiotics appear to be the most effective probiotics in the prevention of necrotizing enterocolitis and mortality: An updated meta-analysis. *PLOS One, 12*(2), 1–14.

Chantry, C. J., Eglash, A., Labbok, M., & The Academy of Breastfeeding Medicine (2015). ABM Position on Breastfeeding – Revised 2015. *Breastfeeding Medicine, 10*(9), 407–411.

Chuang, J., Gutmark-Little, I., & Rose, S. R. (2015). Thyroid disorders in the neonate. In R. J. Martin, A. A. Fanaroff, & M. C. Walsh (Eds.), *Neonatal-perinatal medicine: Diseases of the fetus and infant* (10th ed.). St Louis: Elsevier.

Colditz, M. J., Lai, M. M., Cartwright, D. W., et al. (2015). Subgaleal haemorrhage in the newborn: A call for early diagnosis and aggressive management. *Journal of the Paediatrics & Child Health, 51*(2), 140–146.

Committee on Approaching Death. (2015). *Addressing key end of life issues*; Institute of Medicine, *3*, 1–4.

Committee on Injury and Poison Prevention and Committee on Fetus and Newborn. (1991). American academy of pediatrics safe transportation of premature infants. *Pediatrics, 87*, 120–122.

Conner, S. N., Carter, E. B., Tuuli, M. G., et al. (2015). Maternal marijuana use and neonatal morbidity. *American Journal of Obstetrics and Gynecology, 213*(3), 422–425.

Cortese, F., Scicchitano, P., Gesualdo, M., et al. (2016). Early and late infections in newborns: Where do we stand? A review. *Pediatr Neonatal, 57*(4), 265–273.

Cotten, M., Murtha, A., Goldberg, R., et al. (2014). Feasibility of autologous cord blood cells for infants with hypoxic-ischemic encelphalopathy. *Journal of Pediatrics, 164*, 973–979.

Dani, C., Mosca, F., Vento, G., et al. (2018). Effects of surfactant treatment in late preterm infants with respiratory distress syndrome. *The Journal of Maternal-Fetal and Neonatal Medicine, 31*(10), 1259–1266.

Daniels, B., Ireland, C., Kraus, S., et al. (2016). Magnetic resonance–guided nasogastric feeding tube placement for neonates: A preclinical study. *Journal of Parenteral and Enteral Nutrition*, 1–7.

Davis, N. L. (2015). Care seat screening for low birth weight term neonates. *Pediatrics, 136*(1), 89–96.

Deng, Q., Li, Q., Wang, H., et al. (2018). Early father-infant skin-to-skin contact and its effect on the neurodevelopmental outcomes of moderately preterm infants in China: Study protocol for a randomized controlled trial. *Trials, 19*(1), 1–11.

Dennison, B. A., Nguyen, T. Q., Gregg, D. J., et al. (2016). The impact of hospital resources and availability of professional lactation support on maternity care: Results of breastfeeding surveys 2009-2014. *Breastfeed Medicine, 11*, 479–486.

Denny, L., Coles, S., & Blitz, R. (2017). Fetal alcohol syndrome and fetal alcohol spectrum disorders. *American Family Physician, 96*(8), 515–522.

Dhar, V. (2020). Cleft lip and palate. In R. M. Kliegman, J. W. St. Geme, N. J. Blum, et al. (Eds.), *Nelson textbook of pediatrics* (21st ed.). Philadelphia: Elsevier.

Durbin, D. R., & Committee on Injury, Violence, and Poison Prevention. (2011). Child passenger safety. *Pediatrics, 127*(4), e1050–e1066.

Dying in America. (2014). *Improving quality and honoring individual preferences near the end of life*. Institute of Medicine of the National Academies Report; September17.

Edris, A. A., Ghany, E. A., Razek, A. R., et al. (2014). The role of intensive phototherapy in decreasing the need for exchange transfusion in neonatal jaundice. *The Journal of Pakistan Medical Association, 64*(1), 5–8.

Ellett, M. L., Cohen, M. D., Croffie, J. M., et al. (2014). Comparing bedside methods of determining placement of gastric tubes in children. *The Journal of Pediatric Nursing, 19*(1), 68–79.

El-Metwally, A., Yousef Al-Ahaidib, L., et al. (2018). The prevalence of phenylketonuria in Arab countries, Turkey, and Iran: A systematic review. *BioMed Research International, 18*, 1–13.

Ericson, J. E., Gostelow, M., Autmizguine, J., et al. (2017). Safety of high-dose acyclovir in infants with suspected and confirmed neonatal herpes simplex virus infections. *The Pediatric Infectious Disease Journal, 36*(4), 369–373.

Evereklian, M., & Posmontier, B. (2017). The impact of kangaroo care on premature infant weight gain. *The Journal of Pediatric Nursing, 34*, 10–16.

Fastman, B. R., Howell, E. A., Holzman, I., et al. (2014). Current perspectives on temperature management and hypothermia in low birth weight infants. *Newborn & Infant Nursing Reviews* (14), 50–55.

Finnegan, L. P. (1985). Neonatal abstinence. In N. Nelson (Ed.), *Current therapy in neonatal perinatal medicine* (pp. 1985–1986). Toronto: Decker.

Fry, T. J., Marfurt, S., & Wengier, S. (2018). Systematic review of quality improvement initiatives related to cue-based feeding in preterm infants. *Neonatal Network, 32*(2), 132–137.

Furuta, S., Sato, H., Tsuji, S., et al. (2016). Effective treatment for infantile hemangioma with long-pulsed dye laser with oral propranolol medication: A preliminary report. *Pediatric Surgery International, 32*(9), 857–862.

Gardner, S. L., & Carter, B. S. (2016). Grief and perinatal loss. In S. L. Gardner, B. S. Carter, M. Enzman-Hines, et al. (Eds.), *Merenstein and Gardner's handbook of neonatal intensive care* (8th ed.). St Louis: Mosby/Elsevier.

Gardner, S. L., & Hernandez, J. A. (2016a). Heat balance. In S. L. Gardner, B. S. Carter, M. Enzman-Hines, et al. (Eds.), *Merenstein and Gardner's handbook of neonatal intensive care* (8th ed.). St Louis: Elsevier.

Gardner, S. L., & Hernandez, J. A. (2016b). Initial nursery care. In S. L. Gardner, B. S. Carter, M. Enzman-Hines, et al. (Eds.), *Merenstein and Gardner's handbook of neonatal intensive care* (8th ed.). St Louis: Mosby/Elsevier.

Gardner, S. L., & Lawrence, R. A. (2016). Breast-feeding the neonate with special needs. In S. L. Gardner, B. S. Carter, M. Enzman-Hines, et al. (Eds.), *Merenstein & Gardner's handbook of neonatal intensive care* (8th ed.). St. Louis: Mosby.

Gardner, S. L., Enzman-Hines, M., & Nyp, M. (2016). Respiratory diseases. In S. L. Gardner, B. S. Carter, M. Enzman-Hines, et al. (Eds.), *Merenstein and Gardner's handbook of neonatal intensive care* (8th ed.). St Louis: Mosby/Elsevier.

Gardner, S. L., Goldson, E., & Hernandez, J. A. (2016). The neonate and the environment: Impact on development. In S. L. Gardner, B. S. Carter, M. Enzman-Hines, et al. (Eds.), *Merenstein and Gardner's handbook of neonatal intensive care* (8th ed). St Louis: Mosby/Elsevier.

Gennattasio, A., Perri, E. A., Baranek, D., & Rohan, A. (2015). Oral feeding: Readiness assessment in premature infants. *MCN The American Journal of Maternal Child Nursing, 40*(2), 96–104.

Gilfillan, M., & Bhandari, V. (2017). Biomarkers for the diagnosis of neonatal sepsis and necrotizing enterocolitis: Clinical practice guidelines. *Early Human Development, 105*, 25–33.

Grange, D. K., Hillman, R. E., Burton, B. K., et al. (2014). Phenylketonuria demographics outcomes and safety (PKUDOS) registry; maternal phenylketonuria observational program (PKU MOMS) sub-registry. *Molecular Genetics and Metabolism, 112*(1), 9–16.

Gunn, J. K., Rosales, C. B., Center, K. E., et al. (2016). Prenatal exposure to cannabis and maternal and child health outcomes: A systematic review and meta-analysis. *BMJ, 6*(4), 1–8.

Hale, T. W. (2019). *Medications and mother's milk* (18th ed.). Springer Publishing.

Harding, C., Frank, L., Van Someren, V., Hilari, K., & Botting, N. (2014). How does non-nutritive sucking support infant feeding? *Infant Behavior and Development, 37*(4), 457–464.

Hartnett, M. E. (2014). Vascular endothelial growth factor antagonist therapy for retinopathy of prematurity. *Clinics in perinatology, 41*(4), 925–943.

Horgan, M. J. (2015). Management of the late preterm infant. *Pediatric Clinics of North America, 62*(2), 439–451.

Hudak, M. L. (2015). Infants with antenatal exposure to drugs. In R. J. Martin, A. A. Fanaroff, & M. C. Walsh (Eds.), *Fanaroff and Martin's neonatal-perinatal medicine: Diseases of the fetus and infant* (10th ed.). St Louis: Elsevier.

Human Milk Banking Association. (2015). *2015 guidelines for the establishment and operation of a donor human milk bank*. http://www.hmbana.org/publications.

International Human Genome Sequencing Consortium. (2004). Finishing the euchromatic sequence of the human genome. *Nature, 431*(7011), 931–945.

James, S. H., Sheffield, J. S., & Kimberlin, D. W. (2014). Mother-to-child transmission of herpes simplex virus. *Journal of the Pediatric Infectious Diseases Society, 3*(1), 19–23.

Jasani, B., Simmer, K., Patole, S. K., et al. (2017). Long chain polyunsaturated fatty acid supplementation in infants born at term. *The Cochrane Database of Systematic Reviews, 10*(3), CD000376.

Ji, Y., Chen, S., Li, K., et al. (2014). Signaling pathways in the development of infantile hemangioma. *The Journal of Hematology & Oncology, 7*, 13.

Johnson, T. J., Patra, K., Greene, M. M., et al. (2019). NICU human milk dose and health care use after NICU discharge in very low birth weight infants. *Journal of perinatology, 39*(1), 120–128.

Kamath-Rayne, B. D., Thilo, E. H., Deacon, J., et al. (2016). Jaundice. In S. L. Gardner, B. S. Carter, M. Enzman-Hines, et al. (Eds.), *Merenstein and Gardner's handbook of neonatal intensive care* (8th ed.). St Louis: Mosby/Elsevier.

Kimberlin, D. W., Brady, M. T., & Jackson, M. A. (Eds.). (2018). American Academy of Pediatrics, Committee on Infectious Diseases, *Red book. 2018 report of the Committee on Infectious Diseases* (31th ed.). Elk Grove, IL: American Academy of Pediatrics.

Kishnani, P. S., & Chen, Y. (2020). Defects in galactose metabolism. In R. M. Kliegman, J. W. St. Geme, N. J. Blum, et al. (Eds.), *Nelson textbook of pediatrics* (21st ed.). Philadelphia: Elsevier.

Kochanek, K. D., Murphy, S. L., & Xu, J. (2015). Deaths: Final data for 2011. *National Vital Statistics Reports, 63*(3), 1–120.

Kor, D., Yilmaz, B. S., Bulut, F. D., et al. (2017). Improved metabolic control in tetrahydrobiopterin (bh4), responsive phenylketonuria with sapropterin administered in two divided doses vs. a single daily dose. *The Journal of Pediatric Endocrinology and Metabolism, 30*(7), 713–718.

Lai, N. M., Ahmad, K. A., Choo, Y. M., et al. (2017). Fluid supplementation for neonatal unconjugated hyperbilirubinaemia (Review). *Cochrane Database Systematic Review*, No.: CD011891.

Lau, C. S., & Chamberlain, R. S. (2015). Probiotic administration can prevent necrotizing enterocolitis in preterm infants: A meta-analysis. *Journal of Pediatric Surgery, 50*.

Lawrence, R. A., & Lawrence, R. M. (2016a). *Breastfeeding infants with problems, Breastfeeding: A guide for the medical profession* (8th ed.). Philadelphia, PA: Elsevier.

Lawrence, R. A., & Lawrence, R. M. (2016b). *Premature infants and breastfeding, Breastfeeding: A guide for the medical profession* (8th ed.). Philadelphia, PA: Elsevier.

Lee, B. S., Hwang, L. S., Doumit, G. D., et al. (2017). Management options of non-syndromic sagittal craniosynostosis. *Journal of Clinical Neuroscience, 39*, 28–34.

Lemmon, M. E., Bidegain, M., & Boss, R. D. (2016). Palliative care in neonatal neurology: Robust support for infants, families and clinicians. *Journal of Perinatology, 36*, 331–337.

Lester, B. M., Tronick, E. Z., & Brazelton, T. B. (2004). The Neonatal Intensive Care Unit Network Neurobehavioral Scale procedures. *Pediatrics, 113*(3 Pt 2), 641–667.

Liao, G. J., Gronowski, A. M., & Zhao, Z. (2014). Non-invasive prenatal testing using cell-free fetal dna in maternal circulation. *Clinica Chimica Acta, 428*, 44–50.

Lindqvist, P. G., Ajne, G., Cooray, C., et al. (2014). Identification of pregnancies at increased risk of brachial plexus birth palsy—the construction of a weighted risk score. *The Journal of Maternal-Fetal and Neonatal Medicine, 27*(3), 252–256.

Liu, Y., Cromeens, B. P., Wang, Y., et al. (2018). Comparison of different in vivo incubation sites to produce tissue-engineered small intestines. *Tissue Engineering, 24*(13-14), 1138–1147.

Liu, M., Zhao, L., & Li, X. F. (2015). Effect of skin contact between mother and child in pain relief of full-term newborns during heel blood collection. *Clinical and Experimental Obstetrics & Gynecology, 42*(3), 304–308.

Liu, Y., Huang, X., Luo, B., et al. (2017). Effects of combined oral sucrose and nonnutritive sucking (nns) on procedural pain of NICU newborns, 2001 to 2016: A prisma-compliant systematic review and meta-analysis. *Medicine, 96*(6), 1–9.

Looker, K. J., Magaret, A. S., May, M. T., et al. (2017). First estimates of the global and regional incidence of neonatal herpes infection. *Lancet Glob Health, 5*(3), 300–309.

Lorenz, L., Marulli, A., Dawson, J. A., et al. (2018). Cerebral oxygenation during skin-to-skin care in preterm infants not receiving respiratory support. *Archives of Disease in Childhood, 103*(2), 137–142.

Lund, C. H., & Kuller, J. M. (2014). Integumentary system. In C. Kenner, & J. Lott (Eds.), *Comprehensive neonatal care: An interdisciplinary approach* (5th ed.). New York: Springer.

Lyu, Y., Shah, P. S., Ye, X. Y., et al. (2015). For the Canadian neonatal network: Association between admission temperature and mortality and major morbidity in preterm infants born at fewer than 33 weeks' gestation. *The Journal of the American Medical Association, 169*(4), 1–8.

Malcolm, W. (2015). *Beyond the NICU: Comprehensive care of the high-risk infant* (1st ed.). McGraw-Hill.

Malhotra, Y., Nzegwu, N., Harrington, J., et al. (2016). Identifying barriers to initiating minimal enteral feedings in very low birth weight infants: A mixed methods approach. *American Journal of Perinatology, 33*(1), 47–56.

Mangurten, H. H., Puppala, B. L., & Prazad, P. A. (2015). Birth injuries. In R. J. Martin, A. A. Fanaroff, & M. C. Walsh (Eds.), *Fanaroff and Martin's neonatal-perinatal medicine: Diseases of the fetus and infant* (10th ed.). St Louis: Elsevier/Mosby.

Manley, B. J., Owen, L. S., Hooper, S. B., et al. (2017). Towards evidence-based resuscitation of the newborn infant. *Lancet, 389*(10079), 1639–1648.

Marc-Aurele, K. L., & English, N. K. (2016). Primary palliative care in neonatal intensive care. *Seminars in Perinatology*, 1–7.

Markham, K. B., & Fanaroff, A. A. (2015). Obstetric management of prematurity. In R. J. Martin, A. A. Fanaroff, & M. C. Walsh (Eds.), *Fanaroff and martin's neonatal-perinatal medicine: Diseases of the fetus and infant* (10th ed.). St Louis: Elsevier/Mosby.

Martin, K. L. (2020). Vascular disorders. In R. M. Kliegman, J. W. St. Geme, N. J. Blum, et al. (Eds.), *Nelson textbook of pediatrics* (21st ed.). Philadelphia: Elsevier.

Maree, C., & Downes, F. (2016). Trends in family-centered care in neonatal intensive care. *The Journal of Perinatal and Neonatal Nursing, 30*(3), 265–269.

McCall, E. M., Alderdice, F. A., Halliday, H. L., et al. (2014). Challenges of minimizing heat loss at birth: A narrative overview of evidence-based thermal interventions. *Newborn and Infant Nursing Reviews, 14* 56–53.

McCance, K., & Huether, S. (2010). *Pathophysiology: The biological basis for disease in infants and children* (6th ed.). St Louis: Mosby/Elsevier.

McCarty, D. B., O'Donnell, S., Goldstein, R. F., et al. (2018). Use of a midliner positioning system for prevention of dolichocephaly in preterm infants. *Pediatric Physical Therapy, 30*(2), 126–134.

McCarty, D. B., Peat, J. R., Malcolm, W. F., et al. (2017). Dolichocephaly in preterm infants: Prevalence, risk factors, and early outcomes. *The American Journal of Perinatology, 34*(4), 372–378.

Mikati, M. A., & Tchapjnikov, D. (2020). Neonatal seizures. In R. M. Kliegman, J. W. St. Geme, N. J. Blum, et al. (Eds.), *Nelson textbook of pediatrics* (21st ed.). Philadelphia: Elsevier.

Minnes, S., Singer, L., Min, M. O., et al. (2014). Effects of prenatal cocaine/polydrug exposure on substance use by age 15. *Drugs Alcohol Dependence, 134*, 201–210.

Moise, K. J. (2017). Red cell alloimmunization. In S. G. Gabbe, J. R. Niebyl, & K. L. Simpson (Eds.), *Obstetrics: Normal and problem pregnancies* (7th ed.). London: Churchill Livingstone.

Muchowski, K. E. (2014). Evaluation and treatment of neonatal hyperbilirubinemia. *American Family Physician, 89*(11), 873–878.

Mukhopadhyay, S., & Puopolo, K. M. (2017). Clinical and microbiologic characteristics of early-onset sepsis among very low birth weight infants: Opportunities for antibiotic stewardship. *Pediatric Infectious Diseases, 36*(5), 477–481.

Natarajan, G., & Shankaran, S. (2016). Short- and long-term outcomes of moderate and late preterm infants. *American Journal of Perinatology, 33*(3), 305–317.

Niss, O., & Ware, R. E. (2020). Hemolytic disease of the newborn: Erythroblastosis fetalis. In R. M. Kliegman, J. W. St. Geme, N. J. Blum, et al. (Eds.), *Nelson textbook of pediatrics* (21st ed.). Philadelphia: Elsevier.

Nour, I., Eldegla, H. E., Nasef, N., et al. (2017). Risk factors and clinical outcomes for carbapenem-resistant gram-negative late-onselt sepsis in a neonatal intensive care unit. *The International Journal of Infectious Diseases, 97*(1), 52–58.

Nyp, M., Brunkhorst, J. L., Reavey, D., et al. (2016). Fluid and electrolyte management. In S. L. Gardner, B. S. Carter, M. Enzman-Hines, et al. (Eds.), *Merenstein & Gardner's handbook of neonatal intensive care* (8th ed.). St. Louis: ELSEVIER.

Office of AIDS Research Advisory Council. (2014). *Recommendations for use of antiretroviral drugs in pregnant hiv-1-infected women for maternal health and interventions to reduce perinatal hiv transmission in the United States*. http://aidsinfo.nih.gov/Guidelines/HTML/3/perinatal_guidelines/0/.

Oh, S., Salas-Wright, C. P., Vaughn, M. G., et al. (2017). Marijuana use during pregnancy: A comparison of trends and correlated among married and unmarried pregnant women. *Drug and Alcohol Dependence, 12*(1), 229–233.

Pammi, M., & Suresh, G. (2017). Enteral lactoferrin supplementation for prevention of sepsis and necrotizing enterocolitis in preterm infants. *Cochrane Database Sytematic Reviews, 28*(6), CD007137.

Pammi, M., Brand, M. C., & Weisman, L. E. (2016). Infection in the neonate. In S. L. Gardner, B. S. Carter, M. Enzman-Hines, et al. (Eds.), *Merenstein & Gardner's handbook of neonatal intensive care* (8th ed.). St. Louis: Mosby.

Pammi, M., Flores, A., Versalovic, J., et al. (2017). Molecular assays for the diagnosis of sepsis in neonates. *Cochrane Database Sytematic Reviews, 25*(2), CD011926.

Parcianello, R. R., Mardini, V., Cereser, K. M., et al. (2018). Increased cocaine and amphetamine-regulated transcript cord blood levels in the newborns exposed to crack cocaine in utero. *Psychopharmacology, 235*(1), 215–222.

Parker, L. A., Withers, J. H., & Talaga, E. (2018). Comparison of neonatal nursing practices for determining feeding tube insertion length and verifying gastric placement with current best evidence. *Advances in Neonatal Care, 18*(4), 307–317.

Parsons, J. A., Seay, A. R., & Jacobson, M. (2016). Neurologic disorders. In S. L. Gardner, B. S. Carter, M. Enzman Hines, et al. (Eds.), *Merenstein and Gardner's handbook of neonatal intensive care* (8th ed.). St Louis: Mosby/Elsevier.

Poindexter, B., & Ehrenkranz, R. A. (2015). Nutrient requirements and provision of nutritional support in the premature infant. In R. J. Martin, A. A. Fanaroff, & M. C. Walsh (Eds.), *Neonatal-perinatal medicine: Diseases of the fetus and infant* (10th ed.). St Louis: Elsevier.

Polin, R. A., Carlo, W. A., & American Academy of Pediatrics, & Committee on Fetus and Newborn. (2014). Surfactant-replacement therapy for preterm and term neonates with respiratory distress. *Pediatrics, 133*(1), 156–163.

Radmacher, P. G., & Adamkin, D. H. (2017). Fortification of human milk for preterm infants. *Seminars in Fetal & Neonatal Medicine, 22*(1), 30–35.

Rayfield, S., Oakley, L., & Quigley, M. A. (2015). Association between breastfeeding support and breastfeeding rates in the UK: A comparison of late preterm and term infants. *BMJ Open, 5*(11), 1–10.

Reedy, N. J. (2014). Preterm labor and birth. In K. R. Simpson (Ed.), *Perinatal nursing* (4th ed.). Philadelphia: Lippincott Williams & Wilkins.

Resch, B., Renoldner, B., & Hofer, N. (2016). Comparison between pathogen associated laboratory and clinical parameters in early-onset sepsis of the newborn. *The Open Microbiology Journal, 10*, 133–139.

Reilly, S., Reid, J., Skeat, J., & The Academy of Breastfeeding Medicinew. (2013). ABM clinical protocol #17: Guidelines for breastfeeding infants with cleft lip, cleft palate, or cleft lip and palate, revised 2013. *Breastfeeding Medicine, 8*(4), 349–353.

Rey-Santano, C., Meilgo, V. E., López-de-Heredia-y-Goya, J., et al. (2016). Cerebral effect of intratracheal aerosolized surfactant versus bolus therapy in preterm lambs. *Critical Care Medicine* (44), 218–226 4.

Roland, E., & Hill, A. (2016). Neurologic problems of the newborn. In R. B. Daroff, G. M. Fenichel, J. Jankovic, et al. (Eds.), *Neurology in clinical practice* (7th ed.). Philadelphia: Elsevier/Saunders.

Ross, E. J., Graham, D. L., Money, K. M., et al. (2015). Developmental consequences of fetal exposure to drugs: What we know and what we still must learn. *Neuropsychopharmacology, 40*, 61–87.

Rövekamp-Abels, L. W., Hogewind-Schoonenboom, J. E., de Wijs-Meijler, D. P., et al. (2015). Intermittent bolus or semicontinuous feeding for preterm infants? *Journal of Pediatric Gastroenterology and Nutrition, 61*(6), 659–664.

Sainio, S., Nupponen, I., Kuosmanen, M., et al. (2015). Diagnosis and treatment of severe hemolytic disease of the fetus and newborn: A 10-year nationwide retrospective study. *Acta Obstetricia et Gynecologica Scandinavica, 94*(4), 383–390.

Salzwedel, A. P., Grewen, K. M., Goldman, B. D., et al. (2016). Thalamocortical functional connectivity and behavioral disruptions in neonates with prenatal cocaine exposure. *Neurotoxicology and Teratology, 56*, 16–25.

Shabuj, M. H., Hossain, J., & Dey, S. (2019). Accuracy of transcutaneous bilirubinometry in the preterm infants: A comprehensive meta-analysis. *The Journal of Maternal-Fetal and Neonatal Medicine, 32*(5), 734–741.

Shaughnessy, E. E., & Goyal, N. K. (2020a). Jaundice and hyperbilirubinemia in the newborn. In R. M. Kliegman, J. W. St. Geme, N. J. Blum, et al. (Eds.), *Nelson textbook of pediatrics* (21st ed.). Philadelphia: Elsevier.

Shaughnessy, E. E., & Goyal, N. K. (2020b). Kernicterus. In R. M. Kliegman, J. W. St. Geme, N. J. Blum, et al. (Eds.), *Nelson textbook of pediatrics* (21st ed.). Philadelphia: Elsevier.

Shchelochkov, O. A., & Venditti, C. P. (2020). Defects in metabolism of amino acids. In R. M. Kliegman, J. W. St. Geme, N. J. Blum, et al. (Eds.), *Nelson textbook of pediatrics* (21st ed.). Philadelphia: Elsevier.

Sheanon, N. M., & Muglia, L. J. (2020). The endocrine system. In R. M. Kliegman, J. W. St. Geme, N. J. Blum, et al. (Eds.), *Nelson textbook of pediatrics* (21st ed.). Philadelphia: Elsevier.

Sherman, J. (2015). Perinatal substance abuse. In M. T. Verklan, & M. Walden (Eds.), *Core curriculum for neonatal intensive care nursing* (5th ed.). St Louis: Saunders/Elsevier.

Singer, L. T., Minnes, S., Min, M. O., et al. (2015). Prenatal cocaine exposure and child outcomes: A conference report based on a prospective study from Cleveland. *Human Psychopharmacology, 30*, 285–289.

Soltanizadeh, N., & Mirmoghtadaie, L. (2014). Strategies used in production of phenylalanine-free foods for pku management. *Comprehensive Reviews in Food Science and Food Safety, 13*(3), 287–299.

Sperling, M. A. (2020). Hypoglycemia. In R. M. Kliegman, J. W. St. Geme, N. J. Blum, et al. (Eds.), *Nelson textbook of pediatrics* (21st ed.). Philadelphia: Elsevier.

Steele, C. (2018). Best practices for handling and administration of expressed human milk and donor human milk for hospitalized preterm infants. *Frontiers in Nutrition, 3*(5), 1–5.

Stokowski, L. A. (2014). Endocrine system. In C. Kenner, & J. Lott (Eds.), *Comprehensive neonatal care: An interdisciplinary approach* (5th ed.). New York: Springer.

Tappero, E. (2015). Musculoskeletal system assessment. In E. Tappero, & M. A. Honeyfield (Eds.), *Physical assessment of the newborn* (5th ed.). Petaluma, CA: NICU Ink.

Taylor, S. J., Allan, K., McWilliam, H., et al. (2014). Nasogastric tube depth: the 'NEX' guideline is incorrect. *British Journal of Nursing, 23*(12), 641–644.

Tieu, J., McPhee, A. J., Crowther, C. A., et al. (2017). Screening for gestational diabetes mellitus based on different risk profiles and settings for improving maternal and infant health. *Cochrane Database System Reviews, 3*(8), CD007222.

Uberos, J., Aguilera-Rodríguez, E., Jerez-Calero, A., et al. (2017). Probiotics to prevent encrotising enterocolities and nosocomial infection in very low birth weight preterm infants. *British Journal of Nutrition, 117*(7), 994–1000.

Valdivielso-Ramos, M., Torrelo, A., Martin-Santiago, A., et al. (2018). Infantile hemangioma with minimal or arrested growth as the skin manifestation of phace syndrome. *Pediatric Dermatology, 35*(5), 622–627.

Vento, M. (2015). Oxygen therapy. In R. J. Martin, A. A. Fanaroff, & M. C. Walsh (Eds.), *Fanaroff and Martin's neonatal-perinatal medicine: Diseases of the fetus and infant* (10th ed.). St Louis: Elsevier/Mosby.

Waite, W. M., & Taylor, J. A. (2016). Phototherapy for the treatment of neonatal jaundice and breastfeeding duration and exclusivity. *Breastfeeding Medicine, 11*(4), 180–185.

Wallace, T., & Steward, D. (2014). Gastric tube use and care in the NICU. *Newborn & Infant Nursing Review* (14), 103–108.

Weiner, G. M., & Zaichkin, J. (2015). *Textbook of Neonatal Resuscitation* (7th ed.). American Academy of Pediatrics and the American Heart Association.

Weiner, S. M., & Finnegan, L. P. (2016). Drug withdrawal in the neonate. In S. L. Gardner, B. S. Carter, M. Enzman-Hines, et al. (Eds.), *Merenstein and Gardner's handbook of neonatal intensive care* (8th ed.). St Louis: Mosby/Elsevier.

Weitzman, C. (2020). Fetal alcohol exposure. In R. M. Kliegman, J. W. St. Geme, N. J. Blum, et al. (Eds.), *Nelson textbook of pediatrics* (21st ed.). Philadelphia: Elsevier.

Whetten, C. H. (2016). Cue-based feeding in the NICU. *Nursing for Womens Health, 20*(5), 507–510.

Wilson, E., Maier, R. F., Norman, M., et al. (2016). Admission hypothermia in very preterm infants and neonatal mortality and morbidity. *The Journal of Pediatrics, 175*, 61–67.

Witt, C. (2015). Skin assessment. In E. P. Tappero, & M. E. Honeyfield (Eds.), *Physical assessment of the newborn* (5th ed.). Santa Rosa, CA: NICU Ink.

Wright, T. E., Schuetter, R., Tellei, J., et al. (2015). Methamphetamines and pregnancy outcomes. *Journal Addict Medicine, 9*(2), 111–117.

Wyckoff, M. H., Aziz, K., Escobedo, M. B., et al. (2015). Part 13: Neonatal resuscitation, 2015 American Heart Association guidelines update for cardiopulmonary resuscitation and emergency cardiovascular care. *Circulation, 132*(18 Suppl. 2), 543–560.

Yang, L. J. S. (2014). Neonatal brachial plexus palsy—management and prognostic factors. *Seminars in Perinatology, 38*(4), 222–234.

Young, L., Embleton, N. D., & McGuire, W. (2016). Nutrient-enriched formula versus standard formula for preterm infants following hospital discharge. *The Cochrane Database of Systematic Reviews* (12), CD004696.

Zahorodny, W., Rom, C., Whitney, W., et al. (1998). The neonatal withdrawal inventory: A simplified score of newborn withdrawal. *The Journal of Developmental & Behavioral Pediatrics, 19*(2), 89–93.

Zaichkin, J. (2017). Part 15: Neonatal resuscitation: American Heart Association guidelines for cardiopulmonary resuscitation and emergency cardiovascular care. *Circulation, 122*(18 Suppl. 3), S909–S919.

Zaichkin, J., Weiner, G., & Loren, D. J. (2017). *Understanding the NICU: What parents of preemies and other hospitalized newborns need to know know.* Elk Grove, IL: American Academy of Pediatrics.

Zhao, X., Liu, Q., Cao, S., et al. (2018). A meta-analysis of selective serotonin reuptake inhibitors (SSRIs) use during prenatal depression and risk of low birth weight and small for gestational age. *The Journal of Affective Disorders, 12*(1), 563–570.

Zullino, S., & Simoncini, T. (2018). Impact of selective serotonin reuptake inhibitors (SSRIs) during pregnancy and lactation: A focus on short and long-term vascular effects. *Vascular Pharmacology, 108*, 74–76.

Zwiers, C., Scheffer-Rath, M. E. A., Lopriore, E., et al. (2018). Immuniglobulin for alloimmune hemolytic disease in neonate. *The Cochrane Database of Systematic Reviews* (3), CD003313.

9

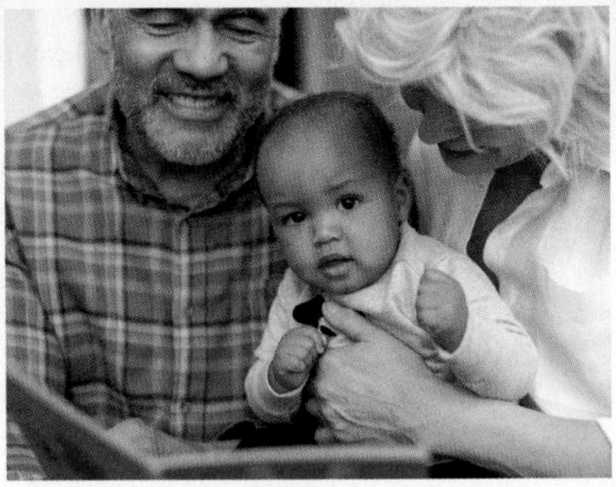

Health Promotion of the Infant and Family

R. Elizabeth Fisher

http://evolve.elsevier.com/wong/essentials

CONCEPTS

- Development
- Functional Ability
- Nutrition
- Safety

PROMOTING OPTIMAL GROWTH AND DEVELOPMENT

BIOLOGIC DEVELOPMENT

At no other time in life are physical changes and developmental achievements as dramatic as during infancy. All major body systems undergo progressive maturation, and there is concurrent development of skills that increasingly allow infants to respond to and cope with the environment. Acquisition of these fine and gross motor skills occurs in an orderly head-to-toe and center-to-periphery (cephalocaudal-proximodistal) sequence.

Proportional Changes

During the first year of life, especially the initial 6 months, growth is very rapid. Infants gain 150 to 210 g (≈5 to 7 oz) weekly until they are approximately 5 to 6 months old, which is when the birth weight has at least doubled. An average weight for a 6-month-old child is 7.3 kg (16 pounds). Weight gain slows during the second 6 months. By 1 year old, the infant's birth weight has tripled, for an average weight of 9.75 kg (21.5 pounds). Infants who are breastfed beyond 4 to 6 months old typically gain less weight than those who are bottle-fed, yet their head circumference is more than adequate. There is evidence that breastfed infants tend to self-regulate energy intake. This self-regulation of intake with breastfeeding (vs. formula [bottle] feeding) is believed to have further significance in the development of childhood obesity and subsequent cardiovascular disease (Fewtrell, 2011). Researchers also found that infants who were breastfed in early infancy were more likely to regulate their appetite in late infancy and childhood than infants who were bottle-fed (DiSantis, Collins, Fisher, et al., 2011).

Height increases by 2.5 cm (1 inch) a month during the first 6 months of life and also slows during the second 6 months. Increases in length occur in sudden spurts rather than in a slow, gradual pattern. The average height is 65 cm (25.5 inches) at 6 months old and 74 cm (29 inches) at 12 months old. By 1 year old, the birth length has increased by almost 50%. This increase occurs mainly in the trunk rather than in the legs and contributes to the characteristic physique of the infant.

Head growth is also rapid. Head circumference increases approximately 2 cm (0.75 inch) per month for the first 3 months, then 1 cm (0.4 inch) per month from 4 to 6 months; then the rate of growth declines to only 0.5 cm (0.2 inch) per month during the second 6 months. The average size is 43 cm (17 inches) at 6 months and 46 cm (18 inches) at 12 months. By 1 year, head size has increased by almost 33%. Closure of the cranial sutures occurs, with the posterior fontanel fusing by 6 to 8 weeks old and the anterior fontanel closing by 12 to 18 months old (average, 14 months old).

Expanding head size reflects the growth and differentiation of the nervous system. By the end of the first year, the brain has increased in weight about 2.5 times. Maturation of the brain is exhibited in the dramatic developmental achievements of infancy (Table 9.1). Primitive reflexes are replaced by voluntary, purposeful movement, and new reflexes that influence motor development appear.

The chest assumes a more adult contour, with the lateral diameter becoming larger than the anteroposterior diameter. The chest circumference approximately equals the head circumference by the end of the first year. The heart grows less rapidly than does the rest of the body. Its weight is usually doubled by 1 year old in comparison with body weight, which triples during the same period. The size of the heart is still large in relation to the chest cavity; its width is approximately 55% of the chest width.

It is important to note that genetic, metabolic, environmental, and nutritional factors strongly influence infant growth; thus the previous statements are general guidelines only. Use the appropriate infant growth charts reflecting weight for length and head circumference in each case to determine appropriate growth parameters. The World Health Organization growth charts released in 2006 are now recommended as reference growth charts in children 0 to 59 months old (Turck, Michaelsen, Shamir, et al., 2013).

TABLE 9.1 Growth and Development During Infancy

Physical	Gross Motor	Fine Motor	Sensory	Vocalization	Socialization and Cognition
1 Month Old					
Weight gain of 150-210 g (5-7 oz) weekly for first 6 months Height gain of 2.5 cm (1 inch) monthly for first 6 months Head circumference increases by 1.5 cm (0.5 inch) monthly for first 6 months Primitive reflexes present and strong Doll's eye reflex and dance reflex fading Obligatory nose breathing (most infants)	• Assumes flexed position with pelvis high but knees not under abdomen when prone (at birth, knees flexed under abdomen) • Can turn head from side to side when prone; lifts head momentarily from bed (see Fig. 9.3A) Has marked head lag, especially when pulled from lying to sitting position (see Fig. 9.2A) Holds head momentarily parallel and in midline when suspended in prone position Assumes asymmetric tonic neck flex position when supine When held in standing position, body is limp at knees and hips In sitting position, back is uniformly rounded, with absence of head control	Hands predominantly closed Grasp reflex strong Hand clenches on contact with rattle	• Able to fixate on moving object in range of 45 degrees when held at a distance of 20-25 cm (8-10 inches) Visual acuity approaches 20/100[a] Follows light to midline Quiets when hears a voice	Cries to express displeasure Makes small, throaty sounds Makes comfort sounds during feeding	Is in sensorimotor phase—stage I, use of reflexes (birth to 1 month old), and stage II, primary circular reactions (1-4 months old) Watches parent's face intently as she or he talks to infant
2 Months Old					
Posterior fontanel closed Crawling reflex disappears	• Assumes less flexed position when prone—hips flat, legs extended, arms flexed, head to side Less head lag when pulled to sitting position (see Fig. 9.2B) Can maintain head in same plane as rest of body when held in ventral suspension When prone, can lift head almost 45 degrees off table When moved to sitting position, head is held up but bends forward (see Fig. 9.5B) Assumes symmetric tonic neck position intermittently	Hands often open Grasp reflex fading	Binocular fixation and convergence to near objects beginning When supine, follows dangling toy from side to point beyond midline Visually searches to locate sounds Turns head to side when sound is made at level of ear	• Vocalizes, distinct from crying Crying becomes differentiated Coos Vocalizes to familiar voice	• Demonstrates social smile in response to various stimuli
3 Months Old					
Primitive reflexes fading	Able to hold head more erect when sitting but still bobs forward Has only slight head lag when pulled to sitting position Assumes symmetric body positioning Able to raise head and shoulders from prone position to a 45- to 90-degree angle from table; bears weight on forearms When held in standing position, able to bear slight fraction of weight on legs Regards own hand	• Actively holds rattle but will not reach for it Grasp reflex absent Hands kept loosely open Clutches own hand; pulls at blankets and clothes	• Follows objects to periphery (180 degrees) • Locates sound by turning head to side and looking in same direction Begins to have ability to coordinate stimuli from various sense organs	• Squeals aloud to show pleasure Coos, babbles, chuckles Vocalizes when smiling "Talks" a great deal when spoken to Less crying during periods of wakefulness	Displays considerable interest in surroundings Ceases crying when parent enters room Can recognize familiar faces and objects, such as feeding bottle Shows awareness of strange situations

Continued

TABLE 9.1 Growth and Development During Infancy—cont'd

Physical	Gross Motor	Fine Motor	Sensory	Vocalization	Socialization and Cognition
4 Months Old					
Drooling begins Moro, tonic neck, and rooting reflexes have disappeared	• Has almost no head lag when pulled to sitting position (see Fig. 9.2C) • Balances head well in sitting position (see Fig. 9.5C) Back less rounded, curved only in lumbar area Able to sit erect if propped up Able to raise head and chest off surface to angle of 90 degrees (see Fig. 9.3B) Assumes predominant symmetric position • Rolls from back to side	• Inspects and plays with hands; pulls clothing or blanket over face in play Tries to reach objects with hand but overshoots Grasps object with both hands Plays with rattle placed in hand and shakes it but cannot pick it up if dropped Can carry objects to mouth	Able to accommodate to near objects Binocular vision fairly well established Can focus on a 1.25-cm (0.5-inch) block Beginning eye–hand coordination	Makes consonant sounds *n, k, g, p, b* • Laughs aloud Vocalization changes according to mood	Is in stage III, secondary circular reactions Demands attention by fussing; becomes bored if left alone Enjoys social interaction with people Anticipates feeding when sees bottle or mother if breast-feeding Shows excitement with whole body, squeals, breathes heavily Shows interest in strange stimuli Begins to show memory
5 Months Old					
Beginning signs of tooth eruption Birth weight doubles	No head lag when pulled to sitting position When sitting, able to hold head erect and steady Able to sit for longer periods when back is well supported Back straight When prone, assumes symmetric positioning with arms extended • Can turn over from abdomen to back When supine, puts feet to mouth	• Able to grasp objects voluntarily Uses palmar grasp, bi-dextrous approach Plays with toes Takes objects directly to mouth Holds one cube while regarding a second one	Visually pursues a dropped object Is able to sustain visual inspection of an object Can localize sounds made below ear	Squeals Makes cooing vowel sounds interspersed with consonant sounds (e.g., *ah-goo*)	Smiles at mirror image Pats bottle or breast with both hands More enthusiastically playful but may have rapid mood swings Is able to discriminate strangers from family Vocalizes displeasure when object is taken away Discovers parts of body
6 Months Old					
Growth rate may begin to decline Weight gain of 90-150 g (3-5 oz) weekly for next 6 months Height gain of 1.25 cm (0.5 inch) monthly for next 6 months • Teething may begin with eruption of two lower central incisors • Chewing and biting occur	When prone, can lift chest and upper abdomen off surface, bearing weight on hands (see Fig. 9.3C) When about to be pulled to a sitting position, lifts head Sits in high chair with back straight Rolls from back to abdomen When held in standing position, bears almost all of weight Hand regard absent	Re-secures a dropped object Drops one cube when another is given Grasps and manipulates small objects Holds bottle Grasps feet and pulls to mouth	Adjusts posture to see an object Prefers more complex visual stimuli Can localize sounds made above ear Will turn head to the side and then look up or down	• Begins to imitate sounds • Babbling resembles one-syllable utterances—*ma, mu, da, di, hi* Vocalizes to toys, mirror image Takes pleasure in hearing own sounds (self-reinforcement)	Recognizes parents; begins to fear strangers Holds arms out to be picked up Has definite likes and dislikes Begins to imitate (cough, protrusion of tongue) Excites on hearing footsteps • Briefly searches for a dropped object (object permanence beginning) Frequent mood swings, from crying to laughing, with little or no provocation
7 Months Old					
Eruption of upper central incisors	When supine, spontaneously lifts head off surface • Sits, leaning forward on both hands (see Fig. 9.5D) When prone, bears weight on one hand Sits erect momentarily Bears full weight on feet (see Fig. 9.6A) When held in standing position, bounces actively	• Transfers objects from one hand to the other (see Fig. 9.5E) Has unidextrous approach and grasp Holds two cubes more than momentarily Bangs cubes on table Rakes at a small object	• Can fixate on very small objects Responds to own name Localizes sound by turning head in a curving arch Beginning awareness of depth and space Has taste preferences	• Produces vowel sounds and chained syllables—*baba, dada, kaka* Vocalizes four distinct vowel sounds "Talks" when others are talking	• Increasing fear of strangers; shows signs of fretfulness when parent disappears Imitates simple acts and noises Tries to attract attention by coughing or snorting Plays peek-a-boo Demonstrates dislike of food by keeping lips closed Exhibits oral aggressiveness in biting and mouthing Demonstrates expectation in response to repetition of stimuli

TABLE 9.1 Growth and Development During Infancy—cont'd

Physical	Gross Motor	Fine Motor	Sensory	Vocalization	Socialization and Cognition
8 Months Old					
Begins to show regular patterns in bladder and bowel elimination Parachute reflex appears (see Fig. 9.4)	• Sits steadily unsupported (see Fig. 9.5E) Readily bears weight on legs when supported; may stand holding on to furniture Adjusts posture to reach an object	Has beginning pincer grasp using index, fourth, and fifth fingers against lower part of thumb Releases objects at will Rings bell purposely Retains two cubes while regarding third cube Secures an object by pulling on a string Reaches persistently for toys out of reach		Makes consonant sounds *t, d, w* Listens selectively to familiar words Utterances signal emphasis and emotion Combines syllables, such as *dada,* but does not ascribe meaning to them	Increasing anxiety over loss of parent, particularly mother, and fear of strangers Responds to word "no" Dislikes dressing, diaper change
9 Months Old					
Eruption of upper lateral incisor may begin	Creeps on hands and knees Sits steadily on floor for prolonged time (10 minutes) Recovers balance when leaning forward but cannot do so when leaning sideways • Pulls self to standing position and stands holding on to furniture (see Fig. 9.6B and C)	• Uses thumb and index finger in crude pincer grasp (see Fig. 9.1) Preference for use of dominant hand now evident Grasps third cube Compares two cubes by bringing them together	Localizes sounds by turning head diagonally and directly toward sound Depth perception increasing	Responds to simple verbal commands Comprehends "no-no"	Parent (mother) is increasingly important for own sake Shows increasing interest in pleasing parent Begins to show fears of going to bed and being left alone Puts arms in front of face to avoid having it washed
10 Months Old					
Labyrinth-righting reflex is strongest when infant is in prone or supine position; is able to raise head	Can change from prone to sitting position Stands while holding on to furniture; sits by falling down Recovers balance easily while sitting While standing, lifts one foot to take a step (see Fig. 9.6D)	Crude release of an object beginning Grasps bell by handle		• Says "dada," "mama" with meaning Comprehends "bye-bye" May say one word (e.g., "hi," "bye," "no")	Inhibits behavior to verbal command of "no-no" or own name Imitates facial expressions; waves bye-bye Extends toy to another person but will not release it • Develops object permanence Repeats actions that attract attention and cause laughter Pulls clothes of another to attract attention Plays interactive games, such as pat-a-cake Reacts to adult anger; cries when scolded Demonstrates independence in dressing, feeding, locomotive skills, and testing of parents Looks at and follows picture in a book

Continued

TABLE 9.1 Growth and Development During Infancy—cont'd

Physical	Gross Motor	Fine Motor	Sensory	Vocalization	Socialization and Cognition
11 Months Old					
Eruption of lower lateral incisor may begin	When sitting, pivots to reach toward back to pick up an object • Cruises or walks holding on to furniture or with both hands held	Explores objects more thoroughly (e.g., clapper inside bell) Has neat pincer grasp Drops object deliberately for it to be picked up Puts one object after another into a container (sequential play) Able to manipulate an object to remove it from tight-fitting enclosure		Imitates definite speech sounds	Experiences joy and satisfaction when a task is mastered Reacts to restrictions with frustration Rolls ball to another on request Anticipates body gestures when a familiar nursery rhyme or story is being told (e.g., holds toes and feet in response to "This little piggy went to market") Plays games up-down, "so big," or peek-a-boo Shakes head for "no"
12 Months Old					
• Birth weight tripled • Birth length increased by 50% Head and chest circumference equal (head circumference 46 cm [18 inches]) Has six to eight deciduous teeth Anterior fontanel almost closed Landau reflex fading Babinski reflex disappears Lumbar curve develops; lordosis evident during walking	• Walks with one hand held Cruises well • May attempt to stand alone momentarily; may attempt first step alone Can sit down from standing position without help	Releases cube in cup Attempts to build two-block tower but fails Tries to insert a pellet into a narrow-necked bottle but fails Can turn pages in a book, many at a time	Discriminates simple geometric forms (e.g., circle) Amblyopia may develop with lack of binocularity Can follow rapidly moving object Controls and adjusts response to sound; listens for sound to recur	• Says three to five words besides "dada," "mama" Comprehends meaning of several words (comprehension always precedes verbalization) Recognizes objects by name Imitates animal sounds Understands simple verbal commands (e.g., "Give it to me," "Show me your eyes")	Shows emotions, such as jealousy, affection (may hug or kiss on request), anger, fear Enjoys familiar surroundings and explores away from parent Is fearful in strange situation; clings to parent May develop habit of "security blanket" or favorite toy Has increasing determination to practice locomotor skills • Searches for an object even if it has not been hidden but searches only where object was last seen

•Milestones that represent essential integrative aspects of development that lay the foundation for the achievement of more advanced skills.
[a]Degree of visual acuity varies according to vision measurement procedure used.

Maturation of Systems

Other organ systems also change and grow during infancy. The respiratory rate slows somewhat and is relatively stable. Respiratory movements continue to be abdominal. Several factors predispose infants to more severe and acute respiratory problems than older children. The close proximity of the trachea to the bronchi and its branching structures rapidly transmits infectious agents from one anatomic location to another. The short, straight eustachian tube closely communicates with the ear, allowing infection to ascend from the pharynx to the middle ear. In addition, the inability of the immune system to produce immunoglobulin A (IgA) in the mucosal lining provides less protection against infection in infancy than during later childhood.

The heart rate slows, and the rhythm is often **sinus arrhythmia** (rate increases with inspiration and decreases with expiration). Blood pressure also changes during infancy. Systolic pressure rises during the first 2 months as a result of the increasing ability of the left ventricle to pump blood into the systemic circulation. Diastolic pressure decreases during the first 3 months and then gradually rises to values close to those at birth. Fluctuations in blood pressure occur during varying states of activity and emotion.

Significant **hematopoietic changes** occur during the first year of life. Fetal hemoglobin (HgbF) is present for the first 5 months, with adult hemoglobin steadily increasing through the first half of infancy. Fetal hemoglobin results in a shortened survival of red blood cells (RBCs) and thus a decreased number of RBCs. A common result at 3 to 6 months old is **physiologic anemia**. High levels of fetal hemoglobin depress the production of erythropoietin, a hormone released by the kidneys that stimulates RBC production.

Maternally derived iron stores are present for the first 5 to 6 months of life and gradually diminish, which also accounts for lowered hemoglobin levels toward the end of the first 6 months. The occurrence of physiologic anemia is not affected by an adequate supply of iron. However, when erythropoiesis is stimulated, iron stores are necessary for the formation of hemoglobin.

The digestive processes are relatively immature at birth. Although term newborn infants have some limitations in digestive function, human milk has properties that partially compensate for decreased digestive enzymatic activity, thus enabling breastfed infants to receive optimal nutrition during the first several months of life. The enzyme amylase (also called *ptyalin*) is present in small amounts but usually has little effect on the foodstuffs because of the small amount of time the food stays in the mouth. Gastric digestion in the stomach consists primarily of the action of hydrochloric acid and rennin, an enzyme that acts specifically on the casein in milk to cause the formation of **curds**—coagulated semisolid particles of milk. The curds cause the milk to be retained in the stomach long enough for digestion to occur.

Digestion also takes place in the duodenum, where pancreatic enzymes and bile begin to break down protein and fat. Secretion of the pancreatic enzyme **amylase**, which is needed for digestion of complex carbohydrates, is deficient until about the fourth to sixth month of life. **Lipase** is also limited, and infants do not achieve adult levels of fat absorption until 4 to 5 months old. **Trypsin** is secreted in sufficient quantities to catabolize protein into polypeptides and some amino acids.

The immaturity of the digestive processes is evident in the appearance of stools. During infancy, solid foods (e.g., peas, carrots, corn, raisins) are passed incompletely broken down in the feces. An excess quantity of fiber easily disposes infants to loose, bulky stools.

During infancy, the stomach enlarges to accommodate a greater volume of food. By the end of the first year, infants are able to tolerate three meals a day and an evening bottle and may have one or two bowel movements daily. However, with any type of gastric irritation, infants are vulnerable to diarrhea, vomiting, and dehydration (see Chapter 22).

The liver is the most immature of all the gastrointestinal organs throughout infancy. The ability to conjugate bilirubin and secrete bile is achieved after the first couple of weeks of life. However, the capacities for gluconeogenesis, formation of plasma protein and ketones, storage of vitamins, and deaminization of amino acids remain relatively immature for the first year of life.

Maturation of the sucking, swallowing, and breathing reflexes and the eruption of teeth (see the Teething section later in the chapter) parallel the changes in the gastrointestinal tract and prepare infants for the introduction of solid foods.

The immunologic system undergoes numerous changes during the first year. Full-term newborns receive significant amounts of maternal immunoglobulin G (IgG), which for approximately 3 months confers immunity against antigens to which their mothers were exposed. During this time, infants begin to synthesize IgG but in limited amounts. Approximately 40% of adult levels are reached by 1 year old; therefore infants are at higher risk for infection during the first 12 months of life. Significant amounts of immunoglobulin M (IgM) are produced at birth, and adult levels are reached by 9 months old. Prebiotic oligosaccharides found in breast milk produce probiotic bacteria such as bifidobacteria and lactobacilli, which in turn stimulate synthesis and secretion of secretory IgA. Secretory IgA is present in large amounts in colostrum; IgA confers protection to the mucous membranes of the gastrointestinal tract (Durand, Ochoa, Bellomo, et al., 2013) against many bacteria, such as *Escherichia coli,* and viruses such as rubella, poliovirus, and the enteroviruses. The development of the mucosa-associated lymphoid tissue occurs during infancy; in part, this system is believed to prevent colonization and passage of bacteria across the infant's mucosal barrier. The function and quantity of T lymphocytes, lymphokines, interferon-γ, interleukins, tumor necrosis factor–α, and complement are reduced in early infancy, thus preventing optimal response to certain bacteria and viruses. The production of IgA and immunoglobulins D and E (IgD and IgE) is much more gradual, and maximum levels are not attained until early childhood. **Probiotics** may have a significant role in helping the gastrointestinal tract establish a "good" bacterial colonization in the gut to prevent many illnesses, including antibiotic-induced diarrhea and possibly *Helicobacter pylori* gastritis (Szajewska, Canani, Guarino, et al., 2016; Yu, Liu, Chang, et al., 2015).

Evidence indicates that **vernix caseosa**, a white oily substance that coats term infants' bodies and is often found in abundance in the creases of the axilla and groin, has innate immunologic properties that serve to protect newborns from infection (Visscher & Narendran, 2014). Vernix also appears to have a role in maintaining the integrity of the stratum corneum and facilitating acid mantle development (Visscher & Narendran, 2014). The epidermis of a full-term infant undergoes maturation during the first month of life; the newborn's skin acts as a barrier to infection, assists in thermal regulation, and prevents transepidermal water loss in term infants.

During infancy, **thermoregulation** becomes more efficient; the ability of the skin to contract and of muscles to shiver in response to cold increases. The peripheral capillaries respond to changes in ambient temperature to regulate heat loss. The capillaries constrict in response to cold, conserving core body temperature and decreasing potential evaporative heat loss from the skin surface. The capillaries dilate in response to heat, decreasing internal body temperature through evaporation, conduction, and convection. Shivering (**thermogenesis**) causes the muscles and muscle fibers to contract, generating metabolic heat, which is distributed throughout the body. Increased adipose tissue during the first 6 months insulates the body against heat loss.

A shift in the total body fluid occurs; at birth, 78% of a term infant's body weight is water, and there is an abundance of extracellular fluid (ECF). As the percentage of body water decreases, so does the amount of ECF—from 44% at term to 20% in adulthood. The high proportion of ECF, which is composed of blood plasma, interstitial fluid, and lymph, predisposes the infant to a more rapid loss of total body fluid and, consequently, dehydration. The loss of 5% to 10% of term newborns' initial birth weight in the first 5 days of life is attributed to ECF compartment contraction, enhanced renal tubular function, and rapidly increasing glomerular filtration rate (Blackburn, 2017).

The immaturity of the renal structures also predisposes infants to dehydration and electrolyte imbalance. Complete maturity of the kidneys occurs during the latter half of the second year, which is when the cuboidal epithelium of the glomeruli becomes flattened. Before this time, the filtration capacity of the glomeruli is reduced. Urine is voided frequently and has a low specific gravity (1.008 to 1.012). At term, most infants produce and excrete approximately 15 to 60 ml/kg/24 hours, and an output of less than 0.5 ml/kg/hour after 48 hours of age is considered to be oliguria (Blackburn, 2017).

Auditory acuity is at adult levels during infancy. Visual acuity begins to improve, and binocular fixation is established. **Binocularity**, or the fixation of two ocular images into one cerebral picture (**fusion**), begins to develop by 6 weeks old and should be established by 4 months old. **Depth perception (stereopsis)** begins to develop by 7 to 9 months old but may not be fully mature until 2 or 3 years old, thus increasing infants' and younger toddlers' risk of falling.

Fine Motor Development

Fine motor behavior includes the use of the hands and fingers in the **prehension** (grasp) of objects. Grasping occurs during the first 2 to 3 months as a reflex and gradually becomes voluntary. At 1 month old, the hands are predominantly closed, and by 3 months old, they are mostly open. By this time, infants demonstrate a desire to grasp objects, but they "grasp" objects more with the eyes than with the

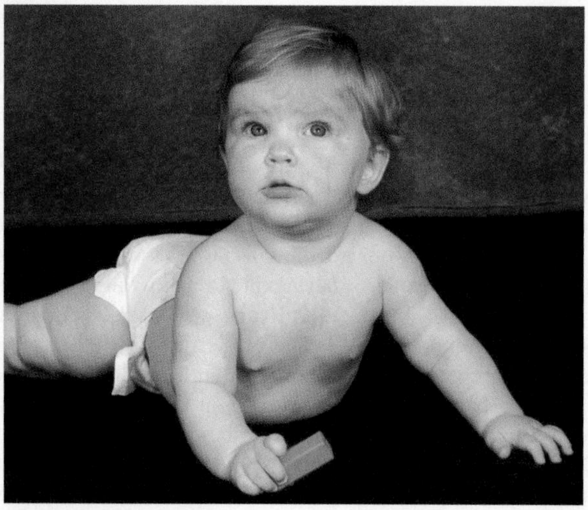

Fig. 9.1 Crude pincer grasp at 8 to 10 months old. (Photo by Paul Vincent Kuntz, Texas Children's Hospital, Houston, TX.)

hands. If a rattle is placed in the hand, infants will actively hold on to it. By 4 months old, infants regard both a small pellet and the hands and then look from the object to the hands and back again. By 5 months old, infants are able to voluntarily grasp objects.

By 6 months old, infants have increased manipulative skill. They hold their bottles, grasp their feet and pull them to their mouths, and feed themselves crackers. By 7 months old, they transfer objects from one hand to the other, use one hand for grasping, and hold a cube in each hand simultaneously. They enjoy banging objects and explore the movable parts of toys.

Gradually, the **palmar grasp** (using the whole hand) is replaced by a **pincer grasp** (using the thumb and index finger). By 8 to 9 months old, infants use a crude pincer grasp, and by 10 months old, they have progressed to a neat pincer grasp sufficient to pick up raisins and other finger foods (Fig. 9.1). They can deliberately let go of an object and offer it to someone. By 11 months old, they put objects into containers and like to remove them. By 1 year old, infants try to build towers of two blocks but fail.

Gross Motor Development

Head Control

Full-term newborns can momentarily hold their heads in midline and parallel when their bodies are suspended ventrally, and can lift and turn their heads from side to side when they are prone (see Chapter 7, Fig. 7.7). This is not the case when infants are lying prone on a pillow or soft surface; infants do not have the head control to lift their heads out of the depression of the object and therefore risk suffocation in the prone position early in infancy (see Chapter 10, Sudden Infant Death Syndrome). Marked head lag is evident when infants are pulled from a lying to a sitting position. By 3 months old, infants can hold their heads well beyond the plane of their bodies. By 4 months old, infants can lift their heads and front portion of their chests approximately 90 degrees above the table, bearing their weight on the forearms. Only slight head lag is evident when infants are pulled from a lying to a sitting position, and by 4 to 6 months old, head control is well established (Figs. 9.2 and 9.3).

Rolling Over

Newborns may roll over accidentally because of their rounded backs. The ability to willfully turn from the abdomen to the back occurs around 5 months old, and the ability to turn from the back to the abdomen occurs at approximately 6 months old. Infants put to sleep on their sides may easily roll over to a prone (face-down) position, thus placing them at higher risk for sudden infant death syndrome (SIDS). It is therefore important to place infants in a supine position for sleep. While infants are awake, a prone position (tummy time) is acceptable to enhance achievement of milestones, such as head control, crawling, creeping, and turning over. It is noteworthy that the parachute reflex (Fig. 9.4), a protective response to falling, appears at approximately 7 months old.

> **! NURSING ALERT**
>
> In the first several months of life, before the infant can roll over, the head should be positioned on alternating sides to prevent positional plagiocephaly (when asleep or awake in the supine position) (see Chapter 10).

Sitting

The ability to sit follows progressive head control and straightening of the back (Fig. 9.5). For the first 2 to 3 months, the back is uniformly rounded. The convex cervical curve forms at approximately 3 to 4 months old, when head control is established. The convex lumbar curve appears when the child begins to sit, at about 4 months old. As the spinal column straightens, infants can be propped in a sitting position. By 7 months old, infants can sit alone, leaning forward on their hands for support. By 8 months old, they can sit well while unsupported and begin to explore their surroundings in this position rather than in a lying position. By 10 months old, they can maneuver from a prone to a sitting position.

Locomotion

Locomotion involves acquiring the ability to bear weight; propel forward on all four extremities; stand upright with support; cruise by holding on to furniture; and finally, walk alone (Fig. 9.6). Following a cephalocaudal pattern, infants who are 4 to 6 months old have increasing coordination in their arms. Initial locomotion results in infants propelling themselves backward by pushing with their arms. By 6 to 7 months old, they are able to bear all of their weight on their legs with assistance. **Crawling** (propelling forward with the belly on the floor) progresses to **creeping** on hands and knees (with the belly off the floor) by 9 months old. At this time, they stand while holding on to furniture and can pull themselves to the standing position, but they are unable to maneuver back down except by falling. By 11 months old, they walk while holding on to furniture or with both hands held; and by 1 year old, they may be able to walk with one hand held. A number of infants attempt their first independent steps by their first birthday.

> **! NURSING ALERT**
>
> An infant who does not pull to a standing position by 11 to 12 months old should be further evaluated for possible developmental dysplasia of the hip (see Chapter 29).

PSYCHOSOCIAL DEVELOPMENT: DEVELOPING A SENSE OF TRUST (ERIKSON)

Erikson's phase I (birth to 1 year old) is concerned with **acquiring a sense of trust** while **overcoming a sense of mistrust**. The trust that

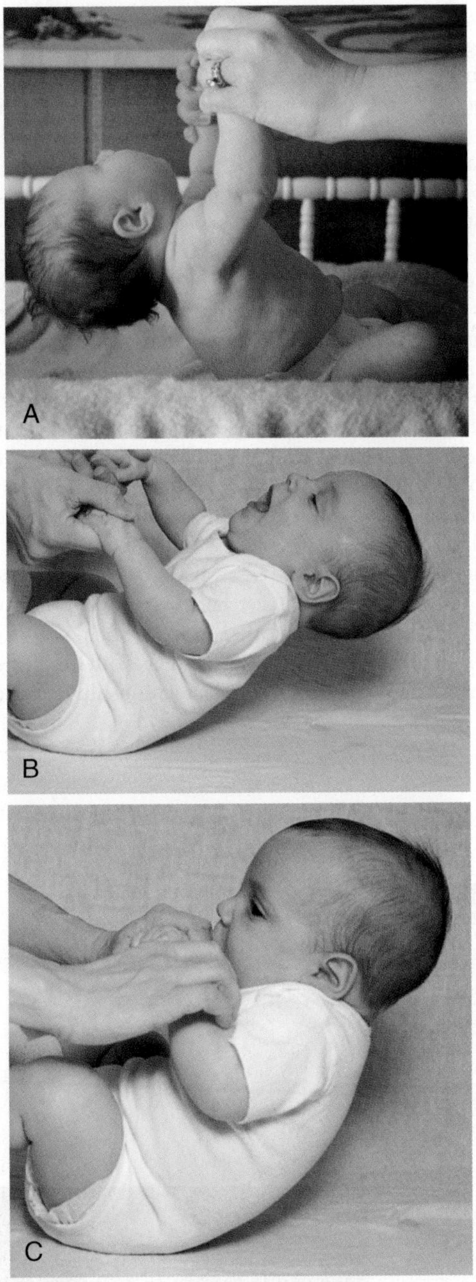

Fig. 9.2 Head control while pulled to sitting position. **A,** Complete head lag at 1 month old. **B,** Partial head lag at 2 months old. **C,** Almost no head lag at 4 months old.

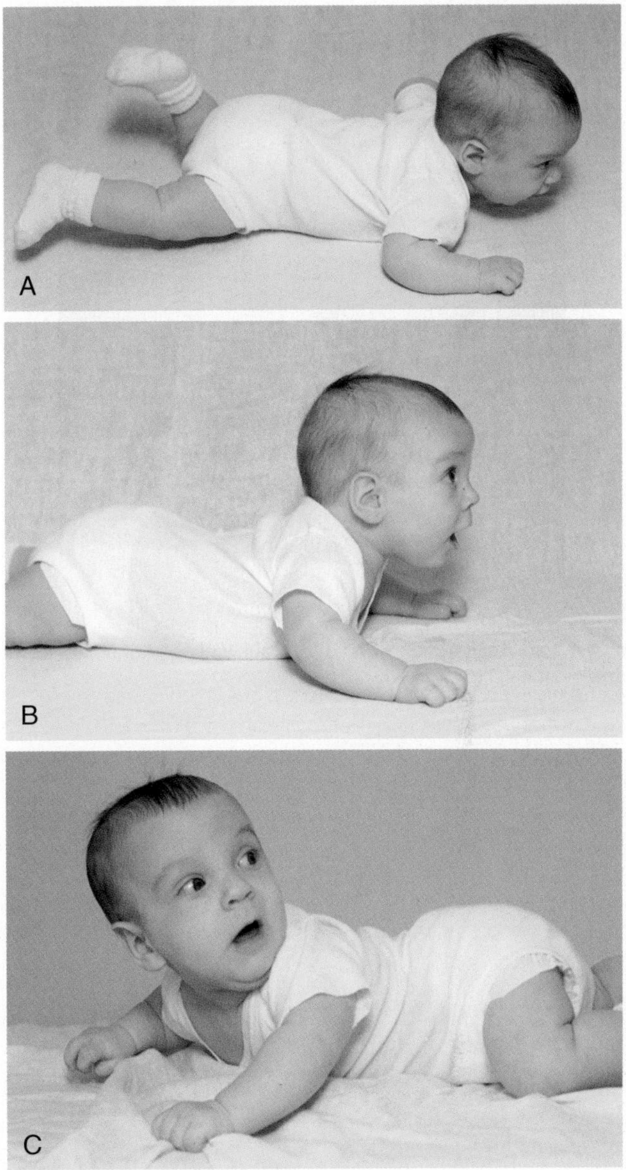

Fig. 9.3 Head control while prone. **A,** The infant momentarily lifts the head at 1 month old. **B,** The infant lifts the head and chest 90 degrees and bears weight on the forearms at 4 months old. **C,** The infant lifts head, chest, and upper abdomen and can bear weight on the hands at 6 months old. Note how this position facilitates turning from the abdomen to the back.

develops is a trust of self, of others, and of the world. Infants "trust" that their feeding, comfort, stimulation, and caring needs will be met. The crucial element for the achievement of this task is the quality of both the parent (caregiver)–child relationship and the care the infant receives. The provision of food, warmth, and shelter by itself is inadequate for the development of a strong sense of self. The infant and parent must jointly learn to satisfactorily meet their needs for mutual regulation of frustration to occur. When this synchrony fails to develop, mistrust is the eventual outcome.

Failure to learn delayed gratification leads to mistrust. Mistrust can result from either too much or too little frustration. If parents always meet their children's needs before the children signal their readiness, infants will never learn to test their ability to control the environment. If the delay is prolonged, infants will experience constant frustration and eventually mistrust others in their efforts to satisfy them. Therefore consistency of care is essential.

The trust acquired in infancy provides the foundation for all succeeding phases. Trust allows infants a feeling of physical comfort and security, which assists them in experiencing unfamiliar, unknown situations with a minimum of fear. Erikson has divided the first year of life into two oral–social stages. During the first 3 to 4 months, food intake is the most important social activity in which the infant engages. Newborns can tolerate little frustration or delay of gratification. Primary **narcissism** (total concern for oneself) is at its height. However, as bodily processes (such as vision, motor movements, and vocalization) become better controlled, infants use more advanced behaviors to interact with others. For example, rather than cry, infants may put their arms up to signify a desire to be held.

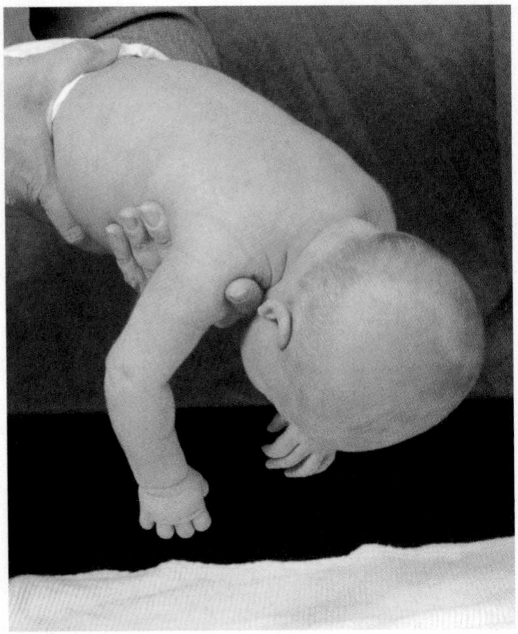

Fig. 9.4 Parachute reflex. (Photo by Paul Vincent Kuntz, Texas Children's Hospital, Houston, TX.)

The next social modality involves a mode of reaching out to others through **grasping**. Grasping is initially reflexive, but even as a reflex, it has a powerful social meaning for the parents. The reciprocal response to the infant's grasping is the parents' holding on and touching. There is pleasurable tactile stimulation for both the child and the parents.

Tactile stimulation is extremely important in the total process of acquiring trust. The degree of mothering skill, the quantity of food, or the length of sucking does not determine the quality of the experience. Rather, the total nature of the quality of the interpersonal relationship influences the infant's formulation of trust.

During the second stage, the more active and aggressive modality of biting occurs. Infants learn that they can hold on to what is their own and can more fully control their environment. During this stage, infants may be confronted with one of their first conflicts. If they are breastfeeding, they quickly learn that biting causes the mother to become upset and withdraw the breast. Yet biting also brings internal relief from teething discomfort and a sense of power or control.

This conflict may be solved in a variety of ways. The mother may wean the infant from the breast and begin bottle-feeding, or the infant may learn to bite substitute nipples, such as a pacifier, and retain pleasurable breastfeeding. The successful resolution of this conflict strengthens the mother-child relationship because it occurs

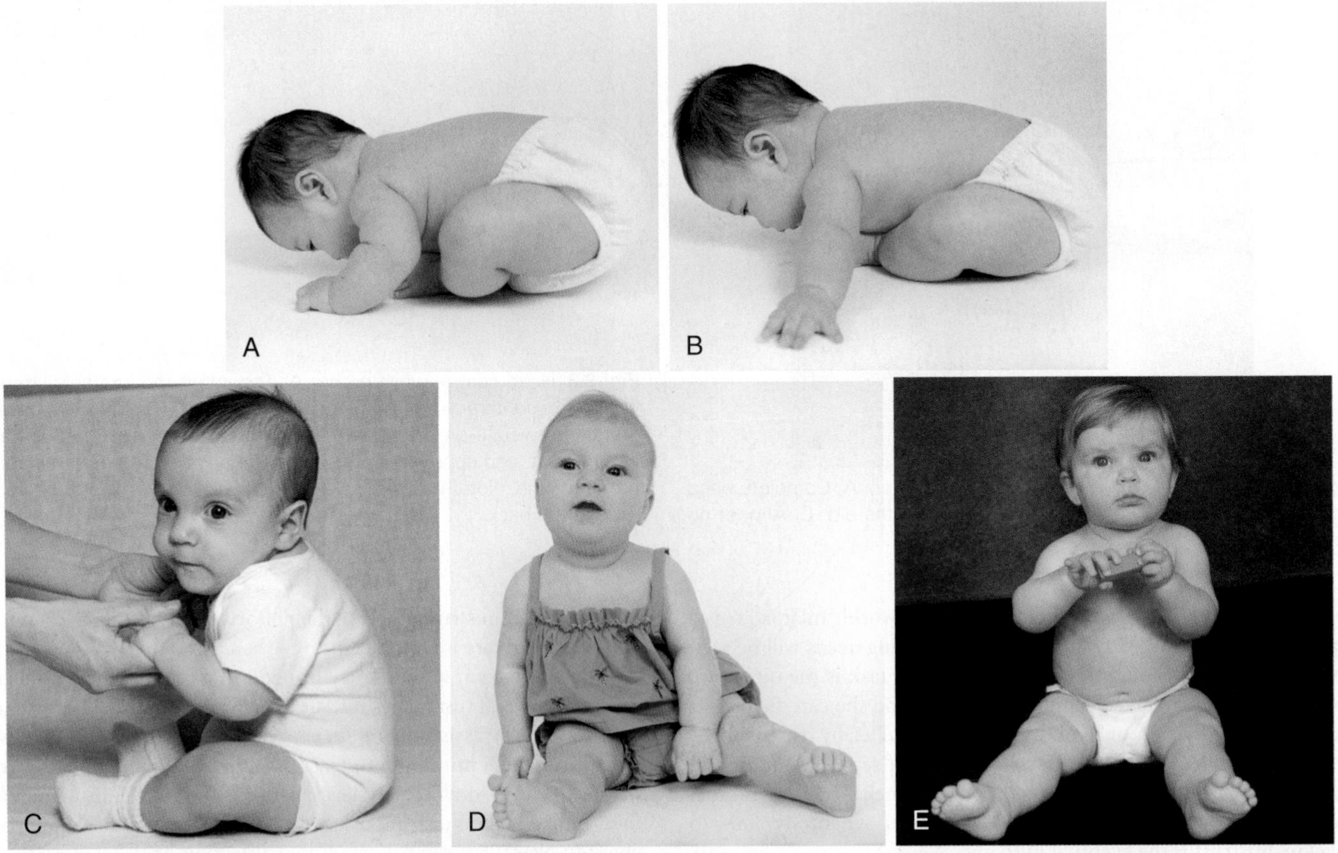

Fig. 9.5 Development of sitting. A, The back is completely rounded, and the infant has no ability to sit upright at 1 month old. B, At 2 months old, the infant exhibits more control; the back is still rounded, but the infant can try to pull up with some head control. C, The back is rounded only in the lumbar area, and the infant is able to sit erect with good head control at 4 months old. D, The infant can sit alone, leaning on the hands for support, at 7 months old. E, The infant sits without support at 8 months old. Note the transferring of objects that occurs at 7 months old. (B, D, and E, Photos by Paul Vincent Kuntz, Texas Children's Hospital, Houston, TX.)

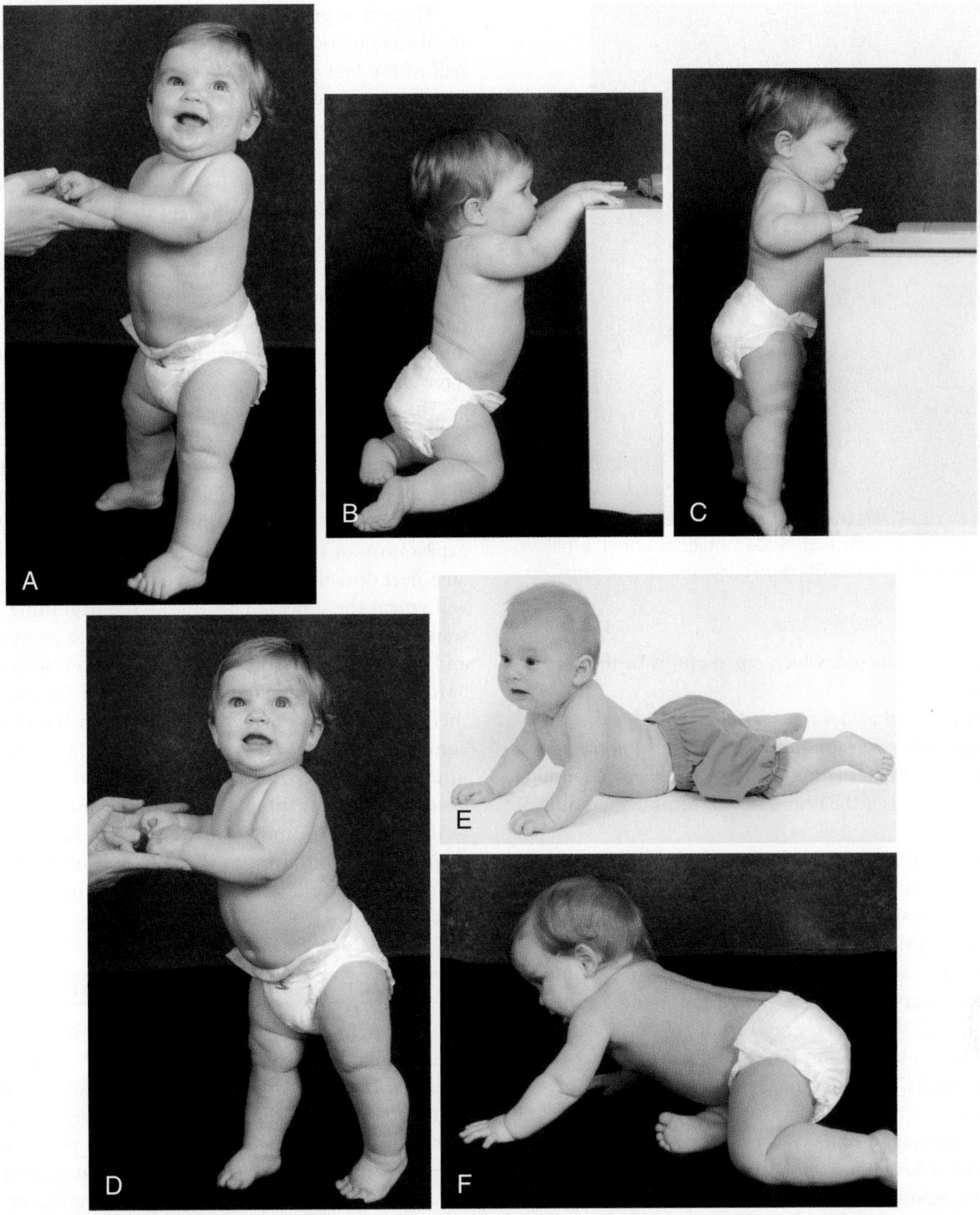

Fig. 9.6 Development of locomotion. **A,** The infant bears full weight on the feet by 7 months old. **B,** The infant can maneuver from a sitting to a kneeling position. **C,** The infant can stand holding on to furniture at 9 months old. **D,** While standing, the infant takes a deliberate step at 10 months old. **E,** The infant crawls with the abdomen on the floor and pulls self forward at about 7 months old and then **(F)** creeps on hands and knees at 9 months old. (Photos by Paul Vincent Kuntz, Texas Children's Hospital, Houston, TX.)

at a time when infants are recognizing the mother as the most significant person in their life.

COGNITIVE DEVELOPMENT: SENSORIMOTOR PHASE (PIAGET)

The theory most commonly used to explain **cognition**, or the ability to know, is that of Piaget. The period from birth to 24 months old is called the **sensorimotor phase** and is composed of six stages; however, because this discussion is concerned with ages birth to 12 months old, only the first four stages are discussed. The last two stages occur during the toddler period of 12 to 24 months old and are discussed in Chapter 11.

During the sensorimotor phase, infants progress from reflexive behaviors to simple repetitive acts to imitative activity. Three crucial events take place during this phase. The first event involves separation, in which infants learn to separate themselves from other objects in the environment. They realize that others besides themselves control the environment and that certain readjustments must take place for mutual satisfaction to occur. This coincides with Erikson's concept of the formation of trust.

The second major accomplishment is achieving the concept of **object permanence**, or the realization that objects that leave the visual field still exist. A typical example of the development of object permanence is when infants can pursue objects they observe being hidden under a pillow or behind a chair (Fig. 9.7). This skill develops at

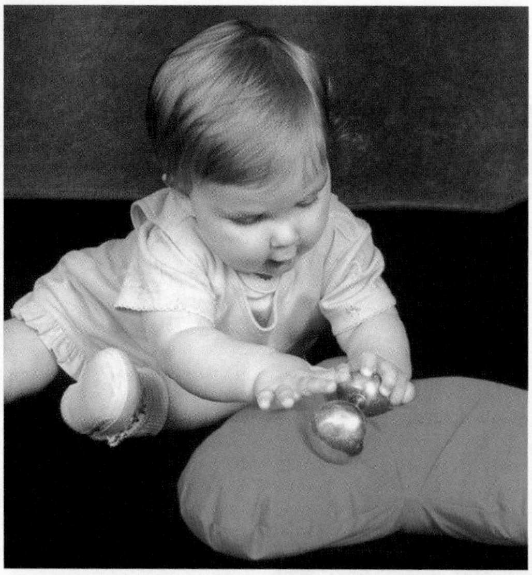

Fig. 9.7 A 9-month-old infant can find hidden objects under a pillow. (Photo by Paul Vincent Kuntz, Texas Children's Hospital, Houston, TX.)

approximately 9 to 10 months old, which corresponds to the time of increased locomotion skills.

The last major intellectual achievement of this period is the ability to use symbols, or **mental representation**. The use of symbols allows infants to think of an object or situation without actually experiencing it. The recognition of symbols is the beginning of the understanding of time and space.

The first stage, from birth to 1 month old, is identified by infants' **use of reflexes**. At birth, infants' individuality and temperament are expressed through the physiologic reflexes of sucking, rooting, grasping, and crying. The repetitious nature of the reflexes is the beginning of associations between an act and a sequential response. When infants cry because they are hungry, a nipple is put in the mouth, and they suck, feel satisfaction, and sleep. They are assimilating this experience while perceiving auditory, tactile, and visual cues. This experience of perceiving certain patterns, or "ordering," provides a foundation for the subsequent stages.

The second stage, **primary circular reactions**, marks the beginning of the replacement of reflexive behavior with voluntary acts. During the period from 1 to 4 months old, activities such as sucking and grasping become deliberate acts that elicit certain responses. The beginning of accommodation is evident. Infants incorporate and adapt their reactions to the environment and recognize the stimulus that produced a response. Previously, they cried until the nipple was brought to the mouth. Now they associate the nipple with the sound of the parent's voice. They accommodate this new piece of information and adapt by ceasing to cry when they hear the voice—before receiving the nipple. What is taking place is realization of causality and recognition of an orderly sequence of events. The environment is taken in with all of the senses and with whatever motor ability is present.

The **secondary circular reactions** stage is a continuation of primary circular reactions and lasts until 8 months old. In this stage, the primary circular reactions are repeated and prolonged for the response that results. Grasping and holding now become shaking, banging, and pulling. Shaking is performed to hear a noise, not solely for the pleasure of shaking. The quality and quantity of an act become evident. "More" or "less" shaking produces different responses. Causality, time, deliberate intention, and separateness from the environment begin to develop.

Three new processes of human behavior occur. **Imitation** requires the differentiation of selected acts from several events. By the second half of the first year, infants can imitate sounds and simple gestures. **Play** becomes evident as they take pleasure in performing an act after they have mastered it. Much of infants' waking hours are absorbed in sensorimotor play. **Affect** (outward manifestation of emotion and feeling) is seen as infants begin to develop a sense of permanence. During the first 6 months, infants believe that an object exists only for as long as they can visually perceive it. In other words, out of sight, out of mind. Affect to external objects is evident when the object continues to be present or remembered even though it is beyond the range of perception. Object permanence is a critical component of parent-child attachment and is seen in the development of stranger anxiety at 6 to 8 months old.

During the fourth sensorimotor stage, **coordination of secondary schemas and their application to new situations**, infants use previous behavioral achievements primarily as the foundation for adding new intellectual skills to their expanding repertoire. This stage is largely transitional. Increasing motor skills allow for greater exploration of the environment. They begin to discover that hiding an object does not mean that it is gone but that removing an obstacle will reveal the object. This marks the beginning of intellectual reasoning. Furthermore, they can experience an event by observing it, and they begin to associate symbols with events (e.g., "bye-bye" with "Mommy or Daddy goes to work"), but the classification is purely their own. In this stage, they learn from the object itself; this is in contrast to the second stage, in which infants learn from the type of interaction between objects or individuals. Intentionality is further developed in that infants now actively attempt to remove a barrier to the desired (or undesired) action (see Fig. 9.7). If something is in their way, they attempt to climb over it or push it away. Previously, an obstacle would cause them to give up any further attempt to achieve the desired goal.

DEVELOPMENT OF BODY IMAGE

The development of body image parallels sensorimotor development. Infants' kinesthetic and tactile experiences are the first perceptions of their bodies, and the mouth is the principal area of pleasurable sensations. Other parts of their bodies are primarily objects of pleasure—the hands and fingers to suck and the feet to play with. As their physical needs are met, they feel comfort and satisfaction with their bodies. Messages conveyed by their caregivers reinforce these feelings. For example, when infants smile, they receive emotional satisfaction from others who smile back.

Achieving the concept of object permanence is basic to the development of self-image. By the end of the first year, infants recognize that they are distinct from their parents. At the same time, they have increasing interest in their image, especially in the mirror (Fig. 9.8). As motor skills develop, they learn that parts of their bodies are useful; for example, their hands bring objects to their mouths, and their legs help them move to different locations. All of these achievements transmit messages to them about themselves. Therefore it is important to transmit positive messages to infants about their bodies.

SOCIAL DEVELOPMENT

Infants' social development is initially influenced by their reflexive behavior, such as the grasp, and eventually depends primarily on the interaction between them and their principal caregivers. Attachment to their parents is increasingly evident during the second half of the

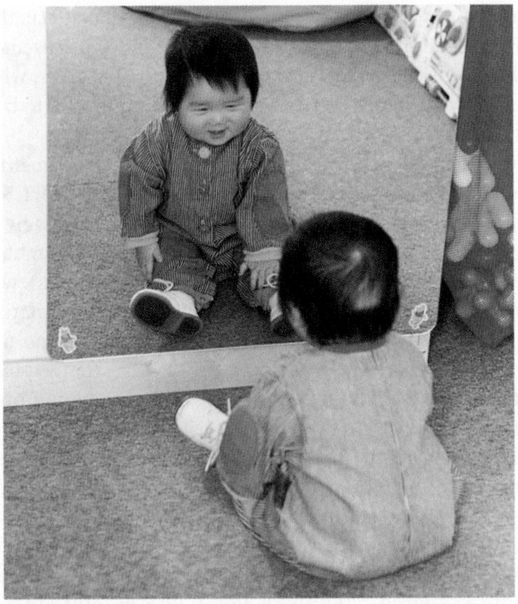

Fig. 9.8 A 9-month-old infant enjoying own image in mirror.

first year. In addition, tremendous strides are made in communication and personal–social behavior. Whereas crying and reflexive behavior are methods to meet one's needs in early infancy, the social smile is an early step in social communication. This has a profound effect on family members and is a tremendous stimulus for evoking continued responses from others. By 4 months old, infants laugh aloud.

Play is a major socializing agent and provides stimulation needed to learn from and interact with the environment. By 6 months old, infants are very personable. They play games such as peek-a-boo when their heads are hidden in a towel, they signal their desire to be picked up by extending their arms, and they show displeasure when a toy is removed or their faces are washed.

Attachment

The importance of human physical contact to infants cannot be overemphasized. Parenting is not an instinctual ability but a learned, acquired process. The attachment of parent and child, which often begins before birth and assumes even more importance at birth (see Chapter 7), continues during the first year (Fig. 9.9). In the following discussion of attachment, the term *mother* is used in the broad context of the consistent caregiver with whom the child relates more than anyone else. However, with society's changing social climate and sex-role stereotypes, this person may well be the father or a grandparent. Studies on father-infant attachment demonstrate that stages similar to maternal attachment occur and that fathers are more involved in child care when mothers are employed (although mothers continue to do the majority of infant care). Additional research has shown that inexperienced, first-time fathers are as capable as experienced fathers of developing a close attachment with their infants. Fathers verbalized more positive feelings of love and affection toward their newborns when they were able to have close physical contact, such as holding their infant (Feeley, Sherrard, Waitzer, et al., 2013). Fathers have also been reported to have a significant role in supporting mothers in the perinatal period. Fathers' involvement at birth has been cited as a strong predictor of continued parental involvement through age 5 years. Fathers' involvement in the prenatal period shows a positive correlation with mother's prenatal care, decreased incidence of prematurity, and decreased infant mortality (Yogman & Garfield, 2016).

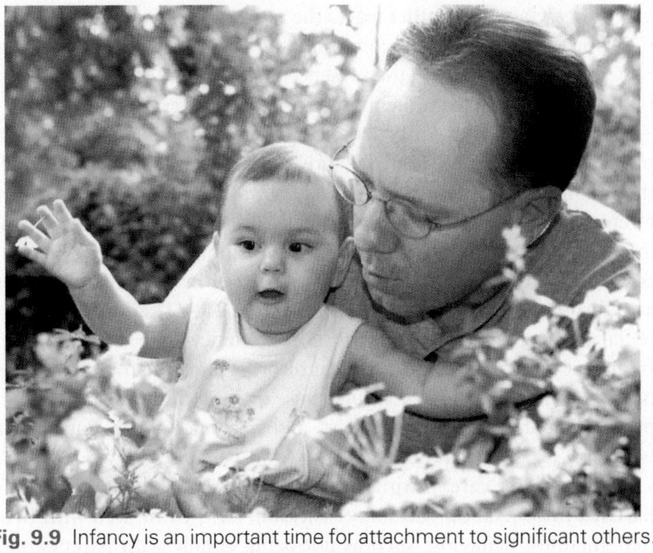

Fig. 9.9 Infancy is an important time for attachment to significant others. (Photo by Paul Vincent Kuntz, Texas Children's Hospital, Houston, TX.)

Research demonstrates that fathers develop feelings of attachment with their offspring and that their relationship with the infant is an important factor in the mother's emotional well-being. With many single-parent families existing today, a grandmother (or other significant caretaker) may become the primary caretaker. It is important for nurses to recognize that infant-parent attachments may be present or absent in situations where caretaker roles are less well defined by those involved.

When infants are not provided a safe haven and consistent and loving care, an insecure attachment develops; such infants do not feel they can trust the world in which they live. This insecure attachment may result in psychosocial difficulties as the child grows and may persist even into adulthood. Insecure attachment may also exist in homes where there is domestic violence and maternal postnatal depression.

Attachment progresses during infancy, with the infant assuming an increasingly significant role in the family. Two components of cognitive development are required for attachment: (1) the ability to discriminate the mother from other individuals and (2) the achievement of object permanence. Both of these processes prepare infants for an equally important aspect of attachment—separation from the parent. Separation-individuation should occur as a harmonious, parallel process with emotional attachment.

During the formation of attachment to the parent, the infant progresses through four distinct but overlapping stages. For the first few weeks of life, infants respond indiscriminately to anyone. Beginning at approximately 8 to 12 weeks old, they cry, smile, and vocalize more to the mother than to anyone else but continue to respond to others, whether familiar or not. At approximately 6 months old, infants show a distinct preference for the mother. They follow her more, cry when she leaves, enjoy playing with her more, and feel most secure in her arms. About 1 month after showing attachment to the mother, many infants begin attaching to other members of the family, most often the father.

Infants acquire other developmental behaviors that influence the attachment process. These include:

- Differential crying, smiling, and vocalization (more to the mother than to anyone else)
- Visual-motor orientation (looking more at the mother, even if she is not close)

- Crying when the mother leaves the room
- Approaching through locomotion (crawling, creeping, or walking)
- Clinging (especially in the presence of a stranger)
- Exploring away from the mother while using her as a secure base

Severe attachment disorders are psychologic and developmental problems that stem from maladaptive or absent attachment between the infant and parent (Zeanah & Gleason, 2015). There are two different patterns of attachment disorders: the emotionally withdrawn–inhibited pattern and an indiscriminate-disinhibited pattern (Zeanah & Gleason, 2015). These two subtypes have been classified into separate disorders: reactive attachment disorder (RAD) and disinhibited social engagement disorder (DSED) of infancy or early childhood. Infants at risk for severe attachment disorders include those who have been victims of physical or sexual abuse or neglect; infants exposed to parental alcoholism, mental illness, and substance abuse; and infants who have experienced the absence of a consistent primary caregiver as a result of foster care, institutionalization, parental abandonment, or parental incarceration (Zeanah & Gleason, 2015). Children with RAD may manifest behaviors such as not being cuddly with parents, failing to seek and respond to comfort when distressed, minimal social and emotional reciprocity, and emotional deregulation such as unexplained fearfulness or irritability (Zeanah & Gleason, 2015). Children with DSED may exhibit behaviors such as inappropriate approach to unfamiliar adults, lack of suspicion of strangers, and poor impulse control (Zeanah & Gleason, 2015). Either or both of these complex disorders are diagnosed with maltreated and orphaned children. Without early intervention, some of these children fail to develop a conscience and develop an antisocial personality disorder that may lead to criminal acts. Children with autism or other pervasive developmental disorders have behaviors that are categorically different from those with RAD (Zeanah & Gleason, 2015).

Separation Anxiety

Between 4 and 8 months old, infants progress through the first stage of separation-individuation and begin to have some awareness of themselves and their mothers as separate beings. At the same time, object permanence is developing, and infants are aware that their parents can be absent. Therefore separation anxiety develops and is manifested through a predictable sequence of behaviors.

During the early second half of the first year, infants protest when placed in their cribs, and a short time later, they object when their mothers leave the room. Infants may not notice the mother's absence if they are absorbed in an activity. However, when they realize her absence, they protest. From this point on, they become alert to her activities and whereabouts. By 11 to 12 months old, they are able to anticipate her imminent departure by watching her behaviors, and they begin to protest *before* she leaves. At this point, many parents learn to postpone alerting the child to their departure until just before leaving.

Stranger Fear

As infants demonstrate attachment to one person, they correspondingly exhibit less friendliness to others. Between 6 and 8 months old, fear of strangers and stranger anxiety become prominent and are related to infants' ability to discriminate between familiar and unfamiliar people. Behaviors such as clinging to the parent, crying, and turning away from the stranger are common.

Language Development

Infants' first means of verbal communication is crying. Crying as a biologic sign conveys a message of urgency and signals displeasure, such as hunger. However, crying is also a social event that affects the development of the parent-infant relationship—either by its absence, which usually has a positive effect on parents, or by its presence, which may evoke a negative response or persuade parents to minister to the child's physical or emotional needs.

In the first few weeks of life, crying has a reflexive quality and is mostly related to physiologic needs. Infants cry for 1 to 1.5 hours a day up to 3 weeks old and then build up to 2 to 4 hours by 6 weeks old. Crying tends to decrease by 12 weeks old. It is thought that the increase in crying for no apparent reason during the first few months may be related to the discharge of energy and the maturational changes in the central nervous system. At the end of the first year, infants cry for attention; from fear (especially stranger fear); and from frustration, usually in response to their developing but inadequate motor skills.

Vocalizations heard during crying eventually become syllables and words (e.g., the "mama" heard during vigorous crying). Infants vocalize as early as 5 to 6 weeks old by making small throaty sounds. By 2 months old, they make single vowel sounds, such as *ah, eh,* and *uh*. By 3 to 4 months old, the consonants *n, k, g, p,* and *b* are added, and infants coo, gurgle, and laugh aloud. By 6 months old, they imitate sounds; add the consonants *t, d,* and *w;* and combine syllables (e.g., "dada"), but they do not ascribe meaning to the words until 10 to 11 months old. By 9 to 10 months old, they comprehend the meaning of the word "no" and obey simple commands. By 1 year old, they can say 3 to 5 words with meaning and may understand as many as 100 words. Because language development is based on expressive skills (ability to make thoughts, ideas, and desires known to others) and receptive skills (ability to understand the words being spoken), it is important that infants are exposed to expressive speech and that infants with delays in achieving milestones are carefully evaluated for potential hearing loss (see Chapter 7, Universal Newborn Hearing Screening).

Play

Play during infancy represents the various social modalities observed during cognitive development. The activity of infants is primarily narcissistic and revolves around their own bodies. As discussed under Development of Body Image earlier in the chapter, body parts are primarily objects of play and pleasure.

During the first year, play becomes more sophisticated and interdependent. From birth to 3 months old, infants' responses to the environment are global and largely undifferentiated. Play is dependent; pleasure is demonstrated by a quieting attitude (1 month old), a smile (2 months old), or a squeal (3 months old). From 3 to 6 months old, infants show more discriminate interest in stimuli and begin to play alone with rattles or soft stuffed toys or with someone else. There is much more interaction during play. By 4 months old, they laugh aloud, show preference for certain toys, and become excited when food or a favorite object is brought to them. They recognize images in a mirror, smile at them, and vocalize to them.

By 6 months to 1 year old, play involves sensorimotor skills. Games such as peek-a-boo and pat-a-cake are played. Verbal repetition and imitation of simple gestures occur in response to demonstration. Play is much more selective, not only in terms of specific toys, but also in terms of "playmates." Although play is solitary or one sided, infants choose with whom they will interact. At 6 to 8 months old, they usually refuse to play with strangers. Parents are definite favorites, and infants know how to attract their attention. At 6 months old, they extend their arms to be picked up; at 7 months old, they cough to make their presence known; at 10 months old, they pull their parents' clothing; and at 12 months old, they call their parents by name. This represents a tremendous advance from the newborn who signaled biologic needs by crying to express displeasure.

Stimulation is as important for psychosocial growth as food is for physical growth. Knowledge of developmental milestones allows nurses to guide parents regarding proper play for infants. It is not sufficient to place a mobile over a crib and toys in a play yard for a child's optimum social, emotional, and intellectual development. Play must provide interpersonal contact and recreational and educational stimulation. Infants need to be *played with,* not merely *allowed to play.* Although the type of play infants engage in is called *solitary,* this is a figurative, not literal, term to denote one-sided play. The type of toys given to children is much less important than the quality of personal interaction that occurs.

TEMPERAMENT

An infant's temperament or behavioral style influences the type of interaction that occurs between the child and parents, especially the mother, and other family members (see Chapter 3, Temperament). In assessing a child's temperament, the parents' perception of the child and the degree of fit between their expectations and the child's actual temperament are important. The more dissonance or lack of harmony between the child's temperament and the parents' ability to accept and deal with the behavior, the greater risk for subsequent parent-child conflicts.

Although most behavioral researchers agree that there is a strong biologic component to temperament, researchers also suggest that the environment, particularly the family, may modify temperament (Bates & Pettit, 2015). Family interaction with the infant is perceived as a circular process wherein each family member affects the others and the family as a unit. With these concepts in mind, the nurse has an important role in helping the family understand the infant's temperament as it relates to family dynamics and the eventual well-being of the child and family unit.

Some researchers speculate that infant temperament may contribute to depression. Depressed mothers and fathers (vs. nondepressed mothers and fathers) rate their infant's temperament as more difficult at 3 and 18 months old (Kerstis, Engström, Edlund, et al., 2013). The researchers stress that depressed parents need to be identified early and provided with supportive programs to enhance the parent-infant relationship. When there is a lack of reciprocity between the infant and parents or when the infant's behavior does not meet parental expectations, there is increased risk for discord. Researchers have correlated fussy infant temperament with the introduction of complementary feedings at 3 months old (Wasser, Bentley, Borja, et al., 2011) and feeding infants foods that may contribute to obesity (Vollrath, Tonstadt, Rothbart, et al., 2011).

Several instruments can measure infant temperament. These include the Revised Infant Temperament Questionnaire (Carey & McDevitt, 1978), the Infant Behavior Questionnaire (Gartstein & Rothbart, 2003), and the Early Infancy Temperament Questionnaire (Medoff-Cooper, Carey, & McDevitt, 1993). In discussing test results with parents, it is best to avoid descriptors (such as "difficult"); instead, infants can be described in terms of characteristics (such as "intense" or "less predictable").

Childrearing Practices Related to Temperament

With knowledge of the infant's temperament, nurses are better able to (1) provide parents with background information that will help them see their child in a better perspective, (2) offer a more organized picture of their child's behavior and possibly reveal distortions in their perceptions of the behavior, and (3) guide parents on appropriate childrearing techniques.

Knowledge of the developmental sequence allows the nurse to assess normal growth and minor or abnormal deviations. It also helps parents gain realistic expectations of their child's ability and provides guidelines for suitable play and stimulation. Parents who lack knowledge of child growth and development may set inappropriate behavioral expectations for their child. Emphasizing the child's developmental rather than chronologic age strengthens the parent-child relationship by fostering trust and lessening frustration. Therefore thorough understanding and appreciation of children's growth and development are essential.

Because of the complexity of the developmental process during the first 12 months, Table 9.1 is presented to help organize and clarify the data already discussed. Although all milestones are important, some represent essential integrative aspects of development that lay the foundation for achievement of more advanced skills. These essential milestones are designated by a black dot (•) in the table. The table represents the average monthly age at which various skills are attained. It must be remembered that although the sequence is the same, the rate will vary among children.

COPING WITH CONCERNS RELATED TO NORMAL GROWTH AND DEVELOPMENT

Separation and Stranger Fear

A number of fears can appear during infancy. However, the fear that causes parents the most concern is fear related to strangers and separation. Although erroneously interpreted by some as a sign of undesirable, antisocial behavior, stranger fear and separation anxiety are important components of a strong, healthy parent-child attachment. Nevertheless, this period can present difficulties for the parent and child. Parents may be more confined to the home because the infant violently protests having babysitters. To accustom the infant to new people, parents are encouraged to have close friends or relatives visit often. This provides other persons with whom the child is comfortable and can give parents time for themselves.

Infants also need opportunities to safely experience strangers. Usually toward the end of the first year, infants begin to venture away from the parent and demonstrate curiosity about strangers. If allowed to explore at their own rate, many infants eventually "warm up." If parents hold the child away from their face, the infant can observe while maintaining close physical contact.

The best approach for the stranger (including nurses) is to talk softly; meet the child at eye level (to appear smaller); maintain a safe distance from the infant; and avoid sudden, intrusive gestures, such as holding out the arms and smiling broadly.

Parents also may wonder whether they should encourage the child's clinging, dependent behavior, especially if there is pressure from others who view this as "spoiling" (see the following discussion). Parents need to be reassured that such behavior is healthy, desirable, and necessary for the child's optimal emotional development. If parents can reassure the infant of their presence, the infant will learn to realize that they are still there even if not physically present. Talking to infants when leaving the room, allowing them to hear one's voice on the telephone, and using transitional objects (e.g., a favorite blanket or toy) reassure the continued presence of the parent.

Alternate Child Care Arrangements

For many parents, especially working mothers, locating safe and competent child care facilities for infants is an increasingly difficult problem, one that is compounded by the number of mothers working outside the home. Over the past 40 years, there have been variable shifts in child care arrangements; whereas the majority of children are cared for in group centers or other settings, increasingly more children are being cared for in home settings.

The basic types of care are in-home care, either in the parents' or caregivers' home (family daycare), and center-based care, usually in a daycare center. In-home care may consist of a full-time babysitter who lives in the home, a full-time babysitter who comes to the home, cooperative arrangements such as exchange babysitting, or family daycare. A licensed small family child care home typically provides care and protection for up to six children for part of a 24-hour day and does not include informal arrangements, such as exchange babysitting or caregivers in the child's own home. The six children may include the family daycare provider's own children younger than 5 years old living in the home. Large family child care homes may provide care for 8 to 12 children. Unfortunately, many family daycare homes operate without a license and may care for large numbers of infants without adequate staff and facilities.

Child center–based care usually refers to a licensed daycare facility that provides care for six or more children for 6 or more hours in a 24-hour day. Work-based group care is another option that is becoming increasingly popular as employers recognize the benefit of providing high-quality and convenient child care to their employees. Sick-child care may also be available for times when children are ill. Such programs are often located in community hospitals or in work settings.

Nurses may fulfill a unique role in guiding parents in locating suitable facilities that have a well-qualified staff. State licensing agencies can help parents identify daycare centers that accept children of specific age-groups and are convenient to home and work. Their records are available to the public and provide reports from the health, safety, and fire departments; periodic evaluations from the licensing agency; complaints filed against the center; and qualification of the center's employees. State-licensed programs are supposed to abide by established standards, which represent the minimum requirements and safeguards. However, enforcement of the standards is sometimes inadequate.

Early childhood programs may also belong to a voluntary accreditation system sponsored by National Association for the Education of Young Children, which serves as a model for optimum care. References from other parents are also helpful, provided that they have investigated the center carefully and have remained involved with the agency's activities.

The same conscientious attention should be applied to locating competent babysitters. References from other employers are essential, and there is no substitute for observing the interaction between the individual and the child.

Important areas for parents to evaluate are the center's daily program, teacher qualifications, the nurturing qualities of caregivers, student-to-staff ratio, discipline policy, environmental safety precautions, provision of meals, sanitary conditions, adequate indoor and outdoor space per child, and fee schedule. Although fees vary considerably, a program that charges a minimum fee may also be providing minimum services. Parents should arrange to meet the director and some of the employees, especially those who would be caring for the child. Resources to familiarize parents with characteristics of quality child care and checklists to systematically evaluate the center and compare it with other facilities can help parents make successful choices. At all times, the parent should have the right to visit the child, and regular conferences should occur to review the child's progress.

One area that is increasingly important in selecting child care is the center's health practices; however, parents often do not check the center for health and safety features. Evidence shows that children, especially those younger than 6 years old in daycare centers, have more illnesses—especially diarrhea, otitis media, respiratory tract infections (especially if the caregiver smokes), hepatitis A, meningitis, and cytomegalovirus—than children cared for in their homes. The strongest predictor of risk of illness is the number of unrelated children in the room. Proactive infection control measures and education of staff have been effective in reducing the incidence of upper respiratory tract infections, diarrhea, and rotavirus. It has been reported that families that have children in out-of-home child care lose on average 1.5 days of work per illness episode (Peetom, Crutzen, Bohnen, et al., 2018). Children under the age of 5 years, being cared for in an early childhood education center or daycare setting, acquire higher rates of infectious diseases that may require parents to miss work (Donoghue, 2017). Parents should inquire about the center's policy on the attendance and care of sick children.

Limit Setting and Discipline

As infants' motor skills advance and mobility increases, parents are faced with the need to set safe limits to protect the child and establish a positive and supportive parent-child relationship (see the Safety Promotion and Injury Prevention section later in the chapter). Although there are numerous disciplinary techniques, some are more appropriate for this age than others. An effective approach used in disciplining a child is the use of time-out. For example, a play yard is better for most infants than a chair. Although parents may be concerned about instituting discipline during infancy, it is important to stress that the earlier effective disciplinary methods are used, the easier it is to continue these approaches.

Parents must recognize the infant's cognitive and behavioral limitations; adequate protection from hazards must be implemented because infants and toddlers do not understand a cause-and-effect relationship between dangerous objects and physical harm. In addition, parents may need reassurance that their infant's behavior is exploratory in nature, not oppositional (at this age) and primarily centered on the infant's basic needs of warmth, love, food, security, and comfort. Parents may verbalize that comforting the infant too much or meeting his or her needs will result in a spoiled child; there is no substantial evidence that meeting the infant's basic needs will result in such behaviors later in life. Children innately test limits and explore during the exploratory phase of growth; instead of discouraging exploration, parents should provide safe alternatives, put dangerous household items away, and give children consistent discipline and nurturing.

Effective teaching for injury prevention optimally begins in infancy by helping parents understand the nature of their child's normal development. It must be reiterated continually that infants cry because a need is not being met, not to intentionally irritate an adult. A fussy or irritable infant is a potential victim of shaken baby syndrome (or other bodily harm) because adults and caretakers may not understand the nature of the infant's crying.

Thumb Sucking and Use of a Pacifier

Sucking is infants' chief pleasure and may not be satisfied by breastfeeding or bottle-feeding. It is such a strong need that infants who are deprived of sucking, such as those with a cleft lip repair, suck on their tongues. Some newborns are born with sucking blisters on their hands from in utero sucking activity.

Problems arise when parents are overly concerned about the sucking of the fingers, thumb, or pacifier and attempt to restrain this natural tendency. Before giving advice, nurses should investigate the parents' feelings and base guidance on this information.

Pacifier use, particularly in the early days after birth and in the birth hospital, has gained considerable attention in the scientific literature (see Research Focus box). Nelson (2012) suggests that it cannot be stated with absolute certainty that pacifier use is bad in every situation. A recent review by Zimmerman and Thompson (2015) found evidence suggesting that nipple confusion happens predominantly with bottle use and is not as likely with pacifier use in breastfed infants. Health care workers must be informed on potential harm and benefits in pacifier use and provide parents with the highest level of evidence in order to make an informed decision on usage.

RESEARCH FOCUS

Pacifier Use and Breastfeeding

The association of pacifier use and decreased breastfeeding duration was found only in observational studies, whereas no effect of pacifier use on breastfeeding duration was noted in randomized control trials (Nelson, 2012). These studies further concluded that the greatest impact on pacifier use and breastfeeding occurred early in the infant's life when learning effective sucking and stimulating the mother's milk.

Pacifier use has been associated with an increased risk of otitis media in several studies (Salah, Abdel-Aziz, Al-Farok, et al., 2013). Because of this, the American Academy of Pediatrics Subcommittee on the Management of Acute Otitis Media recommended that parents reduce pacifier use in the second 6 months of life (Nelson, 2012). However, the American Academy of Pediatrics' (2011) Task Force on Sudden Infant Death Syndrome cites strong evidence for a protective effect in SIDS reduction when pacifiers are used at bedtime and nap time. The exact mechanism involved in the protection for SIDS is not known. Still, pacifiers should be cleaned and replaced regularly, and there should be an emphasis on allowing the infant to control the pace, frequency, and termination of feeding rather than allowing the pacifier (or anything else) to become the focus of the interaction. Pacifier use during painful procedures in neonates has been shown to produce an analgesic effect (see Chapter 5).

A systematic review found an association between pacifier use in infancy and a reduction in breastfeeding and exclusive breastfeeding (Nelson, 2012). However, the author concluded that pacifier use and poor breastfeeding outcomes may not have a causal effect; rather, it may be related to a marker for socioeconomic, demographic, psychosocial, and cultural factors that determine pacifier use and breastfeeding. A recent Cochrane review found that pacifier use in full-term healthy infants started from birth or after lactation did not significantly affect the prevalence of duration of exclusive and partial breastfeeding up to 4 months old (Jaafar, Jahanafar, Angolkar, et al., 2011). At the time of this writing, there is no evidence that pacifier use and nonnutritive sucking in *preterm infants* has any effect on the initiation and length of breastfeeding. Nonnutritive sucking should not be withheld from preterm infants, especially when used in conjunction with concentrated sucrose for pain management.

To decrease dependence on nonnutritive sucking in young infants, sucking pleasure can be increased by prolonging feeding time. Also, the parents' excessive use of the pacifier to calm the child should be explored. It is not unusual for parents to place a pacifier in the infant's mouth as soon as crying begins, thus reinforcing a pattern of distress–relief.

If the child uses a pacifier, stress safety considerations in purchasing one. During infancy and early childhood, there is no need to restrain nonnutritive sucking of the fingers. Malocclusion may occur if thumb sucking persists past approximately 4 years old or when the permanent teeth erupt. Some parents may perceive pacifiers as less damaging because they are discarded by 2 to 3 years old, whereas thumb sucking may persist well into the school-age years. Because of the limited number of studies correlating pacifier use and increased risk of infections or dental malocclusion, there are no recommendations for or against pacifier use related to oral health (Nelson, 2012). Both pacifier use and thumb sucking may also have significant cultural variations. Thumb sucking reaches its peak at age 18 to 20 months and is most prevalent when children are hungry, tired, or feeling insecure. Persistent thumb sucking in a listless, apathetic child always warrants investigation. It may be a sign of an emotional problem between the parent and child or of boredom, isolation, and lack of stimulation.

Teething

One of the more difficult periods in infants' (and parents') lives is the eruption of the deciduous (primary) teeth, often referred to as *teething*. The age of tooth eruption shows considerable variation among children, but the order of tooth appearance is fairly regular and predictable (Fig. 9.10). The first primary teeth to erupt are the lower central incisors, which appear at approximately 6 to 10 months old (average, 8 months old). These are followed closely by the upper central incisors. A quick guide to assessment of deciduous teeth during the first 2 years is: Age of the child in months − 6 = Number of teeth. For example: 8 months of age − 6 = 2 teeth at this age.

Teething is a physiologic process; some discomfort is common as the crown of the tooth breaks through the periodontal membrane. Some children show minimum evidence of teething, such as drooling, increased finger sucking, or biting on hard objects. Others are irritable, have difficulty sleeping, ear rubbing, and decreased interest in solid foods. Generally, signs of illness such as fever (>39° C), vomiting, or

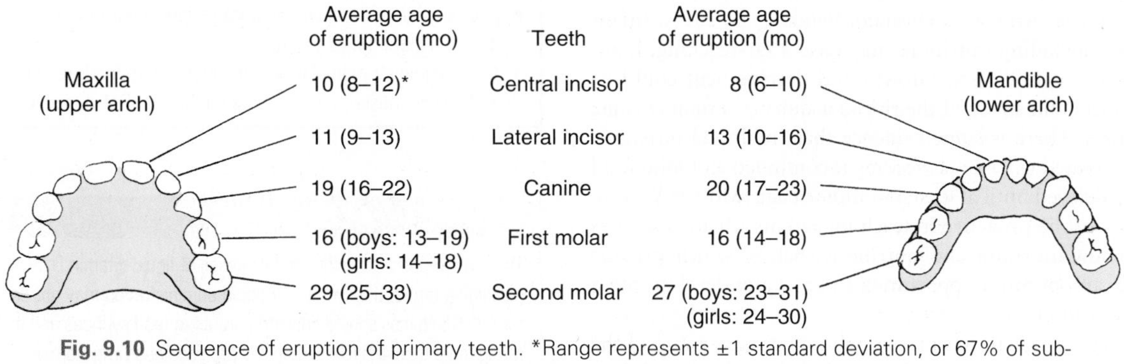

Fig. 9.10 Sequence of eruption of primary teeth. *Range represents ±1 standard deviation, or 67% of subjects studied. (Data from American Dental Association. [2014]. *Eruption charts.* Retrieved from http://www.ada.org/2930.aspx?currentTab=1)

diarrhea are not symptoms of teething but of illness and may warrant further investigation. Because teething pain is a result of inflammation, cold is soothing. Giving the child a frozen teething ring helps relieve the inflammation, but do not freeze teething rings filled with gels or nonsterile water because they may crack and leak into the infant's mouth. Several nonprescription topical anesthetic ointments are available, although the active ingredient in most of them is benzocaine, which may cause a rare but serious disorder called *methemoglobinemia.* Therefore the US Food and Drug Administration (2018) recommends use of such products only under the advice and supervision of a health care provider. In the event of persistent irritability that affects sleeping and feeding, systemic analgesics (such as, acetaminophen or ibuprofen) can be given (if age appropriate) for no more than 3 days; however, parents should know that this is a temporary measure, and they should contact the practitioner if symptoms persist or if the child's condition changes.

The use of teething powders or procedures such as cutting or rubbing the gums with salicylates (aspirin) is discouraged because ingestion of the powder, infection or irritation of the tissue, and ingestion or aspiration of the aspirin can occur. Hard candy may cause accidental choking or aspiration and should be avoided at this age.

PROMOTING OPTIMAL HEALTH DURING INFANCY

NUTRITION

Ideally, discussion of optimal nutrition should begin prenatally to address maternal intake of adequate nutrition in the form of a balanced diet and adequate amounts of protein, vitamins, and minerals—all of which have an impact on the growing fetus. Nurses should encourage and provide information for parents to discuss the options of breastfeeding or bottle-feeding the infant well in advance of the delivery date. The choice is highly individual and is discussed in Chapter 7. This section is primarily concerned with infant nutrition during the months when growth needs and developmental milestones ready the child for the introduction of solid foods.

Despite adequate availability of optimum nutrient sources, experts are concerned that infants are not fed appropriately. Infants may be given solid foods when their digestive systems are not ready to completely absorb such foods. In addition, drinks that are inappropriate for growing infants may be given in place of enriched infant milk and may provide only "empty" calories; contribute to childhood and adult obesity; and place infants at risk for iron-deficiency anemia, vitamin D deficiency, and rickets. A survey of infant feeding practices found that about 20% of infants had consumed solid foods before 4 months of age despite recommendations that such foods not be introduced until 4 to 6 months of age (Aronsson, Uusitalo, Vehik, et al., 2015). Infant health practices, including nutrition, may have a far-reaching, long-term impact on the child's life. Growth and development could be negatively affected, and so could the risk of acquiring certain chronic health conditions. There is some evidence that childhood obesity is significantly decreased when breastfeeding is continued and solid food introduction is delayed until at least 4 months of age (Moss & Yeaton, 2014). Nurses must be proactive in teaching parents what constitutes appropriate infant nutrition and nutritional habits, which provide the infant with an optimum opportunity to grow and develop into a healthy child and adult.

Health care professionals have recently become more aware of the use of complementary and alternative medical therapies in children that may not be as beneficial as touted in various media sources. One concern is children's intake of megavitamins and herbs; parents may assume that the word *natural* in reference to ingredients means that the product is safe when this may not be the case. It is important for nurses to be aware of the effects, availability, and practice of complementary therapies and to be able to cogently discuss their use with parents.

The First 6 Months

Human milk is the most desirable complete diet for infants during the first 6 months. A healthy term infant receiving breast milk from a well-nourished mother usually requires no specific vitamin and mineral supplements with a few exceptions. Daily supplements of vitamin D and vitamin B_{12} may be indicated if the mother's intake of these vitamins is inadequate. The American Academy of Pediatrics (Wagner, Greer, American Academy of Pediatrics Section on Breastfeeding, et al., 2008) recommends that all infants (including those exclusively breastfed) receive a daily supplement of 400 IU of vitamin D beginning in the first few days of life to prevent rickets and vitamin D deficiency. Vitamin D supplementation should occur until the infant is consuming at least 1 L/day (or 1 qt/day) of vitamin D–fortified formula (Wagner et al., 2008). Nonbreastfed infants who are taking less than 1 L/day of vitamin D–fortified formula should also receive a daily vitamin D supplement of 400 IU (see Safety Alert). If the infant is being exclusively breastfed after 4 months old (when fetal iron stores are depleted), iron supplementation (1 mg/kg/day) is recommended until appropriate iron-containing complementary foods (such as iron-fortified cereal) are introduced (Baker & Greer, 2010) (see Community Focus box). Infants, whether breastfed or bottle-fed, do not require additional fluids, especially water or juice, during the first 4 months of life. Excessive intake of water in infants may result in water intoxication and hyponatremia.

COMMUNITY FOCUS

Administration of Iron Supplements

- Ideally, iron supplements should be administered between meals for greater absorption.
- Liquid iron supplements may stain the teeth; therefore administer them with a dropper toward the back of the mouth (side). In older children, administer liquid iron supplements through a straw or rinse the mouth thoroughly after ingestion.
- Avoid administration of liquid iron supplements with whole cow's milk or milk products, because they bind free iron and prevent absorption.
- Educate parents that iron supplements will turn stools black or tarry green.
- Iron supplements may cause transient constipation. Caution parents not to switch to a low-iron formula or whole milk, which are both poor sources of iron and may lead to iron-deficiency anemia (see Chapter 24, Iron-Deficiency Anemia).
- In older children, follow liquid iron supplement with a citrus fruit or juice drink (no more than 3 to 4 oz).
- Avoid administration of iron supplements with foods or drinks that bind iron and prevent absorption (see Chapter 24, Iron-Deficiency Anemia).

SAFETY ALERT

There are reports of accidental overdoses of liquid vitamin D in infants caused by packaging errors; the syringe for liquid administration may not be labeled clearly for 400 IU. Nurses should educate parents to read syringes and to avoid administering more than 400 IU of vitamin D (US Food and Drug Administration Consumer Health Information, 2010).

Fluoride supplementation in exclusively breastfed children is not required for the first 6 months because of the risk of dental fluorosis. However, fluoride supplementation may be necessary if the breastfeeding mother's water supply does not contain the required amount of fluoridation (see discussion later in the chapter). Employed mothers can continue breastfeeding with guidance and encouragement.[a] Mothers are encouraged to set realistic goals for employment and breastfeeding, with accurate information regarding the costs, risks, and benefits of available feeding options. Barriers encountered by working breastfeeding mothers include lack of employer or coworker support, unavailable or inadequate facilities for pumping and storing milk, lack of time to express milk while at work, real or perceived low milk supply, and insufficient time allowed to pump during work. Many mothers may find that a program of breast pumping when away from home and bottle-feeding the infant the expressed milk with or without formula supplementation is successful. Expressed breast milk may be stored in the refrigerator (4°C [39°F]) without danger of bacterial contamination for up to 5 days (Lawrence & Lawrence, 2016). Although feeding the infant at home may occur on a demand basis, pumping milk away from home may be needed every 3 to 4 hours to maintain adequate supply. Breast milk may be expressed by hand or pump (manual or electric) and stored in an appropriate airtight glass or plastic container. Expressed breast milk may be frozen (−18°C [0°F] or lower) for up to 6 months (depending on the type of freezer used), but care should be taken to prevent freezer burn (see *Breastfeeding: A Guide for the Medical Profession* [Lawrence & Lawrence, 2016] for further guidelines on storing and freezing human milk).

In addition to efficient breast pumping, mothers also need child care by a trusted individual or agency and support and assistance from significant others. As with all breastfeeding mothers, these women must have proper nutrition and rest for adequate lactation. Maternal fatigue is considered the biggest threat to successful breastfeeding in employed mothers.

! NURSING ALERT

Warming expressed milk in a microwave decreases the availability of anti-infective properties and nutrients (Labiner-Wolfe & Fein, 2013). To prevent oral burns from uneven warming of the milk, breast milk should never be thawed or rewarmed in a microwave oven. To thaw the frozen milk, either place the container under a lukewarm water bath (<40.5°C [105°F]) or place it in a refrigerator overnight.

There are reports of an increase in the use of herbs by lactating mothers to increase breast milk supply. The **galactogogues**, including fenugreek, blessed thistle, fennel, and chaste tree, have been purported to increase maternal milk supply, but a recent systematic review found insufficient evidence for the use of any type of galactogogues (Mortel & Mehta, 2013). For a discussion of galactogogues, including those mentioned here, see Appendix P, Protocol 9, in *Breastfeeding: A Guide for the Medical Profession* (Lawrence & Lawrence, 2016).

An acceptable alternative to breastfeeding is commercial iron-fortified formula. Similar to human milk, it supplies all nutrients needed by infants for the first 6 months. Unmodified whole cow's milk, low-fat cow's milk, skim milk, other animal milks, and imitation milk drinks are not acceptable as major sources of nutrition for infants because of their limited digestibility, increased risk of contamination, and lack of components needed for appropriate growth. Whole milk can cause iron-deficiency anemia in infants, possibly as a result of occult gastrointestinal blood loss. Pasteurized whole cow's milk is deficient in iron, zinc, and vitamin C and has a high renal solute load, which makes it undesirable for infants younger than 12 months old (American Academy of Pediatrics, 2014, Committee on Nutrition).

! NURSING ALERT

Dietary fat in infants younger than 6 months old should not be restricted unless on specific medical advice. Substituting skim or low-fat milk is unacceptable because the essential fatty acids are inadequate and the solute concentration of protein and electrolytes, such as sodium, is too high.

The amount of formula per feeding and the number of feedings per day vary among infants. Infants being fed on demand usually determine their own feeding schedule, but some infants may need a more planned schedule based on average feeding patterns to ensure sufficient nutrients. In general, the number of feedings decreases from six at 1 month old to four or five at 6 months old. Regardless of the number of feedings, the total amount of formula ingested will usually level off at about 32 ounces (946 ml) per day.

Honey should be avoided in the first 12 months because of the risk of botulism (see Chapter 30); pacifiers should not be coated with honey to encourage the infant to take it. Socializing the infant to food flavors of the family's culture is common in addition to continuing breastfeeding for 2 to 4 years (see Cultural Considerations box).

CULTURAL CONSIDERATIONS

Multicultural Feeding Practices

Cultural beliefs and values often influence infant-feeding practices. Health care professionals may benefit from understanding the multicultural feeding practices that parents choose for their infants. Traditional feeding practices include offering a variety of liquids or foods (such as sugared wine, water, or honey) during the first few days of life and thereafter.

Bottled water for mixing powdered or concentrated formula is a relatively safe alternative to tap water if available. Tap water has a high content of contaminants, such as lead. Do not assume, however, that bottled water is sterile unless specifically stated on the container. Fluoridated bottled water is not necessary for mixing powdered formula unless the local water source is low in fluoride, in which case fluoride supplementation is recommended after 6 months of age (see Dental Health later in this chapter).

The addition of solid foods before 4 to 6 months old is not recommended. During the early months, solid foods are not compatible with the ability of the gastrointestinal tract and infant's nutritional needs. Feeding solids to young infants exposes them to food antigens that may produce food protein allergy. New peanut guidelines from the American Academy of Pediatrics (AAP) (2017), recommend early introduction of peanut proteins for infants who are at highest risk of allergy should be done at 4-6 months of age in an effort to decrease the risk of severe lifetime allergies. Specific guidelines based on the infant's risk factors issued by the AAP can be found at https://www.aap.org/en-us/about-the-aap/aap-press-room/Pages/AAP-Clinical-Report-Highlights-Early-Introduction-of-Peanut-Based-Foods-to-Prevent-Allergies.aspx

Developmentally, infants are not ready for solid food. The extrusion (protrusion) reflex is strong and often causes them to push food out of the mouth. Infants instinctively suck when given food. Because of their

[a]See also *The CDC Guide to Strategies to Support Breastfeeding Mothers and Babies,* which includes information for breastfeeding in the workplace. This guide was updated in 2013 and can be downloaded at http://www.cdc.gov/breastfeeding/pdf/BF-Guide-508.PDF.

limited motor abilities, infants are unable to deliberately push food away or avoid feeding. Therefore, early introduction of solids is a type of forced feeding that may lead to excessive weight gain and increased predisposition to allergies and iron-deficiency anemia. Parents should be cautioned concerning the use of juices and nonnutritive drinks such as fruit-flavored drinks or carbonated beverages (soda or pop) during this period. Many juices and nonnutritive drinks, although readily available to consumers, do not provide sufficient and appropriate caloric intake for infants younger than 12 months old; such drinks may replace the nutrients in breast milk or formula and lead to growth or health problems. Fruit juices offer no nutritional benefit for infants younger than 1 year (Heyman & Abrams, 2017).

The Second 6 Months

During the second half of the first year, human milk or formula should continue to be the primary source of nutrition. The use of fluoride supplementation depends on the infant's intake of fluoride tap water (see the Dental Health section later in the chapter). If breastfeeding is discontinued, a commercial iron-fortified formula should be substituted. Follow-up or transition formulas marketed for older infants offer no special advantages over other infant formulas and provide excessive protein (American Academy of Pediatrics, Committee on Nutrition, 2014).

The major change in feeding habits is the addition of solid foods to the infant's diet. Physiologically and developmentally, infants 4 to 6 months old are in a transition period. By this time, the gastrointestinal tract has matured sufficiently to handle more complex nutrients and is less sensitive to potentially allergenic foods. Tooth eruption is beginning and facilitates biting and chewing. The extrusion reflex has disappeared, and swallowing is more coordinated to allow infants to accept solids easily. Head control is well developed, which permits infants to sit with support and purposely turn their heads away to communicate lack of interest in food. Voluntary grasping and improved eye–hand coordination gradually allow infants to pick up finger foods and feed themselves. Their increasing sense of independence is evident in their desire to hold their bottles and try to "help" during feeding.

Selection and Preparation of Solid Foods

The choice of solid foods to introduce first is variable but should meet the reasons for feeding solids, such as supplying nutrients not found in formula or breast milk. Iron-fortified infant cereal is generally introduced first because of its high iron content (7 mg/3 Tbsp of prepared dry cereal). Commercially prepared ready-to-serve dry cereals for infants include rice, barley, oatmeal, and high-protein cereals; rice is usually suggested as an initial food because of its easy digestibility and low allergenic potential. Cereals (such as cream of farina) are not used because infant commercial cereals are a better source of iron. Some of the commercial baby cereals are combined with fruit. There is little nutritional benefit from these preparations, and they are more expensive. New foods should be added one at a time; therefore parents should avoid cereal combinations when beginning a new grain.

Infant cereal (iron fortified) may be mixed with expressed breast milk or water until whole milk is given. After 12 months of age, small amounts of 100% fruit juices can be mixed with the dry cereal; the vitamin C content of the juice enhances the absorption of iron in the cereal. Because of their benefit as a source of iron, infant cereals should be continued until the child is 18 months old.

Fruit juice can be offered from a cup for its rich source of vitamin C and as a substitute for milk for one feeding a day. Large quantities of certain juices (e.g., apple, pear, prune, sweet cherry, peach, and grape) are avoided because they may cause abdominal pain, diarrhea, or bloating in some children. Avoid fruit-flavored drinks, which may be marketed as juices but contain high concentrations of complex sugars. White grape juice (no more than 5 oz/day) may be better absorbed and safe for infants this age without causing gastrointestinal distress. The American Academy of Pediatrics, Committee on Nutrition (2014) recommends that fruit juice intake not exceed 4 to 6 ounces per day and that juices not be given to infants younger than 4 to 6 months old. Because vitamin C is naturally destroyed by heat, juice is not warmed. Juice containers are always kept covered and refrigerated to prevent further vitamin loss.

The addition of other foods is arbitrary. A common sequence is to introduce strained fruits followed by vegetables and, finally, meats; however, some clinicians prefer to add vegetables before fruit. If foods are introduced early, citrus fruits, meats, and eggs are delayed until after 6 months of age because of their potential to result in allergy. At 6 months, foods such as a cracker or zwieback can be offered as finger and teething foods. By 8 to 9 months of age, junior foods and nutritious finger foods such as firmly cooked vegetable, raw pieces of fruit, or cheese can be given. By 1 year of age, well-cooked table foods are served.

The introduction of solid foods into the infant's diet at this age is primarily for taste and chewing experience, not for growth. The majority of infants' caloric needs are derived from the primary milk source (human or formula); therefore solids should not be perceived as a substitute for milk until the child is older than 12 months. Portion sizes may vary according to the infant's taste. In general, 1 Tbsp per year of age (i.e., ½ to ¾ Tbsp for most infants under 12 months old) is adequate for most infants. In most cases, 2 Tbsp may be served, but because of infants' focus on the texture and feel of the food, smaller amounts will be consumed. Another reason for smaller portions is the concern over feeding habits in early childhood and obesity; early feeding of smaller portions may help prevent the "clean your plate" or "eat all your food or you can't get down from the table" concepts, which are known to contribute to overeating in later life. The addition of solid foods to exclusively breastfed infants' diet does not significantly increase overall caloric intake or weight gain.

Commercially prepared baby foods are the most common type of food served to infants in the United States. They are convenient and usually contain no added salt or sugar but can be relatively expensive. An alternative is to prepare baby foods at home, which is a simple and inexpensive process.

In general, low-calorie milk and foods should be avoided in infants and toddlers unless a strict medically prescribed diet is required. Infants' growth during this phase is crucial to future development, and dietary fat should be curtailed with great caution. At the same time, it is important to recognize that certain types of dietary fat are unacceptable for infants; fried potatoes, candy, ice cream, cake, soda pop and other sweetened drinks, and other such items do not constitute an appropriate amount of fat intake and may contribute to childhood obesity. One suggestion is to limit the *amount* (serving size) of dietary fat in foods provided rather than eliminate them altogether, especially during infancy.

Parents are cautioned to avoid reliance on foods and supplements marketed as iron or vitamin fortified as primary sources of minerals. Instead, encourage parents to offer the child a variety of fruits, vegetables, and whole grains, including those known to naturally be rich in iron.

Introduction of Solid Foods

When the spoon is first introduced, infants often push it away and appear dissatisfied. Food that is placed on the front of the tongue and pushed out is simply scooped up and refed. As infants become accustomed to the spoon, they will more eagerly accept the food and eventually open the mouth in anticipation (or keep it closed in dislike).

One food item is introduced at intervals of 4 to 7 days to allow for identification of food allergies. New foods are fed in small amounts. As the amount of solid food increases, the quantity of milk is decreased to less than 1 L/day to prevent overfeeding.

Because feeding is a learning process, as well as a means of nutrition, new foods are given alone to allow the child to learn new tastes and textures. Food should not be mixed in the bottle and fed through a nipple with a large hole. This deprives the child of the pleasure of learning new tastes and developing a discriminating palate. It can also cause problems with poor chewing of food later in life because of lack of experience. Guidelines for the introduction of new foods are given in the Family-Centered Care box.

FAMILY-CENTERED CARE

Feeding During the First Year

Birth to 6 Months Old (Breastfeeding or Bottle-Feeding)

Breastfeeding

- Most desirable complete diet for the first half of the first year.[a]
- A recommended supplement is oral vitamin D (400 IU/day).
- In exclusively breastfed infants 4 months old and older, recommend an iron supplement of 1 mg/kg/day until iron-rich complementary foods are introduced.

Formula

- Iron-fortified commercial formula is a complete food for the first half of the first year.[a]
- Requires fluoride supplements (0.25 mg) when the concentration of fluoride in the drinking water is below 0.3 ppm after 6 months old.
- Evaporated milk formula requires supplements of vitamin C, iron, and fluoride (in accordance with the fluoride content of the local water supply after 6 months old).

4 to 12 Months Old (Solid Foods)

- May begin to add solids by 4 to 6 months old.
- First foods are strained, pureed, or finely mashed.
- Finger foods such as teething crackers, raw fruit, or vegetables can be introduced by 6 to 7 months old.
- Chopped table food or commercially prepared junior foods can be started by 9 to 12 months old.
- With the exception of cereal, the order of introducing foods is variable; a recommended sequence is fruit, then vegetables, and then meat.
- Introduce one food at a time, usually at intervals of 4 to 7 days, to identify food allergies.
- Introduce solids when the infant is hungry.
- Begin spoon feeding by pushing food to back of tongue because of infants' natural tendency to thrust the tongue forward.
- Use a small spoon with a straight handle; begin with 1 or 2 tsp of food; gradually increase to 2 to 3 Tbsp per feeding.
- As the quantity of solids increases, decrease the quantity of milk to prevent overfeeding. Limit formula or milk to approximately 960 ml (32 oz) daily and fruit juice to less than 180 ml (6 oz) daily.
- Never introduce foods by mixing them with the formula in the bottle.

Cereal—Start at 4 to 6 Months Old

- Introduce commercially prepared iron-fortified infant cereals and administer daily until 18 months old.
- Rice cereal is usually introduced first because of its low allergenic potential.
- Parents can discontinue supplemental iron when iron-fortified cereal is given.

Fruits and Vegetables—Start at 6 to 8 Months Old

- Applesauce, bananas, and pears are usually well tolerated.
- Avoid fruits and vegetables marketed in cans that are not specifically designed for infants because of variable and sometimes high lead content and addition of salt, sugar, or preservatives.
- Offer fruit juice only from a cup, not a bottle, to reduce the development of early childhood caries. Limit to 4 ounces per day or less.

Meat, Fish, and Poultry—Start at 8 to 10 Months Old

- Avoid fatty meats.
- Prepare by baking, broiling, steaming, or poaching.
- Include organ meats such as liver, which has a high iron, vitamin A, and vitamin B complex content.
- If soup is given, be certain all ingredients are familiar to child's diet.
- Avoid commercial meat and vegetable combinations because their protein content is low.

Eggs and Cheese—Start at 12 Months Old

- Serve egg yolk hard boiled and mashed, soft cooked, or poached.
- Introduce egg white in small quantities (1 tsp) toward the end of the first year to detect an allergy.
- Use cheese as a substitute for meat and as finger food.

[a]Breastfeeding or commercial formula feeding for up to 12 months old is recommended. After 1 year, whole cow's milk can be given.

Weaning

Defined as the process of giving up one method of feeding for another, **weaning** usually refers to relinquishing the breast or bottle for a cup. In Western societies, this is generally regarded as a major task for infants and is often seen as a potentially traumatic experience. It is psychologically significant because infants are required to give up a major source of oral pleasure and gratification.

Other cultural groups define weaning in relation to significant life events (e.g., teething) or reaching a specific age. No one time for weaning is best for every child, but generally, most infants show signs of readiness during the second half of the first year. It is recommended that weaning occur with the infant's needs as a guide (Lawrence & Lawrence, 2016). Their increasing desire for freedom of movement may lessen their desire to be held close for feedings. They are acquiring more control over their actions and can easily manipulate a cup to their lips (even if it is held upside down!). Imitation becomes a powerful motivator by 8 or 9 months of age, and they enjoy using a cup or glass like others do.

Weaning should be gradual by replacing one bottle or breastfeeding session at a time. The nighttime feeding is usually the last feeding to be discontinued. It is advisable to never allow a child to take a bottle of milk to bed; this is a major cause of caries in deciduous teeth. If breastfeeding is terminated before 5 or 6 months of age, weaning should be to a bottle (not in bed) to provide for the infant's continued sucking needs. If discontinued later, weaning can be directly to a cup, especially by 12 to 14 months of age. Any sweet liquid, such as fruit juice, should be given in a cup and should not be given at bedtime.

SLEEP AND ACTIVITY

Sleep patterns vary among infants, with active infants typically sleeping less than placid children. The total daily sleep for 2-month-old infants is approximately 15 hours (range, 10 to 20 hours), whereas the total daily sleep for 6- to 12-month-old infants is approximately 13 hours (range, 9 to 17 hours) (Galland, Taylor, Elder, et al., 2012). Sleeping through the night usually occurs between 3 and 4 months of age. Consolidation of nocturnal sleep hours occurs during the first 12 months, with decreasing daytime sleep and increasing nighttime sleep. Generally, by 12 months of age, most infants have developed a nocturnal pattern of sleep that lasts at least 8 hours. The number of naps per day varies, but infants typically take two naps by the end of the first year. Breastfed infants usually sleep for shorter periods, especially during the night, compared with bottle-fed infants (Middlemiss, Yaure, & Huey, 2015). A discussion of sleep problems is found in Chapter 10.

Most infants are naturally active and need no encouragement to be mobile. Problems can arise when devices such as play yards, strollers, commercial swings, and mobile walkers are used excessively. These items restrict movement and prevent infants from exploring and developing gross motor skills. Contrary to popular belief, mobile walkers do not enhance coordination and are dangerous if tipped over or placed near the top of stairs, porches, in-ground pools, furnaces, and other hazardous surfaces.

DENTAL HEALTH

Good dental hygiene begins with appropriate maternal dental health before and during the pregnancy, and counseling during early infancy regarding dietary intake for the promotion of optimum oral hygiene. Counsel parents early regarding feeding practices that increase the risk of poor dental health. Some of these, as previously mentioned, include avoiding propping the milk bottle; giving the milk bottle in the bed; or giving fruit juices in a bottle for as long as possible. These contribute to enamel erosion and **early childhood caries** (previously called *baby bottle tooth decay*).

When the primary teeth erupt, cleaning should begin. The teeth and gums are initially cleaned by wiping them with a damp cloth; toothbrushing is too harsh for the tender gingiva. The caregiver can stabilize the infant by cradling the child with one arm and using the free hand to cleanse the teeth. Oral hygiene can be made pleasant by singing or talking to the infant. It is recommended that the infant have a brief oral health examination by 6 months of age from a qualified pediatric health practitioner; infants at high risk for caries are identified, and oral health counseling is implemented. It is also recommended that the infant have an established dental home by 1 year of age (American Academy of Pediatric Dentistry, 2016). It is generally recommended that a small, soft-bristled toothbrush be used as more teeth erupt and the infant adjusts to the routine of cleaning. Water is preferred to toothpaste, which the infant will swallow (and if the toothpaste is fluoridated, the infant may ingest excessive amounts of fluoride). The American Academy of Pediatric Dentistry (2016) recommends a "smear" of toothpaste for children younger than 3 years old and a pea-size amount for those 3 to 6 years old.

Fluoride, an essential mineral for building caries-resistant teeth, is needed beginning at 6 months of age if the infant does not receive water with adequate fluoride content. The American Academy of Pediatric Dentistry (2016) recommends that the determination of fluoride administration be based on the individual needs of each child. Systemic fluoride administration should be considered for all children at risk for dental caries who drink fluoride-deficient water (<0.6 ppm) but only after determining all dietary sources of fluoride.

Dietary considerations are also important because habits begun during infancy tend to continue into later years. Avoid foods with concentrated sugar (sucrose) in the infant's diet. Dietary considerations are also important because habits begun during infancy tend to continue into later years. Foods with concentrated sugar are used sparingly (if at all) in the infant's diet. The practice of coating pacifiers with honey or using commercially available hard-candy pacifiers is discouraged. Besides being cariogenic, honey also may cause infant botulism, and parts of the candy pacifier can be aspirated (Box 9.1). Parents need to be counseled regarding the detrimental effects of frequent and

BOX 9.1 Safety Promotion and Injury Prevention During Infancy

Birth to 4 Months Old

Major Developmental Accomplishments

Exhibits involuntary reflexes (e.g., crawling reflex may propel infant forward or backward; startle reflex may cause the body to jerk)

May roll over

Has increasing eye–hand coordination and voluntary grasp reflex

Injury Prevention

Aspiration

Aspiration is not as great a danger to this age-group, but parents should begin practicing safeguarding early (see 4 to 7 Months Old later in this box).

Never shake baby powder directly on infant; place powder in hand and then on infant's skin; store container closed and out of the infant's reach.

Hold infant for feeding; do not prop bottle.

Know emergency procedures for choking.

Use pacifier with one-piece construction and loop handle.

Burns

Install smoke detectors in home.

Do not use microwave oven to warm formula; always check temperature of liquid before feeding.

Check bathwater.

Do not pour hot liquids when infant is close by, such as sitting on lap.

Beware of cigarette ashes that may fall on infant.

Do not leave infant in sun for more than a few minutes; keep exposed areas covered.

Wash flame-retardant clothes according to label directions.

Use cool-mist vaporizers.

Do not leave child in parked car.

Check surface heat of car restraint before placing child in seat.

Suffocation and Drowning

Keep all plastic bags stored out of infant's reach; discard large plastic garment bags after tying in a knot.

Do not cover mattress with plastic.

Use firm mattress and loose blankets with no pillows.

Make certain crib design follows federal regulations and mattress fits snugly—crib slats 2.375 inches (6 cm) apart.[a]

Position crib away from other furniture and away from radiators.

Do not tie pacifier on a string around infant's neck.

Remove bibs at bedtime.

Never leave infant alone in bath.

Do not leave infant younger than 12 months old alone on adult or youth mattress or beanbag-type seats.

Motor Vehicles

Transport infant in federally approved, rear-facing car seat, preferably in back seat.

Do not place infant on seat (of car) or in lap.

BOX 9.1 Safety Promotion and Injury Prevention During Infancy—cont'd

Do not place child in a carriage or stroller behind a parked car.
Do not place infant or child in front passenger seat with an air bag.
Do not leave infant unattended in car.

Falls
Use crib with fixed, raised rails.
Never leave infant alone on a raised, unguarded surface.
When in doubt as to where to place child, use floor.
Restrain child in infant seat, and never leave child unattended while the seat is resting on a raised surface.
Avoid using a high chair until child can sit well with support.

Accidental Poisoning
Poisoning is not as great a danger to this age-group, but parents should begin practicing safeguards early (see 4 to 7 Months Old later in this box).

Bodily Damage
Keep sharp or jagged objects, such as knives and broken glass, out of child's reach.
Keep diaper pins closed and away from infant.

4 to 7 Months Old
Major Developmental Accomplishments
Rolls over
Sits momentarily
Grasps and manipulates small objects
Re-secures a dropped object
Has well-developed eye–hand coordination
Can focus on and locate small objects
Has prominent mouthing (oral fixation)
Can push up on hands and knees
Crawls backward

Injury Prevention
Aspiration
Keep buttons, beads, syringe caps, and other small objects out of infant's reach.
Keep floor free of any small objects.
Do not feed infant hard candy, nuts, food with pits or seeds, or whole or circular pieces of hot dog.
Exercise caution when giving teething biscuits because large chunks may be broken off and aspirated.
Do not feed infant while he or she is lying down.
Inspect toys for removable parts.
Keep baby powder, if used, out of reach.
Avoid storing cleaning fluid, paints, pesticides, and other toxic substances within infant's reach.
Know telephone number of local poison control center (800-222-1222) (usually listed in front of telephone directory).

Suffocation
Keep all latex balloons out of reach.
Remove all crib toys that are strung across crib or play yard when child begins to push up on hands or knees or is 5 months old.

Burns
Keep water faucets out of reach.
Place hot objects (cigarettes, candles, incense) on high surface out of child's reach.
Limit exposure to sun; apply sunscreen.

Falls
Restrain in a high chair.
Keep crib rails raised to full height.

Motor Vehicles
See Birth to 4 Months Old earlier in this box.

Accidental Poisoning
Make certain that paint for furniture or toys does not contain lead.
Place toxic substances on a high shelf or in a locked cabinet.
Hang plants or place on high surface rather than on floor.
Know telephone number of local poison control center (800-222-1222) (usually listed in front of telephone directory).

Bodily Damage
Give toys that are smooth and rounded, preferably made of wood or plastic.
Avoid long, pointed objects as toys.
Avoid toys that are excessively loud.
Keep sharp objects out of infant's reach.

8 to 12 Months Old
Major Developmental Accomplishments
Crawls or creeps
Stands holding on to furniture
Stands alone
Cruises around furniture
Walks
Climbs
Pulls on objects
Throws objects
Picks up small objects; has pincer grasp
Explores by putting objects in mouth
Dislikes being restrained
Explores away from parent
Increasingly understands simple commands and phrases

Injury Prevention
Aspiration
Keep small objects off floor, off furniture, and out of reach of children.
Take care when feeding solid table food to give very small pieces.
Do not use beanbag toys or allow child to play with dried beans.
See also 4 to 7 Months Old earlier in this box.

Bodily Damage
See 4 to 7 Months Old earlier in this box.
Avoid placing televisions or other large objects on top of furniture, which may be overturned when infant pulls self to standing position.

Falls
Avoid walkers, especially near stairs.[a]
Ensure that furniture is sturdy enough for child to pull self to standing position and cruise.
Fence stairways at top and bottom if child has access to either end.[a]
Dress infant in safe shoes and clothing (soles that do not "catch" on floor, tied shoelaces, pant legs that do not touch floor).

Suffocation and Drowning
Keep doors of ovens, dishwashers, refrigerators, coolers, and front-loading clothes washers and dryers closed at all times.
If storing an unused large appliance, such as a refrigerator, remove the door.
Supervise contact with inflated balloons; immediately discard popped balloons and keep uninflated balloons out of reach.
Fence swimming pools and other bodies of standing water, such as decorative fountains; lock gate to swimming pools so that only adult can access.

Continued

BOX 9.1 Safety Promotion and Injury Prevention During Infancy—cont'd

Always supervise when near any source of water, such as cleaning buckets, drainage areas, toilets.
Keep bathroom doors closed.
Eliminate unnecessary pools of water.
Keep one hand on child at all times when in tub.

Accidental Poisoning

Administer medications as a drug, not as a candy.
Do not administer medications unless prescribed by a practitioner.
Return medications and poisons to safe storage area immediately after use; replace caps properly if a child-protector cap is used.
Have poison control center number (800-222-1222) on telephone and refrigerator.

Burns

Place guards in front of or around any heating appliance, fireplace, or furnace.
Keep electrical wires hidden or out of reach.
Place plastic guards over electrical outlets; place furniture in front of outlets.
Keep hanging tablecloths out of reach (child may pull down hot liquids or heavy or sharp objects).

[a]Information on many items such as cribs or walkers is available from US Consumer Product Safety Commission, 800-638-2772; http://www.cpsc.gov/.

prolonged bottle-feeding or breastfeeding during sleep, when the sweet milk or other fluid (such as juice) bathes the teeth, producing early childhood caries. In addition, carbonated beverages should be avoided in infancy. (See Chapter 11 for a more extensive discussion of dental health, including early childhood caries.)

SAFETY PROMOTION AND INJURY PREVENTION

Injuries are a major cause of death during infancy, especially for children 6 to 12 months old. The three leading causes of accidental death injury in infants are suffocation, motor vehicle–related injuries, and drowning (Dellinger & Gilchrist, 2019). According to a Cochrane study, one-third of all injuries occur in the home, yet there is insufficient evidence to demonstrate that modification of the home environment has an impact on the rate of injuries (Turner, Arthur, Lyons, et al., 2011). Constant vigilance, awareness, and supervision are essential as children gain increased locomotor and manipulative skills that are coupled with an insatiable curiosity about the environment. Box 9.1 lists the major developmental achievements of each period during infancy and the appropriate injury prevention plan. Table 9.2 lists common types of injuries and associated objects that predispose to such injuries. Suggestions for promoting safety in the home environment are given for specific types of injuries. The acronym SAFE PAD, described in Table 9.2, may be used to identify common types of injuries to infants and older children.

Motor Vehicle Injuries

A significant number of infants are injured or die from improper restraint within vehicles, most often from riding on the lap of another occupant. Child restraint use decreases with increasing age of children and increasing number of occupants. Lack of proper child restraint continues to be a major factor in fatal accidents involving children. One observational report of newborns being placed in a car seat restraint by their family found a 52% incidence of newborn infants placed incorrectly in car seat restraints and a 48% incidence of errors in the placement of infant car seat restraints, with 29% of the car seat restraints not attached to the vehicle (Rogers, Gallo, Saleheen, et al., 2012). All infants must be secured in federally approved restraints rather than held or placed on the seat of the car. There is no safe alternative. Car seat restraints have an expiration date on the seat or in the owner's manual, which indicates the date when it should be destroyed and a new model purchased. If the car seat is in a motor vehicle accident, it may need to be replaced.

Infant restraints are designed either as an infant-only model or as a convertible infant–toddler model. Either restraint is a semireclined seat that faces the rear of the car. A rear-facing car seat provides the best protection for the disproportionately heavy head and weak neck of an infant. This position minimizes the stress on the neck by spreading the forces of a frontal crash over the entire back, neck, and head; the spine is supported by the back of the car seat. If the seat were faced forward, the head would whip forward because of the force of the crash, creating enormous stress on the neck (Fig. 9.11). It is now recommended that all infants and toddlers ride in rear-facing car safety seats for as long as possible or until they surpass the maximum height and weight recommended for the car seat (American Academy of Pediatrics, 2018).[b] Studies indicate that toddlers are safer riding in car seats in the rear-facing position (Truong, Hill, & Cole, 2013).

The restraint is anchored to the vehicle with the vehicle's seat belt, and the restraint has a harness system for securing the infant. Some harness systems require a clip to keep the shoulder straps correctly positioned. Newer vehicles (manufactured after 1999) have tether straps that attach to anchors in the car seat to better secure the seat and minimize forward movement of the forward-facing convertible seats in the event of an accident. The LATCH (lower anchor and tether for children) system provides car seat anchors between the front cushion and backrest so that the seat belt does not have to be used. Some automobiles have tether straps for rear-facing infant-only seats as well (see Fig. 9.11). Although many infant restraints can be recliners, they are used in the car only in the position specified by the manufacturer. In 2014 the National Highway Traffic Safety Administration changed the LATCH system rule, which now states that if the combined weight of the child and the car seat is more than 65 pounds, parents will be instructed to use the shoulder-lap belt restraint to restrain the child in the car seat instead of relying on the LATCH system for maximum protection.

Severe injuries and deaths in children have occurred from air bags deploying on impact in the front passenger seat. The back seat is the safest area of the car for children. For restraints to be effective, they must be used properly. Dressing the infant in an outfit with sleeves and legs allows the harness to hold the child securely in the seat. A small blanket or towel rolled tightly can be placed on either side of the head to minimize movement and keep the infant's hips against the back of the seat. Padding between the infant's legs and crotch is added to prevent slouching. Thick, soft padding is not placed under the infant or behind the back because during the impact, the padding will compress, leaving the harness straps loose. Preterm infants being discharged home from the hospital should be placed in appropriate

[b]Car seat information is available from the American Academy of Pediatrics at https://healthychildren.org/English/safety-prevention/on-the-go/Pages/Car-Safety-Seats-Information-for-Families.aspx and from the Insurance Institute for Highway Safety, 1005 N. Glebe Road, Suite 800, Arlington, VA 22201; 703-247-1500; http://www.iihs.org. The National Highway Traffic Safety Administration, http://www.nhtsa.gov, also provides child passenger safety and air bag safety information for parents.

TABLE 9.2 Common Infant Injuries, Associated Risk Factors, and Safety Promotion

Safe Pad Acronym	Risk Factors	Suggested Safety Interventions
Suffocation, sleep position	Latex balloons	Avoid latex balloons except with close adult supervision.
	Plastic bags	Tie unused plastic bags in a knot and dispose of them in a safe container.
	Bed surface (noninfant), such as sofa or adult bed	Avoid placing infants to sleep on sofas, soft bedding, or adult bed.
	Pillows	Avoid use of pillows for sleep.
	Soft cushions and blankets	Clear bedding of soft cushions and blankets.
	Prone sleeping	Place infant to sleep on back at all times.
Asphyxia, animal bites	Food items: Cylindrical items, such as hot dogs, hard candy, peanuts, almonds	Cut hot dogs lengthwise; avoid hard candy in infants and toddlers. Infants should completely chew each food item in mouth; do not feed more until item is swallowed.
	Toys: Small toys, such as Legos	As a general rule, if the toy fits into a toilet paper cardboard roll, it can be swallowed by a small child.
	Small objects: Batteries, buttons, beads, dried beans, syringe caps, safety pins	Keep out of reach of infants, who are naturally inquisitive.
	Pacifiers	Pacifiers should be one piece.
	Baby (talc) powder	Avoid shaking powder over infant; if used, place on adult's hand and then place on infant's skin.
	Domestic dogs, cats	Supervise child around domestic animals; teach not to approach dog that is eating, has puppies, or is not feeling well. Animals that are "tame" can be unpredictable. Small children are the right size for most domesticated animals to come face to face. Closely supervise child around visiting pets.
Falls	Stairs	Infants like to climb; place childproof gate at top and bottom of stairs.
	Diaper changing table	Infants do not have depth perception and cannot perceive a dangerous height from one that is safe. Never leave infants unattended on a flat surface even if not rolling over.
	Crib, bed-crib sides can fall when infant leans on them	In 2011 a mandate was issued to stop selling drop-side infant cribs.[a]
	Infant carriers	Never leave infant unattended in a carrier on top of a surface, such as a shopping cart, clothes dryer, washer, kitchen cabinet; place carrier on floor.
	Car seat restraints	Secure infant in car seat restraint securely and never leave unattended if unrestrained.
	High chair	Restrain infant in high chair; avoid using high chair except for feeding and only if adult supervision is adequate; even restrained infants can squirm out of some restraints and fall.
	Infant walkers	Use only stationary walkers. There is no evidence that walkers help infants "walk" any sooner. Wheeled walkers can easily be propelled off stairs and other platforms, such as porches or decks, causing significant injury.
	Windows, screens	Avoid placing furniture next to a window. Infants learn to climb and can fall out of open windows, even with screens.
	Television, stereos, sound systems	These must be secured to the stand; infants can pull the stand over, causing the TV or sound system to land on their heads, causing significant injury.
Electrical burns or burns	Electrical outlets	Place safety cap over electrical outlets; infants may be burned by placing conductive object into outlet.
	Hot hair combs, curlers	Keep out of reach of infant and keep turned off when not in use.
	Water	Infants may turn on tap or faucet in bathtub and burn self. Lower the water heater to a safe temperature of 49°C (120°F). Before placing infant in tub, check temperature of water and completely turn off faucet so child cannot alter temperature of water. *Never* leave infant unattended in tub or sink of water.
	Fireplace	Place a childproof screen in front of fireplace.
	Stove, hot liquids	Keep top front burners off and keep pot handles turned toward back to avoid infant pulling hot pot onto self and causing burn injuries.
	Cigarettes	Avoid smoking and holding infant on lap while smoking cigar or cigarette.
Poisoning, ingestions	Medication, ointments, cream, lotions	Medications left in purses or handbags or on a tabletop can often be ingested by the curious infant. Keep poison control center number readily available (800-222-1222).
	Plants: Household plants may be a source of accidental poisoning	Keep plants out of child's reach.
	Cleaning solutions	Store in locked cabinet or in top cabinet where there are no drawers or shelves for infant to climb on. Avoid storing cleaning and caustic solutions in containers such as a soda bottle or jar—infants and toddlers cannot differentiate a soda from a caustic drain cleaner.
	Inhalation or oral or nasal ingestion of poisonous or harmful chemicals such as methamphetamine, gasoline, turpentine	Keep gasoline and turpentine stored in a locked cabinet or closet out of child's reach. Avoid storing in containers that are also used to keep drinks or food.

Continued

TABLE 9.2 Common Infant Injuries, Associated Risk Factors, and Safety Promotion—cont'd

Safe Pad Acronym	Risk Factors	Suggested Safety Interventions
Automobile safety	Car or truck and hot weather	An automobile-related hazard for infants is overheating (hyperthermia) and subsequent death when left in a vehicle in hot weather (>26.4°C [80°F]). Infants dissipate heat poorly, and an increase in body temperature may cause death in a few hours. Caution parents against leaving infants in a vehicle alone for *any reason*.
	Air bags	Avoid placing infant in a car restraint behind an air bag. Deactivate the air bag (available in certain models) or place the infant in the back seat in a proper car seat restraint.
	Car seat restraint	See discussion earlier in the chapter.
Drowning	Bath tub	*Never* leave infant unattended in tub or sink of water.
	Swimming pools, bird baths, decorative ponds of water, splash pads	Place fence around pools with gate lock that is out of child's reach. Supervise infants in water at *all* times; an infant may drown in as little as 2 inches of water. Swimming lessons are encouraged but are not foolproof for drowning if infant or child hits head on hard object and becomes unconscious as falling into water.
	5-gallon buckets	Keep 5-gallon buckets empty of water or elevated out of child's reach.

[a]A number of parent education pamphlets (such as *Crib Safety Tips* and *Is Your Used Crib Safe?*) are available in English and Spanish from the US Consumer Product Safety Commission, 4330 East West Highway, Bethesda, MD 20814; 800-638-2772; http://www.cpsc.gov.

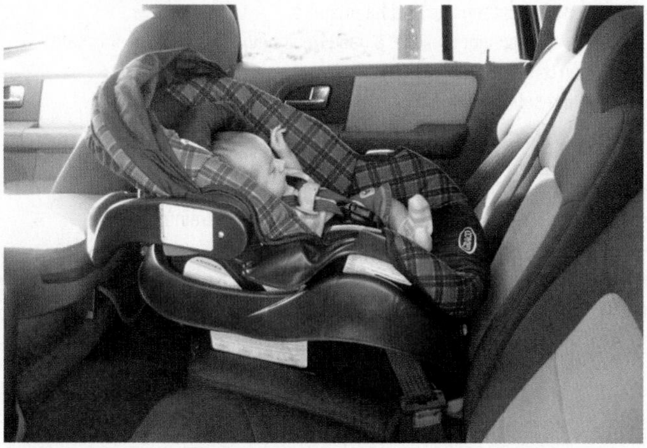

Fig. 9.11 Rear-facing infant seat in rear seat of car. The infant is placed in the seat when going home from the hospital. (Courtesy Brian and Mayannyn Sallee, Anchorage, AK.)

car seat restraints as they would be placed in the car prior to discharge, and their heart rate and oxygen saturation should be monitored for 90 to 120 minutes to detect any potential problems with airway occlusion. (For further discussion of car seat restraints, see Chapter 11.)

! NURSING ALERT

Rear-facing infant safety seats must not be placed in the front seats of cars equipped with an air bag on the passenger side. If an infant safety seat is placed in the passenger seat with an air bag, the child could be seriously injured if the air bag is released because rear-facing infant seats extend closer to the dashboard.

Nurse's Role in Injury Prevention

The task of injury prevention begins to be appreciated only when the potential environmental dangers to which infants are vulnerable are considered. Injury prevention and parent education should be handled on a growth and developmental basis. It is simply impossible to completely protect infants and small children from all potential dangers without placing them in a sterile, impractical environment. However, many childhood deaths continue to occur as a result of preventable injuries. Nurses must be aware of the possible causes of injury in each age-group to provide anticipatory, preventive teaching. For example, the nurse should discuss guidelines for injury prevention during infancy (see Box 9.1) before the child reaches the susceptible age-group. Preventive teaching ideally begins during pregnancy.

One-third of all injuries to children occur in the home, and therefore the importance of safety cannot be overemphasized. The Family-Centered Care box summarizes a home safety checklist that can be presented to parents to increase their awareness of danger areas in the home and assist them in implementing safety devices and practices *before* their absence can inflict injury on infants. Hands-on displays (such as cabinet latches or toilet seat locks) can familiarize parents with inexpensive, commercial devices that can be used in the home to prevent injuries.

Injury prevention requires protection of the child and education of the caregiver. Nurses in ambulatory care settings, health maintenance centers, and visiting nurse agencies are in a most favorable position for injury education. Although early postpartum discharge may be restrictive for parent teaching, this is an excellent opportunity to introduce the family to infant safety and safety for other children as well. One approach to teaching injury prevention is to relate why children in various age-groups are prone to specific types of injuries. However, injury prevention must also be practical. For instance, parents are taught that bathroom cleaning agents, cosmetics, and personal care items can be placed on a top shelf in the linen closet and towels or sheets can be stored on the lower shelves and floor. In addition, parents should be encouraged to take an infant cardiopulmonary resuscitation (CPR) class to deal effectively with potential problems.

Parents need to remember that infants and young children cannot anticipate danger or understand when it is or is not present. When small children are in the home, dangerous objects must be removed or placed out of reach. In addition, infants have no cognitive concept of cause and effect and therefore cannot relate meaning to experiences or potential dangers. A dead electrical wire may present no actual harm, but if the child is allowed to play with it, a poor behavior is enforced and will be practiced when the child encounters a live wire. Although it is always wise to explain why something is dangerous, it must be remembered that small children need to be physically removed from the situation.

It is not easy to teach safety, supervise closely, and refrain from saying "no" a hundred times a day. Parents become acutely aware of

FAMILY-CENTERED CARE

Child Safety Home Checklist

Safety: Fire, Electrical, Burns

- Guards in front of or around any heating appliance, fireplace, or furnace (including floor furnace)[a]
- Electrical wires hidden or out of reach[a]
- No frayed or broken wires; no overloaded sockets
- Plastic guards or caps over electrical outlets; furniture in front of outlets[a]
- Hanging tablecloths out of reach away from open fires[a]
- Smoke detectors tested and operating properly
- Kitchen matches stored out of child's reach[a]
- Large, deep ashtrays throughout house (if used)
- Small stoves, heaters, and other hot objects (cigarettes, candles, coffee pots, slow cookers) placed where they cannot be tipped over or reached by children
- Hot water heater set at 49°C (120°F) or lower
- Pot handles turned toward back of stove and the center of table
- No loose clothing worn near stove
- No cooking or eating hot foods or liquids with child standing nearby or sitting in lap
- All small appliances, such as iron, turned off, disconnected, and placed out of reach when not in use
- Cool, not hot, mist vaporizer used
- Fire extinguisher available on each floor and checked periodically
- Electrical fuse box and gas shutoff accessible
- Family escape plan in case of a fire practiced periodically; fire escape ladder available on upper-level floors
- Telephone number of fire or rescue squad and address of home with nearest cross street posted near phone

Safety: Suffocation and Aspiration

- Small objects stored out of reach[a]
- Toys inspected for small removable parts or long strings[a]
- Hanging crib toys and mobiles placed out of reach
- Plastic bags stored away from young child's reach; large plastic garment bags discarded after tying in knots[a]
- Mattress or pillow not covered with plastic or in manner accessible to child[a]
- Crib design according to federal regulations (crib slats <2.375 inches [6 cm] apart) with snug-fitting mattress[a,b]
- Crib positioned away from other furniture or windows[a]
- Portable play yard sides up and locked at all times while in use[a]
- Accordion-style gates not used[a]
- Bathroom doors kept closed and toilet seats down[a]
- Faucets turned off firmly[a]
- Pool fenced with locked gate
- Proper safety equipment at poolside
- Electronic garage door openers stored safely and garage door adjusted to rise when door strikes object
- Doors of ovens, trunks, dishwashers, refrigerators, and front-loading clothes washers and dryers kept closed[a]
- Unused appliance, such as a refrigerator, securely closed with lock or doors removed[a]
- Food served in small, noncylindrical pieces[a]
- Toy chests without lids or with lids that securely lock in open position[a]
- Buckets and wading pools kept empty when not in use[a]
- Clothesline above head level
- At least one member of household trained in basic life support (cardiopulmonary resuscitation [CPR]), including first aid for choking

Safety: Poisoning

- Toxic substances, including batteries, placed on a high shelf, preferably in locked cabinet
- Toxic plants hung or placed out of reach[a]
- Excess quantities of cleaning fluid, paints, pesticides, drugs, and other toxic substances not stored in home
- Used containers of poisonous substances discarded where child cannot obtain access
- Telephone number of local poison control center (800-222-1222) and home address with nearest cross street posted near phone
- Medicines clearly labeled in childproof containers and stored out of reach
- Household cleaners, disinfectants, and insecticides kept in their original containers separate from food and out of reach
- Smoking in areas away from children

Safety: Falls

- Nonskid mats, strips, or surfaces in tubs and showers
- Exits, halls, and passageways in rooms kept clear of toys, furniture, boxes, and other items that could be obstructive
- Stairs and halls well lighted with switches at both top and bottom
- Sturdy handrails for all steps and stairways
- Nothing stored on stairways
- Treads, risers, and carpeting in good repair
- Glass doors and walls marked with decals
- Safety glass used in doors, windows, and walls
- Gates on top and bottom of staircases and elevated areas, such as porch or fire escape[a]
- Guardrails on upstairs windows with locks that limit height of window opening and access to areas such as fire escape[a]
- Crib side rails raised to full height; mattress lowered as child grows[a]
- Restraints used in high chairs, walkers, or other baby furniture; preferably, walkers not used[a]
- Scatter rugs secured in place or used with nonskid backing
- Walks, patios, and driveways in good repair

Safety: Bodily Injury

- Knives, power tools, and unloaded firearms stored safely or placed in locked cabinet
- Garden tools returned to storage racks after use
- Pets properly restrained and immunized for rabies
- Swings, slides, and other outdoor play equipment kept in safe condition
- Yard free of broken glass, nail-studded boards, and other litter
- Cement birdbaths placed where young child cannot tip them over[a]
- Furniture anchored so child cannot pull down on top of self when climbing or pulling to stand

[a]Safety measures are specific for homes with young children. All safety measures should be implemented in homes where children reside and visit frequently, such as those of grandparents and babysitters.
[b]Federal regulations are available from the US Consumer Product Safety Commission, 800-638-2772; http://www.cpsc.gov.

this dilemma as soon as their infants learn to crawl. When children are taught the meaning of "no," they should also be taught what "yes" means. Children should be praised for playing with suitable toys, their efforts at behaving or listening should be reinforced, and innovative and creative recreational toys should be provided for them. Infants love to tear paper and avidly pursue books, magazines, or newspapers left on the floor. Instead of always scolding them for destroying a valued book, parents should provide child-safe books (e.g., those constructed of fabric) for them to play with. If they enjoy pots and pans, a cabinet can be arranged with safe utensils for them to explore.

One additional factor must be stressed concerning injury prevention and education. Children are imitators; they copy what they see and hear. *Practicing safety teaches safety,* which applies to parents and their children and to nurses and their clients. Saying one thing but doing another confuses children and can lead to difficulties as the child grows older.

ANTICIPATORY GUIDANCE—CARE OF FAMILIES

Childrearing is no easy task; it presents challenges to both new parents and seasoned parents. With society's changing roles, combined with a highly mobile population, traditional role models and time-honored methods of raising children are declining. As a result, parents look to professionals for guidance. Nurses are in an advantageous position to render assistance and suggestions. Every phase of a child's life has its particular traumas—toilet training for toddlers, unexplained fears for preschoolers, and identity crises for adolescents. For parents of infants, some challenges center around dependency, discipline, increased mobility, and safety. Major areas for parental guidance during the first year are listed in the Family-Centered Care box.

FAMILY-CENTERED CARE

Guidance During Infant's First Year

First 6 Months

- Teach parents car safety with use of federally approved restraint, facing rearward, in the middle of the back seat—not in a seat with an air bag.
- Understand each parent's adjustment to newborn, especially mother's postpartum emotional needs.
- Teach care of infant and help parents understand his or her individual needs and temperament and that the infant expresses wants through crying.
- Reassure parents that infant cannot be spoiled by too much attention during the first 4 to 6 months.
- Encourage parents to establish a schedule that meets needs of child and themselves.
- Help parents understand infant's need for stimulation in environment.
- Support parents' pleasure in seeing child's growing friendliness and social response, especially smiling.
- Plan anticipatory guidance for safety.
- Stress need for immunizations.
- Prepare for introduction of solid foods.

Second 6 Months

- Prepare parents for child's "stranger anxiety."
- Encourage parents to allow child to cling to them and avoid long separation from either parent.
- Guide parents concerning discipline because of infant's increasing mobility.
- Encourage use of negative voice and eye contact rather than physical punishment as a means of discipline.
- Encourage showing most attention when infant is behaving well, rather than when infant is crying.
- Teach injury prevention because of child's advancing motor skills and curiosity.
- Encourage parents to leave child with suitable caregiver to allow some free time.
- Discuss readiness for weaning.
- Explore parents' feelings regarding infant's sleep patterns.

CLINICAL JUDGMENT AND NEXT-GENERATION NCLEX® EXAMINATION-STYLE QUESTIONS

1. The nurse is seeing a 5-month-old full-term infant for a well child visit. The nurse is assessing the developmental tasks that a child this age should be able to perform while completing the physical assessment. Select each development task appropriate for a 5-month old infant. **Select all that apply.**
   - **A.** Has slight head lag when pulled to sitting position
   - **B.** When sitting, able to hold head erect and steady
   - **C.** Sits steadily unsupported
   - **D.** Turns over from abdomen to back
   - **E.** When supine, can put feet to mouth
   - **F.** Bears full weight on feet

2. At a 4-month-old full-term well child visit the nurse determines the mother is exclusively breastfeeding. The infant is doing well and there are no issues. What would the nurse discuss with the mother regarding the infant's nutritional needs? **Use an X for the health teaching below that is Indicated (appropriate or necessary), Contraindicated (could be harmful), or Non-Essential (makes no difference or not necessary)**

Health Teaching	Indicated	Contraindicated	Non-Essential
The infant will be taking a Vitamin D supplement daily			
The infant will be receiving fluoride supplement			
The infant will be receiving an Iron supplement			
The infant's head will be covered when breastfeeding.			
Breast milk can be stored in the refrigerate for up to 5 days			

3. A 6-month-old full-term infant is brought to the well-child clinic. The mother indicates that based on her sister's recommendations she has stopped feeding him iron-fortified formula. The history reveals the infant often strains to have a bowel movement, so the mother has been giving him honey. **Choose the most likely options for the information missing from the statements below by selecting from the lists of options provided.**

   The nurse recognizes that the infant is at risk for the development of ____1____. When discussing solid foods with the mother, the nurses should state that solid food can be introduced, with one new food being given every ____2____ to allow for identification of ____3____.

Options for 1	Options for 2	Options for 3
obesity	1 – 2 days	food allergies
iron-deficiency anemia	10 – 12 days	infection
rickets	4 – 7 days	growth delay
infant botulism	14 days	urinary tract infection

4. A 4-month old full-term infant is brought to the clinic and the nurse is reviewing safety promotion and injury prevention strategies for the child's age with the mother. **Indicate which nursing education number listed in the far-left column is appropriate for the potential injury listed in the middle column. Place the number in the far-right column. Note that not all nursing actions will be used.**

Nursing Education	Potential Injury	Appropriate Nursing Action to Promote Safety
1. Keep buttons, beads or other small objects out of infant's reach.	Falls	
2. Restrain in a highchair	Aspiration	
3. Know the local poison control number	Suffocation	
4. Keep out of reach of water faucets	Poisoning	
5. Keep latex balloons out of reach	Burns	
6. Keep bathroom doors closed		
7. Keep large objects that could be overturned off furniture		

REFERENCES

American Academy of Pediatric Dentistry. (2016). *Guideline on infant oral health care*. https://www.aapd.org/globalassets/media/policies_guidelines/bp_perinataloralhealthcare.pdf.

American Academy of Pediatrics: Updates Recommendations on Car Seats fro Children. (2018). https://www.aap.org/en-us/about-the-aap/aap-press-room/Pages/AAP-Updates-Recommendations-on-Car-Seats-for-Children.aspx.

American Academy of Pediatrics. (2014). *Committee on nutrition: Pediatric nutrition handbook* (7th ed). Elk Grove Village, IL: American Academy of Pediatrics.

American Academy of Pediatrics. (2011). Task force on sudden infant death syndrome: SIDS and other sleep-related infant deaths: Expansion of recommendations for a safe infant sleeping environment. *Pediatrics, 128*(5), 1030–1039.

Aronsson, C. A., Uusitalo, U., Vehik, K., et al. (2015). Age at first introduction to complementary foods is associated with sociodemographic factors in children with increased genetic risk of developing type 1 diabetes. *Maternal & Child Nutrition, 11*(4), 803–814.

Baker, R. D., Greer, F. R., & American Academy of Pediatrics. (2010). Committee on nutrition: Diagnosis and prevention of iron deficiency and iron-deficiency anemia in infants and young children (0–3 years of age). *Pediatrics, 126*(5), 1040–1050.

Bates, J., & Pettit, G. (2015). Temperament, parenting, and social development. In J. Grusec, & P. Hastings (Eds.), *Handbook of socialization: Theory and research* (2nd ed) (p. 373). New York, New York: Guilford Press.

Blackburn, S. T. (2017). *Maternal, fetal, and neonatal physiology: A clinical perspective* (5th ed). Philadelphia: Saunders/Elsevier.

Carey, W. B., & McDevitt, S. C. (1978). Revision of the infant temperament questionnaire. *Pediatrics, 61*(5), 735–739.

Dellinger, A., & Gilchrist, J. (2019). Leading causes of fatal and nonfatal unintentional injury for children and teens and the role of lifestyle clinicians. *American Journal of Lifestyle Medicine, 13*(1), 7–21.

DiSantis, K. I., Collins, B. N., Fisher, J. O., et al. (2011). Do infants fed directly from the breast have improved appetite regulation and slower growth during early childhood compared with infants fed from a bottle? *International Journal of Behavioral Nutrition and Physical Activity, 8*, 89.

Donoghue, E. A., & AAP Council on Early Childhood. (2017). Quality early education and child care from birth to kindergarten. *Pediatrics, 140*(2), 1–10.

Durand, D., Ochoa, T. J., Bellomo, S. M. E., et al. (2013). Detection of secretory immunoglobulin A in human colostrum as mucosal immune response against proteins of the type III secretion system of Salmonella, Shigella and enteropathogenic Escherichia coli. *The Pediatric Infectious Disease Journal, 32*(10), 1122–1126.

Feeley, N., Sherrard, K., Waitzer, E., et al. (2013). The father at the bedside: Patterns of involvement in the NICU. *The Journal of Perinatal and Neonatal Nursing, 27*(1), 72–80.

Fewtrell, M. S. (2011). Breastfeeding and later risk of CVD and obesity: evidence from randomized trials. *The Proceedings of the Nutrition Society, 70*(4), 472–477.

Galland, B. C., Taylor, B. J., Elder, D. E., et al. (2012). Normal sleep patterns in infants and children: a systematic review of observational studies. *Sleep Medicine Reviews, 16*(3), 213–222.

Gartstein, M. A., & Rothbart, M. K. (2003). Studying infant temperament via the revised infant behavior questionnaire. *Infant Behavior & Development, 26*(1), 64–86.

Heyman, M. B., & Abrams, S. A. (2017). Fruit juice in infants, children, and adolescents: Current recommendations. *Pediatrics, 139* (6), e20170967.

Jaafar, S. H., Jahanafar, S., Angolkar, M., et al. (2011). Pacifier use versus no pacifier use in breastfeeding term infants for increasing duration of breastfeeding. *The Cochrane Database of Systematic Reviews* (3), CD007202.

Kerstis, B., Engström, G., Edlund, B., et al. (2013). Association between mothers' and fathers' depressive symptoms, sense of coherence and perception of their child's temperament in early parenthood in Sweden. *Scandinavian Journal of Public Health, 41*(3), 233–239.

Labiner-Wolfe, J., & Fein, S. B. (2013). How US mothers store and handle their expressed breast milk. *Journal of Human Lactation : Official Journal of International Lactation Consultant Association, 29*(1), 54–58.

Lawrence, R. A., & Lawrence, R. M. (2016). *Breastfeeding: A guide for the medical profession* (8th ed). St Louis: Elsevier.

Medoff-Cooper, B., Carey, W. B., & McDevitt, S. C. (1993). The early infancy temperament questionnaire. *Journal of Developmental & Behavioral Pediatrics, 14*(4), 230–235.

Middlemiss, S., Yaure, R., & Huey, E. (2015). Translating research-based knowledge about infant sleep into practice. *Journal of the American Association of Nurse Practitioners, 27*(6), 328–337.

Mortel, M., & Mehta, S. D. (2013). Systematic review of the efficacy of herbal galactogogues. *Journal of Human Lactation : Official Journal of International Lactation Consultant Association, 29*(2), 154–162.

Moss, B. G., & Yeaton, W. H. (2014). Early childhood healthy and obese weight status: potentially protective benefits of breastfeeding and delaying solid foods. *Journal of Maternal and Child Health, 18*(5), 1224–1232.

Nelson, A. M. (2012). A comprehensive review of evidence and current recommendations related to pacifier usage. *The Journal of Pediatric Nursing: Nursing, 27*(6), 690–699.

Rogers, S. C., Gallo, K., Saleheen, H., et al. (2012). Wishful thinking: safe transportation of newborns at hospital discharge. *Journal of Trauma and Acute Care Surgery, 73*(4 Suppl. 3), S262–S264.

Peetom, K. K. B., Crutzen, R., Bohnen, H. J. M. G., Verhoeven, R., Nelissen-Vrancken, H. J. M. G, Winkens, B., Dinant, G. J., et al. (2018). Optimising decision making on illness absenteeism due to fever and common infections within childcare centres: Development of a multicomponent intervention and study protocol of a cluster randomized controlled trial. *BioMed Central Public Health, 18*(61), 1–10.

Salah, M., Abdel-Aziz, M., Al-Farok, A., et al. (2013). Recurrent acute otitis media in infants: analysis of risk factors. *International Journal of Pediatric Otorhinolaryngology, 77*(10), 1665–1669.

Szajewska, H., Canani, R. B., Guarino, A., Hojsak, I., Indrio, F., Kolacek, S., et al. (2016). Probiotics for the prevention of antibiotic associated diarrhea in children. *Journal of Pediatric Gastroenterology and Nutrition, 62*(3), 495–506.

Truong, W. H., Hill, B. W., & Cole, P. A. (2013). Automobile safety in children: A review of North American evidence and recommendations. *Journal of the American Academy of Orthopaedic Surgeons, 21*(6), 323–331.

Turck, D., Michaelsen, K. F., Shamir, R., et al. (2013). World Health Organization 2006 child growth standards and 2007 growth reference charts: A discussion paper by the committee on Nutrition of the European Society for Pediatric Gastroenterology, Hepatology, and Nutrition. *Journal of Pediatric Gastroenterology and Nutrition, 57*(2), 258–264.

Turner, S., Arthur, G., Lyons, R. A., et al. (2011). Modification of the home environment for the reduction of injuries. *Cochrane Database of Systematic Reviews* (2), CD003600.

US Food and Drug Administration. (2018). *Safely Soothing Teething pain and Sensory Needs in Babies and Older Children*. https://www.fda.gov/consumers/consumer-updates/safely-soothing-teething-pain-and-sensory-needs-babies-and-older-children.

US Food and Drug Administration Consumer Health Information. (2010). *Infant overdose risk with liquid vitamin D*. https://www.fda.gov/consumers/consumer-updates/infant-overdose-risk-liquid-vitamin-d.

Visscher, M., & Narendran, V. (2014). The ontogeny of skin. *Advanced Wound Care, 3*(4), 291–303.

Vollrath, M. E., Tonstad, S., Rothbart, M. K., et al. (2011). Infant temperament is associated with potentially obesogenic diet at 18 months. *International Journal of Obesity, 6*(2–2), e408–e414.

Wagner, C. L., Greer, F. R., American Academy of Pediatrics, section on breastfeeding, et al. (2008). Prevention of rickets and vitamin D deficiency in infants, children, and adolescents. *Pediatrics, 122*(5), 1142–1152.

Wasser, H., Bentley, M., Borja, J., et al. (2011). Infants perceived as "fussy" are more likely to receive complementary foods before 4 months. *Pediatrics, 127*(2), 229–237.

Yogman, M., Garfield, C. F., & Committee on psychosocial aspects of child and family. (2016). Fathers' roles in the care and development of their children: The role of pediatricians. *Pediatrics, 138*, e1–e15.

Yu H. J, Liu W, Chang Z, Shen H, He L. J, Wang, S. S, et al. (2015). Probiotic BIFICO cocktail ameliorates heliocobacter pylori induced gastritis. *World Journal of Gastroenterology*, 21(21), 6561–6571.

Zeanah, C. H., & Gleason, M. M. (2015). Attachment disorders in early childhood—clinical presentation, causes, correlates, and treatment. *Journal of Child Psychology and Psychiatry's, 56*(3), 207–222.

Zimmerman, E., & Thompson, K. (2015). Clarifying nipple confusion. *Journal of Perinatology, 35*, 895–899.

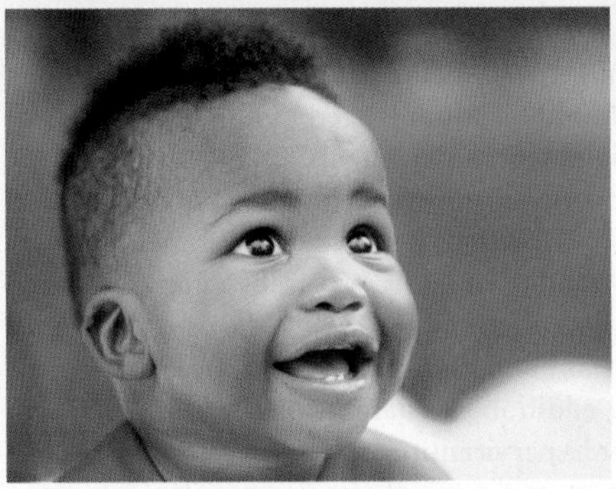

10

Health Problems of Infants

Kristina Miller

http://evolve.elsevier.com/wong/essentials

CONCEPTS

- Development
- Nutrition
- Cellular Regulation
- Safety

NUTRITIONAL IMBALANCES

Reports of children with severe nutritional disorders in most developed countries are uncommon, yet there often exist small numbers of children who may experience a nutritional deficiency of some kind. According to recent National Health and Nutrition Examination Surveys, children in the United States who are 2 years old or younger have an adequate intake of most nutrients (Ahluwalia, Herrick, Rossen, et al., 2016). However, only 21% of these children had a vitamin D intake that met or exceeded the recommended Adequate Intake (AI), and 10% had an iron intake below the Estimated Average Requirement (EAR). The 2016 Feeding Infants and Toddlers Study (FITS) found that fewer older infants are consuming iron-fortified baby cereal, formula, and pureed baby meats, which leads to concerns about the adequacy of iron intake in infants (Dwyer, 2018). Once children reached toddlerhood, more deficiencies were seen; fat intake was lower than recommended in 25% of toddlers, and most had vitamin E (82%) and vitamin D (74%) intakes that were below the EAR (Ahluwalia et al., 2016). Furthermore, very few toddlers (1%) met or exceeded the AI for fiber and potassium. On the other hand, 16% had excessive vitamin A intake, 41% exceeded recommendations for zinc intake, and 50% had sodium intakes that were above the Tolerable Upper Intake Level.

Current trends do show that toddlers are consuming healthy foods, but only in small quantities, and that they continue to prefer larger amounts of calorie-dense items that include unfavorable amounts of sodium and saturated fats (Dwyer, 2018). Although amounts of fruit juice consumed by toddlers continues to decline, studies show that juice is still being introduced in excess before 12 months of age and that toddlers are being given more than the American Academy of Pediatrics (2017) recommendation of 4 ounces (118 ml) per day. Many toddlers lack variety in their intake of vegetables, with white potatoes being most commonly eaten, and whole grain consumption is mostly in the form of cereals. The findings of these studies and other similar reports are important for nurses who work with infants and children. In 2020 the United States Dietary Guidelines will be revised to include infants and toddlers (Bailey, Catellier, Jun, et al., 2018). Nurses must work to promote healthy nutrition habits early in children's lives through proper education of families and children about healthy lifestyle habits, which include diet and exercise for health promotion and prevention of morbidities associated with poor micronutrient intake and sedentary lifestyle.

VITAMIN IMBALANCES

Although true vitamin deficiencies are rare in the United States, subclinical deficiencies are commonly seen in population subgroups in which either maternal or child dietary intake is imbalanced and contains inadequate amounts of vitamins. **Vitamin D–deficiency rickets**, once rarely seen because of the widespread commercial availability of vitamin D–fortified milk, increased before the turn of the century. Populations at risk include:

- Children who are exclusively breastfed by mothers with an inadequate intake of vitamin D or who are exclusively breastfed for longer than 6 months without adequate maternal vitamin D intake or supplementation
- Children with dark skin pigmentation who are exposed to minimal sunlight because of socioeconomic, religious, or cultural beliefs or housing in urban areas with high levels of pollution or who live above or below a latitude of 33 degrees north and south where sunlight does not produce vitamin D (Misra, 2018)
- Children with diets that are low in sources of vitamin D and calcium
- Individuals who use milk products not supplemented with vitamin D (e.g., yogurt,[a] raw cow's milk) as their primary source of milk
- Children who are overweight or obese (Antonucci, Locci, Clemente, et al., 2018)

The findings of population-based studies in the United States show that childhood rates of vitamin D deficiency are two to three times higher in children who are obese and that obese children are at increased risk for inadequate vitamin D intake (Moore & Liu, 2016). Abdominal pain, seizures, limb pain, and weakness are all signs and symptoms of vitamin D deficiency in children. One study by Esposito and Lelii (2015) found a correlation between the incidence of childhood upper respiratory infection and vitamin D deficiency, but the implications of the research findings have yet to be completely understood.

Infants who are exclusively breastfed may also be at risk for vitamin D deficiency. Therefore the American Academy of Pediatrics recommends that infants who are exclusively breastfed receive 400 IU of vitamin D beginning shortly after birth to prevent rickets and

[a]Yogurt does not contain adequate amounts of vitamins A and D yet is an acceptable source of calcium and phosphorus.

vitamin D deficiency (Kleinman & Greer, 2014). Vitamin D supplementation should continue until the infant is consuming at least 1 L/day (or 1 quart/day) of vitamin D–fortified formula. Despite these recommendations, national studies indicate that only one in five breastfed US infants receive this recommended vitamin D supplementation (Furman, 2015). One factor contributing to infants not receiving this supplement could be parental nonadherence. A clinical trial was conducted to determine the feasibility and efficacy of mothers supplementing their diets with vitamin D as a way to address this issue and to ensure that infants had adequate intake of vitamin D if they were exclusively breastfed. Researchers learned that 6400 IU of daily maternal vitamin D_3 supplementation for 6 months successfully supported maternal vitamin D status and was effective in producing sufficient vitamin D levels in breastfeeding infants. Increasing maternal vitamin D intake has the added benefit of improving both maternal and infant health (Furman, 2015).

Nonbreastfed infants who are taking less than 1 L/day of vitamin D–fortified formula should also receive a daily vitamin D supplement of 400 IU. The National Institutes of Health Office of Dietary Supplement (2016) recommends a daily intake of 400 IU for infants (with an upper limit of 1000 to 1500 IU/day) and 600 IU for children older than 1 year (with an upper limit of 2500 to 3000 IU). Salmon, sardines, tuna, and cod liver oil are food sources considered high in vitamin D. There are also several vitamin D–fortified foods such as orange juice, oatmeal, whole milk, yogurt, and certain breakfast cereals (Antonucci et al., 2018).

Children may also be at risk for vitamin deficiencies secondary to disorders, special diets, or medical treatment. For example, vitamin deficiencies of the fat-soluble vitamins A and D may occur in malabsorptive disorders, such as cystic fibrosis and short bowel syndrome. Preterm infants may develop rickets in the second month of life as a result of inadequate intake of vitamin D, calcium, and phosphorus. Children receiving high doses of salicylates may have impaired vitamin C storage. Although scurvy (which is caused by a deficiency in vitamin C) is rare in developed countries, cases have been reported in children who have reduced intake of vitamin C due to poor oral intake, oral motor dysfunction, or feeding problems (Brambilla, Pizza, & Lasagni, 2018; Perry, Page, Manthey, et al., 2018). In addition, children on vegetarian diets, especially vegan diets, are at risk for vitamin B_{12} deficiency, so it must be ensured that an adequate source of this vitamin is consumed (Pawlak, Lester, & Babatunde, 2014). Breastfed infants of mothers who are strict vegetarians are also at risk for vitamin B_{12} deficiency, especially if the mother is vitamin B_{12} deficient (Bousselamti, Hasbaoui, Echahdi, et al., 2018). Children with chronic illnesses resulting in anorexia, decreased food intake, or possible nutrient malabsorption as a result of multiple medications should be carefully evaluated for adequate vitamin and mineral intake in some form (parenteral or enteral).

Children with sickle cell disease (SCD) are reported to have suboptimal intakes of calcium, iron, and vitamins B_1 and C. This is concerning because low intake of calcium and vitamin B_1 has been correlated with an increase in severity of SCD symptoms (Mandese, Marotti, Bedetti, et al., 2016). One study found that children with intestinal failure who received parenteral nutrition at home had significant vitamin D deficiencies. Therefore routine screening and addition of vitamin D supplementation is recommended for children receiving parenteral nutrition (Wozniak, Bechtold, Reyen, et al., 2015).

Vitamin A deficiency can occur in children as a result of diarrhea or infection. Vitamin A deficiency has also been associated with an increased risk of blindness in children who also have measles. However, a recent Cochrane review of studies assessing the efficacy of vitamin A in children with measles found no information specifically related to ocular morbidities (Bello, Meremikwu, Ejemot-Nwadiaro, et al., 2016). Despite the lack of evidence, vitamin A supplementation has minimal side effects and should be administered to children with measles (Bello, Meremikwu, Ejemot-Nwadiaro, et al., 2014).

Excessive doses of vitamins can be alarming as well. An excessive dose of a vitamin is generally defined as 10 or more times the Recommended Dietary Allowance (RDA). Fat-soluble vitamins, especially vitamins A and D, tend to cause toxic reactions at lower doses, while the water-soluble vitamins, primarily niacin, B_6, and C, cause toxicity once higher doses are consumed. With the addition of vitamins to commercially prepared foods, the potential for **hypervitaminosis** has increased, especially when combined with the excessive use of vitamin supplements. Hypervitaminosis of vitamins A and D presents the greatest problems because these fat-soluble vitamins are stored in the body and severe anemia and thrombocytopenia have resulted from megadoses of vitamin A. High intake of vitamin A can also cause anorexia, increased intracranial pressure, painful bone lesions, desquamative dermatitis, and hepatotoxicity (Kleinman & Greer, 2014). Hypercalcemia has been reported in children receiving therapeutic doses of vitamin D for the prevention of rickets (Talarico, Barreca, Galiano, et al., 2016) and in children who are taking high doses of vitamin A for the treatment of autism (Boyd & Moondambail, 2016). Vitamin D is the most likely of all vitamins to cause toxic reactions in relatively small overdoses.

One vitamin supplement that is recommended for all women of childbearing age is a daily dose of 0.4 mg of folic acid, the usual RDA. Folic acid taken before conception and during early pregnancy can reduce the risk of neural tube defects such as spina bifida by as much as 70%. Drugs such as oral contraceptives and antidepressants may decrease folic acid absorption; thus adolescent girls taking such medications should consider supplementation (see Chapter 30, Spina Bifida).

MINERAL IMBALANCES

A number of minerals are essential nutrients. The **macrominerals** refer to those with daily requirements greater than 100 mg and include calcium, phosphorus, magnesium, sodium, potassium, chloride, and sulfur. **Microminerals**, or **trace elements**, have daily requirements of less than 100 mg and include several essential minerals and those whose exact role in nutrition is still unclear. The greatest concern with minerals is deficiency, especially iron-deficiency anemia (see Chapter 24). However, other minerals that may be inadequate in children's diets, even with supplementation, include calcium, phosphorus, magnesium, and zinc. Low levels of zinc can cause nutritional failure to thrive (FTT). Some of the macrominerals may be inadvertently overlooked when a child with intestinal failure or recent surgery is making the transition from total parenteral intake to enteral intake.

An imbalance in the intake of calcium and phosphorous may occur in infants younger than 1 year old who are given whole cow's milk instead of infant formula; neonatal tetany may be observed in such cases (see Chapter 8). Whole cow's milk is also a poor source of iron, and inadequate intake of iron from other food sources (such as iron-fortified cereal) may cause iron-deficiency anemia.

The regulation of mineral balance in the body is a complex process. Dietary extremes of mineral intake can cause a number of mineral–mineral interactions that could result in unexpected deficiencies or excesses. Poor outcomes in infants (e.g., fatal hypermagnesemia) have been associated with megavitamin therapy with high doses of magnesium oxide. Further, excessive amounts of one mineral, such as zinc, can result in a deficiency of another mineral, such as copper, even if sufficient amounts of copper are ingested. Thus megadose intake of one mineral may cause an inadvertent deficiency of another essential mineral by blocking its absorption in the blood or intestinal wall or by competing with binding sites on protein carriers needed for metabolism.

Deficiencies can also occur when various substances in the diet interact with minerals. For example, iron, zinc, and calcium can form insoluble complexes with **phytates** or **oxalates** (substances found in plant proteins), which impair the bioavailability of the mineral. This type of interaction is important in vegetarian diets because plant foods (such as soy) are high in phytates. Contrary to popular opinion, spinach is not an ideal source of iron or calcium because of its high oxalate content.

Children with certain illnesses are at greater risk for growth failure, especially in relation to bone mineral deficiency resulting from medical treatments, decreased nutrient intake, or decreased absorption of necessary minerals. Those at risk for such deficiencies include children who have (1) human immunodeficiency virus (HIV), (2) sickle cell disease, (3) cystic fibrosis, (4) gastrointestinal (GI) malabsorption, or (5) nephrosis. Extremely low birth weight (ELBW) and very low birth weight (VLBW) preterm infants and children who are receiving or have received radiation and/or chemotherapy for cancer are also at risk.

NURSING CARE MANAGEMENT

A vital goal of pediatric nursing is to ensure adequate nutrition in children. This requires a nutritional assessment based on a dietary history and physical examination for signs of deficiency or excess. After assessment data are collected, this information is evaluated against standard intakes to identify areas of concern. One source of standard nutrient intakes is the Dietary Reference Intakes (DRIs) (see Chapter 4).

Standardized growth reference charts are used in infants, children, and adolescents to compare and assess growth parameters such as height and head circumference with the percentile distribution of other children at the same ages. The World Health Organization's growth charts represent the standardized growth reference now recommended for infants and toddlers up to 24 months old. These growth charts include head circumference, height, and weight references, which were derived from healthy children in six different countries around the world. These growth standards are based on the growth of healthy infants who were predominately breastfed for at least 4 months and are still breastfeeding to some extent at 12 months (World Health Organization, 2017a). The Centers for Disease Control and Prevention also offers a set of growth charts for children; however, these charts are recommended only for children 2 to 19 years of age (Kleinman & Greer, 2014).

Current recommendations for the feeding of infants include exclusive breastfeeding for the first 6 months with continued breastfeeding for at least 1 year or longer, if desired, with the addition of age-appropriate complementary foods (Chantry, Eglash, & Labbok, 2015). The addition of some complementary solid foods may begin around 4 to 6 months, and infants should receive iron-fortified cereal for at least 18 months (see Chapter 9). The introduction of solid foods for vegetarian infants may occur using the same guidelines as for other children (see Chapter 11, Nutrition). A variety of foods should be introduced during the early years to ensure a well-balanced intake. Infants who have particular nutritional deficits should be identified. A multidisciplinary approach should be taken to identify the deficiency, determine its etiology, and establish a plan with the caregiver to promote adequate growth and development.

HEALTH PROBLEMS RELATED TO NUTRITION

SEVERE ACUTE MALNUTRITION (PROTEIN-ENERGY MALNUTRITION)

Malnutrition continues to be a major health problem in the world today, particularly in children younger than 5 years old. However, lack of food is not always the primary cause of malnutrition. In many developing and underdeveloped nations, diarrhea (gastroenteritis) is a major factor. Additional factors are (1) bottle-feeding (in poor sanitary conditions), (2) inadequate knowledge of proper child care practices, (3) parental illiteracy, (4) economic and political factors, (5) climate conditions, (6) cultural and religious food preferences, and (7) lack of adequate food. Poverty and food insecurity, which is the lack of a consistent and reliable food source, play an integral role in worldwide malnutrition (US Department of Agriculture, 2016). The most extreme forms of malnutrition, or **protein-energy malnutrition (PEM)**, are kwashiorkor and marasmus. Some authorities suggest that severe malnutrition encompasses more than protein-energy deficits and thus prefer the term *severe childhood undernutrition* (SCU). However, other organizations such as the World Health Organization (2017b) now use the term *severe acute malnutrition* (SAM). SAM may be subdivided into edematous (kwashiorkor) and nonedematous with severe wasting (marasmus) types. A third type, marasmic kwashiorkor, includes both features of marasmus and kwashiorkor (Ashworth, 2020).

In the United States, milder forms of SAM are seen as a result of primary malnutrition, although the classic cases of marasmus and kwashiorkor may also occur but are rare. Unlike in developing countries, where the main reason for SAM is inadequate food, in the United States SAM occurs despite ample dietary supplies (see the Failure to Thrive section later in this chapter). SAM may also be seen in children with chronic health problems, such as (1) cystic fibrosis, (2) renal disease, (3) cancer, (4) bone marrow transplantation, (5) HIV, (6) inborn errors of metabolism, (7) GI malabsorption, and (8) prolonged, untreated anorexia nervosa. Kwashiorkor has been reported in the United States in children fed only a rice beverage diet (Rice Dream) and few solids foods (Ashworth, 2020). The rice drink contains 0.13 g of protein per ounce (compared with the 0.5 g found in human milk and infant formulas) and is an inadequate source of nutrition for children. Therefore it is important that health care workers not assume that SAM cannot occur in developed countries; a comprehensive dietary history should be obtained in any child with clinical features resembling SAM.

Kwashiorkor

Kwashiorkor is taken from the Ga language (Ghana) and means "the sickness the older child gets when the next baby is born." It clearly describes the syndrome that develops in the first child, usually between 1 and 4 years of age, when weaned from the breast after the second child is born. Kwashiorkor has been defined as primarily a deficiency of protein with an adequate supply of calories. A diet consisting mainly of starch grains or tubers provides adequate calories in the form of carbohydrates but an inadequate amount of high-quality proteins. Some evidence, however, supports a multifactorial etiology, including cultural, psychologic, and infective factors that may interact to place the child at risk for kwashiorkor. Further, kwashiorkor may result from the interplay of nutrient deprivation and infectious or environmental stresses, which produces an imbalanced response to such insults (Trehan & Manary, 2015). For example, kwashiorkor often occurs subsequent to an infectious outbreak of measles and dysentery.

The child with kwashiorkor has thin, wasted extremities and a prominent abdomen from edema (ascites). The edema often masks severe muscular atrophy, making the child appear less debilitated than he or she actually is. The skin is scaly and dry and has areas of depigmentation. Several dermatoses may be evident, partly resulting from the vitamin deficiencies. Permanent blindness often results from the severe lack of vitamin A. Mineral deficiencies are common, especially iron, calcium, and zinc. Acute zinc deficiency is a common complication of severe SAM and results in (1) skin rashes, (2) loss of hair, (3) impaired immune response and susceptibility to infections, (4) digestive problems, (5) night blindness, (6) changes in affective behavior, (7) defective wound healing, and (8) impaired growth. Its depressant effect on appetite further limits food intake.

Diarrhea (persistent diarrhea malnutrition syndrome) commonly occurs from a lowered resistance to infection and further complicates the often-concurrent electrolyte imbalance seen in children with kwashiorkor. This can lead to fatal deterioration and circulatory collapse. Low levels of cytokines (i.e., protein cells involved in the primary response to infection) have been reported in children with kwashiorkor, suggesting that such children have a blunted immune response to infection. Protein deficiency increases the child's susceptibility to infection, which eventually results in death. A large number of deaths in children with kwashiorkor occur in those who develop HIV infection. GI disturbances such as fatty infiltration of the liver and atrophy of the acini cells of the pancreas are additional complications of kwashiorkor. Anemia is also a common finding in these children.

Marasmus

Marasmus results from general malnutrition of both calories and protein. It is common in underdeveloped countries during times of drought, especially in cultures where adults eat first. The remaining food is often insufficient in quality and quantity for the children. Marasmus is usually a syndrome of physical and emotional deprivation and is not confined to geographic areas where food supplies are inadequate. It may be seen in children with growth failure in whom the cause is not solely nutritional but primarily emotional. Marasmus may be seen in infants as young as 3 months old if breastfeeding is not successful and there are no suitable alternatives.

Marasmic kwashiorkor is a form of SAM in which clinical findings of both kwashiorkor and marasmus are evident; the child has edema, severe wasting, and stunted growth. In marasmic kwashiorkor, the child has inadequate nutrient intake and superimposed infection. Co-occurring fluid and electrolyte disturbances, hypothermia, and hypoglycemia are associated with a poor prognosis.

Marasmus is characterized by gradual wasting and atrophy of body tissues, especially of subcutaneous fat. The child has an aged appearance, with loose and wrinkled skin, unlike the child with kwashiorkor, who appears more rounded from the edema. Fat metabolism is less impaired than in kwashiorkor; thus deficiency of fat-soluble vitamins is usually minimal or absent. In general, the clinical manifestations of marasmus are similar to those seen in kwashiorkor. However, with marasmus there is no edema from hypoalbuminemia or sodium retention, which contributes to a severely emaciated appearance. There are also no dermatoses caused by vitamin deficiencies, little or no depigmentation of hair or skin, moderately normal fat metabolism and lipid absorption, a smaller head size, and a slower recovery after treatment. The child is fretful, apathetic, withdrawn, and so lethargic that collapse frequently occurs. Concurrent infection with debilitating diseases such as tuberculosis, parasitosis, HIV, and dysentery is common.

Therapeutic Management

The treatment of SAM includes providing a diet with high-quality proteins, carbohydrates, vitamins, and minerals. When SAM occurs as a result of persistent diarrhea, three management goals are identified:

1. Rehydration with an oral rehydration solution that also replaces electrolytes
2. Administration of antibiotics to prevent concurrent infections
3. Provision of adequate nutrition by either breastfeeding or a proper weaning diet

Local protocols are used in developing countries to deal with SAM, but experts recommend a three-phase treatment protocol. In phase one, called the **acute or initial phase**, which occurs in the first 2 to 10 days, management involves initiation of oral rehydration and treatment of diarrhea and intestinal parasites. Other tasks during the first phase include prevention of hypoglycemia and hypothermia and subsequent dietary management. Phase two, **recovery or rehabilitation**, occurs during the next 2 to 6 weeks, and treatment is focused on increasing dietary intake and weight gain. Finally, in phase three, or the **follow-up phase**, the focus shifts to care after discharge in an outpatient setting to prevent relapse and promote weight gain, provide developmental stimulation, and evaluate cognitive and motor development.

Extreme care must be taken in the acute phase to prevent fluid overload, and the child should be observed closely for signs of food or fluid intolerance. **Refeeding syndrome** may occur if caloric intake progresses too rapidly. The resulting cardiac failure may cause sudden death in a child who has been malnourished and is fed too rapidly (Ashworth, 2020). Because severely malnourished children cannot tolerate a high-protein, high-energy diet, a modest-energy food source is given initially and then children are slowly progressed to high-protein and high-energy foods as tolerated (Ashworth, 2020). They include oral rehydration solutions (ReSoMal), amino acid–based elemental food, and ready-to-feed foods that do not require the addition of water, to minimize contaminated water consumption (Jones & Berkley, 2014). In addition, parenteral and oral antibiotics are often part of the standard treatment for SAM (Ashworth, 2020).

Vitamin and mineral supplementation are required in most cases of SAM, with vitamin A, zinc, and copper being recommended. In contrast, iron supplementation is not recommended until the child is able to tolerate a steady food source. During recovery, the child is observed for signs of skin breakdown, which should be treated to prevent infection. Breastfeeding is encouraged if the mother and child are able to do so effectively; however, in some cases partial supplementation with a modified cow's milk–based infant formula may be necessary (Ashworth, 2020).

The World Health Organization issued a statement recognizing the importance of breastfeeding for the first 6 months in developing countries where HIV is prevalent among childbearing women and children (World Health Organization, 2016). The World Health Organization recognizes that appropriate sources of food and water for infants may not be available after the 6 months are concluded and that the risk for malnutrition is greater among such children than the theoretical risk of HIV. Furthermore, the organization recommends that breastfeeding continue after 6 months with the introduction of complementary foods, provided they are safe for child consumption.

Nursing Care Management

Because SAM appears early in childhood, primarily in children 6 months to 2 years old, and is associated with early weaning, maternal illiteracy, poverty, a large family size, and incomplete vaccinations (Mishra, Kumar, Basu, et al., 2014), it is essential that nursing care focus on *prevention* of SAM through parent education about feeding practices and infant care during this critical period. Prevention should also focus on the nutritional health of pregnant women because this will directly affect the health of their unborn children. Breastfeeding is the optimal method of feeding for the first 6 months. The immune properties naturally found in breast milk not only nourish infants but also help prevent opportunistic infections, which may contribute to SAM. Providing for essential physiologic needs, including appropriate nutrition and hydration, protection from infection, and appropriate skin care, is paramount. Additional nursing care should focus on educating parents about the importance of (1) childhood vaccinations to prevent illness, (2) nutrition and well-being for lactating mothers,

(3) attending well-child visits for infants and toddlers, (4) appropriate food sources for children being weaned from breastfeeding, and (5) sanitation practices to prevent childhood GI illnesses.

Nursing care of young infants should also include appropriate skin care because poor skin integrity contributes to infection, hypothermia, water loss, and skin breakdown. Tube feedings may be required for infants too weak to breastfeed or bottle-feed. Oral rehydration with an approved oral rehydration solution is commonly used in cases of SAM in which diarrhea and infection are not immediately life threatening.

Further, infants may be treated with higher calorie (24 to 27 kcal/oz) commercial infant formulas when appropriate. One potential drawback from using therapeutic milks (F75 and F100 formulas) is that they require water for mixing and could be contaminated during mixing. One approach that has gained acceptance for treating childhood malnutrition in developing countries is the use of ready-to-use therapeutic food (RUTF), which is a peanut-based paste containing dried skim milk, vitamins, and minerals and having little water content (UNICEF, 2013). The packaged RUTF can be stored without refrigeration, has a long shelf life, and improves survival rates in malnourished children (UNICEF, 2013). Further, RUTF can be administered by community health workers and offers the added advantage of home-based treatment of SAM, which has been shown to be successful in 80% of children with SAM. Treatment in the home can prevent exposure to hospital-acquired infections in children who are already vulnerable. This rapid and appropriate care management can lower case-fatality rates to as low as 5% in both the community and health care setting (UNICEF, 2013).

It is imperative that nurses be at the forefront in educating and reinforcing healthy nutrition habits in parents of small children to prevent malnutrition. Because children with marasmus may experience emotional starvation as well, care should be consistent with the typical, age-appropriate, developmentally supportive care provided for children with failure to thrive (discussed later in this chapter).

The World Health Organization has published guidelines for the dietary treatment and management of children with SAM (available at https://www.who.int/elena/titles/full_recommendations/sam_management/en/). These guidelines include 11 recommendations for the management of SAM in infants 6 to 59 months of age, as well as hospital admission and discharge criteria for these infants (World Health Organization, 2017b).

FOOD SENSITIVITY

In 2010 the National Institute of Allergy and Infectious Diseases, working with 34 other professional organizations, published new evidence-based guidelines for the diagnosis and management of food allergy (Boyce, Assa'ad, Burks, et al., 2010). **Food allergies** are adverse immunologic reactions to foods (Nowak-Węgrzyn, Sampson, & Sicherer, 2020). They can further be defined as specific components of a food or ingredients in a food, such as a protein, that are recognized by allergen-specific immune cells, eliciting an immune reaction that results in the characteristic symptoms of an allergic response. On the other hand, a **food intolerance** occurs when a food or food component elicits a reproducible adverse reaction but does not have an established or likely immunologic mechanism (Nowak-Węgrzyn et al., 2020). For example, a person with a milk allergy may have an immune-mediated response to cow's milk protein; however, a person who is unable to digest the lactose in cow's milk is intolerant to cow's milk, not allergic to it. Anaphylaxis, GI food allergies, and cutaneous reactions to food are all seen with food allergies (Nowak-Węgrzyn et al., 2020). The exact prevalence of food allergies in children is reported to be much lower than what parents report. Approximately 6% of children may experience food allergic reactions in the first 2 to 3 years of life; 1.5% will have an allergy to eggs, 2.5% to cow's milk, and 1% to peanuts (Nowak-Węgrzyn et al., 2020). Food allergy symptoms are most common in infants and young children but can occur at any age. Clinical manifestations of food allergies are described as follows (Nowak-Węgrzyn et al., 2020):

Systemic: Anaphylaxis, growth failure
GI: Abdominal pain, vomiting, cramping, diarrhea
Respiratory: Cough, wheezing, rhinitis, infiltrates
Cutaneous: Urticaria, rash, atopic dermatitis

Approximately 90% of adverse reactions to food are caused by eight types of foods: eggs, milk, peanuts, tree nuts, fish, shellfish, wheat, and soy (American College of Allergy, Asthma & Immunology, 2014). In children with food allergies, peanuts are the most common allergen followed by milk and then shellfish (American Academy of Allergy, Asthma & Immunology, 2017). A National Institute of Allergy and Infectious Diseases report further points out that most children will eventually be able to tolerate milk, eggs, soy, and wheat, but far fewer will ever tolerate tree nut and peanuts (Nowak-Węgrzyn et al., 2020). Children (50%) will typically outgrow milk and egg allergies by the time they are school age; however, 80% to 90% of children with peanut, nut, or seafood allergies will retain them for life. Further, it is important to note that peanut allergy prevalence has tripled over the past decade (Nowak-Węgrzyn et al., 2020), and in the United States the leading cause of death due to food-induced anaphylaxis is from a peanut allergy (Togias, Cooper, Acebal, et al., 2017).

According to the National Institute of Allergy and Infectious Diseases *Guidelines for the Diagnosis and Management of Food Allergy in the United States* (Boyce et al., 2010), recommendations for the prevention of food allergies in young children include:

- Exclusively breastfeed children for the first 4 to 6 months of life.
- Soy-based infant formulas will not prevent the development of food allergy.
- Introduce complementary solid foods only after 4 to 6 months of exclusive breastfeeding.
- Introduce high allergy-causing foods (eggs, nut products, fish, milk, and wheat) soon after low allergy-causing foods. Delaying the introduction of these foods will not prevent food allergies. Further, avoiding allergy-causing foods during pregnancy or lactation will not prevent food allergy.
- Children, even those with an egg allergy, should be vaccinated with the measles, mumps, and rubella (MMR) or measles, mumps, rubella, and varicella (MMRV) vaccines.
- Patients with severe egg allergy reactions should be referred to an allergist before considering receiving the influenza vaccine (see also Chapter 6, Immunizations).

In 2017 an addendum to the 2010 National Institute of Allergy and Infectious Diseases *Guidelines for the Diagnosis and Management of Food Allergy in the United States* (Boyce, et al., 2010) was published to specifically address prevention of peanut allergy in the United States (Togias et al., 2017). The guidelines were developed based on a landmark clinical trial that provided data suggesting that peanut allergy can be prevented by introducing peanut-containing food early in infancy. The addendum provides three separate guidelines for clinicians to use to determine the risk level for development of peanut allergy and discusses interventions for each risk level. The first guideline states that infants who have an egg allergy, severe eczema, or both need to be introduced to peanut-containing food that is age appropriate by the age of 4 to 6 months in order to reduce the risk of a peanut allergy. Infants with mild to moderate eczema are included in the second guideline, which recommends introducing age-appropriate peanut-containing food by the age of 6 months. Finally, the third guideline suggests that infants who do not have eczema or any food allergy incorporate age-appropriate peanut-containing foods with their regular solid food diet as the family wishes, as there is no evidence for restricting peanut-containing foods and the probability of developing a peanut allergy is very low.

Also provided in the 2017 addendum (Togias et al., 2017) are guidelines about allergy testing using peanut-specific immunoglobulin E (IgE) or skin prick tests and how to analyze those results to guide identification of peanut allergies, referral needs, and whether the introduction of peanut-containing foods can occur in the home or if it is necessary to complete it in the health care provider's office. If after testing and referrals a child is identified as having an allergy to peanuts, the guidelines recommend strict peanut avoidance instead of early introduction. In each guideline recipes are provided to help guide clinicians and parents in how to prepare peanut-containing foods, and it is also recommended that infants be fed other solid foods before peanut-containing foods in order to establish that the infant is developmentally ready for solid foods.

Food allergies usually occur as either an IgE-mediated or a non–IgE-mediated immune response. Some toxic reactions may occur as a result of a toxin found within the food. Food allergy is caused by exposure to **allergens**, usually proteins (but not the smaller amino acids), that are capable of inducing IgE antibody formation (sensitization) when ingested. **Sensitization** refers to the initial exposure of an individual to an allergen, resulting in an immune response. Subsequent exposure induces a much stronger response that is clinically apparent. Consequently, food allergy typically occurs after the food has been ingested one or more times. Sensitization alone is not sufficient to be classified as a food allergy. Rather, an immune-mediated response *and* manifestation of specific signs and symptoms are necessary to categorize an individual as having a food allergy (Boyce et al., 2010). The most common food allergens are listed in Box 10.1.

Oral allergy syndrome occurs when a food allergen (commonly fruits and vegetables) is ingested and there is subsequent edema and pruritus involving the lips, tongue, palate, and throat. Recovery from symptoms is usually rapid. **Immediate GI hypersensitivity** is an IgE-mediated reaction to a food allergen that can result in nausea, abdominal pain, cramping, diarrhea, vomiting, anaphylaxis, or all of these. Additional food allergies seen in young children include allergic eosinophilic esophagitis, allergic eosinophilic gastroenteritis, food protein–induced proctocolitis, and food protein–induced enterocolitis.

Food allergy or hypersensitivity may also be classified according to the interval between ingestion and the manifestation of symptoms: immediate (within minutes to hours) or delayed (2 to 48 hours). Further, food allergies can occur at any time but are common during infancy because the immature intestinal tract is more permeable to proteins than the mature intestinal tract, thus increasing the likelihood of an immune response. Allergies in general demonstrate a genetic component: children who have one parent with allergy have a 50% or greater risk of developing allergy; children who have both parents with allergy have up to a 100% risk of developing allergy. Allergy with a hereditary tendency is referred to as **atopy**. Some infants with atopy can be identified at birth from elevated levels of IgE in umbilical cord blood.

Deaths have been reported in children who experienced an anaphylactic reaction to food. Onset of the reactions occurred shortly after ingestion (5 to 30 minutes). In most of the children, the reactions did not begin with skin signs, such as hives, red rash, and flushing, but rather mimicked an acute asthma attack (wheezing, decreased air movement in airways, dyspnea). Watch children with food anaphylaxis closely, because a biphasic response has been recorded in as many as 35% of children (Keet & Wang, 2014). This may manifest as an immediate response to treatment, apparent recovery, and then acute recurrence of symptoms. Children with extremely sensitive food allergies should wear a medical identification bracelet and have an injectable epinephrine cartridge (EpiPen) readily available (see Chapter 23, Anaphylaxis). Any child with a history of food allergy or previous severe reaction to food should have a written emergency treatment plan, as well as an EpiPen. Note that diphenhydramine (Benadryl) and cetirizine (Zyrtec) are effective for cutaneous and nasal manifestations but not for airway manifestations (Keet & Wang, 2014).

Although the reason is unknown, many children "outgrow" their food allergies (Nowak-Węgrzyn et al., 2020). Therefore allergenic foods should be reintroduced into the diet after a period of abstinence to evaluate whether the food can be safely added back to the diet. There is evidence that children may tolerate foods to which they were previously allergic when these foods are extensively heated as in muffins or bread. The prolonged or complete avoidance of foods to prevent food allergy is not recommended, and there is some evidence that a lack of exposure to antigens may actually be detrimental (Kleinman & Greer, 2014; Togias et al., 2017).

BOX 10.1 Hyperallergenic Foods and Sources

Nuts[a]: Some chocolates, candy, baked goods, cherry soda (may be flavored with a nut extract), walnut oil
Eggs[a]: Mayonnaise, creamy salad dressing, baked goods, egg noodles, some cake icing, meringue, custard, pancakes, French toast, root beer
Wheat[a]: Almost all baked goods, wieners, bologna, pressed or chopped cold cuts, gravy, soy sauce, malt, pasta, some canned soups
Legumes: Peanuts,[a] peanut butter or oil, beans, peas, lentils
Fish or shellfish[a]: Cod liver oil, pizza with anchovies, Caesar salad dressing, any food fried in same oil as fish
Soy[a]: Soy sauce, teriyaki or Worcestershire sauce, tofu, baked goods using soy flour or oil, soy nuts, soy infant formulas or milk, soybean paste, tuna packed in vegetable oil, many margarines
Chocolate: Cola beverages, cocoa, chocolate-flavored drinks
Milk[a]: Ice cream, butter, margarine (if it contains dairy products), yogurt, cheese, pudding, baked goods, wieners, bologna, canned creamed soups, instant breakfast drinks, powdered milk drinks, milk chocolate
Buckwheat: Some cereals, pancakes
Pork, chicken: Bacon, wieners, sausage, pork fat, chicken broth
Strawberries, melon, pineapple: Gelatin, syrups
Corn: Popcorn, cereal, muffins, cornstarch, cornmeal, corn bread, corn tortillas; many processed foods also contain corn syrup
Citrus fruits: Orange, lemon, lime, grapefruit; any of these in drinks, gelatin, juice, or medicines
Tomatoes: Juice, some vegetable soups, spaghetti, pizza sauce, catsup
Spices: Chili, pepper, vinegar, cinnamon

[a]Most common allergens.

! NURSING ALERT

Indications for the administration of **intramuscular** epinephrine in a child with a life-threatening anaphylactic reaction or one who is experiencing severe symptoms is indicated when the child has any one of the following symptoms (Keet & Wang, 2014):

- Itching sensation or tightness in throat; hoarseness, difficulty swallowing
- "Barky" cough, wheezing, dyspnea, cyanosis, respiratory arrest
- Mild cardiac dysrhythmia or mild hypotension
- Severe bradycardia, hypotension, cardiac arrest, or loss of consciousness

DRUG ALERT

Emergency Management of Anaphylaxis

- **Drug:** Epinephrine 0.01 mg/kg up to maximum of 0.5 mg
- **Dosage:** EpiPen Jr 0.15 mg intramuscularly (IM) for child weighing 8 to 25 kg (17.5 to 55 pounds)
  EpiPen 0.3 mg IM for child weighing 25 kg (55 pounds) or more
- **Observe for adverse reactions:** Tachycardia, hypertension, irritability, headache, nausea, and tremors

Data from Sampson, H. A., Wang, J., & Sicherer, S. H. (2020). Anaphylaxis. In R. M. Kliegman, J.W. St. Geme, N.J. Blum, et al, (Eds.), *Nelson textbook of pediatrics* (21st ed.). Philadelphia: Elsevier.

Diagnosis and Therapeutic Management

The diagnosis of food allergy is made based on a number of factors, including the occurrence of anaphylaxis or any combination of 37 symptoms listed in the National Institute of Allergy and Infectious Diseases guidelines within minutes to hours of ingesting food or if such symptoms have occurred after the ingestion of a specific food on one or more occasions. The gold standard is the double-blind, placebo-controlled food challenge. The skin prick test and serum IgE measurements may be used as an adjunct to diagnose food allergy but singly should not be used for diagnosis (Nowak-Węgrzyn et al., 2020). The atopy patch test, intradermal test, and serum IgE test are not recommended for establishing a diagnosis. A single oral food challenge may be used in certain circumstances (Bock & Sampson, 2016).

The traditional management of food allergy consists of avoiding the specific food or ingredient that causes the manifestations. However, oral immunotherapy (OIT) is gaining increasing interest as a potential way to treat food allergies, with treatment of cow's milk allergy, eggs, and peanuts being the most extensively studied (Nowak-Węgrzyn, 2018). OIT consists of administering small amounts of the allergic food to the child in daily doses that are then increased over several months to achieve a maintenance dose. Allergic reactions (e.g. oral and GI symptoms) during this process are common, especially when doses are increasing. Up to 75% of OIT-treated patients experience desensitization (a state of temporary hyporesponsiveness to the food allergen resulting in an increased threshold for reactions). Unfortunately, in many children when the OIT is stopped the state of desensitization goes away, and sustained unresponsiveness is rarely achieved. Most studies that have examined OIT have only involved treatment with a single food, even though many children have multiple food allergies. Further research is examining the efficacy, safety, and use of combined treatments in OIT (Nowak-Węgrzyn, 2018).

Because children with food allergies (usually two or more) are at risk for inadequate nutrient intake and growth failure, it is recommended that they have an annual nutritional assessment to prevent such problems. Dietary restrictions of milk may lead to calcium, vitamin D, calorie, and protein deficiencies in young children. Further, elimination of wheat may result in inadequate intake of the B vitamins, iron, and calories.

Nursing Care Management

A primary prevention strategy for avoiding food atopy in children includes parent education about the importance of exclusive breastfeeding for at least 4 to 6 months. There is no evidence that maternal avoidance (during pregnancy or lactation) of common food allergens (eggs, peanuts) prevents food allergies in children (Kleinman & Greer, 2014). Moreover, researchers have found that delaying the introduction of highly allergenic foods past 4 to 6 months of age may not be as protective against food allergy as previously believed (Nowak-Węgrzyn et al., 2020). Further, there is no evidence that soy formulas prevent allergic disease in infants and children (Kleinman & Greer, 2014).

Nursing care of children with potential food allergy consists of assisting in collecting vital health assessment data for the establishment of a diagnosis and assisting with diagnostic tests. It is important for nurses to be informed about food allergy and provide parents and caregivers, as well as older children, with accurate information regarding food allergy. Education of parents, teachers, and daycare workers regarding signs and symptoms of food allergy and reactions is vital (see Critical Thinking Case Study box). Children with diagnosed food allergy should avoid unfamiliar foods and restaurants that do not disclose food ingredients. New labeling guidelines require that food additives (such as spices and flavoring) be clearly labeled on commercially sold, store-bought foods. Hidden ingredients in prepared foods are also potential sources of food allergy. Nutritional consultation is imperative for children who are diagnosed with allergies to certain foods in order to develop a dietary plan that includes sufficient nutrients for growth and development while avoiding the offending food.

Children with a history of food allergy may spend a considerable amount of time in daycare; therefore persons working in daycare centers and other children's settings need to be properly educated regarding recognition and management of severe anaphylactic reactions. It is also important for schools to ensure that children who have potentially life-threatening food allergies are recognized so that plans can be implemented to prevent contact with allergy-producing foods. A written emergency action or food-allergy plan should be kept for the child and a self-injectable epinephrine device should be readily available for these children (Keet & Wang, 2014). Some strategies included by schools to help manage food allergies include allergen-safe zones on campus, a ban on specific foods on campus, food allergy training for foodservice staff, and keeping ingredient records for all foods served on campus (Sauer, Patten, Roberts, et al., 2018). Unfortunately, there is increasing evidence that children labeled as having a food allergy are falling victim to increased rates of bullying and victimization (Egan & Sicherer, 2016; Rocheleau & Rocheleau, 2019), demonstrating the need for increased education for students on the seriousness of food allergies. Families of children with life-threatening food allergies are also at risk for increased psychosocial distress, so health care workers should be prepared to meet the families' psychosocial as well as physical needs regarding their children.

CRITICAL THINKING CASE STUDY

Food Allergy Anaphylaxis

A group of nursing students is holding a health promotion fair at a local elementary school for first-, second-, and third-graders. The nursing students have several booths set up in the school cafeteria. Three second-grade boys are engaging in horseplay in front of one of the booths when one of the boys, Jason, an 8-year-old child, suddenly starts coughing and clutching his throat. The students also observe that he is developing red splotches on his face, neck, and throat that he is scratching. Jason says, "I'm having trouble breathing!" The school nurse is nearby and comes over to see what the commotion is about. One of the boys with Jason says, "We didn't mean any harm! We were just goofing around when we put peanuts in his trail mix." One of the student nurses says, "He's in obvious distress—what should we do?"

Initial Assessment. What signs and symptoms that Jason is experiencing lead you to believe he is having an anaphylactic reaction to peanuts?

Expected Nursing Action. What interventions are appropriate for an anaphylactic reaction to a food allergy?

Continued

CRITICAL THINKING CASE STUDY—cont'd

Food Allergy Anaphylaxis

Teaching Points

- Treatment of an anaphylactic reaction through the administration of intramuscular epinephrine is indicated if a child is experiencing a "barky" cough, itching sensation or tightness in the throat, difficulty swallowing or breathing, wheezing, or hoarseness.
- Any child who has an extremely sensitive food allergy should wear a medical identification bracelet and have an injectable epinephrine cartridge (EpiPen) readily available. A written emergency treatment plan should be created and discussed with parents, teachers, and school health care personnel.
- Diphenhydramine (Benadryl) and cetirizine (Zyrtec) can be effective for skin and nasal symptoms but will not help with airway symptoms.

Critical Thinking Answers

Initial Assessment. Jason is experiencing the signs and symptoms of coughing, clutching his throat, red splotches on his face/neck/throat, scratching his skin, and experiencing trouble breathing. These signs and symptoms are consistent with an anaphylactic reaction to a food allergy.

Expected Nursing Action. The priority nursing intervention for Jason is administration of intramuscular epinephrine (EpiPen). This can be followed by monitoring his airway and for further symptoms of respiratory distress, as well as following the other steps of his emergency action plan. Someone should also call 911 and wait for emergency personnel to arrive, as Jason will need to go to the hospital for further monitoring, especially for a biphasic reaction.

Cow's Milk Allergy

Cow's milk allergy (CMA) is a multifaceted disorder representing adverse systemic and local GI reactions to cow's milk protein. Approximately 2.5% of infants develop cow's milk hypersensitivity, with 60% being IgE mediated. It is estimated that 50% of those children may outgrow the hypersensitivity by 3 to 4 years of age (Groetch & Sampson, 2016). (This discussion centers on cow's milk protein contained in commercial infant formulas. Whole milk is not recommended for infants younger than 12 months of age.) The allergy may be manifested within the first 4 months of life through a variety of signs and symptoms that may appear within 45 minutes of milk ingestion or after several days (Box 10.2). The diagnosis may initially be made from the history, although the history alone is not diagnostic. The timing and diversity of clinical manifestations vary greatly. For example, CMA may be manifested as colic (see information later in the chapter), diarrhea, vomiting, GI bleeding, gastroesophageal reflux, chronic constipation, or sleeplessness in an otherwise healthy infant.

Diagnostic Evaluation

A number of diagnostic tests may be performed, including stool analysis for blood (both frank and occult bleeding can occur from colitis), eosinophils, and leukocytes; serum IgE levels; and skin prick testing. Skin testing may help identity the offending food, but the results are not always conclusive. No single diagnostic test is considered definitive for diagnosis (Kleinman & Greer, 2014).

The most definitive diagnostic strategy is elimination of cow's milk from the diet followed by challenge testing after improvement of symptoms. Challenge testing involves reintroducing small quantities of milk to the diet to detect resurgence of symptoms. It may also include the use of a placebo so that the parent is unaware of (or "blind" to) the timing of allergen ingestion. A double-blind, placebo-controlled food challenge is the gold standard for diagnosing food allergies such as CMA. Careful observation of the child is required during a challenge test because of the possibility of anaphylactic reaction. A clinical diagnosis is made when symptoms improve after removal of milk from the diet and two or more challenge tests produce symptoms (Groetch & Sampson, 2016).

BOX 10.2 Common Clinical Manifestations of Cow's Milk Sensitivity

Gastrointestinal

Diarrhea
Vomiting
Colic
Wheezing
Gastroesophageal reflux
Bloody stools
Rectal bleeding

Respiratory

Rhinitis
Bronchitis
Asthma
Sneezing
Coughing
Chronic nasal discharge

Other Signs and Symptoms

Eczema
Excessive crying
Pallor (from anemia secondary to chronic blood loss in gastrointestinal tract)
Fussiness, irritability

Therapeutic Management

Treatment of CMA involves elimination of cow's milk–based formula and all other dairy products. For infants fed commercial cow's milk formula, this primarily involves changing the formula to a casein hydrolysate milk formula (Pregestimil, Nutramigen, or Alimentum) in which the protein has been broken down into its amino acids through enzymatic hydrolysis. Although the American Academy of Pediatrics (Kleinman & Greer, 2014) recommends the use of extensively hydrolyzed formulas for CMA, many practitioners may start a soy-based infant formula instead because of the expense of the hydrolyzed formulas. Unfortunately, approximately 50% of infants who are sensitive to cow's milk protein also demonstrate sensitivity to soy-based formulas. Other choices for children who are intolerant to cow's milk–based formulas include amino acid–based formulas, Neocate or EleCare, but their cost is a major consideration. Infants with CMA usually remain on a cow's milk–free diet for 12 months, after which time small quantities of milk are reintroduced.

Nursing Care Management

The principal nursing objectives are identification of potential CMA and appropriate counseling of parents regarding substitute infant formulas. Parents often interpret GI symptoms such as spitting up, loose stools, or fussiness as CMA and switch the infant to a variety of formulas in an attempt to resolve the problem. Parents need reassurance regarding the needs of nonverbal infants who have an array of symptoms. Endless nights of lost sleep and a crying infant may promote feelings of parenting inadequacy and role conflict, thus aggravating the situation. Nurses can reassure parents that many of these symptoms are common and the reasons are often never discovered, yet the child does achieve appropriate growth and development. Parents should be advised to report acute symptoms to the practitioner for further evaluation. They should be reassured that the infant will receive complete nutrition from the new formula and will have no ill effects from the absence of cow's milk–based formula.

When solid foods are introduced, parents need guidance in avoiding cow's milk products. Carefully reading all food labels helps avoid exposure to prepared foods containing milk products. Although labeled as nondairy, cream and butter substitutes may contain cow's milk protein.

FAILURE TO THRIVE

Failure to thrive (FTT) is a term used to describe inadequate growth resulting from an inability to obtain or use calories required for growth. FTT has no universal definition; however, the objective parameter is usually the deceleration of growth in both height and weight. If FTT is severe, poor brain growth could occur as evidenced by a smaller than normal head circumference. The diagnosis is based on growth parameters that (1) drop more than two percentiles from baseline, (2) are persistently below the 3rd to 5th percentiles, or (3) are less than the 80th percentile of median weight for height measurement. The term *growth failure* is now generally considered to be overly simplistic and obsolete (Sirotnak & Chiesa, 2016). Weight for length is reported to be a more accurate indicator of undernutrition (Becker, Carney, Corkins, et al., 2015).

The finding of a pattern of persistent deviation from established growth parameters is used in the diagnosis of FTT, rather than just growth measurements alone. In addition to the lack of consensus on the exact definition of FTT, some advocate for a change in the terminology used to describe FTT; thus terms such as *growth faltering* and *pediatric undernutrition* are starting to be seen in the literature for FTT. Further, some experts suggest that the previously used classifications of *organic FTT* and *nonorganic FTT* are too simplistic because most cases of growth failure have mixed causes. Therefore experts suggest that FTT be classified by pathophysiology into the following categories (Sirotnak & Chiesa, 2016):

Inadequate caloric intake: Incorrect formula preparation, neglect, food fads, excessive juice consumption, poverty, breastfeeding problems, behavioral problems affecting eating, parental restriction of caloric intake, or central nervous system problems affecting intake

Inadequate absorption: Cystic fibrosis, celiac disease, Crohn disease, vitamin or mineral deficiencies, cow's milk allergy, biliary atresia, or hepatic disease

Increased metabolism: Hyperthyroidism, congenital heart disease, or chronic immunodeficiency

Defective utilization: Genetic anomaly such as trisomy 21 or 18, congenital infection, or metabolic storage diseases

Rates of true FTT in US children are not clearly known. However, poverty is believed to be the greatest risk factor for FTT in developed and developing countries (Sirotnak & Chiesa, 2016). Nearly 20% of children younger than 4 years old live in poverty and are unable to obtain adequate food on a regular basis (Sirotnak & Chiesa, 2016). The cause of FTT is often multifactorial and involves a combination of infant organic disease, dysfunctional parenting behaviors, subtle neurologic or behavioral problems, and disturbed parent-child interactions (Sirotnak & Chiesa, 2016). However, the primary etiology of FTT is inadequate caloric intake regardless of the cause.

Infants who are born preterm with VLBW or ELBW and those with intrauterine growth restriction (IUGR) are often seen for FTT within the first 2 years of life. This is because they typically do not grow physically at the same rate as term cohorts even after discharge from the hospital. Catch-up growth has been shown to be much more difficult to achieve in ELBW and VLBW infants. As children, infants who experience FTT are more likely to have small stature and demonstrate lower cognitive and academic achievement scores when compared to infants who did not experience FTT (Feifer & Walker-Descartes, 2017). Children with congenital heart disease are also more likely to develop FTT in infancy due to inadequate caloric intake, malabsorption, increased energy expidenture that supersedes caloric intake, and pulmonary hypertension.

Other factors that can lead to inadequate caloric intake in infancy include (1) health or childrearing beliefs such as fad diets, (2) child neglect, (3) child abuse, (4) inadequate nutritional knowledge, (5) financial difficulties, (6) family stress, (7) feeding resistance, and (8) insufficient breast milk intake. In infants younger than 8 weeks old, breastfeeding problems as a result of inadequate latch or uncoordinated sucking and swallowing may occur (Sirotnak & Chiesa, 2016).

Diagnostic Evaluation

Diagnosis of FTT is initially made clinically through identification of signs and symptoms. If FTT is acute, the weight, but not the length or height, is below accepted standards (usually the 5th percentile). If FTT is chronic, both weight and length or height are low, indicating ongoing malnutrition. The use of weight velocities (according to the World Health Organization growth charts at http://www.who.int/childgrowth/standards/height_for_age/en/) may be a better indicator of acute growth failure while considering age-dependent changes in growth. Perhaps as important as anthropometric measurements is a complete health and dietary history (including perinatal history), physical examination for evidence of organic causes, developmental assessment, and family assessment. A dietary intake history, either in the form of a 24-hour dietary recall or a history of food consumed over a 3- to 5-day period, is also essential. In addition, explore the child's activity level, parental stature, perceived food allergies, and dietary restrictions.

An assessment of household organization and mealtime behaviors and rituals is an important component in the collection of pertinent data. It is often helpful to obtain the growth patterns of the affected child's parents and siblings because these can be compared with norm-referenced standards to evaluate the child's growth. An assessment of the home environment and parent-child interaction may be helpful as well. Other tests (e.g., lead toxicity, anemia, stool-reducing substances, occult blood, ova and parasites, alkaline phosphatase, and zinc levels) are selected only as indicated to rule out organic problems. To prevent the overuse of diagnostic procedures, consider FTT early in the differential diagnosis. To avoid the social stigma of FTT during the early investigative phase, some health care workers use the term *growth delay* (or *growth failure*) until the actual cause is established.

Therapeutic Management

The primary management of FTT is aimed at reversing the cause of the growth failure. If malnutrition is severe, the initial treatment is directed at reversing the malnutrition while avoiding refeeding syndrome (see information earlier in the chapter). The goal is to provide sufficient calories to support "catch-up" growth, which is a rate of growth greater than the expected rate for age. A suggested goal for catch-up growth is two to three times the average rate of weight gain for the child's corrected age (Kleinman & Greer, 2014). In addition to adding caloric density to feedings, the child may require multivitamin supplementation. Finally, any coexisting medical problems must be addressed.

In most cases of FTT, an interprofessional team consisting of physicians, nurses, dietitians, child life specialists, occupational therapists, pediatric feeding specialists, and social workers or mental health professionals is needed to help address the patient's complex needs. Care providers should make efforts to relieve any additional stresses on the family by offering referrals for public assistance or supplemental food programs. In some cases, family therapy may be helpful. Behavior modification focused on mealtime rituals (or lack thereof) and family social time may also be helpful. Hospitalization is indicated for (1) evidence (anthropometric) of SAM, (2) child abuse or neglect, (3) significant dehydration, (4) caretaker substance abuse or psychosis, (5) outpatient management that does not result in weight gain, or (6) serious concurrent infection (Sirotnak & Chiesa, 2016). Depending on the cause of the growth failure and the child's response to nutritional intervention, many children can be treated on an outpatient basis.

Prognosis

The prognosis for children with FTT is related to the cause. If the parents lack knowledge of the infant's needs, teaching may remedy the child's limited caloric intake and permanently reverse the growth failure. Inadequate or infrequent feedings by the infant's primary caretaker, in conjunction with family disorganization, are often the underlying cause of FTT.

There are few long-term studies to provide data on the prognosis of children with FTT; however, some researchers have found that children who had FTT as infants had shorter statures, lower weights, and lower scores on measures of psychomotor and socioemotional development than their peers (Feifer & Walker-Descartes, 2017). Factors that are related to poor prognosis include (1) severe feeding resistance, (2) lack of awareness in parents, (3) poor parental cooperation, (4) low family income, (5) low maternal educational level, (6) adolescent mothers, (7) preterm birth, (8) IUGR, and (9) early age of onset of FTT. Because later cognitive and motor function is affected by malnourishment in infancy, many of these children are below normal in intellectual development with childhood intelligence quotient (IQ) scores significantly lower than their peers who have no history of malnourishment (Romano, Hartman, Privitera, et al., 2015). In addition, there is a higher likelihood of eating and behavioral issues among children with a history of malnutrition when compared with their peers (Romano et al., 2015). These findings indicate that a long-term plan and follow-up care are needed for the optimum development of these children.

BOX 10.3 Clinical Manifestations of Failure to Thrive

- Growth failure
- Developmental delays—social, motor, adaptive, language
- Undernutrition
- Apathy
- Withdrawn behavior
- Feeding or eating disorders, such as vomiting, feeding resistance, anorexia, pica, rumination
- No fear of strangers (at age when stranger anxiety is normal)
- Avoidance of eye contact
- Wide-eyed gaze and continual scan of the environment ("radar gaze")
- Stiff and unyielding or flaccid and unresponsive
- Minimal smiling

Nursing Care Management

Nurses play a critical role as part of the interprofessional team in the diagnosis of FTT through their assessment of the child, parents, and family interactions. Knowledge of the characteristics of children with FTT and their families is essential in the identification of these children and the rapid confirmation of a diagnosis (Box 10.3). The accurate assessment of initial weight, head circumference, length or height, and daily weight is an essential component of nursing care for children with FTT. Further, keeping a record of all food intake is imperative. The nurse documents the child's feeding behaviors, as well as the parent-child interaction during feedings, and assesses other caregiving activities, including play.

Children with FTT may have a history of difficult feeding, vomiting, sleep disturbance, and excessive irritability. Patterns such as crying during feedings, vomiting, hoarding food in the mouth, ruminating after feeding, refusing to switch from liquids to solids, and displaying aversion behavior, such as turning from food or spitting food, can become attention-seeking behaviors to prolong interaction with caregivers at mealtime. Besides showing signs of malnutrition and delayed social development, children with FTT may exhibit altered behavioral interactions with others. In some cases, the child may use feeding as a control mechanism in a poorly organized or chaotic family situation. Parents may allow the child to dictate the norms for behavior and feeding because of inexperience with parenting or poor parenting role models. Thus refusing to eat or only eating sweets and snacks with nonnutritive value may be the child's norm based on food availability and family tradition. In these cases, family therapy is indicated to address this trend and improve the parent-child relationship.

Some of the relationship strain that may occur between parent and child may be the result of dissatisfaction and frustration; therefore the child should have a consistent core team of primary nurses (Fig. 10.1). These nurses caring for the child can learn to perceive his or her cues and address the cycle of dissatisfaction, especially around feeding.

Because many children with FTT are responding to stimuli that have led to the negative feeding patterns, an important primary intervention is to structure the feeding environment to encourage healthful eating. Initially, staff members and a feeding specialist may need to feed these children to

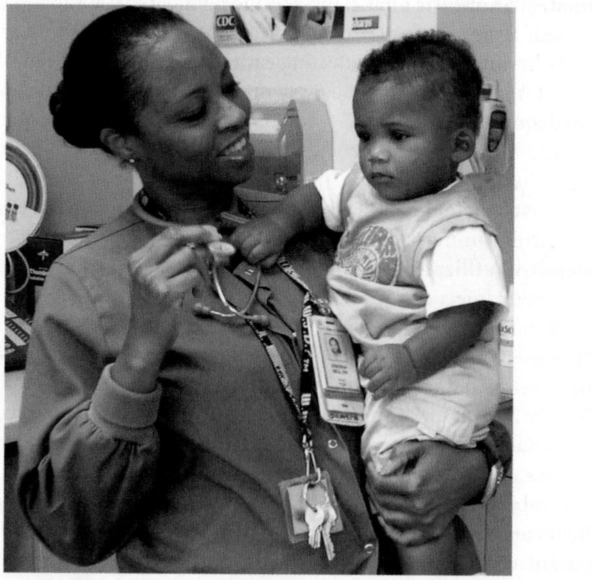

Fig. 10.1 A consistent nurse is important in developing trust in infants who have failure to thrive.

thoroughly assess the difficulties encountered during the feeding process and to devise strategies that eliminate or minimize these problems.

There are four primary goals in the nutritional management of children with FTT: (1) correcting nutritional deficiencies and achieving ideal weight for height, (2) providing adequate calories for catch-up growth, (3) restoring optimum body composition, and (4) educating the parents or primary caregivers about the child's nutritional requirements and age-appropriate feeding methods. For infants, higher calorie formulas (24 kcal/oz) may be provided to increase caloric intake. Older children (1 to 6 years old) may benefit from a 30-kcal/oz milk formula (Kleinman & Greer, 2014). For example, toddlers may be given a high-calorie milk drink such as PediaSure to increase caloric intake. The nurse should carefully monitor for signs of intolerance to the formula. Usually only in extreme cases of malnourishment are tube feedings or intravenous therapy required. Finally, carbohydrate additives, including fortified cereals and vegetable oil, may be indicated. Because vitamin and mineral deficiencies may occur, multivitamin supplementation, including zinc and iron, is recommended.

Maladaptive feeding practices often contribute to growth failure; therefore parents should be given specific, step-by-step directions for formula preparation, as well as a written schedule of feeding times. Fruit juice is restricted in children with FTT until adequate weight gain has been achieved using appropriate milk sources. At that time, juice may be reintroduced but limited to no more than 4 oz/day.

Behavior modification techniques may be used with older infants and toddlers to interrupt maladaptive feeding patterns. Feeding times can become a "war of wills," resulting in food refusal and eventually FTT. These behaviors are different from the occasional toddler behavior of food refusal, which is primarily developmental, not pathologic.

In addition to attending to the child's physical needs, the interdisciplinary team must plan care for appropriate developmental stimulation. After an approximate developmental age is established, a planned program of play should be initiated. Ideally, a child life specialist is involved in this plan to implement and supervise the child's play activities. Every effort should be made to educate parents about how to play and interact with their child at a developmentally appropriate level. A pediatric nutrition specialist should also be involved in planning and implementing a diet specifically tailored for the child's growth needs.

Nursing care of children with FTT involves a "family systems" approach. Therefore if the goal is for the entire family to become healthy, all members should be engaged in the change process. Nursing care of the child's parents is focused on improving their self-esteem and supporting them as they acquire positive, successful parenting skills. Initially, this necessitates providing an environment in which they feel welcomed and accepted.

SKIN DISORDERS

DIAPER DERMATITIS

Diaper dermatitis is common in infants and one of several acute inflammatory skin disorders caused either directly or indirectly by wearing diapers. The peak age of occurrence is 9 to 12 months of age, and the incidence is greater in bottle-fed infants than in breastfed infants.

Pathophysiology and Clinical Manifestations

Diaper dermatitis is caused by prolonged and repetitive contact with an irritant (e.g., urine, feces, soaps, detergents, ointments, friction). Although the irritant in the majority of cases is urine and feces, a combination of factors contributes to irritation.

Prolonged contact of the skin with diaper wetness produces higher friction, greater abrasion damage, increased transepidermal permeability, and increased microbial counts. Healthy skin is less resistant to potential irritants.

Although ammonia was once thought to cause diaper rash because of the association between the strong odor on diapers and dermatitis, ammonia alone is not sufficient. The irritant quality of urine is related to an increase in pH from the breakdown of urea in the presence of fecal urease. The increased pH promotes the activity of fecal enzymes, principally the proteases and lipases, which act as irritants. Fecal enzymes also increase the permeability of skin to bile salts, another potential irritant in feces.

The eruption of diaper dermatitis is manifested primarily on convex surfaces or in folds. The lesions represent a variety of types and configurations. Eruptions involving the skin in most intimate contact with the diaper (e.g., the convex surfaces of buttocks, inner thighs, mons pubis, scrotum) but sparing the folds are likely caused by chemical irritants, especially from urine and feces (Fig. 10.2). Other causes are detergents or soaps from inadequately rinsed cloth diapers or the chemicals in disposable wipes. Perianal involvement is usually the result of chemical irritation from feces, especially diarrheal stools. *Candida albicans* infection produces perianal inflammation and a maculopapular rash with satellite lesions that may cross the inguinal fold (Fig. 10.3). It is seen in up to 90% of infants with chronic diaper dermatitis and should be considered in diaper rashes that are recalcitrant to treatment.

Nursing Care Management

Nursing interventions are aimed at altering the three factors that produce dermatitis: wetness, pH, and fecal irritants. The most significant factor amenable to intervention is the moist environment created in the diaper area. Changing the diaper as soon as it becomes wet eliminates a large part of the problem, and removing the diaper to expose healthy skin to air facilitates drying. The use of a hair dryer or heat lamp is not recommended because these devices can cause burns.

Diaper construction has a significant impact on the incidence and severity of diaper dermatitis. Superabsorbent disposable paper diapers reduce diaper dermatitis. They contain an absorbent gelling material that binds water tightly to decrease skin wetness, maintains pH control by providing a buffering capacity, and decreases skin irritation by preventing mixing of urine and feces in the diaper.

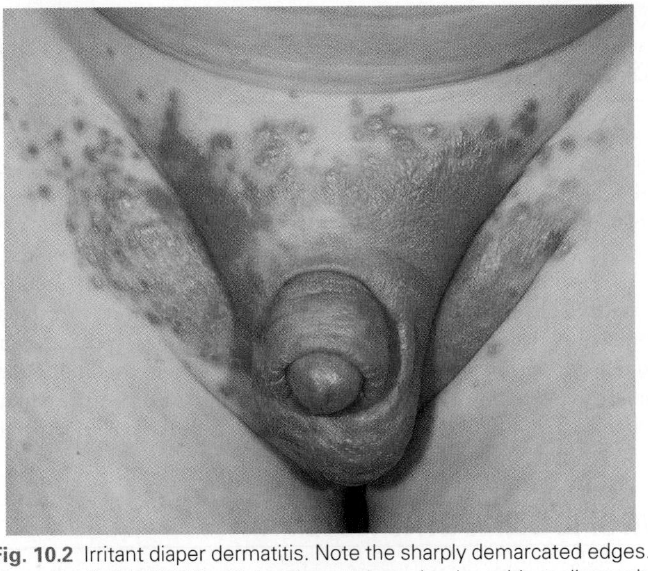

Fig. 10.2 Irritant diaper dermatitis. Note the sharply demarcated edges. (From Habif, T. P. [2010]. Clinical dermatology: A color guide to diagnosis and therapy [5th ed.]. St Louis, MO: Mosby.)

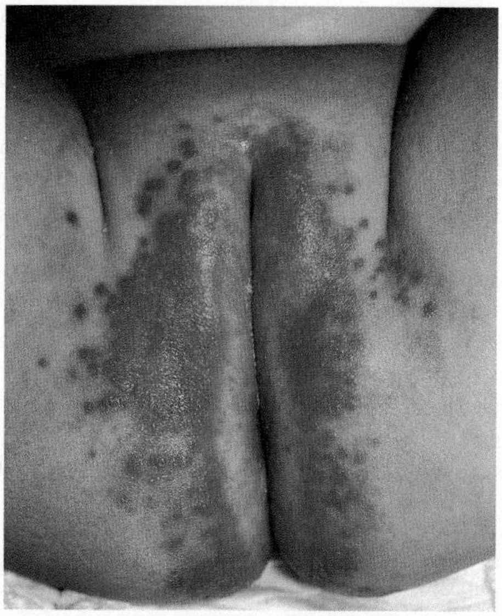

Fig. 10.3 Candidiasis of diaper area. Note the beefy red central erythema with satellite pustules. (From Paller, A. S., & Mancini, A. J. [2011]. *Hurwitz clinical pediatric dermatology* [4th ed.]. St Louis, MO: Saunders Elsevier.)

FAMILY-CENTERED CARE

Controlling Diaper Rash

Keep skin dry.[a]

- Use superabsorbent disposable diapers to reduce skin wetness.
- Change diapers as soon as soiled—especially with stool—whenever possible, preferably once during the night.
- Expose healthy or only slightly irritated skin to air, not heat, to dry completely.

Apply ointment, such as zinc oxide or petrolatum, to protect skin, especially if skin is very red or has moist, open areas.

- Avoid removing skin barrier cream with each diaper change; remove waste material and reapply skin barrier cream.
- To completely remove ointment, especially zinc oxide, use mineral oil; do not wash vigorously.

Avoid overwashing the skin, especially with perfumed soaps or commercial wipes, which may be irritating.

- May use a moisturizer or nonsoap cleanser, such as cold cream or Cetaphil, to wipe urine from skin.
- Gently wipe stool from skin using a soft cloth and warm water.
- Use disposable diaper wipes that are detergent- and alcohol-free.

[a] Powder helps keep the skin dry, but talcum powder is dangerous if breathed into the lungs. Plain cornstarch or cornstarch-based powder is safer. When using any powder product, first shake it into your hand and then apply it to the diaper area. Store the container away from the infant's reach; keep the container closed when not in use.

Guidelines for controlling diaper rash are presented in the Family-Centered Care box. A common misconception about using cornstarch on skin is that it promotes the growth of *C. albicans.* Neither cornstarch nor talcum promotes the growth of fungi under conditions normally found in the diaper area. On the basis of these properties and its safety in terms of inhalation injury, cornstarch is the preferred product. Talcum powder should not be used.

ATOPIC DERMATITIS (ECZEMA)

Atopic dermatitis (AD), also referred to as eczema, refers to a descriptive category of dermatologic diseases and not to a specific etiology. AD is a chronic relapsing inflammatory skin disorder that results in itching and lesions (Grey & Maquiness, 2016). It occurs in 20% of children (Page, Weston, & Loh, 2016). AD manifests in three forms based on the child's age and the distribution of lesions:

1. **Infantile (infantile eczema):** Usually begins at 2 to 6 months of age; generally undergoes spontaneous remission by 3 years of age
2. **Childhood:** May follow the infantile form; occurs at 2 to 3 years of age; 90% of children have manifestations by 5 years of age
3. **Preadolescent and adolescent:** Begins at about 12 years of age; may continue into the early adult years or indefinitely

The diagnosis of AD is based on a combination of history and morphologic findings (Box 10.4). Although symptoms can vary

BOX 10.4 Clinical Manifestations of Atopic Dermatitis

Distribution of Lesions

Infantile form: Generalized, especially face, scalp, neck, and extensor surfaces of extremities

Childhood form: Flexural areas (antecubital and popliteal fossae, neck), wrists, ankles, and feet

Preadolescent and adolescent form: Face, sides of neck, hands, feet, and antecubital and popliteal fossae (to a lesser extent)

Appearance of Lesions

Infantile Form

Erythema
Vesicles
Papules
Weeping
Oozing
Crusting
Scaling
Often symmetric

Childhood Form

Symmetric involvement
Clusters of small erythematous or flesh-colored papules or minimally scaling patches
Dry and may be hyperpigmented
Lichenification (thickened skin with accentuation of creases)
Keratosis pilaris (follicular hyperkeratosis) common

Adolescent or Adult Form

Same as childhood manifestations
Dry, thick lesions (lichenified plaques) common
Confluent papules

Other Physical Manifestations

Intense itching
Unaffected skin dry and rough
African American children likely to exhibit more papular or follicular lesions than white children
May exhibit one or more of the following:

- Lymphadenopathy, especially near affected sites
- Increased palmar creases (many cases)
- Atopic pleats (extra line or groove of lower eyelid)
- Prone to cold hands
- Pityriasis alba (small, poorly defined areas of hypopigmentation)
- Facial pallor (especially around nose, mouth, and ears)
- Bluish discoloration beneath eyes ("allergic shiners")
- Increased susceptibility to unusual cutaneous infections (especially viral)

among children, one symptom that is common is pruritus. Itching can be mild, moderate, or severe, and can intensify the inflammation and erythema associated with the lesions; itching can become so severe that the lesions bleed. This also increases the risk for secondary infection. Lesions gradually disappear when the scratching is stopped.

Although the cause is not fully understood, AD is believed to have genetic and environmental factors (Nguyen, Leonard, & Eichenfield, 2015). The majority of children with infantile AD have a family history of eczema, asthma, food allergies, or allergic rhinitis, which strongly supports a genetic predisposition. The cause is unknown but appears to be related to abnormal function of the skin, including alterations in perspiration, peripheral vascular function, and heat tolerance. Manifestations of the chronic disease improve in humid climates and get worse in the fall and winter, when homes are heated and environmental humidity is lower. The disorder can be controlled but not cured. A recent study of 250 patients with AD showed that the severity of AD significantly affected their quality of life, with more severe disease resulting in a lower quality of life (Holm, Agner, Clausen, et al., 2016). The study also reported a lower quality of life among females and among patients with eczema on their face (Holm et al., 2016).

Therapeutic Management

The major goals in managing AD are to (1) hydrate the skin, (2) relieve pruritus, (3) reduce flare-ups or inflammation, and (4) prevent and control secondary infection. The general measures for managing AD focus on reducing pruritus and other aspects of the disease. Management strategies include avoiding exposure to skin irritants or allergens; avoiding overheating; and administrating medications such as antihistamines, topical immunomodulators, topical steroids, and (sometimes) mild sedatives as indicated.

Enhancing skin hydration and preventing dry, flaky skin are accomplished in a number of ways, depending on the child's skin characteristics and individual needs. A tepid bath with a mild soap (Dove or Neutrogena), no soap, or an emulsifying oil followed immediately by application of an emollient (within 3 minutes) assists in trapping moisture and preventing its loss. Bubble baths and harsh soaps should be avoided. The bath may need to be repeated once or twice daily, depending on the child's status; excessive bathing without emollient application only dries out the skin. Some lotions are not effective, and emollients should be chosen carefully to prevent excessive skin drying. Aquaphor, Cetaphil, and Eucerin are acceptable lotions for skin hydration. A nighttime bath followed by emollient application and dressing in soft cotton pajamas may help alleviate most nighttime pruritus.

Sometimes colloid baths, such as the addition of 2 cups of cornstarch to a tub of warm water, provide temporary relief of itching and may help the child sleep if given before bedtime. Cool, wet compresses are soothing to the skin and provide antiseptic protection.

Oral antihistamine drugs (such as hydroxyzine or diphenhydramine) usually relieve moderate or severe pruritus. Nonsedating antihistamines, such as loratadine (Claritin) or fexofenadine (Allegra), may be preferred for daytime pruritus relief. Because pruritus increases at night, a mildly sedating antihistamine may be needed.

Occasional flare-ups require the use of topical steroids to diminish inflammation. Low-, moderate-, or high-potency topical corticosteroids are prescribed, depending on the degree of involvement, the area of the body to be treated, the child's age, the potential for local side effects (striae, skin atrophy, and pigment changes), and the type of vehicle to be used (e.g., cream, lotion, ointment). Patients receiving topical corticosteroid therapy for chronic conditions should be evaluated for risk factors for suboptimal linear growth and reduced bone density. Topical immunomodulators, a nonsteroidal treatment for AD, are best used at the beginning of a "flare-up" just as the skin becomes red and itches. Second-line management for children with AD includes immunomodulator medications such as tacrolimus and pimecrolimus (Grey & Maquiness, 2016). These medications are approved for use in children 2 years of age and older (Grey & Maquiness, 2016). Both drugs can be used freely on the face without worrying about steroid side effects.

If secondary skin infections occur in children with AD, these infections are managed with appropriate systemic antibiotics. Obtaining cultures from affected areas and the child's nares is helpful to ensure appropriate therapy (Page et al., 2016).

Nursing Care Management

Assessment of the child with AD includes a family history for evidence of atopy, a history of previous involvement, and any environmental or dietary factors associated with the present and previous exacerbations. The skin lesions are examined for type, distribution, and evidence of secondary infection. Parents are interviewed regarding the child's behavior, especially in relation to scratching, irritability, and sleeping patterns. Exploration of the family's feelings and methods of coping is also important.

The nursing care of the child with AD is challenging. Controlling the intense pruritus is imperative if the disorder will be successfully managed because scratching leads to new lesions and may cause secondary infection. In addition to the medical regimen, other measures can be taken to prevent or minimize the scratching. Fingernails and toenails are cut short, kept clean, and filed frequently to prevent sharp edges. Gloves or cotton stockings can be placed over the hands and pinned to shirtsleeves. One-piece outfits with long sleeves and long pants also decrease direct contact with the skin. If gloves or socks are used, the child needs time to be free from such restrictions. An excellent time to remove gloves, socks, or other protective devices is during the bath or after receiving sedative or antipruritic medication.

Conditions that increase itching are eliminated when possible. Woolen clothes or blankets, rough fabrics, and furry stuffed animals are removed from the child's environment. Because heat and humidity cause perspiration (which intensifies itching), proper dress for climatic conditions is essential. Pruritus is often precipitated by exposure to the irritant effects of certain components of common products, such as soaps, detergents, fabric softeners, perfumes, and powders. During cold months, synthetic fabrics (not wool) should be used for overcoats, hats, gloves, and snowsuits. Exposure to latex products, such as gloves and balloons, should also be avoided.

Clothes and sheets are laundered in a mild detergent and rinsed thoroughly in clear water (without fabric softeners or antistatic chemicals). Putting the clothes through a second complete wash cycle without using detergent reduces the amount of residue remaining in the fabric.

! NURSING ALERT

If the child is being treated with baths, it is imperative that the emollient preparation be applied immediately after bathing (while the skin is still slightly moist) to prevent drying.

Preventing infection is usually accomplished by preventing scratching. Baths are given as prescribed; the water is kept tepid; and soaps (except as indicated), bubble baths, oils, and powders are avoided. Skinfolds and diaper areas need frequent cleansing with plain water. A room humidifier or vaporizer may benefit children with extremely dry skin. Skin lesions are examined for signs of infection—usually honey-colored crusts or pustules with surrounding erythema. Any signs of infection are reported to the practitioner.

Wet soaks and compresses are applied, and medications for pruritus or infection are administered as directed. The family is given explicit instructions on the preparation and use of soaks, special baths, and topical medications, including the order of application if more than one is prescribed. It is important to emphasize that one thick application of topical medication is *not* equivalent to several thin applications and that excessive use of an agent (particularly steroids) can be hazardous. If children have difficulty remaining still for a 10- or 15-minute soak, bath, or dressing application, these can be carried out at naptime or when the child is engrossed in watching television, listening to a story, or playing with tub toys.

Diet modification may prevent skin exacerbations. When a hypoallergenic diet is prescribed, parents need help to understand the reason for the diet and the guidelines for avoiding hyperallergenic foods. Because hypoallergenic diets take time before visible effects are apparent, parents need reassurance that results may not be seen immediately. If airborne allergens make eczema worse, the family is counseled about "allergy proofing" the home (see Chapter 21, Asthma).

Parents are assured that the lesions will not produce scarring (unless secondarily infected) and that the disease is not contagious. However, the child may have repeated exacerbations and remissions. Spontaneous and permanent remission takes place at approximately 2 to 3 years old in most children with the infantile disorder.

During acute phases, emotional stress can become intense for the family. They need time to discuss negative feelings and to be reassured that these feelings are normal. Stress tends to aggravate the severity of the condition. Therefore efforts to relieve as much anxiety as possible in both the parents and the child have a beneficial emotional and physical effect.

SEBORRHEIC DERMATITIS

Seborrheic dermatitis is a chronic, recurrent, inflammatory reaction of the skin that occurs most commonly on the scalp (cradle cap) but may involve the eyelids (blepharitis), external ear canal (otitis externa), nasolabial folds, and inguinal region. The cause is unknown, although it is more common in early infancy, when sebum production is increased. The lesions are characteristically thick, adherent, yellowish, scaly, oily patches that may or may not be mildly pruritic. Unlike AD, seborrheic dermatitis is not associated with a positive family history for allergy and is common in infants shortly after birth and in adolescents after puberty. Diagnosis is made primarily on the basis of the appearance and the location of the crusts or scales.

Nursing Care Management

Cradle cap may be prevented with adequate scalp hygiene. Frequently, parents omit shampooing the infant's hair for fear of damaging the "soft spots," or fontanels. The nurse should discuss how to shampoo the infant's hair and emphasize that the fontanel is similar to skin anywhere else on the body; it does not puncture or tear with mild pressure.

When seborrheic lesions are present, direct the treatment at removing the scales or crusts. Parents are taught the appropriate procedure to clean the scalp. Education may need to include a demonstration. Shampooing should be done daily with a mild soap or commercial baby shampoo; medicated shampoos are not necessary, but an antiseborrheic shampoo containing sulfur and salicylic acid may be used. Shampoo is applied to the scalp and allowed to remain on the scalp until the crusts soften. Then the scalp is thoroughly rinsed. A fine-tooth comb or a soft facial brush helps remove the loosened crusts from the strands of hair after shampooing.

SPECIAL HEALTH PROBLEMS

COLIC (PAROXYSMAL ABDOMINAL PAIN)

Colic is believed to occur in 15% to 20% of all infants (Camilleri, Park, Scarpato, et al., 2017; Savino, Ceratto, Poggi, et al., 2015), yet an organic cause may be identified in less than 5% of infants seen by practitioners for excessive crying (Camilleri et al., 2017). The condition is generally described as abdominal pain or cramping that is manifested by loud crying and drawing the legs up to the abdomen. Parents typically express dissatisfaction with the amount of time the infant spends crying each day. Colic can be characterized by crying (1) more than 3 hours per day, (2) for more than 3 days per week, and (3) for more than 3 weeks. Symptoms may increase in the late afternoon or evening (Deshpande, 2015); however, in some infants the onset of symptoms occurs at varying times. Colic is more common in infants younger than 3 months old and in infants with difficult temperaments.

Despite the obvious behavioral indications of pain, the infant with colic gains weight and usually thrives. There is no evidence of a residual effect of colic on older children, except perhaps a strained parent-child relationship in some cases. Typically, colicky infants grow up to be normal children and adults. Colic is self-limiting and usually resolves as the infant matures, generally around 12 to 16 weeks of age (Akhnikh, Engelberts, van Sleuwen, et al., 2014).

Etiology

The potential causes of colic include (1) feeding too rapidly, (2) overfeeding, (3) swallowing excessive air, (4) improper feeding technique (especially positioning and burping), and (5) emotional stress or tension between parent and infant. Although all of these may occur, there is no evidence that one factor is consistently present. Infants with CMA symptoms have a high rate of colic (44%), and eliminating cow's milk products from their diet can reduce the symptoms.

Although the exact cause of colic is not fully understood, some experts believe maternal smoking, inadequate parent-infant interaction, firstborn status, lactase deficiency, difficult infant temperament, difficulty self-regulating, and abnormal GI motility are potential causes of colic (Camilleri et al., 2017). Some experts have suggested that inadequate amounts of lactobacilli in the GI tract influence gut motor function and gas production and that administration of probiotics to infants can help reduce colic (Sung, D'Amico, Cabana, et al., 2018). The consensus of many experts who study colic is that it is multifactorial and that no single treatment for every colicky infant will be effective in alleviating the symptoms.

Therapeutic Management

Management of colic should begin with an investigation of possible organic causes, such as CMA, intussusception, or other GI problem. If a sensitivity to cow's milk is strongly suspected, a trial substitution of another formula such as an extensively hydrolyzed (Nutramigen, Alimentum, Pregestimil), whey hydrolysate or amino acid (Neocate, EleCare) formula is warranted. Soy formulas are frequently prescribed for infants who do not tolerate cow's milk–based formulas, although 10% to 14% of those infants will develop a sensitivity to soy protein as well (Kleinman & Greer, 2014). The addition of lactase to infant formula has produced mixed results as far as reduction of overall symptoms. A recent meta-analysis examined the administration of *Lactobacillus reuteri* to colicky infants, regardless of feeding type, to determine if there was symptom reduction within 21 days of initiation (Sung et al., 2018). It was found that breastfed infants who received the probiotic had less crying and fussing throughout the 21 days compared to the placebo group, resulting in the authors recommending its use in breastfed infants with colic. Further research is needed to determine the benefit of probiotic use in formula-fed infants. When no specific cause can be found, the supportive measures discussed in the Nursing Care Management section are used.

The use of medications such as antispasmodics, antihistamines, and antiflatulents are sometimes recommended. Simethicone (Mylicon) may help relieve the symptoms of colic; however, in most controlled studies no medications completely resolved the symptoms of colic. Behavioral interventions have not proven effective at reducing symptoms of colic either but have helped parents deal with the crying infant in a more positive manner.

Nursing Care Management

The initial step in managing colic is to take a thorough, detailed history of the usual daily events. Areas that should be stressed include (1) the infant's diet; (2) the diet of the breastfeeding mother; (3) timing of the crying; (4) relationship of crying to feedings; (5) presence of specific family members during crying; (6) habits of family members, such as smoking; (7) activity of the mother or usual caregiver before, during, and after crying; (8) characteristics of the cry (e.g., duration, intensity); (9) measures used to relieve crying and their effectiveness; and (10) the infant's stooling, voiding, and sleeping patterns. Of particular importance is a careful assessment of the feeding process via demonstration by the parent.

> **! NURSING ALERT**
>
> To date, there is no evidence to support one remedy that will relieve symptoms in every infant. Dietary changes, including the elimination of cow's milk protein in the infant's diet, may be effective in reducing the infant's crying, yet these interventions have been found to be only moderately effective (Camilleri et al., 2017).
>
> If cow's milk sensitivity is suspected, breastfeeding mothers should follow a milk-free diet for a minimum of 3 to 5 days to see if this is effective in reducing the infant's symptoms. Caution mothers that some nondairy creamers may contain calcium caseinate, a cow's milk protein. If a milk-free diet is helpful, lactating mothers may need calcium supplements to meet requirements. Formula-fed infants may improve with the same dietary modifications as for infants with CMA.

One important nursing intervention is to reassure parents that they are not to blame for their infant's discomfort. Parents, especially mothers, may become frustrated with their infant's crying and perceive this as a sign that something is horribly wrong. Caregivers express feelings of helplessness and frustration at being unable to console the crying infant (Fakhri, Hasanpoor-Azghady, Farahani, et al., 2019). In addition, colicky infants may be at increased risk for being shaken by their caregivers and experiencing traumatic brain injury. An empathetic, gentle, and reassuring attitude, in addition to suggestions for treatment, will help allay parents' anxieties, which are usually exacerbated by loss of sleep and preoccupation over the infant's welfare. Colic disappears spontaneously, usually by 3 to 4 months old, although guarantees should never be made because it may continue for much longer.

Helping caregivers understand the nature of the infant's crying and methods to effectively cope may be more important than finding a specific cause or treatment for colic. Because excessive infant crying increases the risk for abusive head trauma, disrupted caregiver-infant relationships, strained marital relationships, and maternal and paternal depression, the nurse should provide understanding and encourage parents to seek support from family members and friends.

SLEEP PROBLEMS

A number of sleep problems can occur in small children, and they can be fairly common. The two major categories are the **dyssomnias** and **parasomnias**. With dyssomnias, the child either has trouble falling or staying asleep at night or has difficulty staying awake during the day. Parasomnias consist of confusional arousals, sleepwalking, sleep terrors, nightmares, and rhythmic movement disorders. These typically occur in children 3 to 8 years old (Carter, Hathaway, & Lettieri, 2014). This discussion focuses on minor sleep issues in infants, such as refusal to go to sleep and frequent waking during the night (Table 10.1). Other sleep disturbances, such as obstructive sleep-disordered breathing and sleep terrors, are discussed in Chapters 12 and 21.

Concerns regarding sleep are common during infancy. Sometimes these concerns are as basic as parents' questioning whether the infant needs additional sleep. In this case, it is best to investigate the reason for their concern, stressing the individual needs of each child. Infants who are active during wakeful periods and growing normally are typically receiving adequate sleep.

However, several more serious concerns require intervention. Sleep disturbances of physiologic origin are less common in infants, with the exception of colic. The more common sleep disturbances are a learned pattern of developmental characteristics of some infants (see Table 10.1). Although many families may report sleep problems typical of these patterns, interventions are offered only when the pattern is disruptive to the family. Sleep problems in early infancy have been positively correlated with higher maternal depression scores (Muscat, Obst, Cockshaw, et al., 2014); therefore nurses should discuss infant sleep problems with the mother (and family) in addition to other developmental aspects of newborn care.

When a sleeping problem is presented, a careful assessment is essential. Charting sleep habits both before and after interventions is also an important strategy. Questions regarding the frequency and duration of waking, the usual bedtime routine, the number of nighttime feedings, the perceived problem (e.g., how much disruption the behavior generates), and the attempted interventions are important in planning effective approaches designed for the specific sleep problem. The common suggestion given to parents for any type of sleep problem, "Let the child cry until falling asleep," is difficult to implement and is inappropriate for certain conditions.

The best way to prevent sleep problems is to encourage parents to establish bedtime routines that do not foster problematic patterns. One of the most constructive routines consists of placing infants in their crib while still awake. When infants become accustomed to falling asleep somewhere else, such as in a parent's arms, and then being transferred to their crib, they awaken in unfamiliar surroundings and may be unable to fall back to sleep until the routine is repeated. Also, the bed should be used for sleeping only, not play. Although the interventions described previously and in Table 10.1 are usually successful, it is much easier to prevent the problem with appropriate counseling during the early months of the infant's life.

TABLE 10.1 Selected Sleep Disturbances During Infancy and Early Childhood

Disorder and Description	Management
Nighttime Feeding	
Child has a prolonged need for middle-of-night bottle-feeding or breastfeeding. Child goes to sleep at breast or with bottle. Awakenings are frequent (may be hourly). Child returns to sleep after feeding; other comfort measures (e.g., rocking or holding) are usually ineffective.	Increase daytime feeding intervals to >4 h (may need to be done gradually). Offer last feeding as late as possible at night; may need to gradually reduce amount of formula or length of breastfeeding. Offer no bottles in bed. Put to bed awake. When child is crying, check at progressively longer intervals each night; reassure child but do not hold, rock, take to parent's bed, or give bottle or pacifier.
Developmental Night Crying	
Child ages 6-12 months with undisturbed nighttime sleep now awakens abruptly; may be accompanied by nightmares.	Reassure parents that this phase is temporary. Enter room immediately to check on child but keep reassurances brief. Avoid feeding, rocking, taking to parent's bed, or any other routine that may initiate trained night crying.
Refusal to Go to Sleep	
Child resists bedtime and comes out of room repeatedly. Nighttime sleep may be continuous, but frequent awakenings and refusal to return to sleep may occur and become a problem if parent allows child to deviate from usual sleep pattern.	Evaluate whether hour of sleep is too early (child may resist sleep if not tired). Assist parents in establishing consistent before-bedtime routine and enforcing consistent limits regarding child's bedtime behavior. If child persists in leaving bedroom, close door for progressively longer periods. Use reward system with child to provide motivation.
Trained Night Crying (Inappropriate Sleep Associations)	
Child typically falls asleep in place other than own bed (e.g., rocking chair, parent's bed) and is brought to own bed while asleep; on awakening, cries until usual routine is instituted (e.g., rocking).	Put child in own bed when awake. If possible, arrange sleeping area separate from other family members. When child is crying, check at progressively longer intervals each night; reassure child but do not resume usual routine.
Nighttime Fears	
Child resists going to bed or wakes during the night because of fears. Child seeks parent's physical presence and falls asleep easily with parent nearby, unless fear is overwhelming.	Evaluate whether hour of sleep is too early (child may fantasize when nothing to do but think in dark room). Calmly reassure frightened child; keeping night-light on may be helpful. Use reward system with child to provide motivation to deal with fears. Avoid patterns that can lead to additional problems (e.g., sleeping with child, taking child to parent's room). If child's fear is overwhelming, consider desensitization (e.g., progressively spending longer time alone; consult professional help for protracted fears). Distinguish between nightmares and sleep terrors (confused partial arousals).

Modified from Ferber, R. (1987). Behavioral "insomnia" in the child. *Psychiatric Clinics of North America, 10*(4), 641–653.

SUDDEN INFANT DEATH SYNDROME

Sudden infant death syndrome (SIDS) is defined as the sudden death of an infant younger than 1 year of age that remains unexplained after a complete postmortem examination (autopsy), including an investigation of the death scene and a review of the case history. An autopsy is essential to identify any possible natural explanations for sudden unexpected death such as congenital anomalies or infection and to identify a death that resulted from child abuse. The autopsy typically cannot distinguish between SIDS and intentional suffocation, but the scene investigation and medical history may be of help if inconsistencies are discovered.

There has been much debate over the term *SIDS,* yet the definition noted earlier remains for the time being. Other terms have been developed to explain sudden deaths in infants. Sudden unexpected early neonatal death (SUEND) and sudden unexpected infant death (SUID) share similar features but differ regarding the timing of death: whereas SUID is considered a death in the postneonatal period, SUEND occurs in the first week of life. The American Academy of Pediatrics Task Force on Sudden Infant Death Syndrome considers SIDS to be a component of SUID.

SIDS is the third leading cause of infant mortality in the United States, accounting for approximately 8% of all infant deaths and claiming the lives of 3500 US infants each year (Centers for Disease Control and Prevention, 2016). It is the most common cause of postneonatal infant mortality, accounting for 40% to 50% of all deaths between 1 month and 1 year of age (Hauck, Carlin, Moon, et al., 2020). Since 1994, the incidence of SIDS in the United States has steadily decreased due to the Back to Sleep campaign (now called Safe to Sleep).[b] Despite dramatic decreases in SIDS rates, African American, American Indian, and Alaskan Native infants are disproportionately affected by higher rates than the rest of the population. According to the Centers for Disease Control and Prevention (2016), between 2010 and 2013

[b]Safe to Sleep materials may be ordered by contacting the National Institute of Child Health and Human Development Information Resource Center, Safe to Sleep, PO Box 3006, Rockville, MD 20847; 800-505-CRIB (2742); http://www.nichd.nih.gov/sts/.

TABLE 10.2 Epidemiology of Sudden Infant Death Syndrome

Factor	Occurrence
Incidence	3500 US infants each year (Centers for Disease Control and Prevention, 2016)
Peak age	2-3 months old; 95% occur by 6 months; preterm infants die of sudden infant death syndrome (SIDS) at mean age of 6 weeks later than mean age of death from SIDS for term infants
Sex	Higher percentage of boys affected
Time of death	During sleep
Time of year	Increased incidence in winter
Racial	Greater incidence in African American, American Indian, and Alaskan Native infants
Socioeconomic	Increased occurrence in lower socioeconomic class
Birth	Higher incidence in: Preterm infants, especially infants of extremely and very low birth weight Multiple births[a] Neonates with low Apgar scores Infants with central nervous system disturbances and respiratory disorders such as bronchopulmonary dysplasia Increasing birth order (subsequent siblings as opposed to firstborn child)
Health status	Infants with a recent history of illness; lower incidence in immunized infants
Sleep habits	Highest risk associated with prone position; use of soft bedding; overheating (thermal stress); co-sleeping with adult, especially on sofa or noninfant bed; higher incidence in co-sleeping with adult smoker Infants co-sleeping with adult at higher risk if younger than 11 weeks
Feeding habits	Lower incidence in breastfed infants
Pacifier	Lower incidence in infants put to sleep with pacifier
Siblings	May have greater incidence in siblings of SIDS victims
Maternal	Young age; cigarette smoking, especially during pregnancy; poor prenatal care; substance abuse (heroin, methadone, cocaine). A few studies have shown an increased risk in infants exposed to secondhand environmental tobacco smoke.

[a]Although a rare event, simultaneous death of twins from SIDS can occur.

Data from American Academy of Pediatrics, Task Force on Sudden Infant Death Syndrome. (2016). SIDS and other sleep-related infant deaths: Updated 2016 recommendations for a safe infant sleeping environment. *Pediatrics, 138*(5), 1–14.

SIDS rates for infants in these groups were more than twice those of non-Hispanic white infants. See Table 10.2.

Etiology

There are numerous theories regarding the etiology of SIDS, but the cause remains unknown. One hypothesis is that SIDS is related to brainstem abnormalities in the neurologic regulation of cardiorespiratory control. This maldevelopment affects arousal and physiologic responses to a life-threatening challenge during sleep (Hauck, Carlin, Moon, et al., 2020). Abnormalities include prolonged sleep apnea, increased frequency of brief inspiratory pauses, excessive periodic breathing, and impaired arousal responsiveness to increased carbon dioxide or decreased oxygen. However, *sleep apnea is not the cause of SIDS.* The vast majority of infants with apnea do not die, and only a minority of SIDS victims have documented apparent life-threatening events (ALTEs) (see the Apparent Life-Threatening Event section later in the chapter). Further, the findings of numerous studies indicate that no association exists between SIDS and any childhood vaccine.

A **genetic predisposition** to SIDS has been suspected as a potential cause. Differences in genes pertinent to immune system functioning and the development of the autonomic nervous system have been discovered in infants who died of SIDS compared with typical infants (Hauck, Carlin, Moon, et al., 2020). Several "triple-risk factor" models have been proposed to explain the etiology of SIDS. The proposed risk factors include an underlying infant vulnerability such as a brain abnormality, a critical incident in the fetal developmental period or in early neonatal life, and an exogenous stressor such as prone sleep positioning (Moon, 2016).

Risk Factors for Sudden Infant Death Syndrome

Maternal smoking during pregnancy is a major modifiable risk factor for SIDS. The incidence of SIDS is approximately three times greater among infants whose mothers smoked during pregnancy, and risk of death is progressively greater as daily cigarette use increases (Hauck, Carlin, Moon, et al., 2020). The effects of smoking by the father and other household members are more difficult to interpret because they are highly correlated with maternal smoking. There appears to be a small independent effect of paternal smoking, but data on other household members have been inconsistent. It is also difficult to assess the independent effect of infant exposure to environmental tobacco smoke because parental smoking behaviors during and after pregnancy are also highly correlated. However, an increased risk for SIDS has been found in infants exposed only to postnatal maternal environmental tobacco smoke (Hauck, Carlin, Moon, et al., 2020).

Co-sleeping, or an infant sharing a bed with an adult or older child on a noninfant bed, is associated with SIDS. Current studies and guidelines state that there is a significant increase in the risk of SIDS among infants who bed-shared compared with infants who slept alone and recommend that parents avoid bed-sharing (Das, Sankar, Agarwal, et al., 2014; Moon, 2016). The findings of a retrospective analysis of infant deaths showed a twofold increase of accidental suffocation or strangulation when infants were sleeping on a sofa compared to other locations. This is likely due to sharing the sleeping area with another person (Rechtman, Colvin, Blair, et al., 2014).

Prone sleeping may cause oropharyngeal obstruction or affect thermal balance or arousal state. Rebreathing of carbon dioxide by infants due to sleeping in the prone position is also a possible cause of SIDS. Infants sleeping prone and on soft bedding may be unable to move their heads to the side, thus increasing the risk of suffocation and lethal rebreathing. Therefore the side-lying position is no longer recommended for infants sleeping at home, daycare, or hospitals (unless medically indicated). Further, most preterm infants being discharged from the hospital should be placed in a supine sleeping position unless special factors predispose them to airway obstruction.

Another potential cause of SIDS has been a **prolonged Q-T interval** or other cardiac arrhythmias (Hauck, Carlin, Moon, et al., 2020). Recently cardiac ion channelopathies, which occur as a result of gene mutations and may result in lethal arrhythmias, have been proposed as a possible risk factor for SIDS (Hauck, Carlin, Moon, et al., 2020).

Soft bedding (waterbeds, sheepskins, beanbags, pillows, and quilts) should be avoided for infant sleeping surfaces. Bedding items, such as stuffed animals and toys, should be removed from the crib while the infant is asleep. Head covering by a blanket has also been found to be a risk factor for SIDS, thus supporting the recommendation to avoid extra bed linens and other items (Hauck, Carlin, Moon, et al., 2020). Further, crib bumper pads should not be used (American Academy of Pediatrics, 2016).

Protective Factors for Sudden Infant Death Syndrome

The findings of a meta-analysis indicate that SIDS rates may be reduced by up to 45% for infants who are breastfed and that this protective effect increases with exclusive breastfeeding (Hunt & Hauck, 2016). Pacifier use has also been associated with a lower risk of SIDS. Although it is uncertain if this is a direct effect of the pacifier itself or from associated infant or parental behavior, there is increasing evidence that pacifier use even with dislodgment can increase the arousability of infants during sleep. There has been some concern about recommending pacifiers for reducing the risk of SIDS out of fear this may interfere with breastfeeding. The findings of rigorous studies have failed to show an association between pacifier use and breastfeeding duration (Hauck, Carlin, Moon, et al., 2020).

The American Academy of Pediatrics, Task Force on Sudden Infant Death Syndrome (2016) recommends that *all infants* be placed to sleep in the **supine (on the back) position**. They also recommend that medically stable preterm infants and infants diagnosed with gastroesophageal reflux (GER) be placed in a supine sleep position unless they have a specific upper airway disorder that places them at greater risk of death than the risk of death from SIDS. Further, in the new Safe to Sleep recommendations, the American Academy of Pediatrics recommends that infants share a bedroom with parents but not the same sleeping surface, preferably until the infant is 1 year old but at least for the first 6 months. Room-sharing decreases the risk of SIDS by as much as 50% (American Academy of Pediatrics, Task Force on Sudden Infant Death Syndrome, 2016).

Since the 1994 Back to Sleep campaign began advocating for non-prone sleeping for infants, an increased incidence of positional plagiocephaly has been observed (see discussion later in the chapter). Therefore it is recommended that an infant's head position be alternated during sleep time to prevent plagiocephaly. Infants should also be placed prone in "tummy time" during awake periods for 10 to 15 minutes, three times a day, to prevent positional plagiocephaly and to encourage development of upper shoulder girdle strength (Hauck, Carlin, Moon, et al., 2020). Updated childhood immunization status has also been shown to be protective against SIDS.

Although the cause of SIDS is unknown, autopsies reveal consistent pathologic findings, such as pulmonary edema and intrathoracic hemorrhages that confirm the diagnosis. Consequently, autopsies should be performed on all infants suspected of dying of SIDS, and findings should be shared with the parents as soon as possible after the death. Postmortem findings in SIDS and accidental suffocation or intentional suffocation, such as in Munchausen syndrome by proxy (see Chapter 13, Child Maltreatment), are practically the same. Individuals with less experience and training in performing autopsies, such as coroners instead of medical examiners, may not correctly identify some deaths as SIDS. Therefore mortality statistics can vary in different regions.

Infant Risk Factors

Certain groups of infants are at increased risk for SIDS:

- Low birth weight or preterm birth (<37 weeks)
- Low Apgar scores
- Recent viral illness
- Siblings of two or more SIDS victims
- Male gender
- Infants of American Indian or African American ethnicity

No diagnostic tests exist to predict which infants, including those in the above-listed groups, will die of SIDS. The next-born siblings of firstborn infants who died of any noninfectious natural cause are at significantly increased risk for infant death from the same cause, including SIDS. The increased risk for recurrent SIDS in families is consistent with genetic risk factors interacting with environmental risk factors (Hauck, Carlin, Moon, et al., 2020). Home monitoring is not recommended for this group of children, but it is often used by practitioners and may even be requested by parents. There is no evidence that home apnea monitoring prevents SIDS (Hauck, Carlin, Moon, et al., 2020).

Nursing Care Management

Nurses have a vital role in preventing SIDS by educating families about the risk of prone sleeping in infants from birth to 6 months of age. This education should include the use of appropriate bedding surfaces, the association between SIDS and maternal smoking, and the dangers of co-sleeping on noninfant surfaces with adults or other children. In addition, nurses have an important role in modeling behaviors for parents that decrease the risk of SIDS, such as placing infants in a supine sleeping position while in the hospital. Unfortunately, research shows that some nurses still place healthy infants in a side-lying position in the hospital due to a belief in safety concerns if the infant is placed supine (Patton, Stiltner, Wright, et al., 2015). However, research shows that establishing current, evidence-based hospital policies, as well as providing education for both nurses and parents, can change practice (Naugler & DiCarlo, 2018).

Role modeling safe sleep practices and providing education to parents is imperative before hospital discharge because limited opportunities exist for parents to receive information about caring for their infant (Naugler & DiCarlo, 2018). Nurses must be proactive in further decreasing the incidence of SIDS through providing education during postpartum discharge planning, newborn discharge teaching, follow-up home visits, well-baby clinic visits, and immunization visits. Further, nurses must continue to take every opportunity to advocate for infants by providing information for parents and caretakers about the modifiable risk factors for SIDS that can be implemented to prevent its occurrence across all sectors of the population.

Care of the Family of a Sudden Infant Death Syndrome Infant

Loss of a child from SIDS presents several crises for the infant's parents. In addition to grief and mourning the death of their child, the parents must face a tragedy that was sudden, unexpected, and unexplained. This discussion focuses primarily on the objectives of care for families experiencing SIDS rather than on the process of grief and mourning, which is explored in Chapter 17.

The first people to arrive at the scene may be the police and emergency medical service personnel. They should handle the situation by (1) asking few questions; (2) giving no indication of wrongdoing, abuse, or neglect; (3) making sensitive judgments concerning any resuscitation efforts for the child; and (4) comforting the family members as much as possible. A compassionate, sensitive approach to the family may help minimize some of the overwhelming guilt and anguish that commonly follow this type of loss.

The medical examiner or coroner may go to the home or place of death and make the death pronouncement. Until then, the sleep environment should remain as it was when the infant was initially found. If the infant is not pronounced dead at the scene, he or she may be transported to the emergency department to be pronounced dead by a physician. Usually there is no attempt at resuscitation in the emergency department. While they are in the emergency department, the parents should be asked only factual questions, such as when they found the infant, how he or she looked, and whom they called for help. The nurse avoids any remarks that may suggest responsibility, such as "Why didn't you go in earlier?" or "Didn't you hear the infant cry out?" It is the coroner's responsibility to document findings at the scene rather than have parents recount the experience in the emergency department. Parents may also express feelings of guilt about administering cardiopulmonary resuscitation (CPR) correctly or the timing of CPR in relation to finding the infant.

The physician should initiate the discussion of an autopsy, often with the nurse being present to support the family. The physician or medical examiner, depending on the circumstances, should emphasize that a diagnosis cannot be confirmed until the postmortem examination is completed. Instructions about the autopsy and funeral arrangements may need to be repeated or put in writing. If the mother was breastfeeding, she will need information about abrupt discontinuation of lactation. The nurse or physician should contact the primary care practitioner for the infant and the mother to avoid any miscommunications or telephone calls later inquiring about the child's health status.

Parents experiencing perinatal death perceive health care workers' responses as having a significant impact on their grieving process. A family-centered approach that involves the sociocultural context and unique needs of the family is essential for perinatal bereavement care (Flenady, Boyle, Koopmans, et al., 2014). Health care workers require adequate training and support in order to deliver appropriate care and prevent burnout (Flenady et al., 2014).

An important aspect of compassionate care for parents is allowing them to say goodbye to their child. These are the parents' last moments with their child, and they should be as quiet, meaningful, peaceful, and undisturbed as possible. Encourage parents to hold their infant before leaving the emergency department. Because the parents will be leaving the hospital without their infant, it may be helpful to accompany them to the car or arrange for someone to take them home. A debriefing session may help health care workers who cared for the family to cope with troubling emotions.

When the parents return home, a competent, qualified professional should visit them as soon after the death as possible. They should receive printed material that contains excellent information about SIDS (available from several national organizations[c]). During the initial visit, help the parents gain an intellectual understanding of the condition. The nursing objectives are to assess what the parents have been told about SIDS; what they think happened; and how they explained this to the infant's siblings, family members, and friends. One question that the nurse will never be able to answer and therefore should not attempt to is, "Why did this happen to our baby?" or "Who is responsible for this tragedy?" These and other questions may linger in the parents' minds for months or even years.

When the unexpected death of a child occurs, it is common for one parent to blame the other. Parents may also experience guilt over the child's death. For example, they may feel that if they had checked on the child earlier, he or she might still be alive. It is important that the nurse assist parents in working through these feelings to prevent marital disruption in addition to the loss of the loved child.

Some parents are able to discuss their feelings openly, and the nurse should support this coping skill. However, others may be reluctant to express their grief, and the nurse can encourage the expression of emotions by asking about crying and feeling sad, angry, or guilty. During their interaction, the nurse can help the parents to explore their typical coping strategies and, if these are ineffectual, to investigate new approaches. For example, one parent may refrain from discussing the death for fear of upsetting the other parent, but each may need to hear how the other feels.

Ideally, the number of visits and plans for subsequent intervention need to be flexible. Parents facing the question of having a subsequent child will need support. Both the birth of a subsequent child and the survival of that child, especially past the age of death of the previous child, are important transitional stages for parents.

POSITIONAL PLAGIOCEPHALY

Since the Back to Sleep campaign that advocated nonprone sleeping for infants to prevent SIDS began in 1994, an increase in the incidence of positional plagiocephaly has been reported (Myers et al., 2020). Approximately 20% of infants have this type of skull deformity that is most prevalent between 2 and 4 months of age (van Wijk, van Vlimmeren, Groothuis-Oudshoorn, et al., 2014). The term **plagiocephaly** connotes an oblique or asymmetric head. Positional plagiocephaly, deformational plagiocephaly, or nonsynostotic plagiocephaly implies an acquired skull deformity that occurs as a result of cranial molding during infancy, usually as a result of lying in the supine position (van Wijk et al., 2014). Because infants' sutures are not yet fused, the skull is pliable, so when infants are placed on their backs to sleep, the posterior occiput flattens over time (Fig. 10.4A).

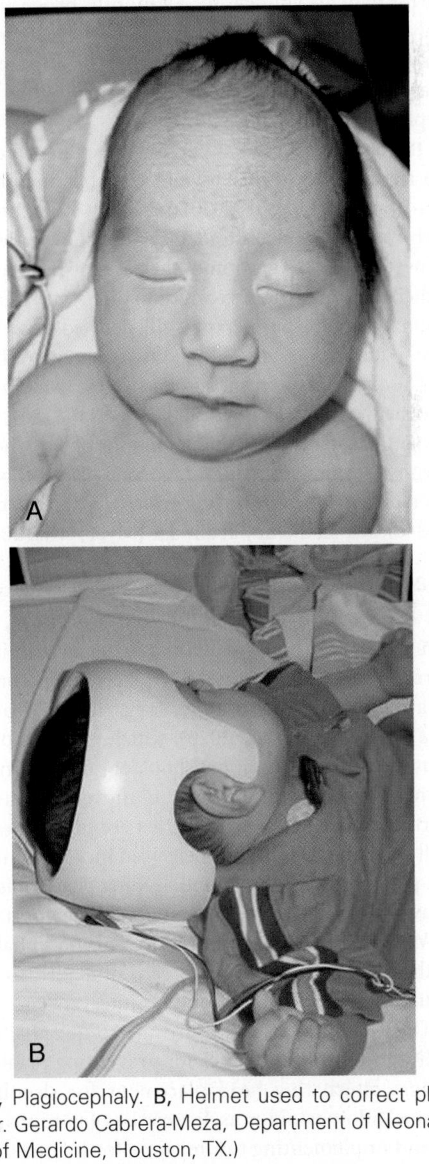

Fig. 10.4 A, Plagiocephaly. B, Helmet used to correct plagiocephaly. (Courtesy Dr. Gerardo Cabrera-Meza, Department of Neonatology, Baylor College of Medicine, Houston, TX.)

[c]American SIDS Institute, 528 Ravens Way, Naples, FL 34110; 239-431-5425; http://www.sids.org; First Candle, 1314 Bedford Ave., Suite 210, Baltimore, MD 21208; 800-221-7437; http://www.firstcandle.org; National Sudden and Unexpected Infant/Child Death and Pregnancy Loss Resource Center, Georgetown University, Box 571272, Washington, DC 20057-1272, 866-866-7437, 202-687-7466, http://sidscenter.org.

A typical bald spot develops over the area, which is usually transient. Prolonged pressure on one side of the skull can result in that side becoming misshapen. Mild facial asymmetry may also develop. The sternocleidomastoid muscle may tighten on the preferential side, resulting in a condition called torticollis. Congenital or acquired torticollis may also cause plagiocephaly. Other causes of deformational plagiocephaly include certain craniofacial syndromes. This discussion focuses only on positional plagiocephaly (PP) caused by supine sleeping position.

Therapeutic Management

Prevention of PP should begin shortly after birth by placing the infant to sleep supine and alternating the infant's head position nightly, avoiding prolonged placement in car safety seats and swings, and using prone positioning or "tummy time" for approximately 10 to 15 minutes, three times per day, while the infant is awake (Myers et al., 2020).

The watch and wait method of treatment for torticollis and plagiocephaly is not recommended (Myers et al., 2020). Repositioning and physical therapy (RPPT), which includes providing counseling and teaching for parents as to positional changes and tummy time for their child, is recommended. A referral to physical therapy may be needed in the case of congenital torticollis. RPPT is the optimal treatment choice for patients younger than 4 months of age who have mild to moderately severe PP. The earliest types of behavioral modifications can be as simple as increasing tummy time or repositioning the infant's crib such that everything interesting in the room is on the side opposite the plagiocephaly (Myers et al., 2020).

Molding therapy (helmet therapy) is the use of an orthotic helmet to promote the resolution of cranial asymmetry while the infant's head is still rapidly growing (Myers et al., 2020) (see Fig. 10.4B). Orthotic helmets do not actively mold the skull; instead, they protect the areas that are flattened and allow the child to "grow into" the flat spots. Studies have shown that helmet therapy alone achieves correction three times faster and better than repositioning alone. This therapy is still debated, however, due to its expense, time requirements, and side effects (irritation, rashes, and pressure sores). The findings of recent studies suggest that combined treatment with helmet therapy and physical therapy is the most beneficial for the management of infants older than 4 months of age who are severely affected or with worsening of mild or moderate plagiocephaly who have been trialed on physical therapy. Infants with severe plagiocephaly should be considered for helmet therapy at any age (Myers et al., 2020).

Nursing Care Management

Minor skull deformation is not considered significant, but parents should learn to prevent plagiocephaly by altering the infant's head position during sleep. Infants should be placed prone on a firm surface during awake time (tummy time) for at least 10 to 15 minutes, three times a day (Myers et al., 2020), which prevents plagiocephaly and facilitates development of upper shoulder girdle strength. The latter helps in the progressive development of movements such as rolling over and starting to rise up on all fours that are precursors to crawling and eventually walking. Despite the perceived increase in the incidence of positional plagiocephaly, the supine sleeping position is still recommended because it has led to a significant decrease in loss of infant lives from SIDS. When a nurse or parent notices plagiocephaly, a consultation with the primary practitioner is recommended to evaluate the head shape and ascertain the need for early intervention.

Nurses in well-child care settings are in a unique position to assess parents' ability to follow guidelines for preventing plagiocephaly by observing them alternating head placement for sleeping, demonstrating sternocleidomastoid muscle exercises (as appropriate to the condition), and implementing tummy time for infants during awake periods. Most important, nurses should continue to encourage parents to place the infant in a supine sleep position despite the development of plagiocephaly. Nurses can also assist parents in the proper use of a skull-molding helmet and reassure them of the high rate of success with the helmet. Allowing parents to verbalize concerns and feelings related to the health status of their child, as well as the provision of current best practice, is an important nursing function.

APPARENT LIFE-THREATENING EVENT

An **apparent life-threatening event (ALTE)**, formerly referred to as an *aborted SIDS death* or a *near-miss SIDS*, generally refers to an event that is sudden and frightening to the observer in which the infant exhibits a combination of apnea; change in color (e.g., pallor, cyanosis, redness); change in muscle tone (usually hypotonia); and choking, gagging, or coughing that usually involves a significant intervention such as CPR provided by the caregiver who witnesses the event (Carolan, 2016). The definition of ALTE may include apnea, but ALTE may occur without apnea (Carolan, 2016). In 2016 the American Academy of Pediatrics released a clinical practice guideline that recommended the replacement of the term *ALTE* with a new term, *brief resolved unexplained event (BRUE)*. The American Academy of Pediatrics defines BRUE as an event observed in infants younger than 1 year of age during which an observer reports a sudden, brief (less than 1 minute), but then resolved episode that includes at least one of the following: (1) cyanosis or pallor; (2) absent, decreased, or irregular breathing; (3) marked change in muscle tone (hypertonia or hypotonia); or (4) altered responsiveness. Per the guidelines, a BRUE can be diagnosed only when there is no explanation for a qualifying event after completion of a through history and physical examination (Carolan, 2016).

It is erroneous to characterize ALTE as a near-miss SIDS incident. A history of an unexplained ALTE occurs in 5% to 9% of SIDS victims, and the risk of SIDS appears to be higher with two or more unexplained events, but no definite incidence rates are available. Compared with healthy control infants, the risk for SIDS may be as much as three to five times greater in infants having experienced an ALTE.

Results from the Collaborative Home Infant Monitoring Evaluation (CHIME) study showed that apnea and bradycardia occurred at conventional and extreme alarm thresholds in all groups of infants studied: siblings of SIDS infants, infants with ALTEs, symptomatic (of apnea and bradycardia) and asymptomatic preterm infants weighing less than 1750 g (3.8 pounds) at birth, and healthy term infants. Many infants experience apnea and bradycardia in each of these groups yet do not die (Hauck, Carlin, Moon, et al., 2020).

Diagnostic Evaluation

An essential component of the diagnostic process includes a detailed description of the event, including who witnessed it, where the infant was during the event, and what, if any, activities were involved (e.g., during or after a feeding, riding in a car seat restraint, presence of siblings or any minor children, what clothing the infant was wearing). In addition, a prenatal and postnatal history must be obtained. A short period of observation in the emergency department may be appropriate to monitor the infant's respiratory pattern and response to feeding. Further, a careful evaluation of late-preterm and preterm infants in the car seat restraint is essential. Upper airway occlusion and subsequent apnea and cyanosis may occur if the infant is not positioned properly. Reported diagnoses in infants with ALTE include (1) neurologic events such as seizures (30% of cases seen); (2) GI problems, including GER (50%); (3) respiratory conditions (20%); (4) cardiac conditions (5%); (5) metabolic or endocrine conditions (<5%); or (6) other problems such as child abuse (Aminiahidashti, 2015).

If an underlying diagnosis cannot be established, home monitoring may be recommended. The most commonly used monitoring is continuous recording of cardiorespiratory patterns (cardiopneumogram or pneumocardiogram). Four-channel pneumocardiograms (or multichannel pneumograms) monitor heart rate, respirations (chest impedance), nasal airflow, and oxygen saturation. A more sophisticated test, polysomnography (sleep study), also records brain waves, eye and body movements, esophageal manometry, and end-tidal carbon dioxide measurements. However, none of these tests can predict risk. Some children with normal results may still have subsequent apneic episodes.

Therapeutic Management

The treatment of an infant with an ALTE depends on the underlying condition. Several diagnostic tests may be carried out to determine the cause of the ALTE; however, a cause may not be determined in up to 50% of cases. Further, testing for seizures, GER, or sepsis is not recommended unless signs were present on the physical examination and history. However, testing for a urinary tract infection is recommended (Aminiahidashti, 2015).

Nursing Care Management

The diagnosis of an ALTE causes great anxiety and concern in parents, and the institution of home monitoring presents additional physical and emotional burdens. Parents of infants on home apnea monitors report experiencing emotional distress, especially depression and hostility, during the first few weeks after hospital discharge. For parents of a SIDS victim who have a new infant on home apnea monitoring, the anxiety is compounded by the uncertainty of the future of the living child and grief for the lost child. Home apnea monitoring may offer some predictability and control over the current child's survival through the period of uncertainty.

If home monitoring is required, the nurse can be a major source of support to the family in terms of education about the equipment, education regarding observation of the infant's status, and instructions regarding immediate intervention during apneic episodes, including CPR. To help the family cope with the numerous procedures they must learn, adequate preparation before discharge and written instructions are essential. In the first few weeks after discharge, parents may benefit from having a practitioner readily available to answer questions regarding false alarms and for other technical assistance.

Several types of home monitors are available and are set up by either a home monitor equipment company or home health staff. Nurses, especially those involved in the care at home, must become familiar with the equipment, including its advantages and disadvantages. Safety is a major concern because monitors can cause electrical burns and electrocution. The following precautions are recommended:

- Remove leads from infant when not attached to the monitor.
- Unplug the power cord from the electrical outlet when the cord is not plugged into the monitor.
- Use safety covers on electrical outlets to discourage children from inserting objects into sockets.

Additional home use instructions should focus on troubleshooting the monitor alarms. Parents should be encouraged to always look at the infant first if an alarm goes off and ensure that the infant is breathing, then determine the cause of the alarm. Parents also need information about traveling or running errands with an infant on an apnea monitor, what to do in case of power failure, and whom to contact if the monitor alarm goes off continuously but the infant appears well. Siblings should be supervised when near the infant and taught that the monitor is not a toy. Other safety practices include informing local utility and rescue squads (fire and/or emergency services) of the home monitoring in case of an emergency, especially if the family lives in a remote, rural area. Telephone numbers for these services should be posted in the home or set up as speed dial on certain phones if a universal 911 system is not available. Instructions for infant CPR should also be posted in a central location of the house. Parents are encouraged to tell visitors and other family members about the location of these instructions. If a cellular phone is the main house phone, make sure it stays in a central location for all family members to access in an emergency.

! NURSING ALERT

If the infant is apneic, gently stimulate the trunk by patting or rubbing it. Call loudly for help even if alone. If the infant is prone, turn to the supine position and flick the heels of the feet. If there is still no response, immediately begin cardiopulmonary respiration (CPR) starting with chest compressions. After approximately 2 minutes of CPR, activate the emergency medical service—"Call 911"—and then resume CPR until emergency responders arrive or the infant starts breathing. Never vigorously shake the child. No more than 10 to 15 seconds is spent on stimulation before implementing CPR (American Heart Association, 2015).

Caregivers need detailed information regarding proper attachment of the electrodes to the infant's chest with impedance monitors that detect chest movement. The electrodes are placed in the midaxillary line at a space one or two fingerbreadths below the nipple. For home use, electrodes attached to a belt that is placed around the child's trunk are preferred (Fig. 10.5). The belt is positioned so that the electrodes contact the skin in the same area. Monitors may have memory chips that allow for event recording, which can be an effective tool in evaluating the use of the monitor, events immediately before and after the ALTE, and reported frequency of alarms. Monitors are effective only if they are used. They do not prevent death but alert the caregiver to the ALTE in time to intervene. The need to use the monitor and to respond appropriately to alarms must be stressed. Noncompliance can result in the infant's death.

Many of the stresses observed during the home monitoring period are characteristic of families with chronically ill children. The child with an apnea or cardiorespiratory monitor may have additional health care needs such as a gastrostomy, tracheostomy, and multiple medications or treatments that exacerbate the parents' stress. Parents report increased stress, including concern for the child's survival, fear

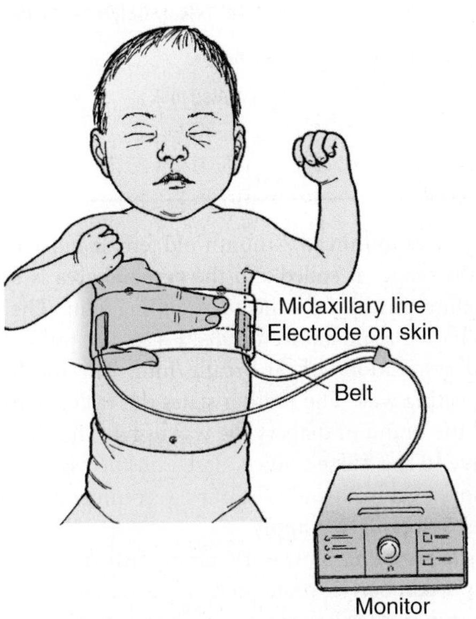

Fig. 10.5 Electrode placement for apnea monitoring. In small infants, one fingerbreadth may be used.

of incompetence in assuming home responsibility, inadequate respite care, lack of time for other children and spouse, social isolation from friends and extended family, constant work, and fatigue. To deal with these potential stressors, nurses need to use the same interventions as those discussed for children with chronic illness and be aware of the need for referral when difficulties are suspected.

To lessen the continuous responsibility of monitoring, other family members, such as grandparents and other immediate family members, should be taught how to assess the infant for responsiveness, manipulate the equipment, read and interpret the signals, and administer CPR (if needed). They are encouraged to stay with the infant for regular periods to allow the parents respite. Support groups of other families who have successfully completed monitoring can also be of benefit. Because reliable babysitters are difficult to locate, support group members and nursing students may be potential sources of qualified caregivers.

CLINICAL JUDGMENT AND NEXT-GENERATION NCLEX® EXAMINATION-STYLE QUESTIONS

1. An 11-month-old infant being seen in the emergency department is experiencing difficulty breathing. The mother states the 5-year-old brother had given the infant peanuts while riding in the back of the car without the mother knowing it. On examination the nurse notices the symptoms listed below. Which of these findings is an indication of a possible anaphylactic reaction? **Select all that apply.**
   A. Wheezing
   B. Flushing
   C. Headache
   D. Trouble breathing
   E. Urticaria
   F. Temperature of 98.2 F (36.8 C)
   G. Decreased bowel signs

2. A 9-month-old full-term infant is being seen in the clinic and the mother states she thinks the infant has cow's milk allergy. She thinks this because her mother told her that she had it when she was an infant. **Choose the most likely options for the information missing from the statements below by selecting from the list of options provided.**
   The nurse is aware that common signs and symptoms of cow's milk allergy involving the gastrointestinal track include ____1____.
   An infant with a cow's milk allergy is placed on ____2____ to prevent further problems.

Options for 1	Options for 2
diarrhea	goat's milk
eczema	soy milk or a hydrolyzed formula
sneezing	whole milk
urticaria	evaporated milk
fever	milk
swelling	eggs

3. The nurse is examining a 7-month-old female full-term infant and notices the diaper is soiled and the perianal area is extremely red with satellite pustules on the surrounding skin. The child's vital signs include a temperature of 98.2 F (26. C), pulse of 100 beats/min and respirations of 30 breaths/min. The mother states the infant is eating well. The mother states the rash occurred after she changed the brand of diapers she was using. The child is alert and responsive to the nurse's voice. Based on the assessment findings, what priority actions would the nurse recommend to the mother at this time? **Select all that apply.**
   A. Using a hair dryer blow warm air on rash area
   B. Apply a skin barrier paste such as zinc oxide.
   C. Keep skin surface irritants such as urine and stool off skin.
   D. Expose skin to air.
   E. Use only cloth diapers.
   F. Educate the mother on how to treat the rash

4. The mother of a 2-month-old male who was premature is extremely concerned about Sudden Infant Death Syndrome (SIDS). She tells the nurse she has read that preterm infants with lower Apgar scores who have older siblings are more at risk. She also states that she believes that keeping the infant in bed with her allows her to watch him more closely. She states she puts him on his side and her waterbed allows him to easily fall asleep. **Use an X for the health teaching below that is Indicated (appropriate or necessary), Contraindicated (could be harmful), or Non-Essential (makes no difference or not necessary).**

Nursing Action: Health Teaching	Indicated	Contraindicated	Non-Essential
Reassure the mother that she is correct in keeping the infant on his side.			
Discuss with the mother that keeping the infant in bed with her can actually increase the risk of SIDS.			
Advise the mother that the waterbed is a type of "soft bedding" and the infant should not sleep on the waterbed.			
Discuss with the mother that a warm bath before bedtime can help minimize risk.			
Advise the mother to keep stuffed animals and toys in the crib to provide comfort.			

REFERENCES

Ahluwalia, N., Herrick, K. A., Rossen, L. M., et al. (2016). Usual nutrient intakes of US infants and toddlers generally meet or exceed Dietary Reference Intakes: Findings from NHANES 2009-2010. *The American Journal of Clinical Nutrition, 104*, 1167–1174.

Akhnikh, S., Engelberts, A. C., van Sleuwen, B. E., et al. (2014). The excessively crying infant: Etiology and treatment. *Pediatric Annals, 43*(4), e69–e75.

American Academy of Pediatrics. (2016). *American Academy of Pediatrics announces new safe sleep recommendations to protect against SIDS, sleep-related infant deaths.* Retrieved from https://www.aap.org/en-us/about-the-aap/aap-press-room/pages/american-academy-of-pediatrics-announces-new-safe-sleep-recommendations-to-protect-against-sids.aspx.

American Academy of Pediatrics. (2017). Fruit juice in infants, children, and adolescents: Current recommendations. *Pediatrics, 139*(6), 1–10.

American Academy of Pediatrics, Task Force on Sudden Infant Death Syndrome. (2016). SIDS and other sleep-related infant deaths: Updated 2016 recommendations for a safe infant sleeping environment. *Pediatrics, 138*(5), 1–14.

American College of Allergy, Asthma and Immunology. (2014). *Types of allergies, food allergies.* Retrieved from http://acaai.org/allergies/types/food-allergy.

American Heart Association. (2015). *Highlight of the 2015 American Heart Association guidelines update for CPR and ECC.* Retrieved from http://eccguidelines.heart.org/wp-content/uploads/2015/10/2015-AHA-Guidelines-Highlights-English.pdf.

Aminiahidashti, H. (2015). Infantile apparent life-threatening events, an educational review. *Emergency, 3*(1), 8–15.

Antonucci, R., Locci, C., Clemente, M. G., et al. (2018). Vitamin D deficiency in childhood: Old lessons and current challenges. *Journal of Pediatric Endocrinology and Metabolism, 31*(3), 247–260.

Ashworth, A. (2020). Nutrition, food security, and health. In R. M. Kliegman, J. W. St. Geme, N. J. Blum, et al. (Eds.), *Nelson textbook of pediatrics* (21st ed.). Philadelphia: Elsevier.

Bailey, R. L., Catellier, D. J., Jun, S., et al. (2018). Total usual nutrient intakes of US children (Under 48 months): Findings from the Feeding Infants and Toddlers Study (FITS) 2016. *The Journal of Nutrition, 148*(3), 1557s–1566s.

Becker, P., Carney, L. N., Corkins, M. R., et al. (2015). Consensus statement of the Academy of Nutrition and Dietetics/American Society for Parenteral and Enteral Nutrition: Indicators recommended for the identification and documentation of pediatric malnutrition (undernutrition). *Nutrition in Clinical Practice, 30*(1), 147–161.

Bello, S., Meremikwu, M. M., Ejemot-Nwadiaro, R. I., et al. (2014). Routine vitamin A supplementation for the prevention of blindness due to measles infection in children. In *The Cochrane Database of Systematic Reviews,* Retrieved from http://onlinelibrary.wiley.com/doi/10.1002/14651858.CD007719.pub3/full.

Bello, S., Meremikwu, M. M., Ejemot-Nwadiaro, R. I., et al. (2016). Vitamin A for preventing blindness in children with measles. In *The Cochrane Database of Systematic Reviews,* Retrieved from http://www.cochrane.org/CD007719/ARI_vitamin-preventing-blindness-children-measles.

Bock, A. S., & Sampson, H. A. (2016). Evaluation of food allergy. In D. Y. Leung, S. J. Szefler, F. A. Bonilla, et al. (Eds.), *Pediatric allergy: Principles and practice* (3rd ed.). New York: Elsevier.

Bousselamti, A., Hasbaoui, B. E., Echahdi, H., et al. (2018). Psychomotor regression due to vitamin B12 deficiency. *PanAfrican Medical Journal, 30*, 1–6.

Boyce, J. A., Assa'ad, A., Burks, A. W., et al. (2010). Guideline for the diagnosis and management of food allergy in the United States: Summary of the NIAID-sponsored expert panel report. *Journal of Allergy and Clinical Immunology, 126*(6), 1005–1118.

Boyd, C., & Moondambail, A. (2016). Severe hypercalcemia in a child secondary to use of alternative therapies. *BMJ Case Reports 2016.*

Brambilla, A., Pizza, C., & Lasagni, D. (2018). Pediatric scurvy: When contemporary eating habits bring back the past. *Frontiers in Pediatrics, 6*(126), 1–4.

Camilleri, M., Park, S. Y., Scarpato, E., et al. (2017). Exploring hypotheses and rationale for causes of infantile colic. *Neurogastroenterology & Motility, 29*(2), 1–11.

Carolan, P. L. (2016). Brief resolved unexplained events (apparent life-threatening events). In M. L. Windle, & G. D. Sharma (Eds.), *Pediatric, general medicine,* Retrieved from http://emedicine.medscape.com/article/1418765-overview.

Carter, K. A., Hathaway, N. E., & Lettieri, C. F. (2014). Common sleep disorders in children. *American Family Physician, 89*(5), 368–377.

Centers for Disease Control and Prevention. (2016). *Sudden unexpected infant death and sudden infant death syndrome, data and statistics.* Retrieved from https://www.cdc.gov/sids/data.htm.

Chantry, C. J., Eglash, A., & Labbok, M. (2015). ABM position on breastfeeding – Revised 2015. *Breastfeeding Medicine: The Official Journal of the Academy of Breastfeeding Medicine, 10*(9), 407–411.

Das, R. R., Sankar, M. J., Agarwal, R., et al. (2014). Is "bed sharing" beneficial and safe during infancy? A systematic review. *International Journal of Pediatrics,* 1–16 *2014.*

Deshpande, P. G. (2015). Colic. In M. L. Windle, S. Guandalini, & C. Cuffari (Eds.), *Pediatrics: General medicine,* Retrieved from http://emedicine.medscape.com/article/927760-overview.

Dwyer, J. T. (2018). The Feeding Infants and Toddlers Study (FITS) 2016: Moving forward. *The Journal of Nutrition, 148*(3), 1575s–1580s.

Egan, M., & Sicherer, S. (2016). Doctor, my child is bullied: Food allergy management in schools. *Current Opinion in Allergy & Clinical Immunology, 16*(3), 291–296.

Esposito, S., & Lelii, M. (2015). Vitamin D and respiratory tract infections in childhood. *BMC Infectious Diseases, 16*, 487.

Fakhri, B., Hasanpoor-Azghady, S. B., Farahani, L. A., et al. (2019). The relationship between social support and perceived stress in the mothers of infants with colic. *Iranian Journal of Pediatrics, 29*(1), 1–6.

Feifer, A., & Walker-Descartes, I. (2017). Abuse or neglect as cause for disability. *International Journal of Child Health and Human Development, 10*(3), 253–265.

Flenady, V., Boyle, F., Koopmans, L., et al. (2014). Meeting the needs of parents after a stillbirth or neonatal death. *BJOG: An International Journal of Obstetrics and Gynaecology, 121*(Suppl. 4), 137–140.

Furman, L. (2015). Maternal vitamin D supplementation for breastfeeding infants: Will it work? *Pediatrics, 136*(4), 763–764.

Grey, K., & Maquiness, S. (2016). Atopic dermatitis: Update for pediatricians. *Pediatric Annals, 45*(8), e280–e286.

Groetch, M., & Sampson, H. A. (2016). Management of food allergy. In D. Y. Lueng, S. J. Szefler, F. A. Bonilla, et al. (Eds.), *Pediatric allergy principles and practice* (3rd ed.). Philadelphia: Elsevier.

Holm, J. G., Agner, T., Clausen, M. L., et al. (2016). Quality of life and disease severity in patients with atopic dermatitis. *Journal of the European Academy of Dermatology and Venereology, 30*(1), 1760–1767.

Hauck, F. R., Carlin, R. F., Moon, R. Y., et al. (2020). Sudden infant death syndrome. In R. M. Kliegman, J. W. St. Geme, N. J. Blum, et al. (Eds.), *Nelson textbook of pediatrics* (21st ed.). Philadelphia: Elsevier.

Jones, K. D., & Berkley, J. A. (2014). Severe acute malnutrition and infection. *Paediatrics and International Child Health, 34*(Suppl. 1), S1–S29.

Keet, C., & Wang, J. (2014). Acute reactions and anaphylaxis. In S. H. Sicherer (Ed.), *Food allergy practical diagnosis and management* (1st ed.). Florida: CRC Press.

Kleinman, R. E., & Greer, R. F. (Eds.). (2014). *Pediatric nutrition* (7th ed.). Elk Grove Village, IL: American Academy of Pediatrics.

Mandese, V., Marotti, F., Bedetti, L., et al. (2016). Effects of nutritional intake on disease severity in children with sickle cell disease. *Nutrition Journal, 15*(1), 1–6.

Misra, M. (2018). Vitamin D insufficiency and deficiency in children and adolescents. In K. J. Motil, & M. K. Drezner (Eds.), *UpToDate.* Retrieved from https://www.uptodate.com/contents/vitamin-d-insufficiency-and-deficiency-in-children-and-adolescents.

Mishra, K., Kumar, P., Basu, S., et al. (2014). Risk factors for severe acute malnutrition in children below 5 y of age in India: A case-control study. *Indian Journal of Pediatrics, 81*(8), 762–765.

Moon, R. Y. (2016). SIDS and other sleep-related infant deaths: evidence base for the 2016 updated recommendations for a safe sleeping environment. *Pediatrics, 138*(5), 1–34.

Moore, C. E., & Liu, Y. (2016). Low serum 25-hydroxyvitamin D concentrations are associated with total adiposity of children in the United States: National Health and Examination Survey 2005 to 2006. *Nutrition Research, 36*(1), 72–79.

Muscat, T., Obst, P., Cockshaw, W., et al. (2014). Beliefs about infant regulation, early infant behaviors and maternal postnatal depressive symptoms. *Birth, 41*(2), 206–213.

Myers, R. P., Fahrenkopf, M. P., Adams, N. S., Mann, R. J., et al. (2020). Deformational plagiocephaly. In R. M. Kliegman, J. W. St. Geme, N. J. Blum, et al. (Eds.), *Nelson textbook of pediatrics* (21st ed.). Philadelphia: Elsevier.

National Institutes of Health Office of Dietary Supplement. (2016). *Strengthening knowledge and understanding of dietary supplements.* Retrieved from https://ods.od.nih.gov/factsheets/VitaminD-Consumer/.

Naugler, M. R., & DiCarlo, K. (2018). Barriers to and interventions that increase nurses' and parents' compliance with safe sleep recommendations for preterm infants. *Nursing for Women's Health, 22*(1), 24–39.

Nguyen, T. A., Leonard, S. A., & Eichenfield, L. F. (2015). An update on pediatric atopic dermatitis and food allergies. *The Journal of Pediatrics, 167*(3), 752–756.

Nowak-Węgrzyn, A., Sampson, H. A., & Sicherer, S. H. (2020). Food allergy and adverse reactions to foods. I. In R. M. Kliegman, J. W. St. Geme, N. J. Blum, et al. (Eds.), *Nelson textbook of pediatrics* (21st ed.). Philadelphia: Elsevier.

Nowak-Węgrzyn, A. (2018). Investigational therapies for food allergy: Oral immunotherapy. In S. H. Sicherer, & E. TePass (Eds.), *UpToDate*.Retrieved from https://www.uptodate.com/contents/investigational-therapies-for-food-allergy-oral-immunotherapy.

Page, S. S., Weston, S., & Loh, R. (2016). Atopic dermatitis in children. *Australian Family Physician, 45*(5), 293–296.

Patton, C., Stiltner, D., Wright, K. B., et al. (2015). Do nurses provide a safe sleep environment for infants in the hospital setting? An integrative review. *Clinical Issues in Neonatal Care, 15*(1), 8–22.

Pawlak, R., Lester, S. E., & Babatunde, T. (2014). The prevalence of cobalamin deficiency among vegetarians assessed by serum vitamin B12: A review of the literature. *European Journal of Clinical Nutrition, 68*, 541–548.

Perry, M., Page, N., Manthey, D. E., et al. (2018). Scurvy: Dietary discretion in a developed country. *Clinical Practice and Cases in Emergency Medicine, 2*(2), 147–150.

Rechtman, L. R., Colvin, J. D., Blair, P. S., et al. (2014). Sofas and infant mortality. *Pediatrics, 134*(5), e1293–e1300.

Rocheleau, G. ,C., & Rocheleau, B. N. (2019). The mark of a food allergy label: School accommodation policy and bullying. *Journal of School Violence.* https://doi.org/10.1080/15388220.2019.1566072.

Romano, C., Hartman, C., Privitera, C., et al. (2015). Current topics in the diagnosis and management of the pediatric non organic feeding disorders (NOFEDs). *Clinical Nutrition, 34*(2), 195–200.

Sauer, K., Patten, E., Roberts, K., et al. (2018). Management of food allergies in schools. *Journal of Child Nutrition and Management, 42*(2), 1–9.

Savino, F., Ceratto, S., Poggi, E., et al. (2015). Preventive effects of oral probiotic on infantile colic: A prospective, randomized blinded, controlled trial using Lactobacillus reuteri DSM 17938. *Beneficial Microbes, 6*(3), 245–251.

Sirotnak, A. P., & Chiesa, A. (2016). Failure to thrive. In M. L. Windle, & C. Pataki (Eds.), *Pediatrics: Developmental and behavioral articles* Retrieved from http://emedicine.medscape.com/article/915575-overview.

Sung, V., D'Amico, F., Cabana, M. D., et al. (2018). *Lactobacillus reuteri* to treat infant colic: A meta-analysis. *Pediatrics, 141*(1), 1–12.

Talarico, V., Barreca, M., Galiano, R., et al. (2016). Vitamin D and risk for vitamin A intoxication in an 18-month-old boy. *Case Reports in Pediatrics, 2016* (article id 1395718), 1–3.

Togias, A., Cooper, S., Acebal, M. L., et al. (2017). *Addendum guidelines for the prevention of peanut allergy in the United States: Report of the NIAID-Sponsored Expert Panel.* Retrieved from https://www.niaid.nih.gov/sites/default/files/addendum-peanut-allergy-prevention-guidelines.pdf.

Trehan, I., & Manary, M. J. (2015). Management of severe acute malnutrition in low-income and middle-income countries. *Archives of Disease in Childhood, 100*(3), 283–287.

UNICEF. (2013). Position paper, ready-to-use therapeutic food for children with severe acute malnutrition. Retrieved from https://www.unicef.org/media/files/Position_Paper_Ready-to-use_therapeutic_food_for_children_with_severe_acute_malnutrition__June_2013.pdf.

US Department of Agriculture. (2016). *Economic Research Service: Definitions of food security.* Retrieved from https://www.ers.usda.gov/topics/food-nutrition-assistance/food-security-in-the-us/definitions-of-food-security.aspx.

van Wijk, R. M., van Vlimmeren, L. A., Groothuis-Oudshoorn, C. G., et al. (2014). Helmet therapy in infants with positional skull deformation: Randomized controlled trial. *BMJ (Clinical Research Ed.), 348*, g2741.

World Health Organization. (2016). *Guideline: Updates on HIV and infant feeding.* Retrieved from https://www.who.int/maternal_child_adolescent/documents/hiv-infant-feeding-2016/en/.

World Health Organization. (2017a). Length/height-for-age, weight-for-age, weight-for-length, weight-for-height and body mass index-for-age methods and development. Retrieved from http://www.who.int/childgrowth/standards/technical_report./en/.

World Health Organization. (2017b). *Management of severe acute malnutrition in infants and children.* Retrieved from http://www.who.int/elena/titles/full_recommendations/sam_management/en/.

Wozniak, L. J., Bechtold, H. M., Reyen, L. E., et al. (2015). Vitamin D deficiency in children with intestinal failure receiving home parenteral nutrition. *Journal of Parenteral Enteral Nutrition, 39*(4), 471–475.

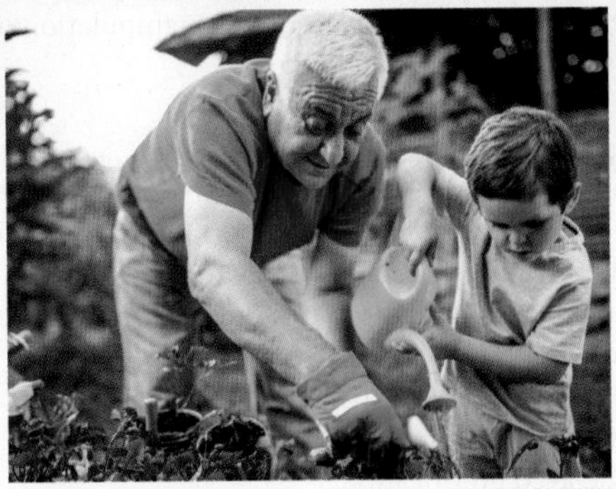

11

Health Promotion of the Toddler and Family

Elizabeth A. Duffy

http://evolve.elsevier.com/wong/essentials

CONCEPTS

- Development
- Functional Ability
- Communication
- Nutrition
- Safety

PROMOTING OPTIMAL GROWTH AND DEVELOPMENT

The term *terrible twos* has often been used to describe the toddler years, the period from 12 to 36 months old. It is a time of intense exploration of the environment as children attempt to find out how things work; what the word "no" means; and the power of temper tantrums, negativism, and obstinacy. "Getting into things" is their way of learning about their world, especially relationships. Successful mastery of the tasks of this age requires a strong foundation of trust during infancy and frequently necessitates guidance from others when parents and toddlers face the struggles of toilet training, limit setting, and sibling rivalry. Nurses who understand the dynamics of growth and development of toddlers can help families deal effectively with the tasks of this age.

BIOLOGIC DEVELOPMENT

Proportional Changes

Physical growth slows considerably during toddlerhood. The average weight gain is 1.8 to 2.7 kg (4 to 6 pounds) per year. The average weight at 2 years old is 12 kg (26.5 pounds). The birth weight is quadrupled by 2½ years old. The rate of increase in height also slows. The usual increment is an additional 7.5 cm (3 inches) per year and occurs mainly in elongation of the legs rather than the trunk. The average height of a 2-year-old child is 86.6 cm (34 inches). In general, adult height is about twice the 2-year-old child's height. Accurate measurement of height and weight during the toddler years should reveal a steady growth curve that is steplike rather than linear (straight), which is characteristic of the growth spurts during the early childhood years.

The rate of increase in head circumference slows somewhat by the end of infancy, and head circumference is usually equal to chest circumference by 1 to 2 years old. The usual total increase in head circumference during the second year is 2.5 cm (1 inch). Then the rate of increase slows until at age 5 years the increase is less than 1.25 cm (0.5 inch) per year. The anterior fontanel closes between 12 and 18 months old.

Chest circumference continues to increase in size and exceeds head circumference during the toddler years. The chest's shape also changes as the transverse, or lateral, diameter exceeds the anteroposterior diameter. After the second year, the chest circumference exceeds the abdominal measurement, which in addition to the growth of the lower extremities makes the child appear taller and leaner. However, toddlers retain a squat, "pot-bellied" appearance because of their less developed abdominal musculature and short legs. The legs retain a slightly bowed or curved appearance during the second year from the weight of the relatively large trunk.

Sensory Changes

Visual acuity of 20/40 is considered acceptable during the toddler years. Full binocular vision is well developed, and any evidence of persistent strabismus requires professional attention as early as possible to prevent amblyopia. Depth perception continues to develop, but because of toddlers' lack of motor coordination, falls from heights continue to be a persistent danger.

The senses of hearing, smell, taste, and touch become increasingly well developed, coordinated with each other, and associated with other experiences. All senses are used to explore the environment. Toddlers visually inspect an object by turning it over; they may taste it, smell it, and touch it several times before they are satisfied with their investigation. They shake it to see if it makes noise and vigorously test its durability.

Another example of the integrated function of the senses is toddlers' development of specific taste and texture preferences. Toddlers are much less likely than infants to try new foods because of their appearance, texture, or smell, not just their taste.

Maturation of Systems

Most of the physiologic systems are relatively mature by the end of toddlerhood. By the end of the first year, all brain cells are present but continue to increase in size. Myelination of the spinal cord is almost complete by 2 years old, which parallels the completion of most of the gross motor skills. Brain growth is 75% completed by the end of 2 years.

The volume of the respiratory tract and growth of associated structures continue to increase during early childhood, lessening some of the factors that predisposed children to frequent and serious infections during infancy. The internal structures of the ear and throat continue to be short and straight, and the lymphoid tissue of the tonsils and adenoids continues to be large. As a result, otitis media, tonsillitis, and upper respiratory tract infections are common. The respiratory and heart rates slow, and the blood pressure increases. Respirations continue to be abdominal.

The digestive processes are fairly complete by the beginning of toddlerhood. The acidity of the gastric contents continues to increase and has a protective function because it can destroy many types of bacteria. Stomach capacity increases to allow for the usual schedule of three meals a day.

One of the more prominent changes of the gastrointestinal system is the voluntary control of elimination. With complete myelination of the spinal cord, control of the anal and urethral sphincters is gradually achieved. The physiologic ability to control the sphincters probably occurs somewhere between 18 and 24 months old. Bladder capacity also increases considerably. By 14 to 18 months old, children can retain urine for up to 2 hours or longer.

Under conditions of moderate variation in temperature, the toddler rarely has the difficulties of young infants in maintaining body temperature. The capillaries can conserve core body temperature by constricting in response to cold and dilating in response to heat.

The defense mechanisms of the skin and blood, particularly phagocytosis, are much more efficient in toddlers than in infants. The production of antibodies is well established. However, many young children demonstrate a sudden increase in colds and minor infections when entering daycare or preschool because of their exposure to new pathogens.

Rapid growth in neurobehavioral organization contributes to greater regularity of sleep–wake cycles, the diminishing of crying and unexplained fussiness, and the enhanced predictability in mood. Valuable stimulants of early brain development include the various interactions (talking, singing, and playing) between the toddler and caregivers. Adequate nutrition; protection from environmental toxins, such as lead, various drugs, and stress; and promotion of good health care all contribute to healthy brain growth.

Gross and Fine Motor Development

The major gross motor skill during the toddler years is the development of locomotion. By 12 to 13 months old, toddlers walk alone using a wide stance for extra balance, and by 18 months old, they try to run but fall easily. At 2 years old, toddlers can walk up and down stairs, and by 2½ years old, they can jump using both feet, stand on one foot for a second or two, and manage a few steps on tiptoe. By the end of the second year, they can stand on one foot, walk on tiptoe, and climb stairs with alternate footing.

Fine motor development is demonstrated in increasingly skillful manual dexterity. For example, by 12 months old, toddlers can grasp a very small object. At 15 months old, they can drop a raisin into a narrow-necked bottle. Casting or throwing objects and retrieving them become almost obsessive activities at about 15 months old. By 18 months old, toddlers can throw a ball overhand without losing their balance. Mastery of gross and fine motor skills is evident in all phases of toddlers' activity, such as play, dressing, language comprehension, response to discipline, social interaction, and propensity for injuries. Activities occur less in isolation and more in conjunction with other physical and mental abilities to produce a purposeful result. For example, the toddler walks to reach a new location, releases a toy to pick it up or to choose a new one, and scribbles to look at the image produced. The possibilities of the exploration, investigation, and manipulation of the environment—and its hazards—are endless.

PSYCHOSOCIAL DEVELOPMENT

Toddlers are faced with the mastery of several important tasks. If the need for basic trust has been satisfied, they are ready to give up dependence for control, independence, and autonomy. Some of the specific tasks to be dealt with include:

- Differentiation of self from others, particularly the mother
- Toleration of separation from parent
- Ability to withstand delayed gratification
- Control over bodily functions
- Acquisition of socially acceptable behavior
- Verbal means of communication
- Ability to interact with others in a less egocentric manner

Mastery of these goals is only begun during late infancy and the toddler years; tasks such as developing interpersonal relationships with others may not be completed until adolescence. However, crucial foundations for successful completion of such developmental tasks are laid during these early formative years.

Developing a Sense of Autonomy (Erikson)

According to Erikson (1963), the developmental task of toddlerhood is acquiring a sense of autonomy while overcoming a sense of doubt and shame. As infants gain trust in the predictability and reliability of their parents, environment, and interactions with others, they begin to discover that their behavior is their own and that it has a predictable, reliable effect on others. Although they are aware of their will and control over others, they are confronted with the conflict of exerting autonomy and relinquishing the much-enjoyed dependence on others. Exerting their will has definite negative consequences, whereas retaining dependent, submissive behavior is generally rewarded with affection and approval. On the other hand, continued dependency creates a sense of doubt regarding their potential capacity to control their actions. This doubt is compounded by a sense of shame for feeling this urge to revolt against others' will and a fear that they will exceed their own capacity for manipulating the environment. Skillful monitoring and balance of controls by parents allows a growing rate of realistic successes and the emergence of autonomy.

Just as infants have the social modalities of grasping and biting, toddlers have the newly gained modality of holding on and letting go. Holding on and letting go are evident in how the toddler uses the hands, mouth, eyes, and eventually the sphincters, when toilet training is begun. Children constantly express these social modalities in play activities, such as throwing objects; taking objects out of boxes, drawers, or cabinets; holding on tighter when someone says, "No; don't touch"; and refusing to eat certain foods as taste preferences become strong.

Several characteristics, especially **negativism** and **ritualism**, are typical of toddlers in their quest for autonomy. As toddlers attempt to express their will, they often act with negativism, giving a negative response to requests. The words "no" or "me do" can be their sole vocabulary. Emotions become strongly expressed, usually in rapid mood swings. One minute, toddlers can be engrossed in an activity, and the next minute they might be angry because they are unable to manipulate a toy or open a door. If scolded for doing something wrong, they can have a temper tantrum and almost instantaneously pull at the parent's legs to be picked up and comforted. Understanding and coping with these swift changes is often difficult for parents. Many parents find the negativism exasperating and, instead of dealing constructively with it, give in to it, which further threatens children in their search for learning acceptable methods of interacting with others (see the Temper Tantrums and Negativism sections later in the chapter).

In contrast to negativism, which frequently disrupts the environment, ritualism, the need to maintain sameness and reliability, provides a sense of comfort. Toddlers can venture out with security when they know that familiar people, places, and routines still exist. One can easily understand why any change in the daily routine represents such a threat to these children. Without comfortable rituals, they have little opportunity to exert autonomy. Consequently, dependency and regression occur (see the Regression section later in the chapter).

Erikson focuses on the development of the **ego**, which may be thought of as reason or common sense, during this phase of psychosocial development. The child struggles to deal with the impulses of the **id**, tolerate frustration, and learn socially acceptable ways of interacting with the environment. The ego becomes evident as children develop the ability to tolerate delayed gratification.

Toddlers also have a rudimentary beginning of the **superego**, or conscience, which is the incorporation of the morals of society and the process of acculturation. With the development of the ego, children further differentiate themselves from others and expand their sense of trust in self. But as they begin to develop awareness of their own will and capacity to achieve, they also become aware of their ability to fail. This ever-present awareness of potential failure creates doubt and shame. Successful mastery of the task of autonomy necessitates opportunities for self-mastery while withstanding the frustration of necessary limit setting and delayed gratification. Opportunities for self-mastery are present in appropriate play activities, toilet training, the crisis of sibling rivalry, and successful interactions with significant others.

COGNITIVE DEVELOPMENT: SENSORIMOTOR AND PREOPERATIONAL PHASE (PIAGET)

The period from 12 to 24 months old is a continuation of the final two stages of the sensorimotor phase. During this time, the cognitive processes develop rapidly and at times seem similar to those of mature thinking. However, reasoning skills are still primitive and need to be understood to effectively deal with the typical behaviors of a child of this age.

In the fifth stage of the sensorimotor phase, **tertiary circular reactions** (13 to 18 months old), the child uses active experimentation to achieve previously unattainable goals. Newly acquired physical skills are increasingly important for the function they serve rather than for the acts themselves. The child incorporates the old learning of secondary circular reactions with new skills and applies the combined knowledge to new situations, with emphasis on the results of the experimentation. In this way, there is the beginning of rational judgment and intellectual reasoning. During this stage, the child further differentiates self from objects. This is evident in the child's increasing ability to venture away from his or her parents and to tolerate longer periods of separation.

Awareness of a **causal relationship** between two events is apparent. After flipping a light switch, toddlers are aware that a reciprocal response occurs. However, they are not able to transfer that knowledge to new situations. Therefore every time they see what appears to be a light switch, they must reinvestigate its function. Such behavior demonstrates the beginning of categorizing data into distinct classes and subclasses. Innumerable examples of this type of behavior occur as toddlers continuously explore the same object each time it appears in a new place.

Because classification of objects is still basic, the appearance of an object indicates its function. For example, if the child's toys are stored in a paper bag or large container, the toddler does not perceive a difference between the toy receptacle and the garbage pail or laundry basket. If allowed to turn over the toy receptacle, the child will just as quickly do the same to other similar containers because, in the child's mind, there is no difference. Expecting the child to judge which receptacles are permissible to explore and which are not is inappropriate for this age-group. Instead, the forbidden object, such as the garbage pail, should be placed out of reach. This has significant implications for prevention of accidents and accidental ingestion of injurious agents.

The discovery of objects as objects leads to the awareness of their **spatial relationships**. Children can recognize different shapes and their relationships to each other. For example, they can fit slightly smaller boxes into each other (nesting) and can place a round object into a hole even if the board is turned around, upside down, or reversed. Children are also aware of space and the relationship of their bodies to dimensions, such as height. They will stretch, stand on a low stair or stool, and pull a string to reach an object.

Object permanence has also advanced. Although they still cannot find an object that has been invisibly displaced and is no longer visible or moved from under one pillow to another without their seeing the change, toddlers are increasingly aware of the existence of objects behind closed doors, in drawers, and under tables. Parents are usually acutely aware of this developmental achievement and find high places and locked cabinets the only places that are inaccessible to toddlers.

During ages 19 to 24 months, the child is in the final sensorimotor stage, invention of new means through mental combinations. This stage completes the more primitive, autistic thought processes of infancy and prepares the way for more complex mental operations that occur during the phase of preoperational thought. One of the most dramatic achievements of this stage is in the area of object permanence. Toddlers will now actively search for an object in several potential hiding places. In addition, they can infer a cause when only experiencing the effect. They can infer that an object was hidden in any number of places even if they only saw the original hiding place.

Imitation displays deeper meaning and understanding. There is greater symbolization to imitation. Children are acutely aware of others' actions and attempt to copy them in gestures and in words. **Domestic mimicry** (imitating household activities) and sex-role behavior become increasingly common during this period and during the second year. Identification with the parent of the same gender becomes apparent by the second year and represents the child's intellectual ability to differentiate different models of behavior and to imitate them appropriately (Fig. 11.1).

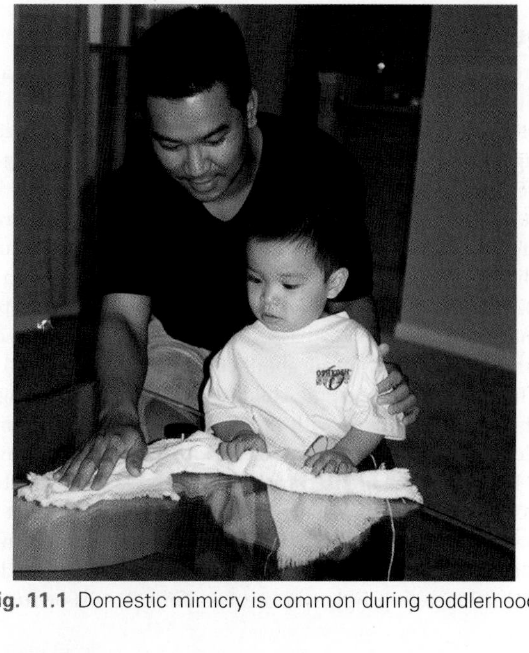

Fig. 11.1 Domestic mimicry is common during toddlerhood.

BOX 11.1 Characteristics of Preoperational Thought

Egocentrism: Inability to envision situations from perspectives other than one's own

Example: If a person is positioned between the toddler and another child, the toddler (who is facing the person) will explain that both children can see the middle person's face. The young child is unable to realize that the other person views the middle person from a different perspective, the back.

Implication: Avoid moralizing about "why" something is wrong if it requires an understanding of someone else's feelings or opinion. Telling a child to stop hitting because hitting hurts the other person is often ineffective because, to the aggressor, it feels good to hit someone else. Instead, emphasize that hitting is not allowed.

Transductive reasoning: Reasoning from the particular to the particular

Example: Child refuses to eat a food because something previously eaten did not taste good.

Implication: Accept child's reasoning; offer refused food at different time.

Global organization: Reasoning that changing any one part of the whole changes the entire whole

Example: Child refuses to sleep in his or her room because location of bed has changed.

Implication: Accept child's reasoning; use same bed position or introduce change slowly.

Centration: Focusing on one aspect rather than considering all possible alternatives

Example: Child refuses to eat a food because of its color even though its taste and smell are acceptable.

Implication: Accept child's reasoning.

Animism: Attributing lifelike qualities to inanimate objects

Example: Child scolds stairs for making child fall down.

Implication: Join child in the "scolding." Keep frightening objects out of view.

Irreversibility: Inability to undo or reverse the actions initiated physically

Example: When told to stop doing something (such as talking), child is unable to think of a positive activity.

Implication: State requests or instructions positively (e.g., "Be quiet.").

Magical thinking: Believing that thoughts are all-powerful and can cause events

Examples: Child wishes someone died; then if the person dies, child feels at fault because of the "bad" thought that made the death happen. Calling children "bad" because they did something wrong makes them feel as if they are bad.

Implication: Clarify that thoughts do not make things happen and that child is not responsible.

- Use "I" messages rather than "you" messages to communicate thoughts, feelings, expectations, or beliefs without imposing blame or criticism. Emphasize that the act, not the child, is bad.

Inability to conserve: Inability to understand the idea that a mass can be changed in size, shape, volume, or length without losing or adding to the original mass (instead, children judge what they see by the immediate perceptual clues given to them)

Example: If two lines of equal length are presented in such a way that one appears longer than the other, child will state that one line is longer even if child measures both lines with a ruler or yardstick and finds that each has the same length.

Implication: Change the most obvious perceptual clue to reorient child's view of what is seen.

- Give medicine in a small medicine cup rather than a large cup because the child will imagine that the large vessel contains more liquid. If child refuses the medicine in the small cup, pour it into a large cup because the liquid will appear to be less in a tall, wide container.
- Give a large, flat cookie rather than a thick, small one or do the reverse with meat or cheese; child will usually eat larger size of favorite food and smaller size of less favorite food.

The concept of time is still embryonic, but children have some sense of timing in terms of anticipation, memory, and a limited ability to wait. They may listen to the command, "Just a minute," and behave appropriately. However, their sense of timing is exaggerated—1 minute can seem like an hour. Toddlers' limited attention spans also indicate their sense of immediacy and concern for the present.

Preoperational Phase (Piaget)

At approximately 2 years old, children enter the preconceptual phase of cognitive development, which lasts until about 4 years old. The preconceptual phase is a subdivision of the preoperational phase, which spans ages 2 to 7 years. The preconceptual phase is primarily one of transition that bridges the purely self-satisfying behavior of infancy and the rudimentary socialized behavior of latency. **Preoperational thinking** implies that children cannot think in terms of operations—the ability to manipulate objects in relation to each other in a logical fashion. Rather, toddlers think primarily based on their perception of an event. Problem solving is based on what they see or hear directly rather than on what they recall about objects and events (Box 11.1).

Within the second year, the child increasingly uses language symbolically and is concerned with the "why" and "how" of things. For example, a pencil is "something to write with," and food is "something to eat." However, such **mental symbolization** is closely associated with prelogical reasoning. For instance, a needle is "something that hurts." Such painful experiences take on new significance because memory is associated with the specific event, and fears are likely to develop, such as resistance to people who wear uniform scrubs or rooms that look like the practitioner's office. Because of the vulnerability of these early years, it is essential to prepare children for any new experience, whether it is a new babysitter or a visit to the dentist.

SPIRITUAL DEVELOPMENT

Spiritual development in children is often discussed in terms of the child's developmental level because the evolution of spirituality often parallels cognitive development (Lima, do Nascimento, de Carvalho, et al., 2013). The child's family and environment strongly influence the child's perception of the world around him or her, and this often includes spirituality. Furthermore, family values, beliefs, customs, and expressions of these influence the child's perception of his or her spiritual self (Lima et al., 2013). Neuman (2011) proposes that Fowler's (1981) stages of faith be used to better understand children and spirituality; she provides an excellent overview of the stages of faith in childhood. The relationship between spirituality, illness in childhood, and nursing has been studied in the context of suffering, terminal illness such as cancer, and end-of-life care. In the past decade, there has been an increased interest in and focus on spiritual care in adults and children as further understanding of the influence of one's spirituality on health, illness, and well-being has progressed.

Toddlers learn about God through the words and the actions of those closest to them. They have only a vague idea of God and religious teachings because of their immature cognitive processes; however, if God is spoken about with reverence, young children associate God with something special. During this period, the assignment of powerful religious symbols and images is strongly influenced by the way these symbols and images are presented, usually in the form of rituals, games, and songs (Lima et al., 2013). Toddlers are said to be in the intuitive-projective phase of Fowler's (1981) faith construct wherein thinking is largely based on fantasy and rather fluid in relation to reality and fantasy. God may be described as being around like air by the toddler because of the fluidity in dividing fantasy and reality (Neuman, 2011).

Toddlers begin to assimilate behaviors associated with the divine (folding hands in prayer). Routines such as saying prayers before meals or at bedtime can be important and comforting. Because toddlers tend to find solace in ritualistic behavior and routines, they incorporate routines associated with religious practices into their behavioral patterns without understanding all of the implications of the rituals until later. Near the end of toddlerhood, when children use preoperational thought, there is some advancement of their understanding of God. Religious teachings, such as reward or fear of punishment (heaven or hell) and moral development (see Chapter 3), may influence their behavior.

DEVELOPMENT OF BODY IMAGE

As in infancy, the development of body image closely parallels cognitive development. With increasing motor ability, toddlers recognize the usefulness of body parts and gradually learn their respective names. They also learn that certain parts of the body have various meanings; for example, during toilet training, the genitalia become significant, and cleanliness is emphasized. By 2 years old, toddlers recognize gender differences and refer to themselves by name and then by pronoun. Gender identity is developed by 3 years old. Also by this time, children begin to remember events with reference to their personal significance, forming an autobiographic memory that helps establish a continuous identity throughout life's events.

Once they begin preoperational thought, toddlers can use symbols to represent objects, but their thinking may lead to inaccuracies. For example, if someone who is pregnant is called "fat," they will describe all "fat" women as having babies. They begin to recognize words used to describe physical appearance, such as "pretty," "handsome," or "big boy." Such expressions eventually influence how children view their own bodies.

It is evident that body integrity is poorly understood and that intrusive experiences are threatening. For example, toddlers forcefully resist procedures such as examining their ears or mouths and having their axillary temperature taken. The procedure itself (e.g., taking vital signs) does not hurt the child, but it represents an intrusion into the child's personal space, which elicits a strong protest. Toddlers also have unclear body boundaries and may associate nonviable parts, such as feces, with essential body parts. This can be seen in a toddler who is upset by flushing the toilet and watching the stool disappear.

Nurses can assist parents in fostering a positive body image in their child by encouraging them to avoid negative labels, such as "skinny arms" or "chubby legs"; such self-perceptions are internalized and can last a lifetime. Body parts, especially those related to elimination and reproduction, should be called by their correct names. Respect for the body should be practiced.

DEVELOPMENT OF GENDER IDENTITY

Just as toddlers explore their environment, they also explore their bodies and find that touching certain body parts is pleasurable. Genital fondling (masturbation) can occur and involves manual stimulation, as well as posturing movements (especially in young girls) such as tightening of the thighs or mechanical pressure applied to the pubic or suprapubic area. Other demonstrations of pleasurable activities include rocking, swinging, and hugging people and toys. Parental reactions to toddlers' behavior influence the children's own attitudes and should be accepting rather than critical. If such acts are performed in public, parents should not condone or bring attention to the behavior but should teach the child that it is more acceptable to perform the behavior in private.

Children in this age-group are learning vocabulary associated with anatomy, elimination, and reproduction. Certain associations between words and functions become significant and can influence future sexual attitudes. For example, if parents refer to the genitalia as dirty, especially in the context of elimination, this association between "genitalia" and "dirty" may be transferred to sexual functions later in life. Sex-role differences become obvious to children and are evident in much of toddlers' imitative play. Although current research indicates that prenatal exposure to testosterone strongly influences the individual's gender identity, researchers also indicate that there are sensitive periods (e.g., puberty) that may also have an influence on the development of gender identity (Hines, Constantinescu, & Spencer, 2015: Stortelder, 2014). A sense of maleness or femaleness, or **gender identity**, begins by 24 months old when children can label their own and others' gender (Steensma, Kreukels, de Vries, et al., 2013). Early attitudes are formed about affectionate behaviors between adults from observing parental and other adult intimate or sensual activities (see also Chapters 12 and 14, Sex Education). The quality of relationships with parents is important to the child's capacity for sexual and emotional relationships later in life.

SOCIAL DEVELOPMENT

A major task of the toddler period is differentiation of the self from significant others, usually the mother. The differentiation process consists of two phases: **separation**, children's emergence from a symbiotic fusion with the mother; and **individuation**, those achievements that mark children's expression of their individual characteristics in the environment. Although the process begins during the latter half of infancy, the major achievements occur during the toddler years.

Toddlers have an increased understanding and awareness of object permanence and some ability to withstand delayed gratification and tolerate moderate frustration. As a result, toddlers react differently to strangers than do infants. The appearance of unfamiliar people does not represent such a significant threat to their attachment to their mothers. They have learned from experience that parents exist when physically absent. Repetition of events such as going to bed without the parents but waking to find them there again reinforces the reliability of such brief separations. Consequently, toddlers can venture away from their parents for brief periods because of the security of knowing that the parents will be there when they return. Verbal and visual reassurance from the parents gradually replaces some of the previous need to be physically close for comfort.

The separation-individuation phase of the toddler encompasses the phenomenon of **rapprochement**; as a toddler separates from the mother and begins to make sense of experiences in the environment, the child is drawn back to the mother for assistance in identifying the meaning of the experiences (Zimmer-Gembeck, Webb, Thomas, et al., 2015). Developmentally, the term *rapprochement* means that the child moves away and returns for reassurance. If the mother's response to the toddler is inappropriate, the toddler may experience insecurity and confusion.

Transitional objects, such as a favorite blanket or toy, provide security for children, especially when they are separated from their parents, dealing with a new stress, or just fatigued (Fig. 11.2). Security objects often become so important to toddlers that they refuse to let them be taken away. Such behavior is normal; there is no need to discourage this tendency. During separations, such as daycare, hospitalization, or even staying overnight with a relative, transitional objects should be provided to minimize any fear or loneliness.

Learning to tolerate and master brief periods of separation are important developmental tasks for children in this age-group. In addition, it is a necessary component of parenting because brief periods of separation allow parents to restore their energy and patience and to minimize directing their irritations and frustrations at the children.

Language Development

The most striking characteristic of language development during early childhood is the increasing level of comprehension. Although the number of words acquired—from about 4 at 1 year old to approximately 300 at 2 years old—is notable, the ability to understand speech is much greater than the number of words the child can say. Bilingual children can also achieve their early linguistic milestones in each of the languages at the same time and produce a substantial number of semantically corresponding words in each of their two languages from the very first words or signs (Estes & Hay, 2015).

At 1 year old, children use one-word sentences or holophrases. The word "up" can mean "pick me up" or "look up there." For children, the one word conveys the meaning of a sentence, but to others, it may mean many things or nothing. At this age, about 25% of the vocalizations are intelligible. By 2 years old, children use multiword sentences by stringing together two or three words, such as the phrases "mama go bye-bye" or "all gone," and approximately 65% of the speech is understandable. By 3 years old, children put words together into simple sentences, begin to master grammatical rules, know their age and gender, and can count three objects correctly (Feigelman, 2016). Reading books together during this period provides an ideal setting for further language development. Language development among infants and toddlers is positively affected by adult-child conversations, including reading, storytelling, and interactive adult-child communication. Because of their immature symbolic, memory, and attentional skills, infants and toddlers cannot learn from traditional digital media as they do from interactions with caregivers, and they have difficulty transferring that knowledge to their three-dimensional experience (Barr, 2013). Emerging evidence shows that at 24 months of age, children can learn words from live video-chatting with a responsive adult or from an interactive touchscreen interface that scaffolds the child to choose the relevant answers (Kirkorian, Choi, & Pempek, 2016; Roseberry, Hirsh-Pasek, & Golinkoff, 2014). The American Academy of Pediatrics, Council on Communications and Media (2016) discourages the use of screen media other than video-chatting for children younger than 18 months. However, children 18 to 24 months of age can be introduced to digital media consisting of high-quality programming or apps, but these should be viewed together by parents and children. Allowing children to use media alone should be avoided.

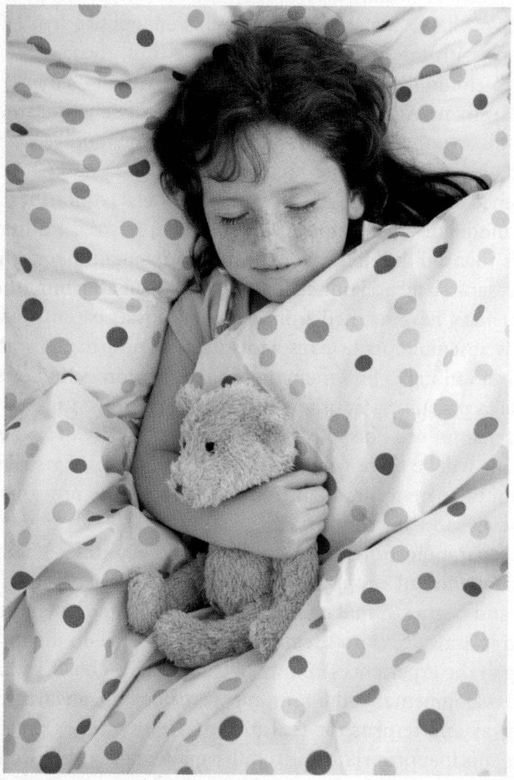

Fig. 11.2 Transitional objects, such as a warm and fuzzy stuffed animal, are sources of security to a toddler. (©2011 Photos.com, a division of Getty Images. All rights reserved.)

Furthermore, educational programs have not been shown to increase cognitive skills in young children.

Gestures precede or accompany each of the language milestones up to 30 months old (putting phone to ear, pointing). After sufficient language development, gestures phase out, and the pace of word learning increases.

Personal-Social Behavior

One of the most dramatic aspects of development in the toddler is personal-social interaction. Personal-social behaviors are evident in such areas as dressing, feeding, playing, and establishing self-control. Parents frequently wonder why their manageable, docile, lovable infant has turned into a determined, strong-willed, volatile little tyrant. In addition, the tyrant of the terrible twos can swiftly and unpredictably revert to the adorable infant. All of this is part of growing up as toddlers acquire a more sophisticated awareness that others' feelings and desires can be different from their own. Through interactions with caregivers, children can explore these differences and their consequences.

Toddlers are developing skills of independence, which are evident in all areas of behavior. By 15 months old, children feed themselves, drink well from a covered cup, and manage a spoon with considerable spilling. By 2 years old, they use a spoon well, and by 3 years old, they may be using a fork. Between 2 and 3 years old, they eat with the family and like to help with chores such as setting the table or removing dishes from the dishwasher, but they lack table manners and may find it difficult to sit through the family's entire meal.

In dressing, toddlers also demonstrate strides in independence. The 15-month-old child helps by putting the arms or feet out for dressing and pulling off shoes and socks. The 18-month-old child removes gloves, helps with pullover shirts, and may be able to unzip. By 2 years old, toddlers remove most articles of clothing and put on socks, shoes, and pants without regard for right or left and back or front. Help is still needed to fasten clothes.

Toddlers also begin to develop concern for the feelings of others and develop an understanding of how adult expectations for behavior apply to specific situations (e.g., causing a sibling to cry while playing rough). As their understanding increases, they develop control. Age-appropriate discipline contributes to healthy social and emotional development. Positive reinforcement, redirection, and time-outs are appropriate for most toddlers. Social and emotional problems can develop in the youngest children. Early screening and intervention promote more positive outcomes as young children grow and develop.

Play

Play magnifies toddlers' physical and psychosocial development. Interaction with people becomes increasingly important. The solitary play of infancy progresses to **parallel play**; toddlers play alongside, not with, other children. Although sensorimotor play is still prominent, there is much less emphasis on the exclusive use of one sensory modality. The toddler inspects toys, talks to toys, tests toys' strength and durability, and invents several uses for toys.

Imitation is one of the most distinguishing characteristics of play and enriches children's opportunity to engage in fantasy. With less emphasis on gender-stereotyped toys, play objects such as dolls, carriages, dollhouses, dishes, cooking utensils, child-size furniture, trucks, and dress-up clothes are suitable for both genders (Fig. 11.3); however, boys may be more interested than girls in activities related to trucks, trailers, action figures, and building blocks; girls may prefer doll-related activities.

Increased locomotive skills make push–pull toys, straddle trucks or cycles, a small gym and slide, balls of various sizes, and riding toys appropriate for energetic toddlers. Finger paints, thick crayons, chalk, blackboard, paper, and puzzles with large, simple pieces use toddlers' developing fine motor skills. Interlocking blocks in various sizes (but large enough to avoid aspiration) and shapes provide hours of fun and, during later years, are useful objects for creative and imaginative play. The most educational toy is the one that fosters the interaction of an adult with a child in supportive, unconditional play. Parents and other providers are encouraged to allow children to play with a variety of toys that foster creative thinking (such as blocks, dolls, and clay), rather than passive toys that the child observes (battery-operated or mechanical). Active play time should be encouraged over the use of computer or video games. Toys should not be substitutes for the attention of devoted caregivers, but toys can enhance these interactions.

Certain aspects of play are related to emerging linguistic abilities. Talking is a form of play for toddlers, who enjoy musical toys such as "talking" dolls and animals and toy telephones. Children's television programs are appropriate for some children over 2 years old, who learn to associate words with visual images. However, total media time should be limited to 1 hour or less of quality programming per day. Parents are encouraged to allow the child to engage in unstructured playtime, which is considered much more beneficial than any electronic media exposure (American Academy of Pediatrics, Council on Communications and Media, 2016). Toddlers also enjoy "reading" stories from a picture book and imitating the sounds of animals.

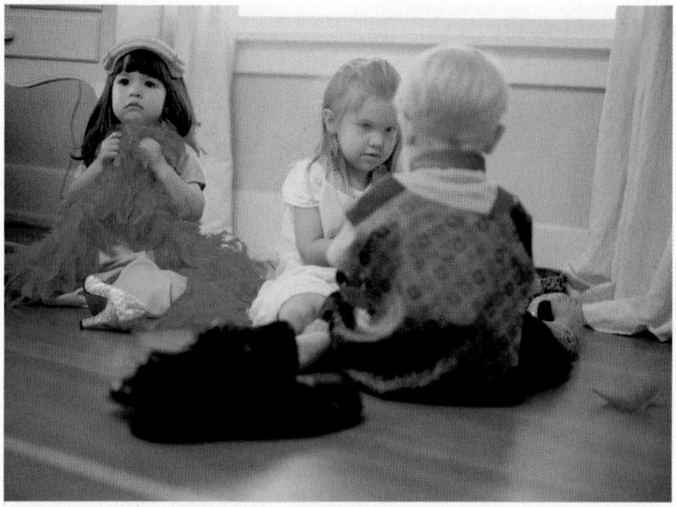

Fig. 11.3 Young children enjoy dressing up. (©2011 Photos.com, a division of Getty Images. All rights reserved.)

Tactile play is also important for exploring toddlers. Water toys, a sandbox with a pail and shovel, finger paints, soap bubbles, and clay provide excellent opportunities for creative and manipulative recreation. Adults sometimes forget the fascination of feeling textures, such as slippery cream, mud, or pudding; catching air bubbles; squeezing and reshaping clay; or smearing paints. These types of unstructured activities are as important as educational play to allow children the freedom of expression.

Selection of appropriate toys must involve safety factors, especially in relation to size and sturdiness. The oral activity of toddlers puts them at risk for aspirating small objects and ingesting toxic substances. Parents need to be especially vigilant of toys played with in other children's homes and toys of older siblings. Toys are a potential source of serious bodily damage to toddlers, who may have the physical strength to manipulate them but not the knowledge to appreciate their danger. Ball pits have been associated with transmission of bacteria, often found to be contaminated with visible dirt, vomit, feces, or urine, providing a permissive environment for contamination (Oesterle, Wright, Fidler, et al., 2019). Ride-on toys (i.e., tricycles, wagons, scooters) and early exploratory toys (i.e., blocks, stacking toys, building sets) were the most common type of toy causing injury to children younger than 5 years old (Abraham, Gaw, Chounthirath, et al., 2015). Government agencies do not inspect and police all toys on the market. Therefore adults who purchase play equipment, supervise purchases, or allow children to use play equipment need to evaluate its safety, including toys that are gifts or those that are purchased by the children themselves. Adults should also be alert to notices of toys determined to be defective and recalled by the manufacturers. Parents and health care workers can obtain information on a variety of recalled products and can report potentially dangerous toys and child products to the US Consumer Product Safety Commission[a] or, in Canada, the Canadian Toy Testing Council.[b] Printable tips on toy safety are also available from Safe Kids Worldwide (http://www.safekids.org).

COPING WITH CONCERNS RELATED TO NORMAL GROWTH AND DEVELOPMENT

Table 11.1 summarizes the major features of growth and development for the age-groups of 15, 18, 24, and 30 months.

Toilet Training

One of the major tasks of toddlerhood is toilet training. Anticipatory guidance and clinical intervention for families surrounding toilet training should begin during routine well-child visits before the child's developmental readiness to toilet train. Preparation and education reveal and allay misconceptions; lead to the development of appropriate expectations; and provide information, guidance, and support to parents for managing this potentially frustrating process.

Voluntary control of the anal and urethral sphincters is achieved sometime after the child is walking, probably between 18 and 24 months old. However, complex psychophysiologic factors are required for readiness. The child must be able to recognize the urge to let go and hold on and be able to communicate this sensation to the parent. In addition, some motivation is probably involved in the desire to please the parent by holding on rather than pleasing oneself by letting go. Cultural beliefs may also affect the age at which children demonstrate readiness (Feigelman, 2016).

Trends in toilet training have changed, likely due to the availability of disposable diapers. In the 1920s, toilet training began around

[a]800-638-2772; http://www.cpsc.gov.
[b]613-228-3155; http://www.toy-testing.org.

TABLE 11.1 Growth and Development During the Toddler Years

Physical	Gross Motor	Fine Motor	Sensory	Language	Socialization
15 Months Old					
Steady growth in height and weight Head circumference, 48 cm (19 inches) Weight, 11 kg (24 pounds) Height, 78.7 cm (31 inches)	Walks without help (usually since 13 months old) Creeps up stairs Kneels without support Cannot walk around corners or stop suddenly without losing balance without support Cannot throw ball without falling	Constantly casting objects to floor Builds tower of two cubes Holds two cubes in one hand Releases a pellet into narrow-necked bottle Scribbles spontaneously Uses cup well but often rotates spoon before it reaches mouth	Able to identify geometric forms; places round object into appropriate hole Binocular vision well developed Displays an intense and prolonged interest in pictures	Uses expressive jargon Says four to six words, including names "Asks" for objects by pointing Understands simple commands May shake head to denote "no" Uses "no" even while agreeing to the request Uses common gestures, such as putting cup to mouth when empty	Tolerates some separation from parent Less likely to fear strangers Beginning to imitate parents, such as cleaning house (sweeping, dusting), folding clothes May discard bottle Kisses and hugs parents; may kiss pictures in a book Expresses emotions; has temper tantrums
18 Months Old					
Physiologic anorexia from decreased growth needs Anterior fontanel closed Physiologically able to control sphincters	Runs clumsily; falls often Walks up stairs with one hand held Pulls and pushes toys Jumps in place with both feet Seats self on chair Throws ball overhand without falling	Builds tower of three or four cubes Release, prehension, and reach well developed Turns two or three pages in a book at a time In a drawing, makes stroke imitatively Manages spoon without rotation		Says 10 or more words Points to common object, such as a shoe or ball, and to two or three body parts Forms word combinations Forms gesture–word combinations (points while naming) Forms gesture–gesture combinations	Great imitator (domestic mimicry) Takes off gloves, socks, and shoes and unzips zippers Temper tantrums may be more evident Beginning awareness of ownership ("my toy") May develop dependence on transitional objects, such as security blanket
24 Months Old					
Head circumference, 49-50 cm (19.5-20 inches) Chest circumference exceeds head circumference Lateral diameter of chest exceeds anteroposterior diameter Usual weight gain of 1.8-2.7 kg (4-6 pounds) per year Usual gain in height of 10-12.5 cm (4-5 inches) per year Adult height approximately double height at 2 years old Primary dentition of 16 teeth May demonstrate readiness for beginning daytime control of bowel and bladder	Goes up and down stairs alone with two feet on each step Runs fairly well, with wide stance Picks up object without falling Kicks ball forward without overbalancing	Builds tower of six or seven cubes Aligns two or more cubes like a train Turns pages of book one at a time In drawing, imitates vertical and circular strokes Turns doorknobs; unscrews lids	Accommodation well developed in geometric discrimination; able to insert square block into oblong space	Has a vocabulary of approximately 300 words Uses two- or three-word phrases Uses pronouns "I," "me," "you" Understands directional commands Gives first name; refers to self by name Verbalizes need for toileting, food, or drink Talks incessantly Able to remember and imitate arbitrary sequences of manual actions and gestures	Stage of parallel play Has sustained attention span Temper tantrums decreasing Pulls people to show them something Increased independence from parent Dresses self in simple clothing Develops visual recognition and verbal self-reference ("me big") Develops awareness that feelings and desires of others may be different and begins to explore implications and consequences
30 Months Old					
Birth weight quadrupled Primary dentition (20 teeth) completed May have daytime bowel and bladder control	Jumps with both feet Jumps from chair or step Stands on one foot momentarily Takes a few steps on tiptoe	Builds tower of eight cubes Adds chimney to train of cubes Good hand–finger coordination; holds crayon with fingers rather than fist In drawing, imitates vertical and horizontal strokes; makes two or more strokes for cross; draws circles		Gives first and last name Refers to self by appropriate pronoun Uses plurals Names one color	Separates more easily from parent In play, helps put things away; can carry breakable objects; pushes with good steering Begins to notice gender differences; knows own gender May attend to toilet needs without help except for wiping Emotions expand to include pride, shame, guilt, embarrassment

12 months old, which changed to at least 18 months old in the 1960s and is now initiated around 21 months old, with approximately half of children toilet trained by 36 months old (Rogers, 2013).

Three markers signal a child's readiness to toilet train: (1) being aware of the urge to void or stool, (2) interest in and/or motivation to use the toilet, and (3) being dry for at least 2 hours during the day (Kimball, 2016). According to some experts, physiologic and psychologic readiness is not complete until 24 to 30 months old (Rogers, 2013); however, parents should begin preparing their children for toilet training earlier than 30 months old. By this time, children have mastered most essential gross motor skills, can communicate intelligibly, are in less conflict with their parents in terms of self-assertion and negativism, and are aware of the ability to control the body and please their parents. There is no universal right age to begin toilet training or an absolute deadline to complete training. An important role for the nurse is to help parents identify the readiness signs in their children (see Nursing Care Guidelines box).[c] On average, girls are developmentally ready to begin toilet training before boys (Elder, 2016).

NURSING CARE GUIDELINES

Assessing Toilet Training Readiness

Physical Readiness

- Voluntary control of anal and urethral sphincters, usually by 24 to 30 months old
- Ability to stay dry for 2 hours; decreased number of wet diapers; waking dry from nap
- Regular bowel movements
- Gross motor skills of sitting, walking, and squatting
- Fine motor skills to remove clothing

Mental Readiness

- Recognizes urge to defecate or urinate
- Verbal or nonverbal communicative skills to indicate when wet or has urge to defecate or urinate
- Cognitive skills to imitate appropriate behavior and follow directions

Psychologic Readiness

- Expresses willingness to please parent
- Able to sit on toilet for 5 to 8 minutes without fussing or getting off
- Curiosity about adults' or older sibling's toilet habits
- Impatience with soiled or wet diapers; desire to be changed immediately

Parental Readiness

- Recognizes child's level of readiness
- Willing to invest the time required for toilet training
- Absence of family stress or change, such as a divorce, moving, new sibling, or imminent vacation

Nighttime bladder control normally takes several months to years after daytime training begins. This is because the sleep cycle needs to mature so that the child can awake in time to urinate. Feigelman (2016) indicates that bedwetting is normal in girls up to 4 years old and in boys up to 5 years old. Few children have night wetting episodes after daytime dryness is totally achieved; however, children who do not have nighttime dryness by 6 years old are likely to require intervention.

[c]A helpful book is *The American Academy of Pediatrics Guide to Toilet Training*, 847-434-4000; http://shop.aap.org.

Bowel training is usually accomplished before bladder training because of its greater regularity and predictability. The sensation for defecation is stronger than that for urination and easier for children to recognize. A well-balanced diet that includes dietary fiber helps keep stool soft and supports the development and maintenance of regular bowel movements.

A number of techniques are helpful when initiating training, and cultural differences should be considered (see Cultural Considerations box). In the United States, some of the options recommended by practitioners include the Brazelton child-oriented approach, the American Academy of Pediatrics guidelines (which are similar to the Brazelton method), Dr. Spock's training method, and the intensive "toilet-training-in-a-day" (operant conditioning) approach by Azrin and Foxx (Wu, 2010). A systematic review by the Agency for Healthcare Research and Quality in 2006 concluded that the child-oriented method and the Azrin and Foxx methods were effective at toilet training healthy children (Kiddoo, 2012). The following discussion of toilet training methods includes suggestions from the child-oriented approach.

CULTURAL CONSIDERATIONS

Toilet Training

Cultural practices influence the timing, method, and significance of toilet training. For many families in China, the timing is liberal, the method is distinct, and the significance is low. Children are diapered during infancy. Once they are walking, they wear loose pants with a long slit between the legs, and they eliminate on the ground. This practice may continue until the child is 5 years old. In cold weather, a piece of cloth, like a "curtain," may be inserted. However, the Chinese have a concept that the buttocks are not susceptible to cold, so this is not a common practice.

Parents should begin the readiness phase of toilet training by teaching the child about how the body functions in relation to voiding and having a stool. Parents can talk about how adults and animals perform such functions on a routine basis. Toilet training should be as easy and simple as possible. Important considerations are the selection of the child's clothing and the potty chair or use of the toilet. A freestanding potty chair allows children a feeling of security (Fig. 11.4A). Planting the feet firmly on the floor also facilitates defecation. Another option is a portable seat attached to the regular toilet, which may ease the transition from potty chair to regular toilet. Placing a small bench under the feet helps stabilize the child's position. It is probably best to keep the potty in the bathroom and to let the child observe the excreta being flushed down the toilet to associate these activities with usual practices. If a potty chair is not available, having the child sit facing the toilet tank provides added support (see Fig. 11.4B). Practice sessions should be limited to 5 to 8 minutes, and a parent should stay with the child, practicing sanitary habits after every session. Children should be praised for cooperative behavior and successful evacuation. Dressing children in easily removed clothing; using training pants, "pull-on" diapers, or underwear; and encouraging imitation by watching others are other helpful suggestions.

When the child begins to experience regular daytime dryness, parents may experiment with underwear during the day. Daytime accidents are common, particularly during periods of intense activity. Young children become so engrossed in play activity that, if they are not reminded, they will wait until it is too late to reach the bathroom. Therefore frequent reminders and trips to the toilet are necessary. Parents often forget to plan ahead when their toddlers are being toilet trained; before trips outside the house, it is important to remind children to at least try to urinate to decrease the chance of needing to use the toilet while the car is stuck in traffic.

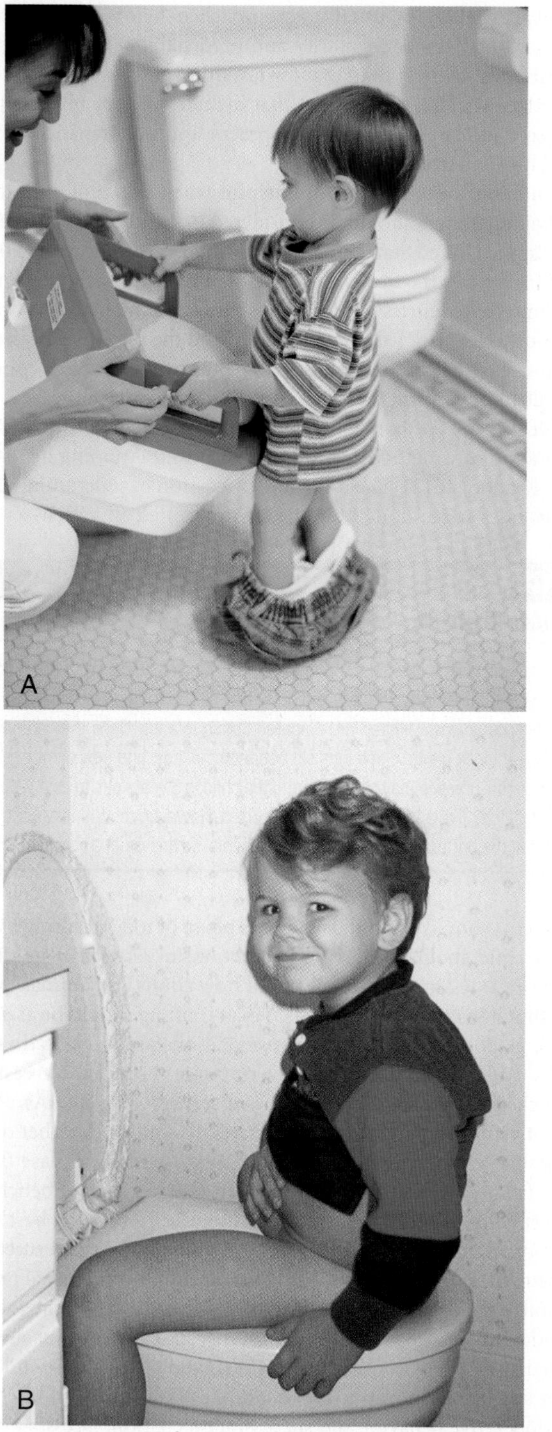

Fig. 11.4 A, Children may begin toilet training sitting on a small potty chair. B, Sitting in reverse fashion on a regular toilet provides additional security to a young child. (A, ©2011 Photos.com, a division of Getty Images. All rights reserved.)

As the child masters each step of toileting (discussion, undressing, going, wiping, dressing, flushing, and hand washing), he or she gains a sense of accomplishment that parents should reinforce. If the parent-child relationship becomes strained, both may need a break to focus on enjoyable activities together. Regression may coincide with a stressful family situation or the child being pushed too hard and too fast. Regression is a normal part of toilet training and does not mean failure but should be viewed as a temporary setback to a more comfortable place for the child.

Daycare providers also play a role in the support and education of parents regarding toilet training practices. It is important for parents to inform all caregivers of their individual family values and the child's specific needs when planning for training away from home. Ensuring consistency in care of toddlers and ensuring healthy practices in a sanitary environment allow for safe and effective toilet practices in all settings.

Sibling Rivalry

The term *sibling rivalry* refers to a natural jealousy and resentment toward a new child in the family or toward other children in the family when a parent turns his or her attention from them and interacts with their brother or sister.

The arrival of a new infant represents a crisis for even the best-prepared toddlers. They do not hate or resent the infant; rather, they hate the changes that this additional sibling produces, especially the separation from mother during the birth. The parents now share their love and attention with someone else, the usual routine is disrupted, and toddlers may lose their crib or room—all at a time when they thought they were in control of their world. Sibling rivalry tends to be most pronounced in firstborn children, who experience **dethronement** (loss of sole parental attention). It also seems to be most difficult for young children, particularly in terms of mother-child interaction.

Preparation of children for the birth of a sibling is individual but is dictated to some extent by age. For toddlers, time is a vague concept. A good time to start talking about the baby is when toddlers become aware of the pregnancy and the changes taking place in the home in anticipation of the new member. To avoid additional stresses when the newborn arrives, parents should perform anticipated changes, such as moving the toddler to a different room or bed, well in advance of the birth.

Toddlers need to have a realistic idea of what the newborn will be like. Telling them that a new playmate will come home soon sets up unrealistic expectations. Rather, parents should stress the activities that will take place when the baby arrives home, such as diapering, bottle-feeding or breastfeeding, bathing, and dressing. At the same time, parents should emphasize which routines will stay the same, such as reading stories or going to the park. If toddlers have had no contact with an infant, it is a good idea to introduce them to one, if feasible. Providing a doll with which toddlers can imitate parental behaviors is another excellent strategy. They can tend to the doll's needs (diapering, feeding) at the same time the parent is performing similar activities for the infant.

When the new baby arrives, toddlers keenly feel the changed focus of attention. Visitors may initiate problems when they inadvertently shower the infant with attention and presents while neglecting the older child. Parents can minimize this by alerting visitors to the toddler's needs, having small presents on hand for the toddler, and including the child in the visit as much as possible. The toddler can also help with the care of the newborn by getting diapers and doing other small tasks (Fig. 11.5).

How children exhibit jealousy is complex. Some will hit the infant, push the child off the mother's lap, or pull the bottle or breast from the infant's mouth. For this reason, infants must be protected by parental supervision of the interaction between the siblings. More often the expressions of hostility and resentment are more subtle and covert. Toddlers may verbally express a wish that the infant "go back inside mommy," or they will revert to more infantile forms of behavior, such as demanding a bottle, soiling their underpants, clinging for attention, using baby talk, or aggressively acting out toward others. The latter is particularly common in preschoolers, who may seem accepting of the new sibling at home but behave poorly in daycare or preschool.

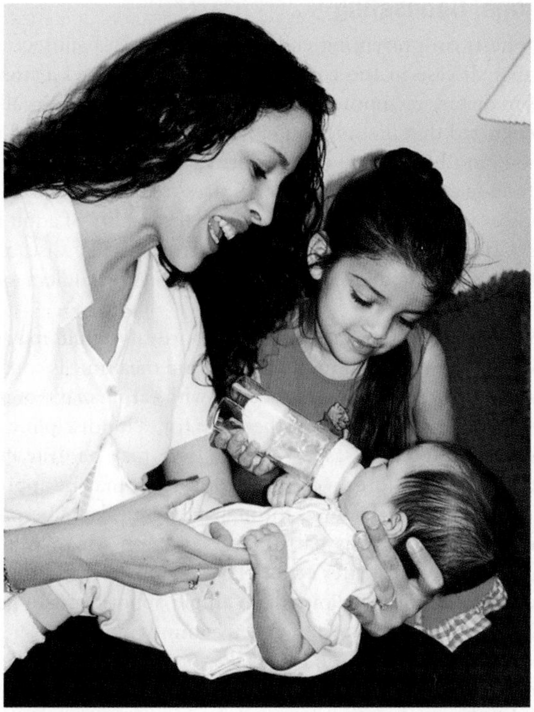

Fig. 11.5 To minimize sibling rivalry, parents should include the toddler during caregiving activities.

This is a form of displacement that says, "I can't let my parents know how I feel, so I will tell you." Encouraging parents to explore how their older child is acting with other caregivers is an important aspect of intervention.

Temper Tantrums

Toddlers may assert their independence by violently objecting to discipline. They may lie down on the floor, kick their feet, and scream at the top of their lungs. Some have learned the effectiveness of holding their breath until the parent relents. Although holding one's breath may cause fainting from the lack of oxygen, the accumulation of carbon dioxide will stimulate the respiratory control center, resulting in no physical harm. Tantrums are an indication of the child's inability to control emotions; toddlers are particularly prone to tantrums because their strong drive for mastery and autonomy is frustrated by adult figures or lack of motor and cognitive skills.

The best approach to tapering temper tantrums requires consistency and developmentally appropriate expectations and rewards. Ensuring consistency among all caregivers in expectations, prioritizing what rules are important, and developing consequences that are reasonable for the child's level of development help manage the behavior. For example, a popular time for a tantrum is before bed. Active toddlers often have trouble slowing down and, when placed in bed, resist staying there. Parents can reinforce consistency and expectations by stating, "After this story, it is bedtime." Starting at 18 months old, time-outs work well for managing temper tantrums.

During tantrums, stay calm and ignore the behavior, provided the behavior is not injurious to the child, such as violently banging the head on the floor. Continue to be present to provide a feeling of control and security to the child when the tantrum has subsided. During periods of no tantrums, practice developmentally appropriate positive reinforcement.

Other suggestions for preventing tantrums include the following (El-Radhi, 2015):

- Offer the child options instead of an "all or none" position.
- Set clear boundaries and expectations with all caregivers.
- Ensure a consistent response to child's behavior by all caregivers.
- Praise the child for positive behavior when he or she is not having a tantrum or provide a reward system (i.e., sticker chart).

Temper tantrums are common during the toddler years and essentially represent normal developmental behaviors. However, temper tantrums can be signs of serious problems. Temper tantrums that occur past 5 years old, last longer than 15 minutes, or occur more than five times a day are considered abnormal and may indicate a serious problem (Eisbach, Cluxton-Keller, Harrison, et al., 2014). Nurses should be alert to situations that require further evaluation.

Negativism

One of the more difficult aspects of rearing children in this age-group is their persistent negative response to every request. The negativism is not an expression of being stubborn or insolent but a necessary assertion of self-control. One method of dealing with the negativism is to reduce the opportunities for a "no" answer. Asking the child, "Do you want to go to sleep now?" is an example of a question that will almost certainly be answered with an emphatic "no." Instead, tell the child that it is time to go to sleep and proceed accordingly. In their attempt to exert control, children like to make choices. When confronted with appropriate choices, such as "You may have a peanut butter and jelly sandwich or chicken noodle soup for lunch," they are more likely to choose one rather than automatically say no. However, if their response is negative, parents should make the choice for the child.

Nurses working with children and parents can assist parents in understanding this concept by role modeling. For example, when the nurse approaches the toddler to take vital signs, instead of asking, "Can I listen to your heart?" the nurse can say, "I am going to listen to your heart." Because of normal developmental behavior, toddlers first resist having their vital signs taken because it is an intrusion on their bodies. Second, toddlers are most likely going to answer "no," not because they necessarily fear the procedure itself but because of the tendency to answer all questions with a negative response. If the nurse asks the question and the toddler says, "No" but the nurse proceeds anyway, the toddler starts to mistrust the nurse's actions because they contradict his or her words.

Regression

The retreat from one's present pattern of functioning to past levels of behavior is referred to as **regression**. It usually occurs in instances of discomfort or stress when one attempts to conserve psychic energy by reverting to patterns of behavior that were successful in earlier stages of development. Regression is common in toddlers because almost any additional stress hinders their ability to master present developmental tasks. Any threat to their autonomy, such as illness, hospitalization, separation, disruption of established routines, or adjustment to a new sibling, represents a need to revert to earlier forms of behavior, such as increased dependency. This can include refusal to use the potty chair; temper tantrums; demand for the bottle or pacifier; and loss of newly learned motor, language, social, and cognitive skills.

At first, such regression appears acceptable and comfortable for children, but the loss of newly acquired achievements is frightening and threatening because children are aware of their helplessness. Parents become concerned about regressive behavior and frequently force the child to cope with an additional source of stress—the pressure to live up to expected standards. Brazelton (1999) suggests that these predictable times of regression, or **touchpoints**, are an opportunity to prepare parents for the next step in their child's development.

When regression does occur, the best approach is to ignore it while praising existing patterns of appropriate behavior. Regression is a child's way of saying, "I can't cope with this present stress and perfect this skill as well, but I will eventually if given patience and understanding." For this reason, it is advisable not to attempt new areas of learning when an additional crisis is present or expected, such as beginning toilet training shortly before a sibling is born or during a brief period of hospitalization.

PROMOTING OPTIMAL HEALTH DURING TODDLERHOOD

NUTRITION

During the period from 12 to 18 months old, the growth rate slows, decreasing the child's need for calories, protein, and fluid. However, the protein (13 g/day) and energy requirements are still relatively high to meet the demands for muscle tissue growth and high activity level. The need for minerals (such as iron, calcium, and phosphorus) may be difficult to meet, considering the characteristic food habits of children in this age-group. Parents may be tempted to rely on vitamin supplementation, rather than a well-balanced diet, to meet these requirements. Toddlers usually require three meals and two snacks per day; however, the portions consumed are generally smaller compared with those of older children.

The Feeding Infants and Toddlers Study (FITS) (Saavedra, Denning, Dattilo, et al., 2013) found that, in general, toddlers met or exceeded the requirements for daily energy and protein requirements. However, intake of a variety of foods was seen with advancing age in toddlers as their food preferences changed. FITS recommended that toddlers be fed a more balanced diet of vegetables, fruits, and whole grains.

At approximately 18 months old, most toddlers manifest this decreased nutritional need with a decreased appetite, a phenomenon known as **physiologic anorexia**. They become picky, fussy eaters with strong taste preferences. They may eat large amounts one day and almost nothing the next. Toddlers are increasingly aware of the nonnutritive function of food (i.e., the pleasure of eating, the social aspect of mealtime, and the control of refusing food). They are influenced by factors other than taste when choosing food. If a family member refuses to eat something, toddlers are likely to imitate that response. If the plate is overfilled, they are likely to push it away, overwhelmed by its size. If food does not appear or smell appetizing, they will probably not agree to try it. In essence, mealtime is more closely associated with psychologic components than with nutritional ones. Toddlers like to eat with their fingers and enjoy foods of different colors and shapes.

The **ritualism** of this age also dictates certain principles in feeding practices. Toddlers like to have the same dish, cup, or spoon every time they eat. They may reject a favorite food simply because it is served in a different dish. If one food touches another, they often refuse to eat it. Mixed foods, such as stews or casseroles, are rarely favorites. Because toddlers have unpredictable table manners, it is best to use plastic dishes and cups for both economic and safety reasons. For some children, a regular mealtime schedule also contributes to their desire and need for predictability and ritualism.

Developmentally, by 12 months old most children eat many of the same foods prepared for the rest of the family. Some may have mastered using a cup with occasional spilling, although most cannot use a spoon until 18 months old or later and generally prefer using their fingers.

Nutritional Counseling

The emphasis on preventing childhood obesity and subsequent cardiovascular disease in the United States has prompted a number of changes in dietary recommendations for children and adults alike. It is now recognized that lifetime eating habits may be established in early childhood, and health care workers are increasingly emphasizing the role of food selection choices, exercise, stress reduction, and other lifestyle choices (tobacco and alcohol use) on the quality of adult life and survival. Conditions such as obesity and cardiovascular disease can be prevented by encouraging healthy eating habits in toddlers and their families.

If food is used as a reward or sign of approval, a child may overeat for nonnutritive reasons. If food is forced and mealtime is consistently unpleasant, the usual pleasure associated with eating may not develop. Mealtimes should be enjoyable rather than times for discipline or family arguments. The social aspect of mealtime may be distracting for young children; therefore an earlier feeding hour may be appropriate. Young children are unable to sit through a long meal and become restless and disruptive. This is particularly common when children are brought to the table just after active play. Calling them in from play 15 minutes before mealtime allows them ample opportunity to get ready for eating while settling down their active minds and bodies.

The method of serving food also takes on more importance during this period. Toddlers need to have a sense of control and achievement in their abilities. Giving them large, adult-size portions can overwhelm them. In general, what is eaten is much more significant than how much is consumed. Toddlers usually restrict their food preference to four or five main foods and rarely try new foods; in some cases, a toddler may insist on one food such as mashed potatoes for lunch and dinner. Small amounts of meat and vegetables supply greater food value than a large consumption of bread or potato. Serving sizes need to be appropriate for age. Young children tend to like less spicy, bland food, although this is a culturally determined preference. Substitutions can be provided for foods that they do not enjoy, although parents need not cater to all of their desires. Frequent nutritious snacks can replace a meal. **Grazing** (i.e., nibbling and snacking) is a good way to ensure proper nutrition, provided that appropriate foods are offered.

To determine serving size for young children, use the following guidelines:

- A general guide to serving sizes for toddlers is 1 tablespoon of solid food per year of age, or one-fourth to one-third of the adult portion size.
- Use the tablespoon guide for easily measured foods, such as vegetables or rice.
- Use the fraction guide for bread or milk.

Mastication skills continue to mature, putting children at risk for choking; therefore large, round foods (e.g., hot dogs, grapes, peas, carrots, popcorn, fruit gel snacks) should be avoided until the child is able to chew them effectively. Active play while eating should be discouraged to prevent choking. Appetite and food preferences are sporadic. Often the interest in food parallels a growth spurt; thus periods of good eating are interspersed with phases of poor eating. If exposed to the same food every day, a young toddler does not learn how to manage the complex sensory information needed to eat new, more difficult foods (e.g., vegetables with a different texture vs. pureed, slippery fruits). To help prevent "food jags," it is recommended that parents present food in various physical forms. The child may need to progress to eating new foods in a stepwise fashion, such as visually tolerating the food, interacting with the food, smelling the food, touching the food, tasting the food, and then eating the food.

Many authorities consider this period of picky eating to be a developmental phase, and growth charts can be used to demonstrate growth to parents who are often concerned (Parks, Shaikhkhalil, Groleau, et al., 2016). Parents should be encouraged to plan a nutritionally balanced week instead of day because of the way toddlers restrict food intake in their effort to exert control over their environment (Schwartz & Benuck, 2013).

Dietary Guidelines

Dietary guidelines are necessary to promote adequate energy and nutrient intake to support physical, emotional, psychologic, and cognitive development. New dietary guidelines have been developed to address the issue of childhood obesity, sedentary lifestyles, and increase in cardiovascular disease mortality in the United States.

The National Academies of Medicine (2017) has developed guidelines for nutritional intake that encompass the Recommended Dietary Allowances (RDAs) yet extend their scope to include additional parameters related to nutritional intake. The Dietary Reference Intakes (DRIs)[d] are composed of four categories. These include Estimated Average Requirements (EARs) for age and gender categories, Tolerable Upper Intake Levels (ULs) that are associated with a low risk of adverse effects, Adequate Intakes (AIs) of nutrients, and new standard RDAs. The guidelines present information about lifestyle factors that may affect nutrient function, such as caffeine intake and exercise, and about how the nutrient may be related to chronic disease. An important factor in the development of the DRIs that affects children, particularly infants from birth to 6 months old, is that the AIs are based on the nutrient intake of full-term, healthy, breastfed infants (by well-nourished mothers), which now represents the gold standard for infant nutrition in this age-group. In 2010 new DRIs for vitamin D and calcium were released by the Institute of Medicine.

The 2015–2020 Dietary Guidelines for Americans may also be used to encourage healthy dietary intakes and regular exercise designed to decrease obesity, cardiovascular risk factors, and subsequent cardiovascular disease, which is now known to occur in both young children and adults. As an example, the 2015–2020 Dietary Guidelines recommend a caloric intake for a moderately active boy, ages 2 to 3 years, of 1000 to 1400 calories per day. The emphasis in the Dietary Guidelines is on decreasing overall fat and sodium intakes, and increasing the amount of daily exercise to reduce the incidence of obesity and cardiovascular disease. The 2015–2020 Dietary Guidelines[e] are for children ages 2 years and older. They encourage a variety of fruits, vegetables, whole grains, and low-fat dairy and nonfat dairy products in addition to fish, beans, and lean meat.

Additional resources for dietary counseling include MyPlate[f], developed by the US Department of Agriculture to replace MyPyramid. This colorful plate shows the five main food groups (i.e., fruits, grains, vegetable, protein, and dairy) with the intended purpose of involving children and their families in making appropriate food choices for meals and decreasing the incidence of overweight and obesity in the United States. MyPlate provides an online interactive feature that allows the individual to select (click on) an individual food group and see choices for foods in that group. Approximate serving sizes are suggested, and vegetarian substitutions are also provided.

Nutrition during toddlerhood involves a transition as a young toddler is weaned off milk- or formula-based diets. Milk intake, the chief source of calcium and phosphorus, should average two or three servings (24 to 30 oz) a day. Consuming more than a quart of milk daily considerably limits the intake of solid foods, resulting in a deficiency of dietary iron and other nutrients. After 2 years of age, children can be given low-fat milk to reduce daily total fat to less than 30% of calories, saturated fatty acids to less than 10% of calories, and cholesterol to less than 300 mg. Other measures to reduce dietary fat include using lean meats, fat-modified products (e.g., low-fat cheese), and low-fat cooking. Because less fat in children's diets can also mean fewer calories and nutrients, caregivers must know what kinds of food to choose. However, trans fatty acids and saturated fats should be avoided.

Iron-fortified cereals and iron-rich foods are recommended for all children older than 6 months of age. Parents should be encouraged to provide an iron-rich diet that includes heme and nonheme iron sources (red meats, poultry, fish, green leafy vegetables, dried fruit, and beans) and limit whole-milk consumption. Iron supplementation may be necessary in some cases. Calcium and vitamin D are essential for healthy bone development. Adequate intake of calcium for children 1 to 3 years old is 500 mg per day. Whole milk, cheese, yogurt, legumes (beans), and vegetables (broccoli, collard greens, and kale) are good sources of calcium. Popular calcium-fortified foods include waffles, cereals and cereal bars, orange juice, and some white breads. Adequate vitamin D intake is essential to prevent rickets; it is now recommended that children and adolescents have an intake of at least 400 IU of vitamin D daily (US Department of Health and Human Services, 2016). Multivitamin preparations containing 400 IU of vitamin D (by tablet or liquid) are adequate if food intake is poor or exposure to sunlight is minimal; vitamin D–only preparations containing 400 IU are also available commercially. Sources of vitamin D include fish, fish oils, and egg yolks. Fortified cereals, dairy products, and meat are also good sources of zinc and vitamin E.

Juice should not be introduced into the diet of infants before 12 months of age unless clinically indicated. Toddlers should not be given juice from bottles or easily transportable covered cups that allow them to consume juice easily throughout the day. Toddlers should not be given juice at bedtime. The intake of juice should be limited to, at most, 4 ounces/day in toddlers 1 through 3 years of age (Heyman & Abrams, 2017). Fruit-flavored drinks advertised as juices may not actually contain 100% juice and should be avoided.

VEGETARIAN DIETS

Vegetarian diets have become increasingly popular in the United States because people are concerned about hypertension; cholesterol; obesity; cardiovascular disease; cancer of the stomach, intestine, and colon; and the influence of the animal rights movement. The American Dietetic Association and the American Academy of Pediatrics endorse vegetarian diets for adults and children (Schürmann, Kersting, & Alexy, 2017). Well-planned vegetarian diets are adequate for all stages of the life cycle; promote normal growth; and have been shown to have lower intakes of cholesterol, saturated fat, and total fat and higher intakes of fruits, fiber, and vegetables than nonvegetarian diets. However, vegetarian diets may vary considerably, and assessment of dietary adequacy is essential to ensure that children are receiving adequate nutrients (Schürmann et al., 2017)

The major types of vegetarianism are:

Lacto-ovo vegetarians, who exclude meat from their diet but consume dairy products and rarely fish

Lactovegetarians, who exclude meat and eggs but drink milk

Pure vegetarians (vegans), who eliminate all foods of animal origin, including milk and eggs

Macrobiotics, who are even more restrictive than pure vegetarians, allowing only a few types of fruits, vegetables, and legumes

[d]http://www.nationalacademies.org/hmd/Home/Global/News%20Announcements/DRI

[e]https://health.gov/dietaryguidelines/2015/guidelines/

[f]http://www.choosemyplate.gov/

BOX 11.2 Factors That Affect Iron Absorption

Increase

Acidity (low pH): Administer iron between meals (gastric hydrochloric acid).
Ascorbic acid (vitamin C): Administer iron with juice, fruit, or multivitamin preparation.
Vitamin A
Tissue (cellular) need
Meat, fish, poultry
Cooking in cast iron pots

Decrease

Alkalinity (high pH): Avoid any antacid preparation.
Phosphates: Milk is unfavorable vehicle for iron administration.
Phytates—found in cereals
Oxalates—found in many fruits and vegetables (plums, currants, green beans, spinach, sweet potatoes, tomatoes)
Tannins—found in tea, coffee
Tissue (cellular) saturation
Malabsorptive disorders
Disturbances that cause diarrhea or steatorrhea
Infection

Semi-vegetarians, who consume a lacto-ovo vegetarian diet with some fish and poultry: This is an increasingly popular form of vegetarianism and poses little or no nutritional risk to infants unless dietary fat and cholesterol intake is severely restricted.

Many individuals who are concerned about healthy diets subscribe to vegetarian diets that may not be typified by the above categories. Therefore during nutritional assessment, it is necessary to clearly list exactly what the diet includes and excludes.[g]

The major deficiencies that may occur in the stricter vegan diets are inadequate protein for growth; inadequate calories for energy and growth; poor digestibility of many of the bulky natural, unprocessed foods, especially for infants; and deficiencies of vitamin B_6, niacin, riboflavin, vitamin D, iron, calcium, and zinc. Vitamin D is essential if exposure to sunlight is inadequate (≈5 to 15 min/day on the hands, arms, and face of light-skinned persons; slightly more in darker pigmented individuals) or in persons who are dark skinned or who live in northern latitudes or cloudy or smoky areas. Many of these deficiencies can be avoided in children who are not consuming 100% of the RDA of vitamins and minerals with a multivitamin and mineral supplement.

Evaluate for iron-deficiency anemia and rickets in children who are on strict vegetarian and macrobiotic diets; these problems may occur as a result of consuming plant foods such as unrefined cereals, which impair the absorption of iron, calcium, and zinc. The American Academy of Pediatrics, Committee on Nutrition (2014) recommends iron supplementation of 1 mg/kg/day in infants exclusively breastfed after 4 to 6 months old by vegetarian mothers and no dietary fat restrictions in vegetarian children younger than 2 years old. Other factors that affect iron absorption are listed in Box 11.2.

Achieving a nutritionally adequate vegetarian diet is not difficult (except with the strictest diets), but it requires careful planning and knowledge of nutrient sources (American Academy of Pediatrics, Committee on Nutrition, 2014). For children, the lacto-ovo vegetarian diet is nutritionally adequate; however, the vegan diet requires supplementation with vitamins D and B_{12} for children 2 to 12 years old.

To ensure sufficient protein in the diet, foods with incomplete proteins (those that do not have all of the essential amino acids) must be eaten at the same meal with other foods that supply the missing amino acids. The three basic combinations of foods consumed by vegetarians that generally provide the appropriate amounts of essential amino acids are:

1. Grains (cereal, rice, pasta) and legumes (beans, peas, lentils, peanuts)
2. Grains and milk products (milk, cheese, yogurt)
3. Seeds (sesame, sunflower) and legumes

Additional dietary considerations for young children are found in Chapter 12.

COMPLEMENTARY AND ALTERNATIVE MEDICINE

There are four complementary and alternative medicine (CAM) domains according to the National Center for Complementary and Integrative Health; this discussion centers on only one of those—biologically based practices, which include herbs, vitamins, and foods. The National Center for Complementary and Integrative Health (2018) classifies probiotics as a type of natural product and CAM. Many CAM products are sold over the counter as dietary supplements, but the use of some dietary supplements such as calcium for bone health or a multivitamin supplement are not considered to be CAM (National Center for Complementary and Integrative Health, 2018). The National Center for Complementary and Integrative Health (2018) reports that natural products are the most commonly used CAM products in children and that most often these products are used for chronic conditions (such as neck and back pain) and for head and chest colds. Other surveys confirm that CAM is often used for children's chronic remedies for which traditional therapy is not effective (National Center for Complementary and Integrative Health, 2018).

The misuse of CAM has the potential for placing some children at risk for health problems. Although 55% of children have used CAM at least once, only 4.4% of CAM use was reported to emergency department physicians, primarily because the parent or child did not think it was important to inform the physician and/or the physician did not ask about CAM use (Taylor, Dhir, Craig, et al., 2015). A survey in a Women, Infants, and Children clinic found that child herbal use was common, especially among Hispanic children attending the clinic. Some herbs used by the children (ma huang, foxglove, anise tea, and mistletoe) have questionable safety (Kemper and Gardiner, 2016). A survey of four pediatric emergency departments found that child herbal use was common, especially among children 6 years of age and older (Taylor, Dhir, Craig, et al., 2015). Some of the herbs used by the children in the survey included chamomile, cranberry, parsley, ginger, celery, amino acids, and green tea, and herbal therapies with known toxicity included garlic, licorice, belladonna, and ginkgo biloba.

There is concern that terms often used to market supplements (such as megavitamins) may mislead parents about the actual benefits (or harm) of such therapies. The intention here is not to discredit the use of CAM such as vitamin supplements but rather to ensure safety and efficacy in children who may experience inadvertent harm. The use of various herbal therapies, or intake of herbs, is also becoming more popular; many of these have been a part of medicine since early days and are beneficial in some cases. Growing evidence from clinical samples suggests that CAM therapies are desired by families and

[g]Additional information on vegetarian diets may be found at the Vegetarian Resource Group; 410-366-8343; http://www.vrg.org. Another helpful resource is the KidsHealth website: http://kidshealth.org/parent/nutrition_center/dietary_needs/vegetarianism.html

may benefit some children with pain conditions (Groenewald, Beals-Erickson, Ralston-Wilson, et al., 2017)

Herbs known to have adverse effects in children include ephedra, comfrey, and pennyroyal; some herbs may not be harmful taken alone but may counteract or potentiate prescription medications when taken together. Parents should be fully informed of the use of herbs to ensure that there is more benefit than potential harm in the ingredients being used. Health care workers also need to be knowledgeable of the benefits or potential harm in herbs to appropriately counsel parents and address their concerns. Little research has been performed in children on many over-the-counter herbal medicines, yet some herbs are known to cause harm in children (Kemper & Gardiner, 2016). Parents should be cautioned not to exceed the upper limits of vitamin intake according to the new DRIs.[h]

SLEEP AND ACTIVITY

Total sleep decreases only slightly during the second year and averages about 11 to 12 hours a day. Most children take one nap a day but may relinquish this habit by the end of the second or third year.

Toddlers are more prone to having bedtime resistance (refusal to go to bed) and frequent night waking. Fears can be provoked by a child's daily stressors, such as pressure to toilet train, moves, sibling birth, experiences of loss, or separation from parents. A recent study found that a consistent nightly bedtime routine is associated with better sleep patterns, such as shorter sleep onset latency, decreased waking, longer total sleep, and decreased daytime behavior problems (Mindell, Li, Sadeh, et al., 2015). In addition, providing transitional objects, such as a favorite stuffed animal or blanket, can ease the child's insecurity at bedtime (see Fig. 11.2). Children may need a light snack before bedtime; a heavy meal immediately before bedtime may interfere with sleep. Other suggestions to help small children sleep better include keeping the television out of the child's room, making the hour before bedtime a quiet time of reading stories, and avoiding stimulating activities, such as computer games and roughhousing (Owens, 2016). Toddlers no longer sleeping in a crib may come out of their rooms after being put to bed. Limit prolonged bedtime rituals by defining a length of time and set of activities (one more story, one more drink). Toddlers who are too immature to respond to the measures identified may need their doorways gated.

A toddler's activity level is high, and there is rarely a problem with too little physical exercise, provided inappropriate restrictions are not instituted. Recently, however, there has been concern that decreased time spent in actual physical play and more time involved with computers and television watching have increased the tendency toward being overweight. This is especially true in large urban centers during the winter months where there may not be adequate "safe" play and physical exercise space. With increasing numbers of young children being cared for outside the home, attention to the kinds of activity provided is important. For example, children with high activity levels may benefit from an environment that encourages vigorous play whether outside or in a large indoor play area.

[h]Helpful websites for health care and consumer information concerning herbs are National Center for Complementary and Integrative Health, https://nccih.nih.gov/; American Botanical Council, http://abc.herbalgram.org; and Herb Research Foundation, http://www.herbs.org/hrfinfo.html.

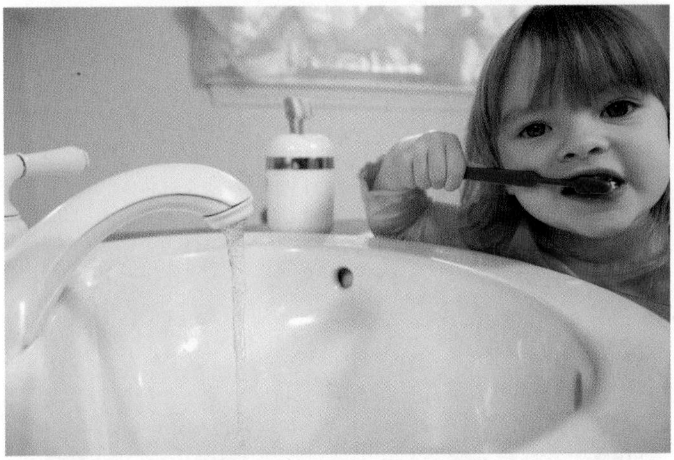

Fig. 11.6 Young children can participate in tooth brushing, but parents need to brush all of the child's teeth thoroughly. (©2011 Photos.com, a division of Getty Images. All rights reserved.)

DENTAL HEALTH

Regular Dental Examinations

The American Academy of Pediatric Dentistry (2016) recommends that every child have an oral health examination by a practitioner by 6 months old; if the child is in a high-risk category for caries, it is recommended that an initial visit to a dentist or pedodontist (pediatric dentist) occur by 6 months old or within 6 months of the eruption of the first tooth. Every child should have an established dental home by 12 months old (American Academy of Pediatric Dentistry, 2016). Initial visits to the dentist should be nontraumatizing. Because toddlers react negatively to new and potentially frightening experiences, the initial visit can center around meeting the dentist, seeing the equipment, and sitting in the chair. If the child is cooperative, the dentist may just look at the teeth but reserve a more thorough examination for another visit. Modeling, in which the child observes procedures performed on the parent or a cooperative sibling, can also be effective but may not work on all toddlers.

Plaque Removal

Oral hygiene measures should be implemented in toddlers to remove plaque, soft bacterial deposits that adhere to the teeth and cause dental caries (decay or cavities) and periodontal (gum) disease. Poor oral hygiene and poor dietary habits are associated with the development of caries in children.

The most effective methods for plaque removal are brushing and flossing. Several brushing techniques exist, although there is no universal agreement on the best method. One that is suitable for cleaning the primary teeth is the scrub method. The tips of the bristles are placed firmly at a 45-degree angle against the teeth and gums and moved back and forth in a vibratory motion. The ends of the bristles should be wiggling but not moving forcefully back and forth, which can damage the gums and enamel. All surfaces of the teeth are cleaned in this manner except the lingual (inner) surfaces of the anterior teeth. To clean these surfaces, the toothbrush is placed vertical to the teeth and moved up and down. Only a few teeth are brushed at one time, using six to eight strokes for each section. A systematic approach is used so that all surfaces are thoroughly cleaned (Fig. 11.6).

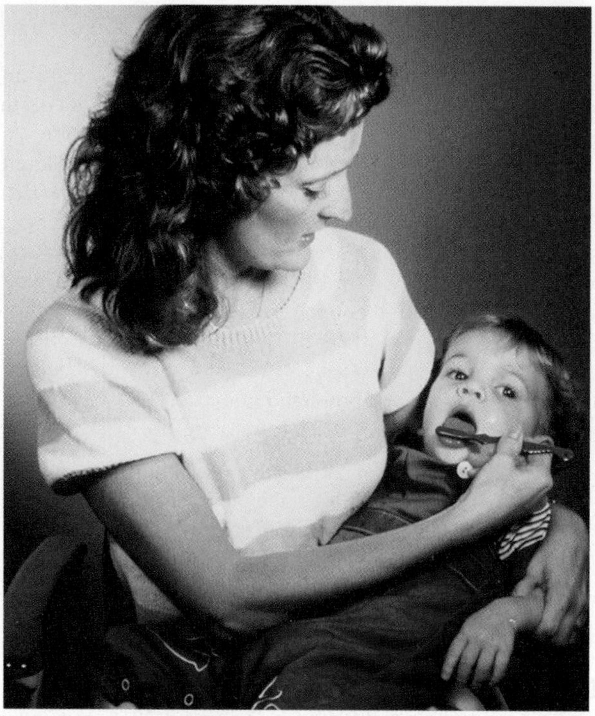

Fig. 11.7 The most effective cleaning of teeth is done by parents.

For young children, the most effective cleaning is done by parents (Fig. 11.7). Several positions can be used that facilitate access to the mouth and help stabilize the head for comfort:

- Stand with the child's back toward the adult. (When performed in front of a bathroom mirror, both the child and the adult can see what is being done in the mirror.)
- Sit on a couch or bed with the child's head resting in the adult's lap.
- Sit on the floor or a stool with the child's head resting between the adult's thighs.

Use one hand to cup the chin and one to brush the teeth. For easier access to back teeth, hold the mouth partially open. After brushing with a fluoridated paste or gel, avoid rinsing the mouth to maximize the beneficial effects of the fluoride.

NURSING TIP

- To encourage children to open their mouths, ask them to "tweet like a bird" or say "cheese" to brush the front teeth and to "roar like a lion" to brush the back teeth.
- Sing, tell stories, or talk to children during teeth cleaning to prevent boredom.

For effective cleaning, a small toothbrush with soft, rounded, multitufted nylon bristles that are short and uniform in length is recommended. Nylon bristles dry more rapidly after use and retain their shape better than natural bristles. Toothbrushes are replaced as soon as the bristles are frayed or bent. With young children, brushing may be more easily accomplished using only water because many children dislike the foam from toothpaste, and the foam interferes with visibility. Use a "smear" or "rice-size" amount of toothpaste for children younger than 3 years old (apply across the narrow width of the toothbrush, rather than along its length, to decrease the chance of applying an excessive amount); a "pea-size" amount of toothpaste should be used in children 3 to 6 years old (American Academy of Pediatric Dentistry, 2018).

After the teeth have been cleaned, they are flossed to remove plaque and debris from between the teeth and below the gum margin, where brushing is ineffective. Because young children do not have the dexterity to manipulate dental floss, parents must perform the procedure.

Ideally, the teeth should be cleaned after each meal and especially before bedtime, and the child should be given nothing to eat or drink after the night brushing except water. At times when brushing is impractical, the "swish-and-swallow" method of cleaning the mouth is taught; with a mouthful of water the child rinses the mouth and swallows, repeating the procedure three or four times.[i]

Fluoride

Fluoride supplementation should be considered for any child. Fluoride, a mineral, is found in water, foods, or drinks in which fluoridated water was used as part of the processing system. Because the water fluoridation process and manufacturing of fluoride toothpaste are almost impossible to standardize in the United States, the dosage of fluoride supplements should be determined in consultation with a medical professional (American Academy of Pediatric Dentistry, 2018). Increased fluoride ingestion leads to enamel protein retention, hypomineralization of the enamel and dentin, and disturbance of crystal formation. The effects caused by this change range from barely discernible white fiberlike lines or spots to gray-brown stains or pitted areas. Parents should be cautioned against regular use of fluoridated water or beverages such as bottled water containing fluoride if the community water supply already has an adequate amount of fluoride. Topical fluoride treatments (e.g., fluoride varnish) performed in the dental home is also effective in decreasing caries (American Academy of Pediatric Dentistry, 2018).

Dietary Factors

Diet is critical to developing good teeth because the carious process depends primarily on fermentable sugars, especially sucrose, and other carbohydrates. Refined table sugar, honey, molasses, corn syrup, and dried fruits (such as raisins) are highly cariogenic. Complex carbohydrates, such as breads, potatoes, and pasta, also contribute to caries because they lower the plaque pH. Beverages that are commonly consumed by children and adolescents and snacks are also highly cariogenic and may contribute to the incidence of overweight and obesity (American Academy of Pediatric Dentistry, 2018).

Ideally, highly cariogenic foods, especially those containing complex sugars, should be eliminated. However, because this is impractical, some suggestions can be helpful. First, *the frequency with which sugar is consumed is more important than the total amount eaten.* Therefore when sweets are eaten, they are less damaging if consumed immediately after a meal rather than as a snack between meals. When sweets are served as the dessert, the teeth can be cleaned afterward, decreasing the amount of time the sugar is in the mouth.

Second, the form of sugar (sucrose) is important. The more cariogenic foods are those that are sticky or hard because they remain in the mouth longer. Consequently, sucking on lollipops is more cariogenic than eating a chocolate bar. Sometimes the source of the sugar is "hidden," as in numerous prescription and nonprescription drugs and in many popular cereals, including the "all-natural" variety. Reading food labels is essential in eliminating sources of sucrose.

Some snacks do not contribute to tooth decay. Aged cheeses, such as cheddar, may alter the pH and delay bacterial growth. Sugarless gum chewed after eating may protect against cavities by stimulating saliva that neutralizes acid.

A special form of tooth decay in children between 18 months and 3 years old is **early childhood caries** (ECC) (historically called *nursing*

[i]More detailed information can be obtained from the American Academy of Pediatric Dentistry, http://www.aapd.org.

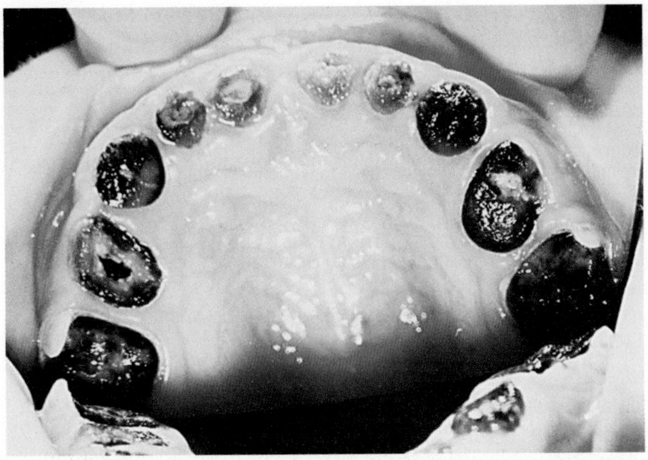

Fig. 11.8 Early childhood caries (ECC). (Courtesy of Bruce Carter, DDS, Texas Children's Hospital, Houston, TX.)

caries or *baby bottle tooth decay*) (Fig. 11.8). This often occurs when a child is routinely given a bottle of milk or juice at naptime or bedtime or uses the bottle as a pacifier while awake. Frequent nocturnal breastfeeding for prolonged periods also leads to extensive destruction of the teeth. The practice of coating pacifiers in honey can also contribute to caries and may be a potential source of botulism. As the sweet liquid pools in the mouth, the teeth are bathed for several hours in this cariogenic environment. Prolonged bottle-feeding, fruit juice consumption, lack of periodic dental examination, and nocturnal feeding contribute to significant ECC (Ozen, Van Strijp, Ozer, et al., 2016). The maxillary (upper) incisors and molars are affected most because the mandibular (lower) incisors are protected by the lower lip, tongue, and saliva. Severely decayed teeth may require the application of stainless steel bands to preserve the spacing until the permanent teeth erupt.

ECC is now considered to be an infectious disease of childhood. There is evidence that *Streptococcus mutans* is a highly cariogenic bacteria (American Academy of Pediatric Dentistry, 2016). One of the early origins of *S. mutans* is the mother's saliva; infants of mothers with high counts of the bacteria have a greater incidence of ECC. Therefore it is important to discuss oral hygiene with pregnant women because of its impact on their children's tooth development.

Prevention involves eliminating the bedtime bottle completely, feeding the last bottle before bedtime, substituting a bottle of water for milk or juice, not using the bottle as a pacifier, and never coating pacifiers in sweet substances. Juice in bottles, especially commercially available ready-to-use bottles, is discouraged; these beverages are especially damaging because the sugar is more readily converted to acid. Juice should always be offered in a cup to avoid prolonging the bottle-feeding habit. Toddlers should be encouraged to drink from a cup at the first birthday and weaned from a bottle by 14 months old. Nurses are in an excellent position to counsel parents on the dangers of this habit and other aspects of dental care.[j]

[j]Sources of information about nursing caries and other aspects of child dental health include the National Institute of Dental and Craniofacial Research, National Institutes of Health, Bethesda, MD 20892-2190; 301-496-4261; http://www.nidcr.nih.gov; American Academy of Pediatric Dentistry, 211 E. Chicago Ave., Suite 1600, Chicago, IL 60611; 312-337-2169; http://www.aapd.org; American Dental Association, 211 E. Chicago Ave., Chicago, IL 60611; 312-440-2500; http://www.ada.org/; and Canadian Dental Association, 1815 Alta Vista Drive, Ottawa, ON K1G 3Y6; 613-523-1770; http://www.cda-adc.ca.

SAFETY PROMOTION AND INJURY PREVENTION

Unintentional childhood injury was the leading cause of death among children 1 to 4 years old in 2013, accounting for 32% of all deaths in this age-group (Centers for Disease Control and Prevention, 2016). Leading causes of accidental death include suffocation for children less than 1 year of age and drowning for children 1 to 4 years of age (Centers for Disease Control and Prevention, 2016). Falls are the leading cause of nonfatal injuries among children. These deaths and injuries are preventable, and they highlight the need for public health action and education. There is evidence that one-on-one and face-to-face education in the home, safety interventions, and safety equipment are effective in reducing the number of unintentional childhood injuries that can have catastrophic results (Folger, Bowers, Dexheimer, et al., 2017).

A major factor in the critical increase of injuries during early childhood is the unrestricted freedom achieved through locomotion combined with a lack of awareness of danger within the environment. Toddlers delight in the repetitive use of gross motor skills, and with increasing age, these skills are refined. This age-group is also very curious about how things work, and exploration of previously unknown or unseen objects and places is common. Toddlers also have not fully developed an understanding of cause-and-effect principles and often are unable to gauge danger; poorly developed depth perception may also contribute to falls and tumbles, as does the general body structure of toddlers. Specific categories of injuries and appropriate prevention are best understood by associating them with the major growth and developmental achievements of this age (Table 11.2). The discussions of injuries in Chapter 13 are also relevant to safety concerns at this age.

Motor Vehicle Safety

Motor vehicle injuries cause more accidental deaths in children ages 5 to 19 years than any other type of injury and are responsible for a significant number of all accidental deaths among children ages 1 to 4 years (Centers for Disease Control and Prevention, 2016). Many of the deaths are caused by injuries within the car when restraints have not been used or age-related guidelines have not been properly followed. Unrestrained children riding in the vehicle's front seat are at the highest risk for injury. Approved restraints properly installed and applied can reduce most fatalities and injuries.

Car Restraints

Nurses are responsible for educating parents regarding the importance of car restraints and their proper use. Five types of restraints are available: (1) infant-only devices, (2) convertible models for both infants and toddlers, (3) booster seats, (4) safety belts, and (5) devices for children with special needs (see Chapter 17). Chapter 9 discusses the infant-type restraints; convertible restraints and boosters are included here. Convertible restraints are suitable for infants and toddlers in the rear-ward-facing position (Fig. 11.9). The American Academy of Pediatrics (2015) and National Highway Traffic Safety Administration now recommend that children up to 2 years old ride in rear-facing car safety seats for as long as possible or until they have outgrown the manufacturer's weight and height recommendation, then transition the child to a forward-facing safety seat with a harness in the back seat of the vehicle (Rivara & Grossman, 2016). Many rear-facing car safety seats can accommodate children weighing up to a maximum of 35 pounds (according to manufacturer specifications). Studies indicate that toddlers are safer riding in convertible seats in the rear-facing position (American Academy of Pediatrics, 2018). Another study confirmed that children 0 to 3 years of age riding properly restrained in the rear seat had significantly less risk of death than passengers in the front seats (Durbin, Jermakian, Kallan, et al., 2015).

TABLE 11.2 Injury Prevention During Early Childhood

Developmental Abilities Related to Risk of Injury	Injury Prevention
Motor Vehicles	
Walks, runs, and climbs Able to open doors and gates Can ride tricycle Can throw ball and other objects	Use federally approved car restraint per manufacturer's recommendations for weight and height. Supervise child while playing outside. Do not allow child to play on curb or behind a parked car. Do not permit child to play in pile of leaves, snow, or large cardboard container in trafficked area. Supervise tricycle riding; have child wear helmet. Limit playing in driveways with parked cars or provide physical barriers limiting access. Lock fences and doors if not directly supervising children. Teach child to obey pedestrian safety rules: • Obey traffic regulations; cross only at crosswalks and only when traffic signal indicates it is safe. • Stand back a step from the curb until it is time to cross. • Look left, right, and left again, and check for turning cars before crossing street. • Use sidewalks; when there is no sidewalk, walk on the left, facing traffic. • Wear light colors at night and attach fluorescent material to clothing.
Drowning	
Able to explore if left unsupervised Has great curiosity Helpless in water; unaware of its danger; depth of water has no significance	Supervise closely when near any source of water, including buckets. Never, under any circumstance, leave unsupervised in bathtub. Keep bathroom doors closed and lid down on toilet. Have fence around swimming pool and lock gate.[a]
Burns	
Able to reach heights by climbing, stretching, and standing on toes Pulls objects Explores any holes or opening Can open drawers and closets Unaware of potential sources of heat or fire Plays with mechanical objects	Turn pot handles toward back of stove. Place electric appliances, such as coffee maker and popcorn machine, toward back of counter. Place guardrails in front of radiators, fireplaces, and other heating elements. Store matches and cigarette lighters in locked or inaccessible area; discard carefully. Place burning candles, incense, hot foods, and cigarettes out of reach. Do not let tablecloth hang within child's reach. Do not let electric cord from iron or other appliance hang within child's reach. Cover electrical outlets with protective plastic caps. Keep electrical wires hidden or out of reach. Do not allow child to play with electrical appliance, wires, or lighters. Stress danger of open flames; teach what "hot" means. Always check bathwater temperature; adjust water heater temperature to 49°C (120°F) or lower; do not allow children to play with faucets. Apply a sunscreen when child is exposed to sunlight (all year round).
Accidental Poisoning	
Explores by putting objects in mouth Can open drawers, closets, and most containers Climbs Cannot read labels Does not know safe dose or amount	Place all potentially toxic agents, including cosmetics, personal care items, cleaning products, pesticides, and medications, out of reach or in a locked cabinet. Caution against eating nonedible items, such as plants. Replace medications or poisons immediately in locked cabinet; replace child-guard caps promptly. Administer medications as a drug, not as a candy. Do not store large surplus of toxic agents. Promptly discard empty poison containers; never reuse to store a food item or other poison. Teach child not to play in trash containers. Never remove labels from containers of toxic substances. Know number of nearest poison control center: **800-222-1222.**
Falls	
Able to open doors and some windows Goes up and down stairs Depth perception unrefined	Use window guards; do not rely on screens to stop falls. Place gates at top and bottom of stairs. Keep doors locked or use childproof doorknob covers at entry to stairs, high porch, or other elevated area, including laundry chute. Ensure safe and effective barriers on porches, balconies, decks. Remove unsecured or scatter rugs.

TABLE 11.2 Injury Prevention During Early Childhood—cont'd

Developmental Abilities Related to Risk of Injury	Injury Prevention
	Apply nonskid decals in bathtub or shower. Keep crib rails fully raised and mattress at lowest level. Place carpeting under crib and in bathroom. Keep large toys and bumper pads out of crib or play yard (child can use these as "stairs" to climb out) and then move to youth bed when child is able to climb out of crib. Avoid using mobile walker, especially near stairs. Dress in safe clothing (soles that do not "catch" on floor, tied shoelaces, pant legs that do not touch floor). Keep child restrained in vehicle; never leave unattended in vehicle or shopping cart. Never leave child unattended in high chair. Supervise at playgrounds; select play areas with soft ground cover and safe equipment.
Choking and Suffocation Puts things in mouth May swallow hard or inedible pieces of food	Avoid large, round chunks of meat, such as whole hot dogs (slice lengthwise into short pieces). Avoid fruit with pits, fish with bones, hard candy, chewing gum, nuts, popcorn, grapes, and marshmallows. Choose large, sturdy toys without sharp edges or small removable parts. Discard old refrigerators, ovens, and so on, and remove the door. Install smoke and carbon monoxide alarms; change batteries every 6 months. Develop a fire escape plan for the entire family and have drills. Keep automatic garage door transmitter in an inaccessible place. Select safe toy boxes or chests without heavy, hinged lids. Keep venetian blind cords out of child's reach. Remove drawstrings from clothing; shorten essential drawstrings to 15.24 cm (6 inches) or less. Avoid contact with round, hollow, semirigid plastic items such as half of a plastic ball.
Bodily Injury Still clumsy in many skills Easily distracted from tasks Unaware of potential danger from strangers or other people	Avoid giving sharp or pointed objects (e.g., knives, scissors, toothpicks), especially when walking or running. Do not allow lollipops or similar objects in mouth when walking or running. Teach safety precautions (e.g., to carry knife or scissors with pointed end away from face). Store all dangerous tools, garden equipment, and firearms in locked cabinet. Be alert to danger of unsupervised animals and household pets. Use safety glass on large glassed areas, such as sliding glass doors. Teach child name, address, and phone number and to ask for help from appropriate people (cashier, security guard, police officer) if lost; have identification on child (sewn in clothes, inside shoe). Teach stranger safety: • Avoid personalized clothing in public places. • Never go with a stranger. • Tell parents if anyone makes child feel uncomfortable in any way. • Always listen to child's concerns regarding others' behavior. • Teach child to say "no" when confronted with uncomfortable situations.

[a]Detailed guidelines for swimming pool safety may be found at http://www.poolsafely.gov.

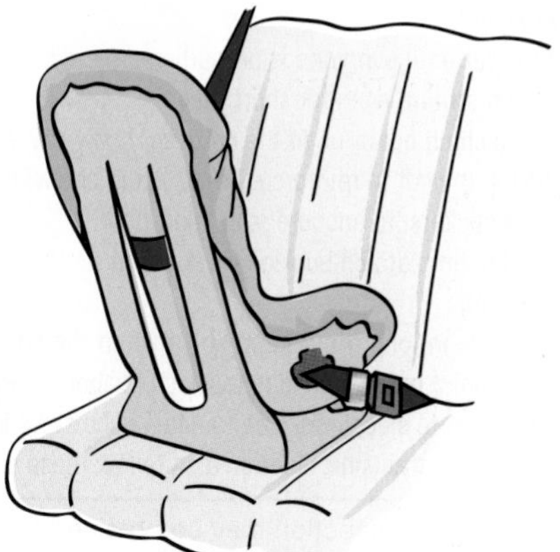

Fig. 11.9 Rear-facing convertible car seat.

Convertible restraints use different types of harness systems: a **five-point harness** that consists of a strap over each shoulder, one on each side of the pelvis, and one between the legs (all five come together at a common buckle), as well as a **padded overhead shield** that uses shoulder straps attached to a shield that is held in place by a crotch strap. With both infant and toddler restraints, it is important not to add extra blankets, head cushions, or padding between the child and the restraint straps that did not come as original equipment because these "add-ons" create spaces of air between the child and the restraint and decrease support for the back, head, and neck. Cars with free-sliding latch plates on the lap or shoulder belt require the use of a metal locking clip to keep the belt in a tight-holding position. The locking clip is threaded onto the belt above the latch plate (Fig. 11.10A). If parents have newer cars with automatic lap and shoulder belts, they need to have additional lap belts installed to properly secure the restraint.

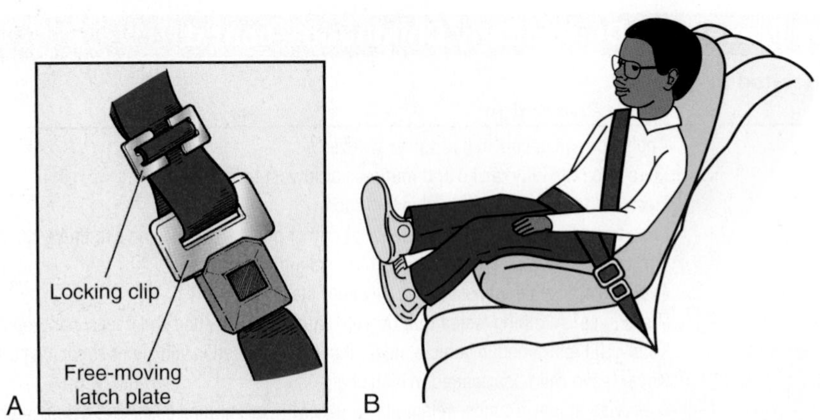

Fig. 11.10 A, Locking clip used with free-sliding lap or shoulder belt to keep the belt in a tight-holding position. B, Automobile booster seat. Note placement of the shoulder strap (away from the neck and face.)

Booster seats are not restraint systems like the convertible devices, because they depend on the vehicle belts to hold the child and booster seat in place. Three booster models have been approved by the National Highway Traffic Safety Administration: the high-back belt-positioning seat (see Fig. 11.10B), which provides head and neck support for the child riding in a vehicle seat without a head rest; the no-back belt-positioning seat, which should be used only if the vehicle seat has a head rest; and a combination seat, which converts from a forward-facing toddler seat to a booster seat. This last model is equipped with a harness for use by toddlers; the harness may be removed and a shoulder-lap belt used when the child outgrows the harness. The belt-positioning booster seats are used for children who are less than 145 cm (4 feet, 9 inches) tall and who weigh 15.9 to 36.3 kg (35 to 80 pounds), depending on the type of booster seat. In general, school-age children should ride in a belt-positioning booster seat until approximately 7 to 8 years old. Note, however, that because children's sizes vary considerably, manufacturer's recommendations should be followed regarding height and weight limitations. A booster seat should be used until the child is able to sit against the back of the seat with feet hanging down and legs bent at the knees. The belt-positioning booster model raises a child higher in the seat, moving the shoulder part of the belt off the neck and the lap portion of the belt off the abdomen onto the pelvis. Children who outgrow the convertible restraint may still be able to ride safely in a booster seat until the midpoint of the head is higher than the vehicle seat back.

Children should use specially designed car restraints until they are 145 cm (4 feet, 9 inches) in height and are between 8 and 12 years old (American Academy of Pediatrics, 2015). **Shoulder-lap safety belts** should be worn low on the hips, snug, and not on the abdominal area. Children should be taught to sit up straight to allow for proper fit. The shoulder belt is used only if it does not cross the child's neck or face.

Shoulder-only automatic belts are designed to protect adults. Children should use the manual shoulder belts in the rear seat. Air bags do not take the place of child safety seats or seat belts and can be lethal to young children. The safest area of the car for children is the back seat. Children who must ride in the passenger side of the front seat with an air bag should be positioned as far back as possible or have the air bag disabled.

For any restraint to be effective, it must be used consistently and properly. Examples of misuse include misrouting the vehicle seat belt through the restraint; failing to use the vehicle seat belt to secure the restraint; failing to use a tether strap; failing to use the restraint's harness system; and incorrectly positioning the child, especially by facing infants forward instead of rearward. To address these issues, nurses must stress correct use of car restraints and rules that ensure compliance (see Family-Centered Care box). Children riding in car safety seats are generally much better behaved than children left unrestrained, which can be a major benefit to parents and should be emphasized as an additional advantage of restraints.

The LATCH (lower anchors and tethers for children) universal child safety seat system was implemented starting in 2002 as a requirement for all new automobiles and child safety seats. This system provides uniform anchorage consisting of two lower anchorages and one upper anchorage in the rear seat of the vehicle (Fig. 11.11). When used appropriately, the top anchor (tether) strap prevents the child from pitching forward in a crash. If the tether strap is not used, up to 90% of the restraint's protection is lost. Instructions for proper installation of the tether strap and permanent bracket are included with the car restraint. New child safety seats will have a hook, buckle, strap, or other connector that attaches to the anchorage. Seat belts will no longer be used to anchor child safety seats to newer vehicles. After Fall 2002, all new cars were required to have the entire LATCH system.

FAMILY-CENTERED CARE

Using Car Safety Restraints

- Read manufacturer's directions and follow them exactly.
- Provide favorite toy, stuffed animal, or snack for child while in car seat.
- Anchor car safety seat securely to car's anchoring system and apply harness snugly to child.[a]
- Do not start the car until everyone is properly restrained.
- Always use the restraint, even for short trips.
- If child begins to climb out or undo the harness, firmly say, "No." It may be necessary to stop the car to reinforce the expected behavior. Use rewards, such as stars or stickers, to encourage cooperation.
- Encourage child to help attach buckles, straps, and shields but always double-check fastenings.
- Decrease boredom on long trips. Keep soft toys in the car for quiet play, talk to child, and point out objects and teach child about them. Stop periodically. If child wishes to sleep, make certain he or she stays in the restraint.
- Insist that others who transport children also follow these safety rules.

[a] A free car seat restraint inspection may be obtained from a SafeKids inspector. Check for local inspection SafeKids clinics or access website for information: http://www.safekids.org.

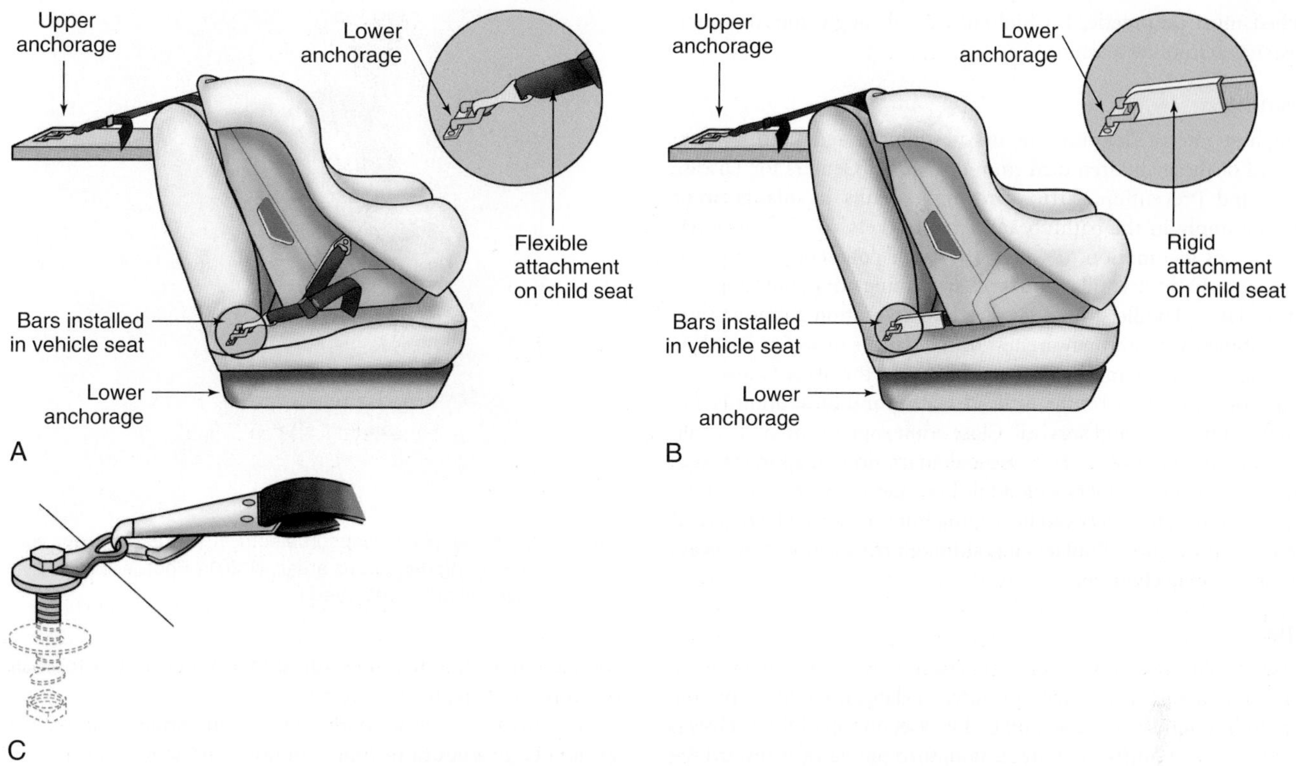

Fig. 11.11 LATCH (lower anchors and tethers for children) universal child safety seat system. **A,** Flexible two-point attachment with top tether. **B,** Rigid two-point attachment with top tether. **C,** Top tether. (Courtesy US Department of Transportation, National Highway Traffic Safety Administration.)

Children with disabilities may require a restraint system that secures them appropriately in the event of a crash. Examples of such devices include car bed restraints for infants who cannot tolerate a semireclining position and specially adapted molded-plastic chairs for children who have spica casts. The EZ-On vest is a special safety harness for larger children with poor trunk control. A HIPPO (Spica Cast) car seat is available for transporting children with spica casts; these are sold only in the United States. Additional safety restraints and a list of distributors are available at the SafetyBeltSafe U.S.A. website.[k] See also Chapter 8 for a discussion of preterm infants being discharged home and car seat evaluation.

Children should not ride in the open back of a truck. The danger of falls can be compounded by another vehicle striking the child or by the truck rolling over. In addition, leaving children unsupervised in a parked vehicle provides an opportunity for a child to release the brake or put the car in gear.

Motor Vehicle–Related Injuries

Toddlers are often involved in pedestrian traffic injuries. Because of their gross motor skills of walking, running, and climbing, and their fine motor skills of opening doors and fence gates, they are likely to be in hazardous areas when unsupervised. Unaware of danger and unable to approximate the speed of cars, they are hit by moving vehicles. Running after a ball, riding a tricycle, and playing behind a parked car are common activities that may result in a vehicular tragedy.

Toddlers playing in driveways or farmyards are at risk of back-over injury from vehicles in reverse gear. A precaution when children are playing in driveways is to attach a pole to tricycles with a bright flag that is high enough to see through an automobile's back window. Another safeguard is the use of a device that beeps when the vehicle is driven in reverse to alert children to the moving car, van, tractor, or truck. Many vehicles now include a rearview motion camera so that the driver can see the driveway clearly while backing out. Physical barriers (fences or barricades) limiting children from playing near vehicles help prevent these injuries.

A type of injury that has become more commonplace occurs when children crawl into an open trunk and pull it closed. Asphyxia may occur in such cases; therefore car trunks should not be left open when children are unsupervised. Some cars are equipped with a safety switch that can be activated from inside the trunk to open a closed trunk door.

Another automobile-related hazard for toddlers is overheating (hyperthermia) and subsequent death when left in a vehicle in hot weather (>27°C [80°F]). Small children dissipate heat poorly, and an increase in body temperature can cause death in a few hours. Since 1998, a total of 661 children have died from hyperthermia when left alone in parked cars; in 2014 the number of child deaths was 41, and it is estimated that an average of 37 children die each year from overheating in cars (Null, 2015). It is estimated that with the ambient temperature at 22° to 35.5°C (72° to 96°F), the vehicle interior temperature rises by 10.5° to 11°C (19° to 20°F) each 10 minutes, even with a window cracked (Duzinski, Barczyk, Wheeler, et al., 2014). Approximately 50% of adults who left a child in a car either forgot or were unaware that the child was still in the car (Duzinski et al., 2014). Parents are cautioned against leaving infants alone in a vehicle for *any reason.*

Preventing vehicular injuries involves protecting and educating children about the danger of moving and parked vehicles. Although preschool children are too young to be trusted to always obey, parents should emphasize looking for moving vehicles before crossing the street, recognizing the stop and go colors of traffic lights, and following traffic officers' signals. Physical barriers limiting children from playing near vehicles help prevent these injuries. Most important, what is

[k]http://www.carseat.org.

preached must be practiced. Children learn through imitation, and consistency reinforces learning.

Drowning

The highest rate of drowning occurs in children ages 1 to 4 years; one-third of these children died from drowning (Centers for Disease Control and Prevention, 2016). Drowning deaths in infants occur most commonly in the bathtub and large buckets. With well-developed skills of locomotion, toddlers can reach potentially dangerous areas, such as bathtubs, toilets, buckets, swimming pools, hot tubs, and ponds or lakes. Toddlers' intense drive for exploration and investigation combined with an unawareness of the danger of water and their helplessness in water makes drowning a viable threat. It is also one category of injury that results in death within minutes, diminishing the chance for rescue and survival. Close adult supervision of children when near any source of water is essential; many drownings in this age-group occur when a supervising adult becomes distracted. Teaching swimming and water safety can be helpful, but this cannot be regarded as sufficient protection. Pool fencing, although critical, does not always deter fast-moving children.

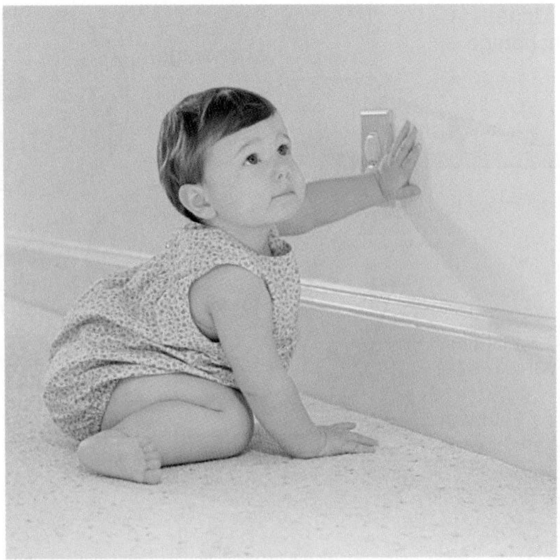

Fig. 11.12 Special plastic caps in electrical sockets prevent young fingers from exploring dangerous areas. (©2011 Photos.com, a division of Getty Images. All rights reserved.)

Burns

Toddlers' ability to climb, stretch, and reach objects above their heads makes any hot surface a potential source of danger. Children pulling pots with hot liquids, especially oil and grease, on top of themselves is a major source of burns. As a precaution, turn pot handles toward the back of the stove, and electric pots and their cords should be placed out of reach.

Other sources of heat, such as radiators, fireplaces, accessible furnaces, kerosene heaters, and wood-burning stoves, should have guards placed in front of them. Portable electric heaters must be placed in a high area, well out of reach of climbing young children. Hair curling irons and hot curlers may also be easily reached and can burn the hands of curious toddlers.

Hot objects such as candles, incense, cigarettes, pots of tea or coffee, and irons must be placed away from children. Flame burns are one of the most fatal types of burns and commonly occur when children play with matches and accidentally set themselves (and the home) on fire. To prevent flame burns, matches and lighters must be stored safely away from children, and parents need to teach children the dangers of playing with such objects. In addition, all homes should have smoke detectors installed to alert the occupants of a fire. A safety plan for immediate escape is also essential.

Electrical burns represent an immediate danger to children. Young toddlers may explore outlets with conductive articles and wires by mouthing them. Because water is an excellent conductor, the chance for a severe circumoral electrical burn is great. Electrical outlets should have protective guards plugged into them when not in use (Fig. 11.12) or be made inaccessible by having furniture placed in front of them when feasible. Children should not be allowed to play with electrical cords, appliances, or batteries.

Scald burns are the most common type of thermal injury in children. A scalding burn is often caused by high-temperature tap water, which children come in contact with as a result of turning on the hot-water faucet, falling into a bathtub of hot water, pulling hot pots onto themselves, or suffering deliberate abuse. Limiting household water temperatures to less than 49°C (120°F) is highly recommended. At this temperature, it takes 10 minutes of exposure to the water to cause a full-thickness burn. Conversely, water temperatures of 54°C (130°F), the usual setting of most water heaters, expose household members to the risk of full-thickness burns within 30 seconds. Nurses can help prevent such burns by advising parents of this common household danger and recommending that they adjust their water heaters to a safe temperature (see Chapter 31, Burns).

Sunburns are a year-round concern in certain regions. Children spend a large amount of time outdoors, and their increased mobility makes it difficult to prevent sun exposure. Sunburn can be prevented by applying a sunscreen with a sun protection factor (SPF) of 15 or greater, dressing in protective clothing (wide-brimmed hat, protective cotton clothing with a tight weave), and avoiding sun exposure between 10 AM and 2 PM.

Accidental Poisoning

Toddlers are at the highest risk for accidental poisoning because of the innate curiosity and ability to open "childproof" containers. Mouthing activity continues to be prevalent after 1 year old, and exploring objects by tasting them is part of children's curious investigation. Toddlers' curiosity and inability to understand logical consequences further place them at risk for ingesting harmful substances. Many household products, medications, and plants can be poisonous if swallowed, if they come in contact with the skin or eyes, or if they are inhaled. Although in many instances poisoning does not result in death, it may cause significant morbidity, such as esophageal stricture from lye ingestion. Toddlers can climb most heights, open most drawers or closets, and unscrew most lids. By trial and error, younger children also manage to undo tops of bottles, plastic containers, aerosol cans, and jars, including those with child-resistant lids. Newer forms of drugs, such as transdermal patches and cough-suppressant lozenges, have created additional dangers because they are not packaged with safety caps and the lozenges look like candy.

The major reason for poisoning is improper storage (Fig. 11.13). The guidelines suggested in Chapter 13 apply to children in this age-group as well. However, unlike infants, who are confined to certain heights and unable to unlatch childproof locks, young children manage to find access to many high-level, tight-security places. For this age-group, only a locked cabinet is safe.

Recent attention has focused on the use of over-the-counter medications used for cough and colds as a common cause of accidental poisonous ingestion in toddlers. Ingestion of acetaminophen is also a common cause of morbidity because it is found in many combination over-the-counter products; caregivers may unknowingly administer a dose of acetaminophen in addition to an over-the-counter drug containing the product without knowing the danger.

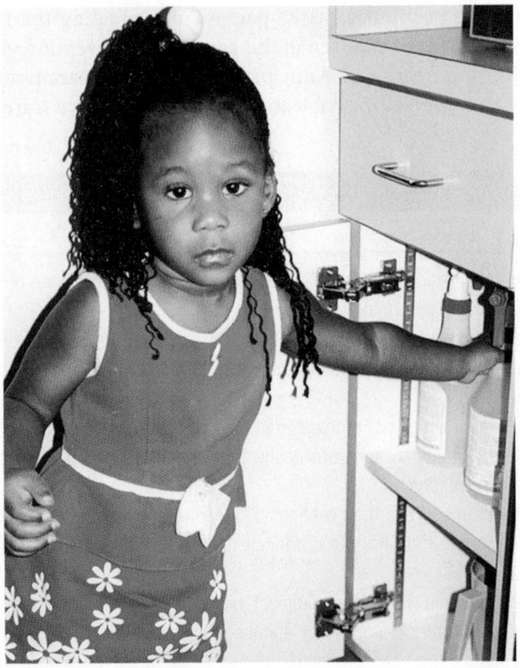

Fig. 11.13 Children are most likely to ingest substances that are on their level, such as household cleaning agents stored under sinks, rat poison, or plants.

Emergency and preventive measures for accidental poisoning are discussed in Chapter 13. Parents should have ready access to the telephone number for the poison control center (National Poison Center, 800-222-1222) and be prepared to act on the advice of the center.

Falls

Falls are still a hazard to children in this age-group, although by the later part of early childhood, gross and fine motor skills are well developed, decreasing the incidence of falls down stairs and from chairs. However, playground injuries are common. Children need to learn safety at play areas, such as no horseplay on high slides or jungle gyms, sitting on swings, and staying away from moving swings. Passive prevention includes placement of grass, sand, or wood chips under play equipment. Swing seats should be made of plastic, canvas, or rubber and have smooth or rounded edges. Slides should have inclines of no more than 30 degrees and have evenly spaced rungs for climbing.

The climbing and running of the typical toddler are complicated by the child's total disregard and lack of appreciation for danger, immature coordination, and a high center of gravity. Gates must be placed at both ends of stairs. Accessible windows must have window guards, not screens, to prevent falls to the ground below. Falling from furniture is a major cause of injury, with more children in this age-group sustaining head injuries than older children. Doors leading to stairwells or porches must be locked. A convenient type of lock is a sliding bar or hook that can be attached to the door and frame at a level higher than the child can reach. The manufacture and sale of drop-side cribs has been banned by the Consumer Product Safety Commission (2010).

Children can fall from high chairs, shopping carts, carriages, car seats, and strollers if not properly restrained or if balance changes from the placing of heavy objects. Therefore proper restraint and adequate supervision are essential. Children, especially older infants who are mobile, should not be placed in an infant seat on top of a shopping cart because the infant seat may fall off the cart; the safest place for an infant seat is inside the cart's bed.

Aspiration and Suffocation

Suffocation death rates are the leading cause of accidental death among infants less than 1 year of age (Centers for Disease Control and Prevention, 2016). Suffocation deaths usually occur in this age-group by choking on food items; other causes include choking on undersize infant pacifiers, small balls, and latex balloons (Rivara & Grossman, 2016). As noted earlier, the Consumer Pubic Safety Commission issued a ban on the manufacture of drop-side cribs in 2010 because of deaths attributed to infants becoming trapped between the crib mattress and side rail and suffocating.

Usually by 1 year old, children chew well, but they may have difficulty with large pieces of food, such as meat and whole hot dogs, and with hard foods, such as nuts. Young children cannot discard pits from fruit or bones from fish. Gel snacks that are sealed in plastic wrappers can be difficult to manage, and the plastic wrapper can be aspirated. Therefore parents must implement the same precautions as discussed for infants regarding food selection (see Chapter 9).

Play objects for toddlers must still be chosen with an awareness of danger from small parts. Large, sturdy toys without sharp edges or removable parts are safest. Balloons, coins, paper clips, pins, bells, button batteries, pull-tabs on cans, thumbtacks, nails, screws, jewelry (especially pierced earrings), and all types of pins are common household objects that can cause significant harm if swallowed or aspirated. Because of the danger of aspiration, parents should be taught emergency procedures for choking.

Suffocation from causes seen during infancy is less frequent, but old refrigerators, car trunks, ovens, and other large appliances are an ever-present threat. Toddlers can climb inside these appliances and, if they close the door behind them, be trapped inside. Removing all doors before discarding or storing old appliances prevents such tragic deaths. Toddlers may also suffocate when toy boxes with heavy, hinged lids accidentally close on their heads or necks. Advise parents of this danger and encourage them to buy storage chests with lightweight, removable covers.

Bodily Harm

Toddlers are still clumsy in many of their skills and can seriously harm themselves when walking while holding a sharp or pointed object or having food or objects (such as spoons) in their mouths. Preventing such occurrences is the best approach with toddlers. The child should be taught that when walking with a pointed object such as a knife or scissors, the pointed end is held away from the face. Dangerous garden or workshop equipment and all firearms should be stored in locked cabinets. Power lawn mowers and weed eaters are especially dangerous because they can throw rocks and other solid items (projectiles); young children should not be allowed in an area where such tools are in use, nor should they be taken for a ride on a mower or allowed to operate the device.

Toddlers are often unable to understand that all pets are not as safe as their own; because of the toddlers' height, they are often at the eye level of some dogs and may be bitten on the face. It is imperative to teach pet safety to toddlers and keep animals at a safe distance.

Safety education should include respect for firearms and their appropriate use, including nonpowder guns, such as air guns, rifles (BB and pellet), and paintball guns, which can cause serious penetrating injuries. Firearm safety devices (such as trigger locks, gun safes, and personalized locks) should be used to prevent unintentional firing of guns and subsequent injuries or fatalities.

An additional safeguard for young children is the use of safety glass in doors, windows, and tabletops, and the application of decals on glass doors and windows to reduce the likelihood of running through glass. Also, children should not be allowed to run, jump, wrestle, or play ball near glass structures.

ANTICIPATORY GUIDANCE—CARE OF FAMILIES

Understanding toddlers is fundamental to successful childrearing. Nurses, particularly those in ambulatory or child health centers, are in a favorable position to assist parents in facilitating the tasks and meeting the needs of children in this age-group. Prevention yields better results than treatment. Anticipatory guidance is paramount if one wishes to prevent future problems (see Family-Centered Care box).

FAMILY-CENTERED CARE

Guidance During the Toddler Years

12 to 18 Months Old

Prepare parents for expected behavioral changes of toddlers, especially negativism and ritualism.

Assess present feeding habits and encourage gradual weaning from bottle and increased intake of solid foods.

Stress expected feeding changes of physiologic anorexia, food fads and strong taste preferences, need for scheduled routine at mealtimes, inability to sit through an entire meal, and lack of table manners.

Assess sleep patterns at night, particularly habit of a bedtime bottle, which is a major cause of early childhood caries (ECC), and procrastination behaviors that delay hour of sleep.

Prepare parents for potential dangers of the home and motor vehicle environment, particularly motor vehicle injuries, drowning, accidental poisoning, and falling injuries; give appropriate suggestions for childproofing the home.

Discuss need for firm but gentle discipline and ways to deal with negativism and temper tantrums; stress positive benefits of appropriate discipline.

Emphasize importance for both child and parents of brief, periodic separations.

Discuss toys that use developing gross and fine motor, language, cognitive, and social skills.

Emphasize need for dental supervision, types of basic dental hygiene at home, and food habits that predispose to caries; stress importance of supplemental fluoride.

18 to 24 Months Old

Stress importance of peer companionship in play.

Explore need for preparation for additional sibling; stress importance of preparing child for new experiences.

Discuss present discipline methods, their effectiveness, and parents' feelings about child's negativism; stress that negativism is an important aspect of developing self-assertion and independence and is not a sign of spoiling.

Discuss signs of readiness for toilet training; emphasize importance of waiting for physical and psychologic readiness.

Discuss development of fears, such as darkness or loud noises, and of habits, such as security blanket or thumb sucking; stress normalcy of these transient behaviors.

Prepare parents for signs of regression in time of stress.

Assess child's ability to separate easily from parents for brief periods under familiar circumstances.

Allow parents to express their feelings of weariness, frustration, and exasperation; be aware that it is often difficult to love toddlers at times when they are not asleep!

Point out some of the expected changes of the next year, such as longer attention span, somewhat less negativism, and increased concern for pleasing others.

24 to 36 Months Old

Discuss importance of imitation and domestic mimicry and need to include child in activities.

Discuss approaches toward toilet training, particularly realistic expectations and attitude toward accidents.

Stress uniqueness of toddlers' thought processes, especially through their use of language, poor understanding of time, causal relationships in terms of proximity of events, and inability to see events from another's perspective.

Stress that discipline still must be structured and concrete and that relying solely on verbal reasoning and explanation leads to injuries, confusion, and misunderstanding.

Discuss investigation of preschool or daycare center toward completion of second year.

Advice is sometimes not the sole answer. Actual assistance, such as being available for home visiting or telephone consulting, should be part of the nurse's flexible repertoire of interventions. Whether parents are experiencing the dilemmas of rearing a first or a subsequent child, they benefit from sharing their feelings, frustrations, and satisfactions. They need adult companionship, freedom from childrearing responsibilities, and periodic separations from their children. Part of a nurse's responsibility is to provide opportunities for parents to express their feelings and to meet their physical, mental, and spiritual needs.

CLINICAL JUDGMENT AND NEXT-GENERATION NCLEX® EXAMINATION-STYLE QUESTIONS

1. The nurse is examining a 4-year-old child and is discussing the child's development with the mother. What findings would require the nurse to intervene? **Select the findings that demonstrate this period of preoperational thought in a 4-year-old child. Select all that apply.**
   A. Child may refuse to eat a food because something previously did not taste good
   B. Child will not sleep in his room because the bed was moved
   C. Child wants to be with friends to affirm their self-image
   D. Child may scold the stairs because they made him fall down
   E. Child may think he is bad because they had bad thoughts
   F. Child has a rich fantasy life

2. Parents of an 18-month-old boy is worried that he is not yet potty trained. The mother states all of her friend's children were potty trained at this age. **In discussing potty training readiness with the parents, select the findings below that indicate the toddler is ready to begin toilet training. Select all that apply.**
   A. Recognizes urge to let go and hold on and is able to communicate this sensation
   B. Has a wet diaper in the morning after sleeping through the night
   C. Demonstrates mastery of dressing and undressing self
   D. Asks parent to have wet or soiled diaper changed
   E. Says 10 or more words

3. When discussing eating practices with a mother of a 3-year-old child, which of the following actions for feeding toddlers would be included in the teaching plan so that adequate amounts of nutrients for growth and development are consumed? **Use an X for the health teaching below that is Indicated (appropriate or necessary), Contraindicated (could be harmful), or Non-Essential (makes no difference or not necessary).**

Health Teaching	Indicated	Contraindicated	Non-Essential
Avoid placing large food portions on the toddler's plate.			
Allow the child to graze on snacks during the day.			
Insist that the child sit at the table until all persons have completed their meals.			
Allow the child to make certain food choices (within reasonable limits)			
Provide meals at the same time of day as much as possible so that the toddler has a sense of consistency.			
Offer the child oranges or applies each day.			
Make the child eat all of the food provided and use disciplinary actions if the plate is not cleaned.			

4. A common cause of accidental death in children 1 to 19 years old involves motor vehicle crashes. A nurse is preparing to discharge a young infant and is reviewing the use of a care restraint seat with the parents. **Choose the most likely options for the information missing from the statements below by selecting from the lists of options provided.**
Placing a young child in a ______1______ weight-appropriate car restraint seat reduces the risk of death from a motor vehicle accident. This type of care restraint seat should be used ______2______ to assure child passenger safety.

Options for 1	Options for 2
rear-facing	until the child is 2 years of age
front seat	for as long as possible
forward-facing	until the child can sit in the front seat
booster that is a	until the child weighs 50 pounds

REFERENCES

Abraham, V. M., Gaw, C. E., Chounthirath, T., et al. (2015). Toy-related injuries among children treated in US emergency departments, 1990-2011. *Clinical Pediatrics, 54*(2), 127–137.

American Academy of Pediatric Dentistry. (2016). Policy on early childhood caries (ECC): Classifications, consequences, and preventive strategies. http://www.aapd.org/media/Policies_Guidelines/P_ECCClassifications.pdf.

American Academy of Pediatric Dentistry. (2018). Policy on use of fluoride. http://www.aapd.org/media/Policies_Guidelines/P_FluorideUse.pdf.

http://www.aapd.org/media/Policies_Guidelines/P_DietaryRec.pdf.

American Academy of Pediatrics: Updates Recommendations on Car Seats fro Children. (2018). https://www.aap.org/en-us/about-the-aap/aap-press-room/Pages/AAP-Updates-Recommendations-on-Car-Seats-for-Children.aspx.

American Academy of Pediatrics, Committee on Nutrition. (2014). *Pediatric nutrition handbook* (7th ed.). Elk Grove Village, IL: American Academy of Pediatrics.

American Academy of Pediatrics, Council on Communications and Media. (2016). Media use by young minds. *Pediatrics, 138*(5).

Barr, R. (2013). Memory constraints on infant learning from picture books, television, and touchscreens. *Child Developmental Perspective, 7*(4), 205–210 e by children younger than 2 years. *Pediatrics, 128*(5), 1040–1045.

Brazelton, T. B. (1999).How to help parents of young children: The touchpoints model. *Journal of perinatology, 19*(6 Pt 2), S6–S7.

Centers for Disease Control and Prevention. (2016). Deaths: Leading causes for 2013. *National Vital Statistics Reports, 65*(2), 1–95.

Consumer Product Safety Commission. (2010). Full-size baby cribs and non-full size baby cribs: Safety standards. *The Federal Register, 75*(248), 81766–81788.

Durbin, D. R., Jermakian, J. S., Kallan, M. J., et al. (2015). Rear seat safety: Variation in protection by occupant, crash and vehicle characteristics. *Accident Analysis and Prevention, 80*, 185–192.

Duzinski, S. V., Barczyk, A. N., Wheeler, T. C., et al. (2014). Threat of paediatric hyperthermia in an enclosed vehicle: A year-round study. *Injury prevention, 20*(4), 220–225.

Eisbach, S. S., Cluxton-Keller, F., Harrison, J., et al. (2014). Characteristics of temper tantrums in preschoolers with disruptive behavior in a clinical setting. *Journal of Psychosocial Nursing and Mental Health Services, 52*(5), 32–40.

Elder, J. S. (2016). Enuresis and voiding dysfunction. In R. M. Kliegman, B. F. Stanton, J. W. St. Geme, et al. (Eds.), *Nelson textbook of pediatrics* (20th ed). Philadelphia: Saunders/Elsevier.

El-Radhi, A. S. (2015). Management of common behavior and mental health problems. *British Journal of Nursing, 24*(11), 586–590.

Erikson, E. H. (1963). *Childhood and society* (2nd ed.). New York: Norton.

Estes, K. G., & Hay, J. F. (2015). Flexibility in bilingual infants' word learning. *Child Development, 86*(5), 1371–1385.

Feigelman, S. (2016). The second year. In R. M. Kliegman, B. F. Stanton, J. W. St. Geme, et al. (Eds.), *Nelson textbook of pediatrics* (20th ed). Philadelphia: Saunders/Elsevier.

Folger, A., Bowers, K. A., Dexheimer, J. W., et al. (2017). Education of early childhood home visiting to prevent medically attended unintentional injury. *Annals of Emergency Medicine, 70*(3), 302–310.

Fowler, J. W. (1981). *Stages of faith: The psychology of human development and the quest for meaning.* San Francisco: Harper & Row.

Groenewald, C. B., Beals-Erickson, S. E., Ralston-Wilson, J., et al. (2017). Complementary and alternative medicine use by children with pain in the United States. *Academic Pediatrics, 17*(7), 785–793.

Heyman, M. B., & Abrams, S. A. (2017). Fruit juice in infants, children, and adolescents: Current recommendations. *Pediatrics, 139*(6), e20170967.

Hines, M., Constantinescu, M., & Spencer, D. (2015). Early androgen exposure and human gender development. *Biology of Sex Differences, 6*(3).

Kemper, K. J., & Gardiner, P. M. (2016). Complementary therapies and integrative medicine. In R. M. Kliegman, B. F. Stanton, J.W. St. Geme, et al. (Eds.), *Nelson textbook of pediatrics* (20th ed). Philadelphia: Saunders/Elsevier.

Kiddoo, D. A. (2012). Toilet training children: When to start and how to train. *CMAJ, 184*(5), 511–512.

Kimball, V. (2016). The perils and pitfalls of potty training. *Pediatric Annals, 45*(6), e199–e201.

Kirkorian, H. L., Choi, K., & Pempek, T. A. (2016). Toddlers' word learning from contingent and noncontingent video on touch screens. *Child Development, 87*(2), 405–413.

Lima, N. N. R., do Nascimento, V. B., de Carvalho, S. M. F., et al. (2013). Spirituality in childhood cancer care. *Neuropsychiatric Disease and Treatment, 9*, 1539–1544.

Mindell, J. A., Li, A. M., Sadeh, A., et al. (2015). Bedtime routines for young children: a dose-dependent association with sleep outcomes. *Sleep, 38*(5), 717–722.

National Academies of Medicine. (2017). Dietary reference intakes tables and application, Washington DC. http://www.nationalacademies.org/hmd/Activities/Nutrition/SummaryDRIs/DRI-Tables.aspx.

National Center for Complementary and Integrative Health. (2018). What is complementary and alternative medicine? http://nccam.nih.gov-/health/whatiscam.

Neuman, M. E. (2011). Addressing children's beliefs through Fowler's stages of faith. *Journal of Pediatric Nursing, 26*(1), 44–50.

Null, J. (2015). Heatstroke deaths of children in vehicles. http://noheatstroke.org/.

Oesterle, M. E., Wright, K., Fidler, M., et al. (2019). Are ball pits in physical therapy clinical settings a source of pathogenic microorganisms? *American Journal of Infection Control, 47*(4).

Owens, J. A. (2016). Sleep medicine. In R. M. Kliegman, B. F. Stanton, J. W. St. Geme, et al. (Eds.), *Nelson textbook of pediatrics* (20th ed). Philadelphia: Saunders/Elsevier.

Ozen, B., Van Strijp, A. J., Ozer, L., et al. (2016). Evaluation of possible associated factors for early childhood caries and severe early childhood caries: A multicenter cross-sectional survey. *The Journal of Clinical Pediatric Dentistry, 40*(2), 118–123.

Parks, E. P., Shaikhkhalil, A., Groleau, V., et al. (2016). Feeding healthy infants, children, and adolescents. In R. M. Kliegman, B. F. Stanton, J. W. St. Geme, et al. (Eds.), *Nelson textbook of pediatrics* (20th ed). Philadelphia: Saunders/Elsevier.

Rivara, F. P., & Grossman, D. C. (2016). Injury control. In R. M. Kliegman, B. F. Stanton, J. W. St. Geme, et al. (Eds.), *Nelson textbook of pediatrics* (20th ed). Philadelphia: Elsevier/Saunders.

Rogers, J. (2013). Daytime wetting in children and acquisition of bladder control. *Nursing Children and Young People, 25*(6), 26–33.

Roseberry, S., Hirsh-Pasek, K., & Golinkoff, R. M. (2014). Skype me: Socially contingent interactions to help toddlers learn. *Child Development, 85*(3), 956–970.

Saavedra, J. M., Deming, D., Dattilo, A., et al. (2013). Lessons from the Feeding Infants and Toddlers Study in North America: What children eat, and implications for obesity prevention. *Annals of Nutrition and Metabolism, 62*(Supp.3), 27–36.

Schürmann, S., Kersting, M., & Alexy, U. (2017). Vegetarian diets in children: A systematic review. *European Journal of Nutrition, 56*(5), 1797–1817.

Schwartz, S., & Benuck, I. (2013). Strategies and suggestions for a healthy toddler diet. *Pediatric annals, 42*(9), 181–183.

Steensma, T. D., Kreukels, B. P., de Vries, A. L., et al. (2013). Gender identity development in adolescence. *Hormones and behavior, 64*(2), 288–297.

Stortelder, F. (2014). Varieties of male-sexual identity development in clinical practice: A neuropsychoanalytic model. *Frontiers in Psychology, 5*(1512).

Taylor, D. M., Dhir, R., Craig, S. S., et al. (2015). Complementary and alternative medicine use among paediatric emergency department patients. *Journal of Paediatrics and Child Health, 51*(9), 895–900.

US Department of Health and Human Services. (2016). 2015–2020 Dietary Guidelines for America. Available at https://health.gov/dietaryguidelines/2015/guidelines/.

Wu, H. Y. (2010). Achieving urinary continence in children. *Nature Reviews Urology, 7*(7), 371–377.

Zimmer-Gembeck, M. J., Webb, H. J., Thomas, R., et al. (2015). A new measure of toddler-parenting practices and associations with attachment and mothers' sensitivity, competence, and enjoyment of parenting. *Early Child Development and Care, 185*(9).

12

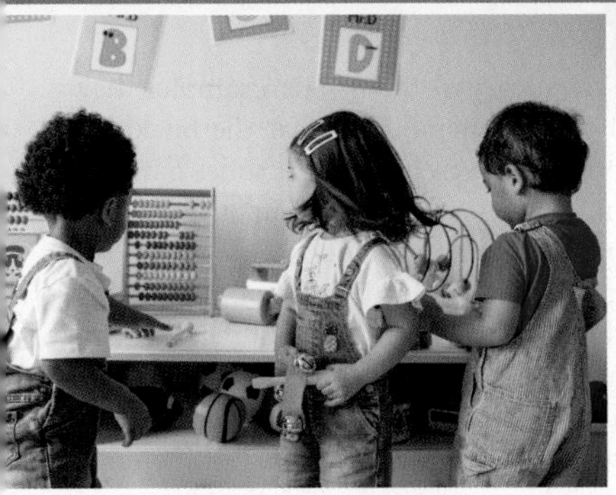

Health Promotion of the Preschooler and Family

Rebecca A. Monroe

http://evolve.elsevier.com/wong/essentials

CONCEPTS

- Development
- Behavior
- Temperament

PROMOTING OPTIMAL GROWTH AND DEVELOPMENT

BIOLOGIC DEVELOPMENT

The rate of physical growth slows and stabilizes during the preschool years. The average weight is 14.5 kg (32 pounds) at 3 years old, 16.7 kg (36.8 pounds) at 4 years old, and 18.7 kg (41.5 pounds) at 5 years old. The average weight gain per year remains approximately 2 to 3 kg (4.5 to 6.5 pounds).

Growth in height also remains steady, with a yearly increase of 6.5 to 9 cm (2.5 to 3.5 inches), and generally occurs by elongation of the legs rather than of the trunk. The average height is 95 cm (37.5 inches) at 3 years old, 103 cm (40.5 inches) at 4 years old, and 110 cm (43.5 inches) at 5 years old.

Physical proportions no longer resemble those of the squat, pot-bellied toddler. Preschoolers are slender but sturdy, graceful, agile, and posturally erect. There is little difference in physical characteristics according to gender except as dictated by such factors as dress and hairstyle.

Most organ systems can adjust to moderate stress and change. During this period, most children are toilet trained. For the most part, motor development consists of increases in strength and refinement of previously learned skills, such as walking, running, and jumping. However, muscle development and bone growth are still far from mature. Excessive activity and overexertion can injure delicate tissues. Good posture, appropriate exercise, and adequate nutrition and rest are essential for optimal development of the musculoskeletal system.

Gross and Fine Motor Skills

Walking, running, climbing, and jumping are well established by 36 months old. Refinement in eye–hand and muscle coordination is evident in several areas. At 3 years old, preschoolers can ride a tricycle, walk on tiptoe, balance on one foot for a few seconds, and do broad jumps. By 4 years old, children can skip and hop proficiently on one foot (Fig. 12.1) and catch a ball reliably. By 5 years old, children can skip on alternate feet and jump rope and begin to skate and swim.

Fine motor development is evident in the child's increasingly skillful manipulation, such as in drawing and dressing. These skills provide readiness for learning and independence for entry into school.

PSYCHOSOCIAL DEVELOPMENT

Developing a Sense of Initiative (Erikson)

After preschoolers have mastered the tasks of the toddler period, they are ready to face the developmental endeavors of the preschool period. Erikson maintained that the chief psychosocial task of this period is acquiring a sense of initiative. Children are in a stage of energetic learning. They play, work, and live to the fullest and feel a real sense of accomplishment and satisfaction in their activities. Conflict arises when children overstep the limits of their ability and inquiry and experience a sense of guilt for not having behaved appropriately. Feelings of guilt, anxiety, and fear may also result from thoughts that differ from expected behavior.

A particularly stressful thought is wishing one's parent dead. As a sense of rivalry or competition develops between the child and same-sex parent, the child may think of ways to get rid of the interfering parent. In most situations, this rivalry is resolved when the child strongly identifies with the same-sex parent and peers during the school years. However, if that parent dies before the identification process is completed, the preschooler may be overwhelmed with feelings of guilt for having wished and therefore "caused" the death. Clarifying for children that wishes cannot and do not make events occur is essential in helping them overcome their guilt and anxiety.

Development of the **superego**, or **conscience**, begins toward the end of the toddler years and is a major task for preschoolers (see Cultural Considerations box). Learning right from wrong and good from bad is the beginning of morality (see the Moral Development section later in the chapter).

COGNITIVE DEVELOPMENT

One of the tasks related to the preschool period is readiness for school and scholastic learning. Many of the thought processes of this period are crucial for achieving such readiness, and it is intentional that

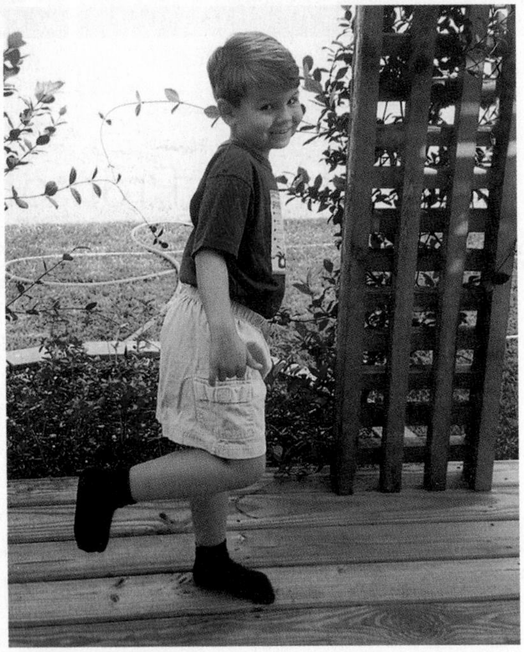

Fig. 12.1 A 4-year-old child has enough balance to stand or hop on one foot.

CULTURAL CONSIDERATIONS

Learning Sociocultural Mores

Developing a conscience implies learning the sociocultural mores of the family's heritage. Depending on the type of attitudes conveyed, children will learn not only appropriate behaviors but also tolerant, biased, or prejudicial values concerning their ethnic, religious, and social background and those of other groups. Much of this influence may remain dormant until they associate with children or adults of a different heritage. Then, depending on the group, they may be accepted or ostracized for their attitudes.

children begin school between 5 and 6 years old rather than at an earlier age.

Preoperational Phase (Piaget)

Piaget's cognitive theory does not include a period specifically for children who are 3 to 5 years old. The preoperational phase covers the age span from 2 to 7 years old and is divided into two stages: the preconceptual phase, ages 2 to 4 years, and the phase of intuitive thought, ages 4 to 7 years. One of the main transitions during these two phases is the shift from totally egocentric thought to social awareness and the ability to consider other viewpoints. However, egocentricity is still evident. (For a review of the characteristics of preoperational thought, see Chapter 11.)

Language continues to develop during the preschool period. Speech remains primarily a vehicle of egocentric communication. Preschoolers assume that everyone thinks as they do and that a brief explanation of their thinking makes the entire thought understood by others. Because of this self-referenced, egocentric verbal communication, it is often necessary to explore and understand young children's thinking through other, nonverbal approaches. For children in this age-group, the most enlightening and effective method is **play**, which becomes children's way of understanding, adjusting to, and working out life's experiences.

Preschoolers increasingly use language without comprehending the meaning of words, particularly concepts of left and right, causality, and time. Children may use the concepts correctly but only in the circumstances in which they have learned them. For example, they may know how to put on shoes by remembering that the buckle is always on the outside of the foot. However, if different shoes have no buckles, they cannot reason which shoe fits which foot. In other words, they do not understand the concept of *left* and *right.*

Superficially, **causality** resembles logical thought. Preschoolers explain a concept as they heard it described by others, but their understanding is limited. An example is the concept of time. Because time is still incompletely understood, the child interprets it according to his or her own frame of reference, such as "*a long time* means until Christmas." Consequently, time is best explained in relationship to an event, such as "Your mother will visit you after you finish your lunch." Avoiding words such as *yesterday, tomorrow, next week,* or *Tuesday* to express when an event is expected to occur and instead associating time with expected daily events help children learn about temporal relationships while increasing their trust in others' predictions.

Preschoolers' thinking is often described as **magical thinking**. Because of their egocentrism and transductive reasoning, they believe that thoughts are all-powerful. Such thinking places them in the vulnerable position of feeling guilty and responsible for bad thoughts, which may coincide with the occurrence of a wished event. Their inability to logically reason the cause and effect of illness or an injury makes it especially difficult for them to understand such events.

! NURSING ALERT

Counseling children whose parents are going through a separation or divorce should involve a discussion with the child about his or her role. Because of magical thinking, the child may believe that he or she wished the other parent away. The child should be reassured that this is not the case.

Preschoolers believe in the power of words and accept their meaning literally. An example of this type of thinking is calling children "bad" because they did something wrong. In the preschooler's mind, calling him or her "bad" means that he or she is a bad person; thus it is better to say that the child's actions were bad by saying, for example, "That was a bad thing to do."

MORAL DEVELOPMENT

Preconventional or Premoral Level (Kohlberg)

Young children's development of moral judgment is at the most basic level. They have little, if any, concern about why something is wrong. They behave because of the freedom or restriction that is placed on actions. In the punishment and obedience orientation, children (about 2 to 4 years old) judge whether an action is good or bad depending on whether it results in a reward or a punishment. If children are punished for it, the action is bad. If they are not punished, the action is good, regardless of the meaning of the act. For example, if parents allow hitting, the child will perceive that hitting is good because it is not associated with punishment.

From approximately 4 to 7 years old, children are in the stage of **naive instrumental orientation** in which actions are directed toward satisfying their needs and, less frequently, the needs of others. They have a concrete sense of justice and fairness during this period of development.

SPIRITUAL DEVELOPMENT

Children generally learn about faith and religion from significant others in their environment, usually from parents and their religious beliefs and practices. However, young children's understanding of spirituality is influenced by their cognitive level. Preschoolers have a concrete concept of a god with physical characteristics, often similar to an imaginary friend. They understand simple Bible stories, memorize short prayers, and imitate the religious practices of their parents without fully understanding the significance of these rituals. Preschoolers benefit from concrete representations of religious practices, such as picture Bible books and small statues, such as those of the Nativity scene.

Development of the conscience is strongly linked to spiritual development. At this age, children are learning right from wrong and behaving correctly to avoid punishment. Wrongdoing provokes feelings of guilt, and preschoolers often misinterpret illness as a punishment for real or imagined transgressions. It is important that children view God as one who bestows unconditional love, rather than as a judge of good or bad behavior. Spirituality and participation in religious traditions often help children cope during illness and hospitalization (Drutchas & Anandarajah, 2014).

DEVELOPMENT OF BODY IMAGE

The preschool years play a significant role in the development of body image. With increasing comprehension of language, preschoolers recognize that individuals have desirable and undesirable appearances. They recognize differences in skin color and racial identity and are vulnerable to learning prejudices and biases. They are aware of the meaning of words such as *pretty* or *ugly,* and they reflect the opinions of others regarding their own appearance. By 5 years old, children compare their size with that of their peers and can become conscious of being large or short, especially if others refer to them as "so big" or "so little" for their age. Research indicates that children as young as preschool age experience body dissatisfaction (Tatangelo, McCabe, Mellor, et al., 2016). Because these are formative years for both boys and girls, parents should instill positive principles on body image, give their children encouraging feedback regarding their appearance, and emphasize the importance of accepting individuals no matter their differences in appearance.

Despite the advances in body image development, preschoolers have poorly defined body boundaries and little knowledge of their internal anatomy. Intrusive experiences are frightening, especially those that disrupt the integrity of the skin, such as injections and surgery. They fear that if their skin is "broken," all of their blood and "insides" can leak out. Therefore bandages are critical to "keep everything from coming out."

DEVELOPMENT OF SEXUALITY

Sexual development during these years is an important phase in a person's overall sexual identity and beliefs. Preschoolers are forming strong attachments to the opposite-sex parent while identifying with the same-sex parent. Sex typing, or the process by which an individual develops the behavior, personality, attitudes, and beliefs appropriate for his or her culture and sex, occurs through several mechanisms during this period. Probably the most powerful mechanisms are childrearing practices and imitations. Gender identification is a result of complex prenatal and postnatal psychologic factors, as well as biologic, social, and genetic factors. Most children are aware of their gender and the expected sets of related behaviors by 1½ to 2½ years of age.

As sexual identity develops beyond gender recognition, modesty may become a concern. Sex-role imitation and dressing up like Mommy or Daddy are important activities. Attitudes and the responses of others to role-playing can condition children to views of themselves and others. For example, comments such as "Boys shouldn't play with dolls" can influence a boy's self-concept of masculinity.

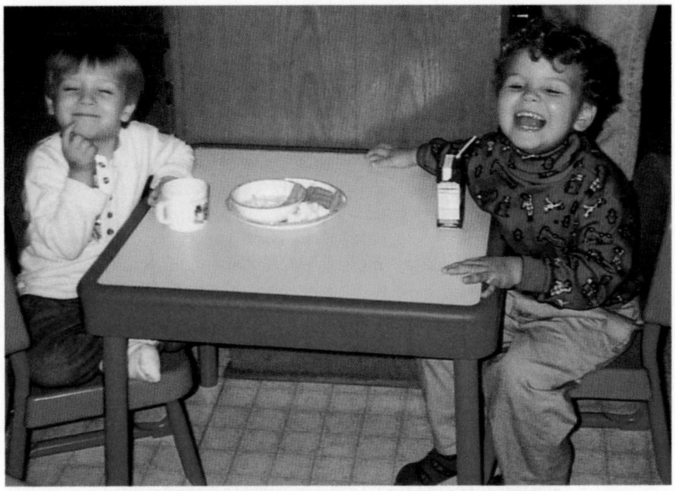

Fig. 12.2 Preschool children enjoy friends and often use nonverbal messages to communicate.

Sexual exploration may be more pronounced now than ever before, particularly in terms of exploring and manipulating the genitalia. Questions about sexual reproduction may come to the forefront in preschoolers' search for understanding (see the Sex Education sections later in this chapter and in Chapter 14).

SOCIAL DEVELOPMENT

During the preschool period, the separation-individuation process is completed. Preschoolers have overcome much of the anxiety associated with strangers and the fear of separation of earlier years. They relate to unfamiliar people easily and tolerate brief separations from their parents with little or no protest. However, they still need parental security, reassurance, guidance, and approval, especially when entering preschool or elementary school. Prolonged separation, such as that imposed by illness and hospitalization, is difficult, but preschoolers respond to anticipatory preparation and concrete explanation. They can cope with changes in daily routine much better than toddlers, although they may develop more imaginary fears. Preschoolers gain security and comfort from familiar objects, such as toys, dolls, or photographs of family members. They are able to work through many of their unresolved fears, fantasies, and anxieties through play, especially if guided with appropriate play objects (e.g., dolls, puppets) that represent family members, health care professionals, and other children.

Language

During the preschool years, language becomes more sophisticated and complex and becomes a major mode of communication and social interaction (Fig. 12.2). Through language, preschool children learn to express feelings of frustration or anger without acting them out. Both cognitive ability and environment—particularly consistent role models—influence vocabulary, speech, and comprehension. Vocabulary increases dramatically, from 300 words at 2 years old to more than 2100 words at the end of 5 years. Sentence structure, grammatical usage, and intelligibility also advance to a more adult level. Language development during these early years predicts school readiness and sets the stage for later success in school (Hammer, Morgan, Farkas, et al., 2017).

Children between 3 and 4 years old form sentences of about three or four words and include only the most essential words to convey a meaning. Such speech is often termed **telegraphic** for its brevity. Three-year-old children ask many questions and use plurals, correct

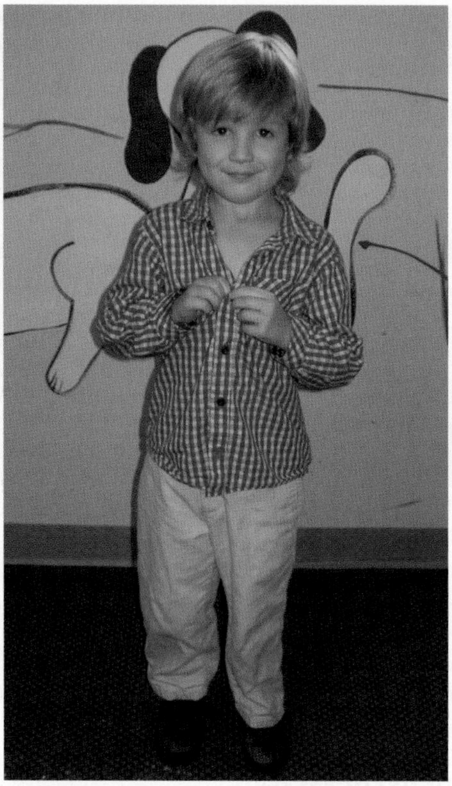

Fig. 12.3 Most preschoolers can dress themselves but need help with more difficult items of clothing.

pronouns, and the past tense of verbs. They name familiar objects, such as animals, parts of the body, relatives, and friends. They can give and follow simple commands. They talk incessantly regardless of whether anyone is listening or answering them. They enjoy musical or talking toys or dolls and imitate new words proficiently.

From 4 to 5 years old, preschoolers use longer sentences of four or five words and use more words to convey a message, such as prepositions, adjectives, and a variety of verbs. They follow simple directional commands, such as "Put the ball on the chair," but can carry out only one request at a time. They answer questions such as "What do you do when you are hungry?" by describing the appropriate action. The pattern of asking questions is at its peak, and children usually repeat a question until they receive an answer.

Personal-Social Behavior

The pervasive ritualism and negativism of toddlerhood gradually diminish during the preschool years. Although self-assertion is still a major theme, preschoolers demonstrate their sense of autonomy differently. They are able to verbalize their request for independence and perform independently because of their much-refined physical and cognitive development. By 4 or 5 years old, they need little if any assistance with dressing, eating, or toileting (Fig. 12.3). They can also be trusted to obey warnings of danger; however, 3- or 4-year-old children may exceed their boundaries at times.

Preschoolers are also much more sociable and willing to please. They have internalized many of the standards and values of the family and culture. However, by the end of early childhood, they begin to question parental values and compare them with those of their peer group and other authority figures. As a result, they may be less willing to abide by the family's code of conduct. Preschoolers become increasingly aware of their position and role within the family. Although this is a more secure age for experiencing the addition of another sibling, relinquishing the position of only or youngest child is still difficult and requires appropriate preparation (see Chapter 11, Sibling Rivalry).

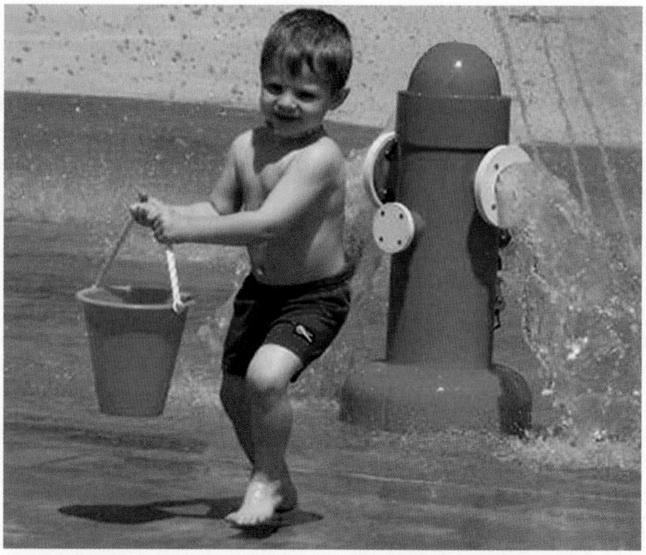

Fig. 12.4 Preschoolers enjoy play activities that promote motor skills, such as jumping and running. Water play is an exciting activity for preschoolers.

Play

Various types of play are typical of this period, but preschoolers especially enjoy associative play—group play in similar or identical activities but without rigid organization or rules. Play should provide for physical, social, and mental development.

Play activities for physical growth and refinement of motor skills include jumping, running, and climbing. Tricycles, wagons, gym and sports equipment, sandboxes, wading pools, and activities at water parks can help develop muscles and coordination (Fig. 12.4). Activities such as swimming and skating teach safety as well as muscle development and coordination. Children involved in the work of play do not require expensive toys and gadgets to keep them entertained but often enjoy playing with common household items such as a broom handle or even items adults consider junk (boxes, sticks, rocks, and dirt). The imaginative mind of the preschooler enjoys playing for play's sake.

Manipulative, constructive, creative, and educational toys provide for quiet activities, fine motor development, and self-expression. Easy construction sets, blocks of various sizes and shapes, a counting frame, alphabet or number flash cards, paints, crayons, simple carpentry tools, musical toys, illustrated books, simple sewing or handicraft sets, large puzzles, and clay are suitable toys. Electronic games and computer programs can be valuable in helping children learn basic skills, such as letters and simple words.

Probably the most characteristic and pervasive preschool activity is **imitative**, **imaginative**, and **dramatic play**. Dress-up clothes, dolls, housekeeping toys, dollhouses, play store toys, telephones, farm animals and equipment, village sets, trains, trucks, cars, planes, hand puppets, and medical kits provide hours of self-expression (Fig. 12.5). Probably at no other time is the reproduction of adult behavior so faithful and absorbing as in 4- and 5-year-old children. Toward the end of the preschool period, children are less satisfied with make-believe or pretend objects and enjoy doing the actual activity, such as cooking and carpentry.

Television and other media also have their place in children's play, although each should be only one part of children's total repertoire of social and recreational activities. Time spent watching television

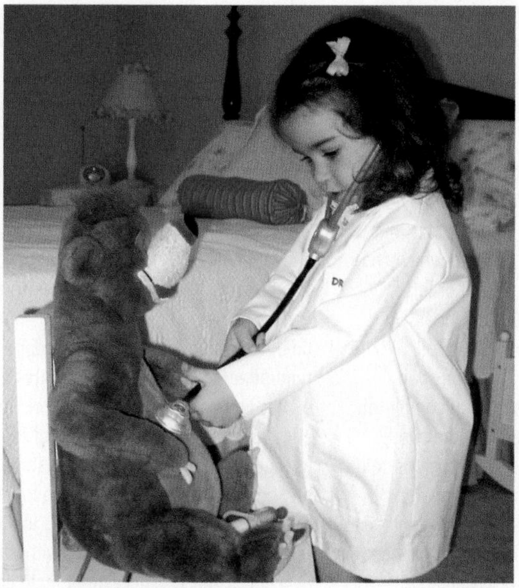

Fig. 12.5 Imaginative and imitative play is typical of preschoolers.

or engaging in digital play may limit time spent in other meaningful activities, such as reading, physical activity, and socialization (American Academy of Pediatrics Council on Communications and Media, 2016). Considering the significant increase in media accessibility through various portable electronic devices and smart phones, parents need to be aware of the potential positive and negative effects of media exposure. Parents and other caregivers should supervise the selection of programs and applications, co-view and discuss programs with their children, play games with their children, limit media exposure to 1 hour per day for children 2 to 5 years of age, and set a good example of media use (American Academy of Pediatrics Council on Communications and Media, 2016). When parents view media with their children and discuss program content, the activity can become interactive and educational.

Play is so much a part of young children's lives that reality and fantasy become blurred. Make-believe is reality during play and only becomes fantasy when the toys are put away or the dress-up clothes are removed. It is no wonder that imaginary playmates are so much a part of this age period. The appearance of imaginary companions usually occurs between 2½ and 3 years old, and for the most part, such playmates are relinquished when the child enters school.

Imaginary companions serve many purposes. They become friends in times of loneliness, they accomplish what the child is still attempting, and they experience what the child wants to forget or remember. It is not unusual for the "friend" to have myriad vices and to be blamed for wrongdoing. Sometimes the child hopes to escape punishment by saying, "My friend George broke the glass." At other times, the child may fantasize that the companion misbehaved and play the role of the parent. This becomes a way of assuming control and authority in a safe situation.

Parents often worry about the imaginary playmates, not realizing how normal and useful they are. Parents need to be reassured that the child's fantasy is a sign of health that helps differentiate make-believe and reality. Parents can acknowledge the presence of the imaginary companion by calling him or her by name and even agreeing to simple requests such as setting an extra place at the table, but they should not allow the child to use the playmate to avoid punishment or responsibility. For example, if the child blames the companion for messing up a room, parents need to state clearly that the child is the only one they see; therefore the child is responsible for cleaning up.

Children also benefit from play that occurs between them and a parent. **Mutual play** fosters development from birth through the school years and provides enriched opportunities for learning. Through mutual play, parents can provide tactile and kinesthetic experiences, maximize verbal and language abilities, and offer praise and encouragement for exploration of the world. In addition, mutual play encourages positive interactions between the parent and child, strengthening their relationship.

Table 12.1 summarizes the major developmental achievements for children 3, 4, and 5 years old.

COPING WITH CONCERNS RELATED TO NORMAL GROWTH AND DEVELOPMENT

Preschool and Kindergarten Experience

Some children are home-schooled, but many children attend some type of early childhood program, usually preschool or a daycare center. Group care has become commonplace with the large number of parents currently employed outside the home (see Chapter 9, Alternate Child Care Arrangements). The effects of early education and stimulation on children have increasingly gained recognition. (For a discussion of the effects of daycare on young children, see Chapter 2, Working Mothers). Because social development widens to include age-mates and other significant adults, preschool provides an excellent vehicle for expanding children's experiences with others. It is also excellent preparation for entrance into elementary school.

In preschool or daycare centers, children are exposed to opportunities for learning group cooperation; adjusting to sociocultural differences; and coping with frustration, dissatisfaction, and anger. If activities are tailored to provide mastery and achievement, children increasingly have feelings of success, self-confidence, and personal competence. Whether structured learning is imposed is less important than the social climate, type of guidance, and attitude toward the children that is fostered by the teacher or leader. With a teacher who is aware of preschoolers' developmental abilities and needs, children will learn from the activity that is provided. Most programs incorporate a daily schedule of quiet play, active outdoor activity, group activities such as games and projects, creative or free play, and snack and rest periods. Preschool is particularly beneficial for children who lack a peer-group experience, such as only children, and for children from impoverished homes.

One of the issues that parents face is their children's readiness for preschool or kindergarten. School readiness is influenced by many factors, including a child's social and emotional maturity, self-regulation, physical development, health status, ability to maintain attention, desire to learn, family environment, and parental support. These elements are as important as a child's academic readiness. Using a developmental screening tool that addresses cognitive (especially language), social, and physical milestones can identify children who may benefit from diagnostic testing and early intervention programs before starting school. Parents play an integral role in their children's school readiness. They can promote school readiness by engaging in the 5 Rs recommended by the American Academy of Pediatrics Early Brain and Child Development (2018) program: **R**ead with their children daily; **R**hyme, play, and cuddle with their children daily; maintain family **R**outines for meals, playtime, and sleeping; **R**eward their children with praise for successes; and establish strong, nurturing **R**elationships with their children.

Nurses and other health care workers can guide parents in selecting enriched social and educational early intervention programs, schools, and child care centers. Careful selection of early childhood education is intrinsic to future learning and development. Licensed and regulated

TABLE 12.1 Growth and Development During the Preschool Years

Physical	Gross Motor	Fine Motor	Language	Socialization	Cognition	Family Relationships
3 Years Old						
Usual weight gain of 1.8-2.7 kg (4-6 pounds) Average weight of 14.5 kg (32 pounds) Usual gain in height of 7.5 cm (3 inches) per year Average height of 95 cm (3 feet, 1½ inches) May have achieved nighttime control of bowel and bladder	Rides tricycle Jumps off bottom step Stands on one foot for few seconds Goes up stairs using alternate feet; may still come down using both feet on step Broad jumps May try to dance, but balance may not be adequate	Builds tower of 9-10 cubes Builds bridge with three cubes Adeptly places small pellets in narrow-necked bottle In drawing, copies circle, imitates cross, names what has been drawn; cannot draw stick figure but may make circle with facial features	Has vocabulary of about 900 words Uses primarily "telegraphic" speech Uses complete sentences of three or four words Talks incessantly regardless of whether anyone is paying attention Repeats sentence of six syllables Asks many questions	Dresses self almost completely if helped with back buttons and told which shoe is right or left Pulls on shoes Has increased attention span Feeds self completely Can prepare simple meals, such as cold cereal and milk Can help set table; can dry dishes without breaking any May have fears, especially of dark and going to bed Knows own gender and gender of others Play is parallel and associative; begins to learn simple games but often follows own rules; begins to share	Is in preconceptual phase Is egocentric in thought and behavior Has beginning understanding of time; uses many time-oriented expressions, talks about past and future as much as about present, pretends to tell time Has improved concept of space, as demonstrated by understanding of prepositions and ability to follow directional command Has beginning ability to view concepts from another perspective	Attempts to please parents and conform to their expectations Is less jealous of younger sibling; may be opportune time for birth of additional sibling Is aware of family relationships and sex-role functions Boys tend to identify more with father or other male figure Has increased ability to separate easily and comfortably from parents for short periods
4 Years Old						
Pulse and respiration rates decrease slightly Growth rate is similar to that of previous year Average weight of 16.5 kg (36.5 pounds) Average height of 103 cm (3 feet, 4½ inches) Length at birth is doubled Maximum potential for development of amblyopia	Skips and hops on one foot Catches ball reliably Throws ball overhead Walks downstairs using alternate footing	Uses scissors successfully to cut out picture following outline Can lace shoes but may not be able to tie bow In drawing, copies square, traces cross and diamond, adds three parts to stick figure	Has vocabulary of 1500 words or more Uses sentences of four or five words Questioning is at peak Tells exaggerated stories Knows simple songs May be mildly profane if associates with older children Obeys prepositional phrases, such as "under," "on top of," "beside," "in back of," or "in front of" Names one or more colors Comprehends analogies, such as "If ice is cold, fire is ___"	Very independent Tends to be selfish and impatient Aggressive physically as well as verbally Takes pride in accomplishments Has mood swings Shows off dramatically, enjoys entertaining others Tells family tales to others with no restraint Still has many fears Play is associative Imaginary playmates common Uses dramatic, imaginative, and imitative devices Sexual exploration and curiosity demonstrated through play, such as being "doctor" or "nurse"	Is in phase of intuitive thought Causality is still related to proximity of events Understands time better, especially in terms of sequence of daily events Unable to conserve matter Judges everything according to one dimension, such as height, width, or order Immediate perceptual clues dominate judgment Is beginning to develop less egocentrism and more social awareness May count correctly but has poor mathematic concept of numbers Obeys because parents have set limits, not because of understanding of right or wrong	Rebels if parents expect too much, such as impeccable table manners Takes aggression and frustration out on parents or siblings Do's and don'ts become important May have rivalry with older or younger siblings; may resent older sibling's privileges and younger sibling's invasion of privacy and possessions May "run away" from home Identifies strongly with parent of opposite sex Is able to run simple errands outside the home

TABLE 12.1 Growth and Development During the Preschool Years—cont'd

Physical	Gross Motor	Fine Motor	Language	Socialization	Cognition	Family Relationships
5 Years Old						
Pulse and respiration rates decrease slightly Average weight of 18.5 kg (41 pounds) Average height of 110 cm (3 feet, 7½ inches) Eruption of permanent dentition may begin Handedness is established (about 90% are right-handed)	Skips and hops on alternate feet Throws and catches ball well Jumps rope Skates with good balance Walks backward with heel to toe Jumps from height of 12 inches and lands on toes Balances on alternate feet with eyes closed	Ties shoelaces Uses scissors, simple tools, or pencil well In drawing, copies diamond and triangle; adds seven to nine parts to stick figure; prints a few letters, numbers, or words, such as first name	Has vocabulary of about 2100 words Uses sentences of six to eight words, with all parts of speech Names coins (e.g., nickel, dime) Names four or more colors Describes drawing or pictures with much comment and enumeration Knows names of days of week, months, and other time-associated words Knows composition of articles, such as "A shoe is made of ____" Can follow three commands in succession	Less rebellious and quarrelsome than at 4 years old More settled and eager to get down to business Not as open and accessible in thoughts and behavior as in earlier years Independent but trustworthy, not fool-hardy; more responsible Has fewer fears; relies on outer authority to control world Eager to do things right and to please; tries to "live by the rules" Has better manners Cares for self totally, occasionally needing supervision in dress or hygiene Not ready for concentrated close work or small print because of slight farsightedness and still unrefined eye–hand coordination Play is associative; tries to follow rules but may cheat to avoid losing	Begins to question what parents think by comparing them with age-mates and other adults May notice prejudice and bias in outside world Is more able to view other's perspective but tolerates differences rather than understanding them May begin to show understanding of conservation of numbers through counting objects regardless of arrangement Uses time-oriented words with increased understanding Cautious about factual information regarding world	Gets along well with parents May seek out parent more often than at 4 years old for reassurance and security, especially when entering school Begins to question parents' thinking and principles Strongly identifies with parent of same sex, especially boys with their fathers Enjoys activities such as sports, cooking, and shopping with parent of same sex

programs are mandated to abide by established standards, which represent minimum requirements and safeguards. Regulation is important to protect children from harm and to promote the conditions essential for a child's healthy development and learning. The National Association for the Education of Young Children serves as the model for optimal care of small children.[a]

Areas for parents to evaluate include the facility's daily program, teacher qualifications, staff-to-student ratio, discipline policy, environmental safety precautions, provision of meals, sanitary conditions, adequate indoor and outdoor space per child, and fee schedule.

[a]Information about accreditation criteria and procedures of the National Association for the Education of Young Children Accreditation of Programs for Young Children is available from the National Association for the Education of Young Children, 1313 L St. NW, Suite 500, Washington, DC 20005; 800-424-2460 or 202-232-8777; fax: 202-328-1846; http://www.naeyc.org. These criteria are excellent guidelines for evaluating preschools and daycare centers.

References from other parents help in evaluating a facility, but personal observation of the facility is recommended. Encourage parents to meet the director and some of the employees at a few facilities to make an informed choice.

Evaluation of the facility's health practices is extremely important. Preschoolers in child care centers have more illnesses than those not in child care centers, especially gastrointestinal tract and respiratory tract infections (Sacri, De Serres, Quach, et al., 2014). Nurses play an important role in infection control. Not only can they advise parents on the evaluation of a facility's sanitary practices, but they can also take an active part in educating staff in measures to minimize transmission of infection (Fig. 12.6).

Children need preparation for the preschool or kindergarten experience. For young children, it represents a change from their usual home environment and prolonged separation from their parents. Before children begin school, parents should present the idea as exciting and pleasurable. Talking to children about activities (such as painting, building with blocks, or enjoying swings and other outdoor equipment) allows children to fantasize about

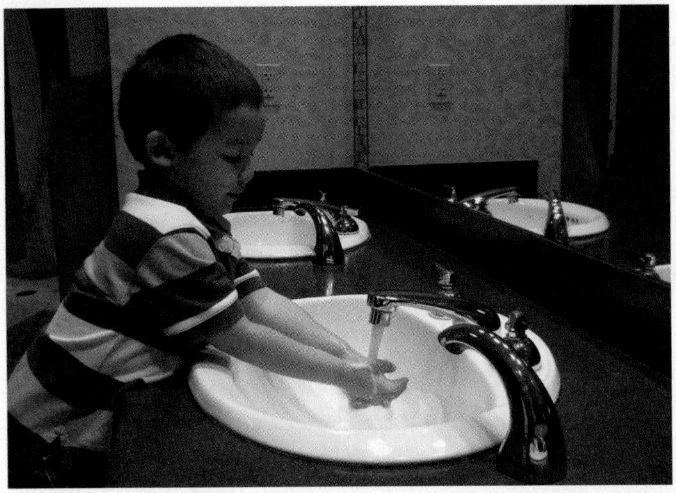

Fig. 12.6 Thorough hand washing is the single most effective method of preventing infection.

the forthcoming event in a positive manner. When the first day of school arrives, parents should behave confidently. Such behavior requires parents to have resolved their own feelings about the experience.

Parents should introduce their child to the teacher and the facility. In some instances, it is helpful for parents to remain with the child for at least part of the first day until the child is comfortable and at ease. Other specific actions that can help reduce separation anxiety include providing the school with detailed information about the child's home environment, such as familiar routines, favorite activities, food preferences, names of siblings or pets, and personal habits. Such information helps the child feel comfortable in the strange surroundings. When schools automatically request this information, the parent has a valuable clue to evaluating the quality of the program because the request represents the staff's awareness of each child's needs. Transitional objects, such as a favorite toy, may also help the child bridge the gap from home to school.

Sex Education

Preschoolers have assimilated a tremendous amount of information during their short lifetimes. Although their thinking may not be mature, they search constantly for explanations and reasons that are logical and reasonable to them. The word "why" seems to supplant the word "no," which was common in toddlerhood. It is only natural that as they learn about "me," they will also want to know "Why me?" and "How me?" Questions such as "Where do babies come from?" are as casual as "What makes it rain?" or "Who is that?" It is the way in which questions about procreation are answered that conditions children, even the youngest, to separate these questions from others about their world.

Two rules govern answering sensitive questions about topics such as sex. The first is to *find out what children know and think.* After investigating the theories children have produced as a reasonable explanation, parents can give correct information but can also help children understand why their explanation is inaccurate. Another reason for ascertaining what the child thinks before offering any information is that the "unasked for" answer may be given. For example, 4-year-old Emma asked her father, "Where did I come from?" Both parents quickly took this inquiry as a clue for offering sex education. After the explanation, Emma exclaimed, "I don't know about all that! All I know is Katie came from New York, and I want to know where I came from."

The second rule for giving information is to *be honest.* It is true that much of the correct information will be forgotten or misunderstood by the preschooler, but the correct information can be restated until the child absorbs and comprehends the facts. Even though the correct anatomic words may be hard to pronounce or even more difficult to remember, they become foundational content for explaining other concepts later on.

Honesty does not imply imparting to children every fact of life or allowing excessive permissiveness in sexual curiosity. When children ask one question, they are looking for one answer. When they are ready, they will ask about the other "unfinished" parts of the story. Sooner or later they will wonder how the "sperm meets the egg" and "how the baby gets out," but during this period it is best to wait until they ask.

Regardless of whether children are given sex education, they will engage in games of sexual curiosity and exploration. At about 3 years old, children are aware of the anatomic differences between the sexes and are curious about how the other works. This is not really "sexual" curiosity because many children are still unaware of the reproductive function of the genitalia. Their curiosity is for the eliminative function of the anatomy. Little boys wonder how girls can urinate without a penis, so they watch girls go to the bathroom. Because they cannot see anything but the stream of urine coming out, they want to observe further. "Doctor play" is often a game invented for such investigation. Little girls are no less curious about boys' anatomy. It is intriguing to closely inspect this "thing" that girls do not have.

One question that parents often have is how to handle such sexual curiosity. A positive approach is to neither condone nor condemn the sexual curiosity but to express that if children have questions, they should ask their parents. Then parents can answer their questions and encourage them to engage in some other activity. In this way, children can be helped to understand that there are ways that their sexual curiosity can be satisfied other than through playing investigative games. This in no way condemns the act but stresses alternate methods to seek solutions and answers. Allowing children unrestricted permissiveness only intensifies their anxiety and concern because exploring and searching usually yield little evidence to satisfy their curiosity.

Many excellent books on sex education are available for preschool children at public libraries. The Sexuality Information and Education Council of the United States[b] and the American Academy of Pediatrics[c] have bibliographies of suggested reading material. Parents should read the books themselves *before* giving or reading them to their children.

Another concern for some parents is **masturbation**, or self-stimulation of the genitalia. This occurs at any age for a variety of reasons and, if not excessive, is normal and healthy. It is most common at 4 years old and during adolescence. For preschoolers, it is a part of sexual curiosity and exploration. If parents are concerned about their child masturbating, it is essential for nurses to investigate the circumstances associated with the activity. Masturbation can be an expression of anxiety, boredom, or stress. In the case of excessive masturbation, it may be associated with physical or sexual abuse, exposure to sexual content, or sexual exposure (Wilkinson & John, 2018). Management of normal childhood masturbation includes parent education and reassurance, redirection of the child to other activities, and discussion with the child regarding appropriate boundaries (Wilkinson & John, 2018). In

[b]Sexuality Information and Education Council of the United States (SIECUS), 1012 14th St. NW, Suite 1108, Washington, DC 20005; 202-265-2405; http://www.siecus.org.

[c]American Academy of Pediatrics, 345 Park Blvd., Itasca, IL 60143; 800-433-9016; http://www.aap.org.

addition, parents should emphasize that masturbation is a private act, thus teaching children socially acceptable behavior.

Fears

A great number and variety of real and imagined fears are present during the preschool years, including fear of the dark, being left alone (especially at bedtime), animals (particularly large dogs), ghosts, sexual matters (castration), and objects or persons associated with pain. The exact cause of children's fears is unknown. Parents often become perplexed about handling the fears because no amount of logical persuasion, coercion, or ridicule will send away the ghosts, bogeymen, monsters, and devils. Inappropriate television viewing by preschoolers may increase fears and anxieties because of the inability to separate reality-based experiences from fantasy portrayed on television.

The concept of **animism**, ascribing lifelike qualities to inanimate objects, helps explain why children fear objects. For example, a child may refuse to use the toilet after watching a television commercial in which the toilet bowl is portrayed as turning into a monster and swallowing a child.

Preschoolers also experience fear of annihilation. Because of poorly defined body boundaries and improved cognitive abilities, young children develop concerns related to loss of body parts. They fear losing body parts with certain medical procedures (such as an intravenous insertion or cast application on a limb) and may see these procedures as real threats to their existence.

The best way to help children overcome their fears is by actively involving them in finding practical methods to deal with the frightening experience. This may be as simple as keeping a night-light on in the child's bedroom for assurance that no monsters lurk in the dark. Exposing children to the feared object in a safe situation also provides a type of conditioning, or **desensitization**. For instance, children who are afraid of dogs should never be forced to approach or touch one, but they may be gradually introduced to the experience by watching other children play with the animal. This type of modeling, with others demonstrating fearlessness, can be effective if the child is allowed to progress at his or her own rate.

Usually by 5 or 6 years old, children relinquish many of their fears. Explaining the developmental sequence of fears and their gradual disappearance may help parents feel more secure in handling preschoolers' fears. Sometimes fears do not subside with simple measures or developmental maturation. When children experience severe fears that disrupt family life, professional help is necessary.

Stress

Although for parents the preschool years generally are less troublesome than toddlerhood, this period of life presents children with many unique stresses. Some, such as fears, are innate and stem from preschoolers' unique understanding of the world. Others are imposed, such as beginning school. Although minimal amounts of stress are beneficial during the early years to help children develop effective coping skills, excessive stress is harmful. Young children are especially vulnerable because of their limited capacity to cope. Expression of frustration, fear, or anxiety is hampered by inadequate expressive language.

To help parents deal with stress in their children's lives, they must be aware of signs of stress and be helped to identify the source. Any number of stressors may be present, such as the birth of a sibling, marital discord, separation and divorce, relocation, or illness.

The best approach to dealing with stress is prevention—monitoring the amount of stress in children's lives so that levels do not exceed their coping ability. In many instances, structuring children's schedules to allow rest and preparing them for change, such as entering school, are sufficient measures.

Aggression

The term **aggression** refers to behavior that attempts to hurt a person or destroy property. Aggression differs from anger, which is a temporary emotional state, but anger may be expressed through aggression. Hyperaggressive behavior in preschoolers is characterized by unprovoked physical attacks on other children and adults, destruction of others' property, frequent intense temper tantrums, extreme impulsivity, disrespect, and noncompliance. Aggression is influenced by a complex set of biologic, sociocultural, and familial variables. Factors that tend to increase aggressive behavior are gender, frustration, modeling, and reinforcement.

Aggressive behavior is exhibited by both boys and girls; however, research indicates that types of aggression differ between genders. Physical aggression peaks in both genders during the second year of life (Dayton & Malone, 2017), but boys exhibit more physical aggression than girls during preschool years (Kung, Li, Golding, et al., 2018). Relational aggression is exhibited at similar rates in boys and girls (Casper & Card, 2017). However, relational aggression has been shown to be the more typical form of aggression in girls, when assessing the proportion of relational aggression to total aggression exhibited (Björkqvist, 2018).

Frustration, or the continual thwarting of self-satisfaction by disapproval, humiliation, punishment, or insults, can lead children to act out against others as a means of release. Especially if they fear their parents, these children will displace their anger on others, particularly peers and other authority figures. This type of aggression often applies to children who are well behaved at home but have a discipline problem at school or are bullies among their playmates.

Modeling, or imitating the behavior of significant others, is a powerful influencing force in preschoolers. Children who see their parents being physically aggressive, through discipline or abuse, are observing behavior they come to know as acceptable and therefore may exhibit this behavior with others (Fleckman, Drury, Taylor, et al., 2016). Another aspect of modeling is the "double standard" for acceptable conduct. For example, in some families, aggression is synonymous with masculinity, and boys are encouraged to defend themselves. Media exposure is also a significant source for modeling at this impressionable age. Studies have found a positive correlation between violent media exposure and aggressive behavior; therefore parents should be encouraged to supervise programming and protect young minds from virtual violence (Hill, 2016). The American Academy of Pediatrics Council on Communications and Media (2016) offers recommendations for healthy media exposure.

Reinforcement can also shape aggressive behavior. Sometimes the reward for aggression is negative (e.g., punishment) yet reinforcing, because it brings attention. For example, children who are ignored by a parent until they hit a sibling or the parent learn that this act garners attention.

When children exhibit extreme behaviors, such as aggression, parents may be concerned about the need for professional help. Generally, the difference between normal and problematic behavior is not the behavior itself but its **quantity** (number of occurrences), **severity** (interference with social or cognitive functioning), **distribution** (different manifestations), **onset** (when behavior started), and **duration** (at least 4 weeks).[d]

[d]Information on child development and behavior can be obtained through the American Academy of Pediatrics, Section on Developmental and Behavioral Pediatrics, http://www.aap.org/en-us/about-the-aap/Sections/Section-on-Developmental-and-Behavioral-Pediatrics/Pages/SODBP.aspx.

Speech Problems

The most critical period for speech development occurs between 2 and 4 years of age. During this period, children are using their rapidly growing vocabulary faster than they can produce the words. Failure to master sensorimotor integrations results in stuttering or stammering as children try to say the word they are already thinking about. This dysfluency in speech pattern is common during language development in children 2 to 5 years old (Nelson, 2013). Stuttering affects boys more frequently than girls, has been shown to have a genetic link, and usually resolves during childhood (Perez & Stoeckle, 2016). The National Institute on Deafness and Other Communication Disorders (2016) encourages parents and caregivers of children who stutter to speak slowly and in a relaxed manner, refrain from interrupting the child's speech, resist completing the child's sentences, and take time to listen attentively.

The best therapy for speech problems is prevention and early detection. Common causes of speech problems include hearing deficits, developmental delay, and physical conditions that impede normal speech production. Referral for further evaluation and treatment may be necessary to prevent a problem from interfering with learning. Anticipatory preparation of parents for expected developmental norms may allay caregiver concerns.

Children pressured into producing sounds ahead of their developmental level may develop **dyslalia** (articulation problems) or revert to using infantile speech. Prevention involves educating parents on the usual achievement of speech production during childhood. The **Denver Articulation Screening Exam** is an excellent tool for assessing articulation skills of a child and for explaining to parents the expected progression of sounds.

PROMOTING OPTIMAL HEALTH DURING THE PRESCHOOL YEARS

Well-child visits during the preschool years are essential to provide guidance for health promotion and disease prevention. Table 12.2 defines the National Quality Forum's pediatric quality indicator for well-child visits.

TABLE 12.2 Pediatric Quality Indicator: Well-Child Visits

Well-Child Visits in the Third, Fourth, Fifth, and Sixth Years of Life[a]	
Measure	The percentage of children 3-6 years of age who received one or more well-child visits during the measurement year.
Numerator	At least one well-child visit during the measurement year.
Denominator	Number of children ages 3-6 years as of December 31 of the measurement year who had well-child visits This measure supports regular well-care visits and provides opportunities for nurses to share information with the child's parents or guardian on health and safety issues, nutrition and physical activity, and how to handle illness and emergencies.

[a]Endorsed by the National Quality Forum NQF #1516 and 2019 Core Set of Children's Health Care Quality Measures for Medicaid and CHIP, https://www.medicaid.gov/federal-policy-guidance/downloads/cib112018.pdf.

Nutrition

Healthy nutrition during childhood should include consuming a variety of nutrient-dense foods, ensuring sufficient energy to promote growth and development, and balancing energy intake with energy expenditure to maintain a healthy weight (American Academy of Pediatrics Committee on Nutrition, 2014). Nutritional needs vary depending on age, gender, activity level, and state of health. For moderately active preschoolers, the estimated daily caloric requirement ranges from 1200 to 1400 calories (US Department of Health and Human Services & US Department of Agriculture, 2015). Fluid requirements depend on activity level, climatic conditions, and state of health. Protein requirements increase during childhood, and the recommended intake for preschoolers is 13 to 19 g/day (US Department of Health and Human Services & US Department of Agriculture, 2015).

The American Academy of Pediatrics Committee on Nutrition (2014) recommends that the total fat intake, averaged over several days, be reduced to 30% of total caloric intake for children 2 years old and older. This recommendation is important in the prevention of childhood obesity and the development of other morbidities. Research has shown that the development of obesity, cardiovascular disease, diabetes, and cancer can be influenced by early eating patterns (Macaulay, Donovan, Leask, et al., 2014).

While limiting fat consumption, it is also important to ensure that diets contain adequate nutrients. This can be done simultaneously, as in the following example regarding calcium. The Recommended Dietary Allowance for calcium for children 1 to 3 years old is 700 mg/day, and the recommendation for children 4 to 8 years old is 1000 mg/day (US Department of Health and Human Services & US Department of Agriculture, 2015). Milk and dairy products are excellent sources of calcium. Low-fat and nonfat milk may be substituted for higher fat choices, so that the quantity of milk may remain the same while limiting fat intake overall.

Excessive consumption of fruit juices and sugar-sweetened beverages has been associated with dental caries, obesity, and adverse cardiometabolic effects (Rader, Mullen, Sterkel, et al., 2014). The American Academy of Pediatrics (2017) recommends limiting the intake of 100% fruit juice to 4 oz/day for children 1 to 3 years of age and 4 to 6 oz/day for children 4 to 6 years of age. Parents should be educated regarding nonnutritious fruit drinks, which usually contain less than 10% fruit juice yet are often advertised as healthy and nutritious. While counseling parents regarding moderation in fruit juice consumption, providers should offer suggestions for more appropriate sources of nutrients, such as ascorbic acid, folate, and potassium. In young children, intake of carbonated beverages that are acidic or that contain high amounts of sugar is also known to contribute to dental caries; large amounts of nonnutritive calories in such beverages may also displace or preclude intake of nutrients necessary for growth.

In 2011 the US Department of Agriculture released a new food guide system called MyPlate (US Department of Agriculture, 2018). This system is comprehensive and provides information for developing a healthy lifestyle at an early age. Parents can develop customizable food plans created specifically for children 2 to 5 years old and access information on growth during the preschool years, healthy eating habits, physical activity, and food safety at http://www.ChooseMyPlate.gov. Parents can use this information to assist their children in making healthy lifestyle choices and to help prevent adverse health

! NURSING ALERT

Obesity in young children has increased significantly over the past 3 decades, so efforts to provide a healthy diet and to encourage physical activity should begin early to help children achieve optimal health (Khalsa, Kharofa, Ollberding, et al., 2017). The 5-2-1-0 framework provides a foundation for patient education regarding healthy lifestyle choices. This framework refers to five or more servings of fruits and vegetables per day, 2 hours or less of screen time per day, a minimum of 1 hour of physical activity per day, and 0 servings of sugar-sweetened beverages (Khalsa, Kharofa, Ollberding, et al., 2017).

conditions secondary to poor nutrition. The importance of role modeling by parents cannot be overemphasized in regard to food intake and dietary habits; if parents will not eat a particular food or if their dietary habits are poor, their children are likely to develop the same habits.

Some preschoolers still have food habits that are typical of toddlers, such as food fads and strong taste preferences. When children reach 4 years of age, they seem to enter another period of finicky eating, which is generally characteristic of the more rebellious behavior of children in this age-group. As with toddlers, small portions of each item being served should be offered. The practice of having children remain at the table until the plate is clean should be avoided, because this may contribute to overeating and the development of poor eating habits that contribute to poor health later in life. By 5 years old, children are more agreeable to trying new foods, especially if they are encouraged by an adult who allows them to help with food preparation or experiment with a new taste or different dish (Fig. 12.7). Mealtimes can become battlegrounds if parents expect perfect table manners.[e] Usually 5-year-old children are ready for the social side of eating, but 3- or 4-year-old children still have difficulty sitting quietly through long family meals.

The amount and variety of foods consumed by young children vary greatly from day to day. Consequently, parents sometimes worry about the quantity and quality of food that preschoolers consume. In general, the quality is much more important than the quantity, a fact that should be stressed during nutritional counseling.

One way to reduce parental concern is advising parents to keep a weekly record of everything the child eats. In particular, the parents can measure the amount of food, such as setting aside a half cup of vegetables and serving the child from this premeasured amount, to provide a more accurate estimate of food intake at each meal. When parents look at the food record at the end of the week, they are usually amazed by how much the child has consumed. In general, preschoolers consume only slightly more than toddlers, or about half an adult's portion.

SLEEP AND ACTIVITY

Sleep patterns vary widely, but the average preschooler sleeps about 12 hours a night and infrequently takes daytime naps. Waking during the night is common throughout early childhood. An appropriate and consistent bedtime, nap schedule (as needed), and bedtime routine can help prevent and treat common sleep problems and night wakings experienced by young children (Honaker & Meltzer, 2014).

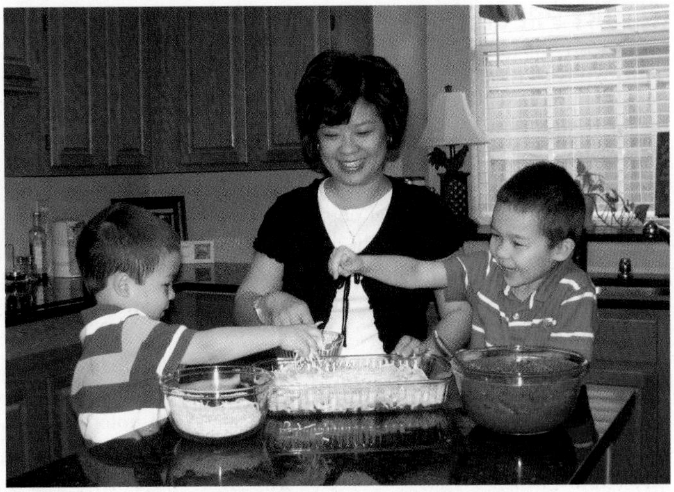

Fig. 12.7 Preschool-age children enjoy helping adults and are more likely to try new foods if they can assist in the preparation.

Motor activity levels continue to be high and allow preschoolers to explore their environment, begin learning physical games and sports, and interact with others. Sedentary activities, such as television and video or computer games, are increasingly appealing and can become unhealthy substitutes for active play.

Preschoolers' increased gross motor abilities and coordination allow them to engage in many physical activities, if only at a novice level. At this age, children benefit from a variety of both structured and unstructured play activities. Whether young children should begin formalized training in an activity at this early age is controversial. Training programs must consider the child's physical and psychologic immaturity, and readiness to participate in organized sports should be determined individually. The decision to participate should be based on the child's, not the parents', motivation and enjoyment. Another key aspect of organized play for preschoolers is that the activity is developmentally appropriate and occurs in a nonthreatening, fun, and safe environment.

DENTAL HEALTH

By the beginning of the preschool period, the eruption of the deciduous (primary) teeth is complete. Dental care is essential to preserve these temporary teeth and to teach good dental habits (see Chapter 11). Although preschoolers' fine motor control is improved, they still require assistance and supervision with brushing, and flossing should be performed by parents. Professional care and prophylaxis, especially fluoride supplements (if needed), should be continued. The frequency of professional dental care should be based on a child's individual needs and risk assessment, including family oral health habits, dental development, presence or absence of dental disease, special health care needs, and dietary habits (American Academy of Pediatric Dentistry, 2016). For children cared for away from home, parents should be encouraged to monitor the dental care provided by others, including minimizing cariogenic food and beverages in the diet. Trauma to teeth during this period is common, and prompt evaluation by a dentist is warranted if oral trauma occurs. Preservation of the space previously occupied by an avulsed tooth is necessary for proper eruption of the secondary tooth.

---

[e]Excellent resources for parents related to mealtimes with toddlers and preschoolers include Jana, L. A., & Shu, J. (2012). *Food fights: Winning the nutritional challenges of parenthood armed with insight, humor, and a bottle of ketchup* (2nd ed.). Elk Grove Village, IL: American Academy of Pediatrics; and Satter, E. (1987). *How to get your kid to eat: but not too much.* Boulder, CO: Bull Publishing Co.

INJURY PREVENTION

Because of improved gross and fine motor skills, coordination, and balance, preschoolers are less prone to falls than toddlers. They tend to be less reckless; listen more to parental rules; and are aware of potential dangers, such as hot objects, sharp instruments, and dangerous heights. Putting objects in the mouth as part of exploration has all but ceased, although accidental poisoning is still a danger. Pedestrian motor vehicle injuries increase because of activities such as playing in parking lots, driveways, or streets; riding tricycles, bicycles, and other play vehicles; running after balls; or forgetting safety regulations when crossing streets.

In general, the guidelines suggested for injury prevention in Chapter 11, Table 11.2 apply to children in this age-group as well. However, emphasis is now on education concerning safety and potential hazards in addition to appropriate protection. This period is an excellent time for enforcing the use of safety items, such as bicycle helmets to prevent head trauma; children are less likely to warm to the idea later in life because of peer pressure. Because preschoolers are great imitators, it is essential that parents set a good example by "practicing what they preach." Children quickly observe discrepancies in what they are told to do and what they see others do. Establishing good habits at this time, such as wearing protective equipment, can create long-term safety behaviors.

ANTICIPATORY GUIDANCE—CARE OF FAMILIES

The preschool years present fewer childrearing difficulties than do the earlier years, and this stage of development is facilitated by appropriate anticipatory guidance in the areas already discussed (see Family-Centered Care box). There is a shift in childrearing practices from protection to education. Whereas injury prevention previously focused on safeguarding the immediate environment with less emphasis on reasoning, now the protective guardrails or electrical outlet caps may be replaced by verbal explanations of why danger exists and how to avoid it.

During this period, an emotional transition between parent and child occurs. Although children are still attached to their parents and accept all of their values and beliefs, they are nearing the period of life when they will question previous teachings and prefer the companionship of peers. Entry into school marks a separation from home for parents as well as for children. Parents may need help in adjusting to this change, particularly if one parent has focused his or her daily activities primarily on home responsibilities. All family members must adjust to changes, which is part of the process of growth and development.

FAMILY-CENTERED CARE

Guidance During Preschool Years

3 Years Old

Prepare parents for child's increasing interest in widening relationships.
Encourage enrollment in preschool.
Emphasize importance of setting limits.
Prepare parents to expect exaggerated tension-reduction behaviors, such as need for a "security blanket."
Encourage parents to offer child choices.
Prepare parents to expect marked changes at 3½ years old when child becomes insecure and exhibits emotional extremes.
Prepare parents for normal dysfluency in speech and advise them to avoid focusing on the pattern.
Prepare parents to expect extra demands on their attention as a reflection of child's emotional insecurity and fear of loss of love.
Warn parents that the equilibrium of a 3-year-old child will change to the aggressive, out-of-bounds behavior of a 4-year-old child.
Inform parents to anticipate a more stable appetite with more food selections.
Stress need for protection and education of child to prevent injury (see Chapter 11, Safety Promotion and Injury Prevention).

4 Years Old

Prepare parents for more aggressive behavior, including motor activity and offensive language.
Prepare parents to expect resistance to parental authority.
Explore parental feelings regarding child's behavior.
Suggest some type of respite for primary caregivers, such as placing child in preschool for part of the day.
Prepare parents for child's increasing sexual curiosity.
Emphasize the importance of realistic limit setting on behavior and appropriate disciplinary techniques.
Prepare parents for the highly imaginative 4-year-old child who indulges in "tall tales" (to be differentiated from lies) and develops imaginary playmates.
Prepare parents to expect nightmares or an increase in them.
Provide reassurance that a period of calmness begins at 5 years of age.

5 Years Old

Inform parents to expect a tranquil period at 5 years of age.
Help parents prepare the child for entrance into school environment.
Make certain that immunizations are up to date before child enters school.
Suggest that unemployed parental caregivers consider own activities when children begin school.
Suggest swimming lessons for the child.

CLINICAL JUDGMENT AND NEXT-GENERATION NCLEX® EXAMINATION-STYLE QUESTIONS

1. During a routine visit for a girl who is 3 years of age, the nurse notices the child is withdrawn and does not interact even when asked direct questions. The nurse performs a history and assessment and notes the following. **Select all the child's history and assessment findings that would require the nurse to further investigate. Select all that apply.**
   A. Able to say about 100 words.
   B. Unable to form sentences.
   C. Knows familiar objects.
   D. Can follow simple commands.
   E. The mother states the child is unable to express feelings

2. When a 4-year-old is in the hospital for pneumonia, the parent tells the nurse, "I think there is something wrong with him because he is so skinny." The mother asks the nurse to explain what a healthy preschooler of this age should look like. The nurse provides health teaching on specific growth parameters for a preschooler to the parent. **Use an X for the health teaching statement below that is Indicated (appropriate or necessary), Contraindicated (could be harmful), or Non-Essential (makes no difference or not necessary).**

Health Teaching	Indicated	Contraindicated	Non-Essential
Most preschoolers weigh between 10 and 12 kilograms.			
The legs of a preschooler, rather than the trunk, increase in length, which may make him look thinner.			
Preschoolers usually keep that pot-bellied appearance until about 6 years old.			
Most preschoolers gain 1/2 to 1 pound per year.			
Most preschoolers do not like to get their weight and height checked.			

3. At the clinic appointment, a 5-year-old's mother wants to discuss several concerns about her daughter with the nurse. The daughter weighs 41 pounds; the mother thinks she is too thin. The mother also states the child questions everything she says and often talks back to her at home. She is worried that the child is becoming a "bad child" and will not follow the conservative views of their family. The child seems withdrawn and quiet, but when the nurse asks a direct question, she readily answers it. **Choose the most likely options for the information missing from the statements below by selecting from the lists of options provided.**
   Based on the mother's concern and the child's assessment, the nurse teaches the mother that children this age begin to ____1____ what parents think and notice ____2____ in the outside world. They begin to view other's ____3____ as well as their own.

Options for 1	Options for 2	Options for 3
understand	prejudice	perspective
wonder	change	likeness
question	colors	family
fear	hardship	status
realize	temperature	parents

4. A five- year old boy is being seen by the nurse for a well-child exam. The mother states the child is gaining weight and is concerned. The nurse's assessment findings include the following. **Select all the child's history and assessment findings that would require the nurse to further investigate. Select all that apply.**
   A. A nutrition intake assessment reveals an average daily intake of 1700 calories.
   B. The child sometimes eats less at one meal and then compensates at another meal or with a snack.
   C. The child drinks fruit juice at every meal and often has a juice box between meals.
   D. The nutrition intake assessment reveals 40% of his calories are from fat consumption.
   E. The child does not want to try new foods at home.

REFERENCES

American Academy of Pediatric Dentistry. (2016). Guideline on periodicity of examination, preventive dental services, anticipatory guidance/counseling, and oral treatment for infants, children, and adolescents. *Pediatric Dentistry, 38*(6), 133–141.

American Academy of Pediatrics. (2017). *Fruit juice and your child's diet*. Retrieved from https://www.healthychildren.org/English/healthy-living/nutrition/Pages/Fruit-Juice-and-Your-Childs-Diet.aspx.

American Academy of Pediatrics Committee on Nutrition. (2014). Carbohydrate and dietary fiber. In R. E. Kleinman F. R., & Greer (Eds.), *Pediatric nutrition* (7th ed.). Elk Grove Village, IL: American Academy of Pediatrics.

American Academy of Pediatrics Council on Communications and Media. (2016). Media and young minds. *Pediatrics, 138*(5), e20162591.

American Academy of Pediatrics Early Brain and Child Development. (2018). *Early education – the 5 R's*. Retrieved from https://www.aap.org/en-us/advocacy-and-policy/aap-health-initiatives/EBCD/Pages/Five.aspx.

Björkqvist, K. (2018). Gender differences in aggression. *Current Opinion in Psychology, 19*, 39–42.

Casper, D. M., & Card, N. A. (2017). Overt and relational victimization: A meta-analytic review of their overlap and associations with social-psychological adjustment. *Child Development, 88*(2), 466–483.

Dayton, C. J., & Malone, J. C. (2017). Development and socialization of physical aggression in very young boys. *Infant Mental Health Journal, 38*(1), 150–165.

Drutchas, A., & Anandarajah, G. (2014). Spirituality and coping with chronic disease in pediatrics. *Rhode Island Medical Journal, 97*(3), 26–30.

Fleckman, J. M., Drury, S. S., Taylor, C. A., et al. (2016). Role of direct and indirect violence exposure on externalizing behavior in children. *Journal of Urban Health, 93*(3), 479–492.

Hammer, C. S., Morgan, P., Farkas, G., et al. (2017). Late talkers: A population-based study of risk factors and school readiness consequences. *Journal of Speech, Language, and Hearing Research, 60*(3), 607–626.

Hill, D. L. (2016). *How virtual violence impacts children's behavior: Steps for parents*. HealthyChildren.org. Retrieved from https://www.healthychildren.org/English/family-life/Media/Pages/Virtual-Violence-Impacts-Childrens-Behavior.aspx.

Honaker, S. M., & Meltzer, L. J. (2014). Bedtime problems and night wakings in young children: An update of the evidence. *Paediatric Respiratory Reviews, 15*(4), 333–339.

Khalsa, A. S., Kharofa, R., Ollberding, N. J., et al. (2017). Attainment of '5-2-1-0' obesity recommendations in preschool-aged children. *Preventive Medicine Reports, 8*, 79–87.

Kung, K. T. F., Li, G., Golding, J., et al. (2018). Preschool gender-typed play behavior at age 3.5 years predicts physical aggression at age 13 years. *Archives of Sexual Behavior, 47*(4), 905–914.

Macaulay, E. C., Donovan, E. L., Leask, M. P., et al. (2014). The importance of early life in childhood obesity and related diseases: A report from the 2014 Gravida Strategic Summit. *Journal of Developmental Origins of Health and Disease, 5*(6), 398–407.

National Institute on Deafness and Other Communication Disorders. (2016). National Institutes of Health. Stuttering. Retrieved from https://www.nidcd.nih.gov/health/stuttering.

Nelson, A. (2013). *Stuttering. KidsHealth*. Retrieved from https://kidshealth.org/en/parents/stutter.html#.

Perez, H. R., & Stoeckle, J. H. (2016). Stuttering: Clinical and research update. *Canadian Family Physician, 62*(6), 479–484.

Rader, R. K., Mullen, K. B., Sterkel, R., et al. (2014). Opportunities to reduce children's excessive consumption of calories from beverages. *Clinical Pediatrics, 53*(11), 1047–1054.

Sacri, A. S., De Serres, G., Quach, C., et al. (2014). Transmission of acute gastroenteritis and respiratory illness from children to parents. *The Pediatric Infectious Disease Journal, 33*(6), 583–588.

Tatangelo, G., McCabe, M., Mellor, D., et al. (2016). A systematic review of body dissatisfaction and sociocultural messages related to the body among preschool children. *Body Image, 18*, 86–95.

US Department of Agriculture. (2018). *A brief history of USDA food guides*. Retrieved from https://www.choosemyplate.gov/brief-history-usda-food-guides.

US Department of Health & Human Services and U.S. Department of Agriculture.. (2015). *2015-2020 Dietary guidelines for Americans* (8th ed.). Retrieved from. http://health.gov/dietaryguidelines/2015/guidelines/.

Wilkinson, B., & John, R. M. (2018). Understanding masturbation in the pediatric patient. *Journal of Pediatric Health Care, 32*(6), 639–643.

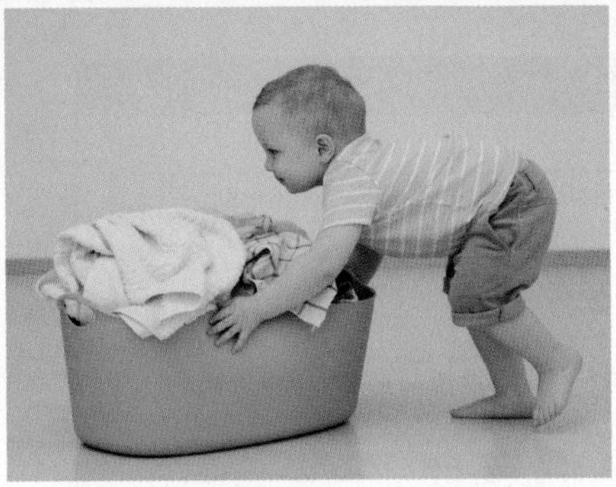

13

Health Problems of Toddlers and Preschoolers

Elizabeth A. Duffy

http://evolve.elsevier.com/wong/essentials

CONCEPTS

- Sleep
- Ingestion of Injurious Agents
- Abuse

SLEEP PROBLEMS

The preschool years are a prime time for sleep disturbances. Children may have trouble going to sleep, wake during the night, have difficulty resuming sleep after waking during the night, have nightmares or sleep terrors, or prolong the inevitable bedtime through elaborate rituals. Such sleep disturbances are typically related to increasing autonomy, negative sleep associations, nighttime fears, inconsistent bedtime routines, and lack of limit setting (Mindell & Williamson, 2018).

Media use can also contribute to sleep disturbances. Research has revealed a direct correlation between sleep problems in preschool children and evening media use, as well as daytime exposure to violent media content (Bathory & Tomopoulus, 2017). Specific sleep problems associated with media use include delayed sleep onset, nightmares, night wakings, daytime tiredness, and difficulty waking in the morning (Bathory & Tomopoulus, 2017). In addition to limiting the duration of television viewing and other media exposure, parents should ensure that all types of media are age appropriate and are not too frightening or overstimulating.

Consequences of inadequate sleep include daytime tiredness, behavior changes, hyperactivity, difficulty concentrating, impaired learning ability, poor control of emotions and impulses, and strain on family relationships (Bathory & Tomopoulus, 2017). Nurses should incorporate assessment of sleep patterns and education about the development of healthy sleep behaviors into every well-child visit. Recommendations for handling a sleep disturbance are offered only after a thorough assessment. Cultural traditions may dictate sleep practices contrary to certain well-accepted professional recommendations. Thus parents may not perceive particular sleep habits as problematic (see Cultural Considerations box).

Interventions differ greatly; for example, **nightmares** and **sleep terrors** require different approaches (Table 13.1). For children who delay going to bed, a recommended approach involves counseling consistent bedtime ritual and emphasizing the normalcy of this type of behavior in young children. Parents should ignore attention-seeking behavior, and the child should not be taken into the parents' bed or allowed to stay up past a reasonable hour. Other measures that may be helpful include keeping a light on in the room, providing transitional objects such as a favorite toy, or leaving a drink of water by the bed.

CULTURAL CONSIDERATIONS

Co-Sleeping

Many experts recommend that infants and children be trained to always sleep in their own crib or bed. However, co-sleeping, or the "family bed" (in which parents allow the children to sleep with them), is an accepted cultural practice among many African American and Asian families (Ward & Doering, 2014; Ward, Robb, & Kanu, 2016). Others who have adopted co-sleeping include parents who believe that co-sleeping promotes parent-child bonding, parents who think that co-sleeping diminishes their child's nighttime fears or other sleep disturbances, and mothers who are breastfeeding. Co-sleeping may be a practical solution to limited numbers of bedrooms or beds in lower-socioeconomic families. Controversy exists regarding the medical, developmental, and social advantages and disadvantages of co-sleeping. Studies have indicated that co-sleeping is associated with sleep problems, such as frequent night wakings, poor sleep quality, and decreased length of sleep (Covington, Armstrong, & Black, 2018). Parents who are considering co-sleeping should fully investigate the potential risks and benefits. Health care providers should be proactive in discussing sleeping arrangements with families at each visit to ensure children's safety and healthy sleep habits.

Helping children slow down before bedtime also reduces resistance to going to bed. One approach is to establish soothing, limited rituals that signal readiness for bed, such as a bath or story. Parents can reinforce the pattern by stating, "After this story, it is bedtime," and consistently carrying through the routine. If anticipated extra stimulation (e.g., having visitors arrive at the children's bedtime) disrupts this routine, it is advisable to settle children in bed beforehand.

INGESTION OF INJURIOUS AGENTS

Since the passage of the Poison Prevention Packaging Act of 1970, which requires that certain potentially hazardous drugs and household products be sold in child-resistant containers, the incidence of poisonings in children has decreased dramatically. However, despite these advances, poisoning remains a significant health concern, with most cases occurring between 1 and 5 years of age (Lee, Connolly, & Calello, 2017). Although pharmaceuticals (such as analgesics, cough and cold

TABLE 13.1 Comparison of Nightmares to Sleep Terrors

Characteristics	Nightmares	Sleep Terrors
Description	A scary dream; takes place during rapid eye movement (REM) sleep and is followed by full waking	A partial arousal from very deep sleep (state IV, non-REM sleep)
Time of distress	After dream is over, not during nightmare itself, child wakes and cries or calls	During terror itself, child screams and thrashes; afterward is calm
Time of occurrence	In second half of night, when dreams are most intense	Usually 1-4 h after falling asleep, when non-REM sleep is deepest
Child's behavior	Crying in younger children, fright in all; behaviors persistent even though child is awake	Initially may sit up, thrash, or run in bizarre manner, with eyes bulging, heart racing, and profuse perspiring; may cry, scream, talk, or moan; shows apparent fright, anger, or obvious confusion, which disappears when child is fully awake
Responsiveness to others	Is aware of and reassured by another's presence	Is not very aware of another's presence, is not comforted, and may push person away and scream and thrash more if held or restrained
Return to sleep	May be considerably delayed because of persistent fear	Usually rapid; often difficult to keep child awake
Description of dream interventions	Yes (if old enough) Accept dream as real fear Sit with child; offer comfort, assurance, and sense of protection Avoid forcing child back to his or her own bed Consider professional counseling for recurrent nightmares unresponsive to above approaches	No memory of dream or of yelling or thrashing Observe child for a few minutes, without interfering, until child becomes calm or wakes fully Intervene only if necessary to protect child from injury Guide child back to bed if needed Stress to parents that sleep terrors are a normal, common phenomenon in preschoolers that requires relatively little intervention

Modified from Haupt, M., Sheldon, S. H., & Loghmanee, D. (2013). Just a scary dream? A brief review of sleep terrors, nightmares, and rapid eye movement sleep behavior disorder. *Pediatric Annals, 42*(10), 211–216.

preparations, topical preparations, antibiotics, vitamins, gastrointestinal preparations, hormones, and antihistamines) are frequently the agents of poisonings, a variety of other substances can also poison children. The most frequently ingested poisons include the following (Lee et al., 2017)[a]

- Cosmetics and personal care products (deodorants, makeup, perfume, cologne, mouthwash)
- Medications (acetaminophen, acetylsalicylic acid, ibuprofen, opioid analgesics, benzodiazapines, amphetamines)
- Household cleaning products (bleaches, laundry pods, disinfectants)
- Foreign bodies, toys, and miscellaneous substances (desiccants, thermometers, bubble-blowing solutions)

Many poisonings reflect the ready accessibility of the products in the home, which is where more than 90% of poisonings occur (Lee et al., 2017). In a recent review of the American Association of Poison Control Centers, more than 60% of exposures to plants occurred in children 5 years old and younger (Bronstein, Spyker, Cantilena, et al., 2012; Petersen, 2011). Box 13.1 lists common poisonous and nonpoisonous plants.

The developmental characteristics of young children predispose them to poisoning by ingestion. Infants and toddlers explore their environment through oral experimentation. Because their sense of taste is not discriminating at this age, they ingest many unpalatable substances. In addition, toddlers and preschoolers are developing autonomy and initiative, which increases their curiosity and noncompliant behavior. Imitation is also a powerful motivator, especially when combined with a lack of awareness of danger.

This section is primarily concerned with the immediate emergency treatment of ingestion of injurious agents. Box 13.2 summarizes

[a]The most common substances in each category are in parentheses. Substances ingested are not necessarily the most toxic but often are readily available.

BOX 13.1 Poisonous and Nonpoisonous Plants

Poisonous Plants (Toxic Parts)

Apple (leaves, seeds)
Apricot (leaves, stem, seed pits)
Azalea (all parts)
Buttercup (all parts)
Castor oil plant (bean or seeds—extremely toxic)
Cherry (wild or cultivated) (twigs, seeds, foliage)
Daffodil (bulbs)
Dumb cane (dieffenbachia) (all parts)
Elephant ear (all parts)
Foxglove (leaves, seeds, flowers)
Holly (berries)
Hyacinth (bulbs)
Ivy (leaves)
Mistletoe[a] (berries, leaves)
Oak tree (acorn, foliage)
Philodendron (all parts)
Plum (pit)
Poinsettia[b] (leaves)
Poison ivy, poison oak (leaves, stems, sap, fruit, smoke from burning plants)
Pokeweed, pokeberry (roots, berries, leaves [when eaten raw])
Pothos (all parts)
Rhubarb (leaves)
Tulip (bulbs)
Wisteria (seeds, pods)
Yew (all parts)

Nonpoisonous Plants

African violet
Aluminum plant
Asparagus fern
Begonia
Boston fern
Christmas cactus
Coleus
Gardenia
Grape ivy
Jade plant
Piggyback plant
Poinsettia[b]
Prayer plant
Rose
Rubber tree
Snake plant
Spider plant
Swedish ivy
Wax plant
Weeping fig
Zebra plant

[a]Eating one or two berries or leaves is probably nontoxic.
[b]Mildly toxic if ingested in massive quantities.

BOX 13.2 Selected Poisonings in Children

Corrosives (Strong Acids or Alkalis)

Drain, toilet, and oven cleaners
Electric dishwasher detergent (liquid because of higher pH, is more hazardous than granular)
Mildew remover
Batteries
Clinitest tablets
Denture cleaners
Bleach

Clinical Manifestations

Severe burning pain in the mouth, throat, and stomach
White, swollen mucous membranes; edema of the lips, tongue, and pharynx (respiratory obstruction)
Coughing, hemoptysis
Drooling and inability to clear secretions
Signs of shock
Anxiety and agitation

Comments

Household bleach is a frequently ingested corrosive but rarely causes serious damage.
Liquid corrosives are easily ingested and cause more damage than granular or solid preparations. Liquids may also be aspirated, causing upper airway injury.
Solid products tend to stick to and burn tissues, causing localized damage.

Treatment

Inducing emesis is contraindicated (vomiting redamages the mucosa).
Contact the PCC immediately. If the PCC or medical advice and treatment not immediately available, it may be appropriate to dilute corrosive with water or milk (usually ≤120 ml [4 oz]).
Do not neutralize. Neutralization can cause an exothermic reaction (which produces heat and causes increased symptoms or produces a thermal burn in addition to a chemical burn).
Maintain patent airway as needed.
Administer analgesics.
Give oral fluids when tolerated.
Esophageal stricture may require repeated dilations or surgery.

Hydrocarbons

Gasoline
Kerosene
Lamp oil
Mineral seal oil (found in furniture polish)
Lighter fluid
Turpentine
Paint thinner and remover (some types)

Clinical Manifestations

Gagging, choking, and coughing
Burning throat and stomach
Nausea
Vomiting
Alterations in sensorium, such as lethargy
Weakness
Respiratory symptoms of pulmonary involvement

- Tachypnea
- Cyanosis
- Retractions
- Grunting

Comments

Immediate danger is aspiration (even small amounts can cause bronchitis and chemical pneumonia).
Gasoline, kerosene, lighter fluid, mineral seal oil, and turpentine cause severe pneumonia.

Treatment

Inducing emesis is generally contraindicated.
Gastric decontamination and emptying are questionable even when the hydrocarbon contains a heavy metal or pesticide; if gastric lavage must be performed, a cuffed endotracheal tube should be in place before lavage because of a high risk of aspiration.
Symptomatic treatment of chemical pneumonia includes high humidity, oxygen, hydration, and acetaminophen.

Acetaminophen

Clinical Manifestations

Occurs in four stages post ingestion:

1. 0 to 24 hours
   - Nausea
   - Vomiting
   - Sweating
   - Pallor
2. 24 to 72 hours
   - Patient improves
   - May have right upper quadrant abdominal pain
3. 72 to 96 hours
   - Pain in right upper quadrant
   - Jaundice
   - Vomiting
   - Confusion
   - Stupor
   - Coagulation abnormalities
   - Sometimes renal failure, pancreatitis
4. More than 5 days
   - Resolution of hepatoxicity or progress to multiple organ failure
   - May be fatal

Comments

This is the most common accidental drug poisoning in children.
Toxicity occurs from acute ingestion. Toxic dose is 150 mg/kg or greater in children.

Treatment

Antidote *N*-acetylcysteine (Mucomyst) is equally effective given intravenously or orally. When given orally may first be diluted in fruit juice or soda because of the antidote's offensive odor. An antiemetic may be given if vomiting occurs.
Given as 1 loading dose followed by 17 additional doses in different dosages. IV administration is given as a continuous infusion.

Aspirin (Acetylsalicylic Acid)

Clinical Manifestations

Acute poisoning (early symptoms):

- Nausea
- Hyperventilation
- Vomiting
- Tinnitus

Acute poisoning (later symptoms):

- Hyperactivity
- Fever

Continued

BOX 13.2 Selected Poisonings in Children—cont'd

- Confusion
- Seizures
- Renal failure
- Respiratory failure

Chronic poisoning:

- Same as listed above but subtle onset and nonspecific symptoms (often mistaken for viral illness)
- Bleeding tendencies

Comments

May be caused by acute ingestion (severe toxicity occurs with 300 to 500 mg/kg).

May be caused by chronic ingestion (i.e., >100 mg/kg/day for ≥2 days); can be more serious than acute ingestion.

Time to peak serum salicylate level can vary with enteric aspirin or the presence of concretions (bezoars).

Treatment

Hospitalization is necessary for severe toxicity.

Activated charcoal is given as soon as possible (unless contraindicated by altered mental status). If bowel sounds are present, may be repeated every 4 hours until charcoal appears in the stool.

Lavage will not remove concretions of ASA.

Sodium bicarbonate transfusions are used to correct metabolic acidosis, and urinary alkalinization may be effective in enhancing elimination; hypokalemia may interfere with achieving urinary alkalinization.

Be aware of the risk for fluid overload and pulmonary edema.

Use external cooling for hyperpyrexia.

Administer anticonvulsants if seizures present.

Provide oxygen and ventilation for respiratory depression.

Administer vitamin K for bleeding.

In severe cases, hemodialysis (not peritoneal dialysis) is used.

Iron

Mineral supplement or vitamin containing iron

Clinical Manifestations

Occurs in five stages (may have significant variation in symptoms and their progression):

1. Within 6 hours (if child does not develop gastrointestinal symptoms in 6 hours, toxicity is unlikely)
   - Vomiting
   - Hematemesis
   - Diarrhea
   - Hematochezia (bloody stools)
   - Abdominal pain
   - Severe toxicity may have tachypnea, tachycardia, hypotension, coma
2. Latency period—up to 24 hours of apparent improvement
3. 12 to 24 hours
   - Metabolic acidosis
   - Fever
   - Hyperglycemia
   - Bleeding
   - Seizures
   - Shock
   - Death (may occur)
4. 2 to 5 days
   - Jaundice
   - Liver failure
   - Hypoglycemia
   - Coma
5. 2 to 5 weeks
   - Pyloric stenosis or duodenal obstruction may occur secondary to scarring.

Comments

Factors related to frequency of iron poisoning include:

- Widespread availability
- Packaging of large quantities in individual containers
- Lack of parental awareness of iron toxicity
- Resemblance of iron tablets to candy (e.g., M&Ms)

Toxic dose is based on the amount of elemental iron ingested. Common preparations include ferrous sulfate (20% elemental iron), ferrous gluconate (12%), and ferrous fumarate (33%). Ingestions of 20 to 60 mg/kg are considered mildly to moderately toxic, and >60 mg/kg is severely toxic and may be fatal.

Treatment

Hospitalization is required when more than mild gastroenteritis is present.

Use whole bowel irrigation if radiopaque tablets are visible on abdominal x-ray; may need to be given via nasogastric tube.

Emesis empties the stomach more effectively than lavage.

Activated charcoal does not absorb iron.

Chelation therapy with deferoxamine should be used in severe intoxication (may turn urine red to orange).

If IV deferoxamine is given too rapidly, hypotension, facial flushing, rash, urticaria, tachycardia, and shock may occur; stop the infusion, maintain the IV line with normal saline, and notify the practitioner immediately.

Plants

Poisonous plants listed in Box 13.1

Clinical Manifestations

Depends on type of plant ingested.

May cause local irritation of oropharynx and entire gastrointestinal tract.

May cause respiratory, renal, and central nervous system symptoms.

Topical contact with plants can cause dermatitis.

Comments

Plants are some of the most frequently ingested substances.

They rarely cause serious problems, although some plant ingestions can be fatal.

Plants can also cause choking and allergic reactions.

Treatment

Wash from skin or eyes.

Provide supportive care as needed.

ASA, Acetylsalicylic acid; *IV*, intravenous; *PCC*, poison control center.

specific management of corrosive, hydrocarbon, acetaminophen, salicylate, iron, and plant poisoning. Because of the importance of lead poisoning among young children, ingestion of lead is discussed separately. Appropriate suggestions for poison prevention are discussed later in the chapter.

PRINCIPLES OF EMERGENCY TREATMENT

A poisoning may or may not require emergency intervention, but in every instance medical evaluation is necessary to initiate appropriate action. Advise parents to call the **poison control center (PCC)** *before* initiating any intervention. Parents should post the local PCC telephone number (usually listed in the front of the telephone directory) near each phone in the house[b] (see Emergency Treatment box).

EMERGENCY TREATMENT

Poisoning

1. Assess the victim:
   - Initiate cardiorespiratory support if needed (circulation, airway, breathing).
   - Assess mental status; reevaluate routinely.
   - Take vital signs; reevaluate routinely.
   - Evaluate for possibility of concomitant trauma or illness; treat prior to initiation of gastric decontamination.
2. Terminate exposure:
   - Empty mouth of pills, plant parts, or other material.
   - Flush any body surface (including the eyes) exposed to a toxin with large amounts of moderately warm water or saline.
   - Remove contaminated clothes, including socks and shoes, and jewelry. Ensure protection of rescuers and health care workers from exposure.
   - Bring victim of an inhalation poisoning into fresh air.
3. Identify the poison:
   - Question the victim and witnesses.
   - Observe the circumstances surrounding the poisoning (e.g., location, activity before ingestion).
   - Look for environmental clues (empty container, nearby spill, odor on breath) and save all evidence of poison (container, vomitus, urine).
   - Be alert to signs and symptoms of potential poisoning in the absence of other evidence, including symptoms of ocular or dermal exposure.
   - Call the poison control center (PCC) or other competent emergency facility for immediate advice regarding treatment.
4. Prevent poison absorption:
   - Place the child in a side-lying, sitting, or kneeling position with the head below the chest to prevent aspiration.

Based on the initial telephone assessment, the PCC counsels the parents to begin treatment at home or to take the child to an emergency facility. When a call is taken, the name and telephone number of the caller are recorded to reestablish contact if the connection is interrupted. Because most poisonings are managed in the home, expert advice is essential in minimizing adverse effects. When the exact quantity or type of ingested toxin is not known, admission to a health care facility with pediatric emergency treatment services for laboratory evaluation and surveillance during the time after ingestion is critical.

Assessment

The first and most important principle in dealing with a poisoning is to treat the child first, not the poison. This requires an immediate concern for life support. Vital signs are taken, mental status is assessed, and respiratory or circulatory support is instituted as needed. The child's condition is routinely reevaluated. Because shock is a complication of several types of household poisons, particularly corrosives, measures to reduce the effects of shock are important, beginning with the CABs (circulation, airway, and breathing support measures) of resuscitation. Establishing and maintaining vascular access for rapid intravascular volume expansion is vital in the treatment of pediatric shock.

The emergency department nurse's responsibility is to be prepared for immediate intervention with all of the necessary equipment. Because time and speed are critical factors in recovery from serious poisonings, anticipating potential problems and complications may mean the difference between life and death.

Gastric Decontamination

Although pediatric poison ingestions are common, they rarely result in significant morbidity or mortality (Mowry, Spyker, Brooks, et al., 2016). Consider using gastrointestinal decontamination (GID) only after careful evaluation of the potential toxicity of the poison and the risks versus benefits. GID (such as ipecac, activated charcoal, and gastric lavage) is not routinely recommended for most childhood poisonings. Because of continuing controversy regarding the use of these methods, treat each toxic ingestion individually (Mowry et al., 2016). Specific antidotes may be administered for certain poisonings.

Syrup of ipecac, an emetic that exerts its action through irritation of the gastric mucosa and by stimulation of the vomiting center, is no longer recommended for routine treatment of poison ingestion (Albertson, Owen, Sutter, et al., 2011; Theurer & Bhavsar, 2013).

NURSING ALERT

Syrup of ipecac is not recommended for routine poison treatment intervention in the home (Albertson et al., 2011; Theurer & Bhavsar, 2013).

A common method of GID is the use of **activated charcoal**, an odorless, tasteless, fine black powder that absorbs many compounds, creating a stable complex (Frithsen & Simpson, 2010). The use of activated charcoal has become less common and was used in only 1.1% of pediatric toxic exposures in 2015 (Mowry et al., 2016). Activated charcoal may be considered in the following situations:

- Child may have ingested large amounts of carbamazepine, dapsone, phenobarbital, quinine, or theophylline.
- Time to activated charcoal administration is within 1 hour after the poison ingestion.
- Child has an intact or protected airway.

Activated charcoal is mixed with water or a saline cathartic to form a slurry. Slurries are neither gritty nor distasteful but resemble black mud. To increase the child's acceptance of activated charcoal, the nurse should mix it with small amounts of chocolate milk, fruit syrup, or cola drinks and serve it through a straw in an opaque container with a cover (e.g., a disposable coffee cup and lid) or an ordinary cup covered with aluminum foil or placed inside a small paper bag. Super-activated charcoal has three to four times the surface area and can absorb greater quantities of poison (Olson, 2010). For small children, a nasogastric tube may be required to administer activated charcoal. Potential complications from the use of activated charcoal include vomiting and potential aspiration, constipation, and intestinal obstruction (in multiple doses) (Albertson et al., 2011).

If the child is admitted to an emergency facility, **gastric lavage** may be performed to empty the stomach of the toxic agent; however, this procedure can be associated with serious complications (gastrointestinal perforation, hypoxia, aspiration). There is no conclusive evidence that gastric lavage decreases morbidity, and it is no longer recommended to be performed routinely, if at all (Albertson et al., 2011; Benson, Hoppu, Troutman, et al., 2013). In addition, gastric lavage may be of little benefit if used later than 1 hour after ingestion (Albertson et al., 2011; McGregor, Parkar, & Rao, 2009). Conditions that may be appropriate for the use of gastric lavage include presentation within 1 hour of ingestion of a toxin, ingestion in a patient who has decreased gastrointestinal motility, the ingestion of a toxic amount of sustained-release medication, and a large or life-threatening amount

[b]Also available by calling 800-222-1222 or online at American Association of Poison Control Centers, http://www.aapcc.org.

of poison (Albertson et al., 2011). When gastric lavage is used, the patient requires a protected airway, possible sedation, and the largest diameter tube that can be inserted to facilitate passage of gastric contents. Gastric lavage should only be performed by medical personnel with proper training and expertise (Benson et al., 2013).

In a minority of poisonings, specific **antidotes** are available to counteract the poison. They are highly effective and should be available in all emergency facilities. The supply of antidotes should be checked routinely and replaced as used or according to expiration dates. Antidotes available to treat toxin ingestion include *N*-acetylcysteine for acetaminophen poisoning, oxygen for carbon monoxide inhalation, naloxone for opioid overdose, flumazenil (Romazicon) for benzodiazepine (diazepam [Valium], midazolam [Versed]) overdose, digoxin immune fab (Digibind) for digoxin toxicity, amyl nitrate for cyanide, and antivenin for certain poisonous bites.

Prevention of Recurrence

The ultimate objective is to prevent poisonings from occurring or recurring. Home safety education improves poison prevention practices (Lee et al., 2017). Research supports the effectiveness of parent education on preventing unintentional injuries (Patel, Magnusen, & Sandell, 2017). One effective counseling method is first to discuss the difficulties of constantly watching and safeguarding young children (see Family-Centered Care box). In this way, the challenging task of raising children can lead to a discussion of injury prevention as part of the parental role. This approach also incorporates contributory causes for the incident, such as inadequate support systems; marital discord; discipline techniques (especially use of physical punishment); and any disruption in the family or family activities, such as vacations, moves, visitors, illnesses, or births. A visit to the home, especially after repeat poisonings, is recommended as part of the follow-up care to assess hazards, including family factors, and to evaluate appropriate injury-proofing measures. One method of identifying risk areas is to ask specific questions or to have the parent complete a questionnaire designed to isolate factors that predispose children to poisoning. Another approach is to encourage parents to bend down to the child's eye level and survey the home environment for potential hazards. Have the parents try to open cabinets and reach shelves to access poisons.

FAMILY-CENTERED CARE

Poisoning

A poisoning is more than a physical emergency for the child; it also usually represents an emotional crisis for the parents, particularly in terms of guilt, self-reproach, and insecurity in the parenting role. The emergency department is no place to admonish the family for negligence, lack of appropriate supervision, or failure to injury-proof the home. Rather, it is a time to calm and support the child and parents while unaccusingly exploring the circumstances of the injury. If the nurse prematurely attempts to discuss ways of preventing such an incident from recurring, the parents' anxiety will block out any suggestions or offered guidance. It is preferable for the nurse to delay the discussion until the child's condition is stabilized or, if the child is discharged immediately after emergency treatment, to make a public health referral or send a packet of information.

Passive measures (those that do not require active participation) have been the most successful in preventing poisoning and include using child-resistant closures and limiting the number of tablets in one container. However, these measures alone are not sufficient to prevent poisoning, because most toxic agents in the home do not have safety closures. **Active measures** (those that require participation) are essential. The Nursing Care Guidelines box lists the guidelines for preventing the occurrence or recurrence of a poisoning.

NURSING CARE GUIDELINES

Poison Prevention

- Assess possible contributing factors in occurrence of injury, such as discipline, parent-child relationship, developmental ability, environmental factors, and behavior problems.
- Institute anticipatory guidance for possible future injuries based on child's age and developmental level.
- Initiate referral to appropriate agency to evaluate home environment and need for injury-proofing measures.
- Provide assistance with environmental manipulation, such as lead removal, when necessary.
- Educate parents regarding safe storage of toxic substances.
- Advise parents to take drugs out of sight of children.
- Teach children the hazards of ingesting nonfood items.
- Advise parents against using plants for teas or medicine.
- Discuss problems of discipline and children's noncompliance and offer strategies for effective discipline.
- Instruct parents regarding correct administration of drugs for therapeutic purposes and to discontinue drug if there is evidence of mild toxicity.
- Advise parents to contact the poison control center (PCC; 800-222-1222) or practitioner immediately when a poisoning occurs.
- Tell them to post the number of the regional PCC with an emergency phone list by the telephone.
- Include by the telephone the home address with nearest cross street in case an ambulance is needed. (In an emergency, family members may not remember the house address, and babysitters may not be aware of the information.)

HEAVY METAL POISONING

Heavy metal poisoning can occur from the ingestion of a variety of substances, the most common being lead. Other sources that are important in terms of children are iron and mercury. **Mercury toxicity**, a rare form of heavy metal poisoning, has occurred in children from a variety of sources, such as predator fish (king mackerel, shark, swordfish, tilefish), broken thermometers or thermostats, broken fluorescent light bulbs, disk batteries, topical medications, gas regulators, cathartics, and interior latex house paint (Carman, Tutkun, Yilmaz, et al., 2013). Elemental mercury (also called *metallic mercury* or *quicksilver*) is nontoxic if ingested and if the gastrointestinal tract is healthy (e.g., has no fistulas). However, mercury is volatile at room temperature and enters the bloodstream after it is inhaled. Chronic exposure produces symptoms ranging from nonspecific (e.g., anorexia, weight loss, memory loss, insomnia, gingivitis, diarrhea) to severe (e.g., tremors, extreme behavior changes, delirium). The classic form of mercury poisoning is called **acrodynia** (or "painful extremities").

! NURSING ALERT

Mercury thermometers are no longer recommended because if they are broken, the inhaled vapors can cause toxicity. To prevent inhalation, clean up spilled mercury quickly, using disposable towels and rubber gloves and washing the hands well afterward.

Heavy metals have an affinity for certain essential tissue chemicals, which must remain free for adequate cell functioning. When metals are bound to these substances, cellular enzyme systems are inactivated. Treatment involves **chelation**, use of a chemical compound that combines with the metal for rapid and safe excretion.

BOX 13.3 Sources of Lead[a]

Lead-based paint in deteriorating condition
Lead solder
Lead crystal
Battery casings
Lead fishing sinkers
Lead curtain weights
Lead bullets
Some of these may contain lead:

- Ceramic ware
- Water
- Pottery
- Pewter
- Dyes
- Industrial factories
- Vinyl miniblinds
- Playground equipment
- Collectible toys
- Some imported toys or children's metal jewelry
- Artists' paints
- Pool cue chalk

Occupations and hobbies involving lead:

- Battery and aircraft manufacturing
- Lead smelting
- Brass foundry work
- Radiator repair
- Construction work
- Furniture refinishing
- Bridge repair work
- Painting contracting
- Mining
- Ceramics work
- Stained-glass making
- Jewelry making

[a]The US Consumer Product Safety Commission issues alerts and recalls for products that contain lead and may unexpectedly pose a hazard to young children. Additional information is available from Alliance for Healthy Homes, https://nchh.org/who-we-are/afhh/.

LEAD POISONING

Poisoning from lead has been a problem throughout history and throughout the world. In the United States, the problem became apparent in the early 1900s when white lead was added to paints and when tetraethyl lead was added to gasoline as an antiknock compound. Lead content in paint was decreased in 1950, and in 1978 the use of lead in household paint was banned. The use of lead in paint and leaded gasoline has been banned in the United States. After this change in policy, the average blood lead level (BLL) in the United States for people 1 to 74 years old dropped from 12.8 mcg/dl in 1980 to 1.3 mcg/dl in 2010 (Centers for Disease Control and Prevention, 2012, 2017). However, children continue to be exposed to lead; an estimated 0.8% of children in the United States 1 to 5 years old had BLLs of more than 10 mcg/dl in 2010, and more than 5% had BLLs of 5 mcg/dl or higher (Centers for Disease Control and Prevention, 2017). There are no safe blood levels in children.

Causes of Lead Poisoning

Although there are numerous sources of lead (Box 13.3), in most instances of acute childhood lead poisoning, the source is nonintact lead-based paint in an older home or lead-contaminated bare soil in the yard. Microparticles of lead gain entrance into a child's body through ingestion or inhalation and, in the case of an exposed pregnant woman, by placental transfer. When measured, a mother's lead level is nearly the same as that of her unborn child. Although the level of lead may not be harmful to adult women, it can be harmful to fetuses.

Whereas inhalation exposure usually occurs during renovation and remodeling activities in the home, ingestion happens during normal day-to-day play and mouthing activities. Sometimes a child will swallow loose chips of lead-based paint because it has a sweet taste. Water and food may also be contaminated with lead. A child does not need to eat loose paint chips to be exposed to the toxin; normal hand-to-mouth behavior, coupled with the presence of lead dust in the environment that has settled over decades, is the usual method of poisoning (Bellinger, Chen, & Lanphear, 2017).

Because of family, cultural, or ethnic traditions, a source of lead may be a routine part of life for a child. Nurses must educate themselves about the practices of their patients and identify when such products may be a source of lead. The use of pottery or dishes containing lead may be an issue, as may the use of folk remedies for stomach aches or the use of some cosmetics (see Cultural Considerations box). Children of immigrants and internationally adopted children may have been exposed to sources of lead before arrival in the United States and should also be carefully evaluated for lead exposure (Raymond, Kennedy, & Brown, 2013). Other risk factors for having an elevated BLL include living in poverty, being younger than 6 years old, dwelling in urban areas, and living in older rental homes where lead decontamination may not be a priority. Nurses are often in a position to observe or elicit information about these practices and educate families about their potential harm.

CULTURAL CONSIDERATIONS

Sources of Lead

In some cultures, the use of traditional ethnic remedies that contain lead may increase children's risk of lead poisoning. These remedies include:

Azarcon (Mexico): For digestive problems; a bright orange powder; usual dose is 0.25 to 1 tsp, often mixed with oil, milk, or sugar or sometimes given as a tea; sometimes a pinch is added to a baby bottle or tortilla dough for preventive purposes

Greta (Mexico): A yellow-orange powder used in the same way as azarcon

Paylooah (Southeast Asia): Used for rash or fever; an orange-red powder given as 0.5 tsp straight or in a tea

Surma (India and Pakistan): Black powder used as a cosmetic and as teething powder

Unknown ayurvedic (Tibet): Small, gray-brown balls used to improve slow development; two balls are given orally three times a day

Tamarind jellied, fruit candy (Mexico): Fruit candy packaged in paper wrappers that contain high lead levels

Lozeena (Iraq): A bright orange powder used to color meat and rice

Litargirio (Dominican Republic): Yellow or peach-colored powder used as a folk remedy and as an antiperspirant or deodorant

Ba-Baw-San (China): Herbal medicine used to treat colic pain

Data from Centers for Disease Control and Prevention. (1993). Lead poisoning associated with use of traditional ethnic remedies—California, 1991–1992. *Morbidity and Mortality Weekly Report, 42*(27), 521–524; Centers for Disease Control and Prevention (1998). Lead poisoning associated with imported candy and powdered food coloring—California and Michigan. *Morbidity and Mortality Weekly Report,* 47(48), 1041–1043; Centers for Disease Control and Prevention. (2002). Childhood lead poisoning associated with tamarind candy and folk remedies—California, 1992–2000. *Morbidity and Mortality Weekly Report,* 51(31), 684–686; Centers for Disease Control and Prevention. (2005). Lead poisoning associated with use of litargirio—Rhode Island. *Morbidity and Mortality Weekly Report,* 54(09), 227–229.

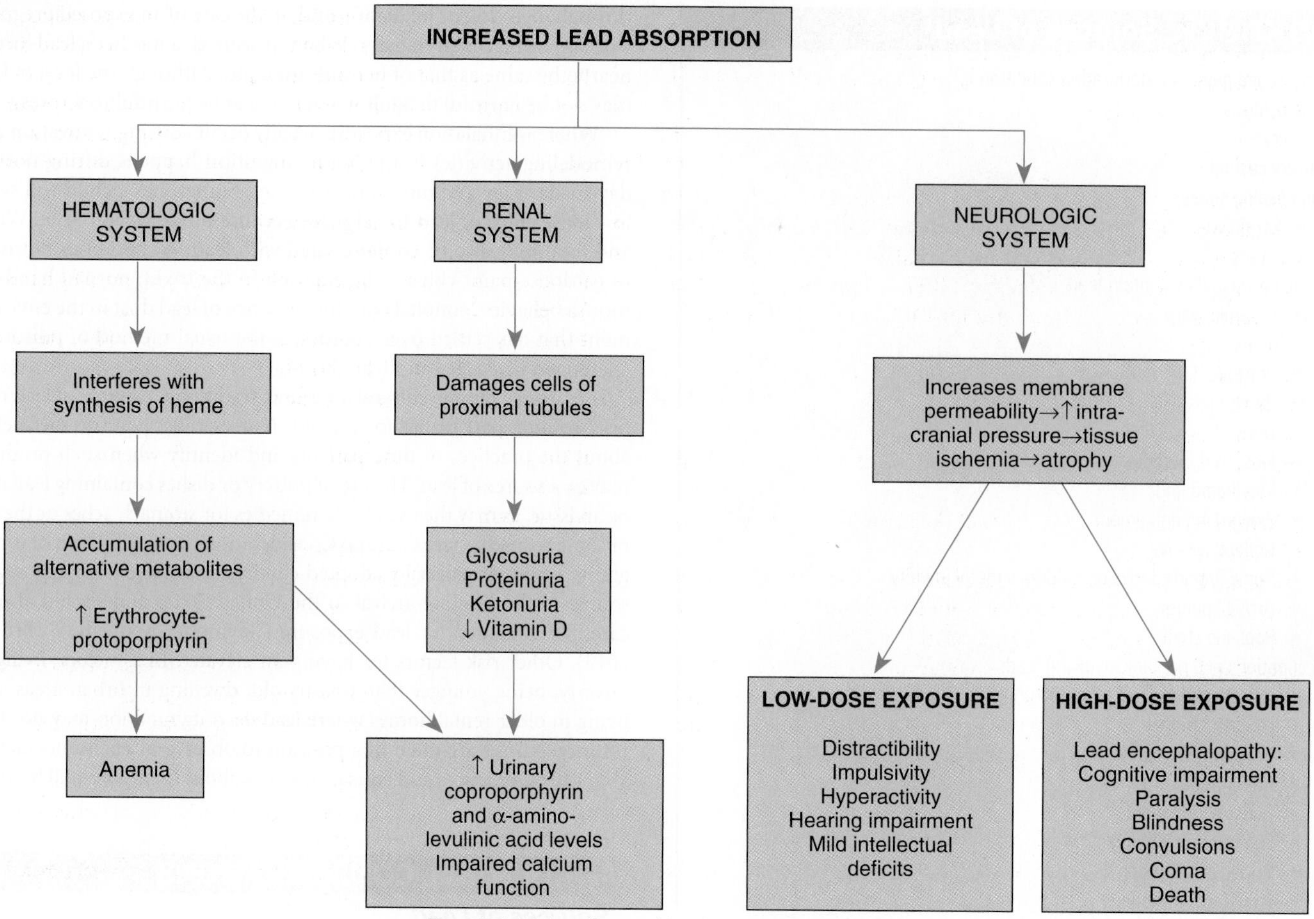

Fig. 13.1 Main effects of lead on body systems.

Pathophysiology and Clinical Manifestation

Lead can affect any part of the body, including the renal, hematologic, and neurologic systems (Fig. 13.1). Of most concern for young children is the developing brain and nervous system, which are more vulnerable than those of older children and adults. Lead in the body moves via an equilibration process between the blood, the soft tissues and organs, and the bones and teeth. Lead ultimately settles in the bones and teeth, where it remains inert and in storage. This makes up the largest portion of the body burden, approximately 75% to 90%. At the cellular level, it competes with molecules of calcium, interfering with the regulating action of calcium. In the brain, lead disrupts the biochemical processes and may have a direct effect on the release of neurotransmitters, may cause alterations in the blood-brain barrier, and may interfere with the regulation of synaptic activity (Cunningham, 2012; Jones, 2009).

There is a relationship between anemia and lead poisoning. Children who are iron deficient absorb lead more readily than those with sufficient iron stores. Lead can interfere with the binding of iron onto the heme molecule. This sometimes creates a picture of anemia even though the child is not iron deficient. Lead toxicity to the erythrocytes leads to the release of the enzyme erythrocyte protoporphyrin (EP). Because EP is not sensitive to BLLs of less than about 16 to 25 mcg/dl, it is no longer used as a screening test. The BLL test is currently used for screening and diagnosis. However, elevation of the EP level (>35 mcg/dl of whole blood) is a good indicator of toxicity from lead and reflects the length of exposure and body burden of lead in an individual child.

Although adults have been shown to experience adverse renal effects from occupational lead exposure, few studies document renal effects in children except at extremely high lead levels. One can hypothesize that lead can affect the renal integrity of children as well as adults. The renal system of a child is still considered a potential target for the harmful effects of lead.

The lead levels identified in children have declined since the initiation of screening for children at risk for lead poisoning. With earlier intervention, the most prevalent effects have changed. Since the late 1960s, children have rarely died of lead poisoning, and seizures or cognitive impairment have become less likely. However, even mild and moderate lead poisoning can cause a number of cognitive and behavioral problems in young children, including aggression, hyperactivity, impulsivity, delinquency, disinterest, and withdrawal. Long-term neurocognitive signs of lead poisoning include developmental delays, lowered intelligence quotient (IQ), reading skill deficits, visual-spatial problems, visual-motor problems, learning disabilities, and lower academic success. Chronic lead toxicity may also affect physical growth and reproductive efficiency (Burns & Gerstenberger, 2014).

Diagnostic Evaluation

Children with lead poisoning rarely have symptoms even at levels requiring chelation therapy. A diagnosis of lead poisoning is based only on the lead testing of a venous blood specimen from a venipuncture. The collection process is important. Blood must be collected carefully to avoid contamination by lead on the skin. The acceptable BLL has dropped from 40 mcg/dl in 1970 to 5 mcg/dl today (Centers for Disease Control and Prevention Advisory Committee on Childhood Lead Poisoning Prevention, 2012).

Anticipatory Guidance

The most effective prevention of lead exposure is ensuring that environmental exposures are reduced before children are exposed. The following information should be made available to families beginning during prenatal and postnatal care (Centers for Disease Control and Prevention Advisory Committee on Childhood Lead Poisoning Prevention, 2012):

- Hazards of lead-based paint in older housing
- Ways to control lead hazards safely
- How to choose safe toys
- Hazards accompanying repainting and renovation of homes built before 1978
- Other exposure sources, such as traditional remedies, that might be relevant for a family

There has been recent concern regarding toys and other imported items children play with that were found to contain lead. Parents should carefully evaluate the source of the toy (manufacturer) or item the child may play with and not assume it is safe because it is sold in a US market. The US Consumer Product Safety Commission (http://www.cpsc.gov) is an excellent resource for parents and caregivers concerned about the safety of a given toy or product that may be harmful.

Screening for Lead Poisoning

When primary prevention fails, secondary prevention screening efforts for elevated BLLs can identify children much earlier than in the past. This need is established using BLL surveillance and other risk factor data collected over time to establish the status and risk of children throughout each state. Universal screening should be done at 1 and 2 years old. Any child between 3 and 6 years old who has not been previously screened should also be tested. All children with risk factors should be screened more often.

Targeted screening is acceptable when an area has been determined by existing data to have less risk. Children should be screened when they live in a high-risk geographic area or are members of a group determined to be at risk (e.g., Medicaid recipients) or if their family cannot answer "no" to the following personal risk questions:

- Does your child live in or regularly visit a house that was built before 1950?
- Does your child live in or regularly visit a house that was built before 1978 with recent or ongoing renovations or remodeling within the past 6 months?
- Does your child have a sibling or playmate who has or had lead poisoning?

Therapeutic Management

The degree of concern, urgency, and need for medical intervention change as the lead level increases. Education is one of the most important elements of the treatment process. Areas that the nurse needs to discuss with the family of every child who has an elevated BLL (≥5 mcg/dl) include the following (Centers for Disease Control and Prevention Advisory Committee on Childhood Lead Poisoning Prevention, 2012):

- The child's BLL and what it means
- Potential adverse health effects of an elevated BLL
- Sources of lead exposure and suggestions on how to reduce exposure, such as the importance of wet cleaning to remove lead dust on floors, windowsills, and other surfaces
- Importance of good nutrition in reducing the absorption and effects of lead; for persons with poor nutritional patterns, adequate intake of calcium and iron and importance of regular meals
- Need for follow-up testing to monitor the child's BLL
- Results of an environmental investigation if applicable
- Hazards of improper removal of lead paint (dry sanding, scraping, or open-flame burning)

Treatment actions vary depending on the child's BLL. Based on a diagnosis from a venous BLL test, the Centers for Disease Control and Prevention (2002) recommends the following actions:

Blood Lead Level (mcg/dl)	Action
<5	Provide family with lead education. Reassess or rescreen in 1 year. If exposure status changes, do this sooner.
5-14	Provide family with lead education, regular developmental and behavioral surveillance, and social service referral if necessary. Provide follow-up testing within 1 month, then every 3 to 4 months.
15-19	Provide family with lead education, regular developmental and behavioral surveillance, and social service referral if necessary. Provide follow-up testing within 1 month, then every 3 to 4 months. Initiate professional environmental cleanup. Follow guidelines for BLL of 20-44 mcg/dl if BLL remains ≥15 mcg/dl on two samples obtained at least 3 months apart.
20-44	Provide family with lead education, regular developmental and behavioral surveillance, and social service referral if necessary. Refer to clinical center specializing in lead poisoning. Provide both clinical and environmental management. Consider treating with appropriate chelation therapy.
45-69	Provide lead education. Refer to clinical center specializing in lead poisoning; provide coordination of care. Provide diagnostic testing within 24-48 h. Perform clinical evaluation and management within 48 h. Provide appropriate chelation therapy. Ensure aggressive environmental intervention. Follow-up testing at least once per month.
≥70	*Immediately* provide diagnostic testing and initiate chelation therapy. Begin other activities (listed above).

Chelation Therapy

Chelation is the term used for removing lead from circulating blood and, theoretically, some lead from organs and tissues. It is unclear whether chelation affects lead stores in bones. Although not an antidote in the truest sense, it does serve a similar purpose in that the toxic substance or poison is removed from the body. However, chelation does not counteract any effects of the lead.

Historically, three chelating agents have been used consistently: calcium disodium edetate ($CaNa_2EDTA$, or calcium EDTA), British anti-Lewisite (BAL; dimercaprol, dimercaptopropanol), and Meso-2,3-dimercaptosuccinic acid (DMSA, Chemet, Succimer). BAL (dimercaprol, dimercaptopropanol) is used in conjunction with EDTA with high lead levels or the presence of lead encephalopathy. All of the agents have potential toxic side effects and contraindications. Renal, hepatic, and hematologic parameters should be monitored.

Because of the equilibration process between blood, soft tissues, and other sites in the body, there is often a rebound of the BLL after chelation. After the body burden of lead is reduced enough to stabilize the BLL, rebound will cease. Multiple chelation treatments may be necessary. Adequate hydration is essential during therapy because the chelates are excreted via the kidneys.

Severe lead toxicity (lead level ≥70 mcg/dl) requires immediate inpatient treatment, whether symptoms are present or not. BAL is contraindicated in children with peanut allergies or hepatic insufficiency, nor should it be given in conjunction with iron. Also, use with caution in children with renal impairment or hypertension; monitor for hemolysis with presence of glucose-6-phosphate dehydrogenase deficiency. It must be given only at a deep intramuscular site, in repeated doses over several days. Calcium EDTA should be given intravenously or intramuscularly (in a different site from BAL). The intravenous route should not be used in children with cerebral edema.

For lead levels of 45 to 69 mcg/dl and an absence of symptoms, DMSA can be used. The capsule is opened and sprinkled on a small amount of food or may be swallowed whole. DMSA can be used in conjunction with iron. Adverse effects include nausea, vomiting, diarrhea, loss of appetite, rash, elevated liver function tests, and neutropenia. Because the chelates are excreted via the kidneys, adequate hydration is essential.

A less used oral chelating agent, D-penicillamine, is sometimes used to treat lead poisoning, but the medication is not approved by the US Food and Drug Administration for use in the United States (Dapul & Laraque, 2014).

Prognosis

Although most of the pathophysiologic effects of lead are reversible, the most serious consequences of both high and low lead exposure are the effects on the central nervous system. In children with lead encephalopathy, permanent brain damage can result in cognitive impairment, behavior changes, possible paralysis, and seizures. However, low-dose exposure may also cause permanent neurologic deficits. Increased distractibility, short attention span, impulsivity, reading disabilities, and school failure have been associated with lead exposure (Centers for Disease Control and Prevention Advisory Committee on Childhood Lead Poisoning Prevention, 2012).

Nursing Care Management

The primary nursing goal in lead poisoning is to prevent the child's initial or further exposure to lead. For children with low-level exposure, this requires identifying the sources of lead in the environment. Careful history taking is the most useful and most valuable tool and should concentrate on the personal risk questions. Suggestions for reducing lead in the child's environment are listed in the Community Focus box.

COMMUNITY FOCUS

Reducing Blood Lead Levels

- Make certain children do not have access to peeling paint or chewable surfaces painted with lead-based paint, especially windowsills and wells.
- If a house was built before 1978 and has hard-surface floors, wet mop them at least once per week. Wipe other hard surfaces (e.g., windowsills, baseboards). If there are loose paint chips in an area, such as a window well, use a wet disposable cloth to pick up and discard them. Do not vacuum hard-surfaced floors or windowsills or wells because this spreads dust. Use vacuum cleaners with agitators to remove dust from rugs rather than vacuum cleaners with suction only. If a rug is known to contain lead dust and cannot be washed, it should be discarded.
- Wash and dry children's hands and faces frequently, especially before eating.
- Wash toys and pacifiers frequently.
- Wipe your feet on mats before entering the home, especially if you work in occupations where lead is used. Removing your shoes when you are entering the home is a good practice to control lead.
- If soil around home is or is likely to be contaminated with lead (e.g., if the home was built before 1978 or is near a major highway), plant grass or other ground cover; plant bushes around outside of the house so that children cannot play there.
- During remodeling of older homes, follow correct procedures. Be certain children and pregnant women are not in the home, day or night, until the process is completed. After deleading, thoroughly clean the house using cleaning solution to a damp mop and dust before inhabitants return.
- In areas where lead content of water exceeds the drinking water standard and a particular faucet has not been used for 6 hours or more, "flush" the cold-water pipes by running the water until it becomes as cold as it will get (30 seconds to 2 minutes). The more time water has been sitting in pipes, the more lead it may contain.
- *Use only cold water* for consumption (drinking, cooking, and especially for reconstituting powder infant formula). Hot water dissolves lead more quickly than cold water and thus contains higher levels of lead. It is acceptable to use first-flush water for nonconsumption uses (e.g., bathing).
- Have water tested by a competent laboratory. This action is especially important for apartment dwellers; flushing may not be effective in high-rise buildings and in other buildings with lead-soldered central piping.
- Do not store food in open cans, particularly if cans are imported.
- Do not use pottery or ceramic ware that was inadequately fired or is meant for decorative use for food storage or service. Do not store drinks or food in lead crystal.
- Avoid folk remedies or cosmetics that contain lead.
- Avoid candy imported from Mexico (e.g., tamarind hard candy).
- Avoid imported toys and toy jewelry that may contain lead.
- Make certain that home exposure is not occurring from parental occupations or hobbies. Household members employed in occupations such as lead smelting should shower and change into clean clothing before leaving work. Construction and lead abatement workers may also bring home lead contaminants.
- Ensure that children eat regular meals because more lead is absorbed on an empty stomach.
- Ensure that children's diets contain sufficient iron and calcium and not excessive fat.
- Consider iron supplementation if child does not regularly consume foods rich in iron.

Modified from Centers for Disease Control and Prevention. (2013). *Lead home*. Retrieved from http://www.cdc.gov/nceh/lead/

For children who undergo chelation therapy, the nurse prepares them for the injections and makes all efforts to reduce injection pain. Chelating agents are administered deeply into a large muscle mass (see Atraumatic Care box). To lessen the pain from calcium EDTA, the local anesthetic procaine is injected with the drug. Rotation of sites is essential to prevent the formation of painful areas of fibrotic tissue. Because calcium EDTA and lead are toxic to the kidneys, keep records of intake and output, and assess the results of urinalysis to monitor renal functioning.

ATRAUMATIC CARE

Lead Chelation Therapy

To lessen the pain from intramuscular injection of calcium disodium edetate ($CaNa_2EDTA$ or calcium EDTA), the local anesthetic procaine is injected with the drug. Apply topical anesthetic cream such as eutectic mixture of local anesthetics (e.g., lidocaine-prilocaine [EMLA]) or LMX4 (4% lidocaine) over the puncture site before the injection of EDTA and British anti-Lewisite (BAL) (time per manufacturer's guidelines).

! NURSING ALERT

Use extreme caution with chelating agents. Incidences of child death from hypocalcemia have been recorded when Na_2EDTA was substituted for $CaNa_2EDTA$ and used as a chelating agent (Fountain & Reith, 2014).

! NURSING ALERT

Adequate urinary output must be ensured with administration of calcium EDTA. Children receiving the drug intramuscularly must be able to maintain adequate oral intake of fluids.

Discharge planning for children with lead poisoning must include thorough education of families on safety from lead hazards, clear instructions regarding medication administration and follow-up, and confirmation that the child will be discharged to a home without lead hazards. Although the nurse must use caution to avoid alarming parents unnecessarily, it is important that they know the risk implications for their child's behavior and cognitive functions. Nurses should observe the development and behavior of children who are hospitalized. Thoroughly evaluate any concerns that are identified. Referral to a child development or speech and language specialist may be necessary.

As in any situational crisis, parents need support and understanding if their child is treated for lead poisoning. Many families at the highest risk for lead poisoning have the fewest resources to comply with measures such as relocation or removal of lead from the environment where the child experiences exposure.

CHILD MALTREATMENT

The broad term *child maltreatment* includes intentional physical abuse or neglect, emotional abuse or neglect, and sexual abuse of children, usually by adults. It is one of the most significant social problems affecting children. In 2015 Child Protective Service agencies in the United States confirmed that an estimated 683,000 children were victims of one or more types of child maltreatment. Of the confirmed cases, about 17.2% suffered physical abuse, 8.4% sexual abuse, 75.3% neglect, and 6.9% psychologic maltreatment or emotional abuse. In 2015 there were an estimated 1585 child fatalities as a result of child abuse and neglect (US Department of Health and Human Services, 2015). Reported statistics only partially represent the actual incidence of child maltreatment because many cases are believed to go unreported.[c]

CHILD NEGLECT

Child neglect is the most common form of maltreatment, and 74.8% of reported neglect cases involve children 3 years old or younger (US Department of Health and Human Services, 2015). Of the children who died, 72.9% suffered from neglect either exclusively or in combination with another type of maltreatment (US Department of Health and Human Services, 2015). **Neglect** is generally defined as the failure of a parent or other person legally responsible for the child's welfare to provide for the child's basic needs and an adequate level of care.

Important contributing factors for child neglect are lack of knowledge of child's needs, lack of resources, and caregiver substance abuse. For example, neglectful parents often demonstrate poor parenting skills. They may be unaware that an infant needs to be fed every 3 to 4 hours, may not know what to feed the child, and may have insufficient funds to buy food. The most serious lack of knowledge is failure to recognize emotional nurturing as an essential need of children (see also Chapter 10, Failure to Thrive).

Types of Neglect

Neglect takes many forms and can be classified broadly as physical or emotional maltreatment. **Physical neglect** involves the deprivation of necessities, such as food, clothing, shelter, supervision, medical care, and education. **Emotional neglect** generally refers to failure to meet the child's needs for affection, attention, and emotional nurturance.

Neglect may also include lack of intervention for or fostering of maladaptive behavior, such as delinquency or substance abuse. **Emotional abuse** or **psychologic maltreatment**, an even more difficult aspect of maltreatment to define, refers to the deliberate attempt to destroy or significantly impair a child's self-esteem or competence. Emotional abuse may take the form of rejecting, isolating, terrorizing, ignoring, corrupting, verbally assaulting, or overly pressuring the child (Hibbard, Barlow, MacMillan, et al., 2012).

PHYSICAL ABUSE

The deliberate infliction of physical injury on a child, usually by the child's caregiver, is called *physical abuse.* Physical abuse can include anything from bruises and fractures to brain damage. Minor physical injury is responsible for more reported cases of maltreatment than major physical injury, but major physical abuse causes more deaths. In 2015, 43.9% of fatalities from abuse suffered physical abuse alone or in combination with other types of maltreatment (US Department of Health and Human Services, 2015). Despite the importance of the problem, a universally accepted definition of what constitutes minor and major physical abuse does not exist. Rather, each state in the United States defines abuse according to its individual reporting laws.

---

[c]Additional information is available from the Children's Bureau, Administration for Children and Families, 370 L'Enfant Promenade SW, Washington, DC 20447; http://www.acf.hhs.gov/programs/cb.

Abusive Head Trauma

Abusive head trauma (AHT) is a serious form of physical abuse caused by violent shaking of infants and young children. Other commonly used terms include *shaken baby syndrome, inflicted head injury,* or *neuro-inflicted brain injury.* This violent shaking would be easily recognized by others as dangerous (American Academy of Pediatrics Committee on Child Abuse and Neglect, 2009; Kemp, 2011) and is most often a result of the caregiver's frustration with crying, maternal stress, or depression (Kemp, 2011). Every year in the United States, an estimated 1200 to 1400 children are shaken, and of these victims, 25% to 30% die as a result of their injuries. The rest have lifelong complications (National Center on Shaken Baby Syndrome, n.d.).

It is important to understand what happens in AHT. Infants have a large head-to-body ratio, weak neck muscles, and a large amount of water in the brain. Violent shaking causes the brain to rotate within the skull, resulting in shearing forces that tear blood vessels and neurons. The characteristic injuries that occur are intracranial bleeding (subdural and subarachnoid hematomas) and, in approximately 80% of cases, bilateral retinal hemorrhages, which are classic results of repetitive acceleration–deceleration head trauma (Maguire, Watts, Shaw, et al., 2013). Injuries may also include fractures of the ribs and long bones. Most often, there are no signs of external injury, making diagnosis difficult. Clinicians base an abusive diagnosis on patterns of injuries to the infant, but this can be subjective. PredAHT, a prediction tool, assists clinicians with an AHT diagnosis by listing six key clinical features of AHT obtained from high-quality publications (Cowley, Morris, Maguire, et al., 2015). The PredAHT has high sensitivity and specificity in estimating the probability of AHT when three or more of the six features are present in the patient (Cowley et al., 2015).

Traumatic brain injury is often not an isolated event, with a large number of children showing evidence of a previous injury (Kemp, 2011). Victims of AHT can be seen with a variety of symptoms, from generalized flulike symptoms to unresponsiveness with impending death (Altimier, 2008). Many of the presenting symptoms, such as vomiting, irritability, poor feeding, and listlessness, are often mistaken for common infant and childhood ailments. In more severe forms, presenting symptoms may include seizures, posturing, alterations in level of consciousness, apnea, bradycardia, or death. The long-term outcomes of AHT include seizure disorders; visual impairments, including blindness; developmental delays; hearing loss; cerebral palsy; and mild to profound mental, cognitive, or motor impairments (Altimier, 2008). Nurses can take an active role in prevention of AHT by teaching caregivers about care for infants and techniques to cope with inconsolable crying (Barr, 2012).

> **! NURSING ALERT**
>
> Stress to parents the danger of shaking infants (shaking can cause abusive head trauma [AHT]). Education must include coping mechanisms to care for children with inconsolable crying.

Munchausen Syndrome by Proxy

Munchausen syndrome by proxy (MSBP), also known as *medical child abuse* or *factitious disorder by proxy,* is a rare but serious form of child abuse in which caregivers deliberately exaggerate or fabricate histories and symptoms or induce symptoms. It is a form of child maltreatment that may include physical, emotional, and psychologic abuse for the gratification of the caregiver. In most cases, the perpetrator is the biologic mother with some degree of health care knowledge and training. Health care providers can become easily misled and unknowingly enable the perpetrator (Skarsaune & Bondas, 2015; Squires & Squires, 2013). Because of the history of symptoms provided by the caregiver, the child endures painful and unnecessary medical testing and procedures. Common symptoms presented are seizures, nausea and vomiting, diarrhea, and altered mental status; they are usually witnessed only by the perpetrator.

Considerations when determining whether a child is a victim of MSBP include:

- Is the child's condition consistent with the reported history?
- Does diagnostic evidence support the reported history?
- Has anyone other than the caregiver witnessed the symptoms?
- Is treatment being provided primarily because of the caregiver's demands?

The resolution of symptoms after separation from the perpetrator confirms the diagnosis.

Factors Predisposing to Physical Abuse

The causes of child abuse are multifaceted. Child maltreatment occurs across all socioeconomic, religious, cultural, racial, and ethnic groups (US Department of Health and Human Services, 2015). Three risk factors are commonly identified in child abuse: (1) parental characteristics, (2) characteristics of the child, and (3) environmental characteristics. However, no single factor or group of factors is predictive of abuse. Rather, the interaction of these factors is thought to increase the risk of abuse occurring in a particular family.

Parental Characteristics

Some identified characteristics occur more frequently in parents who abuse their children and are therefore considered risk factors. Younger parents more often are abusers of their children. Single-parent families are at higher risk for abuse, and in single-parent families that include an unrelated partner, the partner is sometimes the abuser, although a biologic parent is most commonly the perpetrator (US Department of Health and Human Services, 2015).

Abusive families are often socially isolated and have few supportive relationships. They often have additional stressors, such as low-income circumstances with little education. Parents with substance abuse problems pose a greater risk for abuse and neglect because of a variety of factors. The additional stressors of substance abuse with the demands of normal care of children create situations in which abuse and neglect can occur, because these parents have impaired judgment and may react with violence while under the influence of drugs or alcohol (Lyden, 2011). With little or no available support system and concurrent stressors imposed by the child or environment, these parents are vulnerable to additional crises of any nature and may strike out at the child as a method of releasing their frustration and anxiety.

Other factors identified in abusive parents include low self-esteem and little knowledge of appropriate parenting skills. Parenting skills are learned behaviors, and parents who grew up with poor parental role models may have difficulty parenting their own children. Often child abusers were abused or observed some types of abuse in their home (Lyden, 2011).

Characteristics of the Child

The onus for child abuse is always on the abuser. However, children who are abused do have some common characteristics. Children from birth to 1 year old are at highest risk for being abused (US Department of Health and Human Services, 2015). Infants and small children require constant attention and must have all their needs met by others. This can result in parental or caregiver fatigue that may result in striking out at the child with physical force, shaking the child, or ignoring the child's needs.

The physical and emotional demands placed on the parents or caregiver of an unwanted, brain-damaged, hyperactive, or physically disabled child may overwhelm them, resulting in abuse. Children with disabilities may not understand that abusive behaviors are not appropriate, so they may not tell others or defend themselves. Premature infants may be at risk for maltreatment because of failure of parent-child bonding during early infancy, increased physical needs, or irritability. One child may be singled out in an abusive family. Removing that child from the home often places the other siblings at risk for abuse. No child is safe if left in the abusive environment unless the parents can be helped to learn new parenting skills, to meet the children's needs, and to release their frustration through alternatives other than attacking their children.

Environmental Characteristics

The environment is a significant part of the potentially abusive situation. A typical environment is one of chronic stress, including problems of divorce, poverty, unemployment, poor housing, frequent relocation, alcoholism, and drug addiction. Increased exposure between children and parents, such as that which occurs in crowded living conditions, also increases the likelihood of abuse.

Although most reporting of abuse has been from lower socioeconomic populations, as stated earlier, child abuse is not a problem of any one societal group. Stresses imposed by poverty predispose lower socioeconomic families to abusive situations, and abuse in these groups is more likely to be reported. However, concealed crises may also be present in upper-class families. Families who have substitute caregivers (such as daycare providers and babysitters) may also be at risk for child abuse, especially if the family has not fully evaluated the caregiver. Nurses need to be aware of all these factors to identify the less obvious examples of child abuse and neglect.

SEXUAL ABUSE

Sexual abuse is one of the most devastating types of child maltreatment, and estimates indicate that it has increased significantly during the past decade (US Department of Health and Human Services, 2015). Some of the apparent increase is due to increased awareness and increased reporting (Evans, 2011).

As with all forms of child maltreatment, no universal definition for sexual abuse exists. The Child Abuse Prevention and Treatment Act (CAPTA), amended by the CAPTA Reauthorization Act of 2010, defines **sexual abuse** as "the employment, use, persuasion, inducement, enticement, or coercion of any child to engage in, or assist any other person to engage in, sexually explicit conduct or any simulation of such conduct; or the rape, molestation, prostitution, or other form of sexual exploitation of children, or incest with children" (US Department of Health and Human Services, 2015).

Sexual abuse includes the following types of sexual maltreatment (see also Chapter 16, Sexual Violence):

Incest: Any physical sexual activity between family members; blood relationship is not required (abusers can include stepparents, unrelated siblings, grandparents, uncles, and aunts); does not include sexual relations between legally sanctioned partners, such as spouses

Molestation: A vague term that includes "indecent liberties," such as touching, fondling, kissing, single or mutual masturbation, or oral-genital contact

Exhibitionism: Indecent exposure, usually exposure of the genitalia by an adult man to children or women

Child pornography: Arranging and photographing, in any media, sexual acts involving children, alone or with adults or animals, regardless of consent by the child's legal guardian; also may denote distribution of such material in any form with or without profit

Child prostitution: Involving children in sex acts for profit and usually with changing partners

Pedophilia: Literally means "love of child" and does not denote a type of sexual activity but rather the preference of an adult for prepubertal children as the means of achieving sexual excitement

Characteristics of Abusers and Victims

Anyone, including siblings and mothers, can be sexual abusers, but a typical abuser is a man whom the victim knows. Offenders come from all levels of society; however, a higher risk of child abuse has been noted among families with incomes below the poverty level (Breyer & MacPhee, 2015). In addition, parents with a high school education are more likely than parents with a college education to be abusers (Breyer & MacPhee, 2015). Many offenders hold full-time jobs, are active in community affairs, and may not have prior criminal records. Offenders often are employed (or volunteer) in positions such as teaching or coaching that bring them into contact with young girls and boys. Offenders may commit many assaults before being caught.

Incestuous relationships between father or stepfather and daughter are generally prolonged, and the victims are usually reluctant to report the situation because of fear of retaliation and fear that they will not be believed. Typically, incestuous relationships begin later than other forms of child abuse. The eldest daughter is usually abused, but in her absence another sister may be substituted. Sibling incest may also occur. Sexual abuse by relatives with a strong emotional bond with the victim, such as a parent, is often the most devastating to the child.

Boys are also victims of both intrafamilial and extrafamilial abuse. Compared with female victims, male victims are much less likely to report abuse, and they may suffer much greater emotional harm from incestuous relationships. Boys are likely to be subjected to anal penetration and oral-genital contact. They often have subtle physical findings and are abused by a father, stepfather, or mother's boyfriend.

Significant risk factors for child sexual abuse include parental unavailability, lack of emotional closeness and flexibility, social isolation, emotional deprivation, and communication difficulties. Most sexual abuse is committed by men and by persons known to the child, such as family members (Forsdike, Tarzia, Hindmarsh, et al., 2014). Around 20% to 25% of child sexual abuse cases involve penetration or oral-genital contact. In 2011 more than 26% of sexual abuse victims were between 12 and 14 years old, and nearly 22% were between 15 and 17 years old (US Department of Health and Human Services, 2015).

Initiation and Perpetuation of Sexual Abuse

The cycle of sexual abuse often starts insidiously unless it involves an isolated attack, such as rape. Often offenders spend time with the victims to gain their trust before initiating any sexual contact. Most victims are then pressured into being an accessory to the sexual activity through various means (Box 13.4) and may be unaware that sexual activity is part of the offer. Children may not reveal the truth for fear that their parents would not believe them if they told, especially if the offender is a trusted member of the family. Some fear that they will be blamed for the situation, and many young children with limited vocabulary have difficulty describing the activity when they do have the courage or opportunity to reveal the abuse.

Incest most frequently occurs between siblings, but it may also be between fathers or stepfathers and daughters or between grandfather and granddaughter. Sibling incest has been found to have adverse outcomes during childhood that extend into adulthood and are just as damaging as father-daughter abuse (Krienert & Walsh, 2011). Victims

BOX 13.4 Methods Used to Pressure Children Into Sexual Activity

- The child is offered gifts or privileges or has privileges withheld.
- The adult misrepresents moral standards by telling the child that it is "okay to do."
- Isolated and emotionally and socially impoverished children are enticed by adults who meet their needs for warmth and human contact.
- The successful sex offender pressures the victim into secrecy by describing it as a "secret between us" that other people would take away if they found out.
- The offender plays on the child's fears, including fear of punishment by the offender, fear of repercussions if the child tells, and fear of abandonment or rejection by the family.

may take years to disclose this abuse. However, not all incestuous relationships follow this pattern of silence. Reports of father-daughter incest during child custody conflicts have become more common and have raised serious concerns regarding the possibility of false accusation. Rather than tolerating or denying the child's sexual abuse, the other parent (usually the mother) is typically the chief accuser.

NURSING CARE OF THE MALTREATED CHILD

A critical responsibility of health professionals is identifying abusive situations as early as possible. Nurses who increase their knowledge of the different types of abuse and neglect and underlying causes will enhance their ability to identify, intervene, and prevent children from maltreatment and neglect (Lyden, 2011). The characteristics that may predispose members of some families to commit abuse can serve as a framework for assessing vulnerability but are never predictive of actual abuse. A careful, detailed history and interview combined with a thorough physical examination are the diagnostic tools needed to identify abuse. Nurses have a special role because they may be the first person to see the child and parent and are the consistent caregivers if the child is hospitalized (see Nursing Care Guidelines box).

NURSING CARE GUIDELINES

Talking With Children Who Reveal Abuse

- Provide a private time and place to talk.
- Do not promise not to tell; tell them that you are required by law to report the abuse.
- Do not express shock or criticize their family.
- Use their vocabulary to discuss body parts.
- Avoid using any leading statements that can distort their report.
- Reassure them that they have done the right thing by telling.
- Tell them that the abuse is not their fault and that they are not bad or to blame.
- Determine their immediate need for safety.
- Let the child know what will happen when you report.

In interviewing the child and family, the nurse must be careful to avoid biasing the child's retelling of the events. Some experts suggest that health professionals limit the interview to the child's physical and mental health concerns and leave topics of the family's social, legal, or other problems to the police or Child Protective Services (Mollen, Goyal, & Frioux, 2012). If this is not possible, try to coordinate the interview process so that all pertinent health care professionals can be present for the interview.

BOX 13.5 Warning Signs of Abuse

- Child has physical evidence of abuse or neglect, including previous injuries.
- History is incompatible with the pattern or degree of injury, such as bilateral skull fractures after being dropped.
- Explanation of how injury occurred is vague or the parent or guardian is reluctant to provide information.
- The patient is brought in with a minor, unrelated complaint, and significant trauma is found.
- Histories are contradictory among caregivers.
- The mechanism of injury provided is not possible given age or developmental level of the patient, such as 6-month-old turning on hot water.
- Bruising or other injury is present in a nonmobile patient.
- The patient's affect is inappropriate in relation to the extent of injury.
- Evidence of abusive or neglectful parent-child interaction is present.
- The parent, guardian, or custodian disappears after bringing in the patient for trauma, or a patient with suspicious injury is brought in by an unrelated adult.
- The patient has multiple fractures of differing ages.
- There was a delay in seeking care.
- The parent or caregiver discloses that abuse has or may have occurred.
- The patient makes an outcry of abuse or neglect.

Recognition of abuse or neglect necessitates a familiarity with both physical and behavioral signs that suggest maltreatment (Box 13.5). No one indicator can be used to diagnose maltreatment. It is a pattern or combination of indicators that should arouse suspicion and lead to further investigation. It is important to note that some situations (such as bleeding disorders, osteogenesis imperfecta, or sudden infant death syndrome) may be misinterpreted as abuse. Also, some cultural practices, such as cupping or coin rubbing, may mimic physical abuse. Unintentional injuries, such as burns from metal buckles on car seats, bruising from seat belts, or spiral fractures from a twist and fall injury, may also be wrongly diagnosed as abuse. Normal variants, such as mongolian spots and congenital anomalies of genitalia, can be mistaken for abuse.

Caregiver-Child Interaction

The nurse can use the initial contact with the family to assess the interaction between the caregiver and the child. Observations of the caregivers should include emotional support for the child, attentiveness to the child's needs, and concern for the child's injury. Although caregivers and children may vary in responses to a stressful event, note an unusual caregiver-child relationship and factor this into the overall evaluation of the child.

Certain behavioral responses of the parents to their child and to the interviewer should alert the nurse to the possibility of maltreatment. Abusive parents may have difficulty showing concern toward their child. They may be unable or unwilling to comfort the child. Abusers may blame the child for the injuries or belittle him or her for being clumsy or stupid. When interacting with health care workers, the parent may become hostile or uncooperative. During the child's hospitalization, they may not participate in the child's care and may show little concern for his or her progress, eventual discharge, or need for follow-up care.

Abused children's responses to their parents or the injury may also support the suspicion of abuse. Although no one pattern is typical, extremes of behavior may be observed. Children may be unresponsive to the parent or excessively clinging and intolerant of separation. They may be overly attached to the abusive parent, possibly in the hope of preventing any upset that may precipitate anger and another attack.

During care of the injury, children may be passive and accepting of the discomfort or uncooperative and fearful of any physical contact. They may avoid eye contact. Some children maintain a wary watchfulness of all strangers; some shy away from strangers as if frightened; others are unusually affectionate and outgoing.

History and Interview

Child Physical Abuse

It is often difficult to distinguish child maltreatment from accidental injuries. Caregivers whose history of events may be deceptive or incomplete and children who are nonverbal may make the assessment more complex. A purposeful, skilled history and appropriate interview questions help the nurse ensure the right course of action. Knowledge of mechanism of injury and child development is essential. Cases of abuse are often detected when the child or caregiver history of events does not match the physical findings. Children who are verbal can often give a history of the injury. Separating the child from the caregiver may provide a more reliable history. It is important to ask nonleading, open-ended questions. The history should include a narrative of the injury from both caregiver and child (if verbal). Date, time, and location where the injury took place along with who was present at the time of the injury are essential questions. Family history for bleeding and bone disorders is important. Box 13.5 outlines areas of history that are concerning for abuse.

Neglect and Emotional Abuse

Each child may manifest different responses to neglect, depending on the situation and developmental age of the child. The goal of the interview is to determine whether the child is in a safe environment and whether the caregiver has the skills and resources to care for the child. It is often difficult to determine whether the circumstances constitute poor parenting skills or true neglect. Box 13.6 lists flags for behaviors to look for in neglected and abused children.

Sexual Abuse

An essential component to identifying sexual abuse is the interview. Several dynamics may impede the child's revelation of sexual abuse. Child sexual abuse is often perpetrated by someone known to the child, including family members. In some cases, the child may have been sworn to secrecy. The child may have been told that no one will believe the story or that his or her family would be harmed if he or she told someone about the abuse. Small children may imitate behaviors they have had perpetrated on themselves or have seen others do. The nurse must be able to recognize normal, age-related sexual curiosity and self-stimulating behaviors. Typically, children do not act out specific details of the sexual act or perform intrusive acts on others unless they have sexual knowledge beyond their normal age-related development (Dubowitz & Lane, 2016).

Children's reports of sexual abuse may vary from contradictory stories to unwavering versions of the experience. Stories that sound contradictory may reflect the child's experiences in several instances of abuse. Also, children who repeatedly tell identical facts may have been prompted to do so.

Increasing evidence suggests that the types of interrogation children are exposed to after reports of sexual abuse shape their thinking. To avoid biasing the interaction, nurses must be skillful interviewers when questioning children who may be victims of abuse. Medical records should include verbatim statements made by the child and interviewer that reflect appropriate nonleading questions and statements (Lyden, 2011). The child may not be emotionally ready to discuss the abuse. Establishing rapport with the child is essential to gaining his or her trust. Interviews should not be rushed. Engaging the child in play activities while encouraging conversation may help the child discuss the abuse. It may take several interviews or psychologic counseling for the child to be forthcoming about the abuse. Information regarding the last sexual contact is important because it determines the need for a forensic evaluation. Children who have been sexually abused within the past 72 to 96 hours should be considered for forensic testing.

Unfortunately, there is no typical profile of the victim, and the nurse must have a high index of suspicion to identify these children. Physical signs vary and may include any of those listed for sexual abuse. The victim may exhibit various behavioral manifestations, but none of these behaviors is diagnostic. When abused children exhibit these behaviors, the signs may be incorrectly attributed to the normal stresses of childhood, especially in older school-age children or adolescents. Even signs considered most predictive of sexual abuse (such as certain genital findings, sexually inappropriate behavior for age, enactment of adult sexual activity, and intense focus on sexual activity [e.g., masturbation]) do not always indicate that sexual abuse has occurred. Conversely, abused children may not demonstrate more knowledge of sexual activity than nonabused children. However, one difference in the abused children's explanation of sexual activity may be unusual affective responses. For example, abused children have an increased risk for conduct disorders, aggressive behavior, and poor academic performance (Dubowitz & Lane, 2016).

> **! NURSING ALERT**
>
> When children report potentially sexually abusive experiences, take their reports seriously but also cautiously to avoid alarming the child or falsely accusing someone.

PHYSICAL ASSESSMENT

Child Physical Abuse

The goal of the physical assessment for child physical abuse is identification of all injuries. A system approach ensures that the whole body is evaluated. In instances of severe abuse and injuries, the assessment should begin with a rapid assessment of airway, breathing, circulation, and neurologic systems. A systematic head-to-toe examination follows. Attention to areas often overlooked, such as the scalp, behind the ears, and the frenulum, is essential. The child's exterior genital area and posterior surface should be completely examined.

Record the location and a detailed description of all injuries. Note the color, size, and location of all bruising. Burn documentation should include the location, pattern, demarcation lines, and presence of eschar or blisters. Diagrams of the injuries using a body diagram form are helpful. If possible, obtain photographs of the injuries using a measurement tool.

Not all forms of physical abuse have obvious signs. Intra-abdominal organ injury from blunt trauma to the abdomen can occur without signs of external abdominal bruising. Nurses should consider intra-abdominal injury in infants and children who have any other signs of abuse.

> **! NURSING ALERT**
>
> Incompatibility between the history and the injury is probably the most important criterion on which to base the decision to report suspected abuse.

BOX 13.6 Clinical Manifestations of Potential Child Maltreatment

Physical Neglect

Suggestive Physical Findings

Growth failures

Signs of malnutrition, such as thin extremities, abdominal distention, lack of subcutaneous fat

Poor personal hygiene

Unclean or inappropriate dress

Evidence of poor health care, such as delayed immunization, untreated infections, frequent colds

Frequent injuries from lack of supervision

Suggestive Behaviors

Dull and inactive affect; excessively passive or sleepy

Self-stimulatory behaviors, such as finger sucking or rocking

Begging or stealing food

Absenteeism from school

Substance abuse

Vandalism or shoplifting

Emotional Abuse and Neglect

Suggestive Physical Findings

Growth failure (failure to thrive)

Eating or feeding disorder

Enuresis

Sleep disorder

Suggestive Behaviors

Self-stimulatory behaviors, such as biting, rocking, or sucking

During infancy, lack of social smile and stranger anxiety

Withdrawal from environment and people

Unusual fearfulness

Antisocial behavior, such as destructiveness, stealing, cruelty to animals or people

Extremes of behavior, such as overly compliant and passive or aggressive and demanding

Lags in emotional and intellectual development, especially language

Suicide attempts

Physical Abuse

Suggestive Physical Findings

Bruises and welts (may be in various stages of healing)

- On face, lips, mouth, back, buttocks, thighs, or areas of torso
- Regular patterns descriptive of object used, such as belt buckle, hand, wire hanger, chain, wooden spoon, squeeze or pinch marks
- May be present in various stages of healing

Burns

- On soles, palms, back, or buttocks
- Patterns descriptive of object used, such as round cigar or cigarette burns; sharply demarcated areas from immersion in scalding water; rope burns on wrists or ankles from being bound; burns in the shape of an iron, radiator, or electric stove burner
- Absence of "splash" marks and presence of symmetric burns
- Stun gun injury: Lesions circular, fairly uniform (≤0.5 cm), and paired about 5 cm apart

Fractures and dislocations

- Skull, nose, or facial structures
- Injury denoting type of abuse, such as spiral fracture or dislocation from twisting of an extremity or whiplash from shaking the child
- Multiple new or old fractures in various stages of healing

Lacerations and abrasions

- On backs of arms, legs, torso, face, or external genitalia
- Unusual symptoms, such as abdominal swelling, pain, and vomiting from punching
- Descriptive marks, such as from human bites or pulling out of hair

Chemical

- Unexplained repeated poisoning, especially drug overdose
- Unexplained sudden illness, such as hypoglycemia from insulin administration

Suggestive Behaviors

Wary of physical contact with adults

Apparent fear of parents or going home

Lying very still while surveying environment

Inappropriate reaction to injury, such as failure to cry from pain

Lack of reaction to frightening events

Apprehensive when hearing other children cry

Indiscriminate friendliness and displays of affection

Superficial relationships

Acting-out behavior, such as aggression, to seek attention

Withdrawal behavior

Sexual Abuse

Suggestive Physical Findings

Bruises, bleeding, lacerations, or irritation of external genitalia, anus, mouth, or throat

Torn, stained, or bloody underclothing

Pain on urination or pain, swelling, and itching of genital area

Penile discharge

Sexually transmitted disease, nonspecific vaginitis

Difficulty in walking or sitting

Unusual odor in the genital area

Recurrent urinary tract infections

Presence of sperm

Pregnancy in young adolescent

Suggestive Behaviors

Sudden emergence of sexually related problems, including excessive or public masturbation, age-inappropriate sexual play, promiscuity, or overtly seductive behavior

Withdrawn behavior, excessive daydreaming

Preoccupation with fantasies, especially in play

Poor relationships with peers

Sudden changes, such as anxiety, loss or gain of weight, clinging behavior

In incestuous relationships, excessive anger at mother for not protecting daughter

Regressive behavior, such as bedwetting or thumb sucking

Sudden onset of phobias or fears, particularly fears of the dark, men, strangers, or particular settings or situations (e.g., undue fear of leaving the house or staying at the daycare center or the babysitter's house)

Running away from home

Substance abuse, particularly of alcohol or mood-elevating drugs

Profound and rapid personality changes, especially extreme depression, hostility, and aggression (often accompanied by social withdrawal)

Rapidly declining school performance

Suicidal attempts or ideation

All evidence collected must adhere to strict guidelines for legal purposes; the chain of custody must be appropriately maintained with local law enforcement personnel. Documentation on the chain of custody form should include the names of persons collecting and receiving evidence (e.g., photographs, DNA samples), types of evidence collected and received, and date of receipt (Lyden, 2011).

Neglect and Emotional Abuse

Neglect from deprivation of necessities is easier to identify than emotional neglect or psychologic maltreatment because physical signs are usually evident. Assessment of the child's height, weight, nutritional status, hygiene, and age-appropriate interactions is important for the overall picture of potential neglect. Emotional maltreatment may be readily suspected, but it is difficult to substantiate. Physical signs are often nonspecific, and nurses must rely on behavioral indicators, which range from depression to acting-out behavior, to help identify a possibly abusive situation. Any persistent and unexplained change in the child's behavior is an important clue to possible emotional abuse.

Sexual Abuse

Identifying instances of sexual abuse is particularly difficult because, often, few if any obvious physical indications of the activity exist. Physical signs vary and may include any of those listed in Box 13.6 for sexual abuse. The goal of the physical examination is to document genital findings. In most cases, the genital examination findings are normal, which does not mean that sexual abuse did not occur. Fondling or genital-to-genital contact without penetration may leave no physical findings. Forensic evidence obtained directly from a prepubertal victim's body diminishes greatly after 24 hours, with the best chance for evidence collection coming from bed linens or the child's underwear (Girardet, Bolton, Lohoti, et al., 2011). The female genital examination should include a description of the vulva, hymen, and surrounding tissue. Abnormal findings of concern are injuries to the posterior vulva or the lower half of the hymeneal ring or abrasions, bruising, or bleeding of the genital or anal tissue. It is often helpful to use a magnifying instrument (colposcope) to detect subtle injuries. There are many variants of normal findings for female genital anatomy, so it is recommended that the examination be done by a practitioner experienced with these types of cases. Contrary to popular myth, the size of the hymeneal opening is not predictive of the likelihood of sexual abuse (Adams, 2011). For male victims, swelling, abrasions, or bruising of the genital tissue raises concerns for abuse. Examine the anal area for symmetry, tone, fissures, or scars. Genital tissue heals very quickly and most often without scars. Therefore unless the child is seen within a few days of injury, the genital tissue may appear normal. In addition, the vaginal and anal mucosa is elastic; therefore penetration without disruption of tissue is possible. This defies another myth that there is always evidence of female virginity. Consider the collection of specimens for determining the presence of sexually transmitted infections, which may have been contracted during the sexual contact.

Nursing Care Management

Protect the Child From Further Abuse

Initially, identification of instances of suspected abuse or neglect is essential. The nurse may come in contact with abused children in an emergency department, practitioner's office, home, daycare center, or school.

> **! NURSING ALERT**
>
> The priority is to remove the child from the abusive situation to prevent further injury.

All states and provinces in North America have laws for mandatory reporting of child maltreatment. Suspected child abuse is reported to the local authorities.[d] Referrals usually come to the state child welfare department and are assigned to a caseworker in an agency, such as Child Protective Services. After a referral has been made, a caseworker is assigned to investigate the report. Based on the findings, the child is left in the home or temporarily removed.

A court proceeding may be necessary before the child can be placed outside the home or when parental rights are to be terminated. When the courts are involved, they usually require firsthand testimony by the referring parties. Nurses may be subpoenaed to appear in court, or their notes may be introduced as evidence in court hearings. Accurate and factual documentation is essential. Behaviors are described, not interpreted, and are recorded daily to establish a progress record (see Nursing Care Guidelines box). Conversations among the nurse, child, and parent are recorded verbatim as much as possible.

> **NURSING CARE GUIDELINES**
>
> ***Recording Assessment Data in Suspected Abuse***
>
> **History of Injury**
>
> Date, time, and place of occurrence
> Sequence of events with recorded times
> Presence of witnesses, especially person caring for child at time of incident
> Time lapse between occurrence of injury and initiation of treatment
> Interview with child when appropriate, including verbal quotations and information from drawing or other play activities
> Interview with parent, witnesses, and other significant persons, including verbal quotations
> Description of parent-child interactions (verbal interactions, eye contact, touching, parental concern)
> Name, age, and condition of other children in home (if possible)
>
> **Physical Examination**
>
> Location, size, shape, and color of bruises; approximate location, size, and shape on drawing of body outline
> Distinguishing characteristics, such as a bruise in the shape of a hand or a round burn (possibly caused by cigarette)
> Symmetry or asymmetry of injury; presence of other injuries
> Degree of pain; any bone tenderness
> Evidence of past injuries; general state of health and hygiene
> Developmental level of child; screening test (see Chapter 3, Developmental Assessment)

Support the Child

Children suspected of being abused are often hospitalized for medical management of their injuries and to allow further assessment of their safety needs. The needs of these children are the same as those of any hospitalized child. The child should be treated as a child with the usual physical needs, developmental tasks, and play interests—not as a victim of abuse. The goal of the nurse-child relationship is to provide a role model for the parents in helping them to relate positively and constructively to their child and to foster a therapeutic environment for the child in his or her reprieve from the abusing situation.

---

[d]Telephone numbers are usually listed under "Child Abuse" in the business white pages of the local directory, or you can call the emergency child abuse hotline: 800-422-4453 (800-4-A-CHILD).

Support the Family

The nurse also encourages the child's relationship with nonoffending parents. The nurse does not become a substitute parent but rather acts as a role model for parents in helping them to relate positively and constructively to their child. When parental ignorance of childrearing practices has played a part in the abuse, the nurse can educate the parents on children's physical and emotional needs. Because of the parents' own childrearing, they may not be aware of nonviolent methods of discipline, such as time-outs. They may also need help in dealing with their frustration so that they do not vent anger on the child. Because these parents may be sensitive to criticism or resistant to authority figures, teaching is implemented through demonstration and example rather than through lecturing. Praise any competent parenting abilities they demonstrate to promote their sense of parental adequacy.

Advise family members to encourage the child to resume normal activities and observe the child for signs of distress (see Chapter 16, Posttraumatic Stress Disorder). Children express their feelings primarily through behavior. Parents should be alert for changes in behavior that indicate distress resulting from the incident, such as remaining in the house, refusing to go to school, changes in sleeping patterns, and frequency of dreams and nightmares.

Referral to appropriate social service agencies is also essential. Many abusive parents live in poverty, and the daily stresses imposed by their circumstances are overwhelming. Seek resources for financial aid, improved housing, and child care. Self-help groups also provide important services. Groups such as Parents Anonymous[e] (a group for parents who have abused or fear that they may abuse their child but only in terms of physical abuse, not sexual abuse) are accepting and nonjudgmental.

Plan for Discharge

Discharge planning should begin as soon as the legal disposition for placement has been decided, which may be temporary foster home placement, return to the parents, or permanent termination of parental rights. The latter is the most drastic solution, but it is necessary in situations of life-threatening abuse. Whenever children are sent to a foster home or juvenile institution, they must be allowed an opportunity to express their feelings. No matter how severe the abuse, they usually mourn the loss of their parents. They need help to understand why they must not return home and that this new home is in no way a punishment. Whenever possible, foster parents are encouraged to visit in the hospital, and the nurse should take an active role in helping the new parents understand the child, as well as the child's health care needs, because studies have shown that the health care needs of children in foster care often go unmet (Schneiderman, Smith, & Palinkas, 2012).

Prevent Abuse

Prevention of child maltreatment has been an extremely difficult goal. However, nurses have played an important role in such programs. For example, home visits based on identified risk factors (such as mothers who are teenagers, unmarried, or of low socioeconomic status) were noted to be an effective preventive measure (Selph, Bougatsos, Blazina, et al., 2013). The nurses provided information on normal child growth and development and routine health care needs, served as informal support persons, and referred families to appropriate services when a need for assistance was identified. The Nurse-Family Partnership is one program that has demonstrated evidence-based interventions resulting in the prevention of child maltreatment (Lane, 2014).

Nurses in a variety of settings can implement similar activities. For example, nurses in prenatal clinics can prepare expectant families for adjustment to parenthood. Nursery and postpartum nurses can foster the attachment process by encouraging parents to hold and look at their infant, as well as teach coping mechanisms for prolonged crying. Nurses in neonatal intensive care units can minimize the effects of separation by encouraging parents to visit and can help parents become comfortable caring for their child. Nurses in ambulatory settings can teach parents appropriate methods of bathing, feeding, toileting, disciplining, and preventing injuries while stressing the normal needs and developmental characteristics of children. Nurses must be sensitive to parental needs for attention, reassurance, and reinforcement, and should refer parents to community services and self-help groups.

Unlike preventive efforts for neglect and physical abuse, which have been aimed at the potential offender, prevention of child sexual abuse has centered on education of children to protect themselves. Materials that describe sexual abuse and its prevention are available for parents.[f] Helpful games such as "What if the babysitter wants to wrestle and hug but tells you to keep it a secret?" can be used to explore dangerous situations in advance and help children learn the importance of saying "no." They need reassurance that no matter what the other person says or does, the parents want to know about it and will not punish them. Even if children participate in the activity before telling their parents, they must be reassured that it was not their fault. It is equally important to teach children safety in terms of potential risk situations. Several suggestions for parents regarding protecting and educating children against possible molestation are presented in the Family-Centered Care box. The nurse is frequently in a position to discuss the topic of abuse with parents and to provide guidelines. In addition, parents need to be made aware that "nice" people, including friends and relatives, can be offenders; parents should carefully observe how others act toward the child. A sudden change in the child's behavior and a response such as "I don't like Uncle Bob anymore" are clues to investigate the relationship. In the event of any doubt, prevent further solitary encounters with this person and the child. It is sometimes to the child's great misfortune that parents do not take certain comments seriously, such as "He hugs me too tight" or "I don't want to go with him." Casual parental statements such as "He just loves you" or "You do whatever adults tell you to do" can place children in jeopardy. Health professionals must alert parents to such dangers and guide them toward an appreciation of the problem, providing concrete guidelines toward child education and protection.

---

[e]250 West First Street, Suite 250, Claremont, CA 91711; 909-621-6184; http://www.parentsanonymous.org.

[f]Sources of information are Prevent Child Abuse America, 228 S. Wabash Ave., 10th Floor, Chicago, IL 60604; 312-663-3520 or 800-Children (800-244-5373); http://www.preventchildabuse.org.

FAMILY-CENTERED CARE

Preventing and Dealing With Sexual Abuse of Children

Sexual assault of children is much more common than most people realize. It may be preventable if children have good preparation. *To provide protection and preparation:*

- Pay careful attention to who is around children. (Unwanted touch may come from someone liked and trusted.)
- Back up a child's right to say no.
- Encourage communication by taking seriously what children say.
- Take a second look at signals of potential danger.
- Refuse to leave children in the company of those who are not trusted.
- Include information about sexual assault when teaching about safety.
- Provide specific definitions and examples of sexual assault.
- Remind children that even "nice" people sometimes do mean things.
- Urge children to tell about *anybody* who causes them to be uncomfortable.
- Prepare children to deal with bribes, threats, and possible physical force.
- Virtually eliminate secrets between children and parents.
- Teach children how to say no, ask for help, and control who touches them and how.
- Model self-protective and limit-setting behavior for children.

If it ever becomes necessary to help a child recover from a sexual assault:

- Listen carefully to understand the child.
- Support the child for telling through praise, belief, sympathy, and lack of blame.
- Know local resources and choose help carefully.
- Provide opportunities to talk about the assault.
- Provide opportunities for the entire family to go through a recovery process.

Sexual assault affects everyone. To help deal with this social problem:

- Provide care and support to those who have been victimized.
- Recognize that offenders may not change behavior even with intervention.
- Organize neighborhood programs to support each other's efforts to protect children.
- Encourage schools to provide information about sexual assault as a problem of health and safety.
- Organize community groups to support educational treatment and law enforcement programs.

Modified from Adams, C., & Fay, J. (1981). *No more secrets: Protecting your child from sexual assault.* San Luis Obispo, CA: Impact.

CLINICAL JUDGMENT AND NEXT-GENERATION NCLEX® EXAMINATION-STYLE QUESTIONS

1. A mother expresses concerns about her 4-year-old son experiencing "terrible dreams". The nurse conducts a health history and assessment on the child relating to the mother's concern and notes the findings below. **Select all the history and assessment findings that require follow-up. Select all that apply.**
   A. The child awakens at night, cries and screams while being unaware of his mother by his side.
   B. The mother believes the child will grow out of this stage when he is a little older.
   C. The child has a specific nighttime routine that is helpful in calming the child.
   D. The mother watches frightening TV shows with him to help him understand what is real.
   E. The mother admits giving the child a "medication" to help him calm down when this occurs.
   F. The child likes to color and draw pictures of his dreams.

2. A 3-year-old boy is brought to the emergency department by his parents after he was noted to be "acting differently than normal" a few hours ago while he was being cared for by his grandmother. When she went to take her evening medication, the grandmother noted that her pill container had been opened and some pills were missing. The parents state that the grandmother has a heart condition. The nurse conducts a history and assessment and notes the findings below. **Select all the history and assessment findings that would require the nurse to follow-up immediately. Select all that apply.**
   A. The child has nausea and vomiting that began an hour ago
   B. Temperature is 36.8°C (98.4°F).
   C. Pulse is 48 beats/min
   D. Respiration rate is 20 breaths/min
   E. Heart rate is irregular
   F. Child is irritable

3. The nurse is working with the family of a 4-year-old girl and have concerns about possible exposure to lead poisoning. The mother states they live in an old house, built in 1975 that has paint that is peeling off the side. The child frequently plays in the dirt where there were loose paint chips found. A lead blood level was obtained with a result of 8 mcg/dL. **Choose the most likely options for the information missing from the statements below by selecting from the lists of options provided.**
   Based on the child's history and assessment data, the nurse determines that the laboratory findings reflect the need for ____1____.
   The nurse would educate the mother to complete follow-up lead testing within ____2____.

Options for 1	Options for 2
surveillance	1 month
treatment	1 week
chelation	6 months
nutrition	6 weeks
iron supplements	1 year

4. An 8-month-old infant girl is seen in the Emergency Department (ED), because the mother states the child fell down the stairs yesterday and hit her head. The infant presents with vomiting for the past 2 hours, refusing to eat or drink, and has become more listless and tired since the fall. While reading the infant's electronic medical record, the nurse notes a previous ED visit two months for a burn incident, and there is a history of maternal drug abuse also documented. **Select all the additional history and assessment findings below that require the nurse to intervene. Select all that apply.**
   A. Bruises on her arms and legs
   B. No other siblings
   C. Mother is unable to provide details on how the infant fell down the stairs
   D. Infant is wrapped warmly in a blanket and being held by the mother
   E. Weight loss since last visit

REFERENCES

Adams, J. A. (2011). Medical evaluation of suspected child sexual abuse: 2011 update. *Journal of Child Sexual Abuse, 20*(5), 588–605.

Albertson, T. E., Owen, K. P., Sutter, M. E., et al. (2011). Gastrointestinal decontamination in the acutely poisoned patient. *International Journal of Emergency Medicine, 4*, 65.

Altimier, L. (2008). Shaken baby syndrome. *The Journal of Perinatal and Neonatal Nursing, 22*(1), 68–76.

American Academy of Pediatrics Committee on Child Abuse and Neglect. (2009). Abusive head trauma in infants and children. *Pediatrics, 123*(5), 1409–1411.

Barr, R. G. (2012). Preventing abusive head trauma resulting from a failure of normal interaction between infants and their caregivers. *Proceedings of the National Academy of Sciences of the United States, 109*(Suppl. 2), 17294–17301.

Bathory, E., & Tomopoulus, S. (2017). Sleep regulation, physiology, and development, sleep duration and patterns, and sleep hygiene in infants, toddlers, and preschool-age children. *Current Problems in Pediatrics and Adolescent Health Care, 47*(2), 29–42.

Bellinger, D. C., Chen, A., & Lanphear, B. P. (2017). Establishing and achieving national goals for preventing lead toxicity and exposure in children. *JAMA Pediatrics, 17*(7), 616–618.

Benson, B. E., Hoppu, K., Troutman, W. G., et al. (2013). Position paper update: gastric lavage for gastrointestinal decontamination. *Clinical Toxicology (Philadelphia, Pa.), 51*(3), 140–146.

Breyer, R. J., & MacPhee, D. (2015). Community characteristics, conservative ideology, and child abuse rates. *Child Abuse & Neglect, 41*, 126–135.

Bronstein, A. C., Spyker, D. A., Cantilena, L. R., Jr., et al. (2012). 2011 Annual report of the American Association of Poison Control Centers' National Poison Data System (NPDS): 29th annual report. *Clinical Toxicology (Philadelphia, Pa.), 50*(10), 911–1164.

Burns, M. S., & Gerstenberger, S. L. (2014). Implications of the new Centers for Disease Control and Prevention blood lead reference value. *The American Journal of Public Health, 104*(6), e27–e33.

Carman, K. B., Tutkun, E., Yilmaz, et al. (2013). Acute mercury poisoning among children in two provinces of Turkey. *European Journal of Pediatrics, 172*(6), 821–827.

Centers for Disease Control and Prevention. (2002). *Managing elevated blood lead levels among young children: Recommendations from the Advisory Committee on Childhood Lead Poisoning Prevention*. Atlanta: Author.

Centers for Disease Control and Prevention Advisory Committee on Childhood Lead Poisoning Prevention. (2012). *CDC response to Advisory Committee on Childhood Lead Poisoning Prevention recommendations in "low level lead exposure harms children: A renewed call of primary prevention"*. http://www.cdc.gov/nceh/lead/acclpp/final_document_030712.pdf.

Centers for Disease Control and Prevention. (2017). Lead. https://www.cdc.gov/nceh/lead/. Updated 9 February 2017.

Covington, L. B., Armstrong, B., & Black, M. (2018). Perceived toddler sleep problems, co-sleeping, and maternal sleep and mental health. *Journal of Developmental and Behavioral Pediatrics, 39*(3), 238–245.

Cowley, L. E., Morris, C. B., Maguire, S. A., et al. (2015). Validation of a prediction tool for abusive head trauma. *Pediatrics, 136*(2), 290–298.

Cunningham, E. (2012). What role does nutrition play in the prevention or treatment of childhood lead poisoning? *The Journal of the Academy of Nutrition and Dietetics, 112*(11), 1916.

Dapul, H., & Laraque, D. (2014). Lead poisoning in children. *Advances in Pediatrics, 61*(1), 313–333.

Dubowitz, H., & Lane, W. (2016). Abused and neglected children. In R. M. Kliegman, B. F. Stanton, J. W. St Geme, et al. (Eds.), *Nelson textbook of pediatrics* (20th ed.). Philadelphia: Saunders/Elsevier.

Evans, H. (2011). Pediatrics tackles child sexual abuse. *The Archives of Pediatrics & Adolescent Medicine, 165*(9), 783–784.

Forsdike, K., Tarzia, L., Hindmarsh, E., et al. (2014). Family violence across the life cycle. *Australian Family Physician, 43*(11), 768–774.

Fountain, J. S., & Reith, D. M. (2014). Dangers of "EDTA". *New Zealand Medical Journal, 127*(1398), 126–127.

Frithsen, I., & Simpson, W. (2010). Recognition and management of acute medication poisoning. *American Family Physician, 81*(3), 316–323.

Girardet, R., Bolton, K., Lohoti, S., et al. (2011). Collection of forensic evidence from pediatric victims of sexual assault. *Pediatrics, 128*(2), 233–238.

Hibbard, R., Barlow, J., MacMillan, H., et al. (2012). Psychological maltreatment. *Pediatrics, 130*(2), 372–378.

Jones, A. L. (2009). Emerging aspects of assessing lead poisoning in childhood. *Emerging Health Threats Journal, 2*, e3.

Kemp, A. M. (2011). Abusive head trauma: Recognition and the essential investigation. *Archives of Disease in Childhood: Education & Practice edition, 96*(6), 202–208.

Krienert, J. L., & Walsh, J. A. (2011). Sibling sexual abuse: An empirical analysis of offender, victim, and event characteristics in National Incident-based Reporting System (NBRS) data, 2000–2007. *Journal of Child Sexual Abuse, 20*(4), 353–372.

Lane, W. G. (2014). Prevention of child maltreatment. *Pediatric Clinics of North America, 61*(5), 873–888.

Lee, V. R., Connolly, M., & Calello, D. P. (2017). Pediatric poisoning by ingestion: Developmental overview and synopsis of national trends. *Pediatric Annals, 46*(12), e443–e448.

Lyden, C. (2011). Uncovering child abuse. *Nursing Management, 42*(Suppl), 1–5.

Maguire, S. A., Watts, P. O., Shaw, A. D., et al. (2013). Retinal hemorrhages and related findings in abusive and non-abusive head trauma: A systematic review. *Eye, 27*(1), 28–36.

McGregor, T., Parkar, M., & Rao, S. (2009). Evaluation and management of common childhood poisonings. *American Family Physician, 79*(5), 397–403.

Mindell, J. A., & Williamson, A. A. (2018). Benefits of a bedtime routine in young children: Sleep development and beyond. *Sleep Medicine Reviews, 40*, 93–108.

Mollen, C. J., Goyal, M. K., & Frioux, S. M. (2012). Acute sexual abuse. *Pediatric Emergency Care, 28*(6), 584–590.

Mowry, J. B., Spyker, D. A., Brooks, D. E., et al. (2016). Annual report of the American Association Of Poison Control Centers' National Poison Data System (NPDS): 33rd annual report. *Clinical Toxicology (Philadelphia, Pa.), 54*(10), 924–1109. https://doi.org/10.1080/15563650.2016.1245421.

National Center on Shaken Baby Syndrome.(n.d.). Facts & Info. https://www.dontshake.org/learn-more/item/114-facts-and-info.

Olson, K. R. (2010). Activated charcoal for acute poisoning: One toxicologist's journey. *The Journal of Medical Toxicology, 6*(2), 190–198.

Patel, O., Magnusen, E., & Sandell, J. M. (2017). Prevention of unintentional injury in children. *Paediatrics and Child Health, 27*(9), 420–426.

Petersen, D. D. (2011). Common plant toxicology: A comparison of national and southwest Ohio data trends in plant poisonings in the 21st century. *Toxicology and Applied Pharmacology, 254*(2), 148–153.

Raymond, J. S., Kennedy, C., & Brown, M. J. (2013). Blood lead level analysis among refugee children resettled in New Hampshire and Rhode Island. *Public Health Nursing, 30*(1), 70–79.

Schneiderman, J. U., Smith, C., & Palinkas, L. A. (2012). The caregiver as gatekeeper for accessing health care for children in foster care: A qualitative study of kinship and unrelated caregivers. *Children and Youth Services, 34*(10), 2123–2130.

Selph, S. S., Bougatsos, C., Blazina, I., et al. (2013). Behavioral interventions and counseling to prevent child abuse and neglect: A systematic review to update the US Preventative Services Task Force recommendations. *Annals of Internal Medicine, 158*(3), 179–190.

Skarsaune, K., & Bondas, T. (2015). Neglected nursing responsibility when suspecting child abuse. *Clinical Nursing Studies, 4*(1).

Squires, J. E., & Squires, R. H. (2013). A review of Munchausen syndrome by proxy. *Pediatric Annals, 42*(4), 67–71.

Theurer, W. M., & Bhavsar, A. K. (2013). Prevention of unintentional childhood injury. *American Family Physician, 87*(7), 502–509.

US Department of Health and Human Services. (2015). *The Child Abuse Prevention and Treatment Act (CAPTA) 2010*. Washington, DC: US Government Printing Office.

Ward, T. C., & Doering, J. J. (2014). Application of a socio-ecological model to mother infant bed sharing. *Health Education & Behavior, 41*(6), 577–589.

Ward, T. C. S., Robb, S. W., & Kanu, F. A. (2016). Prevalence and characteristics of bed-sharing among black and white infants in Georgia. *Maternal and Child Health Journal, 20*, 347–362.

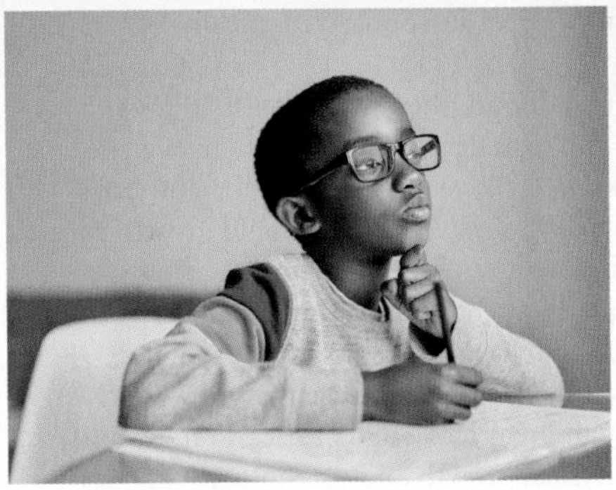

14

Health Promotion of the School-Age Child and Family

Alice M. Burch

http://evolve.elsevier.com/wong/essentials

CONCEPTS

- Development
- Functional Ability
- Culture
- Family Dynamics
- Sexuality
- Stress
- Safety

PROMOTING OPTIMAL GROWTH AND DEVELOPMENT

The segment of the life span that extends from age 6 to approximately age 12 has a variety of labels, each of which describes an important characteristic of the period. These middle years are most often referred to as *school-age years* or *the school years.* This period begins with entrance into the school environment, which has a significant impact on development and relationships.

Physiologically, the middle years begin with the shedding of the first deciduous tooth and end at puberty with the acquisition of the final permanent teeth (with the exception of the wisdom teeth). Before 5 or 6 years old, children have progressed from helpless infants to sturdy, complicated individuals with an ability to communicate, conceptualize in a limited way, and become involved in complex social and motor behaviors. Physical growth has been equally rapid during the preschool-age years. In contrast, the period of middle childhood, between the rapid growth of early childhood and the prepubescent growth spurt, is a time of gradual growth and development with more even progress in both physical and emotional aspects.

BIOLOGIC DEVELOPMENT

During middle childhood, growth in height and weight assumes a slower but steady pace as compared with the earlier years. Between 6 and 12 years old, children grow an average of 5 cm (2 inches) per year to gain 30 to 60 cm (1 to 2 feet) in height and almost double their weight, increasing 2 to 3 kg (4.4 to 6.6 pounds) per year. The average 6-year-old child is about 116 cm (46 inches) tall and weighs about 21 kg (46 pounds); the average 12-year-old child is about 150 cm (59 inches) tall and weighs approximately 40 kg (88 pounds). During this age, girls and boys differ little in size, although boys tend to be slightly taller and somewhat heavier than girls. Toward the end of the school-age years, both boys and girls begin to increase in size, although most girls begin to surpass boys in both height and weight, to the acute discomfort of both girls and boys.

Physical Changes

School-age children are more graceful than they were as preschoolers, and they are steadier on their feet. Their body proportions take on a slimmer look, with longer legs, varying body proportion, and a lower center of gravity. Posture improves over that of the preschool period to facilitate locomotion and efficiency in using the arms and trunk. These proportions make climbing, bicycle riding, and other activities easier. Fat gradually diminishes, and its distribution patterns change, contributing to the thinner appearance of children during these middle years, although as previously stated they continue to gain weight.

Accompanying the skeletal lengthening and fat diminution is an increase in the percentage of body weight represented by muscle tissue. By the end of this age period, both boys and girls double their strength and physical capabilities, and their steady and relatively consistent development of coordination increases their poise and skill. However, this increased strength is often misleading. Although strength increases, muscles are still functionally immature when compared with those of adolescents, and they are more readily damaged by muscular injury caused by overuse. Thus caution must be used in sports activities for children in this age-group.

The most pronounced changes that indicate increasing maturity in children are a decrease in head circumference in relation to standing height, a decrease in waist circumference in relation to height, and an increase in leg length in relation to height. These indicators often provide a clue to a child's degree of physical maturity. There appears to be a correlation between physical indications of maturity and success in school.

Certain physiologic and anatomic characteristics are typical of school-age children. Facial proportions change as the face grows faster in relation to the remainder of the cranium. The skull and brain grow very slowly

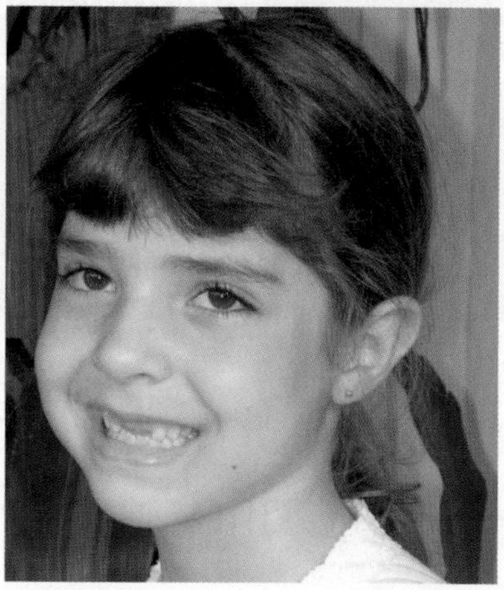

Fig. 14.1 Middle childhood is the stage of development when deciduous teeth are shed.

during this period and increase little in size thereafter. Because all of the primary (deciduous) teeth are lost during this age span, middle childhood is sometimes known as the age of the loose tooth (Fig. 14.1). The early years of middle childhood, when the new secondary (permanent) teeth appear too large for the face, are known as the ugly duckling stage.

Maturation of Systems

Maturity of the gastrointestinal system is reflected in fewer stomach upsets, better maintenance of blood glucose levels, and an increased stomach capacity, which permits retention of food for longer periods. School-age children do not need to be fed as promptly or as frequently as preschool-age children. Caloric needs (kcal/kg) are less than they were in the preschool years and lower than they will be during the coming adolescent growth spurt.

Physical maturation is evident in other body tissues and organs. Bladder capacity, although differing widely among individual children, is generally greater in girls than in boys. The heart grows more slowly during the middle years and is smaller in relation to the rest of the body than at any other period of life. Heart and respiratory rates steadily decrease, and blood pressure increases from 6 to 12 years old.

The immune system becomes more competent in its ability to localize infections and to produce an antibody-antigen response. However, children commonly have several infections in the first 1 to 2 years of school because of increased exposure to others in their school classes.

Bones continue to ossify throughout childhood but yield to pressure and muscle pulls more readily than with mature bones. Children need ample opportunity to move around, but they should observe caution in carrying heavy loads. For example, they should shift books or tote bags from one arm to the other. Backpacks, when worn correctly, distribute weight more evenly.

Wider differences between children are observed at the end of middle childhood than at the beginning. These differences become increasingly apparent and, if they are extreme or unique, may create emotional problems. The associated characteristics of height and weight relationships, rapid or slow growth, and other important features of development should be explained to children and their families. Physical maturity is not necessarily correlated with emotional and social maturity. Seven-year-old children who look like 10-year-old children will think and act like 7-year-olds. To expect behaviors appropriate for an older age is unrealistic and can be detrimental to their development of competence and self-esteem. Conversely, to treat 10-year-old children who look young physically as though they were younger is an equal disservice to them.

Prepubescence

Preadolescence is the period that begins toward the end of middle childhood and ends with the 13th birthday. **Puberty** signals the beginning of the development of secondary sex characteristics, and **prepubescence**, the 2-year period that precedes puberty, typically occurs during preadolescence.

Toward the end of middle childhood, the discrepancies in growth and maturation between boys and girls become apparent. On average, there is a difference of approximately 2 years between girls and boys in the age of onset of pubescence. This is a period of rapid growth in height and weight, especially for girls.

There is no universal age at which children assume the characteristics of prepubescence. The first physiologic signs appear at about 9 years old (particularly in girls) and are usually clearly evident in 11- to 12-year-old children. Although preadolescent children do not want to be different, variability in physical growth and physiologic changes among children of the same sex and between the two sexes is often striking at this time. This variability, especially in relation to the onset of secondary sex characteristics, is of great concern to preadolescents. Either early or late appearance of these characteristics is a source of embarrassment and uneasiness to both sexes.

Preadolescence is a time when considerable overlapping of developmental characteristics occurs, with elements of both middle childhood and early adolescence apparent. However, several unique characteristics set this period apart from others. In general, puberty begins at 10 years old in girls and at 12 years old in boys, but it can be normal for either sex after 8 years old. Boys experience little visible sexual maturation during preadolescence, whereas girls' bodies may change quite visibly.

PSYCHOSOCIAL DEVELOPMENT: DEVELOPING A SENSE OF INDUSTRY (ERIKSON)

Freud described middle childhood as the **latency period**, a time of tranquility between the Oedipal phase of early childhood and the eroticism of adolescence. During this time, children experience relationships with same-sex peers following the indifference of earlier years and preceding the heterosexual fascination that occurs for most boys and girls in puberty.

Successful mastery of Erikson's first three stages of psychosocial development is important in terms of development of a healthy personality. Successful completion of these stages requires a loving environment within a stable family unit. These experiences prepare the child to engage in experiences and relationships beyond the intimate family group. Children who do not experience a stable family life often have a difficult time establishing relationships.

A **sense of industry**, or a sense of accomplishment, occurs somewhere between 6 years old and adolescence. School-age children are eager to develop skills and participate in meaningful and socially useful work. Interests expand in the middle years, and with a growing sense of independence, children want to engage in tasks that can be carried through to completion (Fig. 14.2). Failure to develop a sense of accomplishment may result in a feeling of inferiority.

Many aspects of industry contribute to the child's sense of competence and mastery. Children gain satisfaction from independent behavior in exploring and manipulating their environment and from interaction with peers. Reinforcement in the form of grades, material rewards, additional privileges, and recognition provides encouragement and stimulation.

A sense of accomplishment also involves the ability to cooperate, to compete with others, and to cope effectively with people. Middle childhood is the time when children learn the value of doing things with others and the benefits derived from division of labor in the accomplishment of goals. Peer approval is a strong motivating power.

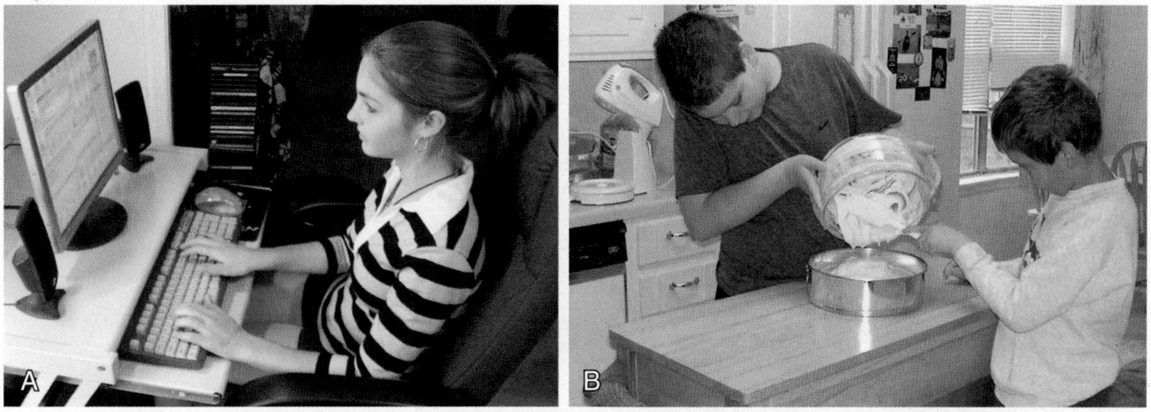

Fig. 14.2 School-age children are motivated to complete tasks. **A**, Working alone. **B**, Working with others.

The danger inherent in this period of development is the occurrence of situations that might result in a sense of inadequacy or **inferiority**. This may happen if the previous stages have not been successfully mastered or if a child is incapable of or unprepared to assume responsibilities associated with developing sense of accomplishment. Children with physical and mental limitations may be at a disadvantage in the acquisition of certain skills. When the reward structure is based on evidence of mastery, children who are incapable of developing these skills risk feeling inadequate and inferior.

Even children without chronic disabilities may experience feelings of inadequacy in some areas. No child is able to do everything well, and children must learn that they will not be able to master every skill they attempt. All children, even children who usually have positive attitudes toward work and their own abilities, will feel some degree of inferiority when they encounter specific skills that they cannot master.

Children need and want real achievement. Children achieve a sense of industry when they have access to tasks that need to be done and they are able to complete the tasks well despite individual differences in their innate capacities and emotional development.

COGNITIVE DEVELOPMENT (PIAGET)

When children enter the school years, they begin to acquire the ability to relate a series of events to mental representations that can be expressed both verbally and symbolically. This is the stage Piaget describes as **concrete operations**, when children can use thought processes to experience events and actions. The rigid, egocentric view of the preschool years is replaced by thought processes that allow children to see things from another's point of view. Their steady reduction in egocentricity helps form the basis for logical thought and the development and maturation of morality.

During this stage, children develop an understanding of relationships between things and ideas. They progress from making judgments based on what they see (perceptual thinking) to making judgments based on what they reason (conceptual thinking). They are increasingly able to master symbols and to use their memories of past experiences to evaluate and interpret the present.

One of the major cognitive tasks of school-age children is mastering the concept of **conservation** (Fig. 14.3). There is a developmental sequence in children's capacity to understand conservation. Children usually grasp conservation of numbers (ages 5 to 6) before conservation of substance. For example, they first recognize that 7 remains 7 whether it is represented by 3 + 4, 2 + 5, 7 buttons, or 7 stars. Conservation of liquids, mass, and length usually is accomplished at about ages 6 to 7. At this time, they recognize that changing the shape of a substance, such as a lump of clay, does not alter its total mass. They learn conservation of weight sometime later (ages 9 to 10) and conservation of volume or displacement last (ages 9 to 12). For example, they no longer perceive a tall, thin glass of water as containing a greater volume than a short, wide glass; they can distinguish between the weights of items regardless of their size. School-age children also develop classification skills. They can group and sort objects according to the attributes these objects share, place things in a sensible and logical order, and hold a concept in mind while making decisions based on that concept. In middle childhood, children derive a great deal of enjoyment from classifying and ordering their environment. They become occupied with collections of objects, such as stickers, shells, dolls, cars, cards, and stuffed animals. They may even begin to order friends and relationships (e.g., best friend, second best friend).

They develop the ability to understand relational terms and concepts, such as yesterday and tomorrow, bigger and smaller, darker and paler, heavier and lighter, to the right of and to the left of, and more than and less than. They view family relationships in terms of reciprocal roles (e.g., to be a brother, one must have a sibling).

School-age children learn the alphabet and the world of symbols called *words,* which can be arranged in terms of structure and their relationship to the alphabet. They learn to tell time, to see the relationship of events in time (history) and places in space (geography), and to combine time and space relationships (geology and astronomy).

The ability to read is acquired during the school years and becomes the most significant and valuable tool for independent inquiry. Children's capacity to explore, imagine, and expand their knowledge is enhanced by reading.

MORAL DEVELOPMENT (KOHLBERG)

As children move from egocentrism to more logical patterns of thought, they also move through stages in the development of conscience and moral standards. Young children do not believe that standards of behavior come from within themselves but that rules are established and set down by others. During the preschool years, children perceive rules as definite and require no reason or explanation. They learn standards for acceptable behavior, act according to these standards, and feel guilty when they violate them. Although children 6 or 7 years old know the rules and behaviors expected of them, they do not understand the reasons behind them. Rewards and punishments guide their judgment; a "bad act" is one that breaks a rule or causes harm. Young children believe that what other people tell them to do is right and that what they themselves think is wrong. Consequently, children 6 or 7 years old may interpret accidents or misfortunes as punishment for "bad" acts.

Older school-age children are able to judge an act by the intentions that prompted it rather than just its consequences. Rules and judgments become less absolute and authoritarian and begin to be founded

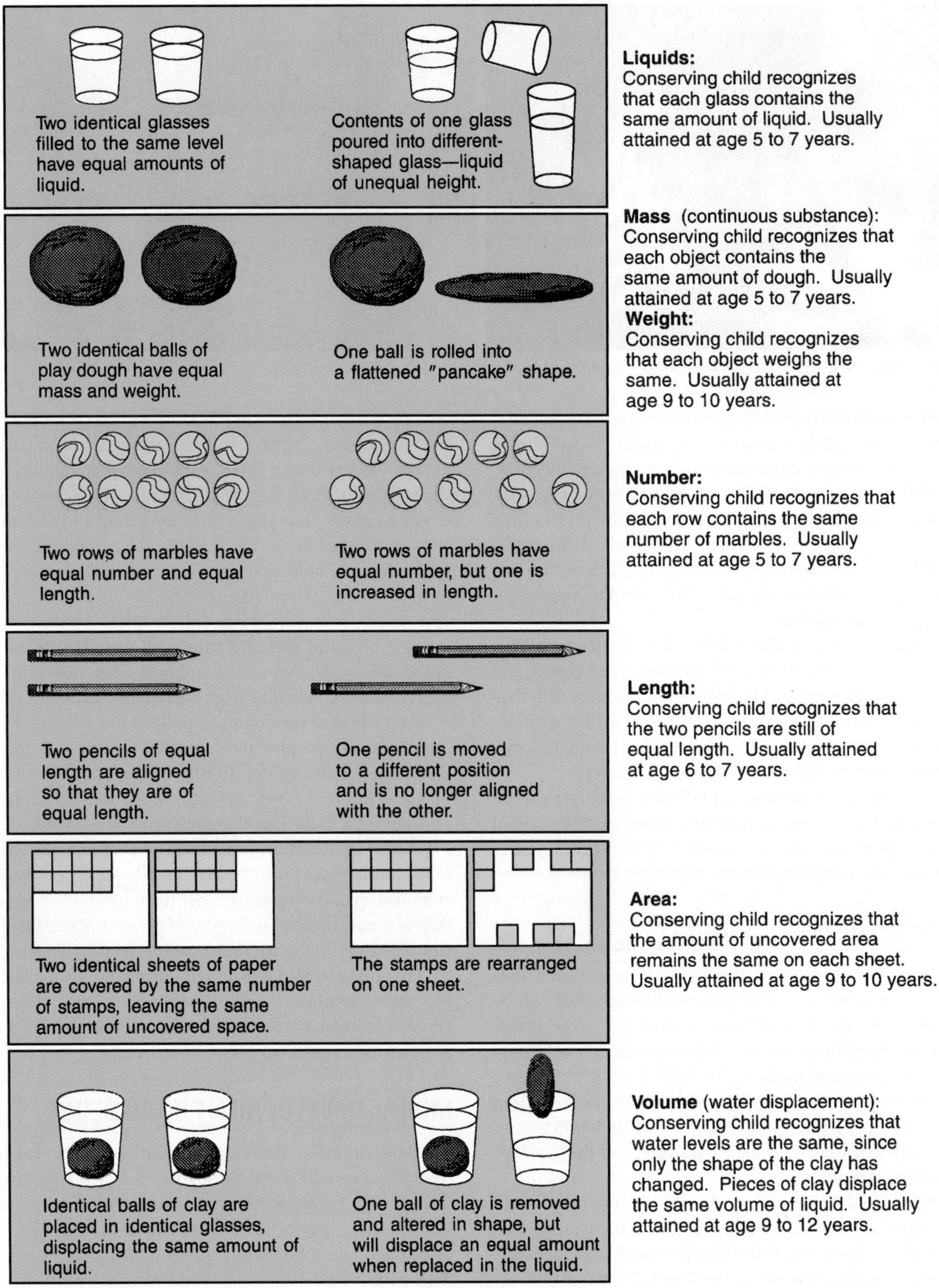
Two identical glasses filled to the same level have equal amounts of liquid.
Contents of one glass poured into different-shaped glass—liquid of unequal height.
Liquids:
Conserving child recognizes that each glass contains the same amount of liquid. Usually attained at age 5 to 7 years.
Two identical balls of play dough have equal mass and weight.
One ball is rolled into a flattened "pancake" shape.
Mass (continuous substance):
Conserving child recognizes that each object contains the same amount of dough. Usually attained at age 5 to 7 years.
Weight:
Conserving child recognizes that each object weighs the same. Usually attained at age 9 to 10 years.
Two rows of marbles have equal number and equal length.
Two rows of marbles have equal number, but one is increased in length.
Number:
Conserving child recognizes that each row contains the same number of marbles. Usually attained at age 5 to 7 years.
Two pencils of equal length are aligned so that they are of equal length.
One pencil is moved to a different position and is no longer aligned with the other.
Length:
Conserving child recognizes that the two pencils are still of equal length. Usually attained at age 6 to 7 years.
Two identical sheets of paper are covered by the same number of stamps, leaving the same amount of uncovered space.
The stamps are rearranged on one sheet.
Area:
Conserving child recognizes that the amount of uncovered area remains the same on each sheet. Usually attained at age 9 to 10 years.
Identical balls of clay are placed in identical glasses, displacing the same amount of liquid.
One ball of clay is removed and altered in shape, but will displace an equal amount when replaced in the liquid.
Volume (water displacement):
Conserving child recognizes that water levels are the same, since only the shape of the clay has changed. Pieces of clay displace the same volume of liquid. Usually attained at age 9 to 12 years.

Fig. 14.3 Common examples that demonstrate the child's ability to conserve (ages are only approximate).

on the needs and desires of others. For older children, a rule violation is likely to be viewed in relation to the total context in which it appears. The situation, as well as the morality of the rule itself, influences reactions. Although younger children judge an act only according to whether it is right or wrong, older children take into account different points of view. They are able to understand and accept the concept of treating others as they would like to be treated.

SPIRITUAL DEVELOPMENT

Children at this age think in concrete terms but are avid learners and have a great desire to learn about their God or deity. They picture God as human and use adjectives such as "loving" and "helping" to describe their deity. They are fascinated by the concepts of hell and heaven, with a developing conscience and concern about rules, and they may fear going to hell for misbehavior. School-age children want and expect to be punished for misbehavior and, when given the option, tend to choose a punishment that "fits the crime." Often they view illness or injury as a punishment for a real or imagined misdeed. The beliefs and ideals of family and religious persons are more influential than those of their peers in matters of faith.

School-age children begin to learn the difference between the natural and the supernatural but have difficulty understanding symbols. Consequently, religious concepts must be presented to them in concrete terms. Prayer or other religious rituals comfort them, and if these activities are a part of their daily lives, they can help them cope with threatening situations. Their petitions to their God in prayers tend to be for tangible rewards. Although younger children expect their prayers to be answered, as they get older they begin to recognize that this does not always occur, and they become less concerned when their prayers are not answered. They are able to discuss their feelings about their faith and how it relates to their lives (see Cultural Considerations box).

CULTURAL CONSIDERATIONS

Religious Orientation

Many schools and communities have a Judeo-Christian orientation toward prayer, holidays, and values. This may result in conflict and discomfort for children of other religious or ethnic groups. Sensitivity must be exercised so as not to offend and confuse children from other religious backgrounds, such as the Buddhist, Hindu, and Muslim faiths, and those with no religious backgrounds.

SOCIAL DEVELOPMENT

Peer group identification is an important factor in gaining independence from parents. Peer groups have a culture of their own with secrets, traditions, and codes of ethics that promote feelings of solidarity and detachment from adults. Through peer relationships, children learn how to deal with dominance and hostility, how to relate to persons in positions of leadership and authority, and how to explore ideas and the physical environment. The aid and support of the group provide children with enough security to risk the moderate parental rejection brought about by small victories in the development of independence.

A child's concept of the appropriate sex role is acquired through relationships with peers. During the early school years, few gender differences exist in the play experiences of children. Both girls and boys share games and other activities. However, in the later school years, the differences in the play of boys and girls become more marked.

Social Relationships and Cooperation

Daily relationships with peers provide important social interactions for school-age children. For the first time, children join group activities with unrestrained enthusiasm and steady participation. Previous interactions were limited to short periods under considerable adult supervision. With increased skills and wider opportunities, children become involved with one or more peer groups in which they can gain status as respected members.

Valuable lessons are learned from daily interaction with age-mates. First, children learn to appreciate the numerous and varied points of view that are represented in the peer group. As children interact with peers who see the world in ways that are somewhat different from their own, they become aware of the limits of their own point of view. Because age-mates are peers and are not forced to accept each other's ideas as they are expected to accept those of adults, other children have a significant influence on decreasing the egocentric outlook of the child. Consequently, children learn to argue, persuade, bargain, cooperate, and compromise to maintain friendships.

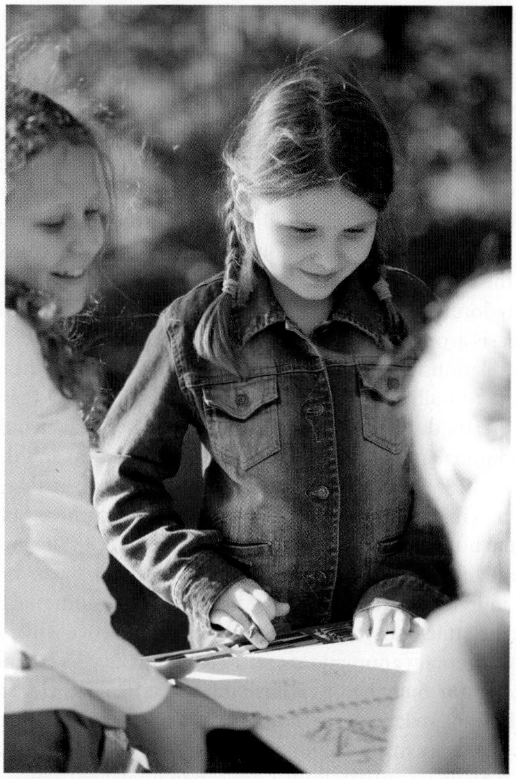

Fig. 14.4 School-age children enjoy engaging in activities with a "best friend."

Second, children become increasingly sensitive to the social norms and pressures of the peer group. The peer group establishes standards for acceptance and rejection, and children are often willing to modify their behavior to be accepted by the group. The need for peer approval becomes a powerful influence toward conformity. Children learn to dress, talk, and behave in a manner acceptable to the group. A variety of roles, such as class joker or class hero, may be assumed by individual children to gain approval from the group.

Third, the interaction among peers leads to the formation of intimate friendships between same-sex peers. The school-age period is the time when children have "best friends" with whom they share secrets, private jokes, and adventures; they come to one another's aid in times of trouble. In the course of these friendships, children also fight, threaten each other, break up, and reunite. These dyadic relationships, in which the child experiences love and closeness with a peer, seem to be important as a foundation for relationships in adulthood (Fig. 14.4).

Clubs and Peer Groups

One of the outstanding characteristics of middle childhood is the formation of formalized groups, or clubs. A prominent feature of these groups is the code of rigid rules imposed on the members. There is exclusiveness in the selection of persons who have the privilege of joining. Acceptance in the group is often determined on a pass–fail basis according to social or behavioral criteria. Conformity is the core of the group structure. There are often secret codes, shared interests, special styles of dress, and special words that signify membership in the group. Each child must abide by a standard of behavior established by the members. Conforming to the rules provides children with feelings of security and relieves them of the responsibility of making decisions. By merging their identities with those of their peers, children are able to move from the family group to an outside group as a step toward seeking further independence. Peer groups and clubs allow children to substitute conformity to a peer group for conformity to a family at a time when children are still too insecure to function independently.

During the early school years, groups are usually small and loosely organized, with changing membership and no formal structure. They do not demonstrate the elements of cooperation and order that are seen in groups of older children. In general, girls' groups are less formalized than boys' are, and although there may be a mixture of both sexes in the early school years, the groups of later school years are composed predominantly of children of the same sex. Common interests are the basis around which the group is structured.

Poor relationships with peers and a lack of group identification can contribute to bullying. **Bullying** is any recurring activity that intends to cause harm, distress, or control toward another in which there is a perceived imbalance of power between the aggressor(s) and the victim (Hensley, 2013). Although bullying can occur in any setting, it most often occurs in school hallways or on the playground where supervision is minimal but peers are present to witness the attack (Shetgiri, 2013). Cyber-bullying involves an electronic medium to harm or bother another individual and can be more harmful than traditional bullying, because the attack can instantly reach a wider audience while allowing the bully to remain anonymous (Sticca & Perren, 2013). Children who are targeted for bullying often have internalizing characteristics such as withdrawal, anxiety, depression, low self-esteem, and reduced assertiveness that may make them an easy target for bullying (Arseneault, Bowes, & Shakoor, 2010). Bullies are generally defiant toward adults, manipulative, and likely to break school rules. They have aggressive attitudes, a positive view of violence, and a lack of empathy and may experience or witness violence or abuse at home (Hensley, 2013). Boys who bully tend to use physical force, referred to as *direct bullying*, but girls usually use bullying methods, such as exclusion, gossip, or rumors, which are referred to as *indirect bullying* (Shetgiri, 2013).

The long-term consequences of bullying are significant. Future problems of bullies include a higher risk for conduct problems, hyperactivity, school dropout, unemployment, and participation in criminal behavior (Shetgiri, Lin, & Flores, 2012). Chronic bullies seem to continue their behaviors into adulthood, negatively influencing their ability to develop and maintain relationships. Victims of bullying are at increased risk for low self-esteem, anxiety, depression, feelings of insecurity, loneliness, poor academic performance, and psychosomatic complaints, such as feeling tense, tired, or dizzy (Giesbrecht, Leadbeater, & Macdonald, 2011). School personnel play an important role in implementing anti-bullying interventions in schools; however, research has recognized that involving the whole family in anti-bullying programs greatly increases success (Arseneault et al., 2010).

There are also dangers in peer group attachments that are too strong. Peer pressures force some children to take risks or engage in behaviors that are against their better judgment. A child's membership in a gang is associated with marked increases in serious delinquent behavior (Bradshaw, Waasdorp, Goldweber, et al., 2013). Peer group activities that result in unlawful or criminal **gang violence** are increasing in the United States (US Department of Justice, 2011). An integration of family-centered and school-based programs is needed to reduce the influences for children to become affiliated with gangs.

Relationships With Families

Although the peer group is influential and necessary for normal child development, parents are the primary influence in shaping their children's personalities, setting standards for behavior, and establishing value systems. Family values usually take precedence over peer value systems. Although children may appear to reject parental values while testing the new values of the peer group, ultimately they retain and incorporate into their own value systems the parental values they have found to be of worth.

In the middle school years, children want to spend more time in the company of peers, and they often prefer peer group activities to family activities. This can be disturbing to parents. Children become intolerant and critical of their parents, especially when their parents' ways deviate from those of the group. They discover that parents can be wrong, and they begin to question the knowledge and authority of their parents, who were previously considered to be all-knowing and all-powerful. Parents can best serve the interests of their children through tolerant understanding and support.

Although increased independence is the goal of middle childhood, children are not prepared to abandon all parental control. They need and want restrictions placed on their behavior, and they are not prepared to cope with all of the problems of their expanding environment. They feel more secure knowing there is an authority figure to implement controls and restrictions. Children may complain loudly about restrictions and try to break down parental barriers, but they are uneasy if they succeed in doing so. They respect adults who prevent them from acting on every urge. Children view this behavior as an expression of love and concern for their welfare.

Children also need their parents to be adults, not "pals." Sometimes parents, hurt by their children's rejection, attempt to maintain their love and gratitude by assuming the role of pal. Children need the stable, secure strength provided by mature adults to whom they can turn during troubled relationships with peers or stressful changes in their world. With a secure base in a loving family, children are able to develop the self-confidence and maturity needed to break loose from the group and stand independently.

Play

Play takes on new dimensions that reflect a new stage of development in the school years. Play involves increased physical skill, intellectual ability, and fantasy. In addition, children develop a sense of belonging to a team or club by forming groups and cliques. Belonging to a group is of vital importance.

Rules and Rituals

The need for conformity in middle childhood is strongly manifested in the activities and games of school-age children. In the preschool years, children's games were either invented for them or played in the company of a friend or an adult, and rules evolved with the game. Now children begin to see the need for rules, and their games have fixed and unvarying rules that may be bizarre and extraordinarily rigid. Part of the enjoyment of the game is knowing the rules because knowing means belonging. Conformity and ritual permeate their play and are also evident in their behavior and language. Childhood is full of chants and taunts, such as "Eeeny, meeny, miney, mo," "Last one is a rotten egg," and "Step on a crack, break your mother's back." Children derive a sense of pleasure and power from such sayings, which have been handed down with few changes through generations.

Team Play

A more complex form of play that evolves from the need for peer interaction is team games and sports. A referee, umpire, or person of authority may be required so that the rules can be followed more accurately. Team play teaches children to modify or exchange personal goals for goals of the group; it also teaches them that division of labor is an effective strategy for attaining a goal.

Team play can also contribute to children's social, intellectual, and skill growth (Eime, Young, Harvey, et al., 2013). Children work hard to

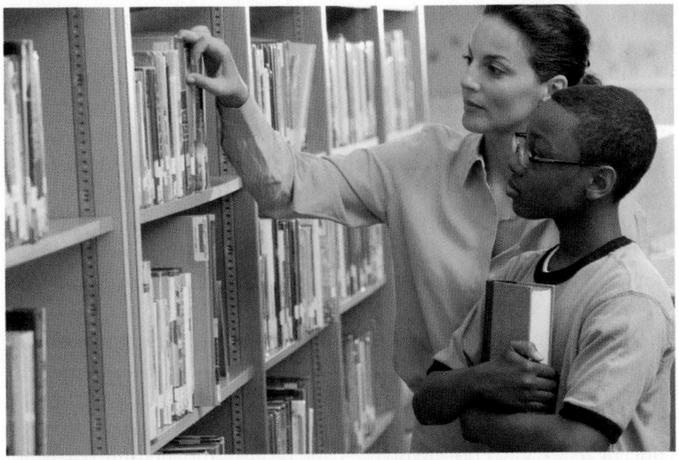

Fig. 14.5 Selecting a book with the assistance of an adult.

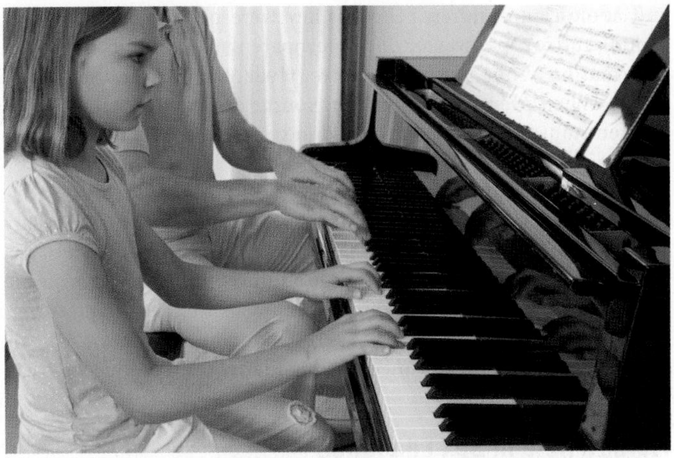

Fig. 14.6 School-age children take pride in learning new skills.

develop the skills needed to become team members, to improve their contribution to the group, and to anticipate the consequences of their behavior for the group. Team play helps stimulate cognitive growth because children are called on to learn many complex rules, make judgments about those rules, plan strategies, and assess the strengths and weaknesses of members of their own team and members of the opposing team.

Quiet Games and Activities

Although the play of school-age children can be highly active, they also enjoy many quiet and solitary activities. The middle years are the time for collections, and young school-age children's collections are an odd assortment of unrelated objects in messy, disorganized piles. Collections of later school years are more orderly and selective and often are organized in scrapbooks, on shelves, or in boxes.

School-age children become fascinated with complex board, card, or computer games that they can play alone or in groups. As in all games, adherence to the rules is fanatic. Disagreements over rules can cause much discussion and argument but are easily resolved by reading the rules of the game.

The newly acquired skill of reading becomes increasingly satisfying as school-age children expand their knowledge of the world through books (Fig. 14.5). School-age children never tire of stories and, as with preschool children, love to have stories read aloud. They also enjoy sewing, cooking, carpentry, gardening, and creative activities, such as painting. Many creative skills, such as music and art, as well as athletic skills such as swimming, karate, dancing, and skating, are learned during these years and continue to be enjoyed into adolescence and adulthood (Fig. 14.6).

Ego Mastery

Play affords children the means to acquire representational mastery over themselves, their environment, and others. Through play, children can feel as big, as powerful, and as skillful as their imaginations will allow. They can also feel in control and attain vicarious mastery and power over whomever and whatever they choose. School-age children still need the opportunity to use large muscles in exuberant outdoor play and the freedom to exert their newfound autonomy and initiative. They need space in which to exercise large muscles and to deal with tensions, frustrations, and hostility. Physical skills practiced and mastered in play help to develop a feeling of personal competence, which contributes to a sense of accomplishment and provides status in their peer group.

DEVELOPING A SELF-CONCEPT

The term self-concept refers to a conscious awareness of self-perceptions, such as one's physical characteristics, abilities, values, self-ideals and expectancy, and idea of self in relation to others. It also includes one's body image, sexuality, and self-esteem. Although primary caregivers continue to exert influence on children's self-evaluation, the opinions of peers and teachers provide valuable input during middle childhood. With the emphasis on skill building and broadened social relationships, children are continually engaged in the process of self-evaluation.

Body Image

Body image is what children think about their bodies and is influenced, but not solely determined, by significant others. The number of significant others that influences children's perception of themselves increases with age. Children are acutely aware of their own bodies, the bodies of their peers, and those of adults. They are also aware of deviations from the norm. Physical impairments, such as hearing or visual defects, ears that "stick out," or birthmarks, assume great importance. Increasing awareness of these differences, especially when accompanied by unkind comments and taunts from others, may cause a child to feel inferior and less desirable. This is especially true if the defect interferes with the child's ability to participate in games and activities.

DEVELOPMENT OF SEXUALITY

Many children experience some form of sex play during or before preadolescence as a response to normal curiosity, not as a result of love or sexual urges. Children are experimentalists by nature, and sex play is incidental and transitory. Any adverse emotional consequences or guilt feelings depend on how the behavior is managed by the parents. Many parents discourage sexual exploration, either through subtle cues or expressions of anger or disgust at their child's behavior. These tactics clearly communicate to children that they should not engage in such activities, discourage questions about sex, and limit the sources of information.

Sex Education

An important component of ongoing sex education is effective communication with parents. If parents either repress the child's sexual curiosity or avoid dealing with it, the sexual information that the child receives may be acquired almost entirely from peers. A recent study found that the majority of parents of preadolescent and adolescent children believed they were open with sex education discussions; however, only a few parents communicated direct information about safe sex practices (Hyde, Drennan, Butler, et al., 2013). When peers are the primary source of sexual information, it is often transmitted and exchanged in secret conversation and contains misinformation.

Although middle childhood is an ideal time for formal sex education, this subject has created considerable controversy. Many parents and groups are unconditionally opposed to the inclusion of sex education in schools. When sex education is presented from a life span perspective and treated as a normal part of growth and development, the information is less likely to contain overtones of uncertainty, guilt, or embarrassment that could in turn produce anxiety in children.

Nurse's Role in Sex Education

No matter where nurses practice, they can provide information on human sexuality to both parents and children. To discuss the topic adequately, nurses must have an understanding of the physiologic aspects of sexuality, know the common myths and misconceptions associated with sex and the reproductive process, understand cultural and societal values, and be aware of their own attitudes, feelings, and biases about sexuality.

When presenting sexual information to school-age children, nurses should treat sex as a normal part of growth and development. Questions should be answered honestly, in a matter-of-fact manner, and at the child's level of understanding. There may be times when boys and girls should be taught content separately; however, each group needs information about both sexes.

Children need help to differentiate sex and sexuality. Exercises on clarifying values, identifying role models, engaging in problem-solving skills, and practicing responsibility are important to prepare children for early adolescence and puberty. In addition, children need explanations of sexual information that is provided via the media or jokes. Information about anatomy, pregnancy, contraceptives, and sexually transmitted infections, including human immunodeficiency virus and human papillomavirus, should be presented in simple, accurate terms. Preadolescents need precise and concrete information that will allow them to answer questions such as, "What if I start my period in the middle of class?" or "How can I keep people from telling I have an erection?" It is important to tell children what they want to know and what they can expect to happen as they become mature sexually.

During encounters with parents, nurses can be open and available for questions and discussion. They can set an example by the language they use in discussing body parts and their function and by the way in which they deal with problems that have emotional overtones, such as exploratory sex play and masturbation. Parents need help to understand normal behaviors and to view sexual curiosity in their children as a part of the developmental process. Assessing the parents' level of knowledge and understanding of sexuality provides cues to their need for supplemental information that will prepare them for the increasingly complex explanations they will need to provide as their children grow older.

COPING WITH CONCERNS RELATED TO NORMAL GROWTH AND DEVELOPMENT

Table 14.1 summarizes the major developmental achievements of the school-age years.

School Experience

School serves as the agent for transmitting the values of society to each succeeding generation of children and as a setting for many peer relationships. After the family, schools are the second most important socializing agent in the lives of children.

Entrance into school causes a sharp break in the structure of the child's world. For many children, it is their first experience in conforming to a group pattern imposed by an adult who is not a parent and who has responsibility for too many children to be constantly aware of each child as an individual. Children want to go to school and usually adapt to the new conditions with little difficulty. Successful adjustment is related to the child's physical and emotional maturity and the parent's readiness to accept the separation associated with school entrance. Unfortunately, some parents express their unconscious attempts to delay the child's maturity by clinging behavior, particularly with their youngest child.

By the time they enter school, most children have a fairly realistic concept of what school involves. They receive information regarding the role of a student from parents, siblings, playmates, and the media. In addition, most children have had some experience with daycare, preschool, or kindergarten. Middle-class children have fewer adjustments to make and less to learn about expected behavior because schools tend to reflect dominant middle-class customs and values. If the child has attended a preschool program, the focus of the preschool program also affects the child's adjustment. Some preschool programs provide custodial care only, but others emphasize emotional, social, and intellectual development.

Role of Teachers

Teachers, like parents, are concerned about the child's psychologic and emotional welfare. Although the functions of teachers and parents differ, both place constraints on behavior and both are in a position to enforce standards of conduct. However, the teacher's primary responsibility involves stimulating and guiding children's intellectual development, as opposed to providing for their physical welfare beyond the school setting.

Children respond best to teachers who possess the characteristics of a warm, loving parent. Teachers in the early grades perform many of the activities formerly assumed by the parent, such as recognizing the child's personal needs (e.g., the need to go to the bathroom, need for help with clothing) and helping to develop their social behavior (e.g., manners).

Teachers serve as models with whom children can identify and whom they try to emulate. Children seek their teachers' approval and avoid their disapproval. The teacher is a significant person in the life of the early school-age child, and hero worship of a teacher may extend into late childhood and preadolescence. Teachers who make supportive statements that reassure or commend children, use accepting and clarifying statements that help children refine ideas and feelings, and provide assistance that aids children with their own problem solving contribute to the development of a positive self-concept in the school-age child.

Role of Parents

Parents share responsibility for helping children achieve their maximum potential. Parents can supplement the school program in numerous ways (see Family-Centered Care box). Cultivating responsibility is the goal of parental assistance. Being responsible for schoolwork helps children learn to keep promises, meet deadlines, and succeed at their jobs as adults. Responsible children may occasionally ask for help (e.g., with a spelling list), but usually they prefer to think through their work by themselves. Excessive pressure or lack of encouragement from parents may inhibit the development of these desirable traits.

TABLE 14.1 Growth and Development During the School-Age Years (ages are approximate)

Physical and Motor	Mental	Adaptive	Personal-Social
Age 6 Years			
Height and weight gain continues slowly Weight: 16-26.3 kg (35.5-58 pounds) Height: 106.7-123.5 cm (42-49 inches) Central mandibular incisors erupt Loses first tooth Demonstrates gradual increase in dexterity Active age; constant activity Often returns to finger feeding More aware of hand as a tool Likes to draw, print, color Vision reaches maturity	Develops concept of numbers Can count 13 pennies Knows whether it is morning or afternoon Defines common objects (such as fork and chair) in terms of their use Obeys triple commands in succession Knows right and left hands Says which is pretty and which is ugly of a series of drawings of faces Describes the objects in a picture rather than simply enumerating them Attends first grade	At table, uses knife to spread butter or jam on bread At play, cuts, folds, pastes paper; sews crudely if needle is threaded Takes bath without supervision; performs bedtime activities alone Reads from memory; enjoys oral spelling game Likes table games, checkers, simple card games Giggles a lot Sometimes steals money or attractive items Has difficulty owning up to misdeeds Tries out own abilities	Can share and cooperate better Has great need for children of own age Will cheat to win Often engages in rough play Often jealous of younger brother or sister Does what adults are seen doing May have occasional temper tantrums Is a boaster Is more independent, probably an influence of school Has own way of doing things Increases socialization
Age 7 Years			
Begins to grow at least 5 cm (2 inches) in height per year Weight: 17.7-30 kg (39-66 pounds) Height: 111.8-129.5 cm (44-51 inches) Maxillary central incisors and lateral mandibular incisors erupt More cautious in approaches to new performances Repeats performances to master them Jaw begins to expand to accommodate permanent teeth	Notices that certain items are missing from pictures Can copy a diamond Repeats three numbers backward Develops concept of time; reads ordinary clock or watch correctly to nearest quarter-hour; uses clock for practical purposes Attends second grade More mechanical in reading; often does not stop at the end of a sentence; skips words such as "it," "the," and "he"	Uses table knife for cutting meat; may need help with tough or difficult pieces Brushes and combs hair acceptably without help May steal Likes to help and have a choice Is less resistant and stubborn	Is becoming a real member of the family group Takes part in group play Boys prefer playing with boys; girls prefer playing with girls Spends a lot of time alone; does not require a lot of companionship
Ages 8 to 9 Years			
Continues to gain 5 cm (2 inches) in height per year Weight: 19.6-39.6 kg (43-87 pounds) Height: 116.8-141.8 cm (46-56 inches) Lateral incisors (maxillary) and mandibular cuspids erupt Movement fluid; often graceful and poised Always on the go; jumps, chases, skips Increased smoothness and speed in fine motor control; uses cursive writing Dresses self completely Likely to overdo; hard to quiet down after recess More limber; bones grow faster than ligaments	Gives similarities and differences between two things from memory Counts backward from 20 to 1; understands concept of reversibility Repeats days of the week and months in order; knows the date Describes common objects in detail, not merely their use Makes change out of a quarter Attends third and fourth grades Reads more; may plan to wake up early just to read Reads classic books but also enjoys comics More aware of time; can be relied on to get to school on time Can grasp concepts of parts and whole (fractions) Understands concepts of space, cause and effect, nesting (puzzles), conservation (permanence of mass and volume) Classifies objects by more than one quality; has collections Produces simple paintings or drawings	Makes use of common tools such as hammer, saw, screwdriver Uses household and sewing utensils Helps with routine household tasks, such as dusting, sweeping Assumes responsibility for share of household chores Looks after all of own needs at table Buys useful articles; exercises some choice in making purchases Runs useful errands Likes pictorial magazines Likes school; wants to answer all questions Is afraid of failing a grade; is ashamed of bad grades Is more critical of self Takes music and sports lessons	Is easy to get along with at home Likes the reward system Dramatizes Is more sociable Is better behaved Is interested in boy-girl relationships but will not admit it Goes about home and community freely, alone or with friends Likes to compete and play games Shows preference in friends and groups Plays mostly with groups of own sex but is beginning to mix Develops modesty Compares self with others Enjoys organizations, clubs, and group sports

Continued

TABLE 14.1 Growth and Development During the School-Age Years (ages are approximate)—cont'd

Physical and Motor	Mental	Adaptive	Personal-Social
Ages 10 to 12 Years			
Weight: 24.3-58 kg (54-128 pounds) Height: 127-162.5 cm (50-64 inches) Remainder of teeth will erupt and tend toward full development (except wisdom teeth) **Girls:** Pubescent changes may begin to appear; body lines soften and round out **Boys:** Slow growth in height and rapid weight gain; may become obese in this period	Writes brief stories Attends fifth to seventh grades Writes occasional short letters to friends or relatives on own initiative Uses telephone for practical purposes Responds to magazine, radio, or other advertising Reads for practical information or own enjoyment—stories or library books of adventure or romance, animal stories	Makes useful tools or does easy repair work Cooks or sews in small ways Raises pets Washes and dries own hair; is responsible for a thorough job of cleaning hair but may need reminding to do so Is sometimes left alone at home for an hour or so Is successful in looking after own needs or those of other children left in his or her care	Loves friends; talks about them constantly Chooses friends more selectively; may have a "best friend" Enjoys conversation Develops beginning interest in opposite sex Is more diplomatic Likes family; family really has meaning Likes mother and wants to please her in many ways Demonstrates affection Likes father, who is admired and may be idolized Respects parents

FAMILY-CENTERED CARE

Helping Children in School

General Guidelines

Be supportive: Provide companionship; share ideas and thoughts.
Be positive: Every child should experience some success each day.
Share an interest in reading: Use the library; discuss books they are reading.
Support and encourage activity rather than passivity.
Encourage originality: Help children make their own projects from discarded articles or other available materials.
Foster the development of hobbies and collections.
Encourage children to wonder and reflect during free time.
Encourage family experiences and trips to places of interest.
Encourage questions: Help children discover sources for information or places to explore and investigate.
Stimulate creative thinking and problem solving: Help children try out new solutions to problems without fear of making mistakes.
Use rewards rather than punishment.

Specific Guidelines

Meet the teacher at the beginning of school and plan to visit the school to see what is taught and expected.
Send the child to school every day. Teachers are concerned when parents make other plans for their children; it conveys the impression that school is unimportant.
Demonstrate an interest in what the child is learning.
Demonstrate an interest in content and growth more than in grades.
Make it clear to the child that schoolwork is between the child and the teacher; the teacher and child should set goals for better school performance to allow the child to feel responsible for school successes and failures.
Take advantage of situations that support and reinforce school learning.
Share information with teachers that will help them understand the child better.
Communicate with the teacher if there appears to be a problem; avoid waiting for a scheduled conference.
Provide a quiet, well-lit area for study that is safe from interruption; do not allow television or music.
Avoid dictating a study time but do enforce rules, such as no video games until homework is done; accept the child's word that work is complete.
Help with homework should focus on explaining the question, not giving the answer.
Teach the child to break large tasks (such as a report) into smaller, manageable tasks spread over the allotted time rather than attempting the entire project the night before it is due.
Request special help for children with learning problems.
Support the school staff by showing respect for both the school system and the teacher, at least in the child's presence.

Latchkey Children

The term latchkey children is used to describe children in elementary school who are left to care for themselves before or after school without the supervision of an adult. The large numbers of single-parent families and working parents, together with the lack of available child care, have created a stress-provoking situation for many school-age children. Some of these children may have a chronic illness as well.

Inadequate adult supervision after school leaves children at greater risk for injury and delinquent behavior. In some instances, outside activities are curtailed, and relationships with peers may be significantly diminished. Most school-age children feel more lonely, isolated, and fearful when left home alone than children who have someone to care for them (Ruiz-Casares, Rousseau, Currie, et al., 2012). To cope with their fears and anxieties while alone, these children may devise strategies, such as hiding (in a bathroom, in a closet, or under a bed), playing the television loudly to drown out noises, and using pets for comfort.

Many communities and persons concerned about the welfare of latchkey children are trying to help these children and their parents deal with this potentially serious problem. Some communities and employers have implemented after-school programs. Other types of programs include those designed to teach self-help skills to children, hotlines to provide telephone check-in and reassurance programs for children, and programs that link latchkey children with reassuring older persons in their community. Nurses should be aware of these community services and encourage parents to teach self-help skills to these children.

Discipline

Many factors influence the amount and manner of discipline and limit setting imposed on school-age children, including the parents' psychosocial maturity, their own childrearing experiences during childhood, the children's temperaments, the context of the children's misconduct, and the children's responses to rewards and punishments. Discipline serves many purposes: (1) to help the child interrupt or inhibit a forbidden action; (2) to point out a more acceptable form of behavior so that the child knows what is right in a future situation; (3) to provide some reason, understandable to the child, that explains why one action is inappropriate and another action is more desirable; and (4) to stimulate the child's ability to empathize with the victim of a misdeed.

To be effective, discipline should take place in a positive, supportive environment with the use of strategies to instruct and guide desired behaviors and eliminate undesired behaviors (Owen, Slep, & Heyman, 2012). Physically aggressive practices, such as spanking, are linked to children with poor internalizing behaviors, including depression, anxiety, hopelessness, and poor external behaviors, such as aggression and violence (Ferguson, 2013). Reasoning, on the other hand, is an effective disciplinary technique for school-age children. With advancing cognitive skills, they are able to benefit from more complex disciplinary strategies. For example, withholding privileges, requiring compensation, imposing penalties, and contracting can be used with great success. Problem solving is the best approach to limit setting, and children themselves can be included in the process of determining appropriate disciplinary measures.

Dishonest Behavior

During middle childhood, children may engage in what is considered to be antisocial behavior. Previously well-behaved children may engage in lying, stealing, and cheating. Such behaviors are disturbing and challenging to parents.

Lying can occur for a number of reasons. By the time children enter school, they still "tell stories," often exaggerating a story or situation as a means of impressing their family or friends, but can distinguish between fact and fantasy. If children do not develop this characteristic, parents need to teach them what is real and what is make-believe.

Young children may lie to escape punishment or to get out of some difficulty even when their misbehavior is evident. Older children may lie to meet expectations set by others to which they have been unable to measure up. However, most children know that lying and cheating are wrong, and they are concerned when it is observed in their friends. They are quick to tell on others when they detect cheating.

Parents need to be reassured that all children lie occasionally and that sometimes children may have difficulty separating fantasy from reality. Parents should be helped to understand the importance of their own behavior as role models and of being truthful in their relationships with children.

Cheating is most common in young children 5 to 6 years old. They find it difficult to lose at a game or contest, so they may cheat to win. They have not yet realized that this behavior is wrong, and they do it almost automatically. This behavior usually disappears as they mature. However, when children observe parental behaviors such as boasting about cheating, they assume this to be appropriate behavior. When parents set examples of honesty, children are more likely to conform to these standards.

As with other ethically related behavior, stealing is not unexpected in younger children. Between 5 and 8 years old, children's sense of property rights is limited, and they tend to take things simply because they are attracted to them or to take money for what it will buy. They are equally likely to give away something valuable that belongs to them. When young children are caught and punished, they are penitent—they "didn't mean to" and "promise to never do it again"—but they may repeat the performance the following day. Often they not only steal but also lie about their behavior or attempt to justify it with excuses. It is seldom helpful to trap children into admission by asking directly if they committed the offense. Children do not take responsibility for these behaviors until the end of middle childhood. Stealing can sometimes be an indication that something is seriously wrong or lacking in the child's life. For example, children may steal to make up for love or another satisfaction that they feel is lacking. In most situations, it is wise not to attempt to attach a hidden or deep meaning to the stealing. An admonition, together with an appropriate and reasonable punishment, such as having the older child pay back the money or return the stolen items, will ordinarily take care of most cases. Most children can be taught to respect the property rights of others with little difficulty despite numerous temptations and opportunities. If children's personal rights are respected, they are likely to respect the rights of others. Some children simply need more time to learn the rules regarding private property.

Stress and Fear

Children today experience significant amounts of stress. Stress in childhood comes from a variety of sources, such as conflict within the family, parental criminality or psychiatric disorder, and low socioeconomic status (Riley, Scaramella, & McGoron, 2014). The school environment and participation in multiple organized activities can be additional sources of stress. The demands from teachers and parents with school work and standardized proficiency testing, in addition to peer pressure, can cause stress on school-age children (White, 2012). In addition, children in the middle school years are often overcommitted with activities such as dance, music, athletics, and other activities until the cumulative effect is overwhelming.

The increasing violence in society has infiltrated the school setting. In the present information age, in which tragedy is broadcast daily in the media, children come to school knowing more about the latest world events than any previous generation of children. Many children know other children who have been killed or children who have brought weapons to school. School-age children can be victims of bullying, verbal insults, unwanted sexual remarks, damaged or stolen property, and physical abuse in the school environment (King, 2014). Furthermore, children are stressed by conflict within the home, and the high number of single-parent families result in altered relationships and increasing responsibilities for children.

To help children cope with stress, parents, teachers, and health care providers must recognize signs that indicate a child is undergoing stress, identify the source of the stress promptly, and refer those children who need specialized treatment. They need to frequently reassure children that they are safe, have honest and open communication, and encourage children to express their feelings.

! NURSING ALERT

The nurse who observes the following signs of stress in a child should explore the situation further:

- Stomach pains or headache
- Sleep problems
- Bedwetting
- Changes in eating habits
- Aggressive or stubborn behavior
- Withdrawal or reluctance to participate
- Regression to earlier behaviors (e.g., thumb sucking)
- Trouble concentrating or changes in academic performance

Children 7 to 12 years old are capable of identifying their own physiologic responses to stress. Children should be taught to recognize the signs as indicators of stress and to use techniques to manage their stress. Children can learn relaxation techniques such as deep-breathing exercises, progressive relaxation of muscle groups, yoga, and positive imagery to reduce stress (Bothe, Grignon, & Olness, 2014; White, 2012). Encouraging them to "blow off steam" through physical activity reduces tension and anxiety. Children can be encouraged to observe effective coping strategies in others and adopt them for their own use. When an effective strategy has been developed for one situation, parents and teachers can show the child how to transfer the coping strategy or technique to other situations.

In addition to stress, school-age children experience a wide variety of fears, including fear of the dark, excessive worry about past behavior, self-consciousness, social withdrawal, and an excessive need for reassurance. These fears are considered normal for children this age. During the middle-school years, children become less fearful of body safety than they were as preschoolers, but they still fear being hurt, being kidnapped, or having to undergo surgery. They also fear death and are fascinated by all aspects of death and dying. The fears of noises, darkness, storms, and dogs lessen, but new fears related predominantly to school and family bother children (e.g., fear of failing, fear of bullies, fear of something bad happening to their parents) during this time.

PROMOTING OPTIMAL HEALTH DURING THE SCHOOL YEARS

Nutrition

Although caloric needs are diminished in relation to body size during middle childhood, resources are being laid down at this time for the increased growth needs of adolescence. Parents and children need to be aware of the value of a balanced diet to promote growth. The quality of the child's diet depends on the family's pattern of eating.

Likes and dislikes established at an early age continue in middle childhood, although preferences for single foods subside, and children develop a taste for a variety of foods. However, the easy availability of fast-food restaurants, the influence of the mass media, and the temptation of "junk food" make it easy for children to fill up on empty calories. Foods that do not promote growth, such as sugars, starches, and excess fats, are common in school-age children's diets. The easy availability of high-calorie foods, combined with the tendency toward more sedentary activities, has also contributed to an epidemic of childhood obesity. This problem is discussed further in Chapter 16.

Parents are unable to monitor what their children eat when they are away from home. A parent may pack a lunch for school but is unaware of how much is eaten, traded, sold, or thrown away. Nutrition education can and should be integrated in the curriculum throughout the school years. Important aspects of nutrition education include the US Food and Drug Administration's MyPlate; elements of a wholesome diet; and how food products are grown, processed, and prepared. School cafeterias may not always provide healthy, nutritious meals; however, parents should advocate for the availability of nutritious food options and the elimination of unhealthy foods at schools.

SLEEP AND REST

The amount of sleep and rest required during middle childhood is highly individualized. The amount of sleep depends on the child's age, activity level, and other factors, such as health status. The growth rate slows in the school-age years, and less energy is expended in growth than during preceding years.

School-age children usually do not require naps, but they do need to sleep approximately 11.5 hours at 5 years old and 9 hours at 11 years old each night (Galland, Taylor, Elder, et al., 2012). Although fewer bedtime problems occur during these years, occasional difficulties are still associated with the bedtime ritual. Usually children 6 or 7 years old exhibit few bedtime problems, and encouraging quiet activity before bedtime (such as coloring or reading) facilitates the task of going to bed. However, most children in middle childhood must be reminded frequently to go to bed; 8- to 9-year-old children and 11-year-old children are particularly resistant (Bhargava, 2011). Often these children are unaware that they are tired; if they are allowed to remain awake later than usual, they are fatigued the following day. Sometimes bedtime resistance can be resolved by allowing a later bedtime as the child gets older. Twelve-year-old children usually offer no resistance at bedtime; some even retire early to read or listen to music.

EXERCISE AND ACTIVITY

The improved capabilities and adaptability of school-age children permit greater speed and effort in motor activities. Larger, stronger muscles permit longer and increasingly strenuous play without exhaustion. School-age children acquire the coordination, timing, and concentration that are required to participate in adult-type activities, but they may lack the strength, stamina, and control of adolescents and adults. They can engage in a greater amount of physical activity during the school years. However, parents, teachers, and coaches must remember that although children this age are large and appear strong, they may not be ready for strenuous competitive athletics.

All growing children need regular exercise and opportunities for satisfying experiences consistent with individual likes and dislikes. Appropriate activities during the school-age years include running, jumping rope, swimming, roller skating, ice skating, dancing, and bicycle riding. Positive reinforcement achieved by experiencing increasingly smooth, rhythmic, and efficient use of the body conditions the child toward regular physical activity. Exercise is essential for muscle development and tone, refinement of balance and coordination, increased strength and endurance, and stimulation of body functions and metabolic processes. Children need ample space to run, jump, skip, and climb in addition to safe indoor and outdoor facilities and equipment. Most children have abundant energy and need little encouragement to engage in physical activity. Children with disabling conditions or those who hesitate to become involved in active play (e.g., obese children) require special assessment and help so that activities appeal to them and are compatible with their limitations while also meeting their developmental needs.

Sports

Considerable controversy surrounds the trend toward early participation in competitive athletics and the amount and type of competitive sports that are appropriate for children in the elementary grades. The current view is that virtually every child is suited for some sport, and authorities do not discourage participation if children are matched to the type of sport appropriate to their abilities and to their physical and emotional constitution. School-age children enjoy competition (Fig. 14.7). However, teachers and coaches must understand the physical limitations of children this age and teach them the proper techniques and safety measures needed to avoid injuries. A safe and appropriate sport can be identified for even the most unskilled and uncompetitive child, including children with chronic illnesses and intellectual disability. Common sporting activities for school-age children include baseball, soccer, gymnastics, and swimming. Equipment must be

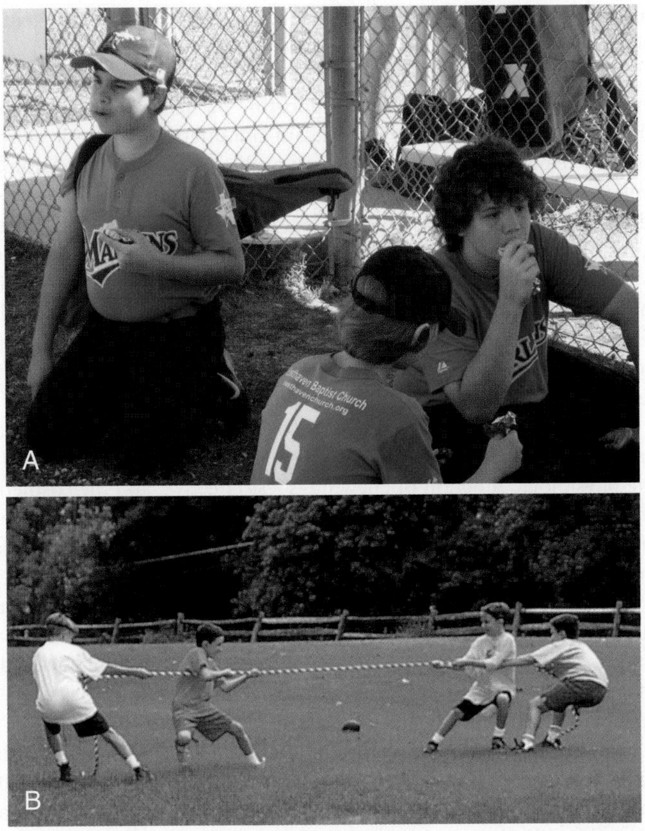

Fig. 14.7 The activities engaged in by school-age children vary according to interest and opportunity. **A,** Little League competitors. **B,** Playing tug-of-war.

maintained in safe condition, and protective apparatus should be worn to prevent serious injury (see Chapter 29, Traumatic Injury).

During the school-age years, girls have the same basic body structure as boys and have a similar response to systematic exercise training. However, at puberty, boys become larger and have more muscle mass, and at this stage, it is usually recommended that girls compete only against other girls. Before puberty, there is no essential difference in strength and size between girls and boys, making these precautions unnecessary.

Preadolescence is a time to teach fundamental motor skills; develop fitness in a practical, safe, and gradual manner; and promote healthy attitudes and values. Activities should include both practice sessions and unstructured play; the actual game or event should be managed in a manner that stresses mastery of the sport and enhancement of self-image rather than winning or pleasing others. All children should have an opportunity to participate, and special ceremonies should recognize all participants, not just individuals who excel in sports or athletics.

Acquisition of Skills

School-age children demonstrate increasing fine motor abilities and complex artistic skills. Handedness is well established by the beginning of the school years, and children make great strides in writing and drawing during this period. It is a time of energetic and vibrant creative productivity. With the tools of language and reading, children create poems, stories, and plays. With more advanced fine motor skills, they are able to master an unlimited variety of handicrafts, such as ceramics, needlework, woodworking, and beadwork. They avidly pursue these skills in solitude, with a friend, or through organized groups such as boys' or girls' clubs or special interest groups that use crafts or other activities as a means to occupy, entertain, and educate children.

School-age children are capable of assuming responsibility for their own needs, although their distaste for soap and water and "dress" clothes is legendary. School-age children can and want to assume their share of household tasks, which usually are related to the male and female roles that have been defined by their culture. Many children also assume responsibility for tasks outside the home, such as babysitting, yard work, or paper routes.

Television, Video Games, and the Internet

Children spend a significant amount of time each day involved in media-related activities, including the use of tablets, video games, and cell phones. Children 8 to 10 years old spend at least 8 hours every day with various forms of media, and teenagers spend more than 11 hours per day (American Academy of Pediatrics, Council on Communications and Media, 2013). Because of the long periods of exposure, media have more time to develop children's attitudes than do parents and teachers.

There is no doubt that children learn from various forms of media, but the values and attitudes depicted on these are not always realistic and may conflict with previously taught values. Violence is common in various forms of media, and significant exposure to media violence increases aggressive behavior in some children (American Academy of Pediatrics, Council on Communications and Media, 2013). In addition, repeated exposure to violence can desensitize children to violence, convey a message that violence is acceptable, and teach children that initiating violent behavior is an appropriate form of protection (Brown & Tierney, 2011). Parents should make the ultimate decision about which programs their child will watch, which video games they are allowed to play, and what Internet sites they can access. These forms of media have valuable educational opportunities, but there are also risks that parents must acknowledge.

DENTAL HEALTH

The first permanent (secondary) teeth erupt at about 6 years old, beginning with the 6-year molar, which erupts posterior to the deciduous molars. Other permanent teeth appear in approximately the same order as eruption of the primary teeth and follow shedding of the deciduous teeth (Fig. 14.8). With the appearance of the second permanent (12-year) molar, most permanent teeth are present. Permanent dentition is more advanced in girls than in boys.

Because the permanent teeth erupt during the school-age years, dental hygiene and regular attention to dental caries are important parts of health supervision during this period. Correct brushing techniques should be taught or reinforced, and the role that fermentable carbohydrates play in production of dental caries should be emphasized. It is important to be alert to possible malocclusion problems that may result from irregular eruption of permanent teeth and that may impair function. Regular dental supervision and continued fluoride supplementation are integral parts of the health maintenance program.

The most effective means of preventing dental caries is proper oral hygiene. Children should be taught to perform their own dental care with the supervision and guidance of the parents. Parents should learn the correct brushing technique with their children, and they should monitor their child's efforts until the child can assume full responsibility.

Teeth should be brushed after meals, after snacks, and at bedtime. Children who brush their teeth frequently and become accustomed to the feel of a clean mouth at an early age usually maintain the habit throughout life. For school-age children with mixed and permanent dentition,

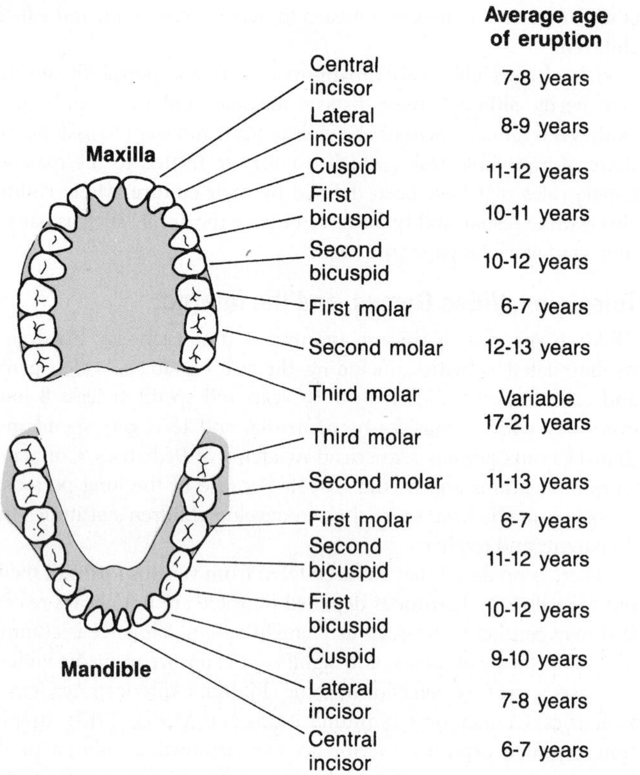

Fig. 14.8 Sequence of eruption of the secondary teeth. (Data from Dean, J. A. [2016]. *McDonald and Avery's dentistry for the child and adolescent* [10th ed.]. St Louis, MO: Mosby/Elsevier.)

the best toothbrush is one with soft nylon bristles and an overall length of about 21 cm (8 inches). Several methods of brushing have been described and recommended for children, but there is no conclusive evidence that one method is superior to another. Thorough cleaning is more important than the specific technique used. The dentist should assess factors, such as the manipulative skills and special needs of the child, and suggest the most appropriate brushing technique and regimen. Flossing follows brushing. Parents should perform the flossing until children acquire the manual dexterity required (usually at about 8 or 9 years old).

Dental Problems

Limited or inadequate dental care results in the most common dental problems: dental caries, malocclusion, and periodontal disease. Trauma, especially tooth avulsion, is another important dental problem. All of these conditions benefit from early intervention to prevent tooth loss.

Dental caries (cavities) is the principal oral problem in children and adolescents. Reducing the incidence and consequences of dental caries is extremely important in childhood. If untreated, dental caries can result in total destruction of the involved teeth. The prevalence rate of caries increases steadily across the life span; whereas 25% of children younger than 5 years old have caries, 68% of children have caries by 19 years old (Mahat, Lyons, & Bowen, 2014).

Dental caries is a multifactorial disease involving susceptible teeth, cariogenic microflora, and an appropriate oral environment. The incidence of lesions and the likelihood of progressive invasion vary considerably and depend on a number of factors being present in the right combination. Because many children are exposed to health care but not dental care, oral inspection is an integral part of the physical assessment of every child. If there is any evidence of dental caries or other unhealthy dental state, the child should be referred for dental services. An alarming number of children do not receive regular dental supervision, and a significant number reach adulthood without dental examinations or treatment by a dentist.

Periodontal disease, an inflammatory and degenerative condition involving the gums and tissues supporting the teeth, often begins in childhood and accounts for a significant amount of tooth loss in adulthood. The more common periodontal problems are **gingivitis** (simple inflammation of the gums) and **periodontitis** (inflammation of the gums and loss of connective tissue and bone in the supporting structures of the teeth). Gingivitis, the most prevalent periodontal disease, is a reversible inflammatory disease that can begin in early childhood and is most often associated with the buildup of plaque on the teeth. Management is directed toward prevention by conscientious brushing and flossing, including the use of fluoride. Children should see a dentist at any signs of inflammation or irritation.

Malocclusion occurs when teeth of the upper and lower dental arches do not approximate in the proper relationships. As a result, the physiologic function of chewing is less effective, and the cosmetic effect is displeasing. Teeth that are uneven, crowded, or overlapping are unable to meet their counterparts in the opposite jaw in the appropriate relationships and may be predisposed to disease in later years.

Orthodontic treatment is most successful when it is started in the late school-age or early teenage years after the last primary teeth have been shed and before growth ceases. However, referral should be made as soon as malocclusion is evident because some deformities can be corrected at an earlier age.

Dental injury may occur in childhood and includes fractures of varying degrees of severity, chipping, dislocation, or avulsion. All tooth injuries require prompt treatment by a competent dentist to prevent permanent displacement or loss. Delayed examination and diagnosis of tooth damage can result in infection or pulp involvement. Because it can affect the remaining teeth, replacement of the lost tooth is needed to maintain normal alignment and position of the other teeth.

A tooth that is **avulsed** (exarticulated, or "knocked out") should be replanted by the child, parent, or nurse and stabilized as soon as possible so that the blood supply to the tooth can be reestablished and the tooth kept alive (see Emergency Treatment box). A tooth that is replanted promptly has a good survival rate. Avulsed primary teeth are usually not reimplanted.

EMERGENCY TREATMENT

Avulsed Permanent Tooth

Recover tooth.
Hold tooth by crown; avoid touching root area.
If tooth is dirty, rinse it gently under running water or saline; be certain to insert stopper in sink or basin (to avoid tooth loss).

To Reimplant the Tooth

Insert tooth into socket; be certain that the lip side (or convex surface) is facing front.
Have child maintain tooth in place by slowly biting down on a piece of gauze.
Transport child to dentist immediately.
Avoid sudden stops or sharp turns to prevent dislodging tooth.

If Reluctant to Reimplant the Tooth

Place avulsed tooth in suitable medium for transport:

- Cold milk
- Saliva—under child's or parent's tongue

If child is holding tooth in the mouth, avoid sudden stops to prevent swallowing tooth.

Do not forget to take the tooth.

As with all injuries to the mouth, an avulsed tooth causes a large amount of bleeding, which is frightening to children and their families; therefore the nurse or anyone faced with dental trauma should be prepared to provide support and reassurance during the trauma.

SCHOOL HEALTH

Child health maintenance is ultimately the responsibility of the parents; however, the public schools and health departments in the United States have contributed to the improvement of child health by providing a healthful school environment, health services, and health education that emphasize sound health practices. Most of these functions constitute major components of community health services and involve large amounts of public funds and large numbers of health professionals, including nurses.

A school health program is involved in ongoing health maintenance through assessment, screening, and referral activities. Routine health services provided by most schools include health appraisal, emergency care, safety education, communicable disease control, counseling, and follow-up care. Health education of school-age children is directed toward providing knowledge of health and influencing habits, attitudes, and conduct in relation to health and injury prevention.

Traditionally, school nurses were viewed from a limited perspective as the individuals who detected diseases in the school, applied bandages, and cared for students who were ill or injured. Although these are important functions, this traditional role has acquired much broader dimensions. School nurses develop, implement, and evaluate health care plans and programs. In some settings, school health services have enlarged into family health centers that meet the needs of not only school-age children but also their families and the community. In these settings, school nurse practitioners provide health care that includes assessment of physical, psychomedical, psychoeducational, behavioral, and learning problems, as well as comprehensive well-child care.

The passage of Public Laws 94-142 and 99-457 requires the integration of children with chronic illnesses and disabilities into the least restrictive environments, including regular classrooms whenever possible. School nurses are responsible for the medical and nursing needs of these children while they are in the school setting. School nurses develop, implement, and evaluate individualized health care plans for these children. Not all schools have a school nurse, and unlicensed assistive personnel (UAP) are used in some cases. After appropriate training and certification, UAP can provide standardized routine health care to students but must be overseen by a school nurse (Resha, 2010). Delegation and supervision of UAP requires skillful nursing assessment, effective communication, and professional judgment.

INJURY PREVENTION

Because school-age children have developed more refined muscular coordination and control and can apply their cognitive capacities to their behavior, the number of injuries in middle childhood is diminished compared with the number in early childhood. The most common cause of severe injury and death in children older than 4 years of age is motor vehicle crashes—either as a pedestrian or passenger (National Highway Traffic Safety Administration, 2013). It is important that nurses continue to emphasize three automobile safety measures that have been found to reduce the severity of injuries: effective car restraint systems, door-lock mechanisms, and appropriate passenger seating locations in the motor vehicle. The rear vehicle seat is the safest place for children younger than 13 years old, and booster seats should be used until the child is 57 inches tall (Centers for Disease Control and Prevention, National Center for Injury Prevention and Control, 2015).

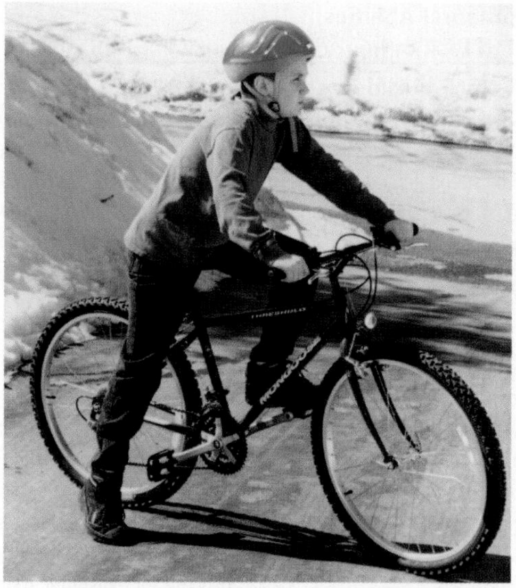

Fig. 14.9 The right-size bike is important. The child should be able to sit on the bike and place the balls of both feet on the ground. Each foot should comfortably reach and manipulate the pedal in the down position. Wearing a protective helmet is mandatory. The helmet should be positioned so that it sits low on the forehead and parallel to the ground when the head is held upright. It should not rock back and forth or shift from side to side. The strap should fasten securely under the chin.

School-age children's desire for riding bicycles increases the risk of injury on streets. Other serious injuries include accidents on skateboards, roller skates, in-line skates, scooters, and other sports equipment. All-terrain vehicles (ATVs) are responsible for a large number of childhood injuries because they are unstable, not easily seen by others, and able to obtain substantial speed. Several national organizations have developed policy and position statements to discourage the use of ATVs in any child younger than 16 years old (Campbell, Kelliher, Borrup, et al., 2010).

Most injuries occur in or near the home or school. The most effective means of prevention is education of the child and family regarding the hazards of risk taking and the improper use of equipment. Safety helmets, protective eye and mouth shields, and protective padding are strongly recommended for children engaging in active sports, even though they may not be required equipment. Falls from bicycles are the cause of a significant number of head injuries in school-age children, and the most important aspect of bicycle safety is to encourage children to wear protective helmets (Fig. 14.9) (Meehan, Lee, Fischer, et al., 2013).

Physically active school-age children are also highly susceptible to cuts and abrasions, and the incidence of childhood fractures, strains, and sprains is high. Trampoline injuries are highest in children 5 through 14 years old and account for numerous fractures, sprains, and head injuries. Trampolines in the home environment, routine physical education classes, or outdoor playgrounds are not recommended for children younger than 6 years old (American Academy of Pediatrics, Council on Sports Medicine and Fitness, 2012). Serious injuries are discussed elsewhere in the book: burns (Chapter 31), eye trauma (Chapter 18), submersive injury (Chapter 27), and head injuries (Chapter 27). The prevalence of injuries depends on the dangers present in the environment, the protection offered by adults, and children's behavior patterns. Table 14.2 lists characteristics of school-age children that make them prone to injury and suggestions for injury prevention. Family-Centered Care boxes provide safety guidelines for bicycle, skateboard, in-line skate, and scooter guidance during the school years.

TABLE 14.2 Injury Prevention During the School-Age Years

Developmental Abilities Related to Risk of Injury	Injury Prevention
Motor Vehicle Accidents	
Is increasingly involved in activities away from home Is excited by speed and motion Is easily distracted by environment Can be reasoned with	Educate child on proper use of seat belts while a passenger in a vehicle. Maintain discipline while the child is a passenger in a vehicle (e.g., ensure that children keep arms inside, do not lean against doors, and do not interfere with driver). Remind parents and children that no one should ride in the bed of a pickup truck. Emphasize safe pedestrian behavior. Insist on child wearing safety apparel (e.g., helmet) when applicable, such as while riding bicycle, motorcycle, moped, or ATV (see Family-Centered Care boxes).
Drowning	
Is apt to overdo May work hard to perfect a skill Has cautious, but not fearful, gross motor actions Likes swimming	Teach child to swim. Teach basic rules of water safety. Select safe and supervised places to swim. Check sufficient water depth for diving. Caution child to swim with a companion. Ensure that child uses an approved flotation device in water or boat. Advocate for legislation requiring fencing around pools. Learn cardiopulmonary resuscitation.
Burns	
Has increasing independence Is adventurous Enjoys trying new things	Make certain home has smoke detectors. Set water heaters to 48.9°C (120°F) to avoid scald burns. Instruct child on behavior in areas involving contact with potential burn hazards (e.g., gasoline, matches, bonfires or barbecues, lighter fluid, firecrackers, cigarette lighters, cooking utensils, chemistry sets). Instruct child to avoid climbing or flying kite around high-tension wires. Instruct child in proper behavior in the event of fire (e.g., fire drills at home and school). Teach child safe cooking (use low heat; avoid any frying; be careful of steam burns, scalds, or exploding foods, especially from microwaving).
Poisoning	
Adheres to group rules May be easily influenced by peers Has strong allegiance to friends	Educate child on hazards of taking nonprescription drugs and chemicals, including aspirin and alcohol. Teach child to say "no" if offered illegal or dangerous drugs or alcohol. Keep potentially dangerous products in properly labeled receptacles, preferably out of reach.
Bodily Damage	
Has increased physical skills Needs strenuous physical activity Is interested in acquiring new skills and perfecting attained skills Is daring and adventurous, especially with peers Frequently plays in hazardous places Confidence often exceeds physical capacity Desires group loyalty and has strong need for friends' approval Delights in physical activity Attempts hazardous feats Accompanies friends to potentially hazardous facilities Is likely to overdo Growth in height exceeds muscular growth and coordination	Help provide facilities for supervised activities. Encourage playing in safe places. Keep firearms safely locked up except under adult supervision. Teach proper care of, use of, and respect for potentially dangerous devices (e.g., power tools, firecrackers). Teach children not to tease or surprise dogs, invade their territory, take dogs' toys, or interfere with dogs' feeding. Stress use of eye, ear, or mouth protection when using potentially hazardous objects or devices or when engaging in potentially hazardous sports. Do not permit use of trampolines except as part of supervised training. Teach safety regarding use of corrective devices (glasses); if child wears contact lenses, monitor duration of wear to prevent corneal damage. Stress careful selection, use, and maintenance of sports and recreation equipment, such as skateboards and in-line skates (see Family-Centered Care boxes). Emphasize proper conditioning, safe practices, and use of safety equipment for sports or recreational activities. Caution against engaging in hazardous sports, such as those involving trampolines. Use safety glass and decals on large glassed areas, such as sliding glass doors. Use window guards to prevent falls. Teach name, address, and phone number, and emphasize that child should ask for help from appropriate people (e.g., cashier, security guard, police) if lost; have identification on child (e.g., sewn in clothes, inside shoe). Teach safety and stranger safety: Avoid personalized clothing in public places. Never go with a stranger. Have child tell parents if anyone makes child feel uncomfortable in any way. Teach child to say "no" when confronted by uncomfortable situations. Always listen to child's concerns regarding others' behavior.

ATV, All-terrain vehicle.

FAMILY-CENTERED CARE

Bicycle Safety

- Always wear a properly fitted bicycle helmet that is approved by the US Consumer Product Safety Commission; replace a damaged or outgrown helmet.
- Ride bicycles with traffic and away from parked cars.
- Ride single file.
- Walk bicycles through busy intersections only at crosswalks.
- Give hand signals well in advance of turning or stopping.
- Keep as close to the curb as practical.
- Watch for drain grates, potholes, soft shoulders, loose dirt, and gravel.
- Keep both hands on handlebars except when signaling.
- Never ride double on a bicycle.
- Do not carry packages that interfere with vision or control; do not drag objects behind a bike.
- Watch for and yield to pedestrians.
- Watch for cars backing up or pulling out of driveways; be especially careful at intersections.
- Look left, right, and then left before turning into traffic or roadway.
- Never hitch a ride on a truck or other vehicle.
- Learn rules of the road and respect for traffic officers.
- Obey all local ordinances.
- Wear shoes that fit securely while riding.
- Wear light colors at night and attach fluorescent material to clothing and bicycle.
- Equip the bicycle with proper lights and reflectors.
- Be certain the bicycle is the correct size for rider (see Fig. 14.9).
- Equip the bicycle with proper lights and reflectors.
- Children riding as passengers must wear appropriate-size helmets and sit in specially designed protective seats.

Modified from American Academy of Pediatrics, Committee on Injury and Poison Prevention. (2008). Bicycle helmets. *Pediatrics, 122*(2), 450.

FAMILY-CENTERED CARE

Skateboard, In-Line Skate, and Scooter Safety

- Children younger than 5 years old should not use skateboards or in-line skates because they are not developmentally prepared to protect themselves from injury. Children ages 6 to 10 years should use these only with close adult supervision.
- The age when children are ready to use in-line skates safely is not known because of differences in the ability to acquire the skills needed to participate in the sport. Novice skaters should learn indoors on a flat, smooth surface. Children who ride skateboards, in-line skates, or scooters should wear helmets and other protective equipment, especially on their knees, wrists, and elbows, to prevent injury.
- Skateboards, in-line skates, and scooters should never be used near traffic or in streets. Their use should be prohibited on streets and highways. Activities that bring skateboards together (e.g., "catching a ride") are especially dangerous.
- Some types of use, such as riding homemade ramps on hard surfaces, may be particularly hazardous.

Data from Brudvik, C. (2006). Injuries caused by small wheel devices. *Prevention Science, 7*, 313–320; and American Academy of Pediatrics, Committee on Injury and Poison Prevention. (2009). In-line skating injuries in children and adolescents. *Pediatrics, 123*(5), 1421–1422.

FAMILY-CENTERED CARE

Guidance During School Years

Age 6 Years

Prepare parents to expect strong food preferences and frequent refusal of specific food items.

Prepare parents to expect an increasingly ravenous appetite.

Prepare parents for emotional reactions as child experiences erratic mood changes.

Help parents anticipate continued susceptibility to illness.

Teach injury prevention and safety, especially bicycle safety.

Encourage parents to respect child's need for privacy and to provide a separate bedroom for child, if possible.

Prepare parents for child's increasing interests outside the home.

Help parents understand the need to encourage child's interactions with peers.

Ages 7 to 10 Years

Prepare parents to expect improvement in health with fewer illnesses but warn them that allergies may increase or become apparent.

Prepare parents to expect an increase in minor injuries.

Emphasize caution in selecting and maintaining sports equipment and reemphasize safety.

Prepare parents to expect increased involvement with peers and interest in activities outside the home.

Emphasize the need to encourage independence while maintaining limit setting and discipline.

Prepare mothers to expect more demands at 8 years old.

Prepare fathers to expect increasing admiration at 10 years old; encourage father-child activities.

Prepare parents for prepubescent changes in girls.

Ages 11 to 12 Years

Help parents prepare child for body changes of pubescence.

Prepare parents to expect a growth spurt in girls.

Make certain child's sex education is adequate with accurate information.

Prepare parents to expect energetic but stormy behavior at 11 years old and child becoming more even-tempered at 12 years old.

Encourage parents to support child's desire to "grow up" but to allow regressive behavior when needed.

Prepare parents to expect an increase in child's masturbation.

Instruct parents that the child may need more rest.

Help parents educate child on experimentation with potentially harmful activities.

Health Guidance

Help parents understand the importance of regular health and dental care for the child.

Encourage parents to teach and model sound health practices, including diet, rest, activity, and exercise.

Stress the need to encourage children to engage in appropriate physical activities.

Emphasize providing a safe physical and emotional environment.

Encourage parents to teach and model safety practices.

ANTICIPATORY GUIDANCE—CARE OF FAMILIES

Parents of the school-age child must share their child's time with the increasingly important peer group. Experiences with the peer group prepare school-age children for the broader world of relationships and increased independence from their parents. Parents must learn to provide support as unobtrusively as possible without feeling rejected, hurt, or angry. The nurse can help parents of the school-age child by providing anticipatory guidance and reassurance throughout this period (see Family-Centered Care box).

CLINICAL JUDGMENT AND NEXT-GENERATION NCLEX® EXAMINATION-STYLE QUESTIONS

1. An 8-year-old boy and his family have recently moved, and he is attending a new school. He states he is unhappy and has difficulty with his classes. He has made no new friends. The mother has talked with his teachers and they are not concerned; he is engaged in the classroom. The nurse performs a complete history and physical examination and finds no areas of concern except that he is in a new school with no friends. Using the principles of Piaget's cognitive development, the nurse would discuss which of the following? **Use an X for the health teaching statement below that is Indicated (appropriate or necessary), Contraindicated (could be harmful), or Non-Essential (makes no difference or not necessary).**

Health Teaching	Indicated	Contraindicated	Non-Essential
"Children this age are able to see things from another's point of view and it is important to keep communication open with your son."			
"He may be having difficulty making judgments about his surroundings and may need further evaluation."			
"It would be helpful to sit beside him and watch a favorite movie to show support."			
"School-age children often use their past experiences to evaluate their present situation and moving to a new school is a tough adjustment for him ."			

2. A 9-year-old boy is seen by the school nurse for the third time this week with reports of a stomachache and requests to go home. The child tells the nurse that he has been bullied for the past month by a group of boys in the school because his father is out of work and he has no money for lunch. The group found this out and continues to make fun of him in the cafeteria and on the playground. The nurse determines it would be important to talk with his teacher, cafeteria staff, and playground staff about bullying. Which characteristic of bullying would the nurse share with the teacher, cafeteria staff, and playground staff? **Select all the apply.**
   - **A.** Unintentional harm is inflicted upon another person that is part of the socialization process in childhood.
   - **B.** The infliction of repetitive physical, verbal, or emotional abuse upon another person with intent to harm.
   - **C.** Attempt to gain acceptance and be liked by same-sex peers.
   - **D.** Attempt to intimidate someone who is seen as vulnerable.
   - **E.** An early sign of a severely disturbed personality disorder that escalates in adulthood.
   - **F.** Emotional abuse can be as harmful as any other type of abuse.

3. A school nurse in middle school (grades 6, 7, and 8) is preparing an outline for a sex education class. Which statements represent important concepts to be covered in discussing this topic with this age group? **For each nursing action, use an X to indicate whether it was Effective (helped to meet expected quality patient outcomes), Ineffective (did not help to meet expected quality patient outcomes), or Unrelated (not related to the quality patient outcomes).**

Sex Education Nursing Action	Effective	Ineffective	Unrelated
Separating the boys and girls into same-sex groups with a leader of the same sex.			
Answer questions in a matter-of-fact way that is honest and appropriate to the children's level of understanding.			
Use vernacular or slang terms to describe human physiologic functions.			
Avoid discussing sexually transmitted diseases in this age group.			
Discuss what it is like to have your first boyfriend or girlfriend.			
Discuss common myths and misconceptions associated with sex and the reproductive process.			

4. A 10-year-old boy's mother says he is "prone" to injury because he is always taking chances on his skateboard and bicycle. Injury prevention is an important area for nursing education. **Choose the most likely options for the information missing from the statements below by selecting from the lists of options provided.**
The nurse educates the mother that injury primarily occurs because of ____1____ and ____2____.

Options for 1	Options for 2
peer pressure	bullying
physical awkwardness	clumsiness
parents' lack of supervision	feeling small
wanting to impress the opposite sex	risk-taking behaviors
hormones	feeling invincible
underdeveloped skeletal muscles	showing off

REFERENCES

American Academy of Pediatrics, Council on Communications and Media. (2013). Media education. *Pediatrics, 132*(5), 958–961.

American Academy of Pediatrics, Council on Sports Medicine and Fitness. (2012). Trampoline safety in childhood and adolescence. *Pediatrics, 130*(6), 1102–1109.

Arseneault, L., Bowes, L., & Shakoor, S. (2010). Bullying victimization in youths and mental health problems: 'Much ado about nothing'? *Psychological Medicine, 40*, 717–729.

Bhargava, S. (2011). Diagnosis and management of common sleep problems in children. *Pediatrics in Review, 32*(3), 91–98.

Bothe, D. A., Grignon, J. B., & Olness, K. N. (2014). The effects of a stress management intervention in elementary school children. *The Journal of Developmental and Behavioral Pediatrics, 35*(1), 62–67.

Bradshaw, C. P., Waasdorp, T. E., Goldweber, A., et al. (2013). Bullies, gangs, drugs, and school: Understanding the overlap and the role of ethnicity and urbanicity. *Journal of Youth and Adolescence, 42*(2), 220–234.

Brown, P., & Tierney, C. (2011). Media role in violence and the dynamics of bullying. *Pediatrics in Review, 32*(10), 453–454.

Campbell, B. T., Kelliher, K. M., Borrup, K., et al. (2010). All-terrain vehicle riding among youth: How do they fair? *Journal of Pediatric Surgery, 45*(5), 925–959.

Centers for Disease Control and Prevention, National Center for Injury Prevention and Control. (2015). *Child passenger safety*. http://www.cdc.gov/MotorVehicleSafety/Child_Passenger_Safety/CPS-Factsheet.html.

Eime, R. M., Young, J. A., Harvey, J. T., et al. (2013). A systematic review of the psychological and social benefits of participation in sport for children and adolescents: Informing development of a conceptual model of health through sport. *International Journal of Behavioral Nutrition and Physical Activity, 10*, 98.

Ferguson, C. J. (2013). Spanking, corporal punishment and negative long-term outcomes: A meta-analytic review of longitudinal studies. *Clinical Psychology Review, 33*(1), 196–208.

Galland, B. C., Taylor, B. J., Elder, D. E., et al. (2012). Normal sleep patterns in infants and children: A systemic review of observational studies. *Sleep Medicine Reviews, 16*(3), 213–222.

Giesbrecht, G. F., Leadbeater, B. J., & Macdonald, S. W. (2011). Child and context characteristics in trajectories of physical and relational victimization among early elementary school children. *Development and Psychopathology, 23*(1), 239–252.

Hensley, V. (2013). Childhood bullying: A review and implications for health care professionals. *Nursing Clinics of North America, 48*(2), 203–213.

Hyde, A., Drennan, J., Butler, M., et al. (2013). Parents' constructions of communication with their children about safer sex. *The Journal of Clinical Nursing, 22*(23–24), 3438–3446.

King, K. K. (2014). Violence in the school setting: A school nurse perspective. *The Online Journal of Issues in Nursing*. http://www.nursingworld.org/MainMenuCategories/ANAMarketplace/ANAPeriodicals/OJIN/TableofContents/Vol-19-2014/No1-Jan-2014/Violence-in-School.html.

Mahat, G., Lyons, R., & Bowen, F. (2014). Early childhood caries and the role of the pediatric nurse practitioner. *The Journal for Nurse Practitioners, 10*(3), 189–193.

Meehan, W. P., 3rd, Lee, L. K., Fischer, C. M., et al. (2013). Bicycle helmet laws are associated with a lower fatality rate from bicycle-motor vehicle collisions. *The Journal of Pediatrics, 163*(3), 726–729.

National Highway Traffic Safety Administration. (2013). *Traffic safety facts 2011 data: Children*. http://www-nrd.nhtsa.dot.gov/pubs/811767.pdf.

Owen, D. J., Slep, A. M., & Heyman, R. E. (2012). The effect of praise, positive nonverbal response, reprimand, and negative nonverbal response on child compliance: A systematic review. *Clinical Child and Family Psychology Review*, *15*(4), 364–385.

Resha, C. (2010). Delegation in the school setting: Is it a safe practice? *The Online Journal of Issues in Nursing*. http://www.nursingworld.org/MainMenuCategories/ANAMarketplace/ANAPeriodicals/OJIN/TableofContents/Vol152010/No2May2010/Delegation-in-the-School-Setting.html.

Riley, M. R., Scaramella, L. V., & McGoron, L. (2014). Disentangling the associations between contextual stress, sensitive parenting, and children's social development. *Family Relations*, *63*, 287–299.

Ruiz-Casares, M., Rousseau, C., Currie, J. L., et al. (2012). 'I hold on to my teddy bear really tight': Children's experiences when they are home alone. *American Journal of Orthopsychiatry*, *82*(1), 97–103.

Shetgiri, R. (2013). Bullying and victimization among children. *Advances in Pediatrics*, *60*(1), 33–51.

Shetgiri, R., Lin, H., & Flores, G. (2012). Identifying children at risk for being bullies in the United States. *Academic Pediatrics*, *12*(6), 509–522.

Sticca, F., & Perren, S. (2013). Is cyberbullying worse than traditional bullying? Examining the differential roles of medium, publicity, and anonymity for the perceived severity of bullying. *Journal of Youth and Adolescence*, *42*(5), 739–750.

US Department of Justice. (2011). *Highlights of the 2009 national youth gang survey*. https://www.ncjrs.gov/pdffiles1/ojjdp/233581.pdf.

White, L. S. (2012). Reducing stress in school-age girls through mindful yoga. *The Journal of Pediatric Health Care*, *26*(1), 45–56.

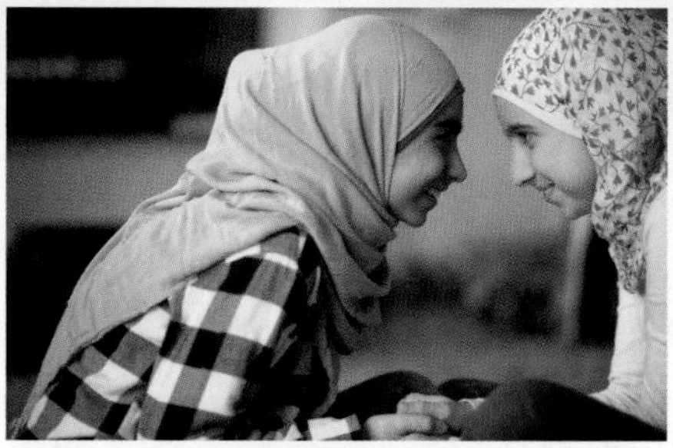

15

Health Promotion of the Adolescent and Family

Elizabeth A. Duffy

http://evolve.elsevier.com/wong/essentials

CONCEPTS

- Development
- Functional Ability
- Family Dynamics
- Reproduction
- Sexuality
- Mood and Affect
- Safety
- Health Promotion

PROMOTING OPTIMAL GROWTH AND DEVELOPMENT

Adolescence is a period of transition between childhood and adulthood—a time of rapid physical, cognitive, social, and emotional maturation.

Several terms are used to refer to this stage of growth and development. **Puberty** refers to the maturational, hormonal, and growth process that occurs when the reproductive organs begin to function and the secondary sex characteristics develop. This process is sometimes divided into three stages: **prepubescence**, the period of about 2 years immediately before puberty when the child is developing preliminary physical changes that herald sexual maturity; **puberty**, the point at which sexual maturity is achieved, marked by the first menstrual flow in girls but by less obvious indications in boys; and **postpubescence**, a 1- to 2-year period after puberty during which skeletal growth is completed and reproductive functions become fairly well established. **Adolescence**, which literally means "to grow into maturity," is generally regarded as the psychologic, social, and maturational process initiated by the pubertal changes. It involves three distinct subphases: **early adolescence** (ages 11 to 14), **middle adolescence** (ages 15 to 17), and **late adolescence** (ages 18 to 20). The term **teenage years** is used synonymously with *adolescence* to describe ages 13 through 19 years. The changes that occur during the early, middle, and late phases of adolescence are summarized in Table 15.1.

BIOLOGIC DEVELOPMENT

The physical changes of puberty are primarily the result of hormonal activity and are controlled by the anterior pituitary gland in response to a stimulus from the hypothalamus. The obvious physical changes are noted in increased physical growth and in the appearance and development of secondary sex characteristics; less obvious are physiologic alterations and neurogonadal maturity, accompanied by the ability to procreate. Physical distinction between the sexes is made on the basis of distinguishing characteristics. **Primary sex characteristics** are the external and internal organs that carry out the reproductive functions (e.g., ovaries, uterus, breasts, penis). **Secondary sex characteristics** are the changes that occur throughout the body as a result of hormonal changes (e.g., voice alterations, development of facial and pubertal hair, fat deposits) but that play no direct part in reproduction.

Neuroendocrine Events of Puberty

The events of puberty are caused by a cluster of events that trigger the production of gonadotropin-releasing hormone (GnRH) by the hypothalamus. GnRH travels to the anterior pituitary gland, where it stimulates the production and secretion of follicle-stimulating hormone (FSH) and luteinizing hormone (LH). Increasing levels of FSH and LH stimulate a gonadal response, which for females consists of growth of ovarian follicles, production of estrogen, and initiation of ovulation; for males, it consists of maturation of the testicles and testosterone and stimulation of sperm production.

The ovaries, testes, and adrenals secrete sex hormones. These hormones are produced in varying amounts by both sexes throughout the life span. The adrenal cortex is responsible for the small amounts secreted before the pubescent years, but the sex hormone production that accompanies maturation of the gonads is responsible for the biologic changes observed during puberty.

Estrogen, the feminizing hormone, is found in low quantities during childhood. Beginning in early puberty, FSH stimulates estrogen production by the ovaries; however, estrogen levels are not high enough to cause ovulation until mid-puberty. The increasing quantity of estrogen in early puberty causes a building of the endometrial lining of the uterus and first menstruation, or menarche. As puberty progresses, one ovarian follicle becomes dominant during each menstrual cycle and produces increasing amounts of estrogen that releases an ovum, a process called *ovulation.* After ovulation, the follicle involutes and estrogen production decreases. The pituitary gland responds to the decreased estrogen production by increasing production of FSH, which initiates a new menstrual cycle. **Androgens**, the masculinizing hormones, are also secreted in small and gradually increasing amounts up to about 7 or 9 years old, at which time there is a more

TABLE 15.1 Growth and Development During Adolescence

Early Adolescence (11 to 14 Years Old)	Middle Adolescence (15 to 17 Years Old)	Late Adolescence (18 to 20 Years Old)
Growth		
Rapidly accelerating growth Reaches peak velocity Secondary sex characteristics appear	Growth decelerating in girls Stature reaches 95% of adult height Secondary sex characteristics well advanced	Physically mature Structure and reproductive growth almost complete
Cognition		
Explores newfound ability for limited abstract thought Clumsy groping for new values and energies Comparison of "normality" with peers of same sex	Developing capacity for abstract thinking Enjoys intellectual powers, often in idealistic terms Concern with philosophic, political, and social problems	Established abstract thought Can perceive and act on long-range options Able to view problems comprehensively Intellectual and functional identity established
Identity		
Preoccupied with rapid body changes Trying out various roles Measurement of attractiveness by acceptance or rejection of peers Conformity to group norms Decline in self-esteem	Modifies body image Self-centered; increased narcissism Tendency toward inner experience and self-discovery Has a rich fantasy life Idealistic Able to perceive future implications of current behavior and decisions; variable application	Body image and gender role definition nearly secured Mature sexual identity Phase of consolidation of identity Increase in self-esteem Comfortable with physical growth Social roles defined and articulated
Relationships With Parents		
Defining independence–dependence boundaries Strong desire to remain dependent on parents while trying to detach No major conflicts over parental control	Major conflicts over independence and control Low point in parent-child relationship Greatest push for emancipation; disengagement Final and irreversible emotional detachment from parents; mourning	Emotional and physical separation from parents completed Independence from family with less conflict Emancipation nearly secured
Relationships With Peers		
Seeks peer affiliations to counter instability generated by rapid change Upsurge of close, idealized friendships with members of the same sex Struggle for mastery within peer group	Strong need for identity to affirm self-image Behavioral standards set by peer group Acceptance by peers extremely important—fear of rejection Exploration of ability to attract opposite sex	Peer group recedes in importance in favor of individual friendship Testing of romantic relationships against possibility of permanent alliance Relationships characterized by giving and sharing
Sexuality		
Self-exploration and evaluation Limited dating, usually group Limited intimacy	Multiple plural relationships Internal identification of heterosexual, homosexual, or bisexual attractions Exploration of "self appeal" Feeling of "being in love" Tentative establishment of relationships	Forms stable relationships and attachment to another Growing capacity for mutuality and reciprocity Dating as a romantic pair May publicly identify as gay, lesbian, or bisexual Intimacy involves commitment rather than exploration and romanticism
Psychologic Health		
Wide mood swings Intense daydreaming Anger outwardly expressed with moodiness, temper outbursts, and verbal insults and name calling	Tendency toward inner experiences; more introspective Tendency to withdraw when upset or feelings are hurt Vacillation of emotions in time and range Feelings of inadequacy common; difficulty in asking for help	More constancy of emotion Anger more likely to be concealed

rapid increase in both sexes, especially boys, until about 15 years old. These hormones have tremendous growth-promoting properties that result in rapid increases of muscle mass, skeletal growth, and bone density. Androgens are responsible for the development of pubic, axillary, facial, and body hair; acne; body odor; and an increase in height.

Boys do not experience a discrete event analogous to menstruation or ovulation in girls; however, FSH and LH act on testicular cells to stimulate production of testosterone and sperm. The production of viable sperm tends to follow boys' first ejaculation. The capacity to ejaculate occurs approximately 1 year after initial testicular enlargement and pubic hair appearance.

Sexual Maturation

The visible evidence of sexual maturation is achieved in an orderly sequence, and the state of maturity can be estimated on the basis of the appearance of these external manifestations. The age at which these

BOX 15.1 Tanner Stages

The Tanner stages were developed by Dr. J. M. Tanner and colleagues. Tanner stages describe the stages of pubertal growth and are numbered from stage 1 (immature) to stage 5 (mature) for both males and females. In girls and young women, the Tanner stages describe pubertal development based on breast size and the shape and distribution of pubic hair. In boys and young men, the Tanner stages describe pubertal development based on the size and shape of the penis and scrotum and the shape and distribution of pubic hair.

Data from Tanner, J. M. (1962). *Growth of adolescents.* Oxford, England: Blackwell Scientific Publications.

BOX 15.2 Usual Sequence of Maturational Changes

Girls

Breast changes
Rapid increase in height and weight
Growth of pubic hair
Appearance of axillary hair
Menstruation (usually begins 2 years after first signs)
Abrupt deceleration of linear growth

Boys

Enlargement of testicles
Growth of pubic hair, axillary hair, hair on upper lip, hair on face and elsewhere on body (facial hair usually appears about 2 years after appearance of pubic hair)
Rapid increase in height
Changes in the larynx and consequently the voice (usually take place along with growth of penis)
Nocturnal emissions
Abrupt deceleration of linear growth

changes are observed and the time required to progress from one stage to another may vary among children. The time from the appearance of breast buds to full maturity may be 1½ to 6 years for adolescent girls. It may take 2 to 5 years for male genitalia to reach adult size. The stages of development of secondary sex characteristics and genital development have been defined as a guide for estimating sexual maturity and are referred to as the **Tanner stages** (Box 15.1). The usual sequence of appearance of maturational changes is presented in Box 15.2.

Sexual Maturation in Girls

In most girls, the initial indication of puberty is the appearance of breast buds, an event known as **thelarche**, which occurs between 8 and 13 years old (Fig. 15.1). In a minority of normally developing girls, however, pubic hair may precede breast development. The average age of thelarche varies among ethnic groups: African American girls have an average age of 8.8 years, white girls' average is 9.7 years, and Hispanic girls' average is 9.3 years (Herman-Giddens, 2013). This is followed in approximately 2 to 6 months by growth of pubic hair on the mons pubis, known as **adrenarche** (Fig. 15.2).

The initial appearance of menstruation, or **menarche**, occurs about 2 years after the appearance of the first pubescent changes, approximately 9 months after attainment of peak height velocity, and 3 months after attainment of peak weight velocity. The mean age of menarche ranges from 10½ to 15 years, with the average age being 12 years, 8 months for non-Hispanic white girls, and 12 years, 2 months for African American girls (Cabrera, Bright, Frane, et al., 2014). Ovulation and regular menstrual periods usually occur 6 to 14 months after menarche. Girls may be considered to have **pubertal delay** if breast development has not occurred by 13 years old (Villanueva & Argente, 2014).

There is evidence that the mean age of menarche has gradually decreased over the past century in the United States and other developing countries. Females are experiencing puberty at younger ages, with differences noted between white and African American girls. The explanation for this is not yet clear but appears to be influenced by complex physiologic, psychologic, and environmental interrelationships and the reduced rates of disease as technology and medicine advances. This decline in the average age of menarche appears to have leveled off in recent years but continues to be studied (Papadimitriou, 2016).

Sexual Maturation in Boys

The first pubescent changes in boys are testicular enlargement accompanied by thinning, reddening, and increased looseness of the scrotum (Fig. 15.3). These events usually occur between 9½ and 14 years old. Early puberty is also characterized by the initial appearance of pubic hair. Penile enlargement begins, and testicular enlargement and pubic hair growth continue throughout mid-puberty. During this period, there is also increasing muscularity, early voice changes, and development of early facial hair. Temporary breast enlargement and tenderness, **gynecomastia**, are common during early to mid-puberty, occurring in up to 70% of boys (Ali & Donohoue, 2020). The spurts in height and weight occur concurrently toward the end of mid-puberty. For most boys, breast enlargement disappears within 2 years; however, gynecomastia may persist in obese individuals. By late puberty, there is a definite increase in the length and width of the penis, testicular enlargement continues, and first ejaculation occurs. Axillary hair develops, and facial hair extends to cover the anterior neck. Final voice changes occur secondary to the growth of the larynx. Concerns about **pubertal delay** should be considered for boys who exhibit no enlargement of the testes or scrotal changes by 14 years old (Villanueva & Argente, 2014).

Physical Growth During Puberty

Along with increases in reproductive hormones and sexual maturation, a dramatic increase in growth occurs. The final 20% to 25% of linear growth is achieved during puberty, and up to 50% of ideal adult body weight is gained during this time as well. Most of this growth of skeletal muscles and internal organs occurs during a 24- to 36-month period—the adolescent **growth spurt**. This accelerated growth occurs in all children but, as in other areas of development, is highly variable in age of onset, duration, and extent. The growth spurt begins earlier in girls, usually between 9½ and 14½ years old; on average it begins between 10½ and 16 years old in boys. During this period, the average boy gains 10 to 30 cm (4 to 12 inches) in height and 7 to 30 kg (15.5 to 66 pounds) in weight. The average girl, in whom the growth spurt is slower and less extensive, gains 5 to 20 cm (2 to 8 inches) in height and 7 to 25 kg (15.5 to 55 pounds) in weight. Growth in height typically ceases 2 to 2½ years after menarche in girls and at 18 to 20 years old in boys.

This increase in size is acquired in a characteristic sequence. Growth in length of the extremities and neck precedes growth in other areas, and because these parts are the first to reach adult length, the hands and feet appear larger than normal during adolescence. Increases in hip and chest breadth take place in a few months, followed several months later by an increase in shoulder width. These changes are followed by increases in length of the trunk and depth of the chest. This sequence of changes is responsible for the characteristic long-legged, gawky appearance of early adolescent children.

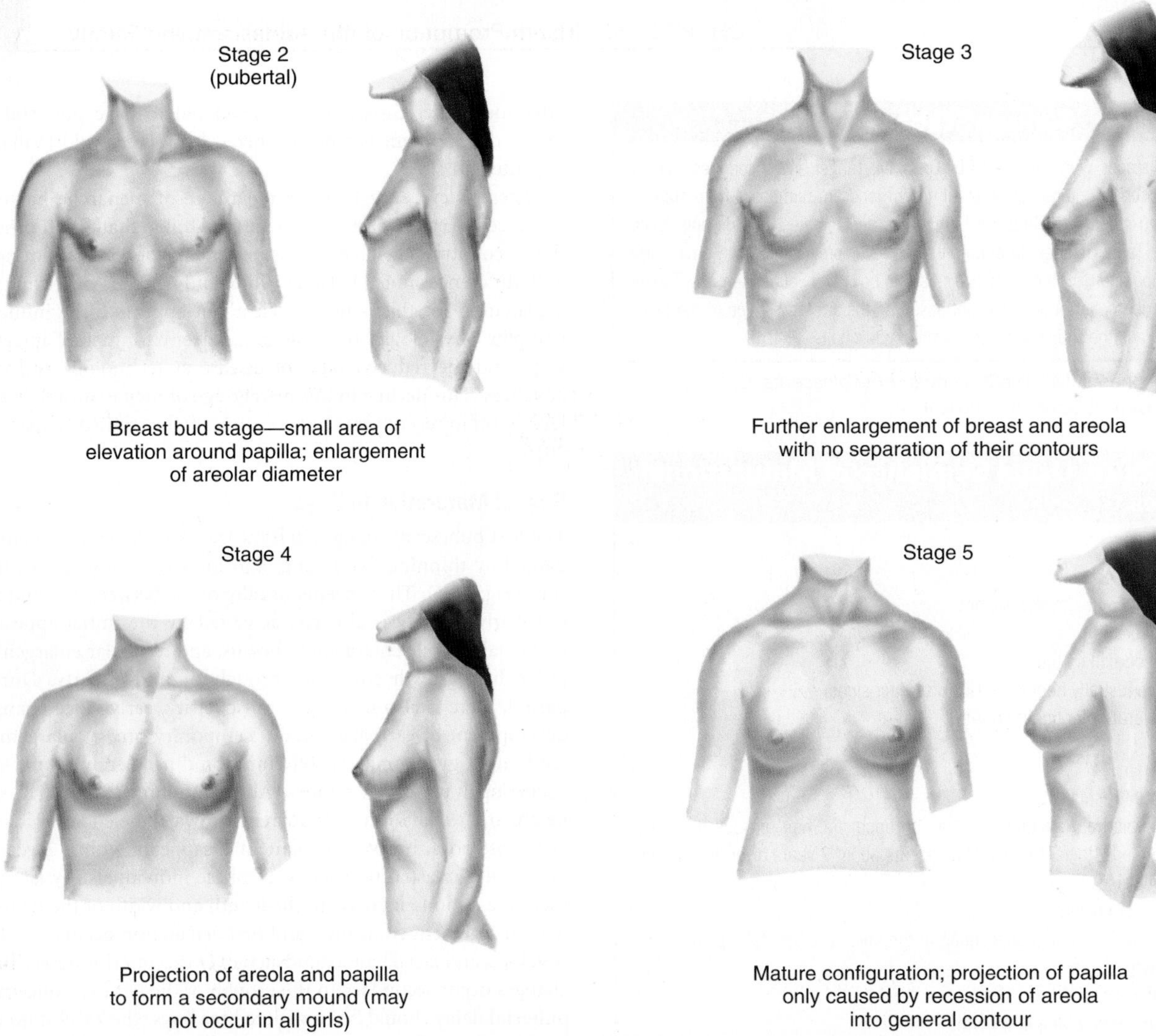

Fig. 15.1 Development of breasts in girls. Stage 1 (prepubertal—elevation of papilla only) is not shown. (Modified from Marshall, W. A., & Tanner, J. M. [1969]. Variations in pattern of pubertal changes in girls. *Archives of Disease in Childhood, 44*[235], 291–303; and Daniel, W. A., & Paulshock, B. Z. [1979]. A physician's guide to sexual maturity. *Patient Care, 13*, 122–124.)

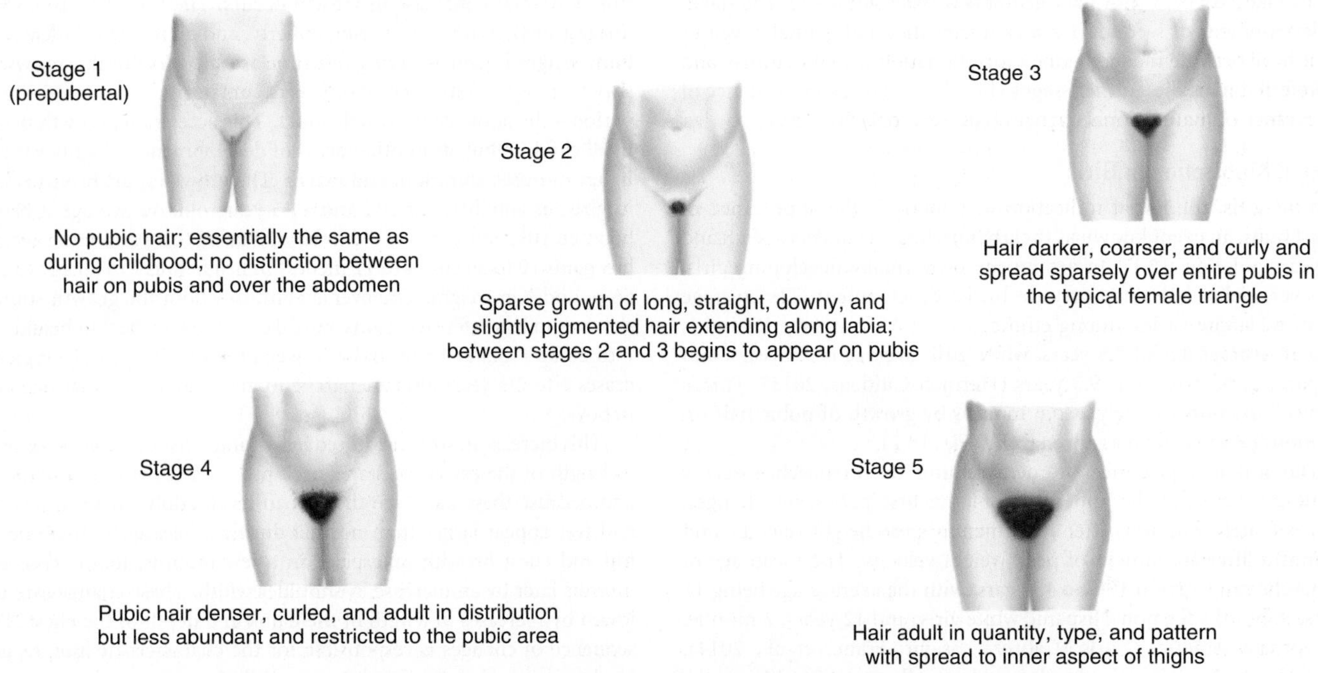

Stage 1
(prepubertal)
No pubic hair; essentially the same as during childhood; no distinction between hair on pubis and over the abdomen
Stage 2
Breast bud stage—small area of elevation around papilla; enlargement of areolar diameter
Sparse growth of long, straight, downy, and slightly pigmented hair extending along labia; between stages 2 and 3 begins to appear on pubis
Stage 3
Hair darker, coarser, and curly and spread sparsely over entire pubis in the typical female triangle
Stage 4
Projection of areola and papilla to form a secondary mound (may not occur in all girls)
Pubic hair denser, curled, and adult in distribution but less abundant and restricted to the pubic area
Stage 5
Mature configuration; projection of papilla only caused by recession of areola into general contour
Hair adult in quantity, type, and pattern with spread to inner aspect of thighs

Fig. 15.2 Growth of pubic hair in girls. (Modified from Marshall, W. A., Tanner, J. M. [1969]. Variations in pattern of pubertal changes in girls. *Archives of Disease in Childhood, 44*[235], 291–303; and Daniel, W. A., & Paulshock, B. Z. [1979]. A physician's guide to sexual maturity. *Patient Care, 13*, 122–124.)

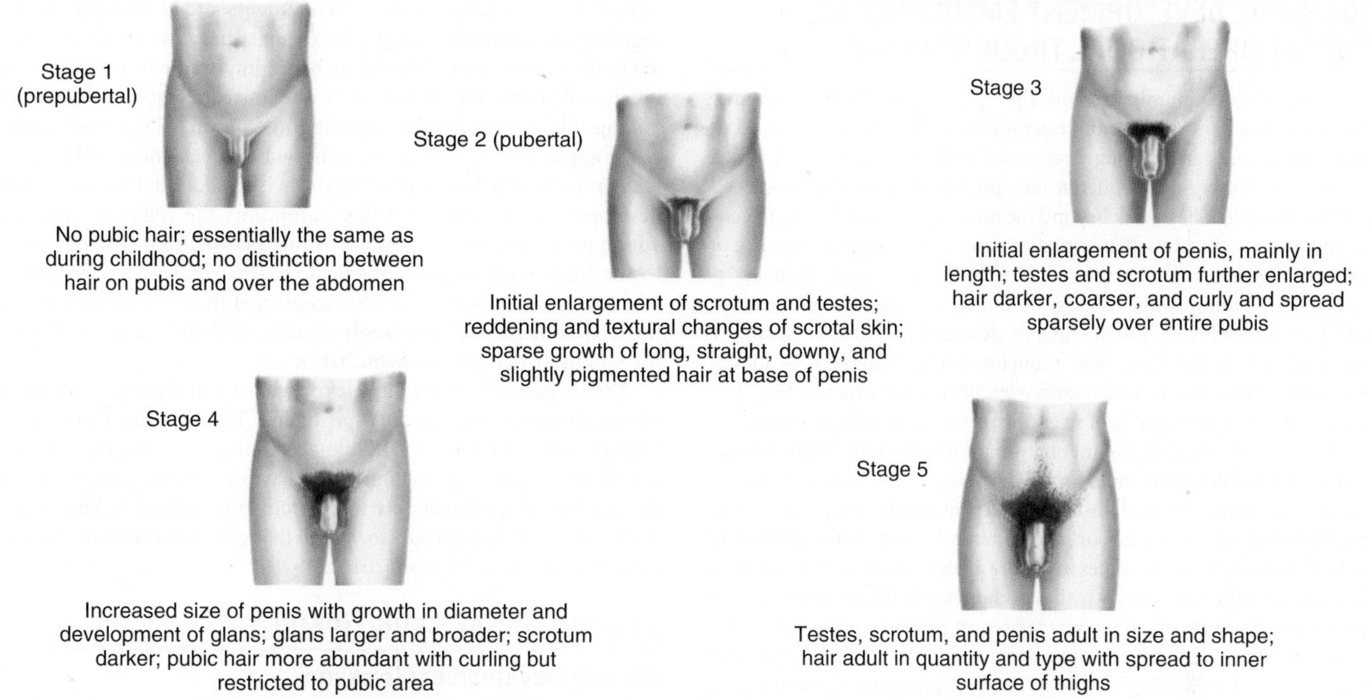
Stage 1
(prepubertal)
No pubic hair; essentially the same as during childhood; no distinction between hair on pubis and over the abdomen
Stage 2 (pubertal)
Initial enlargement of scrotum and testes; reddening and textural changes of scrotal skin; sparse growth of long, straight, downy, and slightly pigmented hair at base of penis
Stage 3
Initial enlargement of penis, mainly in length; testes and scrotum further enlarged; hair darker, coarser, and curly and spread sparsely over entire pubis
Stage 4
Increased size of penis with growth in diameter and development of glans; glans larger and broader; scrotum darker; pubic hair more abundant with curling but restricted to pubic area
Stage 5
Testes, scrotum, and penis adult in size and shape; hair adult in quantity and type with spread to inner surface of thighs

Fig. 15.3 Developmental stages of secondary sex characteristics and genital development in boys. (Modified from Marshall, W. A., & Tanner, J. M. [1970]. Variations in pattern of pubertal changes in boys. *Archives of Disease in Childhood, 45*[239], 13–23; and Daniel, W. A., & Paulshock, B. Z. [1979]. A physician's guide to sexual maturity. *Patient Care, 13*, 122–124.)

Sex Differences in General Growth Patterns

Sex differences in general growth and distribution patterns are apparent in skeletal growth, muscle mass, adipose tissue, and skin. **Skeletal growth** differences between boys and girls are apparently a function of hormonal effects at puberty. The earlier cessation of growth in girls is caused by epiphyseal unity under the potent effect of estrogen secretion, and the hormonal effect on female bone growth is much stronger than the similar effect of testosterone in boys. In boys, the prolonged growth period before puberty and the less rapid epiphyseal closure are reflected in their greater overall height and longer arms and legs. Other skeletal differences are increased shoulder width in boys and broader hip development in girls.

Hypertrophy of the laryngeal mucosa and enlargement of the larynx and vocal cords occur in both boys and girls to produce **voice changes**. Girls' voices become slightly deeper and considerably fuller, but the effect in boys is striking. The change in the voice of adolescent boys occurs between Tanner stages 3 and 4, with the voice often shifting uncontrollably from deep to high tones in the middle of a sentence. The average lengthening of the vocal cords is 10.9 mm (0.4 inch) for boys and 4.2 mm (0.17 inch) for girls.

Growth of **lean body mass**, principally muscle, which tends to occur after the bone growth spurt, takes place steadily during adolescence. Lean body mass is both quantitatively and qualitatively greater in boys than in girls at comparable stages of pubertal development. **Nonlean body mass**, primarily fat, is also increased but follows a less orderly pattern. There may be a transient increase in subcutaneous fat just before the skeletal growth spurt, especially in boys. This is followed 1 to 2 years later by a modest to marked decrease, which is again more marked in boys. Later, variable amounts of fat are deposited to fill out and contour the mature physique in patterns characteristic of the adolescent's sex, particularly in the regions over the thighs, hips, and buttocks and around the breast tissue. It should be noted, however, that pediatric obesity is steadily on the increase in the United States, and obesity can change the timing and sequence of puberty. This may have long-term effects for increased risk of adult adiposity and obesity (Nokoff, Thurston, Hilkin, et al., 2019). A review of recent evidence indicates an association between obesity and onset of early puberty in girls rather than a causal relationship, and other factors such as hormones and insulin resistance may account for early onset puberty as well. A large, racially diverse sample of boys found evidence of earlier puberty for overweight boys compared with normal or obese boys, and later puberty for obese boys compared with normal or overweight boys (Lee, Wasserman, Kaciroti, et al., 2016)

Other Physiologic Changes

A number of physiologic functions are altered in response to some of the pubertal changes. The size and strength of the heart, blood volume, and systolic blood pressure increase, whereas the heart rate decreases. Blood volume, which has increased steadily during childhood, reaches a higher value in boys than in girls, a fact that may be related to the increased muscle mass in pubertal boys. Adult values are reached for all formed elements of the blood. The lungs increase in both diameter and length during puberty. Respiratory rate decreases steadily throughout childhood and reaches the adult rate in adolescence. Respiratory volume and vital capacity are increased, and to a far greater extent in males than in females. The rate of steady decline in basal metabolic rate from birth to adulthood slows during puberty. During this period, physiologic responses to exercise change drastically: performance improves, especially in boys, and the body is able to make the physiologic adjustments needed for normal functioning after exercise is completed. These capabilities are a result of the increased size and strength of muscles and the increased level of cardiac, respiratory, and metabolic functioning.

COGNITIVE DEVELOPMENT EMERGENCE OF FORMAL OPERATIONAL THOUGHT (PIAGET)

Cognitive thinking culminates with the capacity for abstract thinking. This stage, the period of formal operations, is Piaget's fourth and last stage. Adolescents are no longer restricted to the real and actual, which was typical of the period of concrete thought; now they are also concerned with the possible. They think beyond the present. Without having to center attention on the immediate situation, they can imagine a sequence of future events that might occur, including college and occupational possibilities; how things might change in the future, such as relationships with parents; and the consequences of their actions, such as dropping out of school. At this time, their thoughts can be influenced by logical principles rather than just their own perceptions and experiences. They become increasingly capable of scientific reasoning and formal logic.

Adolescents are capable of mentally manipulating more than two categories of variables at the same time. For example, they can consider the relationship between speed, distance, and time in planning a trip. They can detect logical consistency or inconsistency in a set of statements and evaluate a system or set of values in a more analytic manner. For instance, they question the parent who insists on honesty in the youngster but at the same time cheats on an income tax report or expense account.

In adolescence, young people begin to consider both their own thinking and the thinking of others. They wonder what opinion others have of them, and they are able to imagine the thoughts of others. With this capacity comes the ability to differentiate between others' thoughts and their own and to interpret the thoughts of others more accurately. They are able to understand that few concepts are absolute or independent of other influencing factors. As they become aware that other cultures and communities have different norms and standards from their own, it becomes easier for them to accept members of these other cultures, and the decision to behave in their own culture in an accepted manner becomes a more conscious commitment.

MORAL DEVELOPMENT (KOHLBERG)

Although younger children merely accept the decisions or points of view of adults, adolescents question absolutes and rules, and they view moral standards as subjective and based on points of view that are subject to disagreement. There are occasions when social conventions are questioned and principles of justice, caring, and quality of life take precedence over established social norms. Aspects of conventional and principled moral reasoning are present in adolescence and used at different times in different situations.

Late adolescence is characterized by serious questioning of existing moral values and their relevance to society and the individual. Adolescents can easily take the role of another. They understand duty and obligation based on reciprocal rights of others and the concept of justice that is founded on making amends for misdeeds and repairing or replacing what has been spoiled by wrongdoing. However, they seriously question established moral codes, often as a result of observing that adults verbally ascribe to a code but do not adhere to it.

SPIRITUAL DEVELOPMENT

Religious beliefs also become more abstract and principled during the adolescent years. Specifically, adolescents' beliefs become more oriented toward spiritual and ideological matters and less oriented toward rituals, practice, and the strict observance of religious customs. Compared to children, adolescents place more emphasis on the internal aspects of religion and less emphasis on external manifestations.

Generally, the stated importance of participation in organized religion declines somewhat during the adolescent years. More high school students than postsecondary students attend religious services regularly, and, not surprisingly, the younger the adolescents, the more likely they are to view religion as being important to them. Among older adolescents, the importance of organized religion declines more among college students than among those not in college. Late adolescence appears to be a time when individuals reexamine and reevaluate many of the beliefs and values of their childhood. Consistent with developmental changes in value autonomy, the religious beliefs of young people are likely to become more personalized and less bound to the traditional religious practices they may have been exposed to when they were younger. As adolescents mature and form an identity, they may either reject their family's traditional beliefs or decide to conform to those beliefs (Neuman, 2011).

Nurses play an important role for teens by providing an opportunity to discuss issues regarding spirituality. These aspects are especially important to younger and middle-age adolescents who may be contemplating or participating in risky behaviors because greater levels of religiosity and spirituality are associated with protective, health-promoting behaviors, especially for youth living in environments that lack positive influences (Horton, 2015).

PSYCHOSOCIAL DEVELOPMENT

Identity Development (Erikson)

The task of identity formation is to develop a stable, coherent picture of oneself that includes integrating one's past and present experiences with a sense of where one is headed in the future. Throughout childhood, individuals have been going through the process of identification as they concentrate on various parts of the body at specific times. During infancy, children identify themselves as being separate from the mother; during early childhood, they establish gender role identification with the appropriate-sex parent; and in later childhood, they establish who they are in relation to others. In adolescence, they come to see themselves as distinct individuals, somehow unique and separate from every other individual.

Adolescence begins with the onset of puberty and extends to relative physical and emotional stability at or near graduation from high school. During this time, adolescents are faced with the crisis of group identity versus alienation. In the period that follows, individuals strive to attain autonomy from the family and develop a sense of personal identity as opposed to role diffusion. A sense of group identity appears to be essential to the development of a personal identity. Young adolescents must resolve questions concerning relationships with a peer group before they are able to resolve questions about who they are in relation to family and society.

Group Identity

During the early stage of adolescence, pressure to belong to a group is intensified. Teenagers find it essential to belong to a group from which they can derive status. Belonging to a crowd helps adolescents establish the differences between themselves and their parents. They dress as the group dresses and wear makeup and hairstyles according to group criteria, all of which are different from those of the parental generation. Language, music, and dancing reflect a culture that is exclusive to adolescents. If adults begin to emulate these fashions and interests, the style changes immediately. The evidence of adolescent conformity to the peer group and nonconformity to the adult group provides teenagers with a frame of reference for self-assertion and rejection of the identity of their parents' generation. To be different is to be unaccepted and alienated from the group.

Individual Identity

The quest for personal identity is part of the ongoing identification process. As adolescents establish identity within a group, they also attempt to incorporate multiple body changes into a concept of the self. Body awareness is part of self-awareness. In their search for identity, adolescents consider the relationships that have developed between themselves and others in the past, as well as the directions they hope to take in the future.

Significant others hold expectations for the behavior of adolescents. Often these expectations or demands are persistent enough that individuals make certain decisions that they would not make if they were solely responsible for identity formation. Adolescents may find it too easy to slip into the roles expected by others without incorporating their own personal goals or questioning decisions. Thus individuals may become what parents or others wish them to be based on these premature decisions. Young persons might form a negative identity when society or their culture provides them with a self-image that is contrary to the values of the community. Labels such as "juvenile delinquent," "hoodlum," or "failure" are applied to certain adolescents, who then accept and live up to these labels with behaviors that validate and strengthen them.

The process of evolving a personal identity is time consuming and fraught with periods of confusion, depression, and discouragement. Parents provide models for coping during stressful encounters, which likely influence adolescent's social relationships within and outside the family setting (Marceau, Zahn-Waxler, Shirtcliff, et al., 2015). Adolescents still need monitoring and input from parents during their search for identity; total abandonment during this phase is undesirable and may leave the adolescent feeling fragmented, alone, and adrift, resulting in the development of psychopathology. Determining an identity and a place in the world is a critical and perilous feature of adolescence (see Critical Thinking Case Study box). However, as the pieces gradually shift and settle into place, a positive identity emerges. Role diffusion results when the individual is unable to formulate a satisfactory identity from the multiplicity of aspirations, roles, and identifications.

CRITICAL THINKING CASE STUDY

Discussing the Future

Jeremy, 17 years old, will be graduating from high school in the spring. His mother, a single parent, tells you that she is concerned because graduation is quickly approaching, and Jeremy has made no plans for what he will do with his life after graduation. Whenever Jeremy mentions the topic, his mother tells him, "This is what you must do" and begins to outline the steps he must take. Jeremy just walks away. She asks, "What should I do?" What advice should you give Jeremy's mother?

Initial Assessment. What could be occurring in this family as Jeremy nears graduation?

Clinical Reasoning. What developmental considerations are important for the nurse to understand before responding to the mother?

Teaching Points

- High school graduation is an important milestone for an adolescent.
- Uncertainty about the future is commonly experienced by adolescents, and parents should be made aware of this.
- Parents often need support in helping their adolescents to develop their future goals without pressuring them and increasing their stress.

Critical Thinking Answers

Initial Assessment. Jeremy could be anxious about graduation and feeling pressure from his mother. The mother may be feeling the loss of her son as he nears this important milestone in his life.

Clinical Reasoning. The following should be considered before responding to Jeremy's mother:

- Adolescents and the search for personal identity
- The influence of others on the adolescent's search for personal identity
- Ways to communicate with adolescents

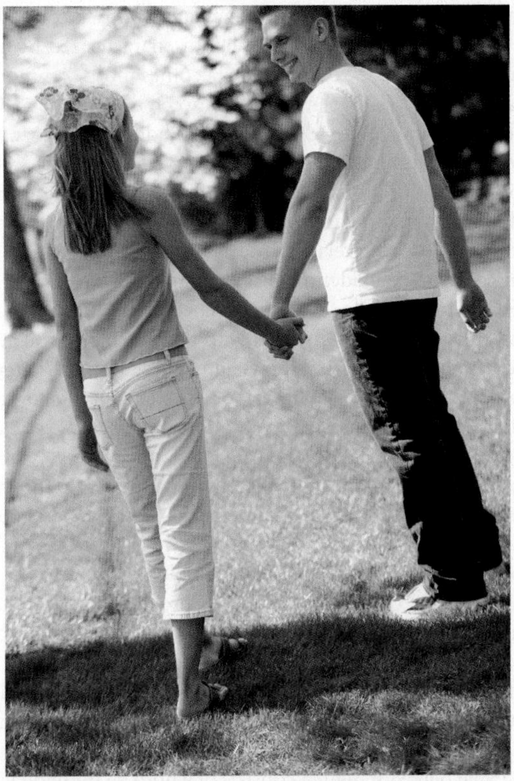

Fig. 15.4 Romantic relationships are important for most adolescents. (©2011 Photos.com, a division of Getty Images. All rights reserved.)

Sex-Role Identity

Adolescence represents a critical time in the development of sexuality and a sex-role identity. Hormonal, physical, cognitive, and social changes that occur during adolescence all have an impact on sexual development. Of all the developmental changes that affect adolescent sexuality, none is more obvious than the impact of puberty. Adolescents must come to terms with hormonal influences, physiologic manifestations such as menstruation and ejaculation, and physical changes such as breast and genital development. All of these changes have a profound impact on the way teenagers perceive their bodies (i.e., body image). In addition to transitions in body image, increasing levels of pubertal hormones contribute to increased levels of sexual motivation among both boys and girls. The emergence of formal operational thinking also increases adolescents' decision-making capabilities concerning sexual issues. As they mature, teenagers become better able to think through potential risks and benefits of sexual behaviors before they engage in any behavior. Older adolescents may also be able to conceptualize more long-term consequences of present behaviors. One of the important tasks of adolescence is to incorporate sexuality successfully into close, intimate relationships. This task is made possible by the advanced cognitive abilities that emerge over the course of adolescence.

Part of adolescent identity formation involves the development of sexual identity. As they begin to integrate changes involved with puberty, young adolescents also develop emotional and social identities separate from their families'. For young adolescents, the process of sexual identity development usually involves forming close friendships with same-sex peers. Many teenagers begin to make a shift from relationships with same-sex peers to intimate relationships with members of the opposite sex during middle adolescence (Fig. 15.4). Opposite-sex relationships typically begin with peer activities involving both boys and girls. Pairing off as couples becomes more common as middle adolescence progresses. The type and degree of seriousness of partner relationships vary. Initial relationships are usually noncommittal, extremely mobile, and seldom characterized by any deep romantic attachments. Sexual activity becomes more common during middle adolescence. The relationship between love and sexual expression is brought into focus during middle adolescence. Most young people oppose exploitation, pressure, or force in sex, as well as sex solely for the sake of physical enjoyment without a personal relationship. Adolescents find it hard to believe that sex can exist without love; therefore they view each relationship as real love.

An integrated sexual identity often emerges during late adolescence as individuals incorporate sexual experiences, feelings, and knowledge. For most, this identity is consistent with their own physical and mental capacities and with societal limits and expectations. Whatever their sexual orientation, most teenagers possess the capacity to have intimate relationships that satisfy the emotional and sexual needs of both partners.

Sexual orientation is an important aspect of sexual identity. **Sexual orientation** is defined as a pattern of sexual arousal or romantic attraction toward persons of the opposite gender (heterosexual), of the same gender (homosexual, often called gay, lesbian, or queer), or of both genders (bisexual), or it may involve the process of gender transition (transgender) or an asexual orientation (not sexually aroused by either gender). Sexual orientation encompasses several dimensions: (1) sexual orientation identity, which consists of how an individual defines his or her sexual orientation; (2) sexual attraction, which includes the gender to which the individual is romantically and physically attracted; and (3) sexual behavior, which consists of whom an individual has sexual relationships with (O'Neill & Wakefield, 2017). In individuals, the direction and intensity of each dimension are not necessarily consistent with any of the others. For example, individuals may be attracted most strongly to their same gender, fantasize about both genders, have sexual activity only with the opposite gender, and identify as gay or lesbian. Other individuals may engage in same-gender sexual behavior and fantasize about both genders but identify as heterosexual. As with all aspects of sexual identity, the dimensions of sexual orientation are influenced by cultural meaning and expectation, by gender, by peer groups, and by other environmental contexts.

Adolescence is the period during which individuals commonly begin to identify their sexual orientation as part of their developing sexual identity. However, this identification process can be profoundly influenced by cultural beliefs and values, by societal and family pressures, or by a lack of similar peers. Most adolescents eventually report an orientation toward exclusively heterosexual relationships. For adolescents whose orientation encompasses any same-gender dimensions, the identity process during adolescence can be complicated, especially when community norms disapprove of orientations other than heterosexual. Adolescents who have witnessed harassment or violence directed at gay, lesbian, and bisexual people, for example, may be reluctant to self-identify with these orientations even when their attractions and behaviors are exclusively same-gender or bisexual.

The development of sexual orientation as part of sexual identity includes several developmental milestones during late childhood and throughout adolescence. These milestones do not necessarily occur in the same order for everyone, nor are they completed in the same amount of time. They include (1) the realization of romantic or erotic attraction to people of one (or both) genders; (2) erotic daydreaming about one or both genders; (3) romantic partners or dates without sexual activity; (4) sexual activity with people of the preferred gender or genders (also, for some teens, sexual activity with a nonpreferred gender, out of curiosity or through social pressure); (5) self-identification of the orientation that best fits one's current circumstances and understanding; (6) publicly self-identifying that orientation, usually to intimate friends and family first and then the wider social group; and (7) an intimate, committed sexual relationship with a person of the gender appropriate to one's orientation.

There is no evidence that homosexual or bisexual adults are more or less likely to create long-term, stable relationships than are heterosexual couples. It should be noted that bisexual adolescents and adults do not generally engage in sexual relationships with both genders concurrently; self-identification as bisexual usually refers to the ability to be attracted to either gender but does not imply that such a person requires partners of both genders or that one must be equally attracted to and have sexual experience with both genders in order to be bisexual.

Although the order of these milestones varies greatly among adolescents, adolescents who identify as gay, lesbian, or bisexual tend to publicly self-identify later than heterosexual peers. Without positive gay, lesbian, or bisexual role models or a supportive peer group, sexual-minority teens can feel isolated, and they may not share their orientation with anyone for fear of rejection or violence.

SOCIAL ENVIRONMENTS

The biologic, cognitive, and social changes of adolescence are shaped by the social environment in which the changes take place. The social environment provides opportunities, barriers, role models, and support for individuals' development and health. Systems within the social environment, including family, peers, schools, community (including the Internet-based community), and the larger society, all contribute uniquely to an adolescent's development and health.

Families

During adolescence, the parent-child relationship changes from one of protection and dependency to one of mutual affection and equality. The process of achieving independence often involves turmoil and ambiguity as both parent and adolescent learn to play new roles and work toward establishing the ultimate relationship. As teenagers assert their rights for grown-up privileges, they frequently create tensions within the home. They resist parental control, and conflicts can arise from almost any situation or any subject. Favorite topics of dispute include Internet use, the need for a personal cell phone, manners, dress, chores and duties, homework, disrespectful behavior, friendships, dating and relationships, money, automobiles, alcohol and other substance abuse, and time schedules.

Teenagers' earliest attempts to achieve emancipation from parental controls are manifested in a period of rejection of the parents. They absent themselves from home and family activities and spend an increasing amount of time with the peer group. They confide less in their parents, but parents continue to play an important role in the personal and health-related decision making of adolescents. With advancing adolescence, teenagers become more competent, and with this competence comes a need for more autonomy. Although they may be psychologically prepared for independence, they are often thwarted in their efforts by lack of money or other parental barriers. Conflict arises in relation to the teenagers' outside activities and the elements of privacy and trust. Parental monitoring remains important throughout adolescence and may have a direct influence on adolescent sexual and substance use behavior. Parents should be guided toward **authoritative parenting** in which authority is used to guide the adolescent while allowing developmentally appropriate levels of freedom and providing clear, consistent messages regarding expectations. However, to gain the trust of adolescents, parents must respect their adolescent's privacy and show an honest and sincere interest in what the adolescent believes and feels (see Family-Centered Care box).

FAMILY-CENTERED CARE

Communication With Adolescents: The Art of Listening

Conflicts between parents and their adolescents are often a result of a natural characteristic of parenthood: the desire to protect one's offspring from harm or from simply doing something "stupid," something embarrassing, or something they may later regret. Teens sometimes bounce their thoughts and ideas off adults. At times, they really want some feedback, but sometimes they simply want to elicit a reaction.

I found it easy to listen openly, thoughtfully, and without interrupting when my teenagers' friends discussed troublesome topics. However, one day, when one of my own teenagers had a similar conversation with me, the parent part kicked in. I felt responsible and spoke my piece on the spot. This brought communication to a halt and resulted in defensiveness. It was a long time before my child tried to talk to me about anything controversial again.

The next time one of my teenagers started a similar conversation, I decided to try to trick myself. Throughout the entire conversation, I told myself over and over again to act as if this were not my teenager but rather someone else's child. I found this actually worked quite well, and I was able to listen without interrupting. I continue to use the system, sometimes with more success than at other times.

—Mother of four

Over the past several decades, changes have taken place within the family microsystem that have important implications for adolescent health. Higher rates of divorce and remarriage, increasing numbers of single-parent or blended families, and greater percentages of working mothers have become characteristic of contemporary US society. Changes in family structure and parent employment have resulted in adolescents having more time unsupervised by adults and increased time alone or with peers. Decreased adult supervision may result in more risk-taking behaviors, such as substance use and sexual intercourse, and decreased opportunities to develop a supportive relationship with parents. Consistently, adolescents with a sense of family belonging along with connectedness with school and community show less susceptibility to negative peer pressure and lower tendencies to be involved in risk-taking behaviors (Brooks, Magnusson, Spencer, et al., 2012).

Peer Groups

For most teenagers, peers assume a more significant role in adolescence than they did during childhood. The peer group serves as a strong support to adolescents, individually and collectively, providing them with a sense of belonging and a feeling of strength and power. The peer group forms the transitional world between dependence and autonomy.

The peer group has an intense influence on adolescents' self-evaluation and behavior. Peers serve as credible sources of information, role models of new social behaviors, sources of social reinforcement, and bridges to alternative lifestyles. To gain acceptance by a group, younger adolescents tend to conform completely in such things as mode of dress, hairstyle, taste in music, and vocabulary. Peers can also be a positive force in health promotion by encouraging healthy behaviors, serving as role models, and promoting positive health norms.

Schools

In contemporary society, schools play an increasingly important role in preparing young people for adulthood. Schooling is essential for a successful future. Failure to complete high school reduces employment opportunities and the probability of earning an adequate income. The dropout rate among minority students is higher than that among nonminority students; however, in 2016, 94.8% of white individuals and 93.8% of African American individuals16 to 24 years old had graduated from high school (Child Trends Data Bank, 2018).

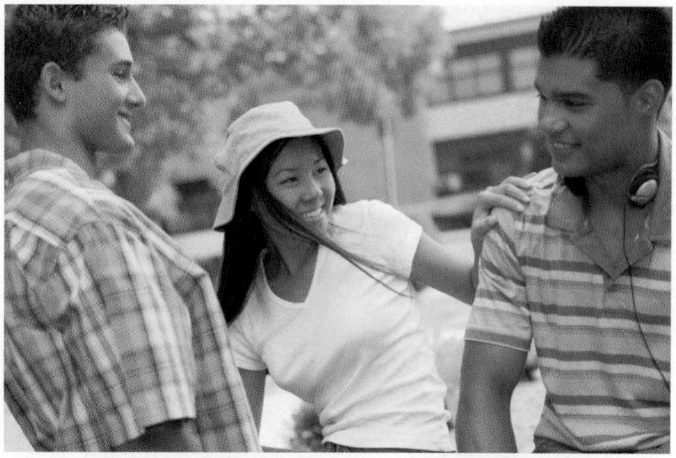

Fig. 15.5 Teenagers like to gather in small groups. (©2011 Photos.com, a division of Getty Images. All rights reserved.)

The school is psychologically important to adolescents as a focus of social life. Teenagers usually distribute themselves into a relatively predictable social hierarchy. They know to which groups they and others belong. A sense of school connectedness and optimal social connectedness is associated with positive outcomes for school completion, positive mood, and decreased high-risk behavior in adolescents (Chapman, Buckley, Reveruzzi, et al., 2014). School connectedness is correlated with caring teachers and the absence of prejudice or discrimination from peers.

Within the larger groups are smaller, distinct, and exclusive crowds or cliques of selected close friends who are emotionally attached to one another. The selection is based on common tastes, interests, and background. Although cliques may become formalized, most remain informal and small. However, each has an identifying feature that proclaims its difference from others and its solidarity within itself in much the same manner as the adolescent generation as a whole sets itself apart from the adult generation. Cliques are usually made up of one sex, and girls tend to be more cliquish than boys and to have a greater need for close friendships (Fig. 15.5). Within the intimacy of the group, adolescents gain support in learning about themselves, consideration for the feelings of others, and increased ego development and self-reliance. To belong is of utmost importance; thus adolescents behave in a way that will ensure their establishment in a group. Adolescents are highly susceptible to social approval, acceptance, and demands. To be ignored or criticized by peers creates feelings of inferiority, inadequacy, and incompetence.

Work

For the majority of young people in the United States, the workplace becomes a fourth microsystem. Most adolescents are employed in an array of jobs as restaurant workers, cashiers, sales clerks, clerical assistants, and unskilled laborers. The jobs tend to require little initiative or decision making and rarely use skills learned in school. Adolescent work may negatively affect development, as it fails to link adolescents to vocational mentors; is not intellectually stimulating; may take time away from other activities that could contribute to identity development; and can lead to fatigue, decreased interest in school, and poorer grades. These detrimental effects are likely to affect adolescents who work more than 20 hours a week.

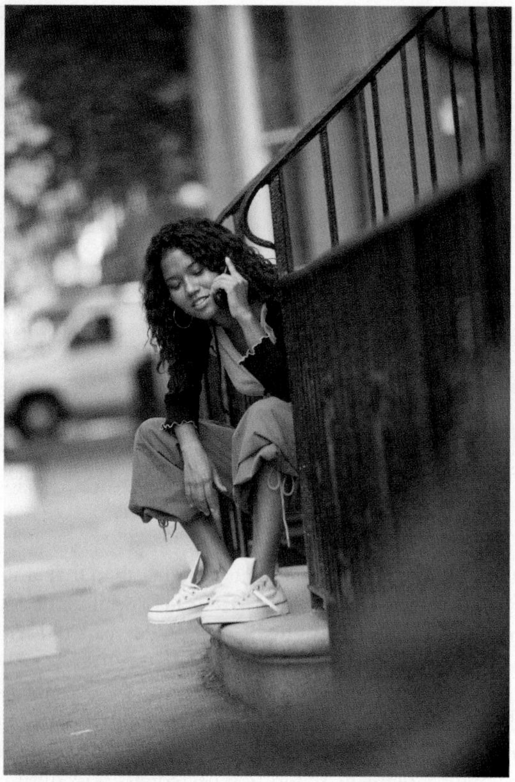

Fig. 15.6 Cell phones allow adolescents to talk for hours with their peers. (©2011 Photos.com, a division of Getty Images. All rights reserved.)

Interests and Activities

Adolescents spend a large amount of time engaged in leisure-time activities. These leisure-time activities move from being family centered to being peer centered. In addition to providing teenagers with fun and enjoyment, leisure-time activities assist in the development of social, physical, and cognitive skills. Leisure-time activities also allow teenagers the opportunity to learn to set priorities and structure their time.

The role of social media and advanced technology are nowhere more prominent than in the lives of today's adolescents. The widespread availability of the Internet and access to social networking websites such as Facebook, Snapchat, Instagram, email, blogs, and Twitter have created "virtual" communities and ways for young people to interact with others; web cameras even allow those interactions to include real-time video communication. Cellular telephones offer more mobile opportunities to talk on the phone, send text messages or instant messaging, send photos, or use video phone capabilities (Fig. 15.6).

Social networking websites have created a more public arena for trying out identities and developing interpersonal skills with a wider network of people, occasionally with anonymity. This can create opportunities for young people who have limited access to friends (because of rural location, shyness, or rare chronic conditions) to interact with people like themselves. However, most adolescents appear to be using the online social environment to interact with the same peers that they spend their day with at school.

Text messaging has become a common activity and can sometimes be disruptive. In addition, both the online and the text environment can create opportunities for **cyberbullying**, where teens engage in insults, harassment, and publicly humiliating statements online or on cell phones. There is a recognized danger of adolescents coming in contact and sharing personal information with sexual predators who pose as adolescents in an attempt to make personal contact with underage victims or engage them in "sexting" (i.e., sending sexually explicit or suggestive pictures or messages online). Adolescent sexting, rather than being an innocent anonymous activity, has been linked to risky sexual behaviors (Morelli, Bianchi, Baiocco, et al., 2016). Studies have noted not only that adolescents are enthusiastic technology users, but also that they frequently use multiple types of media at the same time. They may be listening to music on their digital music player while the television is on and they are surfing the Internet and texting friends on their cell phone. In addition, there are some demonstrated affective and behavioral effects among adolescents who are exposed to high levels of violence or sexual content in the technology sources they use, which can become a cause of concern for health promotion (Jacobson, Bailin, Milanaik, et al., 2016). There is increased concern focusing on adolescent vehicle driving and distractions, such as texting or cell phone usage. In 2017, 39.2% of adolescents reported having texted or emailed someone while driving on at least 1 day in the 30 days before the survey (Kann, McManus, & Harris, 2018). Many states have outlawed the use of handheld mobile devices while actively operating a vehicle (Chase, 2014).

PROMOTING OPTIMAL HEALTH DURING ADOLESCENCE

For adolescents, health promotion involves helping youth acquire the power (including knowledge, attitudes, and skills), authority (permission to use their power), and opportunities to make choices that increase the likelihood of positive expressions of health for themselves. A comprehensive approach to health promotion combines activities aimed at individuals with interventions focused on changing norms, attitudes, and behaviors of peer groups, families, communities, and society at large.

The rationale for focusing on health issues becomes obvious when one examines the major sources of mortality and morbidity during adolescence. The leading causes of mortality during adolescence in the United States are motor vehicle crashes, other accidental injuries, homicide, and suicide, which together are responsible for approximately 70% of all adolescent deaths (Kann, McManus, Harris, et al., 2016). The sources of morbidity in adolescence include injury (primarily motor vehicle related), depression, eating disorders, substance use, sexually transmitted infections (STIs), and pregnancy; obesity may begin in childhood or adolescence, with secondary health consequences becoming evident in adolescence. Health promotion for this age-group consists mainly of teaching and guidance to avoid risk-taking activities and health-damaging behaviors. Adolescence provides an opportunity for teenagers to incorporate healthy lifestyle behaviors that will benefit them not only during the teenage years but also throughout the life span.

Effective health promotion for adolescents should incorporate a developmentally appropriate, multifaceted approach and incorporate adolescents' perspectives on what health means. One strategy for health promotion used by nurses and other professionals in health care settings is the one-on-one health screening (see Nursing Care Guidelines box). Through a health screening interview, the health professional can identify both assets and threats to an adolescent's health and well-being; this interview also provides an opportunity to build a trusting relationship with the adolescent. In addition, the health screening interview provides an opportunity for teaching adolescents self-advocacy skills.

ADOLESCENTS' PERSPECTIVES ON HEALTH

To be most effective, adolescent health promotion efforts must incorporate adolescents' perspectives on what health means. Such efforts also must focus on adolescents' concerns and priorities related to health and health care services. From a positive perspective, adolescents' developmentally based sense of curiosity and movement toward autonomy provide opportunities for health promotion.

Adolescents' health-related interests and concerns include stress and anxiety, relationships with adults and peers, weight, acne, and feelings of sadness or depression. Health concerns are often consistent with the immediate developmental task that teenagers face. For example, younger adolescents have a particular interest in issues related to growth and development, whereas middle adolescents have questions and concerns related to peer-group acceptance, relationships with friends, and physical appearance. Older adolescents focus increasingly on school performance, future career and employment plans, and emotional health issues.

Among the behaviors that adolescents view as risky are substance use, sexual activity, and the use of recreational and motor vehicles. Adolescents identify health threats that primarily involve psychologic issues, such as clinical depression and eating or weight problems. The availability of confidential services is particularly important to adolescents, especially when they have concerns related to sensitive issues. Adolescents are more likely to participate in health care services when services are delivered by caring, respectful providers.

HEALTH CONCERNS OF ADOLESCENCE

As adolescents develop, they are able to assume additional responsibility for their own health, including maintaining health practices, taking prescribed medications, keeping appointments, and performing procedures when necessary. Health professionals who work with adolescents should consider their increasing independence and responsibility while maintaining privacy and ensuring confidentiality (see Nursing Care Guidelines box). Parents should also respect their teenager's independence and move toward the role of consultant about health issues while maintaining some level of involvement throughout adolescence.

Several professional organizations have published guidelines aimed at improving and maintaining health care for adolescents and young adults. The American Academy of Pediatrics, American Academy of Family Physicians, American Medical Association, and US Preventive Services Task Force have similar guidelines for health supervision of adolescents. These guidelines emphasize the need to provide health services to adolescents that meet their physical and emotional needs. They place great importance on the provision of health care by providers who are trained in meeting the adolescents' needs. Bright Futures (American Academy of Pediatrics, 2017a) emphasizes that the following issues should be addressed with adolescents over the course of multiple visits:

- Emotional well-being (coping, mood regulation, mental health, sexuality)
- Physical growth and development (physical and dental health, body image, healthy nutrition, physical activity)
- Social and academic competence (relationships with peers and family, school performance, interpersonal relationships)
- Risk reduction (tobacco, alcohol, other drugs, pregnancy, STIs)
- Violence and injury prevention (safety belt and helmet use, substance abuse and riding in a vehicle, interpersonal violence, bullying)

The following sections focus on some of the Bright Futures topics; other adolescent health issues are discussed later in the chapter.

NURSING CARE GUIDELINES

Interviewing Adolescents

- Ensure confidentiality and privacy; interview adolescent without parents.
- Explain the limits of confidentiality (e.g., legal duty to report physical or sexual abuse or to get others involved if patient is suicidal).
- Show concern for adolescent's perspective, saying, "First, I'd like to talk about your main concerns" and "I'd like to know what you think is happening."
- Offer a nonthreatening explanation for the questions you ask, such as "I'm going to ask a number of questions to help me better understand your health."
- Maintain objectivity; avoid assumptions, judgments, and lectures.
- Ask open-ended questions when possible; move to more directive questions if necessary.
- Begin with less sensitive issues and proceed to more sensitive ones.
- Use language that both the adolescent and you understand.
- Restate: Reflect back to adolescents what they have said, along with feelings that may be associated with their descriptions.

Emotional Well-Being

Adolescents vacillate in their emotional states between considerable maturity and childlike behavior. One minute they are exuberant and enthusiastic; the next minute they are depressed and withdrawn. Unpredictable but essentially normal, mood swings are common during this time. As the tension is relieved, emotion is brought under control, and individuals retreat to review what has happened, to attempt to master their anger and to grow in their ability to control their emotions and gain from the new experience. Because of these mood swings, adolescents are frequently labeled as unstable, inconsistent, and unpredictable. Little things can cause an emotional upheaval and, depending on the teenager's interpretation, can mean a great deal.

Teenagers are better able to control their emotions in later adolescence, when they can approach problems more calmly and rationally. Although they are still subject to periods of sadness, their feelings are less vulnerable, and they begin to demonstrate the more mature emotions of later adolescence. Whereas early adolescents react immediately and emotionally, older adolescents can control their emotions until socially acceptable times and places for expression present themselves. They are still subject to heightened emotion, and when it is expressed, their behavior reflects feelings of insecurity, tension, and indecision.

As sources of credible information, support, and encouragement, nurses can help adolescents cope with the changes and challenges they face. To promote both emotional health and psychosocial adjustment, nurses and other health care professionals can encourage adolescents to develop (1) skills to cope with stress and change and, (2) skills to become involved in personally meaningful activities.

Intentional and Unintentional Injury

The rationale for focusing on health issues becomes obvious when one examines the major sources of mortality and morbidity during adolescence. Motor vehicle crashes are the single greatest source of unintentional injury and death in young people. Many factors contribute to the higher rate of crashes among teen drivers, including the lack of driving experience and maturity, driving too fast, using alcohol, and using cell phones to talk or text. Suicide, a form of intentional injury, is the second leading cause of death among all adolescents in the United States. Homicide is the third leading cause of death among adolescents, mostly involving firearms; many adolescents report easy access to a gun (Centers for Disease Control and Prevention, 2017a).

Injuries also account for substantial morbidity among adolescents. During adolescence, peak physical, sensory, and psychomotor

BOX 15.3 Injury Prevention During Adolescence

Developmental Abilities Related to Risk of Injury

Need for independence and freedom
Testing independence
Age permitted to drive a motor vehicle (varies from state to state)
Inclination for risk taking
Feeling of indestructibility
Need for discharging energy, often at expense of logical thinking and other control mechanisms
Strong need for peer approval
Attempting hazardous maneuvers
Peak incidence for practice and participation in sports
Access to more complex tools, objects, and locations
Can assume responsibility for own actions

Injury Prevention

Motor or Nonmotor Vehicles

Pedestrian

Emphasize and encourage safe pedestrian behavior.
- Use crosswalks.
- At night, walk with a friend.
- If someone is following you, go to nearest public place with people.
- Do not walk in secluded areas; take well-traveled walkways.

Passenger

Promote appropriate behavior while riding in a motor vehicle. Refuse to ride with an impaired person or one who is driving recklessly.

Driver

Provide competent driver education; encourage judicious use of vehicle; discourage drag racing or playing chicken; maintain vehicle in proper condition (e.g., brakes, tires).
Teach and promote safety and maintenance of two- and three-wheeled vehicles.
Promote and encourage wearing of safety apparel, such as a helmet and long trousers.
Reinforce the dangers of drugs, including alcohol, when operating a motor vehicle.
Discourage distractions while driving—cell phone talking or texting, eating, smoking, or reading.

Drowning

Teach nonswimmers to swim.
Teach basic rules of water safety.
- Judicious selection of places to swim
- Sufficient water depth for diving
- Swimming with a companion
- No alcohol with water sports

Burns

Reinforce proper behavior in areas with burn hazards (gasoline, electric wires, and fires).
Advise against excessive exposure to natural or artificial sunlight (ultraviolet burn).
Discourage smoking.
Encourage use of sunscreen.

Poisoning

Educate in hazards of drug use, including alcohol.

Falls

Teach and encourage general safety measures in all activities.

Bodily Damage

Promote acquisition of proper instruction in sports and use of sports equipment.
Instruct in safe use of and respect for firearms and other devices with potential danger (e.g., power tools, firecrackers).
Provide and encourage use of protective equipment when using potentially hazardous devices.
Promote access to or provision of safe sports and recreational facilities.
Be alert for signs of depression (potential suicide).
Instruct regarding proper use of corrective devices (e.g., glasses, contact lenses, hearing aids).
Encourage and foster judicious application of safety principles and prevention.

function gives teenagers a feeling of strength and confidence that they have never experienced before. Their propensity for risk-taking behavior plus feelings of indestructibility make adolescents especially prone to injuries. The leading causes of injury-related morbidity among adolescents include vehicular crashes, firearms, drowning, poisoning, burns, and falls. Some of the developmental characteristics of teenagers and injury prevention suggestions are outlined in Box 15.3.

Dietary Habits, Eating Disorders, and Obesity

Puberty marks the beginning of accelerated physical growth, which can double some adolescents' nutritional requirements. At the same time, growing independence, the need for peer acceptance, concern with physical appearance, and an active lifestyle may affect eating habits, food choices, nutrient intake, and nutritional status.

Pressure for time and commitments to activities adversely affect teenagers' eating habits. Omitting breakfast or eating a breakfast that is nutritionally poor in quality is frequently a problem. Snacks, usually selected for accessibility rather than nutritional merit, become increasingly a part of the habitual eating pattern during adolescence (Fig. 15.7). Excess intake of calories, sugar, fat, cholesterol, and

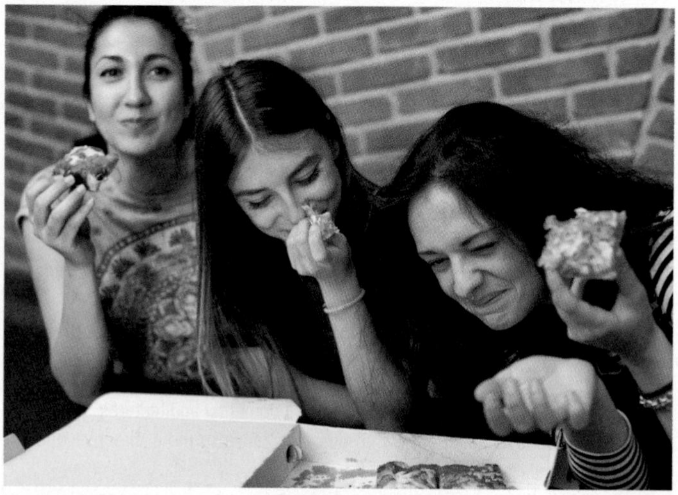

Fig. 15.7 Snacking on empty calories is common among adolescents, especially during inactivity. (©2015 iStock.com.)

sodium is common among adolescents and is found in all income and racial or ethnic groups and both genders. Inadequate intake of certain vitamins (folic acid, vitamin B_6, vitamin A) and minerals (iron, calcium, zinc) is also evident, particularly among girls and teenagers of low socioeconomic status. In combination with other factors, these dietary patterns could result in increased risk for obesity and chronic diseases, such as heart disease, osteoporosis, and some types of cancer later in life. Maximum bone mass is also acquired during adolescence; the calcium deposited during these years determines the risk of osteoporosis. Milk is usually passed over in favor of soft drinks.

Overeating or undereating during adolescence presents special problems. When they experience the normal increase in weight and fat deposition of the growth spurt, teenage girls often resort to dieting. The desire for a slim figure and a fear of becoming "fat" prompt teenage girls to embark on nutritionally inadequate reducing regimens that drain their energy and deprive their growing bodies of essential nutrients. Nationwide, 47.1% of adolescents are trying to lose weight (Kann et al., 2018). Although most teens try to lose weight through exercise and diet, a small percentage engage in risky weight loss practices such as vomiting after meals or taking laxatives. Boys are less inclined to undereat or adopt risky weight loss practices. They are more concerned about gaining size and strength. However, they tend to eat foods high in calories but low in other essential nutrients.

Obesity is increasing among both children and adolescents in the United States. Poor dietary habits and increasingly sedentary lifestyles have caused this obesity epidemic. Results from the 2015–16 National Health and Nutrition Examination Survey (NHANES) estimate that 18.5% of US children and adolescents ages 2 to 19 years are obese, including 5.6% who are severely obesity, and another 16.6% are overweight (Fryar, Carrol, & Ogden, 2018).

Health problems traditionally thought of as adult comorbidities of obesity, including type 2 diabetes mellitus, obstructive sleep apnea, and nonalcoholic steatohepatitis, are occurring in adolescents. Routine nutrition screening for all adolescents should include questions about meal patterns, dieting behaviors, consumption of high-fat and high-salt foods, and recent changes in weight. Discuss healthy dietary habits with all adolescents, including the benefits of a healthy diet; ways to consume foods rich in calcium, iron, and other vitamins and minerals; and safe weight management. Lifestyle changes necessary for adolescents to lose weight require the involvement of family members who provide support and encourage active participation.

Physical Fitness

Although today's youth are less fit than children 20 years ago, adolescents probably spend more time and energy practicing and participating in sports activities than members of any other age-group. In 2017 nearly one-half (46.5%) of all high school students reported that they participated in activities that made them "sweat and breathe hard for at least 20 minutes" three or more times in the past week (Kann et al., 2018). Many adolescents participate in sports within school settings (Fig. 15.8). School-based, health-oriented physical education may provide both immediate effects of the activity and sustained effects through encouragement of lifelong activity patterns. Participation in school physical education classes declines with age because schools often do not have mandatory requirements past grade 9 or 10. Health care organizations such as the American Academy of Pediatrics (2017b) recommend discussing the emotional, social, and physical benefits of exercise with all adolescents. Furthermore, encourage all adolescents to engage in physical activity on a regular basis.

The practice of sports, games, and even dancing contributes significantly to growth and development, the education process, and better health. These activities provide exercise for growing muscles, interactions with peers, and a socially acceptable means of enjoying stimulation and conflict. In addition, competitive activities help teenagers in the process of self-appraisal and the development of self-respect and concern for others. Because physical fitness appears to be a major influence on one's lifelong health status, children should be encouraged to participate in activities that contribute to lifelong physical fitness. Nurses can encourage participation as a way to promote health and build self-esteem. However, adolescents should not be encouraged to engage in physical activities that are beyond their physical or emotional capacity.

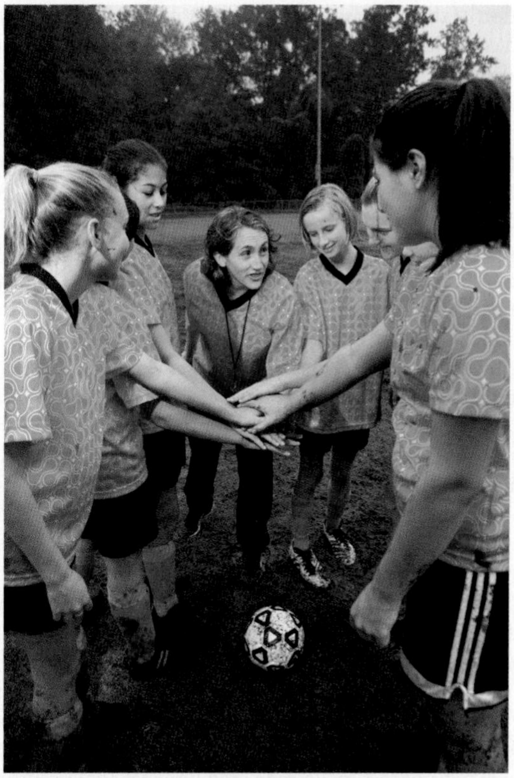

Fig. 15.8 Adolescents should be encouraged to participate in activities that contribute to lifelong physical fitness. (©2011 Photos.com, a division of Getty Images. All rights reserved.)

Sexual Behavior, Sexually Transmitted Infections, and Unintended Pregnancy

Sexual activity significantly decreased among US youth in the 1990s and through 2015, with 61.8 live births per 1000 teens in 1991, 39.1 live births per 1000 teens in 2009, and 22.3 live births per 1000 teens in 2015 (Centers for Disease Control and Prevention, 2017b). Despite this decline, less than 5% of teens use the most effective types of birth control (long-acting reversible contraceptives) and instead rely on condoms or birth control pills, which require consist and correct use (Centers for Disease Control and Prevention, 2017b). Rates of STIs and human immunodeficiency virus (HIV) infection among teens have increased, although this may be due to increased testing and better sensitivity of STI testing. However, many sexually active young people engage in behaviors that put them at risk for STIs or pregnancy, such as having sex with multiple partners and having sex without using contraception.

Obtaining a sexual history can be an important step in promoting sexual health and preventing STIs and unintended pregnancies among young people. Questions about sexuality should be prefaced by an explanation of the purpose and limits of confidentiality. Initially questions can cover less sensitive topics, such as pubertal development, and then address dating behaviors, gender attractions, and sexual activity. Screening questions regarding sexual attractions and experiences should be phrased in ways that allow adolescents to discuss same- and opposite-gender attractions, such as using the term *partner* instead of *boyfriend* or *girlfriend.* Sexually active youth should be asked about their motivation to use condoms or other barrier methods to prevent STIs and their consistency in doing so; use of birth control pills or other forms of hormonal contraception; the number of sexual partners over the past 6 months; and the use of alcohol or other substances in connection with sexual activity.

Sexually active adolescents should be screened for STIs with laboratory tests for gonorrhea, chlamydia, and, if applicable, syphilis. For females, a Papanicolaou (Pap) test should be done to detect human papillomavirus (HPV) infection or other cervical dysplasia. Both males and females should be evaluated for HPV by visual inspection and should also be asked about whether they have received the HPV vaccine series. Adolescents at risk for HIV infection should be offered confidential HIV screening tests. The frequency of laboratory screening for STIs and HIV depends on sexual practices and STI history of individual adolescents.

All adolescents should receive medically accurate health guidance regarding responsible sexual behaviors, including abstinence. Counsel sexually active adolescents about ways to reduce their risk of STIs and unwanted pregnancy and provide positive reinforcement for responsible sexual behaviors. Gay, lesbian, and bisexual adolescents need the same sexuality education and information as heterosexual adolescents. All adolescents should be counseled on ways to reduce their risk of sexual exploitation.

Gay, Lesbian, and Bisexual Adolescents

The population of gay, lesbian, and bisexual adolescents has unique developmental issues and health challenges. Although adolescents may participate in same-gender sexual activity or have same-gender attractions, they do not necessarily become gay, lesbian, or bisexual adults. Assigning sexual orientation labels to adolescents is complex and should be approached cautiously.

Most of the health challenges of sexual minority teens are responses to negative societal attitudes and messages about homosexual or bisexual orientation. They may use alcohol and other substances to escape their anxieties, and they are at much greater risk for suicidal behaviors than their heterosexual peers. Although nurses should screen all youth for suicidal thoughts and history of suicide attempts, it is especially critical for an adolescent who identifies as gay, lesbian, or bisexual or one who is questioning his or her orientation.

Publicly disclosing a gay, lesbian, or bisexual orientation during adolescence ("coming out") brings additional challenges. Many adolescents disclose their orientation to a close peer, then to a sibling, and finally to a parent (Steever, Francis, Gordon, et al., 2014). Adolescents face hostility, violence, and even rejection from their families. Nurses should not encourage teens to disclose their sexual orientation to their families without first forming a safety plan in case the reaction is not supportive. For most young people, referral to an agency that provides support services or social opportunities for gay, lesbian, and bisexual adolescents is appropriate. Parents who seek assistance in adjusting to their child's disclosure can be referred to a local chapter of Parents, Families and Friends of Lesbians and Gays. Adolescents who acknowledge same-gender attractions or relationships are also at risk for violence and harassment from schoolmates, neighbors, and even strangers. Sexual minority adolescents may fear similar uncaring attitudes among health care providers and might avoid disclosing their orientation during health assessments. To provide sensitive, professional care for gay, lesbian, and bisexual adolescents, nurses should be sensitive in their choice of language and be nonjudgmental and caring in their communication.

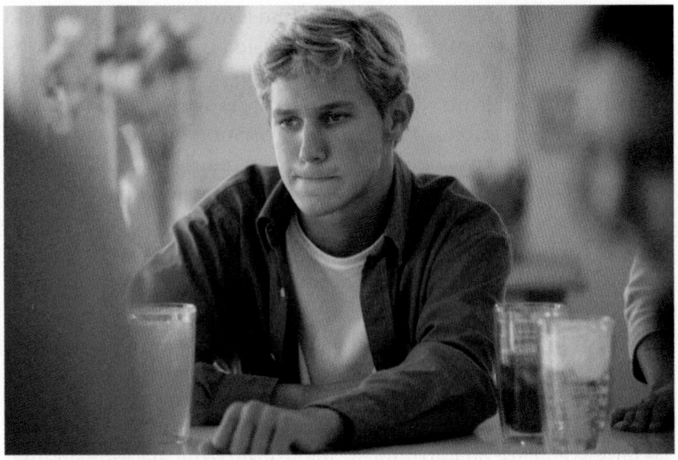

Fig. 15.9 Adolescents use being alone as a method of coping with stress. Health care professionals need to assess whether this indicates clinical depression. (©2011 Photos.com, a division of Getty Images. All rights reserved.)

BOX 15.4 Areas of Stress in Adolescence

- Body image
- Sexuality conflicts
- Academic pressures
- Competitive pressures
- Relationships with parents
- Relationships with siblings
- Relationships with peers
- Finances
- Decisions about present and future roles
- Career planning
- Ideologic conflicts

Use of Tobacco, Alcohol, and Other Substances

Statistically, experimentation with substances is common among US adolescents. By the 12th grade, 60.4% of students have used alcohol, 28.9% have smoked cigarettes, and 35.6% have tried cannibus in the past 30 days (Kann et al., 2018). Many adolescents use these substances because they provide an opportunity to challenge authority, demonstrate autonomy, gain entry into a peer group, or simply relieve stress. There are many documented consequences of early experimentation with alcohol, tobacco, and other drugs, such as becoming heavier smokers, lower academic achievement, dropping out of school, and early sexual behavior.

Depression and Suicide

A national survey of 9th- through 12th-grade students found that 21.4% of boys and 41.1% of girls reported feeling sad or hopeless (Kann et al., 2018) due to real or perceived stress (Fig. 15.9 and Box 15.4). Nearly 17.2% of high school students reported seriously considering suicide during the past year, with female students being more likely than male students to consider a suicide attempt (Kann et al., 2018).

A brief psychologic screening is necessary during a routine health visit. Screening for depression or suicidal risk should be done with adolescents who note declining school grades; chronic melancholy; family dysfunction; alcohol or other drug use; gay, lesbian, or bisexual orientation; a history of abuse; or previous suicide attempts. Immediate referral for an acute intervention with a psychiatrist or other mental health professional is indicated for any suicidal patient.

School and Learning Problems

Among in-school adolescents, a low grade point average has been associated with higher levels of emotional distress; cigarette, alcohol, and marijuana use; and earlier onset of sexual activity. School problems and dropping out of school can be markers for difficulties, such as learning disabilities, language barriers, family problems, lack of supportive relationships at school, and employment needs. In contemporary American society, education is critical to economic self-sufficiency.

Questions about recent grades, school absences, suspensions, and any history of repeating a grade in school can be used to screen for school-related problems. Specific management plans for youth who note school problems should be coordinated with school personnel and with the adolescent's parents or caregivers if possible.

Hypertension

As adolescents experience sexual maturation, along with increases in height and weight, blood pressure increases from the onset of adolescence and continues to rise until the end of pubertal growth. This trend is especially apparent among males. Approximately 1% of adolescents have sustained hypertension, which is defined as a blood pressure greater than the 95th percentile of standards. The detection of hypertension during adolescence is important because hypertension is one of the major preventable risk factors for adult cardiovascular disease. With increasing levels of obesity, there have been reports of increasing incidence of hypertension among adolescents (Cheung, Bell, Samuela, et al., 2017). Screening for hypertension and associated risk factors should take place annually beginning at 3 years old. Specific guidelines for monitoring and treatment of hypertension in adolescents are found in the National Heart, Lung, and Blood Institute's (2016) Summary Report (see also Chapter 23).

Hyperlipidemia

Along with hypertension, smoking, and obesity, elevated serum cholesterol and triglyceride levels are major risk factors for the development of adult cardiovascular disease. The National Heart, Lung, and Blood Institute (2016) recently issued a recommendation for universal lipid (nonfasting or fasting) screening of all children and adolescents between 9 and 11 years old and again between 17 and 21 years old. Drug therapy to lower low-density lipoprotein (LDL) cholesterol levels is recommended for children and adolescents age 10 years and older whose LDL remains elevated after 6 months to 1 year on a restricted-fat diet, lifestyle modification (exercise), and weight management (National Heart, Lung, and Blood Institute, 2016). Additional information and practice guidelines for monitoring cholesterol levels and initiation of medication to lower LDL cholesterol levels, as well as specific dietary modifications, are found in the 2016 National Heart, Lung, and Blood Institute's Summary Report at http://www.nhlbi.nih.gov/health-pro/guidelines/current/cardiovascular-health-pediatric-guidelines/summary.

Immunizations

An immunization update is an important part of adolescent preventive care. Obtaining a record of the teenager's prior immunizations is important. The Tdap (tetanus, diphtheria, acellular pertussis) vaccine is recommended for adolescents 11 to 18 years old who have not received a tetanus-diphtheria booster (Td) or Tdap dose and have completed the childhood diphtheria, tetanus, and acellular pertussis (DTaP/DTP) series. When Tdap is used as a booster dose, it may be administered at any time earlier than the previous 5-year interval to provide adequate pertussis immunity (regardless of interval from the last Td dose) (Centers for Disease Control and Prevention, 2019). Meningococcal vaccine (Menactra or Menveo) should be given to adolescents 11 to 12 years old with a booster dose at 16 years old. If not previously vaccinated, they should receive one dose at 13 through 18 years old (Centers for Disease Control and Prevention, 2019) (see also Chapter 6, Immunizations).

Vaccination against HPV is recommended to prevent HPV infections and HPV-associated diseases, including cancers. Routine vaccination at age 11 or 12 years has been recommended by the Advisory Committee on Immunization Practices since 2006 for females and since 2011 for males. New recommendations involve the use of a two-dose schedule for girls and boys who initiate the vaccination series at ages 9 through 14 years. For persons initiating vaccination on or after their 15th birthday, the recommended immunization schedule is three doses of HPV vaccine (Centers for Disease Control and Prevention, 2019). Each of the HPV vaccines is administered in a two- or three-dose series; it is important to follow the recommended dose intervals for optimal effectiveness.

All adolescents who have not previously received three doses of hepatitis B vaccine should be vaccinated against hepatitis B virus. The hepatitis A vaccine should be given to adolescents who live in areas where vaccination programs target older children or who are at increased risk for infection or for whom immunity against hepatitis A is desired (Centers for Disease Control and Prevention, 2019). Annual influenza vaccination with either the live attenuated influenza vaccine or the trivalent influenza vaccine is recommended for all children and adolescents (see Chapter 6). All adolescents should also be assessed for previous history of varicella infection or vaccination. Vaccination with the varicella vaccine is recommended for those with no previous history; for those with no previous infection or history, the varicella vaccine may be given in two doses 4 or more weeks apart to adolescents age 13 years and older (Centers for Disease Control and Prevention, 2019). Adolescents should receive a tuberculin skin test if they have been exposed to active tuberculosis (TB), have lived in a homeless shelter, have been incarcerated, have lived in or come from an area with a high prevalence of TB, or currently work in a health care setting.

Body Art

Body art (piercing and tattooing) is an aspect of adolescent identity formation. The skin has become the latest source of parent-adolescent conflict. Adolescents often seek body art as an expression of their personal identity and style. Tattoos may mark significant life events, such as new relationships, births, and deaths. Piercing the ear, nose, nipple, eyebrow, navel, penis, or tongue may sometimes create a health problem. It is a nurse's responsibility to caution girls and boys against having piercing performed by friends, parents, or themselves. Although in most cases piercings have few (if any) serious side effects, there is always a risk of complications such as infection, cyst or keloid formation, bleeding, dermatitis, or metal allergy. Using the same unsterilized needle to pierce body parts of multiple teenagers presents the same risk of HIV, hepatitis C virus, and hepatitis B virus transmission as occurs with other needle-sharing activities.

A qualified operator using proper sterile technique should perform the procedure. This is especially important if an adolescent has a history of diabetes, allergies, or skin disorders. Adolescents should be informed about the approximate time for healing after body piercing and the care of the pierced area during and after healing. Some body sites need extra precautions. For example, cartilage (ear, nose) has a poor blood supply and heals slowly and scars easily; nipple piercing puts adolescents at risk for breast abscesses. Finally, migration of the piercing is common with naval and other flat skin surface piercing. Piercing guns should not be used for piercing anything other than the earlobe, because guns place the piercing too deeply.

The presence of body art in the form of tattoos and branding is common among adolescents and young adults. Professionals, as well as amateur artists, administer tattoos. The risk to adolescents receiving tattoos is low. The greatest risk is for the tattoo artist, who comes in contact with the client's blood. Adolescents who are amateur tattoo artists benefit from discussions about Standard Precautions and hepatitis B vaccination. Many states either have no regulations or do not enforce existing regulations of piercing and tattooing facilities. The local health department is a source of information about local regulatory requirements.

Sleep Deprivation and Insomnia

The changing social environment of adolescents can often change their sleep patterns at a time when their growth and development require additional sleep for health. Although adolescents should generally get around 9 hours of sleep each night, early morning school scheduling, extracurricular activities, homework, employment, and desired social time with peers or on the Internet can make it difficult for them to get sufficient sleep. Sleep deprivation can affect physical and mental health and has been associated with higher rates of overweight and obesity, depression, somatic complaints (such as headaches and stomach aches), fatigue, and difficulties with concentration. These physical and psychologic effects of inadequate sleep can also affect school performance and thus contribute to school problems. Health teaching and health promotion should include information to promote sufficient sleep.

Tanning

The quest for an attractive appearance leads many teenagers to excessive sunbathing and artificial means for tanning. However, this practice has serious long-term risks, and adolescents should be educated on the detrimental effects of sunlight on the skin (see Chapter 31, Sunburn). Long-term effects include premature aging of the skin; increased risk of skin cancer; and, in susceptible individuals, phototoxic reactions.

The increasing popularity of artificial tanning has prompted concern from health professionals regarding the use of sunlamps and tanning machines. The long-term effects of tanning machines are similar to those of the sun; dermatologists do not recommend tanning by this means. Those who insist on using tanning equipment should be warned that goggles must be worn in tanning booths to prevent serious corneal burning. Education on the use of sunscreens, including hypoallergenic products, with a sun protection factor (SPF) of at least 15 and a nonalcohol base without lanolin, parabens, or fragrance is important. Broad-spectrum sunscreens that protect against both ultraviolet A and ultraviolet B (UVA and UVB) are the most effective. Self-tanning creams safely stimulate the appearance of a tan; however, teens using these products should be cautioned that with sun exposure, protection is still required. Targeting health education messages to adolescents and incorporating educational components relating to sun protection behaviors in school health curricula and in health care visits will increase adolescents' knowledge and awareness.

Nursing Care Management

With continued increases in the numbers of adolescents in the United States and rising rates of health-related problems of youth, there is an unprecedented need for adolescent health promotion. Nursing professionals can make significant contributions to health promotion among adolescents and their families. Because nurses understand the biologic, cognitive, psychosocial, and social transitions of adolescence and their impact of health behavior, they can address adolescents' developmental and health needs. Working with colleagues from other disciplines, community members, parents, and adolescents themselves, nurses must become part of a comprehensive approach that delivers consistent messages across clinical, school, and community-based settings. Nurses should be at the forefront of developing and disseminating culturally appropriate health promotion interventions.

Both adolescents and their parents are often confused and perplexed about the changes and behavior of this stage of development. Parents need support and guidance to help them through this trying time. They need to understand the changes taking place and to accept the expected behaviors that accompany the process of detachment. Parents may need help to "let go" and to promote the changed relationship from one of dependence to one of mutuality. Suggestions for anticipatory guidance of parents of adolescents are listed in the Family-Centered Care box.

FAMILY-CENTERED CARE

Guidance During Adolescence

Encourage parents to:

- Accept adolescent as a unique individual.
- Respect adolescent's ideas, likes and dislikes, and wishes.
- Be involved with school functions and attend adolescent's performances, whether it is a sporting event or school play.
- Listen and try to be open to teenager's views even when they disagree with parental views.
- Avoid criticism about no-win topics.
- Provide opportunity for choosing options and accept natural consequences of these choices.
- Allow young persons to learn by doing, even when choices and methods differ from those of adults.
- Provide adolescent with clear, reasonable limits.
- Clarify house rules and consequences for breaking them. Let society's rules and consequences teach responsibility outside the home.
- Allow increasing independence within limitations of safety and well-being.
- Respect adolescent's privacy.
- Try to share adolescent's feelings of joy or sorrow.
- Respond to feelings as well as words.
- Be available to answer questions, give information, and provide companionship.
- Try to make communication clear.
- Avoid comparisons with siblings.
- Assist adolescent in selecting appropriate career goals and preparing for adult roles.
- Welcome adolescent's friends into the home and treat them with respect.
- Provide unconditional love and acceptance.
- Be willing to apologize when mistaken.

Be aware that adolescents:

- Are subject to turbulent, unpredictable behavior.
- Are struggling for independence.
- Are extremely sensitive to feelings and behavior that affect them.
- May receive a different message from what was sent.
- Consider friends extremely important.
- Have a strong need to belong.

CLINICAL JUDGMENT AND NEXT-GENERATION NCLEX® EXAMINATION-STYLE QUESTIONS

1. A 14-year-old boy is being seen in the clinic because of concerns that he is not maturing at the same rate as other boys his age. On examination, he has enlargement of the testes and scrotal changes are observed. **Choose the most likely options for the information missing from the statements below by selecting from the lists of options provided.**
The first pubescent change in boys is ___1___. Temporary___2___ enlargement and tenderness are common and can commonly occur of boys.

Options for 1	Options for 2
facial hair	muscle
height	breast
testicular enlargement	penile
ejaculation	testicular
axillary hair	larynx
voice changes	neck

2. A 16-year-old boy is being seen in the emergency department following a car accident while he was driving. He is not severely injured but is being observed for a head concussion. His mother arrives and is extremely concerned because as she states, "he is such a risk taker and never seems to consider what might happen to him." Which of the following statements describe the most common source of unintentional injury and death in young people and would be shared with the mother? **Select all that apply.**
   A. "The leading cause of death in teenagers is suicide."
   B. "Teenagers can be risk takers because of new feelings of strength and confidence."
   C. "Motor vehicle crashes are a concern in that they are the greatest cause of unintentional injuries in young people."
   D. "Teenagers should avoid distractions while driving including cell phone talking and texting."
   E. "Teaching teenagers at this age about safe driving does little to improve their driving habits."
   F. "Giving your teenager an opportunity to talk about the accident without judging his actions is important."

3. A nurse is interviewing a 16-year-old female who is here for a history and physical examination required for all cheerleaders. Which of the following statements would help the nurse **most effectively** communicate with this teenager? **Select all that apply.**
   A. Ask open-ended questions
   B. Ensure confidentiality and privacy
   C. Maintain objectivity and avoid judgment
   D. Begin with sensitive issues then proceed with less sensitive topic
   E. Assume you understand the adolescent by including your own experiences
   F. Interview the adolescent with the parents to ensure accuracy

4. A 12-year-old adolescent male who has completed all recommended routine childhood vaccinations is being seen for a well child examination before school. He has not received any of the immunizations recommended as part of adolescent preventive care. From the list below, which immunizations would be given today? **Select all that apply.**
   A. DTaP vaccine
   B. Tdap vaccine
   C. Measles vaccine
   D. Meningococcal vaccine
   E. Pneumococcal vaccine
   F. HPV vaccine
   G. Hepatitis B vaccine

REFERENCES

Ali, O., & Donohoue, P. A. (2020). Gynecomastia. In R. M. Kliegman, J. W. St. Geme, N. J. Blum, et al. (Eds.), *Nelson textbook of pediatrics* (21st ed.). Philadelphia: Saunders/Elsevier.

American Academy of Pediatrics. (2017a). *Bright Futures guidelines for health supervision of infants, children, and adolescents, 2017*. http://brightfutures.aap.org/pdfs/Guidelines_PDF/18-Adolescence.pdf.

American Academy of Pediatrics. (2017b). *Bright Futures: Adolescent tools*. https://brightfutures.aap.org/materials-and-tools/tool-and-resource-kit/Pages/adolescence-tools.aspx.

Brooks, F. M., Magnusson, J., Spencer, N., et al. (2012). Adolescent multiple risk behaviour: An asset approach to the role of family, school and community. *Journal of Public Health (Oxford, England)*, *34*(Suppl. 1), 48–56.

Cabrera, S. M., Bright, G. M., Frane, J. W., et al. (2014). Age of thelarche and menarche in contemporary US females: A cross-sectional analysis. *The Journal of Pediatric Endocrinology and Metabolism*, *27*(0), 47–51.

Centers for Disease Control and Prevention. (2017a). *Adolescent health*. https://www.cdc.gov/nchs/fastats/adolescent-health.htm.

Centers for Disease Control and Prevention. (2017b). *Preventing teen pregnancy*. https://www.cdc.gov/vitalsigns/larc/index.html.

Centers for Disease Control and Prevention. (2019). *Table 1: Recommended child and adolescent immunization schedule for ages 18 years and younger*. United States. https://www.cdc.gov/vaccines/schedules/hcp/imz/child-adolescent.html?CDC_AA_refVal=https%3A%2F%2Fwww.cdc.gov%2Fvaccines%2Fschedules%2Fhcp%2Fchild-adolescent.html#vaccines-schedule.

Chapman, R. L., Buckley, L., Reveruzzi, B., et al. (2014). Injury prevention among friends: The benefits of school connectedness. *The Journal of Adolescence*, *37*(6), 937–944.

Chase, C. (2014). US state and federal laws targeting distracted driving. *Annals of Advances in Automotive Medicine*, *58*, 84–98.

Cheung, E. L., Bell, C. S., Samuel, J. P., et al. (2017). Race and obesity in adolescent hypertension. *Pediatrics*, *139*(5), e20161433.

Child Trends Data Bank. (2018). *Dropout rates for 16-24-year-olds by gender, race/hispanic orgin, selected years 1970-2016*. https://www.childtrends.org/indicators/high-school-dropout-rate.

Fryar, C. D., Carroll, M. S., & Ogden, C. L. (2018). *Prevalence of overweight, obesity, and severe obesity among children and adolescents aged 2–19 years:*

United States, 1963–1965 Through 2015–2016. Division of Health and Nutrition Examination Surveys.
Herman-Giddens, M. E. (2013). The enigmatic pursuit of puberty in girls. *Pediatrics, 132*(6), 1125–1126.
Horton, S. E. (2015). Religion and health-promoting behaviors among emerging adults. *Journal of Religion and Health, 54*(1), 20–34.
Jacobson, C., Bailin, A., Milanaik, R., et al. (2016). Adolescent health implications of new age technology. *Pediatric Clinics of North America, 63*(1), 183–194.
Kann, L., McManus, T., Harris, W. A., et al. (2016). Youth risk behavior surveillance – United States, 2015. morbidity and mortality weekly report. *Surveillance Summaries, 65*, 1–177.
Kann, L., McManus, T., & Harris, W. A. (2018). Youth risk behavior surveillance – United States, 2017. Morbidity and Mortality Weekly Report. *Surveillance Summaries, 67*(8), 1–479.
Lee, J. M., Wasserman, R., Kaciroti, N., et al. (2016). Timing of puberty in overweight verses obese boys. *Pediatrics, 137*(2), 1–17.
Marceau, K., Zann-Waxler, Shirtcliff, E. A., et al. (2015). Adolescents', mothers', and fathers' gendered coping strategies during conflict: Youth and parent influences on conflict resolution and psychopathology. *Development and Psychopathology, 27*(4), 1025–1044.
Morelli, M., Bianchi, D., Baiocco, R., et al. (2016). Sexting, psychological distress and dating violence among adolescents and young adults. *Psicothema, 28*(2), 137–142.
National Heart, Lung, & Blood Institute (NHLBI) (2016). *Expert panel on integrated guidelines for cardiovascular health and risk reduction in children and adolescents: Summary report*. Bethesda, MD: U.S. Department of Health and Human Services, NHLBI.
Neuman, M. E. (2011). Addressing children's beliefs through Fowler's stages of faith. *The Journal of Pediatric Nursing, 26*(1), 44–50.
Nokoff, N., Thurston, J., Hilkin, A., et al. (2019). Sex differenes in effects of obesity on reproductive hormones and glucose metabolism in early puberty. *Journal of Clinical Endocrinolgy & Metabolism, 104*(10), 4390–4397.
O'Neill, T., & Wakefield, J. (2017). Fifteen-minute consultation in the normal child: Challenges relating to sexuality and gender identity in children and young people. *Archives of Disease in Childhood; Education and Practice Edition, 102*(6).
Papadimitriou, A. (201). The evolution of the age of menarche from prehistoric to modern times. *Journal of Pediatric and Adolescent Gynecology, 29*(6), 527-530.
Steever, J., Francis, J., Gordon, L. P., et al. (2014). Sexual minority youth. *Primary Care, 41*(3), 651–669.
Villanueva, C., & Argente, J. (2014). Pathology or normal variant: What constitutes a delay in puberty? *Hormone Research in Paediatrics, 82*(4), 213–221.

16

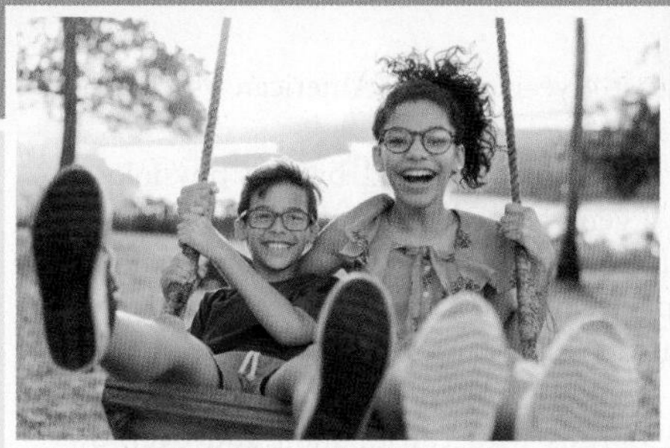

Health Problems of School-Age Children and Adolescents

Kathie Prihoda

http://evolve.elsevier.com/wong/essentials

CONCEPTS

- Nutrition
- Mood and Affect
- Reproduction
- Sexuality
- Addiction
- Safety

HEALTH PROBLEMS OF SCHOOL-AGE CHILDREN

PROBLEMS RELATED TO ELIMINATION

Enuresis

The *Diagnostic and Statistical Manual of Mental Disorders,* Fifth edition (DSM-5; (American Psychiatric Association, 2013) separates elimination disorders into enuresis and encopresis. Enuresis is defined as repeated urination into bed or clothing at least twice a week for a period of at least 3 months that is not due directly to a physiologic condition or substance and occurs in an individual who is at least 5 years of age (American Psychiatric Association, 2013).

Enuresis can happen during the day or at night. It can be a frustrating condition for the caregiver and child. Enuresis is classified into "monosymptomatic" and "nonmonosymptomatic" types, with the former referring to bedwetting plus no other symptoms and the latter referring to bedwetting plus other urinary tract symptoms such as daytime incontinence, infections, or holding maneuvers (Fagundes, Lebl, Soster, et al., 2016). Medical evaluation is recommended when inappropriate voiding of urine occurs at least once a month for a minimum of 3 consecutive months and the chronologic or developmental age of the child is at least 5 years old (Caldwell, Lim, & Nankivell, 2018). In addition, the urinary incontinence must not be related to the direct physiologic effects of a medication (e.g., diuretics) or a general medical condition (e.g., diabetes mellitus or diabetes insipidus, spina bifida, seizure disorder, constipation, sexual abuse).

Enuresis is more common in boys (Fagundes et al., 2016); nocturnal bedwetting usually ceases between 6 and 8 years old. Enuresis can also be defined as **primary** (bedwetting in children who have never been dry for extended periods) or **secondary** (the onset of wetting after a period of established urinary continence).

During the initial phases of evaluation, a routine physical examination is performed to rule out physical causes related to enuresis. These include structural disorders of the urinary tract; urinary tract infection; neurologic deficits; disorders that increase the normal output of urine, such as diabetes; and disorders that impair the concentrating ability of the kidneys, such as chronic renal failure. In addition, the family may be instructed to keep a voiding diary to estimate bladder capacity and urine output. In other cases, enuresis is influenced by psychologic factors. If psychologic difficulties are evident, a routine psychiatric evaluation is warranted.

A detailed history of voiding and bowel habits is obtained, including information about the toilet training process. An important feature of assessment is a baseline count of enuretic incidents and the time of day when each occurs. Despite parental reports that these children sleep more soundly than other children, the depth of sleep has not been identified as the cause of nocturnal enuresis, although defective sleep arousal may contribute to the problem (Elder, 2020). Obstructive sleep apnea (OSA) and nocturnal enuresis (NE) are common clinical problems in children. OSA and NE are thought to be interrelated, but the exact pathophysiologic mechanisms are not yet clear. Nocturnal enuresis has a strong familial tendency in more than 90% of first- and second-degree relatives (Fagundes et al., 2016). Enuresis can persist into adulthood, with prevalence rates of 1% to 3% (American Psychiatric Association, 2013).

The physical examination may be followed by diagnostic evaluation of functional bladder capacity. Normal bladder capacity (in ounces) is calculated as the child's age plus 2 (up to 14 years old); therefore normal bladder capacity for a 6-year-old is 8 ounces (237 ml). A bladder volume of 10 to 12 ounces (300 to 350 ml) is sufficient to hold one night's urine.

Enuresis has been treated in several ways. The first steps of therapy for primary monosymptomatic enuresis include education, behavior modification, and reassurance. No single method has achieved universal endorsement, and more than one technique is often used by families coping with enuresis. Therapeutic techniques used to manage nocturnal enuresis include medications; complementary and alternative medicine techniques, such as hypnotherapy; restriction or elimination of fluids after the evening meal; avoidance of caffeinated and sugar-containing beverages after 4 PM; avoidance of high-protein foods and salt; purposeful interruption of sleep to void; and motivational therapy. Parents should be educated that punishment is not an acceptable treatment for enuresis. Devices designed to establish a conditioned reflex response to waken the child at the initiation of voiding, such as bedwetting alarms, are the first-line treatment for children with nocturnal enuresis (Walle, Rittig, & Tekgul, 2017). The mechanism of alarm therapy is not well understood, but successful resolution of enuresis is thought to be due to changes in sleep arousal associated with voiding. Poor compliance and insufficient duration of therapy are common with alarm therapy (Caldwell et al., 2018).

Drug therapy can be prescribed to treat enuresis. The selection of medication depends on the interpretation of the cause. Desmopressin acetate (DDAVP), an analog of vasopressin, is commonly used to treat nocturnal enuresis. DDAVP works by increasing water reabsorption, thus reducing urine production to a volume less than functional bladder capacity. The medication is available in an oral preparation and is generally well tolerated but may cause dry mouth, headache, or nausea. An advantage of using desmopressin is that a patient will have an immediate response, whereas alarm therapy may take up to 2 weeks to be effective. The drug imipramine (Tofranil) and anticholinergics are not used routinely in primary care to treat enuresis due to their cardiac side effects, including cardiac arrhythmias, hypotension, and hepatotoxicity. Drugs are considered second-line management for enuresis, and parents should be cautioned not to think that these agents will cure the condition; parents are also advised of the drugs' side effects (Elder, 2020). Researchers continue to study interventions for resistant cases of enuresis (Caldwell et al., 2018).

Nursing Care Management

No matter what techniques are used, the nurse can support both children and parents who are coping with the problem of enuresis, the treatment plan, and the difficulties they may encounter in the process. Essential to the success of any method is the supportive management of parents and their children. Both need encouragement and patience. The problem is discussed with both the parent and the child because all treatments involve and require the child's active participation. In some treatment interventions, the child is in charge of the intervention; therefore parents must learn to support the child rather than intervene themselves. Parents should also be taught to observe for side effects of any medications used. Parents should encourage the child to maintain a regular bowel evacuation regimen; constipation can contribute to nocturnal enuresis (Elder, 2020). A calendar with wet and dry nights may be helpful to motivate the child to stay dry and maintain a positive perspective on the problem.

Many parents believe that enuresis is caused by an emotional disturbance and fear that they have somehow produced the situation through improper childrearing practices. They need reassurance that bedwetting does not represent willful misbehavior. Parents need to understand that punishment such as scolding, shaming, and threatening is contraindicated because of its negative emotional impact and limited success in reducing the behavior. Children need to believe that they are helping themselves, and they need to sustain feelings of confidence and hope. Encourage parents to be patient, to be understanding, and to communicate love and support to the child.

Communication with children is directed toward eliminating the emotional impact of the problem, relieving feelings of shame and guilt and the burden of parental disapproval, building self-confidence, and motivating children toward independent control. More important, the nurse can provide consistent support and encouragement to help children through the inconsistent and unpredictable treatment process. Children need to believe that they are helping themselves and to maintain feelings of confidence and hope.

Encopresis

Encopresis is defined as repeated bowel movements into bed or clothing at least one time per month for a period of at least 3 months, is not due directly to a physiologic condition or substance, and occurs in an individual who is at least 4 years of age (American Psychiatric Association, 2013).

The fecal incontinence must not be caused by any physiologic effect, such as a laxative, or a general medical condition. The consistency of the stool may vary from normal to liquid, with a more liquid stool seen in individuals who have overflow incontinence secondary to fecal retention. There are many possible causes of constipation, including behavioral reasons and medical or physiologic reasons. Subtypes of encopresis, including encopresis with constipation and overflow incontinence (which requires the passage of stool less than three times per week) and encopresis without constipation and overflow incontinence (where there is no evidence on physical examination or by history of constipation and soiling is no more than intermittent), continue to be used in diagnosing the condition (American Psychiatric Association, 2013). **Primary encopresis** is identified by 4 years of age when a child has not achieved fecal continence. **Secondary encopresis** is fecal incontinence occurring in a child older than 4 years of age after a period of established fecal continence. One of the most common causes of encopresis is constipation, which may be precipitated by environmental change, such as having a new sibling, moving to a new house, changing schools, or even having to use new or unfamiliar toilet facilities. Chronic, severe constipation has a tendency to impair the usual movement and contractions of the colon, which can lead to fecal obstruction. Abnormalities in the digestive tract (e.g., Hirschsprung disease, anorectal lesions, malformations, rectal prolapse) and medical conditions (such as hypothyroidism, hypokalemia, hypercalcemia, lead intoxication, myelomeningocele, cerebral palsy, muscular dystrophy, and irritable bowel syndrome [IBS]) are also associated with constipation, which can lead to encopresis. Voluntary retention of stool may also follow an incident of painful defecation (e.g., in a child with anal fissures). Involuntary retention may be produced by emotional problems caused by the encopresis, which sets up a fear–pain cycle and results in learned abnormal defecation patterns. **Psychogenic encopresis**, in which the soiling is caused by emotional problems, is often related to a disturbed mother-child relationship.

Normally, children and adolescents have one or two soft-formed stools per day. Children with soiling problems tend to form large-bore stools, which are painful to excrete. Therefore they tend to avoid defecation and withhold stooling. Stool held in the rectum and sigmoid colon loses water and progressively hardens, which causes successively more painful bowel movements and a stretched rectal vault. Over time, the child will lose the urge to defecate on his or her own. A pain–retention–pain cycle is established. Many children have diarrhea or loose leakage in their clothing and pass small amounts of hard stool, which suggests leakage around an impaction.

Children may experience exacerbations with transitions in the school setting. Some reasons for developing retentive tendencies at this time are fear of using school bathrooms, a busy schedule, and the interruption of an established time schedule for bowel evacuation. Children may also react to stress with bowel dysfunction. Children with encopresis have a significantly greater incidence of anxiety and depressive symptoms, attention problems, social problems, disruptive behavior, lower academic performance, and family environments characterized by less expression and poor organization (Olaru, Diaconescu, Trandafir, et al., 2016).

Therapeutic management consists of ruling out a structural issue like congenital megacolon. To determine the cause, a detailed history, including risk factors (negative toilet training, child abuse or neglect, fear of bathrooms), comorbid conditions (such as attention deficit disorder, cognitive delays, oppositional disorders), and associated symptoms of bowel movements (retention, overflow soiling, incontinence), is obtained (Olaru et al., 2016). Next, a thorough physical examination, including a rectal examination, is completed. Abdominal radiography may be done to determine the severity of impaction. Once encopresis is diagnosed, standard therapy involves laxatives, enemas, suppositories, and sometimes manual removal of impacted feces.

Many children require an extensive and invasive bowel cleansing to remove the bowel impaction before starting treatment (Koppen, Vriesman, Saps, et al., 2018). Fecal impaction is relieved by lubricants (such as mineral oil), osmotic laxatives (such as lactulose, sorbitol, or polyethylene glycol [PEG or MiraLax]), probiotics, and magnesium hydroxide (Koppen et al., 2018). Customary dosages are usually insufficient to produce a therapeutic response. Mineral oil should be avoided in children who have dysphagia or vomiting to prevent aspiration.

Children without bowel impaction can start treatment immediately. Dietary modifications, lubricants, and behavior therapy that encourage the child to establish normal defecation are used. Dietary changes, including consumption of increased amounts of high-fiber foods such as fruits, vegetables, and cereals and increased hydration with water, are encouraged. Stool softeners and laxatives are used until stools become soft. Behavior therapy, such as maintaining regular bathroom routines, increasing exercise, and having the child take on more responsibility for the bowel program, is a vital part of the treatment plan (Koppen et al., 2018). Psychotherapeutic intervention with the child and family may become necessary.

Nursing Care Management

A thorough history of the soiling is essential, including when soiling began, how often it occurs and under what circumstances, and whether the child uses the toilet successfully at all. Because the parents and child are reluctant to volunteer information, direct questioning about the soiling is more successful.

Education on the physiology of normal defecation, toilet training as a developmental process, and the treatment outlined for the family is a prerequisite to a successful outcome. Bowel retraining with mineral oil, a high-fiber diet, and a regular toileting routine is essential in treating encopresis or chronic constipation. The toileting routine should consist of the child sitting on the toilet 10 to 15 minutes after meals for intervals of 10 minutes and placing a footstool below the feet to relax the abdomen and make the child more comfortable. Positive reinforcement such as giving stickers, praising the child, and awarding special activities may encourage the child to participate in the bowel regimen.

Family counseling is directed toward reassurance that most problems resolve successfully, although the child may have relapses during periods of stress, such as vacations or illness. If encopresis persists beyond occasional relapses, the condition must be reevaluated. Behavior modification techniques are explained, and the family is assisted with a plan suited to the particular situation.

SCHOOL-AGE DISORDERS WITH BEHAVIORAL COMPONENTS

Attention-Deficit/Hyperactivity Disorder and Learning Disability

Attention-deficit/hyperactivity disorder (ADHD) refers to developmentally inappropriate degrees of inattention, impulsiveness, and hyperactivity (American Psychological Association, 2013). Early identification of affected children is important because the characteristics of ADHD significantly interfere with the normal course of emotional and psychologic development. The behavior of children with ADHD evokes negative responses from others, and repeated exposure to negative feedback adversely affects self-concept. Children with ADHD are at greater risk for conduct disorders, oppositional defiant disorders, depression, anxiety disorders, and developmental disorders (such as speech and language delays and learning disabilities) than are children without ADHD (American Academy of Pediatrics, 2011).

Clinical Manifestations

The behaviors exhibited by the child with ADHD are not unusual aspects of child behavior. The difference lies in the quality of motor activity and developmentally inappropriate inattention, impulsivity, and hyperactivity that the child displays. The manifestations may be numerous or few, may be mild or severe, and vary with the child's developmental level; about half of diagnoses are made by a primary care provider (Canady, 2015). Mild manifestations of the symptoms are apparent in at least two settings, usually educational and family environments. Each child with ADHD is different from all other children with ADHD (American Psychiatric Association, 2013). The American Academy of Pediatrics (2011) recommends that diagnosis incorporate both the use of standardized rating scales based on criteria from the DSM-5 and information from multiple sources such as parents, teachers, and older family members. Current DSM-5 diagnostic criteria include at least six designated symptoms of inattention or hyperactivity-impulsivity (lowered to five symptoms in adolescents over age 17 years) appearing before 12 years of age, with symptoms present for at least 6 months, occurring in more than one setting, and of a degree that impairs functioning or normal development (American Psychological Association, 2013).

Most behavioral manifestations are apparent at an early age, but the associated learning disabilities may not become evident until the child enters school. A major clinical manifestation is distractibility. The stimuli may come from external or internal sources. Children frequently demonstrate immaturity relative to chronologic age. Selective attention in which the child has difficulty attending to "nonpreferred" tasks, such as completing chores or finishing homework, is often seen. The child may not consider the consequences of behavior, may take excessive physical risks (often beginning early in life), and may demonstrate inappropriate social skills.

People with ADHD show a persistent pattern of inattention and/or hyperactivity-impulsivity that interferes with functioning or development. Based on the types of symptoms, different kinds (presentations) of ADHD can occur:

- *Inattentive presentation:* If enough symptoms of inattention but not hyperactivity-impulsivity were present in the past 6 months
- *Hyperactive-impulsive presentation:* If enough symptoms of hyperactivity-impulsivity but not inattention were present in the past 6 months

Diagnostic Evaluation

It is important to emphasize the need for a complete and thorough multidisciplinary evaluation of the child, incorporating the efforts of the primary pediatric health care provider and the family as well as possible support from a psychologist, developmental pediatrician, neurologist, pediatric nurses, classroom teachers, and administrators. The clinicians and professionals must first determine whether the child's behavior is age appropriate or truly problematic. The American Academy of Pediatrics (2011) recommends that children diagnosed with ADHD be assessed for comorbidities of anxiety, depression, oppositional defiant disorder, conduct disorders, language and learning disorders, tics, and sleep apnea.

Prior to diagnosis a complete medical and developmental history is obtained. Descriptions of the child's behavior in the home, school, and social situations are obtained from as many observers of the child as possible, especially the parents and teachers involved in the child's care. A physical examination, including vision and hearing screening and a detailed neurologic evaluation, is completed. Psychologic testing, especially projective tests, is used to identify visual-perceptual difficulties, problems with spatial organization, and other phenomena that suggest cortical or diencephalic involvement, and it helps to identify the child's intelligence and achievement levels.

Behavioral checklists and adaptive scales should be completed by the child's caregivers and educators and scored by the primary care provider. These assessment tools are helpful in measuring social adaptive functioning in children with ADHD as well as providing benchmarks for evaluation of improved or worsening behavioral changes once therapy has begun. Psychiatric disorders, medical problems, and traumatic experiences are ruled out, including lead poisoning, seizures, partial hearing loss, psychosis, and witnessing of sexual activity or violence.

Therapeutic Management

Treatment of ADHD depends on the child's age and severity of symptoms. Evidence supports behavioral therapy as the first-line treatment, but other approaches include family education and counseling, medication, proper classroom placement, environmental manipulation, and psychotherapy for the child. According to McClain and Burks (2015), just over 80% of youth with ADHD receive ongoing treatment.

Behavioral Therapy

Behavioral therapy focuses on the prevention of undesired behavior. Families are helped to identify new appropriate contingencies and reward systems to meet the child's developing needs through different techniques and strategies. Behavior therapy requires both time and effort, but it can lead to improved functioning at home, in school, and in social situations (Centers for Disease Control and Prevention, 2017). Families may also receive instruction in effective parenting skills, such as delivering positive reinforcement, rewarding small increments of desired behaviors, and providing age-appropriate consequences (e.g., time-out, response cost). Additional interventions include skill building, social skills training, and intensive summer-camp treatment programs. Through collaborative teamwork parents learn techniques to help the child become more successful at home and in school.

Pharmacologic Therapy

The choice of medication is determined by age. For children (age 5 years and over) and young people, the drug of first choice is methylphenidate (either long acting or immediate release). If symptoms and impairment are not sufficiently reduced after methylphenidate at an adequate dose, a switch to lisdexamfetamine should be considered (Frampton, 2018).

Children are given a small dosage initially, and the dosage is gradually increased until the desired response is achieved. Children who receive stimulants should be monitored carefully for side effects of the medication: appetite loss, abdominal pain, headaches, sleep disturbances, and growth velocity. Stimulants should be avoided in children who have a history of ticlike behaviors, a family history of Tourette syndrome (TS), or ADHD combined with TS, because these medications may exaggerate tics.

Other medications, including tricyclic antidepressants and extended-release clonidine, may be used as adjunct therapy for ADHD, primarily for children with coexisting conditions, such as sleep disturbances (American Academy of Pediatrics, 2011). The use of stimulants requires special consideration. They are controlled drugs and so prescribing and storage must meet specific requirements. Modified-release, once-daily preparations offer convenience and better adherence. They reduce stigma because they can be taken outside school. Modified-release formulas also eliminate the risk of misuse and diversion. Misuse includes cognitive enhancement in adolescents and appetite suppression. It is important to remember that these medications are not prescribed based on the child's weight (except for atomoxetine) but on resolution of the symptoms; therefore it is important to follow the child closely and evaluate for therapeutic effects as well as potential side effects. Regularly scheduled reevaluation of the child is essential with all of these medications to determine medication effectiveness, detect and evaluate any side effects, monitor development and health status (especially growth and blood pressure), and assess family interaction. See Table 16.1 for a description of the Pediatric Quality Indicator for follow-up of children taking ADHD medications (see also Critical Thinking Case Study box).

TABLE 16.1 Pediatric Quality Indicator[a]

Follow-Up Care for Children Prescribed ADHD Medications	
Measure	Children 6-12 years of age who were given a prescription of ADHD medication had at least two follow-up visits within 270 days, including one visit within 30 days after starting the medication.
Numerator	Number of children who had at least one face-to-face visit with a practitioner with prescribing authority within 30 days after starting the medication during the measurement time.
Denominator	Number of children who were dispensed an ADHD medication during the intake period and who had a visit during the measurement period.

[a]Endorsed by the National Quality Forum NQF #0108 and 2019 Core Set of Children's Health Care Quality Measures for Medicare and CHIP. https://www.medicaid.gov/federal-policy-guidance/downloads/cib112018.pdf.
ADHD, Attention-deficit/hyperactivity disorder.

CRITICAL THINKING CASE STUDY

Attention-Deficit/Hyperactivity Disorder (ADHD)

Johnnie, an 8-year-old third-grader, was recently diagnosed with ADHD. He has been taking the drug methylphenidate (Ritalin) for about 1 month. In the short time that Johnnie has been taking this medication, his math teacher has noticed an improvement in his performance in math class. He is receiving a grade of B instead of his previous grades of D on most math quizzes. The math teacher has also noted that Johnnie is socializing more with his classmates and that he now has a "best friend" in math class. Johnnie usually receives his methylphenidate from the school nurse before lunch. Yesterday Johnnie's mother told the school nurse that Johnnie has not eaten his lunch for the past week and that he is not hungry.

Initial Assessment. How would you describe Johnnie's response to ADHD medication?

Clinical Reasoning. What evidence is found in the case study that supports the use of medication for ADHD in this child?

Teaching Points

- Children on ADHD medication must be monitored closely for side effects.
- Lack of appetite is a common symptom related to ADHD medication.

Critical Thinking Answers

Initial Assessment. The assessment shows that Johnnie has had a positive response to ADHD medication. He is performing better in class and socializing more with others.

Clinical Reasoning. ADHD causes symptoms of inattention that leads to a variety of other behaviors. Children often have trouble with social skills. The case study indicates that Johnnie is more attentive at school and making friends.

Multimodal treatment. The results of several studies suggest that multimodal treatment involving the use of pharmacotherapy and behavioral intervention as well as close follow-up and feedback from school personnel is more effective than intensive behavioral treatment alone (Ahmann, 2017). ADHD coaching has been increasingly identified as a useful, important aspect of multimodal treatment for individuals of all ages with ADHD (Roy & Hectman, 2016). According to the Professional Association for ADHD Coaches, this approach empowers individuals to manage their attention, hyperactivity, and impulsivity by developing self-awareness and strategies.

Environmental manipulation. Encourage families to learn how to modify the environment to allow the child to be more successful. Consistency is especially important for children with ADHD. Consistency between families and teachers in terms of reinforcing the same goals is essential. Fostering improved organizational skills requires a more highly structured environment than most children need. Children should be encouraged to make more appropriate choices and to take responsibility for their actions.

Other helpful interventions include teaching parents how to make organizational charts (e.g., listing all activities that must be performed before leaving for school) and decrease distractions in the environment while the child is completing homework (e.g., turning off the television, having a consistent study area equipped with needed supplies) and helping parents to understand ways to model positive behaviors and problem solving. The focus is on strategies to help the child succeed and cope with deficits while emphasizing strengths.

Appropriate classroom placement. Children with ADHD need an orderly, predictable, and consistent classroom environment with clear and consistent rules. Homework and classroom assignments may need to be reduced, and more time may need to be allotted for tests to allow the child to complete them. Verbal instructions should be accompanied by visual references, such as written instructions on the blackboard. Schedules may need to be arranged so that academic subjects are taught in the morning when the child is experiencing the effects of the morning dose of medication. Low-interest and high-interest classroom activities should be intermingled to maintain the child's attention and interest. Regular and frequent breaks in activity are helpful because sitting in one place for an extended time may be difficult. Computers are helpful for children who have difficulty with written assignments and fine motor skills.

If learning disabilities exist, special training activities may be accomplished. These include self-contained classes limited to six to eight children, special resource rooms with equipment and teaching teams, mobile consultants who move from room to room to provide assistance to teachers and children, and first-grade programs in which high-risk children receive special attention to prevent or reduce the need for services as they progress. The purpose of programs for children with learning disabilities is to assist them toward more successful achievement, personal adjustment, and retention in the regular classroom.

Prognosis. With appropriate intervention, ADHD is relatively stable through early adolescence for most children. Some children experience decreased symptoms during late adolescence and adulthood, but a significant number of these children carry their symptoms into adulthood. The goal for children with ADHD is to help them identify their areas of weakness and learn to compensate for them.

Nursing Care Management

Nurses, especially school nurses, are active participants in all aspects of management of children with ADHD. Nurses in the community work with families and school personnel on a long-term basis to help plan and implement therapeutic regimens and to evaluate the effectiveness of therapy. They coordinate services and serve as a liaison between health and education professionals directly involved in the child's therapy program. School nurses understand the child's special needs and work with teachers (see Family-Centered Care box). Nurses in any setting (community, school, hospital, practitioner's office) provide support and guidance to children and families during the difficult period of the child's growing up with a disabling condition.

FAMILY-CENTERED CARE

A Child's Perception of Taking Ritalin at School

I feel embarrassed by having to leave class early to go take my medication. The other kids always ask where I'm going and why. It would be better if we could leave class at the same time as everyone else, go take the medication, and then just be a little late to the next class. Students don't ask why people are late for class, only why they leave early. It also bothers me when kids tell other kids, "Go take a pill" and other mean things just because someone is acting up.

What could nurses and teachers do to help? Most kids do not understand why other kids have to take medication. I think it would help if a nurse or teacher talked with the other kids and explained why some children take the medication and how ADHD affects people. That way there would be more understanding among all the kids.

—Marissa White, age 16 years

Management begins with an explanation to the parents and the child of the diagnosis, including the nature of the problem and the practitioner's concept of the underlying central nervous system (CNS) basis for the disorder. Parents need to be informed of the possible side effects of medications. If decreased appetite is a concern, giving the psychostimulants with or after meals rather than before, encouraging consumption of nutritious snacks in the evening when the effects of the medication are decreasing, and serving frequent small meals with healthy "on-the-go" snacks are helpful interventions. Sleeplessness is reduced by administering medication early in the day.

Children taking tricyclic antidepressants display a dramatic increase in the incidence of dental caries. The marked anticholinergic action of the drugs increases saliva viscosity and produces a dry mouth. Emphasis on rigorous dental hygiene, conscientious home fluoride treatments, regular visits to the dentist, limited intake of refined carbohydrates, and use of artificial saliva is an important nursing function. The child should drink plenty of fluids and be well hydrated.

Parents often express concern that their children will become addicted to the psychostimulants or antidepressant drugs. Both types of drugs have the potential for abuse, and all children taking these drugs should be monitored closely for psychologic dependence, tolerance, depression, and other adverse behavior changes or idiosyncratic effects. Most children with ADHD are not interested in abusing their drugs because the effect of the drugs in these children is opposite that produced in normal individuals. However, caution parents to keep these drugs safely stored away from young children who may inadvertently ingest them and from adolescents who may abuse them.

Parents need information about the prognosis and an understanding of the treatment plan. The greater their understanding of the disorder and its effects, the more likely they will be to carry out the recommended program of therapy. It is important that they understand that the therapy is not necessarily a panacea and that it will extend over a long period. This has particular significance for changes they need to make in environmental management. Reading material to help the child and family can be obtained from a variety of sources.

Posttraumatic Stress Disorder

Characteristic symptoms of posttraumatic stress disorder (PTSD) occur after exposure to an extremely traumatic experience or catastrophic event. The traumatic experience is typically life threatening to self or a significant other and may involve witnessing mutilation or death, experiencing or witnessing a serious injury, or physical coercion. An accident, assault, or victimization; a natural disaster (e.g., earthquake, flood); sexual abuse; or witnessing a suicide, homicide, beating, or shooting can lead to PTSD. It is important to note that PTSD is not limited to children who have lived in "war-torn" countries. Events such as automobile, school, or recreational accidents and bullying have also been identified as causes of PTSD.

The characteristic symptoms are persistent reexperiencing of the traumatic event, persistent avoidance of stimuli associated with the trauma, numbing of general responsiveness, and persistent symptoms of increased arousal. The response to the event takes place in three stages. The initial response involves intense arousal, which usually lasts for a few minutes to 1 or 2 hours. The stress hormones are at maximum level as the individual prepares for "fight or flight." A prolonged arousal phase may indicate psychosis.

The second phase, which lasts approximately 2 weeks, is one in which defense mechanisms are mobilized. It is a period of calm in which the event appears to have produced no impression. The victim feels numb, and stress hormone secretion is absent. Defense mechanisms are less adaptive to specific situations and may not be what the situation demands. Denial that anything is wrong is a frequently observed defense mechanism. Without professional support the victim may develop severe depression, aggression, or psychosis (Meiser-Stedman & McKinnon, et al., 2017).

The third phase is one of coping and consciously directed inquiry, which normally extends over 2 to 3 months. The victims want to know what happened and appear to be getting worse when actually they are getting better. Numerous psychologic symptoms, such as depression, repetitive phenomena, phobic symptoms, anxiety, and conversion reactions, may be apparent. Children frequently display repetitive actions. They play out the situation over and over in an attempt to come to terms with their fear. Flashbacks are common. This phase can be self-perpetuating, and a prolonged reaction can develop into an obsession with the traumatic event. Some traumatic effects remain indefinitely.

Nursing Care Management

Children need to deal with any traumatic event; much hinges on the intensity of the event and their reactions to it. Children's reactions depend heavily on their social environment and the way in which their caretaking adults react to the event. In the second phase of PTSD, the appropriateness of the defense mechanism must be assessed, and children must be assisted in coping with their emotions.

Coping is a learned response, and children in the third phase can be helped to use their coping strategies to deal with their fears. Children usually are willing to accept reasoning. Those who are assisted in their catharsis and allowed expression will survive without serious lasting effects. Encourage them to play out the stress and discuss their feelings about the event.

Children need professional help if any of the phases of PTSD are prolonged. Boys tend to have a prolonged defense phase more often than girls. Occasionally the precipitating event will go unrecognized (bullying and psychologic abuse are most common in school-age children), and the affected child will engage in what is considered to be unusual behavior. Children exhibiting any sudden change in behavior need to be assessed for exposure to a traumatic event. When the change in behavior is traced to a traumatic event, treatment should be implemented immediately to prevent or reduce the long-term emotional and psychologic effects of PTSD (Hagan, Gentry, Ippen, et al., 2017).

School Phobia

Children, other than beginning students, who resist going to school or who demonstrate extreme reluctance to attend school for a sustained period as a result of severe anxiety or fear of school-related experiences are said to have school phobia. The terms *school refusal* and *school avoidance* are also used to describe this behavior. School phobia occurs in children of all ages, but it is more common in children 10 years of age and older. School avoidance behaviors occur in both boys and girls and in children from all socioeconomic levels.

Anxiety that verges on panic is a constant manifestation, and children can develop symptoms as a protective mechanism to avoid facing the situation that distresses them. Physical symptoms are prominent and may affect any part of the body; anorexia, nausea, vomiting, diarrhea, dizziness, headache, leg pains, and abdominal pains are most common. Children may even develop a low-grade fever. A striking feature of school phobia is the prompt subsiding of symptoms when it is evident that the child can remain at home. Another significant observation is absence of symptoms on weekends and holidays unless they are related to other places, such as Sunday school or parties. Occasional mild reluctance to attend school is common among school-age children, but if the fear continues for longer than a few days, it must be considered a serious problem.

The onset is usually sudden and precipitated by a school-related incident. By taking a careful history, nurses can find out whether a poor attendance record is caused by trivial reasons.

Nursing Care Management

Treatment for school phobia depends on the cause. The primary goal is school attendance. The longer a child is permitted to stay out of school, the more difficult it is for the child to reenter. Parents must be convinced gently but firmly that immediate return is essential and that it is their responsibility to insist on school attendance.

A school reentry protocol may be necessary for the child with severe symptoms. In reentry programs, the child role-plays routines involved in getting ready for school and activities that occur at school. Relaxation techniques are also used. The child usually goes to school initially for a half-day and then progresses to a full day. Often the school nurse can provide support to the parents and teacher during the reentry process. If the problem persists, professional help is recommended.

Conversion Reaction

Conversion reaction, also known as hysteria, hysterical conversion reaction, and childhood hysteria, is a psychophysiologic disorder with a sudden onset that usually can be traced to a precipitating environmental event. The disorder is observed with equal frequency in both sexes in childhood, but affected girls outnumber affected boys during adolescence. The manifestations involve primarily the voluntary musculature and special senses and include abdominal pain, fainting, pseudoseizures, paralysis, headaches, and visual field restriction. Once considered rare in childhood, the disorder occurs more frequently than has generally been acknowledged. The most commonly observed symptom is seizure activity, which can be differentiated from symptoms of neurogenic origin by formal tests, the most useful of which is the finding of a normal electroencephalogram.

Many children with conversion reaction have experienced a major family crisis, such as loss of a parent or other significant person through death, divorce, or moving, before the onset of symptoms. The families of children with conversion reaction characteristically display problems in communication and depression or hypochondriasis in a parent.

BOX 16.1 Characteristics of Children With Depression

Behavior

Predominantly sad facial expression with absence or diminished range of affective response
Solitary play or work; tendency to be alone; disinterest in play
Withdrawal from previously enjoyed activities and relationships
Lowered grades in school; lack of interest in doing homework or achieving in school
Diminished motor activity; tiredness
Tearfulness or crying
Dependent and clinging or aggressive and disruptive behavior

Internal States

Utterance of statements reflecting lowered self-esteem, sense of hopelessness, or guilt
Suicidal ideations

Physiologic Manifestations

Constipation
Nonspecific complaints of not feeling well
Change in appetite resulting in weight loss or gain
Alterations in sleeping pattern, sleeplessness, or hypersomnia

Educating the child and family on the cause of emotional stresses or feelings and alternative approaches to coping with stress may alleviate the child's symptoms. If deep personality problems are evident, psychiatric consultation is indicated. Nursing care is similar to that for the child with recurrent abdominal pain.

Childhood Depression

Childhood depression has been shown to lead to an increased risk of poor academic performance, impaired social functioning, suicidal behavior, homicidal ideation, and alcohol or substance abuse. It is also associated with an increased risk of recurrent depressive episodes. Unfortunately, a large proportion of depression in children and adolescents is underdiagnosed and undertreated. Depression in childhood is often difficult to detect because children may be unable to express their feelings and tend to act out their problems and concerns rather than identify them verbally. Children who cannot verbalize their feelings may exhibit irritability, which may manifest as frustration, temper tantrums, and behavioral problems. Other symptoms indicative of depression in children include increased rejection sensitivity.

Adult caregivers, health care professionals, and educators may not recognize early warning signs of depression in children or may delay referral and treatment, believing that symptoms of depression are "just a stage of development" and will resolve with maturation. Authorities agree that childhood depression exists, but the manifestations often differ from those in depressed adults. Depressed children often exhibit a distinctive style of thinking characterized by low self-esteem, hopelessness, poor social engagement with peers, and a tendency to explain negative events in terms of personal shortcomings (Box 16.1).

Some states of depression are temporary, such as acute depression precipitated by a traumatic event. The causative event might include a period of hospitalization; loss of a parent through death or divorce; or loss of a significant relationship with something (a pet), someone (a friend or family member), or a place (move from a familiar home, neighborhood, or city). The easily identified manifestations include a sad face; tearfulness; irritability; and withdrawal from previously enjoyed activities and relationships. The child tends to spend more time in solitary activities, and schoolwork is impaired. Sleeplessness or hypersomnia, changes in appetite or weight (either increased or decreased), constipation, tiredness, and nonspecific complaints of not feeling well are common reactions.

More serious and less common are depressive responses to more chronic stress and loss. These are frequently observed in children with chronic illness or disability. The manifestations are similar to those seen in acute reactions. Major depressive disorders in childhood have a number of similarities with several other psychologic disorders.

Considering the fact that depression symptoms may be attributed to various physical illnesses, a through physical examination must be carried out in all children and adolescents presenting with depressive features. It is difficult to identify depression in the presence of a medical disorder, especially when the medical disorder is associated with change in appetite, sleep disruption, somatic symptoms, and fatigue.

Therapeutic Management

Depressed children are managed by a health team that is specially trained in the care of children with mental disorders. Treatment is highly individualized and undertaken in the least restrictive environment. Suicidal children are admitted to the hospital for protection if the family is unable to provide constant monitoring. Hospitalization may also be advised for children with associated disruptive behavior, such as fighting with peers or family. Most therapeutic regimens focus on various combinations of counseling, psychotherapy, family therapy, cognitive therapy, education (teaching social and life skills that facilitate coping), environmental improvement, and pharmacotherapy.

For mild-to-moderate depression, psychotherapy is considered to be the preferred initial modality of treatment. Cognitive-behavioral therapy (CBT) is preferred in children and adolescents with cognitive distortions and comorbid anxiety disorders (Weersing, Jeffreys, Do, et al., 2017). Antidepressants are usually considered in the presence of moderate depression for which psychotherapy is not feasible, severe depression with or without psychotic symptoms, and depression that fails to respond to an adequate trial of psychotherapy.

Pharmacotherapy may involve tricyclic antidepressants or selective serotonin reuptake inhibitors (SSRIs); fluoxetine should be considered the first choice in children ages 8 years and older.

Escitalopram or sertraline can also be considered in treatment. There have been reports that antidepressant medications may cause increased suicidal thinking and behaviors in pediatric patients. This prompted the US Food and Drug Administration to require black box drug labeling detailing potential suicide-related risks for pediatric patients. Parents and significant others involved in the care of patients should also be informed of the possible role of SSRIs in suicidality. The decision to start an antidepressant or specific psychotherapy should be made jointly by the clinician and adequately informed parents (guardians) with agreement from the child.

Nursing Care Management

One care of the most important aspects of assessment of children and adolescents with depression includes the assessment of suicide risk. Care providers should not underestimate the risk of suicidal behavior in children and adolescents. Caregivers should ask about the presence of suicidal ideation, specific plans for self-injury, and any history of actual self-harm or overt threats or gestures.

Nurses should be aware that depression is a problem that can be easily overlooked in children and one that can interrupt normal growth and development. Recognizing depression and making appropriate referrals are important nursing functions. Identification of a depressed child requires a careful history (health, growth and development, social and family health); interviews with the child; and

TABLE 16.2 Pediatric Quality Indicator[a]

Screening for Depression and Follow-Up Plan	
Measure	Patients 12 years of age and older screened for depression on the date of the encounter using an age-appropriate standardized depression screening tool AND, if positive, a follow-up plan is documented on the date of the positive screen
Numerator	Patients screened for depression on the date of the encounter using an age-appropriate standardized tool AND, if positive, a follow-up plan is documented on the date of the positive screen
Denominator	All patients ages 12 years and older before the beginning of the measurement period with at least one eligible encounter during the measurement period

[a]Endorsed by the National Quality Forum NQF #0418 and 2019 Core Set of Children's Health Care Quality Measures for Medicaid and CHIP. https://www.medicaid.gov/federal-policy-guidance/downloads/cib112018.pdf.

observations by the nurse, parents, and teachers. If antidepressants are prescribed, the child and family need to know that antidepressants must be at a therapeutic level for 2 to 4 weeks to achieve a beneficial effect. The child and family also need to monitor the child for side effects of the specific drug prescribed and any interactions with other drugs. Hospitalization is usually indicated when a child or adolescent poses a serious threat of harm to self or others. See Table 16.2 for the Pediatric Quality Indicator for screening and follow-up in children and adolescents being treated for depression.

Anxiety

Considerable advances have been made in the assessment and treatment of pediatric anxiety disorders. However, children are often unrecognized and never receive suitable treatment recognition. Although they are common among children and adolescents, many parents and health care providers do not realize that anxiety disorders in youth predict anxiety disorders in adulthood. Symptoms include excessive anxiety, unrealistic worries, and fearfulness not related to a specific object or situation. The adolescent finds it difficult to control worry, with comorbid symptoms of restlessness or feeling keyed up or on edge, being easily fatigued, difficulty concentrating or the mind going blank, irritability, muscle tension, and sleep disturbance. Developing and implementing effective early interventions therefore has been a priority for clinical research over the last decades. CBT has robust empirical support for the treatment of youth anxiety disorders. Generic CBT programs for youth anxiety generally involve 10 to 16 therapy sessions, with change of dysfunctional thoughts and gradual exposure to feared situations as core elements (Heiervang, Villabø, & Wergeland, 2018).

Childhood Schizophrenia

Childhood schizophrenia refers to severe deviations in ego functioning and is generally reserved for psychotic disorders that appear in children younger than 15 years old. Childhood schizophrenia is a very rare illness among children in the general population; only about 2 in every 1000 with mental illness have childhood schizophrenia.

Childhood schizophrenia is characterized by symptoms that last at least 6 months and that seriously interfere with the child's functioning in school, at home, or in other social situations. The basic core disturbance is a lack of contact with reality and the subsequent development by the child of a world of his or her own. Young schizophrenic children can and do experience psychosis, which often is preceded by behavioral problems, developmental lags in fine motor and sensory functions, as well as persistence of primitive reflexes. There may be language and motor delays well before the development of actual psychosis. The DSM-5 points out the poorer prognosis for early-onset schizophrenia. The earlier age of onset has been correlated with high social disability. There are now clear distinctions between childhood schizophrenia, autistic disorder, and pervasive developmental disorders (PDDs). In autistic disorder, onset is before age 3 years and, in contrast to childhood schizophrenia, mental retardation is common. The PDDs each have criteria that differ from childhood schizophrenia and are not usually accompanied by psychosis. The longer psychosis continues to be untreated, the worse the eventual long-term prognosis becomes, so early intervention is important. The treatment for childhood schizophrenia needs to be multimodal and possibly include pharmacotherapeutics, family interventions, cognitive therapy, and environmental interventions.

Treatment involves management of symptoms, prevention of relapse, and social and occupational rehabilitation of the young person. Antipsychotic drugs that may be used include haloperidol, clozapine, chlorpromazine, and risperidone. Antipsychotic drugs are used with caution in children because of the risk of extrapyramidal symptoms of acute dyskinesias and dystonic reactions, tardive dyskinesia, parkinsonism, akinesia, akathisia, and neuroleptic malignant syndrome. Extrapyramidal symptoms are caused by dopamine blockade or depletion in the basal ganglia; this lack of dopamine often mimics idiopathic pathologies of the extrapyramidal system.

Family interventions and family therapy often result in improvements in psychotic symptoms, thought disorders, and social functioning among children with schizophrenia. Children may be managed in both inpatient and outpatient settings.

Nursing Care Management

Nursing care of psychotic children is a highly specialized area. However, nurses should be alert to the possibility that schizophrenia can occur in children and refer children who consistently demonstrate abnormal behavior for evaluation. In addition, nurses need to teach family members of children taking antipsychotic drugs to observe for possible side effects. When the child's reality is distorted due to misperceptions of the environment, the nurse must continually clarify these perceptions and correct them. Parents and guardians of children with schizophrenia typically feel out of control and need help to dispel feelings of helplessness. Parents must be taught that they are an integral part of the treatment plan. Nurses play a key role in the support and psychoeducation of family members of the child with schizophrenia.

HEALTH PROBLEMS OF ADOLESCENTS

ACNE

Acne vulgaris is the most common skin problem treated by physicians during adolescence. Acne stimulates the sebaceous glands of the skin to enlarge, or produce oil, and plug the pores. **Comedogenesis** (formation of comedones) results in a noninflammatory lesion that may be either an open comedone ("blackhead") or a closed comedone ("whitehead") (Fig.16.1).

More than half of the adolescent population will experience acne by the end of the teenage years. Although the disorder can appear before 10 years old, the peak incidence occurs in middle to late adolescence (16 to 17 years old in girls and 17 to 18 years old in boys). It is more common in boys than in girls. After this age period, the disease usually decreases in severity, but it may persist into adulthood. Although the disease is self-limiting and is not life threatening, it has

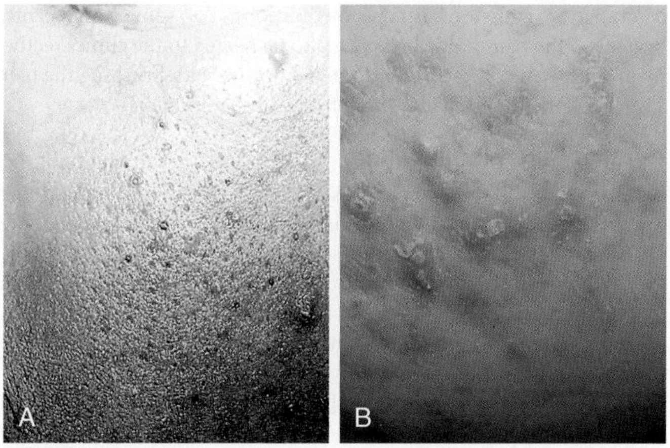

Fig. 16.1 Acne vulgaris. **A,** Acne vulgaris. **B,** Comedones with a few inflammatory pustules. (From Zitelli, B. J., McIntire, S. C., & Nowalk, A. J. [2012]. Zitelli and Davis' atlas of pediatric physical diagnosis [6th ed.]. St Louis, MO: Elsevier.)

great significance to affected adolescents. Health professionals should not underestimate the impact that acne has on teens.

Numerous factors affect the development and course of acne. Its distribution in families and a high degree of concordance in identical twins suggest hereditary factors. Premenstrual flare-ups of acne occur in nearly 70% of adolescent girls, suggesting a hormonal cause. Studies do not indicate a clear association between stress and acne, but adolescents commonly cite stress as a cause for acne outbreaks. Cosmetics containing lanolin, petrolatum, vegetable oils, lauryl alcohol, butyl stearate, and oleic acid can increase comedone production. Exposure to oils in cooking grease can be a precursor in adolescents working in fast-food restaurants. The link between dietary intake and the development or worsening of acne lesions has been a topic of much discussion. There is evidence that there may be an association with the intake of dairy products and high glycemic index foods that may potentiate hormonal and inflammatory factors that contribute to acne severity (Cerman, Aktas, & Altunay, 2016). In patients with features of metabolic syndrome, a low-glycemic diet can be recommended to improve both acne and other metabolic parameters.

Pathophysiology

Acne is a multifactorial inflammatory disease affecting the pilosebaceous follicles of the skin. Four major factors are identified in the pathogenesis of acne: increased sebaceous gland activity, follicular hyperkeratinization, proliferation of *Cutibacterium acnes* (previously *Propionibacterium acnes*), and inflammation (Li, He, & Chen, 2017). Genetic background and environmental factors modulate these factors, driving the flare-ups of acne.

Acne can be categorized as comedonal, inflammatory, or both and can be classified as mild, moderate, or severe based on the number and type of comedones and the extent of affected skin (Eichenfield, Krakowski, Piggott, et al., 2013).

Therapeutic Management

Successful management of acne depends on a cooperative effort between the care provider, adolescent, and parents. Unlike many dermatologic conditions, acne lesions resolve slowly, and improvement may not be apparent for at least 6 weeks. Individual comedones can take several weeks to months to resolve, and papules and pustules usually resolve in about 1 week. The multifactorial causes of acne require a combined approach for successful treatment. Treatment consists of general measures of care and specific treatments determined by the type of lesions involved.

Medications

Treatment success depends on commitment from the adolescent. Before prescribing treatment, the practitioner should determine the adolescent's level of comfort and readiness to begin treatment. The adolescent should be reminded that clinical improvement may take weeks to months. Early intervention, most often with topical medications, may prevent the development of more severe acne.

Tretinoin (Retin-A). Topical retinoids are vitamin A derivatives that normalize keratinization, decrease microcomedone formation, and reduce inflammation. They are strongly recommended for use in all types of acne, as they not only treat active lesions, but also work to prevent recurrences and help with scarring. The US Food and Drug Administration approved adapalene (Differin) 0.1% gel as the first retinoid for sale over the counter (OTC). Now it is possible to have a complete and effective acne regimen, with a retinoid and benzoyl peroxide, available without a prescription (Leyden, Stein-Gold, & Weiss, 2017).

Tretinoin is available as a cream, gel, or liquid. This drug can be extremely irritating to the skin and requires careful patient education for optimal usage. The patient should be instructed to begin with a pea-size dot of medication, which is divided into the three main areas of the face and then gently rubbed into each area. The medication should not be applied for at least 20 to 30 minutes after washing to decrease the burning sensation. The avoidance of the sun and the daily use of sunscreen must be emphasized because sun exposure can result in severe sunburn. Adolescents should be advised to apply the medication at night and to use a sunscreen with a sun protection factor (SPF) of at least 15 in the daytime.

Topical benzoyl peroxide. Benzoyl peroxide is an antibacterial agent that is broadly antimicrobial and inhibits the formation of comedones. Benzoyl peroxide is commonly available as OTC acne washes, gels, foams, or creams in concentrations ranging from 2.5% to 10%. The addition of benzoyl peroxide to acne regimens with other antibiotic therapy enhances results and reduces bacterial resistance.

Benzoyl peroxide is effective against both inflammatory and noninflammatory acne and is an effective first-line agent. Benzoyl peroxide and salicylic acid are the most effective acne treatment kits available OTC. The patient should be informed that the medication may have a bleaching effect on sheets, bedclothes, and towels. The adolescent can be reassured that skin bleaching will not occur. Accommodation to the medication can be gained with a gradual increase in the strength and frequency of application. The current acne guidelines recommend the use of benzoyl peroxide as monotherapy for mild acne or in any combination with topical or topical and oral treatment for mild to severe acne.

When inflammatory lesions accompany the comedones, a **topical antibacterial agent** may be prescribed. These agents are used to prevent new lesions and to treat preexisting acne. Clindamycin, erythromycin-metronidazole, and azelaic acid are currently available for topical antibacterial therapy. Side effects of these medications include erythema, dryness, and burning; using the medications every other day will decrease the adverse effects. A 5% dapsone gel is approved for the treatment of inflammatory acne lesions for children over 12 years of age and is reported to be effective when used in combination with a topical retinoid, such as adapalene or tazarotene. Topical antimicrobials combined with benzoyl peroxide are more effective than either product alone. Retinoids in combination with antimicrobials also improve the penetration of these topical agents and are the only means to address three of the pathogenic causes of acne: keratinization, *C. acnes,* and inflammation.

Systemic antibiotic therapy is initiated when moderate to severe acne does not respond to topical treatments. Recommendations from the American Academy of Dermotology's acne guidelines, as well as other acne guidelines from around the world, emphasize a major change in the role of oral antibiotics in the management of acne. The use of antibiotics is being limited. Systemic antibiotics should be used for the acute management of acne but then discontinued at 3 to 4 months, with the goal of maintaining improvement with a topical retinoid and antimicrobial agent.

Systemic antibiotics are relatively free of side effects, with the exception of occasional gastrointestinal upset, photosensitivity, or vaginal candidiasis. The tetracyclines, doxycycline and minocycline, are preferred over other antibiotics for the treatment of acne in patients older than 8 years of age. With the increase in antibiotic stewardship, patients should be treated systemically for the shortest amount of time possible.

Hormonal. Hormonal treatment is the mainstay systemic treatment in female acne with a significant endocrinologic involvement. Combined oral contraceptives (COCs) are effectively and safely used in combination with other topical and oral antibiotic or hormonal treatment. COCs reduce the endogenous androgen production and decrease the bioavailability of the woman's circulating androgens. COCs containing levonorgestrel, norethindrone, norgestimate, drospirenone, or dienogest decrease acne in women (Powell, 2017).

Isotretinoin, 13-cis-retinoic acid (Accutane), is the only agent available that affects factors involved in the development of acne. Patients who have very severe acne, scarring acne, or significant acne that has not responded to therapy within 3 to 4 months can be prescribed isotretinoin treatment. Pediatric providers typically do not prescribe isotretinoin, but all medical providers of patients who are on it should be familiar with its side effects. These side effects include dry skin and mucous membranes, nasal irritation, dry eyes, decreased night vision, photosensitivity, arthralgia, headaches, mood changes, aggressive or violent behaviors, depression, and suicidal ideation. Many studies, particularly those done prospectively, question the risk of depression or suicide with isotretinoin treatment (Šimić, Babić, & Gunarić, 2017). Given the high risk of depression and suicide in the adolescent and young adult populations, it is judicious for all health care providers to screen patients accordingly, and if depressive or other mood changes develop, isotretinoin use should be discontinued. All systemic retinoids are teratogenic, and the prescription of isotretinoin is strongly regulated by a government prescription program, iPLEDGE, which mandates strict patient counseling and pregnancy testing for all female patients (Henry, Dormuth, Winquist, et al., 2016). The most significant side effects of this drug are the teratogenic effects. Isotretinoin is absolutely contraindicated in pregnant women. Sexually active young women must use an effective contraceptive method during treatment and for 1 month after treatment.

Patients receiving isotretinoin should also be monitored for elevated cholesterol and triglyceride levels. Significant elevation may require discontinuation of the medication.

Health care providers should provide the adolescent with an overall explanation of the disease process, emphasizing the patient's involvement. Improvement of the adolescent's overall health status is part of the general management. Adequate rest, moderate exercise, a well-balanced diet, reduction of emotional stress, and elimination of any foci of infection are all part of general health promotion.

Cleansing

Acne is not caused by dirt or oil on the surface of the skin. Gentle cleansing with a mild cleanser once or twice daily is usually sufficient. Antibacterial soaps are ineffective and may be drying when used in combination with topical acne medications. For some adolescents, hygiene of the hair and scalp appears to be related to the clinical activity of acne. Acne on the forehead may improve with brushing the hair away from the forehead and more frequent shampooing

Nursing Care Management

Because acne is so common and its appearance may seem so mild, the health care provider may underestimate the relative importance of the disease to the adolescent. The nurse should assess the individual adolescent's level of distress, current management, and perceived success of any regimen before initiating a referral. If adolescents do not perceive the acne to be a problem, they may lack motivation to follow the treatment plan.

The nurse can provide ongoing support for the adolescent when a treatment plan is initiated. The family is also encouraged to support the adolescent in his or her efforts. Discuss the use of medications and basic skin care information in detail with the adolescent. Written instructions to accompany the verbal discussion are helpful. Information to dispel myths about the use of abrasive cleansing products can prevent unnecessary costs and trauma to the skin. Adolescents also need education about the factors that aggravate acne and damage the skin, such as too vigorous scrubbing. Picking, squeezing, and manual expression with fingernails break down the ductal walls of lesions and cause the acne to worsen. Mechanical irritation, such as vinyl helmet straps that rub areas predisposed to acne, can also cause the development of lesions.

HEALTH CONDITIONS OF THE MALE REPRODUCTIVE SYSTEM

Because of the physical, mental, and social changes that occur in boys around puberty and into adolescence, and because boys are more likely to initiate sexual behavior, it's important for health care providers to discuss sexual and reproductive health care with their male patients. In younger children, the genital exam provides an opportunity for the health care provider to discuss "safe touch" issues with the child, allowing the parent to reinforce the message. In addition, in preadolescents and adolescents, discussion about testicular self-exam should also be done during the genital exam. Although testicular cancer is rare in teenage boys overall, it is the most common cancer in males between the ages of 15 and 35.

Many obvious anomalies, such as hypospadias, hydrocele, and cryptorchidism, are identified, with corrective measures instituted during infancy or early childhood. Uncircumcised males may encounter problems related to a tight foreskin that cannot be retracted (phimosis) and are at a higher risk for infections, such as balanitis and prostatitis.

Adolescent boys are also self-conscious about their changing bodies and need preparation for a genital examination. The most successful approach is to assume a matter-of-fact attitude toward the examination, explain precisely what will take place, and maintain a continuous commentary about what is being done and the findings at each phase of the examination.

Varicocele

A varicocele is a pathologic enlargement of the testicular veins that is associated with impaired spermatogenesis and infertility. In fact, varicocele is the most common correctable cause of male infertility (Masterson, Ramasamy, & Hotaling, 2017)

Varicoceles are diagnosed by physical examination and are graded I to III. Grade I varicocele is palpable only during the Valsalva maneuver. grade II varicocele is palpable in the standing position. and grade

III varicocele is visible without palpation. Varicoceles are treated with either surgery or embolization. Varicocelectomy is indicated in adolescents when there is growth arrest of the affected testicle or when there is pain associated with the varicocele.

Epididymitis

Epididymitis is an inflammatory response of the epididymis, whereas epididymo-orchitis refers to inflammation of both the epididymis and the testes. Epididymitis may be caused by infectious and noninfectious processes. The etiology of bacterial epididymitis is dependent on age, sexual practices, and the presence of urinary tract abnormalities.

In males younger than 35 years of age, epididymo-orchitis is often associated with sexually transmitted organisms such as *Chlamydia trachomatis* or *Neisseria gonorrhoeae,* whereas in males over 35 years of age, it is often caused by non–sexually transmitted enteric organisms, such as *Escherichia coli* and *Proteus*. The term *men who have sex with men* (MSM) describes a heterogeneous group of men who have varied behaviors, identities, and health care needs. Some MSM are at high risk for human immunodeficiency virus (HIV) infection and other viral and bacterial sexually transmitted infections (STIs) because MSM may practice anal sex and the rectal mucosa is uniquely susceptible to certain STI pathogens.

Clinical presentation is slow and insidious with unilateral scrotal pain, redness, and swelling. Associated symptoms include urethral discharge, dysuria, fever, and pyuria. Treatment consists of analgesics, scrotal support, bed rest, and appropriate antibiotic therapy.

Testicular Torsion

Nurses must be aware of the presentation, timing, and evaluation of testicular torsion because they may triage the pediatric patient with a painful scrotum or be involved in the evaluation in the emergency department or clinic. Pediatric testicular torsion is a surgical emergency that requires a thorough history and physical examination and is, at the outset, a clinical diagnosis. Testicular torsion can occur neonatally, peripubertally, or as an adult. In the pediatric population, approximately 90% of cases occur peripubertally. In a neonate, 70% of torsion occurs prior to birth. Neonatal testicular torsion often presents as a hard mass found on routine examination. Surgical management typically involves orchiectomy with a contralateral orchiopexy. The only known risk factor for peripubertal and adult torsion is the bell clapper deformity, which leaves the testis free to swing and rotate within the tunica vaginalis of the scrotum much like the gong (clapper) inside a bell, predisposing the patient to intravaginal testicular torsion. Peripubertal and adult testicular torsion classically presents with acute-onset severe scrotal pain, nausea and vomiting, a high and horizontal testicular lie, and an absent cremasteric reflex (Hazeltine, Panza, & Ellsworth, 2017, 2018).

In severe torsion, the organ can become swollen and painful; the scrotum becomes red, warm, and edematous and appears to be immobile or fixed as a result of spasm of the cremasteric fibers.

In the pediatric population, testicular torsion has an annual incidence of 3.8 per 100,000 pediatric patients, with the peak incidence occurring between ages 12 and 16 years (Riccabona, Darge, Lobo, et al., 2015). Approximately 10% of testicular torsions occur in neonates; of these, 70% are believed to occur in utero (prenatal torsion), with the remaining 30% occurring within the first 30 days of life (postnatal torsion) (Basta, Courtier, Phelps, et al., 2015).

A prompt diagnosis and definitive surgical management are essential in males of any age to preserve the affected testicle. In patients with a high clinical suspicion, emergent surgical management is warranted.

Gynecomastia

Some degree of bilateral or unilateral breast enlargement occurs frequently in boys during puberty. Approximately half of adolescent boys have transient gynecomastia, usually lasting less than 1 year, which subsides spontaneously with achievement of male development. A careful assessment of the pubertal stage at the onset of gynecomastia; medication history, including anabolic steroids; and the exclusion of renal, liver, thyroid, and endocrine disorders or dysfunction allow the examiner to reassure the adolescent that the changes are pubertal gynecomastia and that no further assessment is indicated. Gynecomastia may also be drug induced; calcium channel blockers, cancer chemotherapeutic agents, histamine$_2$-receptor antagonists, and oral ketoconazole medications have all been shown to cause the condition.

For all adolescents presenting with gynecomastia, a detailed history and physical examination should be performed with the goal of differentiating true pubertal gynecomastia from other causes of breast enlargement. Pertinent information to obtain from the history includes duration of symptoms, presence of nipple discharge or overlying skin changes, reports of below-normal prenatal (less commonly pubertal) androgen effects, and testicular swelling or masses. A careful genitourinary examination is also of particular importance. Attention should be paid to Tanner staging, testicular volume, and masses or irregularities along the testes. Examination for a varicocele should also be undertaken, as recent evidence has shown that gynecomastia is more common in 12- to 14-year-old boys with varicocele than without varicocele.

If gynecomastia persists or is extensive enough to cause embarrassment, plastic surgery is indicated for cosmetic and psychologic considerations. Administration of testosterone has no effect on breast development or regression and may aggravate the condition.

Nursing Care Management

Management usually consists of assurance to the adolescent and his parents that the situation is benign and temporary. However, all adolescents with gynecomastia should receive a careful medical evaluation to rule out pathologic causes. The adolescent may benefit from the knowledge that this condition occurs in more than 50% of all adolescent boys.

HEALTH CONDITIONS OF THE FEMALE REPRODUCTIVE SYSTEM

Amenorrhea

Menarche, or the first menstrual period, occurs relatively late in female pubertal development. Although girls vary in the onset and rate of progression of pubertal development, the sequence and tempo should be the same. When an adolescent is seen with a complaint of absence of menses, a careful history of the timing of her pubertal development will help determine if there is a need for further evaluation or if reassurance is all that is necessary. Amenorrhea can be classified as either primary or secondary depending on the presence (secondary) or absence (primary) of previous menses. Primary amenorrhea is defined as the absence of menses by age 14 years in the absence of secondary sexual characteristics or the absence of menses by age 16 years in the presence of normal secondary sexual characteristics (Austin & Mahmood, 2018).

Irregular menstrual cycles are common within the first year after menarche because these early cycles may be anovulatory, resulting in regular, irregular, or absent bleeding. Girls with a later onset of menarche take longer to establish regular ovulatory cycles. Primary amenorrhea is rare, with less than 5% of adolescent girls presenting to gynecologic services.

It is essential to take a thorough history, particularly focusing on any red-flag symptoms (underweight/eating disorder, raised body mass index [BMI], acne, hirsutism, polycystic ovarian syndrome, short stature, wide-spaced nipples, Turner syndrome) or family history of delayed puberty. An examination should always include height, weight, and an assessment of secondary sexual characteristics (breast development, pubic and axillary hair growth).

Pregnancy is the most common cause of secondary amenorrhea and should be ruled out in both types of amenorrhea even if the adolescent denies sexual activity. Other factors that disturb the hypothalamic–pituitary–gonadal axis and cause amenorrhea include physical or emotional stress; hyperthyroidism or hypothyroidism; polycystic ovary syndrome; sudden and severe weight loss; strenuous exercise; eating disorders; and use of extrinsic pharmacologic agents, especially phenothiazines, contraceptive steroids, and heroin.

Nursing Care Management

When amenorrhea is caused by hypothalamic disturbances, the nurse is an ideal health professional to assist the adolescent because many causes are potentially reversible (e.g., stress, weight loss for nonorganic reasons). Counseling and education are primary interventions and appropriate nursing roles.

Dysmenorrhea

Dysmenorrhea, pain during or shortly before menstruation, is one of the most common gynecologic problems in women of all ages. Approximately 75% of women report some level of discomfort associated with menses, and approximately 15% report severe dysmenorrhea that interferes with work or school (Lentz, 2012). Dysmenorrhea is associated with menarche prior to 12 years of age, nulliparity, heavy menses, pelvic inflammatory disease (PID), BMI greater than 20, smoking, and depression (Roberts, Hodgkiss, DiBenedetto, et al., 2012). Symptoms usually begin with menstruation, although some women may have discomfort several hours before onset of flow. The range and severity of symptoms are different from woman to woman and from cycle to cycle in the same woman. Symptoms of dysmenorrhea may last several hours to several days. Pain is usually located in the suprapubic area or lower abdomen. Women describe the pain as sharp; cramping; or a steady, dull ache.

Dysmenorrhea is differentiated as primary or secondary. Primary dysmenorrhea is a condition associated with ovulatory cycles. Primary dysmenorrhea has a biochemical basis and arises from the release of prostaglandins with menses. The pain begins with the onset of menstruation and lasts 8 to 48 hours (Lentz, 2012). Primary dysmenorrhea usually appears 6 to 12 months after menarche when ovulation is established.

Secondary dysmenorrhea is defined as painful menses associated with a pathologic condition, such as adenomyosis, endometriosis, PID, endometrial polyps, or fibroids. In contrast to primary dysmenorrhea, the pain of secondary dysmenorrhea is often characterized by dull, lower abdominal aching that radiates to the back or thighs and is often associated with feelings of bloating or pelvic fullness. In addition to a history and physical examination, diagnosis may be assisted by ultrasound examination, dilation and curettage (D&C), endometrial biopsy, or laparoscopy. Dysmenorrhea and pelvic pain in adolescent girls should be managed and treated carefully, as this may represent the first sign of a more serious pathology.

Therapeutic Management

Management of dysmenorrhea depends on the severity of the problem and the individual woman's response to various treatments. Heat and exercise minimize cramping by increasing vasodilation and muscle relaxation and minimizing uterine ischemia. Massaging the lower back can reduce pain by relaxing paravertebral muscles and increasing the pelvic blood supply. Soft, rhythmic rubbing of the abdomen (effleurage) is useful because it provides a distraction and alternative focal point. Biofeedback, transcutaneous electrical nerve stimulation (TENS), progressive relaxation, Hatha yoga, acupuncture, and meditation are also used to decrease menstrual discomfort, although evidence is insufficient to determine their effectiveness (Lentz, 2012).

First-line medication treatment for adolescents with dysmenorrhea is the administration of nonsteroidal antiinflammatory drugs (NSAIDs), which block the formation of prostaglandins. Girls should be instructed to begin the medication either at the first sign of symptoms or bleeding or 1 to 2 days before the onset of their menses, and then take it on a regular schedule for 2 to 3 days (Roberts et al., 2012). The medications should be taken with food. If an NSAID such as ibuprofen is not effective, another NSAID should be tried because some women receive relief from different NSAIDs.

Oral contraceptive pills (OCPs) are also effective and a reasonable choice for women who want to use a contraceptive agent. OCPs are effective in relieving symptoms of primary dysmenorrhea for approximately 90% of women, but no single OCP has been shown to be superior to another (Lentz, 2012). However, OCPs may be contraindicated for some women.

Nursing Care Management

All adolescent girls need reassurance that menstruation is a normal function. When nurses are asked for advice on menstrual problems, they have a valuable opportunity to engage in health teaching concerning menstrual physiology; hygiene; and the importance of a well-balanced diet, exercise, and general health maintenance. Health teaching can dispel myths about menstruation and femininity.

A careful history indicates a potential problem and the need for evaluation and referral to an appropriate practitioner, health service, or clinic. The history should include the onset of symptoms; the duration, type of pain, and relationship to menstrual flow; the age at menarche; family history of dysmenorrhea; and sexual history. The nurse should also ask about previous treatments, including dosages of medications. Depending on the results of the history, the physical examination may include a gynecologic examination.

If a gynecologic examination is necessary, the nurse can play a supportive role for the adolescent girl. Whether it is her first experience or not, she is often filled with apprehension. Almost all adolescents are extremely self-conscious about their bodies and the changes taking place. They need continuing support in the form of anticipatory guidance regarding what to expect and suggestions of what to do to relax during the procedure. Most girls favor a semisitting position, which has the additional advantage of allowing eye contact during the procedure. Sometimes a pillow helps the patient feel more comfortable and less vulnerable. The provision of a mirror for the girl to see what is taking place if she so desires helps the examiner explain various aspects of anatomy. When possible, it is important to respect the adolescent's request for a female provider and to have her mother or other supportive person present if she desires.

Premenstrual Syndrome

Approximately 30% to 80% of women experience mood and/or somatic symptoms that occur with their menstrual cycles (Lentz, 2012). Premenstrual syndrome (PMS) is a poorly understood condition that includes one or more of a large number of physical and psychologic symptoms beginning in the luteal phase of the menstrual cycle that occurs to such a degree that lifestyle or work is affected. Symptoms include fluid retention, behavioral or emotional changes, premenstrual cravings, headache, fatigue, and backache. All age-groups are affected.

Premenstrual dysphoric disorder (PMDD) is a more severe variant of PMS. Approximately 3% to 8% of women are affected and experience marked irritability, dysphoria, mood lability, anxiety, fatigue, appetite changes, and a sense of feeling overwhelmed (Lentz, 2012).

Therapeutic Management

There is little agreement on management of PMS. A careful, detailed history and daily log of symptoms and mood fluctuations spanning several cycles may give direction to a plan of management. Education is an important component of management. Nurses advise women that self-help modalities often result in significant symptom improvement. Diet changes can provide symptom relief for some women. Nurses can suggest that women limit their consumption of refined sugar, salt, alcohol, and caffeinated beverages. Three small to moderate-size meals and three small snacks a day that are rich in complex carbohydrates and fiber have been reported to relieve symptoms (American College of Obstetricians and Gynecologists, 2015). Exercise may also provide symptom relief. Aerobic exercise increases beta-endorphin levels to offset symptoms of depression and elevate mood. Stress reduction techniques may also help with symptom management (American College of Obstetricians and Gynecologists, 2015).

If these strategies do not provide significant symptom relief in 1 to 2 months, medication is often added. Medications used in the treatment of PMS include diuretics, prostaglandin inhibitors (NSAIDs), progesterone, and OCPs; however, no single medication alleviates all PMS symptoms (American College of Obstetricians and Gynecologists, 2015).

Vaginal Infections

Vaginal discharge and itching of the vulva and vagina are among the most common reasons that a woman seeks help from a health care provider. Women complain of vaginal discharge more than any other gynecologic symptoms; however, vaginal discharge resulting from an infection must be distinguished from normal secretions. Physiologic leukorrhea is a normal vaginal secretion occurring at ovulation and just before menses. It is clear to cloudy in appearance; is nonirritating; and has a mild, inoffensive odor. On the other hand, inflammatory leukorrhea is caused by physical (e.g., forgotten tampon), chemical (e.g., bubble baths, douching), or infectious (e.g., *Candida* fungi, *Trichomonas* protozoa parasites, bacteria) agents. It is a glutinous, gray-white discharge with an offensive odor. Diagnosis is confirmed with microscopic evaluation of vaginal secretions, vaginal culture, or rapid testing methods.

Treatment varies depending on the cause. Health teaching is important in the management of vaginal discharge. Adolescent girls need reassurance that increased vaginal mucus can occur at the time of ovulation, before menstruation, or with sexual excitement. Many teenage girls mistake these variations as signs of infection. Girls should be taught to wipe from front to back after toileting and to realize that vaginitis can result from irritation, foreign objects, and sexual activity. Nurses should stress the importance of an evaluation to determine the exact cause.

HEALTH CONDITIONS RELATED TO REPRODUCTION

According to the Youth Risk Behavior Survey (YRBS; Centers for Disease Control and Prevention, 2017), the percentage of students who had ever had sex decreased significantly from 2007 (47.8%) through 2017 (39.5%). A significantly higher percentage of male students (41.4%) than female students (37.7%) had ever had sex. A significantly higher percentage of African American students (45.8%) than white students (38.6%) had ever had sex. There was no significant difference between the percentages of white students and Hispanic students who had ever had sex or between the percentages of African American students and Hispanic students who had ever had sex (Youth Risk Behavior Surveillance, 2017). Many serious health consequences are associated with adolescent sexual activity, including unplanned pregnancy and STIs; additional health problems may arise from an increased number of sexual partners over time and incomplete education on sexual practices in adolescents. Health professionals must understand the issues related to adolescent sexual activity and the psychosocial dynamics that influence them.

Adolescent Pregnancy

According to the Centers for Disease Control and Prevention, in 2017 a total of 194,377 babies were born to women ages 15 to 19 years, for a birth rate of 18.8 per 1000 women in this age-group. This is another record low for US teens and a drop of 7% from 2016. Birth rates fell 10% for women ages 15 to 17 years, and 6% for women ages 18 to 19 years.

The decline is attributed to increased condom and contraception use, as well as a delay in the initiation of sexual activity among adolescents. However, the less familiar an adolescent is with his or her partner, the less likely it is that he or she will use contraception during intercourse. Discontinuation of contraception is common; 30% of women 15 to 19 years old and 47% of women 20 to 24 years old have discontinued at least one method because of dissatisfaction (Pazol, Whiteman, Folger, et al., 2015). Teens who postpone the initiation of sexual intercourse decrease their risk for STIs, including HIV.

In most cases, with early prenatal care, teenage pregnancy is no longer considered to be biologically disadvantageous to the child. However, teenage parenting is still regarded as socially, educationally, psychologically, and economically disadvantageous to both mother and child. Predictors of maternal success include participation in a program for pregnant teens, a social support system, and a sense of control over one's life. With better facilities available for care, the mortality associated with teenage pregnancies is decreasing, but morbidity remains high. Teenage girls and their unborn infants are at greater risk for complications of both pregnancy and delivery. Medical concerns of the adolescent include poor maternal weight gain, anemia, and pregnancy-induced hypertension (Cinar & Menekse, 2017). Rates of eclampsia, puerperal endometritis, infections, and caesarean section were higher among adolescent mothers than among older mothers. The age of the adolescent influences complications; the younger the adolescent, the higher risk of preterm birth.

Labor is often prolonged in younger teenagers, particularly those 12 to 16 years old, because of a fetopelvic incompatibility and the teenager's smaller stature and incomplete growth process. Delivery concerns include premature labor and low-birth-weight infants. Information should be provided regarding the pregnant adolescent's nutritional status and health care needs related to the unborn fetus's condition. Because adolescent nutrition habits may vary, it is important to stress that the mother's overall health status will ultimately influence that of her newborn. Myths such as "you can now eat for two" must be addressed. The diet must provide sufficient nutrients to meet the growth needs of both the prospective mother and the unborn child without the threat of excessive weight gain or fetal malnutrition.

Nursing Care Management

A pregnant teenager needs careful assessment by the nurse to determine the level of social support available to her and her partner. The adolescent needs to make many important decisions and may not have the life experience to know how to cope with this stress. Whenever possible, guidance from the adults in her life will be invaluable. Information about options to continue the pregnancy and parent the child, continue the pregnancy with adoption, or terminate the pregnancy with abortion should be given in a nonjudgmental manner. If the adolescent chooses to continue the pregnancy, prenatal care should be initiated as soon as possible.

Basic to the implementation of any care program is communication and the establishment of a trusting relationship. Initially the adolescent may appear apathetic and display little interest in discussing her pregnancy. The nurse must make every effort to put the adolescent at ease and avoid undue pressure. Conveying a nonjudgmental and genuine caring acceptance of the adolescent and her goals will assist the nurse in gaining the adolescent's confidence and trust.

Communication takes time and patience. Asking open-ended questions and listening for cues will help identify physical, emotional, social, and cultural influences that might affect the adolescent's progress through the maternity cycle.

The adolescent needs to know what is happening to her, what is expected of her, and how she can help in developing a care plan. Adolescents have their own ideas about the type of help and support they need. Nurses should consult with them and provide them with an opportunity to share their ideas. Adolescent pregnancy affects families, health care professionals, educators, government officials, children, and adolescents. Implementing comprehensive programs that educate adolescents on sexual behavior, contraceptives, and reproductive health may create a positive change in adolescent reproductive health, especially in low- and middle-income communities.

! NURSING ALERT

All pregnant women should take a vitamin and mineral supplement to ensure that the Recommended Dietary Allowance for folic acid (0.4 mg [400 mcg] daily) is met to help prevent neural tube defects. Initiation before pregnancy has been shown to have the most benefit. Consider a multivitamin for all sexually active women.

Contraception

In 2017, 53.8% of high school students (among the 28.7% of students nationwide who were currently sexually active) used a condom the last time they had sexual intercourse. The percentage of students who used a condom decreased significantly from 2007 to 2017 (Centers for Disease Control and Prevention, 2017). The percentage of male students who used a condom the last time they had sex decreased from 68.5% in 2007 to 61.3% in 2017. The percentage of female students who used a condom the last time they had sex decreased from 54.9% in 2007 to 46.9% in 2017. The YRBS found that in 2017, 29.4% of students used effective hormonal birth control the last time they had sex. A significantly higher percentage of female students (34.6%) used effective hormonal birth control than male students reported their partner using (23.9%). Significantly higher percentages of white students (37.4%) and African American students (22.5%) used effective hormonal birth control than did Hispanic students (16.8%). A significantly higher percentage of white students used effective hormonal birth control than did African American students. Family planning services have developed and expanded during recent years, but the need for contraceptive services as part of adolescents' health care remains great. The birth control pill and condom remain the most popular methods for adolescents; 3-month injectable contraception is more popular among lower income adolescents. Adolescents commonly delay seeking contraceptive information; the typical interval from onset of sexual intercourse until the first visit for contraception is 1 year. A pregnancy scare is usually the precipitating event for the contraception appointment. Counseling about contraceptive options should be conducted in a manner that is consistent with the cognitive level of the adolescent. The adolescent should be given accurate information about the risks and benefits of each method before making a choice.

Many teenagers feel ambivalent about their sexual activity and avoid many contraceptives because their use seems too premeditated and implies that sex is planned rather than a spontaneous activity. Most of these girls believe that sex is all right if it is not planned. This may play a role in adolescents delaying contraception, waiting for a relationship that is "close enough." A close relationship would allow adolescents to accept and acknowledge their sexual activity.

Several evidence-based resources are available to medical professionals when performing a contraceptive consult. These include:

- Centers for Disease Control and Prevention (2016) contraception app, https://www.cdc.gov/reproductivehealth/contraception/mmwr/mec/summary.html?CDC_AA_refVal=https%3A%2F%2Fwww.cdc.gov%2Freproductivehealth%2Fcontraception%2Fusmec.htm
- Bedsider (2016) Method Explorer, https://www.bedsider.org/methods

The choice of a safe and effective contraceptive method must be suited to the individual. The choice is based on preference after the adolescent is informed of the benefits and disadvantages. Motivation is necessary for most methods. For example, the pill is effective if used correctly, but the adolescent must remember to take the pill at approximately the same time every day. For many young women, a medroxyprogesterone injection (Depo-Provera) is an ideal choice because it is extremely effective and is administered every 12 weeks; however, side effects such as weight gain and decreased bone mineralization may make it undesirable. Sexually active adolescents need to know that contraceptive devices other than condoms do not prevent STIs. Condom use is still important and must be discussed with all sexually and non–sexually active adolescents.

Confidentiality is a critical issue when discussing contraception with adolescents. Privacy is important to adolescents as they struggle to forge a personal identity and establish social relationships. Adolescents are particularly concerned about the judgments of others. The predominant belief among many health professionals is that parental notification is important but that the "parents' rights" view is not necessarily sensitive to the health needs and basic rights of youth. No evidence substantiates the belief that providing contraceptive guidance contributes to sexual irresponsibility and promiscuity.

Nursing Care Management

Nurses are often involved in providing education about contraception. Such education is ideally combined with ongoing sex education. Although sexual abstinence is a highly desirable form of contraception for teenagers, nurses working with adolescents must recognize that teens feel multiple pressures to engage in sexual intercourse. Postponing sexual involvement requires effective communication and decision-making skills. Adolescents benefit from role-playing refusal skills and opportunities to practice making decisions in a safe environment. Information about safer sex must be provided, and role-playing how to discuss condom use with a partner is helpful to teenagers.

Education on contraception should be provided in both oral and written form. All available methods, including their benefits, disadvantages, and side effects, should be discussed. Concrete, concise language must be used; demonstrations of how to use the contraceptives should be provided; and adolescents should repeat all instructions in their own words. If teenagers are using OCPs, they should be encouraged to use a daily activity as a reminder or cue to take the pill. A knowledgeable phone triage person should be available for questions and concerns. Parents or other important adults may be included in all discussions, with the adolescent's permission. An organization that provides education and services for adolescents, including both individual and group counseling, is Planned Parenthood Federation of America. It has branches in most cities in the United States.

SEXUALLY TRANSMITTED INFECTIONS

Many young people engage in sexual behaviors that can result in unintended health outcomes, such as unintended pregnancy and STIs, including HIV. In 2016 young people ages 13 to 24 years accounted for an estimated 21% of all new HIV diagnoses in the United States, with most occurring among 20- to 24-year-olds. Half of the nearly 20 million new cases of STIs reported each year are among young people ages 15 to 24 years. Other sexual behaviors, such as condom use and hormonal birth control use, can protect against STIs, including HIV, and unintended pregnancy. Although nearly 210,000 babies were born to teenage girls ages 15 to 19 years in 2016, teenage birth rates are currently at their lowest recorded levels (Centers for Disease Control and Prevention, 2017).

Lack of awareness regarding one's susceptibility to STIs when engaged in unprotected sexual activity, be it oral, anal, or vaginal intercourse, is perhaps one of the greatest dangers adolescents face. Although STIs affect individuals of all ages, they take a particularly heavy toll on young people. The Centers for Disease Control and Prevention estimates that youth ages 15 to 24 years make up just over one-quarter of the sexually active population but account for half of the 20 million new cases of STIs that occur in the United States each year (Centers for Disease Control and Prevention, 2017).

Preventing infection (primary prevention) is the most effective way of reducing the adverse consequences of STIs for adolescents. Despite the high rates of STIs documented in the adolescent population, providers frequently fail to inquire about sexual behaviors, assess STI risks, provide risk reduction counseling, and screen for asymptomatic infections during clinical encounters.

Prompt diagnosis and treatment of current infections (secondary prevention) can prevent personal complications and transmission to others. A critical step in preventing the spread of STIs is including questions about an adolescent's sexual history, sexual risk behaviors, and drug-related risk behaviors in every assessment. When the nurse identifies risk factors, there is an opportunity to provide prevention counseling. Prevention messages should include descriptions of specific actions to prevent contracting or transmitting STIs and should be individualized for each adolescent. To be motivated to take preventive actions, the adolescent must believe that acquiring a disease will be serious and that he or she is at risk for infection. Routine laboratory screening for common STIs is indicated for sexually active adolescents. The following screening recommendations summarize published federal agencies' and medical professional organizations' clinical guidelines for sexually active adolescents (Centers for Disease Control and Prevention, 2017).

Sexually Transmitted Bacterial Infections

C. trachomatis is the most frequently reported infectious disease in the United States, yet most cases remain undiagnosed (Torrone, Papp, Weinstock, et al., 2014). Routine annual screening for *C. trachomatis* is recommended for all sexually active females younger than 25 years of age (LeFevre, 2014). In women, chlamydia infections are difficult to diagnose; the symptoms are nonspecific, and the organism is expensive to culture. These infections are highly destructive, causing PID, increased risk of ectopic pregnancy, and tubal factor infertility. Manifestations, treatment, and nursing considerations of *C. trachomatis* are listed in Table 16.3. See Table 16.4 for the Pediatric Quality Indicator related to chlamydia screening.

Gonorrhea is the oldest communicable disease in the United States, with an estimated 300,000 American men and women contracting gonorrhea each year (Centers for Disease Control and Prevention, 2017). Women are often asymptomatic, therefore the Centers for Disease Control and Prevention recommends screening all women at risk for gonorrhea, including women with previous gonorrhea infection, other STIs, and multiple sex partners with inconsistent condom use and those engaged in commercial sex work and drug use (Centers for Disease Control and Prevention, 2017). Gonococcal infection is concentrated in specific geographic locations and communities. Clinicians should consider the communities they serve and may choose to consult local public health authorities for guidance on identifying groups that are at increased risk. Manifestations, treatment, and nursing considerations of gonorrhea are listed in Table 16.3.

Syphilis is caused by *Treponema pallidum*, a motile spirochete. Transmission occurs by entry through microscopic abrasions in the subcutaneous tissue, kissing, biting, or oral-genital sex. Syphilis is a complex disease that can lead to serious systematic disease and even death when untreated. Manifestations, treatment, and nursing considerations of syphilis are listed in Table 16.3.

Sexually Transmitted Protozoa Infections

Trichomonas vaginalis is a common cause of vaginal infections and is almost always transmitted as an STI. Trichomoniasis is caused by *T. vaginalis*, an anaerobic, one-celled protozoan with characteristic flagella. Manifestations, treatment, and nursing considerations of trichomoniasis are listed in Table 16.3.

Sexually Transmitted Viral Infections

Human papillomavirus (HPV) infection is the most common viral STI seen in ambulatory health care settings. Nearly 80 million Americans are currently infected with some type of HPV. About 14 million Americans, including teens, become infected each year (Centers for Disease Control and Prevention, 2019).

Every year in the United States, HPV causes 33,700 cases of cancer in men and women (Centers for Disease Control and Prevention, 2019). HPV infections can cause cancers of the cervix, vagina, and vulva in women; the penis in men; and the anus and back of the throat, including the base of the tongue and tonsils (oropharynx), in both women and men (Centers for Disease Control and Prevention, 2019).

Herpes simplex virus (HSV) is caused by two different antigen subtypes: HSV type 1 (HSV-1) and HSV type 2 (HSV-2). HSV-1 is commonly associated with gingivostomatitis and oral labial lesions (fever blisters), whereas HSV-2 is transmitted sexually and characterized by genital lesions. During 2015–16, the age-adjusted prevalence of HSV-1 was 48.1% among adolescents and adults ages 14 to 49 years (50.9% for females, 45.2% for males). Prevalence was higher for females than males in most 2-year periods from 1999–2000 to 2015–16. Also during 2015–16, the age-adjusted prevalence of HSV-2 for those ages 14 to 49 years was 12.1% (15.9% for females, 8.2% for males) and was higher for females than males in all 2-year periods (Centers for Disease Control and Prevention, 2019). Adolescents and women between the ages of 15 and 34 years are most likely to become

TABLE 16.3 Selected Sexually Transmitted Infections[a]

Manifestations	Therapy	Nursing Care Management
Gonorrhea *(Neisseria gonorrhoeae)*		
Male: Urethritis (dysuria with profuse yellow discharge, frequency, urgency, nocturia) or pharyngitis *Female:* Cervicitis (postpubertal); may be associated with discharge, dysuria, dyspareunia, vulvovaginitis (prepubertal), or pharyngitis	For uncomplicated urogenital and anorectal gonorrhea: Single intramuscular dose of ceftriaxone *plus* Single oral dose of azithromycin	Instruct patient to abstain from sexual intercourse for 7 days after single-dose treatment. Test and treat for other STIs. Find and treat sexual contacts. Educate young people on facts of the disease and its spread. Encourage use of condoms in sexually active young people.
Chlamydia *(Chlamydia trachomatis)*		
Male: Meatal erythema, tenderness, itching, dysuria, urethral discharge, or no symptoms *Female:* Mucopurulent cervical exudate with erythema, edema, congestion, or no symptoms	Single oral dose of azithromycin *or* 7 days of oral doxycycline administered twice daily If pregnant, azithromycin	Same as above. Rescreen pregnant women 3 wk after treatment. Repeat infection elevates risk for PID.
Syphilis *(Treponema pallidum)*		
Primary stage: Chancre, a hard, painless, red, sharply defined lesion with indurated base, raised border, eroded surface, and scanty yellow discharge; usually located on the penis, vulva, or cervix *Secondary stage:* Systemic influenza-like symptoms; lymphadenopathy; rash; usually appears few weeks to months after healing of chancre	Single intramuscular dose of benzathine penicillin G	Instruct patients to use condoms to avoid spread or infection with other organisms. Identify sexual contacts of infected person. Test women during pregnancy and prior to delivery (VDRL and RPR). Evaluate newborn for presence of disease if mother is untreated.
Herpes Progenitalis (Genital Herpes Simplex Virus)		
Small (usually painful) vesicles on genital area, buttocks, and thighs; itching usually the initial symptom; when vesicles break, shallow, circular, extremely painful lesions remain	No known cure Uncomplicated cases: Acyclovir, famciclovir, or valacyclovir by mouth for 10 days Complicated cases: Acyclovir intravenously May need chronic suppressive therapy for recurrences	Instruct patients to use condoms to avoid spread or infection with other organisms. Infection can be transmitted to infant during birth. Evaluate maternal history and observe infant for signs or symptoms. Cultures may be obtained in newborn.
Trichomoniasis *(Trichomonas vaginalis)*		
Pruritus and edema of external genitalia; foul-smelling, greenish vaginal discharge; sometimes postcoital bleeding May be asymptomatic, especially in men	Single oral dose of metronidazole or tinidazole	Patient should not consume alcohol while taking medication and for at least 48 h after the last dose. Sexual partners should be treated.
Human Papillomavirus		
Warts found on any part of male or female genitalia	Patient applied: Podofilox solution or gel (0.5%) or imiquimod (5%) cream or sinecatechins ointment (15%) Provider applied: Podophyllin resin 10% to 25% in compound tincture of benzoin Freezing with liquid nitrogen (cryotherapy) Trichloroacetic acid or bichloracetic acid 80% to 90% Laser therapy, injectable interferon, or surgical removal	An acceptable alternative is to forgo treatment and await spontaneous resolution. Treatments are usually painful; analgesics may be needed, and steroid cream may provide relief. Vaccine available for prevention (see Chapter 6).

[a]Updated information on specific treatment of STIs may be accessed at http://www.cdc.gov/std/treatment.
PID, Pelvic inflammatory disease; *RPR,* rapid plasma reagin; *STI,* sexually transmitted infection; *VDRL,* Venereal Disease Research Laboratory.

infected with HSV-2, especially if they have multiple partners. Many people are unaware that they are infected and transmit the disease unknowingly.

HIV is a bloodborne pathogen, and transmission of the virus can occur through the perinatal period, sexual intercourse with an infected person, or sharing needles with an infected person. HIV screening should be discussed and offered to all adolescents. Frequency of repeat screenings of those who are at risk for HIV infection should be based on level of risk. HIV is discussed in Chapter 24.

TABLE 16.4 Pediatric Quality Indicator[a]

Chlamydia Screening for Women	
Measure	Assesses the percentage of women 16 to 24 years of age who were identified as sexually active and who had at least one test for chlamydia during the measurement year.
Numerator	At least one chlamydia test during the measurement year as documented through administrative data.
Denominator	Women 16 to 24 years of age.

[a]Endorsed by the National Quality Forum NQF #0033 and 2019 Core Set of Children's Health Care Quality Measures for Medicaid and CHIP. https://www.medicaid.gov/federal-policy-guidance/downloads/cib112018.pdf.
Note: A Healthy People 2020 goal is to reduce the proportion of adolescents and young adults with *Chlamydia trachomatis* infections to 3.0%. In general, females have higher rates of chlamydia, though they also use screening services more often, which may cause misleading statistics. In 2003 the highest age-specific rates of reported chlamydia in women were among 15- to 19-year-olds and 20- to 24-year-olds.

Nursing Care Management

Nursing responsibilities encompass all aspects of STI education, confidentiality, prevention, and treatment. The sex education of young people should include providing information about STIs, including their symptoms and treatment, and dispelling the myths associated with their mode of transmission. Many vulnerable adolescents are uninformed or misinformed about STIs.

Primary prevention efforts for STIs include encouraging abstinence and postponing of sexual involvement, encouraging condom use, and ensuring vaccination for hepatitis A and B and HPV. The Centers for Disease Control and Prevention recommends that all boys and girls get two doses of the HPV vaccine at ages 11 or 12. HPV vaccination can be started at age 9. For the HPV vaccine to be most effective, the series should be given prior to exposure to HPV. HPV vaccine is recommended at ages 11 to 12 to ensure that children are protected long before they are ever exposed to the virus. Children who get the first dose before their 15th birthday only need two doses. Children who get the first dose on or after their 15th birthday need three doses.

Nurses play a role in secondary prevention by helping to identify early cases and referring adolescents for treatment. Nurses can also be involved in tertiary prevention by decreasing the medical and psychologic effects of STIs; conducting support groups for adolescents with HIV, HSV, and HPV infections; and assisting pregnant adolescents in obtaining adequate prenatal screening and treatment of STIs.

Pelvic Inflammatory Disease

PID is an infectious process that most commonly involves the uterine tubes, uterus, and rarely the ovaries and peritoneal surfaces. Multiple organisms have been found to cause PID, and common agents include *N. gonorrhoeae, C. trachomatis,* and a variety of other aerobic and anaerobic bacteria. It is estimated that each year 800,000 women of reproductive age experience an episode of PID, with high rates occurring in adolescents (Trent, 2013). Women younger than 25 years old have a 1 in 8 chance of experiencing PID compared with those older than 25 years of age, whose risk is 1 in 80 (Trent, 2013).

Women who have had PID are at increased risk for ectopic pregnancy, infertility, and chronic pelvic pain. Other problems associated with PID include dyspareunia, pyosalpinx, tubo-ovarian abscess, and pelvic adhesions.

Presenting symptoms in adolescents may be generalized, but pain is a common symptom in all infections. The pain can be dull, cramping, intermittent, persistent, and incapacitating. Women may also report fever, chills, abdominal pain, nausea and vomiting, increased vaginal discharge, urinary tract symptoms, and irregular bleeding. A pelvic examination is indicated for every sexually active woman who complains of lower abdominal pain to evaluate for the possibility of PID.

Prevention is the primary concern of health care professionals. Primary prevention includes education on avoiding contracting STIs; secondary prevention involves preventing a lower genital tract infection from ascending to the upper genital tract. Barrier contraceptive methods, such as condoms, are critical. PID is usually treated with antibiotics to provide empiric, broad-spectrum coverage of likely pathogens. Recommended regimens can be found in the 2015 Sexually Transmitted Diseases Treatment Guidelines (https://www.cdc.gov/std/tg2015/pid.htm).

Treatment for mild to moderate PID may be oral (e.g., ceftriaxone plus doxycycline with or without metronidazole) or parenteral (e.g., cefotetan or cefoxitin plus doxycycline [oral]), and regimens can be administered in inpatient or outpatient settings. Pregnant women should be hospitalized and given parenteral antibiotics. Women should be counseled to comply with therapy and complete all medication, even if symptoms have disappeared. Follow-up after treatment should include endocervical cultures to test for cure.

Sexual Violence

Sexual violence means that someone forces or manipulates someone else into unwanted sexual activity without their consent. Reasons someone might not consent include fear, age, illness, disability, and/or influence of alcohol or other drugs. Anyone can experience sexual violence, including children, teens, adults, and elders. Those who sexually abuse can be acquaintances, family members, trusted individuals, or strangers. This violence includes rape or sexual assault, child sexual assault and incest, intimate partner sexual assault, unwanted sexual contact or touching, sexual harassment, sexual exploitation, showing one's genitals or naked body to others without consent, masturbating in public, and watching someone in a private act without their knowledge or permission.

According to the Centers for Disease Control and Prevention, 1 in 3 women and 1 in 4 men experience sexual violence involving physical contact during their lifetimes. Nearly 1 in 5 women and 1 in 38 men have experienced completed or attempted rape, and 1 in 14 men were made to penetrate someone (completed or attempted) during their lifetime. In addition, 1 in 3 female rape victims experienced rape for the first time between 11 and 17 years old, and 1 in 8 reported that it occurred before age 10 years. Nearly 1 in 4 male rape victims experienced rape for the first time between 11 and 17 years old, and about 1 in 4 reported that it occurred before age 10 years.

Typically, stranger rape is what comes to mind when one thinks of sexual assault; however, more than half of assaults are committed by someone known to the survivor. Although both males and females can be sexually assaulted, females are at greatest risk. Adolescents are at high risk for sexual assault; other high-risk groups include survivors of childhood sexual or physical abuse; persons who are disabled; persons with substance abuse problems; sex workers; persons who are poor or homeless; and persons living in prisons, institutions, or areas of military conflict. Sexual assault remains underreported for multifactorial reasons.

An understanding of the legal definitions of sexual assault, rape, acquaintance rape, and statutory rape is essential for the nurse to identify, treat, and manage adolescent victims (Box 16.2).

Statutory rape laws have been revised in many states across the country. The motivation for tougher laws and greater enforcement is to decrease teen pregnancy, increase male responsibility, and decrease welfare dependency. Traditionally, statutory rape laws have been

BOX 16.2 Definitions of Sexual Assaults

Sexual assault: Comprehensive term that includes various types of forced or inappropriate sexual activity. Sexual assault includes both physical and psychologic coercion as well as touch, penetration, and other sexual contact.

Rape: Forced sexual intercourse that occurs by physical force or psychologic coercion. Rape includes vaginal, anal, or oral penetration by body parts or inanimate objects.

Acquaintance rape (date rape): Applied to situations in which the assailant and victim know each other.

Statutory rape: Consensual sexual contact by a person 18 years old or older with a person under the age of consent or unable to consent because of developmental disability. Age of consent varies by state.

concerned with the protection of girls. In the past 20 years, many laws have been rewritten to be gender neutral. Statutory rape laws require reporting to child protective services or local law enforcement. One risk of strict statutory rape enforcement is that girls may not seek health care for reproductive care, prenatal care, or domestic violence. Young people may fear not only for themselves but also for their partners. However, sexual coercion of teens by adults remains a problem and results in STIs and adolescent pregnancy.

Nurses can obtain information about their state's rape reporting responsibilities from state or local child protective services agencies, legal counsel, rape crisis organizations, state or local law enforcement agencies, or the state nurses' association. The limits of confidentiality should be clearly reviewed with each adolescent patient before beginning an interview about sexual activity.

Sexual assault victims may be targets of sex trafficking. Sex trafficking is a type of human trafficking and is a form of modern-day slavery. It is a serious public health problem that negatively affects the well-being of individuals, families, and communities. Human trafficking occurs when a trafficker exploits an individual with force, fraud, or coercion to make them perform commercial sex or work. Perpetrators of human trafficking often target people who are poor, vulnerable, living in an unsafe situation, or searching for a better life. Victims are trapped and controlled through assault, threats, false promises, perceived sense of protection, isolation, shaming, and debt. Signs and symptoms of sex trafficking can be found at https://humantraffickinghotline.org/human-trafficking/recognizing-signs.

Diagnostic Evaluation

Sexual assault victims may exhibit a variety of reactions (Box 16.3), and the circumstances of the initial medical evaluation may be frightening and stressful. The initial contact with the assault victim must be supportive, because the interrogation and associated activities have the potential to add to the trauma of the sexual assault. First, the victim needs to know that she (or he) is (1) all right and (2) not being blamed for the situation.

It is important to obtain a clear account of the circumstances of an alleged assault without forcing the victim to relive a painful experience. Information includes the date, time, location, and an accurate description of any type of sexual contact. The physical examination is carried out as soon as possible because physical evidence deteriorates rapidly. The victim should not bathe or shower before the examination.

The young person is always told in advance in understandable terms exactly what to expect in the way of tests and procedures, and

BOX 16.3 Clinical Manifestations of Sexual Assault Victims

May display a variety of emotions and behaviors, such as:

- Hysterical crying
- Giggling
- Agitation
- Feelings of degradation
- Anger and rage
- Helplessness
- Nervousness
- Rapid mood swings
- Appearing calm and controlled (masking inner turmoil)
- Confusion
- Self-blame
- Fear—of the rape and of injury

There may be evidence of physical force from the following:

- Roughness
- Nonbrutal beating (slapping)
- Brutal beating (slugging, kicking, beating repeatedly with fists)
- Choking or gagging

Medical examination provides evidence of:

- Penetration
- Ejaculation
- Use of force

! NURSING ALERT

It is common for sexual assault victims to delay seeking help, especially in cases of acquaintance or date rape. Nurses can be most supportive by acknowledging the painful and sometimes confusing feelings that surround such experiences and by focusing on the fact that the victim is seeking assistance now.

the explanation is accompanied by strong emotional support. The victim is examined thoroughly, including nongenital areas, for evidence of injury that might substantiate the use of force.

The forensic examination of a sexual assault victim must follow strict legal requirements. The medical record may provide key evidence for the legal case. Practitioners specially trained for rape examination should be used when possible. Nurses are often members of this group and are known as **sexual assault nurse examiners (SANEs)**. Evaluation for STIs is an important part of the examination. The following procedures are recommended for the initial examination: nucleic acid amplified testing (NAAT) for chlamydia and gonorrhea; wet mount and culture or point-of-care testing of a vaginal swab specimen for trichomoniasis; and a serum sample for HIV infection, hepatitis B, and syphilis. Decisions to perform these tests should be made on an individual basis. Repeat testing for chlamydia and gonorrhea can be done at 2 weeks if prophylactic treatment was not administered. Serologic tests for syphilis and HIV infection can be repeated 6 weeks, 3 months, and 6 months after the assault if infection in the assailant could not be ruled out (Centers for Disease Control and Prevention, 2015).

Prophylactic treatment for chlamydia, gonorrhea, and trichomoniasis is recommended. Vaccination for hepatitis B should be administered if the patient has not been vaccinated previously. Follow-up doses of vaccine should be administered 1 to 2 and 4 to 6 months after the first dose. Female victims should be provided with emergency contraception. The recommendation for HIV prophylaxis varies depending on the geographic area, the circumstances of the assault, and the known HIV status of the perpetrator. The Centers for Disease Control and Prevention (2015) maintains updates and recommendations for treatment of STIs incurred as a result of sexual assault.[a]

Therapeutic Management

Adolescents who have been sexually assaulted arrive at the emergency department or practitioner's office under a variety of circumstances. They are usually brought by parents, friends, or police officers, but some may seek medical help on their own. It is advisable to obtain parental consent for examination, but the examination may be performed without parental consent if the adolescent is mature and the parents are unavailable. A female observer or chaperone should be present during the history and examination of female victims who are examined by a male practitioner. Whether a parent should be present during the examination is determined on an individual basis. The parent's presence is usually encouraged if the parent is supportive and the young person agrees.

Nursing Care Management

Many of the approaches that have been described for sexually abused children (see Chapter 13) also apply to adolescents. Sexual assault is a devastating experience with long-lasting effects. The primary goal of nursing care is to avoid inflicting further stress on the adolescent, who is often angry, confused, frightened, embarrassed, and filled with self-blame. The nurse must do everything possible to reduce the stress of the interrogation and examination. Although most health professionals and law enforcement officers are sensitive to the needs of adolescents and attempt to make the process as nonstressful as possible, the nurse should be alert to cues that indicate that the victim is being overstressed.

The consequences of sexual violence are physical, such as bruising and genital injuries, and psychologic, such as depression, anxiety, and suicidal thoughts. The consequences may also be chronic. Victims may suffer from PTSD and experience recurring gynecologic, gastrointestinal, cardiovascular, and sexual health problems. Sexual violence is also linked to negative health behaviors. For example, victims are more likely to smoke (Centers for Disease Control and Prevention, 2015).

Follow-up care of the assault victim is essential and extends over a long period. Aside from the universal need for emotional support, the needs of assault victims vary widely and depend on the nature of the incident, the victim's age when the assault occurred, the physical and emotional injuries sustained by the victim, the legal actions being considered as a result, the resources available for informal support, and the anticipated reactions of persons in the informal support network (see Family-Centered Care box).[b] https://www.cdc.gov/violenceprevention/pdf/SV-Prevention-Technical-Package.pdf

FAMILY-CENTERED CARE

Supporting the Sexual Assault Victim's Parents

In addition to the needs of the adolescent assault victim, the nurse should also be sensitive to the needs and reactions of the adolescent's parents. Some parents will be angry and blame the adolescent; others will feel guilty and embarrassed. Many reactions can be expected at the time of the incident, ranging from despair to extreme agitation. Frequently the parents require as much support and reassurance as the victim. Agitated, angry, or incapacitated parents are unable to provide support for their adolescent. Meeting their needs can foster their ability to support the teenager during the crisis.

[a]https://www.cdc.gov/std/tg2015/sexual-assault.htm

[b]For information about local organizations, contact National Organization for Victim Assistance, 510 King St., Suite 424, Alexandria, VA 22314; 800-879-6682 or 703-535-6682; http://www.trynova.org.

NUTRITION AND EATING DISORDERS

Obesity

Few problems in childhood and adolescence are so obvious to others, are so difficult to treat, and have such long-term effects on health as obesity. Several different definitions have been proposed for obesity and overweight. **Obesity** has been defined as an increase in body weight resulting from an excessive accumulation of body fat relative to lean body mass. **Overweight** refers to the state of weighing more than average for height and body build. Currently, the **body mass index (BMI)** measurement is recommended as the most accurate method for screening children and adolescents for obesity. The BMI measurement is strongly associated with subcutaneous and total body fat and with skinfold thickness measurements. It is also highly specific for children with the greatest amount of body fat. Pediatric growth charts that include BMI for age and gender are available from the Centers for Disease Control and Prevention.[c] A new classification system recognizes BMI at the 95th percentile or greater as class I obesity, BMI at 120% or greater of the 95th percentile as class II obesity, and BMI at 140% or greater of the 95th percentile as class III obesity. Classes II and III obesity are strongly associated with greater cardiovascular and metabolic risk (Skinner, Perrin, Moss, et al., 2015).

It is important to note that for children with high levels of muscle mass (e.g., athletes), the BMI measurement may misclassify these youth into overweight or obesity. Clinical judgment is needed to understand whether these youth are at risk for obesity.

Numerous studies dating back to the early 1960s have documented childhood overweight through comprehensive evaluations of dietary intake, physical activity, and anthropometric measures; examplies include the National Health and Nutrition Examination Surveys [NHANESs], I, II, III, and IV) (Ogden, Carroll, Kit, et al., 2014; Ogden, Kuczmarski, Flegal, et al., 2002; Ogden, Troiano, Briefel, et al., 1997). In the 1960s and 1970s, the rate of childhood overweight remained fairly constant at approximately 4% to 5.5%. However, surveys conducted during the 1990s and early 2000s demonstrated a steady climb to reach a rate of 17% in both children and adolescents (Flegal, Carroll, Kit, et al., 2012; Ogden et al., 2014). This prevalence has remained stable since 2003, but overall the incidence remains high (Ogden et al., 2014). Non-Hispanic African American and Hispanic children had higher prevalence rates of overweight and all classes of obesity compared with other races. Asian American children had markedly lower rates of overweight and all classes of obesity. The prevalence of overweight and obesity increased with age, with 41.5% of 16- to 19-year-old adolescents having obesity and 4.5% meeting the criteria for class III obesity.

Because adult obesity is associated with increased mortality and morbidity from a variety of complications, both physical and psychologic, adolescent obesity is a serious condition. For the first time in US history, the current generation of children will have a shorter life expectancy than their parents (American Heart Association, 2014). Children, adolescents, and young adults now have obesity-related conditions—type 2 diabetes, liver disease, hypertension, sleep apnea, and more—that were once rarely seen before adulthood and are compromising their current and future health.

Parental obesity increases the risk of overweight by twofold to threefold (Altman & Wilfley, 2015). The probability that overweight children will become obese adolescents is significant. In a large longitudinal study, overweight kindergarteners were four times more likely to become obese by 14 years old than normal-weight kindergarteners (Cunningham, Kramer, & Narayan, 2014).

[c]http://www.cdc.gov/growthcharts

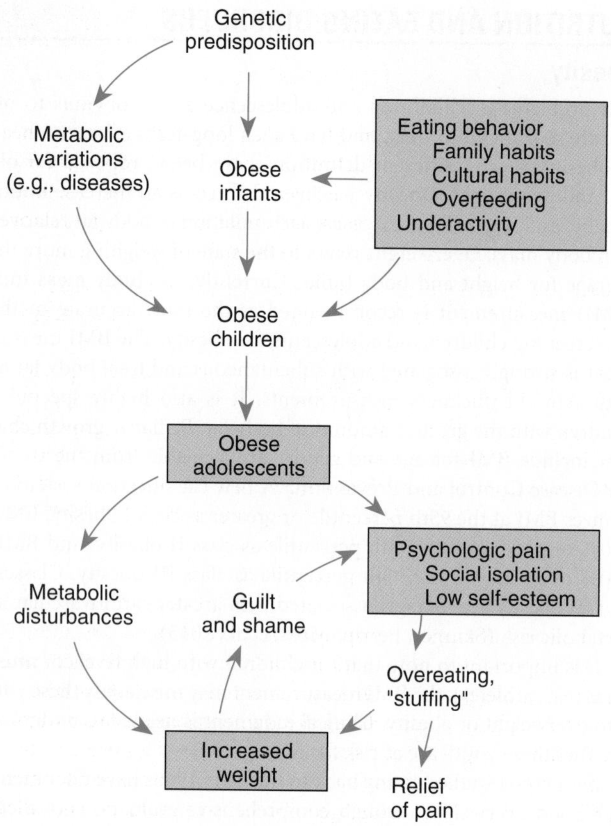

Fig. 16.2 Complex relationships in obesity.

Common emotional consequences of obesity include low self-esteem, social isolation, anxiety, depression, and an increased risk for the development of eating disorders (Altman & Wilfley, 2015).

Etiology and Pathophysiology

Obesity results from a caloric intake that consistently exceeds caloric requirements and expenditure, and may involve a variety of interrelated influences, including metabolic, hypothalamic, hereditary, social, cultural, and psychologic factors (Fig. 16.2). Because the etiology of obesity is multifactorial, the treatment requires multilevel interventions.

A balance between **energy intake** and **energy expenditure** is a critical factor in regulating body weight. For example, eating one small chocolate chip cookie (50 calories) is equivalent to walking briskly for 10 minutes. Factors that raise energy intake or decrease energy expenditure by even small amounts can have a long-term impact on the development of overweight and obesity.

Genetic influence is an epidemiologic consideration regarding children's weight. Genetic mutations, such as FTO (fat mass and obesity), are rare but can predispose individuals to becoming overweight or obese (Gahagan, 2020). Studies have also suggested a tendency for a combination of genetic and environmental factors. Obesity is determined by the genetics as well as the obesogenic environment. Obesogenic environment refers to the cheap and easy availability of a high-calorie diet and sedentary lifestyle. Genetics, the environment, and their complex interaction need to be considered to have a better understanding of obesity. More research is needed to better understand the influences of family behavior and adolescent overweight.

Fewer than 5% of the cases of childhood obesity can be attributed to an underlying disease. Such diseases include hypothyroidism; adrenal hypercorticoidism; hyperinsulinism; and dysfunction or damage to the CNS as a result of tumor, injury, infection, or vascular accident. Obesity is a frequent complication of muscular dystrophy, paraplegia, Down syndrome, spina bifida, and other chronic illnesses that limit mobility.

A major focus of obesity research has been **appetite regulation**. The expression of appetite is chemically coded in the hypothalamus by distinctive circuitry involved in drive and motivation. Orexigenic substances produce signals that increase appetite, and anorexigenic substances promote the cessation of eating behaviors. Feedback loops between signals have been identified where one signal peptide is able to alter the secretion of another signal peptide. No one signal has been identified as the gatekeeper of appetite. It is apparent that an entire network of signals, including their frequency and amplitude, is responsible for triggering eating behaviors.

There is little evidence to support a relationship between obesity and **low metabolism**. Small differences may exist between obese and nonobese children in regulation of dietary intake or metabolic rate that could lead to an energy imbalance and inappropriate weight gain, but these small differences are difficult to accurately quantify. Obese children tend to be less active than lean children, but it is uncertain whether inactivity creates the obesity or obesity is responsible for the inactivity. The tendency toward obesity is manifested whenever environmental conditions are favorable toward excessive caloric intake, such as an abundance of food, limited access to low-fat foods, reduced or minimum physical activity, and snacking combined with excessive screen time (computer, television, video games, cell phone). Family and cultural eating patterns as well as psychologic factors play important roles; many families and cultures consider fat to be an indication of good health. It is common for obese children to have families that emphasize large meals, admonish children for leaving food on their plates, or use food as a reward or punishment. Parents may have an exaggerated concept of the amount of food children require and expect them to eat more than they need.

Particular individuals at increased risk of having low levels of physical activity have been identified and include children who are from ethnic minorities (especially girls) in the preadolescent and adolescent age-groups, children living in poverty, children with disabilities, children residing in apartments or public housing, and children living in neighborhoods where outdoor physical activity is restricted by climate, safety concerns, or lack of facilities (Cradock, Barrett, Kenney, et al., 2017).

Some **community factors** that influence eating and activity patterns include a lack of built environment (food deserts, community gardens, farmers markets, sidewalks, parks, bike paths) or affordable and accessible facilities for low-income youth to be active, thus limiting their opportunities to participate in physical activities or healthful eating. Social policies also contribute to obesity. The increased availability of energy-dense foods, pricing strategies that promote unhealthy food choices, and overzealous food advertising that targets children and adolescents with high-fat and high-sugar foods are some examples (Schwartz & Ustjanauskas, 2012).

Institutional factors also influence patterns of obesity and decreased physical activity. Many school policies allow students to leave school for lunch. Vending machines in school often are filled with high-fat and high-calorie foods and soft drinks. Although well-balanced, nutritious school lunches may be available to students, they often opt for less nutritious choices, such as high-fat and high-sugar snacks.

Physical inactivity has also been identified as an important contributing factor in the development and maintenance of childhood overweight. There is little doubt that physical activity has decreased in elementary and secondary schools in the United States.

The Institute of Medicine recommends that schools take a "whole-of-school approach" to provide students with 60 daily minutes of physical activity, at least half of which should occur during the school day. Many children do not meet the recommended physical activity levels.

Consequently, most of children's physical activity must occur within the family or outside of school, which is often limited by community factors (e.g., unsafe neighborhoods). Decreased physical activity within the family is a powerful influence on children because children imitate their parents and other adults.

The growing attraction and availability of many sedentary activities, including television, video games, computers, and the Internet, have greatly influenced the amount of exercise that children get. Studies have shown the association between screen time and obesity among children (Robinson, Banda, Hale, et al., 2017):

- The American Academy of Pediatrics (2016) issued recommendations for children's media use. For children younger than 18 months of age, avoid use of screen media other than video chatting. Parents of children 18 to 24 months of age who want to introduce digital media should choose high-quality programming and watch it with their children to help them understand what they're seeing.
- For children ages 2 to 5 years, limit screen use to 1 hour per day of high-quality programs. Parents should co-view media with children to help them understand what they are seeing and apply it to the world around them.
- For children ages 6 years and older, place consistent limits on the time spent using media, and the types of media, and make sure that media do not take the place of adequate sleep, physical activity, and other behaviors essential to health.
- Designate media-free times together, such as dinner or driving, as well as media-free locations at home, such as bedrooms.
- Have ongoing communication about online citizenship and safety, including treating others with respect both online and offline.

Psychologic factors also affect eating patterns. Infants experience relief from discomfort through feeding and learn to associate eating with a sense of well-being, security, and the comforting presence of a nurturing person. Eating is soon associated with the feeling of being loved. In addition, the pleasurable oral sensation of sucking provides a connection between emotions and early eating behavior. Many parents use food as a positive reward for desired behaviors. This practice may become a habit, and the child may continue to use food as a reward, a comfort, and a means of dealing with depression or hostility. Many individuals eat when they are not hungry or in response to stress, boredom, loneliness, sadness, depression, or tiredness. Difficulty in determining feelings of satiety can lead to weight problems and may compound the factor of eating in response to emotional rather than physical hunger cues.

Diagnostic Evaluation

A careful history is obtained regarding the development of obesity, and a physical examination is performed to differentiate simple obesity from increased fat that results from organic causes. A family history of obesity, diabetes, coronary heart disease, and dyslipidemia should be obtained for all children who are overweight or at risk for overweight. Specific information from the patient and family about the effects of obesity on daily functioning—for example, problems with nighttime breathing and sleep, daytime sleepiness, joint pain, ability to keep up with family activities and peers at school—is helpful. The physical examination should focus on identifying comorbid conditions and identifiable causes of obesity. For some, psychologic assessment, by interviews and standardized personality tests, may provide insight into the personality and emotional problems that contribute to obesity and that might interfere with therapy.

It is useful to estimate the degree of obesity to determine the component of body weight that can be modified. All of these methods have been used to assess obesity: BMI, body weight, weight-height ratios, weight-age ratios, hydrostatic weight, dual-energy x-ray absorptiometry (DXA), skinfold measurements, bioelectrical analysis, computed tomography (CT), magnetic resonance imaging (MRI), and neutron activation. Each of these methods has advantages and disadvantages. Hydrostatic weighing provides the most accurate measurement of lean body weight.

TABLE 16.5 Pediatric Quality Indicator[a]

Weight Assessment and Counseling for Nutrition and Physical Activity	
Measure	Children and adolescents 3 to 17 years of age who had an outpatient visit and had evidence of the following during the measurement period: height, weight, and body mass index (BMI) percentile documentation, and counseling on nutrition and physical activity.
Numerator	Number of children with BMI percentile documentation, counseling on nutrition, and counseling on physical activity during the measurement time.
Denominator	Number of children 3 to 17 years of age with at least one outpatient visit.

[a]Endorsed by the National Quality Forum NQF #0024 and 2019 Core Set of Children's Health Care Quality Measures for Medicaid and CHIP. https://www.medicaid.gov/federal-policy-guidance/downloads/cib112018.pdf.

BMI is currently considered the best method to assess weight in children and adolescents. The calculation is based on the individual's height and weight. In adults, BMI definitions are fixed measures without regard for sex and age. The BMI in children and adolescents varies to accommodate age- and gender-specific changes in growth. The formula for BMI calculation is weight in kilograms divided by height in meters squared: weight (kg) ÷ (height $[m]^2$). BMI measures in children and adolescents are plotted on growth charts that enable health care professionals to determine BMI for age for the patient.

$$\frac{\text{Weight in pounds} \div \text{Height in inches} \times 703}{\text{Height in inches}}$$

The initial assessment of obese children and adolescents should include screening to evaluate for comorbidities. The history is an important guide to determine the workup. A complete physical examination is important. Some areas to focus on include (1) skin for stretch markings and discolorations (e.g., acanthosis nigricans), (2) joints for swelling and evidence of pain, and (3) airway for evidence of obstruction and enlarged tonsils. Basic laboratory studies include a fasting lipid panel, fasting insulin level, and fasting glucose hepatic enzymes, including gamma-glutamyl transferase (GGT) and, in some institutions, hemoglobin A1c. Other studies, such as a polysomnogram (sleep study), metabolic studies, and radiographic evaluations, may be added based on the history and physical examination. These assessments may determine whether the patient needs a referral to specialty services for more focused evaluation and treatment, such as endocrinology (insulin resistance, diabetes), hepatology (elevated liver enzymes, nonalcoholic fatty liver disease [NAFLD]), orthopedics (Blount disease), or pulmonary medicine (sleep-disordered breathing, continuous positive airway pressure [CPAP]).

Therapeutic Management

The best approach to the management of obesity is a preventive one. The Pediatric Quality Indicator for weight assessment and counseling for nutrition and physical activity is found in Table 16.5. Early recognition and control measures are essential before the child or adolescent

BOX 16.4 Recommended Behaviors for Preventing Obesity

In counseling adolescents whose body mass index (BMI) is between the 5th and 84th percentiles, physicians and health care providers should recommend the following steps to prevent obesity:

- Limit consumption of sugar-sweetened beverages.
- Consume recommended quantities of fruits and vegetables.
- Limit screen time to no more than 2 hours per day.
- Remove television and computer screens from primary sleeping areas.
- Eat breakfast daily.
- Limit eating at restaurants.
- Have frequent family meals in which parents and youth eat together.
- Limit portion sizes.

Adapted from Davis, D. M., Gance-Cleveland, B., Hassink, S., et al. (2007). Recommendations for prevention of childhood obesity. *Pediatrics, 120*(Suppl), S229–S253.

reaches an obese state. Health care providers need to educate families about the medical complications of obesity.

Currently, the only treatments recommended for children are diet, exercise, behavior modification, and in some situations pharmacologic agents, such as orlistat. The treatment of obesity is difficult. Many approaches do not achieve long-term success. The average individual loses only about 5% to 10% of his or her weight with available therapies. Losing weight can have a significant positive effect on many comorbidities, but unfortunately the lost weight is frequently regained in a year or two. A number of multidisciplinary programs offer interventions combining medical, dietary, exercise, and psychologic support. This therapy is labor intensive and costly. **Diet modification** is an essential part of weight reduction programs. Dietary counseling focuses on improving the nutritional quality of the diet rather than on dietary restriction. Children and adolescents should avoid fad diets. Most dietitians and nutrition experts recommend a diet with no trans fats, low in saturated fat, moderate in total fat (≤30%), low in sodium, and with at least nine servings of fruits and vegetables, consistent with the MyPlate[d] food guide for children. Also, promoting high-fiber foods and avoiding highly refined starches and sugars decrease caloric intake. Many programs recommend using a food diary as a helpful tool to increase awareness of food choices and eating behaviors. The goal is to encourage the individual to make healthy choices in food selection and discourage using food by habit or to appease boredom. Box 16.4 contains helpful suggestions.

In patients with severe obesity, strict diets have been used, such as the protein-sparing modified fast, hypocaloric diet, or ketogenic diet (Castaldo, Palmieri, Galdo, et al., 2016; Sukkar, Signori, Borrini, et al., 2013). These diets are designed to provide enough protein to minimize loss of lean body mass during weight loss. Such diets need to be closely monitored and should be used only with multidisciplinary teams that include a physician, nutritionist, and behavioral therapist. Generally, the diet consists of 1.5 to 2.5 g of protein per kilogram. The intake of carbohydrates is low enough to induce ketosis. The benefits of the diet are relatively rapid weight loss and anorexia induced by ketosis. Potential complications include protein losses, hypokalemia, hypoglycemia, inadequate calcium intake, orthostatic hypotension, and increased risk for osteoporosis. It is difficult to sustain these diets over the long term, and the long-term outcomes of using these diets have not been established. Treatment of childhood and adolescent obesity is an active area of research. Comprehensive behavioral interventions including changes in diet, physical activity, and lifestyles involving individual patients or families are commonly used and generally considered primary modes of treatment.

Behavioral modification approaches to weight loss are based on the observation that obese individuals have abnormal eating practices that can be altered. Attention is focused not on food but on the social and behavioral aspects surrounding food consumption. Successful behavior modification weight programs help adolescents identify and eliminate inappropriate eating habits and include a problem-solving component that enables adolescents to identify problems and determine solutions. Programs including family-based behavioral modification, dietary modification, and exercise have been shown to be successful in reducing obesity in some children (Altman & Wilfley, 2015). Behavior modification is an important part of multidisciplinary intervention programs.

Surgical techniques (bariatric surgery) that bypass portions of the intestine or occlude a segment of the stomach to produce a marked diet restriction and weight loss are hazardous and cause many metabolic complications. These complications include severe water and electrolyte depletion, persistent diarrhea, vitamin deficiency, internal herniation, and fatty infiltration and degeneration of the liver. Bariatric surgery may be the only practical alternative for increasing numbers of severely overweight adolescents who have failed organized attempts to lose or maintain weight loss through conventional nonoperative approaches and who have serious life-threatening conditions. Physicians must define clear, realistic, and restrictive guidelines to apply with younger patients when surgery is considered. Candidates for surgery should be referred to centers that offer a multidisciplinary team experienced in the management of childhood and adolescent obesity. The surgery should be performed by surgeons who have participated in subspecialty training in bariatric medical and surgical care as detailed by the American College of Surgeons and the American Society for Metabolic and Bariatric Surgery.

Nursing Care Management

Nurses play a key role in the adherence and maintenance phases of many weight reduction programs. Nurses assess, manage, and evaluate the progress of many overweight adolescents. They also play an important role in recognizing potential weight problems and assisting parents and adolescents in preventing obesity.

The presence of obesity may not be obvious from appearance alone. Regular assessment of height and weight and computation of the BMI facilitate early recognition of risk. Evaluation includes a height and weight history of the adolescent and family members, eating habits, appetite and hunger patterns, and physical activities. A psychosocial history is also helpful in understanding the impact of obesity on the child's life. Steps to approaching behavior change with youth are described in Box 16.5.

Before initiating a treatment plan, it is important to be certain that the family is ready for change. Lack of readiness may result in failure, frustration, and reluctance to address the problem in the future. The nurse should explore with adolescents the reasons behind the desire to lose weight because motivation to lose weight is the key to success. Adolescents need to take personal responsibility for their dietary habits and physical activity. Young persons who are forced by their parents to seek help are seldom motivated, become rebellious, and are unwilling to control their dietary intake.

Nutritional counseling. Preventing an increase in body fat during growth is a realistic approach. This is often accomplished by adjusting four aspects of eating: (1) reducing the quantity eaten by purchasing, preparing, and serving smaller portions; (2) altering

[d]http://www.choosemyplate.gov.

BOX 16.5 Pediatric Obesity Prevention Protocol for Primary Care

Step 1: Assess

Explain and conduct assessments of:

- Weight, height, and body mass index (BMI) percentile
- Dietary intake (fruit, vegetables, sweetened beverages, fast food)
- Activity (screen time, moderate to vigorous activity)
- Eating behaviors (breakfast, portion sizes, family meals)

Provide and elicit feedback on BMI and behaviors found to be inside and outside the optimal range.

Step 2: Set Agenda

Explore interest in changing behaviors not in the optimal range.

Agree on target behaviors with the patient and caregiver.

Step 3: Assess Motivation and Confidence

Regarding interest in changing weight status or behaviors, assess:

- Willingness and ability to make change
- Perceived importance
- Confidence in having success

Probe the patient regarding ratings of willingness, perceived importance, and confidence to explore the advantages and disadvantages of changing.

Step 4: Summarize and Probe Possible Changes

Summarize the advantages and disadvantages of change.

Query possible next steps. Allow the adolescent to suggest ideas.

Provide guidance for getting started in making a change as needed. Encourage achievable goals.

Summarize the change plan.

Provide positive feedback.

Step 5: Schedule Follow-Up Visit

If a change plan is made, agree on a follow-up appointment within a specified number of weeks or months.

If no change plan is made, agree to revisit the topic within a specific number of weeks or months.

Adapted from Davis, D. M., Gance-Cleveland, B., Hassink, S., et al. (2007). Recommendations for prevention of childhood obesity. *Pediatrics, 120*(Suppl), S229–S253.

the quality consumed by substituting low-calorie, low-fat foods for high-calorie foods (especially snacks); (3) eating regular meals and snacks, particularly breakfast; and (4) altering situations by severing associations between eating and other stimuli, such as eating while watching television. Nutrition counseling incorporates health behavior theories to help motivate and maintain behavior change. The most successful changes are those that are attainable, reasonable, and sustainable. The emphasis of counseling should be on health outcomes, not weight. Studies have shown that focusing on weight can be detrimental to therapies and may promote eating disorders (Altman & Wilfley, 2015).

The American Academy of Pediatrics recommends that children older than 2 years of age and adolescents whose weight falls in the overweight category be put on a weight maintenance program to slow the progress of weight gain. This strategy allows the child to add inches in height but not pounds, causing the BMI to drop over time into a healthier range. Children ages 6 to 11 years who are obese might be encouraged to modify their eating habits for gradual weight loss of no more than 1 pound (or about 0.5 kg) a month. Older children and adolescents who are obese or severely obese might be encouraged to modify their eating habits to aim for weight loss of up to 2 pounds (or about 1 kg) a week.

Behavioral therapy. Altering eating behavior and eliminating inappropriate eating habits are essential to weight reduction, especially in maintaining long-term weight control. Most behavioral modification programs include the following concepts:

- A description of the behavior to be controlled, such as eating habits
- Attempts to modify and control the stimuli that govern eating
- Development of eating techniques designed to control speed of eating
- Positive reinforcement for these modifications through a suitable reward system that does not include food
- Creating environments in which the healthy choice is the easy choice

Group involvement. Commercial groups or diet workshops composed primarily of adults may be helpful to some teenagers; however, a peer group is often more effective. Adolescent groups include summer camps designed for obese young people and conducted by health professionals, school groups organized and led by a school nurse or health professional, and groups associated with special clinics.

These groups are concerned not only with weight loss but also with the development of a positive self-image and the encouragement of physical activity. Nutrition education, diet planning, and the improvement of social skills are essential components of these groups. Improvement is determined by positive changes in all aspects of behavior.

Family involvement. There is a definite connection among family environment, interaction, and obesity. The nurse needs to educate parents in the purposes of the therapeutic measures and their role in management. The family needs nutrition education and counseling regarding the reinforcement plan, alterations in the food environment, and ways to maintain proper attitudes. They can support their child in efforts to change eating behaviors, food intake, and physical activity.

Physical activity. The current recommendation for physical activity for children and adolescents is to participate in a combined total of 60 minutes of physical activity daily; this can be moderate- to vigorous-intensive exercise or activity (Centers for Disease Control and Prevention, 2015). Regular physical activity is incorporated into all weight reduction programs. Recommendations for physical activity need to consider the current health status and developmental level of the child or adolescent. The best choice for exercise is any form that is enjoyable and likely to be sustainable. Light exercises, such as walking, may provide an opportunity for the family to increase time together and increase caloric expenditure. Weight training can increase the basal metabolic rate and replace fat mass with muscle mass. However, weight training is not generally recommended for prepubertal children until they have reached physical and skeletal maturity. In prepubertal children, increasing outdoor play time is likely to be beneficial. Limiting sedentary activities such as television viewing while eating snacks is very beneficial.

Prevention. Gradual accumulation of adipose tissue during childhood establishes a pattern of eating that is difficult to reverse in adolescence. Prevention of obesity should begin in early childhood with the development of healthy eating habits, regular exercise patterns, and a positive relationship between parents and children. Prevention of adolescent obesity is best accomplished by early identification of obesity in the preschool, school-age, and preadolescent periods. Health care professionals should encourage frequent health care visits for children who are overweight or obese and incorporate a dietary history and counseling into each well-infant, well-child, and well-adolescent visit.

Anorexia Nervosa and Bulimia Nervosa

Anorexia nervosa (AN) is an eating disorder characterized by a refusal to maintain a minimally normal body weight and by severe weight loss in the absence of obvious physical causes. It is a disorder with social, psychologic, behavioral, cultural, and physiologic components that result in significant morbidity and mortality. The disorder is a clinical diagnosis listed in the DSM-5 (American Psychiatric Association, 2013). Individuals with AN are described as perfectionists, academically high achievers, conforming, and conscientious.

Bulimia (from the Greek meaning "ox hunger") refers to an eating disorder similar to AN. Bulimia nervosa (BN) is characterized by repeated episodes of binge eating followed by inappropriate compensatory behaviors, such as self-induced vomiting; misuse of laxatives, diuretics, or other medications; fasting; or excessive exercise (American Psychiatric Association, 2013). The binge behavior consists of secretive, frenzied consumption of large amounts of high-calorie (or "forbidden") foods during a brief time (usually ≈2 hours). The binge is counteracted by a variety of weight control methods (purging). These binge–purge cycles are followed by self-deprecating thoughts, a depressed mood, and an awareness that the eating pattern is abnormal.

Eating disorder not otherwise specified (EDNOS) is an additional diagnosis for eating disorders. These disorders have components of both AN and BN that are not characteristics of the established diagnostic criteria for AN and BN. Binge eating disorder (BED) is a type of EDNOS. Binge eating disorder (BED) is a distinct diagnostic category that is very similar to BN, with the exception that purging is not involved. EDNOS includes subthresholds of the aforementioned disorders, as well as purging disorder, night eating syndrome, and a residual category for clinically significant problems that meet the definition of a feeding or eating disorder but do not satisfy the criteria for any other disorder or condition (American Psychiatric Association, 2013).

According to eating disorders statistics estimated by the National Eating Disorders Association, in the United States up to 30 million people suffer from an eating disorder such as AN, BN, or BED. Worldwide the figure is more like 70 million sufferers. The problem with statistics on eating disorders is that many sufferers do not come forward for diagnosis due to embarrassment, denial, or confusion as to what their symptoms are. Based on diagnostic interview data from the National Comorbidity Survey Replication Adolescent Supplement (NCS-A), the lifetime prevalence of eating disorders among US adolescents ages 13 to 18 years was 2.7%. Eating disorders were more than twice as prevalent among females (3.8%) than males (1.5%).

These prevalences will likely climb as practitioners begin to use the new DSM-5 criteria. The DSM-5 Feeding and Eating Disorders chapter includes six entities: anorexia nervosa, bulimia nervosa, binge eating disorder, avoidant/restrictive food intake disorder (ARFID), rumination disorder, and pica. Unlike DSM-IV criteria for AN, DSM-5 does not include a requirement for amenorrhea, increasing the applicability of the diagnosis in males, premenarchal females, and postmenopausal females.

Etiology and Pathophysiology

The etiology of these disorders remains unclear. A combination of genetic, neurochemical, psychodevelopmental, sociocultural, and environmental factors appears to cause the disorder (Salafia, Jones, Haugen, et al., 2015). Dieting and body dissatisfaction appear to be common to the initiation of both AN and BN. Also characteristic is a childhood preoccupation with being thin reinforced by sociocultural and environmental factors, supporting the concepts of an ideal body shape. The dominant aspects of AN are a relentless pursuit of thinness and a fear of fatness, usually preceded by a period of mood disturbances and behavior changes.

These causes of anorexia nervosa are not necessarily black and white. Therefore if someone displays several risk factors, this does not guarantee that they will develop an eating disorder. On the other hand, the more of these contributing factors and causes of anorexia that a person possesses, the more likely they are to develop an eating disorder. There is also some evidence to support that some people may be genetically more likely to develop eating disorders. For example, eating disorders tend to run in families. A careful family history is therefore essential when assessing suspected eating disorders in patients

There are no strong empirical data to indicate that one particular family prototype is responsible for the development of an eating disorder. However, many experts have associated the development of an eating disorder with family characteristics, such as an adolescent perception of high parental expectations for achievement and appearance, difficulty managing conflict, poor communication styles, enmeshment and occasionally estrangement among family members, devaluation of the mother or the maternal role, marital tension, and mood and anxiety disorders. Adolescents whose parents focus on weight report higher levels of disordered eating (Salafia et al., 2015). Families struggling with an eating disorder have been characterized as often having difficulties responding positively to the changing physical and emotional needs of the adolescent. Family stress of any kind may become a significant factor in the development of an eating disorder (Salafia et al., 2015)

Individuals with eating disorders commonly have psychiatric problems, including affective disorder, anxiety disorder, obsessive-compulsive disorder (OCD), and personality disorder. Adult women with eating disorders were found to have higher rates of obsessive-compulsive behavior traits in their childhoods. It is important to note that many of the clinical findings are directly related to the state of starvation and improve with weight gain. Research continues in an effort to better understand the etiology and pathogenesis of eating disorders.

Many sports and artistic endeavors that emphasize leanness (e.g., ballet and running) and sports in which the scoring is partly subjective (e.g., figure skating and gymnastics) or where weight class is a prerequisite to participation (e.g., wrestling) have been associated with a higher incidence of eating disorders, as were described by some patients with an eating disorder (Salafia et al., 2015). The term female athlete triad was revised in 2007 to its current meaning to include one or more of the following three components: low energy availability (with or without disordered eating), menstrual dysfunction, and low bone mineral density (Ranson, Patterson, & Colvin, 2018). Published guidelines for determining triad risk stratification and providing guidance for clearance and return to play represent a critical step in the advancement of an evidence-based translation and need to be refined and validated going forward (De Souza, Nattiv, Joy, et al., 2014). It is critical that sports medicine practitioners and researchers continue to work together with these challenges in mind to achieve the goal of reducing the prevalence of the female athlete triad.

Diagnostic Evaluation

Diagnosis is made based on clinical manifestations (Box 16.6) and conformity to the criteria established by the American Psychiatric Association (2013). Characteristics of BN and AN are listed in Table 16.6.

BOX 16.6 Clinical Manifestations of Anorexia Nervosa

- Severe and profound weight loss
- Secondary amenorrhea (if menarche attained)
- Primary amenorrhea (if menarche not attained)
- Sinus bradycardia
- Low body temperature
- Hypotension
- Intolerance to cold
- Dry skin and brittle nails
- Appearance of lanugo hair
- Thinning hair
- Abdominal pain
- Bloating
- Constipation
- Fatigue
- Lightheadedness
- Evidence of muscle wasting (cachectic appearance)
- Bone pain with exercise

A complete history and physical examination are important to rule out other causes of weight loss. The medical assessment of an eating disorder focuses on the complications of altered nutritional status and purging. A careful history assesses weight changes, dietary patterns, and the frequency and severity of purging and excessive exercise. Purging behaviors include vomiting or other methods, such as abuse of laxatives, enemas, diuretics, anorexic drugs, caffeine, or other stimulants. Measure the patient's weight and height and evaluate it for appropriateness according to standard weight for height, age, and sex determined according to the percentile of his or her expected body weight or BMI.

Particularly important parts of the physical examination are vital sign measurement (heart and blood pressure, both supine and standing, and temperature). Hypotension, bradycardia, and hypothermia are often seen in association with extremely low weight. Prolongation of the QT interval may be detected in some patients. Dry skin, lanugo, acrocyanosis, and breast atrophy are findings that have been associated with AN. Distinctive hand lesions (Russell sign) have been observed; the backs of the hands are often scarred and cut from repeated abrasion of the skin against the maxillary incisors during self-induced vomiting.

The diagnosis of eating disorder is made clinically, but additional laboratory diagnostic tests may be obtained to identify malnutrition or other associated complications. Laboratory assessment may include a complete blood count to evaluate for anemia and other hematologic abnormalities; erythrocyte sedimentation rate or C-reactive protein to detect evidence of inflammation; electrolytes as well as calcium, magnesium, phosphorus, blood urea nitrogen, and creatinine; and urinalysis, including specific gravity to detect water loading. In patients with prolonged amenorrhea, human chorionic gonadotropin is assessed to determine the presence of pregnancy. Other tests for patients with amenorrhea include thyroid function tests and measurement of serum prolactin and follicle-stimulating hormone to help rule out prolactinoma (hormone-secreting pituitary tumor), hyperthyroidism, hypothyroidism, and ovarian failure. A bone density study may be ordered to detect bone loss, which is a complication of AN. In addition, a comprehensive cardiac evaluation is often recommended in those with AN. Further diagnostic tests may be required based on the history and findings from these diagnostic tests.

TABLE 16.6 Characteristics of Individuals With Eating Disorders

Factors	Anorexia Nervosa	Bulimia
Food	Turns away from food to cope	Turns to food to cope
Personality	Introverted	Extroverted
	Avoids intimacy	Seeks intimacy
	Negates feminine role	Aspires to feminine role
Behavior	"Model" child	Often acts out
	Obsessive-compulsive	Impulsive
School	High achiever	Variable school performance
Control	Maintains rigid control	Loses control
Body image	Body image distortion	Less frequent body image distortion
Health	Denies illness	Recognizes illness
		Health fluctuates
Weight	Body weight <85% of expected norm	Within 2.3-7 kg (5-15 pounds) of normal body weight or may be overweight
Sexuality	Usually not sexually active	Often sexually active

Screening tools. Annual health supervision examinations and preparticipation sports physicals are ideal screening opportunities. In addition to weight, height, and BMI measurements, a screening tool such as the SCOFF questionnaire can be used to screen for disordered eating. The SCOFF questionnaire has been validated only in adults but suggests an approach that can also be used with children (Rosen, 2010).

The medical history is most important for diagnosing eating disorders because the physical examination findings may be normal, especially early in the illness. A number of screening questionnaires are available to assist with the interview. In the SCOFF questionnaire, 1 point is scored for every "yes." A score of 2 or more indicates a likely case of AN or BN. The questions related to the mnemonic SCOFF (Sick, Control, One, Fat, Food) are (Harrington, Jimerson, Haxton, et al., 2015):

1. Do you make yourself *sick* because you feel uncomfortably full?
2. Do you worry that you have lost *control* over how much you eat?
3. Have you recently lost more than 6.4 kg (14 pounds or *one* stone) in a 3-month period?
4. Do you believe yourself to be *fat* when others say that you are too thin?
5. Do thoughts and fears about *food* and weight dominate your life?

Therapeutic Management

The treatment and management of AN involve three major goals: (1) reinstitution of normal nutrition or reversal of the severe state of malnutrition, (2) resolution of disturbed patterns of family interaction, and (3) individual psychotherapy to correct deficits and distortions in psychologic functioning. Treatment of eating disorders requires interventions of an interdisciplinary team composed of a primary practitioner, nurse, dietitian, and mental health provider with pediatric and adolescent health care experience. Because of the psychogenic nature of the disorder, the treatment may be long.

Most adolescents with AN are treated on an outpatient basis, but those with problems requiring immediate medical attention, such as severe malnutrition, electrolyte disturbances, vital sign abnormalities, or psychiatric disturbances (e.g., severe depression or suicidal ideation), may require hospitalization. Persons with BN may benefit from

CBT, psychotherapy, family-based therapy, and nutritional counseling (Kreipe & Starr, 2020).

Nutrition therapy. The most important goal is to treat any life-threatening malnutrition and to restore dietary stability and weight gain. This may require intravenous or tube feedings if the malnutrition is severe. The patient should avoid rapid weight gain because in some patients this has been associated with severe metabolic abnormalities, such as **refeeding syndrome**, which consists of cardiovascular, neurologic, and hematologic complications that occur when nutritional replacement is given too rapidly. This syndrome can be avoided with slow refeeding and the addition of phosphorus when total body phosphorus is depleted. Treatment goal weights are individualized and based on age, height, stage of puberty, premorbid weight, and previous growth charts. In young women who have reached menarche, resumption of menses is an objective measure of return to biologic health.

Dietary interventions are combined with behavioral therapy to improve the underlying psychologic misconceptions about weight loss. Another aspect of treatment is to relieve the anxiety related to eating and the depression that accompanies the disorder. Weight gain alone cannot be considered a cure for the disease and is an unreliable sign of progress. Relapses are frequent, as the person may revert to previous eating patterns when removed from the therapeutic environment.

Behavioral therapy. Behavioral modification, usually through CBT or motivational interviewing, has met with varying degrees of success. The goal is to increase the patient's feelings of control and responsibility toward achieving recovery. Providing privileges or activities for weight gain or positive eating behaviors may be successful, but treatment should also address the conflict precipitating the disorder. Individual psychotherapy is aimed at helping the young person resolve the adolescent identity crisis, particularly as it relates to a distorted body image. If the disorder is related to a dysfunctional family situation, therapy is most successful when it is started soon after the onset of illness and directed toward disengagement and redirection of malfunctioning processes in the family.

The team responsible for the management of young people with AN arranges a carefully structured environment. First, there must be consistency. The team decides on an approach and adheres to it. The plan is structured with reality testing regarding caloric intake and body image perception as an essential component. The team members provide a unified front to avoid any possibility of manipulation or inconsistency. Second, all team members are involved; responsibility for the program cannot be left to one person. The role and boundaries of each member are clearly spelled out. Third, continuity of team members is important; it is helpful to have the same team members all the time. Fourth, communication among team members is essential. Communication with the patient regarding what is expected is also important. Sometimes the limit setting may seem unreasonable. If the adolescent does not understand the rationale for the limits, he or she may sabotage the entire program. It is also important to communicate with the family. Fifth, the plan must provide for support of the adolescent, the family, and team members. Support the adolescent's efforts and provide positive feedback for accomplishments made in normalizing eating habits. Meetings are held to discuss the feelings and concerns of the patient, immediate caregivers, and team members.

Pharmacotherapy. There is no medication that specifically treats anorexia. However, doctors do sometimes prescribe certain antidepressants or other types of medicines to help some of the symptoms sometimes associated with anorexia, such as depression or anxiety.

The few studies that have been done have primarily evaluated medications' efficacy in the treatment of comorbid disorders, such as OCD and depression. SSRIs such as fluoxetine have not been shown to treat weight loss or prevent relapses in anorexia. Nevertheless, they are sometimes used to treat symptoms of depression or anxiety in people with anorexia.

The SSRI Prozac (fluoxetine) is approved by the US Food and Drug Administration to treat bulimia. There also is some evidence that other SSRIs may also treat symptoms of bulimia.

In addition, there is some evidence that tricyclic antidepressants such as desipramine, imipramine, and amitriptyline; monoamine oxidase inhibitors; and buspirone are more effective compared with a placebo in decreasing bingeing and vomiting in patients with BN. Topiramate, an antiepileptic agent, and the selective serotonin antagonist ondansetron have demonstrated some benefit in treating patients with BN. The American Psychiatric Association's guidelines have discouraged using medication as the only therapy.

The antidepressant bupropion (often marketed as Wellbutrin) has been associated with seizures in patients with purging bulimia and is not recommended for patients with eating disorders.

Medication should generally not be the initial or primary treatment for AN. There is far more evidence supporting nutritional rehabilitation and psychotherapy for treating AN, compared with that supporting medication.

Psychotherapy. Recent guidelines recommend that anorexia nervosa programs should focus on engaging the patient, on nutritional and physical rehabilitation in order to regain weight, and on provision of structured psychologic treatment. In addition, treatment outcome should aim at supporting quality-of-life changes needed for improvement or recovery.

Psychotherapy is central to the treatment of eating disorders. Patients need to be active participants in the treatment process to better understand the impulses, feelings, and needs that have resulted in their eating disorder. The goal is to increase the patient's feelings of control and responsibility toward achieving recovery. Eating disorders are complex and multifaceted. Family therapy addresses dysfunctional roles, conflicts, alliances, and patterns that the eating disorder is precipitating or maintaining, while helping family members to deal with the eating disorder.

Although evidence is yet insufficient to support outpatient versus inpatient programs, the treatment of AN has moved clinically from long-term inpatient programs with outpatient follow-up to a more common model of individual outpatient treatment with hospital backup.

Nursing Care Management

Nurses need to adopt and maintain a kind and supportive yet firm manner in managing the care of the adolescent with eating disorders without creating a passive-dependent attitude. The individual requires sustained support and reassurance to cope with ambivalent feelings related to body concept and the desire to be seen as cooperative, reliable, and worthy of receiving kindness. Encouraging the adolescent with education and activities that strengthen self-esteem facilitates the resocialization process and promotes social acceptance among peers.

It is important for nurses to be aware of the physical side effects of AN. Patients with AN frequently limit their fluid intake. Urinary tract problems are common, and ketones and protein may be detected in the urine as a result of breakdown of fat and protein. Vital sign instability can be severe and can include orthostatic hypotension; the pulse becomes irregular, and the rate decreases markedly. Bradycardia and hypothermia can result in cardiac arrest (see Critical Thinking Case Study box).

CRITICAL THINKING CASE STUDY

Anorexia Nervosa

Jane is a 13-year-old girl whose grades have been excellent and whom the teachers describe as a "model student." Recently, Jane's teacher told the nurse practitioner that Jane's parents were in the middle of a "messy divorce." In addition, several of Jane's friends told the nurse practitioner that they are concerned about Jane because she runs every day at lunchtime and seldom eats lunch with them. Jane told her friends that she gained weight over the winter months and that she is running because she wants to qualify for the track team this spring. At the time of her routine health interview and sports physical examination, the nurse practitioner notes that Jane's oral temperature is 36°C (96.8°F) and she weighs 34 kg (75 pounds). Jane has lost 9 kg (20 pounds) since her last sports physical. Jane tells the nurse practitioner that she has not had her menstrual period for 3 months.

Initial Assessment. What would be your initial concerns for Jane?

Clinical Reasoning. Discuss initial interventions that are appropriate for Jane at this time.

Teaching Points

- Numerous factors can influence the development of anorexia nervosa.
- Indicators for concern in Jane's case include the traumatic family event, concern with qualifying for the track team, and pulling away from her friends.

Critical Thinking Answers

Initial Assessment. Jane has had a traumatic life experience and has lost considerable weight. The absence of her menstrual period causes concern with the effect of rapid weight loss on her body.

Clinical Reasoning. Jane needs immediate support to help her sort through her emotions related to the divorce and actions she is taking regarding her health.

Nursing care of the adolescent with BN is similar to that for the patient with AN. Acute care involves careful monitoring of fluid and electrolyte alterations and observation for signs of cardiac complications. Nutritional consultation and follow-up care are essential. The nurse should encourage the adolescent and family members to structure the environment to reduce the bingeing behavior. Avoiding and eliminating trigger foods that would result in binges; restricting eating to one room of the house to avoid hiding and the shame related to overeating; being mindful and not engaging in other activities while eating; and substituting exercise, crafts, visualization, and relaxation techniques prior to and during urges to binge are helpful interventions.

Nurses, patients, and families can find assistance and information from several organizations. The National Association of Anorexia Nervosa and Associated Disorders[e] provides counseling, referral, and self-help programs for young people with AN. The National Eating Disorders Association[f] provides information and support services for both patients and families.

[e]Helpline 630-577-1330, available 9 AM to 5 PM Central Time, Monday to Friday; email: anadhelp@anad.org; http://www.anad.org.

[f]Referral helpline 800-931-2237, available 9 AM to 9 PM Eastern Time, Monday to Thursday, and 9 AM to 5 PM, Friday; http://www.nationaleatingdisorders.org/.

ADOLESCENT DISORDERS WITH A BEHAVIORAL COMPONENT

Substance Abuse

Monitoring the Future (MTF) is a long-term study of American adolescents, college students, and adult high school graduates through age 55 years. It has been conducted annually by the University of Michigan's Institute for Social Research since its inception in 1975 and is supported under a series of investigator-initiated, competitive research grants from the National Institute on Drug Abuse (Johnston, O'Malley, Miech, et al., 2016). The 2016 survey found that annual marijuana use among 8th-graders increased from 2007 to 2010, decreased slightly from 2010 to 2012, and then declined significantly in 2016. Among 10th-graders, use increased somewhat from 2008 to 2013 and then declined after that. Among 12th-graders, use increased from 2006 to 2011 and then held level through 2016 (Johnston et al., 2016).

Binge drinking (five or more alcoholic drinks at least once in the prior 2 weeks) has been on the decline since the early 1980s; by 2016, proportional declines since the peaks reached in the 1990s were 75%, 60%, and 51% for grades 8, 10, and 12, respectively. The observed prevalence of binge drinking continued its decline from 2015 to 2016 (significant in eighth grade), to 2016 rates of 3%, 10%, and 16% for the three grades (Johnston et al., 2016).

Cigarette use was on a steady decline from the mid-1990s until 2004; by 2016, 30-day prevalence levels had fallen from peak levels by 87%, 84%, and 71% in grades 8, 10, and 12, respectively (Johnston et al., 2016).

Smokeless tobacco use among American young people is almost exclusively a male behavior. Among males, the 30-day prevalence rates in 2016 were 3.6%, 5.8%, and 11.9% in grades 8, 10, and 12, respectively, whereas among females they were 1.4%, 1.3%, and 1.5% (Johnston et al., 2016).

Vaping continues to have higher use among teens than traditional tobacco cigarettes or any other tobacco product. As a point of comparison, prevalence for tobacco cigarettes was 2.6%, 4.9%, and 10.5% among 8th-, 10th-, and 12th-grade students, respectively. In 8th and 10th grades, vaping is more than twice as common as use of regular cigarettes (Johnston et al., 2016).

Between January 2017 and January 2018, the percentage of 12th-graders who reported vaping nicotine (not flavoring or other substances) during the past 30 days nearly doubled, from 11% to nearly 21%; among 10th-graders, the increase was almost as great, from 8.2% to 16.1%. These are the biggest 1-year increases ever seen for any substance in the history of the MTF survey (Johnston et al., 2016). In 2016 the use of illicit drugs, other than marijuana, showed some decline among 8th- and 10th-graders, whereas annual prevalence among 12th-graders showed essentially no change (Johnston et al., 2016).

Drug abuse, **misuse**, and **addiction** are culturally defined and are voluntary behaviors. **Drug tolerance** and **physical dependence** are involuntary physiologic responses to the pharmacologic characteristics of drugs, such as opioids and alcohol. Consequently, an individual can be addicted to a narcotic with or without being physically dependent. A person can also be physically dependent on a narcotic without being addicted (e.g., patients who use opioids to control pain).

Motivation

Most drug use begins with experimentation. The drug may be used only once, may be used occasionally, or may become part of a drug-centered lifestyle. Children and adolescents initiate drug use out of curiosity. Adolescents who use drugs may fall into one of two broad categories—experimenters and compulsive users—or they may fall into a third category somewhere on the continuum between these extremes, referred to as *recreational users*, principally of drugs such as marijuana, cocaine, alcohol, and prescription drugs. For many, the goal is peer acceptance; these users fit more closely with the experimenting, intermittent users. For others, the goal is intoxication or the sustained intense effects from using a particular drug. These users resemble the compulsive users; they may engage in periodic heavy use, or binges. The groups of greatest concern to health care workers are those whose patterns of use involve high doses or mixed drugs with the danger of overdose and compulsive users with the threat of dependence, withdrawal syndromes, and altered lifestyle.

Types of Drugs Abused

Any drug can be abused, and most are potentially harmful to adolescents still going through formative life experiences. Although rarely considered drugs by society, the chemically active substances frequently abused are the xanthines, theobromines, and caffeine contained in such products as chocolate, tea, coffee, colas, and energy drinks. Ethyl alcohol and nicotine are other drugs that are legal and socially sanctioned. Any of these substances can produce mild to moderate euphoric or stimulant effects and can lead to physical and psychologic dependence. Nonmedical use of pharmaceuticals gained renewed attention in the last decade. The increase in deaths from prescription opioids has been called an epidemic, and overdoses from opioids (prescription and illicit) led the US Department of Health and Human Services (2018) to declare a public health emergency in 2017.

In addition, concerns have arisen about nonmedical use of pharmaceuticals other than opioids, such as benzodiazepines, nonbenzodiazepine sleeping aids, stimulants, and cough and cold products.

The primary OTC drug of abuse in the United States is dextromethorphan (DXM), which is found in more than 120 nonprescription cough and cold medications. Using DXM as directed is safe and produces only infrequent side effects. However, it presents a significant potential for abuse, recreational use, and psychologic dependence effects. Individuals who use DXM recreationally primarily are interested in experiencing the dissociative effects associated with consuming large quantities. Prescription cough syrup containing promethazine and codeine is another common medicine-cabinet staple associated with teenage drug abuse. A popular method of consumption involves mixing the cough medicine with a fruit-flavored soda and dropping in a Jolly Rancher candy for coloring and flavor. Teens often call this drink "sizzurp," "purple drank," "syrup" or "lean."

Drugs with mind-altering abilities that are available on the "street" and are of medical and legal concern are the hallucinogenic, narcotic, hypnotic, and stimulant drugs. In addition, health professionals are concerned about the use of alcohol and volatile substances that are inhaled to achieve altered sensation (e.g., gasoline, nail polish remover, household cleaners, deodorant spray cans, liquid paper correction fluid, markers, plastic model cement, organic solvents). Huffing causes a sense of euphoria that lasts about 15 to 45 minutes. Most inhalant users report starting using before age 15 years. The initial euphoria of huffing might be followed by dizziness; headache; slurred speech; and loss of coordination, inhibition, and control. Hallucinations and delusions are possible. If an inhalant causes the heart to work too hard, a dysrhythmia could trigger lethal heart failure, even for first-time inhalers. Chronic inhalant use can cause serious liver and kidney damage.

The online drug trade is also flourishing on a hidden network of websites that are not indexed by normal search engines and are accessible only through special web browsers such as Tor. In January 2016 alone, drug revenues in cryptomarkets totaled between $12 million and $21.1 million, according to an analysis by RAND Europe. Some tech-savvy teens are finding their way to these illicit markets. Adolescents can use numerous methods to get drugs through various avenues. They can use fake IDs, attend parties, or meet dealers on the street. They can also access prescriptions by visiting a physician or by rifling through the cabinets of family members, friends, or neighbors. In addition, medications can be obtained through school, online, and through social media.

Tobacco. Cigarette smoking has been on a slow decline since its peak in 1999 despite multiple efforts, including increased costs, changes in community attitudes about smoking, media campaigns with counteradvertising, and tobacco-free environments. Use of all tobacco products among youth has not changed significantly between 2004 and 2016 (Johnston et al., 2016).

Cigarette smoking is still considered a chief avoidable cause of death. The hazards of smoking at any age are undisputed; however, a preventive approach to teenage smoking is especially important. Because of its addictive nature, smoking begun in childhood and adolescence can result in a lifetime habit, with increased morbidity and early mortality.

The effects of secondhand smoke exposure are well known and include increased incidence of low birth weight and subsequent illness, increased incidence of sudden infant death syndrome (maternal smoking during and after pregnancy), increased incidence of lower respiratory tract infections and ear infections, exacerbation of asthma attacks, sleep disturbances, and intellectual impairment (Al-Sayed & Ibrahim, 2014; Homa, Neff, King, et al., 2015).

Etiology. Teenagers begin smoking for a variety of reasons, including imitation of adult behavior, peer pressure, a desire to imitate behaviors and lifestyles portrayed in movies and advertisements, and a desire to control weight, especially among young women. Teenagers who do not smoke usually have family members and friends who do not smoke or who oppose smoking. Most teens who refrain from smoking have a desire to succeed in academics or athletics and plans to go to college (see Community Focus box). Although smoking among college students has increased in recent years, rates of smoking are highest among adolescents who do not complete high school.

COMMUNITY FOCUS

Early Sexual Maturation, Alcohol, and Cigarettes

Smoking cigarettes and drinking alcohol among adolescents are complex behaviors that are not explained by any one cause or factor. Some theorists and investigators believe that there is a relationship between biologic maturation and risk-taking behaviors. For example, young girls who are sexually mature at an earlier age than their peers are often attracted to older girls and boys who may engage in risk-taking behaviors. If older teens smoke, drink, and drive while under the influence of alcohol with no adverse consequences (e.g., no motor vehicle crashes), young girls may believe that they, too, will be safe while smoking, drinking, or riding in an automobile with friends who are drinking.

Although parents and nurses cannot influence the time of biologic maturation, they can identify young girls who are at risk for the initiation of risk-taking behaviors because of early puberty. Parents need to understand that an early-maturing daughter may be uncomfortable with her body, and they should take advantage of opportunities to build her self-esteem. Parental sensitivity to the importance of peer group acceptance and parental support of a teenage daughter who feels left out or different are crucial. School nurses can provide anticipatory guidance to these girls and help them role-play coping strategies for situations that involve offers to smoke and drink. In addition, school nurses can provide information about physical development during puberty and emphasize the fact that not all teenagers mature at the same time or rate.

Teachers, coaches, and community and church leaders can provide opportunities for these girls to "fit in" with their same-age peers through activities that stress mutual goals. For example, an early-maturing girl is typically taller than her age-mates and can be an asset in sports, such as basketball and track and field events.

Smokeless tobacco. The term *smokeless tobacco* refers to tobacco products that are placed in the mouth but not ignited (e.g., snuff, chewing tobacco). This substitute for cigarettes continues to pose a hazard to adolescents, although use had steadily declined by about 50% since the peak prevalence in 1995. Children and adolescents continue to recognize the risk of smokeless tobacco and have expressed high rates of disapproval (Johnston et al., 2016). These products have also been proven to be carcinogenic, and regular use can cause dental problems, foul-smelling breath, and tooth erosion or loss.

Nursing care management. Prevention of regular smoking in teenagers is the most effective way to reduce the overall incidence of smoking. A variety of methods have been used. Posters, charts, displays, statistics, and the use of examples of actual damaged lungs to communicate the hazards of smoking all have their supporters and doubters. Some schools also use films and demonstrations in science classes.

For the most part, smoking prevention programs that focus on the negative, long-term effects of smoking on health have been ineffective. Youth-to-youth programs and those emphasizing the immediate effects are more effective but primarily in improving teenagers' attitudes toward not smoking. Because smoking and smoking-related behaviors are social symbols, antismoking campaigns must address the norms of potential smokers. Anything that ridicules or threatens the social norms of the peer group can be unproductive or counterproductive. Investigators have found that teaching resistance to peer pressure to smoke is effective in early adolescence. Although the effects of these programs may decrease with time, they can be enhanced in older adolescents by presenting information in class instead of simply handing out written material to the students.

Two areas of focus for antismoking programs are peer-led programs and use of media in smoking prevention (e.g., CDs, videotapes, films). Peer-led programs emphasizing the social consequences of smoking have proved most successful. If a significant number of influential peers can "sell" their classmates on the idea that the habit is not popular, the followers will imitate their behavior. Such programs emphasize short-term rather than long-term consequences (e.g., the effects of smoking on personal appearance, such as unattractive stains on teeth and hands, and unpleasant odor of breath and clothing).

The impact of school-based antismoking programs can be strengthened by expanding these programs to include parents, mass media, youth groups, and community organizations. For example, mass media efforts that involve antismoking radio campaigns have been identified as the most cost-effective mass media intervention.

Smoking bans in schools also accomplish several goals, including discouraging students from starting to smoke, reinforcing knowledge of the health hazards of cigarette smoking and exposure to environmental tobacco smoke, and promoting a smoke-free environment as the norm (see Community Focus box).

Alcohol. Acute or chronic abuse of alcohol (ethanol) is responsible for many acts of violence, suicide, accidental injury, and death. Alcohol drinking is likely to begin in the middle school years and increase with age. By 18 years of age, 80% to 90% of adolescents have tried alcohol. Ethanol is a depressant that reduces inhibitions against aggressive and sexual acting out. Severe physical and psychologic symptoms accompany abrupt withdrawal, and long-term use leads to slow tissue destruction, especially of the brain and liver cells. The most noticeable effects of alcohol occur within the CNS and include changes in cognitive and autonomic functions, such as judgment, memory, learning ability, and other intellectual capacities. Young people with alcoholism often drink alone and cannot control their use of alcohol. They often rely on the substance as a defense against depression, anxiety, fear, or anger. Not all of these characteristics are observed in adolescents who are abusing alcohol, but if several signs are evident, the child or adolescent should be considered at risk. Referral to a health care professional and detoxification therapy may be necessary. Information about alcohol and answers to questions are available through the Alcohol Hotline.[g] Other groups that provide support and counseling for families are Al-Anon, Alateen, Alatot, and Alcoholics Anonymous (an organization that has listings in all local directories).

Cocaine. Although cocaine is not pharmacologically considered a narcotic, it is legally categorized as such. Cocaine is available in two forms: water-soluble cocaine hydrochloride, which is administered by "snorting" or intravenous injection, and nonsoluble alkaloid (freebase) cocaine, which is used primarily for smoking. Crack, or "rock," is a

COMMUNITY FOCUS

Considerations for Nonsmoking Strategies

Nurses who work in schools, hospitals, and community agencies can take advantage of all opportunities to provide education about the dangers of smoking, to discourage smoking initiation by children and adolescents, to encourage smoking cessation, and to promote smoke-free environments. In particular, school nurses must be alert to the vulnerability of young preteens when they enter junior high or middle school. These nurses are in an ideal position to assess stress, personal conflict, weight concerns, peer pressure, and other factors that place preteens at risk for smoking initiation. Nurses should serve as counselors to student, teacher, and parent groups and as advocates for antismoking legislative efforts. The following additional strategies are recommended[a]:

- Provide only brief information about long-term health consequences (e.g., cardiovascular, cancer risks).
- Discuss immediate physiologic consequences (e.g., changes in heart rate, blood pressure, respiratory symptoms, and blood carbon monoxide concentrations).
- Mention alternatives to smoking that also establish a self-image that appears independent, mature, or sophisticated (e.g., weightlifting; jogging; dancing; joining a boys or girls club; volunteering for a hospital or political, religious, or community group).
- Mention the negative effects in detail (e.g., earlier wrinkling of skin; yellow stains on teeth and fingers; tobacco odor on breath, hair, and clothing).
- Mention the increasing ostracism of smokers by nonsmokers, both legal and informal, in the workplace and in public places.
- Mention the increasing evidence that secondhand smoke is injurious to the health of nonsmokers who are regularly exposed, especially small children.
- Acknowledge that many adults who were enticed to start smoking as teenagers because of its social benefits now wish they could stop smoking.
- Give cooperative adolescents effective arguments to deal with peer pressure (e.g., by not smoking, a teenager demonstrates independence and nonconformity, traits normally prized by youth).
- Request posters or pamphlets from local agencies (e.g., American Cancer Society, American Heart Association, American Lung Association) to display in prominent places at school.

[a]The Centers for Disease Control and Prevention has information on the effects of tobacco, smoking cessation, and tobacco control programs: 1600 Clifton Rd., Atlanta, GA 30333; 800-232-4636; email: tobaccoinfo@cdc.gov; http://www.cdc.gov/tobacco.

[g]Toll free 800-331-2900.

purer, more menacing form of the drug. It can be produced cheaply and smoked in either water pipes or mentholated cigarettes.

Cocaine creates a sense of euphoria, or an indefinable high. Withdrawal does not produce the dramatic symptoms observed in withdrawal from other substances. The effects are those commonly seen in depression, including lack of energy and motivation, irritability, appetite changes, psychomotor delay, and irregular sleep patterns. More serious symptoms include cardiovascular manifestations and seizures. Physical withdrawal should not be confused with the so-called crash after a cocaine high, which consists of a long period of sleep. Answers to questions about the risks of using cocaine are available at the National Cocaine Hotline,[h] which also provides referrals to support groups and treatment centers.

Narcotics. Narcotic drugs include opiates, such as heroin and morphine, and opioids (opiate-like drugs), such as hydromorphone (Dilaudid), hydrocodone, fentanyl, meperidine (Demerol), and codeine. These drugs produce a state of euphoria by removing painful feelings and creating a pleasurable experience and a sense of success accompanied by clouding of the consciousness and a dreamlike state. Physical signs of narcotic abuse include constricted pupils, respiratory depression, and often cyanosis. Needle marks may be visible on the arms or legs in chronic users. Physical withdrawal from opiates is extremely unpleasant unless controlled with supervised tapering doses of the opioid or substitution of methadone.

As important as the physical effects are the indirect consequences related to the illegal status of narcotic use and the problems associated with securing the drug (e.g., the time-consuming searches to obtain the drug and the often illegal methods used to meet the high cost of purchasing it). Health problems also result from self-neglect of physical needs (nutrition, cleanliness, dental care); overdose; contamination; and infection, including HIV and hepatitis B and C infection.

Central nervous system depressants. CNS depressants include a variety of hypnotic drugs that produce physical dependence and withdrawal symptoms on abrupt discontinuation. They create a feeling of relaxation and sleepiness but impair general functioning. Drugs in this category include barbiturates, nonbarbiturates, and alcohol. Barbiturates combined with alcohol produce a profound depressant effect. Flunitrazepam (Rohypnol), known as the "date rape drug," is a hypnotic drug abused by adolescents. Many women and men report being raped after unknowingly being given Rohypnol in a drink. Rohypnol is 10 times more powerful than diazepam (Valium). It produces prolonged sedation, a feeling of well-being, and short-term memory loss.

Central nervous system stimulants. Amphetamines and cocaine do not produce strong physical dependence and can be withdrawn without much danger. However, psychologic dependence is strong, and acute intoxication can lead to violent aggressive behavior or psychotic episodes characterized by paranoia, uncontrollable agitation, and restlessness. When combined with barbiturates, the euphoric effects are particularly addictive.

Methamphetamine can be snorted, injected, swallowed, or smoked and produces a burst of energy in its users, along with intense, alternating attacks of boldness and paranoia. It provokes excitement far more intense than that caused by cocaine. The drug, with the street names *crank, meth,* and *crystal,* is inexpensive and has a longer period of action than cocaine. Instead of a short (few minutes) high, as achieved with cocaine, a user can remain "up" for hours on a similar dose of crank.

Health care professionals are concerned about the use of various volatile substances, or **inhalants** such as gasoline, model cement, and organic solvents; these substances are inhaled by the user to achieve an altered sensation, and the most recent surveillance has indicated a modest increase in use after nearly a decade of decline. Adolescents breathe or place these substances in paper or plastic bags or soda cans from which they rebreathe the fumes to produce a feeling of euphoria and altered consciousness. These substances contain chemical solvents and are extremely hazardous. Dusters contain Freon, a substance that can cause fatal cardiac arrhythmias. Inhalants are the only substance that has a higher incidence of use among young adolescents. This is probably related to the fact that the products are readily available and may be the only substances available to young teens. Many young children are unaware of the dangers of "sniffing" or "huffing." In addition to rapid loss of consciousness and respiratory arrest, these substances may cause visual scanning problems, language deficiencies, motor instability, memory deficits, and attention and concentration problems.

Mind-altering drugs. Hallucinogens (psychedelics, psychotomimetics, psychotropics, or illusionogenics) are drugs that produce vivid hallucinations and euphoria. These drugs do not produce physical dependence, and they can be abruptly withdrawn without ill effect. However, the acute and long-term effects are variable, and in some individuals the dissociative behavior may be prolonged. Cannabis (marijuana, hashish) and lysergic acid diethylamide (LSD) are also included in this category of drugs.

Nursing Care Management and Therapeutic Management

Nurses who have contact with children and adolescents are in an excellent position to provide information about substance abuse and to serve as patient advocates. Nurses most often encounter young drug abusers when they are (1) experiencing overdose or withdrawal symptoms, (2) manifesting bizarre behavior or confusion secondary to drug ingestion, (3) worried that they are or will become addicted, or (4) worried about a friend or family member who is addicted.

Nurses who care for hospitalized adolescents need to know if these youths use drugs compulsively. Drug withdrawal can seriously complicate other illnesses. Nurses should be alert for any physical or behavioral clues that indicate the onset of withdrawal or the effects of drugs. School nurses and nurses who work in the community play an essential role in identifying children, adolescents, and families with substance abuse problems. The school nurse may be the first to identify a child or adolescent who has ingested a particular drug by the child's erratic behavior in class or on the school grounds. Early identification of those at risk for substance abuse problems is an essential aspect of prevention. Pediatric health care professionals also prevent substance abuse by creating trusting relationships so that children and adolescents feel comfortable asking questions about drugs, and health professionals can alert them to websites and other aspects of society that encourage experimentation with drugs.

Acute care. Adolescents experiencing toxic drug effects or withdrawal symptoms are usually seen initially in the emergency department. Experienced emergency department personnel are familiar with the management of acute drug toxicity and the signs, symptoms, and behavioral characteristics associated with a variety of substances. When the drug is questionable or unknown, knowledge of these factors facilitates management and treatment. Often observation or description of the child's or adolescent's behavior is more valuable than reports by patients or their friends.

The treatment for drug toxicity or withdrawal varies according to the drug and the method used. Every effort is made to determine the type, time of ingestion, amount of drug taken, mode of administration, and factors related to the onset of presenting symptoms. It is helpful to know the individual's pattern of use. For example, if two types of drugs are involved, they may require different treatments. Historically,

[h]800-COCAINE (800-262-2463).

gastric lavage has been used when the drug has been ingested recently and the cough reflex is intact, but it is of little value when the drug has been administered by the intravenous ("mainlined") or intranasal ("sniffed") route. More commonly, the administration of a drug antidote such as naloxone and the early (within 1 to 2 hours of ingestion) administration of activated charcoal may be used for opioid overdose. Because the actual content of most street drugs is highly questionable, other pharmaceutical agents are administered with caution, except perhaps the narcotic antagonists in cases of suspected opiate overdoses. It is also necessary to assess for possible trauma sustained while the patient was under the influence of the drug.

Long-term management. A major factor in the treatment and rehabilitation of young drug users is careful assessment in the nonacute stage to determine the function that the drug plays in the adolescent's life. The motivation phase is directed toward exploring the factors that influence drug use. It also involves establishing a feeling of self-worth and a commitment to self-help in the teen.

Rehabilitation begins when adolescents decide they can and are willing to change. **Rehabilitation** involves fostering healthy interdependent relationships with caring and supportive adults and exploring alternate mechanisms for problem solving, while simultaneously reducing or eliminating drug use. Persons working with troubled youth must be prepared for **recidivism**, or the tendency to relapse, and maintain a plan for reentry into the treatment process.

Family support. Most treatment programs for substance abusers are based on adult 12-step models, such as Alcoholics Anonymous. Research is needed to determine whether these adult models are effective for adolescents. Tough Love[i] is one program that is based on the conviction that parents have the right and responsibility to be the policymakers in the family, to set limits on the behavior of their children, and to take control of the household from out-of-control adolescents. The premise is that allowing teenagers to experience the negative consequences of their behavior will bring them closer to accepting help or changing their behavior. Another group that provides support and counseling for families experiencing substance abuse and seeking strategies to cope with their children is Parents Anonymous.[j] Another source of information is the Substance Abuse and Mental Health Services Administration's National Clearinghouse for Alcohol and Drug Information.[k]

Prevention. Nurses play an important role in education efforts, as well as in individual observation, assessment, and therapy related to substance abuse. In recent years, a variety of educational programs have been applied with promising results. The most effective prevention strategies are those that are part of a broader, more general effort to promote overall health and success. Health-compromising behaviors are often interconnected and have common antecedents. Prevention efforts that focus on changing only one behavior (e.g., alcohol, other drug use) are less likely to be successful. Successful programs are those that have promoted parenting skills, social skills among distractible children, academic achievement, and skills to resist peer pressure.

Peer pressure is a powerful tool and can be used effectively in substance abuse prevention. A group that has had some success in reducing injury from drunk driving is Students Against Destructive Decisions.[l] Techniques used by this group include peer counseling, parental guidelines for teenage parties, and community awareness. Nurses should encourage the formation of Students Against Destructive Decisions chapters in the high schools in their communities.

[i] https://www.toughlove.com

[j] 675 W. Foothill Blvd., Suite 220, Claremont, CA 91711; 909-621-6184; http://www.parentsanonymous.org.

[k] Choke Cherry Road, Rockville, MD 20857; 877-SAMHSA-7; http://www.samhsa.gov/.

[l] 255 Main St., Marlborough, MA 01752; 877-SADD-INC; http://www.sadd.org.

Suicide

Suicide is defined as the deliberate act of self-injury with the intent that the injury results in death. Most experts distinguish among suicidal ideation, suicide attempt (or parasuicide), and suicide.

Suicidal ideation involves a preoccupation with thoughts about committing suicide and may be a precursor to suicide. Although it is common for adolescents to experience occasional suicidal thoughts, expressions of preoccupation with suicide should be taken seriously, and an assessment should be conducted for appropriate referral. A **suicide attempt** is intended to cause injury or death. The term **parasuicide** is used to refer to behaviors ranging from gestures to serious attempts to kill oneself. *Parasuicide* is a preferred term because it makes no reference to intent and because a person's motive may be too difficult or complex to determine. However, all parasuicidal activity should be taken seriously.

> **! NURSING ALERT**
>
> A history of a previous suicide attempt is a serious indicator for possible suicide completion in the future. Studies of adolescent suicides have found that as many as half of the adolescents had made previous attempts.

Results from the Youth Risk Behavior Surveillance (2017) found that, in 2017, 31.5% of high school students had experienced periods of persistent feelings of sadness or hopelessness (i.e., almost every day for 2 or more consecutive weeks so that the student stopped doing some usual activities) in the past year. The percentage of students who experienced persistent feelings of sadness or hopelessness in the past year increased significantly from 2007 to 2017. That same report found that, in 2017, 17.2% of high school students had seriously considered attempting suicide in the past year. In 2017, 13.6% of high school students had made a suicide plan in the past year. In that same year, 7.4% of high school students had attempted suicide one or more times in the past year.

Suicide is currently the third leading cause of death during the teenage years, surpassed only by death from accidents (unintentional injuries and homicides; see Chapter 1).

Etiology

Environmental, psychologic, and biologic factors play a role in suicide (Cha, Franz, Guzmán, et al., 2017). Some of the environmental factors include a history of child maltreatment, victimization (bullying), and peer and media influence (Cha et al., 2017). Psychologic influences consist of affective issues of worthlessness and low self-esteem, cognitive factors such as impulsivity, and social processes of connectedness and loneliness (Cha et al., 2017). Biologic factors of suicide encompass neural responses, brain circuits, serotonin, and genetics (Cha et al., 2017). The single most important individual factor is the presence of an active psychiatric disorder (depression, bipolar disorder, psychosis, substance abuse, or conduct disorder). For some teenagers, suicide becomes the final pathway for release from their psychiatric and social problems. Child and adolescent suicide victims are reported to have higher rates not only of depression but also of conduct disorders; bipolar disorders; substance abuse; interpersonal problems with parents; and a family history of depression, substance abuse, and suicidal behavior.

Family factors influencing suicide include parental loss; family disruption; a family history of suicide, depression, substance abuse, or emotional disturbance; child abuse or neglect; unavailable parents; poor communication and isolation within the family; family conflict; and unrealistically high parental expectations or parental indifference with low expectations. Families who respect individuality are cohesive and caring, balance discipline with a supportive and understanding relationship, have good systems of communication, and have at least one attentive and caring parent available to the child to protect adolescents from suicidal outcomes. Social or environmental risk factors include incarceration, isolation, acute loss of a boyfriend or girlfriend, lack of future options, and availability of firearms in the home.

! NURSING ALERT

Given what is known about youth suicide, nurses should ask parents, especially those with at-risk teenagers, if firearms are available in the house and, if so, recommend their removal. Parents must ensure that their children—especially those who are depressed, have poor problem-solving skills, or use drugs or alcohol—do not have access to firearms. Parents must also be educated on the warning signs of suicide (Box 16.7).

Motivation

Suicidal ideation is common in adolescents. It represents numerous fantasies, such as relief from suffering, a means of gaining comfort and sympathy, or a means of revenge against those who have hurt them. Adolescents have the erroneous perception that the act of suicide will evoke remorse and pity and that they will be able to return and witness the grief. Angry children or adolescents who are unable to directly punish those who have injured or insulted them may take revenge on those who love them through self-destruction (e.g., "They'll be sorry when they find me dead." "They'll be sorry they were mean to me.").

BOX 16.7 Warning Signs of Suicide

- Preoccupation with themes of death—focuses on morbid thoughts
- Wants to give away cherished possessions
- Talks of own death, desire to die
- Loss of energy, loss of interest, listlessness
- Exhaustion without obvious cause
- Changes in sleep patterns—too much or too little
- Increased irritability, argumentativeness, or stubbornness
- Physical complaints—recurrent stomach aches, headaches
- Repeated visits to physician, nurse practitioner, or emergency department for treatment of injuries
- Reckless behavior
- Antisocial behavior—engages in drinking, uses drugs, fights, commits acts of vandalism, runs away from home, becomes sexually promiscuous
- Sudden change in school performance—lowered grades, cutting classes, dropping out of activities
- Resists or refuses to go to school
- Remains distant, sad, remote—flat affect, frozen facial expression
- Describes self as worthless
- Sudden cheerfulness following deep depression
- Social withdrawal from friends, activities, and interests that were previously enjoyed
- Impaired concentration
- Dramatic change in appetite

For adolescents who are severely depressed, suicide seems to be the only release from their despair. These adolescents rarely provide evidence of their intent and frequently conceal their suicidal thoughts. Many adolescents, however, tell peers of their suicidal thoughts or plans but avoid telling adults. Social isolation is a significant factor in distinguishing adolescents who will kill themselves from those who will not. It is also more characteristic of those who complete suicide than of those who make attempts or threats.

The frequency of **contagion**, or **copycat suicides** (i.e., an increase in youth suicide that occurs after the suicide of one teenager is publicized) is disturbing and may indicate that teenagers perceive suicide as glamorous. In addition, young people may not realize the finality of suicide because they have become desensitized from constantly viewing violence and death on television.

Diagnostic Evaluation

Depression is common among adolescents who attempt suicide. Depression is characterized by both subjective symptoms and objective signs that reflect the adolescent's sadness and despair. Adolescents describe feelings of sadness, despair, helplessness, hopelessness, boredom, loss of interest, and isolation. They may also feel self-reproach, self-deprecation, and guilt. Subjective symptoms of depression or specific changes in behavior place an adolescent at risk for suicide.

Therapeutic Management

Threats of suicide should always be taken seriously. There has been a tendency to dismiss suicide attempts as impulsive acts resulting from temporary crises or depression. If a suicide attempt fails to draw attention to his or her problems or makes them worse, the child or adolescent may conclude that suicide is the only answer. Children and adolescents need to know that someone cares and must be provided with swift and efficient crisis intervention. Although ordinary practitioners can manage an acute depressive reaction without difficulty, the adolescent who has made a serious attempt or has a specific plan for suicide should receive immediate attention and competent psychiatric care.

Youths who are actively suicidal need inpatient care, monitoring, and treatment. Medications for depression and bipolar disorder often take several weeks to reach therapeutic dosages. The time until medications and therapy begin to take effect can be trying for the adolescent and the family. It is important to encourage families to support their teen in adhering to the regimen prescribed. SSRIs are often prescribed for depression, but teens who are taking such medications need careful, frequent monitoring.

! NURSING ALERT

Adolescents who express suicidal feelings and have a specific plan should be monitored at all times. They should not have access to firearms, prescription or over-the-counter drugs, belts, scarves, shoestrings, sharp objects, matches, or lighters. If they are intoxicated, they must be restrained or placed in a protective environment until a psychiatrist or psychologist can assess them.

Nursing Care Management

Nurses play a pivotal role in reducing adolescent suicide. Nurses can provide anticipatory guidance to parents and adolescents. They can teach parents to be supportive and to develop positive communication patterns that help teens feel connected with and loved by their families. To foster healthy development, parents can be encouraged to provide teens with creative outlets and to assist young people in accepting strong emotions—pain, anger, and frustration—as a normal part of the human experience.

Care of suicidal adolescents includes early recognition, management, and prevention. The most important aspect of management is the recognition of warning signs that indicate that an adolescent is troubled and might attempt suicide. The nurse must take any suicidal remarks seriously and not leave the young person alone until the degree of suicidality is assessed. A mnemonic for the assessment process is **SLAP:** **S**pecificity, **L**ethality, **A**ccessibility, and **P**roximity. The first step (specificity) is to ask adolescents whether they feel suicidal or as though they would like to take their own lives. If so, have they chosen a means of suicide, and do they have a specific plan? The second stage of assessment (lethality) involves determining the lethality of the methods available to them. Do they plan to use a gun or knife? Have they chosen highly lethal medications, hanging, or carbon monoxide poisoning? The third stage (accessibility) involves determining the availability of the means of suicide, and the fourth stage (proximity) involves assessing whether they have determined a time to commit suicide and when that time is.

Health professionals must be alert to the signs of depression, and anyone who exhibits such behavior should be referred for thorough psychologic assessment. Depression is manifested differently in children and adolescents than in adults. In teenagers, it may be masked by impulsive aggressive behaviors. Defiance, disobedience, behavior problems, and psychosomatic disturbances can indicate underlying depression, suicidal ideation, and impending suicide attempts.

! NURSING ALERT

No threat of suicide should be ignored or challenged. Threats are a symptom that must be taken seriously. Too often, suicidal threats or minor attempts are confused with bids for attention. It is also a mistake to be lulled into a false sense of security when an adolescent's depression is apparently relieved. The improvement in attitude may mean that the adolescent has made the decision and found the means to carry out the threat.

Peers and other confidants are valuable observers and excellent sources of information about potential suicide attempts. They may not be able to diagnose depression, but they are able to sense when a friend has undergone a marked personality change. It is important to emphasize that the peer who detects any changes in a friend is a potential rescuer and should not remain silent about the observations. Friendship does not imply collusion. A peer who believes that a friend may be suicidal should alert someone who can help (e.g., a parent, teacher, guidance counselor, school nurse).

Routine health assessments of adolescents should include questions that assess the presence of suicidal ideation or intent. There are several assessment tools intended to assist clinicians in the identification and initial management of adolescents with depression in an era of great clinical need and shortage of mental health specialists. These tools cannot replace clinical judgment and are not meant to be the sole source of guidance for depression management in adolescents. Of the many tools available, the most relevant are in publications by Richardson and colleagues (2010), in which they validated the Patient Health Questionnaire–2 (PHQ-2) and the Patient Health Questionnaire–9 (PHQ-9).

Any previous suicide attempt indicates an increased risk for a future attempt. The risk of a suicide attempt in the near future increases as the frequency of suicidal ideation increases.

! NURSING ALERT

The National Suicide Prevention Lifeline (800-273-TALK [8255]; in Spanish, 888-628-9454) offers someone to talk to 24/7.

If children or adolescents express suicidal intent, nurses can make a contract, asking them to sign an agreement that they will not attempt suicide during an agreed-upon period and that they will call the 24-hour crisis line immediately if they feel that they cannot keep to their contract. The amount of time an adolescent feels comfortable contracting to is usually an indication of his or her risk and stability.

Because a suicide attempt is frequently an outgrowth of family distress, it is essential to intervene with the family. It is important to assess family interactions and to recognize disturbed relationships. The most effective approach is recognition of susceptible adolescents during the early stages of family distress so that family counseling can be started. Prevention must be directed toward improving childrearing practices through support and education of parents and changing societal conditions that generate defeat, despair, and maladaptive behavior.

Although confidentiality is an essential part of adolescent counseling, in the case of self-destructive behaviors, it cannot be honored. Suicidal behavior is reported to the family and other professionals, and adolescents are informed that this will be done. Such action conveys an important message to the youth: that the professionals understand and care.

Many schools have instituted suicide prevention programs. These programs include services such as drop-in counseling and a peer counseling telephone line. Information can also be obtained from the American Association of Suicidology.[m]

Adverse Childhood Experiences (ACEs)

From 1995 to 1997 Kaiser Permanente's Health Appraisal Clinic, in collaboration with the Centers for Disease Control and Prevention, implemented one of the largest studies ever conducted on the origins of risk factors that have negative health and social consequences and on the cumulative incidence and influence of psychologic and physical abuse. Risk factors included neglect, sexual abuse, witnessing violence, exposure to substance abuse, mental illness, suicidal behavior, and imprisonment of a family member. The impact of these risk factors on mental health (depression, suicidality), physical health (heart disease, cancer, chronic lung disease, skeletal fractures, liver disease, obesity), health-related behaviors (alcoholism, drug abuse, smoking, high numbers of sexual partners), and poor self-rated health were evaluated (Felitti, Anda, Nordenberg, et al., 1998). The recommendation from the 2012 American Academy of Pediatrics policy statement was to infuse a trauma-informed perspective into pediatrics, and this may be accomplished by introducing caregivers to adverse childhood experiences (ACEs).

An ACE questionnaire[n] (ACE-Q) was constructed using selected questions from published surveys (American Journal of Preventive Medicine, 2017). The findings showed that the more negative events a child experienced, the more likely that child would be to suffer an array of health and behavior problems, including alcoholism, chronic pulmonary disease, depression, illicit drug use, liver disease, and adolescent pregnancy, later in life.

By bringing attention to the powerful impact that negative childhood experiences have on future health and functioning, the ACE study demonstrates the importance of gathering information early in the lives of children and their families and designing early intervention programs that target violence and neglect. It also points to the importance of collecting trauma histories from clients.

[m]5221 Wisconsin Ave. NW, Washington, DC 20015; 202-237-2280; http://www.suicidology.org.

[n]ACE-Q Materials can be found at: https://www.acesconnection.com/g/resource-center/blog/resource-list-extended-aces-surveys

CLINICAL JUDGMENT AND NEXT-GENERATION NCLEX® EXAMINATION-STYLE QUESTIONS

1. A 14-year-old female with severe cystic acne is taking isotretinoin as treatment. She has been on the agent for the past 2 months. During the history assessment by the nurse, the following is noted. She has dry eyes and reports decreased night vision and headaches. She has had increased urination and vomiting the 24 hours. The mother reports that she is depressed and has frequent mood swings. **Highlight the assessment findings in the narrative above that are side-effects of isotretinoin that require follow-up by the nurse.**

2. A 13-year-old female patient visits the clinic for follow-up of a urinary tract infection. The nurse performs a history and physical assessment and notes the adolescent is extremely obese. She has gained considerable weight in the past year. Which of the following conditions listed below are associated with the development of obesity in adolescents and need to be explored further? **Select all that apply.**
   A. Physical inactivity
   B. Hereditary low metabolism
   C. Presence of a chronic illness
   D. Use of food as a positive reinforcer of desired behaviors
   E. Availability of energy-dense foods and drinks
   F. Positive self-esteem

3. A 15-year-old girl is being seen because she is in a relationship and wants to begin a contraceptive. She has had no previous sexual relationships and is healthy with no physical concerns based on her history and physical examination. What information would the nurse need to know to help this teenager make an informed decision about contraception? **Choose the most likely options for the missing information by selecting from the lists of options provided.**

Contraceptive Methods	Advantages	Disadvantages
Withdrawal	No medical visit necessary	High failure rate from noncompliance
Condom	**2**	May decrease sensation, requires consistent use
Spermicidal Foam	Available without a prescription	**3**
1	99% effective is used correctly	Need to follow precise instructions
Diaphragm	Can be fitted in virgins, may be reused	**4**

Option 1	Option 2	Option 3	Option 4
Abstinence	>99% effective	Irregular menstrual bleeding	Not recommended for women >90 kg
Calendar methods	Regulates menses	Latex sensitivity may occur	Risk of perforation
Oral contraceptives	Prevents ovarian cancers	High failure rate unless combined with condom	May cause headaches
Progestin	Easy to use, minimal side effects	May cause nausea	May cause dysmenorrhea
Cervical Cap	Prevents endometriosis	May cause vaginitis	Requires fitting by medical personnel, minimal STI protection

4. A 15-year-old girl visits the clinic with fever, chills, abdominal pain that is dull, cramping and at times incapacitating. She is sexually active and reports vaginal discharge in the past few days. In caring for this adolescent what is **most important** for the nurses to know about sexually transmitted infections? **Choose the most likely options for the information missing from the statements below by selecting from the lists of options provided.**

   ____1____ is the most frequently reported infectious disease in the United States and is often difficult to diagnose because symptoms may be nonspecific. ____2____ presents with warts found on any part of the female genitalia. ____3____ can present with discharge, dysuria and dyspareunia and is the oldest communicable disease in the United States.

Option 1	Option 2	Option 3
Neisseria gonorrhoeae	*Neisseria gonorrhoeae*	*Neisseria gonorrhoeae*
Chlamydia trachomatis	*Chlamydia trachomatis*	*Chlamydia trachomatis*
Treponema pallidum	*Treponema pallidum*	*Treponema pallidum*
Human papillomavirus (HPV)	Human papillomavirus (HPV)	Human papillomavirus (HPV)
Trichomonas vaginalis	Trichomonas vaginalis	Trichomonas vaginalis

REFERENCES

Ahmann, E. (2017). Interventions for ADHD in children and teens: A focus on ADHD coaching. *Pediatric Nursing, 43*(3), 121–131.

Al-Sayed, E. M., & Ibrahim, K. S. (2014). Second-hand tobacco smoke and children. *Toxicology and Industrial Health, 30*(7), 635–644.

Altman, M., & Wilfley, D. E. (2015). Evidence update on the treatment of overweight and obesity in children and adolescents. *Journal of Clinical Child and Adolescent Psychology, 44*(4), 521–537.

American Academy of Pediatrics. (2011). Subcommittee on Attention-Deficit/Hyperactivity Disorder, Steering Committee on Quality Improvement and Management., et al. ADHD: Clinical practice guideline for the diagnosis, evaluation, and treatment of attention-deficit/hyperactivity disorder in children and adolescents. *Pediatrics, 128*(5), 1007–1022.

American Academy of Pediatrics. (2016). *American Academy of Pediatrics announces new recommendations for children's media use*. Retrieved from: https://www.aap.org/en-us/about-the-aap/aap-press-room/Pages/American-Academy-of-Pediatrics-Announces-New-Recommendations-for-Childrens-Media-Use.aspx.

American College of Obstetricians and Gynecologists. (2015). Premenstrual syndrome. Retrieved from: https://www.acog.org/Patients/FAQs/Premenstrual-Syndrome-PMS?IsMobileSet=false.

American Heart Association. (2014). *Overweight in children*. http://www.heart.org/HEARTORG/GettingHealthy/HealthierKids/ChildhoodObesity/Overweight-in-Children_UCM_304054_Article.jsp.

American Journal of Preventive Medicine. (n.d.). Retrieved from https://www.journals.elsevier.com/american-journal-of-preventive-medicine.

American Psychiatric Association. (2013). *Diagnostic and Statistical Manual of Mental Disorders (DSM–5)*. Washington, D.C.: American Psychiatric Association Publishing.

Austin, C. M., & Mahmood, T. (2018). Primary amenorrhoea. *Obstetrics. Gynaecology & Reproductive Medicine, 28*(9), 268–275.

Basta, A. M., Courtier, J., Phelps, A., Copp, H. L., & Mackenzie, J. D. (2015). Scrotal swelling in the neonate. *Journal of Ultrasound in Medicine, 34*(3), 495–505.

Caldwell, P. H., Lim, M., & Nankivell, G. (2018). An interprofessional approach to managing children with treatment-resistant enuresis: An educational review. *Pediatric Nephrology, 33*(10), 1663–1670.

Canady, V. A. (2015). CDC finds best practices guidelines used for most children assessed for ADHD. *Mental Health Weekly, 25*(35), 1–3.

Castaldo, G., Palmieri, V., Galdo, G., et al. (2016). Aggressive nutritional strategy in morbid obesity in clinical practice: Safety, feasibility, and effects on metabolic and haemodynamic risk factors. *Obesity Research and Clinical Practice, 10*(2), 169–177.

Centers for Disease Control and Prevention. (2015). *Sexual assault and abuse and STDs*. Retrieved from: https://www.cdc.gov/std/tg2015/sexual-assault.htm.

Centers for Disease Control and Prevention. (2017). *Youth Risk Behavior Survey Data Summary and Trends Report, 2007-2017*. Retrieved from https://www.cdc.gov/healthyyouth/data/yrbs/results.htm.

Centers for Disease Control and Prevention. (2019). Human papillomavirus. Retrieved from: https://www.cdc.gov/hpv/parents/about-hpv.html.

Cerman, A. A., Aktas, E., & Altunay, I. K. (2016). Dietary glycemic factors, insulin resistance, and adiponectin levels in acne vulgaris. *Journal of the American Academy of Dermatology, 75*, 155–161.

Cha, C. B., Franz, P. J., Guzmán, E. M., et al. (2017). Annual research review: Suicide among youth - epidemiology, (potential) etiology, and treatment. *Journal of Child Psychology and Psychiatry, 59*(4), 460–482.

Cinar, N., & Menekse, D. (2017). Affects of adolescent pregnancy on health of baby. *Open Journal of Pediatrics & Neonatl Care, 2*(1), 20–23.

Cradock, A. L., Barrett, J. L., Kenney, E. L., et al. (2017). Using cost-effectiveness analysis to prioritize policy and programmatic approaches to physical activity promotion and obesity prevention in childhood. *Preventive Medicine, 95*(Suppl.), S17–S27.

Cunningham, S. A., Kramer, M. R., & Narayan, K. M. (2014). Incidence of childhood obesity in the United States. *The New England Journal of Medicine, 370*(5), 403–411.

De Souza, M. J., Nattiv, A., Joy, E., et al. (2014). 2014 Female athlete triad coalition consensus statement on treatment and return to play of the female athlete triad. *Current Sports Medicine Report, 13*(4), 219–232.

Eichenfield, L. F., Krakowski, A. C., Piggott, C., et al. (2013). Evidence-based recommendations for the diagnosis and treatment of pediatric acne. *Pediatrics, 131*(Suppl. 3), S163–S183.

Elder, J. S. (2020). Enuresis and voiding dysfunction. In R. M. Kliegman, J. W. St. Geme, N. J. Blum, et al. (Eds.), *Nelson textbook of pediatrics* (21st ed.). Philadelphia: Elsevier.

Fagundes, S. N., Lebl, A. S., Soster, L. A., et al. (2016). Monosymptomatic nocturnal enuresis in pediatric patients: Multidisciplinary assessment and effects of therapeutic intervention. *Pediatric Nephrology, 32*(5), 843–851.

Felitti, V. J., Anda, R. F., Nordenberg, D., et al. (1998). Relationship of childhood abuse and household dysfunction to many of the leading causes of death in adults. *American Journal of Preventive Medicine, 14*(4), 245–258.

Flegal, K. M., Carroll, M. D., Kit, B. K., et al. (2012). Prevalence of obseity and trends in the distribution of body mass index among US adults, 1999-2010. *The Journal of the American Medical Association, 307*(5), 491–497.

Frampton, J. E. (2018). Lisdexamfetamine dimesylate: A review in paediatric ADHD. *Drugs, 78*(10), 1025–1036.

Gahagan, S. (2020). Overweight and obesity. In R. M. Kliegman, J. W. St. Geme, N. J. Blum, et al. (Eds.), *Nelson textbook of pediatrics* (21st ed.). Philadelphia: Elsevier.

Hagan, M. J., Gentry, M., Ippen, C. G., et al. (2018). PTSD with and without dissociation in young children exposed to interpersonal trauma. *Journal of Affective Disorders, 227*, 536–541.

Harrington, B. C., Jimerson, M., Haxton, C., et al. (2015). Initial evaluation, diagnosis, and treatment of anorexia nervosa and bulimia nervosa. *American Family Physician, 91*(1), 46–52.

Hazeltine, M., Panza, A., & Ellsworth, P. (2017). Testicular torsion: Current evaluation and management. *Urologic Nursing, 372*, 61–93.

Hazeltine, M., Panza, A., & Ellsworth, P. (2018). Testicular torsion: Current evaluation and management. *Urologic Nursing, 37*(2), 61–71.

Heiervang, E. R., Villabø, M. A., & Wergeland, G. J. (2018). Cognitive behavior therapy for child and adolescent anxiety disorders. *Current Opinion in Psychiatry, 31*(6), 484–489.

Henry, D., Dormuth, C., Winquist, B., et al. (2016). Occurrence of pregnancy and pregnancy outcomes during isotretinoin therapy. *Canadian Medical Association Journal, 188*(10), 723–730.

Homa, D. M., Neff, L. J., King, B. A., et al. (2015). Vital signs: Disparities in nonsmokers' exposure to secondhand smoke—United States, 1999-2012. *MMWR Morb Mortal Wkly Rep, 64*(4), 103–108.

Johnston, J. D., O'Malley, P. M., Miech, R. A., et al. (2016). *Monitoring the future national results on adolescent drug use: 1975-2014: Overview, key findings on adolescent drug use*. Ann Arbor, Mi: Institute for Social Research, University of Michigan.

Koppen, I. J., Vriesman, M. H., Saps, M., et al. (2018). Prevalence of functional defecation disorders in children: a systematic review and meta-analysis. *The Journal of Pediatrics, 198*, 121–130.

Kreipe, R. E., & Starr, T. B. (2020). Eating disorders. In R. M. Kliegman, J. W. St. Geme, N. J. Blum, et al. (Eds.), *Nelson textbook of pediatrics* (21st ed.). Philadelphia: Elsevier.

LeFevre, M. L. (2014). *Screening for chlamydia and gonorrhea: U.S. Preventive Services Task Force Recommendation Statement*. Retrieved from https://annals.org/aim/article-abstract/1906843/screening-chlamydia-gonorrhea-u-s-preventive-services-task-force-recommendation.

Lentz, G. M. (2012). Primary and secondary dysmenorrheal, premenstrual syndrome, and premenstrual dysphoric disorder. In G. M. Lentz, R. A. Lobo, D. M. Gershenson, et al. (Eds.), *Comprehensive gynecology* (6th ed.) (pp. 791–803). Philadelpia: Mosby/Elsevier.

Leyden, J., Stein-Gold, L., & Weiss, J. (2017). Why topical retinoids are mainstay of therapy for acne. *Dermatologic Therapy, 7*, 293–304.

Li, X., He, C., & Chen, Z. (2017). A review of the role of sebum in the mechanism of acne pathogenesis. *Journal of Cosmetic Dermatology, 16*, 168–173.

Masterson, T. A., Ramasamy, R., & Hotaling, J. M. (2017). Varicocele: Treatment indications and repair techniques. *Urology Times, 45*(11), 9–11.

McClain, E. K., & Burks, E. J. (2015). Managing attention-deficit/hyperactivity disorder in children and adolescents. *Primary Care: Clinics in Office Practice, 42*(1), 99–112.

Meiser-Stedman, R., McKinnon, A., & Dixon, C. (2017). Acute stress disorder and the transition to posttraumatic stress disorder in children and adolescents: Prevalence, course, prognosis, diagnostic suitability, and risk markers. *Depress Anxiety, 34*(4), 348–355.

Ogden, C. L., Carroll, M. D., Kit, B. K., et al. (2014). Prevalence of childhood and adult obesity in the United States, 2011-2012. *The Journal of the American Medical, 311*(8), 806–814.

Ogden, C. L., Kuczmarski, R. J., Flegal, K. M., et al. (2002). Centers for Disease Control and Prevention 2000 growth charts for the United States: Improvements to the 1977 National Center for Health Statistics version. *Pediatrics, 109*(1), 45–60.

Ogden, C. L., Troiano, R. P., Briefel, R. R., et al. (1997). Prevalence of overweight among preschool children in the United States, 1971 through 1994. *Pediatrics, 99*(4), E1.

Olaru, C., Diaconescu, S., Trandafir, L., et al. (2016). Chronic functional constipation and encopresis in children in relationship with the psychosocial environment. *Gastroenterology Research and Practice*, e7828576.

Pazol, K., Whiteman, M. K., Folger, S. G., et al. (2015). Sporadic contraceptive use and nonuse: Age-specific prevalence and associated factors. *American Journal of Obstetrics and Gynecology, 212*(3), 324.

Powell, A. (2017). Choosing the right oral contraceptive pill for teens. *Pediatric Clinics of North America, 64*, 343–358.

Ranson, W. A., Patterson, D. C., & Colvin, A. C. (2018). Female athlete triad: Past, present, and future directions. *Annals of Joint, 3* 4–4.

Riccabona, M., Darge, K., Lobo, M., et al. (2015). ESPR Uroradiology Taskforce—imaging recommendations in paediatric uroradiology, part VIII: Retrograde urethrography, imaging disorder of sexual development and imaging childhood testicular torsion. *Pediatric Radiology, 45*(13), 2023–2028.

Richardson, L. P., Rockhill, C., Russo, J. E., et al. (2010). Evaluation of the PHQ-2 as a brief screen for detecting major depression among adolescents. *Pediatrics, 125*(5), e1097–e1103.

Roberts, S. C., Hodgkiss, C., DiBenedetto, A., et al. (2012). Managing dysmenorrhea in young women. *The Nurse Practitioner, 37*(7), 47–52.

Robinson, T. N., Banda, J. A., Hale, L., et al. (2017). Screen media exposure and obesity in children and adolescents. *Pediatrics, 140*(Suppl. 2), S97–S101.

Rosen, D. S. (2010). Identification and management of eating disorders in children and adolescents. *Pediatrics, 126*(6), 1240–1253.

Roy, A., & Hechtman, L. (2016). *The Multimodal Treatment of Children with ADHD (MTA) Follow-up Study*. Oxford Medicine Online.

Schwartz, M. B., & Ustjanauskas, A. (2012). Food marketing to youth: Current threats and opportunities. *Childhood Obesity, 8*(2), 85–88.

Šimić, D., Babić, J. Z., & Gunarić, D. (2017). Psychological status and quality of life in acne patients treated with oral isotretinoin. *Psychiatric Danubina, 29*, 104–110.

Skinner, A. C., Perrin, E. M., Moss, L. A., et al. (2015). Cardiometabolic risks and severity of obesity in children and young adults. *New England Journal of Medicine, 373*(14), 1307–1317.

Sukkar, S. G., Signori, A., Borrini, C., et al. (2013). Feasibility of protein-sparing modified fast by tube (ProMoFasT) in obesity treatment: A phase II pilot trial on clinical safety and efficacy (appetite control, body composition, muscular strength, metabolic pattern, pulmonary function test). *The Mediterranean Journal of Nutrition and Metabolism, 6*, 165–176.

Torrone, E., Papp, J., Weinstock, H., & Centers for Disease Control and Prevention (2014). Prevalence of *Chlamydia trachomatis* genital infection among persons aged 14-39 years—United States, 2007-2012. *MMWR Morb Mortal Wkly Rep, 63*(38), 834–838.

Trent, M. (2013). Pelvic inflammatory disease. *Pediatric Review, 34*(4), 163–172.

U.S. Department of Health and Human Services. (2018). *HHS Acting Secretary Declares Public Health Emergency to Address National Opioid Crisis*. Retrieved from https://www.hhs.gov/about/news/2017/10/26/hhs-acting-secretary-declares-public-health-emergency-address-national-opioid-crisis.html.

Walle, J. V., Rittig, S., & Tekgul, S. (2017). Enuresis: Practical guidelines for primary care. *British J General Practice, 67*(660), 328–329.

Weersing, V. R., Jeffreys, M., Do, M. T., Schwartz, K. T., & Bolano, C. (2017). Evidence base update of psychosocial treatments for child and adolescent depression. *Journal of Clinical Child and Adolescent Psychology, 46*(1), 11–43.

Youth Risk Behavior Surveillance - United States, 2017 | MMWR. (n.d.). Retrieved from https://www.cdc.gov/mmwr/volumes/67/ss/ss6708a1.htm

17

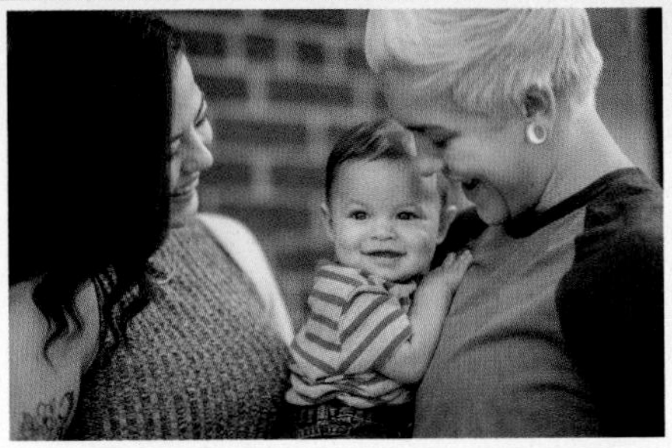

Impact of Chronic Illness, Disability, or End-of-Life Care on the Child and Family

Joy Hesselgrave, Gina Santucci

http://evolve.elsevier.com/wong/essentials

CONCEPTS

- Chronic Illness
- Palliative Care

PERSPECTIVES ON THE CARE OF CHILDREN AND FAMILIES LIVING WITH OR DYING FROM CHRONIC OR COMPLEX CONDITIONS

SCOPE OF THE PROBLEM

A complex chronic condition (CCC) can be defined as any medical condition that persists for more than a year and affects several organ systems or one system critically enough that additional specialty expertise is crucial (Feudtner, Feinstein, Zhong, et al., 2014). With innovations in medical technology, we are seeing a decrease in the mortality of children living with CCCs. These children are living longer, often beyond the age that can be cared for at a pediatric tertiary care center. Many are being discharged to home with sophisticated technology, complex plans of care, and burdensome medication schedules. Transitioning children with medical complexity from hospital to home has some inherent challenges, including determining parent readiness (Leyenaar, O'Brien, Leslie, et al., 2017) and the likelihood of readmission (Bucholz, Toomey, & Schuster, 2019). Advances in neonatology and other subspecialties have increased the viability of premature infants or those who have a congenital or genetic anomaly. Life-sustaining technology that was once available only in a tertiary care center has been adapted for home use, allowing children with complex conditions a chance of living in their community. Families, home care agencies, and schools are being taught how to care for children with increasing technology, complicated treatments, and demanding medication schedules (Feudtner, Dai, & Hexem, 2012). It is not uncommon for a medically fragile child with complex needs to have one or more life-sustaining technologies (e.g., tracheostomy, ventilator, gastrostomy, ventricular peritoneal shunt, parental nutrition), which has increased that child's survival rate (Burke & Alverson, 2010; Elias, Murphy, & Council on Children With Disabilities, 2012; Simon, Berry, Feudtner, et al., 2010). Children with complex conditions require not only multiple medical specialists, but also nurses and therapists (respiratory, physical, occupational, rehabilitative, and speech) with advanced training and expertise who can support their care in the community (Kuo & Houtrow, 2016). The complex high level of skill required to meet their daily health care needs and the continuous nature and potential volatility of their conditions sets this group apart from the broader population of children with special health care needs (Cohen, Kuo, Agrawal, et al., 2011; Kuo, Cohen, Agrawal, et al., 2011; Simon et al., 2010). A range of terms, such as *complex chronic condition, medically complex, technology dependent,* and *multiply handicapped,* have been used to describe this vulnerable population of children (Cohen et al., 2011; Feudtner et al., 2014). Children with complex and chronic conditions are a diverse group, but they share some common characteristics, including high health care use, caregiver burden, and social isolation (Barnert, Coller, Nelso, et al., 2017). Frequent and prolonged hospitalizations, reliance on technology, and care that traverses all settings are key characteristics that differentiate these children from others (Berry, Hall, Hall, et al., 2013; Cohen et al., 2011; Feudtner et al., 2014).

The nature and severity of childhood chronic and complex conditions are widely heterogeneous. Table 17.1 includes a nonexhaustive sampling of conditions, organized by specialty. However, affected children and families are similar in the vulnerability they experience due to the health and developmental consequences of these diagnoses on the child, such as ongoing functional impairment, neurodevelopmental disability, dependence on medical technology, and the need for ongoing skilled and supportive care from health care providers and family members. Although many authors have described the rise in prevalence that has come with advances in medical care (American Academy of Pediatrics, 2019; Simon et al., 2010), accurate estimates of the number of affected families do not exist. The impact of chronic and complex illness in children is wide ranging. Parents report experiencing grief and loss of

TABLE 17.1 Chronic Conditions of Childhood

Specialty	Examples of Chronic Conditions
Cardiology	Complex congenital heart disease, congestive heart failure, cardiac dysrhythmias, Kawasaki disease, rheumatic fever, hyperlipidemia, hypertrophic cardiomyopathy, dilated cardiomyopathy
Endocrinology	Diabetes, congenital adrenal hyperplasia, Cushing syndrome, Turner syndrome
Gastroenterology	Short bowel syndrome, biliary atresia, inflammatory bowel disease, hepatitis, cirrhosis, peptic ulcer disease, celiac disease
Hematology	Sickle cell anemia, thalassemia, aplastic anemia, hereditary anemias, hemophilia
Immunology	Immune deficiency, human immunodeficiency virus, Wiskott-Aldrich syndrome, severe combined immunodeficiency disease
Nephrology	Prune belly syndrome, renal disease
Neurology	Cerebral palsy, ataxia telangiectasia, muscular dystrophy, epilepsy, spina bifida, traumatic brain injury, hydrocephalus, adrenal leukodystrophy, Chiari malformations
Oncology	Brain tumor, leukemia, lymphoma, solid tumors, bone tumors, rare tumors
Pulmonology	Asthma, chronic lung disease, cystic fibrosis, tuberculosis, pulmonary hypertension
Rheumatology	Systemic lupus erythematosus, juvenile rheumatoid arthritis, dermatomyositis

identity once a diagnosis is made; initial feelings of sorrow and self-blame have been reported along with being both physically and emotionally exhausted (Smith, Cheater, & Bekker, 2015). Health care providers have also reported challenges in caring for children with CCCs, including the complexity of care coordination, managing technology, and the persistent and all-encompassing psychosocial needs of the family (Bogetz, Bogetz, Rassbach, et al., 2015). The challenges the family experiences fluctuate with the needs of the child and have been described at times as both frustrating and rewarding and likened to a "roller-coaster ride" with highs and lows (Goudie, Narcisse, Hall, et al., 2014; Kuo et al., 2011; Nurullah, 2013; Smith, Cheater, & Bekker, 2013). Children with CCCs may be at increased risk for behavior or emotional problems. Children lose school days and parents may lose days from work, which compound feelings of physical, emotional, and financial exhaustion.

Many children with CCCs are living at home, and parents are tasked with their care. Even though many children qualify for home nursing, the reality is that parents must assume readiness at any time when nursing is not available (Nageswaran & Golden, 2017).

Siblings are also affected by having a "different" brother or sister, and they may simultaneously feel guilt, anger, or jealousy toward their ill sibling. Clinicians need to know that siblings of children with chronic illnesses are at risk for negative psychologic effects (Hartling, Milne, Tjosvold, et al., 2014). Parents need encouragement and assistance with understanding the reactions of siblings to having a chronically ill family member (e.g., behavioral regression, anxiety, withdrawal, apathy). In addition, secondary losses (such as the ability to participate in extracurricular activities or social events) occur because of routines imposed by the affected child's chronic condition.

TRENDS IN CARE

Developmental Focus

Focusing on the child's developmental level rather than chronologic age or diagnosis emphasizes the child's abilities and strengths rather than their disabilities. Attention is directed to normalizing experiences, adapting the environment, and promoting coping skills. Nurses often are in vital positions to redirect attention from the pathologic model, with its focus on weaknesses and problems, to the developmental model to meet the unique needs of the child and family.

A developmental focus also considers family development. The life cycle of the family unit reflects changing ages and needs of family members, as well as changing external demands. A family member's serious illness can cause significant stress or crisis at any stage of the family life cycle. Just as with individual development, family development may be interrupted or even regress to an earlier level of functioning. Nurses can use the concept of family development to plan meaningful interventions and evaluate care.

Family-Centered Care

Family-centered care is a method of care delivery and a philosophy of care that values the integral role the family plays in the health and well-being of their child (Smith, Swallow, & Coyne, 2015).

Having a child with a chronic condition can be an added source of stress for the family unit, putting additional strain on how a family functions, their cohesiveness, and the family members' relationships with each other (Herzer, Godiwala, Hommel, et al., 2010). A child's physical and emotional health, as well as his or her cognitive and social functioning, is strongly influenced by how well the family functions (Kuhlthau, Bloom, Van Cleave, et al., 2011; Treyvaud, 2014). The importance of family-centered care—a philosophy that considers the family as the constant in the child's life—is especially evident in the care of children with special needs. As parents learn about the child's health care needs, they often become experts in delivering care. Nurses and other health care providers are key to the success of family-centered care and the need to form partnerships with the child's parent and/or caregiver (Coats, Bourget, Starks, et al., 2018). Effective communication and negotiation between parents and nurses are essential to forming trusting and effective partnerships and finding the best ways to meet the needs of the child and family (Corlett & Twycross, 2006; Kuo, Houtrow, Arango, et al., 2012). Collaborative relationships are characterized by communication, dialogue, active listening, awareness, and acceptance of others' differences (Kuhlthau et al., 2011).

Family and Health Care Provider Communication

The disclosure of a serious chronic or complex condition of a child is one of the most stressful aspects of communication between families and health care professionals. Health care providers often struggle with minimizing parental distress and maintaining hope when giving prognostic information, but some parents have reported that honest, clear information can promote hope by clarifying uncertainty. Similarly, being overly optimistic or withholding information was felt to undercut hope (Nyborn, Olcese, Nickerson, et al., 2016). After a diagnosis is made, factors that influence parent dissatisfaction with the way in which information is communicated include disrespectful attitudes, breaking bad news in an insensitive manner, withholding information, and changing a treatment course without preparing the child and family (Barnes, Gardiner,

Gott, et al., 2012). Conversely, parents report satisfaction when they perceive health care providers to be available, demonstrate competence, and engage the child and parent in care decision making. Parents report wanting regular, coordinated team updates on their child's condition (Barnes et al., 2012; Hill, Knafl, & Santacroce, 2017; Kuo, Sisterhen, Sigrest, et al., 2012). Similar factors are important in communicating changes in the child's condition throughout the course of the illness.

Providing information to families with a chronically ill child should be a practice of repeated discussions to allow the family time to process the information. Nurses play an important role in ensuring that families' needs are met during discussions related to the child's diagnosis, condition, and treatment (Kavanaugh, Moro, & Savage, 2010). This requires assessment of how families want to receive information, how much information they are comfortable with, their comprehension of the information given to them, and how they are coping with the information both cognitively and emotionally. Nurses should ensure that the appropriate health care professionals address any concerns or further questions that families may have.

Establishing Therapeutic Relationships

Another important aspect of family-centered care of children with chronic and complex conditions is establishing a therapeutic relationship with the child and family, which has been shown to predict improved health-related outcomes (Kuhlthau et al., 2011). Family members, most often the mother, take on enormous responsibility in providing technical care and symptom management of their child's condition outside of the health care institution (Goudie et al., 2014; Smith et al., 2015). To build successful therapeutic relationships with families, it is necessary for nurses to recognize parents' expertise with regard to their child's condition and needs. Health care environments for children with serious illnesses are fraught with obstacles that serve as barriers to successful therapeutic relationships with families. Individual discussions, especially with the case manager, primary nurse, clinical nurse specialist, or nurse practitioner, help establish a consistent and flexible care plan that can prevent conflicts or deal with these conflicts before they disrupt care.

The Role of Culture in Family-Centered Care

Issues of culture, ethnicity, and race affect access to services, health care use, and follow-through with referrals and recommendations (Coker, Rodriguez, & Flores, 2010; Toomey, Chien, Elliott, et al., 2013). For some ethnic and minority populations, cultural understandings of illness, the structure of family life, social roles for individuals with disabilities, and other factors related to the perception of children may differ from those of mainstream American culture.

Although culture cannot completely explain how an individual will think and act, understanding cultural perspectives can help the nurse anticipate and understand why families may make certain decisions. Cultural attributes such as values and beliefs regarding illness or chronic condition and its causation, social roles for people who are ill or disabled, family structure, the role of children, childrearing practices, self versus group orientation, spirituality, and time orientation also affect a family's response to illness or chronic condition in a child (Wiener, McConnell, Latella, et al., 2013).

When parents are informed of their child's chronic illness, interpreters familiar with both culture and language should be used. Children, family members, and friends of the family should not be used as translators because their presence may prevent parents from openly discussing issues. When working with people of cultural backgrounds different from their own, nurses must listen carefully with an initial goal of understanding and articulating the family's perspective. The ability to interpret the mainstream medical culture to the family is also important. Furthermore, every effort is made to incorporate traditional cultural beliefs of a family into treatment plans. It is important to keep in mind that "cultural norms" may not always apply to every family from a shared background. Developing a care plan in conjunction with the family, considering their preferences and priorities, is an important first step in formulating a plan that best meets the family's needs, no matter what their cultural background may be (Coker et al., 2010; Wiener et al., 2013).

BOX 17.1 Facilitating Shared Decision Making

- Continually assess the impact of the child's illness and treatment on the family.
- Provide honest, accurate information on the trajectory of the disease, anticipated complications, and prognostic information.
- Discuss what the family desires for the child's quality of life.
- Avoid personal opinion or judgment of the family's questions and decisions.
- Be aware of nurses' personal and cultural assumptions and the ways in which these assumptions affect communication, decision making, and judgment.

Shared Decision Making

Shared decision making refers to a model of care in which health care providers and patients share information on treatments and interventions, discuss risks and benefits based on clinical evidence and best practices, and take into account patient preferences and values (Elwyn, Frosch, Thomson, et al., 2012; National Learning Consortium, 2013).

Shared decision making among the child, family, and health care team can result from open, honest, culturally sensitive communication and the establishment of a therapeutic relationship among the family and health care providers. In a shared decision-making model, the health care professionals provide honest, clear information on diagnosis, prognosis, treatment options, and risk–benefit assessment. The patient and family then share information on important family values, acceptable levels of discomfort or inconvenience, and the ability to comply with recommended treatments (Wiener et al., 2013; Wyatt, List, Brinkman, et al., 2015). This process allows for the careful examination of options and consideration of the impact on the child and family. To promote shared decision-making the risks and benefits to the child and family, prognosis or expected course of the illness, and the impact on the family's resources should be discussed (Box 17.1). Together, the parents and health care team can make decisions that are best for the family and child at the time the decision is made (Kon, 2010).

Normalization and Transition

Normalization refers to the effort family members make to create a normal family life, their perceptions of the consequences of these efforts, and the meanings they attribute to their management efforts (Knafl, Darney, Gallo, et al., 2010). For chronically ill children, such efforts may include attending school, pursuing hobbies and recreational interests, and achieving employment and a level of independence. For their families, it may entail adapting the family routine to accommodate the ill or disabled child's health and physical needs (Kuo et al., 2011).

Transition is a term often used when a child's care is transferred to adult care services. However, it is also used to convey the discharge from an acute or chronic care facility to home for children with complex health care needs (Brenner, Larkin, Hilliard, et al., 2015).

Children with chronic and complex conditions and their families face numerous challenges in achieving normalization and transitioning care. Families move between the "normal" of living with the experience of chronic childhood illness and the "normal" of the healthy outside world; they often redefine "normal" based on their particular experiences, needs, and circumstances (Knafl et al., 2010).

Normalization may be an important mediator of illness-related stressors (e.g., treatment demands, uncertainty) on family outcomes.

Nurses can assist families in normalizing their lives by assessing the family's everyday life, social support systems, coping strategies, family cohesiveness, and family and community resources. Interventions include encouraging families to reduce stress through delegation of care and family tasks, identifying ways to incorporate care into current routines, structuring the home environment to encourage the child's engagement in age-appropriate activities, and ensuring that families have access to appropriate community support services (Knafl & Santacroce, 2010). Being supportive of the child's illness and treatment and actively including the family in all aspects of care will improve their self-esteem and promote further development (Jones & Prinz, 2005; Knafl & Santacroce, 2010).

Home care represents the return to a system and set of priorities in which family values are as important in the care of a child with a chronic health problem as they are in the care of other children. Home care seeks to achieve goals that are consistent with the developmental model (Stein, 1985):

- Normalize the life of the child, including those with technologically complex care, in a family and community context and setting.
- Minimize the disruptive impact of the child's condition on the family.
- Foster the child's maximum growth and development.

With appropriate training and support, families provide complex procedures and treatments in the home. Parents are challenged to retain a homelike setting among monitors, ventilators, and other sophisticated equipment. Throughout the text, home care is discussed as appropriate for specific conditions. The process of transition from hospital to home is elaborated on in Chapters 19 and 20.

Paralleling normalization and home care is the process of **mainstreaming**, or integrating children with disabilities into regular classrooms. Children who attend school have the advantages of learning and socializing with a wide group of peers. There is an increased focus on individualization as plans are made to meet the academic needs of these children along with those of the rest of the students.

A variety of supplemental programs have been designed in the school system to accommodate special needs, both at school age and younger, through **early intervention**, which consists of any sustained and systematic effort to assist developmentally vulnerable or disabled children from birth to 3 years old. Increased opportunities for normalization for children with disabilities have resulted in large part from the passage of (1) the Education for All Handicapped Children Act of 1975 (Public Law 94-142) and its 1990 amendments (Public Law 101-476), which changed the name of the Act to the Individuals with Disabilities Education Act (IDEA); (2) the Education of the Handicapped Act Amendments of 1986 (Public Law 99-457), which directs states to develop and implement statewide comprehensive, coordinated, interprofessional interagency programs of early intervention services for infants and toddlers with disabilities, as well as support services for their families; and (3) the Americans with Disabilities Act of 1990. Nurses can provide parents with information about these laws and in some cases may participate in the development of individualized educational programs (IEPs) or individualized family service plans (IFSPs) for children with disabilities.

THE FAMILY OF THE CHILD WITH A CHRONIC OR COMPLEX CONDITION

A major goal in working with the family of a child with a chronic or complex illness is to support the family's coping and promote their optimal functioning throughout the child's life. Long-term, comprehensive care involves forming parent-professional partnerships that can support a family's adaptation across the trajectory of the illness to the many changes that may be necessary in day-to-day life, determine expectations of and for the child, and provide a long-term perspective (Box 17.2).

BOX 17.2 Adaptive Tasks of Parents Having Children With Chronic Conditions

1. Accept the child's condition.
2. Manage the child's condition on a day-to-day basis.
3. Meet the child's normal developmental needs.
4. Meet the developmental needs of other family members.
5. Cope with ongoing stress and periodic crises.
6. Assist family members to manage their feelings.
7. Educate others about the child's condition.
8. Establish a support system.

From Canam, C. (1993). Common adaptive tasks facing parents of children with chronic conditions. *Journal of Advanced Nursing, 18*, 46–53.

Often the impact of a child's medical or developmental condition is first experienced as a crisis at the time of diagnosis, which may occur at birth, after a long period of diagnostic testing, or immediately after a tragic injury. However, the impact may also be felt before the diagnosis is made, when parents are aware that something is wrong with their child but before medical confirmation (Smaldone & Ritholz, 2011).

The diagnosis and initial discharge home are critical times for parents (Coffey, 2006). Several factors can make this particularly difficult, including a long duration of uncertainty in the diagnostic process, negative perceptions of chronic illness, insufficient information, and lack of mutual trust between parents and their child's health care team (Huang, Kenzik, Sanjeev, et al., 2010; LeGrow, Hodnett, Stremler, et al., 2014; Monterosso, Kristjanson, Aoun, et al., 2007; Nuutila & Salanterä, 2006). Parental feelings of shock, helplessness, isolation, fear, and depression are common (Coffey, 2006; Nuutila & Salanterä, 2006). Throughout the first year, parents struggle to accept the child's diagnosis, care, and uncertainty of the future (Coffey, 2006). Optimal support at the time of diagnosis and initial discharge home can be encouraged by providing explicit and uncomplicated information to parents in an empathic way (Nuutila & Salanterä, 2006); assessing the family's daily routine, living conditions, background knowledge, skills and abilities, and coping behaviors; and evaluating the family's understanding of the information. It is also necessary to reassess parents' needs for information and support on a routine basis (Nuutila & Salanterä, 2006).

Other critical times include the exacerbation of the child's physical symptoms, which increases parental care. These crises often involve medical intervention and rehospitalization. Frequently the child does not return to his or her precrisis level of functioning, and parents and family must adapt to new care needs and schedules. Instability may also follow transition points on the illness trajectory. Supporting parents, respecting their stress and emotions, and acknowledging their role as team members in the care of their child are important aspects of nursing care (Coffey, 2006; Nuutila & Salanterä, 2006; Panicker, 2013).

IMPACT OF THE CHILD'S CHRONIC ILLNESS

Each member in the family of a child with a chronic or complex illness is affected by the experience (Goudie et al., 2014; Kuo et al., 2011). The effects on the parents and their responses may be so intense that they directly influence the other members' reactions and the child's own coping.

BOX 17.3 Anticipated Parental Stress Points

Diagnosis of the condition: Parents require considerable education while dealing with an emotional response.
Developmental milestones: Times that children normally achieve walking, talking, and self-care are delayed or impossible for the child.
Start of schooling: Particularly stressful are situations in which appropriate schooling will not be in a regular class placement.
Reaching the ultimate attainment: Parents must handle situations such as realizing that ambulation will be impossible or that the child will not learn to read.
Adolescence: Issues such as sexuality and independence become prominent.
Future placement: Decisions about placement must be made when the child becomes an adult or when the parents can no longer care for the child.
Death of the child

Parents

In addition to the stress of grieving for the loss of hope for a perfect child, parents are affected by whether they receive positive feedback from interactions with their child. Many parents feel satisfaction and fulfillment from the parenting role. For others, parenting may be a series of unrewarding experiences that contribute to feelings of inadequacy and failure (Box 17.3). These responses may be most evident in parents who are responsible for the child's care. For example, parents may become preoccupied with their ability to carry out certain procedures, overlooking the child's personal comfort and satisfaction or failing to offer praise for anything less than perfect cooperation or performance. They may pursue a frustrating activity until they achieve "success"—long after the child has become irritable and uncooperative. As a result, parents can become caught in a pattern of interaction that is mutually unrewarding and minimally productive. This situation may become exacerbated by disagreements or lack of support from other family members and judgment from caregivers and others in the community. For these parents, several strategies may be helpful, including education about what can reasonably be expected of their child, assistance in identifying the child's strengths, praise for a parental job well done, and respite care so that parents can renew their energies.

Parental Roles

Parenting a child with a CCC requires attending to the routine aspects of parenting with the added responsibilities of performing complex technical care, symptom management, and advocating for their child (Morawska, Calam, & Fraser, 2015; Woodgate, Edwards, Ripat, et al., 2015). These added responsibilities must then be balanced with the needs of other family members, extended family and friends, and personal health and obligations to minimize consequences to the overall functioning of the family (Cousino & Hazen, 2013; Pinquart, 2018). Measures to help decrease the stress of parenting a child with a CCC include providing mental health support and teaching parents how to deal with stressors.

Often one parent or partner remains at home to manage existing family responsibilities while the other remains with the ill child. The partner who is not included in the caregiving activities may feel neglected because all of the attention is directed toward the child and may be resentful that he or she is not sufficiently informed to be competent in the care. Without active participation in the child's care, the parent has little appreciation of the time and energy involved in performing care activities. When this partner does attempt to participate, the other parent may criticize the less skillful efforts. As a result, communication and support for each other may be adversely affected.

The nurse can assist parents in avoiding role conflicts by providing anticipatory guidance early on. Teaching should address stressors often identified as having an impact on the marriage, including (1) the burden of care at home assumed by primarily one parent, (2) the financial burden, (3) the fear of the child dying, (4) pressure from relatives, (5) the hereditary nature of the disease (if applicable), and (6) fear of pregnancy. Other causes of tension may center on the inconveniences associated with care, such as long waits for an appointment, lack of parking near care facilities, or lack of overnight accommodations.

Mother-Father Differences

Mothers and fathers of a child with a complex condition often adjust and cope differently. Mothers are often the primary caregiver and are more likely than fathers to give up their jobs to care for their children, often resulting in social isolation (Coffey, 2006). Mothers often have greater needs for social support and positive appraisal of the situation than do fathers.

Fathers of children with disabilities struggle with issues that may be distinct from those of the mothers (Swallow, Macfadyen, Santacroce, et al., 2012). Fathers may think that their role as protector is challenged, because they do not know how to help and cannot protect their family from the seemingly overwhelming recurring problems. The extensive stresses in the family can leave fathers feeling depressed, weak, guilty, powerless, isolated, embarrassed, and angry. Fearful that they will lose control or be viewed as weak or ineffectual, however, fathers often hide their feelings and display an outward confidence that may lead others to believe that everything is fine. Fathers worry about what the future holds for their children, their ability to manage the increasing financial burden, and the daily disruptions of the entire family (Nicholas, Beune, Barrera, et al., 2016; Swallow et al., 2012).

Single-Parent Families

Single-parent families are of special concern. As the only parent of a child who may require extensive, sophisticated, and lifelong care, the single parent may feel an enormous burden. Available financial and emotional resources may already be stretched to the limit. A special effort should be made to assist the single parent in finding financial and support services that can ease the burden of care. Nurses can also assist the single parent in identifying helping roles that may be acceptable to relatives and friends.

Siblings

Results of studies are less clear regarding the ways in which siblings are affected by having a brother or sister with a complex condition (Anderson & Davis, 2011; Hartling et al., 2014). Some evidence shows a negative effect on siblings of children with chronic illnesses compared with siblings of healthy children (Gold, Treadwell, Weissman, et al., 2011; Hartling et al., 2014). Siblings of children with chronic illnesses report psychosocial problems more often than their peers (Gold et al., 2011). A number of factors increase the risk of negative effects for siblings of ill children. Responsibility for caregiving, less attention from parents, and limitations on family resources and recreational time are often the experiences of siblings of ill or disabled children (Barr & McLeod, 2010) (Box 17.4). Siblings may experience a decrease in school attendance and academic functioning, which may be somewhat ameliorated by the support of teachers and peers (Gan, Lum, Wakefield, et al., 2017). An important factor in sibling adjustment and coping is information and knowledge regarding the

BOX 17.4 Supporting Siblings of Children With Special Needs

Promote Healthy Sibling Relationships

Value each child individually and avoid comparisons. Remind each child of his or her positive qualities and contribution to other family members.

Help siblings see the differences and similarities between themselves and the child with special needs. Create a climate in which children can achieve successes without feeling guilty.

Teach siblings ways to interact with the child.

Seek to be fair in terms of discipline, attention, and resources; require the affected child to do as much for himself or herself as possible.

Let siblings settle their own differences; intervene only to prevent siblings from hurting one another.

Legitimize reasonable anger. Even children with special needs behave badly sometimes.

Respect a sibling's reluctance to be with or to include the child with special needs in activities.

Help Siblings Cope

Listen to siblings to let them know that their thoughts and suggestions are valued.

Praise siblings when they have been patient, have sacrificed, or have been particularly helpful. Do not expect siblings to always act in this manner.

Acknowledge the personal strengths that siblings have and their ability to cope with stress successfully.

Provide age-appropriate information about the child's condition and update it when appropriate.

Let teachers know what is happening so that they can be understanding and helpful.

Recognize special stress times for siblings and plan to minimize negative effects.

Schedule special time with siblings; have a friend or family member substitute when parent is unavailable.

Encourage siblings to join or help establish a sibling support group.

Use the services of professionals when needed. If parent feels that such a service is necessary, it should be provided in as vigorous a manner as a service for the child with special needs.

Involve Siblings

Seek out ways to realistically include siblings in the care and treatment of the child with special needs.

Limit caregiving responsibilities and give recognition when siblings perform them.

Develop a library of children's books on special needs.

Invite siblings to attend meetings to develop plans for the child with special needs (e.g., individualized educational program [IEP], individualized family service plan [IFSP]).

Discuss future plans with them.

Solicit their ideas on treatment and service needs.

Have them visit professionals who work with the child.

Help them develop competencies to teach the child new skills.

Provide opportunities for siblings to advocate for the child.

Allow siblings to set their own pace for learning and involvement.

Data from Powell, T., & Ogle, P. (1985). *Brothers and sisters—A special part of exceptional families.* Baltimore, MD: Paul H. Brooks; Spokane Washington Deaconess Medical Center, Pediatric Oncology Unit. (1987); Carlson, J., Leviton, A., & Mueller, M. (1993). Services to siblings: An important component of family-centered practice. *ACCH Advocate, 1*(1), 53–56.

brother's or sister's illness or complex condition. What siblings piece together or overhear is often much worse than the truth. Often they imagine gruesome things regarding the experiences related to the illness, treatment, and hospitalization (Knafl & Santacroce, 2010). Hispanic siblings have reported less accurate information about their siblings' condition than non-Hispanic siblings (Lobato, Kao, & Plante, 2005). Parents are usually in the best position to impart information, although they are often overwhelmed by the medical crisis at hand (Fleitas, 2000). Nurses can encourage parents to talk with the siblings about how they perceive their sick brother or sister, and to be accepting of the siblings' feelings. Nurses can be ideal educators and counselors of siblings during the course of their brother's or sister's illness.

COPING WITH ONGOING STRESS AND PERIODIC CRISES

Professionals can help families cope with stress by providing anticipatory guidance, providing emotional support, assisting the family in assessing and identifying specific stressors, aiding the family in developing coping mechanisms and problem-solving strategies, and working collaboratively with parents so that they become empowered in the process (Anderson & Davis, 2011).

Concurrent Stresses Within the Family

The ability to deal with the overwhelming stress of a chronic illness is challenged further when additional stresses are present. Stressors may be situational or developmental. They may be related to marital difficulties, sibling needs, homelessness, or social isolation. Some families may simultaneously be struggling with a family member's alcohol or other drug problem. Even relatively minor stressors, such as arranging care for siblings, managing the home, and traveling to distant treatment centers, can challenge a family's ability to cope successfully.

Most families, regardless of their income or insurance coverage, have financial concerns. The costs of caring for a child with a complex illness can be overwhelming. Nurses and social workers can help a family review various options for financial assistance, including insurance, managed care, or health maintenance organization policies; Medicaid; Supplemental Security Income; Women, Infants, and Children program; the state Program for Children with Special Health Needs; disease-related associations; and local philanthropic organizations.

Coping Mechanisms

Coping mechanisms are behaviors aimed at reducing the tension caused by a crisis. **Approach behaviors** are coping mechanisms that result in movement toward adjustment and resolution of the crisis. **Avoidance behaviors** result in movement away from adjustment and represent maladaptation to the crisis. Several approach and avoidance behaviors used in coping with a chronic illness are listed in the Nursing Care Guidelines box. Each behavior must be viewed in the context of all of the variables affecting the family. For example, the observation of several avoidance behaviors in an emotionally healthy family may denote significantly less risk to the successful resolution of the crisis than an equal number of avoidance behaviors in an individual who has few available supports.

NURSING CARE GUIDELINES

Assessing Coping Behaviors

Approach Behaviors

Asks for information on diagnosis and child's present condition
Seeks help and support from others
Anticipates future problems; actively seeks guidance and answers
Endows the chronic illness or complex condition with meaning
Shares burden of disorder with others
Plans realistically for the future
Acknowledges and accepts child's awareness of diagnosis and prognosis
Expresses feelings (such as sorrow, depression, and anger) and realizes reason for the emotional reaction
Realistically perceives child's condition; adjusts to changes
Recognizes own growth through passage of time, such as earlier denial and nonacceptance of diagnosis
Verbalizes possible loss of child

Avoidance Behaviors

Fails to recognize seriousness of child's condition despite physical evidence
Refuses to agree to treatment
Intellectualizes about the illness but in areas unrelated to child's condition
Is angry and hostile to members of the staff regardless of their attitude or behavior
Avoids staff, family members, or child
Entertains unrealistic future plans for child with little emphasis on the present
Is unable to adjust to or accept a change in progression of disease
Continually looks for new cures with no perspective toward possible benefit
Refuses to acknowledge child's understanding of disease and prognosis
Uses magical thinking and fantasy; may seek "occult" help
Places complete faith in religion to point of relinquishing own responsibility
Withdraws from outside world; refuses help
Punishes self because of guilt and blame
Makes no change in lifestyle to meet needs of other family members
Resorts to excessive use of alcohol or drugs to avoid problems
Verbalizes suicidal intents
Is unable to discuss possible loss of child or previous experiences with death

Parental Empowerment

Empowerment can be seen as a process of recognizing, promoting, and enhancing competence. For parents of children with chronic conditions, empowerment may occur gradually as strength and capabilities are drawn on to master the child's care, manage family life, and plan for the future. Advocating for the child and developing parent-professional partnerships are part of taking charge (Panicker, 2013).

ASSISTING FAMILY MEMBERS IN MANAGING THEIR FEELINGS

Although some previous research has postulated stages of adaptation to a chronic illness, there is a great deal of individual variation in responses to the diagnosis, adjustments made, and time frames for coming to terms with a diagnosis. It is important that professionals recognize and respect a wide range of reactions and coping mechanisms. In fact, members of the family of a child with a CCC may experience a number of difficult emotions, including fear, guilt, anger, resentment, and anxiety. Learning to manage these emotions promotes adaptive coping (see Nursing Care Guidelines box). Support from professionals, other family members, and friends can assist family members in managing their feelings. The following discussion examines some common phases of adjustment and emotional reactions.

Shock and Denial

The initial diagnosis of a chronic illness or complex condition is often met with intense emotion and is characterized by shock, disbelief, and sometimes denial. Denial as a defense mechanism is a necessary cushion to prevent disintegration and is a normal response to grieving for any type of loss. Probably all family members experience various degrees of adaptive denial as they learn of the impact the diagnosis has on their lives.

Shock and denial can last from days to months, sometimes even longer. Examples of denial that may be exhibited at the time of diagnosis include:

- Physician shopping
- Attributing the symptoms of the actual illness to a minor condition
- Refusing to believe the diagnostic tests
- Delaying consent for treatment
- Acting happy and optimistic despite the revealed diagnosis
- Refusing to tell or talk to anyone about the condition
- Insisting that no one is telling the truth, regardless of others' attempts to do so
- Denying the reason for admission
- Asking no questions about the diagnosis, treatment, or prognosis

Generally, these mechanisms should be respected as short-term responses that allow individuals to distance themselves from the tremendous emotional impact and to collect and mobilize their energies toward goal-directed, problem-solving behaviors.

In children, the importance of denial has repeatedly been demonstrated as a factor in their positive coping with the diagnosis. Denial allows the child to maintain hope in the face of overwhelming odds and to function adaptively and productively. Similar to hope, denial may be an adaptive mechanism for dealing with loss that persists until a family or patient is ready or needs other responses.

Denial is probably the least understood and most poorly dealt-with reaction. If denial is labeled as maladaptive, it can lead to inappropriate attempts to strip away the reaction by repeated and sometimes blunt explanations of the prognosis. However, denial becomes maladaptive only when it prevents recognition of treatment or rehabilitative goals necessary for the child's optimal survival or development.

Adjustment

For most families, adjustment gradually follows shock and is usually characterized by an open admission that the condition exists. This stage may be accompanied by several responses, which are normal parts of the adaptation process. Probably the most universal of these feelings are **guilt** and **self-accusation**. Guilt is often greatest when the cause of the disorder is directly traceable to the parent, as in genetic diseases or accidental injury. However, it can occur even without any scientific or realistic basis for parental responsibility. Frequently the guilt stems from a false assumption that the child's condition is a result of personal failure or wrongdoing, such as not doing something correctly during pregnancy or the birth. Guilt may also be associated with cultural or religious beliefs. Some parents are convinced that they are being punished for some previous misdeed. Others may see the illness as a trial sent by God to test their religious strength and faith. With correct information, support, and time, most parents master guilt and self-accusation.

Children, too, may interpret their serious illness as retribution for past misbehavior. The nurse should be particularly sensitive to the child who passively accepts all painful procedures. This child may believe that such acts are inflicted as deserved punishment. It is vital that parents and health care professionals reassure children that their illnesses are not their fault.

Other common and normal reactions to a diagnosis are bitterness and anger. Anger directed inward may be evident as self-reproaching or punitive behavior, such as neglecting one's health and verbally degrading oneself. Anger directed outward may be manifested in either open arguments or withdrawal from communication and may be evident in the person's relationship with any number of individuals, such as the spouse, the child, and siblings. Passive anger toward the ill child may be evident in decreased visiting, refusal to believe how sick the child is, or an inability to provide comfort. Health care providers are among the most common targets for parental anger. Parents may complain about the nursing care, the insufficient time physicians spend with them, or the lack of skill of those who draw blood or start intravenous infusions.

Children are apt to respond with anger as well, and this includes the affected child and the well siblings. Children are aware of the loss engendered by their illness or complex condition and may react angrily to the restrictions imposed or the feelings of being different. Siblings may also feel anger and resentment toward the ill child and parents for the loss of routine and parental attention. It is difficult for older children and almost impossible for younger children to comprehend the plight of the affected child. Their perception is of a brother or sister who has the undivided attention of their parents, is showered with cards and gifts, and is the focus of everyone's concern.

During the period of adjustment, four types of parental reactions to the child influence the child's eventual response to the disorder:

- **Overprotection:** The parents fear letting the child achieve any new skill, avoid all discipline, and cater to every desire to prevent frustration.
- **Rejection:** The parents detach themselves emotionally from the child but usually provide adequate physical care or constantly nag and scold the child.
- **Denial:** The parents act as if the disorder does not exist or attempt to have the child overcompensate for it.
- **Gradual acceptance:** The parents place necessary and realistic restrictions on the child, encourage self-care activities, and promote reasonable physical and social abilities.

Reintegration and Acknowledgment

For many families, the adjustment process culminates in the development of realistic expectations for the child and reintegration of family life with the illness or complex condition in a manageable perspective. Because a large portion of this phase is one of grief for a loss, total resolution is not possible until the child dies or leaves home as an independent adult. One can regard adjustment as "increased comfort" with everyday living rather than a complete resolution.

This adjustment phase also involves social reintegration in which the family broadens its activities to include relationships outside of the home with the child as an acceptable and participating member of the group. This last criterion often differentiates the reaction of gradual acceptance during the adjustment period from total acceptance or perhaps is more descriptive of the acknowledgment process.

Many parents of children with chronic illnesses experience **chronic sorrow**, which are feelings of sorrow and loss that recur in waves over time. As the child's condition progresses, parents experience repeated losses that represent further declines and new caregiving demands. Even common occurrences can trigger feelings of sorrow well after the initial event; consequently, families must be assessed on an ongoing basis and offered appropriate support and resources as their needs change over time. This represents a critical period because the manner in which the nursing and medical team approach and provide support can directly affect the experience of complicated grief after the death of the child. Complicated grief, which is characterized as persistent distress and chronic stress response, may last for 6 months or longer after the death of a child and has a significant impact on quality of life of the family members left behind (Meert, Shear, Newth, et al., 2011). *Persistent complex bereavement disorder* is a new diagnostic entity included in the fifth edition of the *Diagnostic and Statistical Manual of Mental Disorders* (American Psychological Association, 2013).

BOX 17.5 Concept of Functional Burden

Impact of the Child With Special Needs

The child's need for medical and nursing care
The child's fixed deficits
The child's age-appropriate dependency in activities of daily living
The disruptions in the family routine caused by the care
The psychologic burden of the prognosis on the family

Family Resources and Ability to Cope

The family's physical resources
The family's emotional resources
The family's educational resources
The family's social supports and available help
The competing demands for family members' time and energy

Data from Stein, R. E. K. (1985). Home care: A challenging opportunity. *Child Health Care, 14*(2), 90–95.

ESTABLISHING A SUPPORT SYSTEM

The diagnosis of a child with a CCC is a major situational crisis that affects the entire family system. However, families can experience positive outcomes as they successfully deal with the many challenges that accompany a child with chronic illness (Hungerbuehler, Vollrath, & Landolt, 2011).

One nursing goal is to assess which families are at risk for succumbing to the effects of the crisis. Several variables—available support system, perception of the event, coping mechanisms, reactions to the child, available resources, and concurrent stresses within the family—influence the resolution of a crisis. Although most families cope well, the needs of families at risk are great. If they receive emotional support and guidance early, there is an increased likelihood that they will also cope successfully.

Although it is easy to assume that families of children with the most severe illnesses or disabilities would have the poorest adjustment, the severity of the condition reflects only one part of the overall picture. The level of adjustment is significantly influenced by the **functional burden** on the family (Stein, 1985). This concept considers the issues related to caring for and living with the child in relation to the family's resources and ability to cope (Box 17.5). The family of a child with a high level of technology dependence demanding complex care yet having many resources and coping skills may adjust more successfully to the child's situation than the family of a child with a less serious condition and few resources to counterbalance.

Intrafamilial resources, social support from friends and relatives, parent-to-parent support, parent-professional partnerships, and community resources interweave to provide a flexible web of support for families of children with chronic conditions.

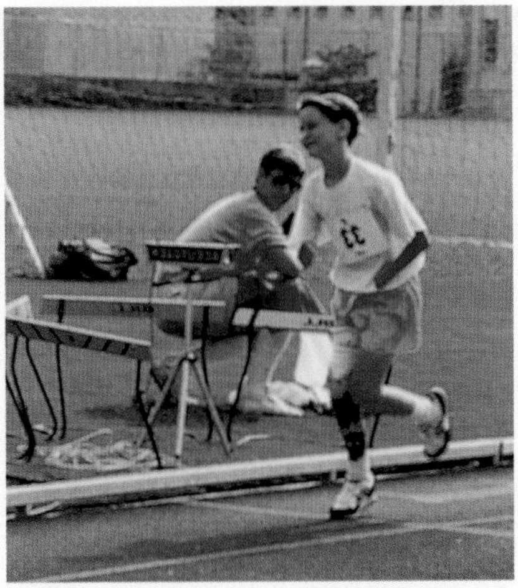

Fig. 17.1 Children with any type of impairment should have the opportunity to develop their skills. (Courtesy Poyo/Hinton Photography.)

THE CHILD WITH A CHRONIC OR COMPLEX CONDITION

The child's reaction to chronic illness depends to a great extent on his or her developmental level, temperament, and available coping mechanisms; on the reactions of family members or significant others; and, to a lesser extent, on the condition itself. A child's conceptual understanding of his or her own illness is based not only on age and developmental level but also on the duration and type of experience accumulated with the disease. Knowledge of these variables is essential to providing the kind of information and support needed by these children to cope with an often overwhelming situation.

DEVELOPMENTAL ASPECTS

The impact of a complex chronic illness is influenced by the age at onset. Chronic illness affects children of all ages, but the developmental aspects of each age-group dictate particular stresses and risks for the child. The nurse must also recognize that children need to redefine their condition and its implications as they develop and grow. For example, appearance, skills, and abilities are highly valued by peers (Fig. 17.1). A teenager who is limited in any of these qualities is subject to rejection. This is especially marked when an illness interferes with sexual attractiveness.

Children's developmental concepts of illness are discussed in Chapter 19. An understanding of these developmental factors facilitates planning care to support the child and minimize the risks. Developmental effects of chronic illness on children are described in Table 17.2.

COPING MECHANISMS

Children with chronic conditions tend to use five distinct patterns of coping (Box 17.6). Children with more positive and accepting attitudes about their chronic illness use a more adaptive coping style characterized by optimism, competence, and compliance. They show fewer behavior problems at home and at school. The two maladaptive coping patterns—"Feels different and withdraws" and "Is irritable, is moody, and acts out"—are associated with poorer adaptation; children using these strategies have poorer self-concepts, more negative attitudes about their conditions, and more behavior problems at home and at school.

Well-adapted children gradually learn to accept their physical limitations and find achievement in a variety of compensatory motor and intellectual pursuits. They function well at home, at school, and with peers. They have an understanding of their disorder that allows them to accept their limitations, assume responsibility for their care, and assist in treatment and rehabilitation regimens. They express appropriate emotions, such as sadness, anxiety, and anger, at times of exacerbations but confidence and guarded optimism during periods of clinical stability (Fig. 17.2). They are able to identify with other similarly affected individuals, promoting positive self-images and displaying pride and self-confidence in their ability to master a productive, successful life despite their illnesses.

Hopefulness

Children, particularly adolescents, are sensitive to the presence or absence of hope. Hopefulness is an internal quality that mobilizes humans into goal-directed action that may be satisfying and life sustaining. Higher levels of hope have been associated with higher levels of resiliency and the ability to see obstacles as opportunities (Griggs & Walker, 2016).

Health Education and Self-Care

Health education is an intervention that promotes coping. Children need information about their condition, the therapeutic plan, and how the disease or the therapy might affect their particular situation. Children nearing puberty also need to understand the maturation process and how their chronic illness may alter this event. For example, a youngster with Crohn disease should understand that this disorder is associated with growth failure and delayed puberty, a child with diabetes needs to know that hormonal changes and increased growth needs will alter food and insulin requirements at this time, and a sexually active girl with sickle cell anemia or systemic lupus erythematosus needs to be aware of the risks of pregnancy. The information should not be given all at once but should be timed appropriately to meet children's changing needs, and it should be described and repeated as often as the situation demands.

RESPONSES TO PARENTAL BEHAVIOR

Parental behavior toward the child is one of the most important factors influencing the child's adjustment. Children's perceptions of their mothers' support and maternal perceptions of the psychosocial impact of the child's chronic illness on the family were shown to be two of the greatest predictors of children's psychologic adjustment (Immelt, 2006). In addition, family organization, illness-related support, and involvement of the parents influence children's adjustment to chronic illness (Schor, 2003). They often display pride and confidence in their ability to cope successfully with the challenges imposed by their disorder. Anticipatory guidance by the nurse and encouragement of normalizing practices may assist parents in facilitating positive adjustment in their children.

TYPE OF ILLNESS OR CONDITION

The type of illness or condition also influences the child's emotional response. Interestingly, children with *more* severe disorders often cope better than those with milder conditions. However, the presence of multiple conditions may place a child at risk for more behavioral problems (Newacheck & Halfon, 1998). Because of children's cognitive

TABLE 17.2 Developmental Effects of Chronic Illness or Disability on Children

Developmental Tasks	Potential Effects of Chronic Illness or Disability	Supportive Interventions
Infancy		
Develop a sense of trust	Multiple caregivers and frequent separations, especially if hospitalized Deprived of consistent nurturing	Encourage consistent caregivers in hospital or other care settings. Encourage parental presence, "rooming in" during hospitalization, and participation in care.
Bond, or attach, to parent	Delayed because of separation; parental grief for loss of "dream" child; parental inability to accept the condition, especially a visible defect	Emphasize healthy, perfect qualities of infant. Help parents learn special care needs of infant for them to feel competent.
Learn through sensorimotor experiences	More exposure to painful experiences than pleasurable ones Limited contact with environment from restricted movement or confinement	Expose infant to pleasurable experiences through all senses (touch, hearing, sight, taste, movement). Encourage age-appropriate developmental skills (e.g., holding bottle, finger feeding, crawling).
Begin to develop a sense of separateness from parent	Increased dependency on parent for care Overinvolvement of parent in care	Encourage all family members to participate in care to prevent overinvolvement of one member. Encourage periodic respite from demands of care responsibilities.
Toddlerhood		
Develop autonomy	Increased dependency on parent	Encourage independence in as many areas as possible (e.g., toileting, dressing, feeding).
Master locomotor and language skills	Limited opportunity to test own abilities and limits	Provide gross motor skill activity and modification of toys or equipment, such as modified swing or rocking horse.
Learn through sensorimotor experience; beginning preoperational thought	Increased exposure to painful experiences	Give choices to allow simple feeling of control (e.g., choice of what book to look at, what kind of sandwich to eat). Institute age-appropriate discipline and limit setting. Recognize that negative and ritualistic behaviors are normal. Provide sensory experiences (e.g., water play, sandbox play, finger painting).
Preschool Age		
Develop initiative and purpose Master self-care skills	Limited opportunities for success in accomplishing simple tasks or mastering self-care skills	Encourage mastery of self-help skills. Provide devices that make tasks easier (e.g., self-dressing).
Begin to develop peer relationships	Limited opportunities for socialization with peers; may appear "like a baby" to age-mates Protection within tolerant and secure family, causing child to fear criticism and withdraw	Encourage socialization (e.g., inviting friends to play, daycare experience, trips to park). Provide age-appropriate play, especially associative play opportunities. Emphasize child's abilities; dress appropriately to enhance desirable appearance.
Develop sense of body image and sexual identification	Awareness of body centering on pain, anxiety, and failure Sex-role identification focused primarily on mothering skills	Encourage relationships with same-sex and opposite-sex peers and adults.
Learn through preoperational thought (magical thinking)	Guilt (thinking he or she caused the illness or disability or is being punished for wrongdoing)	Help child deal with criticisms; realize that too much protection prevents child from realities of world. Clarify that cause of child's illness or disability is not his or her fault or a punishment.
School Age		
Develop a sense of accomplishment	Limited opportunities to achieve and compete (e.g., many school absences, inability to join regular athletic activities)	Encourage school attendance; schedule medical visits at times other than school; encourage child to make up missed work.
Form peer relationships	Limited opportunities for socialization	Educate teachers and classmates about child's condition, abilities, and special needs. Encourage sports activities (e.g., Special Olympics). Encourage socialization (e.g., Girl Scouts, Campfire, Boy Scouts, 4-H Club; having a best friend or club membership).

TABLE 17.2 Developmental Effects of Chronic Illness or Disability on Children—cont'd

Developmental Tasks	Potential Effects of Chronic Illness or Disability	Supportive Interventions
Learn through concrete operations	Incomplete comprehension of the imposed physical limitations or treatment of the disorder	Provide child with information about his or her condition. Encourage creative activities (e.g., VSA Arts).
Adolescence		
Develop personal and sexual identity	Increased sense of feeling different from peers and reduced ability to compete with peers in appearance, abilities, special skills	Help teenager realize that many of the difficulties he or she is experiencing are part of normal adolescence (rebelliousness, risk taking, lack of cooperation, and hostility toward authority).
Achieve independence from family	Increased dependency on family; limited job or career opportunities	Provide instruction on interpersonal and coping skills. Encourage increased responsibility for care and management of the disease or condition (e.g., assuming responsibility for making and keeping appointment [ideally alone], sharing assessment and planning stages of health care delivery, contacting resources). Discuss planning for future and how condition can affect choices.
Form heterosexual relationships	Limited opportunities for heterosexual friendships; less opportunity to discuss sexual concerns with peers Increased concern with issues such as why did he or she get the disorder and whether he or she will marry and have a family	Encourage socialization with peers, including peers with special needs and those without special needs. Encourage activities appropriate for age (e.g., attending mixed-sex parties, sports activities, driving a car). Be alert to cues that signal readiness for information regarding implications of condition on sexuality and reproduction. Emphasize good appearance and wearing stylish clothes, use of makeup. Understand that adolescent has same sexual needs and concerns as any other teenager.
Learn through abstract thinking	Decreased opportunity for earlier stages of cognition impeding achievement of level of abstract thinking	Provide instruction on decision making, assertiveness, and other skills necessary to manage personal plans.

BOX 17.6 Coping Patterns Used by Children With Special Needs

Develops competence and optimism: Accentuates the positive aspects of the situation and concentrates more on what he or she has or can do than on what is missing or on what he or she cannot do; is as independent as possible

Feels different and withdraws: Sees self as being different from other children because of the chronic health condition; views being different as negative; sees self as less worthy than others; focuses on things he or she cannot do and sometimes overrestricts activities needlessly

Is irritable, is moody, and acts out: Uses proactive and self-initiated coping behaviors, although usually counterproductive in that the behaviors are not ego enhancing or socially responsible and do not result in desired outcomes; acts out irritability, which may or may not be associated with condition's symptoms

Complies with treatment: Takes necessary medications and treatments; adheres to activity restrictions; also uses behaviors that indicate developing independence (e.g., assumes responsibility for taking medication)

Seeks support: Talks with adults, children, physicians, and nurses; develops plans to handle problems as they occur; uses downward comparison (i.e., realizes that others have it worse)

Modified from Austin, J., Patterson, J., & Huberty, T. (1991). Development of the coping health inventory for children. *Journal of Pediatric Nursing, 6*(3), 166–174.

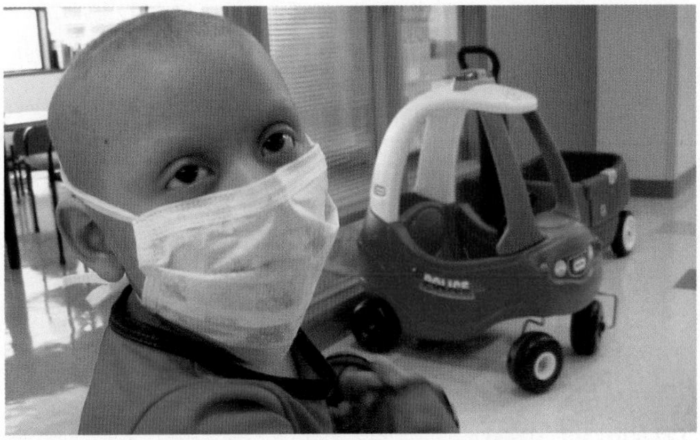

Fig. 17.2 Periods of sadness and anger are appropriate in the child's adjustment to a chronic illness or disability, especially during exacerbations of the disorder.

ability and the timing of onset of abstract thinking in adolescence, an obvious condition may be easier for them to accept because its limitations are concrete.

The onset of a disabling condition may generate a state of confusion for children, who may have trouble differentiating between actual bodily functions and their image of their bodies. They may also experience problems in identifying themselves and those extensions of self (e.g., wheelchairs, braces, crutches, other mechanical or prosthetic devices) and may have difficulty in accepting functional aids.

TABLE 17.3 Assessment of Factors Affecting Family Adjustment

Factors Affecting Adjustment	Assessment Questions
Available Support System	
Status of marital relationship	To whom do you talk when you have something on your mind? (If answer is not the spouse, ask for the reason.)
Alternate support systems	When something is worrying you, what do you do? What helps you most when you are upset?
Ability to communicate	Does talking seem to help when you feel upset?
Perception of the Illness or Disability	
Previous knowledge of disorder	Have you ever heard the word (name of diagnosis) before? Tell me about it (if answer is yes).
Imagined cause of disorder	What are your thoughts about the causes of the disorder?
Effects of illness or disability on family	How has your child's illness or disability affected you and your family? How has your lifestyle changed?
Coping Mechanisms	
Reactions to previous crises	Tell me one time you've had another crisis (problem, bad time) in your family. How did you solve that problem?
Reactions to the child	Do you find yourself being a little more cautious with this child than with your other children?
Childrearing practices	Do you feel as comfortable disciplining this child as your other children?
Influence of religion	Has your religion or faith been of help to you? Tell me how (if answer is yes).
Attitudes	How is this child different from the siblings or other children of similar age? Describe your child's personality. Is it easy, difficult, or in between? When you think of your child's future, what thoughts come to mind?
Available Resources	
	What parts of your child's care are causing the most difficulty for you or your family?
	What services are available to help?
	What services do you need that currently are not available?
Concurrent Stresses	
	What other problems are you facing now? (Be specific; ask about financial, marital, sibling, and extended family or friends concerns.)

NURSING CARE OF THE FAMILY AND CHILD WITH A CHRONIC OR COMPLEX CONDITION

ASSESSMENT

Because the nurse may meet a family during any phase of the adjustment process, several assessment areas are important. The family's ability to cope with previous stresses influences the current situation, and answers to questions about their usual coping skills are enlightening. Knowledge of concurrent stresses, such as financial, marital or nonmarital, and career or unemployment, helps identify families who may have fewer resources to cope with the child's needs.

Finally, awareness of the family members' reactions to the child and the illness or condition is important. Sample questions that the nurse and family can use to evaluate the support system, perception of the illness, coping mechanisms, resources, and concurrent stresses are listed in Table 17.3. Because factors affecting the family's response may change at any point during the illness, assessment must be a continuous process.

Special challenges exist in assessing the child's feelings about having a chronic illness. Though they may develop an understanding of their condition, this may not always translate to an understanding of the long-term implications of their chronic complex diagnosis. Chapter 4 presents several approaches to encourage children to discuss their feelings about their conditions. The nurse should use a variety of communication techniques, such as drawing and play, as assessment tools rather than relying solely on parental reports.

The needs of working parents and siblings also should be assessed; this is a goal that requires flexibility in scheduling appointments. When working parents know that their input is valuable, they will often change their work schedule to meet with a health professional. Because siblings can be of any age, the use of appropriate communication strategies for assessment must be considered. Nonverbal techniques, such as those discussed in Chapter 4, should be considered for these children.

PROVIDE SUPPORT AT THE TIME OF DIAGNOSIS

The diagnosis is a critical time for parents and can influence how they perceive their health care providers across the trajectory of care. Although they may not hear or remember all that is said to them, they frequently sense a certain attitude of acceptance, rejection, hope, or despair that may influence their ability to absorb the shock and begin adapting to the family's altered future.

Parents may be encouraged to be together when they are informed of their child's condition, thus avoiding the problem of one parent having to interpret complex information and deal with the initial emotional reaction of the other. The informing session should take place in a private, comfortable setting free of distractions and interruptions in an atmosphere in which the parents feel free to express their emotions (Fig. 17.3). Their emotional needs are acknowledged by showing acceptance of expressions, such as crying, sadness, anger, and disappointment. Emotional support is offered by having tissues available if a family member cries and demonstrating through facial and body language that indeed this is a difficult and painful period. Although touching is a powerful expression of empathy, it must be used wisely. For example, it can prematurely terminate free expression of feelings, especially when combined with statements such as "Everything will be all right." Nurses should also be aware of cultural issues regarding touching (see Chapter 4).

Parents should receive the kind of information they desire. This can be assessed by asking questions such as "Do you prefer to hear detailed information?" Parents or other family members may have different preferences regarding the amount of information that they wish to hear. Most parents want a clear, simple explanation of the diagnosis; a prediction of possible futures for the child; advice on what to do next; an opportunity to ask questions; a warm, sympathetic listener; and, most important, time. Understanding of explanations is elicited with questions such as "Do you see what I mean?" or "Is this clear to you?" Technical terms are used with simple definitions. If the parents are unaware of the term, they are given written literature or at least a written summary of the diagnosis.

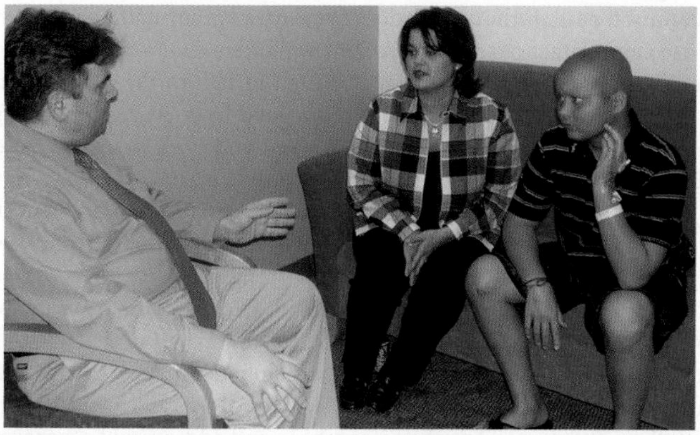

Fig. 17.3 Information sessions should take place in a private, comfortable setting free of distractions and interruptions.

Finally, the informing conference does not end with the presentation of devastating news. Instead, the child's strengths, appealing behaviors, and potential for development are stressed, as are available rehabilitation efforts or treatments. Parents can be encouraged to view their experiences as a series of challenges that they are capable of handling, particularly with available professional feedback. The parents are assured that the nurse will be available to answer questions and to provide further assistance as needed.

The preceding discussion relates primarily to the initial informing interview. However, because of the need for long-term follow-up, it is only one in a series of continuing discussions. In all interactions, the family's input is solicited and incorporated into the care plan. Some situations require consideration of special problems (see Nursing Care Guidelines box).

NURSING CARE GUIDELINES

Situations Requiring Special Consideration

Congenital Anomaly

Tension in the delivery room conveys the sense that something is seriously wrong. Communication is often delayed while the physician is involved with the mother's care. The manner in which the infant is presented may well set the tone for the early parent-child relationship.

Clarify role with physician in regard to revealing information to enable immediate parental support.

Explain to parents briefly in simple language what the defect is and something concerning the immediate prognosis before showing them the infant. Later more information can be given when they are more ready to "hear" what is said.

Be aware of nonverbal communication. Parents watch facial expressions of others for signs of revulsion or rejection.

Present infant as something precious.

Emphasize well-formed aspects of infant's body.

Allow time and opportunity for parents to express their initial response.

Encourage parents to ask questions and provide honest, straightforward answers without undue optimism or pessimism.

Cognitive Impairment

Unless cognitive impairment is associated with other physical problems, it is often easy for parents to miss clues to its presence or to make defensive excuses regarding the diagnosis.

Plan situations that help parents become aware of the problem.

Encourage parents to discuss their observations of child but withhold diagnostic opinions.

Focus on what the child can do and appropriate interventions to promote progress (e.g., infant stimulation programs) to involve parents in their child's care while helping them gain an awareness of the child's condition.

Physical Disability

If loss of motor or sensory ability occurs during childhood, the diagnosis is readily apparent. The challenge lies in helping the child and parents over the period of shock and grief and toward the phase of acceptance and reintegration.

Institute early rehabilitation (e.g., using a prosthetic limb, learning to read braille, learning to read lips).

Be aware that physical rehabilitation usually precedes psychologic adjustment.

When the cause of the disability is accidental, avoid implying that parents or child was responsible for the injury but allow them the opportunity to discuss feelings of blame.

Encourage expression of feelings (see Chapter 4, Communication Techniques).

Chronic Illness

Realization of the true impact may take months or years. Conflict over parents' versus child's concerns may result in serious problems. When condition is inherited, parents may blame themselves or child may blame the parents.

Help each family member gain an appreciation of the others' concerns.

Discuss hereditary aspect of condition with parents at time of diagnosis to lessen guilt and accusatory feelings.

Encourage child to express feelings by using third-person technique (e.g., "Sometimes when a person has an illness that was passed on by the parents, that person feels angry or bitter toward them").

Multiple Disabilities

The child or parent may require additional time for the shock phase and may be able to attend to only one diagnosis before hearing significant information about other disorders.

Acknowledge parents' understanding and acceptance of all diagnoses, especially when an obvious and more hidden disability coexists.

Appreciate the devastating consequences of more than one disability for a child, especially if they interfere with expressive-receptive abilities.

Terminal Illness

Parents require much support to deal with their own feelings and guidance in how to tell the child the diagnosis. They may want to conceal the diagnosis from the child. They may believe that the child is too young to know, will not be able to cope with the information, or will lose hope and the will to live.

Approach the subject of disclosure in a positive way by asking, "How will you tell your child about the diagnosis?"

Help parents understand the disadvantages of not telling the child (e.g., deprives child of the opportunity to discuss feelings openly and ask questions, incurs the risk of child learning the truth from outside and sometimes less tactful sources, may lessen child's trust and confidence in the parents after learning the truth).

Guide parents to see the potential problems involved in fostering a conspiracy.

Offer parents guidelines for how and what to tell the child about the disease or the possibility of death. Explanations should be tailored to child's cognitive ability, be based on knowledge child already has, and be honest. Honesty must be tempered with concern for child's feelings.

Assure parents that telling a child the name of the illness and the reason for treatment instills hope, provides support from others, and serves as a foundation for explaining and understanding subsequent events.

Acknowledge that being honest is not always easy because the truth may prompt the child to ask other distressing questions, such as "Am I going to die?" However, even this difficult question must be answered.

SUPPORT THE FAMILY'S COPING METHODS

For the family to meet the stresses of optimally adjusting to the child's condition, each member must be individually supported so that the family system is strong. Although the family can indefinitely support a member who is in need of assistance, its greatest strength lies in every member supporting each other. The nurse should bear in mind that the family member in greatest need is not necessarily the affected child but may be a parent or sibling who is dealing with stresses that require intervention.

Parents

The nurse can provide support by being attentive to families' responses to their children. Mothers and fathers need to experience success, joy, and pride in their children to give the support they need. It is important for nurses to examine their attitudes to determine their ability to engage in parent-professional partnerships. An essential characteristic is the belief that parents are equal to professionals and are experts on their child (see Nursing Care Guidelines box).

NURSING CARE GUIDELINES

Developing Successful Parent-Professional Partnerships

Promote primary nursing; in nonhospital settings, designate a case manager.
Acknowledge parents' overall competence and their unique expertise with their child.
Respect parents' time as having value equal to that of other members of child's health care team.
Explain or define any medical, technical, or discipline-specific terms.
Tell families, "I am not sure" or "I don't know" when appropriate.
Facilitate family's effectiveness in team meetings (e.g., provide parents with same information as other participants).

Parents can be encouraged to discuss their feelings toward the child, the impact of this event on their marriage, and associated stresses such as financial burdens. For most families, regardless of their income or insurance coverage, financial concerns exist. The costs of caring for a child with special needs can be overwhelming. In addition, one or both parents may have to sacrifice job opportunities to remain close to a medical facility or to avoid losing insurance benefits. Numerous volunteer and community resources that provide assistance, rehabilitation, equipment, and funding for a variety of health problems are available. National and local disease-oriented organizations may provide needed assistance and support to families that qualify. Many of these are discussed elsewhere in the text under the specific diagnosis. State and federal departments of health, mental health, social services, and labor may be able to help locate appropriate regional resources. For example, state programs for Children with Special Health Needs provide financial assistance for children with many disabling conditions. Local and national sources of respite care and medical daycare may be useful to families. Nurses should become acquainted with those in their communities and with vocational programs for special groups.

Parent-to-Parent Support

Just being with another parent who has shared similar experiences is helpful. It may not need to be a parent of a child with the same diagnosis, because parents in the process of adjusting to a child with special needs—or finding respite services, educational or rehabilitative services, special equipment vendors, and financial counseling—tread a common path. If the agency does not have a parent staff position, the nurse can contact parent groups that will often send a representative. Another strategy is to ask another parent to talk to the parents. The nurse should seek out a parent who is a good listener, has a nonjudgmental approach to differences in families, and possesses good advocacy and problem-solving skills.

The parent self-help group can promote parent-to-parent support.[a] Group members feel less alone and have the opportunity to observe both coping and mastery role modeling from other members. Parent groups are rich resources for information. Even if parents are unable to attend meetings, they can still benefit from group newsletters and other literature that often accompany membership. Nurses can assist in starting a group by identifying one or two parents as leaders; sharing with them the names, telephone numbers, and addresses of other families who have expressed both an interest and a willingness to release their phone numbers and addresses; and guiding them in how to initiate a first meeting.

Advocate for Empowerment

Nurses can advocate for methods that foster opportunities for parent empowerment. For example, nurses can suggest reimbursement for travel and child care plus stipends to enable parents' voices to be heard at meetings and conferences. They can encourage parent membership on committees and advisory boards. They can keep parents informed of pending legislation on child health issues or take action when parents inform them.

The Child

Through ongoing contacts with the child, the nurse (1) observes the child's responses to the disorder, ability to function, and adaptive behaviors within the environment and with significant others; (2) explores the child's own understanding of his or her illness or condition; and (3) provides support while the child learns to cope with his or her feelings. Children are encouraged to express their concerns rather than allowing others to express them for them because open discussions may reduce anxiety (see Nursing Care Guidelines box).

NURSING CARE GUIDELINES

Encouraging Expression of Emotion

Describe the behavior: "You seem angry at everyone."
Give evidence of understanding: "Being angry is only natural."
Give evidence of caring: "It must be difficult to endure so many painful procedures."
Help focus on feelings: "Maybe you wonder why this happened to you."

One of the most important interventions is alleviating the child's feeling of being different and normalizing his or her life as much as possible (see Nursing Care Guidelines box). Whenever possible, the nurse assists the family in assessing the child's daily routine for indications of a need for normalizing practices. For example, the child who remains in a bedroom all day requires a restructured daily routine to provide activities in different parts of the house, such as eating in the kitchen or dining room with the family. Such children may also be deprived of social, recreational, and academic activities that can

[a]Information about self-help groups and books and pamphlets are available from the National Self-Help Clearinghouse, 365 Fifth Ave., Suite 3300, New York, NY 10016; 217-817-1822; http://www.selfhelpweb.org.

be better accommodated by applying normalization practices. For example, home and out-of-home health-related treatments should be planned at times that least interfere with normal daily activities.

NURSING CARE GUIDELINES

Promoting Normalization

Preparation: Prepare child in advance for changes that may occur from the chronic or complex condition.

Example: Tell the child in advance the possible side effects of drug therapy.

Participation: Include child in as many decisions as possible, especially those relating to his or her care regimen.

Example: The child is responsible for taking medications or scheduling home treatments.

Sharing: Allow both family members and child's peers to be a part of the care regimen whenever possible.

Examples: Give the child his or her medication when the other siblings receive their vitamins.

The parent cooks the same menu for the whole family.

If the child is invited to another's home, the parent advises the family of the child's dietary restrictions.

Control: Identify areas where child can be in control so that feelings of uncertainty, passivity, and helplessness are decreased.

Example: The child identifies activities that are appropriate to his or her energy level and chooses to rest when fatigued.

Expectation: Apply the same family rules to the child with a complex chronic illness as to the well siblings or peers.

Example: The child is disciplined, is expected to fulfill household responsibilities, and attends school in accordance with abilities.

Children who are concerned that their condition detracts from their physical attractiveness need attention focused on the normal aspects of appearance and capabilities. Health professionals help strengthen and consolidate the self-image by emphasizing the normal while allowing children to express anger, isolation, fear of rejection, feelings of sadness, and loneliness. The children need positive reinforcement for compliance and any evidence of improvement. Anything that might improve attractiveness and contribute to a positive self-image is used, such as makeup for a teenager with a scar, clothing that disguises a prosthesis, or a hairstyle or wig to cover a deformity or lost hair.

Siblings

The presence of a child with special needs in a family may result in parents paying less attention to the other children. Siblings may respond by developing negative attitudes toward the child or by expressing anger in different forms. The nurse can help by using anticipatory guidance, questioning the parents about what they believe is the best way to have siblings respond to the child, and guiding them through ways to meet their other children's needs for attention. This questioning should take place before serious negative effects occur.

Siblings may also experience embarrassment associated with having a brother or sister with a chronic or complex condition. Parents are then faced with the difficulty of responding to this embarrassment in an understanding and appropriate manner without punishing the siblings for how they feel. Parents are encouraged to talk with the siblings about how they view their affected sibling. For example, siblings of a child with developmental disabilities may express fears about their ability to bear normal children. Adolescents in particular may not be able to discuss these vital issues with their parents and may prefer to consult with the nurse. Many siblings benefit from sharing their concerns with other young people who are experiencing a similar situation. Support groups for siblings can help decrease isolation, promote expression of feelings, and provide examples of effective coping skills.

Many parents express concern about when and how to inform the other children in the family about a sibling's illness or disability. The answer depends on each child's level of sophistication and understanding. However, it is usually best to inform the siblings before a neighbor or other nonfamily member does so. Uninformed siblings may fantasize or develop apprehensions that are out of proportion to the child's actual condition. Furthermore, if parents choose to be silent or deceptive about the issue, they are setting a negative precedent for the siblings to follow rather than encouraging the siblings to cope with the experience in a healthy and nurturing way.

The nurse is sensitive to the reactions of siblings and whenever possible intervenes to promote more positive adjustment. For example, siblings often mention that they are expected to take on additional responsibilities to help the parents care for the child. It is not unusual for them to express a positive reaction to assuming the extra duties but a negative response to feeling unappreciated for doing so. Such feelings can often be minimized by encouraging siblings to discuss this with the parents and by suggesting to parents ways of showing gratitude, such as an increase in allowance, special privileges, and, most significantly, verbal praise.

EDUCATE ABOUT THE DISORDER AND GENERAL HEALTH CARE

Educating the family about the disorder is actually an extension of revealing the diagnosis. Education involves not only supplying technical information but also discussing how the condition will affect the child. Parents may only be able to process limited information at any one time. It may be helpful to provide essential information and then follow by asking, "What else would you like to know about your child's condition?" Responding to parents' questions and concerns ensures that their information needs are met.

Activities of Daily Living

Parents also need guidance in how the condition may interfere with or alter activities of daily living, such as eating, dressing, sleeping, and toileting. One area frequently affected is nutrition. Common problems are undernutrition resulting from food being inappropriately restricted or loss of appetite, vomiting, or motor deficits that interfere with feeding; overnutrition may also occur, usually because of a caloric intake in excess of energy expenditure because of boredom and lack of stimulation in other areas. Although the child requires the same basic nutrients as other children, the daily requirements may differ. Special nutritional considerations are discussed as appropriate throughout the text.

Safe Transportation

Modifications may also be needed regarding car safety. Children with conditions such as low birth weight (see Chapter 8, Discharge Planning and Home Care) or orthopedic, neuromuscular, or respiratory impairments often cannot safely use conventional car restraints. For example, children with hip spica casts cannot sit properly in child safety seats (see Chapter 29, Developmental Dysplasia of the Hip). Modifications can be made to some commercial models, and for older children, a special vest that secures the child to the back seat in a lying-down position is available.[b]

If a child requires a wheelchair, the family should consult the wheelchair manufacturer for specific instructions regarding safe car transportation. Considerations for wheelchairs used with vehicle transportation must address securing both the wheelchair and the occupant in the wheelchair. Wheelchairs should be secured facing forward with tie-downs at four points. The tie-down system should be dynamically crash tested, as should the occupant securement system that secures the child in the wheelchair. For example, use of trays is not recommended for transportation. For children who must travel with additional medical equipment, this equipment (e.g., oxygen, monitors, ventilators) should be anchored to the floor or underneath the vehicle seat or wheelchair. Soft padding should be added around the equipment to reduce movement. A second adult should be present to monitor the condition of a medically fragile child while traveling.

Primary Health Care

Children with special needs require all of the usual health care recommended for any child. Attention to injury prevention, immunizations, dental health, and regular physical examinations is essential. Nurses can play an important role in reminding parents of these aspects of care that are so often neglected when the concern is focused on the child's chronic condition. Specific discussions of nutrition, sleep and activity, dental health, and injury prevention are presented in the chapters on health promotion for specific age-groups. Immunizations are discussed in Chapter 6.

Parents also need to be aware of the importance of communicating the child's condition in the event of a medical emergency. Young children are unable to give information about their disorders, and although older children may be reliable sources, after an accident they may be physically unable to speak. All children with any type of chronic condition that may affect medical care should wear some type of identification, such as a MedicAlert bracelet,[c] or carry a card in their wallet that lists the medical condition and a phone number for emergency medical records and other personal information.

PROMOTE NORMAL DEVELOPMENT

Aside from knowledge of the condition and its effect on the child's abilities, the family must be guided toward fostering appropriate development in their child. Although each stage may take longer to achieve, parents are guided toward helping the child fully realize his or her potential in preparation for the next developmental stage. Table 17.2 outlines developmental aspects of complex conditions and supportive interventions. With appropriate planning and knowledge of strategies to improve the child's functional abilities, most children can live fulfilling and productive lives.

One important aspect of promoting normal development is to encourage the child's self-care abilities in both activities of daily living and the medical regimen. An assessment of the child's age and physical, emotional, and mental capacities, as well as the support and structure provided by the family, should be considered in determining the appropriate level of self-care in the medical regimen. Even toddlers can be involved in their own care by holding supplies for the parent during a procedure. Over time, children should be encouraged toward greater autonomy in the self-care arena.

BOX 17.7 Characteristics of Parental Overprotection

- Sacrifices self and rest of family for the child
- Continually helps the child even when the child is capable
- Is inconsistent with regard to discipline or uses no discipline; frequently applies different rules to the siblings
- Is dictatorial and arbitrary, making decisions without considering the child's wishes, such as keeping the child from attending school
- Hovers and offers suggestions; calls attention to every activity; overdoes praise
- Protects the child from every possible discomfort
- Restricts play, often because of fear that the child will be injured
- Denies the child opportunities for growing up and assuming responsibility, such as learning to give own medications or perform treatments
- Does not understand the child's capabilities and sets goals too high or too low
- Monopolizes the child's time, such as sleeping with the child, permitting few friends, or refusing participation in social or educational activities

Early Childhood

During infancy, the child is achieving basic trust through a satisfying, intimate, consistent relationship with his or her parents. However, affected children's early existence may be stressful, chaotic, and unsatisfying. Consequently, they may need more parental support and expressions of affection to achieve trust. Likewise, the parents require assistance in finding ways to meet the infant's needs, such as how to hold a rigid or flaccid infant, how to feed a child with tongue thrust or episodes of dyspnea, and how to stimulate a child who seems incapable of achieving any skills. If hospitalizations are frequent or prolonged, every effort is made to preserve the parent-child relationship (see also Chapter 19).

During early childhood, the goal is to adapt to periods of separation from parents, autonomy, and initiative. However, the natural parental response to having a sick child is overprotection (Box 17.7). Parents need help in realizing the importance of brief separations of the child from them and from others involved in the child's care and of providing social experiences outside the home whenever possible. Respite care, which provides temporary relief for family members, can be essential in allowing caregivers time away from the daily burdens.

Young children also need the opportunity to develop independence. Frequently, the child is able to learn self-help skills, such as finger feeding and removing simple articles of clothing, but the parent continues to perform the act. The nurse can provide parents with anticipatory guidance as to the usual milestones expected from the child. When a child is unable to perform a skill independently, functional aids should be used. With innovation, many adaptations can be implemented in children's environments to increase their mobility and independence and allow them to play like other children their age. For example, with slight modifications, a child with physical limitations may be able to ride a tricycle (Fig. 17.4).

Another critical component for normal child development is discipline. Discipline and guidance serve several purposes, such as providing children with boundaries on which to test out their behavior and teaching them socially acceptable behavior. Resentment and hostility can arise among siblings if different standards are applied to each child. The nurse's responsibility is to help parents learn successful methods

[b]Information on car safety restraints for children with special needs is available from the Automotive Safety Program, 1130 West Michigan Street, Fesler Room 207, Indianapolis, IN 46202; 800-543-6227 or 317-274-2997; http://www.preventinjury.org.

[c]MedicAlert Foundation International, 101 Lander Ave., Turlock, CA 95380; 800-432-5378; http://www.medicalert.org.

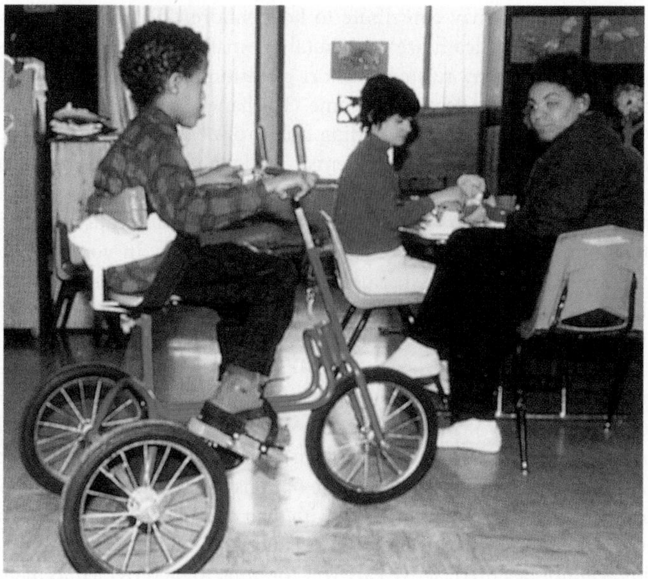

Fig. 17.4 A modified tricycle with block pedals, self-adhesive straps for support, and a modified seat and handlebars can help a child with disabilities gain mobility.

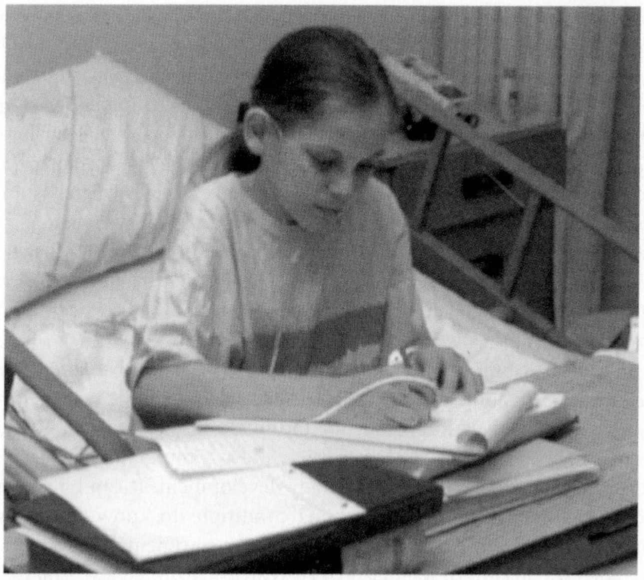

Fig. 17.5 Children with disabilities should continue their schooling as soon as their condition permits.

of managing a child's behaviors before they become problems (see Chapter 2, Limit Setting and Discipline).

School Age

For school-age children, the major tasks are entry into school and achieving a sense of industry. Although the importance of school in the life of all children is well known, school absences are significantly higher among children with chronic illnesses than among their healthy peers. The more school absences the child experiences, the more difficult it is to resume attendance, and school phobia may result. The child should return to school as soon as possible after diagnosis or treatments.

Preparation for entry into or resumption of school is best accomplished through a team approach with the parents, child, teacher, school nurse, and primary nurse in the hospital. Ideally, this planning should begin before hospital discharge, provided that the child is well enough to resume usual activities. A structured plan should be developed, with attention to aspects of care that must be continued during school hours, such as administration of medication or other treatments.

Children also need preparation before entering or resuming school. Having a tutor in the hospital or home as soon as children are physically able helps them realize that school will continue and gives them time to consider this prospect (Fig. 17.5). They need to investigate possible answers to the many questions others will ask. One method of anticipatory preparation is to role-play, with the child as the "returned pupil" and the nurse or parent as "other schoolmates." If the child returns to school with some obvious physical change (such as hair loss, amputation, or a visible scar), the nurse might also ask questions about these alterations to prompt preparatory responses from the child.

Classroom peers also need preparation, and a joint plan created by the teacher, nurse, and child is best. At a minimum, classmates should be given a description of the child's condition, prepared for any visible changes in the child, and allowed an opportunity to ask questions. The child should have the option of attending this session. As the child's condition changes, particularly if the illness is potentially fatal, school personnel, including the students, need periodic appraisal of the child's status and preparation for what to expect.

Children with special needs are encouraged to maintain or reestablish relationships with peers and to participate according to their capabilities in any age-appropriate activities. Alternative activities may be substituted for those that are impossible or that place a strain on the child's condition. Programs such as the Special Olympics[d] offer children an opportunity to compete with their peers and to achieve athletic skill. Summer camps[e] allow children to associate with peers and develop a wide variety of skills. Children with special needs can derive enormous benefits from expressive activities, such as art, music, poetry, dance, and drama. With adaptive equipment and imagination, children can participate in a variety of activities. Organizations such as VSA Arts allow children to celebrate and share their accomplishments.[f] Children need the opportunity to interact with healthy peers and to engage in activities with groups or clubs composed of similarly affected age-mates. Organizations such as ostomy clubs, diabetes clubs, and cerebral palsy groups share information and provide support related to the special problems the members face.

Adolescence

Adolescence can be a particularly difficult period for the teenager and family. All of the needs discussed previously apply to this age-group as well. Developing **independence** or **autonomy**, however, is a major task for the adolescent as planning for the future becomes a prominent concern. Although the emphasis in the past has been on

---

[d]1133 19th St. NW, Washington, DC 20036; 202-628-3630; http://www.specialolympics.org. Several pamphlets on sports and recreation for children with disabilities are available from Easter Seals and American Alliance for Health, Physical Education, Recreation and Dance, 1900 Association Drive, Reston, VA 20191; 703-476-9527 or 800-213-7193; http://www.shapeamerica.org.

[e]A directory of private and paying camps for children with a variety of chronic illnesses and general physical disabilities is available from the American Camp Association, 5000 State Road 67 North, Martinsville, IN 46151-7902; 765-342-8456; http://www.acacamps.org.

[f]VSA Arts has affiliate chapters in all 50 states and in selected sites internationally; yearly festivals are held throughout the world. Information is available from VSA Arts, 2700 F Street NW, Washington, DC 20566; 202-467-4600 or 800-444-1324; https://education.kennedy-center.org/education/vsa/.

achieving independence from physical assistance, recent developments in the fields of special education, adolescent development, and family systems suggest redefining autonomy in terms of individuals' capacities to take responsibility for their own behavior, to make decisions about their own lives, and to maintain supportive social relationships. Given this understanding, even individuals with severe impairments can be viewed as autonomous if they perceive their own needs and take responsibility for meeting them, either directly or by engaging the assistance of others. As adolescents become more autonomous, the nurse can help them articulate their needs, participate in developing their own care plans, and discover and express how others can be of greatest assistance.

Physical symptoms are high on teenagers' list of health-related concerns. Because adolescence is a time of enormous physical and emotional changes, it is important for the nurse to distinguish between body changes that are related to the child's complex condition and those that are a result of normal body development. It can be a great comfort for teenagers with disabling conditions to know that many of the changes they experience are normal developmental outcomes.

A sense of feeling different from peers can lead to loneliness, isolation, and depression. Participation in groups of teenagers with chronic conditions or disabilities can alleviate feelings of isolation and smooth the transition to a meaningful relationship with one person in adulthood.

ESTABLISH REALISTIC FUTURE GOALS

One of the most difficult adjustments is setting realistic future goals for the child that are based on the child's own goals and values.

Planning for the future should be a gradual process. All along, the parents should cultivate realistic vocations for the child. For example, if children have physical disabilities, they can be directed toward intellectual, artistic, or musical pursuits. Children with developmental disabilities can be taught manual skills. In this way, the child's development proceeds in the direction of self-support through gainful employment.

With prolonged survival, young people with chronic illnesses must deal with new decisions and problems, such as marriage, employment, and insurance coverage. With appropriate guidance, individuals with disabilities can attain gainful employment, marriage, and a family. For those whose conditions are genetic, counseling is needed regarding future offspring. Prospective spouses often benefit from an opportunity to discuss their feelings about marriage to an individual with continued health needs and possibly a limited life span. Health insurance coverage is a critical issue for chronically ill children because of their enormous health care costs over time. The Affordable Care Act allows young adults to remain on their parents' insurance until they are 26 years old and prevents private insurance carriers from denying them coverage. Life insurance is another dilemma, especially when children have serious conditions, such as congenital heart anomalies.

PERSPECTIVES ON THE CARE OF CHILDREN AT THE END OF LIFE

Although most childhood illnesses and many injuries and other trauma respond favorably to treatment, some do not. When a child and family face a prolonged and life-limiting illness, health professionals must confront the challenge of providing the best possible care to meet the physical, psychologic, spiritual, and emotional needs of the child and family during the uncertain course of the illness and at the time of death. When death is sudden and unexpected, nurses are challenged to respond to grief and shock in families and provide comfort and support in the absence of a prior relationship.

Many factors may contribute to how children die. In infants, the leading causes of death are congenital anomalies, respiratory distress syndrome, disorders related to short gestation and low birth weight, and sudden infant death syndrome (Kochanek, Murphy, Xu, et al., 2014) (see Chapter 1). The leading causes of death in children 5 to 9 years old include injuries (accidents), malignant neoplasms, congenital anomalies, assault (nonaccidental trauma), and heart disease. In children 10 to 14 years old, suicide is the third leading cause of death after injuries (accidents) and malignant neoplasms. In youths 15 to 19 years old, assault (nonaccidental trauma), suicide, malignant neoplasms, and heart disease follow accidents as the most prevalent causes of death (Cunningham, Walton, & Carter, 2018).

A child who is diagnosed with a life-limiting illness requires thorough medical and nursing assessments and tailored interventions that address his or her symptom burden. When cure is no longer possible and life-prolonging measures result in pain and suffering to the child, parents need information about care options to assist them in deciding how they want the remaining time with their child to be managed by the health care team. It is important to reassure families that although their child cannot be cured, active care will continue to be provided to maintain the child's comfort. Support is provided to assist the child and family during the dying process. As a result, nurses may care for children and families who are making the difficult transition from curative or restorative treatments to palliative care (Kang, Munson, Hwang, et al., 2014).

PRINCIPLES OF PALLIATIVE CARE

Palliative care involves a multidisciplinary and interdisciplinary approach to the care of children living with or dying from chronic, complex, or potentially life-limiting conditions. Need, not prognosis, is the primary reason to consult with a palliative care provider. Pediatric palliative care focuses on providing optimal symptom management, helping families align medical interventions (i.e., proceeding with a tracheostomy) with their goals for their child, assisting with complex decision making, and supporting the family and health care team caring for a child with a CCC throughout the trajectory of their illness. Pediatric palliative care helps families explore the "what ifs," optimizing quality of life as determined by the family (and child) (Field & Behrman, 2004). The World Health Organization (1998) amended the definition of palliative care for children to include:

- Palliative care for children is the active total care of the child's body, mind, and spirit and involves giving support to the family.
- It begins when illness is diagnosed and continues regardless of whether a child receives treatment directed at the disease.
- Health providers must evaluate and alleviate the child's physical, psychologic, and social distress.
- Effective palliative care requires a broad interprofessional approach that includes the family and makes use of available community resources; it can be successfully implemented even if resources are limited.
- It can be provided in tertiary care facilities, in community health centers, and even in children's homes.

Palliative care interventions do not serve to hasten death but rather to ameliorate pain and suffering by providing optimal pain and symptom management, attending to issues faced by the child and family with regard to prolonged illness and, when appropriate, death and dying. Maximizing a child's quality of life as defined by the parent and child is a key principle in pediatric palliative care (Feudtner, Friebert, & Jewell, 2013; Kang et al., 2014). The implementation of neonatal and pediatric palliative care consulting services within hospitals has led to enhanced quality of life and end-of-life care for children and their families and support for their care providers (Blume, Balkin, Aiyagari, et al., 2014;

O'Quinn & Giambra, 2014). The child and family are considered the unit of care. Several principles are hallmarks of pediatric palliative care (National Consensus Project for Quality Palliative Care, 2018):

- Palliative care can be provided in tandem with curative and life-prolonging treatments.
- It is provided based on a child's and family's need, not prognosis.
- It should be offered in all care settings—inpatient, outpatient, home, and long-term facilities—and include assessing all domains (physical, social, and emotional).
- Determining what is most important to the patient and family provides guidance in establishing goals and preferences.

The death of a child is an extremely stressful event for a family because it is out of the natural order of things. Children represent health, hope, and the future. Their death calls into question the understanding of life. An interprofessional and interdisciplinary team of health care professionals consists of physicians, nurses, social workers, chaplains, personal care aides, child life specialists, music and art therapists, and bereavement counselors skilled in caring for dying patients. The team assists the family by focusing care on the complex interactions among physical, emotional, social, and spiritual issues.

Palliative care seeks to create a therapeutic environment that is as homelike as possible, if not in the child's own home. Through education and support of family members, an atmosphere of open communication is provided regarding the child's dying process and its impact on all members of the family (see Translating Evidence Into Practice box).

TRANSLATING EVIDENCE INTO PRACTICE

Pediatric Pain and Symptom Management at the End of Life

Ask the Question

PICOT Question

In children, what is the pain and symptom experience at the end of life?

Search for the Evidence

Search Strategies

Published studies using the subject terms *child, palliative care, pain,* and *symptoms* were identified and examined. Retrospective descriptive studies dominated the findings, describing infants' and children's end-of-life experiences through the use of medical record reviews and provider and parental surveys.

Databases Used

PubMed, CINAHL

Critically Analyze the Evidence

Children experienced an average of 11 symptoms during their last week of life (Drake, Frost, & Collins, 2003). Pain, dyspnea, fatigue, nausea, vomiting, irritability, and anorexia are the most common distressing symptoms reported by children at the end of life (Miller, Jacob, & Hockenberry, 2011). A variety of motives influence parental decision to withhold or withdraw life support. Pain and suffering have been reported as one of the most important factors (Meert, Thurston, & Sarnaik, 2000). Even when their child's condition is ominous, parents want to ensure that they are making decisions in the best interest of their child and within the framework of being a good parent—for example, putting their child's needs above their own, focusing on quality of life and maintaining comfort, making sure their child feels loved, and being their advocate (October, Fisher, Feudtner, et al., 2014).

Morphine remains the most commonly prescribed medication for pain and dyspnea (Masman, van Dijk, Tibboel, et al., 2015), and these continue to be the most frequently reported symptoms by parents at the end of their child's life. Parents also report that their child continues to experience high levels of pain when death is near. Physicians were more likely than nurses or parents to report that a child's pain and symptoms were well managed at the end of life, but the majority of both provider groups believed that the child's physical management was difficult (Andresen, Seecharan, & Toce, 2004; Wolfe, Grier, Klar, et al., 2000). When a child is diagnosed with a life-limiting condition, early integration of pediatric palliative care, ideally before a crisis, provides time to get to know the child and family in order to best facilitate conversations regarding goals of care. The focus of pediatric palliative care is to support the child and family, address pain and other bothersome symptoms, and help maximize quality of life. Although the core of pediatric palliative care is the child and family, it also aims to support the primary care team.

Barriers to the adequate provision of pediatric palliative care include developmental issues specific to infants and children; symptoms, their causes, how they are related, and effective treatment strategies; lack of education; and reimbursement issues (Harris, 2004).

Apply the Evidence: Nursing Implications

There is **moderate-quality evidence** with a **strong recommendation** (Guyatt, Oxman, Vist, et al., 2008) for better pain management at the end of life. Although the philosophy of palliative care encompasses pain and symptom management for infants and children who may not outlive their disease, the provision of that care to ease suffering and provide comfort to those who will die continues to lag. Studies show that children experience significant pain and other distressing symptoms at the end of life that are not well managed. Discrepancies in perceptions of infants' and children's pain and suffering continue to exist between providers and parents. Barriers to the provision of pediatric palliative care exist. Improvements are needed in the management of pain and symptoms at the end of life for infants and children.

Quality and Safety Competencies: Evidence-Based Practice[a]

Knowledge

Differentiate clinical opinion from research and evidence-based summaries.

Describe common symptoms experienced at the end of life.

Skills

Base individualized care plan on patient values, clinical expertise, and evidence.

Integrate evidence into practice by carefully assessing pain and other symptoms in children at the end of life.

Attitudes

Value the concept of evidence-based practice as integral to determining best clinical practice.

Appreciate strengths and weakness of evidence for symptom assessment and management at the end of life.

References

Andresen, E. M., Seecharan, G. A., & Toce, S. S. (2004). Provider perceptions of child deaths. *Archives of Pediatrics and Adolescent Medicine, 158*(5), 430–435.

Drake, R., Frost, J., & Collins, J. J. (2003). The symptoms of dying children. *Journal of Pain and Symptom Management, 26*(1), 594–603.

Guyatt, G. H., Oxman, A. D., Vist, G. E., et al. (2008). GRADE: An emerging consensus on rating quality of evidence and strength of recommendations. *BMJ, 336*(7650), 924–926.

Harris, M. B. (2004). Palliative care in children with cancer: Which child and when? *Journal of the National Cancer Institute Monographs, 32,* 144–149.

Masman, A. D., van Dijk, M., Tibboel, D., Baar, F. P., & Mathôt, R. A. (2015). Medication use during end-of-life care in a palliative care centre. *International Journal of Clinical Pharmacy, 37*(5), 767–775.

Meert, K. L., Thurston, C. S., & Sarnaik, A. P. (2000). End-of-life decision-making and satisfaction with care: Parental perspectives. *Pediatric Critical Care Medicine, 1*(2), 179–185.

Miller, E., Jacob, E., & Hockenberry, M. J. (2011). Nausea, pain, fatigue, and multiple symptoms in hospitalized children with cancer. *Oncology Nursing Forum, 38*(5), E382–E393.

October, T. W., Fisher, K. R., Feudtner, C., & Hinds, P. (2014). The parent perspective: "Being a good parent" when making critical decisions in the PICU. *Pediatric Critical Care Medicine, 15*(4), 291–298.

Wolfe, J., Grier, H. E., Klar, N., et al. (2000). Symptoms and suffering at the end of life in children with cancer. *New England Journal of Medicine, 342*(5), 326–333.

[a]Adapted from the Quality and Safety Education for Nurses website at http://www.qsen.org/.

CONCURRENT CARE

The Patient Protection and Affordable Care Act, now known as the Affordable Care Act (ACA), was passed in 2010 to provide affordable, comprehensive health care. A section of the ACA included a provision to improve health care for children, known as "concurrent care for children." Key points of concurrent care include:

- State Medicaid programs or Children's Health Insurance Program (CHIP) is eligible for both curative and hospice care for children under the age of 21 years.
- Children who receive hospice care can also have other services, including disease-directed treatments.
- Families with children who have life-limiting or life-threatening conditions do not have to choose between disease-directed therapies, palliative care, or hospice (Lindley, Edwards, & Bruce, 2014; National Hospice and Palliative Care Organization, 2010).

DECISION MAKING AT THE END OF LIFE

Discussions about the possibility that a child's illness or condition is not curable and that death is an inevitable outcome cause everyone involved a great deal of stress. Physicians, other members of the health care team, and families must consider all information regarding the child's situation and make decisions that all parties agree to and that will have a profound impact on the child and family.

Ethical Considerations in End-of-Life Decision Making

A number of ethical concerns arise when parents and health care professionals are deciding on the best course of care for the dying child. Many parents and health care providers are concerned that not offering treatment that would cause potential pain and suffering but might extend life would be considered euthanasia or assisted suicide. To eliminate such concerns, it is necessary to understand the various terms. **Euthanasia** involves an action carried out by a person other than the patient to end the life of the patient suffering from a terminal condition. The intent of this action is based on the belief that the act is "putting the person out of his or her misery." **Assisted suicide** occurs when someone provides the patient with the means to end his or her life and the patient uses that means to do so. The important distinction between these two actions involves who is acting to end the person's life.

The American Nurses Association's *Code of Ethics for Nurses* does not support the active intent on the part of a nurse to end a person's life. However, it does permit the nurse to provide interventions to relieve symptoms in the dying patient even when the interventions involve a substantial risk of hastening death. When the prognosis for a patient is poor and death is the expected outcome, it is ethically acceptable to withhold or withdraw treatments that may cause pain and suffering and provide interventions that promote comfort and quality of life (American Nurses Association, 2015).

Physician–Health Care Team Decision Making

Decisions by physicians regarding care are often made on the basis of the progression of the disease or amount of trauma, the availability of treatment options that would provide cure from disease or restoration of health, the impact of such treatments on the child, and the child's overall prognosis (Pousset, Bilsen, Cohen, et al., 2010). Often the main determinants prompting physicians to discuss end-of-life issues and options for children with critical illnesses include the child's age, premorbid cognitive condition and functional status, pain or discomfort, probability of survival, and quality of life (Pousset et al., 2010). When the physician discusses this information openly with families, a shared decision-making process can occur regarding **do not attempt resuscitation (DNaR) orders** and care that is focused on the comfort of the child and family during the dying process (Giannini, Messeri, Aprile, et al., 2008).

Unfortunately, many families are not given the option of terminating treatment and pursuing care that is focused on comfort and quality of life when cure is unlikely, and staff may be reluctant to raise the question of DNaR orders. This occurs for a number of reasons, including the belief that not being able to "save" a child is a "failure." Also, the physician and other members of the health care team may lack knowledge of and experience with the principles of palliative care (Baker, Torkildson, Baillargeon, et al., 2007; Price, Dornan, & Quail, 2013).

Parental Decision Making

Rarely are families prepared to cope with the numerous decisions that must be made when a child is dying. When the death is unexpected, parents are challenged to make difficult choices; this can be especially difficult in emergency settings, as seen in cases of accidents or trauma. If the child has either experienced a life-threatening illness (such as cancer) or lived with a chronic illness that has now reached its terminal phase, parents are often unprepared for the reality of their child's impending death (see Family-Centered Care box). Numerous studies have found that families facing the impending death of a child depend on information provided to them by the health care team, particularly an honest appraisal of the child's prognosis, to make difficult decisions regarding care options for their children (Hinds, Oakes, Furman, et al., 2001; Lipstein, Brinkman, & Britto, 2012; Santoro & Bennett, 2018; Wolfe, Friebert, & Hilden, 2002).

> **FAMILY-CENTERED CARE**
>
> ***Family of the Dying Child***
>
> As the group of health professionals that is most involved with families, nurses are in an excellent position to ensure that families are presented with the options available to them. The nurse's first responsibility is to explore the family's wishes. This is best done in concert with the physician but at times may need to be initiated by the nurse. Statements (such as "Tell me about your thoughts for the type of care you want your child to receive when he is dying" or "Have you considered the types of interventions you would like us to use when your child is near death?") can begin discussion of this sensitive but critical aspect of terminal care.

The Dying Child

Children need honest and accurate information about their illness, treatments, and prognosis. This information needs to be given in clear, simple language. In most situations, this best occurs as a gradual process over time that is characterized by increasingly open dialogue among parents, professionals, and the child (Barnes et al., 2012). Providing an atmosphere of open communication early in the course of an illness facilitates answering difficult questions as the child's condition worsens. Providing appropriate literature about the disease, as well as the experience of illness and possible death, is also helpful. Exactly how and when to involve children in decisions regarding care during their dying process and death is an individual matter. The child's age or developmental level is an important consideration in the process (Table 17.4). In general, parents should be asked how they would like their child to be told of his or her prognosis, and they should be included in his or her care. Some parents may request that their child not be told that he or she is dying even if the child asks. This often places health care providers in a difficult situation. Children, even at a young age, are perceptive. Even if they are not told outright that they are dying, they realize that something is seriously wrong and that it involves them. Often, helping parents understand that honesty and shared decision making between them and their child are important to the child's and family's emotional health will encourage parents to allow discussion of dying with their child. Parents may require professional support and guidance in this process from a nurse, social worker, or child life specialist who has a good relationship with the child and family.

If given the opportunity, children will tell others how much they want to know. Nurses can help children set limits on how much truth they can accept and cope with by asking questions, such as "If the disease came back, would you want to know?" or "Do you want others to tell you everything even if the news isn't good?" or "If someone were not getting better [or more directly, were dying], do you think he would want to know?" Children need time to process feelings and information so that they can assimilate and ideally accept the reality of impending death.

Care of dying adolescents requires the nurse to become knowledgeable about any possible delays or alterations in normal growth and development. Legal and ethical issues also come to the forefront with respect to the age at which an adolescent should have autonomy in decision making with regard to care and treatment. Effective communication among the patient, family, and health care team is an important part of optimal care for dying adolescents (Barnes et al., 2012). See the Next-Generation NCLEX® Examination-Style Unfolding Case Study.

NEXT-GENERATION NCLEX® EXAMINATION-STYLE UNFOLDING CASE STUDY

Care at the End of Life

Mpho Raletshegwana

Day 1, 8:00 am

1. A 9-year-old boy has paravertebral fibrosarcoma of the right lumbosacral area, complicated by paraplegia, urine retention, constipation, and neuropathic pain. He has a 5-month history of progressive lower back pain and swelling and paralysis of the lower limbs. The patient received and responded well to chemotherapy and radiotherapy, with a 40% regression in his tumor. However, the patient continued to suffer severe "burning/piercing" pain in the lower extremities, especially when the limbs are moved. He continues to require oral analgesics daily and remains bedridden with weakness of the lower extremities. Because of the clinically poor response and poor long-term prognosis, a decision was made by him and his family to focus on comfort and consult palliative care. Plans are for him to be discharged on hospice care once the pain is managed. The nursing admission assessment reveals the following results. **Select the assessment findings that need further follow up. Select all that apply.**
   A. Temperature = 98.6 F (37.0 C)
   B. Blood pressure = 100/58mmHg
   C. Heart rate = 124 beats/min
   D. Respirations = 16 breaths/min
   E. Visual pain score 8/10
   F. Persistent localized pain in the vertebrae or lumbar region
   G. Burning/piercing pain in the lower extremities or neuropathic pain
   H. Swelling around the lower lumbar area
   I. Numbness of the lower extremities due to pressure exerted on nerves
   J. Capillary refill <3 sec in left finger
   K. Weight = 60 lbs (27.2 kg)

Day 1, 8:30 am

2. Pain is not being controlled by low-dose oral pain medications and opioids, and the plan is to begin intravenous (IV) pain medications to control his pain. Since it is unclear from the history exactly how much morphine has been given and at what intervals throughout the day, the plan is to use a standard starting dose of IV morphine.
   Choose the most likely options for the information missing from the statements below by selecting from the lists of options provided. (Chapter 5 can be used to answer this question if needed).
   An appropriate standard starting dose of IV morphine to administer is ____1____. This may be given every 10 minutes for three doses until pain relief is achieved, then scheduled every ____2____ hours.

Option 1	Option 2
1–2 mg/kg	4 hours
0.1 to 0.2 mg/kg	15 min
0.5–1.0 mg/kg	2 hours
0.1–1 mg/kg	6 hours
1.0–2.0 mg/kg	10 min

Day 1, 9:15 am

3. IV morphine was started, and the pain assessment revealed a score of 3/10. Because this patient is 9 years old, consideration must be given to the type of pain assessment tool that is most appropriate for a child this age. What specifically would the nurse consider when completing a pain assessment of this 9-year-old? **Select all that apply.**
   A. Self-report should be used
   B. Observe the child's behavior
   C. Evaluate how the patient responds
   D. Use an infant scale since he is in a great deal of pain
   E. Use a verbal intensity scale (less, moderate, or severe pain)
   F. Assess pain once a shift and do not disrupt sleep
   G. If the child is in a great deal of pain use the Wong-Baker FACES Pain Rating Scale

Day 1, 10:00 am

4. The patient is resting comfortably with both parents at his side. The IV morphine dose is relieving the pain. Further discussion with the mother reveals that the child is also taking gabapentin orally due to the burning/piercing pain in his lower extremities. She states that since starting on this medication the burning sensations have resolved. The nurse reports this to the medical team and oral gabapentin is ordered. What potential complications are prevented by the nursing actions listed below?
   Indicate which nursing action number listed in the far-left column is appropriate for the potential complication listed in the middle column. Place the number in the far-right column. Note that NOT all nursing actions will be used.

Continued

NEXT-GENERATION NCLEX® EXAMINATION-STYLE UNFOLDING CASE STUDY—Cont'd

Care at the End of Life

Nursing Action	Potential Complication	Nursing Action for Complication
1. Administer morphine safely. Observe the patient for excessive sedation and respiratory depression.	To reduce unfounded fears.	
2. Monitor for side effects of morphine: decreased respiratory rate, urinary retention, constipation, and pruritus.	To prevent unwanted side effects that may cause additional discomfort.	
3. Educate parents on the safety and effectiveness of the pain-relieving medications.	To ensure optimal pain relief.	
4. Reassess the pain level after administering pain medication. Assess within 1 hour of oral morphine and 30 minutes after IV administration.	To prevent adverse effects and overdose	
5. Recognize when pain is not well controlled on morphine.	To ensure satisfactory pain relief.	
6. Provide appropriate bowel regimen and monitor urine output.		
7. Provide distraction and counseling to assure parents that everything possible is being done.		

2 days later, 9:00 am

5. The parents and child want to go home and want to manage the pain with oral medications. Since the current dose of morphine provides adequate relief, a plan for pain management on discharge is made to switch to oral morphine. The most recent nursing assessment reveals the following:
   - Temperature = 98.6 F (37C)
   - Blood pressure = 104/60mmHg
   - Heart rate = 76 beats/min
   - Respirations = 16 breaths/min
   - Visual pain score 2/10
   - No burning/piercing pain in the lower extremities or neuropathic pain
   - Swelling remains around the lower lumbar area

   The nurse discusses proper administration of the pain medications at home. His regimen will include both oral morphine and gabapentin.

   For each nursing action, use an X to indicate whether it was Effective (helped to meet expected quality patient outcomes), Ineffective (did not help to meet expected quality patient outcomes), or Unrelated (not related to the quality patient outcomes).

Nursing Action	Effective	Ineffective	Unrelated
Assure parents that the IV morphine dose can be the same dose they administer at home			
Instruct parents to continue around-the-clock medications at home			
Encourage parents to communicate any signs of pain; observe patient for nonverbal signs of pain			
A home bowel regimen should be included in the discharge teaching			
Instruct parents to talk to other family members about their feelings toward pain management			
Stress with the parents that escalating doses will not be needed, and that tolerance to pain medications never occur in children			
Discuss appropriate nonpharmacologic options that can relieve pain			

12:00 noon

6. The nurse while obtaining vital signs notes that the patient looks more withdrawn. He no longer talks to the nursing staff and the parents answer all assessment questions. The mother also notices this and asks the nurse why her son is no longer talking to others. She states he seems to be shutting himself off from the world and wants to know if this is what children do when they are dying. The mother confides to the nurse that she is scared to take him home and asks how the hospice nurse will be of support to her during her son's last days. How would the nurse respond to her question? **Select all that apply.**
   A. "The hospice nurse will stay with you in your house until your child dies."
   B. "The hospice nurse will focus on providing comfort for you child."
   C. "The hospice nurse will keep you informed of what is happening to your child."
   D. "The hospice nurse will bring your child to the hospital if he gets worse."
   E. "The hospice nurse will focus on minimizing pain experienced by your child."
   F. "The hospice nurse will begin antibiotics if your child has fever."
   G. "The hospice nurse will answer any questions you have."

TABLE 17.4 Children's Understanding of and Reactions to Death

Concepts of Death	Reactions to Death	Nursing Care Management
Infants and Toddlers		
Death has least significance to children younger than 6 months old. After parent-child attachment and trust are established, the loss, even if temporary, of the significant person is profound. Prolonged separation during the first several years is thought to be more significant in terms of future physical, social, and emotional growth than at any subsequent age. Toddlers are egocentric and can only think about events in terms of their own frame of reference—living. Their egocentricity and vague separation of fact and fantasy make it impossible for them to comprehend absence of life. Instead of understanding death, this age-group is affected more by any change in lifestyle.	With the death of someone else, they may continue to act as though the person is alive. As children grow older, they will be increasingly able and willing to let go of the dead person. Ritualism is important; a change in lifestyle could be anxiety producing. This age-group reacts more to the pain and discomfort of a serious illness than to the probable fatal prognosis. This age-group also reacts to parental anxiety and sadness.	Help parents deal with their feelings, allowing them greater emotional reserves to meet the needs of their children. Encourage parents to remain as near to child as possible yet be sensitive to parents' needs. Maintain as normal an environment as possible to retain ritualism. If a parent has died, encourage having consistent caregiver for child. Promote primary nursing.
Preschool Children		
Preschoolers believe their thoughts are sufficient to cause death; the consequence is the burden of guilt, shame, and punishment. Their egocentricity implies a tremendous sense of self-power and omnipotence. They usually have some understanding of the meaning of death. Death is seen as a departure, a kind of sleep. They may recognize the fact of physical death but do not separate it from living abilities. Death is seen as temporary and gradual; life and death can change places with one another. They have no understanding of the universality and inevitability of death.	If they become seriously ill, they conceive of the illness as a punishment for their thoughts or actions. They may feel guilty and responsible for the death of a sibling. Greatest fear concerning death is separation from parents. They may engage in activities that seem strange or abnormal to adults. Because they have fewer defense mechanisms to deal with loss, young children may react to a less significant loss with more outward grief than to the loss of a very significant person. The loss is so deep, painful, and threatening that the child must deny it for a time to survive its overwhelming impact. Behavior reactions such as giggling, joking, attracting attention, or regressing to earlier developmental skills indicate children's need to distance themselves from tremendous loss.	Help parents deal with their feelings, allowing them greater emotional reserves to meet the needs of their children. Help parents understand behavioral reactions of their children. Encourage parents to remain near the child as much as possible to minimize the child's great fear of separation from parents. If a parent has died, encourage having a consistent caregiver for child. Promote primary nursing.
School-Age Children		
Children still associate misdeeds or bad thoughts with causing death and feel intense guilt and responsibility for the event. Because of their higher cognitive abilities, they respond well to logical explanations and comprehend the figurative meaning of words. They have a deeper understanding of death in a concrete sense. They particularly fear the mutilation and punishment that they associate with death. They personify death as the devil, a monster, or the bogeyman. They may have naturalistic or physiologic explanations of death. By 9 or 10 years old, children have an adult concept of death, realizing that it is inevitable, universal, and irreversible.	Because of their increased ability to comprehend, they may have more fears, for example: • The reason for the illness • Communicability of the disease to themselves or others • Consequences of the disease • The process of dying and death itself Their fear of the unknown is greater than their fear of the known. The realization of impending death is a tremendous threat to their sense of security and ego strength. They are likely to exhibit fear through verbal uncooperativeness rather than actual physical aggression. They are interested in postdeath services. They may be inquisitive about what happens to the body.	Help parents deal with their feelings, allowing them greater emotional reserves to meet the needs of their children. Encourage parents to remain near child as much as possible yet be sensitive to parents' needs. Because of children's fear of the unknown, anticipatory preparation is important. Because the developmental task of this age is industry, interventions of helping children maintain control over their bodies and increasing their understanding allow them to achieve independence, self-worth, and self-esteem and avoid a sense of inferiority. Encourage children to talk about their feelings and provide aggressive outlets. Encourage parents to honestly answer questions about dying rather than avoiding the subject or fabricating euphemisms. Encourage parents to share their moments of sorrow with their children. Provide preparation for postdeath services.

Continued

TABLE 17.4 Children's Understanding of and Reactions to Death—cont'd

Concepts of Death	Reactions to Death	Nursing Care Management
Adolescents		
Adolescents have a mature understanding of death. They are still influenced by remnants of magical thinking and are subject to guilt and shame. They are likely to see deviations from accepted behavior as reasons for their illness.	Adolescents straddle transition from childhood to adulthood. They have the most difficulty in coping with death. They are least likely to accept cessation of life, particularly if it is their own. Concern is for the present much more than for the past or the future. They may consider themselves alienated from their peers and unable to communicate with their parents for emotional support, feeling alone in their struggle. Adolescents' orientation to the present compels them to worry about physical changes even more than the prognosis. Because of their idealistic view of the world, they may criticize funeral rites as barbaric, money making, and unnecessary.	Help parents deal with their feelings, allowing them greater emotional reserves to meet the needs of their children. Avoid alliances with either parent or child. Structure hospital admission to allow for maximum self-control and independence. Answer adolescents' questions honestly, treating them as mature individuals and respecting their needs for privacy, solitude, and personal expressions of emotions. Help parents understand their child's reactions to death and dying, especially that concern for present crises (such as loss of hair) may be much greater than for future ones, including possible death.

Treatment Options for Terminally Ill Children

Based on the child and family's decision regarding their wishes for terminal care, they have several options from which to choose.

Hospital

Families may choose to remain in the hospital to receive care if the child's illness or condition is unstable and home care is not an option or the family is uncomfortable with providing care at home. If a family chooses to remain at the hospital for terminal care, the setting should be made as homelike as possible. Families are encouraged to bring familiar items from the child's room at home. In addition, there should be a consistent and coordinated care plan for the comfort of the child and family.

Home Care

Some families prefer to take their child home and receive services from a home care agency. Generally, these services entail periodic nursing visits to administer a treatment or provide medications, equipment, or supplies. The child's care continues to be directed by the primary physician. Home care is often the option chosen by physicians and families because of the traditional view that a child must be considered to have a life expectancy of less than 6 months to be referred to hospice care. Fortunately, a number of hospice organizations are expanding their services to children based on the presence of a life-limiting disease process for which cure is not possible, rather than on the sole criterion of a limited time-projected prognosis.

Hospice Care

Parents should be offered the option of caring for their child at home during the final phases of an illness with the assistance of a hospice organization. **Hospice**[g] is a community health care organization that specializes in the care of dying patients by combining the hospice philosophy with the principles of palliative care. **Hospice philosophy** regards dying as a natural process and care of dying patients as including management of the physical, psychosocial, and spiritual needs of the patient and family. Care is provided by an interprofessional group in the patient's home or an inpatient facility that uses the hospice philosophy. Hospice care for children was introduced in the 1970s, and a number of community hospice organizations now accept children into their care (Keim-Malpass, Hart, & Miller, 2013; Siden, Chavoshi, Harvey, et al., 2014). However, access to freestanding pediatric hospice services continues to be highly variable (Kassam & Wolfe, 2013). Collaboration between the child's primary treatment team and the hospice care team is essential to the success of hospice care. Families may continue to see their primary care physicians as they choose.

Hospice care is based on a number of important concepts that significantly set it apart from hospital care:

- Family members are usually the principal caregivers and are supported by a team of professional and volunteer staff.
- The priority of care is comfort. The child's physical, psychosocial, and spiritual needs are considered. Pain and symptom control are primary concerns, and no extraordinary efforts are used to attempt a cure or prolong life.
- The family's needs are considered as important as those of the patient.
- Hospice is concerned with the family's postdeath adjustment, and care may continue for a year or more.

The goal of hospice care is for children to live life to the fullest without pain, with choices and dignity, in the familiar environment of their home, and with the support of their family. Hospice care is covered under state Medicaid programs and by most insurance plans. The service provides home visits from nurses, social workers, chaplains, and, in some cases, physicians. Medications, medical equipment, and any necessary medical supplies are all provided by the hospice organization providing care.

With children, the home has been the more common environment for implementing the hospice concept, and this benefits the family in various ways. Children who are dying are allowed to remain with those they love and with whom they feel secure. Many children who were thought to be in imminent danger of death have gone home and lived longer than expected. Siblings can feel more involved

[g]For more information, contact National Hospice and Palliative Care Organization, 1731 King Street, Alexandria, VA 22314; 703-837-1500; fax: 703-837-1233; http://www.nhpco.org; and Children's Hospice International, 1800 Diagonal Road, Suite 600, Alexandria, VA 22314; 703-684-0330; http://www.chionline.org.

in the care and often have more positive perceptions of the death. Parental adaptation is often more favorable, demonstrated by their perceptions of how the experience at home affected their marriage, social reorientation, religious beliefs, and views on the meaning of life and death.

If the home is chosen for hospice care, the child may or may not die in the home. Reasons for final admission to a hospital vary but may be related to the parents' or siblings' wish to have the child die outside the home, exhaustion on the part of the caregivers, and physical problems such as sudden, acute pain or respiratory distress.

NURSING CARE OF THE CHILD AND FAMILY AT THE END OF LIFE

Regardless of where the child is cared for during the terminal stage of illness, both the child and the family usually experience fear of (1) pain and suffering, (2) dying alone (child) or not being present when the child dies (parent), and (3) actual death. Nurses can help families by lessening their fears through attention to the care needs of the child and family.

FEAR OF PAIN AND SUFFERING

The presence of unrelieved pain in a terminally ill child can have detrimental effects on the quality of life experienced by the child and family. Parents feel that having their child in pain is unendurable, and this results in feelings of helplessness and a sense that they must be present and vigilant to get the necessary pain medications. Persistent pain also has an impact on the family as a whole. Nurses can alleviate the fear of pain and suffering by providing interventions aimed at treating the pain and symptoms associated with the terminal process in children.

Pain and Symptom Management

Pain control for children in the terminal stages of illness or injury must be given the highest priority. Despite ongoing efforts to educate physicians and nurses on pain management strategies in children, studies have reported that children continue to be undermedicated for their pain (Wolfe, Grier, Klar, et al., 2000). Nearly all children experience some amount of pain in the terminal phase of their illness. The current standard for treating children's pain follows the World Health Organization's analgesic stepladder, which promotes tailoring the pain interventions to the child's level of reported pain. Children's pain should be assessed frequently and medications adjusted as necessary. Pain medications should be given on a regular schedule, and extra doses for breakthrough pain should be available to maintain comfort. Opioid drugs such as morphine should be given for severe pain, and the dose should be increased as necessary to maintain optimal pain relief (World Health Organization, 2012). Techniques such as distraction, relaxation techniques, and guided imagery (Jibb, Nathan, Stevens, et al., 2015) should be combined with drug therapy to provide the child and family with strategies to control pain (see Chapter 5 for further discussion of pain management strategies).

In addition to pain, children experience a variety of symptoms during their terminal course as a result of their disease process or as a side effect of medicines used to manage pain or other symptoms. These symptoms include fatigue, nausea and vomiting, constipation, anorexia, dyspnea, congestion, seizures, anxiety, depression, restlessness, agitation, and confusion (von Lützau, Otto, Hechler, et al., 2012; Wolfe et al., 2002). Each of these symptoms should be aggressively managed with appropriate medications or treatments and with interventions such as repositioning, relaxation, massage, and other measures to maintain the child's comfort and quality of life.

Occasionally, children require very high doses of opioids to control pain. This may occur for several reasons. Children on long-term opioid pain management can become **tolerant** of the drug, meaning that it is necessary to give more drugs to maintain the same level of pain relief. This should not be confused with **addiction**, which is a psychologic dependence on the side effects of opioids. Addiction is not a factor in managing terminal pain in children. Other obvious reasons for requiring increased doses of opioids include progression of disease and other physiologic experiences of pain. It is important to understand that there is no maximum dose that can be given to control pain. However, nurses often express concern that administering doses of opioids that exceed what they are familiar with will hasten the child's death. The **principle of double effect** (Box 17.8) addresses such concerns. It provides an ethical standard that supports the use of interventions intended to relieve pain and suffering even though there is a foreseeable possibility that death may be hastened (Twycross, 2019). In cases in which the child is terminally ill and in severe pain, using large doses of opioids and sedatives to manage pain is justified when no other treatment options that would relieve the pain but make the risk of death less likely are available (DeGraeff & Dean, 2007; Jacobs, 2005). See Chapter 5 for an extensive discussion of pain assessment and management.

BOX 17.8 Ethical Principle of Double Effect

An action that has one good (intended) and one bad (unintended but foreseeable) effect is permissible if the following conditions are met:

- The action itself must be good or indifferent. Only the good consequences of the action must be sincerely intended.
- The good effect must not be produced by the bad effect.
- There must be a compelling or proportionate reason for permitting the foreseeable bad effect to occur.

Parents' and Siblings' Need for Education and Support

Parents are the primary caregivers when the child is at home, and nurses providing care to the child and family need to teach the family about the medications being given to the child, how to administer them, and the use of nonpharmacologic techniques. This empowers parents and provides a sense of control over the child's comfort and well-being, reducing their fear that the child will be in pain or suffering as he or she is dying. In addition, better bereavement outcomes (e.g., adaptive coping; family cohesion; less anxiety, stress, and depression) have been reported by parents who were actively involved in the care of their child (Goodenough, Drew, Higgins, et al., 2004; Lauer, Mulhern, Schell, et al., 1989). The grief work of fathers in particular seems to be facilitated when their child dies in the home setting. This finding may be related to the increased opportunity of working fathers to provide care to and spend time with their child at home versus the hospital setting.

Siblings may feel isolated and displaced during the time their brother or sister is dying. Parents devote most of their time to the care and comfort of the dying child, causing siblings to feel left out of the parent–sick child relationship. The death of a child affects the entire family, and feelings of loss can also extend into the community.

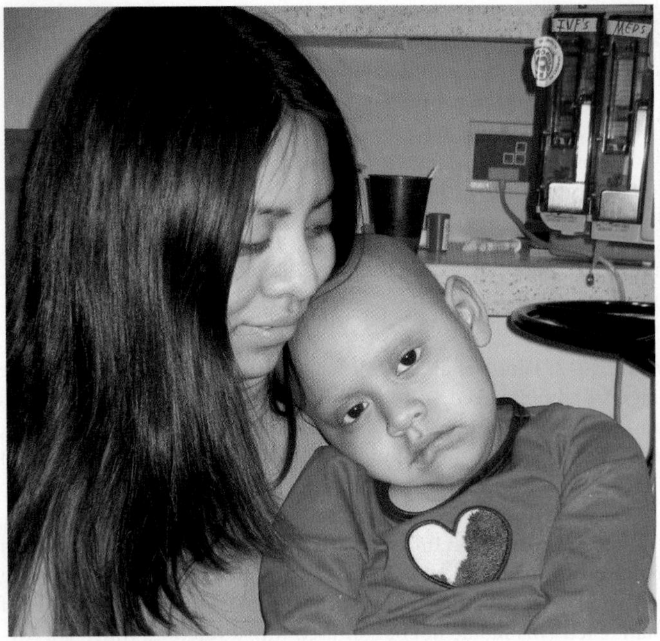

Fig. 17.6 For a dying child, there is no greater comfort than the security and closeness of a parent.

Immediately after a death, siblings may exhibit changes in behavior, but the long-term psychosocial outcomes of bereaved siblings are not known.

Siblings may become resentful of their sick sibling and begin to feel guilty or ashamed about such feelings (Murray, 1999). Nurses can assist the family by helping the parents identify ways to involve siblings in the caring process, perhaps by bringing some supplies or a favorite toy, game, or food item. Parents should also be encouraged to schedule time focusing on the siblings. Helping parents identify a trusted friend or family member who can sit with the ill child for a short period will allow them to attend to their own needs or those of their other children.

FEAR OF DYING ALONE OR OF NOT BEING PRESENT WHEN THE CHILD DIES

When a child is being cared for at home, the burden of care on parents and family members can be great. Often, as the child's condition declines, family members begin the "death vigil." Rarely is a child left alone for any length of time. This can be exhausting for family members, and nurses can assist the family by helping them arrange shifts so that friends or family members can be present with the child and allow others to rest. If the family has limited resources, community organizations, such as hospice or churches, often have volunteers who are willing to visit and sit with children. It is important that whoever is sitting with the child be aware of when the parent(s) would like to be notified to return to the child's bedside (Fig. 17.6).

When a child is dying in the hospital, the parents should be given full access to the child at all times. If the parents need to leave, they should be provided with a pager or other means of immediate communication and alerted if staff members note any change in the child that may indicate imminent death. Nurses should advocate for parents' presence in intensive care and emergency departments and attend to the parents' needs for food, drinks, comfortable chairs, blankets, and pillows.

BOX 17.9 Physical Signs of Approaching Death

Loss of sensation and movement in the lower extremities, progressing toward the upper body
Sensation of heat, although the body feels cool
Loss of senses:
- Tactile sensation decreasing
- Sensitivity to light
- Hearing the last sense to fail

Confusion, loss of consciousness, slurred speech
Muscle weakness
Loss of bowel and bladder control
Decreased appetite and thirst
Difficulty swallowing
Change in respiratory pattern:
- Cheyne-Stokes respirations (waxing and waning of depth of breathing with regular periods of apnea)
- "Death rattle" (noisy chest sounds from accumulation of pulmonary and pharyngeal secretions)

Weak, slow pulse; decreased blood pressure

FEAR OF ACTUAL DEATH

Home Deaths

Most children receiving hospice care die at home; they often die in their own room with family, pets, and loved possessions around them. The physical process of dying can be distressing to parents because often the child slowly becomes less alert in the days before the actual death. The nurse can assist the family by providing them with information about what changes will occur as the child progresses through the dying process (Box 17.9). During this time, nursing visits often become more frequent and longer in duration to provide the family with additional support as the death nears. The most distressing change for parents to observe is the change in the respiratory pattern. In the final hours of life, the dying patient's respirations may become labored, with deep breaths and long periods of apnea, referred to as *Cheyne-Stokes respirations.* Families should be reassured that this is not distressing to the child and that it is a normal part of the dying process. However, the use of opioids can slow the respirations to make the child breathe more easily, and scopolamine, usually applied as a topical patch, can help reduce noisy respirations known as the "death rattle." Noisy respirations are more likely to occur if the child is overhydrated.

All families have the option of admitting their child to the hospital if they feel unable to deal with the death. The child who dies at home must be pronounced dead. Hospice programs typically have provisions so that this proceeds smoothly. In some circumstances, the police may be notified, with an explanation of the circumstances to prevent unnecessary concern regarding abuse. Providing the police with the number of the responsible practitioner is usually all that is necessary to confirm the cause of death.

Hospital Deaths

Children dying in the hospital who are receiving supportive care interventions experience a similar process. Death resulting from accident or trauma or acute illness in settings such as the emergency department or intensive care unit often requires the active withdrawal of some form of life-supporting intervention, such as a ventilator or bypass machine. These situations often raise difficult ethical issues (Sullivan, Monagle, & Gillam, 2014), and parents are often less prepared for the actual moment of death. Nurses can assist these parents by providing detailed information about what will happen as supportive equipment is withdrawn, ensuring that appropriate pain medications are administered to prevent pain during the dying process and allowing the parents time before the start of the withdrawal to be with and speak to their child. It is important that the nurse attempt to control the environment around the family at this time by providing privacy, asking if they would like to play music, softening lights and monitor noises, and arranging for any religious or cultural rituals that the family may want performed.

After the child's death, the family should be allowed to remain with the body and hold or rock the child if they desire. After the nurse has removed all tubes and equipment from the body, the parents should be given the option of assisting with the preparation of the body, such as bathing and dressing. It is important for the nurse to determine whether the family has any specific needs because many cultures have adopted specific methods for coping with and mourning death, and impeding these practices may interfere with the grieving process (Clements, Vigil, Manno, et al., 2003).

At some point, the nurse discusses whether the family has made preparations for the burial service and whether the staff can help in any way. Parents often have concerns about the funeral, such as siblings' involvement in the death rituals. Although no absolute answers exist regarding the question of siblings attending the funeral or burial services, the consensus is that the surviving children benefit from being involved in these events. However, children need preparation for post-death services. They should be told what to expect, particularly how the deceased person will look if the coffin is open; allowed private time to say goodbye; and permitted to stay as long as they wish. Ideally, the parents should prepare the siblings. If the parents' grief prevents this communication, a significant family member or friend should substitute.

ORGAN OR TISSUE DONATION AND AUTOPSY

For some families, organ or tissue donation may be a meaningful act—one that benefits another human being despite the loss of their child. Unfortunately, initiating a discussion about tissue donation is often stressful for staff, and there may be confusion regarding whose responsibility this is. In centers in which transplants are performed, a full-time transplant coordinator is usually available to inform the family about organ donation and to take care of details. If such services are not available, the staff needs to determine which members should discuss this topic with the family. Ideally, the person who knows the family best, knows when the death is expected, or has an opportunity to spend time with the family when the death is unexpected takes the role. Often nurses are in an optimal position to suggest tissue donation after consultation with the attending physician. When possible, the topic should be raised before death occurs. The request should be made in a private and quiet area of the hospital and should be simple and direct with questions such as "Are you a donor family?" or "Have you ever considered organ donation?"

Many states have legislated a mandatory request for organ or tissue donation when a child dies, especially if the patient is brain dead. Written consent from the family is required before donation can proceed. When requests for organ donation are made, health care practitioners must address common misunderstandings families have about brain death and organ donation (Franz, DeJong, Wolfe, et al., 1997). Training health care professionals on sensitive approaches to requests for organ donation has been shown to increase families' willingness to consent to organ donation (Workman, Myrick, Meyers, et al., 2013). The option to donate organs should always be separate from the communication of impending or actual death.

Nurses need to be aware of common questions about organ donation to help families make an informed decision. Healthy children who die unexpectedly are excellent candidates for organ donation. Children with cancer, chronic disease, or infection, and those who have suffered prolonged cardiac arrest may not be suitable candidates, although this is individually determined. The nurse should ask whether organ donation was discussed with the child or whether the child ever expressed such a wish. Any number of body tissues or organs can be donated (skin, corneas, bone, kidney, heart, liver, pancreas), and their removal does not mutilate or desecrate the body or cause any suffering. The family may have an open casket, and there is no delay in the funeral. There is no cost to the donor family, but organ donation does not eliminate funeral or cremation responsibilities. With the exception of Orthodox Judaism, most religions permit organ donation as long as the recipient benefits from the transplant. In cases of unexplained death, violent death, or suspected suicide, autopsy is required by law. In other instances, it may be optional, and parents should be informed of this choice. The procedure, as well as forms that require signing, should be explained. The family should know that the child can be in an open casket after an autopsy.

GRIEF AND MOURNING

Grief is a process, not an event, of experiencing physiologic, psychologic, behavioral, social, and spiritual reactions to the loss of a child. Grief is highly individualized, encompassing a broad range of manifestations from person to person. It is a natural and expected reaction to loss. It is neither orderly nor predictable. Grieving in any form is necessary for healing to occur. When death is the expected or a possible outcome of a disorder, the child and family members may experience **anticipatory grief**. Anticipatory grief may be manifested in varying behaviors and intensities and may include denial, anger, depression, and other psychologic and physical symptoms.

Anticipatory guidance may assist grieving family members. Health care professionals should emphasize that grief reactions such as hearing the dead person's voice, feeling distant from others, or seeking reassurance that they did everything possible for the lost person are normal, necessary, and expected. They in no way signify poor coping, insanity, or an approaching mental breakdown. On the contrary, such behaviors signify that the survivor is working through the acute grief. Anticipatory guidance regarding the mourning process may help families recognize the normalcy of their experiences.

It is important to recognize that some family members may experience complicated grief. **Complicated grief reactions** (>1 year after the loss) include such symptoms as intense intrusive thoughts, pangs of severe emotion, distressing yearnings, feelings of excessive loneliness and emptiness, unusual sleep disturbance, and maladaptive levels of loss of interest in personal activities (Meert et al., 2011). Bereaved persons experiencing such prolonged and complicated grief should be referred to an expert in grief and bereavement counseling.

Another important aspect of grief is the individual nature of the grief experience. Each member of the family will experience the grief of the child's death in his or her own way based on the particular relationship with that child. This can create potential conflict for families, because each family member has expectations that the other family members should feel and grieve as they do. Nurses caring for families experiencing grief should be aware of the different grieving styles and help the family learn to recognize and support the uniqueness of each other's grief.

Parental Grief

Parental grief after the death of a child has been found to be the most intense, complex, long-lasting, and fluctuating grief experience compared with that of other bereaved individuals. Although parents experience the primary loss of their child, many secondary losses are felt, such as the loss of part of one's self, hopes and dreams for the child's future, the family unit, prior social and emotional community supports, and often spousal support. It is common for parents of the same child to experience different grief reactions.

Studies with bereaved parents have shown that grieving does not end with the severing of the bond with the deceased child but rather involves a continuing bond between the parent and the deceased child (Klass, 2001). Parental resolution of grief is a process of integrating the dead child into daily life in which the pain of losing a child is never completely gone but lessens. There are occasions of brief relapse but not to the degree experienced when the loss initially occurred. Thus parental grief work is never completed and is a timeless process of accommodating the new reality of being without a child as it changes over time (Davies, 2004). A child's death can also challenge the marital relationship in several ways. Maternal and paternal reactions often differ (Hendrickson, 2009; Moriarty, Carroll, & Cotroneo, 1996; Scholtes & Browne, 2015; Vance, Najman, Thearle, et al., 1995). Different grieving styles between the couple may hinder communication and support for each other. Differing needs and expectations can place a strain on the marriage.

Sibling Grief

Each child grieves in his or her own way and on his or her own timeline. Children, even adolescents, grieve differently than adults. Adults and children differ more widely in their reactions to death than in their reactions to any other phenomenon. Children of all ages grieve the loss of a loved one, and their understanding and reactions to death depend on their age and developmental level. Children grieve for a longer duration, revisiting their grief as they grow and develop new understandings of death. However, they do not grieve 100% of the time. They grieve in spurts and can be emotional and sad in one instance and then, just as quickly, off and playing. Children express their grief through play and behavior. Children can be exquisitely attuned to their parents' grief and will try to protect them by not asking questions or by trying not to upset them. This can set the stage for the sibling to try to become the "perfect child." Children exhibit many of the grief reactions of adults, including physical sensations and illnesses, anger, guilt, sadness, loneliness, withdrawal, acting out, sleep disturbances, isolation, and search for meaning. Again, nurses should be attentive for signs that siblings are struggling with their grief and provide guidance to parents when possible.

At times, family members may need assistance in their grieving (see Nursing Care Guidelines box). Communication with the bereaved family is essential, but often nurses do not know what to say and feel helpless in offering words of comfort. The most supportive approach is to avoid judging the family's reactions or offering advice or rationalizations and to focus on feelings. Perhaps the most valuable supportive measure the nurse can perform for families is to listen. Families understand that no words will relieve their pain; all they want is acceptance, understanding, and respect for their grief.

It is important for families to understand that mourning takes a long time. Whereas acute grief may last only weeks or months, resolving the loss is measured in years. Holidays and anniversaries can be particularly difficult, and people who previously had been supportive may now expect the family to have "adjusted." Consequently, prolonged mourning is often silent and lonely.

Many families never receive the support and guidance that could help them resolve the loss. A plan for regular follow-up with bereaved families can be beneficial. At minimum, one follow-up phone call or meeting with the family should be arranged. Families can also be referred to self-help groups. When such groups are not available, nurses can be instrumental in bringing families together or facilitating parent and sibling groups. Formal bereavement programs or bereavement counseling can be helpful as well.

NURSING CARE GUIDELINES

Supporting Grieving Families[a]

General

- Stay with the family; sit quietly if they prefer not to talk; cry with them if desired.
- Accept the family's grief reactions; avoid judgmental statements (e.g., "You should be feeling better by now").
- Avoid offering rationalizations for the child's death (e.g., "Your child isn't suffering anymore").
- Avoid artificial consolation (e.g., "I know how you feel," "You are still young enough to have another baby").
- Deal openly with feelings such as guilt, anger, and loss of self-esteem.
- Focus on feelings by using a feeling word in the statement (e.g., "You're still feeling all the pain of losing a child").
- Refer the family to an appropriate self-help group or for professional help if needed.

At the Time of Death

- Reassure the family that everything possible is being done for the child if they want life-saving interventions.
- Do everything possible to ensure the child's comfort, especially relieving pain.
- Provide the child and family with the opportunity to review special experiences or memories in their lives.
- Express personal feelings of loss or frustrations (e.g., "We will miss him so much," "We tried everything; we feel so sorry that we couldn't save her").
- Provide information that the family requests and be honest.
- Respect the emotional needs of family members, such as siblings, who may need brief respites from the dying child.
- Make every effort to arrange for family members, especially the parents, to be with the child at the moment of death if they want to be present.
- Allow the family to stay with the dead child for as long as they wish and to rock, hold, or bathe the child.
- Provide practical help when possible, such as collecting the child's belongings.
- Arrange for spiritual support based on the family's religious beliefs; pray with the family if no one else can stay with them.

Post Death

- Attend the funeral or visitation if there was a special closeness with the family.
- Initiate and maintain contact (e.g., sending cards, telephoning, inviting them back to the unit, making a home visit).
- Refer to the dead child by name; discuss shared memories with the family.
- Discourage the use of drugs and alcohol as a method of escaping grief.
- Encourage all family members to communicate their feelings rather than to remain silent to avoid upsetting another family member.
- Emphasize that grieving is a painful process that often takes years to resolve.

[a] "Family" refers to all significant persons involved in the child's life, such as parents, siblings, grandparents, and other close relatives or friends.

NURSES' REACTIONS TO CARING FOR DYING CHILDREN

The caring for a dying child can be one of the most stressful aspects of nursing, it can also be incredibly rewarding. Even when a child is not expected to live, his or her death seems unnatural. Nurses experience reactions to the death of a patient that are very similar to the responses of family members, including denial, anger, depression, guilt, and ambivalent feelings

Strategies that can assist nurses in maintaining the ability to work effectively in these settings include maintaining good general health, developing well-rounded interests, using distancing techniques such as taking time off when needed, developing and using professional and personal support systems, cultivating the capacity for empathy, focusing on the positive aspects of the caregiver role, and basing nursing interventions on sound theory and empiric observations. Attending shared-remembrance rituals, sharing stories about their patient and experiences, can also help some nurses resolve their grief (Rice, Bennett, & Billingsley, 2014). Similarly, attending the funeral services can be a supportive act for both the family and the nurse and in no way detracts from the professionalism of care.

CLINICAL JUDGMENT AND NEXT-GENERATION NCLEX® EXAMINATION-STYLE QUESTIONS

1. When caring for a 4-year-old with a chronic disability, the nurse notes that while encouraging the child to take part in his own care, the mother constantly gives in to the child, allowing him to have his own way. While in the exam room, the child refused to get on the table and the mother allowed him to remain on the floor making it impossible for the nurse to obtain a blood pressure. What anticipatory guidance can the nurse give to promote normalization in this relationship? **Use an X for the health teaching statement below that is Indicated (appropriate or necessary), Contraindicated (could be harmful), or Non-Essential (makes no difference or not necessary).**

Health Teaching	Indicated	Contraindicated	Non-Essential
"'Giving in' is not a detriment to your child when he or she has a disability and limitations."			
"When parents establish reasonable limits, children are likely to develop independence that is appropriate for their age and achievement equal to their limitations."			
"It is best to wait to explain any procedure to the child until they are at the health care setting or just before the procedure to avoid unduly upsetting your child."			
"I recommend talking to other mothers in your neighborhood about how they parent their children."			
"It is important to realize that it would be unfair to the siblings to expect similar rules to apply to all children in the family."			

2. A 5-year-old boy with cystic fibrosis is hospitalized with pneumonia. His mother remains by his side and confides in the nurses that she is having difficulty coping with her child's chronic illness. She is a single mother and the father is not around. It is important for the nurse to realize that children with disabilities or chronic illness and their families may have different methods of coping than those of healthy children. Often, they have a resilience that is to be admired. Which of these statements reflect ways in which this mother can foster resilience in her young boy? **Select all that apply.**
   - **A.** Accept that chronic illness is part of living.
   - **B.** Home school the child until he is in high school.
   - **C.** Focus on the child's strengths and encourage independence.
   - **D.** The parents should set long-term goals to create a sense of hope.
   - **E.** Protect the child from having to learn about his or her disability or illness on a repeated basis.
   - **F.** Develop relationships with other children and their families who have similar circumstances to build support.

3. A 10-year-old girl is admitted to the hospital with pneumonia. She has acute lymphocytic leukemia and is in relapse. The nurse admitting her is reviewing her pain medications since she has been on oral morphine at home for the past month. Which of the following factors would the nurse consider when managing the pain of a terminally ill child? **Select all that apply.**
   - **A.** Pain medications are given on an as-needed schedule, and extra doses for breakthrough pain are available to maintain comfort.
   - **B.** Opioid drugs, such as morphine, are given for severe pain, and the dosage is increased as necessary to maintain optimum pain relief.
   - **C.** The same dose of morphine should be maintained throughout this hospitalization so she does not become addicted and need a higher dose when discharged.
   - **D.** Addiction is a factor in managing terminal pain in a child, and the nurse plays an important role in educating parents that their child may become addicted.
   - **E.** Nurses often express concern that administering dosages of opioids that exceed those with which they are familiar will hasten the child's death (principle of double effect).
   - **F.** In addition to pain medication, techniques such as music therapy, distraction, and guided imagery should be combined with medications to provide the child and family with strategies to control pain.

4. As the nurse caring for a culturally diverse population, it is important to understand the cultural health beliefs of families. A nurse caring for a child with congenital heart disease whose family is from China has a difficult time communicating with the mother, even though she speaks some English. **Indicate which nursing action number listed in the far-left column is most appropriate for each potential complication that could result from poor communication listed in the middle column. Place the number in the far right column. Note that not all actions will be used.**

Nursing Action	Potential communication problems	Appropriate nursing action for potential communication problem
1. Listen to the mother's perception of the seriousness or severity of the illness.	Lack of support from family and friends	
2. Provide an opportunity for the mother to discuss her concerns and worries.	Nurse unaware of the mother's understanding of the child'	
3. Acknowledge language constraints may make it necessary for the health care team to make some decisions.	Lack of support from health care providers	
4. Ask the mother how her extended family feels about the child's illness.		
5. Tell the mother not to talk to anyone else about her		
6. Explore alternative medicines and therapies.		
7. Explore the mother's support network to find others that can help.		

REFERENCES

American Academy of Pediatrics. (2019). Council on Children with Disabilities. Retrieved February 27, 2019, from Policy Statements, Clinical Reports and Technical Reports: https://www.aap.org/en-us/about-the-aap/Councils/Council-on-Children-with-Disabilities/Pages/Policy-Statements-Clinical-Technical-Reports.aspx.

American Nurses Association. (2015). *Code of ethics for nurses with interpretive statements.* Washington, DC: ANA Publishing.

American Psychological Association. (2013). *Diagnostic and statistical manual of mental disorders (DSM-5)* (5th ed.). Arlington, VA: American Psychological Association.

Anderson, T., & Davis, C. (2011). Evidence-based practice with families of chronically ill children: A critical literature review. *Journal of Evidence-Based Social Work, 8*(4), 416–425.

Baker, J. N., Torkildson, C., Baillargeon, J. G., et al. (2007). National survey of pediatric residency program directors and residents regarding education in palliative medicine and end-of-life care. *The Journal of Palliative Medicine, 10*(2), 420–429.

Barnert, E. S., Coller, R. J., Nelso, B. B., et al. (2017). Experts' perspectives toward a population health approach for children with medical complexity. *Academic Pediatrics, 17*(6), 672–677.

Barnes, S., Gardiner, C., Gott, M., et al. (2012). Enhancing patient-professional communication about end-of-life issues in life-limiting conditions: A critical review of the literature. *Journal of Pain and Symptom Management, 44*(6), 866–879.

Barr, J., & McLeod, S. (2010). They never see how hard it is to be me: Siblings' observations of strangers, peers and family. *International Journal of Speech-Language Pathology, 12*(2), 162–171.

Berry, J. G., Hall, M., Hall, D. E., et al. (2013). Inpatient growth and resource use in 28 children's hospitals: A longitudinal, multi-institutional study. *JAMA Pediatrics, 167*(2), 170–177.

Blume, E. D., Balkin, E. M., Aiyagari, R., et al. (2014). Parental perspectives on suffering and quality of life at end-of-life in children with advanced heart disease: An exploratory study. *Pediatric Critical Care Medicine, 15*(4), 336–342.

Bogetz, J. F., Bogetz, A. L., Rassbach, C. F., et al. (2015). Caring for childen with medical complexity: Challenges and educational opportunities identified by pediatric residents. *Academic Pediatrics, 6*, 621–625.

Brenner, M., Larkin, P. J., Hilliard, C., et al. (2015). Parents' perspectives of the transition to home when a child has complex technological health care needs. *International Journal of Integrated Care, 15.*

Bucholz, E. M., Toomey, S. L., & Schuster, M. A. (2019). Trends in pediatric hospitalizations and readmissions: 2010-2016. *Pediatrics, 143*(2), e20181958.

Burke, R. T., & Alverson, B. (2010). Impact of children with medically complex conditions. *Pediatrics, 126*(4), 789–790.

Clements, P. T., Vigil, G. J., Manno, M. S., et al. (2003). Cultural perspectives of death, grief, and bereavement. *Journal of Psychosocial Nursing and Mental Health Services, 41*(7), 18–26.

Coats, H., Bourget, E., Starks, H., et al. (2018). Nurses' reflection on benefits and challenges of implementing family-centered care in pediatric intensive care units. *American Journal of Critical Care, 27*(1), 52–58.

Coffey, J. S. (2006). Parenting a child with chronic illness: A metasynthesis. *Pediatric Nursing, 32*(1), 51–59.

Cohen, E., Kuo, D. Z., Agrawal, R., et al. (2011). Children with medical complexity: An emerging population for clinical and research initiatives. *Pediatrics, 127*(3), 529–538.

Coker, T. R., Rodriguez, M. A., & Flores, G. (2010). Family-centered care for US children with special health care needs: Who gets it and why? *Pediatrics, 125*(6), 1159–1167.

Corlett, J., & Twycross, A. (2006). Negotiation of parental roles within family-centered care: A review of the research. *Journal of Clinical Nursing, 15*(10), 1308–1316.

Cousino, M. K., & Hazen, R. A. (2013). Parenting stress among caregivers of children with chronic illness: A systematic review. *Journal of Pediatric Psychology, 38*(8), 809–828.

Cunningham, R. M., Walton, M. A., & Carter, P. M. (2018). The major causes of death in children and adolescents in the United States. *The New England Journal of Medicine, 375*, 2468–2475.

Davies, R. (2004). New understandings of parental grief: Literature review. *Journal of Advanced Nursing, 46*(5), 506–513.
DeGraeff, A., & Dean, M. (2007). Palliative sedation therapy in the lasts: A literature review and recommendations for standards. *The Journal of Palliative Medicine, 10*(1), 67–85.
Elias, E. R., Murphy, N. A., & Council on Children with Diabilities (2012). Home care of children and youth with complex health care needs and technology dependencies. *Pediatrics, 129*, 996–1004.
Elwyn, G., Frosch, D., Thomson, R., et al. (2012). Shared decision making: A model for clinical practice. *Journal of General Internal Medicine, 27*(1), 1361–1367.
Feudtner, C., Dai, D., & Hexem, K. (2012). Prevalence of polypharmacy exposure among hospitalizated children in the United States. *Archives of Pediatrics & Adolescent Medicine, 166*(1), 9–16.
Feudtner, C., Feinstein, J. A., Zhong, W., et al. (2014). Pediatric complex chronic conditions classification system version 2: Updated for ICD-10 and complex medical technology dependence and transplantation. *BMC Pediatrics, 14*, 199.
Feudtner, C., Friebert, S., & Jewell, J. (2013). Pediatric palliative and hospice care committments, guidelines and recommendations. *Pediatrics, 132*(5), 966–972.
Field, M. J., & Behrman, R. E. (Eds.). (2004). *When children die: Improving palliative and end-of-life care for children and their families*. Washington, DC: National Academies Press.
Fleitas, J. (2000). When Jack fell down Jill came tumbling after: Siblings in the web of illness and disability. *MCN, The American Journal of Maternal/Child Nursing, 25*(5), 267–273.
Franz, H. G., DeJong, W., Wolfe, S. M., et al. (1997). Explaining brain death: A critical feature of the donation process. *Journal of Transplant Coordination, 7*(1), 14–21.
Gan, L. L., Lum, A., Wakefield, C. E., Nandakumar, B., & Fardell, J. E. (2017). School experiences of siblings of children with chronic illness: A systematic literature review. *The Journal of Pediatric Nursing, 33*, 23–32.
Giannini, A., Messeri, A., Aprile, A., et al. (2008). End-of-life decisions in pediatric intensive care: Recommendations of the Italian Society of Neonatal and Pediatric Anesthesia and Intensive Care (SARNePI). *Paediatric Anaesthesia, 18*(11), 1089–1095.
Gold, J. I., Treadwell, M., Weissman, L., et al. (2011). The mediating effects of family functioning on psychosocial outcomes in healthy siblings of children with sickle cell disease. *Pediatric Blood & Cancer, 57*(6), 1055–1061.
Goodenough, B., Drew, D., Higgins, S., et al. (2004). Bereavement outcomes for parents who lose a child to cancer: Are place of death and sex of parent associated with differences in psychological functioning? *Psychooncology, 13*(11), 779–791.
Goudie, A., Narcisse, M. R., Hall, D. E., et al. (2014). Financial and psychological stressors associated with caring for children with disability. *Families, Systems and Health, 32*(3), 280–290.
Griggs, S., & Walker, R. K. (2016). The role of hope for adolescents with a chronic illness: An integrative review. *The Journal of Pediatric Nursing, 31*(4), 404–421.
Hartling, L., Milne, A., Tjosvold, L., et al. (2014). A systematic review of interventions to support siblings of children with chronic illness or disability. *The Journal of Paediatrics and Child Health, 50*(10), E26–E38.
Hendrickson, K. C. (2009). Morbidity, mortality, and parental grief: A review of the literature on the relationship between the death of a child and the subsequent health of parents. *Palliative and Supportive Care, 7*(1), 109–119.
Herzer, M., Godiwala, N., Hommel, K. A., et al. (2010). Family functioning in the context of pediatric chronic conditions. *Journal of Developmental Behavior Pediatrics, 31*(1), 26–34.
Hill, C., Knafl, K. A., & Santacroce, S. J. (2017). Family-centered care from the perspective of parents of children cared for in a pediatric intensive care unit: An integrated review. *Journal of Pediatric Nursing, 41*, 22–33.
Hinds, P. S., Oakes, L., Furman, W., et al. (2001). End-of-life decision making by adolescents, parents, and healthcare providers in pediatric oncology: Research to evidence-based practice guidelines. *Cancer Nursing, 24*(2), 122–134.
Huang, I. C., Kenzik, K. M., Sanjeev, T. Y., et al. (2010). Quality of life information and trust in physicians among families of children with life-limiting conditions. *Patient Related Outcome Measures, 1*, 141–148.
Hungerbuehler, I., Vollrath, M. E., & Landolt, M. A. (2011). Posttraumatic growth in mothers and fathers of children with severe illnesses. *The Journal of Health Psychology, 16*(8), 1259–1267.
Immelt, S. (2006). Psychological adjustment in young children with chronic medical conditions. *The Journal of Pediatric Nursing, 21*(5), 362–377.
Jacobs, H. H. (2005). Ethics in pediatric end-of-life care: A nursing perspective. *The Journal of Pediatric Nursing, 20*(5), 360–369.
Jibb, L. A., Nathan, P. C., Stevens, B. J., et al. (2015). Psychological and physical interventions for the managment of cancer-related pain in pediatric and young adult patients: An intergrative review. *Oncology Nursing Forum, 42*(6), e339–e357.
Jones, T. L., & Prinz, R. J. (2005). Potential roles of parental self-efficacy in parent and child adjustment: A review. *Clinical Psychology Review, 25*(3), 341–363.
Kang, T. I., Munson, D., Hwang, J., et al. (2014). Integration of palliative care into the care of children with serious illness. *Pediatric Review, 35*(8), 318–325.
Kassam, A., & Wolfe, J. (2013). The ambiguities of free-standing pediatric hospices. *The Journal of Palliative Medicine, 16*(7), 716–717.
Kavanaugh, K., Moro, T. T., & Savage, T. A. (2010). How nurses assist parents regarding life support decisions for extremely premature infants. *Journal of Obstetric Gynecologic, & Neonatal Nursing, 39*(2), 147–158.
Keim-Malpass, J., Hart, T. G., & Miller, J. R. (2013). Coverage of palliative and hospice care for pediatric patients with a life-limiting illness: A policy brief. *The Journal of Pediatric Health Care, 27*(6), 511–516.
Klass, D. (2001). The inner representation of the dead child in the psychic and social narratives of bereaved parents. In R. A. Neimeyer (Ed.), *Meaning reconstruction and the experience of loss*. Washington, DC: American Psychological Association.
Knafl, K. A., Darney, B. G., Gallo, A. M., et al. (2010). Parental perceptions of the outcome and meaning of normalization. *Research in Nursing & Health, 33*(2), 87–98.
Knafl, K. A., & Santacroce, S. J. (2010). Chronic conditions and the family. In P. J. Allen, J. A. Vessey, & N. A. Schapiro (Eds.), *Primary care of the child with a chronic condition* (5th ed.). St Louis: Mosby/Elsevier.
Kochanek, K. D., Murphy, S. L., Xu, J., et al. (2014). Mortality in the United States, 2013. *NCHS Data Brief, 178*, 1–8.
Kon, A. A. (2010). The shared decision-making continuum. *JAMA, 304*(8), 903–904.
Kuhlthau, K. A., Bloom, S., Van Cleave, J., et al. (2011). Evidence for family-centered care for children with special health care needs: A systematic review. *Academic Pediatrics, 11*(2), 136–143.
Kuo, D. Z., Cohen, E., Agrawal, R., et al. (2011). A national profile of caregiver challenges among more medically complex children with special health care needs. *Archives of Pediatrics & Adolescent Medicine, 165*(11), 1020–1026.
Kuo, D., & Houtrow, A. J. (2016). Recognition and managment of medical complexity. *Pediatrics, 138*(6), e20163021.
Kuo, D. Z., Houtrow, A. J., Arango, P., et al. (2012). Family-centered care: Current applications and future directions in pediatric health care. *Maternal and Child Health Journal, 16*(2), 297–305.
Kuo, D. Z., Sisterhen, L. L., Sigrest, T. E., et al. (2012). Family experiences and pediatric health services use associated with family-centered rounds. *Pediatrics, 130*(2), 299–305.
Lauer, M. E., Mulhern, R. K., Schell, M. J., et al. (1989). Long-term follow-up of parental adjustment following a child's death at home or hospital. *Cancer, 63*(5), 988–994.
LeGrow, K., Hodnett, E., Stremler, R., et al. (2014). Bourdieu at the bedside: Briefing parents in a pediatric hospital. *Nursing Inquiry, 21*(4), 327–335.
Leyenaar, J. K., O'Brien, E. R., Leslie, L. K., Lindenauer, P. K., & Mangione-Smith, R. M. (2017). Families' priorities regarding hosptial-to-home transitions for children with medical complexity. *Pediatrics, 139*(1), e20161581.
Lindley, L. C., Edwards, S., & Bruce, D. J. (2014). Factors influencing the implementation of health care reform: A examination of the concurrent care for children provision. *American Journal of Hospice and Palliative Care, 31*(5), 527–533.
Lipstein, E. A., Brinkman, W. B., & Britto, M. T. (2012). What is known about parents' treatment decisions? A narrative review of pediatric decision making. *Medical Decision Making, 32*(2), 246–258.
Lobato, D. J., Kao, B. T., & Plante, W. (2005). Latino sibling knowledge and adjustment to chronic illness. *The Journal of Family Psychology, 19*(4), 625–632.

Meert, K. L., Shear, K., Newth, C. J., et al. (2011). Follow-up study of complicated grief among parents eighteen months after a child's death in the pediatric intensive care unit. *The Journal of Palliative Medicine*, *14*(2), 207–214.

Monterosso, L., Kristjanson, L., Aoun, S., & Phillips, M. B. (2007). Supportive and palliative care needs of families of children with life-threatening illnesses in Western Australia: Evidence to guide the development of a palliative care service. *Palliative Medicine*, *21*(8), 689–696.

Morawska, A., Calam, R., & Fraser, J. (2015). Parenting interventions for childhood chronic illness: A review and recommendations for intervention design and delivery. *Journal of Child Health Care*, *19*(1), 5–17.

Moriarty, H., Carroll, R., & Cotroneo, M. (1996). Differences in bereavement reactions within couples following the death of a child. *Research in Nursing & Health*, *19*(6), 461–469.

Murray, J. S. (1999). Siblings of children with cancer: A review of the literature. *Journal of Pediatric Oncology Nursing*, *16*(1), 25–34.

Nageswaran, S., & Golden, S. L. (2017). Improving the quality of home health care for children with medical complexity. *Academic Pediatrics*, *17*(6), 665–671.

National Consensus Project for Quality Palliatve Care. (2018). *Clinical Practice Guidelines for Qualiity Palliative Care* (4th ed.). Richmond, VA: National Coalition for Hospice and Palliative Care.

National Hospice and Palliative Care Organization. (2010). Retrieved from Concurrent Care for Children. https://www.nhpco.org/palliative-care-overview/pediatric-palliative-and-hospice-care/pediatric-concurrent-care/concurrent-care-for-children/.

National Learning Consortium. (2013). Retrieved February 28, 2019, from Shared decision making fact sheet. https://www.healthit.gov/sites/default/files/nlc_shared_decision_making_fact_sheet.pdf.

Newacheck, P. W., & Halfon, N. (1998). Prevalence and impact of disabling chronic conditions in childhood. *American Journal of Public Health*, *88*(4), 610–617.

Nicholas, D. B., Beaune, L., Barrera, M., Blumberg, J., & Belletrutti, M. (2016). Examining the experiences of fathers of children with a life-limiting illness. *Journal of Social Work In End-Of-Life & Palliative Care*, *12*(1-2), 126–144.

Nurullah, A. S. (2013). "It's really a roller coaster" : Experiences of parenting children with developmental disabilities. *Marriage & Family Review*, *49*(5), 412–445.

Nuutila, L., & Salanterä, S. (2006). Children with a long-term illness: Parents' experiences of care. *Journal of Pediatric Nursing*, *21*(2), 153–160.

Nyborn, J. A., Olcese, M., Nickerson, T., & Mack, J. W. (2016). Don't try to cover the sky with your hands: Parents' experience with prognosis communication about their children with advance cancer. *Journal of Palliative Medicine*, *19*(6), 626–631.

O'Quinn, L. P., & Giambra, B. K. (2014). Evidence of improved quality of life with pediatric palliative care. *Pediatric Nursing*, *40*(6), 284–288 296.

Panicker, L. (2013). Nurses' perceptions of parent empowerment in chronic illness. *Contemporary Nurse*, *45*(2), 210–219.

Pinquart, M. (2018). Parenting stress in caregivers of children with chronic physical condition-A meta-analysis. *Stress Health*, *34*(2), 197–207.

Pousset, G., Bilsen, J., Cohen, J., et al. (2010). Medical end-of-life decisions in children in Flanders, Belgium: A population-based postmortem survey. *Archives Pediatrics &Adolescent Medicine*, *164*(6), 547–553.

Price, J., Dornan, J., & Quail, L. (2013). Seeing is believing—reducing misconceptions about children's hospice care through effective teaching with undergraduate nursing students. *Nurse Education Practice*, *13*(5), 361–365.

Rice, K. L., Bennett, M. J., & Billingsley, L. (2014). Using second life to facilitate peer storytelling for grieving oncology nurses. *The Ochsner Journal*, 14(4), 551–562.

Santoro, J. D., & Bennett, M. (2018). Ethics of end of life decision in pediatrics: A narrative review of the roles of caregivers, shared decision-makers, and patient centered values. *Behavioral Sciences*, *8*(42), 1–9.

Scholtes, D., & Browne, M. (2015). Internalized and externalized continuing bonds in bereaved parents: Their relationship with grief intensity and personal growth. *Death Studies*, *39*(2), 75–83.

Schor, E. L., & American Academy of Pediatrics Task Force on the Family (2003). Family pediatrics: Report of the Task Force on the Family. *Pediatrics*, *111*(6 Pt 2), 1541–1571.

Siden, H., Chavoshi, N., Harvey, B., et al. (2014). Characteristics of a pediatric hospice palliative care program over 15 years. *Pediatrics*, *134*(3), e765–e772.

Simon, T. D., Berry, J., Feudtner, C., Stone, B. L., Sheng, X., Braxton, S. L., et al. (2010). Children with complex chronic conditions in inpatient hospital settings in the United States. *Pediatrics*, *126*(4), 647–655.

Smaldone, A., & Ritholz, M. D. (2011). Perceptions of parenting children with type 1 diabetes diagnosed in early childhood. *Journal of Pediatrics Health Care*, *25*(2), 87–95.

Smith, J., Cheater, F., & Bekker, H. (2013). Parents' experiences of living with a child with a long-term condition: A rapid structured review of the literature. *Health Expectations*, *18*(4), 452–474.

Smith, J., Cheater, F., & Bekker, H. (2015). Parents' experiences of living with a child with a long-term condition: A rapid structured review of the literature. *Health Expect*, *18*(4), 452–474.

Smith, J., Swallow, V., & Coyne, I. (2015). Involving parents in managing their childs long-term condition-A concept synthesis of family centered care and partnership in care. *Journal of Pediatric Nursing*, *30*, 143–159.

Stein, R. E. K. (1985). Home care: A challenging opportunity. *Child Health Care*, *14*(2), 90–95.

Sullivan, J., Monagle, P., & Gillam, L. (2014). What parents want from doctors in end-of-life decision-making for children. *Archives of Disease Childhood*, *99*(3), 216–220.

Swallow, V., Macfadyen, A., Santacroce, S. J., et al. (2012). Fathers' contributions to the management of their child's long-term medical condition: A narrative review of the literature. *Health Expectations*, *15*(2), 157–175.

Toomey, S. L., Chien, A. T., Elliott, M. N., et al. (2013). Disparities in unmet need for care coordination: The national survey of children's health. *Pediatrics*, *131*(2), 217–224.

Treyvaud, K. (2014). Parent and family outcomes following very preterm or very low birth weight birth: A review. *Seminars in Fetal & Neonatal Medicine*, *19*(2), 131–135.

Twycross, R. (2019). Reflections on palliative sedation. *Palliative Care*, *12*, 1–16.

Vance, J. C., Najman, J. M., Thearle, M. J., et al. (1995). Psychological changes in parents eight months after the loss of an infant from stillbirth, neonatal death, or sudden infant death syndrome—A longitudinal study. *Pediatrics*, *96*(5), 933–938.

von Lützau, P., Otto, M., Hechler, T., et al. (2012). Children dying from cancer: Parents' perspectives on symptoms, quality of life, characteristics of death, and end-of-life decisions. *Journal of Palliative Care*, *28*(4), 274–281.

Wiener, L., McConnell, D. G., Latella, L., et al. (2013). Cultural and religious considerations in pediatric palliative care. *Palliative Support Care*, *11*(1), 47–67.

Wolfe, J., Friebert, S., & Hilden, J. (2002). Caring for children with advanced cancer integrating palliative care. *Pediatric Clinics North America*, *49*(5), 1043–1062.

Wolfe, J., Grier, H. E., Klar, N., et al. (2000). Symptoms and suffering at the end of life in children with cancer. *New England Journal of Medicine*, *342*(5), 326–333.

Woodgate, R. L., Edwards, M., Ripat, J. D., Borton, B., & Rempel, G. (2015). Intense parenting: A qualitative study detailing the experiences of parenting children with complex care needs. *BMC Pediatrics*, *15*, 197.

Workman, J. K., Myrick, C. W., Meyers, R. L., et al. (2013). Pediatric organ donation and transplantation. *Pediatrics*, *131*(6), e1723–e1730.

World Health Organization. (1998). Definition of palliative care for children. Retrieved from http://www.who.int/cancer/palliative/definition/en.

World Health Organization. (2012). *Persisting pain in children package: WHO guidelines on the pharmacological.* France: World Health Organization.

Wyatt, K. D., List, B., Brinkman, W. B., et al. (2015). Shared decision making in pediatrics: A systematic review and meta-analysis. *Academy of Pediatrics*, *15*(6), 573–583.

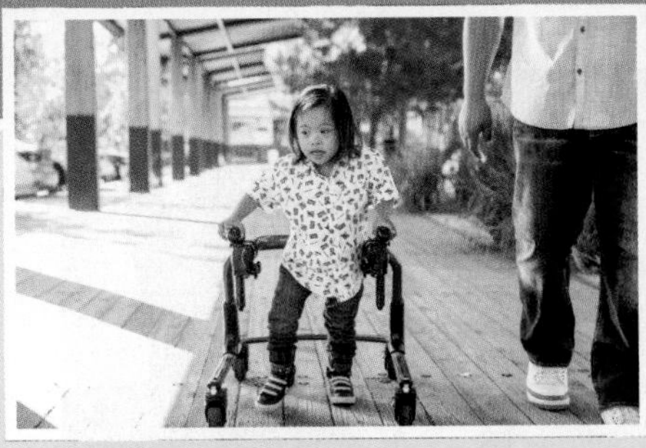

18

Impact of Cognitive or Sensory Impairment on the Child and Family

Rosalind Bryant

http://evolve.elsevier.com/wong/essentials

CONCEPTS

- Cognition
- Sensory Perception

COGNITIVE IMPAIRMENT

GENERAL CONCEPTS

Cognitive impairment (CI) is a general term that encompasses any type of intellectual disability. The term *intellectual disability* (formerly **mental retardation**) has become the most commonly used term internationally (American Association on Intellectual and Developmental Disabilities, 2013; American Psychiatric Association, 2013). In this chapter, the term *CI* is used synonymously with *intellectual disability*.

Intellectual disability, as defined by the American Association on Intellectual and Developmental Disabilities, in children consists of three components: (1) intellectual functioning, (2) adaptive functioning, and (3) the onset of disabilities during childhood or age younger than 18 years. Intellectual functioning is measured by the intelligence quotient (IQ) test, and intellectual disability exists where there is an IQ score of 70 or below or sometimes as high as 75. CI is an umbrella term characterized by significant limitations in intellectual functioning and impairment in a number of different adaptive areas: communication, self-care, home living, social skills, health and safety, self-direction, functional academics, community use, work, and lifelong learning (American Association on Intellectual and Developmental Disabilities, 2013; National Academies of Sciences, Engineering, and Medicine, 2015). The American Psychiatric Association's *Diagnostic and Statistical Manual of Mental Disorders,* Fifth edition (DSM-5) criteria recommend moving away from exclusively relying on IQ testing toward using additional measures of adaptive functioning (American Psychiatric Association, 2013; Moran, 2013). The DSM-5 is the diagnostic standard and states that a child with CI must demonstrate deficits in adaptive functioning that result in failure to meet developmental and sociocultural standards for personal independence and social responsibility (Moran, 2013).

The DSM-5 terminology and diagnostic criteria are consistent with those terms established by the American Association on Intellectual and Developmental Disabilities (Tassé, Luckasson, & Nygren, 2013). Careful evaluation to identify the needs of individuals with CI focuses on promoting habilitation for each person. It is anticipated that the functional capabilities of children with CI will improve over time when appropriate supports are provided.

Diagnosis and Classification

The diagnosis of CI is usually made after professionals or the family suspects that the child's developmental progress is delayed. In some cases, it is confirmed at birth because of recognition of distinct syndromes, such as Down syndrome and fetal alcohol syndrome. At the other extreme, the diagnosis is made when problems such as speech delays or school problems arouse concern. In all cases, a high index of suspicion for developmental delay and behavioral signs are necessary for early diagnosis (Box 18.1), and routine developmental screening can assist in early identification. Delays are typically seen in gross and fine motor and speech development, although the latter is most predictive. **Developmental disability** can be described as any significant lag or delay in a child's physical, cognitive, behavioral, emotional, or social development when compared to developmental norms. CI is an impairment encompassing intellectual ability and adaptive behavior that are functioning significantly below average (see Box 18.1). In the absence of clear-cut evidence of CI, it is more appropriate to use a diagnosis of developmental disability.

Results of standardized tests are helpful in contributing to the diagnosis of CI. Tests for assessing adaptive behaviors include the Vineland Adaptive Behavior Scales (Vineland-3) and the Adaptive Behavior Assessment System (ABS-3). Informal appraisal of adaptive behavior may be made by those fully acquainted with the child (e.g., teachers, parents, other care providers). Usually these behavioral observations lead parents to seek evaluation of the child's development. The Wechsler Intelligence Scale for Children (WISC-V) provides an overall IQ score and aids in the diagnoses of learning disabilities (Na & Burns, 2016).

A more useful approach for clinical application is classification based on educational potential or symptom severity. For educational purposes, the mildly impaired group constitutes about 85% of all people with CI, and the group with moderate levels of CI accounts for about 10% of the intellectually disabled population (Shea, 2012) (Table 18.1).

Etiology

The causes of severe CI are primarily genetic, biochemical, and infectious. Although the etiology is unknown in the majority of cases, familial, social, environmental, and organic causes may predominate. Among individuals with CI, a sizable proportion of the cases are linked to Down syndrome, fragile X syndrome (FXS), or fetal alcohol syndrome. General categories of events that may lead to CI include the

BOX 18.1 Early Signs Suggestive of Cognitive Impairment

Dysmorphic syndromes (e.g., Down syndrome, fragile X syndrome FXS)
Irritability or nonresponsiveness to environment
Major organ system dysfunction (e.g., feeding or breathing difficulties)
Gross motor delay
Fine motor delay
Language difficulties or delay
Behavior difficulties

Modified from Shapiro, B., & O'Neill, M. E. (2020). Intellectual disability. In R. M. Kliegman, J. W. St. Geme, N. J. Blum, et al. (Eds.), *Nelson textbook of pediatrics* (21st ed., pp. 283-293). Philadelphia, PA: Elsevier; Wilks, T., Gerber, J., & Erdie-Lalena, C. (2010). Developmental milestones: Cognitive development. *Pediatrics Review, 31*(9), 364–367.

TABLE 18.1 Cognitive Impairment Intelligence Quotient (IQ) Level

Mild	50–55 to 70–75
Moderate	35–40 to 50–55
Severe	20–25 to 35–40
Profound	<20–25

following (Casanova, Gerstner, Sharp, et al., 2018; Gilissen, Hehir-Kwa, Thung, et al., 2014; Hoyme, Kalberg, Elliot, et al., 2016; Katz & Lazcano-Ponce, 2008; Mefford, Batshaw, & Hoffman, 2012):

- Infection and intoxication, such as congenital rubella, syphilis, maternal drug consumption (e.g., fetal alcohol syndrome), chronic lead ingestion, or kernicterus
- Trauma or physical agent (e.g., injury to the brain experienced during the prenatal, perinatal, or postnatal period)
- Inadequate nutrition and metabolic disorders, such as phenylketonuria or congenital hypothyroidism
- Gross postnatal brain disease, such as neurofibromatosis and tuberous sclerosis
- Unknown prenatal influence, including cerebral and cranial malformations, such as microcephaly and hydrocephalus
- Chromosomal abnormalities resulting from radiation; viruses; chemicals; parental age; and genetic mutations, such as Down syndrome and FXS
- Gestational disorders, including preterm birth, low birth weight, and postterm birth
- Psychiatric disorders with onset during the child's developmental period up to age 18 years, such as autism spectrum disorders (ASDs)
- Environmental influences, including evidence of a deprived environment associated with a history of intellectual disability among parents and siblings

NURSING CARE OF CHILDREN WITH IMPAIRED COGNITIVE FUNCTION

Nurses play a major role in identifying children with CI. In the newborn and early infancy periods, few signs are present, except in such disorders as Down syndrome (discussed later in the chapter). However, delayed developmental milestones are the major clues to CI. In addition, nurses must have a high index of suspicion for early behavior patterns that may suggest CI (see Box 18.1). Parental concerns, such as delayed development compared with siblings, need to be taken seriously. All children should receive regular developmental assessment, and the nurse is often the person responsible for performing such assessments. When delays are found, the nurse must use sensitivity and discretion in revealing this finding to parents.

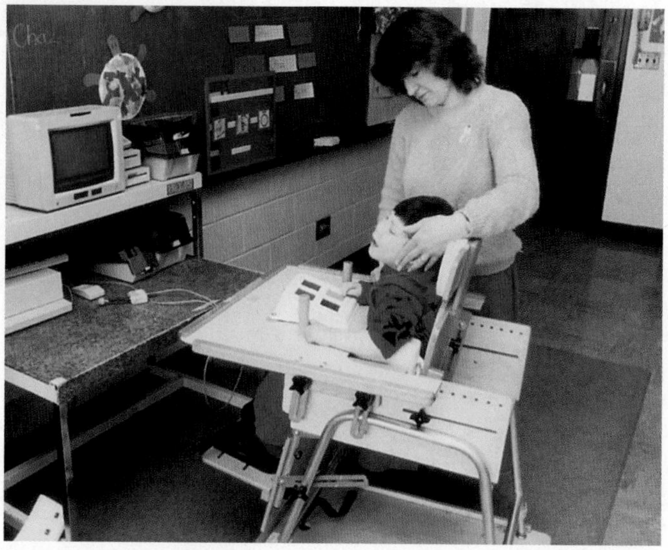

Fig. 18.1 A push panel allows a child with cognitive impairment (CI) to turn a computer on and off.

Educate Child and Family

To teach children with CI, one must investigate their learning abilities and deficits. This is important for the nurse who may be involved in a home care program or who may be caring for the child in a school or health care setting. The nurse who understands how these children learn can effectively teach them basic skills or prepare them for various health-related procedures.

Children with CI have a marked deficit in their ability to discriminate between two or more stimuli because of difficulty in recognizing the relevance of specific cues. However, these children can learn to discriminate if the cues are presented in an exaggerated, concrete form and if all extraneous stimuli are eliminated. For example, the use of colors to emphasize visual cues or the use of singing or rhymes to stress auditory cues can help them learn. Their deficit in discrimination also implies that concrete ideas are learned much more effectively than abstract ideas. Therefore demonstration is preferable to verbal explanation, and learning should be directed toward mastering a skill rather than understanding the scientific principles underlying a procedure.

Another cognitive deficit is in short-term memory. Whereas children of average intelligence can remember several words, numbers, or directions at one time, children with CI are less able to do so. Therefore they need simple, one-step directions. Learning through a step-by-step process requires a **task analysis** in which each task is separated into its necessary components and each step is taught completely before proceeding to the next activity.

One critical area of learning that has had a tremendous impact on education for cognitively impaired individuals is **motivation** or the use of positive reinforcement to encourage the accomplishment of specific tasks or behaviors. Advances in technology have greatly aided in providing reinforcement, especially in children with severe disabilities who may have physical disabilities that limit their range of capabilities. For example, with the use of specially designed switches, children are given control of some event in the environment, such as turning on a computer (Fig. 18.1). Activation of the computer becomes the reinforcement for pushing the switch. Repetitive use of these switches provides an early, simplistic association with a technical device that may progress to increasingly complex aids.

Early intervention program is a systematic program of therapy, exercises, and activities designed to address developmental delays in disabled children to help achieve their full potentials (Bull & Committee on Genetics, 2011; Crnic, Neece, McIntyre, et al., 2017; Guralnick, 2017; National Down Syndrome Society, 2019a). Considerable evidence indicates that these programs are valuable for children with CI. Nurses working with these families need to be aware of the types of programs in their community. Under the Individuals with Disabilities Education Act (IDEA) of 1990 (Public Law 101-476), states are encouraged to provide full early intervention services and are required to provide educational opportunities for all children with disabilities from birth to 21 years of age. Services may be provided under state programs for Children with Special Health Care Needs (CSHCN) or Head Start or by private organizations such as the National Down Syndrome Society,[a] Easter Seals,[b] or The Arc of the United States.[c] Parents should inquire about these programs by contacting the appropriate agencies. The child's education should begin as soon as possible, because it has been shown that early intervention exposure tends to be associated with more positive developmental and behavioral outcomes in children with CI (Crnic et al., 2017; Guralnick, 2017; Wallander, Biasini, Thorsten, et al., 2014). As children grow older, their education should be directed toward vocational training that prepares them for as independent a lifestyle as possible within their scope of abilities.

Teach Child Self-Care Skills

When a child with CI is born, parents often need assistance in promoting normal developmental skills that other children learn easily. There is no way to predict when a child should be able to master self-care skills, such as feeding, toileting, dressing, and grooming, because a wide age variability exists in the child with CI who is able to accomplish such functions.

Teaching self-care skills also necessitates a working knowledge of the individual steps needed to master a skill. For example, before beginning a self-feeding program, the nurse performs a task analysis. After a task analysis, the child is observed in a particular situation, such as eating, to determine what skills are possessed and the child's developmental readiness to learn the task. Family members are included in this process because their "readiness" is as important as the child's. Numerous self-help aids are available to facilitate independence, and these can help eliminate some of the difficulties of learning, such as using a plate with suction cups to prevent accidental spills.

Promote Child's Optimal Development

Optimal development involves more than achieving independence. It requires appropriate guidance for establishing acceptable social behavior and personal feelings of self-esteem, worth, and security. These attributes are not simply learned through a stimulation program. Rather, they must arise from the genuine love and caring that exist among family members. However, families need guidance in providing an environment that fosters optimal development. Often the nurse can provide assistance in these areas of childrearing.

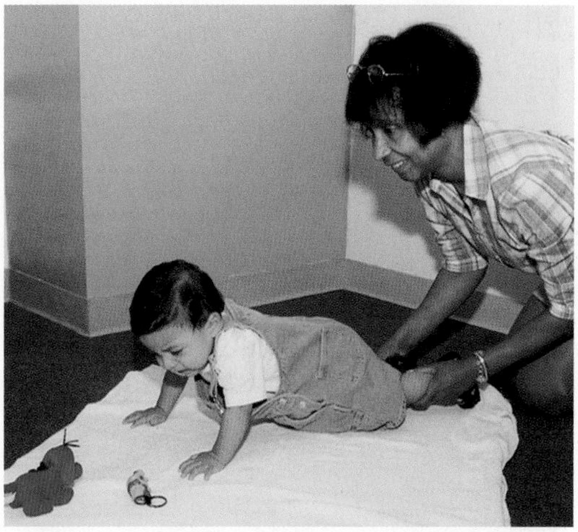

Fig. 18.2 Placing an attractive object outside the child's reach encourages crawling movements. (Courtesy James DeLeon, Texas Children's Hospital, Houston, TX.)

Another important area for promoting optimal development and self-esteem is ensuring the child's physical well-being. Any congenital defects, such as cardiac, gastrointestinal, or orthopedic anomalies, should be repaired. Plastic surgery may be considered when the child's appearance can be substantially improved. Dental health is significant, and orthodontic and restorative procedures can improve facial appearance immensely.

Encourage Play and Exercise

Children who are cognitively impaired have the same need for play and exercise as any other child. However, because of the children's slower development, parents may be less aware of the need to provide such activities. Therefore the nurse will need to guide parents toward selection of suitable play and exercise activities. Because play has been discussed for children in each age-group in earlier chapters, only the exceptions are presented here (Fig. 18.2).

The type of play is based on the child's developmental age, although the need for sensorimotor play may be prolonged. Parents should use every opportunity to expose the child to as many different sounds, sights, and sensations as possible. Appropriate toys include musical mobiles, stuffed toys, floating toys, a rocking chair or horse, a swing, bells, and rattles. The child should be taken on outings, such as trips to the grocery store or shopping center. Other people should be encouraged to visit in the home, and individuals should relate directly to the child through means such as cuddling, holding, rocking, and talking to the child face to face.

Toys are selected for their recreational and educational value. For example, a large inflatable beach ball is a good water toy; it encourages interactive play and can be used to learn motor skills, such as balance, rocking, kicking, and throwing. Attractive toys encourage a child to reach, therefore assisting in the development of motor skills (see Fig. 18.2). Musical toys that mimic animal sounds or respond with social phrases are excellent ways to encourage speech. A doll with removable clothes and different types of closures can help the child learn dressing skills. Toys should be simple in design so that the child can learn to manipulate them without help. For children with severe cognitive and physical impairment, electronic switches can be used to allow them to operate toys (Figs. 18.3 and 18.4).

---

[a]Information on early intervention programs in each state is available from the National Down Syndrome Society, 8E 41st Street, 8th Floor, New York, NY 10017; 800-221-4602; http://www.ndss.org. email: info@ndss.org; https://www.facebook.com/NDSS1979/; https://twitter.com/NDSS.

[b]141 W. Jackson Blvd., 1400A, Chicago, IL 60604; 800-221-6827; TTY: 312-726-4258; fax: 312-726-1494; http://www.easterseals.com; email: info@easterseals.com; https://www.facebook.com/easterseals; https://twitter.com/EasterSealsON.

[c]1825 K Street NW, Suite 1200, Washington, DC 20006; 202-534-3700 or 800-433-5255; fax: 202-534-3731; https://thearc.org; email: info@thearc.org; https://www.facebook.com/thearcus; https://twitter.com/thearcus; https://www.youtube.com/user/thearcoftheus.

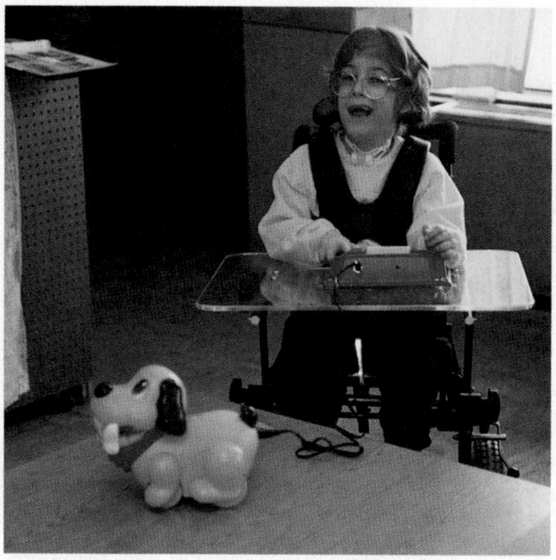

Fig. 18.3 A manual switch allows a child with cognitive impairment (CI) to play with a battery-operated toy.

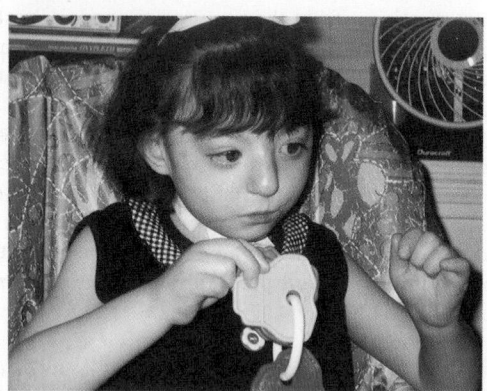

Fig. 18.4 A favorite toy provides stimulation for a young child.

Suitable physical activities are based on the child's size, coordination, physical fitness and maturity, motivation, and health (see Fig. 18.4). Some children may have physical problems that prevent participation in certain sports. These children often have greater success in individual and dual sports than in team sports and enjoy themselves most with children who are at the same developmental level. The Special Olympics[d] provides these children with a unique competitive opportunity.

Safety is a major consideration in selecting recreational and exercise activities. For example, toys that may be appropriate developmentally may present dangers to a child who is strong enough to break them or use them incorrectly.

Provide Means of Communication

Verbal skills are typically delayed more than other physical skills. Speech requires adequate hearing and interpretation (**receptive skills**) and facial muscle coordination (**expressive skills**). Because both receptive and expressive skills may be impaired, these children need

[d]1133 19th St. NW, Washington, DC 20036; 800-700-8585 or 202-628-3630; fax: 202-824-0200; http://www.specialolympics.org (website includes listing of state offices); info@specialolympics.org; https://www.facebook.com/SpecialOlympics/; https://twitter.com/SpecialOlympics. In Canada: Special Olympics Canada, 21 St. Clair Ave. E, Suite 600, Toronto, ON M4T 1N5; 416-927-9050; 888-888-0608; fax: 416-927-8475; http://www.specialolympics.ca.

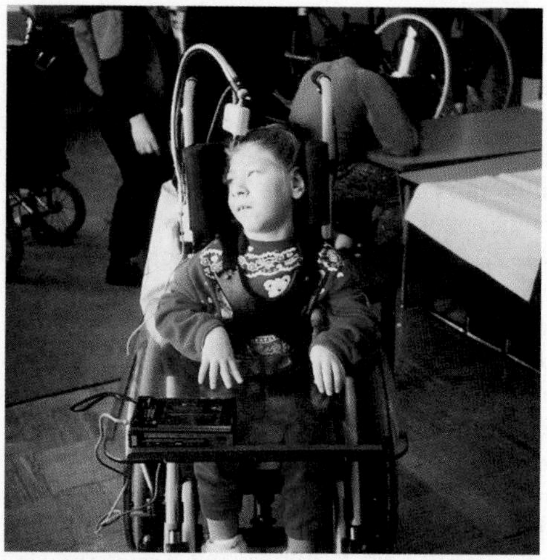

Fig. 18.5 A child with cognitive and physical impairments can activate electronic and communication equipment by moving a device near her head.

frequent audiometric testing and should be fitted with hearing aids if indicated. In addition, they may need help in learning to control their facial muscles. For example, some children may need tongue exercises to correct the tongue thrust or gentle reminders to keep the lips closed.

Nonverbal communication may be appropriate for some of these children, and various devices are available. For children with physical limitations, several adaptations or types of communication devices are available to facilitate selection of the appropriate picture or word (Fig. 18.5). Some children may be taught sign language or **Blissymbols**—a highly stylized system of graphic symbols representing words, ideas, and concepts. Although the symbols require education to learn their meaning, no reading skill is required. The symbols are typically arranged on a board, and the person points or uses some type of selector to convey a message.

Establish Discipline

Discipline must begin early. Limit-setting measures need to be simple, consistently applied, and appropriate for the child's mental age. Control measures are based primarily on teaching a specific behavior rather than on understanding the reasons behind it. Stressing moral lessons is of little value to a child who lacks the cognitive skills to learn from self-criticism or evaluation of previous mistakes. Behavior modification, especially reinforcement of desired actions, and use of time-out procedures are appropriate forms of behavior control.

Encourage Socialization

Acquiring social skills is a complex task, as is learning self-care procedures. Active rehearsals with role-playing, practice sessions, and positive reinforcement for desired behavior have been the most successful approaches. Parents should be encouraged early to teach their child socially acceptable behavior: waving goodbye, saying "hello" and "thank you," responding to his or her name, greeting visitors, and sitting modestly. The teaching of socially acceptable sexual behavior is especially important to minimize sexual exploitation. Parents also need to expose the child to strangers so that he or she can practice manners, because there is no automatic transfer of learning from one situation to another.

Dressing and grooming are also important aspects of self-esteem and social acceptance. Clothes should be clean, age appropriate, and well fitted with self-adhering fasteners and elastic openings to facilitate self-dressing.

Opportunities for social interaction and infant stimulation programs should began at an early age. As soon as possible, parents should enroll their child in early intervention or other appropriate preschool programs. Not only do these programs provide education and training, but they also offer an opportunity for social interaction with other children and adults. As children grow older, they should have peer experiences similar to those of other children, including group outings, sports, and organized activities, such as scouts and Special Olympics. Nurses should assess the child's abilities and encourage others (e.g., parents, teachers) to promote developmentally appropriate peer interaction, such as classroom and school activities, dance classes, clubs, vacations, and family outings (Bull & Committee on Genetics, 2011; National Down Syndrome Society, 2019b; Sanchack & Thomas, 2016; Shapiro & O'Neill, 2020).

Provide Information on Sexuality

Adolescence may be a particularly difficult time for parents, especially in terms of the child's sexual behavior, possibility of pregnancy, future plans to marry, and ability to be independent. Frequently, minimal anticipatory guidance has been offered to parents to prepare the child for physical and sexual maturation. The nurse should help in this area by providing parents with information about sexuality education that is appropriate to the child's developmental level. For example, adolescent girls need a *simple* explanation of menstruation and instructions on personal hygiene during the menstrual cycle.

These adolescents also need practical sexual information on anatomy, physical development, and conception.[e] Because they are easy to persuade and lack judgment, they need a well-defined, concrete code of conduct with specific instructions for handling certain situations. The subtleties of social sexual behavior are less beneficial than specific instructions for handling certain situations. For example, an adolescent should be firmly told never to go alone anywhere with any person that he or she does not know well. To protect the child or adolescent from sexual abuse, parents must closely observe their child's or adolescent's activities and associates. The question of contraceptive protection for these adolescents is often a parental concern.

Parents of these adolescents are often concerned about the advisability of marriage between two individuals with significant CI. There is no conclusive answer; each situation must be judged individually. In some instances, marriage is possible. The nurse should discuss this topic with parents and with the prospective couple, stressing suitable living accommodations and contraceptive methods. If children are conceived, these parents require specialized assistance in learning to meet the needs of their offspring (Brown, Potvin, Lunsky, et al., 2018; Bull & Committee on Genetics, 2011; Homeyard, Montgomery, Chinn, et al., 2016).

Help Family Adjust to Future Care

Not all families are able to cope with home care of children who are cognitively impaired, especially those who have severe or profound CI or multiple disabilities. Older parents may not be able to continue care responsibilities after they reach retirement or older age. The decision regarding residential placement is a difficult one for families, and the availability of such facilities varies widely. The nurse's role includes assisting parents in investigating and evaluating programs and helping parents adjust to the decision for placement.

[e]Sources of information on sexuality and conception include Planned Parenthood Federation of America, 434 W. 33rd St., Floor 12, New York, NY 10001; 212-541-7800 or 800-230-7526; http://www.plannedparenthood.org; https://www.facebook.com/PlannedParenthood/ and also The ARC of the United States (see footnote earlier in this chapter).

Care for Child During Hospitalization

Caring for the child during hospitalization can be a special challenge. Frequently, nurses are unfamiliar with children who are cognitively impaired, and they may cope with their feelings of insecurity and fear by ignoring or isolating the child. Not only is this approach nonsupportive, it may also be destructive to the child's sense of self-esteem and optimum development, and it may impair the parents' ability to cope with the stress of the experience. To prevent engaging in this nontherapeutic approach, nurses should use the mutual participation model in planning the child's care. Parents should stay with their child but not be made to feel as if the responsibility is totally theirs.

When the child is admitted, a detailed history is taken (see Chapter 4), with special focus on all self-care abilities. Questions about the child's abilities are approached positively. For example, rather than asking, "Is your child toilet trained yet?" the nurse may state, "Tell me about your child's toileting habits." The assessment should also focus on any special devices the child uses, effective measures of limit setting, unusual or favorite routines, and any behaviors that may require intervention. If the parent states that the child engages in repetitive behaviors (e.g., overactivity, impulsivity) and self-stimulatory or self-injurious activities (e.g., head banging, self-biting), the nurse should inquire about events that precipitate them and techniques (e.g., distraction, medication) that the parents use to manage them (Davies & Oliver, 2016; Morano, Ruiz, Hwang, et al., 2017).

The nurse also assesses the child's functional level of eating and playing; ability to express needs verbally; progress in toilet training; and relationship with objects, toys, and other children. The child is encouraged to be as independent as possible in the hospital.

Realizing that the child may be lonely in the hospital, the nurse makes certain that toys and other activities are provided. The child is placed in a room with other children of approximately the same developmental age, preferably a room with only two beds to avoid overstimulation. The nurse should treat the child with dignity and respect in a manner that promotes acceptance and understanding by other children, parents, and those with whom the child comes in contact in the hospital.

Explain procedures to the child using methods of communication that are at the appropriate cognitive level. Generally, explanations should be simple, short, and concrete, emphasizing what the child will experience physically. Demonstration either through actual practice or with visual aids is always preferable to verbal explanation. Include parents in preprocedural teaching to aid in the child's learning and to help the nurse learn effective methods of communicating with the child.

During hospitalization, the nurse should also focus on growth-promoting experiences for the child. For example, hospitalization may be an excellent opportunity to emphasize to parents the abilities that the child does have but has not had the opportunity to practice, such as self-dressing. It may also be an opportunity for social experiences with peers, group play, or new educational and recreational activities. For example, one child who had the habit of screaming and kicking demonstrated a definite decrease in those behaviors after he learned to pound pegs and use a punching bag. Through social services, the parents may become aware of specialized programs for the child. Hospitalization may also offer parents a respite from everyday care responsibilities and an opportunity to discuss their feelings with a concerned professional.

Assist in Measures to Prevent Cognitive Impairment

Besides having a responsibility to families with a child with CI, nurses also need to be involved in programs aimed at preventing CI.

Many of the familial, social, and environmental factors known to cause mild impairment are preventable. Counseling and education can reduce or eliminate such factors (e.g., poor nutrition, cigarette smoking, chemical abuse), which increase the risk of prematurity and intrauterine growth restriction. Interventions are directed toward improving maternal health by educating women on the dangers of chemicals, including prenatal alcohol exposure, which affects organogenesis, craniofacial development, and cognitive ability. Other preventive strategies that play an important role include adequate prenatal care; optimal medical care of high-risk newborns; rubella immunization; genetic counseling; and prenatal screening, especially for Down syndrome or FXS. The use of folic acid supplements prevents neural tube defects during pregnancy and during the childbearing years; the use of newborn screening for treatable inborn errors of metabolism (such as congenital hypothyroidism, phenylketonuria, and galactosemia) is appropriate to prevent developmental disabilities in children.

DOWN SYNDROME

Down syndrome is the most common chromosomal abnormality of a generalized syndrome, occurring in 1 in 700 to 733 live births in the United States, with approximately 6000 births annually (Lee, 2020). It occurs in people of all races and economic levels.

Etiology

The cause of Down syndrome is not known, but evidence from cytogenetic and epidemiologic studies supports the concept of multiple causality. Although the cause is unclear, the cytogenetics of the disorder is well established. Approximately 95% of all cases of Down syndrome are attributable to an extra chromosome 21 (group G), hence the name **nonfamilial trisomy 21**. Although children with trisomy 21 are born to parents of all ages, there is a statistically greater risk in older women, particularly those older than 35 years of age. For example, in women 35 years old, the chance of conceiving a child with Down syndrome is about 1 in 350 live births, but in women 40 years old, it is about 1 in 100. However, the majority (≈80%) of infants with Down syndrome are born to women younger than 35 years of age because younger women have higher fertility rates (Arumugam, Raja, Venugopalan, et al., 2016; Lee, 2020). About 4% of cases may be caused by **translocation** of chromosomes 15 and 21 or 22. This type of genetic aberration is usually hereditary and is not associated with advanced parental age. About 1% to 4% of affected persons demonstrate **mosaicism**, which refers to a mixture of normal and abnormal chromosomes in the cells. The degree of cognitive and physical impairment is related to the percentage of cells with the abnormal chromosome makeup.

Diagnostic Evaluation

Down syndrome usually can be diagnosed by the clinical manifestations alone (Box 18.2 and Fig. 18.6), but a chromosome analysis should be done to confirm the genetic abnormality.

Several physical problems are associated with Down syndrome. Many of these children have congenital heart malformations, the most common being septal defects. Respiratory tract infections are prevalent and, when combined with cardiac anomalies, are the chief causes of death, particularly during the first year of life. Hypotonicity of chest and abdominal muscles and dysfunction of the immune system probably predispose the child to the development of respiratory tract infection. Other physical problems include thyroid dysfunction, especially congenital hypothyroidism, and an increased incidence of leukemia.

BOX 18.2 Clinical Manifestations of Down Syndrome

Head and Eyes
- Separated sagittal suture
- Brachycephaly
- Rounded and small skull
- Flat occiput
- Enlarged anterior fontanel
- Oblique palpebral fissures (upward, outward slant)[a]
- Inner epicanthal folds
- Speckling of iris (Brushfield spots)

Nose and Ears
- Small nose[a]
- Depressed nasal bridge (saddle nose)[a]
- Small ears and narrow canals
- Short pinna (vertical ear length)
- Overlapping upper helices
- Conductive hearing loss

Mouth and Neck
- High, arched, narrow palate[a]
- Protruding tongue
- Hypoplastic mandible
- Delayed teeth eruption and microdontia
- Alignment teeth abnormalities common
- Periodontal disease
- Neck skin excess and laxity[a]
- Short and broad neck

Chest and Heart
- Shortened rib cage
- Twelfth rib anomalies
- Pectus excavatum or carinatum
- Congenital heart defects common (e.g., atrial septal defect, ventricular septal defect)

Abdomen and Genitalia
- Protruding, lax, and flabby abdominal muscles
- Rectus abdominus diastasis.
- Umbilical hernia
- Small penis
- Cryptorchidism
- Bulbous vulva

Hands and Feet
- Broad, short hands and stubby fingers
- Incurved little finger (clinodactyly)
- Transverse palmar crease
- Wide space between big and second toes[a]
- Plantar crease between big and second toes[a]
- Broad, short feet and stubby toes

Musculoskeletal and Skin
- Short stature
- Hyperflexibility and muscle weakness[a]
- Hypotonia
- Atlantoaxial instability
- Dry, cracked, and frequent fissuring
- Cutis marmorata (mottling)

Other
- Reduced birth weight
- Learning difficulty (average intelligence quotient [IQ] of 50)
- Hypothyroidism common
- Impaired immune function
- Increased risk of leukemia
- Early-onset dementia (in one-third)

[a] Most common findings in modified chart (Arumugam, Raja, Venugopalan, et al., 2016; Pueschel, 1999).

Therapeutic Management

Although no cure exists for Down syndrome, a number of therapies are advocated, such as surgery to correct serious congenital anomalies (e.g., heart defects, strabismus). These children also benefit from evaluative echocardiography soon after birth and regular medical care. Evaluation of sight and hearing is essential, and treatment of otitis media is required to prevent auditory loss, which can influence cognitive function. Periodic testing of thyroid function is recommended, especially if growth is severely delayed.

About 15% of children with Down syndrome have **atlantoaxial instability**; almost all of these children are asymptomatic. The American Academy of Pediatrics no longer recommends screening asymptomatic children with Down syndrome for atlantoaxial instability with cervical spine x-rays due to the unproven value of detecting patients at risk of developing spinal cord compression injury (Bull & Committee on Genetics, 2011; National Down Syndrome Society,

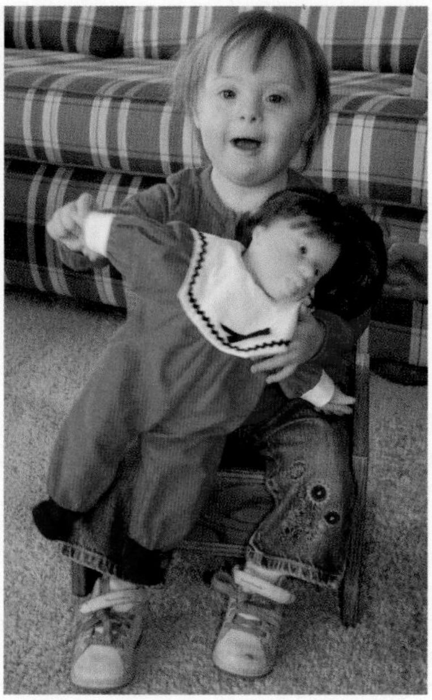

Fig. 18.6 A young child with Down syndrome holds a doll with Down syndrome.

2019d). However, the Special Olympics requires that all athletes with Down syndrome receive neck x-rays and neurologic examination prior to sports participation (Leas, Goldstein, Kellan, et al., 2017; National Down Syndrome Society, 2019d).

! NURSING ALERT

Immediately report any child with the following signs of spinal cord compression:
- Persistent neck pain
- Loss of established motor skills and bladder or bowel control
- Changes in sensation

Prognosis

Life expectancy for those with Down syndrome has improved but remains lower than for the general population. Most individuals with Down syndrome survive to 60 years old and beyond (Englund, Jonsson, Zander, et al., 2013; Weijerman & de Winter, 2010). As the prognosis continues to improve for these individuals, it will be important to provide for their long-term health care and social and leisure needs.

Nursing Care Management

Support the Family at the Time of Diagnosis

Because of the unique physical characteristics, infants with Down syndrome are usually diagnosed at birth, and parents should be informed of the diagnosis at this time. Most parents usually prefer that both of them be present during the informing interview so that they can support one another emotionally. Parents appreciate receiving reading material about the syndrome[f] and being referred to parent groups and/or professional counseling.

Parental responses to the child may greatly influence decisions regarding future care. Whereas some families willingly take the child home, others consider foster care or adoption. The nurse must answer questions about developmental potential carefully, because the responses may influence the parents' decisions. The nurse should share the available informative sources (such as parent groups, professional counseling, and literature) to help the family learn about Down syndrome.

Assist the Family in Preventing Physical Problems

Many of the physical characteristics of infants with Down syndrome present challenges and nursing problems. The hypotonicity of muscles and hyperextensibility of joints complicate positioning. The limp, flaccid extremities resemble the posture of a rag doll; as a result, holding the infant is difficult and cumbersome. Sometimes parents perceive this lack of molding to their bodies as evidence of inadequate parenting. The extended body position promotes heat loss, because more surface area is exposed to the environment. Encourage the parents to swaddle or wrap the infant snugly in a blanket before picking up the child to provide security and warmth. The nurse also discusses with parents their feelings concerning attachment to the child, emphasizing that the child's lack of clinging or molding is a physical characteristic and not a sign of detachment or rejection.

Decreased muscle tone compromises respiratory expansion. In addition, the underdeveloped nasal bone causes a chronic problem of inadequate drainage of mucus. The constant stuffy nose forces the child to breathe by mouth, which dries the oropharyngeal membranes, increasing the susceptibility to upper respiratory tract infections. Measures to lessen these problems include clearing the nose with a bulb-type syringe, rinsing the mouth with water after feedings, increasing fluid intake, and using a cool-mist vaporizer to keep the mucous membranes moist and the secretions liquefied. Other helpful measures include changing the child's position frequently, practicing good hand washing, and properly disposing of soiled articles, such as tissues. If antibiotics are ordered, the nurse stresses the importance of completing the full course of therapy for successful eradication of the infection and prevention of growth of resistant organisms.

Inadequate drainage resulting in pooling of mucus in the nose also interferes with feeding. Because the child breathes by mouth, sucking for any length of time is difficult. When eating solids, the child may gag on the food because of mucus in the oropharynx. Parents are advised to clear the nose before each feeding; give small, frequent feedings; and allow opportunities for rest during mealtime.

The protruding tongue also interferes with feeding, especially of solid foods. Parents need to know that the tongue thrust is not an indication of refusal to feed but a physiologic response. Parents are advised to use a small but long, straight-handled spoon to push the food toward the back and side of the mouth. If food is thrust out, it should be refed.

Dietary intake needs supervision. Decreased muscle tone affects gastric motility, predisposing the child to constipation. Dietary measures, such as increased fiber and fluid, promote evacuation. The child's eating habits may need scrutiny to prevent obesity. Height and weight measurements should be obtained on a serial basis. Because the previously used Down syndrome–specific growth charts no longer reflected the current population styles and body proportions, updated growth charts were developed to provide indications of how growth of an individual child compares with peers of the same age and sex with Down syndrome (Centers for Disease Control and Prevention, 2017; Zemel, Pipan, Stallings, et al., 2015).

During infancy, the child's skin is pliable and soft. However, it gradually becomes rough and dry and is prone to cracking and infection. Skin care involves the use of minimum soap and application of lubricants. Lip balm is applied to the lips, especially when the child is outdoors, to prevent excessive chapping.

Assist in Prenatal Diagnosis and Genetic Counseling

Prenatal diagnosis of Down syndrome through chorionic villus sampling and amniocentesis can detect the presence of trisomy or

[f]For The ARC and National Down Syndrome Society contact information, see the footnotes earlier in the chapter.

translocation in the chromosomal analysis of fetal cells. Advances in development of noninvasive prenatal testing (NIPT) as a measurement of cell-free deoxyribonucleic acid (DNA) from the plasma of pregnant women detects nearly all cases of Down syndrome (Curnow, Sanderson, & Beruti, 2019; Gil, Accurti, Santacruz, et al., 2017; Hui, 2019; Iwarsson, Jacobsson, Dagerhamn, et al., 2017; Lee, 2020; Palomaki & Kloza, 2018). However, invasive fetal karyotyping is still the required diagnostic approach to confirm the presence of a chromosomal abnormality prior to making irreversible decisions relative to the pregnancy outcome (Badeau, Lindsay, Blais, et al., 2017; Gray & Wilkins-Haug, 2018; Iwarsson et al., 2017).

Prenatal testing and genetic counseling should be offered to all women, including those of advanced maternal age, those with a family history of the disorder, and those of younger age because most children with Down syndrome are born to younger mothers due to their higher overall birth rate (Lee, 2020; National Down Syndrome Society, 2019a). If prenatal testing indicates that the fetus is affected, the nurse must allow the parents to express their feelings about whether to proceed with the pregnancy or an elective abortion and support their decision. It is important for nurses to be aware of their own attitudes regarding testing and related decisions.

FRAGILE X SYNDROME

FXS is the most common inherited cause of CI and the second most common genetic cause of CI or intellectual disability after Down syndrome. It has been described in all ethnic groups and races; the incidence of affected boys is 1 in 3600 to 4000, the incidence of affected girls is 1 in 4000 to 6000, the incidence of carrier girls is 1 in 151, and the incidence of carrier boys is 1 in 468 worldwide (Mink, 2016; National Fragile X Foundation, 2019).

The syndrome is caused by an abnormal gene on the lower end of the long arm of the X chromosome. Chromosome analysis may demonstrate a **fragile site** (a region that fails to condense during mitosis and is characterized by a nonstaining gap or narrowing) in the cells of affected males and females and in carrier females. This fragile site has been determined to be caused by a gene mutation that results in excessive repeats of nucleotide in a specific DNA segment of the X chromosome. The number of repeats in a normal individual is between 6 and 50. An individual with 50 to 200 base-pair repeats is said to have a **permutation** and is therefore a carrier. When passed from a parent to a child, these base-pair repeats can expand from 200 or more, which is called a **full mutation**. This expansion occurs only when a carrier mother passes the mutation to her offspring; it does not occur when a carrier father passes the mutation to his daughters.

The inheritance pattern has been termed **X-linked dominant with reduced penetrance**. This is in distinct contrast to the classic X-linked recessive pattern in which all carrier females are normal, all affected males have symptoms of the disorder, and no males are carriers. Consequently, genetic counseling of affected families is more complex than that for families with a classic X-linked disorder, such as hemophilia. Both affected sexes are capable of transmitting the fragile X disorder. Prenatal diagnosis of the fragile X gene mutation is possible with direct DNA testing in a family with an established history using amniocentesis or chorionic villus sampling (Finucane, Lincoln, Bailey, et al., 2017; National Fragile X Foundation, 2019). The FMR1 mutation testing is highly accurate and is being researched for incorporation into the newborn universal screening program (Bailey, Berry-Kravis, Gane, et al., 2017; Riley, Mailick, Berry-Kravis, et al., 2017; Riley & Wheeler, 2017; Tassone, 2014).

BOX 18.3 Clinical Manifestations of Fragile X Syndrome

Physical Features

Increased head circumference
Long, wide, or protruding ears
Long, narrow face with prominent jaw
Strabismus
Mitral valve prolapse, aortic root dilation
Hypotonia
In postpubertal males, enlarged testicles

Behavioral Features

Mild to severe cognitive impairment (CI)
Speech delay; may be rapid speech with stuttering and word repetition
Short attention span, hyperactivity
Hypersensitivity to taste, sounds, and touch
Intolerance to change in routine
Autistic-like behaviors, such as social anxiety and gaze aversion
Possible aggressive behavior

Clinical Manifestations

The classic trend of physical findings in adult men with FXS consists of a long face with a prominent jaw (prognathism); large, protruding ears; and large testes (macroorchidism). In prepubertal children, however, these features may be less obvious, and behavioral manifestations may initially suggest the diagnosis (Box 18.3). In carrier females, the clinical manifestations are extremely varied.

Therapeutic Management

FXS has no cure. Medical treatment may include the use of serotonin agents, such as carbamazepine (Tegretol) or fluoxetine (Prozac), to control violent temper outbursts and the use of central nervous system stimulants or clonidine (Catapres) to improve attention span and decrease hyperactivity and melatonin for sleep difficulties. Treatments of FXS are being investigated in clinical trials; these include targeted therapies as in protein replacement and the identification of blood and tissue biomarkers that quantify brain function (Bagni, Tassone, Neri, et al., 2012; Budimirovic, Berry-Kravis, Erickson, et al., 2017; Hagerman, Berry-Kravis, Hazlett, et al., 2017; Lee, Ventola, Budimirovic, et al., 2018).

All affected children require referral to early intervention programs (speech and language therapy, occupational therapy, and special education assistance) and multidisciplinary assessment, including cardiology, neurology, and orthopedic anomalies.

Prognosis

Individuals with FXS are expected to live a normal life span. Their CI may be improved by behavioral and educational interventions that usually begin in preschool-age children.

Nursing Care Management

Because CI is a fairly consistent finding in individuals with FXS, the care given to these families is the same as for any child with intellectual disability. Because the disorder is hereditary, genetic counseling is important to inform parents and siblings of the risks of transmission. In addition, any male or female with unexplained or nonspecific mental impairment should be referred for genetic testing and, if needed, counseling. Families with a member affected by the disorder should be referred to the National Fragile X Foundation.[g]

SENSORY IMPAIRMENT

HEARING IMPAIRMENT

Hearing impairment is one of the most common disabilities in the United States. An estimated 3 to 6 per 1000 well infants have hearing loss of varying degrees (American Academy of Pediatrics, 2019; Dedhia, Graham, & Park, 2018; Grindle, 2014). For infants admitted to neonatal intensive care units, the incidence rises sharply to approximately 2 to 4 per 100 neonates (Almadhoob & Ohlsson, 2015; American Academy of Pediatrics, Joint Committee on Infant Hearing, 2007; Colella-Santos, Hein, de Souza, et al., 2014). In the United States, there are about 1 million children with hearing impairment ranging in age from birth to 21 years old, and almost one-third of these children have other disabilities, such as visual or cognitive deficits.

Definition and Classification

Hearing impairment is a general term indicating disability that may range in severity from slight to profound hearing loss. *Slight to moderately severe hearing loss* describes a person who has residual hearing sufficient to enable successful processing of linguistic information through audition, generally with the use of a hearing aid. *Severe to profound hearing loss* describes a person whose hearing disability precludes successful processing of linguistic information through audition with or without a hearing aid. Hearing-impaired persons who are speech impaired tend not to have a physical speech defect other than that caused by the inability to hear.

Hearing defects may be classified according to etiology, pathology, or symptom severity. Each is important in terms of treatment, possible prevention, and rehabilitation.

Etiology

Hearing loss may be caused by a number of prenatal and postnatal conditions. These may include a family history of childhood hearing impairment, anatomic malformations of the head or neck, low birth weight, severe perinatal asphyxia, perinatal infection (cytomegalovirus, rubella, herpes, syphilis, toxoplasmosis, bacterial meningitis), maternal prenatal substance abuse, chronic ear infection, cerebral palsy, Down syndrome, prolonged neonatal oxygen supplementation, or administration of ototoxic drugs (Colella-Santos et al., 2014; Gan, Rowe, Benton, et al., 2016; Haddad, Dodhia, & Spitzer, 2020; Neumann, Chadha, & Tavartkiladze, 2019; Singh, 2015).

In addition, high-risk neonates who survive the once fatal prenatal or perinatal conditions may be susceptible to hearing loss from the disorder or its treatment. For example, sensorineural hearing loss may result from continuous humming noises or high noise levels associated with incubators, oxygen hoods, or intensive care units, especially when combined with the use of potentially ototoxic antibiotics.

Environmental noise is a special concern. Sounds loud enough to damage sensitive hair cells of the inner ear can produce irreversible hearing loss. Very loud, brief noise (such as gunfire) can cause immediate, severe, and permanent loss of hearing. Longer exposure to less intense but still hazardous sounds (such as loud, persistent music via headphones, sound systems, concerts, or industrial noises) may also produce hearing loss (Carroll, Eichwald, Scinicariello, et al., 2017; Centers for Disease Control and Prevention, 2018a; Guest, Munro, Prendergast, et al., 2017; Pawlaczyk-Luszczynska, Zamojska-Daniszewska, Dudarewicz, et al., 2017; Sliwinska-Kowalska & Zaborowski, 2017; World Health Organization, 2019). Loud noises combined with toxic substances (such as smoking or secondhand smoke) produce a synergistic effect on hearing that causes hearing loss (Chang, Ryou, Jun, et al., 2016; Fabry, Davila, Arheart, et al., 2011; Hu, Sasaki, & Ogasawara, 2019; Talaat, Metwaly, Khafagy, et al., 2014).

Pathology

Disorders of hearing are divided according to the location of the defect. **Conductive** or **middle-ear hearing loss** results from interference of transmission of sound to the middle ear. It is the most common of all types of hearing loss and most frequently a result of recurrent serous otitis media. Conductive hearing impairment involves mainly interference with loudness of sound.

Sensorineural hearing loss involves damage to the inner ear structures or the auditory nerve. The most common causes are congenital defects of inner ear structures or consequences of acquired conditions, such as kernicterus, infection, administration of ototoxic drugs, or exposure to excessive noise. Sensorineural hearing loss results in distortion of sound and problems in discrimination. Although the child hears some of everything going on around him or her, the sounds are distorted, severely affecting discrimination and comprehension.

Mixed conductive-sensorineural hearing loss results from interference with transmission of sound in the middle ear and along neural pathways. It frequently results from recurrent otitis media and its complications.

Central auditory imperception includes all hearing losses that are not linked to defects in the conductive or sensorineural structures. They are usually divided into organic or functional losses. In the **organic** type of central auditory imperception, the defect involves the reception of auditory stimuli along the central pathways and the expression of the message into meaningful communication. Examples are **aphasia**, the inability to express ideas in any form, either written or verbal; **agnosia**, the inability to interpret sound correctly; and **dysacusis**, difficulty in processing details or discriminating among sounds. In the **functional** type of hearing loss, no organic lesion exists to explain a central auditory loss. Examples of functional hearing loss are conversion hysteria (an unconscious withdrawal from hearing to block remembrance of a traumatic event), infantile autism, and childhood schizophrenia.

Symptom Severity

Hearing impairment is expressed in terms of a **decibel (dB)**, a unit of loudness. Hearing is measured at various frequencies, such as 500, 1000, and 2000 cycles per second, the critical listening speech range. Hearing impairment can be classified according to **hearing threshold level** (the measurement of an individual's hearing threshold by means of an audiometer) and the degree of symptom severity as it affects speech (Table 18.2). These classifications offer only general guidelines regarding the effect of the impairment on any individual child, because children differ greatly in their ability to use residual hearing.

Therapeutic Management

Conductive Hearing Loss

Treatment of hearing loss depends on the cause and type of hearing impairment. Many conductive hearing defects respond to medical or surgical treatment, such as antibiotic therapy for acute otitis media or insertion of tympanostomy tubes for chronic otitis media. When the conductive hearing loss is permanent, hearing can be improved with the use of a hearing aid to amplify sound.

[g]1861 International Drive, Suite 200, McLean, VA 22102; 800-688-8765; email: natlfx@fragilex.org

TABLE 18.2 Classification of Hearing Impairment Based on Symptom Severity

Hearing Level (dB)	Effect
Slight: 16 to 25	Has difficulty hearing faint or distant speech Usually is unaware of hearing difficulty Likely to achieve in school but may have problems No speech defects
Mild to moderate: 26 to 55	May have speech difficulties Understands face-to-face conversational speech at 0.9 to 1.5 m (3 to 5 ft)
Moderately severe: 56 to 70	Unable to understand conversational speech unless loud Considerable difficulty with group or classroom discussion Requires special speech training
Severe: 71 to 90	May hear a loud voice if nearby May be able to identify loud environmental noises Can distinguish vowels but not most consonants Requires speech training
Profound: 91	May hear only loud sounds Requires extensive speech training

dB, Decibels.

The nurse should be familiar with the types, basic care, and handling of hearing aids, especially when the child is hospitalized.[h] Types of hearing aids include those worn in or behind the ear, models incorporated into an eyeglass frame, and types worn on the body with a wire connection to the ear (Fig. 18.7). One of the most common problems with a hearing aid is **acoustic feedback**, an annoying whistling sound usually caused by improper fit of the ear mold. Sometimes the whistling may be at a frequency that the child cannot hear but that is annoying to others. In this case, if children are old enough, they are told of the noise and asked to readjust the aid.

NURSING TIP To reduce or eliminate whistling from a hearing aid, try removing and reinserting the aid, making certain that no hair is caught between the ear mold and the ear canal, cleaning the ear mold or ear, or lowering the volume of the aid.

As children grow older, they may be self-conscious about the device. Efforts may be made to make the aid inconspicuous, such as styling the hair to cover behind-the-ear or in-the-ear models and using attractive frames for glasses with connected hearing aids. Give children responsibility for the care of the device as soon as they are able, because fostering independence is a primary goal of rehabilitation.

! NURSING ALERT

Stress to parents the importance of storing batteries for hearing aids in a safe location out of reach of children and of teaching children not to remove the battery from the hearing aid (or supervising young children when they do so). Battery ingestion requires immediate emergency management.

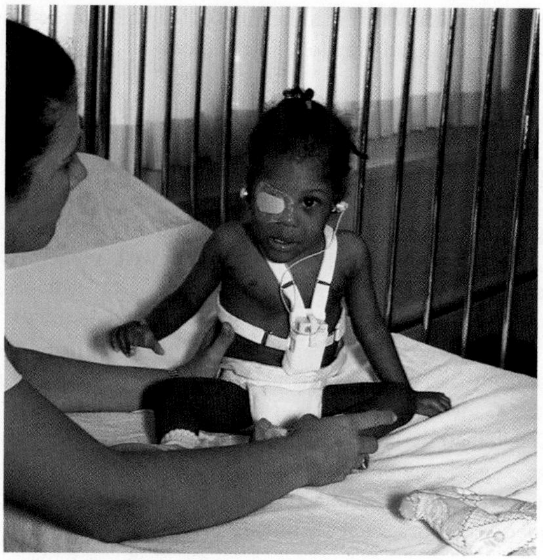

Fig. 18.7 On-the-body hearing aids are convenient for young children, such as this child with severe bilateral hearing loss. Note eye patching for strabismus.

Sensorineural Hearing Loss

Treatment for sensorineural hearing loss is much less satisfactory. Because the defect is not one of intensity of sound, hearing aids are of less value in this type of defect. The use of **cochlear implants**[i] (a surgically implanted prosthetic device) provides a sensation of hearing for individuals who have severe or profound hearing loss (Centers for Disease Control and Prevention, 2018a; Health Quality Ontario, 2018; Korver, Smith, & Van Camp, 2017; Pettinato, De Clerck, Verhoeven, et al., 2017). Children with sensorineural hearing loss have lost or damaged some or all of their hair cells or auditory nerve fibers. Often these children cannot benefit from conventional hearing aids because they only amplify sound that cannot be processed by a damaged inner ear. A cochlear implant bypasses the hair cells to directly stimulate surviving auditory nerve fibers so that they can send signals to the brain. These signals can be interpreted by the brain to produce sound and sensations (Easwar, Yamazaki, Deighton, et al., 2017; Gan et al., 2016; Grindle, 2014; Pettinato et al., 2017).

Multichanneled implants are sophisticated devices that stimulate the auditory nerve at a number of locations with differently processed signals. This type of stimulation allows a person to use the pitch information present in speech signals, leading to better understanding of speech. The trend is toward early use of cochlear implants, usually by 12 months old, to give the child maximum opportunity to develop listening, language, and speaking skills.

Nursing Care Management

Assessment of children for hearing impairment is a critical nursing responsibility. Identification of hearing loss before 3 months of age with intervention no later than 6 months of age is essential to improve the language and educational development of children with hearing impairments (American Academy of Pediatrics, 2019; Centers for

[h]Information about hearing aids is available from the International Hearing Society, 16880 Middlebelt Road, Suite 4, Livonia, MI 48154; 800-521-5247 (hearing help line) or 734-522-7200; fax: 734-522-0200; http://www.ihsinfo.org; http://www.facebook.com/ihsinfo; http://twitter.com/IHSinfo.

[i]Hearing Enrichment Language Program of the Hough Ear Institute as part INTEGRIS Baptist Medical Center Cochlear Implant Clinic, 3300 N.W. Expressway, Oklahoma City, OK 73112; 405-949-3011 or 888-951-2277; http://integrisok.com/baptist-medical-center-oklahoma-city-ok-services-hearing; http://www.facebook.com/integrishealthOK.

BOX 18.4 Clinical Manifestations of Hearing Impairment

Infants

Lack of startle or blink reflex to a loud sound
Failure to be awakened by loud environmental noises
Failure to localize a source of sound by 6 months old
Absence of babble or voice inflections by 7 months old
General indifference to sound
Lack of response to the spoken word; failure to follow verbal directions
Response to loud noises as opposed to the voice

Children

Use of gestures rather than verbalization to express desires, especially after 15 months old
Failure to develop intelligible speech by 24 months old
Monotone and unintelligible speech; lessened laughter
Vocal play, head banging, or foot stamping for vibratory sensation
Yelling or screeching to express pleasure, needs, or annoyance
Asking to have statements repeated or answering them incorrectly
Greater response to facial expression and gestures than to verbal explanation
Avoidance of social interaction; prefer to play alone
Inquiring, sometimes confused facial expression
Suspicious alertness alternating with cooperation
Frequent stubbornness because of lack of comprehension
Irritability at not making themselves understood
Shy, timid, and withdrawn behavior
Frequent appearance of being "in a world of their own" or markedly inattentive

Disease Control and Prevention, 2018a; Grindle, 2014; Lammers, Jansen, Grolman, et al., 2015; World Health Organization, 2012). The Joint Committee on Infant Hearing issued guidelines on auditory screening of newborns and infants to detect early hearing loss and implement intervention programs (American Academy of Pediatrics, 2019; American Academy of Pediatrics, Joint Committee on Infant Hearing, 2007; Centers for Disease Control and Prevention, 2018a; Joint Committee on Infant Hearing of the American Academy of Pediatrics, Muse, Harrison, et al., 2013). Auditory testing is presented in Chapter 4.

At birth, the nurse should observe the neonate's response to auditory stimuli, as evidenced by the startle reflex, head turning, eye blinking, and cessation of body movement. The infant may vary in the intensity of the response, depending on the state of alertness. However, consistent absence of a reaction should lead to suspicion of hearing loss. Box 18.4 summarizes other clinical manifestations of hearing impairment in infants.

Children who are profoundly hearing impaired are much more likely to be diagnosed during infancy than are children who are less severely affected. If the defect is not detected during early childhood, it likely will become evident on entry into school, when the child has difficulty learning. Unfortunately, some of these children are erroneously placed in special classes for students with learning disabilities or CI. Therefore it is essential that the nurse suspect a hearing impairment in any child who demonstrates the behaviors listed in Box 18.4.

! NURSING ALERT

When parents express concern about their child's hearing and speech development, refer the child for a hearing evaluation. Absence of well-formed syllables *(da, na, yaya)* by 11 months old should result in immediate referral.

During early childhood, the primary importance of hearing impairment is the effect on speech development. A child with a mild conductive hearing loss may speak fairly clearly but in a loud, monotone voice. A child with a sensorineural defect usually has difficulty in articulation. Communication may be difficult, leading to frustration when words are not understood. For example, an inability to hear higher frequencies may result in the word "spoon" being pronounced "poon." Children with articulation problems need to have their hearing tested.

Lipreading

Although the child may become an expert at lipreading, only about 40% of the spoken word is understood, or less if the speaker has an accent, mustache, or beard. Exaggerating pronunciation or speaking in an altered rhythm further lessens comprehension. Parents can help the child understand the spoken word by using the suggestions in the Nursing Care Guidelines box. The child learns to supplement the spoken word with sensitivity to visual cues, primarily body language and facial expression (e.g., tightening the lips, muscle tension, eye contact).

NURSING CARE GUIDELINES

Facilitating Lipreading

Attract child's attention before speaking; use light touch to signal speaker's presence.
Stand close to child.
Face child directly or move to a 45-degree angle.
Stand still; do not walk back and forth or turn away to point or look elsewhere.
Establish eye contact and show interest.
Speak at eye level and with good lighting on speaker's face.
Be certain nothing interferes with speech patterns, such as chewing food or gum.
Speak clearly and at a slow and even rate.
Use facial expression to assist in conveying messages.
Keep sentences short.
Rephrase message if child does not understand the words.

Cued Speech

The cued speech method of communication is an adjunct to straight lipreading. It uses hand signals to help the child with hearing impairment to distinguish between words that look alike when formed by the lips (e.g., mat, bat). It is most commonly used by children with hearing impairment who are using speech rather than by those who are nonverbal.

Sign Language

Sign language, such as **American Sign Language** (ASL) or **British Sign Language** (BSL), is a visual-gestural language that uses hand signals that roughly correspond to specific words and concepts in the English language. Encourage family members to learn signing, because using or watching hands requires much less concentration than lipreading or talking. Also, a symbol method enables some children with hearing impairment to learn more and to learn faster.

Speech Language Therapy

The most formidable task in the education of a child who is profoundly hearing impaired is learning to speak. Speech is learned through a multisensory approach using visual, tactile, kinesthetic, and auditory stimulation. Encourage parents to participate fully in the learning process.

Additional Aids

Everyday activities present problems for older children with hearing impairment. For example, they may not be able to hear the telephone, doorbell, or alarm clock. Several commercial devices are available to help them adjust to these dilemmas. Flashing lights can be attached to a telephone or doorbell to signal its ringing. Trained hearing ear dogs can provide great assistance because they alert the person to sounds, such as someone approaching, a moving car, a signal to wake up, or a child's cry. Special teletypewriters or telecommunications devices for the deaf (TDD or TTY) help those who are hearing impaired to communicate with each other over the telephone; the typed message is conveyed via the telephone lines and displayed on a small screen.[j]

Any audiovisual medium presents dilemmas for these children, who can see the picture but cannot hear the message. However, with closed captioning a special decoding device is attached to the television, and the audio portion of a program is translated into subtitles that appear on the screen.[k]

Socialization

Socialization is extremely important to children's development. If children attend a special school for the hearing impaired, they are able to socialize with peers in that setting. Classmates become a potential source of close friendships because they communicate more easily among themselves. Encourage parents to promote these relationships whenever possible.

Children with a hearing impairment may need special help with school or social activities. For children wearing hearing aids, keep background noise to a minimum. Because many of these children are able to attend regular classes, the teacher may need assistance in adapting methods of teaching for the child's benefit. The school nurse is often in an optimal position to emphasize methods of facilitated communication, such as lipreading (see Nursing Care Guidelines box). Because group projects and audiovisual teaching aids may hinder the hearing-impaired child's learning, carefully evaluate the use of these educational methods.

In a group setting, it is helpful for the other members to sit in a semicircle in front of the child with a hearing impairment. Because one of the difficulties in following a group discussion is that the child is unaware of who will speak next, someone should point out each speaker. Speakers can also be given numbers, or their names can be written down as each person talks. If one person writes down the main topic of the discussion, the child is able to follow lipreading more closely. Such practices can increase the child's ability to participate in sports, organizations such as Scouts, and group projects.

Support Child and Family

Once the diagnosis of hearing impairment is made, parents need extensive support to adjust to the shock of learning about their child's disability and an opportunity to realize the extent of the hearing loss. If the hearing loss occurs during childhood, the child also requires sensitive, supportive care during the long and often difficult adjustment to this sensory loss. Early rehabilitation is one of the best strategies for fostering adjustment. Progress in learning communication, however, may not always coincide with emotional adjustment. Depression or anger is common, and such feelings are a normal part of the grieving process.

Care for the Child During Hospitalization

The needs of the hospitalized child with impaired hearing are the same as those of any other child, but the disability presents special challenges to the nurse. For example, verbal explanations must be supplemented by tactile and visual aids, such as books or actual demonstration and practice. Children's understanding of the explanation needs to be constantly reassessed. If their verbal skills are poorly developed, they can answer questions through drawing, writing, or gesturing. For example, if the nurse is attempting to clarify where a spinal tap is done, ask the child to point to where the procedure will be done on the body. Because children with hearing impairments often need more time to grasp the full meaning of an explanation, the nurse needs to be patient and allow ample time for understanding.

When communicating with the child, the nurse should use the same principles as those outlined for facilitating lipreading. The child's hearing aid should be checked to ensure that it is working properly. If it is necessary to awaken the child at night, the nurse should gently shake the child or turn on the hearing aid before arousing the child. The nurse should always make certain that the child can see him or her before any procedures, even routine ones such as changing a diaper or regulating an infusion. It is important to remember that the child may not be aware of the nurse's presence until alerted through visual or tactile cues.

Ideally, parents are encouraged to room with the child. However, the nurse must convey to them that this is not to serve as a convenience to the nurse but as a benefit to the child. Although the parents' aid can be enlisted in familiarizing the child with the hospital and explaining procedures, the nurse should also talk directly to the youngster, encouraging expression of feelings about the experience. If the child's speech is difficult to understand, try to become familiar with his or her pronunciation of words. Parents often can be helpful by explaining the child's usual speech habits. Nonverbal communication devices that use pictures or words that the child can point to are also available. The nurse can make boards by drawing pictures or writing words on cardboard that represent common needs, such as *parent, food, water,* or *toilet.*

The nurse has a special role as child advocate and is in a strategic position to alert other health team members and other patients to the child's special needs regarding communication. For example, the nurse should accompany other practitioners on visits to the child's room to ensure that they speak to the child and that the child understands what is said. Caregivers may forget that the child can perceive and learn despite a hearing loss, and consequently they communicate only with the parents. As a result, the child's needs and feelings remain unrecognized and unaddressed.

Because children with impaired hearing may have difficulty forming social relationships with other children, introduce the child to roommates and encourage them to engage in play activities. The hospital setting can provide growth-promoting opportunities for social relationships. With the assistance of a child life specialist, the child can learn new recreational activities, experiment with group games, and engage in therapeutic play. Playing with puppets or dollhouses, role-playing with dress-up clothes, building with a hammer and nails, finger painting, and water play can help the child express feelings that previously were suppressed.

---

[j]Resources and support network information are provided by the Alexander Graham Bell Association for the Deaf and Hard of Hearing, 3417 Volta Place NW, Washington, DC 20007; voice: 202-337-5220; TTY: 202-337-5221; 866-337-5220; fax: 202-337-8314; email: info@agbell.org; and by Canadian Hearing Society, 271 Spadina Road, Toronto, ON M5R 2V3; voice: 416-928-2535 or 877-347-3427; TTY: 877-216-7310; fax: 416-928-2506; email: info@chs.ca.

[k]Additional information is available from the National Captioning Institute, 3725 Concord Pkwy, Suite 100, Chantilly, VA 20151; voice/TTY: 703-917-7600.

Assist in Measures to Prevent Hearing Impairment

A primary nursing role is prevention of hearing loss. Because the most common cause of impaired hearing is chronic otitis media, it is essential that appropriate measures be instituted to treat existing infections and prevent recurrences (see Chapter 21. Children with a history of ear or respiratory infections or any other condition known to increase the risk of hearing impairment should receive periodic auditory testing.

To prevent the causes of hearing loss that begin prenatally and perinatally, pregnant women need counseling on the need for early prenatal care, including genetic counseling for known familial disorders; avoidance of all ototoxic drugs, especially during the first trimester; tests to rule out syphilis, rubella, or blood incompatibility; medical management of maternal diabetes; strict control of alcohol intake; adequate dietary intake; and avoidance of smoke exposure. Stress the need for routine immunization during childhood to eliminate the possibility of acquired sensorineural hearing loss from rubella, mumps, or measles (encephalitis).

Exposure to excessive noise pollution is a well-established cause of sensorineural hearing loss. The nurse should routinely assess the possibility of environmental noise pollution and advise children and parents of the potential danger. When individuals engage in activities associated with high-intensity noise (e.g., flying model airplanes, loud music, target shooting, snowmobiling), they should protect their hearing by wearing ear protection devices, decreasing music volume, and limiting or avoiding exposure to loud sounds (Centers for Disease Control and Prevention, 2018a). Even common household equipment, such as lawn mowers, vacuum cleaners, and telephones, can be harmful.

> **! NURSING ALERT**
>
> Suspect hazardous noise if the listener experiences (1) difficulty in communication while hearing the sound, (2) ringing in the ears (tinnitus) after exposure to the sound, or (3) muffled hearing after leaving the sound.

VISUAL IMPAIRMENT

Visual impairment is a common problem during childhood. In the United States, the prevalence of serious visual impairment in the pediatric population is estimated to be between 30 and 64 children per 100,000 population. Visual impairment such as refractive error, strabismus, and amblyopia occur in 5% to 10% of all preschoolers, who are usually identified through vision screening programs (American Academy of Pediatrics, Committee on Practice and Ambulatory Medicine, 2016; O'Hara, 2016; US Department of Health and Human Services, Office of Disease Prevention and Health Promotion, 2015; US Preventive Services Task Force, 2017; Ying, Maguire, Cyert, et al., 2014). The nurse's role is one of assessment, detection, prevention, referral, and (in some instances) rehabilitation.

Definition and Classification

Visual impairment is a general term that encompasses both partial sight and legal blindness. **Partial sight** or **partial visual impairment** is defined as a visual acuity between 20/70 and 20/200. The child can generally use normal-size print, because near vision is almost always better than distance vision. **Legal blindness** or **severe permanent visual impairment** is defined as a visual acuity of 20/200 or lower or a visual field of 20 degrees or less in the better eye. It is important to keep in mind that legal blindness is not a medical diagnosis but a legal definition. Educational and governmental agencies in the United States use the legal definition of blindness to determine tax status, eligibility for entrance into special schools, eligibility for financial aid, and other benefits.

Etiology

Visual impairment can be caused by a number of genetic and prenatal or postnatal conditions. These include perinatal infections (herpes, chlamydia, gonococci, rubella, syphilis, toxoplasmosis); retinopathy of prematurity; trauma; postnatal infections (meningitis); and disorders such as sickle cell disease, juvenile rheumatoid arthritis, Tay-Sachs disease, albinism, and retinoblastoma. In many instances, such as with refractive errors, the cause of the defect is unknown.

Refractive errors are the most common types of visual disorders in children. The term **refraction** means bending and refers to the bending of light rays as they pass through the lens of the eye. Normally, light rays enter the lens and fall directly on the retina. However, in refractive disorders, the light rays fall either in front of the retina (**myopia**) or beyond it (**hyperopia**). Other eye problems, such as strabismus, may or may not include refractive errors, but they are important because, if untreated, they result in severe permanent visual impairment from amblyopia.

Trauma

Trauma is a common cause of visual impairment in children. Injuries to the eyeball and adnexa (supporting or accessory structures, such as eyelids, conjunctiva, or lacrimal glands) can be classified as penetrating or nonpenetrating. **Penetrating wounds** are most often a result of sharp instruments (such as sticks, knives, or scissors) or propulsive objects (such as firecrackers, guns, arrows, or slingshots). **Nonpenetrating injuries** may be a result of foreign objects in the eyes, lacerations, a blow from a blunt object such as a ball (baseball, softball, basketball, racquet sports) or fist, or thermal or chemical burns.

Treatment is aimed at preventing further ocular damage and is primarily the responsibility of the ophthalmologist. It involves adequate examination of the injured eye (with the child sedated or anesthetized in severe injuries); appropriate immediate intervention, such as removal of the foreign body or suturing of the laceration; and prevention of complications, such as administration of antibiotics or steroids and complete bed rest to allow the eye to heal and blood to reabsorb (see Emergency Treatment box). The prognosis varies according to the type of injury. It is usually guarded in all cases of penetrating wounds because of the high risk of serious complications.

Infections

Infections of the adnexa and structures of the eyeball or globe may occur in children. The most common eye infection is **conjunctivitis** (see Chapter 6. Treatment is usually with ophthalmic antibiotics. Severe infections may require systemic antibiotic therapy. Steroids are used cautiously because they exacerbate viral infections such as herpes simplex, increasing the risk of damage to the involved structures.

Nursing Care Management

Nursing care of the visually impaired child is a critical nursing responsibility. Discovery of a visual impairment as early as possible is essential to prevent social, physical, and psychologic damage to the child. Assessment involves (1) identifying those children who by virtue of their history are at risk, (2) observing for behaviors that indicate a vision loss, and (3) screening all children for visual acuity and signs of other ocular disorders such as strabismus. This discussion focuses on clinical manifestations of various types of visual problems. Vision testing is discussed in Chapter 6.

EMERGENCY TREATMENT

Eye Injuries

Foreign Object

Examine eye for presence of a foreign body (evert upper eyelid to examine upper eye).
Remove a freely movable object with pointed corner of gauze pad lightly moistened with water.
Do not irrigate eye or attempt to remove a penetrating object (see Penetrating Injuries).
Caution child against rubbing eye.

Chemical Burns

Irrigate eye copiously with tap water for 15 to 20 minutes.
Evert upper eyelid to flush thoroughly.
Hold child's head with eye under a tap of running lukewarm water.
Take child to emergency department.
Have child rest with eyes closed.
Keep room darkened.

Ultraviolet Burns

If skin is burned, patch both eyes (make certain eyelids are completely closed); secure dressing with Kling bandages wrapped around head rather than with tape.
Have child rest with eyes closed.
Refer to an ophthalmologist.

Hematoma ("Black Eye")

Use a flashlight to check for gross hyphema (hemorrhage into anterior chamber; visible fluid meniscus across iris; more easily seen in light-colored than in brown eyes).
Apply ice for first 24 hours to reduce swelling if no hyphema is present.
Refer to an ophthalmologist immediately if hyphema is present.
Have child rest with eyes closed.

Penetrating Injuries

Take child to emergency department.
Never remove an object that has penetrated eye.
Follow strict aseptic technique in examining eye.
Observe for:

- Aqueous or vitreous leaks (fluid leaking from point of penetration)
- Hyphema
- Shape and equality of pupils, reaction to light, prolapsed iris (not perfectly circular)

Apply a Fox shield if available (not a regular eye patch) and apply patch over unaffected eye to prevent bilateral movement.
Maintain bed rest with child in a 30-degree Fowler position.
Caution child against rubbing eye.
Refer to an ophthalmologist.

Infancy

At birth, the nurse should observe the neonate's response to visual stimuli, such as following a light or object and cessation of body movement. The infant may vary in the intensity of the response, depending on the state of alertness.

Of special importance in detecting visual impairment during infancy are the parents' concerns regarding visual responsiveness in their child. Their concerns, such as lack of eye contact from the infant, must be taken seriously. During infancy, the child should be tested for strabismus. Lack of binocularity after 2 to 4 months of age is considered abnormal and must be treated to prevent amblyopia (American Academy of Pediatrics, Committee on Practice and Ambulatory Medicine, 2016; Rogers & Jordan, 2013).

NURSING ALERT

Suspect visual impairment in an infant who does not react to light and in a child of any age if the parents express concern.

Childhood

Because the most common visual impairment during childhood is refractive error, testing for visual acuity is essential. The school nurse usually assumes major responsibility for vision testing in schoolchildren. In addition to assessing for refractive errors, the nurse should be aware of signs and symptoms that indicate other ocular problems. If the family is given a referral requesting further eye testing, the nurse is responsible for follow-up concerning the recommendation.

Learning that their child is visually impaired precipitates an immense crisis for families. Encourage the family to investigate appropriate early intervention and educational programs for their child as soon as possible. Sources of information include state commissions for the visually impaired, local schools for children with visual impairments, the American Foundation for the Blind,[l] the National Federation of the Blind,[m] the National Association for Parents of Children with Visual Impairments,[n] the National Association for Visually Handicapped,[o] the American Council of the Blind,[p] and CNIB.[q]

Promote Parent-Child Attachment

A crucial time in the life of visually impaired infants is when the infant and the parents are getting acquainted with each other. Pleasurable patterns of interaction between the infant and parents may be lacking if there is not enough reciprocity. For example, if the parent gazes fondly at the infant's face and seeks eye contact but the infant fails to respond because he or she cannot see the parent, a troubled cycle of responses may occur. The nurse can help parents learn to look for other cues that indicate the infant is responding to them, such as whether the eyelids blink; whether the activity level accelerates or slows; whether respiratory patterns change, such as faster or slower breathing, when the parents come near; and whether the infant makes throaty sounds when the parents speak to the infant. In time, parents learn that the infant has unique ways of relating to them. Encourage the parents to show affection using nonvisual methods, such as talking or reading, cuddling, and walking the child.

Promote the Child's Optimal Development

Promoting the child's optimum development requires rehabilitation in a number of important areas. These include learning self-help skills and appropriate communication techniques to become independent. Although nurses may not be directly involved in such programs, they can provide direction and guidance to families regarding the availability of programs and the need to promote these activities in their child.

[l]1401 South Clark Street, Suite 730, Arlington, VA 22202; 800-232-5463 or 212-502-7600; fax: 888-545-8331; http://www.afb.org; email: afbinfo@afb.net.
[m]200 E. Wells St. at Jernigan Place, Baltimore, MD 21230; 410-659-9314; http://www.nfb.org.
[n]15 West 65th Street, New York, NY 10023; 212-769-6318 or 800-562-6265; email: napvi@lighthouseguild.org.
[o]111 East 59th St., The Sol and Lillian Goldman Building, New York, NY 10022-1202; 212-821-9200 or 800-284-4422; email: info@lighthouse.org.
[p]1703 N. Beauregard St., Suite 420, Alexandria, VA 22311; 800-424-8666 or 202-467-5081; http://www.acb.org; email: info@acb.org
[q]1929 Bayview Ave., East York, ON M4G 0A1, Canada; 800-563-2642.

Development and Independence

Motor development depends on sight almost as much as verbal communication depends on hearing. From earliest infancy, parents are encouraged to expose the infant to as many visual-motor experiences as possible, such as sitting supported in an infant seat or swing and being given opportunities for holding up the head, sitting unsupported, reaching for objects, and crawling.

Despite visual impairment, the child can become independent in all aspects of self-care. The same principles used for promoting independence in sighted children apply, with additional emphasis on nonvisual cues. For example, the child may need help in dressing, such as special arrangement of clothing for style coordination and braille tags to distinguish colors and prints.

The child with permanent visual impairments also must learn to become independent in navigational skills. The two main techniques are the **tapping method** (use of a cane to survey the environment for direction and to avoid obstacles) and **guides**, such as a sighted human guide or a dog guide, such as a seeing eye dog. Children who are partially sighted may benefit from ocular aids, such as a monocular telescope.

Play and Socialization

Children with severe permanent visual impairments do not learn to play automatically. Because they cannot imitate others or actively explore the environment as sighted children do, they depend much more on others to stimulate and teach them how to play. Parents need help in selecting appropriate play materials, especially those that encourage fine and gross motor development and stimulate the senses of hearing, touch, and smell. Toys with educational value are especially useful, such as dolls with various clothing closures.

Children with severe permanent visual impairments have the same needs for socialization as sighted children. Because they have little difficulty in learning verbal skills, they are able to communicate with agemates and participate in suitable activities. The nurse should discuss with parents opportunities for socialization outside the home, especially regular preschools. The trend is to include these children with sighted children to help them adjust to the outside world for eventual independence.

To compensate for inadequate stimulation, these children may develop self-stimulatory activities, such as body rocking, finger flicking, or arm twirling. Discourage such habits because they delay the child's social acceptance. Behavior modification is often successful in reducing or eliminating self-stimulatory activities.

Education

The main obstacle to learning is the child's total dependence on nonvisual cues. Although the child can learn via verbal lecturing, he or she is unable to read the written word or to write without special education. Therefore the child must rely on **braille**, a system that uses raised dots to represent letters and numbers. The child can then read braille with the fingers and can write messages using a braille writer. However, this system is not useful for communicating with others unless others read braille. A more portable system for written communication is the use of a braille slate and stylus or a microcassette tape recorder. A recorder is especially helpful for leaving messages for others and taking notes during classroom lectures. For mathematic calculations, portable calculators with voice synthesizers are available.[r]

Books on CDs and cassette tapes are significant sources of reading material in addition to braille books, which are large and cumbersome. The Library of Congress[s] has talking books and braille books, which are available at many local and state libraries and directly from the Library of Congress. Currently, there are two types of talking books and book players: digital and cassette, though new books are made only in the digital format with the recorded cassettes being phased out (The New York Public Library, 2019). The talking book machine and cassette tape player are provided at no cost to families, and there is no postage fee for returning the materials. Learning Ally (formally known as Recording for the Blind and Dyslexic)[t] also provides texts and CDs and cassette tapes of books, which are helpful for secondary and college students who are visually impaired. A means of writing is learning to use a home computer with a voice synthesizer that can be adapted to speak each letter or word typed.

Children with partial sight benefit from specialized visual aids that produce a magnified retinal image. The basic methods are accommodative techniques, such as bringing the object closer; devices such as special plus lenses, handheld and stand magnifiers, telescopes, video projection systems, and large print materials are used. Special equipment is available to enlarge print. Information about services for the partially sighted is available from the National Association for Visually Handicapped and American Foundation for the Blind. Children with diminished vision often prefer to do close work without their glasses and compensate by bringing the object very near to their eyes. This should be allowed. The exception is children with vision in only one eye, who should always wear glasses for protection.

Care for the Child During Hospitalization

Because nurses are more likely to care for children who are hospitalized for procedures that involve temporary loss of vision than for children who have severe permanent visual impairments, the following discussion concentrates primarily on the needs of such children. The nursing care objectives in either situation are to (1) reassure the child and family throughout every phase of treatment, (2) orient the child to the surroundings, (3) provide a safe environment, and (4) encourage independence. Whenever possible, the same nurse should care for the child to ensure consistency in the approach.

When sighted children temporarily lose their vision, almost every aspect of the environment becomes bewildering and frightening. They are forced to rely on nonvisual senses for help in adjusting to the visual impairment without the benefit of any special training. Nurses have a major role in minimizing the effects of temporary loss of vision. They need to talk to the child about everything that is occurring, emphasizing aspects of procedures that are felt or heard. They should always identify themselves as soon as they enter the room and before they approach the child. Because unfamiliar sounds are especially frightening, these are explained. Encourage the parents to room with their child and participate in the care. Familiar objects, such as a teddy bear or doll, should be brought from home to help lessen the strangeness of the hospital. As soon as the child is able to be out of bed, orient the child to the immediate surroundings. If the child is able to see on admission, this opportunity is taken to point out significant aspects of the room. Encourage the child to practice ambulating with the eyes closed to become accustomed to this experience.

[r]A catalog of numerous products for people with vision problems is available from Lighthouse International. For contact information, see footnote earlier in the chapter.

[s]National Library Service for the Blind and Physically Handicapped, Library of Congress, 1291 Taylor St. NW, Washington, DC 20011; 202-707-5100 or 888-657-7323; TTD: 202-707-0744; http://www.loc.gov-/nls; email: nis@loc.gov. (State listings of libraries for readers who are visually impaired or physically handicapped, as well as other reference circulars, are available from this office.)

[t]20 Roszel Road, Princeton, NJ 08540; 800-221-4792 or 866-RFBD-585; http://learningally.org; email: info@learningally.org; http://www.facebook.com/LearningAlly.org.

The room is arranged with safety in mind. For example, a stool is placed next to the bed to help the child climb in and out of bed. The furniture is always placed in the same position to prevent collisions. Remind cleaning personnel to keep the room in order. If the child has difficulty navigating by feeling the walls, a rope can be attached from the bed to the point of destination, such as the bathroom. Attention to details (such as well-fitting slippers and robes that do not drag on the floor) is important in preventing tripping. Unlike the child who is visually impaired, these children are not familiar with navigating with a cane.

The child is encouraged to be independent in self-care activities, especially if the visual loss may be prolonged or potentially permanent. For example, during bathing, the nurse sets up all of the equipment and encourages the child to participate. At mealtimes, the nurse explains where each food item is on the tray, opens any special containers, prepares cereal or toast, and encourages the child in self-feeding. Favorite finger foods (such as sandwiches, hamburgers, hot dogs, or pizza) may be good selections. Praise the child for efforts at being cooperative and independent. Any improvements made in self-care, no matter how small, are stressed.

Appropriate recreational activities are provided, and if a child life specialist is available, such planning is done jointly. Because children with temporary visual impairment have a wide variety of play experiences to draw on, they are encouraged to select activities. For example, if they like to read, they may enjoy listening to books on CD or having someone to read to them. If they prefer manual activity, they may appreciate playing with clay or building blocks or feeling different textures and naming them. If they need an outlet for aggression, activities such as pounding or banging on a drum can be helpful. Simple board and card games can be played with a "seeing partner" or an opponent who helps with the game. They should have familiar toys from home to play with because familiar items are more easily manipulated than new ones. If parents want to bring presents, they should be objects that stimulate hearing and touch, such as a radio, music box, or stuffed animal.

Occasionally, children who are visually impaired come to the hospital for procedures to restore their vision. Although this is an extremely happy time, it also requires intervention to help them adjust to sight. They need an opportunity to take in all that they see. They should not be bombarded with visual stimuli. They may need to concentrate on people's faces or their own to become accustomed to this experience. They often need to talk about what they see and to compare the visual images with their mental ones. The children may also go through a period of depression, which must be respected and supported. Encourage the children to discuss how it feels to see, especially in terms of seeing themselves.

Newly sighted children also need time to adjust and engage in activities that were impossible before. For example, they may prefer to use braille to read rather than learning a new "visual approach" because of familiarity with the touch system. Eventually, as they learn to recognize letters and numbers, they will integrate these new skills into reading and writing. However, parents and teachers must be careful not to push them before they are ready. This applies to social relationships and physical activities as well as to learning situations.

Assist in Measures to Prevent Visual Impairment

An essential nursing goal is to prevent visual impairment. This involves many of the same interventions discussed for hearing impairments:

- Prenatal screening for pregnant women at risk, such as those with rubella or syphilis infection and family histories of genetic disorders associated with visual loss
- Adequate prenatal and perinatal care to prevent prematurity
- Periodic screening of all children, especially newborns through preschoolers, for congenital and acquired visual impairments caused by refractive errors, strabismus, and other disorders
- Rubella immunization of all children
- Safety counseling regarding the common causes of ocular trauma, including safe practices when working with, playing with, and carrying objects such as scissors, knives, and balls

> **! NURSING ALERT**
>
> A helmet with a face mask should be required for children playing football, hockey, fencing and baseball (catcher).

After detection of eye problems, the nurse should encourage the family to prevent further ocular damage by undertaking corrective treatment. For the child with strabismus, this often necessitates occlusion patching of the stronger eye. Compliance with the procedure is greatest during the early preschool years. It is more difficult to encourage school-age children to wear the occlusive patch because the poor visual acuity of the uncovered weaker eye interferes with school work and the patch sets them apart from their peers. In school, they benefit from being positioned favorably (closer to the white board or other visual media) and allowed extra time to read or complete an assignment. If treatment of the eye disorder requires instillation of ophthalmic medication, the family is taught the correct procedure (see Chapter 20).

Children who need glasses to correct refractive errors need time to adjust to wearing glasses. Young children who often pull off glasses benefit from temporal pieces that wrap around the ears or an elastic strap attached to the frames and around the back of the head to hold the glasses on securely. Once children appreciate the value of clear vision, they are more likely to wear the corrective lenses.

Glasses should not interfere with any activity. Special protective guards are available during contact sports to prevent accidental injury, and all corrective lenses should be made from safety glass, which is shatterproof. Often, corrective lenses improve visual acuity so dramatically that children are able to compete more effectively in sports. This in itself is a tremendous inducement to continue wearing glasses.

Contact lenses are a popular alternative to conventional glasses, especially for adolescents. Several types are available, such as hard lenses, including gas-permeable ones, and soft lenses, which may be designed for daily or extended wear. Contact lenses offer several advantages over glasses, such as greater visual acuity, total corrected field of vision, convenience (especially with the extended-wear type), and optimal cosmetic benefit. Unfortunately, they are usually more expensive and require much more care than glasses, including considerable practice to learn techniques for insertion and removal. If they are prescribed, the nurse can be helpful in teaching parents or older children how to care for the lenses.

Because trauma is the leading cause of visual impairment, the nurse has the major responsibility of preventing further eye injury until specific treatment is instituted. The major principles to follow when caring for an eye injury are outlined in the Emergency Treatment box earlier in the chapter. Because patients with a serious eye injury fear visual impairment, the nurse should provide the child and family with support and reassurance.

HEARING–VISUAL IMPAIRMENT

The most traumatic sensory impairment is loss of both vision and hearing, which may have profound effects on the child's development. These losses interfere with the normal sequence of physical, intellectual, and psychosocial growth. Although such children often achieve the usual motor milestones, their rate of development is slower. These children learn communication only with specialized training. **Finger spelling** is one desirable method often taught to these children. Words are spelled letter by letter into the hearing–visually impaired child's hand, and the child spells into the other person's hand. Some children with residual hearing or visual impairment can learn to speak. Whenever possible, encourage speech because it allows communication with other individuals.

The future prospects for hearing–visually impaired children are, at best, unpredictable. Congenital hearing and visual impairment are accompanied by other physical or neurologic problems, which further diminish the child's learning potential. The most favorable prognosis is for children who have acquired hearing and visual impairments with few, if any, associated disabilities. Their learning capacity is greatly potentiated by their developmental progress before the sensory impairments. Although total independence, including gainful vocational training, is the goal, some children with hearing–visual impairment are unable to develop to this level. They may require lifelong parental or residential care. The nurse working with such families helps them deal with future goals for the child, including possible alternatives to home care during the parents' advancing years.

COMMUNICATION IMPAIRMENT

AUTISM SPECTRUM DISORDERS

ASDs are complex neurodevelopmental disorders of unknown etiology. The DSM-5 revised the definition of ASD based on two behavior domains: difficulties in social communication and social interaction and unusually restricted, repetitive behavior, interest, or activities (American Psychiatric Association, 2013; Brentani, Paula, Bordini, et al., 2013; Lai, Lombardo, & Baron-Cohen, 2014).

ASD is frequently diagnosed in toddlers because their atypical development is being recognized early (Lai et al., 2014; Sanchack & Thomas, 2016; Zwaigenbaum, Bauman, Stone, et al., 2015). It occurs in 1 in 59 to 68 children in the United States; is about four times more common in boys than in girls; and is not related to race, region, or socioeconomic level (Baio, Wiggins, Christensen, et al., 2018; Centers for Disease Control and Prevention, 2018b; Christensen, Baio, Braun, et al., 2016; National Autism Association, 2017).

Etiology

The cause of ASD is unknown. Researchers are investigating a number of theories, including a link between hereditary, genetic, medical, immune dysregulation or neuroinflammation, oxidative stress (damage to cellular tissue), and environmental factors (Andrews, Sheppard, & Windham, 2018; Feinberg, Bakulski, Jaffe, et al., 2015; Gilbert & Man, 2017: Ng, de Montigny, Ofner, et al., 2017; Posar & Visconti, 2016; Willfors, Carlsson, Anderlid, et al., 2017; Wong, Napoli, Krakowiak, et al., 2016). Individuals with ASD have been associated with early medical events (cerebral hemorrhage, hyperbilirubinemia), abnormal electroencephalograms, epileptic seizures, delayed development of hand dominance, persistence of primitive reflexes, metabolic abnormalities (elevated blood serotonin), cerebellar vermis hypoplasia (part of the brain involved in regulating motion and some aspects of memory), and infantile abnormal head enlargement (Bridgemohan 2020; Gilbert & Man, 2017; Willfors et al., 2017).

The strong evidence for a genetic basis in twins is consistent with an autosomal recessive pattern of inheritance. Twin studies demonstrate a high concordance (60% to 96%) for monozygotic (identical) twins and less than 5% concordance for dizygotic (nonidentical) twins (Tick, Bolton, Happe, et al., 2016).

There is a relatively high risk of recurrence of ASD in families with one affected child (Chawarska, Shic, Macari, et al., 2014; Sandin, Lichtenstein, Kuja-Holkola, et al., 2014; Zwaigenbaum et al., 2015). Several genes have been suggested as possible causative factors in ASD (Gilbert & Man, 2017; Talkowski, Minikel, & Gusella, 2014; Willsey & State, 2015; Wong et al., 2016).

The scientific evidence to date shows no link between measles, mumps, and rubella (MMR); prenatal tetanus, diphtheria, and acellular pertussis (Tdap); and thimerosal-containing vaccines and ASDs (Barile, Kuperminc, Weintraub, et al., 2012; Becerra-Culqui, Getahun, Chiu, et al., 2018; Centers for Disease Control and Prevention, 2017; Goin-Kochel, Mire, Dempsey, et al., 2016; Price, Thompson, Goodson, et al., 2010; Taylor, Swerdfeger, & Eslick, 2014; Uno, Uchiyama, Kurosawa, et al., 2015; US Food and Drug Administration, 2018; Zerbo, Qian, Yoshida, et al., 2017) (see Translating Evidence Into Practice box). ASD has been reported in association with a number of conditions, such as FXS, tuberous sclerosis, Prader-Willie syndrome, metabolic disorders, fetal rubella syndrome, *Haemophilus influenzae* meningitis, and structural brain anomalies (Kaufmann, Kidd, Andrews, et al., 2017; National Autism Association, 2017; Niu, Han, Dy, et al., 2017). Reports have retrospectively tied ASD to prenatal and perinatal events, such as maternal and paternal ages over 40 years old, uterine bleeding during pregnancy, low Apgar score, fetal distress, and neonatal hyperbilirubinemia (Amin, Smith, & Wang, 2011; Hadjkacem,

TRANSLATING EVIDENCE INTO PRACTICE

Thimerosal-Containing Vaccines and Autism Spectrum Disorders

Ask the Question

Is the incidence of autism spectrum disorders (ASDs) increased in children who receive vaccines containing thimerosal?

Search for the Evidence

Search Strategies

Published studies from 2003 to 2018 focused on the pediatric population and restricted to the English language.

Databases Used

PubMed, Cochrane Collaboration, MD Consult, Vaccine Adverse Events Reporting System (VAERS) database, American Academy of Pediatrics, Autism Research Institute.

Critically Analyze the Evidence

Grade criteria: Moderate evidence with strong recommendations for practice (Balshem, Helfand, Schünemann, et al., 2011). Evidence does not support an association between the increased incidence of autism and mercury exposure from the pharmaceutical preservative thimerosal.

- A Cochrane systematic review of 64 studies assessing the effectiveness and adverse effects associated with the trivalent measles, mumps, and rubella (MMR) vaccine on healthy patients up to 15 years old found no significant association between MMR and either autism or other conditions (Demicheli, Rivetti, Debalini, et al., 2012). Previously done studies supported the same conclusion because the studies found no association between thimerosal-containing vaccines and ASD (Demicheli, Jefferson, Rivetti, et al., 2005; Hurley, Tadrous, & Miller, 2010; Parker, Schwartz, Todd, et al., 2004; Schultz, 2010; World Health Organization, 2012).
- Two large studies in Europe found no evidence that childhood vaccination with thimerosal-containing vaccines was associated with the development of ASDs. One longitudinal study evaluated more than 14,000 children in the United Kingdom. The mercury exposure from thimerosal-containing vaccines was recorded and calculated at ages 3, 4, and 6 months and compared with

Continued

TRANSLATING EVIDENCE INTO PRACTICE—cont'd

Thimerosal-Containing Vaccines and Autism Spectrum Disorders

cognitive and behavioral-developmental assessments performed from 6 to 91 months old (Heron, Golding, & ALSPAC Study Team, 2004). The second study, a cohort of 467,450 children in Denmark, compared the incidence of ASDs in children vaccinated with thimerosal-containing vaccines with the incidence of ASDs in children vaccinated with a thimerosal-free formulation of the same vaccine (Hvid, Stellfeld, & Wohlfahrt, 2003).

- Another study that evaluated 1047 children from early life to 7 to 10 years old and their biologic mothers found no statistically significant associations between thimerosal exposure from vaccines early in life. It noted a small but statistically significant association between early thimerosal exposure and the presence of tics in boys and recommended that there be further research in this area (Barile, Kuperminc, Weintraub, et al., 2012). A cohort study that evaluated 196,929 children suggested a possible increased risk of ASD among children whose mothers received an influenza vaccination during their first trimester of pregnancy, although this association was not statistically significant after a post hoc analysis adjusting for multiple comparisons, and there was no association between ASD and influenza vaccination received during any trimester (Zerbo, Qian, Yoshida, et al., 2017).
- Case-control studies have also found no relationships between MMR vaccination and the increased risk of ASDs (Price, Thompson, Goodson, et al., 2010; Uno, Uchiyama, Kurosawa, et al., 2015). Another small case control study investigated the mercury level in maternal prenatal serum and early postnatal newborn serum of children with ASD (n = 84) compared to children with intellectual disability or developmental delay (n = 49) and the general population (n = 159) and found no significant association with the risk of ASD (Yau, Green, Alaimo, et al., 2014). A similar finding was concluded in a meta-analysis of evidence on the impact of prenatal and early infancy exposures to mercury on autism and attention-deficit/hyperactivity disorder (ADHD) with the recommendation of further study to be conducted on the effects of environmental perinatal mercury exposures and increased risk of developmental disorders (Yoshimasu, Kiyohara, Takemura, et al., 2014).
- Review studies by the same first author reported epidemiologic evidence of a suggestive and/or significant relationship between increasing organic mercury exposure from thimerosal-containing vaccines and subsequent risk of neurodevelopmental disorders. The case-controlled studies examined automated records updated through the year 2000 in the Vaccine Safety Datalink (VSD) for organic exposure to hepatitis B vaccine administered in the first 6 months of life with a significant increased risk of neurodevelopmental disorder (Geier, Hooker, Kern, et al., 2014) and also examined organic exposure from *Haemophilus influenzae* type b with suggestive neurodevelopmental outcomes (Geier, Kern, Homme, et al., 2018; Geier, Kern, King, et al., 2015). Conversely, the Global Advisory Committee on Vaccine Safety reviewed both animal and human toxicity studies in which the blood and brain did not attain toxic levels, making it biologically implausible for any relationship between thimerosal in vaccines and neurologic toxicity to exist (World Health Organization, 2012). Another evidence-based meta-analysis of case-controlled studies and cohort studies supported the same conclusion; the findings suggested that vaccinations are not associated with the development of autism or ASD (Taylor, Swerdfeger, & Eslick, 2014).
- In 2004 the Institute of Medicine completed a review and concluded that the epidemiologic evidence supports the rejection of a causal relationship between thimerosal exposure from childhood vaccines and the onset of autism (Institute of Medicine, 2004). In 2013 the Institute of Medicine completed an update to the review of the evidence reported from January 1990 to May 2013 and concluded that the review did not reveal an evidence base, suggesting that the US childhood immunization schedule is linked to learning or developmental disorders or attention-deficit or disruptive disorders. This review was also supported by the Institute of Medicine (2011) in a report on adverse effects of vaccines. The Institute of Medicine, now called the National Academy of Medicine, concluded that the body of evidence favors rejection of a causal relationship between autism and the MMR vaccine and thimerosal-containing vaccines (Institute of Medicine, 2011, 2013) as reported by the US Food and Drug Administration (2018). Based on guidelines established by the US Food and Drug Administration (2018), Centers for Disease Control and Prevention (2017), and other government monitoring agencies, no children will be exposed to excessive mercury from childhood vaccines.

Apply the Evidence: Nursing Implications

There is moderate-quality evidence with a strong recommendation that there is no link between vaccines containing thimerosal and ASDs.

Quality and Safety Competencies: Evidence-Based Practice[a]

Knowledge

Differentiate clinical opinion from research and evidence-based summaries.

Compare research summaries that provide evidence of the lack of association between vaccines containing thimerosal and autism or other neurodevelopmental disorders.

Skills

Base individualized care plan on patient values, clinical expertise, and evidence.

Integrate evidence into practice by sharing results with parents regarding the benefits of vaccinating their children and the evidence regarding lack of association between immunizations and autism disorders.

Attitudes

Value the concept of evidence-based practice as integral to determining best clinical practice.

Appreciate strengths and weaknesses of the evidence that confirms the lack of a link between vaccines containing thimerosal and autism or other neurodevelopmental disorders.

References

Balshem, H., Helfand, M., Schünemann, H. J., et al. (2011). GRADE guidelines: 3. Rating the quality of evidence. *Journal of Clinical Epidemiology, 64*(4), 401–406.

Barile, J. P., Kuperminc, G. P., Weintraub, E. S., et al. (2012). Thimerosal exposure in early life and neuropsychological outcomes 7–10 years later. *Journal of Pediatric Psychology, 37*(1), 106–118.

Centers for Disease Control and Prevention. (2017). Thimersol in flu vaccine. Retrieved from https://www.cdc.gov/flu/protect/vaccine/thimersol.htm.

Demicheli, V., Jefferson, T., Rivetti, A., et al. (2005). Vaccines for measles, mumps and rubella in children. *Cochrane Database of Systematic Reviews*, (4), CD004407.

Demicheli, V., Rivetti, A., Debalini, M. G., et al. (2012). Vaccines for measles, mumps and rubella in children. *Cochrane Database of Systematic Reviews*, (2), CD004407.

Geier, D. A., Hooker, B. S., Kern, J. K., et al. (2014). A dose-response relationship between organic mercury exposure from thimerosal-containing vaccines and neurodevelopmental disorders. *International Journal of Environmental Research and Public Health, 11*(9), 9156–9170.

Geier, D. A., Kern, J. K., Homme, K. G., et al. (2018). The risk of neurodevelopmental disorders following thimerosal-containing Hib vaccine in comparison to thimerosal-free Hib vaccine administered from 1995 to 1999 in the United States. *International Journal of Hygiene and Environmental Health*, (4), 677–683.

Geier, D. A., Kern, J. K., King, P. G., et al. (2015). A case-control study evaluating the relationship between thimerosal-containing *Haemophilus influenzae* type b vaccine administration and the risk for pervasive developmental disorder diagnosis in the United States. *Biological Trace Element Research, 163*(1–2), 28–38.

Heron, J., Golding, J., & ALSPAC Study Team (2004). Thimerosal exposure in infants and developmental disorders: A prospective cohort study in the United Kingdom does not support a causal association. *Pediatrics, 114*(3), 577–583.

Hurley, A. M., Tadrous, M., & Miller, E. S. (2010). Thimerosal-containing vaccines and autism: Review of recent epidemiologic studies. *Journal of Pediatric Pharmacology and Therapeutics, 15*(3), 173–181.

TRANSLATING EVIDENCE INTO PRACTICE—cont'd

Thimerosal-Containing Vaccines and Autism Spectrum Disorders

Hvid, A., Stellfeld, M., & Wohlfahrt, J. (2003). Association between thimersol-containing vaccine and autism. *Journal of the American Medical Association, 290*(13), 1763–1766.
Institute of Medicine. (2004). Immunization safety review: Vaccines and autism. Washington, DC: National Academies Press.
Institute of Medicine. (2011). Adverse effects of vaccines: Evidence and causality. Retrieved from http://www.iom.edu/Reports/2011/Adverse-Effects-of-Vaccines-Evidence-and-Causality.aspx.
Institute of Medicine. (2013). *The childhood immunization schedule and safety: Stakeholder concerns, scientific evidence, and future studies.* Washington, DC: National Academies Press.
Parker, S. K., Schwartz, B., Todd, J., et al. (2004). Thimerosal-containing vaccines and autistic spectrum disorder: A critical review of published original data. *Pediatrics, 114*(3), 793–804.
Price, C. S., Thompson, W. W., Goodson, B., et al. (2010). Prenatal and infant exposure to thimerosal from vaccines and immunoglobulins and risk of autism. *Pediatrics, 126*(4), 656–664.
Schultz, S. T. (2010). Does thimerosal or other mercury exposure increase the risk for autism? A review of current literature. *Acta Neurobiologiae Experimentalis (Wars), 70*(2), 187–195.
Taylor, L. E., Swerdfeger, A. L., & Eslick, G. D. (2014). Vaccines are not associated with autism: An evidence-based meta-analysis of case-control and cohort studies. *Vaccine, 32*(29), 3623–3629.
Uno, Y., Uchiyama, T., Kurosawa, M., et al. (2015). Early exposure to the combined measles-mumps-rubella vaccine and thimerosal-containing vaccines and risk of autism spectrum disorder. *Vaccine, 33*(21), 2511–2516.
US Food and Drug Administration. (2018). Thimerosal and vaccines. Retrieved from http://www.fda.gov/biologicsbloodvaccines/.../vaccinesafety/ucm096228.
World Health Organization. (2012). Global vaccine safety: Global Advisory Committee on Vaccine Safety, report of meeting held 6–7 June 2012. Retrieve from http://www.who.int/vaccine_safety/committee/reports/Jun_2012/en/.
Yau, V. M., Green, P. G., Alaimo, C. P., et al. (2014). Prenatal and neonatal peripheral blood mercury levels and autism spectrum disorders. *Environmental Research, 133*, 294–303.
Yoshimasu, K., Kiyohara, C., Takemura, S., et al. (2014). A meta-analysis of the evidence on the impact of prenatal and early infancy exposures to mercury on autism and attention deficit/hyperactivity disorder in the childhood. *Neurotoxicology, 44*, 121–131.
Zerbo, O., Qian, Y., Yoshida, C., et al. (2017). Association betweenn influenza and vaccination during pregnancy and risk of autism spectrum disorder. *JAMA Pediatrics, 171*(1), e163609.

Rosalind Bryant

[a]Based on the Quality and Safety Education for Nurses website at http://www.qsen.org.

Ayadi, Turki, et al., 2016; Wang, Hua, Weidong, et al., 2017). These same researchers, however, urge caution in interpreting these findings.

Clinical Manifestations and Diagnostic Evaluation

Children with ASD demonstrate core deficits primarily in social interactions, communication, and behavior. Failure of social interaction and communication development is one of the hallmarks of ASD. Parents of autistic children have reported that their child showed less interest in social interaction (e.g., abnormal eye contact, decreased response to own name, decreased imitation, usual repetitive behavior) and had verbal and motor delay (Bolton, Golding, Emond, et al., 2012; Kirchner, Hatri, Heekeren, et al., 2011; National Autism Association, 2017; Sanchack & Thomas, 2016). Children with ASD may have significant gastrointestinal symptoms. Constipation is a common symptom and can be associated with acquired megarectum in children with ASD (National Autism Association, 2017; Neumeyer, Anixt, Chan, et al., 2018).

Children with autism do not always have the same manifestations, from mild forms requiring minimal supervision to severe forms in which self-abusive behavior is common. The majority of children with autism have some degree of CI, with scores typically in the moderate to severe range. Despite their relatively moderate to severe disability, some children with autism (known as **savants**) excel in particular areas, such as art, music, memory, mathematics, or perceptual skills, such as puzzle building.

[a]Additional information on secretin may be found by contacting the Autism Society, 4340 East-West Hwy., Suite 350, Bethesda, MD 20814-3067; 800-3AUTISM or 301-657-0881; http://www.autism-society.org.

NURSING TIP Claims of beneficial results from the use of secretin, a peptide hormone that stimulates pancreatic secretion, have been studied extensively in multiple randomized control trials, denoting clear evidence that it lacks any benefit (Krishnaswami, McPheeters, & Veenstra-Vanderweele, 2011; Lee, Oh, Park, et al., 2014; Lyra, Rizzo, Sunahara, et al., 2017; Williams, Wray, & Wheeler, 2012).[a]

Communication impairments are a common sign in children with ASD that may range from absent to delayed speech. Any child who does not display language skills such as babbling or gesturing by 12 months old, single words by 16 months old, and two-word phrases by 24 months old is recommended for immediate hearing and language evaluation. Autism regression occurs when the child seems to develop normally, then regresses suddenly; this is a red-flag event that has been frequently displayed in expressive language (Fernell, Eriksson, & Gillberg, 2013; National Autism Association, 2017; Pearson, Charman, Happe, et al., 2018).

Early recognition, referral, diagnosis, and intensive early intervention tend to improve outcomes for children with ASD (Adelman & Kubiszyn, 2016; Christensen, Maenner, Bilder, et al., 2019; National Autism Association, 2017; Reichow, Hume, Barton, et al., 2018; Zwaigenbaum et al., 2015). Unfortunately, diagnosis is often not made until 2 to 3 years after symptoms are first recognized. However, in a retrospective study, the majority of parents observed atypical development in their children with ASD before 24 months of age (Lemcke, Juul, Parner, et al., 2013).

The American Academy of Pediatrics has recommended that pediatric health care providers administer two ASD screenings at ages 18 and 24 months using a valid screening tool. Children whose screening results are concerning subsequently should receive a comprehensive developmental evaluation from a developmental pediatrician, child neurologist, child psychiatrist, or child psychologist (Baio et al., 2018; National Autism Association, 2017).

Prognosis

ASD is usually a lifelong condition with often devastating comorbidities. However, with early and intensive interventions, the symptoms associated with autism can be greatly improved, and in some cases reported symptoms were completely overcome (Kerub, Haas, Menashe, et al., 2018; National Autism Association, 2017; Sanchack & Thomas, 2016; Wodka, Mathy, & Kalb, 2013). Some ultimately achieve independence, but most require lifelong adult supervision. Aggravation of psychiatric symptoms occurs in about half of children with ASD during adolescence, with girls having a tendency for continued deterioration.

Early recognition of behaviors associated with ASD is critical to implement appropriate interventions and family involvement. There is a growing body of evidence that parent-delivered interventions are associated with some improved outcomes, yet further research incorporating consistent measures is needed in this area (Bearss, Burrell, Stewart, et al., 2015; Brentani et al., 2013; Oono, Honey, & McConachie, 2013). The prognosis is most favorable for children with higher intelligence, functional speech, and less behavioral impairment (Bridgemohan 2020; Orinstein, Helt, Troyb, et al., 2014; Solomon, Buaminger, & Rogers, 2011).

Nursing Care Management

Therapeutic intervention for children with ASD is a specialized area involving professionals with advanced training. Although there is no cure for ASD, numerous therapies have been used. The most promising results have been through highly structured and intensive behavior modification programs. In general, the objective in treatment is to promote positive reinforcement, increase social awareness of others, teach verbal communication skills, and decrease unacceptable behavior. Providing a structured routine for the child to follow is key in the management of ASD.

ASD is associated with comorbidities (e.g., aggression, explosive outburst, self-injury, asthma, epilepsy, gastrointestinal or digestive disorders, immune disorders, feeding disorders, anxiety disorder, bipolar disorder, sleeping disorders) that have been treated with not only early behavioral modification programs but also medical management (e.g., aripiprazole [Abilify] and risperidone [Risperdal]) and complementary and alternative medicine (Goel, Hong, Findling, et al., 2018; National Autism Association, 2017; Sanchack & Thomas, 2016). Complementary and alternative medicine has emerged as a treatment of ASD ranging from massage and therapeutic horseback riding to the implementation of elimination diets (e.g., gluten-free diet and casein-free diet); vitamin and omega-3 supplementation; and high-fat, low-carbohydrate ketogenic diet. However, there is a need for further research to validate these therapeutic approaches (Adams, Audhya, Geis, et al., 2018; Cheng, Rho, & Masino, 2017; Hopf, Madren, & Santianni, 2016; Ly, Bottelier, Hoekstra, et al., 2017; Nath, 2017; Trzmiel, Purandare, Michalak, et al., 2019).

When these children are hospitalized, the parents are essential to planning care and ideally should stay with the child as much as possible. Nurses should recognize that not all children with ASD are the same and that they require individual assessment and treatment. Decreasing stimulation by using a private room, avoiding extraneous auditory and visual distractions, and encouraging the parents to bring in possessions the child is attached to may lessen the disruptiveness of hospitalization. Because physical contact often upsets these children, minimal holding and eye contact may be necessary to avoid behavioral outbursts. Take care when performing procedures on, administering medicine to, and feeding these children because they may be either fussy eaters who willfully starve themselves or gag to prevent eating or indiscriminate hoarders who swallow any available edible or inedible items, such as a thermometer. The eating habits of children with ASD may be particularly problematic for families and may involve food refusal accompanied by mineral deficiencies, mouthing objects, eating nonedibles, and smelling and throwing food (Herndon, DiGuiseppi, Johnson, et al., 2009; Lazaro & Ponde, 2017; Panerai, Suraniti, Cantania, et al., 2018).

Children with ASD need to be introduced slowly to new situations, with visits with staff caregivers kept short whenever possible. Because these children have difficulty organizing their behavior and redirecting their energy, they need to be told directly what to do. Communication should be at the child's developmental level, brief, and concrete.

Family Support

ASD, as with so many other chronic conditions, involves the entire family and often becomes "a family disease." Nurses can help alleviate the guilt and shame often associated with this disorder by stressing what is known from a biologic standpoint and by providing family support. It is imperative to help parents understand that they are not the cause of the child's condition.

Parents need expert counseling early in the course of the disorder and should be referred to the Autism Society website. The society provides information about education, treatment programs and techniques, and facilities such as camps and group homes. Other helpful resources for parents of children with ASD are the local and state departments of mental health and developmental disabilities; these organizations provide important programs and in-school programs throughout the United States for children with ASD.

As much as possible, the family is encouraged to care for the child in the home. With the help of family support programs in many states, families are often able to provide home care and assist with the educational services the child needs. As the child approaches adulthood and the parents become older, the family may require assistance in locating a long-term placement facility.

CLINICAL JUDGMENT AND NEXT-GENERATION NCLEX® EXAMINATION-STYLE QUESTIONS

1. A mother comments to a nurse working on the pediatric unit, "My second child just does not seem to be acting like or responding the same way as my first child. She is 2 years old and she does not speak." The nurse performs a complete history and assessment and the findings are listed below. **Select the assessment findings that require follow-up by the nurse. Select all that apply.**
   - **A.** Unable to speak
   - **B.** The mother is a single mom
   - **C.** Unable to follow instructions
   - **D.** Sibling was delayed a year in school
   - **E.** History of urinary tract infection at 1year of age
   - **F.** The child was premature; born at 36 weeks' gestation
   - **G.** History of maternal drug consumption during pregnancy
   - **H.** History of irritability and crying without being able to be consoled.

2. When interacting with a parent at a 3-year-old during the child's well visit, which information below provided by the parent would be an indication for a speech referral? **Select all that apply.**
   - **A.** Frequent omission of final consonants
   - **B.** Stuttering or any other type of dysfluency
   - **C.** Failure to use sentences of three or more words
   - **D.** Failure to speak any meaningful words spontaneously
   - **E.** Using different words or nicknames for certain people
   - **F.** Omission of word endings (e.g., plurals, tenses of verbs)

3. A mother of a child with Down syndrome is overwhelmed by thoughts of the future and asks many questions. She is 35 years old and blames herself for waiting so long to get pregnant. She is not sure how to care for the child now that she is turning 1 year of age. The nurse providing teaching would discuss which of the following with the mother? **Use an X for the health teaching statement below that is Indicated (appropriate or necessary), Contraindicated (could be harmful), or Non-Essential (makes no difference or not necessary).**

Health Teaching	Indicated	Contraindicated	Non-Essential
"It is unfortunate that you waited so long to have children, most children with Down syndrome are born to older women."			
"When feeding your infant use a small, straight-handled spoon to push food to the side and back of the mouth."			
"Parents like you believe that the experience of having this special child makes them stronger and more accepting of others."			
"As your child gets older it has been found that school is detrimental to the child with Down syndrome due to lack of one-on-one teaching."			
"I am going to listen closely to your child's heart because congenital heart problems can occur in a child with Down syndrome."			

4. The nurse is caring for a 4-year-old boy who has been diagnosed with Autism Spectrum Disorder (ASD). The mother is convinced that the childhood immunizations he has received have caused his ASD. The child has difficulty making eye contact and has verbal and motor delays. Understanding autism spectrum disorders (ASDs) is very important for those who care for children. What would be the nurse's response to the mother's concerns? **Choose the most likely options for the information missing from the statements below by selecting from the lists of options provided.**

Research studies have found that there is <u>no</u> link between ___1___ containing ___2___ and the development of ASD in children.

Options for 1	Options for 2
antibiotics	thimerosal
vitamins	arsenic
vaccines	penicillin
milk	hormones
fruit juices	amoxicillin

REFERENCES

Adams, J. B., Audhya, T., Geis, E., et al. (2018). Comprehensive nutritional and dietary intervention for autism spectrum disorder-A randomized, controlled 12-month trial. *Nutrients, 10*(3), 369.

Adelman, C. R., & Kubiszyn, T. (2016). Factors that affect age of identification of children with autism spectrum disorder. *Journal of Early Intervention, 39*(1), 18–32.

Almadhoob, A., & Ohlsson, A. (2015). Sound reduction management in the neonatal intensive care unit for preterm or very low birth weight infants. *The Cochrane database of systematic reviews*, (1), CD010333.

American Academy of Pediatrics. (2019). Early hearing detection and intervention, a program of the American Academy of Pediatrics. https://www ,aao.org/en-us/advicacy-and-policy/ aap-health-initiatives/.../pages/early-hearing-detection-and-intervention.aspx.

American Academy of Pediatrics, Committee on Practice and Ambulatory Medicine. (2016). Visual system assessment in infants, children, and young adults by pediatricians. *Pediatrics, 137*(1), 28–30.

American Academy of Pediatrics, Joint Committee on Infant Hearing. (2007). Year 2007 position statement: principles and guidelines for early hearing detection and intervention programs. *Pediatrics, 120*(4), 898–921.

American Association on Intellectual and Developmental Disabilities. (2013). *Intellectual disability: definition, classification, and systems of supports* (11th ed.). Washington, DC: Author.

American Psychiatric Association. (2013). *Diagnostic and statistical manual of mental disorders* (5th ed.). (DSM-V). Arlington, VA: American Psychiatric Association.

Amin, S. B., Smith, T., & Wang, H. (2011). Is neonatal jaundice associated with autism spectrum disorders: a systematic review. *The Journal of Autism and Developmental Disorders, 41*(11), 1455–1463.

Andrews, S. V., Sheppard, B., Windham, G. C., et al. (2018). Case-control meta-analysis of blood DNA methylation and autism spectrum disorder. *Mol Autism, 9*, 40.

Arumugam, A., Raja, K., Venugopalan, M., et al. (2016). Down-syndrome-A narrative review with a focus on anatomical features. *Clinical Anatomy, 29*, 568–577.

Available online: http: //apps.who.int/iris/bitstream/handle/10665/260336/9789241550260- eng.pdf?sequence=1&ua=1. Accessed January 20, 2019.

Badeau, M., Lindsay, C., Blais, J., et al. (2017). Genomics-based non-invasive prenatal testing for detection of fetal chromosomal aneuploidy in pregnant women. *The Cochrane database of systematic reviews, 10*(11), CD011767.

Bagni, C., Tassone, F., Neri, G., et al. (2012). Fragile X syndrome: causes, diagnosis, mechanisms, and therapeutics. *The Journal of Clinical Investigation, 122*(12), 4314–4322.

Bailey, D. B., Jr., Berry-Kravis, E., Gane, L. W., et al. (2017). Fragile X newborn screening: Lessons learned from a multisite screening study. *Pediatrics, 139*(Suppl 3), S216–S225.

Baio, J., Wiggins, L., Christensen, D. L., et al. (2018). Prevalence of autism spectrum disorder among children aged 8 years - Autism and developmental disabilities monitoring network, 11 Sites, United States, 2014. *MMWR Surveillance Summaries, 67*(6), 1–23. https://doi.org/10.15585/mmwr.ss6706a1.

Barile, J. P., Kuperminc, G. P., Weintraub, E. S., et al. (2012). Thimerosal exposure in early life and neuropsychological outcomes 7–10 years later. *The Journal of Pediatric Psychology, 37*(1), 106–118.

Bearss, K., Burrell, T. L., Stewart, L., et al. (2015). Parent training in autism spectrum disorder: What's in a name? *Clinical Child and Family Psychology Review, 18*(2), 170–182.

Becerra-Culqui, T. A., Getahun, D., Chiu, V., et al. (2018). Prenatal tetanus, diphtheria, acellular pertussis vaccination and autism spectrum disorder. *Pediatrics, 142*(3), pii:e20180120.

Bolton, P. F., Golding, J., Emond, A., et al. (2012). Autism spectrum disorder and autistic traits in the Avon Longitudinal Study of Parents and Children: precursors and early signs. *Clinical Child and Family Psychology Review, 51*(3), 249–260.

Brentani, H., Paula, C. S., Bordini, D., et al. (2013). Autism spectrum disorders: an overview on diagnosis and treatment. *Revista Brasileira de Psiquiatria, 35*(Suppl 1), S62–S72.

Bridgemohan, C. F. (2020). Autism spectrum disorder. In R. M. Kliegman, J. W. St. Geme, N. J. Blum, et al. (Eds.), *Nelson textbook of pediatrics* (21th ed). Philadelphia: Elsevier/Saunders.

Brown, H. K., Potvin, L. A., Lunsky, Y., et al. (2018). Maternal intellectual or developmental disability and newborn discharge to protective services. *Pediatrics, 142*(6).

Budimirovic, D. B., Berry-Kravis, E., Erickson, C. A., et al. (2017). Updated report on tools to measure outcomes of clinical trials in fragile X syndrome. *Journal of Neurodevelopmental Disorders, 9*, 14.

Bull, M. J., & Committee on Genetics. (2011). Health supervision for children with Down syndrome. *Pediatrics, 128*(2), 393–406.

Carroll, Y., Eichwald, J., Scinicariello, F., et al. (2017). Vital signs: Noise-induced hearing loss among adults-United States 2011-1012. *MMWR, 66*(5), 139–144.

Casanova, E. L., Gerstner, Z., Sharp, J. L., et al. (2018). Widespread genotype-phenotype correlations in intellectual disability. *Frontiers in Psychiatry, 9*, 535.

Centers for Disease Control and Prevention. (2017). Growth charts for children with Down Syndrome. Available at: http://www.cdc.gov/ncbddd/birthdefects/down syndrome/growth-charts.html. Retrieved 19 January 2019.

Centers for Disease Control and Prevention. (2018a). Hearing loss in children. Available at: https://www.cdc.gov/ncbddd/recommendations.html.

Centers for Disease Control and Prevention. (2018b). Autism Spectrum Disorder. Available at:https://www.cdc.gov/ncbddd/autism/index.html .

Chang, J., Ryou, N., Jun, H. J., Hwang, S. Y., Song, J. J., & Chae, S. W. (2016). Effect of cigarette smoking and passive smoking on hearing impairment: data from a population-based study. *PLoS One, 11*(1), e0146608.

Chawarska, K., Shic, F., Macari, S., et al. (2014). 18-month predictors of later outcomes in younger siblings of children with autism spectrum disorder: A baby siblings research consortium study. *Journal of the American Academy of Child and Adolescent Psychiatry, 53*(12), 1317–1327.

Cheng, N., Rho, J. M., & Masino, S. A. (2017). Metabolic dysfunction underlying autism spectrum disorder and potential treatment approaches. *Frontiers in Molecular Neuroscience, 10*(34).

Christensen, D. L., Baio, J., Braun, K. V., et al. (2016). Prevalence and characteristics of autism spectrum disorder among children aged 8 years—Autism and developmental disabilities monitoring network, 11 sites, United States, 2012. *MMWR Surveillance Summaries, 65*, 1–23 (No.SS-3)(No. SS-3).

Christensen, D. L., Maenner, M. J., Bilder, D., et al. (2019). Prevalence and characteristics of Autism Spectrum Disorder among children aged 4 years-Early autism and developmental disabilities monitoring network, seven sites, United States, 2010, 2012, 2014. *MMWR Surveillance Summaries, 68*(2), 1–19.

Colella-Santos, M. F., Hein, T. A., de Souza, G. L., et al. (2014). Newborn hearing screening and early diagnostic in the NICU. *Biomed Research International*, 845308.

Crnic, K. A., Neece, C. L., McIntyre, L. L., et al. (2017). Intellectual disability and developmental risk: Promoting intervention to improve child and family well-being. *Child Development, 88*(2), 436–445.

Curnow, K. J., Sanderson, R. K., & Beruti, S. (2019). Noninvasive detection of fetal aneuploidy using next generation sequencing. *Methods in Molecular Biology, 1885*, 325–345.

Davies, L. E., & Oliver, C. (2016). Self-injury, aggression and destruction in children with severe intellectual disability: Incidence, persistence and novel, predictive behavioral risk markers. *Research In Developmental Disabilities, 49–50*, 291–301.

Dedhia, K., Graham, E., & Park, A. (2018). Hearing loss and failed newborn hearing. *Clinics in Perinatology, 45*(4), 629–643.

Easwar, V., Yamazaki, H., Deighton, M., et al. (2017). Cortical representation of interaural time difference is impaired by deafness in development: Evidence from children with early long- term access to sound through bilateral cochlear implants provided simultaneously. *The Journal of Neuroscience, 37*(9), 2349–2361.

Englund, C. K., Jonsson, B., Zander, C. S., et al. (2013). Changes in mortality and causes of death in the Swedish Down syndrome population. *The American Journal of Medical Genetics, PartA, 161*, 642–649.

Fabry, D. A., Davila, E. P., Arheart, K. L., et al. (2011). Secondhand smoke exposure and the risk of hearing loss. *Tobacco Control, 20*(1), 82–85.

Feinberg, J. I., Bakulski, K. M., Jaffe, A. E., et al. (2015). Paternal sperm DNA methylation associated with early signs of autism risk in the autism-enriched cohort. *International Journal of Epidemiology, 44*(4), 1199–1210.

Fernell, E., Eriksson, M. A., & Gillberg, C. (2013). Early diagnosis of autism and impact on prognosis: a narrative review. *Clinical Epidemiology, 5*, 33–43.

Finucane, B., Lincoln, S., Bailey, L., & Martin, C. L. (2017). Prognostic dilemmas and genetic counseling for prenatally detected Fragile X gene expansions. *Prenatal Diagnosis, 37*, 37–42.

Gan, R., Rowe, A., Benton, C., et al. (2016). Management of hearing loss in children. *Paediatrics and Child Health, 26*(1), 15–20.

Gil, M. M., Accurti, V., Santacruz, B., et al. (2017). Analysis of cell-free DNA in maternal blood in screening for aneuploides: updated meta-analysis. *Ultrasound in Obstetrics & Gynecology, 50*(3), 302–314.

Gilbert, J., & Man, H. (2017). Fundamental elements in autism: From neurogenesis and neurite growth to synaptic plasticity. *Frontiers in Cellular Neuroscience, 11*, 359.

Gilissen, C., Hehir-Kwa, J., Thung, D. T., et al. (2014). Genome sequencing identifies major causes of severe intellectual disability. *Nature, 11*, 344–347.

Goel, R., Hong, J. S., Findling, R. L., et al. (2018). An update on pharmacotherapy of autism spectrum disorder in children and adolescents. *Int Rev Psychiatry, 30*(1), 78–95.

Goin-Kochel, R. P., Mire, S. S., Dempsey, A. G., et al. (2016). Parental report of vaccine receipt in children with autism spectrum disorder: Do rates differ by pattern of ASD onset? *Vaccine, 34*, 1335–1342.

Gray, K. J., & Wilkins-Haug, L. E. (2018). Have we done our last aminocentesis? Updates on cell-free DNA for Down syndrome screening. *Pediatric Radiology, 48*(4), 461–470.

Grindle, C. R. (2014). Pediatric hearing loss. *Pediatric Reviews, 35*(11), 456–463.

Guest, H., Munro, K. L., Prendergast, G., et al. (2017). Tinnitis with a normal audiogram: Relation to noise exposure but no evidence for cochlear synaptopathy. *Hearing Research, 344*, 265–274.

Guralnick, M. J. (2017). Early intervention for children with intellectual disabilities: an update. *JARID, 30*, 211–229.

Haddad, J., Dodhia, S. N., & Spitzer, J. B. (2020). Hearing loss. In R. M. Kliegman, J. W. St. Geme, N. J. Blum, et al. (Eds.), *Nelson textbook of pediatrics* (21 ed.). Philadelphia: Elsevier Inc.

Hadjkacem, I., Ayadi, H., Turki, M., et al. (2016). Prenatal, perinatal and postnatal factors associated with autism spectrum disorder. *Jornal de pediatria, 92*(6), 595–601.

Hagerman, R. J., Berry-Kravis, E., Hazlett, H. C., Bailey, D. B., Moine, H., Kooy, R. F., et al. (2017). Fragile X syndrome. *Nature Reviews Disease Primers, 3*, 17065.

Health Quality Ontario. (2018). Bilateral cochlear implantation: A health technology assessment. *Ontario Health Technology Assessment Series, 18*(6), 1–139.

Herndon, A. C., DiGuiseppi, C., Johnson, S. L., et al. (2009). Does nutritional intake differ between children and autism spectrum disorders and children with typical development? *The Journal of Autism and Developmental Disorders, 39*(2), 212–222.

Homeyard, C., Montgomery, E., Chinn, D., et al. (2016). Current evidence on antenatal care provision for women with intellectual disabilities: a systematic review. *Midwifery, 32*, 45–57.

Hopf, K. P., Madren, E., & Santianni, K. A. (2016). Use and perceived effectiveness of complementary and alternative medicine to treat and manage the symptoms of autism in children: A survey of parents in a community population. *The Journal of Alternative and Complementary Medicine, 22*(1), 25–32.

Hoyme, H. E., Kalberg, W. O., Elliot, A. J., et al. (2016). Updated clinical guidelines for diagnosing fetal alcohol spectrum disorders. *Pediatrics, 138*(2), pii:e20154256.

Hu, H., Sasaki, N., & Ogasawara, T. (2019). Smoking, smoking cessation, and the risk of hearing loss: Japan epidemiology collaboration on occupational health study. *Nicotine and Tobacco Research, 21*(4), 481–488.

Hui, L. (2019). Noninvasive approaches to prenatal diagnosis: Historical perspective and future directions. *Methods in Molecular Biology, 1885*, 45–58.

Iwarsson, E., Jacobsson, B., Dagerhamn, J., et al. (2017). Analysis of cell-free DNA in maternal blood for detection of trisomy 21,18 and 13 in a general pregnant population and in high risk population-a systemic review and meta-analysis. *Acta Obstetricia et Gynecologica Scandinavica, 96*(1), 7–18.

Joint Committee on Infant Hearing of the American Academy of Pediatrics, Muse, C., Harrison, J., et al. (2013). Supplement to the JCIH 2007 position statement: principles and guidelines for early intervention after confirmation that a child is deaf or hard of hearing. *Pediatrics, 131*(4), e1324–e1349.

Katz, G., & Lazcano-Ponce, E. (2008). Intellectual disability: definition, etiological factors, classification, diagnosis, treatment and prognosis. *Salud Pública de México, 50*(Suppl 2), S132–S141.

Kaufmann, W. E., Kidd, S. A., Andrews, H. F., et al. (2017). Autism spectrum disorder in Fragile X syndrome: Co-occurring conditions and current treatment. *Pediatrics, 139*(Suppl 3), S194–S206.

Kerub, O., Haas, E. J., Menashe, I., et al. (2018). Autism spectrum disorder: Evolution of disorder definition, risk factors and demographic characteristics in Israel. *The Israel Medical Association Journal, 20*(9), 576–581.

Kirchner, J. C., Hatri, A., Heekeren, H. R., et al. (2011). Autistic symptomatology, face processing abilities, and eye fixation patterns. *The Journal of Autism and Developmental Disorders, 41*(2), 158–167.

Korver, A. M. H., Smith, R. J. H., & Van Camp, G. (2017). Congenital hearing loss. *Nature Reviews Disease Primers, 12*(3), 16094.

Krishnaswami, S., McPheeters, M. L., & Veenstra-Vanderweele, J. (2011). A systematic review of secretin for children with autism spectrum disorders. *Pediatrics, 127*(5), e1322–e1325.

Lai, M. C., Lombardo, M. V., & Baron-Cohen, S. (2014). Autism. *Lancet, 383*(9920), 896–910.

Lammers, M. J., Jansen, T. T., Grolman, W., et al. (2015). The influence of newborn hearing screening on the age at cochlear implantation in children. *Laryngoscope, 125*(4), 985–990.

Lazaro, C. P., & Ponde, M. P. (2017). Narratives of mothers of children with autism spectrum disorders: Focus on eating behavior. *Trends in Psychiatry and Psychotherapy, 39*(3), 180–187.

Leas, D. P., Goldstein, J. A., Kellan, J. F., et al. (2017). What activity restrictions are indicated in the treatment of atlantoaxial instability (AAI)? Medscape. http://www.medscape.com/.../what-activity-restrictions-are-indicated-in-the-treatment. Accessed 19 January 2019.

Lee, A. W., Ventola, P., Budimirovic, D., et al. (2018). Clinical development of targeted Fragile X syndrome treatment: an industry perspective. *Brain Sciences, 8*(12).

Lee, B. (2020). Cytogenetics: Down syndrome and other abnormalities of chromosome number. In R. M. Kliegman, J. W. St. Geme, N. J. Blum, et al. (Eds.), *Nelson textbook of pediatrics* (21 ed.). Philadelphia: Elsevier Inc.

Lee, Y. J., Oh, S. H., Park, C., et al. (2014). Advanced pharmacology evidenced by pathogenesis of autism spectrum disorder. *Clinical Psychopharmacology and Neuroscience, 12*(1), 19–30.

Lemcke, S., Juul, S., Parner, E. T., et al. (2013). Early signs of autism in toddlers: a follow-up study in the Danish National Birth Cohort. *The Journal of Autism and Developmental Disorders, 43*(10), 2366–2375.

Ly, V., Bottelier, M., Hoekstra, P. J., et al. (2017). Elimination diet's efficacy and mechanisms in attention deficit hyperactivity disorder and autism spectrum disorder. *European Child and Adolescent Psychiatry, 26*(9), 1067–1079.

Lyra, L., Rizzo, L. E., Sunahara, C. S., et al. (2017). What do Cochrane systematic reviews say about interventions for autism spectrum disorder? *Sao Paulo Medical Journal, 135*(2), 192–201.

Mefford, H. C., Batshaw, M. L., & Hoffman, E. P. (2012). Genomics, intellectual disability, and autism. *The New England Journal of Medicine, 366*, 733–743.

Mink, J. W. (2016). Congenital, developmental, and neurocutaneous disorders: Fragile X syndrome. In M. K. Crow, J. H. Doroshow, J. M. Drazen, et al. (Eds.), *Goldman-Cecil medicine* (25 ed.). Philadelphia: Elsevier-Saunders.

Moran, M. (2013). DSM-5 provides new take on neurodevelopment disorders. *Psychiatric News, 48*(2), 6–23.

Morano, S., Ruiz, S., Hwang, J., et al. (2017). Meta-analysis of single-case treatment effects on self-injurious behavior for individuals with autism and intellectual disabilities. *Autism and Developmental Language Impairments, 2*, 1–26.

Na, S. D., & Burns, T. G. (2016). Wechsler Intelligence Scale for children-V: Test review. *Applied Neuropsychology: Child, 5*(2), 156–160.

Nath, D. (2017). Complementary and alternative medicine in the school-age child with autism. *The Journal of Pediatric Health Care, 31*(3), 393–397.

National Academies of Sciences, Engineering, and Medicine. (2015). *Mental disorders and disabilities among low-income children*. Washington, DC: The National Academies Press. https://doi.org/10.17226/21780.

National Autism Association. (2017). About autism. http://nationalautismassociation.org/resources/autism-fact-sheet/.

National Down Syndrome Society. (2019a). Early intervention. http://www.ndss.org/Resources/Therapies-Development/Early-Intervention/.

National Down Syndrome Society. (2019b). Recreation and friendship. http://www.ndss.org/Resources/Wellness/Recreation-Friendship/.

National Down Syndrome Society. (2019d). Atlantoaxial instability and Down syndrome. http://www.ndss.org/Resources/Health-Care/Associated-Conditions/Atlantoaxial-Instability-Down-Syndrome/.

National Fragile X Foundation. (2019). Fragile X disorders. https://fragilex.org.

Neumann, K., Chadha, S., & Tavartkiladze, G. (2019). Newborn and infant hearing screening facing globally growing numbers of people suffering from disabling hearing loss. *International Journal of Neonatal Screening, 5*(1), 7.

Neumeyer, A. M., Anixt, J., Chan, J., et al. (2018). Identifying associations among co-occuring medical conditions with autism spectrum disorders. *Academic Pediatrics, S1876-2859*(18)30456–X.

Ng, M., de Montigny, J. G., Ofner, M., et al. (2017). Environmental factors associated with autism spectrum disorder: A scoping review for the years 2003-2013, Health Promotion and Chronic Disease Prevention in Canada-Research. *Policy and Practice, 37*(1), 1–23.

Niu, M., Han, Y., Dy, A. B. C., et al. (2017). Autism symptoms in Fragile X syndrome. *Journal of Child Neurology, 32*(10), 903–909.

O'Hara, M. A. (2016). Instrument-based pediatric vision screening. *Current Opinion in Ophthalmology, 27*(5), 398–401.

Oono, I. P., Honey, E. J., & McConachie, H. (2013). Parent-mediated early intervention for young children with autism spectrum disorders (ASD). *The Cochrane Database of Systematic Reviews*, (4), CD009774.

Orinstein, A. J., Helt, M., Troyb, E., et al. (2014). Intervention for optimal outcome in children and adolescents with a history of autism. *The Journal of Developmental & Behavioral Pediatrics, 35*(4), 247–256.

Palomaki, G. E., & Kloza, E. M. (2018). Prenatal cell-free DNA screening test failures: A systematic review of failure rates, risk of Down syndrome and impact of repeat testing. *Genetics in Medicine, 20*(11), 1312–1323.

Panerai, S., Suraniti, G. S., Catania, V., et al. (2018). Improvements in mealtime behaviors of children with special needs following a day-center-based behavioral intervention for feeding problems. *Rivista di Psichiatria, 53*(6), 299–308.

Pawlaczyk-Luszczynska, M., Zamojska-Daniszewska, M., Dudarewicz, A., et al. (2017). Exposure to excessive sounds and hearing status in academic classical music students. *International Journal of Occupational Medicine and Environmental Health, 30*(1), 55–75.

Pearson, N., Charman, T., Happe, F., et al. (2018). Regression in autism spectrum disorder: Reconciling findings from retrospective and prospective research. *Autism Research, 11*(12), 1602–1620 2.

Pettinato, M., De Clerck, I., Verhoeven, J., et al. (2017). Expansion of prosodic abilities at the transition from babble to words: A comparison between children with cochlear implants and normally hearing children. *Ear and Hearing, 38*(4), 475–486.

Posar, A., & Visconti, P. (2016). Autism in 2016: The need for answers. *J Pediatr (Rio J), 93*(2), 111–119.

Price, C. S., Thompson, W. W., Goodson, B., et al. (2010). Prenatal and infant exposure to thimerosal from vaccines and immunoglobulins and risk of autism. *Pediatrics, 126*(4), 656–664.

Pueschel, S. M. (1999). The child with Down syndrome. In M. D. Levine, W. B. Carey, & A. C. Crocker (Eds.), *Developmental-behavioral pediatrics* (3rd ed.). Philadelphia: Saunders.

Reichow, B., Hume, K., Barton, E. E., et al. (2018). Early intensive behavioral intervention (EIBI) for young children with autism spectrum disorders (ASD). *The Cochrane database of systematic reviews, 5*, CD009260.

Riley, C., Mailick, M., Berry-Kravis, E., et al. (2017). The future of Fragile X syndrome: CDC stakeholder meeting summary. *Pediatrics, 139*(Suppl 3), S147–S152.

Riley, C., & Wheeler, A. (2017). Assessing the Fragile X syndrome newborn screening landscape. *Pediatrics, 139*(Suppl 3), S207–S215.

Rogers, G. L., & Jordan, C. O. (2013). Pediatric vision screening. *Pediatrics in Review, 34*(3), 126–133.

Sanchack, K. E., & Thomas, C. A. (2016). Autism spectrum disorder: Primary care principles. *American Family Physician, 94*(12), 972–979.

Sandin, S., Lichtenstein, P., Kuja-Holkola, R., et al. (2014). The familial risk of autism. *JAMA, 2311*(17), 1770–1777.

Shapiro, B. K., & O'Neill, M. E. (2020). Intellectual disability. In R. M. Kliegman, J. W. St. Geme, N. J. Blum, et al. (Eds.), *Nelson textbook of pediatrics* (21 ed.). Philadelphia: Elsevier/Saunders.

Shea, S. E. (2012). Intellectual disability (mental retardation). *Pediatrics in Review, 33*(3), 110–121.

Singh, V. (2015). Newborn hearing screening: Present scenario. *Indian Journal of Community Medicine, 40*(1), 62–65.

Sliwinska-Kowalska, M., & Zaborowski, K. (2017). WHO environmental noise guidelines for the European region: A systematic review on environmental noise and permanent hearing loss and tinnitus. *International Journal of Environmental Research and Public Health, 14*(10).

Solomon, M., Buaminger, N., & Rogers, S. J. (2011). Abstract reasoning and friendship in high functioning preadolescents with autism spectrum disorders. *The Journal of Autism and Developmental Disorders, 41*(1), 32–43.

Talaat, H. S., Metwaly, M. A., Khafagy, A. H., et al. (2014). Dose passive smoking induce sensorineural hearing loss in children? *International Journal of Pediatric Otorhinolaryngology, 78*(1), 46–49.

Talkowski, M. E., Minikel, E. V., & Gusella, J. F. (2014). Autism spectrum disorder genetics: Diverse genes with diverse clinical outcomes. *The Harvard Review of Psychiatry, 22*(2), 65–75.

Tassé, M. J., Luckasson, R., & Nygren, M. (2013). AAIDD proposed recommendations for ICD-11 and the condition previously known as mental retardation. *Intellectual and Developmental Disabilities, 51*(2), 127–131.

Tassone, F. (2014). Newborn screening for Fragile X syndrome. *JAMA Neurology, 71*(3), 355–359.

Taylor, L. E., Swerdfeger, A. L., & Eslick, G. D. (2014). Vaccines are not associated with autism: An evidence-based meta-analysis of case-control and cohort studies. *Vaccine, 32*(29), 3623–3629.

The New York Public Library. (2019). *Talking Book Players*. https://www.nypl.org/about/locations/heiskell/digital-player.

Tick, B., Bolton, P., Happe, F., et al. (2016). Heritability of autism spectrum disorders: A meta-analysis of twin studies. *The Journal of Child Psychology Psychiatry, 57*(5), 585–595.

Trzmiel, T., Purandare, B., Michalak, M., et al. (2019). Equine assisted activities and therapies in children with autism spectrum disorder: A systematic review and meta-analysis. *Complementary Therapies in Medicine, 42*, 104–113.

Uno, Y., Uchiyama, T., Kurosawa, M., et al. (2015). Early exposure to the combined measles-mumps-rubella vaccine and thimerosal-containing vaccines and risk of autism spectrum disorder. *Vaccine, 33*(21), 2511–2516.

US Department of Health and Human Services, Office of Disease Prevention and Health Promotion. (2015). Healthy people 2020: Vision. http://www.healthypeople.gov/2020/topics-objectives/topic/vision.

US Food and Drug Administration. (2018). Thimerosal and vaccines-FDA. http://www.fda.gov/biologicsbloodvaccines/.../vaccinesafety/ucm096228.

US Preventive Services Task Force. (2017). Vision screening for children aged 6 months to 5 years of age: US Preventive Services Task Force Recommendation statement. *JAMA, 318*(9), 836–844.

Wallander, J. L., Biasini, F. J., Thorsten, V., et al. (2014). Dose of early intervention treatment during children's first 36 months of life is associated with developmental outcomes: An observational cohort study in three low/low-middle income countries. *BMC Pediatrics, 14*, 281.

Wang, C., Hua, G., Weidong, L., et al. (2017). Prenatal, perinatal, and postnatal factors associated with autism: A meta-analysis. *Medicine (Baltimore), 96*(18), e6696.

Weijerman, M. E., & de Winter, J. P. (2010). Clinical practice: The care of children with Down syndrome. *The European Journal of Pediatrics, 169*(12), 1445–1452.

Willfors, C., Carlsson, T., Anderlid, B.-M., et al. (2017). Medical history of discordant twins and environmental etiologies of autism. *Translational Psychiatry, 7*, e1014.

Williams, K. J., Wray, J. J., & Wheeler, D. M. (2012). Intravenous secretin for autism spectrum disorder (ASD). *The Cochrane database of systematic reviews* (4), CD003495.

Willsey, A. J., & State, M. W. (2015). Autism spectrum disorders: from genes to neurobiology. *Current Opinion in Neurobiology, 30*, 92–99.

Wodka, E. L., Mathy, P., & Kalb, L. (2013). Predictors of phrase and fluent speech in children with autism and severe language delay. *Pediatrics, 131*(4), e1128–e1134.

Wong, S., Napoli, E., Krakowiak, P., et al. (2016). Role of p53, mitochondrial DNA deletions, and paternal age in autism: a case-control study. *Pediatrics, 137*(4), e20151888.

World Health Organization. (2012). Deafness and hearing loss. http://www.who.int/mediacentre/factsheets/fs300/en/.

World Health Organization. (2019). Addressing the rising prevalence of hearing loss.

Ying, G., Maguire, M., Cyert, et al. (2014). Prevalence of vision disorders by racial and ethnic group among children participating in Head Start. *Ophthalmology, 12*(3), 630–636.

Zemel, B. S., Pipan, M., Stallings, V. A., et al. (2015). Growth charts for children with Down syndrome in the United States. *Pediatrics, 136*(5), e1204–1211.

Zerbo, O., Qian, Y., Yoshida, C., et al. (2017). Association between influenza and vaccination during pregnancy and risk of autism spectrum disorder. *JAMA Pediatrics, 171*(1), e163609.

Zwaigenbaum, L., Bauman, M. L., Stone, W. L., et al. (2015). Early identification of autism spectrum disorder: Recommendations for practice and research. *Pediatrics, 136*, S10–S40.

19

Family-Centered Care of the Child During Illness and Hospitalization

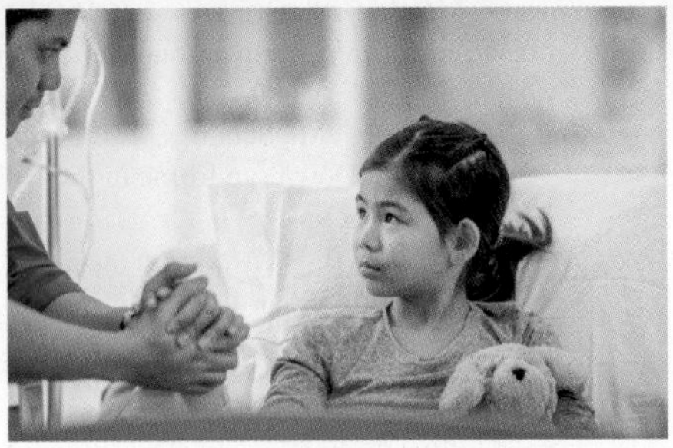

Tara Taneski Merck, Patricia McElfresh

http://evolve.elsevier.com/wong/essentials

CONCEPTS

- Stress
- Coping
- Communications
- Family-Centered Care

STRESSORS OF HOSPITALIZATION AND CHILDREN'S REACTIONS

Often illness and hospitalization are the first crises children must face. Especially during the early years, children are particularly vulnerable to these stressors because stress represents a change from the usual state of health and environmental routine, and children have a limited number of coping mechanisms to resolve **stressors**. Major stressors of hospitalization include separation, loss of control, bodily injury, and pain. Children's reactions to these crises are influenced by their developmental age; their previous experience with illness, separation, or hospitalization; their innate and acquired coping skills; the seriousness of the diagnosis; and the support system available. Children also expressed fears caused by the unfamiliar environment or lack of information; child-staff relations; and the physical, social, and symbolic environment (Samela, Salanterä, & Aronen, 2009).

SEPARATION ANXIETY

The major stress from middle infancy throughout the preschool years, especially for children ages 6 to 30 months, is separation anxiety, also called **anaclitic depression**. The principal behavioral responses to this stressor during early childhood are summarized in Box 19.1. During the stage of **protest**, children react aggressively to the separation from the parent. They cry and scream for their parents, refuse the attention of anyone else, and are inconsolable in their grief (Fig. 19.1). In contrast, through the stage of **despair**, the crying stops, and depression is evident. The child is much less active, is uninterested in play or food, and withdraws from others (Fig. 19.2).

The third stage is **detachment**, also called **denial**. Superficially, it appears that the child has finally adjusted to the loss. The child becomes more interested in the surroundings, plays with others, and seems to form new relationships. However, this behavior is the result of resignation and is not a sign of contentment. The child detaches from the parent in an effort to escape the emotional pain of desiring the parent's presence and copes by forming shallow relationships with others, becoming increasingly self-centered, and attaching primary importance to material objects. This is the most serious stage in that reversal of the potential adverse effects is less likely to occur after detachment is established. In most situations, the temporary separations imposed by hospitalization do not cause such prolonged parental absences that the child enters the detachment stage. In addition, considerable evidence suggests that even with stressors (such as separation) children are remarkably adaptable, and permanent ill effects are rare.

Although progression to the stage of detachment is uncommon, the initial stages are frequently observed even with brief separations from either parent. Unless health team members understand the meaning of each stage of behavior, they may erroneously label the behaviors as positive or negative. For example, they may see the loud crying of the protest phase as "bad" behavior. Because the protests increase when a stranger approaches the child, they may interpret that reaction as meaning that they should stay away. During the quiet, withdrawn phase of despair, health team members may think that the child is finally "settling in" to the new surroundings, and they may see the detachment behaviors as proof of a "good adjustment." The faster this stage is reached, the more likely it is that the child will be regarded as the "ideal patient."

Because children seem to react "negatively" to visits by their parents, uninformed observers feel justified in restricting parental visiting privileges. For example, during the protest stage, children outwardly do not appear happy to see their parents (Fig. 19.3). In fact, they may even cry louder. If they are depressed, they may reject their parents or begin to protest again. Often they cling to their parents in an effort to ensure their continued presence. Consequently, such reactions may be regarded as "disturbing" the child's adjustment to the new surroundings. If the separation has progressed to the phase of detachment, children will respond no differently to their parents than they would to any other person.

Such reactions are distressing to parents, who are unaware of their meaning. If parents are regarded as intruders, they will see their absence as "beneficial" to the child's adjustment and recovery. They may respond to the child's behavior by staying for only short periods, visiting less frequently, or deceiving the child when it is time to leave. The result is a destructive cycle of misunderstanding and unmet needs.

BOX 19.1 Manifestations of Separation Anxiety in Young Children

Stage of Protest

Behaviors observed during later infancy include:

- Cries
- Screams
- Searches for parent with eyes
- Clings to parent
- Avoids and rejects contact with strangers

Additional behaviors observed during toddlerhood include:

- Verbally attacks strangers (e.g., "Go away")
- Physically attacks strangers (e.g., kicks, bites, hits, pinches)
- Attempts to escape to find parent
- Attempts to physically force parent to stay

Behaviors may last from hours to days.

Protest, such as crying, may be continuous, ceasing only with physical exhaustion.

Approach of a stranger may precipitate increased protest.

Stage of Despair

Observed behaviors include:

- Is inactive
- Withdraws from others
- Is depressed, sad
- Lacks interest in environment
- Is uncommunicative
- Regresses to earlier behavior (e.g., thumb sucking, bedwetting, use of pacifier, use of bottle)

Behaviors may last for variable length of time.

Child's physical condition may deteriorate from refusal to eat, drink, or move.

Stage of Detachment

Observed behaviors include:

- Shows increased interest in surroundings
- Interacts with strangers or familiar caregivers
- Forms new but superficial relationships
- Appears happy

Detachment usually occurs after prolonged separation from parent; it is rarely seen in hospitalized children.

Behaviors represent a superficial adjustment to loss.

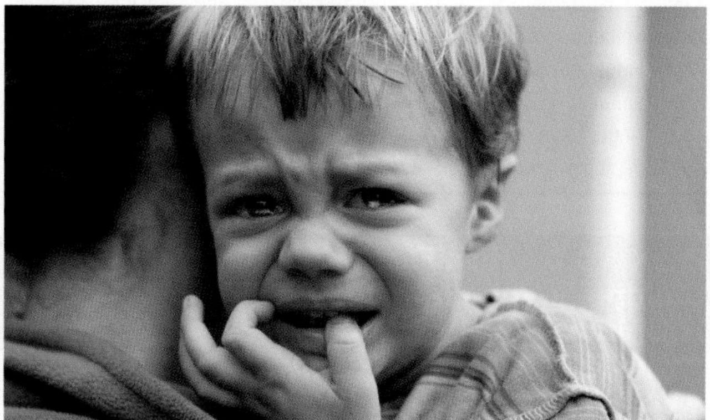

Fig. 19.1 In the protest phase of separation anxiety, children cry loudly and are inconsolable in their grief for the parent. (© 2015 iStock.com.)

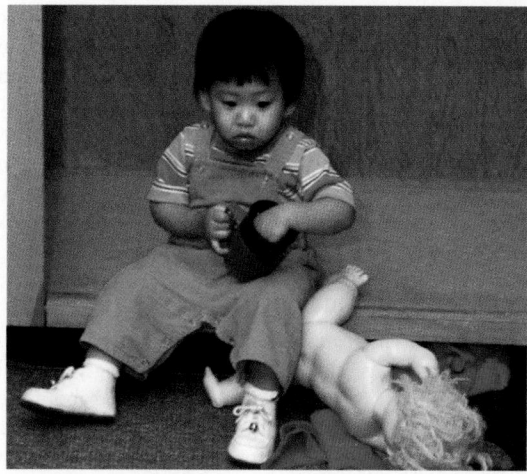

Fig. 19.2 During the despair phase of separation anxiety, children are sad, lonely, and uninterested in food and play.

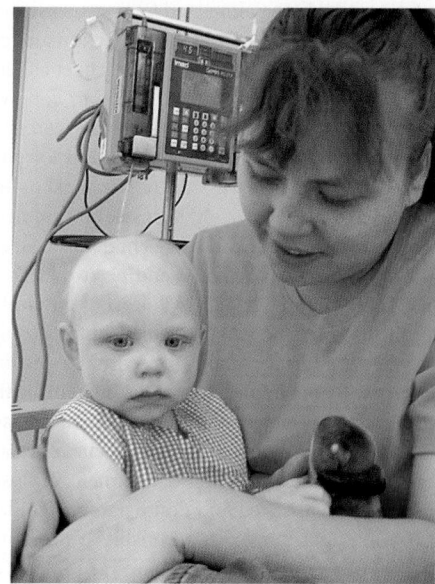

Fig. 19.3 Young children may appear withdrawn and sad even in the presence of a parent. (Courtesy E. Jacob, Texas Children's Hospital, Houston, TX.)

Early Childhood

Separation anxiety is the greatest stress imposed by hospitalization during early childhood. If separation is avoided, young children have a tremendous capacity to withstand any other stress. During this age period, the typical reactions just described are seen. Children in the toddler stage demonstrate more goal-directed behaviors. For example, they may plead with the parents to stay and physically try to keep the parents with them or try to find parents who have left. The child may demonstrate displeasure on the parents' return or departure by having temper tantrums; refusing to comply with the usual routines of mealtime, bedtime, or toileting; or regressing to more primitive levels of development. Temper tantrums, bedwetting, or other behaviors exhibited by children may also be expressions of anger, a physiologic response to stress, or symptoms of illness.

Because preschoolers are more secure interpersonally than toddlers, they can tolerate brief periods of separation from their parents and are more inclined to develop substitute trust in other significant adults. The stress of illness usually renders preschoolers less able to cope with separation; as a result, they manifest many of the stage behaviors of separation anxiety. In general, the protest behaviors are more subtle and passive than those seen in younger children. Preschoolers may demonstrate separation anxiety by refusing to eat, having trouble sleeping, crying quietly for their parents, continually asking when the parents will visit, or withdrawing from others. They may express anger indirectly by breaking toys, hitting other children, or refusing to cooperate during usual self-care activities. Nurses need to be sensitive to these less obvious signs of separation anxiety in order to intervene appropriately.

Later Childhood and Adolescence

Previous research has indicated that the family does not play as important a role for school-age children as it does during the toddler and preschool years. In a prior study, children were asked about their fears when hospitalized, and children listed their greatest fears regarding hospitalization as being separated from family and friends, being in an unfamiliar environment, receiving investigations or treatments, and losing self-determination or choices (Coyne, 2006). In a qualitative study of children 5 to 9 years old, children described hospitalization in stories that focused on being alone and feeling scared, angry, or sad. These children also described the need for protection and companionship while hospitalized (Wilson, Megel, Enenbach, et al., 2010).

Although school-age children are better able to cope with separation in general, the stress and often accompanying regression imposed by illness or hospitalization may increase their need for parental security and guidance. This is particularly true for young school-age children who have only recently left the safety of the home and are struggling with the crisis of school adjustment. School-age children may react more to the separation from their usual activities and peers than to the absence of their parents. These children have a high level of physical and mental activity that frequently finds no suitable outlets in the hospital environment, and even when they dislike school, they admit to missing its routine and worry that they will not be able to compete or "fit in" with their classmates when they return. Feelings of loneliness, boredom, isolation, and depression are common. Such reactions may occur more as a result of separation than of concern over the illness, treatment, or hospital setting.

School-age children may need and desire parental guidance or support from other adult figures but may be unable or unwilling to ask for it. Because the goal of attaining independence is so important to them, they are reluctant to seek help directly, fearing that they will appear weak, childish, or dependent. Cultural expectations to "act like a man" or to "be brave and strong" weigh heavily on these children, especially boys, who tend to react to stress with stoicism, withdrawal, or passive acceptance. Often the need to express hostile, angry, or other negative feelings finds outlets in alternate ways, such as irritability and aggression toward parents, withdrawal from hospital personnel, inability to relate to peers, rejection of siblings, or subsequent behavioral problems in school.

For adolescents, separation from home and parents may produce varied emotions, ranging from difficulty coping to welcoming the event. Loss of peer-group contact may pose a severe emotional threat because of loss of group status, inability to exert group control or leadership, and loss of group acceptance. Deviations within peer groups are poorly tolerated, and although group members may express concern for the adolescent's illness or need for hospitalization, they continue their group activities, quickly filling the gap of the absent member. During the temporary separation from their usual group, ill adolescents may benefit from group associations with other hospitalized teens.

LOSS OF CONTROL

One of the factors influencing the amount of stress imposed by hospitalization is the amount of control a person perceives he or she possesses. Lack of control increases the perception of threat and can affect children's coping skills. Many hospital situations decrease the amount of control a child feels. Although the usual sensory stimulations are lacking, the additional hospital stimuli of sight, sound, and smell may be overwhelming. Without an insight into the type of environment conducive to children's optimal growth, the hospital experience can at best temporarily slow development and at worst permanently restrict it. Because children's needs vary greatly depending on their age, the major areas of loss of control in terms of physical restriction, altered routine or rituals, and dependency are discussed for each age-group.

EFFECTS OF HOSPITALIZATION ON THE CHILD

Children may react to the stressors of hospitalization before admission, during hospitalization, and after discharge. A child's concept of illness is even more important than age and intellectual maturity in predicting the level of anxiety before hospitalization (Clatworthy, Simon, & Tiedeman, 1999). This may or may not be affected by the duration of the condition or prior hospitalizations; therefore nurses should avoid overestimating the illness concepts of children with prior medical experience (Box 19.2).

Individual Risk Factors

A number of risk factors make certain children more vulnerable than others to the stresses of hospitalization (Box 19.3). Rural children

BOX 19.2 Post-Hospital Behaviors in Children

Young Children

They show initial aloofness toward parents; this may last from a few minutes (most common) to a few days.

This is frequently followed by dependency behaviors:

- Tendency to cling to parents
- Demands for parents' attention
- Vigorous opposition to any separation (e.g., staying at preschool or with a babysitter)

Other negative behaviors include:

- New fears (e.g., nightmares)
- Resistance to going to bed, night waking
- Withdrawal and shyness
- Hyperactivity
- Temper tantrums
- Food peculiarities
- Attachment to blanket or toy
- Regression in newly learned skills (e.g., self-toileting)

Older Children

Negative behaviors include:

- Emotional coldness followed by intense, demanding dependence on parents
- Anger toward parents
- Jealousy toward others (e.g., siblings)

BOX 19.3 Risk Factors That Increase Children's Vulnerability to the Stressors of Hospitalization

"Difficult" temperament
Lack of fit between child and parent
Age (especially between 6 months old and 5 years old)
Male gender
Below-average intelligence
Multiple and continuing stresses (e.g., frequent hospitalizations)

may exhibit significantly greater degrees of psychologic upset than urban children, possibly because urban children have opportunities to become familiar with a local hospital. Because separation is such an important issue surrounding hospitalization for young children, children who are active and strong willed tend to fare better when hospitalized than youngsters who are passive. Consequently, nurses should be alert to children who passively accept all changes and requests; these children may need more support than "oppositional" children.

The stressors of hospitalization may cause young children to experience short- and long-term negative outcomes. Adverse outcomes may be related to the length and number of admissions, multiple invasive procedures, and the parents' anxiety. Common responses include regression, separation anxiety, apathy, fears, and sleeping disturbances, especially for children younger than 7 years old (Melnyk, 2000). Supportive practices, such as family-centered care and frequent family visiting, may lessen the detrimental effects of such admissions. Nurses should attempt to identify children at risk for poor coping strategies (Small, 2002).

Changes in the Pediatric Population

The pediatric population in hospitals has changed dramatically over the past 2 decades. With a growing trend toward shortened hospital stays and outpatient surgery, a greater percentage of the children hospitalized today have more serious and complex problems than those hospitalized in the past. Many of these children are fragile newborns and children with severe injuries or disabilities who have survived because of major technologic advances and have been left with chronic or disabling conditions that require frequent and lengthy hospital stays. The nature of their conditions increases the likelihood that they will experience more invasive and traumatic procedures while they are hospitalized. These factors make them more vulnerable to the emotional consequences of hospitalization and result in their needs being significantly different from those of the short-term patients of the past (see Chapter 18 for further discussion on children with special needs). Most of these children are infants and toddlers, which is the age-group most vulnerable to the effects of hospitalization.

Concern in recent years has focused on the increasing length of hospitalization because of complex medical and nursing care, elusive diagnoses, and complicated psychosocial issues. Without special attention devoted to meeting children's psychosocial and developmental needs in the hospital environment, the detrimental consequences of prolonged hospitalization may be severe.

Beneficial Effects of Hospitalization

Although hospitalization can be and usually is stressful for children, it can also be beneficial. The most obvious benefit is the recovery from illness, but hospitalization also can present an opportunity for children to master stress and feel competent in their coping abilities. The hospital environment can provide children with new socialization experiences that can broaden their interpersonal relationships. The psychologic benefits need to be considered and maximized during hospitalization. Appropriate nursing strategies to achieve this goal are presented later in the chapter.

STRESSORS AND REACTIONS OF THE FAMILY OF THE CHILD WHO IS HOSPITALIZED

PARENTAL REACTIONS

The crisis of childhood illness and hospitalization affects every member of the family. Parents' reactions to illness in their child depend on a variety of factors. Although one cannot predict which factors are most likely to influence their response, several variables have been identified (Box 19.4). (See also Chapter 17.)

BOX 19.4 Factors Affecting Parents' Reactions to Their Child's Illness

- Seriousness of the threat to the child
- Previous experience with illness or hospitalization
- Medical procedures involved in diagnosis and treatment
- Available support systems
- Personal ego strengths
- Previous coping abilities
- Additional stresses on the family system
- Cultural and religious beliefs
- Communication patterns among family members

Recent research has identified common themes among parents whose children were hospitalized. These include feelings of an overall sense of helplessness, questioning the skills of staff, accepting the reality of hospitalization, needing to have information explained in simple language, dealing with fear, coping with uncertainty, and seeking reassurance from caregivers. Reassurance from the health care team can be in the form of collaboration, information sharing, preparation for procedures, ensuring formal and informal support for the family, and providing information in an unbiased and culturally sensitive manner (Eichner & Johnson, 2012).

SIBLING REACTIONS

Siblings' reactions to a sister's or brother's illness or hospitalization are discussed in Chapter 17 and differ little when a child becomes temporarily ill. Siblings experience loneliness, fear, and worry, as well as anger, resentment, jealousy, and guilt. Illness may also result in children's loss of status within either their family or their social group. Various factors that influence the effects of the child's hospitalization on siblings have been identified. Recently, it has been found that parents of siblings of children with chronic illness tended to rate sibling health-related quality of life better than the siblings' self-reports, and greater disease severity of the affected child and older sibling age may be risk factors for impaired well sibling quality of life (Limbers & Skipper, 2014). Although these factors are similar to those seen when a child has a chronic illness, Craft (1993) reported that the following factors regarding siblings are related specifically to the hospital experience and increase the effects on the sibling:

- Being younger and experiencing many changes
- Being cared for outside the home by care providers who are not relatives
- Receiving little information about their ill brother or sister
- Perceiving that their parents treat them differently compared with before their sibling's hospitalization

Parents are often unaware of the number of effects that siblings experience during the sick child's hospitalization and the benefit of simple interventions to minimize such effects, such as explicit explanations about the illness and provisions for the siblings to remain at home. Sibling visitation is usually beneficial to the patient, sibling, and parent but should be evaluated on an individual basis. Siblings should be prepared for the visit with developmentally appropriate information and be given the opportunity to ask questions.

NURSING CARE OF THE CHILD WHO IS HOSPITALIZED

PREPARATION FOR HOSPITALIZATION

Children and families require individualized care to minimize the potential negative effects of hospitalization. One method that can decrease negative feelings and fear in children is preparation for hospitalization. The rationale for preparing children for the hospital experience and related procedures is based on the principle that fear of the unknown exceeds fear of the known. When children do not have paralyzing fear to cope with, they are able to direct their energies toward dealing with the other, unavoidable stresses of hospitalization.

Although preparation for hospitalization is a common practice, there is no universal standard or program for all settings. The preparation process may be elaborate, with tours, puppet shows, and playtime with miniature hospital equipment; it may involve the use of books, videos, or films; or it may be limited to a brief description of the major aspects of any hospital stay. No consensus exists on the timing of preparation. Some authorities recommend preparing children 4 to 7 years old about 1 week in advance so that they can assimilate the information and ask questions. For older children, the time may be longer. For young children, who may be unsure about what they observed, 1 or 2 days before admission is sufficient for anticipatory preparation. The length of the session should be tailored to the children's attention span—the younger the child, the shorter the program. The optimal approach is one that is individualized for each child and family.

Regardless of the specific type of program, all children, even those who have been hospitalized previously, benefit from an introduction to the environment and routine of the unit. Sometimes it is not possible to prepare children and families for hospitalization, such as in the event of sudden, acute illness. Care should be taken to orient the child and family to hospital routines, establish expectations, and allow for questions (Abraham & Moretz, 2012).

NURSING TIP: In many hospitals, child life specialists—health care professionals with extensive knowledge of child growth and development and of the special psychosocial needs of children who are hospitalized and their families—help prepare children for hospitalization, surgery, and procedures. Although the structure of a program may vary depending on the size of the pediatric facility, the patient population, and the availability of ancillary services, the two primary program objectives for child life specialists are consistent: (1) to reduce the stress and anxiety related to the hospitalization or health care–related experiences and (2) to promote normal growth and development in the health care setting and at home (Thompson, 2009).

A collaborative effort between the nurse, child life specialist, and other members of the child's health care team helps ensure the best possible hospital experience for the child and family.

Admission Assessment

The nursing admission history refers to a systematic collection of data about the child and family that allows the nurse to plan individualized care. The nursing admission history presented in Box 19.5

BOX 19.5 Nursing Admission History According to Functional Health Patterns[a]

Health Perception/Health Management Pattern

Why has your child been admitted?

How has your child's general health been?

What does your child know about this hospitalization?

- Ask the child why he or she came to the hospital.
- If the answer is "For an operation or for tests," ask the child to tell you about what will happen before, during, and after the operation or tests.

Has your child ever been in the hospital before?

- How was that hospital experience?
- What things were important to you and your child during that hospitalization? How can we be most helpful now?

What medications does your child take at home?

- Why are they given?
- When are they given?
- How are they given (if a liquid, with a spoon; if a tablet, swallowed with water; or other)?
- Does your child have any trouble taking medication? If so, what helps?
- Is your child allergic to any medications?

What, if any, forms of complementary medicine practices are being used?

Nutrition/Metabolic Pattern

What is the family's usual mealtime?

Do family members eat together or at separate times?

What are your child's favorite foods, beverages, and snacks?

- Average amounts consumed or usual size of portions
- Special cultural practices, such as family eats only ethnic food

What foods and beverages does your child dislike?

What are your child's feeding habits (bottle, cup, spoon, eats by self, needs assistance, any special devices)?

How does your child like the food served (warmed, cold, one item at a time)?

How would you describe your child's usual appetite (hearty eater, picky eater)?

- Has being sick affected your child's appetite? In what ways?

Are there any known or suspected food allergies?

Is your child on a special diet?

Are there any feeding problems (excessive fussiness, spitting up, colic); any dental or gum problems that affect feeding?

- What do you do for these problems?

Elimination Pattern

What are your child's toileting habits (diaper, toilet trained—day only or day and night, use of word to communicate urination or defecation, potty chair, regular toilet, other routines)?

What is your child's usual pattern of elimination (bowel movements)?

Do you have any concerns about elimination (bedwetting, constipation, diarrhea)?

- What do you do for these problems?

Have you ever noticed that your child sweats a lot?

Sleep/Rest Pattern

What is your child's usual hour of sleep and awakening?

What is your child's schedule for naps; length of naps?

Is there a special routine before sleeping (bottle, drink of water, bedtime story, night-light, favorite blanket or toy, prayers)?

Is there a special routine during sleep time, such as waking to go to the bathroom?

What type of bed does your child sleep in?

Does your child have a separate room or share a room; if shares, with whom?

Does your child sleep with someone or alone (e.g., sibling, parent, other person)?

What is your child's favorite sleeping position?

Are there any sleeping problems (falling asleep, waking during night, nightmares, sleep walking)?

Are there any problems in awakening and getting ready in the morning?

- What do you do for these problems?

BOX 19.5 Nursing Admission History According to Functional Health Patterns—cont'd

Activity/Exercise Pattern

What is your child's schedule during the day (preschool, daycare center, regular school, extracurricular activities)?

What are your child's favorite activities or toys (both active and quiet interests)?

What is your child's usual television-viewing schedule at home?

What are your child's favorite programs?

Are there any television restrictions?

Does your child have any illness or disabilities that limit activity? If so, how?

What are your child's usual habits and schedule for bathing (bath in tub or shower, sponge bath, shampoo)?

What are your child's dental habits (brushing, flossing, fluoride supplements or rinses, favorite toothpaste); schedule of daily dental care?

Does your child need help with dressing or grooming, such as hair combing?

Are there any problems with these patterns (dislike of or refusal to bathe, shampoo hair, or brush teeth)?

- What do you do for these problems?

Are there special devices that your child requires help in managing (eyeglasses, contact lenses, hearing aid, orthodontic appliances, artificial elimination appliances, orthopedic devices)?

Note: Use the following code to assess functional self-care level for feeding, bathing and hygiene, dressing and grooming, toileting:

0: Full self-care
I: Requires use of equipment or device
II: Requires assistance or supervision from another person
III: Requires assistance or supervision from another person and equipment or device
IV: Is totally dependent and does not participate

Cognitive/Perceptual Pattern

Does your child have any hearing difficulty?

- Does the child use a hearing aid?
- Have "tubes" been placed in your child's ears?

Does your child have any vision problems?

- Does the child wear glasses or contact lenses?

Does your child have any learning difficulties?

What is the child's grade in school?

For information on pain, see Chapter 5.

Self-Perception/Self-Concept Pattern

How would you describe your child (e.g., takes time to adjust, settles in easily, shy, friendly, quiet, talkative, serious, playful, stubborn, easygoing)?

What makes your child angry, annoyed, anxious, or sad? What helps?

How does your child act when annoyed or upset?

What have been your child's experiences with and reactions to temporary separation from you (parent)?

Does your child have any fears (places, objects, animals, people, situations)?

- How do you handle them?

Do you think your child's illness has changed the way he or she thinks about himself or herself (e.g., more shy, embarrassed about appearance, less competitive with friends, stays at home more)?

Role/Relationship Pattern

Does your child have a favorite nickname?

What are the names of other family members or others who live in the home (relatives, friends, pets)?

Who usually takes care of your child during the day and night (especially if other than parent, such as babysitter, relative)?

What are the parents' occupations and work schedules?

Are there any special family considerations (adoption, foster child, stepparent, divorce, single parent)?

Have any major changes in the family occurred lately (death, divorce, separation, birth of a sibling, loss of a job, financial strain, mother beginning a career, other)? Describe child's reaction.

Who are your child's play companions or social groups (peers, younger or older children, adults, or prefers to be alone)?

Do things generally go well for your child in school or with friends?

Does your child have "security" objects at home (pacifier, bottle, blanket, stuffed animal or doll)? Did you bring any of these to the hospital?

How do you handle discipline problems at home? Are these methods always effective?

Does your child have any condition that interferes with communication? If so, what are your suggestions for communicating with your child?

Will your child's hospitalization affect the family's financial support or care of other family members (e.g., other children)?

What concerns do you have about your child's illness and hospitalization?

Who will be staying with your child while hospitalized?

How can we contact you or another close family member outside of the hospital?

Sexuality/Reproductive Pattern

(Answer questions that apply to your child's age-group.)

Has your child begun puberty (developing physical sexual characteristics, menstruation)? Have you or your child had any concerns?

Does your daughter know how to do breast self-examination?

Does your son know how to do testicular self-examination?

How have you approached topics of sexuality with your child?

Do you think you might need some help with some topics?

Has your child's illness affected the way he or she feels about being a boy or a girl? If so, how?

Do you have any concerns with behaviors in your child, such as masturbation, asking many questions or talking about sex, not respecting others' privacy, or wanting too much privacy?

Initiate a conversation about an adolescent's sexual concerns with open-ended to more direct questions and using the terms *friends* or *partners* rather than *girlfriend* or *boyfriend:*

- Tell me about your social life.
- Who are your closest friends? (If one friend is identified, could ask more about that relationship, such as how much time they spend together, how serious they are about each other, if the relationship is going the way the teenager hoped.)
- Might ask about dating and sexual issues, such as the teenager's views on sexuality education, "going steady," "living together," or premarital sex.
- Which friends would you like to have visit in the hospital?

Coping/Stress Tolerance Pattern

(Answer questions that apply to your child's age-group.)

What does your child do when tired or upset?

- If upset, does your child want a special person or object?
- If so, explain.

If your child has temper tantrums, what causes them, and how do you handle them?

Whom does your child talk to when worried about something?

How does your child usually handle problems or disappointments?

Have there been any big changes or problems in your family recently? If so, how have you handled them?

Has your child ever had a problem with drugs or alcohol or tried to commit suicide?

Do you think your child is "accident prone?" If so, explain.

Value/Belief Pattern

What is your religion?

How is religion or faith important in your child's life?

What religious practices would you like continued in the hospital (e.g., prayers before meals or bedtime; visit by minister, priest, or rabbi; prayer group)?

[a]The focus of the admission history is the child's psychosocial environment. Most of the questions are worded in terms of parental responses. Depending on the child's age, they should be addressed directly to the child when appropriate.

BOX 19.6 Complementary Medicine Practices and Examples

Nutrition, diet, and lifestyle or behavioral health changes: Macrobiotics, megavitamins, diets, lifestyle modification, health risk reduction and health education, wellness
Mind-body control therapies: Biofeedback, relaxation, prayer therapy, guided imagery, hypnotherapy, music or sound therapy, massage, aromatherapy, education therapy
Traditional and ethnomedicine therapies: Acupuncture, Ayurvedic medicine, herbal medicine, homeopathic medicine, American Indian medicine, natural products, traditional Asian medicine
Structural manipulation and energetic therapies: Acupressure, chiropractic medicine, massage, reflexology, therapeutic touch, Qigong
Pharmacologic and biologic therapies: Antioxidants, cell treatment, chelation therapy, metabolic therapy, oxidizing agents
Bioelectromagnetic therapies: Diagnostic and therapeutic application of electromagnetic fields (e.g., transcranial electrostimulation, neuromagnetic stimulation, electroacupuncture)

is organized according to the functional health patterns outlined by Gordon (2002) (see Chapter 1, Diagnosis). This assessment framework is a guideline for formulating nursing diagnoses. One of the main purposes of the history is to assess the child's usual health habits at home to promote a more normal environment in the hospital. Questions related to activities of daily living in the nutritional/metabolic, elimination, sleep/rest, and activity/exercise patterns are a major part of the assessment. The questions found under the health perception/health management pattern are directed toward evaluation of the child's preparation for hospitalization and are key factors in determining whether additional preparation is needed. The questions included in the self-perception/self-concept and role/relationship patterns offer insight into the child's potential reaction to hospitalization, especially in terms of separation.

The nurse should also inquire about the use of any medications at home, including complementary medicine practices (Box 19.6). In a study of children with cancer, 42% had used alternative or complementary therapies simultaneously with or after conventional treatments (Fernandez, Pyesmany, & Stutzer, 1999). It is important that the use of any herbal or complementary therapy be noted in a preoperative assessment because of possible anesthesia or surgical complications related to herbal products (Flanagan, 2001) (see Critical Thinking Case Study box).

In addition to completing the nursing admission history, nurses should also perform a physical assessment (see Chapter 4) before planning care. At the very least, the nurse's physical assessment of the child should include observation of the body for any bruises, rashes, signs of neglect, deformities, or physical limitations. The nurse should also listen to the heart and lungs to assess overall physical status. For example, it is impossible to evaluate improvement in respiratory function in a child admitted with pulmonary disease unless there are baseline data with which to compare subsequent findings.

Preparing the Child for Admission

The preparation that children require on the day of admission depends on the kind of pre-hospital counseling they have received. If they have been prepared in a formalized program, they usually know what to expect in terms of initial medical procedures, inpatient facilities, and nursing staff. Pre-hospital counseling does not preclude the need for support during procedures, such as obtaining blood specimens, x-ray tests, or physical examination. For example, undressing young

CRITICAL THINKING CASE STUDY

Complementary and Alternative Medicine

Maria, a 13-year-old Hispanic girl, has had severe nosebleeds. She is admitted to the hospital for a complete workup in an attempt to determine the cause. Her parents and grandparents have gathered around her bed. When you enter her room to begin admitting procedures, you notice an unusual scent. Maria's mother is rubbing the contents from an unfamiliar bottle of liquid on Maria. Meanwhile, the grandmother is rubbing Maria's head. She is startled at your entry and drops something on the floor near your feet. You bend over to pick it up and discover that it is a penny.

Initial Assessment. Is there an external cause for the nosebleeds?

Expected Nursing Action. Determine what interventions are appropriate to use in patients with nosebleeds. Has the family used alternative methods to treat Maria's nosebleeds and why?

Teaching Points

- Most epistaxis in children is minor and is easily managed with direct compression of both nostrils at the bottom of the nose (cartilaginous area) for 5 to 10 minutes.
- In patients with marked nasal hemorrhage, rapid assessment and stabilization is followed immediately by attempts to identify the source of bleeding and initiation of measures to control it.
- Alternative medications are not recommended for the treatment of acute epistaxis, as these medications may have adverse effects such as delayed clotting and/or prolonged bleeding.
- Begin discussions of ethnic or folk remedies in the family's health care practice.

Critical Thinking Answers

Initial Assessment. Maria is experiencing acute epistaxis based on the history and exam.

Expected Nursing Action. Continue to apply pressure for at least 5 minutes while attempting to identify the source of the bleeding. The mother should not administer any alternative medications, including the topical liquid.

children before they feel comfortable in their new surroundings can be upsetting. Causing needless anxiety and fear during admission may adversely affect the nurse's establishment of trust with these children. Nursing assistance during the admission procedure is vital regardless of how well prepared any child is for the experience of hospitalization. In addition, spending this time with the child gives the nurse an opportunity to evaluate the child's understanding of subsequent procedures (Fig. 19.4). Ideally, a primary nurse is assigned whenever possible to allow for individualized care and to provide a substitute support person for the child.

When a child is admitted, nurses follow several universal admission procedures (Box 19.7). The minimum considerations for room assignment are age, sex, and nature of the illness. No absolute rules govern room selection, but in general, placing children of the same age-group and with similar types of illness in the same unit is both psychologically and medically advantageous. There may be exceptions; for example, a child in traction may be therapeutic for another child confined to bed because of a serious illness. A child who is independent despite physical disabilities may help another child with similar or different limitations, and the parents of the child with disabilities may achieve deeper insight into and acceptance of their child's disorder.

Age grouping is especially important for adolescents. Many hospitals try to place teenagers on their own unit or in a separate designated section of the pediatric or general unit whenever possible.

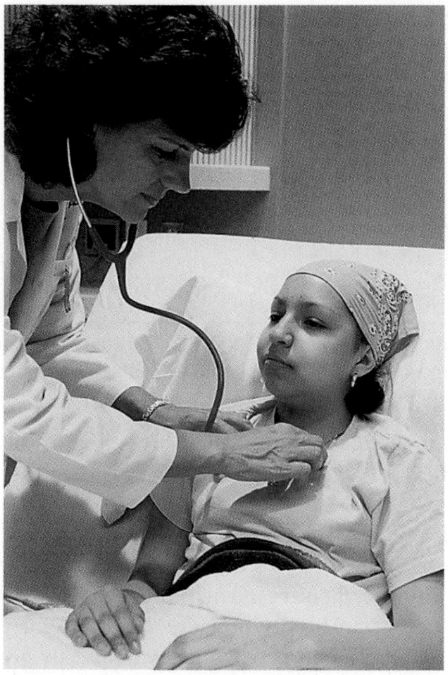

Fig. 19.4 The initial admission procedures give the nurse an opportunity to get to know the child and to assess the child's understanding of the hospital experience.

BOX 19.7 Guidelines for Admission

Preadmission

Assign a room based on developmental age, seriousness of diagnosis, communicability of illness, and projected length of stay.

Prepare roommate(s) for the arrival of a new patient; when children are too young to benefit from this consideration, prepare parents.

Prepare room for child and family, with admission forms and equipment nearby to eliminate need to leave child.

Admission

Introduce primary nurse to child and family.

Orient child and family to inpatient facilities, especially to assigned room and unit; emphasize positive areas of pediatric unit.

Room: Explain call light, bed controls, television, bathroom, telephone, and so on.

Unit: Direct to playroom, desk, dining area, or other areas.

Introduce family to roommate and his or her parents.

Apply identification band to child's wrist, ankle, or both (if not already done).

Explain hospital regulations and schedules (e.g., visiting hours, mealtimes, bedtime, limitations [give written information if available]).

Perform nursing admission history (see Box 19.5).

Take vital signs, blood pressure, height, and weight.

Obtain specimens as needed and order needed laboratory work.

Support child and assist practitioner with physical examination (for purposes of nursing assessment).

NURSING INTERVENTIONS

Preventing or Minimizing Separation

A primary nursing goal is to prevent separation, particularly in children younger than 5 years old. Many hospitals have developed a system of **family-centered care**. This philosophy of care recognizes the integral role of the family in a child's life and acknowledges the family as an essential part of the child's care and illness experience. The family is considered a partner in the care of the child (Smith & Conant Rees, 2000). Family-centered care also supports the family by establishing priorities based on the needs and values of the family unit (Lewandowski & Tesler, 2003). Efforts to collaborate with families and encourage their involvement in the patient's care include optimizing family visitation, family-centered rounding, family presence during procedures or interventions, and opportunities for formal and informal family conferences (Meert, Clark, & Eggly, 2013). Historically, hospitals have had restrictive visiting policies. Family-centered care started in pediatrics with the increased recognition of child and family separation trauma in the inpatient setting. Policies were adapted first in pediatrics to allow for rooming-in, longer visiting hours, sibling visits, and systems to allow families to accompany patients off the unit for procedures (Institute for Patient- and Family-Centered Care, 2010a, 2010b).

Most hospitals welcome parents at any time. Many provide facilities such as a chair or bed for at least one person per child, unit kitchen privileges, and other amenities that create a welcoming atmosphere for parents. Not all hospitals provide such amenities, and parents' own schedules may prevent rooming-in. In such instances, strategies to minimize the effects of separation must be implemented.

Nurses must have an appreciation of the child's separation behaviors. As discussed earlier, the phases of protest and despair are normal. The child should be allowed to cry. Even if the child rejects strangers, the nurse provides support through physical presence. **Presence** is defined as spending time being physically close to the child while using a quiet tone of voice, appropriate choice of words, eye contact, and touch in ways that establish rapport and communicate empathy. If behaviors of detachment are evident, the nurse maintains the child's contact with the parents by frequently talking about them; encouraging the child to remember them; and stressing the significance of their visits, telephone calls, or letters. The use of cellular phones can increase the contact between the hospitalized child and parents or other significant family members and friends. Wireless technology devices may not be compatible with medical equipment, and use may be restricted in certain areas within the hospital.

Parental Absence During Infant Hospitalization

Familiar surroundings also increase the child's adjustment to separation. If the parents cannot stay with the child, they should leave favorite articles from home, such as a blanket, toy, bottle, feeding utensil, or article of clothing, with the child. Because young children associate such inanimate objects with significant people, they gain comfort and reassurance from these possessions. The child makes the association that if the parents left an object, the parents will surely return. Placing an identification band on the toy lessens the chances of its being misplaced and provides a symbol that the toy is experiencing the same needs as the child. Other reminders of home include photographs and recordings of family members reading a story, singing a song, saying prayers before bedtime, relating events at home, or taking a "talking walk" through the home. These reminders can be played at lonely times, such as on awakening or before sleeping. Some units allow pets to visit, which can have therapeutic benefits for a child. Older children also appreciate familiar articles from home, particularly photographs, a radio, a favorite toy or game, and their own pajamas. Often the importance of treasured objects to school-age children is overlooked or criticized. Many school-age children have a special object to which they formed an attachment in early childhood. Therefore such treasured or transitional objects can help even older children feel more comfortable in a strange environment.

The strange sights, smells, and sounds in the hospital that are commonplace for the nurse can be frightening and confusing for children. It is important for the nurse to try to evaluate stimuli in the environment

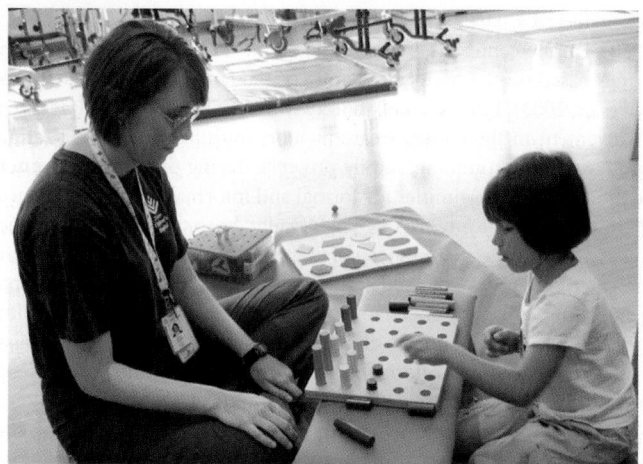

Fig. 19.5 For extended hospitalizations, children enjoy doing projects to occupy time.

from the child's point of view (considering also what the child may see or hear happening to other patients) and to make every effort to protect the child from frightening and unfamiliar sights, sounds, and equipment. The nurse should offer explanations or prepare the child for experiences that are unavoidable. Combining familiar or comforting sights with the unfamiliar can relieve much of the harshness of medical equipment.

Helping children maintain their usual contacts also minimizes the effects of separation imposed by hospitalization. This includes continuing school lessons during the illness and confinement, visiting with friends either directly or through letter writing or telephone calls, and participating in stimulating projects whenever possible (Fig. 19.5). For extended hospitalizations, children enjoy personalizing the hospital room to make it "home" by decorating the walls with posters and cards, rearranging the furniture, and displaying a collection or hobby.

Minimizing Loss of Control

Feelings of loss of control result from separation, physical restriction, changed routines, enforced dependency, and magical thinking. Although some of these cannot be prevented, most can be minimized through individualized planning of nursing care.

Promoting Freedom of Movement

Younger children react most strenuously to any type of physical restriction or immobilization. Although temporary immobilization may be necessary for some interventions such as maintaining an intravenous line, most physical restriction can be prevented if the nurse gains the child's cooperation.

For young children, particularly infants and toddlers, preserving parent-child contact is the best means of decreasing the need for or stress of restraint. For example, almost the entire physical examination can be done in a parent's lap with the parent hugging the child for procedures, such as an otoscopic examination. For painful procedures, the nurse should assess the parents' preferences for assisting, observing, or waiting outside the room.

Environmental factors may also restrict movement. Keeping children in cribs or play yards may not represent immobilization in a concrete sense, but it certainly can limit sensory stimulation. Increasing mobility by transporting children in carriages, wheelchairs, carts, or wagons provides them with a sense of freedom.

In some cases, physical restraint or isolation is necessary because of the child's medical diagnosis. In these cases, the environment can be altered to increase sensory freedom (e.g., moving the bed toward the window; opening window shades; providing musical, visual, or tactile activities).

Eric's Daily Schedule

7:30 AM	– Breakfast, morning bath	3:00 PM	– Tutor (M, W, F) – Study time (T, Th)
9:00	– Medications, dressing change	4:00	– Physical therapy
		5:30	– Dinner
11:00	– Physical therapy	9:00	– Medications, dressing change
12:00 PM	– Lunch	9:15	– Bedtime

Fig. 19.6 Time structuring is an effective strategy for normalizing the hospital environment and increasing the child's sense of control.

Maintaining the Child's Routine

Altered daily schedules and loss of rituals are particularly stressful for toddlers and early preschoolers and may increase the stress of separation. The nursing admission history provides a baseline for planning care around the child's usual home activities. A frequently neglected aspect of altered routines is the change in the child's daily activities. A typical child's day, especially during the school years, is structured with specific times for eating, dressing, going to school, playing, and sleeping. This time structure vanishes when the child is hospitalized. Although nurses have a set schedule, the child is frequently unaware of it, and the new schedules that are imposed may be rigid. For example, some units have uniform nap times and bedtimes for all children, but others allow children to stay up late at night. Many children obtain significantly less sleep in the hospital than at home; the primary causes are a delay in sleep onset and early termination of sleep because of hospital routines. Not only are hours of sleep disrupted, but waking hours are spent in passive activities. For example, few institutions impose any limits on the amount of time the child spends watching television. This may lead to children being less "tired" at bedtime and delay the onset of sleep.

One technique that can minimize the disruption in the child's routine is establishing a daily schedule. This approach is most suitable for non–critically ill school-age and adolescent children who have mastered the concept of time. It involves scheduling the child's day to include all those activities that are important to the child and nurse, such as treatment procedures, schoolwork, exercise, television, playroom, and hobbies. Together, the nurse, parent, and child then plan a daily schedule with times and activities written down (Fig. 19.6). This schedule is left in the child's room, and a clock or watch is available for the child's use. Whenever possible, a calendar is also constructed with special events marked, such as favorite television programs, visits by friends or relatives, events in the playroom, and holidays or birthdays. If specific changes in treatment are expected (e.g., "beginning physical therapy in 2 days"), these are added.

> **NURSING TIP:** Ask the young child to select or draw pictures or symbols to represent daily or weekly fun activities (e.g., favorite television programs, family visits, playroom times). Draw a visual schedule to help plan and prepare the activities of the day. Use your consultation skills to ask child life specialists for assistance.

Encouraging Independence

The dependent role of the hospitalized patient imposes tremendous feelings of loss on older children. Principal interventions should focus on respect for individuality and the opportunity for decision making.

Although these sound simple, their efficacy lies with nurses who are flexible and tolerant. It is also important for the nurse to empower the patient while not feeling threatened by a sense of lessened control.

Enabling children's control involves helping them maintain independence and promoting the concept of self-care. **Self-care** refers to the practice of activities that individuals personally initiate and perform on their own behalf in maintaining life, health, and well-being (Orem, 2001). Although self-care is limited by the child's age and physical condition, most children beyond infancy can perform some activities with little or no help. Whenever possible, these activities are encouraged in the hospital. Other approaches include jointly planning care, time structuring, wearing street clothes, making choices in food selections and bedtime, continuing school activities, and rooming with an appropriate age-mate.

Promoting Understanding

Loss of control can occur from feelings of having too little influence on one's destiny or from sensing overwhelming control or power over fate. Although preschoolers' cognitive abilities predispose them to magical thinking and delusions of power, all children are vulnerable to misinterpreting causes for stresses, such as illness and hospitalization.

Most children feel more in control when they know what to expect because the element of fear is reduced. Anticipatory preparation and provision of information help lessen stress and increase understanding (see Chapter 20, Preparation for Diagnostic and Therapeutic Procedures).

Informing children of their rights while hospitalized fosters greater understanding and may relieve some of the feelings of powerlessness they typically experience. An increasing number of hospitals and organizations have developed a patient "bill of rights" that is prominently displayed throughout the hospital or is presented to children and their families on admission (Box 19.8).

Preventing or Minimizing Fear of Bodily Injury

Beyond early infancy, all children fear bodily injury from mutilation, bodily intrusion, body image change, disability, or death. In general, preparation of children for painful procedures decreases their fears and increases cooperation. Modifying procedural techniques for children in each age-group also minimizes fear of bodily injury. For example, because toddlers and young preschoolers are traumatized by insertion of a rectal thermometer, less invasive axillary temperatures or temperatures taken with electronic or tympanic membrane devices can effectively be substituted. Whenever procedures are performed on young children, the most supportive intervention is to do the procedure as quickly as possible while maintaining parent-child contact.

Because of toddlers' and preschool children's poorly defined body boundaries, the use of bandages may be particularly helpful. For example, telling children that the bleeding will stop after the needle is removed does little to relieve their fears, but applying a small Band-Aid usually reassures them. The size of bandages is also significant to children in this age-group; the larger the bandage, the more importance is attached to the wound. Watching their surgical dressings become successively smaller is one way that young children can measure healing and improvement. Removing a dressing too soon may cause these children considerable concern for their well-being. Remember to consult child life specialists to use therapeutic measures to reduce fear and pain in children. Specific pain management strategies are discussed in Chapter 5.

For children who fear mutilation of body parts, it is essential that the nurse repeatedly stress the reason for a procedure and evaluate the child's understanding. For example, explaining cast removal to preschoolers may seem simple enough, but children's comprehension of the details may vary considerably from the explanation. Asking the child to draw a picture of what they foresee happening presents substantial evidence of how they perceive events.

Children may fear bodily injury from a great variety of sources. Imaging machines, strange equipment used for examination, unfamiliar rooms, and awkward positions can be perceived as potentially hazardous. In addition, thoughts and actions can be imagined sources of bodily damage. Therefore it is important to investigate imagined reasons, particularly of a sexual nature, for illness. Because children may fear revealing such thoughts, using techniques such as drawing or doll play may elicit previously undisclosed misconceptions.

Older children fear bodily injury of both internal and external origins. For example, school-age children are aware of the significance of the heart and may fear the actual operation as much as the pain, the stitches, and the possible scar. Adolescents may express concern about the actual procedure but be much more anxious over the resulting scar.

Children can grasp information if it is presented on or close to their level of cognitive development. This necessitates an awareness of the words used to describe events or processes. For example, young children told that they are going to have a CAT (i.e., CT, computed tomography) scan may wonder, "Will there be cats or something that scratches?" It is clearer to describe the procedure in simple terms and explain what the letters of the common name stand for. Therefore to prevent or alleviate fears, nurses must be keenly aware of the medical terminology and vocabulary that they use every day.

When children are upset about their illness, their perception can be changed by providing a somewhat different and less negative account of the disease or offering an explanation that is characteristic of the next stage of cognitive development. An example of the first strategy is reassuring a preschooler who fears that after a tonsillectomy, another sore throat means a second operation. Explaining that after tonsils are "fixed" they do not need fixing again can help relieve the fear. An example of the latter strategy is to explain that germs made the tonsils sick and even though germs can cause another sore throat, they cannot cause the tonsils to ever be sick again. This higher-level explanation is based on the school-age child's concept of germs as a cause of disease.

Providing Developmentally Appropriate Activities

A primary goal of nursing care for the child who is hospitalized is to minimize threats to the child's development. Many strategies (e.g., minimizing separation) have been discussed and may be all that the short-term patient requires. Children who experience prolonged or repeated hospitalization are at greater risk for developmental delays or regression. The nurse who provides opportunities for the child to participate in developmentally appropriate activities further normalizes the child's environment and helps reduce interference with the child's ongoing development.

BOX 19.8 Bill of Rights for Children and Teens

In this hospital, you and your family have the right to:

- Respect and personal dignity
- Care that supports you and your family
- Information you can understand
- Quality health care
- Emotional support
- Care that respects your need to grow, play, and learn
- Make choices and decisions

From Association for the Care of Children's Health. (1991). *A pediatric bill of rights*. Bethesda, MD: Author.

Interference with normal development may have long-term implications for developing infants and toddlers. The nurse plays a primary role in identifying children at risk and helping to plan, implement, and evaluate developmental intervention (see Chapters 9 and 11).

School is an integral part of the school-age child's and adolescent's development. Accreditation standards for hospitals serving children consider access to appropriate educational services a key factor in the accreditation decision process when a child's treatment requires a significant absence from school (The Joint Commission, 2011). The nurse can encourage children to resume schoolwork as quickly as their condition permits, help them schedule and protect a selected time for studies, and help the family coordinate hospital educational services with their children's schools. Children should have the opportunity to continue art and music classes, as well as their academic subjects.

To meet the unique developmental needs of adolescents, special units may be developed that provide privacy, increased socialization, and appropriate activities for these young people. Typically, these units can be set apart from the general pediatric facility so that the teenagers do not share space with younger children, who are often perceived as a threat to their maturity.

In caring for adolescent patients, it is essential to provide flexible routines and activities, such as more group activity, wearing of street clothes, and access to the items important to adolescents—wireless technology devices and Wi-Fi access for email, electronic video game systems, and streaming technology. Because adolescents' food habits are rarely limited to the three traditional meals a day, a ready supply of snacks should be available. The most important benefit of these units is increased socialization with peers. In addition, staff members usually enjoy working with this age-group and are able to establish the trust that is so essential for communication.

NURSING TIP: When adolescents must share a common activity room with younger patients, referring to the area as the "activity room" rather than the "playroom" may entice them to visit the room and participate in activities.

Although regression is expected and normal for all age-groups, nurses have the responsibility for fostering the child's growth and development. Hospitalization can become a significant opportunity for learning and advancing. Extended hospitalizations for long-term chronic illness or situations of failure to thrive, abuse, or neglect represent instances in which regression must be seen as an adjustment period to be followed by plans for promoting appropriate developmental skills.

Providing Opportunities for Play and Expressive Activities

Play is one of the most important aspects of a child's life and one of the most effective tools for managing stress. Illness and hospitalization constitute crises in a child's life and often involve overwhelming stresses, and children need to act out their fears and anxieties as a means of coping with these stresses. Play is essential to children's mental, emotional, and social well-being. Play does not stop when children are ill or in the hospital. On the contrary, play in the hospital serves many functions (Box 19.9). Of all hospital facilities, the playroom or activity room alleviates the stressors of hospitalization. In the playroom, children temporarily distance themselves from their illness, hospitalization, and the associated stressors. This room should be a safe haven for children, free from medical or nursing procedures (including medication administration), strange faces, and probing questions. The playroom then becomes a sanctuary in an otherwise frightening environment.

Engaging in play activities gives children a sense of control. In the hospital environment, most decisions are made for the child; play and other expressive activities offer the child much-needed opportunities to make choices for themselves. Even if a child chooses not to participate in a particular activity, the nurse has offered the child a choice, perhaps one of only a few real choices the child has had that day.

Hospitalized children typically have lower energy levels than healthy children of the same age. Children may not appear engaged and enthusiastic about an activity even though they are enjoying the experience. Activities may need to be adjusted or limited based on the child's age, endurance, and any special needs.

Diversional Activities

Almost any form of play can be used for diversion and recreation, but the activity should be selected based on the child's age, interests, and limitations (Fig. 19.7). Children do not necessarily need special direction for using play materials. All they require is the raw materials with which to work and adult approval and supervision to help keep their natural enthusiasm or expression of feelings from getting out of control. Small children enjoy a variety of small, colorful toys that they can play with in bed or in their room or more elaborate play equipment, such as playhouses, sandboxes, rhythm instruments, or large boxes and blocks that may be a part of the hospital playroom.

Games that can be played alone or with another child or an adult are popular with older children, as are puzzles; reading material; quiet, individual activities, such as sewing, stringing beads, and weaving; and Lego blocks and other building materials. Assembling models is an excellent pastime, but one should make certain that all pieces and necessary materials are included in the package so that the child is not disappointed and frustrated.

BOX 19.9 Functions of Play in the Hospital

- Provides diversion and brings about relaxation
- Helps the child feel more secure in a strange environment
- Lessens the stress of separation and the feeling of homesickness
- Provides a means for release of tension and expression of feelings
- Encourages interaction and development of positive attitudes toward others
- Provides an expressive outlet for creative ideas and interests
- Provides a means for accomplishing therapeutic goals (see Chapter 20, Use of Play in Procedures)
- Places child in active role and provides opportunity to make choices and be in control

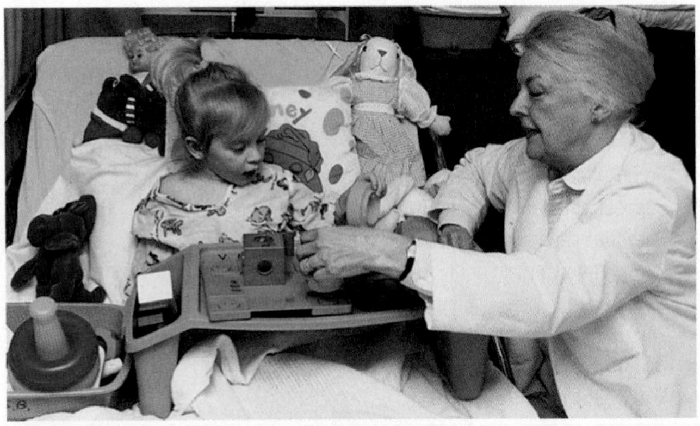

Fig. 19.7 Play materials for children in the hospital need to be appropriate for their age, interests, and limitations.

Well-selected books are of infinite value to children. Children rarely tire of stories; having someone read aloud gives them endless hours of pleasure and is of special value to children who have limited energy to expend in play. Current electronic technology and communication devices should be included in most hospital room amenities as useful tools for entertaining children. Computers with access to the Internet can provide diversion, educational opportunities, and online support groups.

When supervising play for ill or recuperating children, it is best to select activities that are simpler than would normally be chosen for the child's specific developmental level. These children usually do not have the energy to cope with more challenging activities. Other limitations also influence the type of activities. Special consideration must be given to children who are confined in terms of movement, have a restricted extremity, or are isolated. Toys for isolated children must be disposable or need to be disinfected after every use.

Toys

Parents of hospitalized children often ask nurses about the types of toys that would be best to bring for their child. Although parents often want to buy new toys for the hospitalized child to offer cheer and comfort, it is often better to wait to bring new things, especially in the case of younger children. Small children need the comfort and reassurance of familiar things, such as the stuffed animal the child hugs for comfort and takes to bed at night. These familiar items can be a link with home and the world outside the hospital. All toys brought into the hospital should be assessed for safety.

Large numbers of toys often confuse and frustrate small children. A few small, well-chosen toys are usually preferred to one large, expensive one. Children who are hospitalized for an extended time benefit from changes. Rather than a confusing accumulation of toys, older toys should be replaced periodically as interest wanes.

A highly successful diversion for a child who is hospitalized for a length of time and whose parents are unable to visit frequently is having the parents bring a box with several small, inexpensive, brightly wrapped items with a different day of the week printed on the outside of each package. The child will eagerly anticipate the time for opening each one. If the parents know when their next visit will be, they can provide the number of packages that corresponds to the time between visits. In this way, the child knows that the diminishing packages also represent the anticipated visit from the parent.

Expressive Activities

Play and other expressive activities provide one of the best opportunities for encouraging emotional expression, including the safe release of anger and hostility. Nondirective play that allows children freedom for expression can be tremendously therapeutic. Therapeutic play, however, should not be confused with play therapy, a psychologic technique reserved for use by trained and qualified therapists as an interpretative method with emotionally disturbed children. Therapeutic play, on the other hand, is an effective, nondirective modality for helping children deal with their concerns and fears; at the same time, it often helps the nurse gain insights into children's needs and feelings.

Tension release can be facilitated through almost any activity; with younger ambulatory children, large-muscle activity such as use of tricycles and wagons is especially beneficial. Much aggression can be safely directed into pounding and throwing games or activities. Beanbags are often thrown at a target or open receptacle with surprising vigor and hostility. A pounding board is used with enthusiasm by young children; clay and play dough are beneficial for use at any age.

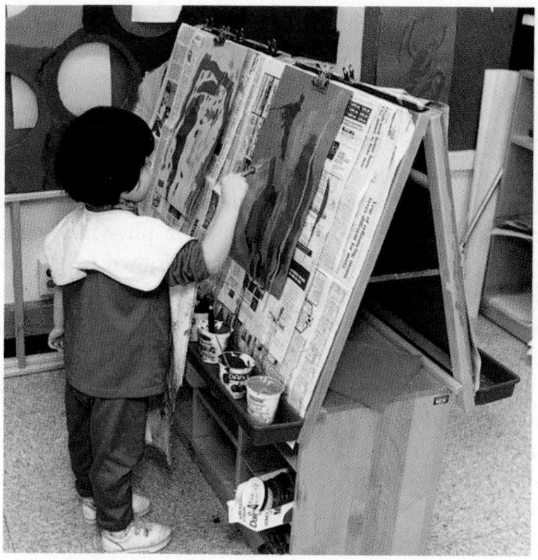

Fig. 19.8 Drawing and painting are excellent media for expression.

Creative Expression

Although all children derive physical, social, emotional, and cognitive benefits from engaging in art and other creative activities, children's need for such activities is intensified when they are hospitalized. Drawing and painting are excellent media for expression. Children are more at ease expressing their thoughts and feelings through art because humans think first in images and later learn to translate these images into words. Children need only be supplied with the raw materials, such as crayons and paper, large brushes, an ample supply of newsprint supported on easels, or materials for finger painting (Fig. 19.8). Children can work individually or together on a group project, such as a mural painted on a long piece of paper.

Although interpretation of children's drawings requires special training, observing changes in a series of the child's drawings over time can be helpful in assessing psychosocial adjustment and coping. The nurse can use children's drawings, stories, poetry, and other products of creative expression as a springboard for discussion of thoughts, fears, and understanding of concepts or events (see Chapter 4, Communication Techniques). A child's drawing before surgery, for example, may reveal unvoiced concerns about mutilation, body changes, and loss of self-control.

Nurses can incorporate opportunities for musical expression into routine nursing care. For example, simple musical instruments, such as bracelets with bells, can be placed on infants' legs for them to shake to accompany mealtime music or dressing changes. Dance and movement suggestions may encourage a child to ambulate.

Holidays provide stimulus and direction for unlimited creative projects. Children can participate in decorating the pediatric unit; making pictures and decorations for their rooms gives children a sense of pride and accomplishment. This is especially beneficial for children who are immobilized and isolated. Making gifts for someone at home helps maintain interpersonal ties.

Dramatic Play

Dramatic play is a well-recognized technique for emotional release, allowing children to reenact frightening or puzzling hospital experiences. Through use of puppets, replicas of hospital equipment, or some actual hospital equipment, children can act out the situations that are a part of their hospital experience. Dramatic play enables children to learn about procedures and events that concern them and to assume the roles of the adults in the hospital environment.

Puppets are universally effective for communicating with children. Most children see them as peers and readily communicate with them. Children will tell the puppet feelings that they hesitate to express to adults. Puppets can share children's own experiences and help them find solutions to their problems. Puppets dressed to represent figures in the child's environment—for example, a physician, nurse, child patient, therapist, and members of the child's own family—are especially useful. Small, appropriately attired dolls are equally effective in encouraging the child to play out situations, although puppets are usually best for direct conversation.

Play must consider medical needs, but at times a procedure can be postponed briefly to allow the child to complete a special activity (see Critical Thinking Case Study box). Play must consider any limitations imposed by the child's condition. For example, small children may eat paste and other creative media; therefore a child who is allergic to wheat should not be given finger paint made from wallpaper paste or modeling dough made with flour. A child on a restricted salt intake should not play with modeling dough because salt is one of its major constituents. At home, the play program can be planned around the therapy regimen. However, play can be satisfactorily incorporated into the child's care if the nurse and others involved allow some flexibility and use creativity in planning for play.

CRITICAL THINKING CASE STUDY

Balancing Diagnostics With Play

Joel, an 8-year-old with cystic fibrosis, has been hospitalized numerous times with complications from the condition. He is playing a board game with his brother, sister, and several other children in the playroom on the pediatric unit. A pediatric phlebotomist enters the playroom and says, "Joel, I need to take some blood. I can see that you are playing a game, so I'll just do it while you play. It will just take a minute." The playroom is usually off limits for invasive procedures. As Joel's nurse, you are aware that Dr. Lung wants the results of the laboratory studies as soon as possible to make a decision about the course of therapy.

Initial Assessment. How would you balance the need for diagnostic interventions with a child's need to play?

Expected Nursing Action. What diagnostics can be delayed to allow a child to play and where is the best location to obtain diagnostic samples?

Teaching Points

- Play is one of the most important aspects of a child's life and one of the most effective tools for managing stress.
- Children derive physical, social, emotional, and cognitive benefits from engaging in play and other creative activities. Children's need for such activities is intensified when they are hospitalized.
- In the playroom, children temporarily distance themselves from their illness, hospitalization, and the associated stressors, and this room should be a safe haven for children, free from medical or nursing procedures (including medication administration), strange faces, and probing questions. The playroom then becomes a sanctuary in an otherwise frightening environment.

Critical Thinking Answers

Initial Assessment. Joel requires a laboratory study to determine the most appropriate course of therapy.

Expected Nursing Action. An appropriate nursing action is to notify Joel that he has to go back to his room to obtain the laboratory study and, upon completion, he can return to the playroom.

Maximizing Potential Benefits of Hospitalization

Although hospitalization generally represents a stressful time for children and families, it also represents an opportunity for facilitating positive change within the child and among family members. For some families, the stress of a child's illness, hospitalization, or both can lead to strengthening of family coping behaviors and the emergence of new coping strategies.

Fostering Parent-Child Relationships

The crisis of illness or hospitalization can mobilize parents into more acute awareness of their child's needs. For example, hospitalization provides opportunities for parents to learn more about their children's growth and development. When parents are helped to understand children's usual reactions to stress, such as regression or aggression, they are not only better able to support the child through the hospital experience but also may extend their insights into childrearing practices after discharge.

Difficulties in parent-child relationships that existed before hospitalization and are characterized by feeding problems, negative behavior, and sleep disturbances may decrease during hospitalization. The temporary cessation of such problems sometimes alerts parents to the role they may be playing in propagating the negative behavior. With assistance from health professionals, parents can restructure ways of relating to their children to foster more positive behavior.

Hospitalization may also represent a temporary reprieve or refuge from a disturbed home. Typically, abused or neglected children's dramatic physical and social improvement during hospitalization is proof of the benefits and potential growth that can occur during hospitalization. These children temporarily can seek support, reassurance, and security from new relationships, particularly with nurses and hospitalized peers.

Providing Educational Opportunities

Illness and hospitalization represent excellent opportunities for children and other family members to learn more about their bodies, each other, and the health professions. For example, during a hospital admission for a diabetic crisis, the child may learn about the disease; the parents may learn about the child's needs for independence, normalcy, and appropriate limits; and each of them may find a new support system in the hospital staff.

Illness or hospitalization can also help older children in choosing a career. Frequently, children have impressions of physicians or nurses that are disproportionately positive or negative. Actual experience with different health professionals can influence their attitude about health professionals and even a decision regarding a career in health care.

Promoting Self-Mastery

The experience of facing a crisis such as illness or hospitalization, coping successfully with it, and maturing as a result of it constitutes an opportunity for self-mastery. Younger children have the chance to test fantasy versus reality fears. They realize that they were not abandoned, mutilated, or punished. In fact, they were loved, cared for, and treated with respect for their individual concerns. It is not unusual for children who have undergone hospitalization or surgery to tell others that "it was nothing" or to display proudly their scars or bandages. For older children, hospitalization may represent an opportunity for decision making, independence, and self-reliance. They are proud of having survived the experience and may feel a genuine self-respect for their achievements. Nurses can facilitate such feelings of self-mastery by emphasizing aspects of personal competence in the child and not focusing on uncooperative or negative behavior.

Providing Socialization

Hospitalization may offer children a special opportunity for social acceptance. Lonely, asocial, and even delinquent children find a sympathetic

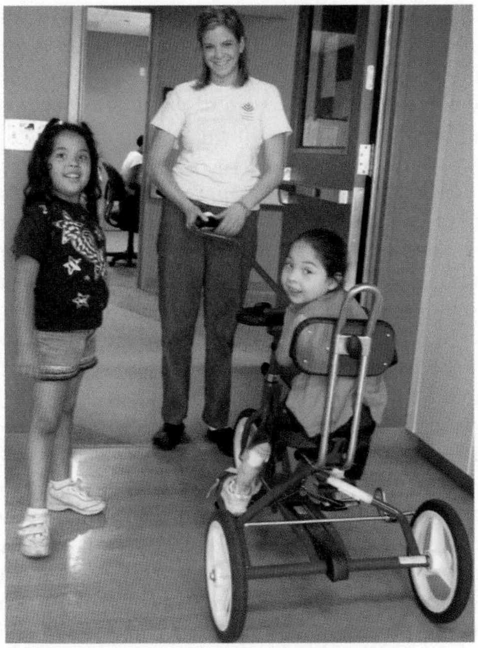

Fig. 19.9 Placing children of the same age-group with similar illnesses near each other on the unit is both psychologically and medically supportive. (Courtesy E. Jacob, Texas Children's Hospital, Houston, TX.)

environment in the hospital. Children who have a physical disability or are in some other way "different" from their age-mates may find an accepting social peer group (Fig. 19.9). Although this does not always occur spontaneously, nurses can structure the environment to foster a supportive child group. For example, the introduction of an age-compatible peer can help children gain a new friend and learn more about themselves. Forming relationships with significant members of the health care team, such as the physician, nurse, child life specialist, or social worker, can greatly enhance children's adjustment in many areas of life.

Parents may also encounter a new social group in other parents who have similar problems. The waiting room or hallway "self-help" groups are inherent to every institution. Parents meet while in the hospital or clinic and discuss their children's illnesses and treatments. Nurses can capitalize on this informal gathering by encouraging parents to discuss collectively their concerns and feelings. Nurses can also refer parents to organized parent groups or can use the help and support of parents of recovered hospitalized patients. It is important that nurses emphasize to families that each child responds differently to disease, treatments, and care. Any questions raised during group discussions should be clarified with a nurse or physician.

NURSING CARE OF THE FAMILY

Although it is not possible to predict exactly which factors are most likely to influence a family's reactions, important variables are the seriousness of the child's illness, the family's previous experience with hospitalization, and the medical procedures involved in the diagnosis and treatment. Important information is also obtained in the nursing admission history (see Box 19.5).

SUPPORTING FAMILY MEMBERS

Support involves the willingness to stay and listen to parents' verbal and nonverbal messages. Sometimes the nurse does not give this support directly. For example, the nurse may offer to stay with the child to allow the parents time alone or may discuss with other family members the parents' need for extra relief. Often relatives and friends want to help but do not know how. Suggesting ways, such as babysitting, preparing meals, doing laundry, or transporting the siblings to school, can prompt others to help reduce the responsibilities that burden parents.

Support may also be provided through the clergy. Parents with deep religious beliefs may appreciate the counsel of a clergy member, but because of their stress, they may not have sufficient energy to initiate the contact. Nurses can be supportive by arranging for clergy to visit, upholding parents' religious beliefs, and respecting the individual meaning and significance of those beliefs (Feudtner, Haney, & Dimmers, 2003).

Support involves accepting cultural, socioeconomic, and ethnic values. For example, health and illness are defined differently by various ethnic groups. For some, a disorder that has few outward manifestations of illness, such as diabetes, hypertension, or cardiac problems, is not a sickness. Consequently, following a prescribed treatment may be seen as unnecessary. Nurses who appreciate the influences of culture are more likely to intervene therapeutically. (See also Chapter 2, Sociocultural Influences on Children and Families.)

Parents need help in accepting their own feelings toward the ill child. If given the opportunity, parents often disclose their feelings of loss of control, anger, and guilt. They often resist admitting to such feelings because they expect others to disapprove of behavior that is less than perfect. Unfortunately, health personnel, including nurses, sometimes do exercise little tolerance for deviation from the norm. This only increases the psychologic impact of a child's illness on family members. Helping parents identify the specific reason for such feelings and emphasizing that each is a normal, expected, and healthy response to stress may reduce the parents' emotional burden.

Family-centered care also addresses the needs of siblings. Support may involve preparing siblings for hospital visits, assessing their adjustment, and providing appropriate interventions or referrals when needed. The Family-Centered Care box suggests ways in which parents can support siblings during hospitalization.

FAMILY-CENTERED CARE

Supporting Siblings During Hospitalization

Trade off staying at the hospital with spouse or have a surrogate who knows the siblings well stay in the home.

Offer information about the child's condition to young siblings as well as older siblings; respect the sibling who avoids information as a means of coping with the situation.

Arrange for children to visit their brother or sister in the hospital if possible.

Encourage phone visits and mail between brothers and sisters; provide children with phone numbers, writing supplies, and stamps.

Help each sibling identify an extended family member or friend to be their support person and provide extra attention during parental absence.

Make or buy inexpensive toys or trinkets for siblings, one gift for each day the child will be hospitalized.

- Wrap each gift separately and place them in a basket, box, or other container at the child's bedside.
- Instruct siblings to open one gift at bedtime and to remember that they are in their parents' thoughts.

If the child's condition is stable and distance is not prohibitive, plan a special time at home with the siblings or have spouse or another relative or friend bring the children to meet parent(s) at a restaurant or other location near the hospital.

- Have extended family members or friends schedule a visit to the child in the hospital during parental absence.
- Arrange to have the child leave the care unit with a staff member to have change of scenery if the child's condition permits.

Modified from Craft, M., & Craft, J. (1989). Perceived changes in siblings of hospitalized children: A comparison of sibling and parent reports. *Child Health Care, 18*(1), 42–48; Rollins, J. (1992). *Brothers and sisters: A discussion guide for families.* Landover, MD: Epilepsy Foundation of America.

PROVIDING INFORMATION

One of the most important nursing interventions is providing information about the disease, its treatment, prognosis, and home care; the child's emotional and physical reactions to illness and hospitalization; and the probable emotional reactions of family members to the crisis.

For many families, the child's illness is the first contact they have with the hospital experience. Often parents are not prepared for the child's behavioral reactions to hospitalization, such as separation behaviors, regression, aggression, and hostility. Providing the parents with information about these normal and expected behavioral responses can lessen the parents' anxiety during the hospital admission. The family is equally unfamiliar with hospital rules, which often compounds their confusion and anxiety. Therefore the family needs clear explanations of what to expect and what is expected of them.

Parents also need to be aware of the effects of illness on the family and strategies to prevent negative changes. Specifically, parents should keep the family well informed and communicate with everyone as much as possible. They should treat all of their children equally and as normally as before the illness occurred. Discipline, which initially may be lessened for the ill child, should be continued to provide a measure of security and predictability. When ill children know that their parents expect certain standards of conduct from them, they feel certain that they will recover. Conversely, when all limits are removed, they fear that something catastrophic will happen.

Helping parents understand the meaning of post-hospitalization behaviors in the sick child is necessary for them to tolerate and support such behaviors. In addition, parents should be forewarned of the common reactions after discharge (see Box 19.2). Parents who do not expect such reactions may misinterpret them as evidence of the child's "being spoiled" and demand perfect behavior at a time when the child is still reacting to the stress of illness and hospitalization. If the behaviors, especially the demand for attention, are dealt with in a supportive manner, most children can relinquish them and assume prior levels of functioning.

Nurses should also prepare parents for the reactions of siblings—particularly anger, jealousy, and resentment. Older siblings may deny such reactions because they provoke feelings of guilt. However, everyone needs outlets for emotions, and the repressed feelings may surface as problems in school or with age-mates, as psychosomatic illnesses, or in delinquent behavior.

Probably one of the most neglected areas of communication involves giving information to siblings. Frequently, age becomes the only factor that leads to an awareness of this problem because older children may begin to ask questions or request explanations. Even in this situation, however, the information may be seriously inadequate. Children in every age-group deserve some explanation of the sibling's illness or hospitalization. In addition, nurses can minimize a sibling's fear of also getting sick or having caused the illness.

ENCOURAGING PARENT PARTICIPATION

Preventing or minimizing separation is a key nursing goal with the child who is hospitalized, but maintaining parent-child contact is also beneficial for the family. One of the best approaches is encouraging parents to be present with their child and to participate in the care whenever possible. Although some health facilities provide special accommodations for parents, the concept of rooming-in can be instituted anywhere. The first requirement is the staff's positive attitude toward parents. A negative attitude toward parent participation can create barriers to collaborative working relationships.

When hospital staff genuinely appreciate the importance of continued parent-child attachment, they foster an environment that encourages parents to stay. When parents are included in the care planning and understand that they are a contributing factor to the child's recovery, they are more inclined to remain with their child and have more emotional reserves to support themselves and the child through the crisis. Family-centered rounds for pediatric patients have shown improved nurse satisfaction and increased family participation (Rappaport, Ketterer, Nilforoshan, et al., 2012). An empowerment model of helping allows the nurse to focus on parents' strengths and seek ways to promote growth and family functioning so that the parents become empowered in caring for their child. Strategies such as bedside family-centered rounds that allow parents to be involved in the discussion of the child's current status are moving health care settings closer to family-centered care (Anderson & Mangino, 2006). Liaison nursing roles—for example, a patient-nurse educator—in tertiary care settings are also focused on improving communication between parents and health care providers (Caffin, Linton, & Pellegrini, 2007).

Because one parent may tend to be the usual family caregiver, they usually spend more time in the hospital than the other parent. Not all parents feel equally comfortable assuming responsibility for their child's care. Some may be under such great emotional stress that they need a temporary reprieve from total participation in caregiving activities or may be insecure about participating in specialized areas of care, such as bathing the child after surgery. On the other hand, some parents may feel a great need to control their child's care. This seems particularly true of young parents, who have recently established their role as a parent; parents of children too young to verbalize their needs; and ethnic-minority parents when the hospital setting is predominantly staffed by nonminority personnel. Individual assessment of each parent's preferred involvement is necessary to prevent the effects of separation while also supporting parents in their needs.

With lifestyles and gender roles changing, some of the usual "parenting" roles in the household may change. Both parents need to be included in the care plan and respected for their parental role. For some parents, the child's hospitalization may represent an opportunity to alter their usual caregiving role and increase their involvement. In single-parent families, the caregiver may not be a parent but an extended family member, such as a grandparent or aunt.

One of the potential problems with continuous parent involvement is neglect of the parent's need for sleep, nutrition, and relaxation. Often the sleeping accommodations are limited to a chair, and sleep is disrupted by hospital care. Encouraging the parents to leave for brief periods, arranging for sleeping quarters on the unit or outside the child's room, and planning a schedule of alternating visits with another family member can minimize the stresses for the parent.

All too often, nurses respond to parent participation by assuming that the parent will take over the care responsibilities. Nurses need to restructure their roles to complement and augment the caregiving functions of parents (Hopia, Tomlinson, Paavilainen, et al., 2005).

Even in units structured to provide care by parents, parents frequently feel anxiety in their caregiving responsibilities; those more involved in direct care may feel more anxiety than those less involved in direct care. Responsibility 24 hours per day may be too much for some parents. Assistance and relief by nursing personnel should always be available to these families, and nurses may need to work diligently to establish the strong bond of trust that some parents need to take advantage of these opportunities.

PREPARING FOR DISCHARGE AND HOME CARE

Most hospitalizations necessitate some type of discharge preparation. Often this involves education of the family for continued care and follow-up in the home. Depending on the diagnosis, this may be relatively simple or highly complex. Preparing the family for home care demands a high degree of competence in planning and implementing discharge instructions.

Nurses are often key individuals in initiating and carrying out the discharge process. They collaborate with others in the planning and implementation phases to ensure appropriate care after hospitalization. Throughout the hospitalization, the nurse should be aware of the need for discharge planning and those assessment factors that affect the family's ability to provide home care. A thorough assessment of the family and home environment should occur to ensure that the family's emotional and physical resources are sufficient to manage the tasks of home care. (For discussion of family and home assessment strategies, see Chapter 4.) In addition to adequate family resources, an investigation of community services, including respite care, is needed to ensure that appropriate support agencies, such as emergency facilities, home health agencies, and equipment vendors, are available. Financial resources and insurance are also a significant consideration. To coordinate the immense task of assessment and to plan implementation, a care coordinator should begin early in the discharge process.

The preparation for hospital discharge and home care begins during the admission stage. Short- and long-term goals are established to meet the child's physical and psychosocial needs. For children with complex care needs, discharge planning focuses on obtaining appropriate equipment and health care personnel for the home. Discharge planning is also concerned with treatments that parents or children are expected to continue at home. In planning appropriate teaching, nurses need to assess the actual and perceived complexity of the skill, the parents' or child's ability to learn the skill, and the parents' or child's previous or present experience with such procedures.

The teaching plan incorporates levels of learning, such as observing, participating with assistance, and finally demonstrating without help or guidance. The skill is divided into discrete steps, and each step is taught to the family member until it is learned. Return demonstration of the skill is requested before new skills are introduced. A record of teaching and performance provides an efficient checklist for evaluation. All families need to receive detailed written instructions about home care, with telephone numbers for assistance, before they leave the hospital. Communication between discharge planning and home health care is essential to ensure a smooth transition for the child and family.

After the family is competent in performing the skill, they are given responsibility for the care. When possible, the family should have a transition or trial period to assume care with minimal health care supervision. This may be arranged on the unit; during a home pass; or in a facility, such as a hotel near the hospital. Such transitions provide a safe practice period for the family, with assistance readily available when needed, and are especially valuable when the family lives far from the hospital.

In many instances, parents need only simple instructions and understanding of follow-up care. The often overwhelming care assumed by some families, coupled with other stressors, necessitates continued professional support after discharge. A follow-up home visit or telephone call gives the nurse an opportunity to individualize care and provide information in perhaps a less stressful learning environment than the hospital. Appropriate referrals and resources may include visiting nurse or home health agencies, private nurse services, the school system, a physical therapist, a mental health counselor, a social worker, and any number of community agencies. Sharing the important issues surrounding the child's and family's needs is essential. Referral summaries should be concise, specific, and factual. When numerous support services are required, collaboration among the professionals involved and the family is an excellent strategy to ensure efficient use and comprehensive delivery of services.

CARE OF THE CHILD AND FAMILY IN SPECIAL HOSPITAL SITUATIONS

In addition to a general pediatric unit, children may be admitted to special facilities, such as an ambulatory or outpatient setting, an isolation room, or intensive care.

AMBULATORY OR OUTPATIENT SETTING

The ambulatory or outpatient setting provides needed medical services for the child while eliminating the necessity of overnight admission. The benefits of ambulatory care are minimized stressors of hospitalization, especially separation from the family; reduced chances of infection; and increased cost savings. Admission to the ambulatory or outpatient hospital setting usually is for surgical or diagnostic procedures.

In the ambulatory or outpatient setting, adequate preparation is particularly challenging. Ideally, the child and parents should receive preadmission preparation, including a tour of the facility and a review of a typical schedule. Parents need information in advance to help prepare the child and themselves for surgery and enable them to care for the child at home afterwards. Parents also appreciate suggestions for personal items to bring to the hospital. When preadmission preparation is not possible, time should be allowed on the day of the procedure for children to become acquainted with their surroundings and for nurses to assess, plan, and implement appropriate teaching.

Explicit discharge instructions are important after outpatient surgery (see Family-Centered Care box and the Preparing for Discharge and Home Care section earlier in this chapter). Parents need guidelines on when to call their provider about a change in the child's condition. A follow-up telephone call system allows for nurses to check on the child's progress within 48 to 72 hours after discharge to review information and answer questions.

FAMILY-CENTERED CARE

Discharge From Ambulatory Settings

1. Explain that all instructions will also be presented in writing for the family to refer to later.
2. Provide an overview of the typical expected pattern of recovery.
3. Discuss expected progression of the child's activity level during the post-discharge period (e.g., "Mary will probably sleep for the rest of the day and feel kind of tired most of tomorrow but will be back to her usual activities on the next day.").
4. Explain which activities the child is allowed and what is not permitted (e.g., bed rest, bathing).
5. Discuss dietary restrictions, being very specific and giving examples of "clear fluids" or what is meant by a "full liquid diet."
6. Discuss nausea and vomiting, if applicable, explaining how much is "normal" and what to do if more occurs (e.g., "Juan may be sick to his stomach and vomit. This is normal. However, if he vomits more than three times, please call us at this number right away.").
7. Discuss fever and appropriate comfort measures, explaining how much fever is considered "acceptable" and specifically what to do if the child goes beyond the range.
8. Explain the amount, location, and kind of pain or discomfort the child may experience.
   - Give any prescribed medication before leaving the facility.
   - Send a pain scale home with the family.
   - Explain how much pain and discomfort is "normal" and what to do if the child surpasses that level or if pain management interventions are unsuccessful.
   - Discuss pain management, including dosage for pain medications and details on how to administer them.
   - Describe appropriate nonpharmacologic comfort measures, such as holding, rocking, or swaddling.
9. Provide information about each medication that the child will be taking at home.
   - Request that all prescriptions be filled and given to the family before discharge
   - Review the details, including dose and route.
   - Demonstrate how to administer medications.
   - Discuss guidelines for requesting other medications.
10. Make certain the family has all equipment and supplies that they will need at home.
11. Discuss complications that may occur and the steps to take if they do.
12. Ensure that appropriate measures are in place for safe transport home.
    - Remind family to use a seat belt or car seat for the child.
    - Determine if there will be one person whose sole responsibility is helping ensure the child's safety and comfort during transport.
13. Provide emergency phone numbers for the family to call with any concerns.
14. Explain that the family may be contacted to follow up on the child but that they should not hesitate to call if concerns arise before then.
15. Ask the family and child if they have any questions and problem solve with family members to meet their unique needs.

NURSING TIP: Help the family prepare for the transportation home by offering these suggestions:
- Have a blanket and pillow in the car. (Always use the car safety restraint system.)
- Take a basin or plastic bag in case of vomiting.
- Use a cup with a cap and straw for the child to drink fluids (except in cases of oral facial surgery in which a straw may be contraindicated).
- Give any prescribed pain medication before leaving facility.
- Provide parents with verbal and written information on potential side effects of pain medication for which they should be vigilant after discharge.

ISOLATION

Admission to an isolation room increases all of the stressors typically associated with hospitalization. There is further separation from familiar persons; additional loss of control; and added environmental changes, such as sensory deprivation and the appearance of strangers. Orientation to time and place is affected. These stressors may be compounded by a child's limited understanding of isolation. Preschool children have difficulty understanding the rationale for isolation, as they cannot comprehend the cause-and-effect relationship between infections and illness. They are likely to view isolation as punishment. Older children understand the causality better but still require information to decrease fantasizing or misinterpretation.

When a child is placed in isolation, preparation is essential for the child to feel in control. With young children, the best approach is a simple explanation, such as "You need to be in this special room to help you get better. The infection made you sick and you could not help that."

All children, but especially younger ones, need preparation in terms of what they will see, hear, and feel in isolation. Therefore they are shown the mask, gloves, and gown and are encouraged to "dress up" in them. Playing with the hospital personal protective equipment can lessen the fear of hospital personnel entering the room. Nurses and other health personnel should introduce themselves and let the child see their faces before donning masks. In this way, the child associates them with significant experiences and gains a sense of familiarity in an otherwise strange and lonely environment.

When the child's condition improves, appropriate play activities are provided to minimize boredom and stimulate the senses. The environment can be manipulated to increase sensory freedom by moving the bed toward the door or window. Opening window shades; providing musical, visual, or tactile toys; and increasing interpersonal contact can substitute mental mobility for the limitations of physical movement. Rather than dwelling on the negative aspects of isolation, the child can be encouraged to view this experience as challenging and positive.

NURSING TIP: Have the child select a place he or she would like to visit. Help the child decorate the bed and equipment to suit the theme (e.g., truck, circus tent, spaceship, sky). At a set time each day, pretend to go with the child to the special place. Consider including props such as a suitcase or picnic basket.

EMERGENCY ADMISSION

One of the most traumatic hospital experiences for the child and parents is an emergency admission. The sudden onset of an illness or the occurrence of an injury leaves little time for preparation and explanation. Sometimes the emergency admission is compounded by admission to an intensive care unit (ICU) or the need for immediate surgery.

In instances requiring only outpatient treatment, the child is exposed to a strange, frightening environment and to experiences that may elicit fear or cause pain.

There is a wide discrepancy between what constitutes a medically defined emergency and a patient-defined emergency. A growing concern is the use of major emergency departments for routine primary care health visits. To offset overcrowding in emergency departments, many facilities have minor emergency units or pediatric minor emergency units for after-hours health care. Telephone triage for minor illnesses for patients is also emerging as a health care delivery mode to differentiate illnesses such as a common cold from true life-threatening conditions that require immediate practitioner attention and intervention. Other factors contributing to the overuse of emergency departments include the increasing number of uninsured persons and households where both parents work full time and cannot afford to take time off during the day to take the sick child to a practitioner.

In pediatric populations, most visits to an emergency department are for respiratory infections; skin conditions, gastrointestinal disorders, and trauma (such as poisoning) account for the remaining cases. The most common reason parents give for bringing the child to the emergency department is concern about the illness worsening. Providers may not think that the progressive symptoms need immediate or emergency care. One of the nurse's primary goals is to assess the parents' perception of the event and their reasons for considering it serious or life threatening.

Emergency situations usually do not allow for lengthy preparatory admission procedures. In such instances, nurses must focus their nursing interventions on the essential components of admission counseling (Box 19.10) and complete the process as soon as the child's condition has stabilized.

Unless an emergency is life threatening, children need to participate in their care to maintain a sense of control. Because emergency departments are frequently hectic, there is a tendency to rush through procedures to save time. The extra few minutes needed to allow children to participate may save many more minutes of useless resistance and uncooperativeness during subsequent procedures. Other supportive measures include ensuring privacy, accepting various emotional responses to fear or pain, preserving parent-child contact, explaining all events before or as they occur, and personally remaining calm. Pain management strategies are discussed in Chapter 5.

BOX 19.10 Guidelines for Special Hospital Admission[a]

Emergency Admission

Lengthy preparatory admission procedures are often impossible and inappropriate for emergency situations.

Focus assessment on airway, breathing, and circulation; weigh child whenever possible for calculation of drug dosages.

Unless an emergency is life threatening, children need to participate in their care to maintain a sense of control.

Focus on essential components of admission counseling, including:

- Appropriate introduction to the family
- Use of child's name, not terms such as "honey" or "dear"
- Determination of child's age and some judgment about developmental age (If the child is of school age, asking about the grade level will offer some evidence of intellectual ability.)
- Information about child's general state of health, any problems that may interfere with medical treatment (e.g., allergies), and previous experience with hospital facilities
- Information about the chief complaint from both the parents and the child

Admission to Intensive Care Unit

Prepare child and parents for elective intensive care unit (ICU) admission, such as for postoperative care after cardiac surgery.

Prepare child and parents for unanticipated ICU admission by focusing primarily on the sensory aspects of the experience and on usual family concerns (e.g., persons in charge of child's care, schedule for visiting, area where family can stay).

Prepare parents regarding child's appearance and behavior when they first visit child in ICU.

Accompany family to bedside to provide emotional support and answer questions.

Prepare siblings for their visit; plan length of time for sibling visitation; monitor siblings' reactions during visit to prevent them from becoming overwhelmed.

Encourage parents to stay with their child:

- If visiting hours are limited, allow flexibility in schedule to accommodate parental needs.
- Give family members a written schedule of visiting times.
- If visiting hours are liberal, be aware of family members' needs and suggest periodic respites.
- Assure family they can call the unit at any time.

Prepare parents for expected role changes and identify ways for parents to participate in child's care without overwhelming them with responsibilities:

- Help with bath or feeding.
- Touch and talk to child.
- Help with procedures.

Provide information about child's condition in understandable language:

- Repeat information often.
- Seek clarification of understanding.
- During bedside conferences, interpret information for family members and child or, if appropriate, conduct report outside room.

Prepare child for procedures even if it involves explanation while procedure is performed.

Assess and manage pain; recognize that a child who cannot talk, such as an infant or child in a coma or on mechanical ventilation, can be in pain.

Establish a routine that maintains some similarity to daily events in child's life whenever possible:

- Organize care during normal waking hours.
- Keep regular bedtime schedules, including quiet times when television or radio is lowered or turned off.
- Provide uninterrupted sleep cycles (60 minutes for infants; 90 minutes for older children).
- Close and open drapes and dim lights to allow for day and night.
- Place curtain around bed for privacy.
- Orient child to day and time; have clocks or calendars in easy view for older children.

Schedule a time when child is left undisturbed (e.g., during naps, visit with family, playtime, or favorite program).

Provide opportunities for play.

Reduce stimulation in environment:

- Refrain from loud talking or laughing.
- Keep equipment noise to a minimum.
- Turn alarms as low as safely possible.
- Perform treatments requiring equipment at one time.
- Turn off bedside equipment that is not in use, such as suction and oxygen.
- Avoid loud, abrupt noises.

[a]See also Box 19.7.

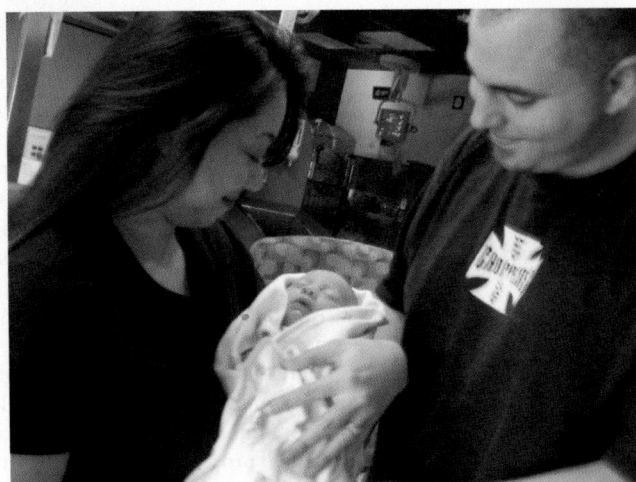

Fig. 19.10 Parental presence during hospitalization provides emotional support for the child and increases the parents' sense of empowerment in the caregiver role. (Courtesy E. Jacob, Texas Children's Hospital, Houston, TX.)

At times, because of the child's physical condition, little or no preparatory counseling for emergency hospitalization can be done. In such situations, counseling subsequent to the event has therapeutic value. The counseling should focus on evaluating children's thoughts on admission and related procedures. Projective techniques such as drawing, doll play, or storytelling are especially effective. The nurse then bases additional information on what has already been understood.

INTENSIVE CARE UNIT

Admission to an ICU can be traumatic for both the child and parents (Fig. 19.10). The nature and severity of the illness and the circumstances surrounding the admission are major factors, especially for parents. Parents experience significantly more stress when the admission is unexpected rather than expected. Stressors for the child and parent are described in Box 19.11. Although several studies have described what parents perceive as most stressful, the most effective strategy may be to simply ask parents what is stressful and implement interventions that will enhance their ability to cope (Board & Ryan-Wenger, 2003). Assessment should be repeated periodically to account for changes in perceptions over time. The use of daily patient goal sheets has been successful in improving communication among health care providers caring for children in the ICU (Agarwal, Frankel, Tourner, et al., 2008; Phipps & Thomas, 2007). By clearly defining daily patient care goals, health care providers believed that care was improved. Standardized rounding structure improved adherence to daily goal sheet use, with the intent of improved communication among caregivers (Seigel, Whelan, et al., 2014).

The family's emotional needs are paramount when a child is admitted to an ICU. A major stressor for parents of a child in the ICU is the child's appearance (Latour, van Goudoever, & Hazelzet, 2008). Although the same interventions discussed earlier for the stressors of separation and loss of control apply here, additional interventions may also benefit the family and child (see Box 19.11). In a qualitative study of 19 parents of 10 children in an ICU, parents reported that they simply wanted nurses to nurture the child in the same way the family would (Harbaugh, Tomlinson, & Kirschbaum, 2004). Nurse behaviors that exemplified caring and affection were perceived as helpful in decreasing stress. Behaviors perceived as not helpful included separating the child from the parents and communicating poorly with parents. Therefore even critical care must be centered on the family.

BOX 19.11 Neonatal or Pediatric Intensive Care Unit Stressors for the Child and Family

Physical Stressors

Pain and discomfort (e.g., injections, intubation, suctioning, dressing changes, other invasive procedures)
Immobility (e.g., use of restraints, bed rest)
Sleep deprivation
Inability to eat or drink
Changes in elimination habits

Environmental Stressors

Unfamiliar surroundings (e.g., crowding)
Unfamiliar sounds

- Equipment noise (e.g., monitors, telephone, suctioning, computer printout)
- Human sounds (e.g., talking, laughing, crying, coughing, moaning, retching, walking)

Unfamiliar people (e.g., health care professionals, patients, visitors)
Unfamiliar and unpleasant smells (e.g., alcohol, adhesive remover, body odors)
Constant lights (disturb day-night rhythms)
Activity related to other patients
Sense of urgency among staff
Unkind or thoughtless comments from staff

Psychologic Stressors

Lack of privacy
Inability to communicate (if intubated)
Inadequate knowledge and understanding of situation
Severity of illness
Parental behavior (expression of concern)

Social Stressors

Disrupted relationships (especially with family and friends)
Concern with missing school or work
Play deprivation

Data primarily from Tichy, A. M., Braam, C. M., Meyer, T. A., et al. (1988). Stressors in pediatric intensive care units. *Pediatric Nursing, 14*(1), 40–42.

It is important that visiting hours be liberal and flexible enough to accommodate parental needs and involvement.

Critically ill children become the focus of their parents' lives, and parents' most pressing need is for information. They want to know if their child will live and, if so, whether the child will be the same as before. They need to know why various interventions are being done for the child, that the child is being treated for pain or is comfortable, and that the child may be able to hear them even though not awake. When parents first visit the child in the ICU, they need preparation regarding the child's appearance. Ideally, the nurse should accompany the parents to the bedside to provide emotional support and answer any questions.

Despite the stresses normally associated with ICU admission, a special security develops from being carefully monitored and receiving individualized care. Therefore planning for transition to the regular unit is essential and should include:

- Assignment of a primary nurse on the regular unit
- Continued visits by the ICU staff to assess the child's and parents' adjustment and to act as a temporary liaison with the nursing staff
- Explanation of the differences between the two units and the rationale for the change to less intense monitoring of the child's physical condition
- Selection of an appropriate room, such as one that is close to the nursing station, and a compatible roommate

CLINICAL JUDGMENT AND NEXT-GENERATION NCLEX® EXAMINATION-STYLE QUESTIONS

1. The nurse is caring for a 5-year-old girl who is newly diagnosed with a seizure disorder. She observes that the child is having separation anxiety when her parents leave the room. What are important aspects of separation anxiety that are specific to this stage of development? **Use an X for the health teaching statement below that is Indicated (appropriate or necessary), Contraindicated (could be harmful), or Non-Essential (makes no difference or not necessary).**

Health Teaching	Indicated	Contraindicated	Non-Essential
"Separation anxiety may be seen in your child by refusing to eat, having trouble sleeping, crying quietly for you when gone, or withdrawing from others."			
"Separation anxiety comes in stages: denial, despair, and detachment."			
"Loss of peer group contact may pose a severe emotional threat because of loss of group status, and loss of group acceptance."			
"Your child may need and desire parental guidance or support from other adult figures as she returns to school."			
"Young children can react "negatively" to their parents during hospitalization; they may cling to you to ensure your continued presence."			

2. A 3-year-old child has been hospitalized for the past week for pneumonia. Since his condition is stable, his mother has returned to work and the child is often alone during the day. The nurse caring for the child reviews the medical record and performs an assessment and findings are listed below. Which findings are reflective of the Stage of Despair that can occur because of separation anxiety? **Select the assessment findings that are reflective of the Stage of Despair in separation anxiety. Select all that apply.**
   A. Appears happy
   B. Refuses to communicate
   C. Withdraws from the nurse
   D. Appears depressed and sad
   E. Verbally attacks the nurse
   F. Attempts to escape the room
   G. Lacks interest in the environment
   H. Cries and screams when the nurse enters the room

3. The nurse is admitting an 8-year-old child to the hospital for further evaluation of a congenital heart disorder. Her mother is with her. What are important aspects of the admission process that the nurse needs to remember during this first encounter with the patient and family? **Select all that apply.**
   A. Introduce yourself
   B. Orient the child and family to the unit
   C. Apply identification band on the child's wrist
   D. Apply identification band to the mother's wrist
   E. Take vital signs, blood pressure, height and weight
   F. Draw extra blood in case labs will be ordered later
   G. Discuss hospital schedules and regulations
   H. Explain how to use the electronic devices in the room such as call light, bed controls, television
   I. Take the child to the cafeteria so family will know where to go for dinner

4. When discharging an 8-year-old boy who was hospitalized for an appendectomy, the nurse reviews the plan for continued care at home. He was hospitalized 4 days ago after a 2-day history of abdominal pain and fever. The patient underwent an emergency appendectomy. What health teaching would the nurse include as part of the discharge instructions? **Select all that apply.**
   A. "Your son can have soft foods at home, examples include Jell-O, pudding, and apple juice."
   B. "You can use other things to help with pain, such as distraction (reading a book, music, or a movie), after the pain medication is given."
   C. "You can get your child's prescription in the next couple of days."
   D. "You can drive your son home without concern; make sure you both wear a seatbelt."
   E. "We will contact you tomorrow for follow-up, but do not hesitate to call if you have any concerns before then."
   F. "If fever develops in the next 10 days, start oral antibiotics again at home."

REFERENCES

Abraham, M., & Moretz, J. G. (2012). Implementing patient- and family-centered care: Part I—understanding the challenges. *Pediatric Nursing, 38*(1), 44–47.

Agarwal, S., Frankel, L., Tourner, S., et al. (2008). Improving communication in a pediatric intensive care unit using daily patient goal sheets. *The Journal of Critical Care, 23*(2), 227–235.

Anderson, C. D., & Mangino, R. R. (2006). Nurse shift report: Who says you can't talk in front of the patient? *Nursing Administration Quarterly, 30*(2), 112–122.

Board, R., & Ryan-Wenger, N. (2003). Stressors and symptoms of mothers with children in the PICU. *The Journal of Pediatric Nursing, 18*(3), 195–201.

Caffin, C. L., Linton, S., & Pellegrini, J. (2007). Introduction of a liaison nurse role in a tertiary paediatric ICU. *Intensive and Critical Care Nursing, 23*(4), 226–233.

Clatworthy, S., Simon, K., & Tiedeman, M. E. (1999). Child drawing: Hospital—an instrument designed to measure the emotional status of hospitalized school-aged children. *The Journal of Pediatric Nursing, 14*(1), 2–9.

Coyne, I. (2006). Children's experiences of hospitalization. *Journal of Child Health Care, 10*(4), 326–336.

Craft, M. J. (1993). Siblings of hospitalized children: Assessment and intervention. *The Journal of Pediatric Nursing, 8*(5), 289–297.

Eichner, J. M., & Johnson, B. H. (2012). Patient- and family-centered care and the pediatrician's role. *Pediatrics, 129*(2), 394–404.

Fernandez, C., Pyesmany, A., & Stutzer, C. (1999). Alternative therapies in childhood cancer. *The New England Journal of Medicine, 340*(7), 569–570.

Feudtner, H. J., Haney, J., & Dimmers, M. A. (2003). Spiritual care needs of hospitalized children and their families: A national survey of pastoral care providers' perceptions. *Pediatric, 111*(1), e67–e72.

Flanagan, K. (2001). Preoperative assessment: Safety considerations for patients taking herbal products. *The Journal of Pediatric Nursing, 16*(1), 19–26.

Gordon, M. (2002). *Manual of nursing diagnosis* (10th ed.). St Louis: Mosby.

Harbaugh, B. L., Tomlinson, P. S., & Kirschbaum, M. (2004). Parents' perceptions of nurses' caregiving behaviors in the pediatric intensive care unit. *Issues in Comprehensive Pediatric Nursing, 27*(3), 163–178.

Hopia, H., Tomlinson, P. S., Paavilainen, E., et al. (2005). Child in hospital: Family experiences and expectations of how nurses can promote family health. *Journal of Clinical Nursing, 14*(2), 212–222.

Institute for Patient- and Family-Centered Care. (2010a). Frequently asked questions: What are the core concepts of patient- and family-centered care? http://www.ipfcc.org/about/pfcc.html.

Institute for Patient- and Family-Centered Care. (2010b). *Advancing the practice of patient- and family-centered care in hospitals: How to get started.* http://www.ipfcc.org/resources/getting_started.pdf.

The Joint Commission. (2011). *Comprehensive accreditation manual for hospitals (CAMH).* Oakbrook Terrace, IL: Author.

Latour, J. M., van Goudoever, J. B., & Hazelzet, J. A. (2008). Parent satisfaction in the pediatric ICU. *Pediatric Clinics of North America, 55*(3), 779–790.

Lewandowski, L. A., & Tesler, M. D. (2003). *Family centered care: Putting it into action.* Washington, DC: American Nurses Association.

Limbers, C., & Skipper, S. (2014). Health-related quality of life measurement in siblings of children with physical chronic illness: A systematic review. *Families, Systems, & Health, 32*(4), 408–415.

Meert, K. L., Clark, J., & Eggly, S. (2013). Family-centered care in the pediatric intensive care unit. *Pediatric Clinics of North America, 60*(3), 761–772.

Melnyk, B. M. (2000). Intervention studies involving parents of hospitalized young children: An analysis of the past and future recommendations. *The Journal of Pediatric Nursing, 15*(1), 4–13.

Orem, D. (2001). *Nursing: Concepts of practice* (5th ed.). New York: Mosby.

Phipps, L. M., & Thomas, N. J. (2007). The use of a daily goals sheet to improve communication in the paediatric intensive care unit. *Intensive and Critical Care Nursing, 23*(5), 264–271.

Rappaport, D. I., Ketterer, T. A., Nilforoshan, V., & Sharif, I. (2012). Family-centered rounds: Views of families, nurses, trainees, and attending physicians. *Clinical Pediatrics, 51*(3), 260–266.

Samela, M., Salanterä, S., & Aronen, E. (2009). Child-reported hospital fears in 4- to 6-year-old children. *Pediatric Nursing, 35*(5), 269–276 303.

Seigel, J., Whelan, L., et al. (2014). Successful implementation of standardized multidisciplinary bedside rounds, including daily goals, in a pediatric ICU. *Joint Commission Journal on Quality and Patient Safety, 40*(2), 83–90.

Small, L. (2002). Early predictors of poor coping outcomes in children following intensive care hospitalization and stressful medical encounters. *Pediatric Nursing, 28*(4), 393–401.

Smith, T., & Conant Rees, H. L. (2000). Making family-centered care a reality. *Seminars for Nurse Managers, 8*(3), 136–142.

Thompson, R. (2009). *The handbook of child life: A guide for pediatric psychosocial care.* Springfield, IL: Charles C Thomas.

Wilson, M. E., Megel, M. E., Enenbach, L., et al. (2010). The voices of children: Stories about hospitalization. *The Journal of Pediatric Health Care, 24*(2), 95–102.

20

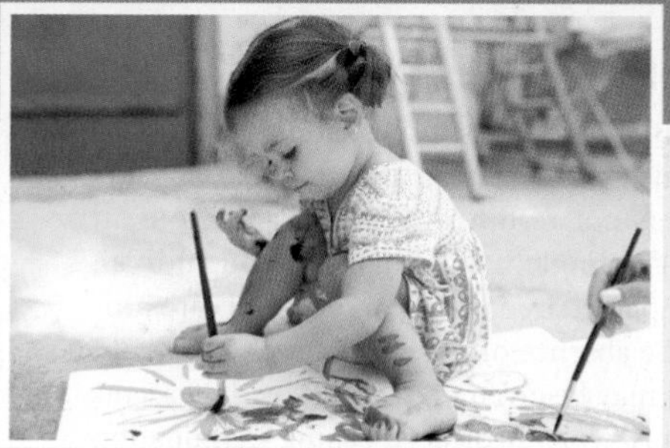

Pediatric Nursing Interventions and Skills

Caroline E. Anderson, Ruth Anne Herring

http://evolve.elsevier.com/wong/essentials

CONCEPTS

- Informed Consent
- Procedure Preparation
- Medication Administration
- Specimen Collection
- Fluid Balance and Nutrition
- Respiratory Support

GENERAL CONCEPTS RELATED TO PEDIATRIC PROCEDURES

INFORMED CONSENT

Before undergoing any invasive procedure, the patient or the patient's legal surrogate must receive sufficient information on which to make an informed health care decision. **Informed consent** should include the nature of the illness or condition, proposed care, or treatment; potential risks, benefits, and alternatives; and what might happen if the patient chooses not to consent. In addition, discussions should include the procedure team roles, including trainees involved in care (Firdouse, Wajchendler, Koyle, et al., 2017). To obtain valid informed consent, health care providers must meet the following three conditions:

1. The person must be capable of giving consent; he or she must be over the age of majority (usually age 18 years) and must be considered competent (i.e., possess the mental capacity to make choices and understand their consequences).
2. The person must receive the information needed to make an intelligent decision.
3. The person must act voluntarily when exercising freedom of choice without force, fraud, deceit, duress, or other forms of constraint or coercion.

The patient has the right to accept or refuse any health care. If a patient is treated without consent, the hospital or health care provider may be charged with assault and held liable for damages. In addition, consent is a two-way process that requires both the health care provider to share all required information and the patient to hear and understand the information. Health care providers must deliver information in the appropriate language and health literacy level for the patient and family. There must also be adequate time for questions and opportunity to clarify concerns. Informed consent and medical decision making is not a one-time event but an ongoing process that requires continual communication among the health care team, patient, and caregivers (American Academy of Pediatrics, Committee on Bioethics, 2016).

REQUIREMENTS FOR OBTAINING INFORMED CONSENT

Written informed consent of the patient, parent, or legal guardian is usually required for medical or surgical treatment of a minor, including many diagnostic procedures. One universal consent is not sufficient. Separate informed permissions must be obtained for each surgical or diagnostic procedure, including the following:

- Major surgery
- Minor surgery (e.g., cutdown, biopsy, dental extraction, suturing a laceration [especially one that may have a cosmetic effect], removal of a cyst, closed reduction of a fracture)
- Diagnostic tests with an element of risk (e.g., bronchoscopy, angiography, lumbar puncture, cardiac catheterization, bone marrow aspiration)
- Medical treatments with an element of risk (e.g., blood transfusion, thoracentesis or paracentesis, radiotherapy)

Other situations that require patient or parental consent include the following:

- Photographs for medical, educational, or public use
- Removal of the child from the health care institution against medical advice
- Postmortem examination, except in unexplained deaths, such as sudden infant death, violent death, or suspected suicide
- Release of medical information

Decision making involving the care of older children and adolescents (older than 7 years of age with appropriate age, maturity, and psychologic state) should include the patient's **assent** (if feasible) as well as the parent's consent (Poston, 2016). Assent means that the child or adolescent has been informed about the proposed treatment, procedure, or research and is willing to permit a health care provider to perform it. If the child or adolescent merely fails to object, this does not equate assent. Assent should include the following:

- Helping the patient achieve a developmentally appropriate awareness of the nature of his or her condition
- Telling the patient what he or she can expect

- Making a clinical assessment of the patient's understanding
- Soliciting an expression of the patient's willingness to accept the proposed procedure

Health care providers should use multiple methods to provide information, including age-appropriate methods (e.g., videos, peer discussion, diagrams, written materials). The nurse should provide an assent form for the child to sign, and the child should keep a copy. By including the child in the decision-making process and gaining his or her acceptance, staff members demonstrate respect for the child. Assent is not a legal requirement but an ethical one to protect the rights of children. Chapter 17 provides further discussion on the dying child's right to refuse treatment.

Eligibility for Giving Informed Consent

Informed Consent of Parents or Legal Guardians

Parents have full responsibility for the care and rearing of their minor children, including legal control over them. As long as children are minors, their parents or legal guardians are required to give informed consent before medical treatment is rendered or any procedure is performed. If the parents are married to each other, consent from only one parent is required for nonurgent pediatric care. If the parents are divorced, consent usually rests with the parent who has legal custody (American Academy of Pediatrics, Committee on Bioethics, 2016). Emergency care of a pediatric patient should never be withheld due to the absence of a parent or legal guardian. Parents also have a right to withdraw consent later. If the legal caregivers disagree on the treatment course, it is within the health care providers' scope to request consultation of a hospital ethics board to determine what care is in the best interest of the patient (Dahl, Sinha, Rosenberg, et al., 2015).

Evidence of Consent

Regulations on obtaining informed consent vary from state to state, and policies differ at each health care facility. It is the physician's legal responsibility to explain the procedure, risks, benefits, and alternatives. The nurse witnesses the patient's, parent's, or legal guardian's signature on the consent form and may reinforce what the patient has been told. A signed consent form is the legal document that signifies that the process of informed consent has occurred. If parents are unavailable to sign consent forms, verbal consent may be obtained via the telephone in the presence of two witnesses. Both witnesses record that informed consent was given and by whom. Their signatures indicate that they witnessed the verbal consent. If the parents or legal guardians cannot be reached for an extended period, the nurse may request the assistance of social work or law enforcement officers to locate a legal guardian.

Informed Consent of Mature and Emancipated Minors

State laws differ with regard to the age of majority, the age at which a person is considered to have all the legal rights and responsibilities of an adult. In most states, 18 years is the age of majority. Competent adults can give informed consent on their own behalf. An **emancipated minor** is one who is legally under the age of majority but is recognized as having the legal capacity or social status of an adult under circumstances prescribed by state law, such as pregnancy, marriage, high school graduation, independent living, or military service. A **mature minor** exception to consent laws is recognized in a few states for children age 14 years and older who possesses the maturity and cognitive abilities to understand all elements of informed consent and make a choice based on the information. Legal action may be required for designation as a mature minor (American Academy of Pediatrics, Committee on Bioethics, 2016).

Treatment Without Parental Consent

Exceptions to requiring parental consent before treating minor children occur in situations in which children need urgent medical or surgical treatment and a parent is not readily available to give consent or refuses to give consent. For example, a child may be brought to an emergency department accompanied by a grandparent, child care provider, teacher, or others. In the absence of parents or legal guardians, persons in charge of the child may be given permission by the parents to give informed consent by proxy. A medical screening examination is required by federal law under the Emergency Medical Treatment and Active Labor Act for all patients presenting to an emergency center. In emergencies, including danger to life or the possibility of permanent injury, appropriate care should not be withheld or delayed because of problems obtaining consent (American Academy of Pediatrics, Committee on Bioethics, 2016). The nurse should document any efforts made to obtain consent.

Parental refusal to give consent for life-saving treatment or to prevent serious harm can occur and requires notification to child protective services to render emergency treatment. For example, Jehovah's Witnesses commonly choose to avoid receiving blood products due to religious beliefs. In cases where a blood product is crucial for the child's survival, it is important to work together with the family, medical team, and child protective services to determine the course of action that is in the best interest of the child. "Parental decision-making should primarily be understood as parents' responsibility to support the interests of their child and to preserve family relationships, rather than being focused on their rights to express their own autonomous choices" (American Academy of Pediatrics, Committee on Bioethics, 2016). Evaluation for child abuse or neglect can occur without parental consent and without notification to the state before evaluation in most states.

Adolescents, Consent, and Confidentiality

The Health Insurance Portability and Accountability Act of 1996 (HIPAA) was passed to help protect and safeguard the security and confidentiality of health information. Because adolescents are not yet adults, parents have the right to make most decisions on their behalf and receive information. Adolescents, however, are more likely to seek care in a setting in which they believe their privacy will be maintained. All 50 states have enacted legislation that entitles adolescents to consent to treatment without the parents' knowledge to one or more "medically emancipated" conditions such as sexually transmitted infections, mental health services, substance abuse and addiction, pregnancy, and contraceptive advice (American Academy of Pediatrics, Committee on Bioethics, 2016). Consent to abortion is controversial, and statutes vary widely by state. The Planned Parenthood Federation of America provides consent and notification law requirements listed by state. State law preempts HIPAA regardless of whether that law prohibits, mandates, or allows discretion about a disclosure.

Informed Consent and Parental Right to the Child's Medical Chart

Some state statutes give parents the unrestricted right to a copy of their children's medical records. In states without statutes, the best practice is to allow parents to review or have a copy of minors' charts under reasonable circumstances. Practitioners should avoid restrictive requirements such as review permitted only in the presence of a clinician. Rather, an appropriate practitioner should be available to answer any questions that parents may have during their reviews. It is important for the nurse to check the state and health care institution's policies surrounding providing printed copies of medical records to patients and families.

PREPARATION FOR DIAGNOSTIC AND THERAPEUTIC PROCEDURES

Technologic advances and changes in health care have resulted in more pediatric procedures being performed in a variety of settings. Many procedures are both stressful and painful experiences. For many procedures, the focus of care is psychologic preparation of the child and family. However, some procedures require the administration of sedatives and analgesics.

The child life specialist is an especially valued member of the health care team when preparing a child for diagnostic and therapeutic procedures. Child life specialists address the psychosocial concerns that accompany stressful life experiences by promoting optimal child development and minimizing adverse effects. Child life specialists receive advanced education and training in the developmental stages of childhood as well as strategies to cope with illness and injury. Therapeutic play, procedural preparation and support, developmentally appropriate education, and promoting normalcy are all significant ways in which the child life specialist can have a positive impact on the health care experience of the child and family. Child life specialists and nursing staff can work together to implement evidence-based interventions to decrease fear, anxiety, and discomfort experienced by children in the health care environment (Association of Child Life Professionals, 2017).

Psychologic Preparation

Preparing children for procedures decreases their anxiety, promotes their cooperation, supports their coping skills and may teach them new ones, and facilitates a feeling of mastery in experiencing a potentially stressful event. Many institutions have developed preadmission teaching programs designed to educate the pediatric patient and family by offering hands-on experience with hospital equipment, the procedure performed, and departments they will visit. Preparatory methods may be formal, such as group preparation for hospitalization. Most preparation strategies are informal, focus on providing information about the experience, and are directed at stressful or painful procedures. The most effective preparation includes the provision of sensory-procedural information and helping the child develop coping skills, such as imagery, distraction, or relaxation.

The Applying Evidence to Practice boxes describe general guidelines for preparing children for procedures along with age-specific guidelines that consider children's developmental needs and cognitive abilities. In addition to these suggestions, nurses should consider the child's temperament, existing coping strategies, and previous experiences in individualizing the preparatory process. Stress point coping can be used to determine the child's most stressful or upsetting part of previous procedural experiences (Thompson, 2018). Once the stress point is identified, coping strategies to address this specific point in the procedure can be discussed with the child. Children who are distractible and highly active or those who are "slow to warm up" may need individualized sessions—shorter for active children and more slowly paced for shy children. Whereas children who tend to cope well may need more emphasis on using their present skills, those who appear to cope less adequately can benefit from more time devoted to simple coping strategies, such as relaxing, breathing, counting, squeezing a hand, or singing. Children with previous health-related experiences still need preparation for repeat or new procedures; however, the nurse must assess what they know, correct their misconceptions, supply new information, and introduce new coping skills as indicated by their previous reactions. Especially for painful procedures, the most effective preparation includes providing sensory-procedural information and helping the child develop coping skills, such as imagery or relaxation (see Applying Evidence to Practice boxes).

All experiences of childhood can affect development and influence the way in which a child responds to the health care environment, even into adulthood. Adverse childhood experiences can include abuse, neglect, substance abuse, or any other traumatic experiences and may result in negative health behaviors, chronic health conditions, and even early death (Centers for Disease Control and Prevention, 2019). While in the health care environment, children can experience medical traumatic stress during difficult or frightening medical events or from simply being present in the hospital environment. As care providers, it is important to practice trauma-informed care; consider the impact that past physical, mental, and emotional trauma may have on a patient; and adapt care appropriately. This may include reducing distress through pain control, offering choices, psychologic preparation for procedures, providing emotional support, and including the family in what health care providers may perceive as routine care (National Child Traumatic Stress Network, 2019).

APPLYING EVIDENCE TO PRACTICE

Preparing Children for Procedures

- Determine details of exact procedure to be performed.
- Review parents' and child's present understanding through open-ended questions.
- Base teaching on developmental age and existing knowledge.
- Incorporate parents in the teaching if they desire, especially if they plan to participate in care.
- Inform parents of their supportive role during the procedure, such as standing near child's head or in child's line of vision and talking softly to child, participating in comfort holding positions, and typical responses of children undergoing the procedure.
- Allow for ample discussion to prevent information overload and ensure adequate feedback.
- Use concrete, not abstract, terms and visual aids to describe procedure. For example, use a simple line drawing of a boy or girl and mark the body part that will be involved in the procedure. Use nonthreatening but realistic models.[a]
- Emphasize that no other body part will be involved.
- If the body part is associated with a specific function, stress the change or noninvolvement of that ability (e.g., after tonsillectomy, child can still speak).
- Use words and sentence length appropriate to child's level of understanding (a rule of thumb for the number of words in a child's sentence is equal to his or her age in years plus 1).
- Avoid words and phrases with dual meanings (see Table 20.1) unless child understands such words.
- Clarify all unfamiliar words (e.g., "Anesthesia is a *different kind of* sleep").
- Emphasize sensory aspects of procedure—what child will feel, see, hear, smell, taste, and touch, and what child can do during procedure (e.g., lie still, count out loud, squeeze a hand, hug a doll).
- Allow child to practice procedures that will require cooperation (e.g., turning, deep breathing, using an incentive spirometer).
- Introduce anxiety-inducing information last (e.g., starting an intravenous line).
- Be honest with child about unpleasant aspects of a procedure but avoid creating undue concern. When discussing that a procedure may be uncomfortable, state that it feels differently to different people.
- Emphasize end of procedure and any pleasurable events afterwards (e.g., going home, seeing parents).
- Stress positive benefits of procedure (e.g., "After your tonsils are fixed, you won't have as many sore throats").
- Provide a positive ending, praising efforts at cooperation and coping.

[a] Soft-sculptured dolls and customized adapters and overlays for preparing children and families about procedures and as teaching models for technical care are available from Legacy Products, Inc., 120 West Main Street, PO Box 267, Cambridge City, IN 47327; 800-238-7951; email: info@legacyproductsinc.com; https://legacyproductsinc.com/.

APPLYING EVIDENCE TO PRACTICE

Age-Specific Preparation of Children for Procedures Based on Developmental Characteristics

Infant—Developing Trust and Sensorimotor Thought

Attachment to Parent

Involve parent in procedure if desired.[a]

Keep parent in infant's line of vision.

If parent is unable to be with infant, place familiar object with infant (e.g., stuffed toy, blanket).

Stranger Anxiety

Have usual caregivers perform or assist with procedure.[a]

Make advances slowly and in a nonthreatening manner.

Limit number of strangers entering room during procedure.[a]

Sensorimotor Phase of Learning

During procedure, use sensory soothing measures (e.g., stroking skin, talking softly, giving pacifier, providing sucrose water solution with pacifier, breastfeeding).

Use analgesics (e.g., topical anesthetic, intravenous opioid) to control discomfort.[a]

Cuddle and hug infant after stressful procedure; encourage parent to comfort infant.

Increased Muscle Control

Expect older infants to resist.

Restrain adequately using comfort holds.

Keep harmful objects out of reach.

Memory for Past Experiences

Realize that older infants may associate objects, places, or persons with prior painful experiences and will cry and resist at the sight of them.

Keep frightening objects out of view.[a]

Perform painful procedures in a separate room, not in crib (or bed).[a]

Use nonintrusive procedures whenever possible (e.g., axillary or tympanic temperatures, oral medications).[a]

Imitation of Gestures

Model desired behavior (e.g., opening mouth).

Toddler—Developing Autonomy and Sensorimotor to Preoperational Thought

Use same approaches as for infant plus the following.

Egocentric Thought

Explain procedure in relation to what child will see, hear, taste, smell, and feel.

Emphasize those aspects of procedure that require cooperation (e.g., lying still).

Tell child it is okay to cry, yell, or use other means to express discomfort verbally.

Designate one health care provider to speak during procedure. Hearing more than one provider can be confusing and overwhelming to a child.[a]

Negative Behavior

Expect treatments to be resisted; child may try to run away.

Use firm, direct approach.

Ignore temper tantrums.

Use distraction techniques (e.g., singing a song *with* child).

Restrain adequately using a comfort hold technique.

Animism

Keep frightening objects out of view (young children believe that objects have lifelike qualities and can harm them).

Limited Language Skills

Communicate using gestures or demonstrations.

Use a few simple terms familiar to child.

Give child one direction at a time (e.g., "Lie down" and then "Hold my hand").

Use small replicas of equipment; allow child to handle equipment.

Use play; demonstrate on doll but avoid child's favorite doll because child may think doll is really "feeling" procedure.

Prepare parents separately to avoid child's misinterpreting words.

Limited Concept of Time

Prepare child shortly or immediately before procedure.

Keep teaching sessions short (about 5 to 10 minutes).

Have preparations completed before involving child in procedure.

Have extra equipment nearby (e.g., alcohol swabs, new needle, adhesive bandages) to avoid delays.

Tell child when procedure is completed.

Striving for Independence

Allow choices whenever possible but realize that child may still be resistant and negative.

Allow child to participate in care and to help whenever possible (e.g., drink medicine from a cup, hold a dressing).

Preschooler—Developing Initiative and Preoperational Thought

Egocentric

Explain procedure in simple terms and in relation to how it affects child (as with toddler, stress sensory aspects).

Demonstrate use of equipment.

Allow child to play with miniature or actual equipment.

Encourage "playing out" experience on a doll both before and after procedure to clarify misconceptions.

Use neutral words to describe the procedure (see Table 20.1).

Increased Language Skills

Use verbal explanation but avoid overestimating child's comprehension of words.

Encourage child to verbalize ideas and feelings.

Limited Concept of Time and Frustration Tolerance

Implement same approaches as for toddler but may plan longer teaching session (10 to 15 minutes); may divide information into more than one session.

Illness and Hospitalization Viewed as Punishment

Clarify why each procedure is performed; child will find it difficult to understand how medicine can make him or her feel better and can taste bad at the same time.

Ask child thoughts regarding why a procedure is performed.

State directly that procedures are never a form of punishment.

Animism

Keep equipment out of sight except when shown to or used on child.

Fears of Bodily Harm, Intrusion, and Castration

Point out on drawing, doll, or child where procedure is performed.

Emphasize that no other body part will be involved.

Use nonintrusive procedures whenever possible (e.g., axillary temperatures, oral medication).

Apply an adhesive bandage over puncture site.

Encourage parental presence.

Realize that procedures involving genitalia provoke anxiety.

APPLYING EVIDENCE TO PRACTICE—cont'd

Age-Specific Preparation of Children for Procedures Based on Developmental Characteristics

Allow child to wear underpants with gown.
Explain unfamiliar situations, especially noises or lights.

Striving for Initiative

Involve child in care whenever possible (e.g., hold equipment, remove dressing).
Give choices whenever possible, but avoid excessive delays.
Praise child for helping and attempting to cooperate; never shame child for lack of cooperation.
Identify one thing the child did well during the procedure.

School-Age Child—Developing Industry and Concrete Thought

Increased Language Skills; Interest in Acquiring Knowledge

Explain procedures using correct scientific and medical terminology.
Explain procedure using simple diagrams and photographs.
Discuss why procedure is necessary; concepts of illness and bodily functions are often vague.
Explain function and operation of equipment in concrete terms.
Allow child to manipulate equipment; use doll or another person as model to practice using equipment whenever possible (doll play may be considered childish by older school-age child).
Allow time before and after procedure for questions and discussion.

Improved Concept of Time

Plan for longer teaching sessions (about 20 minutes).
Prepare up to 1 day in advance of procedure to allow for processing of information.

Increased Self-Control

Gain child's cooperation.
Tell child what is expected.
Suggest several ways of maintaining control the child may select from (e.g., deep breathing, relaxation, counting).

Striving for Industry

Allow responsibility for simple tasks (e.g., collecting specimens).
Include child in decision making when choices are possible (e.g., time of day to perform procedure, preferred site).
Encourage active participation (e.g., removing dressings, handling equipment, opening packages).

Developing Relationships With Peers

Prepare two or more children for same procedure or encourage one to help prepare another.
Provide privacy from peers during procedure to maintain self-esteem.

Adolescent—Developing Identity and Abstract Thought

Increasing Abstract Thought and Reasoning

Discuss why procedure is necessary or beneficial.
Explain long-term consequences of procedures; include information about body systems working together.
Realize adolescent may fear death, disability, or other potential risks.
Encourage questioning regarding fears, options, and alternatives.

Consciousness of Appearance

Provide privacy; describe how the body will be covered and what will be exposed.
Discuss how procedure may affect appearance (e.g., scar) and what can be done to minimize it.
Emphasize any physical benefits of procedure.

Concern More With Present Than With Future

Realize that immediate effects of procedure are more significant than future benefits.

Striving for Independence

Involve adolescent in decision making and planning (e.g., time, place, individuals present during procedure, clothing, whether they will watch procedure).
Impose as few restrictions as possible.
Explore what coping strategies have worked in the past; they may need suggestions of various techniques.
Accept regression to more childish methods of coping.
Realize that adolescent may have difficulty accepting new authority figures and may resist complying with procedures.

Developing Peer Relationships and Group Identity

Same as for school-age child but assumes even greater significance.
Allow adolescents to talk with other adolescents who have had the same procedure.

[a] Applies to any age.

Children differ in their "information-seeking dimension." Some actively ask for information about the intended procedure, but others characteristically avoid information. Parents can often guide nurses in deciding how much information is enough for the child because parents know whether the child is typically inquisitive or satisfied with short answers. Asking older children their preferences about the amount of explanation is also important.

The exact timing of the preparation for a procedure varies with the child's age and developmental level and the type of procedure. No exact guidelines govern timing, but in general, the younger the child, the closer the explanation should be to the actual procedure to prevent undue fantasizing and worrying. Concurrent preparation is a strategy that can be used during a procedure to explain what a child can expect to occur and sense immediately before it happens (Thompson, 2018). This can be helpful for emergency procedures, for a highly anxious child, or for younger age-groups where extensive prior preparation is not possible or beneficial. With complex procedures, more time may be needed for assimilation of information, especially with older children. For example, the explanation for an injection can immediately precede the procedure for all ages, but preparation for surgery may begin the day before for young children and a few days before for older children, although the nurse should elicit older children's preferences.

NURSING TIP Use photographs or videos of children in different areas of the hospital (e.g., radiology department, operating room) to give children a more realistic idea of equipment they may encounter.

Establish Trust and Provide Support

The nurse who has spent time with and established a positive relationship with a child usually finds it easier to gain cooperation. If the relationship is based on trust, the child will associate the nurse with caregiving activities that give comfort and pleasure most of the time rather than discomfort and stress. If the nurse does not know the child, it is best for the nurse to be introduced by another staff person whom the child trusts. The first visit with the child should not include any painful procedure and ideally should focus on the child first and then on an explanation of the procedure. A simple way to begin the process of creating trust is by engaging in play with the patient through favorite activities or toys. Body language is another key element of promoting trust. Positive body language, such as sitting instead of standing, and avoiding the use of technical medical terminology in conversation can enhance the therapeutic caregiver relationship with the child and family (Lidgett, 2016).

Parental Presence and Support

Children need support during procedures, and for young children, the greatest source of support is the parents. They represent security, protection, safety, and comfort. Parental presence has a positive impact on the level of pain and negative behavior experienced by the child, as well as on parental distress and satisfaction (Saglik & Caglar, 2018). In addition, there is no difference in technical complications when parents remain with children. However, controversy exists regarding the role parents should assume during the procedure, especially if discomfort is involved. The nurse should assess the parents' preferences for assisting, observing, or waiting outside the room, as well as the child's preference for parental presence. Respect the child's and parents' choices. Give parents who wish to stay appropriate explanation about the procedure and coach them about where to sit or stand and what to say or do to help the child through the procedure. Support parents who decide they do not want to be present and encourage them to remain close by so that they can be available to support the child immediately after the procedure. It can be helpful for parents to assist the health care team in identifying an alternative support person for their child, such as a child life specialist or nurse, if they are unable to be present during the procedure. Parents should know that someone will be with their child to provide support. Ideally, this person should inform the parents after the procedure about how the child did.

Provide an Explanation

Age-appropriate explanations are one of the most widely used interventions for reducing anxiety in children undergoing procedures. Before performing a procedure, explain what is to be done, what sensations the child may feel, what is expected of the child, and why the procedure is being done. It is important that the child understand that the procedure is not punishment. The explanation should be short, simple, and appropriate to the child's level of comprehension. Long explanations may increase anxiety in a young child. When explaining the procedure to parents with the child present, the nurse uses language appropriate to the child because unfamiliar words can be misunderstood (Table 20.1). If the parents need additional preparation, it is done in an area away from the child. Teaching sessions are planned at times most conducive to the child's learning (e.g., after a rest period) and for the usual span of attention.

Special equipment is not necessary for preparing a child, but for young children who cannot yet think conceptually, using objects to supplement verbal explanation is important. Children often learn through behavior modeling such as seeing a doll experience the procedure, watching a video, or seeing a picture. In addition, allowing children to handle actual items that will be used in their care, such as a stethoscope, sphygmomanometer, or oxygen mask, helps them develop familiarity with these items and reduces the fear often associated with their use. Miniature versions of hospital items such as gurneys and x-ray and intravenous (IV) equipment can be used to explain what the children can expect and permit them to safely experience situations that are unfamiliar and potentially frightening. Written and illustrated materials are also valuable aids to preparation.[a]

[a]Preparatory materials include Berenstain Bears Go to the Doctor and Berenstain Bears Visit the Dentist (New York, NY: Random House).

TABLE 20.1 Selecting Nonthreatening Words or Phrases

Words and Phrases to Avoid	Suggested Substitutions
Shot, bee sting, stick	Medicine under the skin, poke that will feel like a pinch
Organ	Place in body
Test	To see how (specify body part) is working
Incision, cut	Make an opening
Edema	Puffiness
Stretcher, gurney	Rolling bed, bed on wheels
Stool, urine	Child's usual term
Dye	Medicine to help place in your body show up on a picture
Pain	Hurt, discomfort, "owie," "boo-boo," sore, achy, scratchy, pinch
Deaden, numb	Not feel body part as much
Fix	Make better
Take (as in "take your temperature")	See how warm you are
Take (as in "take your blood pressure")	Check your pressure, hug your arm
Put to sleep, anesthesia	Different kind of sleep so you won't feel anything
Catheter	Soft tube, small straw
Monitor	Television screen
Electrodes	Stickers, ticklers
Specimen	Take some blood

NURSING TIP To avoid a delay during a procedure, have extra supplies handy. For example, have tape, bandages, alcohol swabs, and an extra needle when performing an injection or venipuncture.

NURSING TIP Prepare a basket, toy chest, or cart to keep near the treatment area. Items ideal for the basket include a Slinky; a sparkling "magic" wand (sealed, acrylic tube partially filled with liquid and suspended metallic confetti); a soft foam ball; bubble solution; party blowers; pop-up books with foldout, three-dimensional scenes; real medical equipment, such as a syringe, adhesive bandages, and alcohol packets; toy medical supplies or a toy medical kit; marking pens; a notepad; and stickers. Have the child choose an item to help distract and relax during the procedure. After the procedure, allow the child to choose a small gift, such as a sticker, or to play with items, such as medical equipment. Do not allow a child to keep a syringe to play with because it can cause harm (e.g., air embolism or infection) if connected to a needleless infusion port.

Physical Preparation

One area of special concern is the administration of appropriate sedation and analgesia before stressful procedures.

Performance of the Procedure

Supportive care continues during the procedure and can be a major factor in a child's ability to cooperate. Ideally, the same nurse who explains the procedure should perform or assist with the procedure. The child may also benefit from a parent or trusted caregiver who can offer coaching techniques and support during the procedure. Before beginning, all equipment is assembled, and the room is readied to prevent unnecessary delays and interruptions that increase the child's anxiety. Minimizing the number of people present and allowing one person to speak during the procedure also can decrease the child's anxiety.

To promote long-term coping and adjustment, give special consideration to the patient's age, coping skills, and procedure to be performed in determining where a procedure will occur. Treatment rooms should be used for procedures requiring sedation, such as bone marrow aspirates and lumbar punctures in younger children. Traumatic procedures should never be performed in "safe" areas, such as the playroom. If the procedure is lengthy, avoid conversation that could be misinterpreted by the child. As the procedure is nearing completion, the nurse may inform the child "this is the last piece of tape" or simply inform the child when the procedure is completed.

NURSING TIP Help the child select and practice a coping technique before the procedure. Consider having the parent or some other supportive person, such as a child life specialist, "coach" the child in learning and using the coping skill.

Expect Success

Nurses who approach children with confidence and who convey the impression that they expect to be successful are less likely to encounter difficulty. It is best to approach a child as though cooperation is expected. Children sense anxiety and uncertainty in an adult and respond by striking out or actively resisting. Although it is not possible to eliminate such behavior in every child, a firm approach with a positive attitude tends to convey a feeling of security to most children.

Involve the Child

Involving children helps gain their cooperation. Permitting choices gives them some measure of control. However, a choice is given only in situations in which one is available. Asking children, "Do you want to take your medicine now?" leads them to believe they have an option and provides them the opportunity to legitimately refuse or delay the medication. This places the nurse in an awkward, if not impossible, position. It is much better to state firmly, "It's time to drink your medicine now." Children usually like to make choices, but the choice must be one that they do indeed have (e.g., "It's time for your medicine. Do you want to drink it plain or with a little water?").

Many children respond to tactics that appeal to their maturity or courage. This also gives them a sense of participation and achievement. For example, preschool children will be proud that they can hold the dressing during the procedure or remove the tape. The same is true for school-age children, who often cooperate with minimal resistance.

Provide Distraction

Distraction is a powerful coping strategy during painful procedures (Dastgheyb, Fishlock, Daskalakis, et al., 2018). It is accomplished by focusing the child's attention on something other than the procedure. Singing favorite songs, listening to music with a headset, counting aloud, or blowing bubbles to "blow the hurt away" are effective techniques. (For other nonpharmacologic interventions, see Chapter 5.)

Allow Expression of Feelings

The child should be allowed to express feelings of anger, anxiety, fear, frustration, or any other emotion. It is natural for children to strike out in frustration or to try to avoid stress-provoking situations. The child needs to know that it is all right to cry. Behavior is children's primary means of communication and coping and should be permitted unless it inflicts harm on them or those caring for them. Harmful behavior should be acknowledged and appropriate limitations should be set to promote patient and caregiver safety.

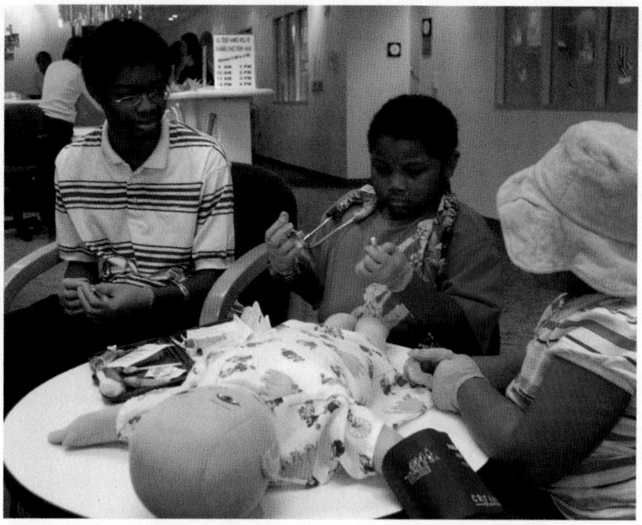

Fig. 20.1 Playing with medical objects provides children with the opportunity to play out fears and concerns with supervision by a nurse or child life specialist.

Postprocedural Support

After the procedure, the child continues to need reassurance that he or she performed well and is accepted and loved. If the parents did not participate, the child is united with them as soon as possible so that they can provide comfort.

Encourage Expression of Feelings

Planned activity after the procedure is helpful in encouraging constructive expression of feelings. For verbal children, reviewing the details of the procedure can clarify misconceptions and garner feedback for improving the nurse's preparatory strategies. Play is an excellent activity for all children. Infants and young children should have the opportunity for gross motor movement. Older children are able to vent their anger and frustration in acceptable pounding or throwing activities. Play-Doh is a remarkably versatile medium for pounding and shaping. Dramatic play provides an outlet for anger and places the child in a position of control, in contrast to the position of helplessness in the real situation. Puppets also allow the child to communicate feelings in a nonthreatening way. One of the most effective interventions is **therapeutic play**, which includes well-supervised activities such as permitting the child to give an injection to a doll or stuffed toy to reduce the stress of injections (Fig. 20.1).

Positive Reinforcement

Children need to hear from adults that they did the best they could in the situation—no matter how they behaved. There should be specific acknowledgment of what aspect of the procedure the child performed well. It is important for children to know that their worth is not being judged based on their behavior in a stressful situation. Reward systems, such as earning stars, stickers, or a supportive care program such as Beads of Courage that celebrates a child's milestones in medical treatment, are appealing to children.[b]

Returning to the child a short while after the procedure helps the nurse strengthen a supportive relationship. Relating with the child in a relaxed and nonstressful period allows him or her to see the nurse not

[b]Beads of Courage information is available at http://www.beadsofcourage.org/.

BOX 20.1 Play Activities for Specific Procedures

Fluid Intake

Make ice pops using child's favorite juice.
Cut gelatin into fun shapes.
Make a game out of taking a sip when turning page of a book or in games such as Simon Says.
Use small medicine cups; decorate the cups.
Color water with food coloring or powdered drink mix.
Have a tea party; pour at a small table.
Cut straws in half and place in a small container (much easier for child to suck liquid).
Use a "crazy" straw.
Make a "progress poster"; give rewards for drinking a predetermined quantity.

Deep Breathing

Blow bubbles with a bubble blower.
Blow bubbles with a straw (no soap).
Blow on a pinwheel, feather, whistle, harmonica, balloon, or party blower.
Practice band instruments.
Have a blowing contest using balloons,[a] boats, cotton balls, feathers, marbles, ping-pong balls, pieces of paper; blow such objects on a tabletop over a goal line, over water, through an obstacle course, up in the air, against an opponent, or up and down a string.
Suck paper or cloth from one container to another using a straw.
Dramatize stories such as "I'll huff and I'll puff, and I'll blow your house down" from the "Three Little Pigs."
Do straw-blowing painting.
Take a deep breath and "blow out the candles" on a birthday cake.
Use a little paintbrush to "paint" nails with water and blow nails dry.

Range of Motion and Use of Extremities

Throw beanbags at a fixed or movable target or throw wadded-up paper into a wastebasket.
Touch or kick Mylar balloons held or hung in different positions (if child is in traction, hang balloon from a trapeze).
Play "tickle toes"; have the child wiggle the toes on request.
Play Twister game or Simon Says.
Play pretend and guessing games (e.g., imitate a bird, butterfly, or horse).
Have tricycle or wheelchair races in safe area.
Play kickball or throw ball with a soft foam ball in a safe area.
Position bed so that child must turn to view television or doorway.
Climb wall with fingers like a "spider."
Pretend to teach aerobic dancing or exercises; encourage parents to participate.
Encourage swimming if feasible.
Play video games or pinball (fine motor movement).
Play hide and seek: hide toy somewhere in bed (or room if ambulatory) and have child find it using specified hand or foot.
Provide clay to mold with fingers.
Paint or draw on large sheets of paper placed on floor or wall.
Encourage combing own hair; play "beauty shop" with "customer" in different positions.

Soaks

Play with small toys or objects (e.g., cups, soap dishes) in water.
Wash dolls or toys.
Pick up marbles or pennies[a] from bottom of bath container.
Make designs with coins on bottom of container.
Pretend a boat is a submarine by keeping it immersed.
Read to child during soaks; sing with child; or play game, such as cards, checkers, or other board game (if both hands are immersed, move board pieces for child).
Sitz bath: give child something to listen to (e.g., music, stories) or look at (e.g., View-Master, book).
Punch holes in bottom of plastic cup, fill with water, and let it "rain" on child.

Injections

Let child handle syringe, vial, and alcohol swab and give an injection to doll or stuffed animal.
Draw a "magic circle" on area before injection; draw smiling face in circle after injection but avoid drawing on puncture site.
If multiple injections or venipunctures are planned, make a "progress poster"; give rewards for predetermined number of injections.
Have child count to 10 or 15 during injection.

Ambulation

Give child something to push:
- Toddler: push-pull toy
- School-age child: wagon or a doll in a stroller or wheelchair
- Adolescent: decorated intravenous stand

Have a parade; make hats, drums, and so on.

Extending Environment (e.g., for Patients in Traction)

Make bed into a pirate ship or airplane with decorations.
Put up mirrors so patient can see around room.
Move bed frequently to playroom, hallway, or outside.

[a]Small objects such as marbles and coins, as well as gloves and balloons, are unsafe for young children because of possible aspiration. Latex products also carry the risk of an allergic reaction.

only as someone associated with stressful situations but also as someone with whom to share pleasurable experiences.

Use of Play in Procedures

The use of play is an integral part of relationships with children. As such, its value in specific situations is discussed throughout this book, such as in Chapter 19 in relation to hospitalization. Many institutions have elaborate and well-organized play areas and programs under the direction of child life specialists. Other institutions have limited facilities. No matter what the institution provides for children, nurses can include play activities as part of nursing care. Play can be used to teach, express feelings, or achieve a therapeutic goal. Consequently, it should be included in preparing children for and encouraging their cooperation during procedures. Play sessions after procedures can be structured, such as directed toward needle play, or general, with a wide variety of equipment available for children to play with.

Routine procedures such as measuring blood pressure and oral administration of medication may be of concern to children. Box 20.1 describes suggestions for incorporating play into nursing procedures and activities for the hospitalized child that facilitate learning and adjustment to a new situation.

Preparing the Family

The process of patient education involves giving the family information about the child's condition, the regimen that must be followed and why, and other health teaching as indicated. The goal of this education is to enable the family to modify behaviors and adhere to the regimen that has been mutually established (see Applying Evidence to Practice box).

APPLYING EVIDENCE TO PRACTICE

General Principles of Family Education

- Establish a rapport with the family.
- Avoid using confusing specialized terms or jargon. Clarify all terms with the family and use the term that is clear to the child.
- When possible, allow family members to decide how they want to be taught (e.g., all at once or over a day or two). This gives the family a chance to incorporate the information at a rate that is comfortable.
- Provide accurate information to the family about the illness.
- Assist family members in identifying obstacles to their ability to comply with the regimen and in identifying the means to overcome those obstacles. Then help family members find ways to incorporate the plan into their daily lives.
- Incorporate teach-back strategies that allow the family to provide return demonstration and discussion of the material taught.

If equipment will be needed at home (e.g., suction machines, syringes), begin making the necessary arrangements in advance so that discharge can proceed smoothly. Whenever possible, make arrangements for the family to use the same equipment in the home that they are using in the hospital. This allows them to become familiar with the items. In addition, the staff can help troubleshoot the equipment in a controlled environment. Plan the teaching sessions well in advance of the time the family will be responsible for performing the care. The more complex the procedure, the more time is needed for training.

Review the instructions with family members (see Applying Evidence to Practice box). Encourage note taking if they desire. Allow ample practice time under supervision. At least one family member, but preferably two members, should demonstrate the procedure before they are expected to care for the child at home. Provide the family with the telephone numbers of resource individuals who are available to assist them in the event of a problem.

APPLYING EVIDENCE TO PRACTICE

Family Preparation for Procedures

Family education for specific procedures is included throughout this unit. General concepts applicable to most family education sessions include the following:

- Name of the procedure
- Purpose of the procedure
- Length of time anticipated to complete the procedure
- Anticipated effects
- Signs of adverse effects
- Assess the family's level of understanding
- Demonstrate and have family return demonstration (if appropriate)

SURGICAL PROCEDURES

Preoperative Care

Children experiencing surgical procedures require both psychologic and physical preparation. An important concern is restriction of food and fluids before surgery to avoid pulmonary aspiration during anesthesia. In addition, fasting for too long can cause discomfort, headache, dehydration, or hypoglycemia and can delay recovery and hospital discharge (Dolgun, Yavuz, Eroğlu, et al., 2017). Infants require special attention to fluid needs. They should not be without oral fluids for an extended period preoperatively to avoid glycogen depletion and dehydration. If surgical procedures are delayed, it is the nurse's responsibility to communicate with the surgical team to adjust fasting guidelines appropriately (Williams, Johnson, Guzzetta, et al., 2014). Table 20.2 contains current preoperative fasting guidelines.

TABLE 20.2 Fasting Recommendations to Reduce the Risk of Pulmonary Aspiration[a]

Ingested Material	Minimum Fasting Period (hr)[b]
Clear liquids[c]	>2
Breast milk	4
Infant formula	6
Nonhuman milk[d]	6
Light meal[e]	6

[a]These recommendations apply to healthy patients who are undergoing elective procedures. They are not intended for women in labor. Following the guidelines does not guarantee that complete gastric emptying has occurred.

[b]Fasting periods noted in chart apply to all ages.

[c]Examples of clear liquids include water, fruit juices without pulp, carbonated beverages, clear tea, and black coffee.

[d]Because nonhuman milk is similar to solids in gastric emptying time, the amount ingested must be considered when determining appropriate fasting period.

[e]A light meal typically consists of toast and clear liquids. Meals that include fried or fatty foods or meat may prolong gastric emptying time. Both the amount and type of foods ingested must be considered when determining an appropriate fasting period.

From American Society of Anesthesiologists, Committee on Standards and Practice Parameters. (2011). Practice guidelines for preoperative fasting and the use of pharmacological agents to reduce the risk of pulmonary aspiration: Application to healthy patients undergoing elective procedures. *Anesthesiology, 114*(3), 495–511.

In general, psychologic preparation is similar to that discussed earlier for any procedure and uses many of the same techniques used in preparing a child for hospitalization, such as films, books, brochures, play, and tours (see Chapter 19). Stress points before and after surgery include the admission process, blood tests, administration of preoperative medication (if prescribed), transport to the operating room, the mask on the face during induction, and the stay in the postanesthesia care unit. Wearing a hospital gown without the security of underpants or pajama bottoms can also be traumatic. Therefore these articles of clothing should be allowed to be worn into the operating room and removed after induction of anesthesia. Children are at higher risk of ineffective response to anesthesia and complications in the recovery period because of higher anxiety in the preoperative period associated with stranger anxiety (infants), separation anxiety (toddlers and preschoolers), and fear of injury or death (adolescents) (Al-Yateem, Brenner, Shorrab, et al., 2016).

Individualized psychologic intervention consisting of systematic preparation, rehearsal of the forthcoming events, and supportive care at each of these points has shown to be more effective than a single-session preparation or consistent supportive care without systematic preparation and rehearsal (Fortier, Kain, & Morton, 2015). A family-centered preoperative preparation program may consist of a tour of the perioperative areas with short explanations of the events 5 to 7 days before surgery, a video to take home and review a couple of times with additional explanations and demonstrations of perioperative processes, a mask to take home and practice with, pamphlets to guide parents on supporting children during induction, phone calls to coach parents on preparing children 1 or 2 days before surgery, toys and supplies in the holding area, and mobile phone applications with interactive tours and videos. In addition, the use of interactive electronic games, tablets, or therapy dogs in the preoperative setting can provide effective alternatives or complements to pharmacologic premedication. Therapeutic play is an effective strategy in preparing children, and increased familiarity with medical procedures can decrease anxiety.

Parental Presence

Some institutions support parental presence during induction of anesthesia. Benefits of well-prepared children and parents along with parental presence during induction of anesthesia include reduced anxiety for children and parents, lower doses of postoperative analgesia, lower incidence of severe emergence delirium symptoms, decreased postoperative maladaptive behaviors, and shorter discharge time for short procedures (Fortier et al., 2015). Other studies have not supported a reduction in children's anxiety (Erhaze, Dowling, & Devane, 2016; Manyande, Cyna, Yip, et al., 2015).

Concern exists regarding the appropriateness of parental presence during induction for all parents. Some parents may become upset by the rapid succession of induction events, by observing their child becoming limp, and by leaving the child in the care of strangers. Although parents who are anxious before surgery tend to become even more anxious after the induction, the reverse is true of parents with little anxiety. There is little evidence to suggest that parental presence during induction provides decreased anxiety for parents and caregivers (Al-Yateem et al., 2016). Appropriate education is essential to help parents understand the stages of anesthesia, what to expect, and how to support their child.

Preoperative Sedation

The goals for using preoperative medications include anxiety reduction, amnesia, sedation, antiemetic effect, and reduction of secretions (Manworren & Fledderman, 2000). (Chapter 5 includes a discussion of pain management strategies for children undergoing surgery.) When drugs are administered, they should be delivered atraumatically via oral, intranasal, or IV routes. Numerous preanesthetic drug regimens are used with children, and no consensus exists on the optimal method. Some institutions promote distraction or parental support instead of medications due to the incidence of postoperative medication delirium (Batawi, 2015).

Intraoperative Care

The role of the pediatric operating room nurse is to advocate for care of the patient in surgery through the verification of procedure and laterality, implants, skin preparation, necessary instrumentation, and supplies. The operating room nurse assesses, recognizes, and intervenes for the pediatric surgical patient at high risk for pressure injury due to patient diagnosis, patient anatomy, general anesthesia, intraoperative positioning, immobility, moisture, and nothing-by-mouth (NPO) status. Clear communication is used through collaboration with the interdisciplinary team (anesthesia, surgeon, scrub technician, nurses, radiology, etc.) to coordinate the intraoperative and postoperative disposition of the surgical patient. Family-centered care is provided through engaging the family in the preoperative procedure verification and updating them throughout the procedure (Herd & Rieben, 2014).

Postoperative Care

Various psychologic and physical interventions and observations help prevent or minimize possible unpleasant effects from anesthesia and the surgical procedure. Although serious postoperative complications in healthy children undergoing surgery are rare, continuous monitoring of the child's cardiopulmonary status is essential during the immediate postoperative period to reduce this risk (Pawar, 2012). Postanesthesia complications such as airway obstruction, postextubation croup, laryngospasm, and bronchospasm make maintaining a patent airway and maximum ventilation critical.

Monitoring the patient's oxygen saturation and providing supplemental oxygen as needed, maintaining body temperature, and promoting fluid and electrolyte balance are important aspects of immediate postoperative care. Vital signs are continuously monitored, and each vital sign is evaluated in terms of side effects from anesthesia, shock, or respiratory compromise (Table 20.3).

A change in vital signs that demands immediate attention in the perioperative period is caused by **malignant hyperthermia (MH)**, a potentially fatal pharmacogenetic disorder of muscle metabolism. In susceptible children, inhaled anesthetics and the muscle relaxant succinylcholine trigger the disorder, producing hypermetabolism. Symptoms of MH include hypercarbia (increasing end-tidal carbon dioxide), elevated temperature, tachycardia, tachypnea, acidosis, muscle rigidity, hyperkalemia, and rhabdomyolysis. A family or previous history of sudden high fever associated with a surgical procedure and myotonia increase the risk for MH. Children who have successfully undergone prior surgery without adverse effects may still be considered susceptible (Salazar, Yang, Shen, et al., 2014).

Treatment of MH includes immediate discontinuation of the triggering agent, hyperventilation with 100% oxygen, and IV dantrolene sodium. If the child is hyperthermic, initiate cooling measures such as ice packs to the groin, axillae, and neck and iced nasogastric (NG) lavage. The surgery may be discontinued, or if it is emergent, it may be continued with a different anesthetic agent. The patient should be transferred to an intensive care unit for at least 36 hours and closely monitored for stabilization of vital signs, metabolic state, and possible recurrence of symptoms.

Managing pain is a major nursing responsibility after surgery. The nurse should assess pain frequently and administer analgesics to provide comfort and facilitate cooperation with postoperative care such as ambulation and deep breathing. Opioids are the most commonly used analgesics. Routinely scheduled IV analgesics, patient-controlled analgesia, regional blocks, and epidural infusions, rather than as-needed orders, provide excellent analgesia in postoperative pediatric patients.

Nonpharmacologic postoperative recovery interventions include the use of distraction, videos, interactive game applications, and therapy dogs. Therapy dogs can facilitate decreased pain perception, increase in activity, and emotional stabilization in the postoperative period (Calcaterra, Veggiotti, Palestrini, et al., 2015).

> **NURSING TIP** Because deep breathing is usually painful after surgery, be certain that the child has received analgesics. Have the child splint the operative site (depending on its location) by hugging a small pillow or a favorite stuffed animal.

Because respiratory tract infections are a potential complication of anesthesia, make every effort to aerate the lungs and remove secretions. The lungs are auscultated regularly to identify abnormal sounds or any areas of diminished or absent breath sounds. To prevent pneumonia, encourage respiratory movement with incentive spirometers or other motivating activities (see Box 20.1). If these measures are presented as games, the child is more likely to comply. The child's position is changed every 2 hours, and deep breathing is encouraged. Patients with preexisting pulmonary disease may be advised to begin incentive spirometry before the day of surgery (Azhar, 2015). Early respiratory movement can decrease the patient's need for supplemental oxygen and promote discharge home sooner (Shaughnessy, White, Shah, et al., 2015).

During the recovery period, spend some time with the child to assess his or her perceptions of surgery. Play, drawing, and storytelling are excellent methods of discovering the child's thoughts. With such information, the nurse can support or correct the child's perceptions and boost his or her self-esteem for having endured a stressful procedure.

Many pediatric patients are discharged shortly after surgery. Preparation for discharge begins with the preadmission preparation visit. Thorough

TABLE 20.3 Potential Causes of Postoperative Vital Sign Alterations in Children

Alteration	Potential Cause	Comments
Heart Rate		
Increase	Decreased perfusion (shock) Elevated temperature Pain Respiratory distress (early) Medications (atropine, morphine, epinephrine) Hypoxia	Heart rate may increase to maintain cardiac output.
Decrease	Vagal stimulation Increased intracranial pressure Respiratory distress (late) Medications (neostigmine [Prostigmin])	Bradycardia is of more concern in young child than tachycardia.
Respiratory Rate		
Increase	Respiratory distress Fluid volume excess Hypothermia Elevated temperature Pain	Body responds to respiratory distress primarily by increasing rate.
Decrease	Anesthetics, opioids Pain	Decreased respiratory rate from opioids may be compensated for by increased depth of respiration.
Blood Pressure		
Increase	Excess intravascular volume Increased intracranial pressure Carbon dioxide retention Pain Medication (ketamine, epinephrine)	This is serious in premature infants because it increases risk of intraventricular hemorrhage.
Decrease	Vasodilating anesthetic agents (halothane, isoflurane, enflurane) Opioids (e.g., morphine)	Decreased blood pressure is late sign of shock because of elasticity and constriction of vessels to maintain cardiac output.
Temperature		
Increase	Shock (late sign) Infection Environmental causes (warm room, excess coverings) Malignant hyperthermia	Fever associated with infection usually occurs later than fever of noninfectious origin. Absence of fever does not rule out infection, especially in infants. Malignant hyperthermia requires immediate treatment.
Decrease	Vasodilating anesthetic agents (halothane, isoflurane, enflurane) Muscle relaxants Environmental causes (cool room) Infusion of cool fluids or blood	Neonates are especially susceptible to hypothermia, with serious or fatal consequences.

discharge processes and education can greatly assist in the prevention of unplanned readmissions (Payne & Flood, 2015). The nurse should discuss instructions for postoperative care and review them throughout the perioperative visit with the strategy that works best for the patient and family. After discharge, the nursing staff often makes phone calls to check the patient's status. Patient education and compliance with discharge instructions can also be assessed during these phone calls (Flippo, NeSmith, Stark, et al., 2015) (see Applying Evidence to Practice box).

APPLYING EVIDENCE TO PRACTICE

Postoperative Care

- Ensure that preparations are made to receive child:
  - Bed or crib is ready.
  - Intravenous pumps and poles, suction apparatus, and oxygen flow meter are at bedside.
- Obtain baseline information:
  - Take vital signs, including blood pressure and pulse oximetry; keep blood pressure cuff in place and deflated to lessen disturbance to child.
  - Take and record vital signs more frequently if any value fluctuates.
- Inspect operative area.
- Check dressing if present.
- Outline any bleeding area on dressing or cast with pen.
- Reinforce, but do not remove, loose dressing.
- Observe areas below or underneath surgical site for blood that may have drained toward bed.
- Assess for compartment syndrome with any restrictive dressings.
- Assess for bleeding and other symptoms in areas not covered with a dressing, such as throat after tonsillectomy.
- Assess skin color and characteristics.
- Assess level of sedation and activity.
- Notify physician of any irregularities in child's condition.
- Assess for evidence of pain. (See Chapter 5, Pain Assessment.)
- Review surgeon's orders after completing initial assessment and check that any preoperative orders, such as seizure or cardiac medications, have been reordered and can be given by available routes (oral preparations may be contraindicated).
- Monitor vital signs as ordered and more often if indicated.
- Check dressings for bleeding or other abnormalities.
- Check bowel sounds.
- Observe for signs of shock, abdominal distention, and bleeding.
- Assess for bladder distention.
- Observe for signs of dehydration.
- Detect presence of infection:
  - Take vital signs every 2 to 4 hours as ordered.
  - Collect or request needed specimens.
  - Inspect wound for signs of infection—redness, swelling, heat, pain, and purulent drainage.

Compliance

Compliance, also called **adherence**, refers to the extent to which the patient's behavior coincides with the prescribed regimen in terms of taking medication, following diets, or executing other lifestyle changes. In developing strategies to improve compliance, the nurse must first assess level of compliance. Because many children are too young to assume partial or total responsibility for their care, parents are usually primarily responsible for home management.

Factors relating to the care setting are important in ensuring compliance and should be considered in planning strategies to improve compliance. Basically, any aspect of the health care setting that increases the family's satisfaction with the physical setting and the relationship with the provider positively influences adherence to the treatment regimen. However, the more complex, expensive, inconvenient, and disruptive the treatment protocol, the less likely the family is to comply. During long-term conditions that involve multiple treatments and considerable rearrangement of lifestyle, compliance is severely affected.

Although it is helpful to know those factors that influence compliance, assessment must include more direct measurement techniques. When inquiring about a patient's compliance, it can be helpful to ask details about how medication administration or other interventions are carried out instead of asking yes-or-no questions. For example, a health care provider could ask about what time of day patients perform their prescribed interventions, what beverages they prefer to take their medications with, or how many doses were missed this week. A number of methods exist, each with advantages and disadvantages. The most successful approach includes a combination of at least two of the following methods:

Clinical judgment—This is subject to bias and inaccuracy unless the nurse carefully evaluates the criteria used in assessment.

Self-reporting—Most people overestimate their compliance even when they admit to lapses.

Direct observation—This is difficult to use outside the health care setting, and awareness of being observed frequently affects performance.

Monitoring appointments—Keeping appointments indirectly indicates compliance with the prescribed care.

Monitoring therapeutic response—Few treatments yield directly measurable results (e.g., decreased blood pressure, weight loss); record on a graph or chart.

Pill counts—The nurse counts the number of pills remaining in the original container and compares the number missing with the number of times the medication should have been taken. Although this is a simple method, families may forget to bring the container or deliberately alter the number of pills to avoid detection. This method is also poorly suited to liquid medication. Another technique is the use of pill container caps that record every opening as a presumptive dose.

Chemical assay—For certain drugs, such as digoxin, measurement of plasma drug levels provides information on the amount of drug recently ingested. However, this method is expensive, indicates only short-term compliance, and requires precise timing of the assay for accurate results.

Compliance Strategies

Strategies to improve compliance involve interventions that encourage families to follow the prescribed treatment regimen. Some evidence suggests that higher levels of self-esteem and increased autonomy favorably affect adolescent compliance (Letitre, DeGroot, Draaisma, et al., 2014). In addition, anxiety, depression, and self-esteem can be negatively affected when treatment regimens are inadequately followed. However, family factors are important, and characteristics associated with good compliance include family support, family reminders, good communication, and expectations for successful completion of the therapeutic regimen. No one approach is always successful, and the best results occur when at least two strategies are used.

Organizational strategies involve the care setting and the therapeutic plan. This may involve increasing the frequency of appointments, designating a primary provider, reducing the cost of medication by prescribing generic brands, reducing the treatment's disruption of the family's lifestyle, and using "cues" to minimize forgetting. Numerous devices are available commercially or can be improvised for cueing, such as pill dispensers; watches with alarms; charts to record completed therapy; messages on the refrigerator or morning coffee pot; mobile phone applications; and individualistic, self-timed schedules that incorporate the treatment plan into the daily routine, such as physical therapy after the evening bath (Britto, Munafo, Schoettker, et al., 2012; Carbone, Zebrack, Plegue, et al., 2013).

The nurse instructs the family about the treatment plan. Although education is an important factor in enhancing compliance, and patients who are more knowledgeable about their condition are more likely to comply, education alone does not ensure compliant behavior. The nurse should incorporate teaching principles known to enhance understanding and retention of material. Written materials are essential, especially in any regimen requiring multiple or complex treatments, and they need to be understandable to the average individual, who reads at about the fourth-grade level. Learning disabilities can negatively affect medication adherence and should be routinely assessed along with health literacy (Dharmapuri, Best, Kind, et al., 2015). Individualized teaching strategies appropriate for developmental and cognitive levels of the individual, as well as involvement of the immediate and extended family (e.g., grandparents) in education sessions, may enhance compliance.

Treatment strategies relate to the child's refusal or inability to take the prescribed medication. The family may also have difficulty following a prescribed treatment regimen. They may remember and understand the instructions but may not be able to give the medicine as prescribed. Assess the reason for refusal. For example, the child may not be able to swallow pills. In this case, perhaps pills could be crushed or a liquid medication substituted (always review medication to ensure that crushing is acceptable before giving this instruction).

Assess the treatment and medication schedule to determine whether it is reasonable for a home situation. Although an every-6-hour or every-8-hour schedule is reasonable for hospitals, a parent would have difficulty getting up once or twice nightly. Instead, the patient could take a medication during the day at times that would be easy to remember.

Behavioral strategies are designed to modify behavior directly. Nurses can use several effective strategies with children to encourage the desired behavior. Positive reinforcement is one strategy that strengthens the behavior. One example of this is the child earning stars or tokens, which can be exchanged for a special privilege or gift. Sticker charts also serve as a visual reminder of positive behavior and motivation to continue compliance. At times, however, disciplinary techniques, such as a time-out for young children or withholding privileges for older children, may be needed to improve compliance. The child life specialist can be especially helpful in determining behavioral compliance strategies across the developmental spectrum.

SKIN CARE AND GENERAL HYGIENE

MAINTAINING HEALTHY SKIN

Maintaining an IV line, removing a dressing, positioning a child in bed, changing a diaper, using electrodes, and using restraints all have the potential to contribute to skin injury. General guidelines for skin care are listed in the Applying Evidence to Practice box. (Specific guidelines for skin care of neonates are provided in Chapter 8, Skin Care.)

Assessment of the skin is easiest to accomplish during the bath. Examine for early signs of injury, including redness, flaking, decreased perfusion, or skin breakdown. Risk factors include impaired mobility, protein malnutrition, edema, incontinence, sensory loss, anemia, infection, failure to turn the patient, and intubation. Identification of risk factors helps determine children who need a more thorough skin assessment. Several risk assessment scales, such as the Braden Q Scale, the Neonatal Skin Risk Assessment Scale, the Waterlow Scale, and the Glamorgan Scale, are available for use in pediatrics (Razmus & Bergquist-Beringer, 2017). Initial assessment should occur on admission to identify pressure ulcers and wounds that occurred before

APPLYING EVIDENCE TO PRACTICE

Skin Care

- Keep skin free of excess moisture (e.g., urine or fecal incontinence, wound drainage, excessive perspiration). All diapered patients should have a barrier cream applied.
- Cleanse skin with mild nonalkaline soap or soap-free cleaning agents for routine bathing.
- Provide daily cleansing of eyes, oral and diaper or perineal areas, and any areas of skin breakdown.
- Apply non–alcohol-based moisturizing agents after cleansing to retain moisture and rehydrate skin.
- Use minimum amount of tape and adhesives. On very sensitive skin, use a protective, pectin-based or hydrocolloid skin barrier between skin and tape or adhesives.
- Place pectin-based or hydrocolloid skin barriers directly over excoriated skin. Leave barrier undisturbed until it begins to peel off or for 5 to 7 days. With wet, oozing excoriations, place a small amount of stoma powder on site, remove excess powder, and apply skin barrier. Hold barrier in place for several minutes to allow barrier to soften and mold to skin surface.
- Alternate electrode and probe placement sites and thoroughly assess underlying skin typically every 8 to 24 hours.
- Eliminate pressure secondary to medical devices such as tracheostomy tubes, wheelchairs, braces, and gastrostomy tubes.
- Be certain fingers or toes are visible whenever extremity is used for intravenous (IV) or arterial line.
- Use a draw sheet to move child in bed or onto a stretcher; do not drag child from under the arms.
- Position in neutral alignment; pillows, cushions, or wedges may be needed to prevent hip abduction and pressure to bony prominences, such as heels, elbows, and sacral and occipital areas. When child is positioned laterally, pillows or cushions between the knees, under the head, and under the upper arm will help promote neutral body alignment. Avoid donut cushions because they can cause tissue ischemia. Elevate the head of bed 30 degrees or less to reduce pressure unless contraindicated.
- Do not massage reddened bony prominences because this can cause deep tissue damage; provide pressure relief to bony prominences with gel pads or pillows.
- Routinely assess the child's nutritional status. A child who is NPO (nothing by mouth) for several days and is receiving only IV fluid is nutritionally at risk, which can also affect the skin's ability to maintain its integrity. Consider parenteral nutrition.

admission. Skin assessment should be repeated every shift and at least every 4 hours in perfusion-compromised patients.

Pressure ulcers, a form of pressure injuries, are localized damage to the skin and/or underlying soft tissue due to decreased perfusion as a result of increased pressure. Pressure ulcers most often occur over bony prominences or related to medical or other devices. Pressure injuries are staged to classify the amount of tissue damage that has occurred.[c] Necrotic tissue must be removed so that the tissue depth can accurately be assessed. Accurate documentation of redness or obvious skin breakdown is essential. Color, size (diameter and depth), location, presence of sinus tracts, odor, exudate, and response to treatment are observed and recorded at least daily.

Pressure ulcers in children typically occur on the occiput, earlobes, sacrum, heels, and scapula (Schober-Flores, 2012); the heels and sacrum are common sites in adults. Critically ill children; children with sensory deficits, mobility deficits, or cardiopulmonary abnormalities; and bariatric patients are at a higher risk of pressure ulcers and skin breakdown because they often have several risk factors combined. Although pressure ulcers in hospitalized children are generally uncommon, the incidence in critically ill children can be significantly higher. Interventions found to prevent pressure ulcers in critically ill children include the following:

- Assessing the patient's skin from head to toe on admission and each shift
- Turning children every 2 hours
- Using pillows, blanket rolls, and positioning devices
- Using draw sheets to minimize shear
- Using pressure reduction surfaces (e.g., foam overlays, gel pads, specialty beds)
- Allowing moisture reduction by using dry-weave diapers and disposable underpads
- Using skin moisturizers
- Conducting nutrition consults

Medical devices such as pulse oximeter probes, bilevel and continuous positive airway pressure masks, oxygen cannulas, tracheostomy tubes, orthotics, and casts can also cause pressure ulcers (Freundlich, 2017). In addition, both medical devices and special garments such as shoes, slippers, jewelry, hair ties, and restraints should be removed to inspect skin at least every shift.

Friction and shear contribute to pressure ulcers. **Friction** occurs when the surface of the skin rubs against another surface, such as bed sheets. The skin may have the appearance of an abrasion. The skin damage is usually limited to the epidermal and upper layers. It most often occurs over the elbows, heels, or occiput. Prevention of friction injury includes the use of foam matresses that redistribute pressure; customized splinting or foam-padded boots over the heels; gel pillows; moisturizing agents; protective, transparent barrier dressings over susceptible areas; and soft, smooth bed linens and clothing (Freundlich, 2017). By itself, friction does not cause tissue necrosis, but when it acts with gravity, it results in shear injury.

Shear is the result of the force of gravity pushing down on the body and friction of the body against a surface, such as the bed or chair. For example, when a patient is in the semi-Fowler position and begins to slide to the foot of the bed, the skin over the sacral area remains in the same place because of the resistance of the bed surface. The blood vessels, bone, and muscle in the area are stretched and slide parallel to the stationary skin, which may cause small-vessel thrombosis and tissue death. Prevention of shear injury includes using lift sheets when repositioning a patient, elevating the bed no more than 30 degrees for short periods, and elevating the knees to interrupt the pull of gravity on the body toward the foot of the bed.

Epidermal stripping results when the epidermis is unintentionally removed when tape is pulled off the skin. These lesions are usually shallow and irregularly shaped. Babies are at increased risk for epidermal injury. Prevention includes using no tape when possible or securing dressings with laced binders (Montgomery straps) or stretchy netting (Spandage or stockinette). Using porous or low-tack tapes (e.g., Medipore, paper, hydrogel), using alcohol-free skin sealants (No Sting Barrier Film), or picture-framing wounds with hydrocolloid or wafer barriers (e.g., DuoDERM, Coloplast, Stomahesive) and then taping on top of the barrier also will reduce epidermal stripping.

Tape should be placed so that there is no tension, traction, or wrinkles on the skin. To remove tape, slowly peel the tape away while stabilizing the underlying skin. Adhesive remover may be used to break the adhesive bond but may be drying to the skin. Avoid adhesive removers in preterm neonates because absorption rates vary and toxicity may

[c]Staging of pressure ulcers and guidelines for prevention and management of pressure ulcers are available online from the National Pressure Ulcer Advisory Panel.

occur. Remove the adhesive with water to prevent absorption and irritation. Wetting the tape with water or alcohol-based foam hand cleansers may facilitate removal.

Chemical factors can also lead to skin damage. Fecal incontinence, especially when mixed with urine; wound drainage; or gastric drainage around gastrostomy tubes can erode the epidermis. The skin can quickly progress from redness to denudement if exposure continues. Moisture barriers, gentle cleansing with alcohol-free cleansers or wipes as soon after exposure as possible, and skin barriers can be used to prevent damage caused by chemical factors. For nonintact skin, a barrier cream with zinc oxide should be applied. It is important to cleanse only the stool and urine during diaper changes, not the paste. In addition, foam dressings that wick moisture away from the skin are helpful around gastrostomy tubes and tracheostomy sites.

BATHING

Most infants and children can be bathed at the bedside or in a standard bathtub or shower. Assess the child's and family's preferences for bath time frequency and family involvement. For infants and young children confined to bed, use commercially available bath cloths or the towel method. Immerse two towels in a dilute soap solution and wring them damp. With the child lying supine on a dry towel, place one damp towel on top of the child and use it to gently clean the body. Discard the towel, dry the child, and turn him or her prone. Repeat the procedure using the second damp towel. If bar soap is used, discard the basin and bar soap after a single bath because they can serve as a reservoir for pathogens in the hospital setting. Chlorhexidine is much less likely to harbor microbes, but it is generally not approved for use in infants younger than 2 months of corrected gestational age. Daily chlorhexidine gluconate bathing in the pediatric population can reduce bacteremia and prevent hospital-acquired infections (Karcz, Kelley, Conrad, et al., 2015; Raulji, Clay, Velasco, et al., 2015).

Infants and small children are never left unattended in a bathtub, and infants who are unable to sit alone are securely held with one hand during the bath. The nurse securely supports the infant's head with one hand or grasps the infant's farther arm while the head rests comfortably on the nurse's arm. Children who are able to sit without assistance need only close supervision and a pad placed in the bottom of the tub to prevent slipping and loss of balance.

School-age children and adolescents may shower or bathe. Nurses need to use judgment regarding the amount of supervision the child requires. Some children can assume this responsibility unaided, but others need someone in constant attendance. Children with cognitive impairments, physical limitations such as severe anemia or leg deformities, or suicidal or psychotic problems (who may commit bodily harm) require close supervision.

Areas that require special attention are the ears, between skinfolds, the neck, the back, and the genital area. The genital area should be carefully cleansed and dried, with particular care given to skinfolds. In uncircumcised boys younger than 3 years of age, the foreskin is not fully retractile. For older males, the foreskin should be gently retracted, the exposed surfaces cleansed, and the foreskin then replaced. If the condition of the glans indicates inadequate cleaning, such as accumulated smegma, inflammation, phimosis (condition in which the foreskin cannot be retracted), or foreskin adhesions, teaching proper hygiene is indicated. Do not forcibly retract the foreskin to avoid trauma and further complications (Hunter, 2012). Notify the provider of abnormal clinical findings during genitourinary assessment. In the Vietnamese and Cambodian cultures, the foreskin is traditionally not retracted until adulthood. Older children have a tendency to avoid cleaning the genitalia; therefore they may need a gentle reminder.

ORAL HYGIENE

Mouth care is an integral part of daily hygiene and should be continued in the hospital. Oral hygiene can prevent infection and promote comfort, adequate nutrition, and verbal communication. For some young children, this is their first introduction to the use of a toothbrush. Infants and debilitated children require the nurse or a family member to perform mouth care. For infants who do not yet have teeth, a soft moistened cloth or swab can be used to gently clean the gums. Children should begin brushing their teeth after the first teeth emerge around 6 months of age. For children younger than 3 years of age, a grain-sized amount of fluoride toothpaste should be used. For children 3 to 6 years of age, a pea-sized amount of fluoride toothpaste should be used (American Dental Association, 2017). Although young children can manage a toothbrush and are encouraged to use it, most need assistance to perform satisfactorily. Older children, although capable of brushing and flossing without assistance, sometimes need to be reminded.

HAIR CARE

Children should have their hair brushed and combed at least once daily for hair and scalp health. The hair is styled for comfort and in a manner pleasing to the child and parents. The hair should not be cut without parental permission, although clipping hair to provide access to a scalp vein for IV insertion may be necessary.

If children are hospitalized for more than a few days, the hair may need shampooing. With infants, the hair may be washed during the daily bath or less frequently. For most children, washing the hair and scalp once or twice weekly is sufficient unless there is an indication for more frequent washing, such as after a high fever and profuse sweating. Adolescents normally have increased oily sebaceous secretions that require frequent hair care and more frequent shampoos.

Almost any child can be transported to an accessible sink for shampooing. Inspect the hair and scalp before shampooing using a fine toothcomb to assess for the presence of lice or other scalp abnormalities. Nits are a gray-white color, the size of a knot of thread, and difficult to remove from the scalp in comparison to dandruff. Adult lice are a red-black color and the size of a sesame seed and can live on the scalp for 3 to 4 weeks if untreated (Cummings, Finlay, & McDonald, 2018). If lice are suspected, an order for a pediculicide treatment and nit combing must be obtained. It is important for the nurse to don personal protective equipment, including a gown and cap, during the lice removal process. In addition, other members of the household should be evaluated for the presence of lice and the family educated on the importance of individual hair care products.

Patients who are unable to be transported can receive a shampoo in their beds with adequate protection, specially adapted equipment or positioning, or dry shampoo caps. Comb or brush the hair before washing. When necessary, a shampoo basin may be used or the child may be positioned near the edge of the bed, towels placed under the shoulders and neck, a large plastic garbage bag draped at the edge of the bed with one open end under the shoulders, and the hair placed inside the opening. The other end is opened and placed in a collection container. Water can be transported in a basin.

For African American children with curly hair, most standard combs are inadequate and may cause hair breakage and discomfort. Use a special comb with widely spaced teeth. It is also much easier to comb the hair after shampooing when it is wet. Use a special hair dressing or pomade, which usually has a coconut oil base. Rub the preparation on the hands and then transfer it to the hair to make it more pliable and manageable. Consult the child's parents regarding the preparation to use on the child's hair and ask if they can provide some for use during the child's hospitalization. Petroleum jelly should not be used. If braiding or plaiting the hair, weave it loosely while the hair is damp. The hair tightens as it dries, which could result in tension folliculitis. Tight braids should be avoided, as braiding can increase pressure on the scalp or hide pressure injuries.

FEEDING THE SICK CHILD

Loss of appetite is a symptom common to most childhood illnesses. Decreased appetite can be a result of pain or discomfort, nausea and vomiting, emotional concerns, or loss of control. Because an acute illness is usually short, the nutritional state is seldom compromised. Urging food on the sick child may precipitate nausea and vomiting. In most cases, children can usually determine their own need for food.

Refusing to eat may also be one way children can exert power and control in an otherwise helpless situation. For young children, loss of appetite may be related to depression caused by separation from their parents. Parents' concern with eating can intensify the problem. Forcing a child to eat meets with rebellion and reinforces the behavior as a control mechanism. Encourage parents to relax any pressure during an acute illness. Although it is best to provide high-quality, nutritious foods, the child may desire foods and liquids that contain mostly empty or nonnutritional calories. Some well-tolerated foods include gelatin, diluted clear soups, carbonated drinks, flavored ice pops, dry toast, and crackers. Even though these substances are not nutritious, they can provide necessary fluid and calories.

Dehydration is always a hazard when children have a fever or anorexia, especially when accompanied by vomiting or diarrhea. Fluids should not be forced, and the child should not be awakened to take fluids. Forcing fluids may create the same difficulties as urging the child to eat unwanted food. Gentle persuasion with preferred beverages will usually meet with success. Using play techniques can also be effective (see Applying Evidence to Practice box).

An understanding of children's feeding habits can also increase food consumption. For example, if children are given all their food at one time, they generally eat the dessert first. Likewise, if they are presented with large portions, they often push the food away because the amount overwhelms them. If young children are not supervised during mealtime, they tend to play with the food rather than eat it. Therefore nurses should present food in the usual order, such as soup first followed by small portions of meat, potatoes, and vegetables, and ending with dessert.

When the child is feeling better, appetite usually begins to improve. It is best to take advantage of any hungry period by serving high-quality foods and snacks. If the child still refuses to eat, offer nutritious fluids, such as prepared breakfast drinks. Parents can help by bringing in food items from home, especially if the family's cultural eating habits differ from the hospital food. A clinical dietitian may be consulted for alternative food choices.

When children are placed on special diets, such as clear liquids after surgery or during episodes of diarrhea, assessment of their intake and readiness to advance to more complex foods is essential.

Regardless of the type of diet, charting the amount consumed is an important nursing responsibility. Descriptions need to be detailed and accurate, such as "4 ounces of orange juice, one pancake, and 8 ounces of milk." Comments such as "ate well" or "ate poorly" are inadequate. Charting the percentage of the meal eaten is also inadequate unless food is measured before serving. For infants, assess the duration, amount, and frequency of breastfeeding or bottle-feeding and the possible addition of solid foods to determine whether nutrition is adequate.

If the parents are involved in the child's care, encourage them to keep a list of everything the child eats. Using a premeasured cup for fluids ensures a more accurate estimate of intake. A comparison of the intake at each meal can isolate food deficiencies, such as insufficient intake of meat or vegetables. Behaviors associated with mealtime also identify possible factors influencing appetite. For example, the observation "Child eats well when with other children but plays with food if left alone in room" helps the nurse plan mealtime activities that stimulate the child's appetite.

Although sick children's appetites may be poor and not characteristic of their home eating habits, the hospital stay provides numerous opportunities for nurses to assess the family's knowledge of good nutrition and to implement teaching as needed to improve nutritional intake.

APPLYING EVIDENCE TO PRACTICE

Feeding a Sick Child

Take a dietary history (see Chapter 4) and use information to make eating time as similar as possible to eating at home.

Encourage parents or other family members to feed child or to be present at mealtimes.

Make mealtimes pleasant; avoid any procedures immediately before or after eating; make certain child is rested and pain free.

Serve small, frequent meals rather than three large meals or serve three meals and nutritious between-meal snacks.

Provide finger foods for young children.

Involve children in food selection and preparation whenever possible.

Serve small portions and serve each course separately, such as soup first, followed by meat, potatoes, and vegetables and ending with dessert. With young children, camouflage size of food by cutting meat thicker so less appears on plate or by folding a cheese slice in half. Offer second helpings.

Ensure a variety of foods, textures, and colors.

Provide food selections that are favorites of most children, such as peanut butter and jelly sandwiches, hot dogs, hamburgers, macaroni and cheese, pizza, spaghetti, tacos, fried chicken, corn, and fruit yogurt.

Avoid foods that are highly seasoned, have strong odors, or are all mixed together unless typical of cultural practices.

Provide fluid selections that are favorites of most children, such as fruit punch, cola, ginger ale, sweetened tea, flavored ice pops, sherbet, ice cream, milk, milkshakes, pudding, gelatin, clear broth, or creamed soups.

Offer nutritious snacks, such as frozen yogurt or pudding, ice cream, oatmeal or peanut butter cookies, hot cocoa, cheese slices, pieces of raw vegetable or fruit, and dried fruit or cereal.

Make food attractive and different—for example:

- Serve a "picnic lunch" in a paper bag.
- Pack food in a Chinese takeout container; decorate container.
- Put a "face" or a "flower" on a hamburger or sandwich with pieces of vegetable.
- Use a cookie cutter to shape a sandwich.
- Serve pudding, yogurt, or juice frozen as an ice pop.
- Make Slurpies or snow cones by pouring flavored syrup on crushed ice.
- Serve fluids through brightly colored or unusually shaped straws.
- Make "bowtie" sandwiches by cutting them in triangles and placing two points together.
- Slice sandwiches into "fingers."
- Grate mounds of cheese.
- Cut apples horizontally to make circles.
- Put a banana on a hot dog bun and spread with peanut butter.
- Break uncooked spaghetti into toothpick lengths and skewer cheese, cold meat, vegetables, or fruit chunks.

Praise children for what they do eat.

Do not punish children for not eating by removing their dessert or putting them to bed.

CONTROLLING ELEVATED TEMPERATURES

An elevated temperature, most frequently from fever but occasionally caused by hyperthermia, is one of the most common symptoms of illness in children. This manifestation is a great concern to parents. To facilitate an understanding of fever versus hyperthermia, the following terms are defined:

Set point—The temperature around which body temperature is regulated by a thermostat-like mechanism in the hypothalamus

Fever (hyperpyrexia)—An elevation in set point such that body temperature is regulated at a higher level; may be arbitrarily defined as rectal temperature above 38°C (100.4°F)

Hyperthermia—Body temperature exceeding the set point, which usually results from the body or external conditions creating more heat than the body can eliminate, such as in heat exhaustion, heatstroke, aspirin toxicity, seizures, or hyperthyroidism

Body temperature is regulated by a thermostat-like mechanism in the hypothalamus. This mechanism receives input from centrally and peripherally located receptors. When temperature changes occur, these receptors relay the information to the thermostat, which either increases or decreases heat production to maintain a constant set point temperature. However, during an infection, pyrogenic substances cause an increase in the body's normal set point, a process that is mediated by prostaglandins. Consequently, the hypothalamus increases heat production until the core temperature reaches the new set point.

During the fever (febrile) state, shivering and vasoconstriction generate and conserve heat during the chill phase of fever, raising central temperatures to the level of the new set point. The temperature reaches a plateau when it stabilizes in the higher range. When the temperature is greater than the set point or when the pyrogen is no longer present, a crisis, or defervescence, of the temperature occurs.

Most fevers in children are of brief duration with limited consequences and are viral in origin (Patricia, 2014). Children may experience warm, flushed skin, chills, aches, malaise, or irritability during a fever. However, children who appear very ill, immunocompromised children, and neonates are at high risk for serious bacterial illness, such as urinary tract infections or bacteremia, and will likely receive a sepsis workup, antibiotics, and hospitalization.

Fever has physiologic benefits, including increased white blood cell activity, interferon production and effectiveness, and antibody production and enhancement of some antibiotic effects such as penicillin (Patricia, 2014). Contrary to popular belief, neither the rise in temperature nor its response to antipyretics indicates the severity or etiology of the infection, which casts doubt on the value of using fever as a diagnostic or prognostic indicator.

Therapeutic Management

Treatment of elevated temperature depends on whether it is attributable to a fever or hyperthermia. Because the set point is normal in hyperthermia but increased in fever, different approaches must be used to lower body temperature successfully.

Fever

The principal reason for treating fever is the relief of discomfort. However, children with cardiopulmonary disease or immunocompromised children may not tolerate the increase in metabolic demand from a fever and should receive antipyretic therapy. Relief measures include pharmacologic and environmental intervention. The most effective intervention is the use of antipyretics to lower the set point.

Antipyretics include acetaminophen, aspirin, and nonsteroidal antiinflammatory drugs (NSAIDs). Acetaminophen is the preferred drug. Aspirin should not be given to children because of its association in children with influenza virus or chickenpox and Reye syndrome. One nonprescription NSAID, ibuprofen, is approved for fever reduction in children as young as 6 months of age.

Another antipyretic, acetaminophen, can be given every 4 hours but no more than five times in 24 hours due to the risk of hepatotoxicity. Because body temperature normally decreases at night, three or four doses in 24 hours will control most fevers. The temperature is usually retaken 30 to 60 minutes after the antipyretic is given to assess its effect but should not be measured repeatedly. The child's level of discomfort is the best indication for continued treatment.

The nurse can use environmental measures to reduce fever if they are tolerated by the child and if they do not induce shivering. Shivering is the body's way of maintaining the elevated set point by producing heat. Compensatory shivering greatly increases metabolic requirements above those already caused by the fever.

Traditional cooling measures, such as wearing minimum clothing; exposing the skin to air; reducing room temperature; increasing air circulation; and applying cool, moist compresses to the skin (e.g., the forehead), are effective if used approximately 1 hour after an antipyretic is given so that the set point is lowered. Cooling procedures such as sponging or tepid baths are ineffective in treating febrile children (these measures are effective for hyperthermia) either when used alone or in combination with antipyretics, and they cause considerable discomfort (Monsma, Richerson, & Sloand, 2015).

Seizures associated with a fever occur in 2% to 5% of all children, usually in those between 6 months and 5 years of age. About 30% to 50% of children have subsequent febrile seizures; a younger age at onset and a family history of febrile seizures are associated with increased incidence of recurring episodes. Evidence does not support the use of antipyretic drugs or anticonvulsants to prevent a second febrile seizure. Nursing interventions should focus on ways to provide care and comfort during a febrile illness. Simple febrile seizures lasting less than 10 minutes do not cause brain damage or other debilitating effects (Patricia, 2014). (See Chapter 27, Febrile Seizures.)

Hyperthermia

Unlike in fever, antipyretics are of no value in hyperthermia because the set point is already normal. Consequently, cooling measures are used. If a child is severely hyperthermic with a core temperature above 40°C, it may be necessary to perform continuous monitoring of vital signs, including core temperature and urinary output, and administer IV fluids in a critical care environment (Chan & Mamat, 2015). Cool applications to the skin help reduce the core temperature. Cooled blood from the skin surface is conducted to inner organs and tissues, and warm blood is circulated to the surface, where it is cooled and recirculated. The surface blood vessels dilate as the body attempts to dissipate heat to the environment and facilitate this cooling process.

Commercial cooling devices, such as cooling blankets or mattresses, are available to reduce body temperature. Place the patient on the bed and cover with a sheet or lightweight blanket. Frequent temperature monitoring is essential to prevent excessive cooling of the body.

Traditionally, cool compresses decrease high temperature. For tepid tub baths, it is usually best to start with warm water and gradually add cool water until the desired water temperature of 37°C (98.6°F) is reached to acclimate the child to the lower water temperature. Generally, the temperature of the water has to be only 1°C (2°F) less than the child's temperature to be effective. The child is placed directly in the tub of tepid water for 15 to 20 minutes while water is gently squeezed from a washcloth over the back and chest or gently sprayed over the body from a sprayer. In the bed or crib, cool washcloths or towels are used, exposing only one area of the body at a time. Continue sponging for approximately 20 minutes.

After the tub or sponge bath, the child is dried; dressed in lightweight pajamas, a nightgown, or a diaper; and placed in a dry bed.

The child is dried by gently rubbing the skin surface with a towel to stimulate circulation. The temperature is retaken 30 minutes after the tub or sponge bath. The tub or sponge bath should not be continued or restarted until the skin surface is warm or if the child feels chilled. Chilling causes vasoconstriction, which defeats the purpose of the cool applications. In this condition, little blood is carried to the skin surface; the blood remains primarily in the viscera to become heated.

Whether a temperature elevation in the critically ill child is caused by fever or hyperthermia, it should be treated aggressively. The metabolic rate increases 10% for every 1°C increase in temperature and three to five times during shivering, thus increasing oxygen, fluid, and caloric requirements. If the child's cardiovascular or neurologic system is already compromised, these increased needs are especially hazardous. In all children with an elevated temperature, attention to adequate hydration is essential. Most children's needs can be met through additional oral fluids.

FAMILY TEACHING AND HOME CARE

Fever is one of the most common problems for which parents seek health care. High levels of parental anxiety (fever phobia) surrounding potential complications of fever such as seizures and dehydration are prevalent and can result in overusing antipyretics. Parents need to know that sponging is indicated for elevated temperatures from hyperthermia rather than fever and that ice water and alcohol are inappropriate, potentially dangerous solutions (Monsma et al., 2015). Parents should know how to take the child's temperature, how to read the thermometer accurately, and when to seek professional care (see Family-Centered Care box). A dedicated thermometer should be used for the rectal route. Oral temperatures should not be taken within 15 minutes of the child eating or drinking hot or cold food. Some of the newer temperature-measuring devices, such as plastic strip or digital thermometers, may be better suited for home use. (See Chapter 4, Temperature.) If the use of acetaminophen or ibuprofen is indicated, the parents need instructions in administering the drug. Emphasize accuracy in both the amount of drug given and the time intervals at which the drug is administered. Along with reduced activity, encourage small, frequent sips of clear liquids. Dress the child in light clothing; use a light blanket for children who are cold or shivering (Monsma et al., 2015).

FAMILY-CENTERED CARE

The Child With Fever

Call the doctor immediately if:

Your child is younger than 3 months old and has a temperature of 38°C (100.4°F) or higher.

The fever is over 40°C (104°F).

Your child looks or acts very sick or sleepy, or has a stiff neck, severe headache, severe ear pain, severe sore throat, repeated vomiting or diarrhea, unexplained rash on the skin, confusion, trouble breathing, or inability to be comforted.

Your child has had a recent seizure.

Your child has a history of immune system problems such as cancer or sickle cell disease.

Your child has been in a very hot place such as a car.

Your child has taken steroid medication.

The fever continues for more than 24 hours in a child younger than 2 years old or more than 3 days in a child older than 2 years of age.

Modified from American Academy of Pediatrics. (2015). When to call the pediatrician: Fever. Retrieved from https://www.healthychildren.org/English/health-issues/conditions/fever/Pages/When-to-Call-the-Pediatrician.aspx

SAFETY

Safety is an essential component of any patient's care, but children have special characteristics that require an even greater concern for safety. Because small children in the hospital are separated from their usual environment and do not possess the capacity for abstract thinking and reasoning, it is the responsibility of everyone who comes in contact with them to maintain protective measures throughout their hospital stay. Nurses need to understand the age level at which each child is operating and plan for safety accordingly.

Identification bands and the use of two patient identifiers are particularly important for children. Infants and unconscious patients are unable to tell or respond to their names. Toddlers may answer to any name or to a nickname only. Older children may exchange places, give an erroneous name, or choose not to respond to their own names as a joke, unaware of the hazards of such practices. In addition, allergy bands for medications and food should be worn by all patients as should bands for other precautions such as fall risks or antineoplastic precautions.

ENVIRONMENTAL FACTORS

All of the environmental safety measures for the protection of adults apply to children, including good illumination, floors that are clear of fluid and objects that might contribute to falls, and nonskid surfaces in showers and tubs. All staff members should be familiar with the area-specific fire plan. Elevators and stairways should be made safe.

All windows should be secured. Window blind and curtain cords should be out of reach, with split cords to prevent strangulation. Pacifiers should not be tied around the neck or attached to an infant by a string.

Electrical equipment should be in good working order and used only by personnel familiar with its use. It should not be in contact with moisture or situated near tubs. Electrical outlets should have covers to prevent burns in small children, whose exploratory activities may extend to inserting objects into the small openings.

Staff members should practice proper care and disposal of small objects such as syringe caps, needle covers, and temperature probes. Staff also must carefully check bathwater before placing the child in it and never leave children alone in a bathtub. Infants are helpless in water, and small children (and some older ones) may turn on the hot water faucet and be severely burned.

Furniture is safest when it is scaled to the child's proportions, is sturdy, and is well balanced to prevent its being easily tipped over. A special hazard for children is the danger of entrapment under an electronically controlled bed when it is activated to descend. Infants and small children must be securely strapped into infant seats, feeding chairs, and strollers. Baby walkers should not be used because they provide access to hazards, resulting in burns, falls, and poisonings. Infants; young children; and children who are weak, paralyzed, agitated, confused, sedated, or cognitively impaired should never be left unattended on treatment tables, on scales, or in treatment areas. Even premature infants are capable of surprising mobility; therefore portholes in incubators must be securely fastened when not in use. For patients at risk of suicide, it is necessary to remove all items such as sharp objects, cords, and plastic bags that can be used to impose self-harm. Depending on patient diagnosis, a one-to-one sitter should also be considered. In addition, visitors, personal items, and Internet access may be restricted to protect the patient.

Crib sides should always be raised and fastened securely. Use cribs that meet federal safety standards (https://www.cpsc.gov/safety-education/safety-education-centers/cribs). Anyone attending to an infant

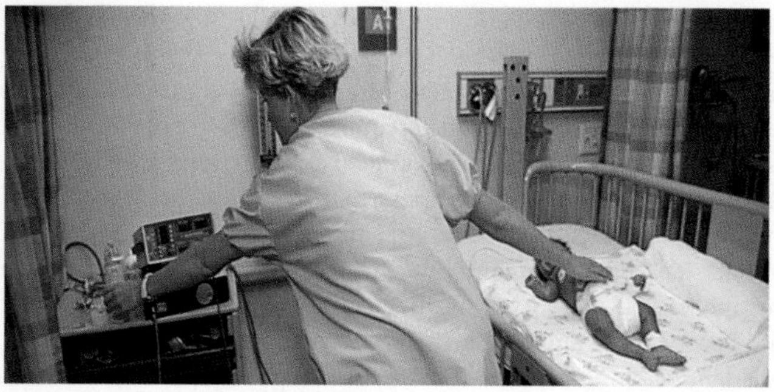

Fig. 20.2 The nurse maintains hand contact when her back is turned.

or small child on a stretcher or table should never turn away without maintaining hand contact with the child—that is, keeping one hand on the child's back or abdomen to prevent rolling, crawling, or jumping from the open crib (Fig. 20.2). A child who is likely to climb over the sides of the crib is safest when placed in a specially constructed crib with a cover over the top. Never tie nets to the movable crib sides or use knots that do not permit quick release.

The safest sleeping position to prevent sudden infant death syndrome is wholly supine until at least 1 year of age (American Academy of Pediatrics, Task Force on Sudden Infant Death Syndrome, 2016). No pillows should be placed in a young infant's crib while the infant is sleeping. A firm sleep surface with no other bedding or any soft items in the crib in a shared room (not a shared bed) and the avoidance of overheating or exposure to tobacco smoke, alcohol, and illicit drugs further increase the safety of an infant's sleeping environment. The use of car seats, strollers, swings, or other sitting devices should not be used for routine sleep. In addition, swaddling is not recommended for infants over 2 months of age due to the risk of death if the infant rolls into the prone position. In accordance with the American Academy of Pediatrics guidelines to avoid extra bedding in the crib, many institutions recommend an infant sleep sack for adequate warmth and safety.

Toys

Toys play a vital role in the everyday lives of children, and they are no less important in the hospital setting. Nurses are responsible for assessing the safety of toys brought to the hospital by well-meaning parents and friends. Toys should be appropriate to the child's age, condition, and treatment. For example, if the child is receiving oxygen, electrical or friction toys or equipment are not safe because sparks can cause oxygen to ignite. Inspect toys to ensure that they are nonallergenic, washable, and unbreakable and that they have no small, removable parts that can be aspirated or swallowed or can otherwise inflict injury on a child. All objects within reach of children younger than 3 years of age should pass the choke tube test. A toilet paper roll is a handy guide. If a toy or object fits into the cylinder (items less than 1¼ inches across or balls less than 1¾ inches in diameter), it is a potential choking danger to the child. Latex balloons pose a serious threat to children of all ages. If the balloon breaks, a child may put a piece of the latex in his or her mouth. If it is aspirated or swallowed, the latex piece is difficult to remove, resulting in choking. Latex balloons should never be permitted in the hospital setting.

Preventing Falls

Although children have a known predisposition to falls based on normal growth and development, falls risk identification and prevention for children with medical conditions is especially important due to greater risk for injury from a fall (Murray, Edlund, & Vess, 2016). Falls prevention begins with identification of children most at risk for falls. Pediatric hospitals use various methods to identify a child's risk of falls. After a risk assessment is performed, multiple interventions are needed to minimize pediatric patients' risk of falling, including education of patient, family, and staff.

To identify children at risk of falling, perform a falls risk assessment on patients on admission and throughout hospitalization. Risk factors for hospitalized children include the following:

- **Medication effects**—Postanesthesia or sedation; analgesics or narcotics, especially in those who have never had narcotics in the past and in whom effects are unknown
- **Altered mental status**—Secondary to seizures, brain tumors, or medications
- **Altered or limited mobility**—Reduced skill at ambulation secondary to developmental age, disease process, tubes, drains, casts, splints, or other appliances; new to ambulation with assistive devices such as walkers or crutches
- **Postoperative children**—Risk of hypotension or syncope secondary to large blood loss, a heart condition, or extended bed rest
- History of falls
- Infants or toddlers in cribs with side rails down or on the daybed with family members
- Changes to the patient's environment

Once children at risk of falls have been identified, alert other staff members by posting signs on the door and at the bedside, applying a special-colored armband labeled "Fall Precautions," labeling the chart with a sticker, or documenting information on the chart.

Prevention of falls requires alterations in the environment, including the following:

- Keep the bed in the lowest position with the breaks locked and the side rails up.
- Place the call bell within reach and orient the patient and caregivers to the bed and room.
- Ensure that all necessary and desired items are within reach (e.g., water, glasses, tissues, snacks).
- Offer toileting on a regular basis, especially if the patient is taking diuretics or laxatives.
- Keep lights on at all times, including dim lights while sleeping.
- Lock wheelchairs before transferring patients.
- Ensure that the patient has an appropriate-size gown and nonskid footwear. Do not allow gowns or ties to drag on the floor during ambulation.
- Keep the floor clean and free of clutter. Post a "wet floor" sign if the floor is wet.
- Ensure that the patient has glasses on if he or she normally wears them.
- Use a gait belt during ambulation.
- Keep the patient's door open unless isolation status prohibits.

Preventing falls also relies on age-appropriate education of patients. Assist the child with ambulation even though he or she may have ambulated well before hospitalization. Patients who have been lying in bed need to get up slowly, sitting on the side of the bed before standing.

The nurse also needs to educate family members:

- Call the nursing staff for assistance and do not allow patients to get up independently.
- Keep the side rails of the crib or bed up whenever patient is in the crib or bed.
- Do not leave infants on the daybed; put them in the crib with the side rails up.
- When all family members need to leave the bedside, notify the staff and ensure that the patient is in the bed or crib with the side rails up and call bell within reach (if appropriate).

In the event of a fall, it is important to immediately respond to the needs of the patient; notify appropriate personnel, including caregivers; and document the event.

INFECTION CONTROL

According to the Centers for Disease Control and Prevention, nosocomial (health care–associated) infections pose a significant threat to patient safety. These infections occur when there is interaction among patients, health care personnel, equipment, and bacteria. Health care–associated infections include infections such as *Clostridium difficile* or hospital-onset methicillin-resistant *Staphylococcus aureus,* as well as central line–associated bloodstream infections (CLABSIs), catheter-associated urinary tract infections (CAUTIs), and some surgical site infections. Health care–associated infections can be preventable if caregivers practice meticulous cleaning and disposal techniques.

Standard Precautions synthesize the major features of Universal (blood and body fluid) Precautions (designed to reduce the risk of transmission of bloodborne pathogens) and body substance isolation (designed to reduce the risk of transmission of pathogens from moist body substances). Standard Precautions involve vigilant hand hygiene and the use of barrier protection, such as gloves, goggles, gown, or mask, to prevent contamination from (1) blood; (2) all body fluids, secretions, and excretions except sweat, regardless of whether they contain visible blood; (3) nonintact skin; and (4) mucous membranes. Standard Precautions are designed for the care of all patients to reduce the risk of transmission of microorganisms from both recognized and unrecognized sources of infection.

Transmission-Based Precautions are designed for patients with documented or suspected infection or colonization (i.e., presence of microorganisms in or on the patient but without clinical signs and symptoms of infection) with highly transmissible or epidemiologically important pathogens for which additional precautions beyond Standard Precautions are needed to interrupt transmission in hospitals. There are three types of Transmission-Based Precautions: Airborne Precautions, Droplet Precautions, and Contact Precautions. They may be combined for diseases that have multiple routes of transmission (Box 20.2). They are to be used in addition to Standard Precautions.

Airborne Precautions reduce the risk of airborne transmission of infectious agents. Airborne transmission occurs by dissemination of either airborne droplet nuclei (small-particle residue [<5 mm] of evaporated droplets that may remain suspended in the air for long periods) or dust particles containing the infectious agent. Microorganisms carried in this manner can be dispersed widely by air currents and may become inhaled by or deposited on a susceptible host within the same room or over a longer distance from the source patient, depending on environmental factors. Individuals who have not had direct face-to-face contact with the source individual may become infected. Special air handling and ventilation are required to prevent airborne transmission. Airborne Precautions apply to patients with known or suspected infection with pathogens transmitted by the airborne route such as measles, varicella, and tuberculosis.

Droplet Precautions reduce the risk of droplet transmission of infectious agents. Droplet transmission involves contact of the conjunctivae or the mucous membranes of the nose or mouth of a susceptible person with large-particle droplets (>5 mm) containing microorganisms generated from a person who has a clinical disease or who is a carrier of the microorganism. Droplets are generated from the source person primarily during coughing, sneezing, or talking, and during procedures such as suctioning and bronchoscopy. Transmission requires close contact between source and recipient persons because droplets do not remain suspended in the air and generally travel only short distances, usually 3 feet or less but up to 10 feet, through the air. Because droplets

BOX 20.2 Types of Precautions and Patients Requiring Them

Standard Precautions for Prevention of Transmission of Pathogens

Use Standard Precautions for the care of all patients.

Airborne Precautions

In addition to Standard Precautions, use Airborne Precautions for patients known or suspected to have serious illnesses transmitted by airborne droplet nuclei. Examples of such illnesses include measles, varicella (including disseminated zoster), and tuberculosis.

Droplet Precautions

In addition to Standard Precautions, use Droplet Precautions for patients known or suspected to have serious illnesses transmitted by large-particle droplets. Examples of such illnesses include the following:

- Invasive *Haemophilus influenzae* type b disease, including meningitis, pneumonia, epiglottitis, and sepsis
- Invasive *Neisseria meningitidis* disease, including meningitis, pneumonia, and sepsis
- Other serious bacterial respiratory tract infections spread by droplet transmission, including diphtheria (pharyngeal), mycoplasma pneumonia, pertussis, pneumonic plague, streptococcal pharyngitis, pneumonia, and scarlet fever in infants and young children
- Serious viral infections spread by droplet transmission, including adenovirus, influenza, mumps, parvovirus B19, and rubella

Contact Precautions

In addition to Standard Precautions, use Contact Precautions for patients known or suspected to have serious illnesses easily transmitted by direct patient contact or by contact with items in the patient's environment. Examples of such illnesses include the following:

- Gastrointestinal, respiratory, skin, or wound infections or colonization with multidrug-resistant bacteria judged by the infection control program, based on current state, regional, or national recommendations, to be of special clinical and epidemiologic significance
- Enteric infections with a low infectious dose or prolonged environmental survival, including *Clostridium difficile;* for diapered or incontinent patients: enterohemorrhagic *Escherichia coli* 0157:H7, *Shigella* organisms, hepatitis A, or rotavirus
- Respiratory syncytial virus, parainfluenza virus, or enteroviral infections in infants and young children
- Skin infections that are highly contagious or that may occur on dry skin, including diphtheria (cutaneous), herpes simplex virus (neonatal or mucocutaneous), impetigo, major (noncontained) abscesses, cellulitis or decubitus, pediculosis, scabies, staphylococcal furunculosis in infants and young children, zoster (disseminated or in the immunocompromised host)
- Multidrug-resistant organisms, infection, or colonization (methicillin-resistant *Staphylococcus aureus,* vancomycin-resistant enterococci)
- Viral or hemorrhagic conjunctivitis
- Viral hemorrhagic infections (Ebola, Lassa, or Marburg)

A complete list of the guidelines for isolation precautions for the prevention of transmission of infectious agents in health care can be found at https://www.cdc.gov/infectioncontrol/guidelines/isolation/index.html.

do not remain suspended in the air, special air handling and ventilation are not required to prevent droplet transmission. Droplet Precautions apply to any patient with known or suspected infection with pathogens that can be transmitted by infectious droplets (see Box 20.2).

Contact Precautions reduce the risk of transmission of microorganisms by direct or indirect contact. Direct-contact transmission involves skin-to-skin contact and physical transfer of microorganisms to a susceptible host from an infected or colonized person, such as occurs when turning or bathing patients. Direct-contact transmission also can occur between two patients (e.g., by hand contact). Indirect contact transmission involves contact of a susceptible host with a contaminated intermediate object, usually inanimate, in the patient's environment. Contact Precautions apply to specified patients known or suspected to be infected or colonized with microorganisms that can be transmitted by direct or indirect contact.

> **! NURSING ALERT**
>
> The most common piece of medical equipment, the stethoscope, can be a potent source of harmful microorganisms and nosocomial infections.

Nurses caring for young children are frequently in contact with body substances, especially urine, feces, and vomitus. Nurses need to exercise judgment concerning those situations when gloves, gowns, or masks are necessary. For example, wear gloves and possibly gowns for changing diapers when there are loose or explosive stools. Otherwise, the plastic lining of disposable diapers provides a sufficient barrier between the hands and body substances. During feedings or oral medication administration, wear gowns if the child is likely to vomit or spit up, which often occurs during burping. When wearing gloves, wash the hands thoroughly after removing the gloves because gloves fail to provide complete protection. The absence of visible leaks does not indicate that gloves are intact.

Another essential practice of infection control is that all needles (uncapped and unbroken) are disposed of in a rigid, puncture-resistant container located near the site of use. Consequently, these containers are installed in patients' rooms. Because children are naturally curious, extra attention is needed in selecting a suitable type of container and a location that prevents access to the discarded needles. Puncture-resistant containers should be changed when three-quarters full or when the fill line marker on the container is reached (US Food and Drug Administration, 2018). The use of needleless systems allows secure syringe or IV tubing attachment to vascular access devices without the risk of needlestick injury to the child or nurse.

TRANSPORTING INFANTS AND CHILDREN

Infants and children need to be transported within the unit and to areas outside the pediatric unit. Infants and small children can be carried for short distances within the unit, but for more extended trips, the child should be securely transported in a suitable conveyance.

Small infants can be held or carried in the horizontal position with the back supported and the thigh grasped firmly by the carrying arm (Fig. 20.3A). In the football hold, the infant is carried on the nurse's arm with the head supported by the hand and the body held securely between the nurse's body and elbow (see Fig. 20.3B). Both of these holds leave the nurse's other arm free for activity. The infant also can be held in the upright position with the buttocks on the nurse's forearm and the front of the body resting against the nurse's chest. The infant's head and shoulders are supported by the nurse's other arm in case the infant moves suddenly (see Fig. 20.3C). Older infants are able to hold their heads erect but are still subject to sudden movements. Medically stable infants can be carried in a variety of ways for transport as long as their head is supported at all times.

The method of transporting children depends on their age, condition, and destination. Older children are safe in wheelchairs or on stretchers. Younger children can be transported in a crib, on a stretcher, in a wagon with raised sides, or in a wheelchair with a safety belt. Stretchers should be equipped with high sides and a safety belt, both of which are secured during transport.

Special care is needed in transporting critically ill patients in the hospital. Critically ill children should always be transported on a stretcher or bed (rather than carried) by at least two appropriately trained staff members with monitoring continued during transport. A blood pressure monitor (or standard blood pressure cuff), pulse oximeter, and cardiac monitor/defibrillator should accompany every patient (Alamanou & Brokalaki, 2014). Airway equipment, oxygen, and emergency medications should accompany the patient. The monitoring and staff members required for transport will vary depending on the acuity and clinical status of the patient. In addition, it is important for the nurse to be familiar with emergency transport of patients

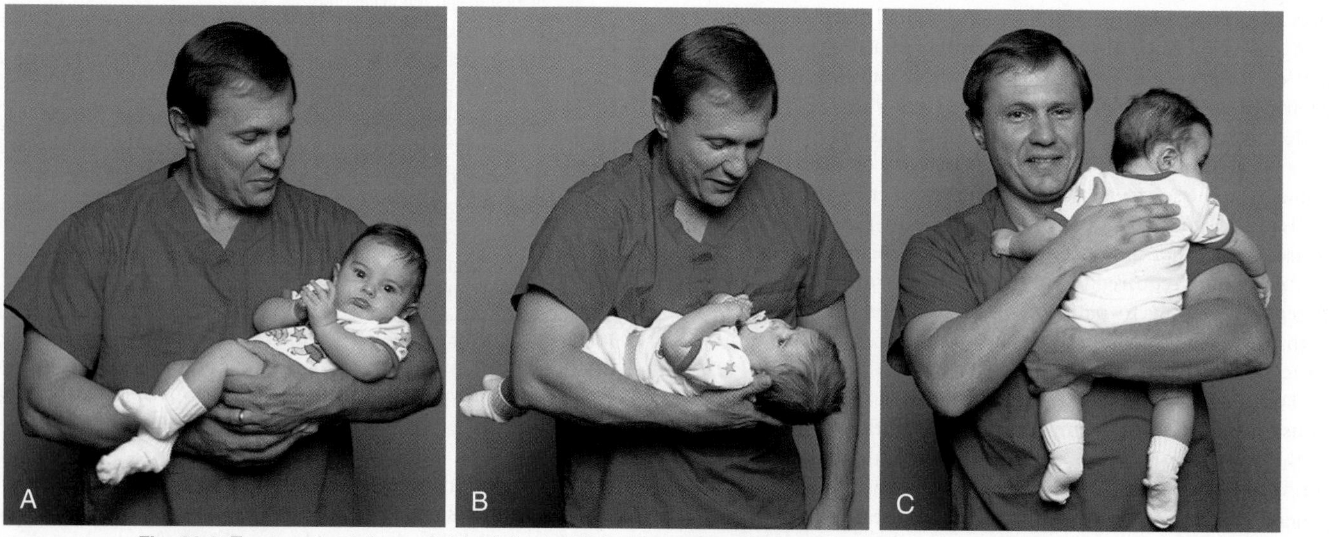

Fig. 20.3 Transporting infants. **A,** The infant's thigh is firmly grasped in the nurse's hand. **B,** Football hold. **C,** Back supported.

in the event of severe weather, fire, or security threats when power or elevators may be unavailable.

RESTRAINING METHODS

The Centers for Medicare and Medicaid Services (2015) has established regulations to minimize the use of and ensure the safety of patients in restraints. It defines *restraint* as "any manual method, physical or mechanical device, material, or equipment that immobilizes or reduces the ability of a patient to move his or her arms, legs, body, or head freely . . . or a drug or medication when it is used as a restriction to manage the patient's behavior or restrict the patient's freedom of movement and is not a standard treatment or dosage for the patient's condition." A restraint should be applied only by a health care team member with demonstrated competency in restraint management. The physical force may be human, mechanical devices, or a combination of the two. Examples of restraints include limb restraints, elbow restraints, vest restraints, and tight tucking of sheets to prevent movement in bed.

Mechanical supports such as immobilizers for fractures, orthopedic devices to maintain proper body alignment, leg braces, protective helmets, and surgical dressings are not considered restraints. An armboard to secure a peripheral IV line is not considered a restraint unless it is tied to the bed or immobilizes the entire limb such that the patient cannot access his or her body. Hand mitts are not considered a restraint unless tied to the bed or used in conjunction with a wrist restraint. Developmentally age-appropriate safety interventions for infants, toddlers, and preschoolers, such as net enclosures on beds, crib domes, crib side rails, and high chair lap safety belts, are generally not considered restraints. Picking up, redirecting, or holding an infant, toddler, or preschooler is not considered restraint. Interventions that typically would be used by a child care provider outside a health care environment to ensure safety in young children are not considered restraints.

Before initiating restraints, the nurse completes a comprehensive assessment of the patient to determine whether the need for a restraint outweighs the risk of not using one. Restraints can result in loss of dignity, violation of patient rights, psychologic harm, physical harm, and even death. Consider alternative methods first and document them in the patient's record. Some examples of alternative measures include bringing a child to the nurses' station for continuous observation, providing diversional activities such as music, and encouraging the participation of the parents. The use of restraints can often be avoided with adequate preparation of the child; parental or staff supervision of the child; or adequate protection of a vulnerable site, such as an infusion device.

The nurse needs to assess the child's development, mental status, potential to hurt others or self, and safety. The nurse is responsible for selecting the least restrictive type of restraint. Using less restrictive restraints is often possible by gaining the cooperation of the child and parents. An order must be obtained as soon as possible (during application or within a few minutes) after the initiation of restraints and specify the time frame in which they can be used, the reason they are being used, and reasons for discontinuation. Discontinuation of restraints should occur as soon as it is safe, even if the order time frame has not expired.

Restraints for violent, self-destructive behavior are limited to situations with a significant risk of patients physically harming themselves or others because of behavioral reasons and when nonphysical interventions are not effective. Before initiating a behavioral restraint, the nurse should assess the patient's mental, behavioral, and physical status to determine the cause for the child's potentially harmful behavior. If behavioral restraints are indicated, a collaborative approach involving the patient (if appropriate), the family, and the health care team should be used. Behavioral restraints can include personal restraints, such as a physical hold, or mechanical restraints, such as secured anklets and wristlets or bilateral arm immobilizers.

Unless state law is more restrictive, behavioral restraints for children must be reordered every 15 minutes for a personal restraint, every 1 hour for children under 9 years of age, and every 2 hours for children 9 to 17 years old; orders for adults 18 years and older are required every 4 hours. A licensed independent practitioner or specially trained nurse must conduct an in-person evaluation within 1 hour and at least every 24 hours to continue restraints.

Children in behavioral restraints must be observed and assessed according to facility policy—typically continuously, every 15 minutes, or every 2 hours. Assessment components include signs of injury associated with applying restraint, nutrition and hydration, circulation and range-of-motion of extremities, vital signs, hygiene and elimination, physical and psychologic status and comfort, and readiness for discontinuation of restraint. The nurse must use clinical judgment in setting a schedule within the facility's policy for when each of these parameters needs to be evaluated.

Nonviolent and non–self-destructive patients may also require restraints to support medical healing. Examples of situations where a nonbehavioral restraint may be necessary for the patient's safety include removal of an artificial airway or airway adjunct for delivery of oxygen, indwelling catheters, tubes, drains, lines, pacemaker wires, or disruption of suture sites. The medical-surgical restraint is used to ensure that safe care is given to the patient. Patient confusion, agitation, unconsciousness, and developmental inability to understand direct requests or instructions may warrant the use of nonbehavioral restraints to maintain patient safety. The potential risks of the restraint are offset by the potential benefit of providing safer care.

Nonbehavioral restraints can be initiated by an individual order or by protocol; the use of the protocol must be authorized by an individual order. The order for continued use of restraints must be renewed each day. Patients are monitored per facility policy, typically at least every 2 hours.

Restraints with ties must be secured to the stationary bed or crib frame, not the side rails. Suggestions for increasing safety and comfort while the child is in a restraint include leaving one fingerbreadth between skin and the device and tying knots that allow for quick release. The nurse can also increase safety by ensuring that the restraint does not tighten as the child moves and by decreasing wrinkles or bulges in the restraint. Placing jacket restraints over an article of clothing; placing limb restraints below waist level, below knee level, or distal to the IV; and tucking in dangling straps also increase safety and comfort. Do not place objects over a patient's face to protect staff from being spit on or bitten. Masks and face shields should be readily available for staff to wear; some facilities also provide bite gloves and arm and hand wraps made of strong barrier materials such as Kevlar for staff to wear to prevent injury from bites and scratches.

Mummy Restraint or Swaddle

When an infant or small child requires short-term restraint for examination or treatment that involves the head and neck (e.g., venipuncture, throat examination, gavage feeding), a papoose board with straps or a mummy wrap effectively controls the child's movements. When used only for the duration of the test or procedure, this is not considered a restraint. The mummy restraint or swaddle should not be used for behavior or long-term restraint. A blanket or sheet is opened on the bed or crib with one corner folded to the center. The infant is placed on the blanket with the shoulders at the fold and feet toward the opposite

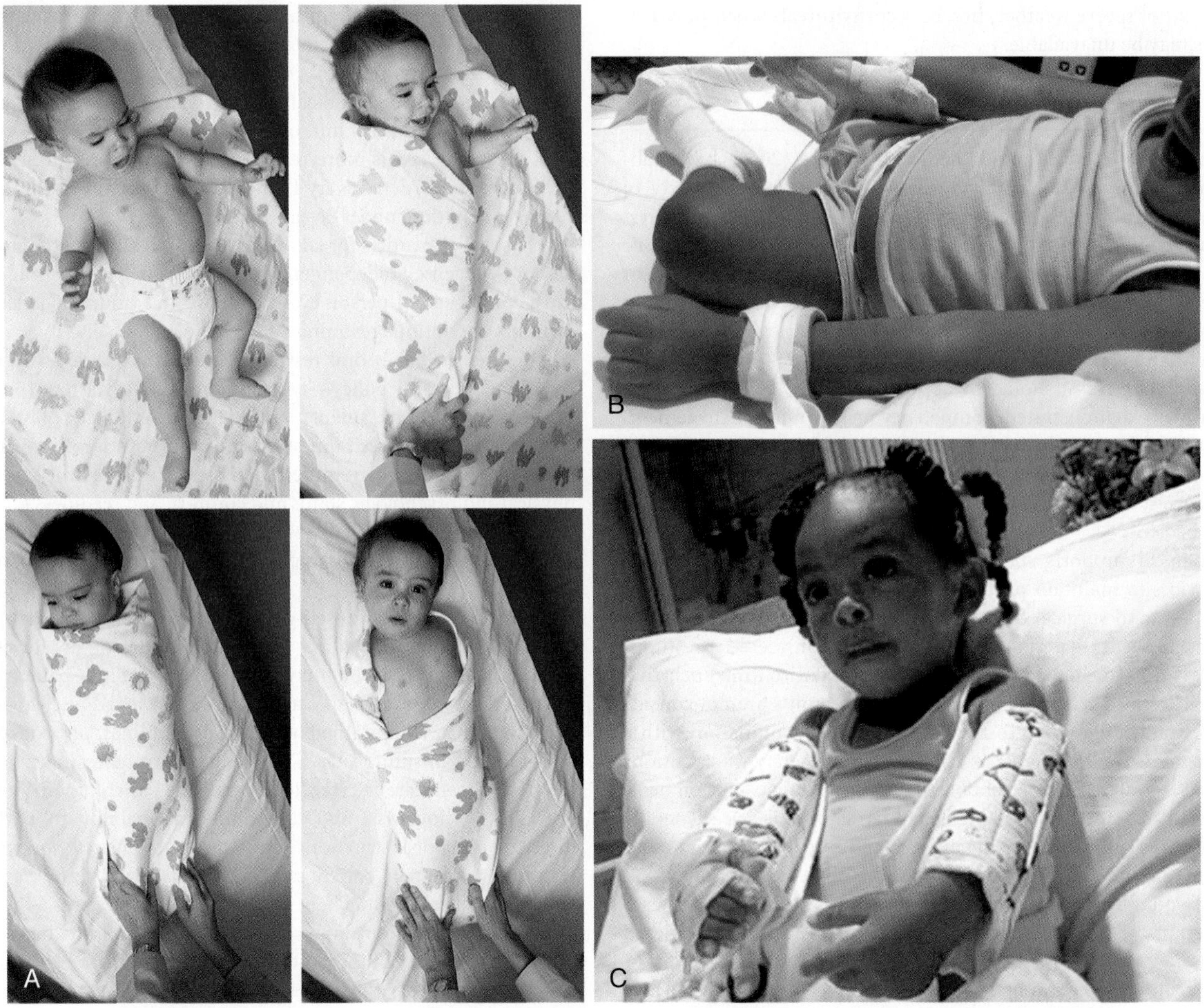

Fig. 20.4 Restraint examples from most restrictive to least restrictive. **A,** Mummy restraint. **B,** Wrist restraints. **C,** Elbow restraints.

corner. With the infant's right arm straight down against the body, the right side of the blanket is pulled firmly across the infant's right shoulder and chest and secured beneath the left side of the body. The left arm is placed straight against the infant's side, and the left side of the blanket is brought across the shoulder and chest and locked beneath the body on the right side. The lower corner is folded and brought over the body and tucked or fastened securely with safety pins. Safety pins can be used to fasten the blanket in place at any step in the process. To modify the mummy restraint for chest examination, bring the folded edge of the blanket over each arm and under the back and then fold the loose edge over and secure it at a point below the chest to allow visualization and access to the chest (Fig. 20.4A).

Arm and Leg Restraints

Occasionally, the nurse needs to restrain one or more extremities or limit their motion. Several commercial restraining devices are available, including disposable wrist and ankle restraints (see Fig. 20.4B). Restraints must be appropriate to the child's size and padded to prevent undue pressure, constriction, or tissue injury, and the extremity must be observed frequently for signs of irritation or impaired circulation. The ends of the restraints are never tied to the side rails because lowering the rail will disturb the extremity, frequently with a jerk that may hurt or injure the child.

Elbow Restraint

Sometimes it is important to prevent the child from reaching the head or face (e.g., after cleft lip or palate surgery, when a scalp vein infusion is in place, or to prevent scratching in skin disorders). Bilateral elbow restraints fashioned from a variety of materials function well (see Fig. 20.4C). Commercial elbow restraints or immobilizers are available. They extend from just below the axilla to the wrist and are sometimes referred to as "no-no's." A shoulder strap to prevent slipping may be used in an awake, active older infant or toddler to prevent slippage but should not be used when sleeping.

POSITIONING FOR PROCEDURES

Infants and small children are unable to cooperate for many procedures. Therefore the nurse is responsible for minimizing their movement and discomfort with proper positioning. It can also be helpful to involve the caregivers or child life specialists during procedures to minimize distress in the child. Older children usually need only minimal, if any, positioning hold or movement restrictions. Careful explanation and preparation beforehand and support and simple guidance during the procedure are usually sufficient. For painful procedures, the child should receive adequate analgesia and sedation to minimize pain and the need for excessive restraint. For local anesthesia, use buffered

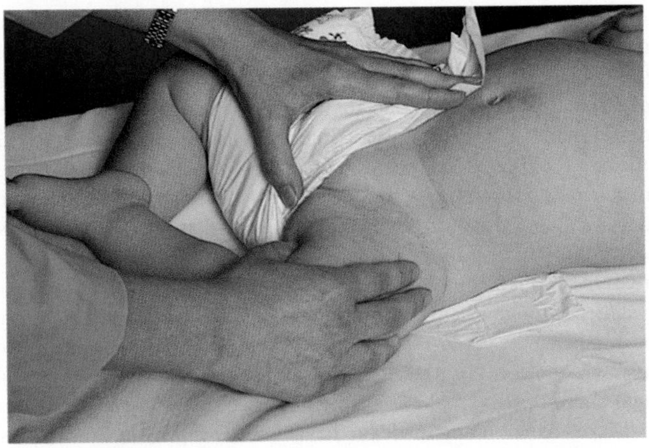

Fig. 20.5 Positioning infant for femoral venipuncture.

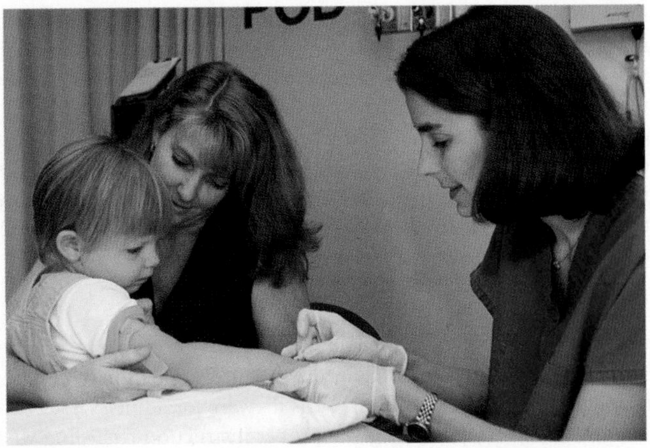

Fig. 20.6 Therapeutic comfort hold of child for extremity venipuncture with parental assistance.

lidocaine to reduce the stinging sensation or a topical anesthetic. (See Chapter 5, Pain Management.)

FEMORAL VENIPUNCTURE

The nurse places the child supine with the legs in a frog position to provide extensive exposure of the groin area. A towel can also be placed under the hips. The infant's legs can be effectively controlled by the nurse's forearms and hands (Fig. 20.5). Only the side used for the venipuncture is uncovered, so the practitioner is protected if the child urinates during the procedure. Apply pressure to the site to prevent oozing from the site.

EXTREMITY VENIPUNCTURE OR INJECTION

The most common sites of venipuncture are the veins of the extremities, especially the arm and hand. A convenient position is to place the child in the parent's (or assistant's) lap with the child facing the parent and in the straddle position. Next, place the child's arm for venipuncture on a firm surface, such as a treatment table. The nurse can partially stabilize the child's outstretched arm and have the parent hug the child's upper body, preventing movement; the nurse can then use the parent's arm to immobilize the venipuncture site. This type of comfort hold also comforts the child because of the close body contact, allows for distraction techniques for the child, and allows each person to maintain eye contact (Fig. 20.6).

LUMBAR PUNCTURE

Pediatric lumbar puncture (LP) sets contain smaller spinal needles, but sometimes the provider will specify a different size or type of needle depending on the child's size or obesity. The technique for the LP procedure in infants and children is similar to that in adults, although modifications are suggested in neonates, who have less distress in a side-lying position with modified neck extension than in flexion or a sitting position.

Children can be positioned in a side-lying or sitting position. Children are usually easiest to control in the side-lying position, with the head flexed and the knees drawn up toward the chest. Even cooperative children need to be held gently under the knees and around the shoulders to prevent possible trauma from unexpected, involuntary movement. They can be reassured that, although they are trusted, holding will serve as a reminder to maintain the desired position. It also provides a measure of support and reassurance to them (Fig. 20.7).

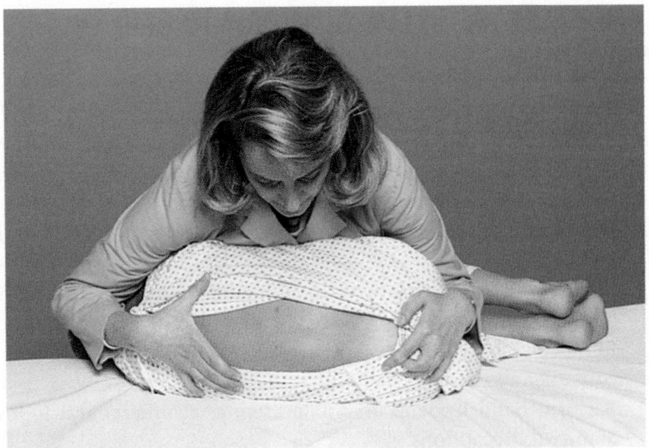

Fig. 20.7 Side-lying position for lumbar puncture.

A flexed sitting position may be used, depending on the child's ability to cooperate and whether sedation will be used. In the sitting position with the hips flexed and spine curved forward, the interspinous space is maximized between L3 and L5. The child is placed with the buttocks at the edge of the table. For an infant, the nurse's hands immobilize the arms and legs. Neck flexion has not been shown to enhance the interspinous space opening in children.

Specimens and spinal fluid pressure are obtained, measured, and sent for analysis in the same manner as for adult patients. Take vital signs as ordered throughout and after the procedure and observe the child for any changes in level of consciousness, motor activity, and other neurologic signs. Post-LP headache may occur and can be related to larger needle size, prior history of headaches, and postural changes. There is insufficient evidence to support the use of bed rest after LP to reduce post-LP headaches (Rusch, Schulta, Hughes, et al., 2014). Treatment generally includes rest and oral analgesics, such as acetaminophen, that do not inhibit platelet function.

BONE MARROW ASPIRATION OR BIOPSY

The position for a bone marrow aspiration or biopsy depends on the chosen site. In children, the posterior or anterior iliac crest is most frequently used, but in infants less than 18 months old, the tibia may be selected because the iliac crest has not yet ossified.

If the posterior iliac crest is used, the child is positioned prone, and if the anterior iliac crest is used, the child is typically positioned side-lying or supine. Sometimes a small pillow or folded blanket is placed under the hips to facilitate obtaining the bone marrow specimen. Children should receive adequate analgesia or anesthesia to relieve pain and should be monitored appropriately throughout the procedure. If the child might awaken, he or she may need to be held, preferably by two people—one person to immobilize the upper body and a second person to immobilize the lower extremities. A pressure dressing is applied to the puncture site on completion of the procedure. The dressing will be removed after 24 hours and the site assessed for infection.

COLLECTION OF SPECIMENS

Many of the specimens needed for diagnostic examination of children are collected in much the same way as they are for adults. Older children are able to cooperate if given proper instruction regarding what is expected of them. Infants and small children, however, are typically unable to follow directions or control body functions sufficiently to help in collecting some specimens.

FUNDAMENTAL STEPS COMMON TO ALL PROCEDURES

The following steps are very important for every procedure and should be considered fundamental aspects of care. These steps, although important, are not listed in each of the specimen collection procedures.

1. Assemble the necessary equipment.
2. Introduce self to the family and verify the specimen that is to be collected.
3. Identify the child using two patient identifiers (e.g., patient name and medical record or birth date; neither identifier can be a room number). Compare the same two identifiers with the specimen container and order.
4. Perform hand hygiene, maintain aseptic technique, and follow Standard Precautions.
5. Explain the procedure to parents and child according to the developmental level of the child; reassure the child that the procedure is not a punishment.
6. Provide atraumatic care and position the child securely.
7. Prepare area with antiseptic agent.
8. Place specimens in appropriate containers with appropriate collection information such as date and time and apply a patient identification label to the specimen container in the presence of the child and family.
9. Discard puncture device in puncture-resistant container near the site of use.
10. Wash the procedural preparation agent off if povidone-iodine is used, if skin is sensitive, and for infants. Check that all collection supplies have been removed from the patient's bed area to ensure patient safety.
11. Remove gloves and perform hand hygiene after the procedure. Have children wash their hands if they have helped.
12. Praise the child for helping.
13. Document pertinent aspects of the procedure, such as number of attempts, site, and amount of blood or urine withdrawn, as well as type of test performed.

URINE SPECIMENS

Many diagnostic situations warrant urine specimens. The age of the child will affect the collection technique, as will developmental considerations. Children will better understand what is expected if the nurse uses familiar terms, such as "pee-pee," "wee-wee," or "tinkle." Preschoolers and toddlers are usually unable to void on request. It is often best to offer them water or other liquids that they enjoy and wait about 30 minutes until they are ready to void voluntarily. Some have difficulty voiding in an unfamiliar receptacle. Potty chairs or a potty hat placed on the toilet is usually satisfactory. Toddlers who have recently acquired bladder control may be especially reluctant because they undoubtedly have been admonished for "going" in places other than those approved by parents. Enlisting the parents' help usually leads to success. School-age children are generally cooperative with collection methods but curious. They are concerned about the reasons behind things and are likely to ask questions about the disposition of their specimen and what one expects to discover from it. Self-conscious adolescents may be reluctant to carry a specimen through a hallway or waiting room and appreciate a paper bag for disguising the container. The presence of menses may be an embarrassment or a concern to teenage girls; therefore it is a good idea to ask them about this and make adjustments as necessary. The specimen can be delayed or a notation made on the laboratory slip to explain the presence of red blood cells.

At times, parents may be asked to bring a urine sample to a health care facility for examination, especially when infants are unable to void during an outpatient visit. In these instances, parents need instructions on applying the collection device and storing the specimen. Ideally, the specimen should be brought to the designated place as soon as possible. If there is a delay, the sample should be refrigerated and the lapsed time reported to the examiner.

Although it is a convenient and noninvasive collection method, direct urine aspiration from a diaper can alter the specimen results. Superabsorbent gel disposable diapers may absorb all urine and may also produce a false crystalluria. Direct aspiration from the diaper may not be suitable for all urine specimen tests. Nurses should verify collection procedures with the laboratory before collection.

Urine Collection Bags

For infants and toddlers who are not toilet trained, special urine collection bags with self-adhering material around the opening at the point of attachment may be used. To prepare the infant, the genitalia, perineum, and surrounding skin are washed and dried thoroughly because the adhesive will not stick to a moist, powdered, or oily skin surface. The collection bag is easiest to apply if attached first to the perineum, progressing to the symphysis pubis (Fig. 20.8). With girls, the perineum is stretched taut during application to ensure a leakproof fit. With boys, the penis and sometimes the scrotum are placed inside the bag. The adhesive portion of the bag must be firmly applied to the skin all around the genital area to avoid leakage. The bag is checked frequently and removed as soon as the specimen is available because the moist bag may become loosened on an active child.

The American Academy of Pediatrics guidelines (American Academy of Pediatrics, Subcommittee on Urinary Tract Infections, 2011) for diagnosis and management of urinary tract infections in infants 2 to 24 months old recommend that any positive screen obtained from a bag specimen be confirmed by culture via bladder catheterization or suprapubic aspiration due to an unacceptably high rate of false-positive results. Although the bag specimen collection method is less invasive and traumatic to an infant, some families and clinicians may prefer to collect only one definitive specimen and avoid additional delay in obtaining a second specimen. Urine bag specimens may be most appropriate for a urine dipstick or urinalysis, not urine cultures (Stein, Dogan, Hoebeke, et al., 2015).

> **NURSING TIP** In infants, wipe the abdomen with an alcohol pad and fan it dry; the cooling effect often causes voiding within 2 minutes. Apply pressure over the suprapubic area or stroke the paraspinal muscles (along the spine) to elicit the Perez reflex. In infants 4 to 6 months of age, this reflex causes crying, extension of the back, flexion of the extremities, and urination.

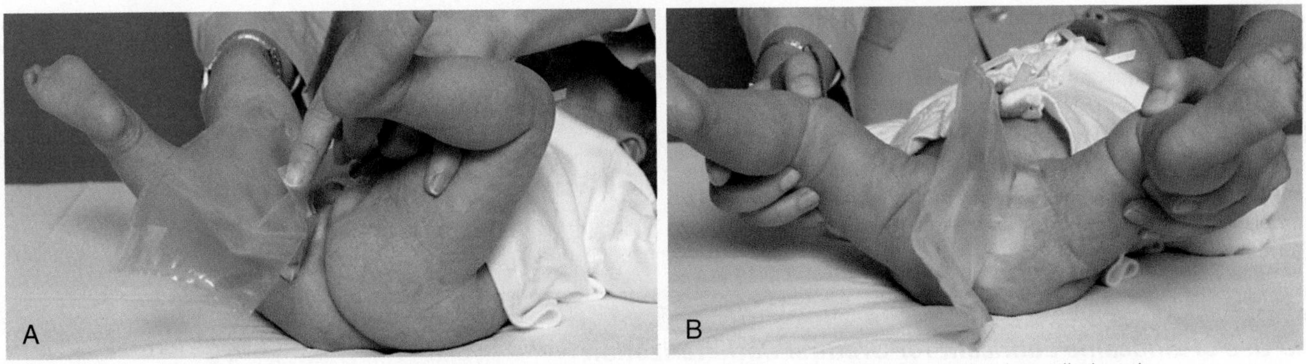

Fig. 20.8 Application of urine collection bag. **A,** On female infants, the adhesive portion is applied to the exposed and dried perineum first. **B,** The bag adheres firmly around the perineal area to prevent urine leakage.

Clean-Catch Specimens

Clean-catch specimen traditionally refers to a urine sample obtained for culture after the urethral meatus is cleaned and the first few milliliters of urine are voided (midstream specimen). In girls, the perineum is wiped with an antiseptic pad from front to back. In boys, the tip of the penis is cleansed. If the boy is uncircumcised, the foreskin is retracted and the glans is cleansed. It is important that the inside of the specimen cup or lid is not touched or contaminated during collection to ensure accurate results.

NURSING TIP When using a urine collection bag, cut a small slit in the diaper and pull the bag through to allow room for urine to collect and to facilitate checking on the contents.

Twenty-Four-Hour Collection

For a 24-hour collection, collection bags are required in infants and small children. Older children require special instruction about notifying someone when they need to void or have a bowel movement so that urine can be collected separately and is not discarded. Some older school-age children and adolescents can take responsibility for collection of their own 24-hour specimens and can keep output records and transfer each voiding to the 24-hour collection container.

The collection period always starts and ends with an empty bladder. At the time the collection begins, instruct the child to void and discard the specimen. All urine voided in the subsequent 24 hours is saved in a container with a preservative or is placed on ice. Twenty-four hours from the time the precollection specimen was discarded, the child is again instructed to void, the specimen is added to the container, and the entire collection is taken to the laboratory.

Infants and small children who are bagged for 24-hour urine collection require a special collection bag. Frequent removal and replacement of adhesive collection devices can produce skin irritation. A thin coating of sealant, such as Skin-Prep, applied to the skin helps protect it and aids adhesion (unless its use is contraindicated, such as in premature infants or children with irritated skin). Plastic collection bags with collection tubes attached are ideal when the container must be left in place for a time. These can be connected to a collecting device or emptied periodically by aspiration with a syringe. When such devices are not available, a regular bag with a feeding tube inserted through a puncture hole at the top of the bag serves as a satisfactory substitute. However, take care to empty the bag as soon as the infant urinates to prevent leakage and loss of contents. An indwelling catheter may also be placed for the collection period.

TABLE 20.4 Straight Catheter or Foley Catheter[a]

	Size (Length of Insertion [cm]) for Girls	Size (Length of Insertion [cm]) for Boys
Term neonate	5-6 (5)	5-6 (6)
Infant to 3 yr	5-8 (5)	5-8 (6)
4-8 yr	8 (5-6)	8 (6-9)
8 yr to prepubertal	10-12 (6-8)	8-10 (10-15)
Pubertal	12-14 (6-8)	12-14 (13-18)

[a]Foley catheters are approximately 1 Fr size larger because of the circumference of the balloon. Example: 10-Fr Foley catheter = approximately 12-Fr calibration.

Bladder Catheterization and Other Techniques

Bladder catheterization or suprapubic aspiration is used when a specimen is urgently needed or a child is unable to void or otherwise provide an adequate specimen. The American Academy of Pediatrics recommends that a urine specimen be obtained by bladder catheterization or suprapubic aspiration in ill-appearing febrile infants with no apparent source of infection before antimicrobial administration and to confirm a positive screen for infection (American Academy of Pediatrics, Subcommittee on Urinary Tract Infections, 2011).

Catheterization is a sterile procedure, and Standard Precautions for body substance protection should be followed. If the catheter is to remain in place, a Foley catheter is used. Table 20.4 gives guidelines for choosing the appropriate-size catheter and length of insertion. The supplies needed for this procedure include sterile gloves, sterile lubricant anesthetic, the appropriate-size catheter, povidone-iodine (Betadine) swabs or an alternative cleansing agent and 4- × 4-inch gauze squares, a sterile drape, and a syringe with sterile water if a Foley catheter is used. It may also be helpful to ensure that an extra catheter is readily available if needed. Many manufacturers no longer recommend testing the balloon of the Foley catheter by injecting sterile water before catheter insertion due to risk of weakening the balloon.

Adolescent boys and children with a history of urethral surgery may be catheterized with a curved, coudé-tipped catheter to assist with guiding the catheter past tight or partially blocked urethral openings. Children with myelodysplasia and those who have been identified as being sensitive or allergic to latex are catheterized with catheters manufactured from an alternative material. When an indwelling catheter is indicated for urinary drainage, a lubricious-coated or silicone catheter is selected because these materials produce less irritation of the urethral mucosa compared with Silastic or latex catheters when left in place for more than 72 hours.

A 2% lidocaine lubricant with applicator is assembled according to the manufacturer's instructions, and several drops of the lubricant are placed at the meatus. The child is advised that the lubricant is used to reduce any discomfort associated with inserting the catheter and that introduction of the catheter into the urethra will produce a sensation of pressure and a desire to urinate (Gray, 1996) (see Translating Evidence Into Practice box).

NURSING TIP: Although lidocaine lubricant may reduce discomfort during urinary catheterization, it is important for the nurse to weigh the benefit of analgesia against a prolonged procedure time. Lidocaine gel lubricant takes approximately 5 to 10 minutes for the anesthetic benefit to take effect. This increase in procedure length may significantly increase the anxiety of a young child. Thus the lidocaine lubricant may be more appropriate in the older child or adolescent age-groups.

TRANSLATING EVIDENCE INTO PRACTICE

The Use of Lidocaine Lubricant for Urethral Catheterization

Ask the Question

PICOT Question

In children, does a lidocaine lubricant decrease the pain associated with urethral catheterization?

Search for the Evidence

Search Strategies

Search selection criteria included English-language publications, research-based studies, and review articles on the use of the lidocaine lubricant before urethral catheterization.

Databases Used

Cochrane Collaboration, PubMed, MD Consult, BestBETs, American Academy of Pediatrics

Critically Analyze the Evidence

- Gray (1996) published a review of strategies to minimize distress associated with urethral catheterization in children and supported intraurethral instillation of a local anesthetic that contains 2% lidocaine before catheter insertion.
- One prospective, double-blind, placebo-controlled trial evaluated the use of lidocaine lubricant for discomfort in 20 children before urethral catheterization. Two doses of lidocaine lubricant instilled into the urethra 5 minutes apart significantly reduced pain and distress during urethral catheterization (Gerard, Cooper, Duethman, et al., 2003).
- Boots and Edmundson (2010) conducted a randomized controlled trial in 200 children in a follow-up to the study by Gerard and colleagues (2003). Conclusions were that a topical application of 2% lidocaine gel followed by urethral instillation of lidocaine gel is effective in reducing discomfort before urinary catheterization, and two urethral instillations offered no significant difference over a single instillation.
- Mularoni and colleagues (2009) found in a three-armed placebo-controlled, double-blind, randomized controlled trial of 43 children younger than 2 years of age that topical and intraurethral lidocaine lubricant was superior to the placebos of topical aqueous lubricant alone and topical and intraurethral aqueous lubricant in lowering distress, but it did not fully alleviate pain.
- A placebo-controlled, double-blind, randomized controlled trial of 115 children younger than 2 years of age found no significant difference when 2% lidocaine gel was compared with a nonanesthetic lubricant. The lubricant was applied to the genital mucosa for 2 to 3 minutes and liberally applied to the catheter but not instilled into the urethra (Vaughn, Paton, Bush, et al., 2005).
- A randomized controlled trial of 126 children ages 4 days to 23 months found a significant decrease in pain response in children who received topical and intraurethral 2% lidocaine gel compared with children who received a nonanesthetic lubricant (Castelo, Li, Taddio, et al., 2014).
- A randomized controlled trial of 133 children ages 0 to 24 months found no difference in pain response in children who received intraurethral 2% lidocaine gel lubricant compared with children who received a nonanesthetic lubricant during urethral catheterization. However, there was significantly increased pain response in children during instillation of the lidocaine lubricant compared with the nonanesthetic lubricant. In addition, there was no difference in parent satisfaction scores between the nonanesthetic lubricant and lidocaine lubricant (Poonai, Li, Langford, et al., 2015).

Apply the Evidence: Nursing Implications

There is moderate-quality evidence with strong recommendations (Guyatt, Oxman, Vist, et al., 2008) for using a lidocaine lubricant to decrease pain associated with urethral catheterization.

Four published research studies were found to support the use of anesthetic before urethral catheterization, one found topical application alone insufficient to reduce pain, and one found no difference in pain response between anesthetic and nonanesthetic application. Several publications support the effectiveness of lidocaine gel lubricant in clinical practice. Topical application followed by one or two transurethral instillations of 2% lidocaine gel before urethral catheterization minimizes distress and reduces pain before urinary catheterization.

Quality and Safety Competencies: Evidence-Based Practice[a]

Knowledge

Differentiate clinical opinion from research and evidence-based summaries.

Describe use of lidocaine gel for pain reduction during urethral catheterization.

Skills

Base individualized care plan on patient values, clinical expertise, and evidence.

Integrate evidence into practice by using lidocaine gel for pain reduction during urethral catheterization in children.

Attitudes

Value the concept of evidence-based practice as integral to determining best clinical practice.

Appreciate the strengths and weakness of evidence for using lidocaine gel for pain reduction during urethral catheterization in children.

References

Boots, B. K., & Edmundson, E. E. (2010). A controlled, randomised trial comparing single to multiple application lidocaine analgesia in paediatric patients undergoing urethral catheterisation procedures. *Journal of Clinical Nursing, 19*(5–6), 744–748.

Castelo, M., Li, J., Taddio, A., et al. (2014). A randomized controlled trial of 2% lidocaine gel compared to current standard of care in infants undergoing urinary catheterization. *Annals of Emergency Medicine, 64*(Suppl. 4), S105.

Gerard, L. L., Cooper, C. S., Duethman, K. S., et al. (2003). Effectiveness of lidocaine lubricant for discomfort during pediatric urethral catheterization. *Journal of Urology, 170*, 564–567.

Gray, M. (1996). Atraumatic urethral catheterization of children. *Pediatric Nursing, 22*(4), 306–310.

Guyatt, G. H., Oxman, A. D., Vist, G. E., et al. (2008). GRADE: An emerging consensus on rating quality of evidence and strength of recommendations. *British Medical Journal, 336*, 924–926.

Mularoni, P. P., Cohen, L. L., DeGuzman, M., et al. (2009). A randomized clinical trial of lidocaine gel for reducing infant distress during urethral catheterization. *Pediatric Emergency Care, 25*(7), 439–443.

Poonai, N., Li, J., Langford, C., et al. (2015). Intraurethral lidocaine for urethral catheterization in children: A randomized controlled trial. *Pediatrics, 136*(4), 880–886.

Vaughn, H., Paton, E. A., Bush, A., et al. (2005). Does lidocaine gel alleviate the pain of bladder catheterization in young children? a randomized, controlled trial. *Pediatrics, 116*(4), 917–920.

[a] Adapted from the Quality and Safety Education for Nurses (QSEN) website at http://www.qsen.org.

In male patients, grasp the penis with the nondominant hand and retract the foreskin. In uncircumcised newborns and infants, the foreskin may be adhered to the shaft; use care when retracting. If the penis is pendulous, place a sterile drape under the penis. Using the sterile hand, swab the glans and meatus three times with povidone-iodine beginning at the meatus and moving outward toward the edge of the glans. If appropriate to use lidocaine lubricant based on the child's age, developmental level, and preference, apply a small amount of lidocaine jelly to the tip of the penis over the urethra. Gently introduce the tip of the lidocaine jelly applicator into the urethra 1 to 2 cm (0.4 to 0.8 inch) so that the lubricant flows only into the urethra; insert 5 to 10 ml 2% lidocaine lubricant into the urethra and hold it in place for 2 to 5 minutes by gently squeezing the distal penis. Lubricate the catheter and insert it into the urethra while gently stretching the penis and lifting it to a 90-degree angle to the body. Resistance may occur when the catheter meets the urethral sphincter. Ask the patient to inhale deeply and advance the catheter. Do not force a catheter that does not easily enter the meatus, particularly if the child has had corrective surgery. For indwelling catheters, after urine is obtained, advance the catheter to the hub, inflate the balloon with sterile water, pull it back gently to test inflation, and connect it to the closed drainage system. Cleanse the glans and meatus and replace the retracted foreskin. If blood is seen at any time during the procedure, discontinue the procedure and notify the provider.

In female patients, place a sterile drape under the buttocks. Use the nondominant hand to gently separate and pull up the labia minora to visualize the meatus. Swab the meatus from front to back three times using a different povidone-iodine swab each time. If appropriate to use lidocaine lubricant based on the child's age, developmental level, and preference, place 1 to 2 ml 2% lidocaine lubricant on the periurethral mucosa and insert the lubricant 1 to 2 ml into the urethral meatus. Delay catheterization for 2 to 5 minutes to maximize absorption of the anesthetic into the periurethral and intraurethral mucosa. Add lubricant to the catheter and gently insert it into the urethra until urine returns; then advance the catheter an additional 2.5 to 5 cm (1 to 2 inches). When using an indwelling Foley catheter, inflate the balloon with sterile water and gently pull back; then connect to a closed drainage system. Cleanse the meatus and labia (see Cultural Considerations box). Because the use of lidocaine jelly can increase the volume of intraurethral lubricant, urine return may not be as rapid as when minimal lubrication is used. For both male and female patients, apply a securement device from the catheter tubing to the patient's thigh to avoid kinks and painful pulling on the catheter. Ensure that the patient can move his or her thigh without pulling on the catheter tubing.

! NURSING ALERT

Do not advance the catheter too far into the bladder to prevent knotting of catheters and tubes within the bladder. Feeding tubes should not be used for urinary catheterization because they are more flexible, longer, and prone to knotting compared with commercially designed urinary catheters.

CULTURAL CONSIDERATIONS

Bladder Catheterization

Parents may be upset when their child is catheterized. Aside from the trauma the child experiences, some parents may fear that the procedure affects their daughter's virginity. To correct this misconception, the family may benefit from a detailed explanation of the genitourinary anatomy, preferably with a model that shows the separate vaginal and urethral openings. The nurse can also indicate that catheterization has no effect on virginity.

Suprapubic aspiration is used mainly when the bladder cannot be accessed through the urethra (e.g., with some congenital urologic birth defects, severe phimosis, or labial adhesions) or to reduce the risk of contamination that may be present when passing a catheter. With the advent of small catheters (5- and 6-Fr straight catheters), the need for suprapubic aspiration has decreased. Access to the bladder via the urethra has a much higher success rate than suprapubic aspiration, in which success depends on the practitioner's skill at assessing the location of the bladder and the amount of urine in the bladder. However, suprapubic aspiration remains a more accurate specimen collection method for urine cultures and should be considered for infants who have unsatisfactory urine collection or inconclusive results (Eliacik, Kanik, Yavascan, et al., 2016).

Suprapubic aspiration involves aspirating bladder contents by inserting a 20- or 21-gauge needle in the midline approximately 1 cm (0.4 inch) above the symphysis pubis and directed vertically downward. The nurse prepares the skin as for any needle insertion, and the bladder should contain an adequate volume of urine. This can be assumed if the infant has not voided for at least 1 hour or the bladder can be palpated above the symphysis pubis or verified via ultrasound. This technique is useful for obtaining sterile specimens from young infants because the bladder is an abdominal organ and is easily accessed. Suprapubic aspiration is painful; therefore pain management during the procedure is important (see Atraumatic Care box).

ATRAUMATIC CARE

Bladder Catheterization or Suprapubic Aspiration

- Use distraction to help the child relax (e.g., blowing bubbles, deep breathing, singing a song).
- Use lidocaine jelly to anesthetize the area before insertion of the catheter. EMLA cream (a eutectic mixture of lidocaine and prilocaine) or LMX cream (lidocaine) may lessen an infant's discomfort as the needle passes through the skin for suprapubic aspiration, but care should be taken that the site is thoroughly cleaned and prepped before the procedure.
- Children often become agitated at being restrained for either procedure. Use comfort measures through touch and voice, both during and after the procedure, to help reduce the child's distress.

STOOL SPECIMENS

Stool specimens are frequently collected from children to identify parasites and other organisms that cause diarrhea, assess gastrointestinal function, and check for occult (hidden) blood. Ideally, stool should be collected without contamination with urine, but in children wearing diapers, this is difficult unless a urine bag is applied. Children who are toilet trained should urinate first, flush the toilet, and then defecate into a bedpan (preferably one that is placed on the toilet to avoid embarrassment) or a commercial potty hat over the toilet. Stool specimens should never be contaminated with toilet water to avoid inaccurate results.

Stool specimens should be large enough to obtain an ample sampling, not merely a fecal fragment. Specimens are placed in an appropriate container, which is covered and labeled. If several specimens are needed, mark the containers with the date and time and keep them in a specimen refrigerator. Exercise care in handling the specimen because of the risk of contamination. If a stool specimen cannot be obtained, some laboratory tests may allow for internal rectal swab.

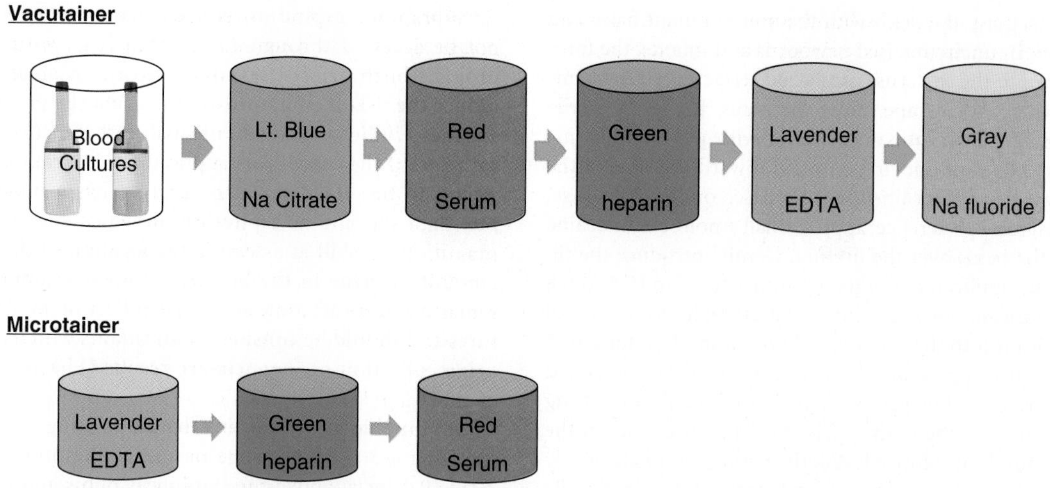

Fig. 20.9 Order of draw for blood collection by vacutainer and microtainer. *EDTA*, Ethylenediaminetetraacetic acid; *Na*, sodium. (Courtesy Cook Children's Medical Center Laboratory.)

> **NURSING TIP:** To obtain a stool specimen, use a tongue depressor or disposable spoon or knife to collect the stool.

BLOOD SPECIMENS

Whether the specimen is collected by the nurse or by others, the nurse is responsible for making certain that specimens, such as serial examinations and fasting specimens, are collected on time and that the proper equipment is available. Collecting, transporting, and storing specimens can have a major impact on laboratory results. For accurate results, blood must be collected in the proper tube for the test. When preparing for blood specimen collection, the nurse should consult the institution's laboratory reference guide to determine appropriate tubes for specimen collection, as well as the volume of blood required for the test, and any special instructions, such as "transport on ice" or "protect from light." Inadequate sample size will result in rejected specimens and may require repeat venipuncture in order to obtain accurate samples, causing additional discomfort for the patient. When multiple blood tests are ordered for a patient and there is concern about the total volume of blood that may be needed, the nurse should be aware that the World Health Organization advises that the maximum volume of blood collected over any 24-hour period should not exceed 3 ml/kg (Clinical Laboratory Standards Institute, 2017; Howie, 2011). When collecting multiple samples via vacutainer system, the order of sample collection also has an impact on test results because the additive from one tube may inadvertently be transferred to subsequent tubes, affecting sample integrity (Clinical Laboratory Standards Institute, 2017). See Fig. 20.9 for proper order of collection. The order of collection is different if collecting blood in capillary tubes or microtainers. Venous blood samples can be obtained by venipuncture or by aspiration from a peripheral or central access device (see Research Focus box). Evidence for best practice supports use of direct venipuncture as the preferred method for venous blood collection because it minimizes risk for hemolysis of the specimen (McCaughey, Vecellio, Lake, et al., 2017). However, when venous access is difficult or repeated specimens are necessary, sampling blood from an indwelling catheter may be warranted. Benefits of sampling blood from an indwelling catheter include decreased anxiety, discomfort, and dissatisfaction associated with venipuncture samples (Infusion Nurses Society, 2016). Withdrawing blood specimens through peripheral lock devices in small peripheral veins has varying degrees of success. Factors influencing successful blood draw through an existing peripheral intravenous (PIV) line include gauge of catheter, location of the PIV catheter, and size of syringe used to obtain the waste sample (Braniff, DeCarlo, Haskamp, & Broome, 2014). When using an IV infusion site for specimen collection, pause the infusion before collecting the blood sample, because the type of fluid being infused may affect test results. For example, a specimen collected for glucose determination would be inaccurate if removed from a catheter through which glucose-containing solution was infusing. Before obtaining laboratory specimens from a PIV catheter, 1 to 2 ml of blood must be withdrawn from the catheter to clear any saline, heparin, or IV fluids from the tubing. Blood cultures should not be obtained through an existing PIV.

RESEARCH FOCUS

Obtaining Blood Samples From Existing Peripheral Intravenous Catheters

Blood specimens collected from existing peripheral intravenous (PIV) catheters in pediatric patients were reviewed for rejected samples. Out of 150 specimens reviewed, successful sample collection occurred in 91.3%. Whether the catheter was heplocked or had fluids infusing did not contribute to sample contamination. There was a low rate of unacceptable specimens (clotted, hemolyzed, insufficient quantity). Only 1.3% of the PIVs were nonfunctional after being used for specimen collection (Braniff et al., 2014).

Central venous catheters can be used to withdraw blood specimens; however, risks include catheter occlusion and catheter-associated bloodstream infection. When collecting blood specimens from a central venous catheter, a small volume of blood must first be withdrawn and discarded to clear the line of any IV fluids, heparin, or other fluids that might erroneously affect test results. The Infusion Nurses Society (2016) recommends withdrawing and discarding 3 ml from the central venous access device (CVAD). Limited research supports using the initial volume obtained as a blood culture specimen (see Research Focus box). The Infusion Nurses Society (2016) recommends not reinfusing the blood obtained as discard sample, due to risk of contamination and clot formation. Some facilities allow reinfusion of the blood initially withdrawn from the CVAD, especially when blood conservation is essential. Another technique that conserves blood is the push-pull method in which blood is withdrawn into a syringe and reinfused into the CVAD three times. A new sterile syringe is then attached, and the specimen is withdrawn; no blood is discarded (Hess & Decker, 2017). If drawing blood from a multilumen central line, ensure that all lumens are clamped, except for the lumen being used to draw blood.

RESEARCH FOCUS

Central Venous Access Device

In 62 pediatric oncology emergency room patients, the initial 5 ml of blood drawn from a central venous access device (CVAD) was used to inoculate blood culture bottles instead of the usual practice of discarding the first 5 ml of blood. A second specimen was obtained (as per standard of care) and used to inoculate separate blood culture bottles. In the 186 paired blood cultures, 4.8% were positive. In all positive cultures, both specimens contained the same organism. In four pairs, the first specimen that is usually discarded grew organisms earlier than the standard of care specimen, allowing for earlier administration of definitive antibiotic. The results of this study could lead to a change in practice, allowing the first 5 to 10 ml of blood obtained from CVADs to be used for blood cultures, rather than discarding this initial sample (Winokur, Pai, Rutledge, et al., 2014).

When venipuncture is performed, the needed specimens are quickly collected, and after the needle is withdrawn, pressure is applied to the puncture site with dry gauze until bleeding stops (see Atraumatic Care box). When the venipuncture site is in the antecubital fossa, pressure should be applied with the arm extended, not flexed, to reduce bruising. The nurse then covers the site with an adhesive bandage. In young children, adhesive bandages pose an aspiration hazard, so avoid using them or remove the adhesive bandage as soon as the bleeding stops. If bruising or hematoma develops after venipuncture, applying warm compresses to the ecchymotic area increases circulation, helps remove extravasated blood, and decreases pain.

Arterial blood samples are sometimes needed for blood gas measurement, although noninvasive techniques such as transcutaneous oxygen monitoring and pulse oximetry are used frequently. Arterial samples may be obtained by arterial puncture using the radial, brachial, or femoral arteries or from indwelling arterial catheters. Assess adequate circulation before arterial puncture by observing capillary refill or performing the **Allen test**, a procedure that assesses the circulation of the radial, ulnar, or brachial arteries. When collecting a blood sample from an established arterial line, use the in-line sampling port and follow institutional policy. Because unclotted blood is required,

ATRAUMATIC CARE

Guidelines for Skin and Vessel Punctures

To reduce the pain associated with heel, finger, venous, or arterial punctures:

- Apply a lidocaine-based topical cream to the site, if time permits: lidocaine-prilocaine (EMLA) cream should be applied at least 60 minutes prior to venipuncture; lidocaine 4% cream (LMX) requires a 30-minute application time. A dollop of cream is applied to the skin and then covered by a transparent dressing for the application time. To remove the transparent dressing atraumatically, grasp opposite sides of the film and pull the sides away from each other to stretch and loosen the film. After the film begins to loosen, grasp the other two sides of the film and pull. As an alternative, the cream can be covered by a 3- to 4-inch piece of kitchen plastic wrap.
- When unable to wait 30 to 60 minutes for EMLA or LMX products to work, a vapocoolant spray or buffered lidocaine (injected intradermally near the vein with a 30-gauge needle) can be used to numb the skin. Buffered lidocaine can also be administered using a J-tip needleless injection system (Stoltz & Manworren, 2017).
- Use nonpharmacologic methods of pain and anxiety control (e.g., ask the child to take a deep breath when the needle is inserted and again when the needle is withdrawn, to exhale a large breath or blow bubbles to "blow hurt away," or to count slowly and then faster and louder if pain is felt).
- Keep all equipment out of sight until used.
- Enlist parental presence or assistance if they wish.
- Restrain child *only as needed* to perform the procedure safely; use comfort positioning.
- Allow the skin preparation to dry completely before penetrating the skin.
- Use the smallest gauge needle (e.g., 23 to 25 gauge) that permits free flow of blood; for neonates and infants, a 27-gauge needle may be sufficient for obtaining 1 to 1.5 ml of blood and for prominent veins (needle length is only 1.25 cm [0.5 inch]).
- If possible, avoid putting an IV catheter in the dominant hand or the hand the child uses to suck the thumb.
- Use an automatic lancet device for precise puncture depth of the finger or heel; press the device lightly against the skin; avoid steadying the finger against a hard surface.
- Have a "two-try-only" policy to reduce excessive insertion attempts—two operators each have two insertion attempts. If insertion is not successful after four punctures, consider alternative venous access, such as a PICC.
- Have a policy for proactively identifying children with difficult access and appropriate interventions (e.g., most experienced operator for the first attempt, use transilluminator or ultrasonography for insertion guidance).

For Multiple Blood Samples

- Use an intermittent infusion device (saline lock) to collect additional samples from an existing IV line.
- Consider PICC lines early, not as a last resort.
- Coordinate care to allow several tests to be performed on one blood sample; use micromethods of collection whenever possible.
- Anticipate tests (e.g., drug levels, chemistry, immunoglobulin levels) and ask the laboratory to save blood for additional testing.
- Maximum blood collection volumes for any 24-hour period should not exceed 3 ml/kg; limits should be lower for children who are acutely or chronically ill (Clinical Laboratory Standards Institute, 2017; Howie, 2011)

For Heel Lancing in Newborns

- Heelsticks have been shown to be more painful than venipuncture (Shah & Ohlsson, 2011).
- Kangaroo care (placing the diapered newborn against the parent's bare chest in skin-to-skin contact) 10 to 15 minutes before and during heel lance reduces pain. (Gao, Xu, Gao, et al., 2015; Johnston, Campbell-Yeo, Disher, et al., 2017)
- Breastfeeding during a neonatal heel lance is effective in reducing pain and has been found to be more effective than sucrose in some studies (Benoit, Martin-Misener, Latimer, et al., 2017). If breast milk is unavailable, administer sucrose and encourage the newborn to suck a pacifier (Stevens, Yamada, Ohlsson, et al., 2016). When commercially manufactured 24% sucrose solution is unavailable, add 1 teaspoon of table sugar to 4 teaspoons of sterile water. Use this solution to coat the pacifier or administer 2 ml to the tongue 2 minutes before the procedure.
- Although safe for use in preterm infants when applied correctly, EMLA has been found to be no more effective than placebo in preventing pain during heel lancing (Anand & Hall, 2006).

EMLA, Eutectic mixture of local anesthetics; *IV,* intravenous; *LMX,* lidocaine; *PICC,* peripherally inserted central catheter.

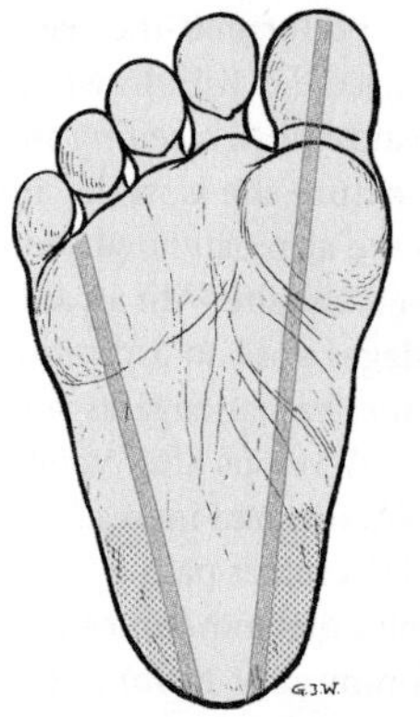

Fig. 20.10 Puncture site *(colored stippled area)* on the sole of an infant's foot.

use only heparinized collection tubes or syringes for arterial blood samples. In addition, no air bubbles should enter the collection tube or syringe because they can alter blood gas concentration. Crying, fear, and agitation affect blood gas values; therefore make every effort to comfort the child. Pack arterial blood samples in ice to reduce blood cell metabolism and transport to the laboratory immediately.

Take capillary blood samples from children by fingerstick or heelstick. When using a finger for capillary blood collection, use the second or third finger. Cleanse the area with alcohol or chlorhexidine and allow to dry. After performing the fingerstick, wipe once with dry gauze before beginning collection. Gently massage the entire finger to maintain blood flow. Avoid squeezing just the tip of the finger. Hold the fingerstick site facing downward to facilitate blood collection. A common method for taking peripheral blood samples from infants younger than 6 months old is by heelstick. Before the blood sample is taken, warm the heel for 3 minutes, then cleanse the area with alcohol or chlorhexidine. Holding the infant's foot firmly with the free hand, the nurse then punctures the heel with an automatic lancet device. An automatic device delivers a more precise puncture depth and is less painful than using a lance (Sorrentino, Fumagalli, Milani, et al., 2017). Several studies demonstrate that the automatic lancet is safer and has been shown to require fewer heel punctures, less collection time, and lower recollection rates. Sorrentino and colleagues (2017) reported that certain automated devices were more effective and that a surgical blade of any kind is contraindicated when obtaining blood by heelstick. Although obtaining capillary venous blood gases is a common practice, these measures may not accurately reflect arterial values.

The most serious complications of infant heel puncture are necrotizing osteochondritis from lancet penetration of the underlying calcaneus bone, resulting in infection and abscess of the heel. To avoid osteochondritis, the puncture should be no deeper than 2 mm and should be made at the outer aspect of the heel. The boundaries of the calcaneus can be marked by an imaginary line extending posteriorly from a point between the fourth and fifth toes and running parallel with the lateral aspect of the heel and another line extending posteriorly from the middle of the great toe and running parallel with the medial aspect of the heel (Fig. 20.10). Repeated trauma to the walking surface of the heel can cause fibrosis and scarring that may interfere with locomotion.

Children do not like the discomfort associated with venous, arterial, and capillary punctures. Children have identified these procedures as the most frequent causes of pain during hospitalization. Arterial puncture was identified as one of the most painful of all procedures experienced. Toddlers are most distressed by venipuncture, followed by school-age children and then adolescents. Consequently, nurses should use developmentally appropriate language when preparing a child for venipuncture (see Table 20.1 and Applying Evidence to Practice: Age-Specific Preparation of Children for Procedures Based on Developmental Characteristics) and use developmentally appropriate pain reduction techniques to lessen the discomfort of these procedures. (See Chapter 5, Pain Management.)

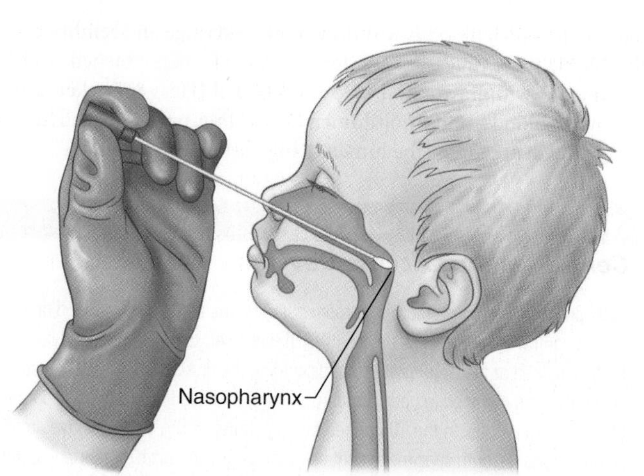

Fig. 20.11 Technique for collecting a nasopharyngeal swab. (From "Standard method for detecting upper respiratory carriage of *Streptococcus pneumonia:* Updated recommendations from the World Health Organization Pneumococcal Carriage Working Group," by C. Satzke, P. Turner, A. Virolainen-Julkunen, P. V. Adrian, M. Antonio, K. M. Hare . . . K. L. O'Brien, 2013, *Vaccine, 32*(1), p. 168. Copyright 2013 by Elsevier Ltd. Reprinted with permission.)

RESPIRATORY SECRETION SPECIMENS

Upper respiratory tract infections are common in children, and about 80% of these infections are due to viruses. Laboratory detection of important viruses such as influenza and respiratory syncytial virus (RSV) can be diagnosed from epithelial cells of the nasopharynx. These respiratory specimens are usually collected by nasopharyngeal swab or nasal wash. The choice of collection method depends on laboratory specifications. The nurse is responsible for confirming which collection method is preferred for the test ordered.

For collection by nasopharyngeal swab, ensure that the appropriate swab is used, as specified in the laboratory manual. The swab should be flocked or rayon. Use only swabs with plastic shafts. Do not use cotton swabs or swabs with wooden shafts, as these will result in inadequate specimen. After gathering the necessary supplies, the nurse should don mask and gloves. If the child has a lot of nasal secretions, have him or her blow the nose prior to the procedure (remember that the nurse is collecting epithelial cells and not nasal discharge). The child should be placed in a sitting position. For younger children or children who may have difficulty holding still, a comfort hold by a second caregiver is strongly recommended to avoid injury. With the child in position, tilt the head up slightly, then gently insert the swab into the nose, aiming toward the ear, parallel to the palate, until it reaches the posterior nares (half the distance from the nostril to the opening of the ear) (Fig. 20.11). Gently rotate the swab for 10 to 15 seconds while withdrawing it from the nose. Be aware that the child may sneeze or cough during this procedure. Once the swab is removed, immediately place it in the transport media tube, then snap off the top part of the plastic shaft so that the cap can be closed securely on the transport tube. Specimens for *Bordetella pertussis* are also collected in this manner, but they must be placed in a different transport media.

For collection by nasal wash, gather supplies and don mask and gloves, then place the child supine, with an additional caregiver providing a comfort hold if needed. Using a sterile syringe without a needle, instill 1 to 3 ml of sterile normal saline into one nostril. Then aspirate the contents using a small, sterile bulb syringe and place them in a sterile container. As an alternate method, use a syringe with 5 cm (2 inches) of 18- to 20-gauge tubing attached. Gently insert the tubing into the nostril, then quickly instill the saline and promptly aspirate while withdrawing the tubing to recover the nasal specimen. To prevent any additional discomfort, all equipment should be ready before beginning the procedure.

Specimens from the oropharynx are collected for diagnosis of streptococcal throat infections, *Bordetella*, and other pathogens. With the child in a sitting position and using the appropriate swab, the nurse should swab both tonsils and the posterior pharynx when obtaining a throat culture. Ideally, the swab should not touch the tongue, teeth, or gums. The swab stick should then be inserted into the culture tube, taking care that the swab does not come in contact with the outside of the container or the hands of the nurse collecting the sample. Some culture kits require squeezing an ampule within the transport tube to release the culture medium. Viral testing usually requires that the specimen be place in a container with special transport medium and be kept on ice. The nurse should ensure that the correct container is on hand before obtaining the specimen.

Infections of the lower respiratory tract, such as pneumonia or tuberculosis, may require sputum collection. Because the infectious organisms are in the lungs and lower airways, the sputum specimen must be produced by deep cough, not just spitting oral secretions into a container. Older children and adolescents can cough as directed and supply sputum specimens when given proper directions. The nurse must make it clear to the patient that a coughed specimen is needed, not merely mucus cleared from the throat. It is helpful to demonstrate a deep cough. Infants and small children are unable to follow directions to cough on command, and often swallow any sputum produced; therefore gastric washings (lavage) may be used to collect a sputum specimen. Gastric washing specimens should be collected in early morning for best results. Sometimes a satisfactory specimen can be obtained using a suction device, such as a mucus trap, if the catheter is inserted into the trachea and the cough reflex is elicited. A catheter inserted into the back of the throat is not sufficient. For children with a tracheostomy, a specimen is easily aspirated from the trachea or major bronchi by attaching a collecting device to the suction apparatus. Sputum collection from a young child can be uncomfortable, so the nurse should be sure to provide developmentally appropriate comfort measures.

ADMINISTRATION OF MEDICATION

DETERMINATION OF DRUG DOSAGE

Nurses must understand the safe dosages of medications that they administer to children, as well as the expected actions, possible side effects, and signs of toxicity. Unlike the standardized doses for adult medications, dosing for pediatric medications is usually presented as a recommended dosage range based on the age, weight, and/or body surface area (BSA) of the child. Differences between adult and pediatric dosing of medications are related to physiologic differences. Factors related to growth and maturation significantly alter an individual's capacity to metabolize and excrete drugs. Immaturity or defects in any of the important processes of absorption, distribution, biotransformation, or excretion can significantly alter the pharmacodynamics of a drug, resulting in increased toxicity or inadequate effect. Newborn and premature infants are particularly vulnerable to the harmful effects of drugs because they have immature enzyme systems in the liver (where most drugs are broken down and detoxified), lower concentrations of plasma proteins (necessary for binding with drugs), and immature functioning of kidneys (where most drugs are excreted). Beyond the newborn period, children metabolize many drugs more rapidly than adults. Consequently, children may require larger doses (per weight) than adults and/or more frequent administration to achieve a therapeutic effect. This is particularly important in pain control, when the dosage of analgesics may need to be increased or the interval between doses decreased to obtain a therapeutic effect.

Nurses are accountable for the medications that they administer. An important part of that responsibility is having a working knowledge of drug actions and potential side effects. In addition, nurses should know the safe dose ranges for the drugs with which they work. Before giving any medication, the pediatric nurse must be vigilant to verify that the drug has been dispensed in a dose that is within the recommended range for the child. Pediatric dosages are most often expressed in units of measure per body weight (mg/kg). Some medications, such as chemotherapy, are more precisely dosed using BSA (expressed as mg/m^2), which historically is believed to be a more accurate reflection of metabolic rate and less affected by adipose tissue than weight-based calculations. The ratio of BSA to weight varies inversely with length; therefore an infant who is shorter and weighs less than an older child or adult has relatively more BSA than would be expected from the weight. BSA can be determined using the **West nomogram** or the commonly used Mosteller formula: BSA = the square root of [height (cm) × weight (kg)] divided by 3600. Conversion programs are widely available on the Internet.

Checking Dosage

Administering the correct dosage of a drug is a shared responsibility between the provider who orders the drug and the nurse who carries out that order. Children react with unexpected severity to some drugs, and ill children may be especially sensitive to drugs. When a dose that is outside the usual range is ordered or when there is some question regarding the preparation or the route of administration, the nurse should check with the prescribing provider before proceeding with the administration, because the nurse is legally liable for any drug administered.

Even when given at the correct dosage, many drugs are potentially hazardous or lethal. For this reason, the Institute for Safe Medication Practices has identified a list of "high-alert" medications (see https://www.ismp.org/recommendations/high-alert-medications-acute-list). Most facilities have regulations requiring that these "high-alert" medications be double-checked by another nurse before giving them to the child. Among drugs that require such additional safeguards to reduce risk of error and minimize harm are antiarrhythmics, anticoagulants, chemotherapeutic agents, and insulin. Other high-alert medications include epinephrine, opioids, and sedation agents (Institute for Safe Medication Practices, 2018; Maaskant, Eskes, van Rijn-Bikker, et al., 2013). A misplaced decimal point could result in a 10-fold or greater dosing error. So even if this precaution is not mandatory, nurses are wise to incorporate this safe practice and take the additional time to independently check and recheck drug dose calculations.

Another category of high-alert medications is the "look-alike, sound-alike" drugs that have similar names but significantly different doses and side effects. To emphasize these differences, Tall Man lettering is recommended by the Institute for Safe Medication Practices and the US Food and Drug Administration (Institute for Safe Medication

Practices, 2016). Examples of Tall Man lettering include DOBUTamine and DOPamine, and predniSONE and prednisoLONE.

Identification

Before the administration of any medication, the child must be correctly identified using two identifiers (e.g., name and medical record number or birth date). With an infant, young child, or nonverbal child, the parent or guardian (if present) can verify the child's identity. After verbal verification of the child's identity (by the parent, guardian, or child), the identification band should be verified using two identifiers. Bedside computers and handheld barcode scanners can be used to verify the identification bracelet directly with the patient's electronic record.

Preparing the Parents

Nearly all parents have given some type of medication to their child and can describe the approaches that they have found successful. In some cases, it is less traumatic for the hospitalized child if a parent gives the medication, provided that the nurse prepares the medication and supervises its administration. Children who take daily medications at home are accustomed to the parent functioning in this capacity and may be less likely to fuss than if a stranger administers the medication. Individual decisions need to be made regarding parental presence and participation in other procedures, such as holding the child during injections.

Preparing the Child

Every child requires developmentally appropriate preparation for parenteral administration of medication and supportive care during the procedure (see discussion earlier in the chapter). Even if the child has received previous injections, rarely does a child become accustomed to the discomfort. With every dose of medication, the nurse should be cognizant of the developmental needs of the child, whether it is the first dose or the 200th dose for that child.

ORAL ADMINISTRATION

The oral route is preferred for giving medications to children because of the ease of administration. Oral medications are available in various dosing formulations, including tablets, capsules, chewable tablets, orally dissolving tablets, sprinkles, and oral liquids. Although some children can swallow or chew solid medications at an early age, solid preparations are not recommended for young children because of the danger of aspiration. Determining when a child is old enough to swallow pills depends on the developmental age of the child, the size of the pill, and the child's past experiences with medications. The nurse should ensure that the formulation of any prescribed medication will be appropriate for the child, based on developmental level, swallowing ability, and available formulations of the medication.

Many pediatric medications come in liquid preparations for added ease of administration. Some of these liquids have a slightly unpleasant aftertaste. The taste can be camouflaged when necessary, by mixing the medication with a small amount of juice or applesauce. In the hospital, pharmacies can provide flavored syrup, known as Syrpalta, for this purpose (see Atraumatic Care box).

Preparation

The most accurate means for measuring small amounts of medication is the plastic disposable calibrated oral syringe (Centers for Disease Control and Prevention, 2017; Paul & Yin, 2012; US Food and Drug Administration, 2011). Not only does the syringe provide a reliable measure, but it also serves as a convenient means for transporting and administering the medication. The medication can be placed directly into the child's mouth from the syringe.

Paper cups are totally unsuitable for liquid medications because they collapse easily, are likely to have irregularly shaped or crumpled bottoms, and retain considerable amounts of thick medication. Molded plastic cups with measuring lines are often supplied with over-the-counter medications for cough and fever, but most families in one study could not accurately measure a 5-ml dose within 0.5 ml (Ryu & Lee, 2012; Yin, Parker, Sanders, et al., 2016). Quantities less than 5 ml are impossible to determine accurately with a medicine cup.

The household teaspoon is also an inaccurate measuring device and is subject to error. Household teaspoons vary greatly in capacity, and different persons using the same spoon will pour different amounts, resulting in potentially dangerous dosing errors (Beckett, Tyson, Carroll, et al., 2012; Torres, Parker, Sanders, et al., 2017).

Because of the risk of inaccurate dosing when using medicine cups and teaspoons, a policy statement issued by the American Academy of Pediatrics recommends that all liquid oral medications, over-the-counter and prescription, should be dosed only in milliliters and never in teaspoons or other nonmetric units (American Academy of Pediatrics, Committee on Drugs, 2015). Syringes are the preferred device for dosing accuracy. Measuring cups with metric markings may be used as an alternative. A convenient hollow-handled medicine spoon with calibrations is available to accurately measure and administer the drug. Household spoons, including measuring spoons, should be avoided.

Another unreliable device for measuring liquids is the dropper, which varies to a greater extent than the teaspoon or measuring cup. The volume of a drop varies according to the viscosity (thickness) of

ATRAUMATIC CARE

Encouraging a Child's Acceptance of Oral Medication

- Give the child a flavored ice pop or small ice cube to suck to numb the tongue before giving the drug.
- Mix the drug with a small amount (about 5 ml) of sweet-tasting substance, such as flavored syrups, jam, fruit purees, sherbet, or applesauce; avoid essential food items because the child may later refuse to eat them.
- Wrap bad-tasting pills (i.e., corticosteroids) in a small piece of fruit-flavored candy roll-up.
- Give a "chaser" of water, juice, or child's drink of choice, or ice pop or frozen juice bar after the drug.
- Avoid dairy products with medication administration due to risk of interfering with absorption
- If nausea is a problem, give a carbonated beverage poured over finely crushed ice before or immediately after the medication.
- When medication has an unpleasant taste, have the child pinch the nose and drink the medicine through a straw. Much of what we taste is associated with smell.
- Commercially available flavorings, such as apple, banana, and bubble gum can be added at many local pharmacies for a nominal additional cost. As an alternative, some pharmacies may be able to prepare the drug in a flavored, chewable troche or lozenge. Infants will suck medicine from a needleless syringe or dropper in small increments (0.25 to 0.5 ml) at a time.
- Use a nipple or a special pacifier with a reservoir for the drug.
- Avoid adding a medication to an infant's regular bottle, as the infant may not drink the entire bottle within a time frame appropriate for one dose of medication.

the liquid measured (Bauters, Claus, Willems, et al., 2012). Viscous fluids produce much larger drops than thin liquids. The Institute for Safe Medication Practices (2017) recommends only using droppers that display a metric scale and describe the medication dose in milliliters, not in drops. In addition, the Institute for Safe Medication Practices recommends using an oral syringe to administer the dose, for better accuracy.

Young children and some older children have difficulty swallowing tablets or pills. For these children, if a liquid formulation is not available, tablets may need to be crushed. Commercial devices for crushing pills are available. Simple methods can also be used, such as crushing a pill between two spoons or placing the pill in a plastic sandwich bag and then crushing it with a spoon. Certain pills may easily be dissolved in a small amount of warm water. Crushed tablets can be mixed with applesauce or a small amount of juice for ease of administration. Some drugs, such as medication with an enteric or protective coating or formulated for slow release, should not be crushed because crushing will alter the amount of drug that is absorbed. In some cases, this might result in overdose of medication. The Institute for Safe Medication Practices maintains a list of oral medications that should not be crushed (http://www.ismp.org/tools/DoNotCrush.pdf). In addition, some drugs may be hazardous if the powder becomes aerosolized while being crushed. These drugs should be prepared in a pharmacy, or the pharmacist or drug label should be consulted for recommendations.

When a child needs to take solid oral medication for an extended period, the nurse can teach the child how to swallow tablets or capsules. Training sessions include verbal instruction, demonstration, reinforcement for swallowing progressively larger candy or capsules, no attention for inappropriate behavior, and gradual withdrawal of guidance after children can swallow their medication. Helpful tips for patients of all ages can be found at http://www.pillswallowing.com.

In some situations, pediatric doses may require splitting pills or tablets. The nurse should be vigilant to ensure that the divided dose is accurate. With tablets, only those that are scored can be halved or quartered accurately. If the medication is soluble, the tablet or contents of a capsule can be mixed in a small premeasured amount of liquid and the appropriate portion given (Valizadeh, Rasekhi, Hamishehkar, et al., 2015). For example, if half a dose is required, the tablet is dissolved in 5 ml of water, and 2.5 ml is given.

Administration

Although administering liquids to infants is relatively easy, the nurse must take care to prevent aspiration. While holding the infant in a semireclining position, place the medication in the mouth using an oral syringe. It is best to place the syringe along the side of the infant's tongue and administer the liquid slowly in small amounts, waiting for the child to swallow between increments.

> **NURSING TIP** In infants up to 11 months old and children with neurologic impairments, blowing a small puff of air in the face frequently elicits a swallow reflex.

Allowing the infant to suck the medication that has been placed in an empty nipple or, for breastfeeding infants, inserting the syringe into the side of the mouth, parallel to the nipple, while the infant nurses are other convenient methods for giving liquid medications to infants. Medication is not added to the infant's formula feeding because the child may subsequently refuse the formula. Dispose of any plastic covers that may be on the ends of syringes because these covers are choking hazards.

Children are more likely to take their oral medication willingly if they feel involved in the process (as opposed to being forced). Giving choices to a child helps them feel involved. Although taking the medicine is not a choice, the child can be offered other options such as whether they want to take the medicine before or after a specific activity, what they would like to drink with their medicine, or if they want to help give the medicine. Allowing a child to push the plunger of the syringe of oral medication while the caregiver holds the syringe in the mouth may improve adherence.

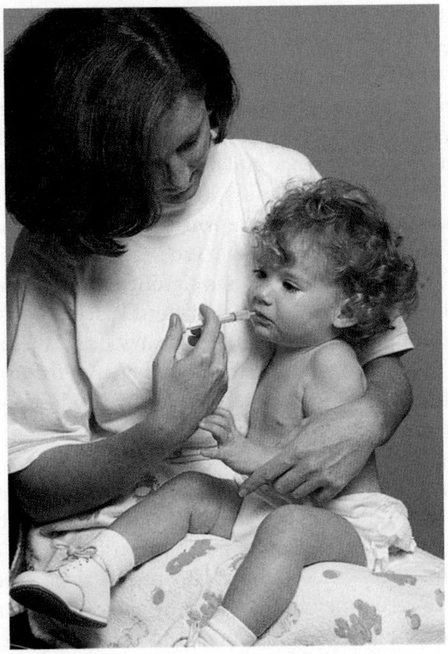

Fig. 20.12 A nurse partially restrains a child for easy and comfortable administration of oral medication.

When giving oral liquids from a syringe, it is often helpful to give the dose in several small increments and allow the child to swallow between squirts. Place the tip of the syringe into the pocket formed between the lower teeth and cheek. Aiming at the back of the throat increases the risk of aspiration. Children who refuse to cooperate or who resist consistently despite explanation and encouragement may require physical holding. If holding is necessary, it should be done in a position of comfort, sitting up or semireclining. Make every effort to reassure the child that holding is for his or her well-being and is not a form of punishment. There is always a risk in using even mild forceful techniques. A crying child can aspirate a medication, particularly when lying on the back. If the nurse holds the child in the lap with the child's right arm behind the nurse, the left hand firmly grasped by the nurse's left hand, and the head securely cradled between the nurse's arm and body, the medication can be slowly administered into the mouth (Fig. 20.12).

Because of the natural outward tongue thrust in infancy, medications may need to be retrieved from the lips or chin and refed. If part of a dose of oral medication is lost due to spitting, drooling, or vomiting, the nurse should discuss with a provider before readministering the dose. There are no evidence-based recommendations regarding a specific time frame for repeating a dose of medication after a patient has vomited (Kendrick, Ma, DeZorzi, et al., 2012). Because it is difficult to accurately estimate the amount of dose that was received, giving additional amounts may result in overdose.

INTRAMUSCULAR ADMINISTRATION

Selecting the Syringe and Needle

The volume of medication prescribed for intramuscular (IM) injections in small children necessitates selection of a syringe that can measure small amounts of solution. For volumes less than 1 ml, the tuberculin syringe, calibrated in 0.01-ml increments, is appropriate. Doses smaller than 0.5 ml may be facilitated by the use of a 0.5-ml, low-dose syringe. These syringes, along with specially constructed needles, minimize the possibility of inadvertently administering incorrect amounts of a drug because of **dead space**, which allows fluid to remain in the syringe and needle after the plunger is pushed completely forward. A minimum of 0.2 ml of solution remains in a standard needle hub; therefore when very small amounts of two drugs are combined in the syringe, such as mixtures of insulin, the ratio of the two drugs can be altered significantly due to dead space. Measures that minimize the effect of dead space are (1) when two drugs are combined in the syringe, always draw them up in the same order to maintain a consistent ratio between the drugs, (2) use the same brand of syringe (dead space may vary between brands), and (3) use one-piece syringe units (needle permanently attached to the syringe).

Dead space is also an important factor to consider when injecting medication because flushing the syringe with an air bubble adds an additional amount of medication to the prescribed dose. This can be hazardous when very small amounts of a drug are given. Consequently, flushing is not recommended, especially when less than 1 ml of medication is given. Syringes are calibrated to deliver a prescribed drug dose, and the amount of medication left in the hub and needle is not part of the syringe barrel calibrations.

Certain drugs (such as iron dextran and diphtheria and tetanus toxoid) may cause irritation if inadvertently tracked into the subcutaneous tissue. To prevent tracking, the Z-track method is recommended to prevent drug leakage (Yilmaz, Khorshid, & Dedeoglu, 2016). The Z-track method is performed by using the nondominant hand to move skin slightly laterally at the injection site just prior to inserting the needle. This action will shift the subcutaneous skin over the muscle below. Maintain the skin in this displaced position while giving the injection, then remove the needle before releasing the skin. The skin and subcutaneous tissue slide back to their original position, creating an interruption in the needle's pathway and minimizing the risk of fluid leaking from the muscle into subcutaneous tissue. Changing the needle after withdrawing the fluid from the vial is another technique to minimize tracking.

The needle length must be sufficient to penetrate the subcutaneous tissue and deliver the medication into the body of the muscle. The needle gauge should be as small as possible to deliver the fluid safely. Smaller-diameter (25- to 30-gauge) needles cause the least discomfort, but larger gauges are needed for viscous medication and prevention of accidental bending of longer needles.

Determining the Site

Factors to consider when selecting a site for an IM injection on an infant or child include:

- The amount and viscosity of the medication to be injected
- The amount and general condition of the muscle mass
- The frequency or number of injections to be given during the course of treatment
- The type of medication being given
- Factors that may impede access to or cause contamination of the site
- The child's ability to assume the required position safely

Older children and adolescents usually pose few problems in selecting a suitable site for IM injections, but infants, with their small and underdeveloped muscles, have fewer available options. It is sometimes difficult to assess the amount of fluid that can be safely injected into a single site. Usually 1 ml is the maximum volume that should be administered in a single site to small children and older infants. The muscles of small infants may not tolerate more than 0.5 ml. As the child approaches adult size, the nurse can use volumes approaching those given to adults. However, the larger the amount of solution, the larger the muscle at the injection site must be.

Injections must be placed in muscles large enough to accommodate the medication, while avoiding major nerves and blood vessels. The IM immunization site recommended by the Centers for Disease Control and Prevention, World Health Organization, and American Academy of Pediatrics for infants is the anterolateral thigh or vastus lateralis (Table 20.5). Additional studies have shown that injections at the ventrogluteal site are suitable for children and infants as young as 2 months old (Atay, Kurt, Akkaya, et al., 2017; Yapucu, Ceylan, & Bayindir, 2016). Cook and Murtagh (2006) also found fewer systemic reactions (irritability and persistent crying or screaming) and greater

TABLE 20.5 Intramuscular Injection Sites in Children

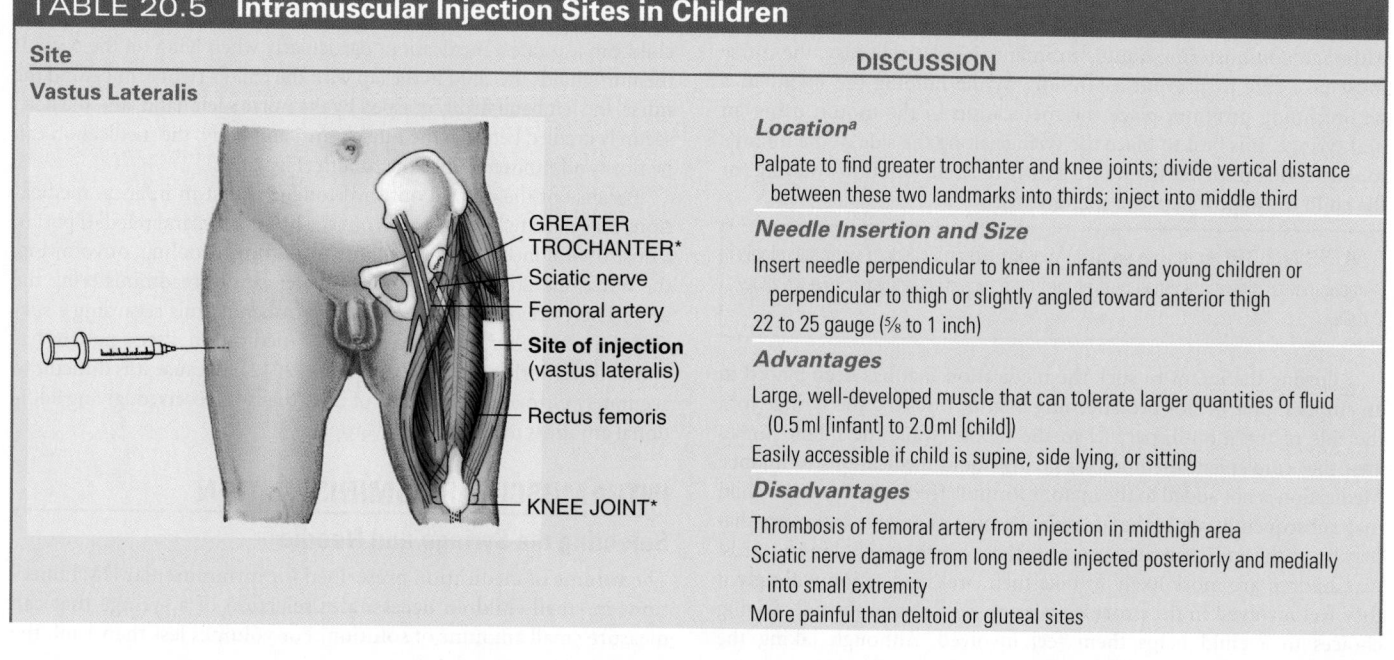

Site	DISCUSSION
Vastus Lateralis 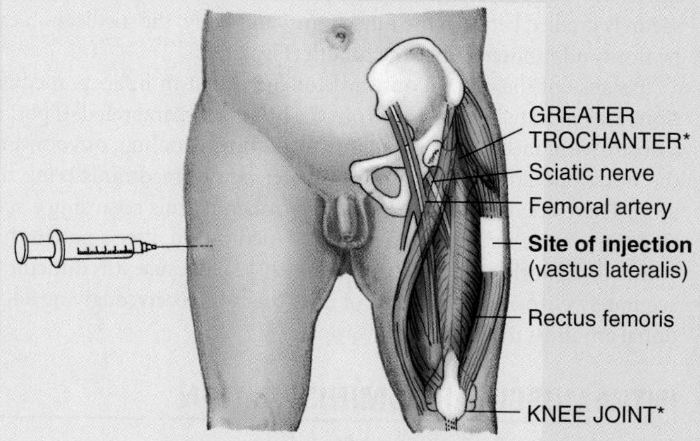 	***Location***[a] Palpate to find greater trochanter and knee joints; divide vertical distance between these two landmarks into thirds; inject into middle third ***Needle Insertion and Size*** Insert needle perpendicular to knee in infants and young children or perpendicular to thigh or slightly angled toward anterior thigh 22 to 25 gauge (⅝ to 1 inch) ***Advantages*** Large, well-developed muscle that can tolerate larger quantities of fluid (0.5 ml [infant] to 2.0 ml [child]) Easily accessible if child is supine, side lying, or sitting ***Disadvantages*** Thrombosis of femoral artery from injection in midthigh area Sciatic nerve damage from long needle injected posteriorly and medially into small extremity More painful than deltoid or gluteal sites

TABLE 20.5 Intramuscular Injection Sites in Children—cont'd

Site | **DISCUSSION**

Ventrogluteal

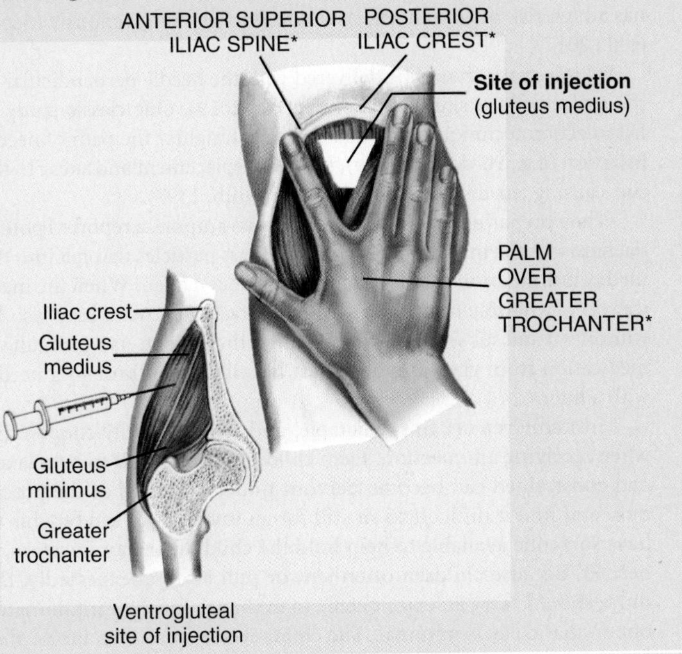

Ventrogluteal site of injection

Location[a]

Palpate to locate greater trochanter, anterior superior iliac tubercle (found by flexing thigh at hip and measuring up to 1 to 2 cm [0.4 to 0.8 inch] above crease formed in groin), and posterior iliac crest; place palm of hand over greater trochanter, index finger over anterior superior iliac tubercle, and middle finger along crest of ileum posteriorly as far as possible; inject into center of V formed by fingers

Needle Insertion and Size

Insert needle perpendicular to site but angled slightly toward iliac crest
22 to 25 gauge (½ to 1 inch)

Advantages

Free of important nerves and vascular structures
Easily identified by prominent bony landmarks
Thinner layer of subcutaneous tissue than in dorsogluteal site, thus less chance of depositing drug subcutaneously rather than intramuscularly
Can accommodate larger quantities of fluid (0.5 ml [infant] to 2.0 ml [child])
Easily accessible if child is supine, prone, or side lying
Less painful than vastus lateralis

Disadvantages

Health professionals' unfamiliarity with site

Deltoid

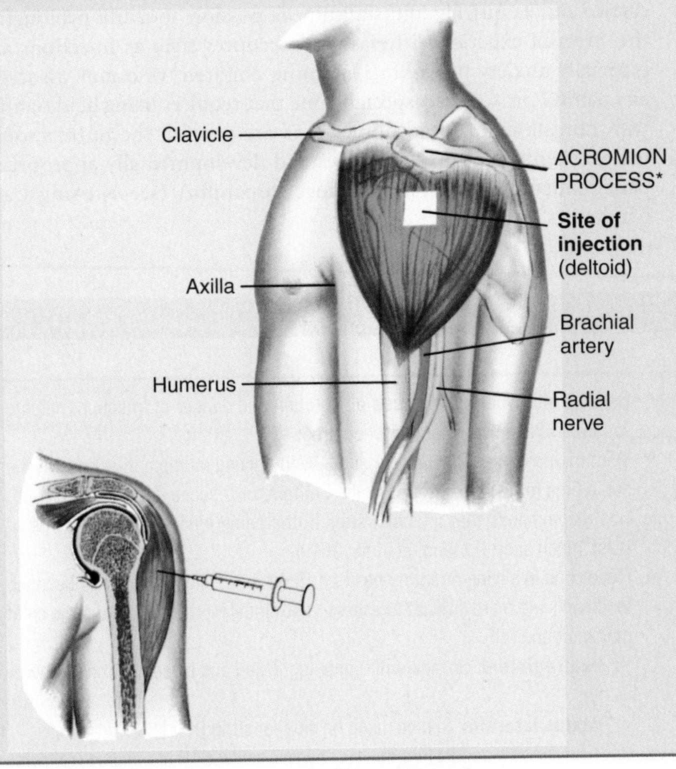

Location[a]

Locate acromion process; inject only into upper third of muscle that begins about two fingerbreadths below acromion

Needle Insertion and Size

Insert needle perpendicular to site but angled slightly toward shoulder
22 to 25 gauge (½ to 1 inch)

Advantages

Faster absorption rates than gluteal sites
Easily accessible with minimal removal of clothing
Less pain and fewer local side effects from vaccines compared with vastus lateralis

Disadvantages

Small muscle mass; only limited amounts of drug can be injected (0.5 to 1.0 ml)
Small margins of safety with possible damage to radial nerve and axillary nerve (not shown; lies under deltoid at head of humerus)

[a]Locations are indicated by asterisks (*) on illustrations.

parental acceptance for the ventrogluteal site. The ventrogluteal site is relatively free of major nerves and blood vessels, is a relatively large muscle with less subcutaneous tissue than the dorsal site, has well-defined landmarks for safe site location, and is easily accessible in several positions. Distraction and prevention of unexpected movement may be more easily achieved by placing the child supine on a parent's lap for ventrogluteal site use (Cook & Murtagh, 2006). The deltoid muscle, a small muscle near the axillary and radial nerves, can be used for small volumes of fluid in children as young as 18 months old. Its advantages are less pain and fewer side effects from the injectate (as observed with immunizations), compared with the vastus lateralis. Table 20.5 summarizes the three major injection sites and the location of the preferred IM injection sites for children.

Administration

Although injections that are executed with care seldom cause trauma to children, there have been reports of serious disability related to IM injections in children. Repeated use of a single site has been associated with fibrosis of the muscle with subsequent muscle contracture. Injections close to large nerves, such as the sciatic nerve, have been responsible for permanent disability, especially when potentially neurotoxic drugs are administered. For this reason, the dorsogluteal muscle (buttocks) is no longer recommended as a site for IM injections for children under the age of 10 years (Brown, Gillespie, & Chard, 2015).

Aspiration prior to injection of IM medications is no longer universally recommended. Traditionally, the absence of blood during aspiration is intended to confirm that the medication is being delivered intramuscularly and not inadvertently being injected into a vein. However, there is insufficient evidence to show that significant adverse reactions have occurred when aspiration has not been performed (Sepah, Samad, Alrag, et al., 2017). In addition, studies have shown that aspiration can increase the pain associated with injection. Aspiration during IM vaccine administration is no longer recommended by the Centers for Disease Control and Prevention, World Health Organization, American Academy of Pediatrics, or Immunization Action Coalition (Ezeanolue, Harriman, Hunter, et al., 2019; Sisson, 2015; Thomas, Mraz, & Rajcan, 2016). Aspiration for routine injections into deltoid or vastus lateralis is not indicated because there are no large blood vessels in these locations. Aspiration may still be indicated before injection of medications such as penicillin into larger muscle groups such as the ventrogluteal site (Crawford & Johnson, 2012). Aspiration should also be considered if the medication has a high risk of adverse effects if administered intravenously (Sepah et al., 2017).

IM injections should be delivered with the needle perpendicular to the surface of the skin (Ezeanolue et al., 2019). One classic study of IM injection techniques revealed that the straighter the path of needle insertion (e.g., 90-degree angle), the less displacement and shear to tissue, causing less discomfort (Katsma & Smith, 1997).

When preparing medication from a glass ampule, a reported potential hazard is the inadvertent creation of glass particles that fall into the medication solution when the ampule is broken open. When the medication is withdrawn into the syringe, the glass particles may also be withdrawn and subsequently injected into the patient. As a precaution, medication from glass ampules must be withdrawn through a needle with a filter.

Most children are unpredictable, and few are totally cooperative when receiving an injection. Even children who appear to be relaxed and constrained can become nervous under the stress of the procedure and find it difficult to sit still for an injection. It is advisable to have someone available to help hold the child during an injection, if needed. Because children often jerk or pull away unexpectedly, the nurse should carry an extra needle to exchange for the contaminated one so that delay is minimal. The child, even a small one, is told that he or she is receiving an injection (preferably using a phrase such as "putting the medicine under the skin"), and then the procedure is carried out as quickly and skillfully as possible to avoid prolonging the stressful experience. Invasive procedures such as injections are especially anxiety provoking in young children, who may associate any painful procedure, especially one that requires being held tightly, with punishment. Because injections are painful, the nurse should use excellent injection techniques and developmentally appropriate pain reduction measures to reduce discomfort (see Nursing Care Guidelines box).

NURSING CARE GUIDELINES

Intramuscular Administration of Medication

- Apply EMLA (a eutectic mix of lidocaine and prilocaine) or LMX cream (lidocaine) topically over injection site if time permits. (See Chapter 5, Pain Management.)
- Prepare medication.
  - Select appropriate-size needle and syringe.
  - If withdrawing medication from an ampule, use a needle equipped with a filter that removes glass particles; then change to a new, nonfilter needle for injection.
  - Maximum volume to be administered in a single site is 1 ml for older infants and small children and 2 ml for older children and adolescents.
  - Have medication at room temperature before injection.
- Determine site of injection (see Table 20.5); make certain that the muscle is large enough to accommodate volume and type of medication.
  - For infants and small or debilitated children, use the vastus lateralis or ventrogluteal muscles; for school-age children and adolescents, use the deltoid or ventrogluteal muscle.
- Obtain sufficient help for restraining child, if needed.
- Explain briefly what is to be done and, if appropriate, what the child can do to help.
- Expose injection site area for unobstructed view of landmarks.
- Select a site where skin is free of irritation and danger of infection; palpate for and avoid sensitive or hardened areas.
- With multiple injections, rotate sites. When giving multiple injections at the same time (e.g., immunizations), the Centers for Disease Control and Prevention recommends that injection sites in the same muscle group must be at least 1 inch apart (Ezeanolue et al., 2019).
- Place child in a lying or sitting position; child is not allowed to stand because landmarks are more difficult to assess, restraint is more difficult, and the child may faint and fall.
  - **Ventrogluteal:** On side with upper leg flexed and placed in front of lower leg
  - **Vastus lateralis:** Supine, lying on side, or sitting
- Use a new, sharp needle (not one that has pierced rubber stopper on vial) with smallest diameter that permits free flow of the medication.
- Grasp muscle firmly between thumb and fingers to isolate and stabilize muscle for deposition of drug in its deepest part; in obese children, spread skin with thumb and index finger to displace subcutaneous tissue and grasp muscle deeply on each side.
- Allow skin preparation to dry completely before penetrating skin.
- Decrease perception of pain.

NURSING CARE GUIDELINES—cont'd

Intramuscular Administration of Medication

- Distract child with conversation.
- Give child something on which to concentrate (e.g., squeezing a hand or side rail, pinching own nose, humming, counting, yelling "Ouch!").
- Spray vapocoolant on site before injection, place a cold compress or wrapped ice cube on site about 1 minute before injection, or apply cold to contralateral site.
- Studies have shown that applying manual pressure to the injection site for 10 seconds before injection can reduce postinjection pain (Derya, Ukke, Taner, et al., 2015; Öztürk, Baykara, Karadag, et al., 2017).
- Have child hold a small adhesive bandage and place it on puncture site after IM injection is given.
- Insert needle quickly using a dart-like motion at a 90-degree angle, unless contraindicated.
- Aspirate for blood return only if indicated.
- Avoid tracking any medication through superficial tissues:
  - Change needle after withdrawing medication from vial.
  - Use the Z-track or air-bubble technique as indicated.
  - Avoid any depression of the plunger during insertion of the needle.
- Administer the medication, then remove the needle quickly; hold gauze firmly against skin near needle when removing it to avoid pulling on tissue.
- Apply firm pressure to site after injection; massage site to hasten absorption unless contraindicated (e.g., if patient has a bleeding disorder or is receiving anticoagulation therapy).
- Place a small adhesive bandage on puncture site; with young children, decorate it by drawing a smiling face or other symbol of acceptance. Remind parents to remove the bandage as soon as bleeding has stopped, because bandages are a choking hazard in younger children.
- Hold and cuddle young child and encourage parents to comfort child; praise older child.
- Allow expression of feelings.
- Discard syringe and uncapped, uncut needle in puncture-resistant container located near site of use.
- Record time of injection, drug, dose, and injection site.

EMLA, Eutectic mixture of local anesthetics; *IM*, intramuscular; *LMX*, lidocaine.

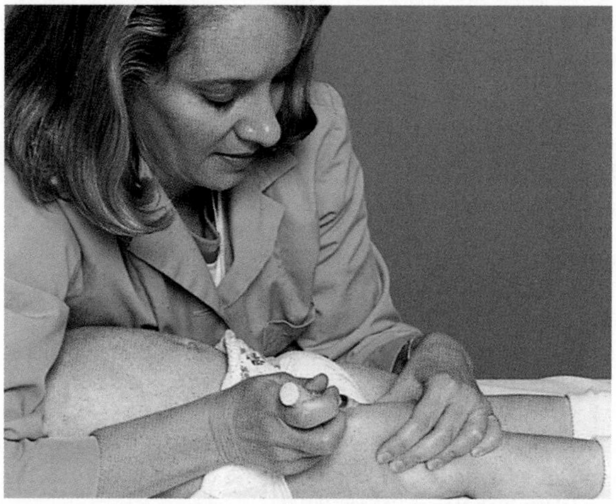

Fig. 20.13 Holding a small child for intramuscular injection. Note how the nurse isolates and stabilizes the muscle.

Small infants usually can be positioned without assistance. A larger infant's body can be securely restrained between the nurse's arm and body. To inject into the body of a muscle, the nurse firmly grasps the muscle mass between the thumb and fingers to isolate and stabilize the site (Fig. 20.13). However, in obese children, it is preferable to first spread the skin with the thumb and index finger to displace subcutaneous tissue and then grasp the muscle deeply on each side.

If medication is given around the clock, the nurse must wake the child. Although it may seem easier to surprise the sleeping child and do it quickly, this can cause the child to fear going back to sleep. When awakened first, children will know that nothing will be done to them unless they are forewarned. The Nursing Care Guidelines box summarizes administration techniques that maximize safety and minimize the discomfort often associated with injections.

SUBCUTANEOUS AND INTRADERMAL ADMINISTRATION

Subcutaneous and intradermal injections are frequently administered to children, but the technique differs little from the method used with adults. Examples of **subcutaneous injections** include insulin, hormone replacement, allergy desensitization, and some vaccines. Tuberculin testing, local anesthesia, and allergy testing are examples of frequently administered **intradermal injections**.

Techniques to minimize the pain associated with these injections include changing the needle if it pierced a rubber stopper on a vial, using 26- to 30-gauge needles (only to inject the solution), and injecting small volumes (≤0.5 ml). The angle of the needle for the subcutaneous injection is typically 90 degrees. In children with little subcutaneous tissue, some practitioners insert the needle at a 45-degree angle. However, the benefit of using the 45-degree angle rather than the 90-degree angle remains controversial.

Although subcutaneous injections can be given anywhere there is subcutaneous tissue, common sites include the center third of the lateral aspect of the upper arm, the abdomen, and the center third of the anterior thigh. Some practitioners believe it is not necessary to aspirate before injecting subcutaneously; for example, this is an accepted practice in the administration of insulin. Automatic injector devices do not aspirate before injecting.

When giving an intradermal injection into the volar surface of the forearm, the nurse should avoid the medial side of the arm, where the skin is more sensitive.

NURSING TIP Families often need to learn injection techniques to administer medications, such as insulin, at home. Begin teaching as early as possible to allow the family the maximum amount of practice time.

INTRAVENOUS ADMINISTRATION

The IV route for administering medications is frequently used in pediatric therapy. For some drugs, it is the only effective route. This method is used for giving drugs to children who:

- Have poor absorption as a result of diarrhea, vomiting, or dehydration
- Need a high serum concentration of a drug
- Have resistant infections that require parenteral medication over an extended time
- Need continuous pain relief
- Require emergency treatment

Intravenous Line Placement

The nurse needs to consider several factors in relation to IV medication. When a drug is administered intravenously, the effect is almost instantaneous and further control is limited. Most drugs for IV administration require a specified minimum dilution, rate of flow, or both, and many drugs are highly irritating or toxic to tissues outside the vascular system. In addition to the precautions and nursing observations commonly related to IV therapy, factors to consider when preparing and administering drugs to infants and children by the IV route include:

- Amount of drug to be administered
- Minimum dilution of drug and whether child is fluid restricted
- Type of solution in which drug can be diluted
- Length of time over which drug can be safely administered
- Rate limitations of child, vascular system, and infusion equipment
- Time that this or another drug is to be administered
- Compatibility of all drugs that child is receiving intravenously
- Compatibility with infusion fluids

Before any IV infusion, check the site of insertion for patency, which includes a brisk blood return and flushing easily without resistance. Never flush against resistance and if encountered, the integrity of the access should be further evaluated (Infusion Nurses Society, 2016). Never administer medications into the same IV tubing with blood products. Only one antibiotic should be administered at a time. Extra fluids needed to administer IV medications can be problematic for infants and fluid-restricted children. Syringe pumps are often used to deliver IV medication because they minimize fluid requirements and more precisely deliver small volumes of medication compared with large-volume infusion pumps. Regardless of the technique, the nurse must know the minimum dilutions for safe administration of IV medications to infants and children.

Peripheral Intermittent Infusion Device

When prolonged access to a vein is required without the need for continuous fluid, a **peripheral lock**, also known as an **intermittent infusion device** or **saline** or **heparin lock**, is an alternative. The peripheral lock allows a child more freedom than being connected to a continuous IV infusion. It is most frequently used for intermittent infusion of medication, such as antibiotics, via peripheral venous route. A short, flexible catheter is used as the lock device, and a site where there will be minimal movement, such as the forearm, is selected. The catheter is inserted and secured in the same manner as for any IV infusion device, but an injection cap or needleless connector is attached to the hub. When it is time for medication administration, the needleless connector is disinfected, the lock is flushed to ensure patency, and then IV tubing, primed with either normal saline or medication, is connected.

The type of device used may vary, and the care and use of the peripheral lock are carried out according to the policy of the institution or unit. However, the general concept is the same. The catheter remains in place and is flushed with saline before and after infusion of the medication. See the Translating Evidence Into Practice box and Table 20.6 on flushing with normal saline or heparin.

TRANSLATING EVIDENCE INTO PRACTICE

Normal Saline or Heparinized Saline Flush Solution in Pediatric Intravenous Lines

Ask the Question

PICOT Question

Is there a significant difference in the longevity of intravenous (IV) intermittent infusion locks in children when normal saline (NS) is used as a flush instead a heparinized saline (HS) solution?

Search for the Evidence

Search Strategies

Selection criteria included evidence during the years 2006 to 2017 with the following terms: saline versus heparin intermittent flush, children's heparin lock flush, heparin lock patency, peripheral venous catheter in children.

Databases Used

CINAHL, PubMed

Critical Appraisal of the Evidence

- No differences in patency were established in a double-blind prospective randomized study in neonates. NS was deemed preferable to HS in peripheral intravenous (PIV) locks in neonates, in consideration of complications associated with heparin (Arnts, Heijnen, Wilbers, et al., 2011).
- Infusion devices flushed with NS lasted longer than those flushed with HS (Cook, Bellini, & Cusson, 2011).
- Peripheral catheters flushed with heparin remained patent longer but were also more likely to develop phlebitis (Tripathi, Kaushik, & Singh, 2008).
- A randomized trial in neonates demonstrated that use of HS for flushing before and after IV antibiotics significantly increased the duration of PIVs when compared to NS flushes (Upadhyay, Verma, Lal, et al., 2015).
- A systematic review of 10 randomized controlled trials in pediatrics found minimal benefit to use of HS as intermittent flush of peripheral catheters compared to NS. The difference was not statistically significant (Kumar, Vandermeer, Bassler, et al., 2013).
- Peripheral catheters in children, ages 1 to 17 years, flushed once every 24 hours with NS did not affect patency when compared to flushing with NS every 12 hours (Schreiber, Zanchi, Ronfani, et al., 2015).
- Either HS or preservative-free NS may be used to flush a PIV line (Arnts et al., 2011; Bellini, 2012; Cook et al., 2011; Infusion Nurses Society, 2016; White, Crawley, Rennie, et al., 2011).
- After each catheter use, peripheral catheters should be locked with either HS (0.5 to 10 units/ml) or preservative-free NS, since outcome data remain equivocal (Infusion Nurses Society, 2016).
- Intermittent flushing with NS results in fewer complications, lower cost, and less time compared with continuous infusion (Stok & Wieringa, 2016).
- The Centers for Disease Control and Prevention recommends use of NS for intermittent flushing to avoid complications (O'Grady, Alexander, Burns, et al., 2011).
- Switching from HS to NS involves educational and administrative interventions (Cook et al., 2011; Thamlikitkul & Indranoi, 2006).
- NS is more cost effective (Thamlikitkul & Indranoi, 2006).
- NS flush has fewer side effects. HS can be associated with anticoagulation, thrombocytopenia, drug interactions, and hypersensitivity (Arnts et al., 2011).
- NS flushes once a day maintained patency of pediatric PIV locks, resulting in reduced costs and increased patient satisfaction (Schreiber et al., 2015).
- Nurses in Italy tend to use HS with smaller-gauge (24-gauge) catheters when access is less frequent (12 hours or more between doses) and when patients are on specific units (hematology/oncology, pediatric surgery, and short-stay units) (Bisogni, Guisti, Ciofi, et al., 2014).

Apply the Evidence: Nursing Implications

There is **low-quality evidence with a weak recommendation** (Guyatt, Oxman, Vist, et al., 2008) for using NS versus HS flush solution in pediatric IV lines. Further research is needed with larger samples of children, especially preterm neonates, using small-gauge catheters (24 gauge) and other gauge catheters flushed with NS

TRANSLATING EVIDENCE INTO PRACTICE—cont'd

Normal Saline or Heparinized Saline Flush Solution in Pediatric Intravenous Lines

and HS as intermittent infusion devices only (no continuous infusions). Variables to be considered include catheter dwell time; medications administered; period between regular flushing and flushing associated with medication administration; pain, erythema, and other localized complications; concentration and amount of HS used; type of needleless connector used (negative pressure, positive pressure, or neutral pressure); flush method (positive-pressure technique vs. no specific technique); reason for IV device removal; and complications associated with either solution. NS is a safe alternative to HS flush in infants and children with intermittent IV locks larger than 24 gauge; smaller neonates may benefit from HS flush (longer dwell time), but the evidence is inconclusive for all weight ranges and gestational ages. Neonates may benefit from a continuous infusion of NS at 5 ml/h to maintain patency.

Quality and Safety Competencies: Evidence-Based Practice[a]

Knowledge

Differentiate clinical opinion from research and evidence-based summaries.

Describe methods for using NS or HS flush solution in pediatric IV lines.

Skills

Base individualized care plan on patient values, clinical expertise, and evidence.

Integrate evidence into practice on NS or HS flush solution in pediatric IV lines.

Attitudes

Value the concept of evidence-based practice as integral to determining best clinical practice.

Appreciate the strength and weakness of evidence for NS or HS flush solution in pediatric IV lines.

References

Arnts, I. J., Heijnen, J. A., Wilbers, H. T., et al. (2011). Effectiveness of heparin solution versus normal saline in maintaining patency of intravenous locks in neonates: A double blind randomized controlled study. *Journal of Advanced Nursing, 67*(12), 2677–2685.

Bellini, S. (2012). Flushing of intravenous locks in neonates: No evidence that heparin improves patency compared with saline. *Evidence-Based Nursing, 15*, 86–87.

Bisogni, S., Guisti, F., Ciofi, D., et al. (2014). Heparin solution for maintaining peripheral venous catheter patency in children: A survey of current practice in Italian pediatric units. *Issues in Comprehensive Pediatric Nursing, 37*(2), 122–135.

Cook, L., Bellini, S., & Cusson, R. M. (2011). Heparinized saline vs normal saline for maintenance of intravenous access in neonates: An evidence-based practice change. *Advances in Neonatal Care, 11*, 208–215.

Guyatt, G. H., Oxman, A. D., Vist, G. E., et al. (2008). GRADE: An emerging consensus on rating quality of evidence and strength of recommendations. *British Medical Journal, 336*(7650), 924–926.

Infusion Nurses Society. (2016). Infusion nursing standards of practice. *Journal of Infusion Nursing, 34*(Suppl. 1), S63–S64.

Kumar, M., Vandermeer, B., Bassler, D., et al. (2013). Low dose heparin use and the patency of peripheral intravenous catheters in children: A systematic review. *Pediatrics, 131*(3), e864–e872.

O'Grady, N. P., Alexander, M., Burns, L. A., et al. (2011). *Guidelines for the prevention of intravascular catheter-related infections.* Atlanta, GA: Healthcare Infection Control Practices Advisory Committee of the Centers for Disease Control and Prevention.

Schreiber, S., Zanchi, C., Ronfani, L., et al. (2015). Normal saline flushes performed once daily maintain peripheral intravenous catheter patency: A randomized controlled trial. *Archives of Disease in Children, 100*(7), 700–703.

Stok, D., & Wieringa, J. W. (2016). Continuous infusion versus intermittent flushing: Maintaining peripheral intravenous access in newborn infants. *Journal of Perinatology, 36*(10), 870–873.

Thamlikitkul, V., & Indranoi, A. (2006). Switching from heparinized saline flush to normal saline flush for maintaining peripheral venous catheter patency. *International Journal for Quality in Health Care, 18*(3), 183–185.

Tripathi, S., Kaushik, V., & Singh, V. (2008). Peripheral IVs: Factors affecting complications and patency—A randomized controlled trial. *Journal of Infusion Nursing, 31*(3), 182–188.

Upadhyay, A., Verma, K. K., Lal, P., Chawla, D., & Sreenivas, V. (2015). Heparin for prolonging peripheral intravenous catheter use in neonates: A randomized controlled trial. *Journal of Perinatology, 35*, 274–277.

White, M. L., Crawley, J., Rennie, E. A., et al. (2011). Examining the effectiveness of 2 solutions used to flush capped pediatric peripheral intravenous catheters. *Journal of Infusion Nursing, 34*, 260–270.

[a] Adapted from the Quality and Safety Education for Nurses (QSEN) website at http://www.qsen.org.

TABLE 20.6 Intravenous Catheter Flushes for Lines Without Continuous Fluid Infusions

Peripheral lines (Hep-Lock or saline locks)	NS[a] after medications or every 8 hours for dormant lines; instill 2½ times tubing volume 24-g catheters: NS[a] or heparin 2 units/ml
Midline	Heparin 10 units/ml; 3 ml in a 10-ml syringe[b] after medications or every 8 hours if dormant Newborns: heparin 1-2 units/ml to run continuously at ordered rate
External central line (nonimplanted, nontunneled, tunneled, or PICC)	Heparin 10 units/ml; 3 ml in a 10-ml syringe[b] after medications or once daily if dormant Newborns: heparin 2 units/ml; 2-3 ml after medications or to check line patency OR heparin 1-2 units/ml to run continuously at ordered rate
Totally implanted central line (TIVAS, implanted port)	Heparin 10 units/ml; 5 ml after medications or once daily if dormant and accessed; if not accessed, heparin 100 units/ml; 5 ml every month
Arterial and central venous pressure continuous monitored lines	Heparin 2 units/ml in 55-ml syringe to run continuously at 1 ml/h

[a] Use 5% dextrose in water when medication is incompatible with saline.
[b] Smaller syringes may be used when flush is delivered by a pump. *NS,* Normal saline; *PICC,* peripherally inserted central catheter; *TIVAS,* totally implantable venous access device.

Children who require medications on a short-term basis may be discharged from the hospital with a peripheral lock in place to continue receiving IV medications at home under the care of a home health infusion company. When IV therapy is needed for more than 6 days, use of a midline catheter or peripherally inserted central catheter is recommended (O'Grady, Alexander, Burns, et al., 2011). Midline catheters are peripheral catheters that are placed in one of the larger veins of the upper arm, with the catheter tip terminating below the axilla. Midline catheters are appropriate for short-term use, usually lasting 2 to 6 weeks (Adams, Little, Vinsant, et al., 2016). A midline catheter is not considered a central venous catheter, so total parenteral nutrition (TPN) or any other drug known to irritate a peripheral vein (e.g., chemotherapy drugs) should not be administered through it. The high concentration of glucose in TPN is irritating to the interior lining of the blood vessel; therefore TPN should always be infused through a central catheter.

Central Venous Access Device

Children with acute or chronic illnesses who require repeated blood sampling or medications, long-term chemotherapy, intensive care, or frequent hyperalimentation or antibiotic therapy are best managed with a central venous catheter. Because the large central veins (such as the subclavian, femoral, or superior vena cava) allow more rapid diffusion of fluids and medications, they offer a more durable venous access than PIV catheters. However, central venous catheters also have a greater risk of bloodstream infection.

Short-term or **nontunneled catheters** are used in acute care, emergency, and intensive care units. These catheters are made of polyurethane and are placed in large veins, such as the subclavian, femoral, or jugular. Insertion is by surgical incision or large percutaneous threading. A chest radiograph should be taken to verify that the catheter tip is properly located in a large central vein before administration of fluids or medications.

Peripherally inserted central catheters (PICCs) can be used for short-term to moderate-length therapy. These catheters consist of silicone or polymer material and are placed by specially trained nurses, physicians, or interventional radiologists. The most common insertion site is above the antecubital area using the median, cephalic, or basilic vein. The catheter is threaded either with or without a guidewire into the superior vena cava.

The decision to insert a PICC needs to be made before several attempts at IV insertion are done. When the antecubital veins have been punctured repeatedly, they are not considered candidates for this type of catheter. Because this catheter is the least costly and has less chance of complications than other CVADs, it is an excellent choice for many pediatric patients who require IV therapies for weeks or months.

Children with chronic illnesses who require long-term venous access, for months or years, are best managed with a CVAD. CVADs have several different characteristics. They can be tunneled or nontunneled, external or internal, inserted peripherally or centrally. Factors that influence selection of the type of CVAD for a child include the reason for placement of the catheter (diagnosis), length of therapy, risk to the patient in placement of the catheter, and availability of resources to assist the family in maintaining the catheter.

> **! NURSING ALERT**
>
> Most peripherally inserted central catheter (PICC) lines are not sutured into place, so great care is needed when changing the dressing to avoid accidental catheter dislodgment.

Long-term CVADs include tunneled catheters and implanted infusion ports (Table 20.7 and Fig. 20.14). They may have single, double, or triple lumens. Several lumens (multilumen) catheters allow more than one therapy to be administered at the same time. Reasons for placement of multilumen catheters include repeated blood sampling, TPN administration, frequent administration of blood products, frequent infusion of large quantities or concentrations of fluids, administration of incompatible drugs or fluids at the same time (through different lumens), and central venous pressure monitoring.

TABLE 20.7 Comparison of Long-Term Central Venous Access Devices

Description	Benefits	Care Considerations
Tunneled Catheter (e.g., Hickman or Broviac Catheter)		
Silicone, radiopaque, flexible catheter with open ends or VitaCuffs (biosynthetic material impregnated with silver ions) on catheter(s) enhances tissue ingrowth May have more than one lumen	Reduced risk of bacterial migration after tissue adheres to cuff One or two Dacron cuffs Easy to use for self-administered infusions Removal requires pulling catheter from site (nonsurgical procedure)	Requires daily heparin flushes Requires semipermeable dressing over exit site at all times; dressing must be changed regularly and whenever it becomes wet or loose Must be clamped or have clamp nearby at all times Must keep exit site dry Heavy activity restricted until tissue adheres to cuff Water sports may be restricted (risk of infection) Risk of infection still present Protrudes outside body; susceptible to damage from sharp instruments and may be pulled out; may affect body image More difficult to repair Patient or family must learn catheter care
Implanted Ports (e.g., Port-a-Cath, Infuse-a-Port, Mediport, NorPort, Groshong Port)		
Totally implantable metal or plastic device that consists of self-sealing injection port with preconnected or attachable silicone catheter that is placed in large blood vessel	Reduced risk of infection Placed completely under the skin and therefore much less likely to be pulled out or damaged No maintenance care and reduced cost for family Heparinized monthly and after each infusion to maintain patency No limitations on regular physical activity, including swimming Dressing needed only when port accessed with Huber needle that is not removed No or only slight change in body appearance (slight bulge on chest)	Must pierce skin for access; pain with insertion of needle; can use local anesthetic (EMLA, LMX) or intradermal buffered lidocaine before accessing port Special noncoring needle (Huber) with straight or angled design must be used to inject into port Skin cleansing preparation needed before injection Difficult to manipulate for self-administered infusions Catheter may migrate internally, especially if child "plays" with port site (twiddler syndrome) Vigorous contact sports generally not allowed Removal requires surgical procedure

EMLA, Eutectic mix of local anesthetics; *LMX,* lidocaine.

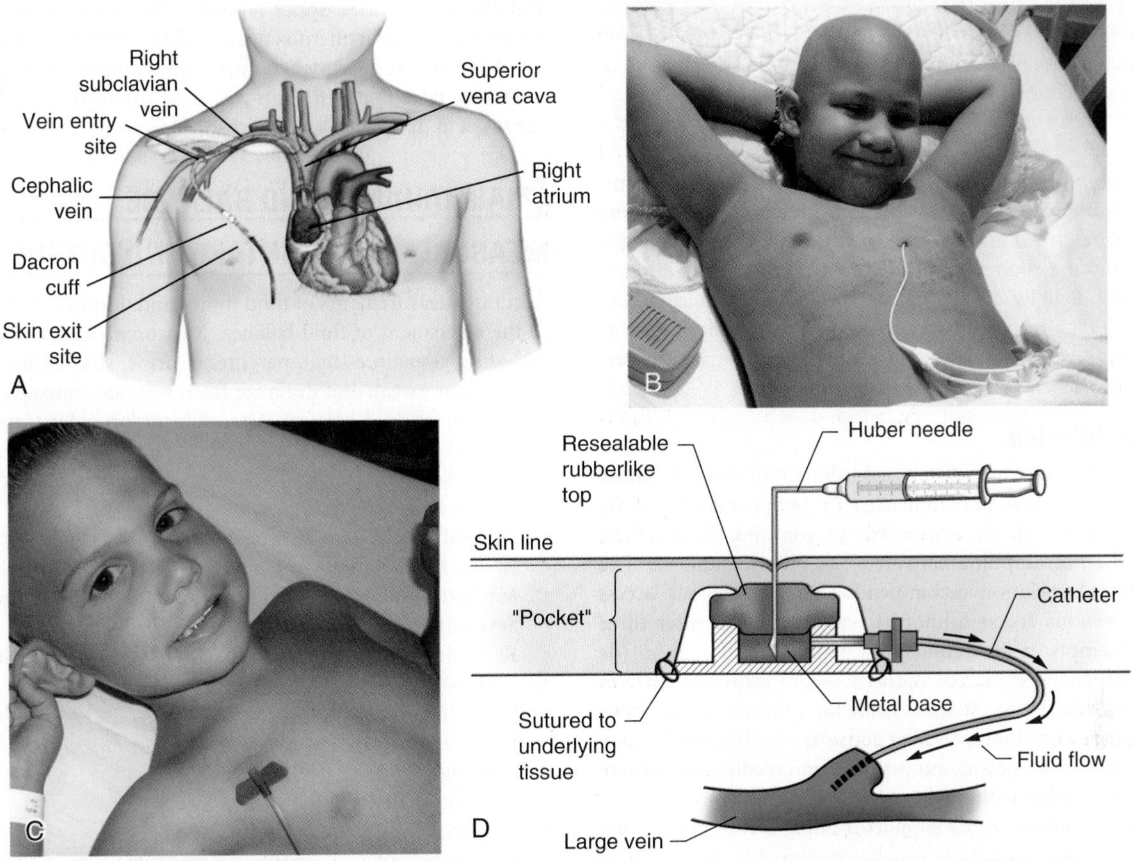

Fig. 20.14 Venous access devices. **A**, External central venous catheter insertion and exit site. **B**, Child with an external central venous catheter (dressing removed for photo). **C**, Child with an implanted port with a Huber needle in place (dressing removed for photo). **D**, Side view of an implanted port.

Maintenance of the catheter includes dressing changes, flushing to maintain patency, and prevention of occlusion or dislodgment.

! NURSING ALERT

When working with tunneled catheters, peripherally inserted central catheters (PICCs), and peripheral intravenous (PIV) lines, avoid the use of any scissors around the tubing or dressing. Removal is best accomplished using fingers and much patience. If a tunneled catheter is cut, use a padded clamp to occlude the catheter between the exit site and the site of damage to avoid blood loss. Repair kits are available, which may save the catheter and avoid surgery to replace a damaged catheter.

To access the implanted CVAD, the port must be palpated for placement and stabilized. The overlying skin should be cleansed. The port should be accessed only with a special noncoring Huber needle. The needle is inserted through the diaphragm of the port, which is usually located on the top of the device. If the port needs to be accessed for several days, a special infusion set with a Huber needle and extension tubing with a Luer connection can be inserted and an occlusive dressing applied to keep the needle in place. When the infusion set is used, the procedure for administration of fluids and medications is the same as for an intermittent infusion device or a central venous catheter. To prevent infection, meticulous aseptic technique must be used any time the CVAD is entered, including instillation of heparin or saline to prevent clotting. Huber needles are changed at established intervals, usually 5 to 7 days (see Research Focus box).

NURSING TIP A pocket sewn on the inside of a T-shirt provides a place in which to coil the catheter line while the child is at play if a dressing is not used.

Infection and catheter occlusion are two of the most common complications of central venous catheters. They require treatment with antibiotics for infection and a fibrinolytic agent, such as alteplase, for thrombus formation (Anderson, Pesaturo, Casavant, & Ramsey, 2013). When the line is not in use, the catheter should be flushed with heparin, then clamped.

Parents are cautioned to keep scissors away from the child with an external central venous catheter, to prevent accidental cutting of the tubing. If the catheter leaks, the parents are instructed to tape it above the leak and then clamp the catheter at the taped site. The child should be taken to the hospital or clinic as soon as possible to prevent infection or clotting after a catheter leak (see Research Focus box).

RESEARCH FOCUS

Dressing Changes

Semipermeable transparent dressings should be changed at least every 5 to 7 days; the interval depends on the dressing material, age, and condition of the patient; infection rate reported by the organization; environmental conditions; and manufacturer labeled uses and directions (Infusion Nurses Society, 2016). In children older than 2 months of age, use of chlorhexidine-impregnated dressing (i.e., BioPatch) should be considered as an extra prevention measure for catheter-related bloodstream infection (Infusion Nurses Society, 2016).

! NURSING ALERT

If a central venous catheter is accidentally removed, apply pressure to the skin overlying the location of vein entry, not the exit site on the skin.

The children and parents are taught the procedure for care of the CVAD before discharge from the hospital, including preparation and injection of the prescribed medication, the flush, and dressing changes. A protective wrap may be recommended for some active children to prevent their accidentally dislodging the needle. Older children and adolescents may take responsibility for preparing and administering medications. Both verbal and written step-by-step instructions are provided for the learners.

Intraosseous Infusion

Situations may occur in which rapid establishment of systemic access is vital and venous access is complicated by peripheral circulatory collapse, hypovolemic shock (secondary to vomiting or diarrhea, burns, or trauma), cardiopulmonary arrest, or other conditions. The American Heart Association recommends that intraosseous access be obtained if venous access cannot be readily achieved after three unsuccessful attempts or 90 seconds in a pediatric resuscitation (de Caen, Berg, Chameides, et al., 2015). **Intraosseous infusion** provides a rapid, safe, and life-saving alternate route for administration of fluids and medications until intravascular access is possible. Health care providers, including physicians, nurses, and paramedics, can secure intraosseous cannulation within 30 to 60 seconds. Some hospitals recommend pediatric advanced life support training before performing this procedure. This procedure is usually reserved for children who are unconscious or for those receiving analgesia because the procedure is painful. Local anesthesia should be used for a semiconscious patient. Contraindications for placement of an intraosseous catheter include concurrent problems involving that extremity, such as previous intraosseous attempt, skin rash, bone fracture, osteogenesis imperfecta, or osteosarcoma.

A large-bore rigid needle, such as an intraosseous needle (e.g., Cook) or a bone marrow aspiration needle (e.g., Jamshidi), is inserted into the medullary cavity of a long bone. The anteromedial aspect of the tibia—1 to 3 cm (0.4 to 1.2 inch) below the tibial tuberosity—is the preferred site for children of all ages because it is flat and has a large marrow cavity. In newborns, the distal third of the femur may be used. The distal tibia is an alternative site. Local anesthesia should be used for semiconscious patients. Spring-loaded and battery-powered intraosseous needle drivers are available for use (Bielski, Szarpak, Smereka, et al., 2017).

Once the bone marrow needle is in place, the needle should stand alone and feel secure. The needle should be stabilized and secured with tape and gauze. If a bone marrow aspirate needle is used, gauze should be built up around the needle to provide support and prevent trauma or dislodgment (Lewis, Crapo, & Williams, 2013). Drugs may be pushed and fluids delivered via an infusion pump. The intraosseous line may be discontinued after IV access has been achieved, typically within 24 to 48 hours.

Once established, the intraosseous route can be used during resuscitation to administer the same medications that could be given through the IV route. During infusion through an intraosseous needle, monitor the extremity closely for swelling or oozing of fluid at the insertion site. Give particular attention to the dependent tissue of the leg. Extravasation of fluid from the bone marrow may be hidden under the leg. Check for swelling of the entire lower leg when the intraosseous bone marrow needle is in the tibia or ankle, and check the entire upper leg when the intraosseous needle is in the femur. Compartment syndrome has resulted from an infiltrated intraosseous line. Other complications, although rare, include fractures, fat embolism, skin necrosis, osteomyelitis, and cellulitis (Lewis et al., 2013).

MAINTAINING FLUID BALANCE

MEASUREMENT OF INTAKE AND OUTPUT

Accurate measurements of fluid intake and output (I&O) are essential to the assessment of fluid balance. Measurements from all sources—including gastrointestinal, parenteral, urine, stools, vomitus, fistulas, NG suction, sweat, and drainage from wounds—must be included in assessment of fluid balance. Although the provider usually indicates when I&O measurements are to be recorded, it is a nursing responsibility to keep an accurate I&O record on certain children, including those with any of the following:

- Current IV therapy
- Recent major surgery
- Medications that include diuretic or corticosteroid therapy
- Severe thermal burns or injuries
- Renal disease or damage
- Congestive heart failure
- Dehydration
- Diabetes mellitus
- Oliguria
- Respiratory distress
- Chronic lung disease

Wet diapers or pads should be carefully weighed to ascertain the amount of fluid lost. This includes liquid stool, vomitus, and other losses. The applicaton of a collection bag may be useful for monitoring urine output in diapered infants and small children who have bowel movements with every void. The volume of fluid in milliliters is equivalent to the weight of the fluid measured in grams. The specific gravity as a measure of urine osmolality assists in assessing the degree of hydration.

NURSING TIP 1 g of wet diaper weight = 1 ml of urine

In infants with diapers, weigh all dry diapers to be used and note in an indelible marker the dry weight of the diaper; when there is fluid (urine or liquid stool) in the diaper, the amount of output can be approximated by subtracting the weight of the dry diaper from the weighed amount of the wet diaper.

Disadvantages of the weighed-diaper method of fluid measurement include (1) an inability to differentiate one type of loss from another because of admixture, (2) loss of urine or liquid stool from leakage or evaporation (especially for infants under a radiant warmer), and (3) additional fluid in the diaper (superabsorbent disposable type) from absorption of atmospheric moisture (in high-humidity incubators).

Special Needs When the Child Is Not Permitted to Take Fluids by Mouth

Infants or children who are unable or not permitted to take fluids by mouth (NPO) have special needs. To ensure that they do not receive fluids, a sign can be placed in some obvious place, such as over their beds or on their shirts, to alert caregivers and other hospital personnel to the NPO status. To prevent the temptation to drink, fluids should not be left at the bedside. Older children may try to sneak a drink when out of sight of caregivers, so nurses would be wise to keep an eye on

NPO children if they go into bathrooms or other locations where they are not easily observed.

Oral hygiene, a part of routine hygienic care, is especially important when fluids are restricted or withheld. For young children who cannot brush their teeth or rinse their mouth without swallowing fluid, the mouth and teeth can be cleaned and kept moist by swabbing with saline-moistened gauze.

NURSING TIP To keep the mouth feeling moist when the child is not permitted to take fluids by mouth, give ice chips (if this is permitted by the provider) or spray the mouth from an atomizer. To meet the need to suck, infants are provided with a safe commercial pacifier.

The child who is fluid restricted presents an equal challenge. Limiting fluids is often more difficult for the child than being NPO, especially when IV fluids are also eliminated. To make certain the child does not drink the entire amount allowed early in the day, the daily amount is calculated, then divided to provide fluids at periodic intervals throughout the child's waking hours. Serving the fluids in small containers gives the illusion of larger servings. No extra liquid is left at the bedside.

PARENTERAL FLUID THERAPY

Site and Equipment

The site selected for PIV infusion depends on accessibility and convenience. Current evidence also supports choosing the site that is most likely to last the duration of time needed (Infusion Nurses Society, 2016). The child's developmental, cognitive, and mobility needs must be considered when selecting a site. Ideally, in older children, the superficial veins of the forearm should be used, leaving the hands free. An older child can help select the site and thereby maintain some measure of control. For veins in the extremities, it is best to start with the most distal site and avoid the child's favored hand to reduce the temporary disability created by having an IV in the hand. Avoid placing peripheral IVs over joints (wrist, antecubital fossa, ankle), if possible, as these are areas of flexion and are more prone to accidental dislodgement, infiltration, and phlebitis (Infusion Nurses Society, 2016). In small infants, a superficial vein of the hand, wrist, forearm, foot, or ankle is usually most convenient and most easily stabilized (Fig. 20.15). Foot veins should be avoided in children learning to walk and in children already walking. Superficial veins of the scalp have no valves, are easily accessed, and can be used in infants up to about 9 months old, but they should be used only after attempts at other sites have failed.

The Infusion Nurses Society (2016) recommends use of vein-locating devices for assistance in starting PIVs on infants and children with difficult venous access. Vein-locating devices include ultrasound, transilluminators, and near-infrared light technology. Although not as powerful as ultrasound, a transilluminator requires minimal training and experience to use (Bahl, Pandurangadu, Tucker, et al., 2016). Small veins that may not be visible or palpable (especially in infants and toddlers) are often more readily visualized using a transilluminator. The cephalic vein in the proximal forearm may be the optimal vein for ultrasound-guided placement (Takeshita, Nakayama, Nakajima, et al., 2015). Because veins stand out so clearly with transillumination, they appear more superficial than they really are. Although visualization of veins is improved with transillumination, an increase in successful venipuncture is not guaranteed (Rothbart, Yu, Müller-Lobeck, et al., 2015). Some devices require assistance to hold in place. Commercial devices have not caused burns in infants

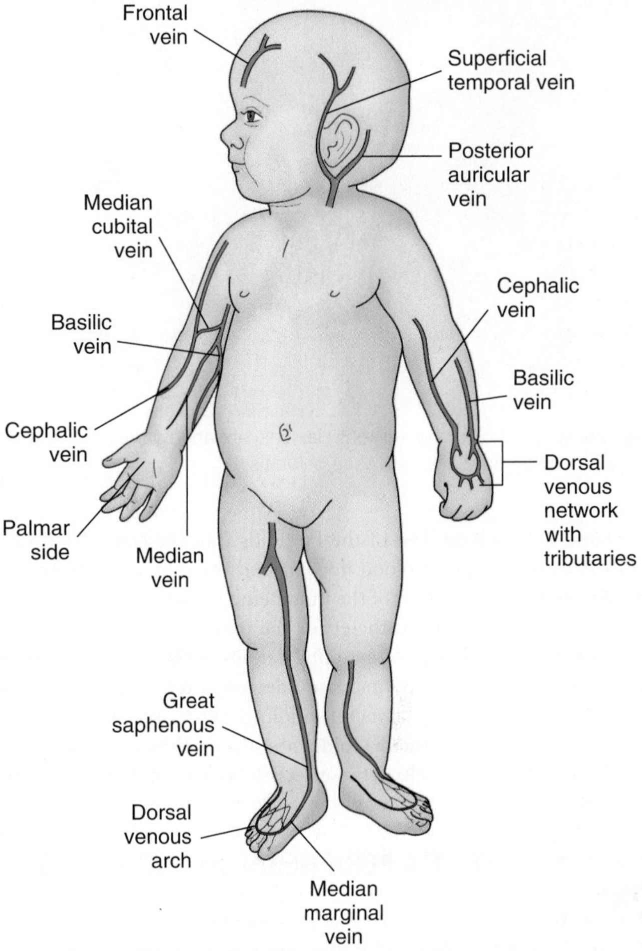

Fig. 20.15 Preferred sites for venous access in infants.

or children. Practice in this technique is necessary for optimal outcomes (Stolz, Cappa, Minckler, et al., 2016).

Selection of a scalp vein may require clipping the hair in the area around the site to better visualize the vein and provide a smoother surface on which to tape the catheter hub and tubing. Clipping a portion of the infant's hair may be upsetting to parents; therefore they should be told what to expect and be reassured that the hair will grow back. Remove as little as possible directly over the insertion site and taping surface. Save the clipped hair because parents often wish to keep it. A rubber band slipped onto the head from brow to occiput will usually suffice as a tourniquet, although if the vein is visible, a tourniquet may not be necessary.

NURSING TIP A tab of tape should be placed on the rubber band to help grasp it when removing it from the infant's head. The rubber band should be cut to avoid accidentally dislodging the catheter when moving the rubber band over the IV insertion site. The tape tab will lift the rubber band and allow it to be cut. Hold the rubber band in two places and cut between these areas to prevent the rubber band from snapping on the head.

For most IV infusions in children, a 20- to 24-gauge catheter may be used if therapy is expected to last 6 days or less. The smallest gauge and shortest length catheter that will accommodate the prescribed therapy should be chosen. The length of the catheter may be directly related to infection or embolus formation; the shorter the catheter, the fewer the complications. The gauge of the catheter should be sufficient

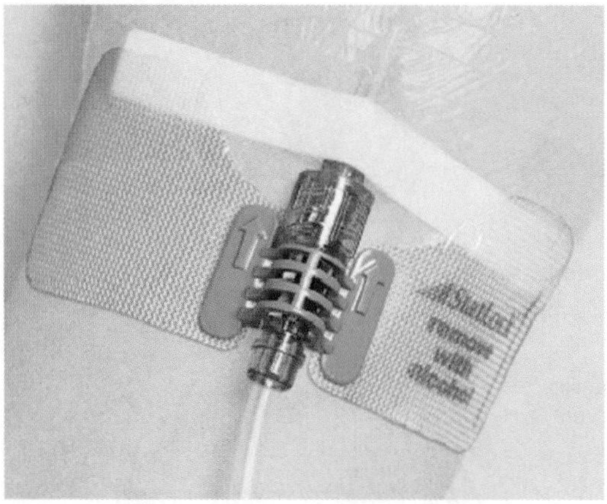

Fig. 20.16 StatLock securement devices enhance peripheral intravenous line dwell time and decrease phlebitis.

to maintain adequate flow of the IV fluids into the cannulated vein, while allowing adequate blood flow around the catheter walls to promote proper hemodilution of the fluid being infused.

Determining the best catheter for the patient early in the therapy provides the best chance of avoiding catheter-related complications. As the duration of therapy increases, decisions regarding the type of infusion device (short peripheral, midline, PICC, or central venous catheter) should be explored. Guidelines such as flow charts and algorithms are available to help in these decisions (Sou, McManus, Mifflin, et al., 2017).

SECUREMENT OF A PERIPHERAL INTRAVENOUS LINE

Catheters must be stabilized for easy monitoring and evaluation of the access site; to promote delivery of therapy; and to prevent damage, dislodgement, or migration of the catheter (Infusion Nurses Society, 2016)

To maintain the integrity of the IV line, adequate protection of the site is required. The catheter hub is firmly secured at the puncture site with a transparent dressing and commercial securement device (e.g., StatLock; Fig. 20.16) or clear nonallergenic tape. Transparent dressings are ideal because the insertion site is easily observed. Minimal tape should be used at the puncture site and on about 1 to 2 inches of skin beyond the site to avoid obscuring the insertion site for early detection of infiltration. The catheter insertion site and 1 to 2 inches along the vein proximal to the site should be readily visible so that the area can be monitored for signs of infiltration, irritation, or leakage.

Current guidelines recommend minimal use of additional tape or securement methods at the PIV site (Infusion Nurses Society, 2016). Plastic site protectors, improvised or commercial, are not recommended. These devices can lead to catheter dislodgement and can cause injury to patients.

It is important to safely secure the IV tubing to prevent infants and children from becoming entangled in the tubing and from accidentally pulling out the catheter or needle. Taping of the IV tubing should not obscure visibility of the catheter site.

Finger and toe areas are left unconcealed by dressings or tape to allow for assessment of circulation. The thumb is never immobilized because of the danger of contractures with prolonged limitation of movement. An extremity should never be encircled with tape, as this can become an unintentional tourniquet if the IV infiltrates. The use of roll gauze, self-adhering stretch bandages (Coban), and ACE bandages is not recommended because these can cause constriction and hide signs of infiltration.

> **! NURSING ALERT**
>
> Opaque covering should be avoided; however, if any type of opaque covering is used to secure the IV line, the insertion site and extremity distal to the site should be visible to detect an infiltration. If these sites are not visible, they must be checked frequently to detect problems early.

Traditionally, padded boards and splints have been used to partially immobilize the joint nearest to the PIV site. Padded boards and splints and restraints were appropriate when metal needles were used for venous access, in order to prevent the sharp tip of the needle from puncturing the vessel, especially at a joint. With the more recent use of soft, pliable catheters, arm or leg boards may not be necessary and have several disadvantages. They obscure the IV site, can constrict the extremity, may excoriate the underlying tissue and promote infection, can cause a contracture of a joint, restrict useful movement of the extremity, and are generally uncomfortable. No research has been conducted to demonstrate the proposed benefit of increasing dwell time and maintaining patency of the IV line. Adequate securement should eliminate the need for padded boards in most circumstances. Older children who are alert and cooperative can usually be trusted to protect the IV site.

SAFETY CATHETERS AND NEEDLELESS SYSTEMS

Needlestick injuries are a serious risk for nurses and other health care professionals who provide IV therapy to their patients. Current technologies, including safety catheters and needleless systems, have minimized the risk of exposure to bloodborne pathogens by needlestick injury. Safety catheters use retractable needle mechanisms to prevent accidental needlesticks when inserting over-the-needle PIV catheters.

Needleless IV systems are designed to prevent needlestick injuries during administration of IV push medications and IV piggyback medications. Needleless IV systems rely on connectors that function as caps. These connectors maintain a closed system until activated by insertion of a syringe or IV tubing set, which opens the fluid pathway. The needleless connectors of most needleless systems have an internal mechanical valve that controls how fluid flows through the connector when IV tubing or syringe is attached. There are three general types of needleless systems, based on how fluid is displaced within the connector. Each system has benefits and risks (Hadaway, 2012):

- Negative displacement systems (including blunt-tip cannulas for use with pre-slit injection caps)—fluid flows straight through the middle of the connector (Fig. 20.17A); these systems can allow a reflux or backflow of blood from the IV catheter when a syringe or IV tubing is disconnected, creating a potential for catheter occlusion.
- Positive displacement systems—the mechanical valve within the connector keeps a small amount of IV fluid in a tiny reservoir separate from the fluid pathway; when disconnecting the syringe or IV tubing, this reserve fluid is automatically released into the connector housing to prevent backflow of blood (see Fig. 20.17B). This action prevents inadvertent catheter occlusion but may allow trace amounts of incompatible fluids to remain within the connector.
- Neutral displacement systems—the mechanical valve within the connector is designed to prevent backflow of blood without the need for a fluid reservoir within the connector (see Fig. 20.17C).

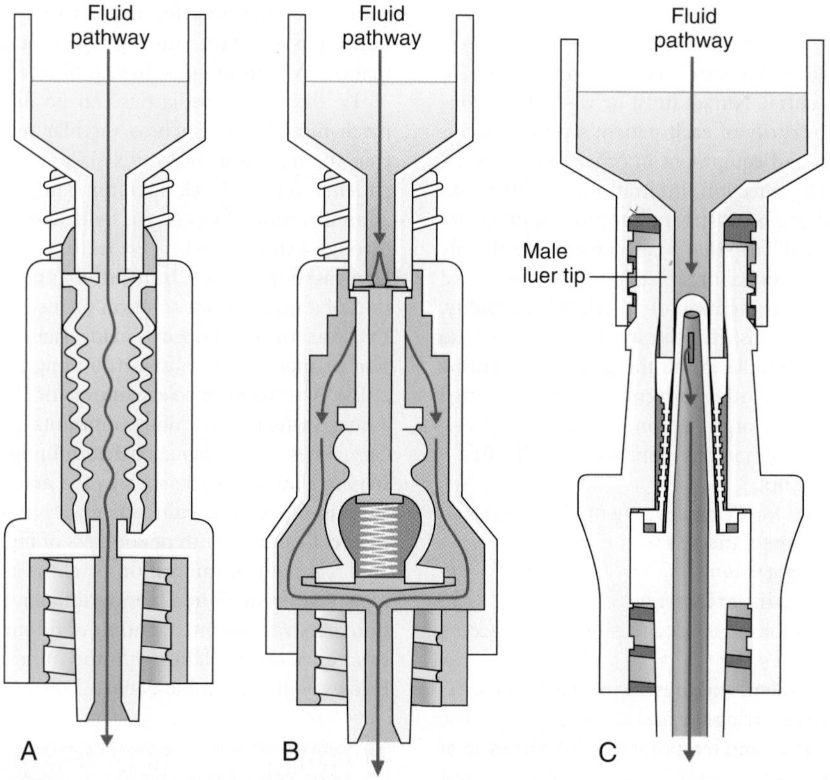

Fig. 20.17 Fluid pathways of needleless connectors. A, Negative displacement. B, Positive displacement. C, Neutral displacement. (**A** and **B,** Copyright by Becton, Dickinson, and Company. Used with permission. **C,** From Hadaway, L. [2012]. Needleless connectors for IV catheters. *American Journal of Nursing, 112*[11], 32–44. Courtesy Lynn Hadaway Associates, Inc.)

Flushing and disconnection procedures are different for each type of system. There is no way to know which type of mechanism is used by simply looking at the connectors. Therefore the nurse must understand the mechanics of the system in use at the institution. Some needleless devices can be used with any tubing, but others require use of an entire brand-specific IV delivery system for compatibility.

! NURSING ALERT

Misconnections of tubing have occurred, resulting in patient deaths. Many needleless IV systems allow other types of tubing, such as blood pressure and oxygen tubing, to connect and instill air directly into the IV line. Before tubing is connected or reconnected to a patient, trace it completely from the patient to the point of origin for verification.

An important potential risk of needleless systems, especially those with mechanical valves, is the possibility of contamination, either on the connector surface or by colonization of the internal valve mechanism. Disinfection of the needleless connector should occur prior to connecting any syringe or IV tubing. Chlorhexidine, 70% isopropyl alcohol, or combination products are all acceptable agents for decontamination, although the time required to adequately disinfect connector surfaces varies between agents. Disinfection is a two-step process: scrubbing the hub, followed by allowing the agent to dry for an appropriate length of time. The time involved in each step of the process depends on the agent used. Nurses should practice strict adherence to their institutional policy for cleansing the connector prior to attaching any syringe or IV tubing. Passive cleansing caps, impregnated with chlorhexidine or 70% isopropyl alcohol, can be applied to needleless connectors when not in use to provide continuous passive disinfection of catheter connectors between uses (Moureau & Flynn, 2015).

INFUSION PUMPS

In infants and children, most IV infusions are delivered via infusion pump in order to accurately administer fluids and medication and minimize the possibility of overloading the circulation. It is important to calculate the amount to be infused in a given length of time, set the infusion rate, and monitor the apparatus frequently (at least every 1 to 2 hours) to make certain that the desired rate is maintained, the integrity of the system remains intact, the venous access site remains intact (free of redness, edema, infiltration, or irritation), and the infusion does not stop.

Smart infusion pump technology provides built-in safety features that can alert nurses when pump settings are outside of programmed parameters, thereby reducing infusion errors and improving patient safety. Smart pump software within the infusion pump is preprogrammed with dose and infusion rate information for commonly used drugs. The smart pump can recognize drug information in its database, check dosing, calculate infusions rates, monitor line pressure, and report errors back to nursing. However, programming the pump for an infusion is a multistep process. The nurse must take great care in ensuring that the pump is properly programmed, especially if the set-up involves secondary infusions or multiple agents (Guiliano, 2018). A hastily programmed pump, bypassed drug libraries, or overridden alerts can result in potential patient safety issues or medication errors. After the pump is programmed, careful periodic reassessments should be performed by the nurse.

MAINTENANCE

Nurses play a significant role in the care and maintenance of IV devices, both peripheral and central. Nurses must be vigilant in monitoring and maintaining the integrity of each patient's venous access site and all associated supplies and equipment in order to prevent IV therapy–related harm, including infection, infiltration, phlebitis, and pain. The occurrence of IV-related bloodstream infections is of particular concern because of the added harm that it can cause to the already hospitalized patient. Many professional organizations have published evidence-based guidelines for the prevention of IV-related morbidity, especially hospital-acquired infections. Health care organizations also establish care guidelines, called bundles, with the goal of preventing IV therapy–related infections and other adverse events. Although most care bundles are unique to the organization, they are always evidence-based and include some common components (Hugull, 2017):

- Decision to insert a device or not
- Device selection considering, for example, patient characteristics, intended purpose, and duration of therapy
- Good hand hygiene for all caregivers
- Skin asepsis before needle or catheter insertion
- Aseptic nontouch techniques for insertion, use, site and line access, and removal
- Effective stabilization, securement, and dressing of the device
- Actions to maintain antisepsis during use and access
- Decisions about removing PIVs and temporary IV lines as soon as they are no longer needed
- Monitoring of the integrity of the device and side effects of use
- Audit of and feedback on essential components of compliance to individuals and teams

There is growing evidence that care bundles are effective in preventing infections, and the nurse should incorporate institutional bundles into daily practice.

COMPLICATIONS

The same precautions regarding maintenance of asepsis, prevention of infection, and observation for infiltration are carried out with patients of any age. However, infiltration may be more difficult to detect in infants and small children than in adults. The increased amount of subcutaneous fat and the amount of tape used to secure the catheter often obscure the early signs of infiltration. When the fluid appears to be infusing too slowly or ceases to infuse, the usual assessment for obstruction within the apparatus—tubing kinks, roller clamps, shutoff valve, and positioning interference (e.g., a bent elbow)—often locates the difficulty. When these actions fail to detect the problem, it may be necessary to carefully remove some of the dressing to obtain a clear view of the venipuncture site. Dependent areas, such as the palm and undersides of the extremity or the occiput and behind the ears, should be examined because infiltrations in these areas may not be readily visible.

Whenever possible, the hospital identification (ID) bracelet should not be placed on the same extremity where a peripheral IV is located. If the ID band fits too snugly, it can act like a tourniquet, preventing adequate venous return, resulting in serious circulatory impairment. To check for return blood flow through the catheter, the tubing is removed from the infusion pump, and the bag is lowered below the level of the infusion site. Using this maneuver, a backflash of blood can usually be observed at the catheter site, if the IV is patent. A good blood return, or lack thereof, is not always an indicator of infiltration in small infants or in smaller-gauge catheters. Flushing the catheter and observing for edema, redness, or streaking along the vein are also appropriate methods for assessment of IV patency. Resistance during flushing or resistance during aspiration for blood return may indicate that the IV infusion may have infiltrated surrounding tissue.

IV therapy in pediatrics can be difficult to maintain because of mechanical factors such as vascular trauma resulting from the catheter, the insertion site, vessel size, vessel fragility, pump pressure, the patient's activity level, operator skill and insertion technique, forceful administration of boluses of fluid, and infusion of irritants or vesicants through a small vessel. These factors increase the risk of infiltration and extravasation injuries. **Infiltration** is defined as inadvertent administration of a nonvesicant solution or medication into surrounding tissue. **Extravasation** is defined as inadvertent administration of vesicant solution or medication into surrounding tissue (Infusion Nurses Society, 2016). A **vesicant** or **sclerosing agent** causes varying degrees of cellular damage when even minute amounts escape into surrounding tissue. Guidelines are available for determining the severity of tissue injury by staging characteristics, such as the amount of redness, blanching, the amount of swelling, pain, the quality of pulses below infiltration, capillary refill, and warmth or coolness of the area (Nickel, 2019).

Treatment of infiltration or extravasation varies according to the type of vesicant. Guidelines outlining nursing management of infiltration or extravasation, including antidotes that could be used in specific situations, are available from the Infusion Nurses Society (Doellman, Hadaway, Bowe-Geddes, et al., 2009).

! NURSING ALERT

When infiltration or extravasation is observed (signs include erythema, pain, edema, blanching, streaking on the skin along the vein, and darkened area at the insertion site), immediately stop the infusion, elevate the extremity, notify the provider, and initiate the ordered treatment as soon as possible. Remove the intravenous (IV) line when it is no longer needed (e.g., after infusing an antidote).

Phlebitis, or inflammation of the vessel wall, may also develop in children receiving IV therapy. There are three types of phlebitis: mechanical (caused by rapid infusion rate, manipulation of the IV), chemical (caused by medications), and bacterial (caused by staphylococcal organisms). The initial sign of phlebitis is erythema (redness) at the insertion site. Pain may or may not be present. Incidence of phlebitis can be minimized by use of conscientious asepsis at site of PIV placement, adequate securement of site to minimize mechanical phlebitis, awareness of medications prone to causing phlebitis and adjusting infusion rates accordingly, and monitoring PIV sites for early signs of phlebitis (Higginson, 2011).

! NURSING ALERT

The most effective ways to prevent infection of an intravenous (IV) site are to cleanse hands between each patient, wear gloves when inserting a catheter, and closely inspect the insertion site and physical condition of the dressing. Proper education of the patient and family regarding signs and symptoms of an infected site can help prevent infections from going unnoticed.

REMOVAL OF A PERIPHERAL INTRAVENOUS LINE

When the time comes to discontinue an IV infusion, many children are distressed by the thought of catheter removal. Therefore they need a careful explanation of the process and suggestions for helping. Encouraging children to remove or help remove the tape from the site provides them with a measure of control and often fosters their cooperation. The procedure consists of turning off any pump apparatus, occluding the IV tubing, removing the tape, pulling the catheter out of the vessel in the opposite direction of insertion, and exerting firm pressure at the site. A dry dressing (adhesive bandage strip) is placed over the puncture site. The use of adhesive-removal pads can decrease the pain of tape removal, but the skin should be washed after use to avoid irritation. To remove transparent dressings (e.g., OpSite, Tegaderm), pull the opposing edges parallel to the skin to loosen the bond. Hand sanitizer can also be applied over the top of the transparent dressing to help loosen the adhesive and allow the dressing to come off more easily. Inspect the catheter tip after removal, to ensure that the catheter is intact and that no portion remains in the vein.

When removing the needle from an implanted port, the line should be flushed with 5 ml of heparin, 100 units/ml, before removal of the needle, to ensure patency during the interim between accesses.

Nontunneled central lines can be removed by specially trained nurses with orders by the provider. Tunneled lines and implanted ports should be removed by the surgical team.

! NURSING ALERT

Consider the child's age, development, and neurologic status, as well as the predictability of the child (how the child responds to painful treatments), when determining the need for assistance to maintain safety. Manual removal of tape is the preferred method. Only if absolutely necessary should a small cut be made in the tape, using bandage scissors, to facilitate its removal. Before cutting the tape:

- Ensure that all digits are visible.
- Remove any barrier that hinders visibility, such as a protective covering.
- Protect the child's skin and digits by sliding own finger(s) between the tape and the child's skin so that the scissors do not touch the patient.
- Cut the tape on the medial aspect (thumb side) of the extremity.

RECTAL ADMINISTRATION

The rectal route for administration of medications is useful when a child is unable to take oral medications due to vomiting, altered gastrointestinal motility, or altered mental status. Advantages to medication administration via the rectal route include no need to coax a child to swallow unpleasant-tasting medications and relative ease of accessibility for giving medications during an emergency if the patient is unconscious or vomiting and there is no venous access. If the patient is neutropenic, immunosuppressed, or thrombocytopenic, the rectal route may be contraindicated due to the risk of introducing bacteria into the bloodstream.

Some of the drugs available in suppository form are acetaminophen, aspirin, sedatives, analgesics (morphine), antiemetics, and laxatives. Absorption by rectal mucosa is dependent on several factors, including gut motility, amount of time the drug remains in the rectum, and amount of stool present at time of drug administration. The difficulty in using the rectal route is that unless the rectum is empty at the time of insertion, the absorption of the drug may be delayed, diminished, or prevented by the presence of feces. Sometimes the drug is later evacuated, securely surrounded by stool.

When preparing to administer medication by the rectal route, first remove the wrapping on the suppository and lubricate the suppository with warm water (water-soluble jelly may affect medication absorption). Have the child lie on the side with top leg flexed; alternatively, the child can lie prone. Provide developmentally appropriate distraction for the child during the procedure. Rectal suppositories are traditionally inserted with the apex (pointed end) foremost. Reverse contractions or the pressure gradient of the anal canal may help the suppository slip higher into the canal. Using a glove or finger cot, quickly but gently insert the suppository into the rectum beyond both of the rectal sphincters. Then hold the buttocks together firmly to relieve pressure on the anal sphincter until the urge to expel the suppository has passed, which occurs within 5 to 10 minutes. Sometimes the amount of drug ordered is less than the dose available. The irregular shape of most suppositories makes the process of dividing them into a desired dose difficult if not dangerous. If it must be halved, the suppository should be cut lengthwise. However, there is no guarantee that the drug is evenly dispersed throughout the glycerin base.

If medication is administered via a retention enema, the same procedure is used. Drugs given by enema are diluted in the smallest amount of solution possible to minimize the likelihood of being evacuated.

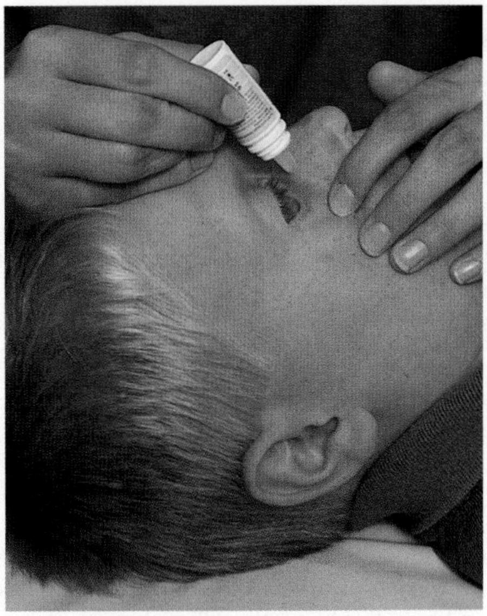

Fig. 20.18 Administering eye drops.

OPTIC, OTIC, AND NASAL ADMINISTRATION

There are few differences in administering eye, ear, and nose medication to children and to adults. The major difficulty is in gaining the child's cooperation. Older children need only an explanation and direction. Although the administration of optic, otic, and nasal medication is not painful, these drugs can cause unpleasant sensations, which can be eliminated with various techniques.

To instill eye medication, place the child supine or sitting with the head extended and ask the child to look up. Use one hand to pull the lower eyelid downward; the hand that holds the dropper rests on the head so that it may move synchronously with the child's head, thus reducing the possibility of trauma to a moving child or dropping medication on the face (Fig. 20.18). When the lower eyelid is pulled down, a small conjunctival sac is formed; apply the solution or ointment to this area, rather than directly on the eyeball. If applying an ointment, start at the inner canthus and move outward. Another effective technique is to pull the lower eyelid down and out to form a cup effect, into which the medication is dropped. Take care not to touch the tip of the dropper to the eyeball. Gently close the eyelids to prevent expression of the medication. Wipe excess medication from the inner canthus outward to prevent contamination to the contralateral eye.

NURSING TIP To reduce unpleasant sensations when administering medications:

- **Eye:** Apply finger pressure to the lacrimal punctum at the inner aspect of the eyelid for 1 minute to prevent drainage of medication to the nasopharynx and the unpleasant "tasting" of the drug.
- **Ear:** Allow medications stored in the refrigerator to warm to room temperature before instillation.
- **Nose:** Position the child with the head hyperextended to prevent strangling sensations caused by medication trickling into the throat rather than up into the nasal passages.

Instilling eye drops in infants can be difficult because they often clench the eyelids tightly closed. One approach is to place the drops in the nasal corner where the eyelids meet. The medication pools in this area, and when the child opens the eyelids, the medication flows onto the conjunctiva. For young children, playing a game can be helpful, such as instructing the child to keep the eyes closed to the count of three and then open them, at which time the drops are quickly instilled. Ointment can be applied by gently pulling down the lower eyelid and placing the ointment in the lower conjunctival sac.

DRUG ALERT

If both eye ointment and drops are ordered, give drops first, wait 3 minutes, and then apply the ointment to allow each drug to work. When possible, administer eye ointments before bedtime or naptime because the child's vision will be blurred temporarily.

Ear drops are instilled with the child in the prone or supine position and the head turned to the appropriate side. To avoid uncomfortable stimulation of vertigo, ensure that ear medications are at room temperature before instilling. For children younger than 3 years old, the external auditory canal is straightened by gently pulling the pinna downward and straight back. The pinna is pulled upward and back in children older than 3 years old. To place the drops deep into the ear canal without contaminating the tip of the dropper, place a disposable ear speculum in the canal and administer the drops through the speculum. Position the dropper so that the drops fall against the side of the ear canal. After instillation, the child should remain lying on the unaffected side for a few minutes. Gentle massage of the area immediately anterior to the ear facilitates the entry of drops into the ear canal. The use of cotton pledgets prevents medication from flowing out of the external canal. However, they should be loose enough to allow any discharge to exit from the ear. Premoistening the cotton with a few drops of medication prevents the wicking action from absorbing the medication instilled in the ear.

The intranasal route can be used for administration of steroids for local relief of the inflammation associated with rhinosinusitis. This route is also being used in emergency departments and in palliative care for the systemic administration of fentanyl for pain, midazolam and ketamine for sedation, lorazepam for seizures, and naloxone for drug overdose (Tucker, Tucker, & Brown, 2018). The intranasal route allows quick absorption of medications across the nasal mucosa, with fairly painless patient preparation and rapid onset of action (Del Pizzo & Callahan, 2014). Intranasal delivery systems include nose drops (low volume, low pressure), intranasal sprays, and atomizers (low volume, high pressure). Nose drops are instilled in the same manner as in the adult patient. Remove mucus from the nose with a clean tissue or a washcloth. Unpleasant sensations associated with medicated nose drops are minimized when care is taken to position the child with the head extended well over the edge of the bed or pillow (Fig. 20.19). Depending on size, infants can be positioned in the football hold (see Fig. 20.3B), in the nurse's arm with the head extended and stabilized between the nurse's body and elbow and the arms and hands immobilized with the nurse's hands, or with the head extended over the edge of the bed or a pillow. When administering a nasal spray, the patient can be either sitting up or lying down. Insert the nasal spray dispenser into the nostril, aiming toward the top of the ear to direct the medication away from the nasal septum and toward the turbinates for rapid absorption. Quickly squeeze the pump sprayer to instill the medication. The patient should inhale slightly as the medication is being delivered. If the patient sniffs, instead of slowly inhaling, the medication will bypass the intended turbinates and end up in the back if the throat, likely resulting in a bad taste and slower absorption. After instillation of the drops or spray, the child should remain in position for 1 minute to allow the medication to come in contact with the nasal surfaces. For intranasal medication administration using an atomizer, the patient can be sitting up or lying down. The atomizer device is attached to the syringe of medication. Maximum volume for intranasal administration is 1 ml per nostril (Tucker et al., 2018). The procedure for administration is similar to that for intranasal spray.

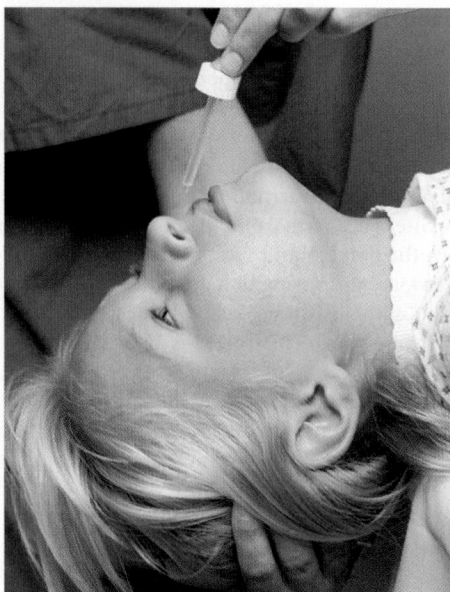

Fig. 20.19 Proper position for instilling nose drops.

AEROSOL THERAPY

Aerosol therapy can be an effective method for administering medication directly into the lower airway (trachea, bronchi, bronchioles). Bronchodilators, steroids, mucolytics, and antibiotics, suspended in particulate form, can be inhaled so that the medication reaches the small airways. This route of administration can be useful in avoiding the systemic side effects of certain drugs and in reducing the amount of drug necessary to achieve the desired effect. Aerosol therapy is particularly challenging in children who are too young to cooperate with controlling the rate and depth of breathing. Administration of this therapy requires skill, patience, and creativity. Because many children with airway diseases, such as asthma, use aerosol therapies on a regular basis, it is important for families to understand the home plan of care, including drugs to use for maintenance and drugs to use for rescue.

DRUG ALERT

Medications can be aerosolized or nebulized with air or with oxygen-enriched gas. Delivery systems include the metered-dose inhaler (MDI) and the nebulizer. The MDI is a self-contained, handheld device that allows for intermittent delivery of a specified amount of medication. Many bronchodilators are available in this form and are successfully used by children with asthma. A spacer device attached to the MDI can help with coordination of breathing and aerosol delivery. It also allows the aerosolized particles to remain in suspension longer. For nebulized administration, a handheld nebulizer discharges a medicated mist through a mouthpiece or a small plastic mask that the child holds over the nose and mouth. To avoid particle deposition in the nose and pharynx, the child is instructed to take slow, deep breaths through an open mouth during the treatment. For home use, an air compressor is necessary to force air through the liquid medication to form the aerosol. Compact, portable units can be obtained from health equipment companies.

Breath sounds and work of breathing should be assessed before and after treatments. Young children who become upset by having a mask held close to the face may become fatigued with fighting the procedure and may appear worse during and immediately after the therapy. It may be necessary to spend a few minutes calming the child after the procedure and allowing the vital signs to return to baseline to accurately assess changes in breath sounds and work of breathing.

FAMILY TEACHING AND HOME CARE

The nurse usually assumes responsibility for preparing families to administer medications at home. The family should understand why the child is receiving the medication and the effects that might be expected, as well as the amount, frequency, and length of time the drug is to be administered. Instruction should be carried out in an unhurried, relaxed manner, preferably in an area away from a busy ward or office.

Instruct the caregiver carefully regarding the correct dosage. Some persons have difficulty understanding medical terminology, and just because they nod or otherwise indicate that they understand, the nurse should not assume that the message is clear. It is important to be certain that they have acceptable devices for measuring the drug. If the drug is packaged with a dropper, syringe, or plastic cup, the nurse should show or mark the point on the device that indicates the prescribed dose and demonstrate how the dose is drawn up into a dropper or syringe, measured, and the bubbles eliminated. To allow an opportunity to demonstrate their understanding of the skills required, caregivers should always perform return demonstration before returning home. This is essential when the drug has potentially serious consequences from incorrect dosage, such as insulin or digoxin, or when more complex administration is required, such as parenteral injections. When teaching a parent to give an injection, the nurse must allot adequate time for instruction and practice.

Home modifications are often necessary because the availability of equipment or assistance can differ from the hospital setting. For example, the parent may need guidance in devising methods that allow one person to hold the child and safely give the drug.

NURSING TIP To administer oral, nasal, or optic medication when only one person is available to hold the child and the child is unable to cooperate, use the following procedure:
- Place child supine on a flat surface (bed, couch, floor).
- Sit facing child so child's head is between operator's thighs and child's arms are under operator's legs.
- Place lower legs over child's legs to restrain lower body, if necessary.
- To administer oral medication, place a small pillow under child's head to reduce risk of aspiration.
- To administer nasal medication, place a small pillow under child's shoulders to aid flow of liquid through nasal passages.

The nurse should clarify with parents the time that the drug is to be administered. For instance, when a drug is prescribed in association with meals, the number of meals that the family is accustomed to eating influences the amount of drug the child receives. Does the family have meals twice a day or five times a day? When a drug is to be given several times during the day, together the nurse and parents can work out a schedule that accommodates the family's routine. This is particularly significant if a drug must be given at equal intervals throughout a 24-hour period. For example, telling parents that the child needs 5 ml of medicine four times a day is subject to misinterpretation, because the parents may routinely schedule the doses at incorrect times. Instead, a preplanned schedule based on 6-hour intervals should be set up with the number of days required for the therapeutic dosage listed. Modification should also be made to accommodate sleep schedules. Written instructions should accompany all drug prescriptions.

NURSING TIP If parents have difficulty reading or if there is a language barrier, use colors and/or pictures to convey instructions. For example, mark each drug with a color and place the appropriate color on a calendar chart or on a drawing of a clock to identify when the drug needs to be given. If a liquid medication and syringe are used, also mark the syringe at the place the plunger needs to be with color-coded tape. Several websites and phone applications are available to help create patient-specific medication calendars.

ALTERNATIVE FEEDING TECHNIQUES

Some children are unable to take nourishment by mouth because of anomalies of the throat, esophagus, or bowel; impaired swallowing capacity; severe debilitation; respiratory distress; or unconsciousness. These children are frequently fed by way of a tube inserted orally or nasally into the stomach (**orogastric [OG]** or **NG gavage**) or duodenum-jejunum (**enteral gavage**) or by a tube inserted directly into the stomach (**gastrostomy**) or jejunum (**jejunostomy**). Such feedings may be intermittent or by continuous drip. Feeding resistance, a problem that may result from any long-term feeding method that bypasses the mouth, is discussed in Chapter 8. During gavage or gastrostomy feedings, infants are given a pacifier. Nonnutritive sucking has several advantages, such as increased weight gain and decreased crying. However, only pacifiers with a safe design can be used to prevent the possibility of aspiration. Using improvised pacifiers made from bottle nipples is not a safe practice.

When a child is concurrently receiving both continuous gastroenteral feedings and parenteral (IV) therapy, the potential exists for inadvertent administration of the enteral formula through the circulatory system. The possibility for harmful error increases when the parenteral solution is a fat emulsion, a milky-appearing substance. Safeguards to prevent this potentially serious error include:

- Be sure that the feeding bag and all enteral tubings are cleaned on a regular basis, according to the manufacturer's recommendations.
- Use enteral-specific connectors (ENFit) that are not compatible with Luer Lock or needleless connections used for IV tubing (Guenter & Lyman, 2016).
- Use a separate, specifically designed enteral feeding pump mounted on a separate pole for continuous-feeding solutions.
- Use specifically designed enteral feeding bags instead of parenteral equipment, such as a burette, to contain the feeding solutions.
- Label all enteral feeding tubing with brightly colored tape or labels.
- Whenever access or connections are made, trace the tubing all the way from the patient to the bag to ensure that the correct tubing source is selected.

NASOGASTRIC, OROGASTRIC, AND GASTROSTOMY ADMINISTRATION

When a child has an indwelling feeding tube or a gastrostomy, oral medications are usually given via that route. An advantage of this method is the ability to administer oral medications around the clock without disturbing the child. A disadvantage is the risk of occluding, or clogging, the tube, especially when giving viscous or incompatible solutions through small-bore feeding tubes. The most important measure to prevent enteral tube occlusions is adequate flushing before and after any medication is instilled (see Nursing Care Guidelines box).

NURSING CARE GUIDELINES

Nasogastric, Orogastric, or Gastrostomy Medication Administration in Children

Use only syringes compatible with the enteral feeding tube; avoid using syringes with Luer Locks, designed for intravenous (IV) medications

Confirm with pharmacist that the medication is suitable to be given through an enteral feeding tube (a drug that is inappropriately given via enteral tube can lead to occluded tubes, decreased drug effect, and increased drug toxicity) (American Society for Parenteral and Enteral Nutrition, 2017):

- Extended-release and enteric-coated medications should not be administered via enteral tube because they may result in inadvertent overdose.
- Some medications, such as lansoprazole delayed-release oral suspension packets, ursodiol, and bulk-forming laxatives cannot be given via enteral feeding route.
- Some medications (i.e., esomeprazole granules) must be administered promptly after they are mixed in water because they deteriorate after only a few minutes and will not be effective.
- Avoid oily medications (e.g., tacrolimus) because they tend to cling to side of tube.
- Some drugs, such as oral iron, warfarin, phenytoin, and digoxin may not be properly absorbed if given through jejunal feeding tubes.
- Medications with high osmolality can cause diarrhea if given via jejunal feeding tube, if not adequately diluted (European Society of Paediatric Gastroenterology, Hepatology, and Nutrition, 2010). Check with pharmacist.

Use elixir or suspension (rather than tablet) preparations of medication whenever possible.

Dilute viscous medication or syrup with a small amount of water if possible.

If administering tablets, crush tablet to a fine powder and dissolve drug in a small amount of warm water. Enteral tubes are easily clogged by incompletely crushed or incompletely dissolved medication.

Never crush enteric-coated or sustained-release tablets or capsules.

Tubing should be flushed with clear water before and after each medication.

Do not add medication directly to the enteral feeding bag.

When administering a medication via nasogastric (NG) tube that is used intermittently (i.e., clamped):

- Check for correct placement of NG or orogastric (OG) tube (see Translating Evidence Into Practice box).
- Flush the NG tube with clear water prior to giving medication.
- Attach medication-filled syringe to the tube and administer the medication.
- Follow the medication with clear water to flush the medication from the tubing, then remove syringe and clamp tubing.

When administering a medication via NG tube with enteral feeding infusing continuously:

- Pause the pump.
- If the feeding tube has medication side port, use this port for administration of medication and any flushes; if the tube does not have a medication port, disconnect the feeding from the NG tube.
- Check for correct placement of NG or OG tube (see Translating Evidence Into Practice box).
- If the medication is not compatible with the enteral formula, attach a syringe filled with clear water and flush the NG tube to remove the formula from the tubing.
- Attach medication-filled syringe to tube and administer the medication.
- Follow the medication with clear water to flush the medication from the tubing before resuming the continuous enteral feeding.

When flushing enteral tubing:

- Always flush with clear water (bottled water, purified water, or tap water, depending on degree of contaminants) (American Society for Parenteral and Enteral Nutrition, 2017).
- Amount of water depends on length and gauge of tubing.
- Before administering any medication, determine amount of water needed by using a syringe to fill completely an unused NG or OG tube with water. Amount of flush solution is usually 1.5 times this volume.
- With certain drug preparations (e.g., suspensions), more fluid may be needed.

If administering more than one drug at the same time, flush tube with clear water between each medication.

GAVAGE FEEDING

Infants and children can be fed simply and safely by a tube passed into the stomach through either the nares or the mouth. The tube can be left in place or inserted and removed with each feeding. In older children, it is usually less traumatic to tape the tube securely to the cheek between feedings. For long-term enteral tube feedings, the tube should be removed and replaced with a new tube at specified intervals according to hospital policy, manufacturer recommendations, specific orders, and the type of tube used. Meticulous hand washing is practiced during the procedure to prevent bacterial contamination of the feeding, especially during continuous feedings.

Preparations

The equipment needed for gavage feeding includes:

- A suitable feeding tube, selected according to the child's size, the viscosity of the solution being fed, and anticipated duration of treatment
- A receptacle for the fluid to be administered; for small amounts, a 10- to 30-ml syringe barrel or Asepto syringe is satisfactory; for

larger amounts, a 60-ml syringe with a catheter tip is more convenient
- A 10-ml syringe to aspirate stomach contents after the tube has been placed
- Water or water-soluble lubricant to lubricate the tube; sterile water is used for infants
- Paper or nonallergenic tape to mark the tube and to attach the tube to the infant's or child's cheek
- pH paper to determine the correct placement in the stomach
- The solution for feeding

Not all feeding tubes are the same. Polyethylene and polyvinylchloride types lose their flexibility and need to be replaced frequently, usually every 3 or 4 days. Polyurethane and silicone tubes remain flexible, so they can remain in place for up to 30 days. Advantages of small-bore tubes include a reduced incidence of pharyngitis, otitis media, aspiration, and discomfort. Disadvantages include difficulty during insertion (may require a stylet or metal guidewire), collapse of the tube during aspiration of gastric contents to test for correct placement, dislodgment during forceful coughing, migration out of position, knotting, occlusion, and unsuitability for thick feedings.

Procedure

Infants are easier to control if they are first wrapped in a mummy restraint (see Fig. 20.4A). Even tiny infants with random movements can grasp and dislodge the tube. Preterm infants do not ordinarily require restraint, but if they do, a small blanket folded across the chest and secured beneath the shoulders is usually sufficient. Be careful that breathing is not compromised.

Whenever possible, the infant should be held and provided with a means for nonnutritive sucking during the procedure to associate the comfort of physical contact with the feeding. When this is not possible, gavage feeding is carried out with the infant or child lying supine or on the right side; the head and chest should be elevated. Feeding the child in a sitting position helps maintain placement of the tube in the lowest position, thus increasing the likelihood of correct placement in the stomach.

Although the most accurate method for testing tube placement is radiography, this practice is not always possible before each feeding. Research indicates that bedside assessment of gastrointestinal aspirate color and pH is useful in predicting feeding tube placement (see Translating Evidence Into Practice box). If doubt exists regarding correct placement, consult the provider. The Nursing Care Guidelines box describes the procedure for gavage feeding.

TRANSLATING EVIDENCE INTO PRACTICE

Confirming Nasogastric Tube Placement in Pediatric Patients

Ask the Question

PICOT Question

In children, how should correct placement of nasogastric (NG) tubes be assessed during hospitalization?

Search for the Evidence

Search Strategies

Search selection criteria included English-language, research-based articles and children and adolescents requiring NG tube placement. Search areas included aspirate, auscultation and radiology methods, NG tube length prediction methods, age-related height-based methods, and accurate NG tube placement. Searches excluded newborns and preterm infants.

Databases Used

PubMed, Cochrane Collaboration, MDConsult, Joanna Briggs Institute, Agency for Healthcare Research and Quality National Guideline Clearinghouse, TRIP Database Plus, PedsCCM, BestBETS

Critical Appraisal of the Evidence

Studies compared various methods used to evaluate correct placement of the NG tube.

Accurate Nasogastric Tube Length Measurement

- Children 8 years, 4 months old or younger: Use age-related height-based equation for NG length predictions.
- Children older than 8 years, 4 months old, short stature, or when you cannot obtain accurate height: Use nose-ear–midway to umbilicus (NEMU) (Beckstrand, Cirgin Ellett, & McDaniel, 2007).
- Use of the nose-ear-xyphoid (NEX) method resulted in increased risk of misplaced tubes (Irving, Rempel, Lyman, et al., 2018).

Radiographs

- Although abdominal x-ray provides confirmation of enteral tube location, the results can sometimes be equivocal. In addition, this method cannot be used for ongoing, frequent placement verification basis due to the risk of radiation exposure to the child (Irving, Lyman, Northington, et al., 2014). Alternate methods of verification have evidence-based support in the literature (Cincinnati Children's Hospital Medical Center, 2011; Emergency Nurses Association, 2019).

Nonradiologic Verification Methods

- A pH of 5 or less supports that the tip of the tube is in the gastric location (Ellett, Croffie, Cohen, et al., 2005; Gilbertson, Rogers, & Ukoumunne, 2011; Nyqvist, Sorell, & Ewald, 2005; Society of Pediatric Nurses Clinical Practice Committee, Society of Pediatric Nurses Research Committee, & Longo, 2011).
- A pH greater than 5 does not reliably predict correct distal tip location. This may indicate respiratory or esophageal placement or the presence of medications to suppress acid secretion. Gastric aspirate pH means are statistically significantly lower compared with means from intestinal and respiratory pH aspirates (Ellett et al., 2005; Gilbertson et al, 2011; Society of Pediatric Nurses Clinical Practice Committee et al., 2011).

Visual Inspection of Aspirate

- Visual inspection is less accurate than pH to confirm placement. Aspirate colors are specific to the intended placement location. Gastric contents are clear, off-white, or tan or may be brown-tinged if blood is present. Respiratory secretions may look the same. Intestinal contents are often bile stained, light to dark yellow, or greenish-brown (Society of Pediatric Nurses Clinical Practice Committee et al., 2011).

Enzyme Testing

- Aspirate testing of enzyme levels for bilirubin, pepsin, and trypsin is highly accurate but limited to laboratory assessment (Ellett et al., 2005).

Carbon Dioxide Monitoring

- Carbon dioxide (CO_2) monitoring (capnography or colorimetric capnometry) is as reliable as radiograph for confirmation of gastrointenstinal (GI) versus respiratory placement of NG tubes but cannot distinguish between gastric and duodenal placement (Erzincanli, Zaybak, & Guler, 2017; Miller, 2013).

Continued

TRANSLATING EVIDENCE INTO PRACTICE—cont'd

Confirming Nasogastric Tube Placement in Pediatric Patients

Gastric Auscultation

- Auscultation as a verification tool is not reliable and should not be used without additional methods (Boeykens, Steeman, & Duysburgh, 2014).
- Although evidence shows auscultation alone is not a reliable confirmatory test, it is still widely used by nurses for evaluation of enteral tube placement (Bourgault, Heath, Hooper, et al., 2015; Lyman, Kemper, Northington, et al., 2016; Metheny, Stewart, & Mills, 2012; Northington, Lyman, Guenter, et al., 2017).
- Using aspirate and nonaspirate NG tube placement verification methods in combination increases the likelihood for accurate NG tube placement to 97% to 99%, similar to the chest radiography gold standard of 99% (Ellett et al., 2005; Society of Pediatric Nurses Clinical Practice Committee et al., 2011).

Electromagnetic Device

- An electromagnetic tracing device demonstrated more than 94% accuracy in enteral feeding tubes in a study of both adults and children (Powers, Luebbehusen, Aguirre, et al., 2018); however, the device requires special training and considerable expertise for proper use (Metheny & Meert, 2017) and cannot detect enteral tubes smaller than 8 French (Bourgault et al., 2015; Bryant, Phang, &Abrams, 2015).

Apply the Evidence: Nursing Implications

There is **good evidence** with **strong recommendations** (Guyatt, Oxman, Vist, et al., 2008) that a combination of verification methods to confirm NG tube placement will reduce the required number of x-rays in children (Society of Pediatric Nurses Clinical Practice Committee et al., 2011). These methods include pH testing and visual inspection of the pH aspirate. There is also good evidence that improving the accuracy of predicting NG tube length before insertion will enhance the precision of successful NG tube placement. Auscultation is used in combination with other NG tube verification methods. Further investigation of additional noninvasive, user-friendly, portable verification methods, including ultrasound and electromagnetic tracer, is warranted (Irving et al., 2018; Powers, Luebbehusen, Spitzer, et al., 2011).

Quality and Safety Competencies: Evidence-Based Practice[a]

Knowledge

Differentiate clinical opinion from research and evidence-based summaries.

Describe the various verification methods to confirm NG tube placement.

Skills

Base individualized care plan on patient values, clinical expertise, and evidence.

Integrate evidence into practice by using the techniques for NG and orogastric (OG) tube placement verification in clinical care.

Attitudes

Value the concept of evidence-based practice as integral to determining best clinical practice.

Appreciate the strengths and weakness of evidence for confirming NG tube placement.

References

Beckstrand, J., Cirgin, Ellett, M, L., & McDaniel, A. (2007). Predicting the internal distance to the stomach for positioning nasogastric and orogastric feeding tubes in children. *Journal of Advanced Nursing, 59*, 274–289.

Boeykens, K., Steeman, E., & Duysburgh, I. (2014). Reliability of pH measurement and the ascultatory method to confirm the position of a nasogastric tube. *International Journal of Nursing Studies, 51*, 1427–1433.

Bourgault, A. M., Heath, J., Hooper, V., Sole, M. L., & Nesmith, E. G. (2015). Methods used by critical care nurses to verify feeding tube placement in clinical practice. *Critical Care Nurse, 35*(1), e1–e7.

Bryant, V., Phang, J., & Abrams, K. (2015). Verifying placement of small-bore feeding tubes: Electromagnetic device images versus abdominal radiographs. *American Journal of Critical Care, 24*, 525–530.

Cincinnati Children's Hospital Medical Center. (2011). Confirmation of nasogastric/orogastric tube (NGT/OGT) placement—BeST evidence statement. Retrieved from https://www.childrensmn.org/departments/webrn/pdf/ng-og-verification-clinical-standard-preview-2015.pdf .

Ellett, M. L., Croffie, J. M., Cohen, M. D., et al. (2005). Gastric tube placement in young children. *Clinical Nursing Research, 14*(3), 238–252.

Emergency Nurses Association. (2019). Clinical practice guideline: Gastric tube placement verification. *Journal of Emergency Nursing, 45*(3) 306.e1–306.e19.

Erzincanli, S., Zaybak, A., & Guler, A. (2017). Investigation of the efficacy of colorimetric capnometry method used to verify the correct placement of the nasogastric tube. *Intensive & Critical Care Nursing, 38*, 46–52.

Gilbertson, H. R., Rogers, E. J., & Ukoumunne, O. C. (2011). Determination of a practical pH cutoff level for reliable confirmation of nasogastric tube placement. *Journal of Parenteral and Enteral Nutrition, 35*(4), 540–544.

Guyatt, G. H., Oxman, A. D., Vist, G. E., et al. (2008). GRADE: An emerging consensus on rating quality of evidence and strength of recommendations. *British Medical Journal, 336*(7650), 924–926.

Irving, S. Y., Lyman, B., Northington, L., et al. (2014). Nasogastric tube placement and verification in children: Review of the current literature. *Critical Care Nurse, 34*(3), 67–78.

Irving, S. Y., Rempel, G., Lyman, B., Sevilla, W. M., Northington, L., & Guenter, P. (2018). Pediatric nasogastric tube placement and verification: Best practice recommendations from the NOVEL project. *Nutrition in Clinical Practice, 33*(6), 921–927.

Lyman, B., Kemper, C., Northington, L., et al. (2016). Use of temporary enteral access devices in hospitalized neonatal and pediatric patients in the United States. *Journal of Parenteral and Enteral Nutrition, 40*(4), 574–580.

Metheny, N. A., & Meert, K. L. (2017). Update on effectiveness of an electromagnetic feeding tube-placement device in detecting respiratory placements. *American Journal of Critical Care, 26*, 157–161.

Metheny, N. A., Stewart, B. J., & Mills, A. C. (2012). Blind insertion of feeding tubes in intensive care units: A national survey. *American Journal of Critical Care, 21*(5) 352–60.

Miller, S. L. (2013). Capnometry vs pH testing in nasogastric tube placement. *Gastrointestinal Nursing, 9*(2), 30.

Northington, L., Lyman, B., Guenter, P., et al. (2017). Current practices in home management of nasogastric tube placement in pediatric patients: A survey of parents and homecare providers. *Journal of Pediatric Nursing, 33*, 46–53.

Nyqvist, K. H., Sorell, A., & Ewald, U. (2005). Litmus tests for verification of feeding tube location in infants: Evaluation of their clinical use. *Journal of Clinical Nursing, 14*(4), 486–495.

Powers, J., Luebbehusen, M., Aguirre, L., et al. (2018). Improved safety and efficacy of small-bore feeding tube confirmation using an electromagnetic placement device. *Nutrition in Clinical Practice, 33*(2), 268–273.

Powers, J., Luebbehusen, M., Spitzer, T., et al. (2011). Verification of an electromagnetic device compared with abdominal radiograph to predict accuracy of feeding tube placement. *Journal of Parenteral and Enteral Nutrition, 35*(4), 535–539.

Society of Pediatric Nurses Clinical Practice Committee, Society of Pediatric Nurses Research Committee, & Longo, M. A. (2011). Best evidence: Nasogastric tube placement verification. *Journal of Pediatric Nursing,* 26(4), 373–376.

[a]Adapted from the Quality and Safety Education for Nurses website at http://www.qsen.org.

NURSING CARE GUIDELINES

Nasogastric Tube Feedings in Children

Place child supine with head slightly hyperflexed or in a sniffing position (nose pointed toward ceiling).

Measure the tube for approximate length of insertion and mark the point with a small piece of tape.

Consider using lidocaine nasal spray to numb the nostril before tube insertion.

Insert a tube that has been lubricated with sterile water or water-soluble lubricant through either the mouth or one of the nares to the predetermined mark. Because most young infants are obligatory nose breathers, insertion through the mouth causes less distress and helps stimulate sucking. In older infants and children, the tube is passed through the nose and alternated between nostrils. An indwelling tube is almost always placed through the nose.

- When using the nose, slip the tube along the base of the nose and direct it straight back toward the occiput.
- When entering through the mouth, direct the tube toward the back of the throat (see Fig. 20.20B).
- If the child can swallow on command, synchronize passing the tube with swallowing.

Confirm placement (see Translating Evidence Into Practice: Confirming Nasogastric Tube Placement in Pediatric Patients box).

Stabilize the tube by holding or taping it to the cheek, not to the forehead, because of possible damage to the nostril. To maintain correct placement, measure and record the amount of tubing extending from the nose or mouth to the distal port when the tube is first positioned. Recheck this measurement before each feeding.

Warm the formula to room temperature. Do not microwave!

For bolus feeds: pour formula into the barrel of the syringe attached to the feeding tube. To start the flow, give a gentle push with the plunger but then remove the plunger and allow the fluid to flow into the stomach by gravity. The rate of flow should not exceed 5 ml every 5 to 10 minutes in premature and very small infants and 10 ml/min in older infants and children to prevent nausea and regurgitation. The rate is determined by the diameter of the tubing and the height of the reservoir containing the feeding and is regulated by adjusting the height of the syringe. A usual feeding may take 15 to 30 minutes to complete.

Flush the tube with sterile water (1 or 2 ml for small tubes to 5 to 15 ml or more for large ones) to clear it of formula, or see discussion of flushing for administering medication through nasogastric (NG) tubes in the Nursing Care Guidelines box earlier in this chapter.

Cap or clamp indwelling tubes to prevent loss of feeding.

If the tube is to be removed, first pinch it firmly to prevent escape of fluid as the tube is withdrawn. Withdraw the tube quickly.

Position the child with the head elevated 30 to 45 degrees or on the right side for 30 to 60 minutes in the same manner as after any infant feeding to minimize the possibility of regurgitation and aspiration. If the child's condition permits, burp the youngster after the feeding.

Record the feeding, including the type and amount of residual, the type and amount of formula, and how it was tolerated.

For most infant feedings, any amount of residual fluid aspirated from the stomach is re-fed to prevent electrolyte imbalance, and the amount is subtracted from the prescribed amount of feeding. For example, if the infant is to receive 30 ml and 10 ml is aspirated from the stomach before the feeding, the 10 ml of aspirated stomach contents is re-fed along with 20 ml of feeding. Another method can be used in children. If residual fluid is more than one-fourth of the last feeding, return the aspirate and recheck in 30 to 60 minutes. When residual fluid is less than one-fourth of the last feeding, give the scheduled feeding. If large amounts of aspirated fluid persist and the child is due for another feeding, notify the practitioner.

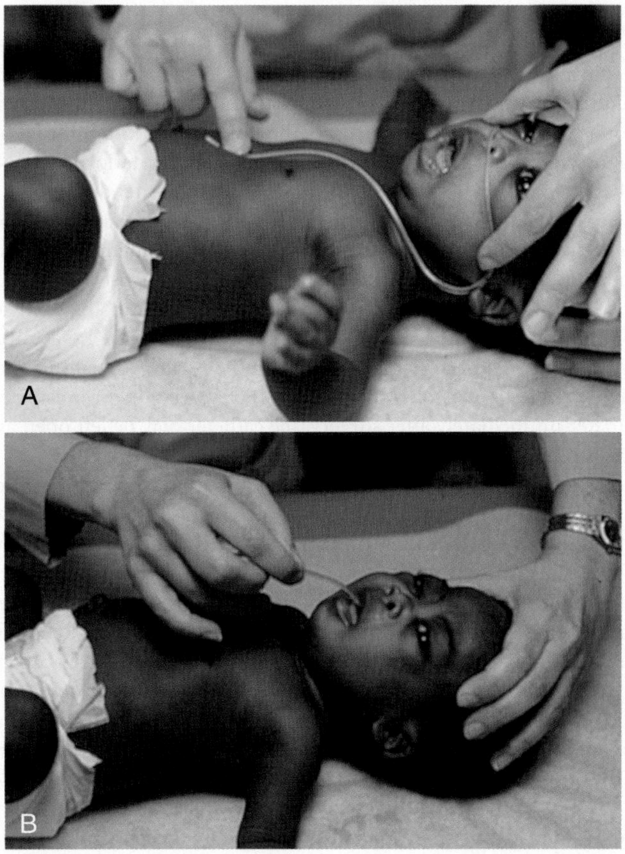

Fig. 20.20 Gavage feeding. **A,** Measuring the tube for orogastric feeding from the tip of the nose to the earlobe and to the midpoint between the end of the xiphoid process and the umbilicus. **B,** Inserting the tube.

Most NG tubes are placed at the bedside by nurses. Proper placement of the tube is essential, and incorrectly placed tubes can result in significant harm to the patient. Correct determination of the length of the tube is a crucial step in the placement procedure. Studies evaluating NG and OG tube length in infants and children found that age-specific methods for predicting the distance based on height is a more accurate estimate of internal distance to the stomach (Beckstrand, Cirgin Ellett, & McDaniel, 2007; Ellett, Cohen, Perkins, et al., 2012), but the calculations are complex and not readily accessible. A convenient and reliable morphologic measurement, the nose-ear–midway to umbilicus (NEMU) span, approached the accuracy of the age-specific prediction equations and is easy to use in a clinical setting (Ellett et al., 2012) (Fig. 20.20A) (see Nursing Care Guidelines box). Research supports radiographs as the gold standard for confirmation of enteral tube placement. Additional methods to check placement, all of which can be done at the bedside, include visual confirmation of aspirate and pH testing of aspirate. Although auscultation is still widely used, multiple sources have documented that it is not an accurate method to confirm enteral tube placement.

NURSING TIP: Enteral feeding tubes may become occluded by debris from medications and/or formulas. Best practice guidelines are aimed at preventing occlusions by adequately flushing between medications and before and after feedings. However, when a feeding tube does become clogged, research shows that warm water is the best choice for initial attempts to unclog (American Society for Parenteral and Enteral Nutrition, 2017). If initial attempts to unclog using water are unsuccessful, a solution of pancreatic enzymes (such as Creon) or commercially available enzyme declogging kits are recommended as a second-line option. Carbonated drinks and cranberry juice are not recommended because these liquids can change the pH of the clogging debris and worsen the occlusion (American Society for Parenteral and Enteral Nutrition, 2017).

GASTROSTOMY FEEDING

Feeding by way of gastrostomy tube, or G-tube, is often used for children in whom passage of a tube through the mouth, pharynx, esophagus, and cardiac sphincter of the stomach is contraindicated or impossible. It is also used to avoid the constant irritation of an NG tube in children who require tube feeding over an extended period. A gastrostomy tube may be placed with the child under general anesthesia or percutaneously using an endoscope with the patient sedated and under local anesthesia (percutaneous endoscopic gastrostomy [PEG]). The tube is inserted through the abdominal wall into the stomach about midway along the greater curvature and secured by a purse-string suture. The stomach is anchored to the peritoneum at the operative site. The gastrostomy tube can be a Foley, wingtip, or mushroom catheter. Immediately after surgery, the catheter may be left open and attached to gravity drainage for 24 hours or more.

Postoperative care of the wound site is directed toward prevention of infection and irritation. Cleanse the area with soap and water, then dry thoroughly, at least daily or as often as needed to keep the area free of drainage. After healing, meticulous care is needed to keep the area surrounding the tube clean and dry to prevent excoriation and infection. Exercise care to prevent excessive tension on the catheter that might cause widening of the opening and subsequent leakage of highly irritating gastric juices. Use barrier ointments such as zinc oxide, and alcohol-free skin barrier film to control leakage; add absorptive powders and pectin-based skin barrier wafers if skin irritation is present (Townley, Wincentak, Krog, et al., 2018). Secure the tube to the abdomen using a commercial stabilizer, polyurethane foam, or the H tape method and leave a small loop of tubing at the exit site to prevent tension on the site.

Granulation tissue may grow around a gastrostomy site (Fig. 20.21). This moist, beefy red tissue is not a sign of infection. However, if it continues to grow, the excess moisture can irritate the surrounding skin. Recommendations for management of hypergranulation include using triamcinolone cream (0.5%) three times daily, applying silver nitrate, stabilizing the tube, and keeping the peristomal area dry by applying polyurethane foam (Fuchs, 2017; Townley et al., 2018). Hydrogen peroxide should not be used because it may dry the tissue too much, leading to additional damage.

For children who require long-term enteral feeding, a low-profile, **skin-level** gastrostomy device (e.g., MIC-KEY, Bard Button) offers several advantages. The small, flexible silicone device protrudes slightly from the abdomen, is cosmetically pleasing, affords increased comfort and mobility to the child, is easy to care for, and is fully immersible in water. The one-way valve at the proximal end minimizes reflux and eliminates the need for clamping. However, the skin-level device requires a well-established gastrostomy site and is more expensive than the conventional tube (Hueschkel, Gottrand, Devarajan, et al., 2015). In addition, the valve may become clogged. When functioning, the valve prevents air from escaping; therefore the child may require frequent bubbling. Some skin-level devices require a special tube to be able to decompress the stomach (to check residual or release air). With some devices, during feedings, the child must remain still, because the tubing easily disconnects from the opening if the child moves. With other devices, extension tubing can be securely attached to the opening (Fig. 20.22). The feeding is instilled at the other end of the tubing in a manner similar to that for a regular gastrostomy. The extension tubing may also have a separate medication port. Both the feeding and the medication ports have plugs attached.

Feeding of water, formula, or pureed foods is carried out in the same manner and rate as for gavage feeding. A mechanical pump may be used to regulate the volume and rate of feeding. After feedings, the infant or child is positioned on the right side or in the Fowler position, and the tube may be clamped or left open and suspended between feedings, depending on the child's condition. A clamped tube allows more mobility but is appropriate only if the child can tolerate intermittent feedings without vomiting or prolonged backup of feeding into the tube. Sometimes a Y tube is used to allow for simultaneous decompression during feeding. If a Foley catheter is used as the gastrostomy tube, apply very slight tension. The tube is securely taped to maintain the balloon at the gastrostomy opening and prevent leakage of gastric contents and the tube's progression toward the pyloric sphincter, where it may occlude the stomach outlet. As a precaution, the length of the tube is measured postoperatively and then remeasured each shift to be certain it has not slipped. The nurse can make a mark above the skin level to further ensure its placement. When the gastrostomy tube is no longer needed, it is removed; the skin opening usually closes spontaneously by contracture.

NASODUODENAL AND NASOJEJUNAL TUBES

Children at high risk for regurgitation or aspiration such as those with gastroparesis, mechanical ventilation, or brain injuries may require placement of a postpyloric feeding tube. A trained provider inserts the nasoduodenal or nasojejunal tube because of the risk of misplacement and potential for perforation in tubes requiring a stylet. Accurate placement is verified by radiography. Small-bore tubes may clog easily. Flush the tube when feeding is interrupted, before and after medication administration, and routinely every 4 hours or as directed by

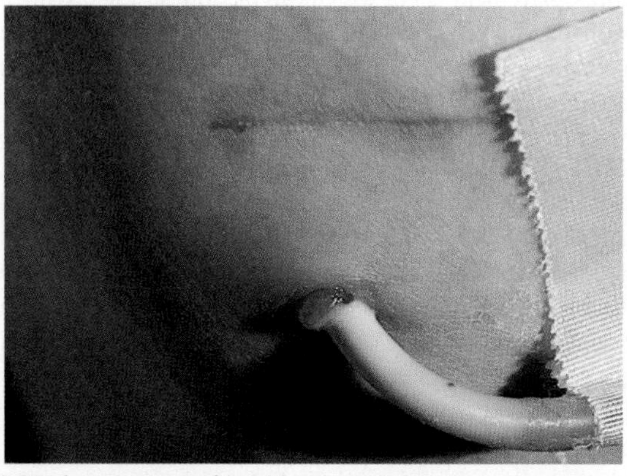

Fig. 20.21 Appearance of healthy granulation tissue around a stoma.

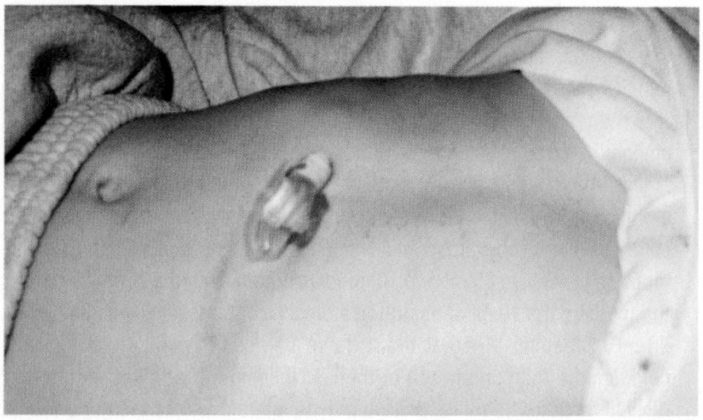

Fig. 20.22 Child with a low-profile gastrostomy device (MIC-KEY), which provides for secure attachment of extension tubing to the gastrostomy opening.

institutional policy. Tube replacement should be considered monthly to ensure optimal tube patency. Continuous feedings are delivered by a mechanical pump to regulate their volume and rate. Bolus feeds are contraindicated. Tube displacement is suspected in children showing signs of feeding intolerance, such as vomiting. In these cases, stop the feedings and notify the provider. Some medications cannot be administered via postpyloric feeding tubes because they will not be absorbed in the duodenum or jejunum.

TOTAL PARENTERAL NUTRITION

TPN provides for the nutritional needs of infants and children whose lives are threatened because feeding by way of the gastrointestinal tract is impossible, inadequate, or hazardous.

TPN therapy involves IV infusion of highly concentrated solutions of protein, glucose, and other nutrients. The solution is infused through conventional IV tubing with a special filter attached to remove particulate matter or microorganisms that may have contaminated the solution. The highly concentrated solutions require infusion into a central vein with sufficient volume and turbulence to allow for rapid dilution. The wide-diameter vessels selected are the superior vena cava and innominate or intrathoracic subclavian veins, approached by way of the external or internal jugular veins. The highly irritating nature of concentrated glucose precludes the use of the small peripheral veins in most instances. However, dilute glucose–protein hydrolysates that are appropriate for infusing into peripheral veins are being used with increasing frequency. When peripheral veins are used, soybean oil (Intralipid) becomes the major calorie source. For long-term alimentation, central venous catheters are usually used.

The major nursing responsibilities are the same as for any IV therapy and include control of sepsis, monitoring of the infusion rate, and assessment of the patient. The TPN solution must be prepared under rigid aseptic conditions, which is best accomplished by specially trained pharmacists and technicians.

Nurses should change the TPN, lipids, and tubing on a frequent basis. More frequent tubing changes are required for TPN and lipids because these solutions can increase the risk of microbial growth. Meticulous aseptic precautions should be used whenever the line is entered or changed. In most institutions, this is a nursing responsibility, and the procedure is carried out according to hospital protocol.

The TPN infusion is maintained at a constant rate by means of an infusion pump to ensure the proper concentrations of glucose and amino acids. Accurate calculation of the rate is required to deliver a measured amount in a given length of time. Because alterations in flow rate are relatively common, the infusion should be checked frequently to ensure an even, continuous administration. The TPN infusion rate should not be increased or decreased without the provider being informed because alterations can cause hyperglycemia or hypoglycemia.

General assessments, such as vital signs, input and output measurements, and checking results of laboratory tests, facilitate early detection of infection or fluid and electrolyte imbalance. Additional amounts of potassium and sodium chloride are often required in hyperalimentation; therefore observation for signs of potassium or sodium deficit or excess is part of nursing care. This is rarely a problem except in children with reduced renal function or metabolic defects. Hyperglycemia may occur during the first day or two as the child adapts to the high-glucose load of the hyperalimentation solution. Although hyperglycemia occurs infrequently, insulin may be required to help the body adjust. When this occurs, nursing responsibilities include blood glucose testing. To prevent hypoglycemia when the hyperalimentation is discontinued, the rate of the infusion and the amount of insulin are decreased gradually.

FAMILY TEACHING AND HOME CARE

When alternative feedings are needed for an extended period, the family needs to learn how to feed the child with an NG, gastrostomy, or TPN feeding regimen. The same principles apply as discussed earlier in this chapter for compliance, especially in terms of education, and in Chapter 19 for discharge planning and home care. Plan ample time for the family to learn and perform the procedures under supervision before they assume full responsibility for the child's care. Refer the family to community agencies that provide support and practical assistance. The Oley Foundation (http://www.oley.org) is a nonprofit research and education organization that assists persons receiving enteral nutrition and home TPN.

PROCEDURES RELATED TO ELIMINATION

ENEMA

Although not common in pediatrics, enemas are sometimes performed in children: as therapeutic treatment for constipation that has not responded to other measures, for administration of barium contrast during radiologic evaluation of the colon, and occasionally for reduction of intussusception. The procedure for giving an enema to an infant or child does not differ essentially from that for an adult except for the type and amount of fluid administered and the distance for inserting the tube into the rectum (Table 20.8). Depending on the volume, use a syringe with rubber tubing, an enema bottle, or an enema bag.

An isotonic solution is used in children. Plain water is not used because, being hypotonic, it can cause rapid fluid shift and fluid overload. The Fleet enema (pediatric or adult size) is not advised for children because of the harsh action of its ingredients (sodium biphosphate and sodium phosphate). Commercial enemas can be dangerous to patients with megacolon and to dehydrated or azotemic children. The osmotic effect of the Fleet enema may produce diarrhea, which can lead to metabolic acidosis. Other potential complications are extreme hyperphosphatemia, hypernatremia, and hypocalcemia, which may lead to neuromuscular irritability and coma.

NURSING TIP: If prepared saline is not available, the nurse can make some by adding 1 tsp of table salt to 500 ml (1 pint) of tap water.

Because infants and young children are unable to retain the solution after it is administered, the buttocks must be held together for a short time to retain the fluid. The enema is administered and expelled

TABLE 20.8 Administration of Enemas to Children

Age	Amount (ml)	Insertion Distance
Infant	120-240	2.5 cm (1 inch)
2-4 years	240-360	5 cm (2 inches)
4-10 years	360-480	7.5 cm (3 inches)
11 years	480-720	10 cm (4 inches)

while the child is lying with the buttocks over the bedpan and with the head and back supported by pillows. Older children are ordinarily able to hold the solution if they understand what to do and if they are not expected to hold it for too long. The nurse should have the bedpan handy or, for ambulatory children, ensure that the bathroom is available before beginning the procedure. An enema is an intrusive procedure and thus threatening to preschool children; therefore a careful explanation is especially important to ease possible fear.

Antegrade continence enemas (ACEs) are used in the treatment of refractory functional constipation or fecal incontinence. After surgical placement of a cecostomy (an ostomy near the cecum at the proximal end of the large bowel), enema solutions can be administered through the cecostomy, stimulating the bowels to empty "from the top down."

A preoperative bowel preparation solution given orally or through an NG tube is increasingly being used instead of an enema. The polyethylene glycol–electrolyte lavage solution (GoLYTELY) mechanically flushes the bowel without significant absorption, thereby avoiding potential fluid and electrolyte imbalances. NuLYTELY, a modification of GoLYTELY, has the same therapeutic advantages as GoLYTELY and was developed to improve on the taste. Another effective oral cathartic is magnesium citrate solution.

OSTOMIES

Children may require stomas for various health problems. The most frequent causes in infants are necrotizing enterocolitis and imperforate anus and, less often, Hirschsprung disease. In older children, the most frequent causes are inflammatory bowel disease, especially Crohn disease (regional enteritis), and ureterostomies for distal ureter or bladder defects.

Care and management of ostomies in older children differ little from the care of ostomies in adult patients. The major emphasis in pediatric care is preparing the child for the procedure and teaching care of the ostomy to the child and family. The basic principles of preparation are the same as for any procedure (see earlier in the chapter). Simple, straightforward language is most effective together with the use of illustrations and a replica model (e.g., drawing a picture of a child with a stoma on the abdomen and explaining it as "another opening where bowel movements [or any other term the child uses] will come out"). At another time, the nurse can draw a pouch over the opening to demonstrate how the contents are collected. Using a doll to demonstrate the process is an excellent teaching strategy, and special books are available.

Children with ileostomies are fitted immediately after surgery with an appliance to protect the skin from the proteolytic enzymes in the liquid stool. Infants may not be fitted with a pouch in the immediate postoperative period. When stomal drainage is minimal, as is often the case in small or preterm infants, gauze dressing will suffice. Give the parents a choice of caring for the colostomy with or without an appliance. Pediatric appliances are available in a variety of sizes to ensure an adequate fit. Several helpful online resources for parents and children exist through websites of the major ostomy supply companies.

Ostomy equipment consists of a one- or two-piece system with a hypoallergenic skin barrier to maintain peristomal skin integrity. The pouch should be large enough to contain a moderate amount of stool and flatus but not so large as to overwhelm the infant or child. A hydrocolloid backing helps minimize the risk of skin breakdown from moisture trapped between the skin and pouch. Avoid small clips and rubber bands to prevent choking in young children.

Protection of the peristomal skin is a major aspect of stoma care. Well-fitting appliances are important to prevent leakage of contents. Before putting on the appliance, prepare the skin with a skin sealant that is allowed to dry. Then apply stoma paste around the base of the stoma or to the back of the wafer. The sealant and paste work together to prevent peristomal skin breakdown.

In infants with a colostomy left unpouched, skin care is similar to that for any diapered child. However, protect the peristomal skin with a barrier substance (e.g., zinc oxide–based ointment [Sensi-Care] or a mixture of zinc oxide ointment and stoma powder [Stomahesive]). A diaper larger than the one usually worn may be needed to extend upward over the stoma and absorb drainage. If the skin becomes inflamed, denuded, or infected, the care is similar to the interventions used for diaper dermatitis. A zinc-based product helps protect healthy skin, heal excoriated skin, and minimize pain associated with skin breakdown. The skin protectant adheres to denuded, weeping skin. The nurse can apply zinc-based products over topical antifungal and antibacterial agents if infection is present. No-sting barrier film is a skin sealant that has no alcohol base and can be used on open skin without stinging.

With young children, preventing them from pulling off the pouch is also an important consideration. One-piece outfits keep exploring hands from reaching the pouch, and the loose waist avoids any pressure on the appliance. Keeping the child occupied with toys during the pouch change is also helpful. As children mature, encourage their participation in ostomy care. Even preschoolers can assist by holding supplies, pulling paper backings from the appliance, and helping clean the stoma area. Toilet training for bladder control needs to begin at the appropriate time as for any other child.

Older children and adolescents should eventually have total responsibility for ostomy care just as they would for usual bowel function. During adolescence, concerns for body image and the ostomy's impact on intimacy and sexuality emerge. The nurse should stress to teenagers that the presence of a stoma need not interfere with their activities. These youngsters can choose which ostomy equipment is best suited to their needs. Attractively designed and decorated pouch covers are well liked by teenagers.

Children with familial adenomatous polyposis may require a colectomy with ileoanal reservoir to prevent or treat carcinoma of the colon. Peristomal skin care for these children is particularly challenging because of increased liquid stools, increased digestive enzymes that may cause skin breakdown, and the stoma being at skin level rather than raised. Additional care with this condition includes close monitoring of fluid and electrolyte status and increased incidence of bowel obstruction.

An enterostomal therapy nurse specialist is an important member of the health care team and will have additional suggestions and assistance with skin care information and ostomy pouching options. The nurse can obtain further information by contacting the Wound, Ostomy and Continence Nurses Society.[d]

FAMILY TEACHING AND HOME CARE

Because these children are almost always discharged with a functioning colostomy, preparation of the family should begin as early as possible in the hospital. The nurse instructs the family in the application of the device (if used), care of the skin, and appropriate action in case skin problems develop. Early evidence of skin breakdown or stomal complications (such as ribbonlike stools, excessive diarrhea, bleeding, prolapse, or failure to pass flatus or stool) is brought to the attention of the physician, nurse, or stoma specialist. The same principles are applied as discussed earlier in this chapter for compliance, especially in terms of education, and in Chapter 19 for discharge planning and home care.

[d]888-224-9626; http://www.wocn.org.

PROCEDURES FOR MAINTAINING RESPIRATORY FUNCTION

INHALATION THERAPY

Oxygen Therapy

Oxygen is administered for hypoxemia and may be delivered by mask, nasal cannula, face tent, hood, face mask, or ventilator. Oxygen therapy is essential in many pediatric cases, yet unnecessary oxygen delivery can increase hospitalization time and cost (Walsh & Smallwood, 2017). The mode of delivery is selected based on the concentration needed and the child's ability to cooperate in its use. Oxygen therapy is frequently administered in the hospital, although increasing numbers of children are receiving oxygen in the home. Oxygen is dry and therefore must be humidified to prevent damage to the mucosa and dehydration.

Although use is becoming infrequent, oxygen delivered to infants is well tolerated by using a **plastic hood**. At least 7 L/min of flow is necessary to maintain oxygen concentrations and remove the exhaled carbon dioxide. The humidified oxygen should not be blown directly into the infant's face. Older, cooperative infants and children can use a **nasal cannula** or **prongs**, which can supply a concentration of oxygen of about 50%. High-flow nasal cannula (2 to 8 L/min for neonates and 4 to 70 L/min for children) can provide specific oxygen concentration with flow rates capable of meeting the child's inspiratory demand (Walsh & Smallwood, 2017). High-flow nasal cannula may be used to avoid intubation, postextubation, in palliative care, and as a mode of ventilatory support in very low-birth-weight infants. Care with prong size, placement, and maintenance is important to prevent breakdown of the nasal alae.

Oxygen masks are available in pediatric sizes but may not be well tolerated in children, because a snug fit is required to ensure adequate oxygen delivery. Several variations are available with specific flow rates and oxygen concentrations as indicated for patient need. **Oxygen tents** (croup tents) are rarely used today in developed countries. Oxygen concentration is difficult to control, and the child's clothing can become saturated with water from the humidification and cause hypothermia. **Blow-by** oxygen is occasionally attempted for young children who are not able to tolerate a directly applied oxygen delivery device. However, blow-by oxygen therapy provides low, and frequently inconsistent, concentrations of oxygen and should be used only for patients with short-term or intermittent oxygen needs (Walsh & Smallwood, 2017). **Continuous positive airway pressure (CPAP)** systems provides noninvasive mechanical respiratory support through nasal canula or a variety of mask devices for neonates and children in respiratory distress without the need for emergency intubation. CPAP provides regulated, constant pressure to keep airways open and prevent obstruction. **Bilevel positive airway pressure (BiPAP)** provides similar respiratory support but with two different pressure settings for inspiration and expiration. Both CPAP and BiPAP systems can be used during inhaler or nebulizer treatments (Behnke, Lemyre, Czernik, et al., 2019).

DRUG ALERT

Oxygen Toxicity

Prolonged exposure to high oxygen tensions can damage some body tissues and functions. The organs most vulnerable to the adverse effects of excessive oxygenation are the retinas of extremely preterm infants and the lungs of persons at any age.

! NURSING ALERT

Inspect all toys for safety and suitability (e.g., vinyl or plastic, not stuffed items that absorb moisture and are difficult to keep dry). The high-level oxygen environment makes any source of sparks (e.g., mechanical or electrical toys) a potential fire hazard.

Oxygen-induced carbon dioxide narcosis is a physiologic hazard of oxygen therapy that may occur in persons with chronic pulmonary disease, such as cystic fibrosis. In these patients, the respiratory center has adapted to the continuously higher arterial carbon dioxide ($PaCO_2$) tension levels, and therefore hypoxia becomes the more powerful stimulus for respiration. When the arterial oxygen (PaO_2) tension level is elevated during oxygen administration, the hypoxic drive is removed, causing progressive hypoventilation and increased $PaCO_2$ levels, and the child rapidly becomes unconscious. Carbon dioxide narcosis can also be induced by the administration of sedation in these patients.

Monitoring Oxygen Therapy

In addition to a patient's respiratory effort and color, **pulse oximetry** is a continuous, noninvasive method of determining arterial oxygen saturation (SaO_2) to guide oxygen therapy. A sensor composed of a light-emitting diode (LED) and a photodetector is placed in opposition around a foot, hand, finger, toe, or earlobe, with the LED placed on top of the nail when digits are used (Fig. 20.23). The diode emits red and infrared lights that pass through the skin to the photodetector. The photodetector measures the amount of each type of light absorbed by functional hemoglobin. Hemoglobin saturated with oxygen (oxyhemoglobin) absorbs more infrared light than does hemoglobin not saturated with oxygen (deoxyhemoglobin). Pulsatile blood flow is the primary physiologic factor that influences accuracy of the pulse oximeter. Reposition the probe at least every 4 to 8 hours to prevent pressure necrosis; poor perfusion and very sensitive skin may necessitate more frequent repositioning.

Another noninvasive method is **transcutaneous monitoring (TCM)**, which provides continuous monitoring of transcutaneous partial pressure of oxygen in arterial blood ($tcPaO_2$) and, with some devices, of transcutaneous partial pressure of carbon dioxide in arterial blood ($tcPaCO_2$). An electrode is attached to the warmed skin to facilitate arterialization of cutaneous capillaries. Because the site of the

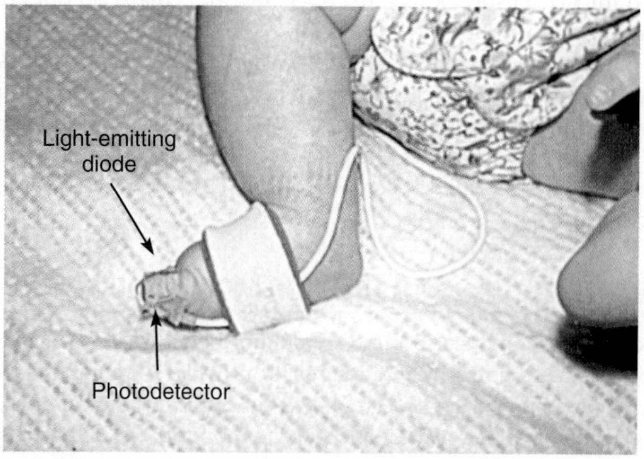

Fig. 20.23 Oximeter sensor on the great toe. Note that the sensor is positioned with a light-emitting diode (LED) opposite the photodetector. The cord is secured to the foot to minimize movement of the sensor.

electrode must be changed every 3 to 4 hours to avoid burning the skin and the machine must be calibrated with every site change, TCM has diminished in use.

Oximetry is insensitive to hyperoxia because hemoglobin approaches 100% saturation for all PaO_2 readings greater than approximately 100 mm Hg, which is a dangerous situation for preterm infants at risk for developing retinopathy of prematurity (see Chapter 8). Therefore preterm infants being monitored with oximetry should have their upper limits identified, such as 90% to 95%, and a protocol should be established for decreasing oxygen when saturations are high.

! NURSING ALERT

It is important to make certain that sensor connectors and oximeters are compatible. Wiring that is incompatible can generate considerable heat at the tip of the sensor, causing second- and third-degree burns under the sensors. Pressure necrosis can also occur from sensors attached too tightly. Therefore inspect the skin under the sensor frequently.

Applying the sensor correctly is essential for accurate SaO_2 measurements. Because the sensor must identify every pulse beat to calculate the SaO_2, movement can interfere with sensing. Some devices synchronize the SaO_2 reading with the heartbeat, thereby reducing the interference caused by motion. Sensors are not placed on extremities used for blood pressure monitoring or with indwelling arterial catheters because pulsatile blood flow may be affected.

NURSING TIP

Infant: Secure the sensor to the great toe and tape the wire to the sole of the foot (or use a commercial holder that fastens with a self-adhering closure). Place a snugly fitting sock over the foot but check the site frequently for color, temperature, and pulse.

Child: Secure the sensor securely to the index finger and tape the wire to the back of the hand.

Ambient light from ceiling lights and phototherapy, as well as high-intensity heat and light from radiant warmers, can interfere with readings. Therefore the sensor should be covered to block these light sources. IV dyes; green, purple, or black nail polish; nonopaque synthetic nails; and possibly ink used for footprinting can also cause inaccurate SaO_2 measurements. The dyes should be removed, or in the case of porcelain nails, a different area should be used for the sensor. Skin color, thickness, and edema do not affect the readings.

Blood gas measurements are sensitive indicators of change in respiratory status in acutely ill patients. They provide valuable information on lung function, lung adequacy, and tissue perfusion. The pH, $PaCO_2$, bicarbonate (HCO_3), and PaO_2 levels can provide information about whether the child is compensating and guide critical treatment decisions.

END-TIDAL CARBON DIOXIDE MONITORING

End-tidal carbon dioxide ($ETCO_2$) monitoring measures exhaled carbon dioxide noninvasively. Capnometry provides a numeric display, and capnography provides a graph over time. Continuous capnometry is available in many bedside physiologic monitors, as well as standalone monitors. $ETCO_2$ differs from pulse oximetry in that it is more sensitive to the mechanics of ventilation rather than oxygenation. Hypoxic episodes can be prevented through the early detection of hypoventilation, apnea, or airway obstruction.

Children who are experiencing an asthma exacerbation, receiving procedural sedation, or are mechanically ventilated may have $ETCO_2$ monitoring. Special sampling cannulas are used for nonintubated patients, and a small device is placed between the endotracheal (ET) tube and the ventilator tubing in intubated patients. Although $ETCO_2$ monitoring is not a substitute for arterial blood gases, it does have the information of providing ventilation information continuously and noninvasively. Normal $ETCO_2$ values are 30 to 43 mm Hg, which is slightly lower than normal partial pressure of carbon dioxide (PCO_2) of 35 to 45 mm Hg. During cardiopulmonary resuscitation (CPR), $ETCO_2$ values consistently below 15 mm Hg indicate ineffective compressions or excessive ventilation. Changes in waveform and numeric display follow changes in ventilation by very few seconds and precede changes in respiratory rate, skin color, and pulse oximetry values.

For years, disposable colorimetric $ETCO_2$ detectors have been used to assess ET tube placement. A color change with each exhaled breath when there is adequate systemic perfusion indicates that the tube is in the lungs. These devices do not provide numbers or graphic representation and do not provide the same early detection of hypoventilation as the continuous quantitative monitors.

Additional uses of $ETCO_2$ monitoring include early detection of opioid-induced respiratory depression, effectiveness of CPR, and severity of asthma exacerbation (Siobal, 2016).

When there is a change in the $ETCO_2$ value or waveform, assess the patient quickly for adequate airway, breathing, and circulation. Sedated patients may be hypoventilating and need stimulation. Intubated patients may need suctioning, have self-extubated or dislodged the tube, or have equipment failure or disconnection. Patients with asthma may have a worsening condition. Problems with the $ETCO_2$ monitoring system can include a kink in the sample line or disconnection. In general, check the patient first and then check the equipment.

BRONCHIAL (POSTURAL) DRAINAGE

Bronchial drainage is indicated whenever excessive fluid or mucus in the bronchi is not being removed by normal ciliary activity and cough. Positioning the child to take maximum advantage of gravity facilitates removal of secretions from the lobes to the larger airways to be expelled. Postural drainage can be effective in children with chronic lung disease characterized by thick mucus, such as cystic fibrosis.

Postural drainage is carried out two to four times daily and is more effective when it follows other respiratory therapy, such as bronchodilator or nebulization medication. Bronchial drainage is generally performed before meals (or 1 to 1½ hours after meals) to minimize the chance of vomiting and is repeated at bedtime. The duration of treatment depends on the child's condition and tolerance; it usually lasts 20 to 40 minutes. Several positions facilitate drainage from all major lung segments. When the child is in each position, the caregiver cups a hand and claps on the chest wall. The child then is encouraged to cough or huff forcefully to move the mucus up and out of the lungs (Cystic Fibrosis Foundation, 2012).

CHEST PHYSICAL THERAPY

Chest physical therapy (CPT) usually refers to the use of postural drainage in combination with adjunctive techniques that are thought to enhance the clearance of mucus from the airway. These techniques include manual percussion, vibration, and squeezing of the chest; cough; forceful expiration; and breathing exercises. Special mechanical devices are also currently used to perform CPT (e.g., vest-type percussors). Postural drainage in combination with forced expiration has been shown to be beneficial.

Common techniques used in association with postural drainage include manual percussion of the chest wall and percussion with mechanical devices, such as a high-frequency handheld chest compression device. A "popping," hollow sound, not a slapping sound, should be the result. The procedure should be done over the rib cage only and should be painless. Percussion can be performed with a soft circular mask (adapted to maintain air trapping) or a percussion cup marketed especially for the purpose of aiding in loosening secretions. CPT is contraindicated when patients have pulmonary hemorrhage, pulmonary embolism, end-stage renal disease, increased intracranial pressure, osteogenesis imperfecta, or minimal cardiac reserves. To enhance patient comfort during CPT, the patient should wear light clothing without zippers, buttons, or pins. CPT should not be painful, and the caregiver should remove watches and rings to minimize discomfort (Cystic Fibrosis Foundation, 2012).

INTUBATION

Rapid-sequence intubation (RSI) is commonly performed in pediatric and neonatal patients to induce an unconscious, neuromuscular blocked condition in order to intubate quickly and reduce complications (Groth, Acquisto, & Khadem, 2018). Atropine, etomidate, midazolam, ketamine, diazepam, propofol, and fentanyl are commonly used to induce sedation while vecuronium, rocuronium, and succinylcholine are used as paralytic agents during RSI (Groth et al., 2018; Pallin, Dwyer, Walls, et al., 2016).

Indications for intubation include:

- Respiratory failure or arrest, agonal or gasping respirations, apnea
- Upper airway obstruction
- Significant increase in work of breathing, use of accessory muscles
- Potential for developing partial or complete airway obstruction—respiratory effort with no breath sounds, facial trauma, and inhalation injuries
- Potential for or actual loss of airway protection, increased risk for aspiration
- Anticipated need for mechanical ventilation related to chest trauma, shock, increased intracranial pressure
- Hypoxemia despite supplemental oxygen
- Inadequate ventilation

In preparation for intubation, the child should be preoxygenated with 100% oxygen using an appropriate-size bag and mask. Historically, uncuffed ET tubes were used in young children to avoid the risk of postintubation stridor and tracheal mucosal injury. However, current literature suggests that there is no significant difference in postintubation stridor, potential trachea mucosa damage, intubation duration, and the need for reintubation between uncuffed and cuffed ET tubes (Shi, Xiao, Xiong, et al., 2016). Air or gas delivered directly to the trachea must be humidified. During intubation, the cardiac rhythm, heart rate, and oxygen saturation should be monitored continuously with audible tones. Video laryngoscopy is a technique increasing in use that can assist the provider in accurately visualizing the airway and is associated with increased first attempt success (Pallin et al., 2016). ET tube placement should be verified by at least one clinical sign and at least one confirmatory technology:

- Visualization of bilateral chest expansion
- Auscultation over the epigastrium (breath sounds should not be heard) and the lung fields bilaterally in the axillary region (breath sounds should be equal and adequate)
- Color change on $ETCO_2$ detector during exhalation after at least three to six breaths or waveform/value verification with continuous capnography
- Chest radiography

Apply a protective skin barrier and secure the ET tube with tape or a securement device. An NG tube is typically inserted after intubation.

MECHANICAL VENTILATION

ET intubation can be accomplished by the nasal (nasotracheal), oral (orotracheal), or direct tracheal (tracheostomy) routes. Although it is more difficult to place and infrequently practiced, nasotracheal intubation is preferred to orotracheal intubation because it facilitates oral hygiene and provides more stable fixation, which reduces the complication of tracheal erosion and the danger of accidental extubation.

Basic ongoing assessment of the mechanically ventilated patient includes observing the chest rise and fall for symmetry, bilateral breath sounds equal or unchanged from last assessment, level of consciousness, capillary refill and skin color, and vital signs. A heart rate that is too fast or too slow is a possible indication of hypoxemia, air leak, or low cardiac output. Pulse oximetry and $ETCO_2$ monitoring is also routine along with periodic arterial blood gas analysis. If sudden deterioration of an intubated patient occurs, the American Heart Association recommends considering the following etiologies:

- DOPE (de Caen et al., 2015)
  - Displacement: the tube is not in the trachea or has moved into a bronchus (right mainstem most common)
  - Obstruction: secretions or kinking of the tube
  - Pneumothorax: chest trauma, barotraumas, or noncompliant lung disease
  - Equipment failure: check the oxygen source, Ambu bag, and ventilator
- Verify placement again during each transport and when patients are moved to different beds

To maintain skin integrity in the mechanically ventilated patient, reposition the patient at least every 2 hours as the patient's condition tolerates. Apply a hydrocolloid barrier to protect the facial cheeks. Place gel pillows under pressure points, such as occiput, heels, elbows, and shoulders. Allow no tubes, lines, wires, or wrinkles in bedding under the patient. Provide meticulous skin care.

Provide analgesia and sedation as needed. Use a system for communication that includes sign boards, pointing, and opening and closing eyes. To maintain safety, use soft restraints if necessary to maintain a critical airway.

Ventilator-associated pneumonia (VAP) is a complication that can be prevented through the use of aggressive hand hygiene, wearing gloves to handle respiratory secretions or contaminated objects, use of closed suctioning systems, routine oral care, elevation of the head of the bed between 30 and 45 degrees (unless contraindicated), and discontinuing the ventilator as soon as possible (Centers for Disease Control and Prevention, 2019). Enteral nutrition is often provided to decrease the risk of bacterial translocation. Routinely assess the patient's intestinal motility (e.g., by auscultating for bowel sounds and measuring residual gastric volume or abdominal girth) and adjust the rate and volume of enteral feeding to avoid regurgitation. In high-risk

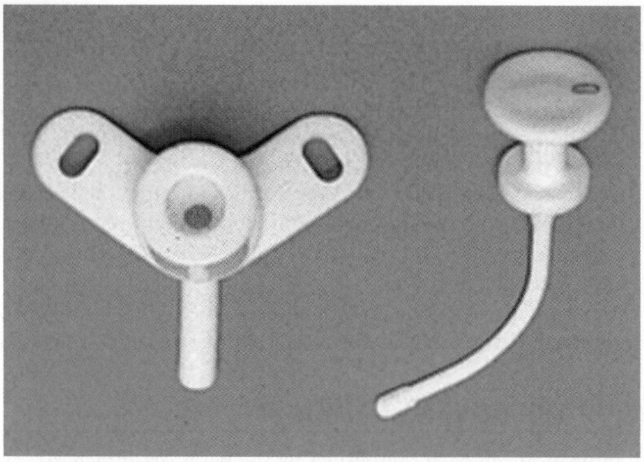

Fig. 20.24 Silastic pediatric tracheostomy tube and obturator.

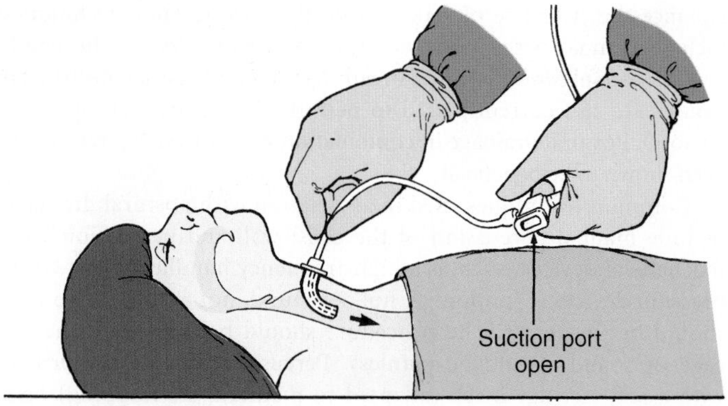

Fig. 20.25 Tracheostomy suction catheter insertion. Note that the catheter is inserted just to the end of the tracheostomy tube.

patients (decreased gag reflex, delayed gastric emptying, gastroesophageal reflux, severe bronchospasm), postpyloric (duodenal or jejunal) feeding tubes are often used. To prevent the aspiration of pooled secretions, suction the hypopharynx before suctioning the ET tube, before repositioning the ET tube, and before repositioning the patient. Prevent ventilator circuits' condensate from entering the ET tube or in-line medication nebulizers.

Assess readiness to extubate daily. Indications that a child is ready to be extubated include an improvement in underlying condition, hemodynamic stability, and mechanical support no longer being necessary. Assess level of consciousness and ability to maintain a patent airway by mobilizing pulmonary secretions through effective coughing. Maintain NPO status 4 hours before extubation. After extubation, monitor for respiratory distress, which may develop within minutes or hours. Signs of postintubation respiratory distress include stridor, hoarseness, increased work of breathing, unstable vital signs, and desaturations.

Tracheostomy

A tracheostomy is a surgical opening in the trachea; the procedure may be done on an emergency basis or may be an elective one, and it may be combined with mechanical ventilation. Indications for tracheostomy placement include upper-airway obstruction or abnormalities, the need for chronic ventilatory support, abnormal ventilatory drive, or neuromuscular conditions affecting ventilation (Watters, 2017). Pediatric tracheostomy tubes are usually made of plastic or silastic (Fig. 20.24). The most common types are the Bivona, Shiley, Tracoe, Arcadia, and Hollinger tubes. These tubes are constructed with a more acute angle than adult tubes, and they soften at body temperature, conforming to the contours of the trachea. Because these materials resist the formation of crusted respiratory secretions, they are made without an inner cannula.

Children who have undergone a tracheostomy must be closely monitored for complications, such as hemorrhage, edema, aspiration, accidental decannulation, tube obstruction, pulmonary infections, skin breakdown, and the entrance of free air into the pleural cavity. The focuses of nursing care are maintaining a patent airway, facilitating the removal of pulmonary secretions, providing humidified air or oxygen, cleansing the stoma, monitoring the child's ability to swallow, and teaching while simultaneously preventing complications.

Because the child may be unable to signal for help, direct observation and use of respiratory and cardiac monitors are essential in the early postoperative period. Respiratory assessments include breath sounds and work of breathing, vital signs, tightness of the tracheostomy ties, skin assessment around the device, and the type and amount of secretions. Large amounts of bloody secretions are uncommon and should be considered a sign of hemorrhage. The practitioner should be notified immediately if this occurs.

The child is positioned with the head of the bed raised or in the position most comfortable to the child with the call light easily available. Suction catheters, suction source, oxygen, bag valve mask, gloves, water-based lubricant, sterile gauze for wiping away secretions, scissors, an extra tracheostomy tube of the same size with ties already attached, another tracheostomy tube one size smaller, and the obturator are kept at the bedside. A source of humidification is provided because the normal humidification and filtering functions of the airway have been bypassed. IV fluids ensure adequate hydration until the child can swallow sufficient amounts of fluids.

Suctioning

The airway must remain patent and may require frequent suctioning to remove mucus plugs and excessive secretions. Proper vacuum pressure and suction catheter size are important to prevent tissue damage, atelectasis, and decrease hypoxia from the suctioning procedure. Vacuum pressure should range from 60 to 80 mm Hg for neonates, 80 to 100 mm Hg for infants and children, and 80 to 120 mm Hg for adolescents (Boroughs & Dougherty, 2015). Unless secretions are thick and tenacious, the lower range of negative pressure is recommended. Tracheal suction catheters are available in a variety of sizes. The catheter selected should be the largest size possible that will fit inside the tracheostomy tube. The catheter should have multiple holes at its distal end to increase secretion removal. Historically, applying suction only when removing the catheter by covering the port with the thumb was the standard recommendation (Fig. 20.25). However, one study found that applying suction while inserting and removing the catheter resulted in fewer secretions by patients over the next 90 minutes when compared to patients suctioned using the traditional method (McClean, 2012). The catheter is inserted just to the end of the tracheostomy tube. Suctioning duration should not last more than 5 seconds. Twisting or twirling the catheter between fingers and thumb rather than stirring can assist in removing secretions (Boroughs & Dougherty, 2015). The practice of instilling sterile saline in the tracheostomy tube before suctioning is not supported by research and is no longer recommended (see Translating Evidence Into Practice box).

TRANSLATING EVIDENCE INTO PRACTICE

Normal Saline Instillation Before Endotracheal or Tracheostomy Suctioning: Helpful or Harmful?

Ask the Question

PICOT Question

In intubated children and those with tracheostomy, is normal saline (NS) instillation before suctioning helpful or harmful?

Search for the Evidence

Search Strategies

All English-language literature from 1980 to 2013 was searched.

Databases Used

PubMed, Cochrane Collaboration, MDConsult, BestBETs, PedsCCM

Critically Analyze the Evidence

There is **moderate evidence** with a **strong recommendation** (Balshem, Helfand, Schunemann, et al., 2011).

- Instillation of NS before endotracheal (ET) tube suctioning has been used for years to loosen and dilute secretions, lubricate the suction catheter, and promote cough. In recent years, the possible adverse effects of this procedure have been explored. Adult studies have found decreased oxygen saturation, increased frequency of nosocomial pneumonia, and increased intracranial pressure after instillation of NS before suctioning (Ackerman, 1993; Ackerman & Gugerty, 1990; Bostick & Wendelgass, 1987; Hagler & Traver, 1994; Kinlock, 1999; O'Neal, Grap, Thompson, et al., 2001; Reynolds, Hoffman, Schlichtig, et al., 1990).
- Two of the first research studies evaluating the effect of NS instillation before suctioning in neonates found no deleterious effects. Shorten, Byrne, and Jones (1991) found no significant differences in oxygenation, heart rate, or blood pressure before or after suctioning in a group of 27 intubated neonates.
- In a second study of nine neonates acting as their own controls, no adverse effects on lung mechanics were found after NS instillation and suctioning (Beeram & Dhanireddy, 1992).
- A study evaluating the effects of NS instillation before suctioning in children found results similar to those in the previously published adult studies. Ridling, Martin, and Bratton (2003) evaluated the effects of NS instillation before suctioning in a group of 24 critically ill children, ages 10 weeks to 14 years old (level 1 evidence). A total of 104 suctioning episodes were analyzed. Children experienced significantly greater oxygen desaturation after suctioning if NS was instilled. Sedigheh and Hossein (2011) also found that instillation of NS before suctioning can cause an adverse effect on oxygen saturation. Another study by Zahran and Abd El-Razik (2011) found a significant increase in arterial carbon dioxide ($PaCO_2$) after suctioning and a reduction in oxygen tension and arterial oxygen saturation (SaO_2) 5 minutes after suctioning. The authors advocate to educate caregivers to avoid using saline to liquefy secretions before suctioning and recommend adequate hydration and humidification, as well as the use of mucolytics.
- The American Thoracic Society states that routine use of NS is not recommended and that adequate humidification should be maintained (Sherman, Davis, Albamonte-Petrick, et al., 2000).
- Gardner and Shirland (2009) evaluated 10 studies on the effects of instilling NS in intubated neonates and concluded that the evidence does not support routine instillation of NS; however, the evidence indicating adverse effect of NS instillation is abundant. Morrow and Argent (2008) suggest that despite evidence indicating the detriment of the use of saline for suctioning in adults, evidence is lacking in the pediatric population. They conclude, however, that saline should not be routinely used for suctioning infants and children.
- Wang and colleagues (2017) evaluated 5 studies on the effects of instilling NS before suctioning in 337 intubated pediatric patients in the intensive care unit. Oxygen saturations remained significantly higher in groups without NS instillation, whereas blood pressure and heart rate did not significantly vary. Overall, the authors conclude that there is no benefit to instilling NS prior to suctioning for pediatric patients.

Apply the Evidence: Nursing Implications

Studies support the contention that the adverse effects of NS instillation before suctioning in children are similar to those found for adults. This technique causes a significant reduction in oxygen saturation that can last up to 2 minutes after suctioning. The evidence does not support the use of NS instillation before ET suctioning in children.

References

Ackerman, M. H. (1993). The effect of saline lavage prior to suctioning. *American Journal of Critical Care, 2*(4), 326–330.

Ackerman, M. H., & Gugerty, B. (1990). The effect of normal saline bolus instillation in artificial airways. *The Journal - Society of Otorhinolaryngology and Head-Neck Nurses, 8*, 14–17.

Balshem, H., Helfand, M., Schunemann, H. J., et al. (2011). GRADE guidelines: Rating the quality of evidence. *Journal of Clinical Epidemiology, 64*(4), 401–406.

Beeram, M. R., & Dhanireddy, R. (1992). Effects of saline instillation during tracheal suction on lung mechanics in newborn infants. *Journal of Perinatology, 12*(2), 120–123.

Bostick, J., & Wendelgass, S. T. (1987). Normal saline instillation as part of the suctioning procedure: Effects of PaO_2 and amount of secretions. *Heart & Lung, 16*(5), 532–537.

Gardner, D. L., & Shirland, L. (2009). Evidence-based guideline for suctioning the intubated neonate and infant. *Neonatal Network, 28*(5), 281–302.

Hagler, D. A., & Traver, G. A. (1994). Endotracheal saline and suction catheters: Sources of lower airway contamination. *American Journal of Critical Care, 3*(6), 444–447.

Kinlock, D. (1999). Instillation of normal saline during endotracheal suctioning: Effects on mixed venous oxygen saturation. *American Journal of Critical Care, 8*(4), 231–240.

Morrow, B. M., & Argent, A. C. (2008). A comprehensive review of pediatric endotracheal suctioning: Effects, indications, and clinical practice. *Pediatric Critical Care Medicine, 9*(5), 465–477.

O'Neal, P. V., Grap, M. J., Thompson, C., et al. (2001). Level of dyspnoea experienced in mechanically ventilated adults with and without saline instillation prior to endotracheal suctioning. *Intensive and Critical Care Nursing, 17*(6), 356–363.

Reynolds, P., Hoffman, L, A., Schlichtig, R., et al. (1990). Effects of normal saline instillation on secretion volume, dynamic compliance, and oxygen saturation (abstract). *American Review of Respiratory Disease, 141*, A574.

Ridling, D. A., Martin, L. D., & Bratton, S. L. (2003). Endotracheal suctioning with or without instillation of isotonic sodium chloride in critically ill children. *American Journal of Critical Care, 12*(3), 212–219.

Sedigheh, I., & Hossein, R. (2011). Normal saline instillation with suctioning and its effect on oxygen saturation, heart rate, and cardiac rhythm. *International Journal of Nursing Education, 3*(1), 42.

Sherman, J. M., Davis, S., Albamonte-Petrick, S., et al. (2000). Care of the child with a chronic tracheostomy. This official statement of the American Thoracic Society was adopted by the ATS Board of Directors, July 1999. *American Journal of Respiratory and Critical Care Medicine, 161*(1), 297–308.

Shorten, D. R., Byrne, P. J., & Jones, R. L. (1991). Infant responses to saline instillations and endotracheal suctioning. *Journal of Obstetric, Gynecologic, & Neonatal Nursing, 20*(6), 464–469.

Wang, C. H., Tsai, J. C., Chen, S. F., Su, C. L., Chen, L., Lin, C. C., & Tam, K. W. (2017). Normal saline instillation before suctioning: A meta-analysis of randomized controlled trials. *Australian Critical Care, 30*(5), 260–265.

Zahran, E. M., & Abd El-Razik, A. A. (2011). Tracheal suctioning with versus without saline instillation. *Journal of American Science, 7*(8), 23–32.

NURSING TIP In a closed suction system, a suction catheter is attached directly to the ventilator tubing. This system has several advantages. First, there is no need to disconnect the patient from the ventilator, which allows for better oxygenation. Second, the suction catheter is enclosed in a plastic sheath, which reduces the risk that the nurse will be exposed to the patient's secretions.

! NURSING ALERT

Suctioning is carried out only as often as needed to keep the tube patent. Signs of mucus partially occluding the airway include an increased heart rate, a rise in respiratory effort, a drop in oxygen saturation, cyanosis, or an increase in the positive inspiratory pressure on the ventilator. If the patient has no signs of secretions, the patient should be suctioned at least in the morning and at night.

The child is allowed to rest for 30 to 60 seconds after each aspiration to allow oxygen saturation to return to normal; then the process is repeated until the trachea is clear. Suctioning should be limited to about three aspirations in one period. If secretions are unable to be cleared after three attempts, the nurse should consider the presence of a mucus plug and possibly perform a tracheostomy tube change. Oximetry is used to monitor suctioning and prevent hypoxia.

In the acute care setting, aseptic technique is used during care of the tracheostomy. Secondary infection is a major concern because the air entering the lower airway bypasses the natural defenses of the upper airway. Gloves are worn during the aspiration procedure, although a sterile glove is needed only on the hand touching the catheter. A new tube, gloves, and sterile saline solution are used each time.

Routine Care

The tracheostomy stoma requires care twice per day. Assessments of the stoma area include observations for signs of infection and breakdown of the skin. The skin is kept clean and dry, and crusted secretions around the stoma may be gently removed with mild soap and water or half-strength hydrogen peroxide. Hydrogen peroxide should not be used with sterling silver tracheostomy tubes, because it tends to pit and stain the silver surface. The nurse should be aware of wet tracheostomy dressings, which can predispose the peristomal area to skin breakdown. Several products are available to prevent or treat excoriation. The Allevyn tracheostomy dressing is a hydrophilic sponge with a polyurethane back that is highly absorptive. Other possible barriers to help maintain skin integrity include the use of hydrocolloid wafers (e.g., DuoDERM CGF, Hollister Restore, Mepilex Lite) under the tracheostomy flanges, as well as extra-thin hydrocolloid wafers under the chin.

The tracheostomy tube is held in place with tracheostomy ties made of a durable, nonfraying material. The ties are changed daily and when soiled. A self-adhering Velcro collar is commonly used. The collar or ties should be tight enough to allow just a fingertip to be inserted between the ties and the neck (Fig. 20.26). It is easier to ensure a snug fit if the child's head is flexed rather than extended while the ties are being secured.

Routine tracheostomy tube changes are usually carried out weekly after a tract has been formed to minimize the formation of granulation tissue. The first change is usually performed by the surgeon; subsequent changes are performed by the nurse or respiratory therapist and, if the child is discharged home with the tracheostomy, by either a parent or a visiting nurse. Ideally, two caregivers participate in the procedure to assist with positioning the child.

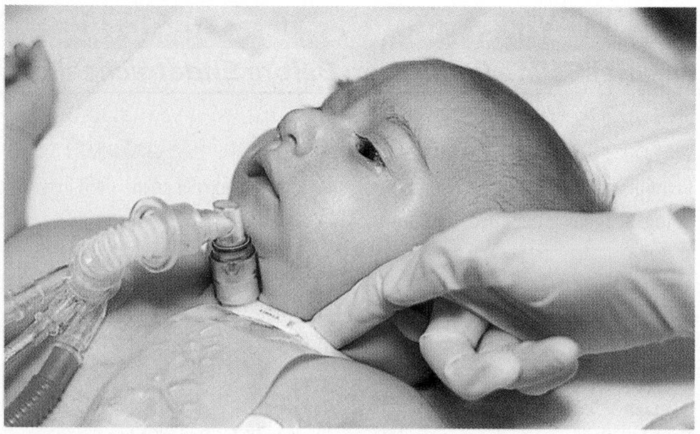

Fig. 20.26 Tracheostomy ties are snug but allow one finger to be inserted.

Changing the tracheostomy tube is accomplished using strict aseptic technique. A gown and eye protection should be worn to change the tracheostomy. Sterile gloves may be worn for insertion of the sterile tracheostomy tube, but clean gloves may be used for tubes that are cleansed and reused. Tube changes should occur before meals or 2 hours after the last meal. Continuous feedings should be turned off at least 1 hour before a tube change. The new sterile tube is prepared by inserting the obturator, applying water-based lubricant, and attaching new ties. The child may be suctioned if necessary, before the procedure and positioned with the neck slightly extended. One caregiver removes the old ties and removes the tube from the stoma. The new tube is inserted gently into the stoma (using a downward and forward motion that follows the curve of the trachea), the obturator is removed, and the ties are secured. Assess for airway placement and adequacy of ventilation to ensure that the tube is not inserted into the soft tissue surrounding the trachea.

Supplemental oxygen is always delivered with a humidification system to prevent drying of the respiratory mucosa. Humidification of room air for an established tracheostomy can be intermittent if secretions remain thin enough to be coughed or suctioned from the tracheostomy. Direct humidification via a heat and moisture exchanger (HME) can be provided to promote thin secretions and improve speech quality. HMEs may not be suitable for all patients, as they can increase the work of breathing or increase the difficulty of clearing large amounts of secretions (Watters, 2017). HMEs are not used routinely at night in order to allow the patient to rest comfortably without increased work of breathing. A tracheostomy collar is another alternative to provide humidification for patients unable to tolerate HMEs and is also the preferred humidification method for use while sleeping. Room humidifiers are also used successfully.

If present, the inner cannula, should be removed twice daily, cleaned per manufacturer guidelines, dried thoroughly, and reinserted. In some cases, the inner cannula is disposable and replaced with each change.

Current literature supports the use of speaking valves to promote language development in infants and children, improve swallowing skills, and provide earlier decannulation (Watters, 2017). One-way speaking valves allow expiratory flow to pass through the vocal cords, resulting in the ability to speak. Speaking valves should be ordered by the provider and initiated through a trial period. The speaking valve should be removed if the patient exhibits any signs of distress. Speech therapy is a key member of the multidisciplinary team when evaluating the patient's tolerance of the speaking valve.

Emergency Care: Tube Occlusion and Accidental Decannulation

Occlusion of the tracheostomy tube is life threatening, and infants and children are at greater risk than adults because of the smaller diameter of the tube. Maintaining patency of the tube is accomplished with suctioning and routine tube changes to prevent the formation of crusts that can occlude the tube.

> **! NURSING ALERT**
>
> Hyperventilating the child with 100% oxygen before and after suctioning (using a bag valve mask or increasing the fraction of inspired oxygen [FiO_2] concentration ventilator setting) may be performed to prevent hypoxia. Closed tracheal suctioning systems that allow for uninterrupted oxygen delivery may also be used.

Accidental decannulation also requires immediate tube replacement. Some children have a rigid trachea, so the airway remains partially open when the tube is removed. However, others have malformed or flexible tracheal cartilage, which causes the airway to collapse when the tube is removed or dislodged. Because many infants and children with upper airway problems have little airway reserve, if replacement of the dislodged tube is impossible, a smaller tube should be inserted. If the stoma cannot be cannulated with another tracheostomy tube, the stoma may be covered with gauze and manual breaths administered through a bag valve mask device until emergency help arrives (Boroughs & Dougherty, 2015).

CHEST TUBE PROCEDURES

A chest tube is placed to remove fluid or air from the pleural or pericardial space. Chest tube drainage systems collect air and fluid while inhibiting backflow into the pleural or pericardial space. Indications for chest tube placement include pneumothorax, hemothorax, chylothorax, empyema, pleural or pericardial effusion, and prevention of accumulation of fluid in the pleural and pericardial space after cardiothoracic surgery. Nursing responsibilities include assisting with chest tube placement, managing chest tubes, and assisting with chest tube removal.

Before chest tube insertion, assess hematologic and coagulation studies for any risk of bleeding during the procedure. Notify the physician of abnormal findings. Prepare the drainage system with sterile water as described in the package insert (some systems may not require this step). Administer pain and sedation medications as ordered. Monitor airway, breathing, circulation, and pulse oximetry throughout the procedure.

After the tube has been inserted and connected to the chest drainage system, secure the tubing to the patient's gown or diaper so that it does not become disconnected. If suction is required, use connection tubing to join the drainage system to a wall suction adapter and adjust suction on the drainage system as ordered (usually −10 to −20 cm H_2O). There should be gentle, continuous bubbling in the suction control chamber. Place occlusive dressing over the chest tube insertion site per hospital policy. Note the date, time, and your initials on the dressing. Ensure that the drainage system is positioned below the patient's chest and secured to the floor or bed. Keep the drainage tubing free of dependent loops. Obtain a chest radiograph to confirm placement of the chest tube. Ensure that daily chest radiographs are scheduled to monitor placement of the chest tube as well as resolution of the pneumothorax or effusion. An emergency kit consisting of clamps, petroleum gauze, sterile gauze, and a transparent occlusive dressing should be kept at the patient's bedside in case of emergency.

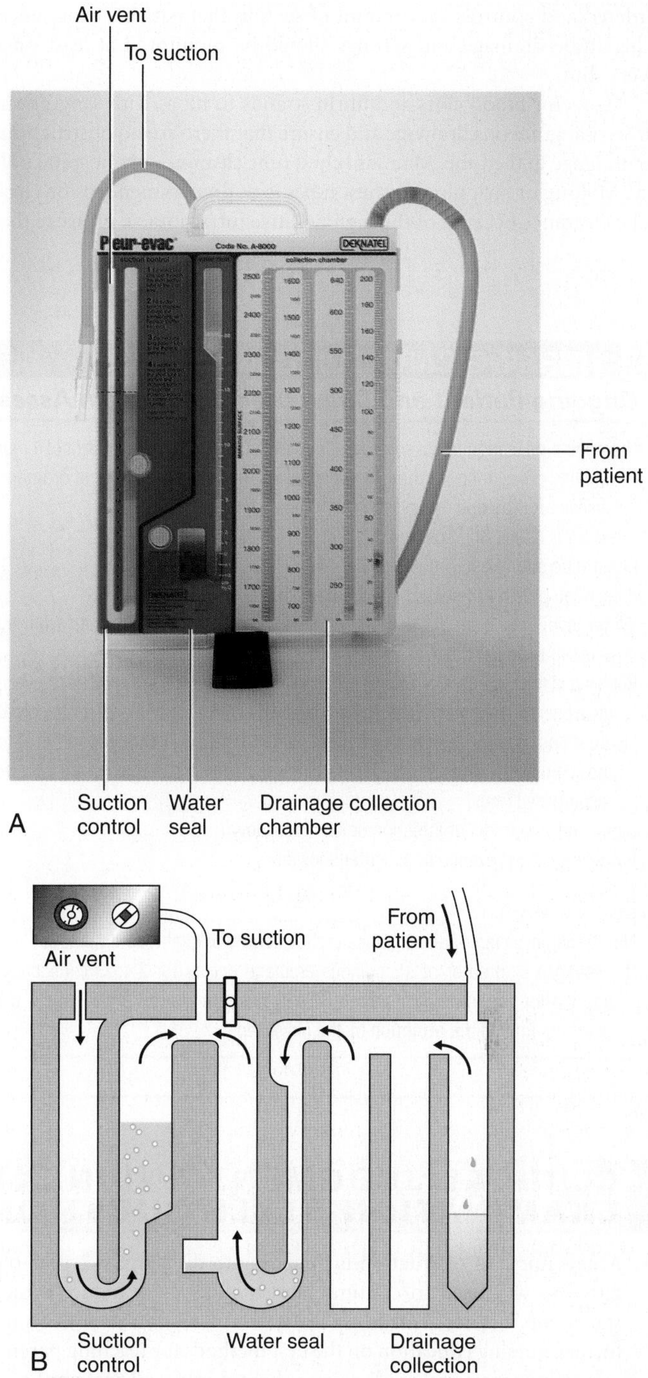

Fig. 20.27 A, The Pleur-Evac drainage system, a commercial three-bottle chest drainage device. B, Schematic of the drainage device. (From Ignatavicius, D. D., & Workman, L. M. [2013]. *Medical-surgical nursing: Patient-centered collaborative care* [7th ed.]. Philadelphia, PA: Saunders/Elsevier.)

Disposable chest drainage systems typically consist of three chambers next to one another in one drainage unit (Fig. 20.27). The fluid collection chamber collects drainage from the patient's pleural or pericardial space. The water seal chamber is directly connected to the fluid collection chamber and acts as a one-way valve, protecting patients from air returning to the pleural or pericardial space. The suction chamber may be a dry suction or calibrated water chamber. It is connected to external vacuum suction set to the amount of suction ordered and controls the amount of suction that patients experience. Chest tube drainage and settings should be monitored at least once every shift.

Assess for blood clots and fibrin strands in tubes with sanguinous or serosanguineous drainage and ensure that there are no obstructions to drainage in the tube. Maintain chest tube clearance per hospital policy. Milking or stripping of chest tubes is not recommended for chest tube clearance because of the high negative intrathoracic pressure that is created. Striping of chest tubes should be performed only with a provider order. However, some special circumstances warrant chest tube clearance with these methods, such as maintaining chest tube patency while a patient is bleeding. Notify the physician immediately if chest tube obstruction is suspected. Generally, chest tubes should not be clamped. However, it may be necessary to clamp a chest tube when exchanging the collection chamber or to determine the site of an air leak (see Nursing Care Guidelines box).

NURSING CARE GUIDELINES

Ongoing Patient and Chest Drainage System Assessment

Drainage type (sanguinous, serosanguineous, serous, chylous, empyemic), color, amount, consistency. If there is a marked decrease in the amount of drainage, assess for drainage around the chest tube insertion site.

Dressing is clean, dry, and intact.

Chest tube sutures are intact.

Prescribed amount of suction is applied.

Water level is at 2 cm. If the water column is too high, the flow of air from the chest may be impeded.

Bubbling in the water seal chamber is normal if the chest tube was placed to evacuate a pneumothorax. The bubbling will stop when the pneumothorax has resolved.

Fluctuations may be seen in the water column because of changes in intrathoracic pressure. Substantial fluctuations may reflect changes in a patient's respiratory status.

Signs and symptoms of infection or skin breakdown.

Palpate for the presence of subcutaneous air.

Interventions

Notify the physician of any changes in the quantity or quality of drainage.

If 3 ml/kg/h or greater of sanguinous drainage occurs for 2 to 3 consecutive hours after cardiothoracic surgery, it may indicate active hemorrhaging and warrants immediate attention by the physician.

Change dressing and perform site care per hospital policy. Typically, a minimal, occlusive dressing is applied.

When the collection chamber is almost full, exchange existing drainage system with a new one per manufacturer's instructions using sterile technique.

To lower the water column, depress the manual vent on the back of the unit until the water level reaches 2 cm. *Do not depress the filtered manual vent when the suction is not functioning or connected.*

If evacuation of a pneumothorax was not the indication for placement of the chest tube, bubbling in the water seal chamber may be the result of a break in the chest drainage system. Identify the break in the system by briefly clamping the system between the drainage unit and the patient. When the clamp is placed between the unit and the break in the system, the bubbling will stop. Tighten any loose connections. If the air leak is suspected to be at the patient's chest wall, notify the physician.

Encourage patient ambulation. Secure chest tube drainage system to prevent chest tube dislodgment from patient or disconnection from drainage system.

CLINICAL JUDGMENT AND NEXT-GENERATION NCLEX® EXAMINATION-STYLE QUESTIONS

1. A new nurse in orientation is preparing to discharge a 2-year-old girl who will need to continue oral antibiotics at home. Which statements below, if made by the new nurse, indicate a need for further nursing education on the best methods for teaching parents to administer an oral medication at home? **Select all that apply.**
   - **A.** The best means for measuring small amounts of medication is a plastic cup.
   - **B.** Using a dropper is acceptable, remembering that thick fluids are easier to measure than viscous fluids.
   - **C.** For more exact measuring, emptying dropper contents into a medicine cup can be helpful.
   - **D.** The most accurate means of measuring small amounts of medication is using a plastic disposable calibrated oral syringe.
   - **E.** A measuring teaspoon is often the unit of measurement for pediatric medication and is especially helpful when working with families.
   - **F.** Household spoons can provide accurate measurement when other devices are not available.

2. The nurse will be giving an intramuscular injection. The infant is 6 months of age and is to receive his scheduled vaccinations. Which principles would the nurse consider when giving the scheduled injections? **Choose the most likely options for the information missing from the statements below by selecting from the lists of options provided.**

   Usually __1__ of fluid is the maximum volume that would be administered intramuscularly in a single site to infants. The __2__ muscle should never be used to administer immunizations.

Option 1	Option 2
5 ml	deltoid
2 ml	dorsogluteal
1 ml	ventrogluteal
8 ml	vastus lateralis

3. A mother of a newborn is extremely upset because blood was obtained by a heelstick. She found bruising at the site and believes that the procedure was performed incorrectly. What statements below are appropriate for the nurse to discuss with the mother? **Select all that apply.**
   A. "Feeding your newborn during the heel lance can reduce pain."
   B. "A heelstick can be performed safely using the outer aspect of the heel."
   C. " We use a device that delivers a precise puncture depth and is less painful."
   D. "We avoid osteochondritis (underlying calcaneus bone, infection, and abscess of the heel), the puncture by going no deeper than 5 mm."
   E. "The heelstick is performed on a newborn because it is less invasive and less painful than a venipuncture."
   F. "Breastfeeding during the heelstick can reduce pain if you would like to try this before the next blood draw."

4. The nurse is preparing to insert a peripheral intravenous line on a 9-year-old girl who has sickle cell disease and experiencing a vaso-occlusive crisis. The child has been stuck numerous times because of the disease and tells the nurse she is not afraid of needles. Which actions would the nurse take? **Use an X for the nursing action statements below that are Indicated (appropriate or necessary), Contraindicated (could be harmful), or Non-Essential (makes no difference or not necessary).**

Nursing Action	Indicated	Contraindicated	Non-Essential
An 18-gauge catheter needs to be inserted.			
A blunt plastic cannula needs to be used because it prevents the need for steel needles.			
An injection port site is used to deliver medications.			
An opaque covering of the IV site needs to be used.			
Music should be played in the background when performing the insertion.			
A padded board would be placed below the hand where the catheter is inserted.			
Fingers are left unoccluded by tape or dressing to assess circulation.			

REFERENCES

Adams, D. Z., Little, A., Vinsant, C., et al. (2016). The midline catheter: A clinical review. *Journal of Emergency Medicine, 51*(3), 252–258.

Alamanou, D. G., & Brokalaki, H. (2014). Intrahospital transport policies: The contribution of the nurse. *Health Science Journal, 8*(2), 166–178.

Al-Yateem, N., Brenner, M., Shorrab, A. A., et al. (2016). Play distraction versus pharmacological treatment to reduce anxiety levels in children undergoing day surgery: A randomized controlled non-inferiority trial. *Child: Care, Health and Development, 42*(4), 572–581.

American Academy of Pediatrics. (2011). Subcommittee on urinary tract infections: Urinary tract infection: Clinical practice guideline for the diagnosis and management of the initial UTI in febrile infants and children 2 to 24 months. *Pediatrics, 128*(3), 595–610.

American Academy of Pediatrics. (2016). Task force on Sudden Infant Death Syndrome: SIDS and other sleep-related infant deaths: Evidence base for 2016 updated recommendations for a safe infant sleeping environment. *Pediatrics, 138*(5), e1–e34.

American Academy of Pediatrics, Committee on Bioethics. (2016). Informed consent in decision-making in pediatric practice. *Pediatrics, 138*(2), e1–e9.

American Academy of Pediatrics, Committee on Drugs. (2015). Metric units and the preferred dosing of orally administered liquid medications. *Pediatrics, 135*(4), 784–787. Retrieved from https://pediatrics.aappublications.org/content/pediatrics/135/4/784.full.pdf.

American Dental Association. (2017). *Mouth healthy: Babies and kids*. Mouth Healthy. http://www.mouthhealthy.org/en/babies-and-kids.

American Society for Parenteral and Enteral Nutrition (ASPEN). (2017). ASPEN safe practices for enteral nutrition therapy. *Journal of Parenteral and Enteral Nutrition, 41*(1), 15–103.

Anand, K. J., & Hall, R. W. (2006). Pharmacological therapy for analgesia and sedation in the newborn. *Archives of Diseases in Childhood Fetal and Neonatal Edition, 91*(6), 448–453.

Anderson, D. M., Pesaturo, K. A., Casavant, J., & Ramsey, E. Z. (2013). Alteplase for the treatment of catheter occlusion in pediatric patients. *Annals of Pharmacotherapy, 47*(3), 405–409.

Association of Child Life Professionals. (2017). *Mission, values, vision*. Association of Child Life Professionals. http://www.childlife.org/child-life-profession/mission-values-vision.

Atay, S., Kurt, F. Y., Akkaya, G., Karatag, G., Demir, S. I., & Calidag, U. (2017). Investigation of suitability of ventrogluteal site for intramuscular injection in children aged 36 months and under. *Journal for Specialists in Pediatric Nursing, 22*(4), e12187.

Azhar, N. (2015). Pre-operative optimisation of lung function. *Indian Journal of Anaesthesia, 59*(9), 550–556.

Bahl, A., Pandurangadu, A. V., Tucker, J., et al. (2016). A randomized controlled trial assessing the use of ultrasound for nurse-performed IV placement in difficult access ED patients. *The American Journal of Emergency Medicine, 34*(10), 1950–1954.

Batawi, H. E. (2015). Effect of preoperative oral midazolam sedation on separation anxiety and emergence delirium among children undergoing dental treatment under general anesthesia. *Journal of International Society of Preventive & Community Dentistry, 5*(2), 88–94.

Bauters, T., Claus, B., Willems, E., De Porre, J., Verlooy, J., Benoit, Y., & Robays, H. (2012). What's in a drop? Optimizing strategies for administration of drugs in pediatrics. *International Journal of Clinical Pharmacy, 34*(5), 679–681.

Beckett, V. L., Tyson, L. D., Carroll, D., et al. (2012). Accurately administering oral medication to children isn't child's play. *Archives of Disease in Childhood, 97*(9), 838–841.

Beckstrand, J., Cirgin Ellett, M. L., & McDaniel, A. (2007). Predicting internal distance to the stomach for positioning NG and OG feeding tubes in children. *Journal of Advanced Nursing, 59*(3), 274–289.

Behnke, J., Lemyre, B., Czernik, C., Zimmer, K. P., Ehrhardt, H., & Waitz, M. (2019). Non-invasive ventilation in neonatology. *Dtsch Arztebl Int, 116*(11), 177–183.

Benoit, B., Martin-Misener, R., Latimer, M., et al. (2017). Breast-feeding analgesia in infants: An update on the current state of evidence. *The Journal of Perinatal & Neonatal Nursing, 31*(2), 145–159.

Bielski, K., Szarpak, L., Smereka, J., Ladny, J. R., Leung, S., & Ruetzler, K. (2017). Comparison of four different intraosseous access devices during simulated pediatric resuscitation. A randomized crossover manikin trial. *European Journal of Pediatrics, 176*(7), 865–871.

Boroughs, D. S., & Dougherty, J. M. (2015). Pediatric tracheostomy care: What home care nurses need to know. *American Nurse Today, 10*(3), 8–10.

Braniff, H., DeCarlo, A., Haskamp, A. C., & Broome, M. E. (2014). Pediatric blood sample collection from a pre-existing peripheral intravenous (PIV) catheter. *Journal of Pediatric Nursing, 29*(5), 451–456.

Britto, M. T., Munafo, J. K., Schoettker, P. J., et al. (2012). Pilot and feasibility test of adolescent-controlled text messaging reminders. *Clinical Pediatrics, 51*(2), 114–121.

Brown, J., Gillespie, M., & Chard, S. (2015). The dorso-ventro debate: In search of empirical evidence. *The British Journal of Nursing, 24*(22), 1132–1139.

Calcaterra, V., Veggiotti, P., Palestrini, C., et al. (2015). Post-operative benefits of animal-assisted therapy in pediatric surgery: A randomised study. *PLoS ONE, 10*(6), 1–13.

Carbone, L., Zebrack, B., Plegue, M., et al. (2013). Treatment adherence among adolescents with epilepsy: What really matters? *Epilepsy & Behavior, 27*(1), 59–63.

Centers for Disease Control and Prevention. (2017). *Protect Initiative: Advancing Children's Medication Safety.* Retrieved from http://www.cdc.gov/medicationsafety/protect/protect_initiative.html.

Centers for Disease Control and Prevention. (2019). *Adverse Childhood Experiences (ACEs),* United States Department of Health and Human Services, https://www.cdc.gov/violenceprevention/childabuseandneglect/acestudy/index.html. Retrieved April 30, 2019.

Centers for Medicare and Medicaid Services. (2015). State operations manual appendix a survey protocol, regulations and interpretive guidelines for hospitals. Revision 151, 11–20. 15 http://www.cms.gov/Regulations-and-Guidance/Guidance/Manuals/downloads/som107ap_a_hospitals.pdf.

Chan, Y. K., & Mamat, M. (2015). Management of heat stroke. *Trends in Anaesthesia and Critical Care, 5*(2–3), 65–69.

Clinical Laboratory Standards Institute. (2017). *Collection of diagnostic venous blood specimens. CLSI standard GP41* (7th ed.). Wayne, PA: Clinical and Laboratory Standards Institute.

Cook, I. F., & Murtagh, J. (2006). Ventrogluteal area—a suitable site for intramuscular vaccination of infants and toddlers. *Vaccine, 24*(13), 2403–2408.

Crawford, C. L., & Johnson, J. A. (2012). To aspirate or not: An integrative review of the evidence. *Nursing, 42*(3), 20–25.

Cummings, C., Finlay, J. C., & MacDonald, N. E. (2018). Head lice infestations: A clinical update. *Paediatrics & Child Health, 23*(1), 18–24.

Cystic Fibrosis Foundation. (2012). *An Introduction to Postural Drainage And Percussion.* Cystic Fibrosis Foundation Education Committee. Retrieved https://www.cff.org/PDF-Archive/Introduction-to-Postural-Drainage-and-Pecussion/. Retrieved 15 May 2019.

Dahl, A., Sinha, M., Rosenberg, D. I., et al. (2015). Assessing physician-parent communication during emergency medical procedures in children: An observational study in a low-literacy Latino patient population. *Pediatric Emergency Care, 31*(5), 339–342.

Dastgheyb, S., Fishlock, K., Daskalakis, C., et al. (2018). Evaluating comfort measures for commonly performed painful procedures in pediatric patients. *Journal of Pain Research* (11), 1383–1390 2018.

de Caen, A. R., Berg, M. D., Chameides, L., Gooden, C. K., Hickey, R. W., Scott, H. F., et al. (2015). Part 12: Pediatric advanced life support: 2015 American Heart Association Guidelines Update for Cardiopulmonary Resuscitation and Emergency Cardiovascular Care. *Circulation, 132*(18 Suppl. 2), S526–S542.

Del Pizzo, J., & Callahan, J. M. (2014). Intranasal medications in pediatric emergency medicine. *Pediatric Emergency Care, 30*, 496–504.

Derya, E. Y., Ukke, K., Taner, Y., et al. (2015). Applying manual pressure before benzathine penicillin injection for rheumatic fever prophylaxis reduces pain in children. *Pain Management Nursing, 16*(3), 328–335.

Dharmapuri, S., Best, D., Kind, T., et al. (2015). Health literacy and medication adherence in adolescents. *The Journal of Pediatrics, 166*(2), 378–382.

Doellman, D., Hadaway, L., Bowe-Geddes, L. A., et al. (2009). Infiltration and extravasation: Update on prevention and management. *Journal of Infusion Nursing, 32*(4), 203–211.

Dolgun, E., Yavuz, M., Eroğlu, B., et al. (2017). Investigation of preoperative fasting times in children. *Journal of Perianesthesia Nursing, 32*(2), 121–124.

Eliacik, K., Kanik, A., Yavascan, O., et al. (2016). A comparison of bladder catheterization and suprapubic aspiration methods for urine sample collection from infants with a suspected urinary tract infection. *Clinical Pediatrics, 55*(9), 819–824.

Ellett, M. L., Cohen, M. D., Perkins, S. M., et al. (2012). Comparing methods of determining insertion length for placing gastric tubes in children 1 month to 17 years. *Journal for Specialists in Pediatric Nursing, 17*(1), 19–32.

Erhaze, E. K., Dowling, M., & Devane, D. (2016). Parental presence at anaesthesia induction: A systematic review. *International Journal of Nursing Practice, 22*(4), 397–407.

European Society of Paediatric Gastroenterology, Hepatology, and Nutrition (ESPGHAN). (2010). Practical approach to paediatric enteral nutrition: A comment by the ESPGHAN Committee on Nutrition. *Journal of Pediatric Gastroenterology and Nutrition, 51*, 110–112.

Ezeanolue, E., Harriman, K., Hunter, P., Kroger, A., & Pellegrini, C. (2019). General Best Practice Guidelines for Immunization. Best practices guidance of the Advisory Committee on Immunization Practices (ACIP). Retrieved from https://www.cdc.gov/vaccines/hcp/acip-recs/general-recs/index.html.

Firdouse, M., Wajchendler, A., Koyle, M., et al. (2017). Checklist to improve informed consent process in pediatric surgery: A pilot study. *Journal of Pediatric Surgery, 52*(5), 859–863.

Flippo, R., NeSmith, E., Stark, N., et al. (2015). Reduction of 30-day preventable pediatric readmission rates with postdischarge phone calls utilizing a patient- and family-centered care approach. *Journal of Pediatric Health Care, 29*(6), 492–500.

Fortier, M. A., Kain, Z. N., & Morton, N. (2015). Treating perioperative anxiety and pain in children: A tailored and innovative approach. *Pediatric Anesthesia, 25*(1), 27–35.

Freundlich, K. (2017). Pressure injuries in medically complex children: A review. *Children (Basel, Switzerland), 4*(4), 1–7.

Fuchs, S. (2017). Gastrostomy tubes: Care and feeding. *Pediatric Emergency Care, 33*, 787–793.

Gao, H., Xu, G., Gao, H., Dong, R., Fu, H., Wang, D., & Zhang, H. (2015). Effect of repeated kangaroo mother care on repeated procedural pain in preterm infants: A randomized controlled trial. *International Journal of Nursing Studies, 7*, 1157–1165.

Gray, M. (1996). Atraumatic urethral catheterization of children. *Pediatric Nursing, 22*(4), 306–310.

Groth, C. M., Acquisto, N. M., & Khadem, T. (2018). Current practices and safety of medication use during rapid sequence intubation. *Journal of Critical Care, 6*(1), 65–70.

Guenter, P., & Lyman, B. (2016). ENFit enteral nutrition connectors. *Nutrition in Clinical Practice, 31*(6), 769–772.

Guiliano, K. K. (2018). Intravenous smart pumps: Usability issues, intravenous medication administration error, and patient safety. *Critical Care Nursing Clinics of North America, 30*(2), 215–224.

Hadaway, L. (2012). Needleless connectors for IV catheters. *American Journal of Nursing, 112*(11), 32–44.

Herd, H. A., & Rieben, M. A. (2014). Establishing the surgical nurse liaison role to improve patient and family member communication. *AORN Journal, 99*(5), 594–599.

Hess, S., & Decker, M. (2017). Comparison of the single-syringe push-pull technique with the discard technique for obtaining blood samples from pediatric central venous access devices. *Journal of Pediatric Oncology Nursing, 34*(6), 381–386.

Heuschkel, R. B., Gottrand, F., Devarajan, K., et al. (2015). ESPGHAN position paper on management of percutaneous endoscopic gastrostomy in children and adolescents. *Journal of Pediatric Gastroenterology and Nutrition, 60,* 131–141.

Higginson, R. P. (2011). Phlebitis: treatment and prevention. *Nursing Times, 107*(36), 18–21.

Howie, S. R. C. (2011). Blood sample volumes in child health research: Review of safe limits. *Bulletin of the World Health Organization, 89,* 46–53.

Hugull, K. (2017). Preventing bloodstream infection in IV therapy. *British Journal of Nursing, 26*(14), S4–S10.

Hunter, D. (2012). Conditions affecting the foreskin. *Nursing Standard, 26*(37), 35–39.

Infusion Nurses Society. (2016). *Infusion therapy standards of practice.* Norwood, MA: Infusion Nurses Society.

Institute for Safe Medication Practices. (2016). *Look-alike drug names with recommended Tall Man letters.* Retrieved from https://www.ismp.org/recommendations/tall-man-letters-list.

Institute for Safe Medication Practices. (2017). ISMP Targeted medication safety best practices for hospitals: Best practice 5. Retrieved from https://www.ismp.org/sites/default/files/attachments/2019-01/TMSBP-for-Hospitalsv2.pdf.

Institute for Safe Medication Practices. (2018). High-alert medications in acute care settings. Retrieved from https://www.ismp.org/recommendations/high-alert-medications-acute-list.

Johnston, C., Campbell-Yeo, M., Disher, T., et al. (2017). Skin-to-skin care for procedural pain in neonates. *Cochrane Database of Systematic Reviews* (2), CD008435.

Karcz, A., Kelley, K., Conrad, J., et al. (2015). Daily bathing of pediatric inpatients with chlorhexidine gluconate to prevent hospital acquired infections. *American Journal of Infection Control, 43*(6), S8.

Katsma, D., & Smith, G. (1997). Analysis of needle path during intramuscular injection. *Nursing Research, 46*(5), 288–292.

Kendrick, J. G., Ma, K., DeZorzi, P., et al. (2012). Vomiting of oral medications by pediatric patients: Survey of medication redosing practices. *The Canadian Journal of Hospital Pharmacy, 65*(3), 196–201.

Letitre, S. L., DeGroot, E. P., Draaisma, E., et al. (2014). Anxiety, depression and self-esteem in children with well-controlled asthma: Case-control study. *Archives of Disease in Childhood, 99*(8), 744–748.

Lewis, G. C., Crapo, S. A., & Williams, J. G. (2013). Critical skills and procedures in emergency medicine: vascular access skills and procedures. *Emergency Medicine Clinics of North America, 31*(1), 59–86.

Lidgett, C. D. (2016). Improving the patient experience through a commit to sit service excellence initiative. *Journal of Patient Experience, 3*(2), 67–72.

Maaskant, J. M., Eskes, A., van Rijn-Bikker, P., Bosman, D., van Aalderen, W., & Vermeulen, H. (2013). High-alert medications for pediatric patients: An international modified Delphi study. *Expert Opinion on Drug Safety, 12*(6), 805–814.

Manworren, R., & Fledderman, M. (2000). Preparation of the child and family for surgery. In B. V. Wise, C. McKenna, G. Garvin, et al. (Eds.), *Nursing Care of the General Pediatric Surgical Patient.* Gaithersburg, MD: Aspen.

Manyande, A., Cyna, A. M., Yip, P., et al. (2015). Non-pharmacological interventions for assisting the induction of anaesthesia in children. *The Cochrane Database of Systematic Reviews, 7,* 1–73.

McCaughey, E. J., Vecellio, E., Lake, R., et al. (2017). Key factors influencing the incidence of hemolysis: a critical appraisal of current evidence. *Critical Reviews in Clinical Laboratory Sciences, 54*(1), 59–72.

McClean, E. B. (2012). Tracheal suctioning in children with chronic tracheostomies: A pilot study applying suction both while inserting and removing the catheter. *Journal of Pediatric Nursing, 27*(1), 50–54.

Monsma, J., Richerson, J., & Sloand, E. (2015). Empowering parents for evidence-based fever management: An integrative review. *Journal of the American Association of Nurse Practitioners, 27*(4), 222–229.

Moureau, N. L., & Flynn, J. (2015). Disinfection of needleless connector hubs: Clinical evidence systematic review. *Nursing research and practice,* 796762 2015.

Murray, E., Edlund, B. J., & Vess, J. (2016). Implementing a pediatric fall prevention policy and program. *Pediatric Nursing, 42*(5), 256–259.

National Child Traumatic Stress Network. (2019). *Trauma Informed Systems: Healthcare, United States Department of Health and Human Services,* https://www.nctsn.org/trauma-informed-care/creating-trauma-informed-systems/healthcare. Retrieved 30 April 2019.

Nickel, B. (2019). Peripheral intravenous access: Applying infusion therapy standards of practice to improve patient safety. *Critical Care Nurse, 39*(1), 61–71.

O'Grady, N. P., Alexander, M., Burns, L. A., et al. (2011). Guidelines for the prevention of intravascular catheter-related infections. *Clinical Infectious Diseases, 52*(9), e162–e193.

Öztürk, D., Baykara, Z. G., Karadag, A., et al. (2017). The effect of the application of manual pressure before the administration of intramuscular injections on students' perceptions of postinjection pain: A semi-experimental study. *Journal of Clinical Nursing, 26*(11–12), 1632–1638.

Pallin, D. J., Dwyer, R. C., Walls, R. M., Brown, C. A., & Brown, C. A., 3rd. (2016). Techniques and trends, success rates, and adverse events in emergency department pediatric intubations: A report from the National Emergency Airway Registry. *Annals of Emergency Medicine, 67*(5), 610–615.

Patricia, C. (2014). Evidence-based management of childhood fever: What pediatric nurses need to know. *Journal of Pediatric Nursing, 29*(4), 372–375.

Paul, I. M., & Yin, H. S. (2012). Out with teaspoons, in with metric units. *AAP News, 33*(3). Retrieved from https://www.aappublications.org/content/aapnews/33/3/10.full.pdf.

Pawar, D. (2012). Common post-operative complications in children. *Indian Journal of Anaesthesia, 56*(5), 496–501.

Payne, N. R., & Flood, A. (2015). Preventing pediatric readmissions: Which ones and how? *The Journal of Pediatrics, 166*(3), 519–520.

Poston, R. D. (2016). Assent described: Exploring perspectives from the inside. *Journal of Pediatric Nursing, 31*(6), 353–365.

Raulji, C. M., Clay, K., Velasco, C., et al. (2015). Daily bathing with chlorhexidine and its effects on nosocomial infection rates in pediatric oncology patients. *Pediatric Hematology and Oncology, 32*(5), 315–321.

Razmus, I., & Bergquist-Beringer, S. (2017). Pressure ulcer risk and prevention practices in pediatric patients: A secondary analysis of data from the national database of nursing quality indicators. *Ostomy/Wound Management, 63*(2), 26–36.

Rothbart, A., Yu, P., Müller-Lobeck, L., et al. (2015). Peripheral intravenous cannulation with support of infrared laser vein viewing system in a pre-operation setting in pediatric patients. *BMC Research Notes, 8,* 463.

Rusch, R., Schulta, C., Hughes, L., et al. (2014). Evidence-based practice recommendations to prevent/manage post-lumbar puncture headaches in pediatric patients receiving intrathecal chemotherapy. *Journal of Pediatric Oncology Nursing, 31*(4), 230–238.

Ryu, G. S., & Lee, Y. J. (2012). Analysis of liquid medication dose errors made by patients and caregivers using alternative measuring devices. *Journal of Managed Care Pharmacy, 18*(6), 439–445.

Saglik, D. S., & Caglar, S. (2018). The effect of parental presence on pain and anxiety levels during invasive procedures in the pediatric emergency department. *Journal of Emergency Nursing,* 1–8, 2018.

Salazar, J. H., Yang, J., Shen, L., et al. (2014). Pediatric malignant hyperthermia: Risk factors, morbidity, and mortality identified from the nationwide inpatient sample and kids' inpatient database. *Pediatric Anesthesia, 24*(12), 1212–1216.

Schober-Flores, C. (2012). Pressure ulcers in the pediatric population. *Journal of the Dermatology Nurses' Association, 4*(5), 295–306.

Sepah, Y., Samad, L., Alrag, A., Halim, M. S., Rahagopalan, N., & Khan, A. J. (2017). Aspiration in injections: Should we continue or abandon the practice? *F1000 Research, 3*(157).

Shah, V., & Ohlsson, A. (2011). Venepuncture versus heel lance for blood sampling in term neonates. *Cochrane Database of Systematic Reviews* (5), CD001452.

Shaughnessy, E. E., White, C., Shah, S. S., et al. (2015). Implementation of postoperative respiratory care for pediatric orthopedic patients. *Pediatrics, 136*(2), 505–512.

Shi, F., Xiao, Y., Xiong, W., Zhou, Q., & Huang, X. (2016). Cuffed versus uncuffed endotracheal tubes in children: A meta-analysis. *Journal of Anesthesia, 30*(1), 3–11.

Siobal, M. S. (2016). Monitoring exhaled carbon dioxide. *Respiratory Care, 61*(10), 1397–1416.

Sisson, H. (2015). Aspirating during the intramuscular injection procedure: A systematic literature review. *Journal of Clinical Nursing, 24*(17–18), 2368–2375.

Sorrentino, G., Fumagalli, M., Milani, S., et al. (2017). The impact of automatic devices for capillary blood collection on efficiency and pain response in newborns: A randomized controlled trial. *International Journal of Nursing Studies, 72*, 24–29.

Sou, V., McManus, C., Mifflin, N., Frost, S. A., Ale, J., & Alexandrou, E. (2017). A clinical pathway for the management of difficult venous access. *BioMed Central nursing Nursing, 16*, 64.

Stein, R., Dogan, H. S., Hoebeke, P., et al. (2015). Urinary tract infections in children: EAU/ESPU guidelines. *European Urology, 67*(3), 546–558.

Stevens, B., Yamada, J., Ohlsson, A., et al. (2016). Sucrose for analgesia in newborn infants undergoing painful procedures. *Cochrane Database of Systematic Reviews* (7), CD001069.

Stoltz, P., & Manworren, R. C. B. (2017). Comparison of children's venipuncture fear and pain: randomized controlled trial of EMLA® and J-Tip needleless injection system®. *Journal of Pediatric Nursing, 37*, 91–96.

Stolz, L. A., Cappa, A. R., Minckler, M. R., et al. (2016). Prospective evaluation of the learning curve for ultrasound-guided peripheral intravenous placement. *The Journal of Vascular Access, 17*(4), 366–370.

Takeshita, J., Nakayama, Y., Nakajima, Y., et al. (2015). Optimal site for ultrasound-guided venous catheterisation in paediatric patients. *Critical Care, 19*(1), 15.

Thomas, C. M., Mraz, M., & Rajcan, L. (2016). Blood aspiration during IM injection. *Clinical Nursing Research, 25*(5), 549–559.

Thompson, R. H. (2018). *The handbook of child life: A guide for pediatric psychosocial care*. Springfield IL: Charles C Thomas Publisher.

Torres, A., Parker, R. M., Sanders, L. M., et al. (2017). Parent preferences and perceptions of milliliters and teaspoons: Role of health literacy and experience. *Academic Pediatrics*, pii: S1876–2879. (17), 30147.

Townley, A., Wincentak, J., Krog, K., et al. (2018). Paediatric gastrostomy stoma complications and treatments: A rapid scoping review. *Journal of Clinical Nursing, 27*, 1369–1380.

Tucker, C., Tucker, L., & Brown, K. (2018). The intranasal route as an alternative method of medication administration. *Critical Care Nurse, 38*(5), 26–32.

US Food and Drug Administration. (2011). *Dosage delivery devices for orally ingested OTC liquid drug products.* Retrieved from https://www.fda.gov-/regulatory-information/search-fda-guidance-documents/dosage-delivery-devices-orally-ingested-otc-liquid-drug-products.

US Food and Drug Administration. (2018). *Sharps Disposal Containers.* Retrieved from https://www.fda.gov/medical-devices/safely-using-sharps-needles-and-syringes-home-work-and-travel/sharps-disposal-containers.

Valizadeh, S., Rasekhi, M., Hamishehkar, H., et al. (2015). Medication errors in oral dosage form preparation for neonates: The importance of preparation technique. *Journal of Research in Pharmacy Practice, 4*(3), 147–152.

Walsh, B. K., & Smallwood, C. D. (2017). Pediatric oxygen therapy: A review and update. *Respiratory Care, 62*(6), 645–661.

Watters, K. F. (2017). Tracheostomy in infants and children. *Respiratory Care, 62*(6), 799–825.

Williams, C., Johnson, P. A., Guzzetta, C. E., et al. (2014). Pediatric fasting times before surgical and radiologic procedures: Benchmarking institutional practices against national standards. *Journal of Pediatric Nursing, 29*(3), 258–267.

Winokur, E. J., Pai, D., Rutledge, D. N., et al. (2014). Blood culture accuracy: Discards from central venous catheters in pediatric oncology patients in the emergency department. *Journal of Emergency Nursing, 40*(4), 323–329.

Yapucu, G. U., Ceylan, B., & Bayindir, P. (2016). Is the ventrogluteal site suitable for intramuscular injection sin children under the age of three? *Journal of Advanced Nursing, 72*(1), 127–134.

Yilmaz, D., Khorshid, L., & Dedeoglu, Y. (2016). The effect of the Z-track technique on pain and drug leakage in intramuscular injections. *Clinical Nurse Specialist, 30*(6), E7–E12.

Yin, H. S., Parker, R. M., Sanders, L. M., et al. (2016). Liquid medication errors and dosing tools: A randomized controlled experiment. *Pediatrics, 138*(4), e20160357.

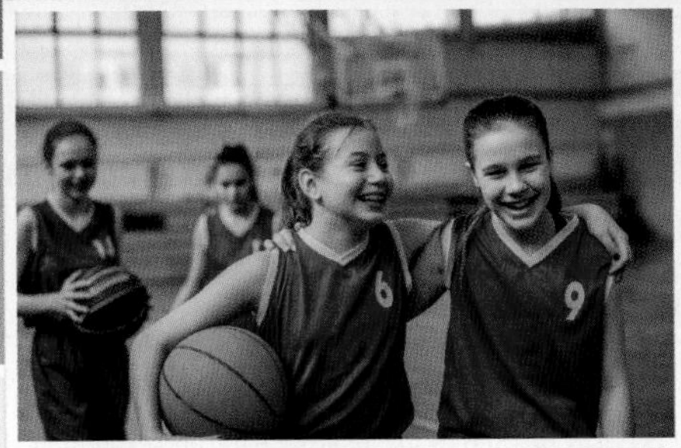

21

The Child With Respiratory Dysfunction

Rosalind Bryant

http://evolve.elsevier.com/wong/essentials

CONCEPTS

- Gas Exchange
- Inflammation
- Infection
- Fluid and Electrolyte Balance
- Patient Education

RESPIRATORY INFECTIONS

Infections of the respiratory tract are described according to the anatomic area of involvement. The upper respiratory tract, or upper airway, consists of the oronasopharynx, pharynx, larynx, and upper part of the trachea. The lower respiratory tract consists of the lower trachea and two cone-shaped lungs including the bronchi, bronchioles, and innumerable small air sacs, or alveoli (see Chapter 4, Lungs). The bronchi and bronchioles are the reactive portion of the lower respiratory tract because they have smooth muscle content and the ability to constrict. Respiratory infections often spread from one structure to another because of the contiguous nature of the mucous membrane lining the entire tract. Consequently, respiratory tract infections involve several areas rather than a single structure, although the effect on one area may predominate in any given illness. The impact of COVID-19 is widespread. Children are less likely to become severely ill than older adults but there are subpopulations of children with an increased risk for more significant illness. Children with underlying pulmonary pathology, immunocompromising conditions, and those who are younger are associated with more severe outcomes (Cruz & Zeichner, 2020). Nursing care for the severely ill child with COVID-19 is similar to the child with acute respiratory distress syndrome found on p. 643 of this chapter.

ETIOLOGY AND CHARACTERISTICS

Respiratory tract infections account for the majority of acute illnesses in children. The age of the child, season, living conditions, and preexisting medical problems influence the cause and course of the infections.

Infectious Agents

The respiratory tract is subject to a wide variety of infective organisms. Most infections are caused by viruses, particularly respiratory syncytial virus (RSV), rhinovirus, nonpolio enterovirus (coxsackievirus A and B), adenovirus, parainfluenza virus, influenza virus, and human metapneumovirus. Other agents involved in primary or secondary invasion include group A beta-hemolytic streptococci (GABHS), staphylococci, *Haemophilus influenzae, Bordetella pertussis, Chlamydia trachomatis, Mycoplasma* organisms, and pneumococci.

Age

Healthy full-term infants younger than 3 months old are presumed to have a lower infection rate because of the protective function of maternal antibodies. However, infants are susceptible to respiratory tract infections, such as pertussis, during this time. The infection rate increases from 3 to 6 months old, which is the period between the disappearance of maternal antibodies and the infant's own antibody production. The viral infection rate remains high during the toddler and preschool years. By 5 years old, viral respiratory tract infections are less frequent, but the incidence of *Mycoplasma pneumoniae* and GABHS infections increases. The amount of lymphoid tissue increases throughout middle childhood, and repeated exposure to organisms confers increasing immunity as children grow older.

Some viral or bacterial agents produce a mild illness in older children but severe lower respiratory tract illness or croup in infants. For example, pertussis causes a relatively harmless tracheobronchitis in childhood but is a serious disease in infancy.

Size

Anatomic differences influence the response to respiratory tract infections. The diameter of the airways is smaller in young children and subject to considerable narrowing from edematous mucous membranes and increased production of secretions. In addition, the distance between structures within the tract is shorter in the young child. Therefore organisms may move rapidly down the shorter respiratory tract, causing more extensive involvement. The relatively short and open eustachian tube in infants and young children allows pathogens easy access to the middle ear.

Resistance

The ability to resist pathogens depends on several factors. Deficiencies of the immune system place the child at risk for infection. Other conditions that decrease resistance are malnutrition, anemia, and fatigue. Conditions

BOX 21.1 Signs and Symptoms Associated With Respiratory Tract Infections in Infants and Small Children

Fever
May be absent in neonates (<28 days)
Greatest at 6 months to 3 years old
Temperature may reach 103°F to 105°F (39.5°C to 40.5°C) even with mild infections
Often appears as first sign of infection
May leave child listless and irritabile, with altered activity pattern (i.e., restless, fatigued)
Tendency to develop high temperatures with infection in certain families
May precipitate febrile seizure (see Chapter 27)

Meningismus
Meningeal signs without infection of the meninges
Occurs with abrupt onset of fever
Accompanied by:
- Headache
- Pain and stiffness in the back and neck
- Presence of Kernig and Brudzinski signs

Subsides as body temperature decreases

Anorexia
Common with most childhood illnesses
Frequently the initial evidence of illness
Persists to a greater or lesser degree throughout febrile stage of illness; often extends into convalescence

Vomiting
Common in small children with illness
A clue to onset of infection
May precede other signs by several hours
Usually short lived but may persist during the illness
Is frequent cause of dehydration

Diarrhea
Usually mild, transient diarrhea but may become severe
Often accompanies viral respiratory infections

Abdominal Pain
Common complaint
Sometimes indistinguishable from pain of appendicitis
May represent referred pain (e.g., chest pain associated with pneumonia)
May be caused by mesenteric lymphadenitis
May be linked to muscle spasms from vomiting, especially in nervous, tense child

Nasal Blockage
Small nasal passages of infants easily blocked by mucosal swelling and exudation
Can interfere with respiration and feeding in infants
May contribute to the development of otitis media and sinusitis

Nasal Discharge
Common sign
May be thin and watery (rhinorrhea) or thick and purulent
Depends on the type and stage of infection
Associated with itching
May irritate upper lip and skin surrounding the nose

Cough
Common sign
May be evident only during acute phase
May persist several months after a disease

Respiratory Sounds
Sounds associated with respiratory disease:
- Cough
- Hoarseness
- Grunting
- Stridor
- Wheezing

Findings on auscultation:
- Wheezing
- Crackles
- Absence of air movement

Sore Throat
Frequent complaint of older children
Young children (unable to describe symptoms) may not complain even when highly inflamed
Increased drooling noted by parents
Refusal to take oral fluids or solids

that weaken defenses of the respiratory tract and predispose children to infection also include allergies (e.g., allergic rhinitis), bronchopulmonary dysplasia (BPD), asthma, history of RSV infection, cardiac anomalies that cause pulmonary congestion, and cystic fibrosis (CF). Daycare attendance and exposure to secondhand smoke increase the likelihood of infection.

Seasonal Variations

The most common respiratory pathogens appear in epidemics during the winter and spring months, but mycoplasmal infections occur more often in autumn and early winter. Infection-related asthma (e.g., asthmatic bronchitis) occurs more frequently during cold weather. Winter and spring are typically RSV season, when children are indoors in close contact and more likely to spread the disease to one another.

CLINICAL MANIFESTATIONS

Infants and young children, especially those between 6 months and 3 years old, react more severely to acute respiratory tract infections than older children. Young children display a number of generalized signs and symptoms and local manifestations that differ from those seen in older children and adults. Signs and symptoms associated with respiratory tract illnesses are outlined in (Box 21.1).

NURSING CARE OF THE CHILD WITH A RESPIRATORY TRACT INFECTION

Assessment of the respiratory system follows the guidelines described in Chapter 4 (for assessment of the ears, nose, mouth and throat, chest, and lungs). The assessment should include respiratory rate, depth and rhythm, heart rate, oxygenation, hydration status, body temperature, level of consciousness, activity level, and level of comfort. Special attention should also be given to the observations outlined in Box 21.1 and the components in Box 21.2 and to assessment of the following:

- Respiratory effort (respiratory rate, rhythm and depth; accessory muscle use; retractions; nasal flaring)

BOX 21.2 Components for Assessing Respiratory Function

Pattern of Respirations

Rate: Rapid (tachypnea), normal, or slow for the particular child

Depth: Normal depth, too shallow (hypopnea), too deep (hyperpnea); usually estimated from the amplitude of thoracic and abdominal excursion (age dependent)

Ease: Effortless, labored (dyspnea), orthopnea (difficult breathing except in upright position), associated with intercostal or substernal retractions (inspiratory "sinking in" of soft tissues in relation to the cartilaginous and bony thorax), pulsus paradoxus (blood pressure falling with inspiration and rising with expiration), nasal flaring, head bobbing (head of sleeping child with suboccipital area supported on caregiver's forearm bobbing forward in synchrony with each inspiration), grunting, wheezing, or stridor

Labored breathing: Continuous, intermittent, becoming steadily worse, sudden onset, at rest or on exertion, associated with wheezing, grunting, and/or chest pain

Rhythm: Variation in rate and depth of respirations

Other Observations

In addition to respirations, particular attention is addressed to:

Evidence of infection: Check for elevated temperature; enlarged cervical lymph nodes; inflamed mucous membranes; and purulent discharges from the nose, ears, or lungs (sputum).

Cough: Observe the characteristics of the cough (if present), when the cough is heard (e.g., night only, on arising), the nature of the cough (paroxysmal with or without wheeze, "croupy" or "brassy"), frequency of the cough, association with swallowing or other activity, character of the cough (moist or dry), productivity.

Wheeze: Note whether it is with expiration or inspiration, high pitched or musical, prolonged, slowly progressive or sudden, association with labored breathing.

Cyanosis: Note distribution (peripheral, perioral, facial, trunk, and face), degree, duration, association with activity.

Chest pain: Older children tend to have this complaint. Note location and circumstances: localized or generalized; referral to base of neck or abdomen; dull or sharp; deep or superficial; association with rapid, shallow respirations or grunting.

Sputum: Older children may provide sputum sample by coughing, whereas young children may need use of bulb suction or early-morning gastric lavage to provide a sample. Note volume, color, viscosity, and odor.

Bad breath (halitosis): May be associated with some throat and lung infections.

- Oxygenation (pulse oximetry, skin color)
- Body temperature
- Child's activity level
- Child's level of comfort

The nursing care of the child with a respiratory tract infection follows established guidelines based on the child's and family's individualized needs (see Next-Generation NCLEX® Examination-Style Unfolding Case Study).

Ease Respiratory Efforts

Many acute respiratory tract infections are mild and cause few symptoms. Although children may feel uncomfortable and have a "stuffy" nose and some mucosal swelling, acute respiratory distress occurs infrequently. Interventions delivered at home are usually sufficient to relieve minor discomfort and ease respiratory efforts. However, in some cases, the infant or child may require hospitalization for close observation and therapy.

Moisturized air is a common therapeutic measure for symptomatic relief of respiratory discomfort. The moisture soothes inflamed membranes and is beneficial when there is hoarseness or laryngeal involvement. Mist tents have been used in the hospital for humidifying the air and relieving discomfort but are seldom used in developed countries. The use of steam vaporizers in the home is often discouraged because of the hazards related to their use and limited evidence to support their efficacy (Lonie, Baker, & Teixeira, 2016; Verma, Lodha, & Kabra, 2013).

A time-honored (but not evidence-based) method of producing steam is the shower. Running a shower of hot water into an empty bathtub or open shower stall with the bathroom door closed produces a quick source of steam. Keeping a child in this environment for approximately 10 to 15 minutes humidifies inspired air and may help ease respiratory efforts. A small child may sit on the lap of a parent or other adult. The use of kettles or bowls of boiling water is strongly discouraged due to the risk of accidental scalding.

Promote Comfort

Children who have an acute febrile illness should be encouraged to drink fluids and rest, but accumulated nasal secretions may interfere with these activities. Older children are usually able to manage nasal secretions with little difficulty. Instruct parents in the correct administration of prescribed nose drops or throat gargles and the correct technique for removing nasal secretions. For very young infants who normally breathe through their noses, an infant nasal aspirator or a bulb syringe is helpful in removing nasal secretions before feeding and sleeping. This practice, in addition to instillation of saline nose drops, may clear nasal passages and promote feeding and rest. Saline nose drops can be prepared at home by dissolving ½ to 1 tsp of salt in 1 cup of warm water. Two to three drops of saline can be put into the nostril, and a bulb syringe can be used to suction it out.

Topical vapor rubs could be considered for children older than 2 years of age to ease nasal congestion. A study by Santhi and colleagues (2017) found that people with the common cold had significantly improved sleep quality when using a vapor rub containing camphor, menthol, and eucalyptus oils compared with placebo. These vapor rubs should never be given orally or placed beneath the nose.

! NURSING ALERT

To avoid rebound nasal congestion, vasoconstrictive nose drops or sprays should not be administered for more than 3 days.

The hospitalized child may be apprehensive; the treatments and tests are frightening and stress producing. It is important to involve the entire family in the care as appropriate and to encourage questions and facilitate effective communication. Reducing anxiety and apprehension reduces psychologic distress in the child, and when the child is more relaxed, the respiratory efforts are reduced. Easing respiratory efforts makes the child less apprehensive, and encouraging the presence of the caregiver provides the child with a source of comfort and support.

NEXT-GENERATION NCLEX® EXAMINATION-STYLE UNFOLDING CASE STUDY

The Child With Acute Respiratory Tract Illness

Day 1, 8:00 am

1. A 7-month-old infant girl is being evaluated in the emergency department for fever and cough. Mom reports over the past 2 days that she has not been as active as usual and is eating less. She started coughing during the night and upon awakening had a temperature of 103°F (39.4°C). The mother states her infant is *"breathing fast and she doesn't seem to be getting enough air."* The nurse performs a complete history and assessment and finds the following. **Select the assessment findings that require follow-up by the nurse. Select all that apply.**
   A. Nasal flaring
   B. Decrease appetite
   C. Skin color—pallor
   D. Irritable and restless
   E. Pulse = 164 beats/min
   F. Retractions visualized
   G. Respiration = 42 breaths/min
   H. SaO_2 on pulse oximeter 88%
   I. Blood pressure = 100/60 mm Hg
   J. Rhonchi and fine crackles in left lung
   K. Axillary temperature = 102.4° F (39.1° C)

2. The nurse understands that common conditions that affect the bronchi in children. The nurse plans care knowing which findings are **most likely** to be noted? **Chose the most likely options for the information missing from the table below by selecting from the lists of option provided.**

Diagnosis	Characteristics	Treatment
Asthma	Wheezing, cough, labored respirations	Inhaled corticosteroids, bronchodilators
Bronchitis	2	Cough suppressants
1	Labored respirations, poor feeding, cough tachypnea, retractions, flaring nares, fever	3

Options for 1	Options for 2	Options for 3
pneumonia	Persistent dry, hacking cough worse at night, more productive in 2-3 days	Inhaled corticosteroids, antibiotics
bronchiolitis	Retractions, labored respirations	Allergen and "triggers control"
emphysema	Poor feeding, inability to sleep, gastrointestinal symptoms	Supplemental oxygen, fluid intake, suctioning as needed
wheezing	Seizures, altered consciousness, inability to focus	Long-term anti-inflammatory medications

Day 1, 3:00 pm

3. The infant has been diagnosed with bronchiolitis and laboratory results confirm it is caused by respiratory syncytial virus (RSV). The infant is resting comfortably on oxygen therapy and receiving intravenous antibiotics and fluids. The nursing assessment reveals the following:
   - Axillary temperature = 99.0° F (37.2° C)
   - Pulse = 92 beats/min
   - Respiration = 24 breaths/min
   - SpO_2 on pulse oximeter 97% room air
   - Blood pressure = 102/54 mm Hg
   - No retractions visualized
   - No nasal flaring
   - Rhonchi and fine crackles in left lung
   - Skin color—no pallor noted
   - Sleeping

   Choose the most likely options for the information missing from the statements below by selecting from the lists of options provided. The nurse realizes that bronchiolitis is the most common infectious disease of the ___1___ airways. RSV affects the ___2___ cells of the respiratory tract. The respiratory illness usually begins with an upper respiratory infection after an incubation of about ___3___ days.

Options for 1	Options for 2	Options for 3
upper	Skin	1-2
middle	Epithelial	2-3
lower	Blood	5-8
extreme	Muscle	10-14
Left	Nasal	14-18
right	Bone	21-24

NEXT-GENERATION NCLEX® EXAMINATION-STYLE UNFOLDING CASE STUDY—cont'd

4. What are the most appropriate immediate nursing interventions for this infant with acute respiratory tract illness? **Indicate which nursing action number listed in the far-left column is appropriate for the potential complication listed in the middle column. Place the number in the far-right column. Note that NOT all nursing actions will be used.**

Nursing Action	Potential Complication	Nursing Action for Complication
1. Position infant for maximum ventilation and airway patency	Inability to identify alterations in temperature, respiratory status, or circulation and need for additional interventions is missed	
2. Monitor vital signs, including temperature and respiratory, cardiac, and oxygen status	Nasal mucosal membrane drying	
3. Provide humidified oxygen as indicated	Fever	
4. Suction airway (nares, mouth, nasopharynx) as indicated	Bronchial constriction and decreased ventilation	
5. Provide gentle chest percussion and chest physiotherapy (CPT) as indicated	Secretions causing lack of airway patency	
6. Administer antipyretics as indicated	Infection	
7. Administer bronchodilators as indicated	Spread of infection	
8. Administer antibiotics if indicated	Dehydration or fluid overload	
9. Obtain specimens (e.g., secretions, blood) as indicated		
10. Maintain appropriate precautions such as Standard Precautions, droplet isolation, and frequent hand washing		
11. Monitor hydration status through strict intake and output and daily weights		
12. Implement comfort measures such as allowing parent presence, parent holding infant, and comfort item such as favorite blanket or stuffed animal		

Day 2, 9:00 am

5. The infant remains hospitalized and the nurse caring for performs the change of shift assessment. Which of the assessment findings support discharge of the infant to home? **Select all that apply.**
   A. SaO_2 of 97% on room air.
   B. Axillary temperature = 102.4° F (39.1° C)
   C. Respiratory rate 24 breaths/ min
   D. Oral intake 100mL/24 hours
   E. Minimal nasal secretions in past 24 hours
   F. Lungs clear to auscultation

Day 3, 10:00 am

6. The infant has been afebrile for 24 hours and has an SpO_2 of 98% on room air. She is now taking oral fluids and there is no longer any nasal discharge. The nurse prepares for discharge teaching and evaluates how prepared the parents are for taking the infant home. **Use an X for the health teaching evaluation below that is Indicated (appropriate or necessary), Contraindicated (could be harmful), or Non-Essential (makes no difference or not necessary).**

Health Teaching Evaluation	Indicated	Contraindicated	Non-Essential
Parents able to verbalize definition and characteristics of acute respiratory tract infection.			
Parents able to verbalize treatment, including medication and interventions that promote ventilation and airway clearance.			
Parents can identify discharge medications, including antipyretics, bronchodilators, and antibiotics as prescribed.			
Parents want to purchase a pulse oximeter before taking the infant home so they can constantly monitor the oxygen level.			
Parents feel that keeping the infant supine will assist with any nasal secretions the infant may have.			
Parents want to purchase another bed for the infant to keep her close to them at night.			

Continued

Prevent Spread of Infection

Perform careful hand washing when caring for children with respiratory tract infections. Children and families should use a tissue or their elbow to cover their mouth or nose when they cough or sneeze, dispose of the used tissues properly, and wash their hands. Used tissues should be immediately thrown into the wastebasket and not allowed to accumulate in a pile. Children with respiratory tract infections should not share drinking cups, eating utensils, washcloths, or towels. To decrease respiratory virus contamination, wash hands frequently and do not touch eyes or noses with the hands.

Parents should try to remove affected children from contact with other children when possible. An effort should be made to teach well children to stay away from ill children, to wash their hands frequently, and to avoid eating and drinking from the same utensils or cups.

Reduce Body Temperature

If the child has a significantly elevated body temperature, controlling the fever is important for comfort. Nurses should verify that family members have a thermometer and know how to correctly take a child's temperature and read a thermometer accurately.

If the practitioner prescribes an antipyretic such as ibuprofen (for children 6 months of age and older) or acetaminophen, parents may need instruction on administering the drug. Most parents can read the label and calculate the desired dosage, but some may require detailed instruction. It is important to emphasize accuracy in both the amount of drug given and the time intervals for drug administration to avoid cumulative effects.

Children with respiratory illnesses will perform activities as appropriate to their energy level. One of the cardinal signs that the child is feeling better is an increase in activity; however, this may be temporary if a high fever returns after a few hours of increased activity. Liquids are encouraged to reduce the temperature and minimize the chances of dehydration (see Chapter 20, Controlling Elevated Temperatures).

> **! NURSING ALERT**
>
> Parents are cautioned about over-the-counter combination "cold" remedies because these often include acetaminophen. Careful calculation of both the acetaminophen given separately and the acetaminophen in combination medications is necessary to avoid an overdose.

Promote Hydration

Dehydration is a potential complication when children have respiratory tract infections and are febrile or anorexic, especially when vomiting or diarrhea is present. Infants are especially prone to fluid and electrolyte deficits when they have a respiratory illness because a rapid respiratory rate that accompanies such illnesses precludes adequate oral fluid intake. In addition, the presence of fever increases the total body fluid turnover in infants. If the infant has nasal secretions, this further prevents adequate respiratory effort by blocking the narrow nasal passages when the infant reclines to bottle-feed or breastfeed and ceases the compensatory mouth breathing effort, thus causing the child to limit intake of fluids. Parents are instructed to encourage adequate fluid intake by offering small amounts of favorite fluids (clear liquids if vomiting) at frequent intervals. Oral rehydration solutions, such as Infalyte or Pedialyte, are beneficial for infants and young children, and water or low-carbohydrate (≤5 g per 8 oz) flavored drinks are appropriate for older children. Fluids with caffeine (tea, coffee) are avoided because these may act as diuretics and promote fluid loss. Carbonated drinks, fruit drinks, and energy drinks are not recommended for oral rehydration (Davies, 2015). Infants who are breastfeeding should continue to be breastfed, because human milk confers some degree of protection from infection (see Chapter 7). Fluids should not be forced. Gentle persuasion with preferred beverages is usually more successful. Intravenous (IV) fluids may be required for a short period to reestablish hydration if the child is dehydrated and not drinking. A nasogastric (NG) tube may be placed to provide enteral hydration using Infalyte or Pedialyte.

To assess their child's level of hydration (see Chapter 22), advise parents to observe the frequency of voiding and to notify the nurse or practitioner if there is insufficient voiding. In the hospital, diapers are weighed to assess output, which should be approximately 1 ml/kg/h in a child who weighs less than 30 kg. It should be at least 30 ml/h in patients weighing more than 30 kg. The practitioner should be notified if the urine output is below normal range for the child's weight.

Observe for Deterioration

Signs of clinical deterioration include increasing respiratory distress, increasing respiratory rate, increasing heart rate, worsening hypoxia, poor perfusion, reduced level of consciousness, and lethargy. The primary service is notified of any deterioration. Some institutions operationalize a rapid response team whereby a designated group of health care providers can be called on to deliver critical care expertise upon deterioration of a patient's condition outside the intensive care unit (ICU).

Provide Nutrition

Loss of appetite is characteristic of children with acute infections. In most cases, children can be permitted to determine their own need for food. Urging foods on anorexic children may precipitate nausea and vomiting and cause an aversion to feeding that may extend into the convalescent period and beyond. Many children show no decrease in appetite, and others respond well to foods such as soup, gelatin, popsicles, and puddings (see Chapter 20, Feeding the Sick Child). In the acute period of the illness, maintaining hydration with encouragement of fluids is of greater importance.

Provide Family Support and Home Care

Young children with respiratory tract infections may be irritable and difficult to comfort. Therefore the family needs support, encouragement, and practical suggestions concerning comfort measures and administration of medication.

In addition to antipyretics and nose drops, the child may require antibiotic therapy. Parents of children receiving oral antibiotics need to understand the importance of administering the drug regularly and continuing it for the prescribed length of time regardless of whether the child appears ill. Parents are cautioned against giving their children any medications that are not approved by the practitioner or prescribed for another child (see Chapter 20 for administration of medications and family teaching). Adverse effects have occurred in children who have received preparations intended for adults (e.g., some long-acting nose drops and dextromethorphan cough squares [mistaken for candy]).

UPPER RESPIRATORY TRACT INFECTIONS

ACUTE VIRAL NASOPHARYNGITIS

Acute nasopharyngitis (equivalent of the "common cold") is caused by a number of viruses such as rhinoviruses, RSV, adenoviruses, influenza virus, and parainfluenza virus. Symptoms are more severe in infants and children than in adults. Fever is common in young children, whereas older children may have low-grade fevers that appear early in the course of the illness. In children 3 months to 3 years old, fevers occur suddenly and are associated with irritability, restlessness, open-mouth breathing, decreased appetite and fluid intake, and decreased activity; these children also may develop vomiting and diarrhea. The initial symptoms in older children are dryness and irritation of nasal passages and the pharynx, followed by chilling sensations, muscular aches, skin-irritating nasal discharge, and occasionally coughing or sneezing. Clinical manifestations are listed in Box 21.3.

The disease is self-limiting, and symptoms typically last 10 to 14 days with a peak on day 2 to 3 of illness. Occasionally, fever recurs and a child (particularly an infant) might experience otitis media (OM), usually early or after the initial phase of nasopharyngitis is past. Pneumonia is less frequent but may occur in some infants.

Therapeutic Management

Children with nasopharyngitis are managed at home. There is no specific treatment, and effective vaccines are not available. Antipyretics may be prescribed for fever and discomfort (see Chapter 20 for management of fever). Fluids and rest are recommended.

Over-the-counter cough suppressants are not routinely recommended and should be prescribed with caution (cough is a protective way of clearing secretions) (Lowry & Leeder, 2015). A cough is normal when the airway is irritated and suppressing it may result in adverse outcomes. Products containing dextromethorphan may be prescribed for a dry, hacking cough, especially at night. Some preparations contain 22% alcohol and can cause adverse effects, such as confusion, hyperexcitability, dizziness, nausea, and sedation. Parents should monitor the child carefully for potential adverse effects.

Recent concerns regarding serious side effects of cough and cold preparations in young children, particularly infants, and lack of convincing evidence that such medications are effective in reducing symptoms have prompted recommendations by health experts to carefully evaluate the benefits and risks of recommending such preparations for children (Lowry & Leeder, 2015). In 2015 the American Academy of Pediatrics stated that over-the-counter cough and cold medications do not work for children under 6 years of age and in some cases may pose a health risk (Clarke, 2017).

Antihistamines are largely ineffective in treatment of nasopharyngitis. These drugs have a weak atropine-like effect that dries secretions, but they can cause drowsiness or, paradoxically, have a stimulatory effect on children. There is no support for the usefulness of expectorants, and antibiotics are usually not indicated because most infections are viral.

BOX 21.3 Clinical Manifestations of Acute Nasopharyngitis and Pharyngitis

Nasopharyngitis

Younger Children

- Fever
- Irritability, restlessness
- Decreased appetite and fluid intake
- Sneezing
- Nasal mucus (abundant) causing mouth breathing
- Vomiting or diarrhea may be present
- Decreased activity

Older Children

- Dryness and irritation of nose and throat initially
- Nasal discharge causing mouth breathing
- Chilling sensations
- Muscular aches
- Cough or sneezing (occasionally)

Physical Assessment Signs

- Edema and vasodilation of mucosa

Pharyngitis

Younger Children

- Fever
- General malaise
- Anorexia
- Moderate sore throat
- Headache

Older Children

- Fever (may reach 104°F [40°C])
- Headache
- Anorexia
- Dysphagia
- Abdominal pain
- Vomiting

Physical Assessment Signs

Younger Children

- Mild to moderate hyperemia

Older Children

- Mild to bright red, edematous pharynx
- Hyperemia of tonsils and pharynx; may extend to soft palate and uvula
- Often abundant follicular exudate that spreads and coalesces to form pseudomembrane on tonsils
- Cervical glands enlarged and tender

Prevention

Nasopharyngitis is so widespread in the general population that it is impossible to prevent. The best methods for preventing transmission of these viruses are frequent hand washing and avoiding touching one's eyes, nose, and mouth. Children are more susceptible because they have not yet developed resistance to many viruses. Very young infants are subject to relatively serious complications; therefore they should be protected from exposure.

Nursing Care Management

The common cold is often the parents' first introduction to an illness in their infant. Most discomfort of nasopharyngitis is related to the nasal obstruction, especially in small infants. Elevating the head of the bed or crib mattress assists with drainage of secretions. Suctioning and vaporization may also provide relief. Saline nose drops and gentle suction with a bulb syringe before feeding and sleep time may be useful.

Maintaining adequate fluid intake is essential during any infectious process. Although a child's appetite for solid foods is usually diminished for several days, it is important to offer appropriate fluids to prevent dehydration. Fluids can be cool (e.g., gelatin, popsicles) or warm (e.g., soups, broths), depending on individual preference.

Because nasopharyngitis is spread from secretions, the best means for prevention is avoiding contact with affected persons. This goal is difficult to accomplish when large numbers of people are confined in a small area for a long time, such as daycare centers and classrooms. Family members with a cold should carefully dispose of tissues; not share towels, glasses, or eating utensils; and avoid direct contact with others if possible. They should cover the mouth and nose with tissues or an elbow when coughing or sneezing and wash hands thoroughly after nose blowing or sneezing. The most frequent carriers of infection are the human hands, which deposit viruses on doorknobs, faucets, and other objects. Children should wash their hands thoroughly or use hand sanitizer and avoid touching their eyes, noses, and mouths.

Family Support

Support and reassurance are important elements of care for families of young children with recurrent upper respiratory infections (URIs). Because URIs are so frequent in children younger than 3 years old, families may need reassurance that frequent colds are a normal part of childhood. Usually by 5 years old, most children will have developed immunity to many viruses. When children spend time in daycare centers, their infection rate is higher than if they are cared for in the home because of increased exposure. Conversely, children who were cared for at home before starting school have an increased infection rate when exposed to more children at school.

Parents should know the signs of respiratory complications and should notify a health professional if such signs appear (e.g., signs of dehydration, the child does not improve within 2 to 3 days) (Box 21.4).

ACUTE STREPTOCOCCAL PHARYNGITIS

Group A beta-hemolytic streptococci (GABHS) infection of the upper airway (strep throat) is not in itself a serious disease, but affected children are at risk for serious sequelae: acute rheumatic fever, which is an inflammatory disease of the heart, joints, and central nervous system (CNS; see Chapter 23), and acute glomerulonephritis, which is an acute kidney infection (see Chapter 26). Permanent damage can result from these sequelae, especially from acute rheumatic fever. GABHS may also cause skin manifestations, including impetigo and pyoderma.

BOX 21.4 Early Evidence of Respiratory Complications

Parents are instructed to notify the health professional if any of the following are noted:

- Evidence of earache
- Respirations faster than 50 to 60 breaths/min
- Fever over 101°F (38.3°C)
- Listlessness
- Crying
- Increasing irritability with or without fever
- Persistent cough for 2 days or more
- Wheezing
- Refusal to eat
- Restlessness and sleep pattern disturbance

Modified from National Association of Pediatric Nurse Practitioners. (2017). *Cold and flu sniffles?* New York, NY: CW Publishing Group; American Academy of Pediatrics. (2018). Children and colds. Retrieved from https://www.healthychildren.org/English/health-issues/conditions/ear-nose-throat/Pages/Children-and-Colds.aspx

Scarlet fever may also occur as a result of a strain of group A streptococcus. The clinical manifestations of scarlet fever include pharyngitis and a characteristic erythematous sandpaper-like rash; otherwise, scarlet fever shares the same clinical manifestations as those mentioned for GABHS, and treatment and sequelae are the same. Severe scarlet fever is rarely seen in the United States.

Clinical Manifestations

GABHS infection is generally a relatively brief illness that varies in severity from subclinical (no symptoms) to severe toxicity. The onset is often abrupt and characterized by pharyngitis, headache, fever, and abdominal pain. The tonsils and pharynx may be inflamed and covered with exudate (Fig. 21.1), which usually appears by the second day of illness. However, streptococcal infections should be suspected in children older than 2 years of age who have pharyngitis even if no exudate is present (Fig. 21.2).

Anterior cervical lymphadenopathy (30% to 50% of cases) usually occurs early, and the nodes are often tender. Pain can be relatively mild to severe enough to make swallowing difficult. Clinical manifestations usually subside in 3 to 5 days unless complicated by sinusitis or parapharyngeal, peritonsillar, or retropharyngeal abscess. Nonsuppurative complications may appear after the onset of GABHS: acute nephritis in about 10 days and rheumatic fever in an average of 18 days.

Children who are GABHS carriers may have a positive throat culture but often experience a coincidental viral illness. Although antibiotic administration is not indicated for most GABHS carriers, some conditions may require antibiotic therapy (American Academy of Pediatrics, Committee on Infectious Diseases, 2018). Transmission to others from a carrier is reportedly minimal.

Diagnostic Evaluation

Although 80% to 90% of all cases of acute pharyngitis are viral, rapid streptococcal antigen testing (obtained by vigorous swabbing of both tonsils and the posterior pharynx) and/or throat culture may be performed to rule out GABHS (American Academy of Pediatrics, Committee on Infectious Diseases, 2018). Rapid identification of GABHS with diagnostic test kits is possible in the office or clinic setting. However, because these kits have questionable sensitivity and depend on a high-quality swab being obtained, a confirmatory throat culture is recommended in patients who have a negative test result with a rapid diagnostic test kit but in whom classic signs of the infection are present (American Academy of Pediatrics, Committee on Infectious Diseases, 2018).

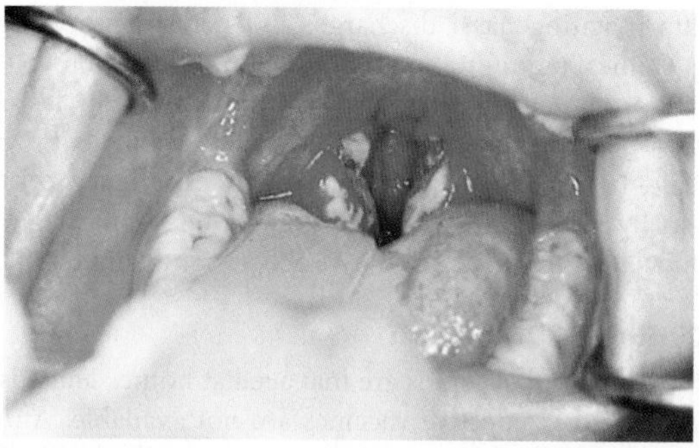

Fig. 21.1 Tonsillitis and pharyngitis. (Courtesy Dr. Edward L. Applebaum, Head, Department of Otolaryngology, University of Illinois Medical Center, Chicago, IL.)

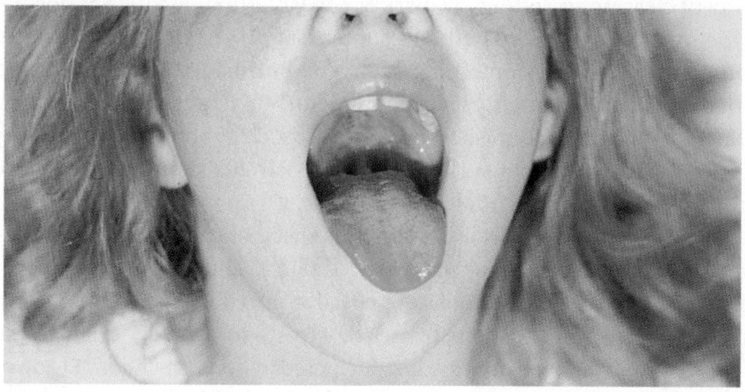

Fig. 21.2 Pharyngitis associated with group A beta-hemolytic streptococci (GABHS) infection. (From Cohen, J., & Powderly, W. G. [2004]. *Infectious diseases* [2nd ed.]. St Louis, MO: Mosby.)

Because some children normally harbor streptococci in their throats, a positive culture or antigen test is not always conclusive evidence of active disease. Most streptococcal infections are short-term illnesses, and antibody (antistreptolysin O) responses appear later than symptoms and are useful only for retrospective diagnosis.

Therapeutic Management

If streptococcal sore throat infection is present, oral penicillin or other antibiotics such as amoxicillin are prescribed for 10 days to control the acute local manifestations and maintain an adequate level to eliminate any organisms that might remain to initiate rheumatic fever symptoms. Penicillin does not prevent the development of acute glomerulonephritis in susceptible children. However, it may prevent the spread of a nephrogenic strain of GABHS to others in the family. Penicillin usually produces a prompt response within 24 hours. Some patients require retreatment if the organism is not eradicated. Amoxicillin given once a day (50 mg/kg; maximum 1000 mg) for 10 days is as effective as penicillin or amoxicillin given multiple times per day (American Academy of Pediatrics, Committee on Infectious Diseases, 2018).

Intramuscular (IM) penicillin G benzathine is also an appropriate therapy. This drug ensures adequate blood concentrations and avoids the problem of compliance, yet it is painful. An oral macrolide or azalide (e.g., erythromycin, azithromycin, clarithromycin) is indicated for children who are allergic to penicillin. Other antibiotics used to treat GABHS are oral cephalosporins, clindamycin, and amoxicillin with clavulanic acid (American Academy of Pediatrics, Committee on Infectious Diseases, 2018).

Nursing Care Management

The nurse often obtains a throat swab for culture and instructs the parents about administering the antibiotic and analgesic as prescribed. Cold or warm compresses to the neck may provide relief. In children old enough to cooperate, warm saline gargles offer relief of throat discomfort.

Ibuprofen (for ages 6 months and older) and acetaminophen may be effective in decreasing throat pain; liquid preparations or chewable forms may be preferable because of the pain associated with swallowing. Pain may interfere with oral intake, and the child should not be forced to eat, but fluid intake is essential. Encourage intake of cool liquids, ice chips, or flavored ice pops that may be tolerated better than solid foods.

Special emphasis is placed on correctly administering oral medication and completing the total course of antibiotic therapy (see Chapter 20, Administration of Medication, and Compliance). If an antibiotic injection is required, it must be administered deep into a large muscle mass (e.g., vastus lateralis or ventrogluteal muscle). To reduce pain, application of a topical anesthetic cream, such as LMX4 (4% lidocaine) or eutectic mixture of local anesthetics (EMLA; lidocaine and prilocaine) over the injection site 30 minutes before the injection may be helpful (see Chapter 20, Intramuscular Administration). Parents need to be aware of the residual tenderness that may develop. Local applications of heat may be helpful in relieving the discomfort. If the child continues to be febrile and/or has not improved within 24 to 48 hours, or appears toxic, further evaluation by the health care provider is important.

Children are considered infectious to others at the onset of symptoms and up to 24 hours after initiation of oral antibiotic therapy. It is generally recommended that the children not return to school or daycare until they have been taking antibiotics for a full 24-hour period. Nurses should remind the children with a streptococcal throat infection and parents to discard the child's toothbrush and replace it with a new one after taking antibiotics for 24 hours. Orthodontic appliances should be washed thoroughly because they may harbor the organisms. Parents are cautioned to prevent other household members, especially if immunocompromised, from having close contact with the sick child and avoid sharing towels and drinking or eating items.

DRUG ALERT

Never administer penicillin G procaine or penicillin G benzathine suspensions intravenously (they may cause embolism or toxic reaction with ensuing death in minutes). Instead, administer these medications deep into the muscle tissue to decrease localized reactions and pain.

TONSILLITIS

The tonsils are masses of lymphoid tissue located in the pharyngeal cavity. The tonsils filter and protect the respiratory and alimentary tracts from invasion by pathogenic organisms and also play a role in antibody formation. Although the size of tonsils varies, children generally have larger tonsils than adolescents or adults. This difference is thought to be a protective mechanism because young children are especially susceptible to URIs.

Pathophysiology

Several pairs of tonsils are part of a mass of lymphoid tissue encircling the nasopharynx and oropharynx, known as the Waldeyer tonsillar ring (Fig. 21.3). The palatine, or faucial, tonsils are located on either side of the oropharynx, behind and below the pillars of the fauces (opening from the mouth). A surface of the palatine tonsils is usually visible during oral examination. The palatine tonsils are those removed during tonsillectomy. The pharyngeal tonsils, also known as the adenoids, are located above the palatine tonsils on the posterior wall of the nasopharynx. Their proximity to the nares and eustachian tubes causes difficulties in instances of inflammation. The lingual tonsils are located at the base of the tongue. The tubal tonsils, found near the posterior nasopharyngeal opening of the eustachian tubes, are not part of the Waldeyer tonsillar ring.

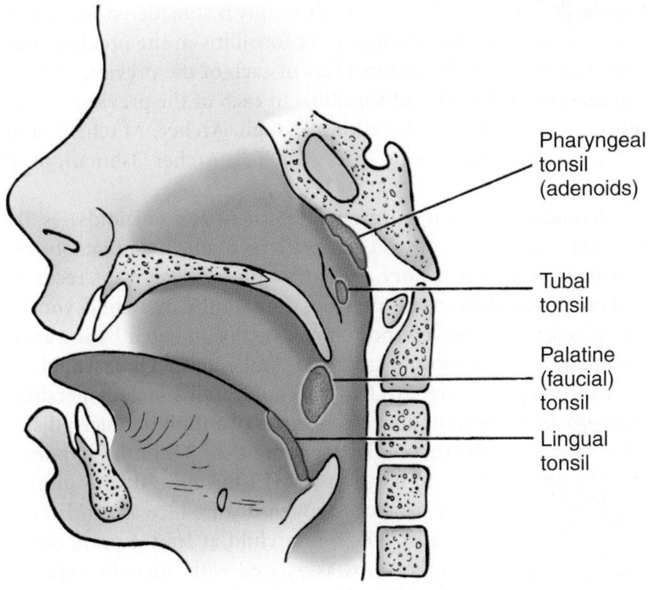

Fig. 21.3 Location of various tonsillar masses.

Etiology

Tonsillitis often occurs with pharyngitis. Because of the abundant lymphoid tissue and the frequency of URIs, tonsillitis is a common cause of illness in young children. The causative agent may be viral or bacterial.

Clinical Manifestations

The manifestations of tonsillitis are caused by inflammation. As the palatine tonsils enlarge from edema, they may meet in the midline (touching or kissing tonsils), obstructing the passage of air or food. The child has difficulty swallowing and breathing. When enlargement of the adenoids occurs, the space behind the posterior nares becomes blocked, making it difficult or impossible for air to pass from the nose to the throat. As a result, the child breathes through the mouth. Chronic enlargement of the tonsils and adenoids may result in obstruction of breathing during sleep.

If mouth breathing is continuous, the mucous membranes of the oropharynx become dry and irritated. There may be an offensive mouth odor and impaired senses of taste and smell. The voice may have a nasal and muffled quality, and a persistent cough is also common. Because of the proximity of the adenoids to the eustachian tubes, this passageway is frequently blocked by swollen adenoids, interfering with normal drainage and frequently resulting in OM or difficulty hearing.

Therapeutic Management

Because tonsillitis is self-limiting, treatment of viral pharyngitis is symptomatic. Throat cultures positive for GABHS infection require antibiotic treatment. It is important to differentiate between viral and streptococcal infection in febrile, exudative tonsillitis. Because most infections are viral, early rapid tests can eliminate unnecessary antibiotic administration.

Tonsillectomy (surgical removal of the palatine tonsils) may be indicated for massive enlargement that results in difficulty breathing or eating. Absolute indications are peritonsillar abcess, PFAPA (periodic fever, aphthous stomatitis, pharyngitis, adenitis), airway obstruction, chronic tonsillitis unresponsive to antimicrobials, multiple antibiotic allergies, and tonsils requiring tissue pathology

(Ingram & Friedman, 2015). Tonsillectomy is considered when there have been seven or more episodes of tonsillitis in the previous year, or at least five episodes of tonsillitis in each of the previous 2 years, or at least three episodes of tonsillitis in each of the previous 3 years and/or sleep-disordered breathing (Baugh, Archer, Mitchell, et al., 2011; Ingram & Friedman, 2015; Mitchell, Archer, Ishman, et al., 2019).

Adenoidectomy (the surgical removal of the adenoids) is recommended for children who have enlarged adenoids that obstruct nasal breathing or a history of four or more episodes of recurrent purulent rhinorrhea in the previous 12 months in a child younger than 12 years old (one episode should be documented by intranasal examination or imaging) (American Academy of Otolaryngology–Head and Neck Surgery, 2011). Other indications include persisting symptoms of adenoiditis after two courses of antibiotics, sleep disturbance with nasal obstruction lasting more than 3 months, hyponasal speech, otitis media with effusion (OME) for more than 3 months, dental malocclusion or orofacial growth disturbance as validated by an orthodontist or dentist, OME in a child at least 4 years old, or cardiopulmonary complications associated with adenoid hypertrophy (American Academy of Otolaryngology–Head and Neck Surgery, 2011).

For some children, the effectiveness of tonsillectomy or adenoidectomy is modest and may not justify the risk of surgery. In practice, many providers rely on individualized decision making and do not subscribe to an absolute set of eligibility criteria for these surgical procedures.

A Cochrane review (Burton, Glasziou, Chong, et al., 2014) concluded that there was a modest benefit to adenotonsillectomy in children with recurrent sore throats; others have reached similar conclusions (Morad, Sathe, Francis, et al., 2017). The American Academy of Otolaryngology–Head and Neck Surgery's recent evidence-based guideline update recommended further research be done to investigate the treatment of recurrent throat infections by tonsillectomy versus antibiotics or watchful waiting in children older than 12 months of age and younger than 12 years of age (Mitchell et al., 2019).

Contraindications to either tonsillectomy or adenoidectomy are (1) cleft palate, because the tonsils help minimize escape of air during speech; (2) acute infections at the time of surgery, because locally inflamed tissues increase the risk of bleeding; and (3) uncontrolled systemic diseases or blood dyscrasias.

Generally, removal of the tonsils should not occur until after 3 or 4 years of age because of the problem of excessive blood loss in young children and the possibility of regrowth or hypertrophy of lymphoid tissue. The tubal and lingual tonsils often enlarge to compensate for the lost lymphoid tissue, resulting in continued pharyngeal and eustachian tube obstruction.

Nursing Care Management

Nursing care of the child with tonsillitis involves providing comfort and minimizing activities or interventions that precipitate bleeding. A soft to liquid diet is generally preferred. Warm saltwater gargles, warm fluids, throat lozenges, and regularly prescribed nonopiods (such as acetaminophen and ibuprofen) are used to promote comfort. Often a combination nonopioid and opioid are needed to reduce pain for the child to drink. The American Academy of Otolaryngology–Head and Neck Surgery's updated guidelines state that clinicians must not administer or prescribe codeine, or any medication containing codeine, after tonsillectomy in children younger than 12 years of age because of the US Food and Drug Administration's 2013 black box warning about codeine-related fatalities (Mitchell et al., 2019).

If surgery is needed, the child requires the same psychologic preparation and physical care as for any procedure (see Chapters 19 and 20). The following discussion focuses on nursing care for tonsillectomy and adenoidectomy (T&A), although both procedures may not be performed.

The nurse takes a complete history, with special notation of any bleeding tendencies because the operative site is highly vascular. Baseline vital signs are important for postoperative monitoring and observation. All patients, especially those with sleep-disordered breathing, require close monitoring of airway and breathing postoperatively. Signs of loose teeth or any URIs are noted and reported, and bleeding and clotting times may be obtained with the usual laboratory work prior to surgery.

After the surgery, until they are fully awake, children are positioned to facilitate drainage of secretions. Suctioning is usually avoided, but when performed, it is done carefully to avoid trauma to the oropharynx. When alert, the child may prefer sitting up. The child is discouraged from coughing frequently, clearing the throat, blowing the nose, and any activities that may aggravate the operative site.

Some secretions, particularly dried blood from surgery, are common. Inspect all secretions and vomitus for evidence of fresh bleeding (some blood-tinged mucus is expected). Dark brown (old) blood is usually present in the emesis, in the nose, and between the teeth. If parents are not prepared regarding the presence of these possible secretions, they may be frightened at a time when they need to be calm and reassuring.

The throat is usually very sore after surgery. An ice collar may provide relief, but many children find it bothersome and refuse to use it. Most children experience moderate pain after a T&A and need pain medication at regular intervals for at least the first 24 to 48 hours. Analgesics may be given rectally or intravenously to avoid the oral route, but liquid analgesics may be given as tolerated. Local anesthetics, such as tetracaine lollipops or ice pops, and antiemetics, such as ondansetron (Zofran) or a Scopolamine transdermal patch (ages 12 years and older), may be administered postoperatively (see Chapter 5, Pain Management).

An integrative review of pain management for pediatric tonsillectomy revealed that preoperative education (child and parent) regarding anxiety and pain were important in the management of the child's postoperative pain (Howard, Finn Davis, Phillips, et al., 2014). In addition, family education on both pharmacologic and nonpharmacologic pain management in the home setting was viewed as being crucial to successful outcomes. An optimal pharmacologic postoperative pain medication regimen was not described, but reviews suggest that acetaminophen, ibuprofen, and hydrocodone may be safe and effective for postoperative pain (Howard et al., 2014; Mitchell et al., 2019).

Food and fluids are restricted until the child is alert and able to swallow with no signs of hemorrhage. Cool water, crushed ice, flavored ice pops, or diluted fruit juice may be given, but fluids with a red or brown color may be avoided to distinguish fresh or old blood in emesis from the ingested liquid. Citrus juice may cause discomfort and is usually not well tolerated. Milk, ice cream, and pudding are usually not offered until clear fluids are retained because milk products coat the mouth and throat, causing the child to clear the throat, which may initiate bleeding.

Children often begin soft foods, particularly gelatin, cooked fruits, sherbet, soup, and mashed potatoes, on the first or second postoperative day or as the child tolerates feeding. The pain from surgery often inhibits oral intake, reinforcing the need for adequate pain control.

Postoperative hemorrhage is unusual but may occur between 5 and 10 days after surgery with the sloughing of the primary eschar as the tonsil bed heals (Mitchell et al., 2019). The nurse observes the throat directly for evidence of bleeding, using a good source of light and, if necessary, carefully inserting a tongue depressor. Other signs of hemorrhage are tachycardia, pallor, frequent clearing of the throat or swallowing by a younger child, and vomiting of bright red blood. Restlessness, an indication of hemorrhage, may be difficult to differentiate from general discomfort after surgery. Decreasing blood pressure is a much later sign of shock.

Surgery may be required to cauterize or ligate a bleeding vessel. Airway obstruction may also occur as a result of edema or accumulated secretions and is indicated by signs of respiratory distress, such as stridor, drooling, restlessness, agitation, increasing respiratory rate, and progressive cyanosis. Suction equipment and oxygen should be available after tonsillectomy.

! NURSING ALERT

The most obvious early sign of bleeding is the child's continuous swallowing of the trickling blood. While the child is sleeping, note the frequency of swallowing. If continuous bleeding is suspected, notify the surgeon immediately.

Family Support and Home Care

Discharge instructions include (1) avoiding irritating and highly seasoned foods, (2) avoiding the use of gargles or vigorous toothbrushing, (3) discouraging the child from coughing or clearing the throat or putting objects in the mouth, (4) using pain medications as prescribed, and (5) limiting activity to decrease the potential for bleeding. Hemorrhage may occur after surgery, therefore any sign of bleeding warrants immediate medical attention. Objectionable mouth odor and slight ear pain with a low-grade fever are common a few days postoperatively. However, persistent severe earache, fever, or cough requires medical evaluation. Most children are ready to resume normal activity within 1 to 2 weeks after the operation.

Most children are admitted to a same-day surgery or ambulatory surgery unit and discharged home after a recovery period. T&A often represents the first hospitalization experience for the child and family. Because the surgery is usually an elective procedure, there is ample opportunity to prepare both the child and parents for this event. Both need reassurance about what to expect at the time of admission, before and after surgery, and at discharge.

INFLUENZA

Influenza (the "flu") is caused by the orthomyxoviruses and classified into three antigenically distinct groups: types A and B, which cause epidemic disease (included in the vaccine), and type C, which causes milder disease and is not included in the vaccine. The viruses undergo significant changes from time to time. Major changes that occur at intervals of usually 5 to 10 years are called antigenic shift; minor variations within the same subtypes, antigenic drift, occur almost annually. Consequently, antigenic drift can alter the virus sufficiently to result in susceptibility of individuals to a type for which they were previously immunized or infected.

Influenza is spread from one individual to another by direct contact (large-droplet infection) usually occurring during talking, sneezing, coughing, or via articles recently contaminated by nasopharyngeal secretions. Attack rates are highest in young children who have had no previous contact with a strain, pregnant women, and patients with chronic medical conditions (e.g., diabetes, asthma). Influenza is frequently most severe in infants and older adults. During epidemics, infection among school-age children is believed to be a major source of transmission in a community.

The disease is more common during the winter months and has a 1- to 4-day incubation period (average of 2 days), and affected persons are most infectious for 24 hours before and 5 to 7 days after the onset of symptoms (Centers for Disease Control and Prevention, 2016, 2018a). The virus has a peculiar affinity for epithelial cells of the respiratory tract mucosa, where it destroys ciliated epithelium with metaplastic hyperplasia of the tracheal and bronchial epithelium with associated edema. The alveoli may also become distended with a hyaline-like material. The viruses can be isolated from nasopharyngeal secretions early after the onset of infection, and serologic tests identify the type by complement fixation or the subgroups by hemagglutination inhibition.

H1N1 (swine flu) is a subtype of influenza type A. In 2009 a pandemic of H1N1 caused significant morbidity and mortality, particularly in Mexico and the United States, lasting until the end of August 2010. A pandemic is defined by the World Health Organization as the spread of a new disease to which the population has little or no immunity and that spreads rapidly from human to human. The H1N1 vaccine has been included in the seasonal influenza vaccination since the 2011–2012 season. Any influenza virus that is novel in nature is reportable to the Centers for Disease Control and Prevention (American Academy of Pediatrics, Committee on Infectious Diseases, 2018).

Clinical Manifestations

The manifestations of influenza may be subclinical, mild, moderate, or severe. In most cases, there is a dry cough and a tendency toward hoarseness. A sudden onset of fever and chills may be accompanied by flushed face, photophobia, myalgia, sore throat, headache, hyperesthesia, fatigue and sometimes prostration, vomiting, and diarrhea. Subglottal croup is common, especially in infants. The symptoms of influenza last for 4 or 5 days. Complications include severe viral pneumonia (often hemorrhagic), febrile seizures, encephalitis, encephalopathy, dehydration, and secondary bacterial infections, such as myocarditis, OM, sinusitis, or pneumonia. Diagnosis is confirmed by analyzing nasopharyngeal secretions for viral culture or rapid detection testing. Influenza A and B can be rapidly detected by direct fluorescent antibody and indirect immunofluorescent antibody staining.

Therapeutic Management

Uncomplicated influenza in children usually requires only symptomatic treatment, including acetaminophen or ibuprofen for fever and sufficient fluids to maintain hydration. Several influenza antiviral drugs were approved by the US Food and Drug Administration for use in the United States, but only oral oseltamivir (Tamiflu), inhaled zanamivir (Relenza), and IV peramivir (Rapivab) are recommended because of widespread resistance to amantadine (Symmetrel) and rimantadine (Flumadine) (American Academy of Pediatrics, Committee on Infectious Diseases, 2018).

Oseltamivir (a neuroaminidase inhibitor) is the antiviral drug of choice that may be administered orally for 5 days to decrease flu symptoms. The medication can be used for infants and children of any age and is effective for types A and B influenza (American Academy of Pediatrics, Committee on Infectious Diseases, 2018). As with other antiviral drugs, for best results the medication should be started within 2 days of the onset of symptoms. Children should not receive aspirin because of its possible link with Reye syndrome.

Zanamivir can be used for treatment of influenza in patients 7 years of age and older or as a prophylaxis for patients 5 years of age and older (American Academy of Pediatrics, Committee on Infectious Diseases, 2018). Zanamivir is an inhaled medication effective for types A and B influenza. The drug is taken twice daily for 5 days and is administered by a specially designed oral inhaler (Diskhaler). Bronchospasm and a decline in lung function can occur when zanamivir is used in patients with underlying airway disease, such as asthma or chronic obstructive pulmonary disease (COPD).

Prevention

The influenza vaccine is now recommended annually for children over 6 months old. Influenza vaccine (inactivated influenza vaccine) may be given to healthy children 6 months of age and older and is administered yearly because different strains of influenza are used each year in the manufacture of the vaccine. The vaccine is safe and effective provided the antigens in the vaccine correlate with the circulating influenza viruses (see Chapter 6, Immunizations). During the 2016–2017 influenza season, the live attenuated influenza vaccine, administered intranasally, was discontinued due to concerns about its effectiveness (Belongia, Karron, Reingold, et al., 2018). See Chapter 6 for guidelines for administering influenza vaccine to patients with a hypersensitivity to eggs.

Nursing Care Management

Nursing care is the same as for any child with a URI, including helping the family implement measures to relieve symptoms. Prolonged fever or the appearance of fever during early convalescence is a sign of secondary bacterial infection and should be reported to the practitioner for antibiotic therapy. Nursing care of the child with influenza also includes educating the parents on the prevention of spread of the disease to other individuals, especially those who are at higher risk for complications, and on the use of antiviral medications. Many institutions have developed protocols to allow nurses to screen patients for eligibility to receive the influenza vaccine.

OTITIS MEDIA

Otitis media (OM) is the presence of fluid in the middle ear along with acute signs of illness and symptoms of middle ear inflammation (Venekamp, Damoiseaux, & Schilder, 2017). The standard terminology used to define OM is outlined in Box 21.5. OM is one of the most prevalent illnesses of early childhood. Its incidence is highest in the winter months. Many cases of bacterial OM are preceded by a viral respiratory infection. Most episodes of acute otitis media (AOM) occur in the first 24 months of life, but the incidence decreases with age except for a small increase at 5 or 6 years old when children enter school. OM occurs infrequently in children older than 7 years of age. Attending daycare is a significant risk factor for OM. Children who have siblings or parents with a history of chronic OM also have a higher incidence of OM.

Children living in households with many members (especially smokers) are more likely to have OM than those living with fewer persons. Passive smoking increases the risk of persistent middle ear effusion by enhancing attachment of the pathogens that cause otitis to the respiratory epithelium in the middle ear space, by prolonging the inflammatory response, and by impeding drainage through the eustachian tube (Kerschner & Preciado, 2020). Family socioeconomic status and extent of exposure to other children are important identifiable risk factors for the occurrence of OM (Kerschner & Preciado, 2020).

BOX 21.5 Standard Terminology for Otitis Media

Otitis media (OM): An inflammation of the middle ear without reference to etiology or pathogenesis

Acute otitis media (AOM): An inflammation of the middle ear space with a rapid onset of the signs and symptoms of acute infection—namely, fever and otalgia (ear pain)

Otitis media with effusion (OME): Fluid in the middle ear space without symptoms of acute infection

Etiology

The most common bacteria causing AOM are *Streptococcus pneumoniae, H. influenzae,* and *Moraxella catarrhalis.* The two viruses most likely to precipitate OM are RSV and influenza, although the adenoviruses, human metapneumoviruses, and picornaviruses (rhinovirus and enterovirus) also cause a significant number of URIs and OM. The etiology of noninfectious OM is unknown but may occur because of blocked eustachian tubes. Predisposing factors include URIs, allergic rhinitis, Down syndrome, cleft palate, daycare attendance, exposure to secondhand smoke, and bottle propping during feeding. Infants fed breast milk have a lower incidence of OM than formula-fed infants (Abrahams & Labbok, 2011; Korvel-Hanquist, Djurhuus, & Homoe, 2017). Breastfeeding may protect infants against respiratory viruses and allergy because breast milk contains secretory immunoglobulin A, which limits the exposure of the eustachian tube and middle ear mucosa to microbial pathogens and foreign proteins. Reflux of milk up the eustachian tubes is less likely in breastfed infants because of the semivertical positioning during breastfeeding compared with bottle-feeding.

Pathophysiology

OM is primarily a result of a dysfunctioning eustachian tube. Mechanical or functional obstruction of the eustachian tube causes accumulation of secretions in the middle ear. Infection or allergy can cause intrinsic obstruction. Extrinsic obstruction is usually a result of enlarged adenoids or nasopharyngeal tumors. Eustachian tube obstruction results in negative middle ear pressure with fluid pulled from the mucosal lining. The sustained negative pressure impairs the ciliary transport within the eustachian tube, inhibiting the fluid drainage that accumulates and tends to become colonized by infectious organisms. When the passage is not totally obstructed, contamination of the middle ear can take place by reflux, aspiration, or insufflation during crying, sneezing, nose blowing, and swallowing when the nose is obstructed.

Diagnostic Evaluation

Careful assessment of tympanic membrane mobility with a pneumatic otoscope is essential to differentiate AOM from OME (Kerschner & Preciado, 2020). A diagnosis of AOM is made with moderate to severe bulging of the tympanic membrane, acute onset of ear drainage not due to acute otitis externa, mild bulging of the tympanic membrane with onset of pain in less than 48 hours, and intense erythema of the tympanic membrane (Kerschner & Preciado, 2020). An immobile tympanic membrane or an orange, discolored membrane indicates OME, with other nonspecific symptoms such as rhinitis, cough, or diarrhea often present. Clinical symptoms of otitis are also helpful in making the diagnosis (Box 21.6). In OME, other symptoms may be manifested through poor balance, behavioral problems, school performance issues, or limited progress with ongoing speech therapy (Rosenfeld, Shin, Schwartz, et al., 2016). Several tests provide an assessment of mobility of the tympanic membrane (see Chapter 4).

BOX 21.6 Clinical Manifestations of Otitis Media

Acute Otitis Media
Follows an upper respiratory tract infection
Otalgia (earache)
Fever—may or may not be present
Purulent discharge (otorrhea)—may or may not be present

Infants and Very Young Children
Crying, fussiness, restlessness, irritability, especially on lying down
Tendency to rub, hold, or pull affected ear
Rolling head from side to side
Difficulty comforting child
Loss of appetite, refusal to feed

Older Children
Crying or verbalizing feelings of discomfort
Irritability
Lethargy
Loss of appetite

Chronic Otitis Media
Hearing loss
Difficulty communicating
Feeling of fullness, tinnitus, or vertigo may be present

Therapeutic Management

Treatment for AOM is one of the most common reasons for antibiotic use in the ambulatory setting. However, concerns about drug-resistant strains have led infectious disease authorities to recommend careful and judicious use of antibiotics for the treatment of this illness. Treatment guidelines for AOM emphasize the need for accurate diagnosis, pain management, and watchful waiting in children with "nonsevere" AOM (Schilder, Marom, Bhutta, et al., 2017). However, the watchful waiting approach is not recommended for children younger than 2 years old who have persistent acute symptoms of fever and severe ear pain (Kerschner & Preciado, 2020). In addition, immediate antibiotic treatment is reserved for high-risk children, including infants younger than 6 months old, because of their immature immune systems and the potential for infection with bacteria.

When antibiotics are necessary, oral amoxicillin in high doses (80 to 90 mg/kg/day divided twice daily) is recommended for 5 to 7 days with children 2 years of age and older and for 10 days with younger children; children with underlying medical conditions, craniofacial anomalies, or tympanic membrane perforation; and children with chronic otitis media.

Second-line antibiotics used to treat OM include amoxicillin/clavulanate, azithromycin, and cephalosporins (such as cefdinir, cefuroxime, and cefpodoxime). IM ceftriaxone is used if the causative organism is a highly resistant pneumococcus or if there is noncompliance with the therapy. An important consideration with the use of single-dose IM injections is the pain involved in this therapy. One strategy to minimize pain at the injection site is to reconstitute the cephalosporin with 1% lidocaine (without epinephrine). A topical analgesic cream such as LMX4 or EMLA can also be applied to the site beforehand to reduce pain.

Supportive care or symptomatic treatment of AOM includes treating the fever and pain. For fever or discomfort associated with OM, analgesic-antipyretic drugs such as acetaminophen or ibuprofen (ibuprofen only if over 6 months of age unless prescribed) may be given. Topical pain relief is recommended by external application of heat or cold, or the practitioner may prescribe topical pain relief drops such as benzocaine drops. Antibiotic ear drops have no value in treating AOM. Children with AOM may be seen after antibiotic therapy is complete to evaluate the effectiveness of the treatment and to identify potential complications, such as effusion or hearing impairment.

Myringotomy, a surgical incision of the eardrum, may be necessary to alleviate the severe pain of AOM. A myringotomy is also performed to drain infected middle ear fluid in the presence of complications (mastoiditis, labyrinthitis, or facial paralysis) or to allow purulent middle ear fluid to drain into the ear canal for culture. A minimally invasive laser-assisted myringotomy procedure may be performed in outpatient settings. These procedures should be performed only by ear, nose, and throat (ENT) specialists.

Tympanostomy tube placement and adenoidectomy are surgical procedures that may be done to treat recurrent chronic OM (three episodes in 6 months or four episodes in 1 year, with one episode during the preceding 6 months) (Kerschner & Preciado, 2020). Tympanostomy tubes are pressure-equalizer (PE) tubes or grommets that facilitate continued drainage of fluid and allow ventilation of the middle ear. They are inserted to treat severe eustachian tube dysfunction, OME, or complications of OM (mastoiditis, facial nerve paralysis, brain abscess, labyrinthitis).

The additive benefit of adenoidectomy to tympanostomy tubes in recurrent AOM and OME is controversial and age dependent (Schilder et al., 2017). The American Academy of Otolaryngology–Head and Neck Surgery guidelines' recommendation is against adenoidectomy for OME in children younger than 4 years old, including those with prior tympanostomy, unless a distinct indication, such as nasal obstruction or chronic adenoiditis, exists (Rosenfeld et al., 2016)

In some children, residual middle ear effusions remain after episodes of AOM. Some children have fluid that persists in the middle ear for weeks or months. Antibiotics are not required for initial treatment of OME (Kerschner & Preciado, 2020; Rosenfeld et al., 2016). Placement of tympanostomy tubes is recommended after a total of 3 to 6 months of bilateral effusion with a bilateral hearing deficit (Kerschner & Preciado, 2020; Rosenfeld et al., 2016). This therapy allows for mechanical drainage of the fluid, which promotes healing of the membrane and prevents scar formation and loss of elasticity. The primary objective is to allow the eustachian tissue a period of recovery while the surgically placed tube performs its functions. The surgery is relatively benign; however, sometimes the tubes become plugged and may require reinsertion. Myringotomy with or without insertion of PE tubes should not be performed for initial management of OME but may be recommended for children who have recurrent episodes of OME with a long cumulative duration. A meta-analysis concluded that tympanostomy tubes had a significant improvement in hearing and a decrease in the incidence of AOM compared with watchful waiting (Steele, Adam, Di, et al., 2017).

Prolonged middle ear disorders may develop several complications such as cholesteatoma (epithelial lining forms scales in middle ear space), tympanosclerosis (eardrum scarring), or adhesive OM (thickening of mucous membranes), but the most frequently associated complication is mild to moderate impairment of hearing. The causes of hearing loss include negative middle ear pressure, effusion in the middle ear, involvement of the eighth cranial nerve, and/or structural damage to the tympanic membrane. Therefore a hearing test should also be performed, especially if OME persists for 3 months or more or if there is evidence of language or learning delays. Follow-up examinations of children with chronic OME should be maintained on a 3- to 6-month basis with repeat hearing test until the OME is resolved (Rosenfeld et al., 2016; Schilder et al., 2017). Children with hearing loss should be referred to a pediatric otolaryngologist and possibly to a pediatric allergist for identification and treatment of the cause. They should receive a speech and language evaluation as necessary.

Prevention

Routine immunization with the pneumococcal vaccine has reduced the incidence of AOM in some infants and children, especially those with frequent episodes of AOM (Kerschner & Preciado, 2020). A conjugate vaccine, Prevnar 13, replaced Prevnar 7 and is approved for use in patients 6 weeks to 17 years old (American Academy of Pediatrics, Committee on Infectious Diseases, 2018). The vaccine is administered as a four-dose series beginning at 2 months of age. Influenza vaccination to children older than 6 months of age is also important (see Chapter 6, Immunizations).

Nursing Care Management

Nursing objectives for children with AOM include relieving pain, facilitating drainage when possible, preventing complications or recurrence, educating the family on care of the child, and providing emotional support to the child and family.

Analgesics (ibuprofen and acetaminophen) are helpful in reducing severe ear pain and controlling fever. Ibuprofen has a longer duration of action (about 6 hours) and is especially beneficial for nighttime comfort but should not be used in children younger than 6 months of age unless directed by a medical provider. Lying on the affected side may reduce pain in some children, as it may facilitate drainage from a ruptured eardrum or myringotomy.

If the ear is draining, the external canal may be cleaned with sterile cotton swabs coupled with topical antibiotic treatment, as directed by the provider. If ear wicks or lightly rolled sterile gauze packs are placed in the ear after surgical treatment, they should be loose enough to allow accumulated drainage to flow out of the ear; otherwise, infection may be transferred to the mastoid process. Parents should be instructed to keep the wicks dry during shampoos and baths. Occasionally, drainage is so profuse that the pinna and surrounding skin become excoriated from the exudate. Frequent cleansing and application of various moisture barriers (e.g., Proshield Plus), zinc oxide–based products, or petrolatum jelly (e.g., Vaseline) can prevent or treat skin irritation.

Tympanostomy tubes may allow water to enter the middle ear, but recommendations for earplugs are inconsistent. Most patients, including very young children, often need no special water precautions. Recent research has indicated that there is no need for water precautions unless the child develops recurrent drainage after swimming (Moualed, Masterson, Kumar, et al., 2016). Health care providers tend to offer recommendations for water precautions.

The tympanostomy tube is eventually pushed out of the eardrum, usually 8 to 18 months after tube placement. Parents should be aware of the appearance of a tympanostomy tube (usually a tiny plastic spool-shaped tube) so that they can recognize it if it falls out. They are reassured that this is normal and requires no immediate intervention, although they should notify the practitioner.

Prevention of recurrence requires adequate parent education on antibiotic therapy. Because the symptoms of pain and fever usually subside within 24 to 48 hours, nurses must emphasize that although the child may appear well, the infection is not completely eradicated until all prescribed medication is taken. It is important to stress the potential complications of OM, especially hearing loss, which can be prevented with adequate treatment and follow-up care.

Parents also need anticipatory guidance regarding methods to reduce the risks of OM, especially in children younger than 2 years old. Reducing the chances of OM is possible with measures such as sitting or holding an infant upright for feedings, maintaining routine childhood immunizations, and exclusively breastfeeding until at least 6 months old. Propping bottles is discouraged to avoid pooling of milk while the child is in the supine position and to encourage human contact during feeding. Eliminating tobacco smoke and known allergens is also recommended. Early detection of middle ear effusion is essential to prevent complications. Infants and preschool children should be screened for effusion, and all schoolchildren, especially those with learning disabilities, should be tested for hearing deficits related to a middle ear effusion.

ACUTE OTITIS EXTERNA

Acute otitis externa is commonly caused by *Pseudomonas aeruginosa* or *Staphylococcus aureus* but may include other pathogens such as *Aspergillus* and *Candida* species. Ordinarily the external ear canal is protected by a waxy, water-repellent coating composed of highly viscid secretions of the sebaceous glands and the watery, pigmented secretions of apocrine glands, in combination with exfoliated surface cells. Inflammation occurs when this environment is altered by swimming or increased environmental humidity; by infection, dermatoses, or insufficient cerumen; or by trauma from a foreign body (FB) or a finger. The ear canal becomes irritated, and maceration takes place. It is most common in 5- to 14-year-olds and peaks in summer (American Academy of Pediatrics, Committee on Infectious Diseases, 2018). It is commonly referred to as swimmer's ear.

The predominant symptom of external ear infection is ear pain accentuated by manipulation of the pinna, especially pressure on the tragus. Conductive hearing loss may be present as a result of the edema, secretions, and accumulation of debris within the canal. Edema, erythema, a cheesy green-blue-gray discharge, tenderness, and fever may appear as the infection progresses. The external canal may be so tender and swollen that visualization is difficult. In advanced cases the pain is intense, constant, and aggravated by jaw motion or ear manipulation.

Therapeutic objectives include relief of pain, edema, and itching, as well as restoration of normal flora, cerumen, and canal epithelium. Analgesics are prescribed for pain. Debris is removed with gentle suction and wisps of cotton on metal cotton carriers. Otic preparations such as polymyxin B sulfate/neomycin sulfate, ciprofloxacin, and gentamycin sulfate, with or without corticosteroids, are instilled in the canal for 7 to 10 days. If the child has tympanostomy tubes, polymyxin B sulfate, neomycin sulfate, or gentamycin should not be used because of the risk of ototoxicity. A gauze wick may be inserted if edema is present to facilitate the medication reaching the site of inflammation. The wick is removed after swelling and pain have subsided, but the drops are continued for at least 3 days after relief of pain. The best management for external ear inflammation is prevention.

Nursing Care Management

Nurses can teach parents or patients simple steps to prevent recurrent infections. Children should limit their stay in the water to less than 1 hour, if possible, and ears should dry completely (1 to 2 hours) before entering the water again. Placing a 50:50 combination of acetic acid (white vinegar) and rubbing alcohol in both ear canals on arising, at bedtime, and at the end of each swim is effective in restoring pH and preventing recurrence. This mixture must not be used if tympanostomy tubes are present. The solution should remain in the ear canal for 5 minutes. The child should be cautioned not to submerge his or her head in water for 7 to 10 days, but well-fitting earplugs can be used if this is not possible. Caution children not to pick at the ears with a pencil, cotton swab, bobby pin, or other object, which can injure or infect the ear canal.

INFECTIOUS MONONUCLEOSIS

Infectious mononucleosis is an acute, self-limiting infectious disease that is common among young people under 25 years old. Symptoms include fever, exudative pharyngitis with petechiae, lymphadenopathy, hepatosplenomegaly, and an increase in atypical lymphocytes. The course is usually mild but occasionally can be severe or, rarely, accompanied by serious complications.

Etiology and Pathophysiology

The Epstein-Barr virus (EBV) is the principal cause of infectious mononucleosis. It appears in both sporadic and epidemic forms, but the sporadic cases are more common. The virus is believed to be transmitted by direct contact (close personal contact is needed to transmit the virus), blood transfusion, or transplantation. It is mildly contagious, and the period of communicability is unknown. The incubation period after exposure is approximately 30 to 50 days (American Academy of Pediatrics, Committee on Infectious Diseases, 2018).

Diagnostic Tests

The diagnosis is established based on clinical manifestations, increase in atypical leukocytes in a peripheral blood smear, and a positive heterophil agglutination test.

Heterophil antibody tests (Monospot or Paul-Bunnell) determine the extent to which the patient's serum will agglutinate sheep red blood cells. The response is primarily to immunoglobulin M (IgM), which is present in the first 2 weeks of the illness and may last for 6 months (American Academy of Pediatrics, Committee on Infectious Diseases, 2018). Because children younger than 4 years of age have a lower rate of heterophil antibody responses, the diagnosis may be overlooked in this group.

The spot test (Monospot) is a slide test of venous blood that has high specificity for the diagnosis of infectious mononucleosis. It is rapid, sensitive, inexpensive, and easy to perform, and it has the advantage that it can detect significant agglutinins at lower levels, thus allowing earlier diagnosis. Blood is usually obtained for the test by finger puncture or venous sampling and is placed on special paper. If the blood agglutinates, forming fragments or clumps, the test result is positive for the infection.

Clinical Manifestations

The onset of symptoms may be acute or insidious and may appear anywhere from 10 days to 6 weeks after exposure. The presenting symptoms vary greatly in type, severity, and duration (Box 21.7). The characteristics of the disease are malaise, sore throat, fatigue, and fever with generalized lymphadenopathy and splenomegaly that may persist for several months. The child's chief complaint is difficulty in maintaining the usual level of activity. The clinical manifestations of infectious mononucleosis are usually less severe (often subclinical or unapparent), and the recovery phase is shorter in younger children than in older children and young adults. Many young children do not develop all of the expected clinical and laboratory findings. The extensive mononuclear infiltration produces symptoms related to any body tissue, and the clinical picture can resemble that of many conditions.

BOX 21.7 Clinical Manifestations of Infectious Mononucleosis

Early Signs
Headache
Epistaxis
Malaise
Fatigue
Chills
Low-grade fever
Loss of appetite
Puffy eyes

Acute Disease
Cardinal Features
Fever
Sore throat
Cervical adenopathy

Common Features
Splenomegaly (may persist for several months)
Palatine petechiae
Macular eruption (especially on trunk)
Exudative pharyngitis or tonsillitis
Hepatic involvement to some degree, often associated with jaundice

Therapeutic Management

No specific treatment exists for infectious mononucleosis. A mild analgesic is usually sufficient to relieve the headache and fever. Rest is encouraged for fatigue and malaise but is not imposed for any specific period. Gargles, warm drinks, analgesic or anesthetic troches, or analgesics, including opioids, can relieve a sore throat. Persons suspected to have infectious mononucleosis should not receive ampicillin or amoxicillin, which may cause a significant nonallergic, maculopapular rash in the presence of active EBV infection. A short course of corticosteroids may have a beneficial effect on some acute symptoms; however, because of the potential adverse effects, their use should be considered only for patients with marked tonsillar inflammation with impending airway obstruction, massive splenomegaly, myocarditis, and hemolytic anemia (American Academy of Pediatrics, Committee on Infectious Diseases, 2018).

Strenuous activity and contact sports should be avoided for 21 days after onset of symptoms of infectious mononucleosis (American Academy of Pediatrics, Committee on Infectious Diseases, 2018). After 21 days, limited noncontact aerobic activity can be allowed if there are no symptoms and there is no overt splenomegaly. Clearance to participate in contact sports is appropriate after 4 to 6 weeks following the onset of symptoms if the athlete is asymptomatic and has no overt splenomegaly (American Academy of Pediatrics, Committee on Infectious Diseases, 2018).

Prognosis

The course of infectious mononucleosis is self-limiting and usually uncomplicated. Acute symptoms often disappear within 7 to 10 days, and persistent fatigue subsides within 2 to 4 weeks. The child is encouraged to maintain limited exercise to prevent deconditioning.

Complications are uncommon but can be serious and require appropriate management. Neurologic complications occur in some outbreaks and vary in severity and outcome. These include seizures, ataxia, aseptic meningitis, encephalitis, optic neuritis, cranial nerve palsies, and perceptual distortions of shapes, spatial relationships, and sizes. Other complications include pneumonitis, orchitis, myocarditis, transverse myelitis, hemolytic anemia, agranulocytosis, thrombocytopenia, hemophagocytic lymphohistiocytosis, and ruptured spleen. Some evidence indicates a depressed cellular immune reactivity during the course of the disease and for some time afterward. Thus it is best to avoid live vaccines until several months after recovery.

Nursing Care Management

Direct nursing responsibilities toward providing comfort measures to relieve the symptoms and helping affected children and adolescents and their families determine appropriate activities for the stage of the disease and their interests. Throat pain may be severe, therefore careful nursing assessment of the airway is imperative to detect serious airway edema and airway compromise. Pain medications in elixir form, such as acetaminophen, ibuprofen, or hydrocodone, may be required during the acute phase so that the young person can maintain an adequate fluid intake. In addition, the nurse should encourage the affected individual to curtail activities that are strenuous until splenomegaly is resolved. Make every effort to prevent a secondary infection by counseling the child and adolescent to limit exposure to persons outside the family, especially during the acute phase of illness.

> **! NURSING ALERT**
>
> Advise the family to seek medical evaluation of the child or adolescent if:
> - Breathing becomes difficult
> - Severe abdominal pain develops
> - Sore throat pain is so severe that the child is unable to eat or drink
> - Respiratory stridor is observed

CROUP SYNDROMES

Croup is a general term applied to a symptom complex characterized by hoarseness, a resonant cough described as "barking" or "brassy" (croupy), varying degrees of inspiratory stridor, and varying degrees of respiratory distress resulting from swelling or obstruction in the region of the larynx and subglottic airway. It occurs primarily in children 6 months to 3 years of age and is rare after 6 years of age. Acute infections of the larynx are of greater importance in infants and small children because of the increased incidence in children in this age-group and the smaller airway diameter that places them at risk for significant narrowing with inflammation. With widespread immunization programs aimed at preventing *H. influenzae* type B (Hib), most cases of croup in the United States are attributed to viruses—namely, influenza types A and B, adenovirus, RSV, and measles (Rodrigues & Roosevelt, 2020). Bacteria such as *M. pneumoniae* can also cause croup.

Croup syndromes affect to varying degrees the larynx, trachea, and bronchi. However, laryngeal involvement often dominates the clinical picture because of the severe effects on the voice and breathing. Croup syndromes are usually described according to the primary anatomic area affected (i.e., epiglottitis [or supraglottitis], laryngitis, laryngotracheobronchitis [LTB], and tracheitis). In general, LTB occurs in very young children, whereas epiglottitis is more common in older children. A comparison of croup syndromes is provided in Table 21.1.

ACUTE EPIGLOTTITIS

Acute epiglottitis, or acute supraglottitis, is a medical emergency that requires immediate medical attention. It is a serious obstructive inflammatory process that occurs predominantly in children 2 to 5 years old but can occur from infancy to adulthood. The obstruction is supraglottic as opposed to the subglottic obstruction of laryngitis. The causative agent is usually *H. influenzae.* However, since the administration of the Hib conjugate vaccine, the incidence of epiglottitis has declined. The disease now is often caused by viral agents. LTB and epiglottitis do not occur together. Epiglottitis (noninfectious) may also be caused by ingestion of caustic agents, smoke inhalation, or foreign bodies (Abdallah, 2012).

Clinical Manifestations

The onset of epiglottitis is abrupt and can rapidly progress to severe respiratory distress. The child usually goes to bed asymptomatic to

TABLE 21.1 Comparison of Croup Syndromes

	Acute Epiglottitis	Acute LTB	Acute Spasmodic Laryngitis	Acute Tracheitis
Age-group affected	2-5 years old but varies	Infant or child younger than 5 years old	1-3 years old	1 month old–6 years old
Etiologic agent	Bacterial	Viral	Viral with allergic component	Viral or bacterial with allergic component
Onset	Rapidly progressive	Slowly progressive	Sudden; at night	Moderately progressive
Major symptoms	Dysphagia Stridor aggravated when supine Drooling High fever Toxic appearance Rapid pulse and respirations	URI Stridor Brassy cough Hoarseness Dyspnea Restlessness Irritability Low-grade fever Nontoxic appearance	URI Croupy cough Stridor Hoarseness Dyspnea Restlessness Symptoms awakening child but disappearing during day Tendency to recur	URI Croupy cough Purulent secretions High fever No response to LTB therapy
Treatment	Airway protection, possible intubation, tracheotomy Humidified oxygen Corticosteroids Fluids Antibiotics Reassurance	Humidified mist if needed Corticosteroids Fluids Reassurance Nebulized epinephrine (possible short-term improvement) Heliox: moderate to severe croup	Cool mist Reassurance	Antibiotics Fluids

LTB, Laryngotracheobronchitis; *URI*, upper respiratory infection.

awaken later, complaining of sore throat and pain on swallowing. The child has a fever and appears sicker than clinical findings suggest. The child insists on sitting upright and leaning forward (tripod position) with the chin thrust out, mouth open, and tongue protruding. Drooling of saliva is common because of the difficulty or pain on swallowing and excessive secretions.

> **! NURSING ALERT**
>
> Three clinical observations that are predictive of epiglottitis are absence of spontaneous cough, presence of drooling, and agitation.

The child is irritable and extremely restless and has an anxious, apprehensive, and frightened expression. The voice is thick and muffled, with a froglike croaking sound on inspiration, but the child is not hoarse. Suprasternal and substernal retractions may be visible. Slow, quiet breathing provides better air exchange. The sallow color of mild hypoxia may progress to frank cyanosis if treatment is delayed. The throat is red and inflamed, and a distinctive large, cherry red, edematous epiglottis is visible on careful throat inspection.

> **! NURSING ALERT**
>
> Throat inspection should be performed only when immediate endotracheal intubation or an emergency tracheotomy can be performed if needed.

Therapeutic Management

Epiglottitis may develop suddenly, with respiratory obstruction appearing rapidly. Progressive obstruction leads to hypoxia, hypercapnia, and acidosis followed by decreased muscular tone and reduced level of consciousness; when obstruction becomes more or less complete, sudden death may ensue.

A lateral neck radiograph of the soft tissues is indicated for diagnosis. Experienced personnel with advanced airway management skills should accompany the child to the radiology department. For a young child who is likely to become more agitated by the procedure, it is preferable that the child remain on the parent's lap if content during transportation and in the examination area during portable radiology.

The child who is suspected of having epiglottitis should be examined in a setting where emergency airway equipment is readily available. Examination of the throat with a tongue depressor is contraindicated until experienced personnel and equipment are available to proceed with immediate intubation or tracheostomy if the examination precipitates further or complete obstruction.

Endotracheal intubation is usually considered for the child with epiglottitis with severe respiratory distress. Nasotracheal intubation is sometimes preferred. It is recommended that the intubation or any invasive procedure, such as starting an IV infusion, be performed in an area where emergency airway maintenance can be easily and quickly accomplished. For patients who are not intubated, humidified oxygen is administered as necessary either via mask in older children or via blow-by in younger children to avoid further agitation (see Translating Evidence Into Practice box, later in the chapter). Whether or not there is an artificial airway, the child requires intensive observation by experienced personnel. The epiglottal swelling usually decreases after 24 hours of antibiotic therapy, and the epiglottis is near normal by the third day. Intubated children are generally extubated at this time.

Children with suspected bacterial epiglottitis are given antibiotics intravenously usually after obtaining culture (blood and an epiglottic in intubated patient) and followed by oral antibiotic administration to complete a 7- to 10-day course. Ceftriaxone/cefotaxime and vancomycin are generally the first antibiotics started. The use of corticosteroids for reducing edema may be beneficial during the early treatment phase.

Nursing Care Management

Epiglottitis is a serious and frightening disease for the child, family, and health professionals. It is important to act quickly but calmly and to provide support without increasing anxiety. The child can remain in the position that provides the most comfort and security and the parents are reassured that everything possible is being done to obtain relief for their child.

> **! NURSING ALERT**
>
> Nurses who suspect epiglottitis should not attempt to visualize the epiglottis directly with a tongue depressor or take a throat culture but should have the child seen by the provider immediately. Resuscitation equipment and suction should be immediately available and ready at the child's bedside.

Droplet isolation precautions are indicated for 24 hours with the initiation of effective antibiotic therapy to control spread of respiratory organisms. Prophylactic antibiotic treatment of household and other contacts may be indicated. Continuous monitoring of respiratory status, including pulse oximetry (and blood gases if the patient is intubated), is an important part of nursing observations, and the IV infusion is maintained as described in Chapter 20 (see Critical Thinking Case Study).

CRITICAL THINKING CASE STUDY

Epiglottitis

Kim, a 4-year-old, is admitted to the emergency department with a sore throat, pain on swallowing, drooling, and a fever of 102.2°F (39°C). She looks ill, is agitated, and prefers to sit up and lean over. According to her mother, she has not had anything to eat or drink since early morning.

Initial Assessment. What immediate concerns do you have about Kim's condition?

Clinical Reasoning. What interventions are appropriate for her immediate care?

Teaching Points

- Infants or children with epiglottis can have severe respiratory distress occur quickly.
- Absence of spontaneous cough, presence of drooling, and agitation are important clinical observations.
- If epiglottitis is suspected, do not attempt to examine the throat without appropriate expertise and equipment available in case intubation or tracheostomy is needed.

Critical Thinking Answers

Initial Assessment. Kim presents with classic symptoms of epiglottitis. Immediate intervention is needed with a focus on respiratory stability.

Clinical Reasoning. An appropriate nursing action is to act quickly and calmly to provide support while rapid assessment and interventions are being implemented. Continuous monitoring of respirations, including pulse oximetry, is the immediate course of action while the diagnosis is established. Examination must occur when emergency airway equipment is readily available.

ACUTE LARYNGOTRACHEOBRONCHITIS

Acute laryngotracheobronchitis (LTB) is the most common type of croup syndrome that primarily affects children 6 months to 3 years old. Organisms responsible for LTB are the parainfluenza virus type 1, followed by parainfluenza virus types 2 and 3, adenoviruses, RSV, and *M. pneumoniae.* Less common causative organisms include influenza A and B, rhinoviruses, enteroviruses, herpes simplex virus. *S. aureus, Streptococcus pyogenes,* and *S. pneumoniae.* The illness is usually preceded by a URI, which gradually descends to adjacent structures. It is characterized by a gradual onset of low-grade fever, and the parents often report that the child went to bed and later awoke with a barky, brassy cough.

Inflammation of the mucosal lining of the larynx and trachea causes a narrowing of the airway. When the airway is significantly narrowed, the child struggles to inhale air past the obstruction and into the lungs, producing the characteristic inspiratory stridor and suprasternal retractions. Other classic manifestations include cough and hoarseness. Respiratory distress in infants and toddlers may be manifested by nasal flaring, intercostal retractions, tachypnea, and continuous stridor. The typical child with LTB is a toddler who develops the classic barking or seal-like cough and acute stridor after several days of rhinitis. When the child is unable to inhale a sufficient volume of air, symptoms of hypoxia become evident. Obstruction that is severe enough to prevent adequate ventilation and exhalation of carbon dioxide can cause respiratory acidosis and eventually respiratory failure.

Therapeutic Management

The major objective in medical management of infectious LTB is maintaining an airway and providing for adequate respiratory exchange. Children with mild croup (no stridor at rest) can be managed at home. Parents should be instructed on the signs of respiratory distress so that they can obtain professional help if needed. Children with progressively worsening respiratory distress (e.g., labored respirations, stridor, other respiratory symptoms) should receive immediate medical attention.

Cool mist may provide relief for children with mild croup, although there is no substantial evidence of its efficacy (Petrocheilou, Tanou, Kalampouka, et al., 2014). In the hospital, mist may be provided with a face mask or as blow-by, but controversy surrounds the use of mist therapy to treat croup. The cool-temperature therapy modalities assist by constricting edematous blood vessels. In the home environment, suggestions to provide cool air include taking the child outside to breathe in cool night air, using a cold-water vaporizer or humidifier, standing in front of the open freezer, or taking the child to a cool basement or garage. Although these are often recommended, there is no evidence to unconditionally support their use. A ride in the car with the window down may help relieve symptoms, and the child often improves on the way to the emergency department (ED) due to exposure to cool air.

Nebulized racemic epinephrine is administered as quickly as possible for moderate to severe cases. The beta-adrenergic effects cause mucosal vasoconstriction and subsequently decrease subglottic edema. The onset of action is rapid, the peak effect is observed within 2 hours, and additional doses may be administered every 20 to 30 minutes as needed. Close observation of patients receiving nebulized racemic epinephrine is critical to detect the reappearance of symptoms, monitor the response to therapy, and note any deterioration in respiratory status. The patient who has received nebulized epinephrine for croup should be observed for 3 to 4 hours for any visible signs of respiratory distress.

Oral steroids (dexamethasone), due to their antiinflammatory effects, have proven effective in the treatment of croup (often as a single dose) and are considered standard treatment for this condition. IV or IM dexamethasone may be given to children who are unable to tolerate oral dosing. The onset of action is clinically detectable as early as 6 hours after administration, with continued improvement over a period of 12 to 24 hours.

Supplemental oxygen with mist may be needed if hypoxemic. On occasion, intubation and ventilation may be required when airway obstruction becomes more severe.

Nursing Care Management

The most important nursing function in the care of children with LTB is continuous, vigilant observation and accurate assessment of respiratory status. Cardiac, respiratory, and pulse oximetry monitoring supplement visual observation. Changes in therapy are frequently based on the nurses' observations and assessments of a child's status, response to therapy, and tolerance of procedures. The trend away from early intubation of children with LTB emphasizes the importance of nursing observations and the ability to recognize impending respiratory failure so that intubation can be implemented without delay. Therefore intubation equipment and bag valve mask equipment should be readily accessible.

> **! NURSING ALERT**
>
> Early signs of impending airway obstruction include increased pulse and respiratory rate; substernal, suprasternal, and intercostal retractions; flaring nares; and increased restlessness.

Infants or small children find that being placed on a face mask, coughing, having laryngeal spasms, and needing IV therapy are additional sources of distress. Infants and small children prefer sitting upright, and most want to be held. Blow-by mist can be administered by a parent while the child is being held. Children need the security of the parent's presence. Because crying increases respiratory distress and hypoxia, the nurse needs to assess a child's individual tolerance for these therapies.

The rapid progression of croup, the alarming sound of the cough and stridor, and the child's apprehensive behavior and ill appearance combine to create a frightening experience for the parents. Parents should be provided with frequent reassurance (provided in a calm, quiet manner), explanation of treatment, and education regarding what they can do to make their child more comfortable. Fortunately, as the crisis subsides and the child responds to therapy, breathing becomes easier and the recovery is generally prompt. Home care after discharge includes monitoring for worsening symptoms, continued humidity, adequate hydration, and nourishment.

ACUTE SPASMODIC LARYNGITIS

Acute spasmodic laryngitis (spasmodic croup, "midnight or twilight croup") is distinct from laryngitis and LTB and characterized by recurrent paroxysmal attacks of laryngeal obstruction that occur chiefly at night. Signs of inflammation are absent or mild with a usual history of previous attacks lasting for 2 to 5 days, followed by an uneventful recovery. The child goes to bed well or with some mild respiratory symptoms but awakens suddenly with the characteristic barking, metallic cough; hoarseness; noisy inspirations; and restlessness. The child appears anxious and frightened. However, there is no fever, the episode subsides in a few hours, and the child appears well the next day, with the exception of slight hoarseness. Some children appear to be predisposed to the condition; allergies or hypersensitivities may be implicated in some cases.

Cool mist is recommended for the child's room. Warm mist provided by steam from hot running water in a closed bathroom may be helpful. Parents are usually advised to have the child sleep in humidified air until the cough has subsided to prevent subsequent episodes. The disease is usually self-limiting.

BACTERIAL TRACHEITIS

Bacterial tracheitis, an infection of the mucosa and soft tissues of the upper trachea, is a distinct entity with features of both croup and epiglottitis. The disease occurs typically at a mean age between 5 and 7 years and may cause severe airway obstruction (Rodrigues & Roosevelt, 2020). It is believed to be a complication of LTB or other viral URIs, and although *S. aureus* is the most frequent organism responsible, *M. catarrhalis, S. pneumoniae, S. pyogenes,* alpha-hemolytic streptococci, and *H. influenzae* have also been implicated. Causes of bacterial tracheitis are often polymicrobial. Viruses such as influenza A and B, RSV, parainfluenza, measles, and enteroviruses have been associated with bacterial tracheitis.

Anteroposterior or lateral neck x-rays show narrowing (steeple sign), and infiltrates may be seen. An endoscopy of the airway performed in the operating room (OR) or intensive care unit (ICU) is usually indicated to remove secretions and obtain cultures.

Many of the manifestations of bacterial tracheitis are similar to those of LTB but are unresponsive to LTB therapy. The child has a history of previous URI with croupy cough, stridor unaffected by position, toxicity, absence of drooling, high fever, and elevated white blood cell count. Thick, purulent tracheal secretions are common, and respiratory difficulties are secondary to these copious secretions.

Therapeutic Management and Nursing Care Management

Bacterial tracheitis requires vigorous management with maintenance of adequate airway and fluid status and treatment with antibiotics and antipyretics. Many children require endotracheal intubation and mechanical ventilation; patients are closely monitored for impending respiratory failure if not intubated. Early recognition is essential to prevent life-threatening airway obstruction.

INFECTIONS OF THE LOWER AIRWAYS

The reactive portion of the lower respiratory tract includes the bronchi and bronchioles in children. Cartilaginous support of the large airways is not fully developed until adolescence. Consequently, the smooth muscle in these structures represents a major factor in the constriction of the airway, particularly in the bronchioles, the portion that extends from the bronchi to the alveoli. Table 21.2 compares some of the major features of bronchial and bronchiolar infections.

BRONCHITIS

Bronchitis (sometimes referred to as tracheobronchitis) is inflammation of the large airways (trachea and bronchi), which is frequently associated with URIs. Viral agents are the primary cause of the disease, including influenza A and B, parainfluenza, coronavirus (types 1 to 3), rhinovirus, respiratory syncytial virus, and human metapneumovirus. The condition is characterized by a dry, hacking, and nonproductive cough that is worse at night, lasting more than 5 days but that can persist for 1 to 3 weeks.

Bronchitis is a mild, self-limiting disease that requires only symptomatic treatment, including analgesics, antipyretics, and humidity. Cough suppressants may be useful to allow rest, especially at night, but can interfere with clearance of secretions. Most patients recover uneventfully in 5 to 10 days. It can be associated with other underlying conditions (such as CF and bronchiectasis) and can become chronic in nature (cough >3 months). Adolescents with chronic bronchitis (>3 months) should be screened for tobacco or marijuana use.

TABLE 21.2 Comparison of Conditions Affecting the Bronchi

	Asthma[a]	Bronchitis	Bronchiolitis
Description	Exaggerated response of bronchi to a trigger such as URI, animal dander, cold air, exercise Bronchospasm, exudation, and edema of bronchi	Usually occurs in association with URI Seldom an isolated entity	Most common infectious disease of lower airways Maximum obstructive impact at bronchiolar level
Age-group affected	Infancy to adolescence or adulthood	First 4 years of life	Usually children 2-12 months old; rare after 2 years old Peak incidence approximately 6 months old
Etiologic agents	Most often viruses such as RSV in infants but may be any of a variety of URI pathogens	Usually viral Other agents (e.g., bacteria, fungi, allergic disorders, airborne irritants) can trigger symptoms	Viruses, predominantly RSV; also adenoviruses, parainfluenza viruses, human metapneumovirus, and *Mycoplasma pneumoniae*
Predominant characteristics	Wheezing, cough, labored respirations	Persistent dry, hacking cough (worse at night) becoming productive in 2-3 days	Labored respirations, poor feeding, cough, tachypnea, retractions and flaring nares, increased nasal mucus, wheezing, may have fever
Treatment	Inhaled corticosteroids, bronchodilators, leukotriene modifiers, allergen control, control of triggers	Cough suppressants if needed	Supplemental oxygen if saturations ≤90%; bronchodilators (optional) Suction nasopharynx Ensure adequate fluid intake Maintain adequate oxygenation

[a]See Asthma later in the chapter.
RSV, Respiratory syncytial virus; *URI,* upper respiratory infection.

RESPIRATORY SYNCYTIAL VIRUS AND BRONCHIOLITIS

Bronchiolitis is an acute viral infection with maximum effect at the bronchiolar level. The infection typically begins with upper respiratory symptoms and occurs primarily in winter and early spring. Most cases of bronchiolitis are caused by RSV, adenoviruses, parainfluenza viruses, and human metapneumovirus, but RSV is the most common cause, resulting in more than 57,000 hospitalizations and 2.1 million outpatient visits each year (Smith, Seales, & Budzik, 2017). Occasionally, *M. pneumoniae* has been associated with bronchiolitis in children.

RSV is transmitted predominantly through direct or close contact with contaminated respiratory secretions. Viable RSV can live on environmental surfaces (e.g., countertops, paper tissues, cloth) for several hours and on hands for 30 minutes or more (American Academy of Pediatrics, Committee on Infectious Diseases, 2018).

RSV occurs less frequently in breastfed infants and more frequently in children who live in crowded conditions. RSV infection is the most frequent cause of hospitalization in children younger than 2 years old. Severe RSV infections in the first year of life represent a significant risk factor for the development of asthma that can persist into adulthood (American Academy of Pediatrics, Committee on Infectious Diseases, 2018; Smith et al., 2017). However, the association between RSV infection early in life and subsequent asthma remains poorly understood (American Academy of Pediatrics, Committee on Infectious Diseases, 2018).

Pathophysiology

RSV infection affects the epithelial cells of the respiratory tract. The ciliated cells swell, protrude into the lumen, and lose their cilia. The walls of the bronchi and bronchioles are infiltrated with inflammatory cells, and peribronchiolar interstitial pneumonitis is usually present. Because luminal epithelial cells are shed into the bronchioles when they die, the lumina are frequently obstructed, particularly on expiration. The varying degrees of obstruction produced in small air passages lead to hyperinflation, obstructive emphysema resulting from partial obstruction, and patchy areas of atelectasis. Dilation of bronchial passages on inspiration allows sufficient space for intake of air, but narrowing of the passages on expiration prevents air from leaving the lungs. Thus air is trapped distal to the obstruction and causes progressive overinflation (emphysema).

Clinical Manifestations

The younger the infant, the greater the likelihood that severe lower respiratory tract disease will develop, requiring hospitalization. The peak incidence for RSV is less than 3 months of age, but it can occur at all ages. Higher rates occur in children who attend a daycare home or daycare center. The severity of RSV tends to diminish with age and repeated infections.

Symptoms such as rhinorrhea and low-grade fever often appear first after an incubation ranging from 2 to 8 days. In time, a cough may develop. If the disease progresses, it becomes a lower respiratory tract infection and manifests typical symptoms (Box 21.8). Infants may have several days of URI symptoms or no symptoms except slight lethargy, poor feeding, or irritability. When the lower airway is involved, classic manifestations include signs of altered air exchange, such as wheezing, retractions, crackles, dyspnea, tachypnea, and diminished breath sounds. Apnea may be the first recognized indicator of RSV infection in very young infants (younger than 1 month old). Children who are infected with RSV have viral shedding for 3 to 8 days, but some infants and patients with weakened immune systems can be contagious for as long as 4 weeks (American Academy of Pediatrics, Committee on Infectious Diseases, 2018).

BOX 21.8 Signs and Symptoms of Respiratory Syncytial Virus Infection

Initial
- Rhinorrhea
- Pharyngitis
- Coughing, sneezing
- Wheezing
- Possible ear or eye drainage
- Intermittent fever

With Progression of Illness
- Increased coughing and wheezing
- Fever
- Tachypnea and retractions
- Refusal to nurse or bottle-feed
- Copious secretions

Severe Illness
- Tachypnea, greater than 70 breaths/min
- Listlessness
- Apneic spells
- Altered air exchange (e.g., retractions, crackles)
- Diminished breath sounds

Diagnostic Evaluation

Routine testing for specific viruses is no longer recommended because bronchiolitis may be caused by many viruses (Smith et al., 2017). Routine x-rays are also not indicated (Smith et al., 2017). If identification is necessary, rapid immunofluorescent antibody–direct fluorescent antibody staining or enzyme-linked immunosorbent assay techniques for RSV antigen detection are performed on nasopharyngeal secretions. The more traditional viral culture is becoming obsolete because it takes several days to get a result (see Chapter 20, Respiratory Secretion Specimens).

Other simultaneous viral or bacterial infections may occur with RSV. The infant should be carefully evaluated for the presence of urinary tract infection, meningitis, and bacteremia; antibiotics are prescribed only for a coexisting bacterial infection.

Therapeutic Management

Most children with bronchiolitis can be managed at home. Uncomplicated cases of bronchiolitis are treated symptomatically with adequate fluid intake, airway maintenance, and medications. Hospitalization is recommended for children with respiratory distress or those with poor feeding, lethargy, dehydration, moderate to severe respiratory distress, apnea, or hypoxemia. Other reasons for hospitalization include complicating conditions, such as underlying lung or heart disease (e.g., prematurity) or caregiver inability to provide adequate care during illness.

The American Academy of Pediatrics recommends that continuous pulse oximetry and supplemental oxygen are not necessary if oxygen saturations are 90% or higher (Smith et al., 2017). Heated high-flow nasal cannula (HHFNC) has been increasingly used for hospitalized infants and young children with bronchiolitis who are at risk of respiratory failure. (Fig. 21.4). HHFNC allows extra humidity blended with oxygen administration and continuous positive airway pressure (CPAP) to be administered. The medical provider indicates the flow rate and percentage of the oxygen therapy. The HHFNC improves functional residual capacity, reducing the work of breathing. If respiratory acidosis is present,

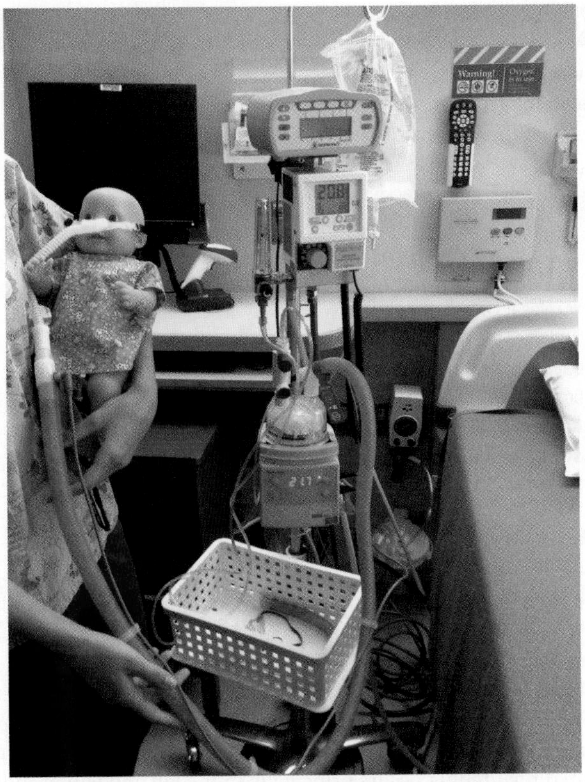

Fig. 21.4 High-flow nasal cannula (HFNC).

CPAP, bilevel positive airway pressure (BiPAP), or intubation may be required.

Routine chest percussion and drainage is not recommended (Smith et al., 2017). Infants with abundant nasal secretions benefit from regular suctioning, especially before feeding. Nasal aspiration of the external nares using an aspirator may be sufficient to remove most secretions. Nasopharyngeal suctioning is traumatic to the airways but can be considered if there are signs of respiratory distress or deoxygenation. Researchers found that the use of deep suctioning on the first day of admission and not suctioning the nose at least every 4 hours results in a longer length of stay for infants (Mussman, Parker, Statile, et al., 2013).

Fluids by mouth may be contraindicated because of tachypnea, weakness, and fatigue. Therefore IV fluids are preferred until the acute stage of the disease has passed. Nasogastric fluids may be required if the infant is unable to tolerate oral fluids and a peripheral IV is difficult to establish.

Clinical assessments, noninvasive oxygen monitoring, and, in severe cases, blood gas values may guide therapy. Medical therapy for bronchiolitis is primarily supportive and aimed at decreasing airway hyperresonance and inflammation and promoting adequate fluid intake. Bronchodilators are not recommended and are rarely beneficial. The use of 3% nebulized (hypertonic) saline is associated with an increase in mucociliary clearance in children with RSV when used for more than 24 hours, but it is recommended for use only in patients hospitalized for more than 3 days (Smith et al., 2017).

The use of systemic corticosteroids is controversial, but they may be used in some centers. Studies have reported prolonged viral shedding with corticosteroid use. Antibiotics are not part of the treatment of RSV unless there is a coexisting bacterial infection such as OM or pneumonia. Additional treatment recommendations are to encourage breastfeeding, avoid passive tobacco smoke exposure, and promote preventive measures, including hand washing and the administration of palivizumab (Synagis) to high-risk infants.

Ribavirin, an inhaled antiviral agent (synthetic nucleoside analog), is the only specific therapy approved for hospitalized children. However, use of this drug in infants with RSV is controversial because of concerns about the high cost, aerosol route of administration, potential toxic effects among exposed health care personnel, and conflicting results of efficacy trials (American Academy of Pediatrics, Committee on Infectious Diseases, 2018; Mejias & Ramilo, 2015).

Prevention of Respiratory Syncytial Virus Infection

The only product available in the United States for prevention of RSV is palivizumab (Synagis), a humanized monoclonal antibody, which is given at the onset of the RSV season and then monthly in an IM injection or IV infusion for a maximum of five doses to prevent hospitalization associated with RSV.

Candidates for this drug include the following (Smith et al., 2017):

- Infants born before 29 weeks of gestation
- Infants in the first year of life with hemodynamically significant heart disease
- Infants in the first year of life for preterm infants (<32 weeks of gestation) with chronic lung disease or children in the second year of life with chronic lung disease who require continued medical intervention

Some children acquire the illness despite palivizumab prophylaxis. Additional age and condition recommendations are outlined in the American Academy of Pediatrics Bronchiolitis Guidelines Committee policy statement (American Academy of Pediatrics, Committee on Infectious Diseases, 2014).

QUALITY PATIENT OUTCOMES: Bronchiolitis

- Oxygen (O_2) saturation 90% or higher
- Respiratory rate less than 60 breaths/min
- Adequate oral fluid intake

Nursing Care Management

Children admitted to the hospital with suspected RSV infection are usually assigned separate rooms or grouped with other RSV-infected children. Contact and Standard Precautions are used with hospitalized patients, and some institutions use Droplet Precautions as well. Proper hand washing is essential to reduce the spread of the illness. Other isolation procedures of potential benefit are those aimed at diminishing the number of hospital personnel, visitors, and uninfected children in contact with the child. Another measure is to organize patient assignments so that nurses assigned to children with RSV are not caring for other patients who are considered high risk for RSV. Staff must be careful to avoid touching the nasal mucosa or conjunctiva.

Due to the copious nasal secretions associated with RSV infection, infants often have difficulty with breathing and feeding. Breastfeeding mothers are encouraged to continue feeding the infant or, if feedings are contraindicated due to severity of the illness, mothers should pump their milk and store it appropriately for later use (see Chapter 7). Parents are taught how to instill normal saline drops into the nares and suction the mucus with bulb syringe before feedings and before bedtime so that the child may more easily eat, rest, and sleep.

To address the issue of decreased fluid intake, parents may offer small amounts of fluids, 5 to 10 ml at a time, using a medication syringe every 10 minutes or so to maintain adequate hydration. Infants' hydration status may also be affected by coughing and/or vomiting as the secretions settle in the throat and stomach.

Nursing care is also aimed at monitoring oxygenation with pulse oximetry as clinically indicated, monitoring IV fluids or NG fluids, monitoring for fever, administering prescribed medications, and providing information for the parent and family regarding the infant's status. In most cases, infants recover quickly from the disease and resume normal daily activities, including fluid intake.

PNEUMONIA

Pneumonia, inflammation of the pulmonary parenchyma, is common in childhood but occurs more frequently in infancy and early childhood. Clinically, pneumonia may occur either as a primary disease or as a complication of another illness.

The most useful classification of pneumonia is based on the etiologic agent (e.g., viral, bacterial, mycoplasmal, or aspiration of foreign substances) (see Aspiration Pneumonia, later in the chapter). The causative agent is usually introduced into the lungs through inhalation or from the bloodstream. Other terms that describe pneumonias are *hemorrhagic, fibrinous,* and *necrotizing.*

Pneumonitis is a localized acute inflammation of the lung without the toxemia associated with lobar pneumonia. The clinical manifestations of pneumonia vary depending on the etiologic agent, the child's age, the child's systemic reaction to the infection, the extent of the lesions, any underlying conditions, and the degree of bronchial and bronchiolar obstruction. The clinical history, the child's age, the general health history, the physical examination, radiography, and the laboratory examination can help identify the etiologic agent. Many organisms can cause pneumonia, and vary according to the child's age:

- **Neonates:** Group B streptococci, gram-negative enteric bacteria, cytomegalovirus, *Ureaplasma urealyticum, Listeria monocytogenes, C. trachomatis*
- **Infants:** RSV, parainfluenza virus, influenza virus, adenovirus, metapneumovirus, *S. pneumoniae, H. influenzae, M. pneumoniae, Mycobacterium tuberculosis,* group A streptococci, *M. catarrhalis*
- **Preschool children:** RSV, parainfluenza virus, influenza virus, adenovirus, metapneumovirus, *S. pneumoniae, H. influenzae, M. pneumoniae, M. tuberculosis,* group A streptococci, *M. catarrhalis*
- **School-age children:** *M. pneumoniae, Chlamydia pneumoniae, M. tuberculosis,* group A streptococci, *S. aureus, M. catarrhalis,* and respiratory viruses

Viral Pneumonia

Viral pneumonias occur more frequently than bacterial pneumonias, are seen in children of all ages, and are often associated with viral URIs. The pathologic changes involve interstitial pneumonitis with mucosal inflammation of the walls of bronchi and bronchioles with possible parenchymal involvement. The onset may be acute or insidious, and symptoms vary from mild fever, slight cough, and malaise to high fever, severe cough, and fatigue. Early in the illness, the cough is likely to be unproductive or productive for small amounts of whitish sputum. Radiography reveals diffuse or patchy infiltration with a peribronchial distribution (Box 21.9).

The prognosis is generally good, although viral infections of the respiratory tract render the affected child more susceptible to secondary bacterial invasion, especially when there is denuded bronchial mucosa. Treatment is symptomatic and includes measures to promote oxygenation and comfort, such as oxygen administration, chest percussion and postural drainage, antipyretics for fever management, monitoring fluid intake, and family support. Antibiotics are reserved for children in whom a bacterial infection is demonstrated.

BOX 21.9 General Signs of Pneumonia

Fever: Usually high
Respiratory
- Cough: unproductive to productive with whitish sputum
- Tachypnea
- Breath sounds: crackles or rhonchi
- Dullness with percussion
- Chest pain
- Retractions
- Nasal flaring
- Pallor to cyanosis (depends on severity)

Chest radiography: Diffuse or patchy infiltration with peribronchial distribution
Behavior: Irritability, restlessness, lethargic
Gastrointestinal: Anorexia, vomiting, diarrhea, abdominal pain

Primary Atypical Pneumonia

Atypical pneumonia refers to pneumonia that is caused by pathogens other than the traditionally most common and readily cultured bacteria (e.g., *S. pneumoniae*). In the category of atypical pneumonias, *M. pneumoniae* is the most common cause of community-acquired pneumonia in children 5 years or older (Jain, Williams, Arnold, et al., 2015). Community-associated methicillin-resistant *Staphylococcus aureus* (CA-MRSA) has become prevalent in certain areas. Community-acquired pneumonia occurs principally in the fall and winter months and is more prevalent in crowded living conditions.

The onset may be sudden or insidious and is usually accompanied by general systemic symptoms, including fever, chills (in older children), headache, malaise, anorexia, and muscle pain (myalgia). These symptoms are followed by rhinitis, sore throat, and a dry, hacking cough. The cough, initially nonproductive, produces seromucoid sputum that later becomes mucopurulent or blood streaked. The degree of fever varies widely, from several days to 2 weeks. Dyspnea occurs infrequently

Radiographic examination may reveal evidence of pneumonia before physical signs are apparent. Most affected persons recover from acute illness in 7 to 10 days with symptomatic treatment followed by 1 week of convalescence. The incubation period is 2 to 3 weeks, but the cough may last several weeks. Hospitalization is rarely necessary. Erythromycin, azithromycin, and clarithromycin are the primary agents used for treating atypical pneumonia.

Bacterial Pneumonia

S. pneumoniae is the most common bacterial pathogen responsible for community-acquired pneumonia in both children and adults. Other bacteria that cause pneumonia in children are group A streptococcus, *S. aureus, M. catarrhalis, M. pneumoniae,* and *C. pneumoniae.*

Pneumonia in the immediate neonatal period is different from other types of pneumonia described. If infection occurs within 3 to 5 days of birth, the pathogen is usually obtained from the mother transplacentally, or through aspiration of infected amniotic fluid intrauterine or during or after birth (e.g., Group B hemolytic, chlamydial, or herpes simplex viral pneumonia). Early symptoms of neonatal pneumonia can be abrupt and nonspecific but may include respiratory distress.

Beyond the neonatal period, bacterial pneumonias display distinct clinical patterns that facilitate their differentiation from other forms of pneumonia. The onset of illness generally follows a viral infection that disturbs the natural defense mechanisms of the upper respiratory tract. In the 3-month to 5-year age-group, *S. pneumoniae, M. catarrhalis,* and group A streptococci are common causes. *H. influenzae* type B causes fewer infections because of the Hib vaccine. *S. aureus* pneumonia is rare but is particularly progressive and must be treated aggressively. The child with bacterial pneumonia usually appears ill. Symptoms include fever, malaise, rapid and shallow respirations, cough, and chest pain. The associated cough may persist for several weeks or months. The pain of pneumonia may be referred to the abdomen in young children. Chills and meningeal symptoms (meningism) without meningitis are common.

Most older children with pneumonia can be treated at home if the condition is recognized and treatment is initiated early. Antibiotic therapy, rest, liberal oral intake of fluid, and administration of an antipyretic for fever are the principal therapeutic measures. Chest percussion and postural drainage may be indicated, but there is a lack of evidence to show that they have benefit to children with pneumonia.

Infants and young children develop more severe symptoms than older children. Cyanosis and apnea are common, and the parent may report that the infant's activity and eating pattern was decreased for a few days. Additional clinical manifestations in infants include abrupt fever, vomiting, diarrhea, and abdominal distention. Because pneumonia in newborns carries a high morbidity and mortality rate, bacterial infection should be suspected in all neonates with respiratory symptoms.

A follow-up examination is recommended for small infants and toddlers. Hospitalization is indicated when pleural effusion or empyema accompanies the disease, when moderate or severe respiratory distress or deoxygenation occurs, in situations in which compliance with therapy is estimated to be poor, in infants younger than 6 months old, and when there are chronic illnesses such as congenital heart disease or BPD (Barson, 2015). IV fluids may be necessary to ensure adequate hydration, and oxygen is required if the child is in respiratory distress; some children may require initial therapy with parenteral antibiotics because of the severity of illness.

Complications

At present, the classic features and clinical course of pneumonia are rarely seen because of early and vigorous antibiotic and supportive therapy. However, some children, especially infants, with staphylococcal pneumonia develop empyema, pyopneumothorax, or tension pneumothorax. AOM and pleural effusion are common in children with pneumococcal pneumonia (Box 21.10) (see Translating Evidence Into Practice box). As previously mentioned, vaccination with pneumococcal vaccines is an important part of preventing pneumococcal pneumonia.

TRANSLATING EVIDENCE INTO PRACTICE

Nursing Interventions for Prevention of Ventilator-Associated Pneumonia in Children

Ask the Question

PICOT Question

What nursing interventions prevent VAP in children?

Search for the Evidence

Search Strategies

Search selection included English-language publications on nursing interventions for prevention of VAP in children and adolescents.

Databases Used

PubMed, AHRQ.

Critically Analyze the Evidence

- Implementation of VAP bundle resulted in a decreased VAP rate from 5.6 infections per 1000 ventilator days at baseline to 0.3 per 1000 ventilator days (Bigham, Amato, Bondurrant, et al., 2009). Another study reported similar results with implementation of a VAP bundle that had a decreased VAP rate from 21.6 per 1000 ventilator days at baseline to 11.6 per 1000 ventilator days (P = 0.01) (Parisi, Gerovasili, Dimopoulos, et al., 2016).
- Common VAP prevention interventions include the following (Bigham et al., 2009; Chinnadurai, Fenlason, Bridges, et al., 2016; Coffin, Klompas, Classes, et al., 2008; Garland, 2010; Kollef, 2004; Morrow, Argent, Jeena, et al., 2009; Norris, Barnes, & Roberts, 2009):
  - Change ventilator circuits and in-line suction catheters only when soiled.
  - Every 2 to 4 hours, drain condensate from ventilator circuit (use heated wire circuits to reduce rainout).
  - Rinse oral suction devices after use and store in a nonsealed plastic bag at the bedside.
  - Hand hygiene should be used before and after contact with ventilator circuit.
  - Wear PPE before providing care to patients when soiling from respiratory secretions is anticipated.
  - Maintenance of ET tube cuff pressure adequate to prevent aspiration of secretions.
  - Minimizing transportation outside the ICU for other procedures.
  - Use of noninvasive ventilation when possible.
  - Every 2 to 4 hours, follow unit mouth care policy.
  - Unless contraindicated, elevate head of bed to 30 to 45 degrees.
  - Before repositioning patient, always drain ventilator circuit.
  - For patients older than 12 years of age, when possible, use ET tube with dorsal lumen above ET cuff to help suction secretions above the cuff.
  - Evaluate daily for possible extubation.
  - Avoid reintubation.
- Infants in supine position (infant lying on back with ET tube held upright in the vertical position) had increased colony counts or new organisms in tracheal aspirate compared to infants in lateral position (infant lying on side with ET tube at same level as the trachea) (Aly, Badawy, El-Kholy, et al., 2008).
- Staff education on VAP and improvements to practice changes can have a substantial impact on reducing VAP (Garland, 2010; Hill, 2016; Richardson, Hines, Dixon, et al., 2010; Turton, 2008).
- A 7-day versus 3-day ventilator circuit change was not associated with increased VAP rates (Samransamruajkit, Jirapaiboonsuk, Siritantiwat, et al., 2010).
- Use of low-sodium solution for airway care was associated with a decrease in VAP as well as chronic lung disease (Christensen, Henry, Baer, et al., 2010).
- In bronchoalveolar lavage fluid, PAI-1 levels can aid in early diagnosis of VAP (Srinivasan, Song, Wiener-Kronish, et al., 2011).
- Reduced mortality rates were observed in patients with VAP when a silver-coated ET tube was used versus an uncoated ET tube (Afessa, Shorr, Anzueto, et al., 2010).

Apply the Evidence: Nursing Implications

There is **moderate evidence** with a **strong recommendation** (Guyatt, Oxman, Vist, et al., 2008) for use of interventions to prevent VAP in children. Some prevention methods included in VAP bundles are hand hygiene, oral hygiene, use of PPE, elevation of head of bed 30 to 45 degrees, and more. Staff education and engagement in VAP prevention initiatives is important.

References

Afessa, B., Shorr, A. F., Anzueto, A. R., et al. (2010). Association between a silver-coated endotracheal tube and reduced mortality in patients with ventilator-associated pneumonia. *Chest, 137*(5), 1015–1021.

Continued

TRANSLATING EVIDENCE INTO PRACTICE—cont'd

Aly, H., Badawy, M., El-Kholy, A., et al. (2008). Randomized, controlled trial on tracheal colonization of ventilated infants: Can gravity prevent ventilator-associated pneumonia? *Pediatrics, 122*(4), 770–774.

Bigham, M. T., Amato, R., Bondurrant, P., et al. (2009). Ventilator-associated pneumonia in the pediatric intensive care unit: Characterizing the problem and implementing a sustainable solution. *Journal of Pediatrics, 154*(4), 582–587.

Chinnadurai, K., Fenlason, L., Bridges, B., et al. (2016). Implementation of sustainable ventilator-associated pneumonia prevention protocol in a pediatric intensive care unit in Managua, Nicaragua. *Dimensions of Critical Care Nursing, 35*(6), 323–331.

Christensen, R. D., Henry, E., Baer, V. L., et al. (2010). A low-sodium solution for airway care: Results of a multicenter trial. *Respiratory Care, 55*(12), 1680–1685.

Coffin, S. E., Klompas, M., Classen, D., et al. (2008). Strategies to prevent ventilator-associated pneumonia in acute care hospitals. *Infection Control & Hospital Epidemiology, 29*(Suppl. 1), S31–S40.

Garland, J. S. (2010). Strategies to prevent ventilator-associated pneumonia in neonates. *Clinics in Perinatology, 37*(3), 629–643.

Guyatt, G. H., Oxman, A. D., Vist, G. E., et al. (2008). GRADE: An emerging consensus on rating quality of evidence and strength of recommendations. *BMJ, 336*(7650), 924–926.

Hill, C. (2016). Nurse-led implementation of a ventilator-associated pneumonia care bundle in a children's critical care unit. *Nursing Children and Young People, 28*(4), 23–27.

Kollef, M. H. (2004). Prevention of hospital-associated pneumonia and ventilator-associated pneumonia. *Critical Care Medicine, 32*(6), 1396–1405.

Morrow, B. M., Argent, A. C., Jeena, P. M., et al. (2009). Guideline for the diagnosis, prevention and treatment of paediatric ventilator-associated pneumonia. *South African Medical Journal, 99*(4 Pt 2), 255–267.

Norris, S. C., Barnes, A. K., & Roberts, T. D. (2009). When ventilator-associated pneumonias haunt your NICU—One unit's story. *Neonatal Network, 28*(1), 59–66.

Parisi, M., Gerovasili, V., Dimopoulos, S., et al. (2016). Use of ventilator bundle and staff education to decrease ventilator-associated pneumonia in intensive care patients. *Critical Care Nurse, 36*(5), e1–e7.

Richardson, M., Hines, S., Dixon, G., et al. (2010). Establishing nurse-led ventilator-associated pneumonia surveillance in paediatric intensive care. *Journal of Hospital Infection, 75*(3), 220–224.

Samransamruajkit, R., Jirapaiboonsuk, S., Siritantiwat, S., et al. (2010). Effect of frequency of ventilator circuit changes (3 vs 7 days) on the rate of ventilator-associated pneumonia in PICU. *Journal of Critical Care, 25*(1), 56–61.

Srinivasan, R., Song, Y., Wiener-Kronish, J., et al. (2011). Plasminogen activation inhibitor concentrations in bronchoalveolar lavage fluid distinguishes ventilator-associated pneumonia from colonization in mechanically ventilated pediatric patients. *Pediatric Critical Care Medicine, 12*(1), 21–27.

Turton, P. (2008). Ventilator-associated pneumonia in paediatric intensive care: A literature review. *Nursing in Critical Care, 13*(5), 241–248.

ET, Endotracheal; *ICU,* intensive care unit; *PAI,* plasminogen activation inhibitor; *PPE,* personal protection equipment; *VAP,* ventilator-associated pneumonia.

BOX 21.10 Pneumothorax

Pneumothorax occurs when air accumulates in the pleural space; this air increases intrapleural pressure, making it more difficult to expand the affected lung. This leads to the clinical manifestations of dyspnea, chest pain and often back pain, labored respirations, tachycardia, and decreased oxygen saturation (SaO_2). In neonates and infants on mechanical ventilation, the first clinical signs of a pneumothorax are oxygen desaturation and hypotension. The three major types of pneumothorax are tension, spontaneous, and traumatic. The definitive diagnosis of pneumothorax is a chest radiograph. The emergent treatment involves needle aspiration of the air within the pleural space; subsequently a chest tube to closed drainage is usually inserted to prevent the reaccumulation of air.

Pleural effusion occurs when there is an excessive accumulation of fluid in the pleural space. The diagnosis is made by chest radiography, and the treatment involves evacuation of the fluid by needle aspiration followed by insertion of a chest tube to closed drainage.

When fluid is either suspected or identified by radiograph in the pleural cavity, a needle aspiration or thoracentesis may be performed. Nonpurulent effusions do not require surgical drainage.

Continuous closed chest drainage may be instituted with complicated pleural effusion. If a large amount of purulent drainage is obtained, an appropriate antibiotic may be instilled into the chest cavity, and chest drainage is discontinued for approximately 1 hour after the instillation. Closed drainage using a chest tube is continued until drainage fluid is minimal and free of pathogens, which rarely requires more than 5 to 7 days. Sometimes repeated pleural taps are sufficient to remove fluid; however, if the purulent drainage accumulates rapidly and is highly viscous, continuous drainage is preferred. Rarely, thoracotomy with open debridement of the infected lung tissue is required.

Additional therapies for empyema may involve instillation of intrapleural fibrinolytics such as urokinase or streptokinase or video-assisted thoracoscopy (Livingston, Colozza, Vogt, et al., 2016; van Loo, van Loo, Selvadurai, et al., 2014). These therapies may preclude the need for open debridement and thoracotomy.

Nursing Care Management

Nursing care of the child with pneumonia is primarily supportive and symptomatic but necessitates thorough respiratory assessment and administration of supplemental oxygen (as required), fluids, and antibiotics. The child's respiratory rate and status, oxygenation, general disposition, and level of activity are frequently assessed. To prevent dehydration, fluids may be needed intravenously during the acute phase. An NG tube may be placed to provide hydration and antibiotics if oral intake is poor.

Nursing care of the child with a chest tube requires close attention to respiratory status, as noted previously. The chest tube and drainage device used are monitored for proper function (e.g., drainage is not impeded, vacuum setting is correct, tubing is free of kinks, dressing covering chest tube insertion site is intact, water seal is maintained [if used], drainage tube is below the chest tube entry site and chest tube remains in place). Movement in bed and ambulation with a chest tube are encouraged according to the child's respiratory status, but children may require frequent doses of analgesia due to possible chest tube discomfort. If needed, supplemental oxygen may be administered by nasal cannula, face mask, blow-by, or face tent. Children are usually more comfortable in a semierect position (Fig. 21.5) but should be allowed to determine the position of comfort. Lying on the affected side if the pneumonia is unilateral ("good lung up") splints the chest on that side and reduces the pleural rubbing that often causes discomfort. Fever is controlled by cooling the environment and administrating antipyretic drugs as prescribed.

Vital signs and oxygenation are monitored to assess the progress of the disease and to detect early signs of complications. Children with ineffectual cough or difficulty handling secretions, especially infants, may require suctioning to maintain a patent airway. A simple bulb suction syringe is usually sufficient for clearing the nares and nasopharynx of infants, but mechanical suction should be readily available if needed. A nasal aspirator device can be attached to wall suction to remove secretions from nares without causing trauma to the nasal mucosa. Older children can usually handle secretions without assistance. Postural drainage, chest percussion, and nebulized bronchodilator therapy may be prescribed, depending on the child's condition. However, there is lack of empirical support on the benefit of chest percussion in children with community-acquired pneumonia.

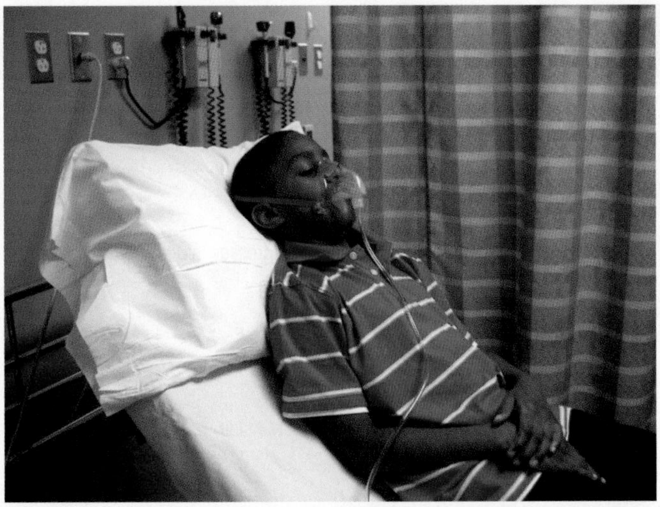

Fig. 21.5 Child placed in semierect position is often more comfortable, and this position enhances diaphragmatic expansion.

The nurse educates the family regarding observation for worsening symptoms, antibiotic and antipyretic administration, and encouragement of oral fluid intake. If the ill child rejects solid foods, fluid intake should be encouraged until the child feels well enough to eat solids. The hospitalized child may be apprehensive because the treatments and tests tend to be frightening and stress producing. It is important to involve the family in the care and to encourage questions and facilitate effective communication. Reducing the child's anxiety, apprehension, and psychologic distress leads to relaxation and decreased respiratory efforts. Easing respiratory efforts further reduces the child's apprehension. Encouraging the presence of the caregiver provides the child with a source of comfort and support.

OTHER INFECTIONS OF THE RESPIRATORY TRACT

PERTUSSIS (WHOOPING COUGH)

Pertussis, or whooping cough, is an acute respiratory tract infection caused by *Bordetella pertussis* that occurs primarily in children younger than 4 years old who were not immunized. It is highly contagious and is particularly threatening in young infants, who have a higher morbidity and mortality rate. Infants younger than 6 months of age may not come to the practitioner with the typical whooping cough yet may present with apnea, but usually the infant tends to look deceptively well with coryza, sneezing, and mild cough (Cherry, 2016). Older children are known to manifest the disease with a persistent cough and the absence of the characteristic whoop (see Table 6.3 for signs, symptoms, and management of pertussis). It presents as a URI, and cough symptoms develop. The cough can be mild but is generally more severe in unimmunized children. It persists for 6 to 10 weeks and can result in encephalopathy, seizures, pneumonia, rib fractures (adolescents), bleeding into the conjunctiva, or even death (infants). The incubation period is 7 to 10 days but can be as long as 21 days (American Academy of Pediatrics, Committee on Infectious Diseases, 2018). The incidence is highest in the spring and summer months, and a single attack confers lifetime immunity.

Pertussis is diagnosed using the *B. pertussis* polymerase chain reaction (PCR) test or culture on specimens obtained with a nasopharyngeal swab. The PCR test has optimal sensitivity during the first 3 weeks of cough, is unlikely to be useful if antimicrobial therapy has been given for more than 5 days, and has lower sensitivity in previously immunized people, but still is more sensitive than culture (American Academy of Pediatrics, Committee on Infectious Diseases, 2018). Antibiotics (e.g., erythromycin, azithromycin, clarithromycin) in the early stage may result in a milder form of the infection and limit the spread to others. Household members, high-risk individuals (immunodeficiency, pregnancy, high-risk contacts, infants, or those who care for infants), and close contacts may be treated to prevent them from developing the infection and should be immunized when indicated (American Academy of Pediatrics, Committee on Infectious Diseases, 2018).

Most children with pertussis can be managed at home with supportive care, including encouraging adequate hydration and administering antibiotic and antipyretics. When coughing spasms occur in small children, they can be frightening for the parent and family in an unvaccinated child. A child is admitted to the hospital if respiratory symptoms are severe or if apnea occurs. Hospitalized patients are placed on Droplet Precautions. Patients are considered infectious until at least 5 days of antibiotics have been completed or for 3 weeks if no antibiotics have been administered.

The resurgence of pertussis in the United States, particularly among children 10 years of age and older, has prompted concerns about the long-term effects of the pertussis vaccine. Consequently, a booster vaccine for pertussis was been approved for older children and adults. Boostrix contains acellular pertussis, diphtheria toxoid, and tetanus toxoid and is indicated as a booster for children 11 years of age and older (American Academy of Pediatrics, Committee on Infectious Diseases, 2018). (See also Chapter 6, Immunizations.)

TUBERCULOSIS

Tuberculosis (TB) along with human immunodeficiency virus (HIV) is the leading cause of death from a single infectious disease (World Health Organization, 2018). In 2017, a total of 9093 new cases of TB were reported in the United States (Stewart, Tsang, Pratt, et al., 2018). TB occurs in all ages but is most common in urban, low-income areas and among nonwhite racial and ethnic groups (American Academy of Pediatrics, Committee on Infectious Diseases, 2018). Children who were born in other countries have accounted for more of the newly diagnosed cases of TB in children living in the United States (American Academy of Pediatrics, Committee on Infectious Diseases, 2018; Stewart et al., 2018). The following groups have the highest rates of latent TB infection: immigrants, international adoptees, refugees from or travelers to high-prevalence regions (Asia, Africa, Latin America, and countries of the former Soviet Union), homeless individuals, people who use alcohol excessively or illicit drugs, and residents of certain correctional facilities and other congregate settings (American Academy of Pediatrics, Committee on Infectious Diseases, 2018). In recent years, more than 65% of all TB cases in the United States have been in people born outside the country (American Academy of Pediatrics, Committee on Infectious Diseases, 2018).

Etiology

TB is caused by *Mycobacterium tuberculosis,* an acid-fast bacillus. Children are susceptible to the human *(M. tuberculosis)* and the bovine *(Mycobacterium bovis)* organisms. In parts of the world where TB in cattle is not controlled or milk is not pasteurized, the bovine type is a common source of infection from dairy products but also can be contacted from airborne transmission.

Other factors that influence the degree to which the organism produces an altered state in the host include heredity (resistance to the infection may be genetically transmitted), gender (higher rates in adolescent girls), age (lower resistance in infants, higher incidence during adolescence), stress (emotional or physical), nutritional state, immunodeficiency (HIV, immunosuppressive medications), IV drug abuse, medical conditions (diabetes mellitus, chronic renal failure, malnutrition), and intercurrent infection (measles and pertussis) (American Academy of Pediatrics, Committee on Infectious Diseases, 2018). The risk is increased for individuals who are born in another country, have a parent who was born in another country, lived outside the United States for 2 months or more, or use tobacco (World Health Organization, 2018).

Adolescents and adults being treated with tumor necrosis factor–alpha (TNF-α) antagonists for conditions such as inflammatory bowel disease or arthritis have been identified as having contracted TB; therefore it is recommended that screening for TB occur in such persons before the use of TNF-α antagonists (American Academy of Pediatrics, Committee on Infectious Diseases, 2018). Children with HIV infection have an increased incidence of TB disease, and all children with TB should be tested for HIV. TB is the leading cause of the mortality of persons infected with HIV.

Pathophysiology

The source of TB infection in children is usually an infected member of the household or a frequent visitor to the home. The airway is the usual portal of entry for the organism as the child inhales microdroplets (usually 1 to 5 mm in size) into the respiratory tract after someone has coughed or sneezed. When the *M. tuberculosis* droplet is inhaled, it passes down the bronchial tree, implants in either a bronchiole or an alveolus, and starts to multiply. In the lungs, a proliferation of epithelial cells surrounds and encapsulates the multiplying bacilli in an attempt to wall off the invading organisms, thus forming the typical tubercle. Extension of the primary lesion at the original site causes progressive tissue destruction as it spreads within the lung, discharges material from foci to other areas of the lungs (e.g., bronchi, pleura), and/or produces pneumonia. Erosion of blood vessels by the primary lesion can cause widespread dissemination of the tubercle bacillus to near and distant sites (miliary TB). Extrapulmonary (miliary) TB may be manifested as meningitis or granulomatosis inflammation of lymph nodes, bones, joints, skin, middle ear, and the mastoid (American Academy of Pediatrics, Committee on Infectious Diseases, 2018). With the exception of meningitis, the treatment for extrapulmonary TB may be the same drug regimen as for pulmonary TB. Infants and children younger than 3 years old are more likely to develop miliary TB.

Clinical Manifestations

The clinical manifestations of the disease are extremely variable (Box 21.11). The disease may be asymptomatic or produce a broad range of symptoms, including general responses such as fever, cough, night sweats, chills, delayed growth, and weight loss or more specific symptoms related to the site of infection (e.g., lungs, bone, brain, kidneys) within 1 to 6 months after infection (American Academy of Pediatrics, Committee on Infectious Diseases, 2018). Lung disease may or may not include cough (which progresses slowly over weeks to months), aching pain and tightness in the chest, and (rarely) hemoptysis. Progression of the infection includes the generalized responses with manifestations such as persistent fever, diminished breath sounds and crackles on auscultation, pallor, anemia, weakness, and weight loss (Box 21.11).

Diagnostic Evaluation

Diagnosis is based on information derived from physical examination, history, tuberculin skin test reaction, organism cultures, and radiographic examinations. In addition, it must be determined whether the lesion is in the active, quiescent, or healed stage.

BOX 21.11 Clinical Manifestations of Tuberculosis

May be asymptomatic or produce a broad range of symptoms:
- Fever
- Malaise
- Anorexia
- Weight loss
- Cough (may or may not be present; progresses slowly over weeks to months)
- Aching pain and tightness in the chest
- Hemoptysis (rare)

With progression:
- Increasing respiratory rate
- Decreased expansion of lung on the affected side
- Diminished breath sounds and crackles
- Dullness to percussion
- Persistent fever
- Generalized symptoms
- Pallor, anemia, weakness, and weight loss

Targeted TB testing is used in children and adolescents at high risk for contracting the disease, and those patients at risk for progression to TB disease are also screened. A risk factor assessment questionnaire for TB facilitates screening of these children and should be performed at the first encounter of a child with a health care provider and then annually if possible (American Academy of Pediatrics, Committee on Infectious Diseases, 2018). Tuberculin skin test (TST) recommendations for children are listed in Box 21.12.

The tuberculin skin test (TST) is the most common test used to determine whether a child has been infected with the tubercle bacillus. Skin tests must be carried out correctly to obtain accurate results. The standard dose of purified protein derivative (PPD) is 5 tuberculin units in 0.1 ml of solution, which is administered using a 27-gauge needle and a 1-ml syringe intradermally into the volar aspect of the forearm. The tuberculin is injected intradermally with the bevel of the needle pointing upward. A wheal 6 to 10 mm in diameter should form between the layers of the skin when the solution is injected properly. If the wheal is not formed, the procedure is repeated. The reaction to the skin test is determined in 48 to 72 hours by a health care professional. Reactions occurring after 72 hours should be measured and considered the result. The size of the transverse diameter of induration, not the erythema, is measured. The diameter transverse to the long axis of the forearm is the only one standardized for measurement purposes (American Academy of Pediatrics, Committee on Infectious Diseases, 2018).

A positive TST reaction indicates that the individual has been infected and has developed sensitivity to the protein of the tubercle bacillus (Fig. 21.6). However, it does not confirm the presence of active disease. The test is usually positive 2 to 10 weeks after initial infection with the organism. Once individuals react positively, they will always react positively. Any negative reaction does not exclude active disease because false negatives can occur due to immunosuppression or certain medications. Guidelines for interpreting the TST are listed in Box 21.13. A clinical examination with a prompt chest radiographic evaluation is recommended if the child has a positive TST reaction.

The term latent tuberculosis infection (LTBI) is used to indicate infection in a person who has a positive TST, no physical findings of disease, and normal chest radiograph findings. A diagnosis of LTBI or TB disease in a young child represents a public health sentinel event often indicating recent transmission of the *M. tuberculosis* organism

BOX 21.12 Tuberculin Skin Test Recommendations for Infants, Children, and Adolescents

Children for Whom Immediate Tuberculin Skin Test Is Indicated

Contacts of persons with confirmed or suspected contagious tuberculosis (TB; contact investigation)

Children with radiographic or clinical findings suggesting TB disease

Children immigrating from endemic countries (e.g., Asia, Middle East, Africa, Latin America, countries of the former Soviet Union), including international adoptees

Children with travel histories to endemic countries or significant contact with indigenous persons from such countries[a]

Children Who Should Have Annual Tuberculin Skin Test[b]

Children infected with human immunodeficiency virus (HIV)

Children at Increased Risk for Progression of Infection to Disease

Children with other medical risk factors, including diabetes mellitus, chronic renal failure, malnutrition, and congenital or acquired immunodeficiencies, deserve special consideration. Without recent exposure, these people are not at increased risk of acquiring TB infection. Underlying immune deficiencies associated with these conditions theoretically would enhance the possibility for progression to severe disease. Initial histories of potential exposure to TB should be included for all of these patients. If these histories or local epidemiologic factors suggest a possibility of exposure, immediate and periodic tuberculin skin test (TST) should be considered. An initial TST should be performed before initiation of immunosuppressive therapy, including prolonged steroid administration, for any child with an underlying condition that necessitates immunosuppressive therapy.

[a]If child is well, TST should be delayed for up to 10 weeks after return.
[b]Initial tuberculin skin testing is done at the time of diagnosis or circumstance, beginning as early as 3 months old.

From American Academy of Pediatrics, Committee on Infectious Diseases, Kimberlin, D. W., Brady, M. T., Jackson, M. A., & Long, S.S. (Eds.). (2018). *Red book: 2018 report of the Committee on Infectious Diseases* (31st ed.). Itaca, IL: American Academy of Pediatrics.

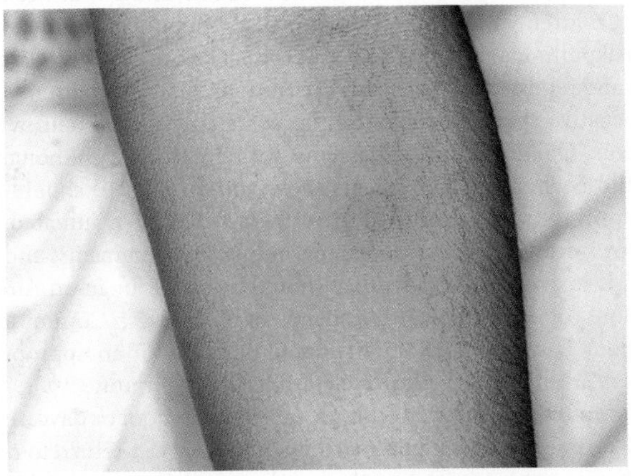

Fig. 21.6 Induration and erythema resulting from a positive tuberculosis (TB) skin test. (From Mullins, J. E. Jr., Ogle, O., & Cottrell, D. A. [2000]. Painless mass in the parotid region. *Journal of Oral and Maxillofacial Surgery, 58*[3], 316–319.)

BOX 21.13 Definition of Positive Tuberculin Skin Test Results in Infants, Children, and Adolescents[a]

Induration ≥5 mm

Children in close contact with known or suspected contagious cases of tuberculosis (TB) disease

Children suspected to have TB disease:

- Findings on chest radiography consistent with active or previously active TB
- Clinical evidence of TB disease[b]

Children receiving immunosuppressive therapy, including immunosuppressive doses of corticosteroids, or who have immunosuppressive conditions, including human immunodeficiency virus (HIV) infection

Induration ≥10 mm

Children at increased risk of disseminated disease:

- Children younger than 4 years old
- Children with other medical risk conditions, including Hodgkin disease, lymphoma, diabetes mellitus, chronic renal failure, or malnutrition

Children at increased risk of exposure to TB:

- Children born in high-prevalence (TB) regions of the world
- Children frequently exposed to adults who are HIV infected, homeless, users of illicit drugs, residents of nursing homes, incarcerated or institutionalized
- Children who travel to high-prevalence (TB) regions of the world

Induration ≥15 mm

Children 4 years old or older without any risk factors

[a]These definitions apply regardless of previous bacillus Calmette-Guérin (BCG) immunization; erythema at the tuberculin skin test (TST) site does not indicate a positive test result. TSTs should be read at 48 to 72 hours after placement.
[b]Evidence by physical examination or laboratory assessment that would include TB in the working differential diagnosis (e.g., meningitis).

From American Academy of Pediatrics, Committee on Infectious Diseases, Kimberlin, D. W., Brady, M. T., Jackson, M. A., & Long, S.S. (Eds.). (2018). *Red book: 2018 report of the Committee on Infectious Diseases* (31st ed.). Itaca, IL: American Academy of Pediatrics.

(American Academy of Pediatrics, Committee on Infectious Diseases, 2018). Most children are asymptomatic when a positive skin test result is found, and most of them do not go on to develop the disease. Children younger than 5 years old who have LTBI often progress rapidly to disease, and complications (such as TB meningitis and miliary TB) are more common in this age-group.

The term TB disease or clinically active TB is used when a child has clinical symptoms or radiographic manifestations caused by the *M. tuberculosis* organism. Prompt evaluation, treatment, and identification and treatment of contacts are key components to managing TB.

Sputum specimens are difficult or impossible to obtain from infants and young children because they tend to swallow any mucus coughed from the lower respiratory tract. The *Mycobacterium* organism is identified from microscopic examination of properly prepared and stained smears from early-morning gastric washings or from sputum, pleural fluid, urine, spinal fluid, draining lymph nodes, and other body fluids. Induced sputum and gastric lavage sputum specimens are often obtained for culture from children who are unable to expectorate a sputum specimen. In some cases, an induced sputum specimen may be obtained by administering aerosolized normal saline for 10 to 15 minutes, followed by CPT and suctioning of the nasopharynx for sputum collection.

The QuantiFERON-TB Gold and T-SPOT.TB are tests of interferon quantification (interferon-gamma release assay [IGRA]). They are the preferred tests to perform on asymptomatic children 2 years and older who have received the bacillus Calmette-Guérin (BCG) vaccine and have a borderline positive or negative TST (American Academy of Pediatrics, Committee on Infectious Diseases, 2018). These tests cannot determine latent infection, but children with a positive IGRA test are considered to be infected with the *M. tuberculosis* bacterium.

Radiographic examinations may be normal or may show lymphadenopathy, pleural effusion, or cavitary TB. However, the lesions of numerous chronic intrathoracic diseases resemble tuberculous lesions, therefore chest radiography is not diagnostic by itself.

Therapeutic Management

Medical management of TB disease in children consists of adequate nutrition, pharmacotherapy, general supportive measures, prevention of unnecessary exposure to other infections that further compromise the body's defenses, prevention of reinfection, and sometimes surgical procedures. Family members and other contacts should also be assessed for symptoms by public health and treated accordingly.

Antituberculosis drugs (e.g., ethambutol, isoniazid, pyrazinamide [PZA], rifampin) are common medications used to treat LTBI or TB disease in children. They are prescribed daily or once or twice weekly with recommended directly observed therapy (DOT). DOT means that a health care worker or other responsible, mutually agreed-on individual is present when medications are administered to the patient. DOT decreases the rates of relapse, treatment failures, and drug resistance, and is recommended for treatment of children and adolescents with TB in the United States.

The duration of treatment depends on the medication, presence of disease versus LTBI, whether multidrug-resistant TB is present, and the patient's immune status. There are several recommended drug regimens for LTBI in children and adolescents, with the three newest treatment options being (1) 12 weeks of weekly isoniazide and rifapentine (long-acting rifamycin) in children older than 2 years of age; (2) 4 months of daily rifampin; or (3) 9 months of daily isoniazid. All of these treatment options are considered adequate (American Academy of Pediatrics, Committee on Infectious Diseases, 2018).

For the child with clinically active pulmonary and extrapulmonary TB, the goal is to achieve sterilization of the tuberculous lesion. There are several alternative regimens, but a 6-month, four-drug regimen consisting of a combination of isoniazid, PZA, and ethambutol daily or twice weekly for 2 months is recommended, followed by isoniazid and rifampicin for 4 months (American Academy of Pediatrics, Committee on Infectious Diseases, 2018). Alternatively, DOT with isoniazid, rifampin, and PZA two to three times per week for 6 months is recommended except in people with HIV-related disease and drug-resistant, disease (American Academy of Pediatrics, Committee on Infectious Diseases, 2018). Alternative treatment regimens may be used when managed by a TB specialist. Infection with *M. bovis* is treated with isoniazid and rifampin for 9 to 12 months.

When drug resistance is suspected, other antimicrobials are added to the therapeutic regimen until drug susceptibility results are available. It is not within the scope of this text to outline the treatment regimen for multiple drug–resistant and extensively drug-resistant TB (American Academy of Pediatrics, Committee on Infectious Diseases, 2018). Optimal therapy for TB in children with HIV infection has not been established, and consultation with a specialist is advised. However, the duration of the present therapy is longer for patients who have HIV infection or who have cavitary lesions or positive sputum analysis after 2 months of antimicrobial therapy (American Academy of Pediatrics, Committee on Infectious Diseases, 2018).

Surgical procedures may be required to remove the source of infection in tissues that are inaccessible to pharmacotherapy or that are destroyed by the disease. Orthopedic procedures may be performed for correction of bone deformities, bronchoscopy may be done for removal of a tuberculous granulomatous polyp, or resection of a portion of a diseased lung may be performed.

Prognosis

Most children recover from primary TB infection and may be unaware of its presence. However, very young children have a higher incidence of disseminated disease. TB is a serious disease during the first 2 years of life and in children infected with HIV. Except in cases of tuberculous meningitis, death seldom occurs in treated children. Antibiotic therapy has decreased the death rate and the hematogenous spread from primary lesions.

Prevention

The only definite means to prevent TB is to avoid contact with the tubercle bacillus. Maintaining an optimal state of health with adequate nutrition and avoiding debilitating infections promote natural resistance but do not prevent infection. Pasteurization and routine testing of milk and elimination of diseased cattle have reduced the incidence of bovine TB.

Limited immunity can be produced by administration of BCG, a live vaccine containing bovine bacilli with reduced virulence (attenuated). In most instances, positive tuberculin reactions develop after inoculation with BCG. The distribution of BCG is controlled by local or state health departments, and the vaccine is not used extensively. The World Health Organization (2018) recommends the administration of the BCG vaccine in countries with a high prevalence of the disease. BCG vaccination is not generally recommended for use in the United States. However, it may be recommended for long-term protection of infants and children with negative TST results who are not infected with HIV and who (1) are at high risk for continuing exposure to persons with infectious pulmonary TB or (2) are continuously exposed to persons with TB who have bacilli resistant to both isonicotinic acid hydrazide (INH) and rifampin (American Academy of Pediatrics, Committee on Infectious Diseases, 2018).

Nursing Care Management

Hospitalization for TB is seldom necessary in the United States. Only children with the more serious forms of the disease are placed in the hospital. Children with TB typically receive their nursing care in ambulatory settings, outpatient departments, schools, and public health settings. Children younger than 10 years old with only chest adenopathy or small pulmonary lesions and nonproductive cough are rarely contagious and require only Standard Precautions. Children with no cough and negative sputum smears can be hospitalized in a room without isolation. Children and adolescents with infectious pulmonary TB (i.e., those whose sputum smears show acid-fast bacilli) should be on Isolation Precautions until effective therapy has been initiated, their sputum smears show a diminishing number of organisms, and their cough is improving. Ideally, they should be cared for in an Airborne Isolation room (American Academy of Pediatrics, Committee on Infectious Diseases, 2018). Staff should be fitted for an appropriately sized N95 or higher-level particulate-filtering respirator.

Asymptomatic children with TB can attend school or daycare facilities if they are receiving pharmacotherapy. They can return to regular activities as soon as effective therapy has been instituted, adherence to therapy has been documented, and clinical symptoms have diminished. Children receiving pharmacotherapy for TB can receive measles and other age-appropriate live virus vaccines unless they are receiving high-dose corticosteroids, are severely ill, or have specific contraindications to immunization.

Nurses assume several roles in management of the disease, including instructing the family on the disease and its ramifications, reducing family and child anxieties, promoting optimal health, explaining the rationale for diagnostic procedures, assisting with radiographic examinations, performing and interpreting skin tests accurately, obtaining specimens for laboratory examination, and educating on the TB pharmacotherapy regimen and the rationale for DOT. Case finding in the community and follow-up of known contacts—individuals from whom the affected child may have acquired the disease and persons who may have been exposed to the child with the disease—are essential control measures. Early diagnosis affords a means for early protection or treatment and prevents further spread of the disease. The health department is notified about TB cases.

PULMONARY DYSFUNCTION CAUSED BY NONINFECTIOUS IRRITANTS

FOREIGN BODY ASPIRATION

Foreign body (FB) aspiration is a life-threatening event due to potential airway obstruction and inability to adequately oxygenate the body. Small children characteristically explore matter with their hands and mouth and are prone to place FBs into air passages (nose and mouth). They also place such objects as beads, toys, paper clips, small magnets, or food items in the nose and mouth, which can easily be aspirated into the trachea. FB aspiration or ingestion can occur at any age but is most common in children 1 to 3 years old. Severity is determined by the location, type of object aspirated, and extent of obstruction. For example, dry vegetable matter, such as a seed, nut, or piece of carrot or popcorn, that does not dissolve and may swell when moistened creates a particularly difficult problem. The high fat content of potato chips and peanuts may cause the added risk of lipoid pneumonia. "Fun foods," such as hard candy and hot dogs, are among the worst offenders. Offending foods include hot dogs, round candies, peanuts or other types of nuts, grapes, cookies or biscuits, pieces of meats, caramels, carrots, apples, peas, celery, popcorn, fruit and vegetable seeds, cherry pits, gum, and peanut butter. Other items include burst latex balloons, plastic or glass beads, marbles, pen or marker caps, button or disc batteries, magnets, and coins. Aspiration of certain medications can cause inflammation and stenosis. Aspirated objects can obstruct the air passage, producing various changes, including atelectasis, emphysema, inflammation, and abscess.

CLINICAL MANIFESTATIONS

Initially, an FB in the air passages can cause choking, gagging, wheezing, or coughing, but symptoms depend on the site of obstruction and on the interval between aspiration and presentation. However, nearly half of all children with FB ingestion may be asymptomatic.

Most inhaled FBs lodge in a mainstem or lobar bronchus, a few find their way into more distal portions of the lung field, and the remaining FBs lodge in the trachea. Laryngotracheal obstruction most commonly causes dyspnea, cough, stridor, and hoarseness because of decreased air entry. Cyanosis may occur if the obstruction becomes worse. Bronchial obstruction usually produces cough (frequently paroxysmal), wheezing, asymmetric breath sounds, decreased airway entry, and dyspnea. When an object is lodged in the larynx, the child is unable to speak or breathe. Nasal FBs often manifest by unilateral purulent drainage that does not improve with time.

If the obstruction progresses, the child's face may become livid, and if the obstruction is total, the child may become unconscious and die of asphyxiation. If obstruction is partial, hours, days, or even weeks may pass without symptoms after the initial period. Secondary symptoms are related to the anatomic area in which the FB is lodged and are usually caused by a persistent respiratory tract infection located distal to the obstruction. FB aspiration should also be suspected in the presence of acute or chronic pulmonary lesions. Often by the time secondary symptoms appear, the parents have forgotten the initial episode of coughing and gagging. The most common symptoms observed in children brought to medical attention are stridor, wheezing, sternal retraction, and cough.

DIAGNOSTIC EVALUATION

The diagnosis of FB obstruction is usually suspected based on the history and physical signs. Radiographic examination reveals opaque FBs but is of limited value in localizing vegetable matter and some plastic items. Bronchoscopy is required for a definitive diagnosis of objects in the larynx and trachea. Fluoroscopic examination is valuable in detecting FBs in the bronchi. The mainstay of diagnosis and management of FBs is endoscopy and bronchoscopy. If there is doubt about the presence of an FB, endoscopy can be diagnostic and therapeutic.

THERAPEUTIC MANAGEMENT

FB aspiration may result in life-threatening airway obstruction, especially in infants because of the small diameters of their airways. Current recommendations for the emergency treatment of the choking child include the use of abdominal thrusts for children older than 1 year of age and back blows and chest thrusts for children younger than 1 year old. An FB is rarely coughed up spontaneously; therefore it must be removed by endoscopy or bronchoscopy. This procedure usually requires sedation with an agent (such as IV propofol or midazolam) and is carried out as quickly as possible because the progressive local inflammatory process triggered by the FB hampers removal. A chemical pneumonia soon develops, and vegetable matter begins to macerate within a few days, making it even more difficult to remove. After removal of the FB, the child is usually observed for any complications such as laryngeal edema and then discharged home within a matter of hours if vital signs are stable and recovery is satisfactory.

NURSING CARE MANAGEMENT

A major role of nurses is to recognize the signs of FB aspiration and implement immediate measures to relieve the obstruction. Choking on food or other material should not be fatal. To aid a child who is choking, nurses must recognize the signs of distress. Back blows or abdominal thrusts performed by both health professionals and properly instructed lay persons can save lives.

However, not every child who gags or coughs while eating is truly choking.

! NURSING ALERT

The child in severe distress (1) cannot speak, (2) becomes cyanotic, and (3) collapses. These three signs indicate that the child is truly choking and requires immediate action. The child can die within 4 minutes. Follow-up care after the foreign body (FB) is removed includes monitoring for respiratory distress and educating the parents.

Prevention

Nurses are able to teach prevention in a variety of settings. They can educate parents singly or in groups about the hazards of aspiration in relation to the developmental level of their children and encourage them to teach their children safety. Caution parents about behaviors that their children might imitate (e.g., holding FBs such as pins, nails, and toothpicks between their lips or in the mouth). (Prevention based on the child's age is discussed in Chapters 9 and 11.) Educate parents on age-appropriate toys and how older siblings' toys could be hazardous for younger siblings.

ASPIRATION PNEUMONIA

Aspiration pneumonia occurs when food, secretions, vomitus, medications, inert materials, volatile compounds, hydrocarbons (e.g., kerosene, gasoline, solvents, lighter fluid, furniture polish, mineral oil), or liquids enter the lung and cause inflammation and a chemical pneumonitis. Aspiration of fluid or food is particularly hazardous in the child who has difficulty with swallowing or is unable to swallow because of paralysis, weakness, debility, congenital anomalies, or absent cough reflex or in the child who is force-fed, especially while crying or breathing rapidly.

Clinical signs of the aspiration of oral secretions may not be distinguishable from those of other forms of acute bacterial pneumonia. For example, if vegetable matter has been aspirated, manifestations may not appear for several weeks after the event. Classic symptoms include an increasing cough or fever with foul-smelling sputum, and other signs of lower airway involvement. Aspiration of objects typically manifest with varying degrees of cyanosis, tachycardia, tachypnea, nasal flaring, retractions, grunting, cough, wheezes, and crackles, and fever may appear within 30 minutes or be delayed for a few hours. Rarely, aspiration causes immediate death from asphyxia; more often, the irritated mucous membrane becomes a site for secondary bacterial infection. However, the severity of the lung injury depends on the pH of the aspirated material, presence of bacteria, and volatility and viscosity of the substance. Endotracheal intubation may be required if the child develops respiratory failure. Severe injury causes hemoptysis, pulmonary edema, severe cyanosis, and death within 24 hours of aspiration.

Nursing Care Management

Care of the child with aspiration pneumonia is the same as that described for the child with pneumonia from other causes. Treatment is the same as for any lower respiratory tract inflammation and consists of high humidity, supplemental oxygen, hydration, and treatment of any secondary infection. However, the major focus of nursing care is on prevention of aspiration. Proper feeding techniques should be carried out for weak, debilitated, and uncooperative children, and measures should be taken to prevent aspiration of any material that might enter the nasopharynx. Feeding tubes should be checked for correct placement before the initiation of enteral feedings, flushes, or medication administration. The child should be maintained with the head elevated during feeding and for 30 minutes after if possible. The presence of an NG feeding tube or a history of gastroesophageal reflux disease places the child at risk of aspiration. Other risk factors include decreased gastrointestinal (GI) motility, ineffective cough, poor gag reflex, impaired swallow, high gastric residual, and trauma or surgery to the neck, face, or mouth.

Children who are at risk for swallowing difficulties as a result of illness, physical debilitation, anesthesia, or sedation are kept on nothing by mouth (NPO) status until they can properly swallow fluids effectively. An evaluation by an occupational or speech therapist may be indicated to assess the child's ability to swallow effectively. The child who is at risk for vomiting and incapable of protecting the airway should be positioned in a side-lying recovery position (see Fig. 21.20). Educating parents on the prevention of aspiration pneumonia is important.

PULMONARY EDEMA

Pulmonary edema (PE) is the movement of excess fluid into the alveoli and interstitium of the lungs caused by extravasation from the pulmonary vasculature (Woods & Mazor, 2020). The two main types of PE are cardiogenic and noncardiogenic.

Cardiogenic (hydrostatic, hemodynamic) PE is caused by an increase in pulmonary capillary pressure because of an increase in pulmonary venous pressure. It can be caused by excessive IV fluid administration, renal failure, left ventricular failure, heart valve disorder (aortic regurgitation, aortic stenosis, mitral regurgitation), myocardial ischemia, myocarditis, acute tachydysrhythmia, or coronary artery disease (Powell, Graham, O'Reilly, et al., 2016). Noncardiogenic PE is caused by various conditions that result in increased pulmonary capillary permeability. Some subtypes of noncardiogenic PE include permeability PE (caused by acute respiratory distress syndrome [ARDS] or acute lung injury [ALI]), high-altitude PE (caused by rapid ascension to heights above 12,000 feet), or neurogenic PE (after CNS insult such as seizures, head injury, or cerebral hemorrhage). Some less common forms of PE are reperfusion PE (after removal of thromboemboli from the lung or a lung transplant), reexpansion PE (caused by rapid reexpansion of a collapsed lung), or PE that results from opiate overdose (e.g., methadone or heroin), salicylate toxicity (chronic), aspiration (FB inhalation), inhalation injuries, near drowning, pulmonary embolism, viral infections, or pulmonary veno-occlusive disease. Other causes include aspiration, traumatic injury, organ dysfunction caused by sepsis, multiorgan failure, alcoholism or substance abuse, pregnancy (eclampsia), chronic renal impairment, malnutrition, hypertension, or a blood transfusion (transfusion-related ALI).

Pathophysiology

Fluid flows from the pulmonary vasculature into the alveolar interstitial space and then returns to the systemic circulation in a normal lung. Movement of this fluid is controlled by the net difference between hydrostatic and osmotic pressures and the permeability of the capillary membrane (Woods & Mazor, 2020). Increased pulmonary hydrostatic pressure or increased permeability of the vascular membrane results in movement of fluid into the alveoli and interstitium of the lung. The pulmonary lymph system normally drains away any fluid from the alveoli, but when the amount of fluid present in the alveoli exceeds lymph drainage, PE occurs.

Symptoms include extreme shortness of breath, cyanosis, tachypnea, diminished breath sounds, anxiety, agitation, confusion, diaphoresis, orthopnea, respiratory crackles, expiratory wheezing (in young infants), heart murmur, third heart sound (S_3) gallop, cool peripheries, jugular venous distention, nocturnal dyspnea, cough, pink frothy sputum (if severe), tachycardia, hypertension, and hypotension (if caused by left ventricle dysfunction).

Therapeutic Management

Management of PE depends on the cause but can include oxygen therapy, positive end-expiratory pressure (PEEP) via CPAP, and intubation with ventilatory support if respiratory failure occurs. If ventricular failure is the cause, medications such as diuretics, digoxin, positive inotropes, and vasodilators (nitroglycerin) may be started, and the child may be placed on fluid and sodium restriction. Morphine may be prescribed to relieve dyspnea. The primary goal of management is to determine why PE occurred and treat the underlying condition.

Nursing Care Management

Nursing care of the child with PE is similar to that for any other acute respiratory condition. Pulse oximetry is monitored, and vital signs are observed closely for any deterioration. The nurse should note changes in oxygen saturation (SaO_2), end-tidal carbon dioxide ($ETCO_2$), and arterial blood gas (ABG) values. An ongoing assessment of the child's cardiopulmonary status is needed by checking lung sounds and observing respiratory rate, rhythm, depth, and effort. Oxygen, medications, and other respiratory treatments are administered as prescribed. Close monitoring of intake and output, electrolytes, and comfort are important. The child should be monitored for restlessness, anxiety, and air hunger. Placing the child in a high Fowler position may help with lung expansion. Because this position places pressure on bony prominences in the sacrum and hips, pressure areas must be relieved at intervals. Most of the care of PE occurs in the ICU, which is anxiety provoking for the child and family. They should be given the opportunity to express their fears and anxieties and to ask questions. (For other nursing care activities, see the Acute Respiratory Distress Syndrome section.)

ACUTE RESPIRATORY DISTRESS SYNDROME AND ACUTE LUNG INJURY

Acute respiratory distress syndrome (ARDS) and *acute lung injury* (ALI) are potentially life-threatening inflammatory lung conditions that may occur in children and adults. They are caused by direct injury to the lungs or by systemic insults that lead indirectly to lung injury with subsequent hypoxemia and respiratory failure due to noncardiogenic PE. Sepsis, trauma, viral pneumonia, aspiration, fat emboli, drug overdose, reperfusion injury after lung transplantation, smoke inhalation, and submersion injury, among others, have been associated with ARDS and ALI. Both are characterized by respiratory distress and hypoxemia that occur within 72 hours of a serious injury or surgery in a person with previously normal lungs. ALI involves a spectrum of inflammatory disease responses to a precipitating event, with ARDS being the more severe form of ALI.

The diagnostic criteria established by the American European Consensus Conference (Bernard, Artigas, Brigham, et al., 1994) have been superseded by the Berlin definition of ARDS (ARDS Definition Task Force, Ranieri, Rubenfeld, et al., 2012). According to the Berlin definition, ARDS occurs within 1 week of a known clinical insult or new or worsening respiratory symptoms; is characterized by bilateral opacities on chest imaging not fully explained by effusions, lobar or lung collapse, or nodules; and manifests as respiratory failure not fully explained by cardiac failure or fluid overload (ARDS Definition Task Force et al., 2012). Hypoxemia is expressed in terms of the ratio of partial pressure of oxygen (PaO_2) to the fraction of inspired oxygen (FiO_2) (P/F ratio). In the setting of a PEEP or CPAP of 5 cm H_2O or greater, mild, moderate, and severe ARDS are defined by P/F ratios between 200 and 300, between 100 and 200, and 100 mm Hg or lower, respectively. In 2015 the Pediatric Acute Lung Injury Consensus Conference Group published pediatric-specific definitions, recommendations regarding treatment, and future research priorities.

Pathologically, the hallmark of ARDS is increased permeability of the alveolar-capillary membrane that results in PE. During the acute phase of ARDS, inflammatory mediators cause damage to the alveolar-capillary membrane, with an increasing pulmonary capillary permeability with resulting interstitial edema. Later stages are characterized by pneumocyte and fibrin infiltration of the alveoli, with the start of either the healing process or fibrosis. In ARDS, the lungs become stiff as a result of surfactant inactivation; gas diffusion is impaired; and eventually, bronchiolar mucosal swelling and congestive atelectasis occur. The net effect is decreased functional residual capacity, pulmonary hypertension, and increased intrapulmonary right-to-left shunting of blood. Surfactant secretion is reduced, and the atelectasis and fluid-filled alveoli provide an excellent medium for bacterial growth. Hypoxemia or increased work of breathing may require ventilatory support.

The child with ARDS may first demonstrate only symptoms caused by an injury or infection, but as the condition deteriorates, hyperventilation, tachypnea, increasing respiratory effort, cyanosis, and decreasing oxygen saturation occur. The hypoxemia may be refractory to oxygen administration.

Treatment involves supportive measures to ensure adequate oxygenation and pulmonary perfusion; treatment of infection (or the precipitating cause); and maintenance of adequate cardiac output and vascular volume, hydration, adequate nutritional support, comfort measures, prevention of complications such as GI ulceration and aspiration, and psychologic support. Specific treatment should be directed at the underlying cause (e.g., antibiotics, source control for infection). Many patients require mechanical ventilatory support. The goal of mechanical ventilation in patients with ARDS is to rest the respiratory muscles and maintain adequate gas exchange while mitigating the deleterious effects of ventilator-induced lung injury (Fan, Brodie, & Slutsky, 2018). This is usually achieved invasively (e.g., with endotracheal intubation), but occasionally noninvasive ventilation is used in milder cases. Patients requiring invasive mechanical ventilation usually require sedation, at least initially, to allow for ventilatory synchrony. Fluid administration to maintain adequate intravascular volume and end-organ perfusion must be balanced against the desire to decrease lung fluid to improve oxygenation. The provision of adequate nutrition, maintenance of patient comfort, and prevention of complications (such as GI ulceration) are essential. Psychologic support of the patient and family is also important.

Definitive therapy is directed toward improvement of oxygenation. The use of endotracheal intubation, PEEP, and low tidal volume may be required to ensure maximum oxygen delivery by increasing functional residual capacity, reducing intrapulmonary shunting, and reducing pulmonary fluid. Inappropriate use of mechanical ventilation may worsen the lung injury by causing volutrauma, barotrauma, atelectrauma, and biotrauma to the injured lungs. Ventilation with low tidal volumes (6 ml/kg ideal body weight) has been associated with lower mortality rates in children with ALI (Wong, Jit, Sultana, et al., 2017). Other supportive strategies include use of the prone position, pharmacologic neuromuscular blockade to facilitate ventilation, administration of inhaled nitric oxide or prostaglandins, and high-frequency oscillatory ventilation. The evidence to support these therapies is variable and evolving. Extracorporeal membrane oxygenation (ECMO) should be considered in cases of severe ARDS when the cause of respiratory failure is believed to be reversible or if the child is likely to be suitable for consideration for lung transplantation (Pediatric Acute Lung Injury Consensus Conference Group, 2015).

Prognosis

The prognosis for patients with ARDS is improving. Nonetheless, the mortality rate remains high and ranges from 14% to 45% in children (Lopez-Fernandez, Azagra, de la Oliva, et al., 2012). The precipitating disorder influences the outcome; the worst prognosis is associated with profound hypoxemia, uncontrolled sepsis, bone marrow transplantation, cancer, and multisystem involvement with hepatic failure.

Children who recover may have persistent cough, exertional dyspnea, and pulmonary function test abnormalities.

Nursing Care Management

The child with ARDS is cared for in the ICU during the acute stages of illness. Nursing care involves close monitoring of oxygenation and respiratory status, cardiac output, perfusion, fluid and electrolyte balance, and renal function (urinary output). Blood gas analysis, acid-base status, and pulse oximetry are important evaluation tools. Most children with ARDS require invasive monitoring with arterial and central venous catheters. Diuretics may be administered to reduce pulmonary fluid, and vasodilators may be administered to decrease pulmonary vascular pressure. Nutritional support is often required because of the prolonged acute phase of the illness. Nursing management also includes monitoring the effects of the numerous parenteral fluids and drugs used to stabilize the child and monitoring for changes in the child's hemodynamic status. To prevent superimposed ventilator-associated pneumonia (VAP), nursing care includes elevation of the head of the bed to between 30 and 35 degrees (crib at 20 degrees) unless contraindicated. Additional strategies to prevent VAP include use of a closed suctioning system, removal of oropharyngeal secretions, and draining breathing circuit condensate periodically. The risk of pressure ulcers is greater with the head of the bed in an elevated position, and this must be balanced with the risk of VAP. Nursing should perform frequent oral care at least every 4 hours with ongoing observation of skin for pressure areas. The multidisciplinary care team performs a daily assessment of readiness to wean or liberate from mechanical ventilation. The child must also be assessed for risk of deep vein thrombosis, and appropriate prophylactic strategies must be initiated (e.g., passive range-of-motion exercises as able, sequential compression devices, anticoagulant therapy, early ambulation). Respiratory distress is a frightening situation for both the child and the parents, and attention to their psychologic needs is a major element in the care of these children. The child is often sedated during the acute phase of the illness, and weaning from sedation requires close monitoring and interventions to promote comfort.

SMOKE INHALATION INJURY

A number of noxious substances that may be inhaled are toxic to humans. They are primarily products of incomplete combustion and cause more deaths from fires than flame injuries. The severity of the injury depends on the nature of the substances generated by the material burned, whether the victim is confined in a closed space, and the duration of contact with the smoke.

Three distinct syndromes of pulmonary complications may occur in children suffering from inhalation injury: (1) early carbon monoxide (CO) poisoning, airway obstruction, and pulmonary edema; (2) ARDS occurring at 24 to 48 hours or later in some cases; and (3) late complications of pneumonia and pulmonary emboli (Antoon, 2020). Smoke inhalation causes three types of injury: heat, chemical, and systemic.

Heat injury causes thermal damage to the upper airway, but because air has low specific heat, the injury goes no farther than the upper airway. Reflex closure of the glottis prevents injury to the lower airway. Heat may reach the middle airway occasionally, but it rarely penetrates to the lungs.

Chemical injury involves gases that may be generated during the combustion of materials, such as clothing, furniture, and floor coverings. Acids, alkalis, and their precursors in smoke can produce chemical burns. These substances can be carried deep into the respiratory tract, including the lower respiratory tract, in the form of insoluble gases. Soluble gases tend to dissolve in the upper respiratory tract. Heated plastics are the source of extremely toxic vapors, including chlorine and hydrochloric acid from polyvinylchloride and hydrocarbons, aldehydes, ketones, and acids from polyethylene. Irritant gases such as nitrous oxide or carbon dioxide combine with water in the lungs to form corrosive acids. Chemical burns to the airways are similar to burns on the skin, except they are painless because the tracheobronchial tree is relatively insensitive to pain.

Inhalation of small amounts of noxious irritants produces alveolar and bronchiolar damage that can lead to obstructive bronchiolitis. Severe exposure causes further injury, including alveolar-capillary damage with hemorrhage, necrotizing bronchiolitis, inhibited secretion of surfactant, and formation of hyaline membranes, which are all manifestations of ARDS.

Systemic injury occurs from gases that are nontoxic to the airways (e.g., CO, hydrogen cyanide). However, these gases cause injury and death by interfering with or inhibiting cellular respiration. CO is responsible for more than half of all fatal inhalation poisonings in the United States. CO is a colorless, odorless, tasteless gas with an affinity for hemoglobin 230 times greater than that of oxygen. When CO enters the bloodstream, it binds readily with hemoglobin to form carboxyhemoglobin (COHb). Because CO is released less readily than oxygen, tissue hypoxia reaches dangerous levels before oxygen is available to meet tissue needs.

! NURSING ALERT

With carbon monoxide (CO) poisoning, the oxygen saturation (SaO_2) obtained by pulse oximetry will be normal because the device measures only oxygenated and deoxygenated hemoglobin; it does not measure dysfunctional hemoglobin, such as carboxyhemoglobin (COHb).

Accidental CO poisoning is most often a result of exposure to fumes of heaters or smoke from structural fires, although poorly ventilated recreational vehicles with improperly operated or maintained gas lamps or stoves and cooking in underventilated areas with charcoal grills are also frequent causes. CO is produced by incomplete combustion of carbon or carbonaceous material, such as wood or charcoal. CO poisoning can also occur in a running vehicle parked in a closed garage for a long period or in a vehicle with inadequate vented exhaust that leaks into the vehicle's passenger (or closed truck bed) compartment.

The signs and symptoms of CO poisoning are secondary to tissue hypoxia and vary with the level of COHb. Mild manifestations include headache, visual disturbances, irritability, and nausea, whereas more severe intoxication causes confusion, hallucinations, ataxia, and coma. CO may increase cerebral blood flow, increase cerebral capillary permeability, and increase cerebrospinal fluid pressure, all of which contribute to CNS signs. The bright, cherry red lips and skin often described are less common than pallor and cyanosis. Patients who have significant exposure to CO can develop a delayed neurologic deficit, which can occur 3 to 240 days after initial exposure. The deficits can last up to 1 year.

Therapeutic Management

Treatment of children with smoke inhalation injury is largely symptomatic. The most widely accepted treatment is placing the child on humidified 100% oxygen as quickly as possible to rapidly reverse tissue hypoxia and to displace CO and cyanide from protein-binding sites. The child is monitored for signs of respiratory distress and impending failure. A laryngoscopy or bronchoscopy evaluation may be done to assess for airway damage. Baseline ABGs and COHb levels are obtained. PaO_2 may be within normal limits unless there is marked respiratory depression. If CO poisoning is confirmed, 100% oxygen is continued until COHb levels fall to the nontoxic range of about 10%. If CO poisoning is severe, the patient may benefit from hyperbaric oxygen therapy. Hyperbaric oxygen therapy may be useful in the treatment of neurologic complications related to CO poisoning. In a hyperbaric oxygen therapy chamber, the air pressure is increased to three times higher than normal air pressure and so lungs can gather more oxygen than would be possible breathing pure oxygen at normal air pressure. Hyperbaric oxygen therapy significantly decreases the half-life of COHb compared with 100% oxygen treatment alone. Pulmonary care may be facilitated by bronchodilators, inhaled corticosteroids, humidification, and CPT to enhance the removal of necrotic material, minimize bronchoconstriction, and avoid atelectasis. Bronchoscopy may be needed to clear heavy secretions.

Respiratory distress may occur early in the course of smoke inhalation as a result of hypoxia, or patients who are breathing well on admission may suddenly develop respiratory distress. Therefore endotracheal intubation equipment should be readily available. Transient edema of the airways can occur at any level in the tracheobronchial tree. Assessment and localization of the obstruction should be accomplished before severe swelling of the head, neck, or oropharynx occurs. Intubation is often necessary when (1) severe burns in the area of the nose, mouth, and face increase the likelihood of developing oropharyngeal edema and obstruction; (2) vocal cord edema causes obstruction; (3) the patient has difficulty handling secretions; and (4) progressive respiratory distress requires artificial ventilation. Controversy surrounds tracheostomy, but many prefer this procedure when the obstruction is proximal to the larynx and reserve nasotracheal intubation for lower tract involvement.

Nursing Care Management

Nursing care of the child with inhalation injury is the same as that for any child with respiratory distress. The initial goal is to maintain a patent airway and effective ventilation status; endotracheal intubation may be required early, depending on the patient's respiratory status and the progression of airway and pulmonary edema. In the acute phase, the nurse should monitor vital signs, oxygenation, work of breathing, and other respiratory assessments frequently. The administration of nebulized bronchodilators, humidified oxygen, and inhaled corticosteroids is often part of the nursing care. Chest percussion and postural drainage are often required. Fluid requirements for children experiencing inhalation injury are greater than for those with surface burns alone, and IV fluids are generally prescribed. However, one concern is the development of pulmonary edema; therefore accurate monitoring of fluid intake and output is essential.

In addition to observation and management of the physical aspects of inhalation injury, the nurse also deals with the psychologic needs of a frightened child and distraught parents. Parents need support, reassurance, and information regarding the child's condition, treatment, and progress. The nurse can provide anticipatory guidance and educate families on prevention of inhalation injuries and the importance of CO detectors in the home.

ENVIRONMENTAL TOBACCO SMOKE EXPOSURE

Numerous investigations indicate that parental or family smoking is an important cause of morbidity in children. Children exposed to passive or environmental tobacco smoke have an increased number of respiratory illnesses, increased respiratory symptoms (i.e., cough, sputum, and wheezing), and reduced performance on pulmonary function tests (PFTs). AOM and OME are also increased in children who have smoking family members. Indoor exposure to tobacco smoke has been linked to asthma in children (Makadia, Roper, Andrews, et al., 2017). Among children with asthma, there is an association between parental or family member cigarette smoking and asthma exacerbations, trips to the ED, medication use, and impaired recovery after hospitalization for acute asthma. Maternal cigarette smoking is associated with increased respiratory symptoms and illnesses in children; decreased fetal growth; increased deliveries of low birth weight, preterm, and stillborn infants; and a greater incidence of sudden infant death syndrome (SIDS). Antenatal maternal smoking has emerged as a significant risk factor for SIDS (Friedmann, Dahdouh, Kugler, et al., 2017). The risk for diagnosis of early-onset asthma in the first years of life is associated with in utero exposure to maternal and paternal smoking (Harju, Keski-Nisula, Georgiadis, et al., 2016). Exposure to tobacco smoke during childhood may also contribute to the development of chronic lung disease in the adult.

Electronic cigarettes (e-cigarettes) have increased in popularity among adolescents and adults. Regular use of electronic cigarettes has increased tenfold among high school students, from 1.5% in 2011 to 16% in 2015 (Chun, Moazed, Calfee, et al., 2017), and 5% of middle school students reported regular use of electronic cigarettes in 2015 (Chun et al., 2017). This increase may be due to adolescents' belief that electronic cigarettes are less harmful and less addictive than cigarettes (Amrock, Lee, & Weitzman, 2016). Although these products are advertised as being safe because they are smokeless, the battery-powered cigarettes still contain nicotine and other chemicals. Recent studies have shown toxic effects on the pulmonary system, including altered airways, increased oxidative stress, interference in lung development, and impaired immune defense against bacterial and viral pathogens (Chun et al., 2017). Electronic cigarettes can also increase the risk for cancer (Canistro, Vivarelli, Cirillo, et al., 2017).

Secondhand smoke consists of passive smoke exposure emitted from a tobacco product. The amount of passive smoke exposure in infants and children is directly related to the number of smokers in a household. Cotinine, a byproduct of nicotine, is considered a valid biochemical marker for smoke exposure. Cotinine levels are increased in children who live in homes with smokers, and these levels increase proportionately with the number of smokers in the home.

In recent years, concern has grown regarding "thirdhand" tobacco exposure—the tobacco toxins that remain in the environment long after the smoker has stopped smoking (Jacob, Benowitz, Destaillats, et al., 2017; Samet, Chanson, & Wipfli, 2015). Thirdhand smoke has been defined as "the four Rs": tobacco chemicals (some toxic) that remain, react, re-emit, and/or are resuspended long after active smoking ends and found in such objects as cars, walls, carpet, furniture, clothing, skin, and hair (Drehmer, Walters, Nabi-Burza, et al, 2017). Reviewed evidence-based research supported advocating for environments free of thirdhand smoke contamination for families and children, therefore it is important to educate and counsel families regarding the harm thirdhand smoke poses to children (Drehmer, Walters, Nabi-Burza, et al, 2017).

Nursing Care Management

Nurses should provide information about the hazards of environmental smoke exposure in all interactions with children and their family members. Nurses and other health care professionals need to include assessments of passive smoke exposure in all children, especially those with respiratory illnesses. In families where smokers refuse to quit, house rules should be established for reducing smoke in the child's environment, such as smoking outside of the home, wearing removable clothing while smoking, and not smoking in vehicles (see Family-Centered Care box). Nurses should set an example for children and families and become advocates for "no smoking" ordinances in public places, prohibition of advertising tobacco products in the media, and inclusion of health warnings of sidestream smoke on tobacco products.[a] Nurses have an important role in offering parents smoking cessation education resources such as counseling and classes. Adolescents should be screened for inhalation of tobacco products or marijuana with counseling on cessation offered.

FAMILY-CENTERED CARE

Decreasing Childhood Exposure to Environmental Tobacco Smoke

- Do not smoke around infants and children.
- Maintain a smoke-free home. Do not allow visitors to smoke in the home.
- Restrict smoking to outside the house where children do not play.
- Encourage exclusive breastfeeding for the first 6 months.
- Change clothing after smoking and before holding an infant in proximity. Suggest wearing a removable outer garment for smoking that is removed on return to the house or when in contact with the child.
- Do not smoke in motor vehicles with children.

LONG-TERM RESPIRATORY DYSFUNCTION

ASTHMA

Asthma is a chronic inflammatory disorder of the airways characterized by recurring symptoms, airway obstruction, and bronchial hyperresponsiveness (Pinfield, Gaskin, Bentley, et al., 2015; Trent, Zimbro, & Rutledge, 2015). Asthma is the most common chronic disease of childhood, the primary cause of school absences, and the third-leading cause of hospitalizations in children under the age of 15 years. More than 25 million people are known to have asthma, and about 7 million of them are children (National Heart, Lung, and Blood Institute, 2014). Although the onset of asthma may occur at any age, 80% to 90% of children have their first symptoms before 4 or 5 years old.

The asthma episodes are associated with airflow limitation or obstruction that is reversible either spontaneously or with treatment. Inflammation causes an increase in bronchial hyperresponsiveness to a variety of stimuli (Liu, Spahn, & Sicherer, 2020). In susceptible children, inflammation causes recurrent episodes of wheezing, breathlessness, chest tightness, and cough, especially at night or in the early morning. Recognition of the key role of inflammation has made the use of antiinflammatory agents, especially inhaled steroids, a major component in the treatment of asthma.

Asthma is classified into four categories based on the symptom indicators of disease severity. These categories are intermittent, mild persistent, moderate persistent, and severe persistent. Symptoms increase in frequency or intensity until the last category of severe persistent asthma (Box 21.14). These categories provide a stepwise approach to the pharmacologic management, environmental control, and educational interventions needed for each category. For example, if control of asthma is not maintained at one level or step, pharmacologic therapy for the next step up should be considered. If control is adequate at one step, a gradual stepwise reduction in therapy may be possible. The stepwise approach is a guide to assist clinical decision making. In addition to pharmacologic management, environmental control and educational interventions are essential at each step (Liu et al., 2020). These categories emphasize the multifaceted aspect of the disease for consideration of effects on present quality of life and functional capacity and the future risk of adverse events.

Asthma prevalence, morbidity, and mortality are increasing in the United States and may result from worsening air pollution, more premature infants with chronic lung disease, poor access to medical care, underdiagnosis, and undertreatment.

BOX 21.14 Asthma Severity Classification in Children[a]

Step 5 or 6: Severe Persistent Asthma

Continual symptoms throughout the day

Frequent nighttime symptoms (greater (>) than 1 time/week ages 0 to 4 and 7 nights/week, ages 5 and older)

Pulmonary expiratory flow (PEF): less (<) than 60%

Forced expiratory volume in 1 second (FEV1): <75% of predicted value

Interference with normal activity: Extremely limited

Use of short-acting β-agonist for symptom control: Several times a day

Step 3 or 4: Moderate Persistent Asthma

Daily symptoms

Nighttime symptoms: Three to four times a month (0 to 4 years old), >1/week but not nightly (5 to 11 years old)

PEF: 60% to 80% of predicted value (ages 5 and older)

FEV1: 75% to 80% (ages 5 and older)

PEF variability: >30%

Interference with normal activity: Some limitation

Use of short-acting β-agonist for symptom control: Daily

Step 2: Mild Persistent Asthma

Symptoms >2 times/week but <1 time/day

Nighttime symptoms: One to two times a month (0 to 4 years old), three or four times a month (5 to 11 years old)

PEF or FEV1: greater or equal (≥) 80% of predicted value

PEF variability: 20% to 30%

Interference with normal activity: Minor limitation

Use of short-acting β-agonist for symptom control: >2 days/week but not daily

Step 1: Intermittent Asthma

Symptoms ≤2 days/week

Nighttime symptoms (awakenings): None (0 to 4 years old); ≤2 nights per month (5 to 11 years old)

PEF or FEV1: ≥80% of predicted value

PEF variability: <20%

Interference with normal activity: None

Use of short-acting β-agonist for symptom control: <2 days/week

[a]The presence of one clinical feature of severity is sufficient to place a patient in that category. An individual should be assigned to the most severe grade in which any feature occurs. The characteristics in this table are general and may overlap because asthma is highly variable. An individual's classification may change over time. Risk factors for each category are not presented in this table. See original reference for additional classification data. Asthma treatment should not be based on this table.

From National Asthma Education and Prevention Program. (2007) *Guidelines for the diagnosis and management of asthma: Summary report 2007.* Retrieved from http://www.nhlbi.nih.gov/guidelines/asthma/index.htm

[a]For a copy of the Environmental Protection Agency report *Respiratory Health Effects of Passive Smoking,* visit http://cfpub.epa.gov/ncea/CFM/recordisplay.cfm?deid=2835.

ETIOLOGY

Studies of children with asthma indicate that allergies influence both the persistence and the severity of the disease. In fact, atopy, or the genetic predisposition for the development of an immunoglobulin E (IgE)–mediated response to common aeroallergens, is the strongest identifiable predisposing factor for developing asthma (Pinfield et al., 2015). Although allergens play an important role in asthma, 20% to 40% of children with asthma have no evidence of allergic disease. In addition to allergens, other substances and conditions can serve as triggers that may exacerbate asthma (Box 21.15). Evidence shows that viral respiratory infections, including RSV infection, may also have a significant role in the development and expression of asthma (Knudson & Varga, 2015; National Heart, Lung, and Blood Institute, 2014).

Risk factors for asthma include the following:

- Atopy (includes a history of allergies or atopic dermatitis)
- Heredity (e.g., parent or sibling with asthma)
- Gender (boys are affected more frequently than girls until adolescence, when the trend reverses)
- Smoking or exposure to secondhand smoke
- Maternal smoking during pregnancy
- Ethnicity (African Americans at greatest risk)
- Low birth weight
- Being overweight

BOX 21.15 Triggers Tending to Precipitate or Aggravate Asthma Exacerbations

- Allergens
  - Outdoor: Trees, shrubs, weeds, grasses, molds, pollens, air pollution, spores
  - Indoor: Dust or dust mites, mold, cockroach antigen
- Irritants: Tobacco smoke, wood smoke, odors, sprays
- Exposure to occupational chemicals
- Exercise
- Cold air
- Changes in weather or temperature
- Environmental change: Moving to new home, starting new school
- Colds and infections
- Animals: Cats, dogs, rodents, horses
- Medications: Aspirin, nonsteroidal antiinflammatory drugs, antibiotics, beta-blockers
- Strong emotions: Fear, anger, laughing, crying
- Conditions: Gastroesophageal reflux, tracheoesophageal fistula
- Food additives: Sulfite preservatives
- Foods: Nuts, milk or other dairy products
- Endocrine factors: Menses, pregnancy, thyroid disease

PATHOPHYSIOLOGY

There is general agreement that inflammation contributes to heightened airway reactivity in asthma. It is unlikely that asthma is caused by either a single cell or a single inflammatory mediator. Rather, it appears that asthma results from complex interactions among inflammatory cells, mediators, and the cells and tissues present in the airways (Liu et al., 2020). However, recognition of the importance of inflammation has made the use of antiinflammatory agents, such as steroids, a key component of asthma therapy.

Another important component of asthma is bronchospasm and obstruction. The mechanisms responsible for the obstructive symptoms in asthma include inflammatory response to stimuli; airway edema and accumulation and secretion of mucus; spasm of the smooth muscle of the bronchi and bronchioles, which decreases the caliber of the bronchioles; and airway remodeling, which causes permanent cellular changes (Pinfield et al., 2015) (Fig. 21.7).

Airflow is determined by the size of the airway lumen, degree of bronchial wall edema, mucus production, smooth muscle contraction, and muscle hypertrophy. Bronchial constriction is a normal reaction to foreign stimuli, but in the child with asthma, it is abnormally severe, producing impaired respiratory function. The smooth muscle arranged in spiral bundles around the airway causes narrowing and shortening of the airway, which significantly increases airway resistance to airflow. Because the bronchi normally dilate and elongate during inspiration and contract and shorten on expiration, the respiratory difficulty is more pronounced during the expiratory phase of respiration.

Increased resistance in the airway causes forced expiration through the narrowed lumen. The volume of air trapped in the lungs increases as airways are functionally closed at a point between the alveoli and the lobar bronchi. This trapping of gas forces the individual to breathe at

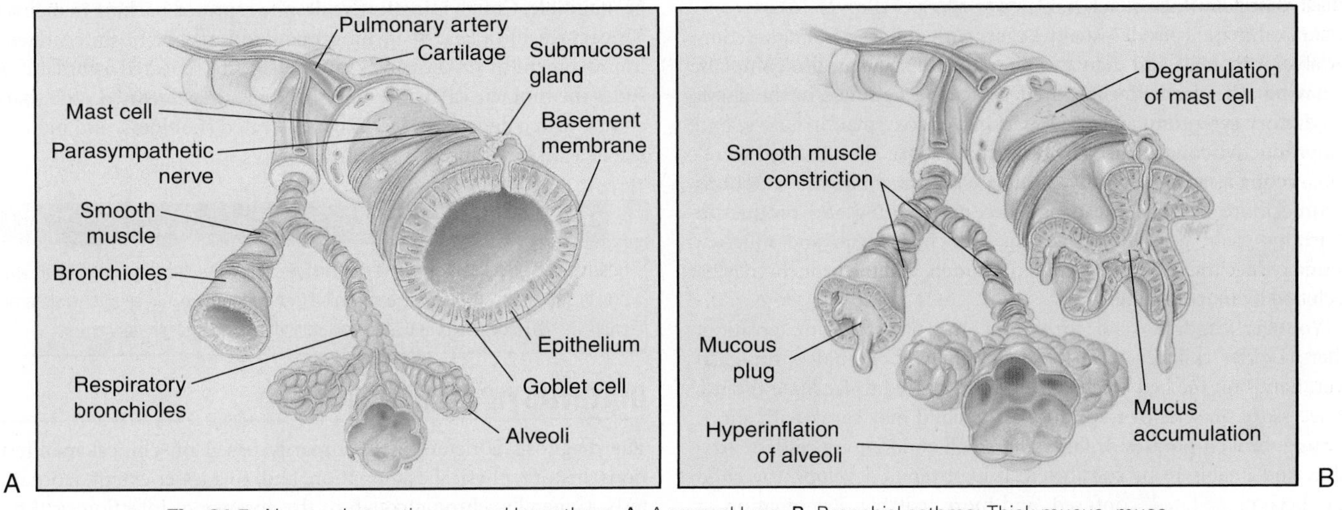

Fig. 21.7 Airway obstruction caused by asthma. **A,** A normal lung. **B,** Bronchial asthma: Thick mucus, mucosal edema, and smooth muscle spasm causing obstruction of small airways; breathing becomes labored, and expiration is difficult. (Modified from Des Jardins, T., & Burton, G. G. [1995]. *Clinical manifestations and assessment of respiratory disease* [3rd ed.]. St Louis, MO: Mosby.)

higher and higher lung volumes. Consequently, the person with asthma fights to inspire sufficient air. This expenditure of effort for breathing causes fatigue, decreased respiratory effectiveness, and increased oxygen consumption. The inspiration occurring at higher lung volumes hyperinflates the alveoli and reduces the effectiveness of the cough. As the severity of obstruction increases, there is a reduced alveolar ventilation with carbon dioxide retention; hypoxemia; respiratory acidosis; and, eventually, respiratory failure. Chronic inflammation may also cause permanent damage (airway remodeling) to airway structures and is difficult to treat successfully with current therapies.

Exacerbations are episodes of progressively worsening shortness of breath, cough, wheezing, chest tightness, or some combination of these changes. A decrease in expiratory airflow is also characteristic. Airways narrow because of bronchospasm, mucosal edema, and mucus plugging, with air being trapped behind occluded or narrowed airways. Functional residual capacity rises because the child is breathing close to total lung capacity; hyperinflation enables the child to keep the airways open and permits gas exchange to occur.

Having an allergy is the strongest epidemiologic risk factor for chronic asthma morbidity and mortality. Many substances in the environment can induce an asthmatic response, but the most significant are those that are antigenic (e.g., that evoke the immune response). The antigen (or foreign substance) is deposited on the respiratory mucosa, where lysozymes immediately digest its outer coating, releasing fragments of foreign protein that initiate the immune sequence. The antibody (immunoglobulin) most active in allergic disorders, including asthma, is IgE, located primarily in skin and mucous membranes and mediating the immediate hypersensitive reaction in the bronchial mucosa.

CLINICAL MANIFESTATIONS

The classic manifestations of asthma are dyspnea, wheezing, and coughing. An attack may develop gradually or appear abruptly and may be preceded by a URI. The age of the child is often a significant factor because the first attack frequently occurs between ages 3 and 8 years, with some children manifesting clinical signs and symptoms in infancy. In infancy, an attack usually follows a respiratory infection. Bronchoconstriction in response to an allergen can have an immediate, histamine type of pattern or a late response with airway hypersensitivity lasting for days, weeks, or months. Some children may experience a prodromal itching at the front of the neck or over the upper part of the back just before an attack, especially if the attack is related to allergies (Box 21.16).

An asthmatic episode usually begins with children feeling uncomfortable or irritable and increasingly restless. They may also complain of having a headache, feeling tired, or feeling tightness in the chest. Respiratory symptoms include a hacking, paroxysmal, irritative, and nonproductive cough caused by bronchial edema. Accumulated secretions, acting as a foreign body, stimulate the cough. As the secretions become more profuse, the cough becomes rattling and productive of frothy, clear, gelatinous sputum. Bronchial spasm and mucosal edema reduce the size of the bronchial lumen, and the bronchi may be occluded by mucous plugs.

Younger children tend to assume the tripod sitting position, whereas older children tend to sit upright with shoulders hunched over, hands on the bed or chair, and arms braced to facilitate the use of accessory muscles of respiration. The child may speak with short, panting, broken phrases. Infants and small children are restless, irritable, and unable to be comforted. If hypoxemia develops, the child may become agitated, confused, and more irritable. Examination of the chest reveals hyperresonance on percussion. Breath sounds are coarse and loud, with sonorous crackles throughout the lung fields.

BOX 21.16 Clinical Manifestations of Asthma

Cough

Hacking, paroxysmal, irritative, and nonproductive
Becomes rattling and productive of frothy, clear, gelatinous sputum

Respiratory-Related Signs

Shortness of breath
Prolonged expiratory phase
Wheezing
May have a malar flush and red ears
Lips deep, dark red color
May progress to cyanosis of nail beds or circumoral cyanosis
Restlessness
Apprehension
Prominent sweating as the attack progresses
Older children sitting upright with shoulders in a hunched-over position, hands on the bed or chair, and arms braced (tripod)
Speaking with short, panting, broken phrases

Chest

Hyperresonance on percussion
Coarse, loud breath sounds
Wheezes throughout the lung fields
Prolonged expiration
Crackles
Generalized inspiratory and expiratory wheezing; increasingly high pitched

With Repeated Episodes

Barrel chest
Elevated shoulders
Use of accessory muscles of respiration
Facial appearance—flattened malar bones, dark circles beneath the eyes, narrow nose, prominent upper teeth

Expiration is prolonged. Coarse rhonchi can be heard, as can generalized inspiratory and expiratory wheezing that becomes more high pitched as obstruction progresses. With minimum obstruction, wheezing may be mild or even absent.

With severe spasm or obstruction, breath sounds and crackles may be inaudible. Cough is ineffective despite repeated hacking maneuvers. This represents a lack of air movement and may be misinterpreted as improvement by unknowing examiners. With repeated asthmatic episodes the thoracic cavity becomes fixed in a hyperaerated state (barrel chest), with a depressed diaphragm, elevated shoulders, and increased use of accessory muscles of respiration.

! NURSING ALERT

Shortness of breath with air movement in the chest restricted to the point of absent breath sounds (silent chest) accompanied by a sudden rise in respiratory rate is an ominous sign indicating ventilatory failure and imminent respiratory arrest.

DIAGNOSTIC EVALUATION

The diagnosis is determined primarily based on clinical manifestations, history, physical examination, and, to a lesser extent, laboratory tests. Generally, chronic cough in the absence of infection or diffuse wheezing during the expiratory phase of respiration is sufficient to establish a diagnosis.

Pulmonary function tests (PFTs) provide an objective method of evaluating the presence and degree of lung disease and the response to therapy. Spirometry can generally be performed reliably on children by 5 or 6 years old and includes either the traditional and simple mechanical spirometer often used in clinics, offices, and the home or new computerized versions. The National Asthma Education and Prevention Program (2007) recommends that spirometry testing be done at the time of initial assessment of asthma, after treatment is initiated and symptoms have stabilized, and at least every 1 to 2 years to assess the maintenance of airway function.

Bronchoprovocation testing (e.g., direct exposure of the mucous membranes to a suspected antigen in increasing concentrations) helps identify inhaled allergens. Exposure to methacholine (methacholine challenge), histamine, or cold or dry air may be performed to assess airway responsiveness or reactivity. Exercise challenges may be used to identify children with exercise-induced bronchospasm (EIB) (Liu et al., 2020). Although these tests are highly specific and sensitive, they place the child at risk for an asthmatic episode and should be done under close observation in a qualified laboratory or clinic.

The peak expiratory flow rate (PEFR) can be measured using a peak expiratory flow meter (PEFM). The PEFR is the maximum flow of air that can be forcefully exhaled in 1 second and is measured in liters per minute. Three zones of measurement, patterned after a traffic light, are typically used to interpret the PEFR. The reliability of the PEFM is controversial because it relies on the child's ability to use the PEFM and willingness to participate. The child's technique on doing the PEFR should be examined on an ongoing basis and reeducation provided when needed. Families are encouraged to record PEFR at regular intervals and to bring the recorded results to the medical appointment for health care providers to review trends. Each child needs to establish his or her personal best value during a 2- to 3-week period when the child's asthma is stable. After the personal best value has been established, the child's current PEFR on any occasion can be compared with the personal best value. PEFR monitoring can be used for short-term monitoring, managing exacerbations, and daily long-term monitoring. However, the PEFM should not be used to diagnose asthma severity. The Expert Panel (National Asthma Education and Prevention Program, 2007) recommends either PEFM or symptom monitoring or a combination of both.

NURSING CARE GUIDELINES

Interpreting Peak Expiratory Flow Rates[a]

- **Green (80% to 100% of personal best)** signals all clear. Asthma is under reasonably good control. No symptoms are present, and the routine treatment plan for maintaining control can be followed.
- **Yellow (50% to 79% of personal best)** signals caution. Asthma is not well controlled. An acute exacerbation may be present. Maintenance therapy may need to be increased. Call the practitioner if the child stays in this zone.
- **Red (<50% of personal best)** signals a medical alert. Severe airway narrowing may be occurring. A short-acting bronchodilator should be administered. Notify the practitioner if the peak expiratory flow rate (PEFR) does not return immediately and stay in yellow or green zones.

[a]These zones are guidelines only. Specific zones and management should be individualized for each child.

Modified from American Lung Association. (2017). Measuring your peak flow rate. Retrieved from http://www.lung.org/lung-health-and-diseases/lung-disease-lookup/asthma/living-with-asthma/managing-asthma/measuring-your-peak-flow-rate.html

A variety of easy-to-use, inexpensive PEFMs are available for use in the home and at school to assess changes in pulmonary function. In general, children 5 years of age and older can use a PEFM successfully. However, young children need to be supervised while they are learning to use the PEFM. Children should use the same PEFM over time, and they should bring it for use at every follow-up visit. Using the same brand of meter is recommended because different brands can give significantly different values. The use of a PEFM provides objective monitoring of the severity of asthma and can decrease asthma episodes, health care visits, and missed school days. Similarly, studies show that PEFM use can improve quality of life and asthma health outcomes in children with asthma (Walter, Sadeque-Igbal, Ulysse, et al., 2015).

Skin testing is useful in identifying specific allergens, and those obtained by the puncture technique correlate better than intracutaneous tests with symptoms and measurements of specific IgE antibody. Since the allergen-specific IgE testing also accurately determines allergic sensitization status to specific allergens, it was selected in a recent study instead of skin testing because of the objectivity of the in vitro test and the lack of the need to discontinue antihistamines (Nagarajan, Ahmad, Quinn, et al., 2018). It is recommended that all patients with year-round asthma symptoms be tested with skin tests or laboratory blood analysis to determine sensitization to perennial allergens (e.g., house dust mites, cats, dogs, cockroaches, molds, and fungus) (Liu et al., 2020; National Heart, Lung, and Blood Institute, 2014; Onell, Whiteman, Nordlund, et al., 2017).

In addition to these tests, other tests include laboratory tests (e.g., complete blood count with differential, allergen-specific IgE) and chest radiographs. Eosinophilia greater than 500/mm^3 suggests the presence of an allergic or inflammatory disorder. Frontal and lateral radiographs may show infiltrates and hyperexpansion of the airways, with the anteroposterior diameter on physical examination indicating an increased diameter (suggestive of barrel chest). Radiography may also assist in ruling out a respiratory tract infection.

THERAPEUTIC MANAGEMENT

The overall goals of asthma management are to maintain normal activity levels, maintain normal pulmonary function, prevent chronic symptoms and recurrent exacerbations, provide optimum drug therapy with minimum or no adverse effects, and assist the child in living as normal and happy a life as possible. This includes facilitating the child's social adjustments in the family, school, and community and normal participation in recreational activities and sports. To accomplish these goals, several treatment principles need to be followed (Pinfield et al., 2015):

- Regular contact with the health care provider is necessary to control symptoms and prevent exacerbations. Registered nurse (RN) care coordinators or case managers can often assist with this and troubleshoot symptoms via phone.
- Prevention of exacerbations includes avoiding triggers, avoiding allergens, and using medications as needed.
- Therapy includes efforts to reduce underlying inflammation and relieve or prevent symptomatic airway narrowing.
- Therapy includes patient and family education, environmental control, pharmacologic management, and the use of objective measures to monitor the severity of disease and guide the course of therapy.

Allergen Control

Nonpharmacologic therapy is aimed at the prevention and reduction of exposure to airborne allergens and irritants. House dust mites and other components of house dust are frequent agents identified in children who are allergic to inhalants. The cockroach, another common household inhabitant, is an important allergen in many locations. Exterminating live cockroaches, carefully cleaning kitchen floors and cabinets, putting food away after eating, and taking trash out in the evening are essential measures to control cockroaches. Other animal-related allergens include mice (especially in the homes of inner-city children) and cat and dog dander. Sensitized persons should carefully evaluate having such pets in the household, but there are inconclusive data on the effects of cat or dog dander on asthma development (Kanchongkittiphon, Mendell, Gaffin, et al., 2015). Additional sources of respiratory irritants include particulate matter produced by tobacco smoke, wood-burning stoves, lead, pesticides, mold spores, and nitrogen dioxide; these are believed to contribute to asthma morbidity in children and should be avoided or minimized (Kanchongkittiphon et al., 2015; Liu et al., 2020). Exposure to tobacco smoke is a significant contributing factor in the development and triggering of asthma in infants and children (Makadia et al., 2017; Skaaby, Taylor, Jacobsen, et al., 2017). Living in damp homes also can be a factor in the development of asthma in infants and small children (Kanchongkittiphon et al., 2015).

Skin testing can identify specific allergens. Steps should be taken to eliminate or avoid them. Often simply removing the offending environmental allergens or irritants (e.g., removing carpeting from the home of a child sensitive to mold and dust particles) decreases the frequency of asthma episodes. Dehumidifiers or air conditioners may control nonspecific factors such as extremes of temperature that trigger an episode. Avoiding known outdoor allergens such as tree, grass, and weed pollen during seasonal elevation may reduce asthma exacerbations as well.

Additional suggestions include the following:

- Cover pillows and mattresses with dustproof covers.
- Wash bedding in hot water once a week. Dry completely.
- Avoid using feather- or down-filled pillows and mattresses.
- Keep child indoors while lawn is being mowed, bushes and trees are being trimmed, or pollen count is high.
- Keep windows and doors closed during pollen season; use air conditioner if possible, or go to places that are air conditioned, such as libraries and shopping malls, when the weather is hot.
- The child should not be present during cleaning activities.
- Wet-mop bare floors weekly; wet-dust and clean child's room weekly.
- Vacuum carpet and fabric-covered furniture every week to reduce dust buildup, using a high-efficiency particulate air filter.
- Limit or prevent child's exposure to tobacco and wood smoke; do not allow cigarette smoking in the house or car; select places such as play and shopping areas that are smoke free.
- Use air conditioners with high-efficiency particulate air filters.
- Use indoor air purifiers with high-efficiency particulate air filters.
- Choose stuffed toys that can be washed in hot water. Dry completely before the child plays with the toy

Drug Therapy

Pharmacologic therapy is used to prevent and control asthma symptoms, reduce the frequency and severity of asthma exacerbations, and reverse airflow obstruction. A stepwise approach is recommended based on the severity of the child's asthma. Because inflammation is considered an early and persistent feature of asthma, therapy is directed toward long-term suppression of inflammation. The National Asthma Education and Prevention Program (2012) highlights that asthma control has two domains:

- Reducing impairment (associated with the frequency and intensity of symptoms and functional limitations experienced by the patient)
- Reducing risk (preventing future attacks, ED visits, and decline in lung function, as well as watching for medication side effects)

Asthma medications are categorized into two general classes: long-term control medications (preventive medications) to achieve and maintain control of inflammation and quick-relief medications (rescue medications) to treat symptoms and exacerbations.

Quick-relief and long-term medications are often used in combination. Inhaled corticosteroids, cromolyn sodium and nedocromil, long-acting β_2-agonists (LABAs), methylxanthines, and leukotriene modifiers are used as long-term control medications. Short-acting β_2-agonists, anticholinergics, and systemic corticosteroids are used as quick-relief medications. Bronchodilators that relax bronchial smooth muscle and dilate the airways include β_2-agonists, methylxanthines, and anticholinergics that can be used as both quick-relief and long-term medications.

Many asthma medications are given by inhalation with a nebulizer or a metered-dose inhaler (MDI). The MDI should always be attached to a spacer when an inhaled corticosteroid is administered to prevent yeast infections in the mouth. Spacers are also important for children who have difficulty coordinating or learning proper inhalation technique. The spacer and holder can be equipped with a mask or a mouthpiece. MDIs that contain propellant chlorofluorocarbons (CFCs) have been banned in the United States due to their linkage with depletion of the Earth's ozone level. An alternative propellant, hydrofluoroalkane, does not cause ozone depletion, delivers more fine particles of the medication, and has less oral deposition. The Diskhaler and Aerosolizer are similar, but with the Aerosolizer, the medication must be loaded into the inhaler before use. Infants and young children who have difficulty using MDIs or other inhalers can receive their asthma medications via a handheld nebulizer. When this device is used, the medication is mixed with saline (also available in premixed form) and nebulized with compressed air. Children are instructed to breathe normally with the mouth open to provide a direct route to the trachea.

Corticosteroids are antiinflammatory drugs used to treat reversible airflow obstruction, control symptoms, and reduce bronchial hyperresponsiveness in chronic asthma. Inhaled corticosteroids are used as first-line therapy in children older than 5 years of age. Clinical studies of corticosteroids have indicated significant improvement of all asthma parameters, including decreases in symptoms, ED visits, hospitalizations, and medication requirements (Bekmezian, Fee, & Weber, 2015; Falk, Hughes, & Rodgers, 2016).

Corticosteroids may be administered parenterally, orally, or by inhalation. Oral medications are metabolized slowly, with an onset of action up to 3 hours after administration and peak effectiveness occurring within 6 to 12 hours. Oral systemic steroids may be given for short periods (e.g., 3- or 10-day "bursts") to gain prompt control of inadequately controlled persistent asthma or to manage severe persistent asthma. These drugs should be given in the lowest effective dose. They have few side effects (cough, dysphonia, and oral thrush), and there is evidence that they improve the long-term outcomes for children of all ages with mild or moderate persistent asthma. Evidence from clinical trials that monitored children for 6 years indicates that the use of inhaled corticosteroids at recommended dosages does not have long-term significant effects on growth, bone mineral density, or suppression of the adrenal-pituitary axis (Falk et al., 2016; Liu et al., 2020). However, primary care providers should frequently monitor (at least every 3 to 6 months) the growth of children and adolescents taking corticosteroids to assess the systemic effects of these drugs and make appropriate reductions in dosages or changes to other types of asthma therapy when necessary. Inhaled corticosteroids include budesonide and fluticasone.

β-Adrenergic agonists (short acting) (primarily albuterol, levalbuterol [Xopenex], and terbutaline) are used for treatment of acute exacerbations and for the prevention of EIB. These drugs bind with the β-receptors on the smooth muscle of airways, where they activate adenylate cyclase and convert adenosine monophosphate (AMP) to cyclic AMP (cAMP). The increased cAMP enhances binding of intracellular calcium to the cell membrane, reducing the availability of calcium and thus allowing smooth muscle to relax. Other effects of the drug help stabilize mast cells to prevent release of mediators. Most β-adrenergics used in asthma therapy affect predominantly the β_2-receptors, which help eliminate bronchospasm. β_1-receptor effects, such as increased heart rate and GI disturbances, have been minimized. Albuterol is given orally or via nebulizer or inhaler, whereas levalbuterol is given only via inhaler or nebulizer. The inhaled drugs have a more rapid onset of action than oral forms. Levalbuterol is more expensive than albuterol but reportedly causes fewer side effects than albuterol. There continues to be some discussion about the administration of β_2-agonists via an MDI versus a nebulizer. However, administration via an MDI is as effective to delivery of medication by a small-volume nebulizer in reversing bronchospasm (Mitselou, Hedlin, & Hederos, 2016).

LABAs are approved as single-ingredient products (Serevent and Foradil) and in combination products containing inhaled corticosteroids (Advair and Symbicort). The National Asthma Education and Prevention Program (2007) recommends use of a LABA with low- or medium-dosage inhaled corticosteroid to improve lung function and asthma symptoms, as well as reduce use of short-acting β_2-agonists. They are used for patients whose symptoms cannot be adequately controlled on asthma controller medications.

LABAs must be added to antiinflammatory therapy and never used as monotherapy (Liu et al., 2020). Inhaled β-adrenergic agents should not be taken more than three or four times daily for acute symptoms without medical supervision. LABAs can increase the risk of severely worsening asthma symptoms, potentially leading to hospitalizations and death. The US Food and Drug Administration has required LABA manufacturers to conduct studies to evaluate the safety of using them with inhaled corticosteroids versus inhaled corticosteroids alone. Salmeterol and Foradil are not used for patients younger than 4 years of age.

Theophylline (a methylxanthine drug) was used for decades to relieve symptoms and prevent asthma attacks; however, it is now used primarily when the child is not responding to maximum therapy (Liu et al., 2020). Therapeutic levels should be obtained with this drug because it has a narrow therapeutic window. Theophylline is not recommended for acute asthma exacerbations.

Cromolyn sodium is a medication used in maintenance therapy for asthma in children older than 2 years of age. It stabilizes mast cell membranes; inhibits activation and release of mediators from eosinophil and epithelial cells; and inhibits the acute airway narrowing after exposure to exercise, cold dry air, and sulfur dioxide. It does not result in immediate relief of symptoms and has minimal side effects (occasional coughing on inhalation of the powder formulation). It is now only available as an oral preparation or via nebulizer. Cromolyn or nedocromil inhaler preparations were discontinued in 2010.

Leukotrienes are mediators of inflammation that cause increases in airway hyperresponsiveness. Leukotriene modifiers (e.g., zafirlukast [Accolate], zileuton [Zyflo], montelukast sodium [Singulair]) block inflammatory and bronchospasm effects. These drugs are not used to treat acute episodes but are given orally in combination with β-agonists and steroids to provide long-term control and prevent symptoms in mild persistent asthma. Montelukast is approved to treat asthma in children 12 months of age and older, whereas zafirlukast is approved for children 5 years of age and older.

Anticholinergics (atropine and ipratropium [Atrovent]) help relieve acute bronchospasm. However, these drugs have adverse side effects that include drying of respiratory secretions, blurred vision, and cardiac and CNS stimulation. The primary anticholinergic drug used is ipratropium, which does not cross the blood-brain barrier and therefore elicits no CNS effects. Ipratropium, when used in combination with albuterol, can be effective during acute severe asthma in significantly improving lung function in children and reducing hospitalizations and ED visits (Liu et al., 2020).

Omalizumab (Xolair) is a monoclonal antibody that is used for patients with moderate to severe persistent allergic asthma whose asthma symptoms are not controlled by inhaled corticosteroids. It blocks the binding of IgE to mast cells to inhibit the inflammation associated with asthma. Many patients with asthma are atopic and possess specific IgE antibodies to allergens responsible for airway inflammation. Xolair has been approved for use in children 12 years of age and older. IgE levels are measured before beginning treatment. Dosage and frequency of administration of Xolair are dependent on the serum total IgE level and body weight. The drug is administered once or twice a month by subcutaneous injection. Efficacy of omalizumab is not immediate and takes 12 to 16 weeks. In early 2007, the US Food and Drug Administration (2007) added a "black box warning" to omalizumab that highlighted the risk of anaphylaxis. Anaphylaxis was observed in 0.14% of patients receiving omalizumab in clinical trials, and 60% of these instances occurred within 2 hours of administration; therefore recommendations include observing the recipient for 2 hours after the first three doses are administered and for 30 minutes thereafter for subsequent doses (Thomson & Chaudhuri, 2012). Some children with severe asthma and a history of severe life-threatening episodes may need a prescription for an EpiPen (subcutaneous injectable epinephrine).

Magnesium sulfate, a potent muscle relaxant that acts to decrease inflammation and improves pulmonary function and peak flow rate, may be used in pediatric patients treated in the ED or ICU with moderate to severe asthma. Studies on the use of IV and inhaled magnesium sulfate offer significant benefits for children with acute asthma exacerbations (Griffiths, Kew, & Normansell, 2016; Schuh, Sweeney, Freedman, et al., 2016).

Exercise

Exercise-induced bronchospasm (EIB) is an acute, reversible, usually self-terminating airway obstruction that develops during or after vigorous activity, reaches its peak 5 to 10 minutes after stopping the activity, and usually stops in another 20 to 30 minutes. Patients with EIB have cough, shortness of breath, chest pain or tightness, wheezing, and endurance problems during exercise, but an exercise challenge test in a laboratory is necessary to make the diagnosis.

The problem occurs rarely in activities that require short bursts of energy (e.g., baseball, sprints, gymnastics, skiing) but more commonly during endurance exercises (e.g., soccer, basketball, distance running). Swimming is well tolerated by children with EIB because they are breathing air fully saturated with moisture and because of the type of breathing required in swimming.

Parents, teachers, and practitioners often exclude children with asthma from exercise, and the children themselves are reluctant to participate because it may provoke an attack. However, doing so can seriously hamper peer interaction and physical health. Exercise is advantageous for children with asthma, and most children can participate in activities at school and in sports with minimal difficulty, provided their asthma is under control. Evaluate participation on an individual basis. Appropriate prophylactic treatment with β-adrenergic agents or cromolyn sodium before exercise usually permits full participation in strenuous exertion.

Breathing Exercises

Breathing exercises and physical training help produce physical and mental relaxation, improve posture, strengthen respiratory musculature, and develop more efficient breathing patterns. For motivated child, breathing exercises and controlled breathing help prevent overinflation and improve efficiency of the cough. However, these exercises are not recommended during acute asthma exacerbations.

Hyposensitization

The role of hyposensitization in childhood asthma is somewhat controversial. In the past, allergen immunotherapy was used for seasonal allergies and when single substances were identified as the offending allergen. It is not recommended for allergens that can be eliminated, such as foods, drugs, and animal dander.

The National Asthma Education and Prevention Program (2007) guidelines recommend allergen immunotherapy for asthma patients in the following situations:

- When there is evidence of a relationship between asthma symptoms and unavoidable exposure to an allergen to which the patient is sensitive
- When symptoms occur all year or at least during a major portion of the year
- When symptom control is difficult with drug therapy because multiple medications are required, the patient is not responsive to available drugs, or the patient refuses to take the medications

Injection therapy is usually limited to clinically significant allergens. The initial dose of the offending allergen(s), based on the size of the skin reaction, is injected subcutaneously. The amount is increased at weekly intervals until a maximum tolerance is reached, after which a maintenance dose is given at 4-week intervals. This may be extended to 5- or 6-week intervals during the off-season for seasonal allergens. Successful treatment is continued for a minimum of 3 years and then stopped. If no symptoms appear, acquired immunity is assumed; if symptoms recur, treatment is reinstituted. Hyposensitization injections should be administered only with emergency equipment and medications readily available in the event of an anaphylactic reaction.

Status Asthmaticus

Status asthmaticus is a medical emergency that can result in respiratory failure and death if unrecognized and untreated. Children who continue to display respiratory distress despite vigorous therapeutic measures, especially the use of sympathomimetics (e.g., albuterol, epinephrine), are in status asthmaticus. The condition may develop gradually or rapidly, often coincident with complicating conditions, such as pneumonia or a respiratory virus, that can influence the duration and treatment of the exacerbation.

> **! NURSING ALERT**
>
> A child with asthma who sweats profusely, remains sitting upright, and refuses to lie down is in severe respiratory distress. Also, a child who suddenly becomes agitated or an agitated child who suddenly becomes quiet may have serious hypoxia and requires immediate intervention.

Therapy for status asthmaticus is aimed at improving ventilation, decreasing airway resistance, relieving bronchospasm, correcting dehydration and acidosis, allaying child and parent anxiety related to the severity of the event, and treating any concurrent infection. Humidified oxygen is recommended and should be given to maintain an oxygen saturation greater than 90%. Inhaled aerosolized short-acting β_2-agonists are recommended for all patients. Three treatments of β_2-agonists spaced 20 to 30 minutes apart are usually given as initial therapy, and continuous administration of β_2-agonists via nebulizer may be initiated. A systemic corticosteroid (oral, IV, or IM) is given to decrease the effects of inflammation. An anticholinergic agent (such as ipratropium bromide) may be added to the aerosolized solution of the β_2-agonist. Anticholinergics have resulted in additional bronchodilation in patients with severe airflow obstruction. An IV infusion is often initiated to provide a means for hydration and to administer medications. Correction of dehydration, acidosis, hypoxia, and electrolyte disturbance is guided by frequent determination of arterial pH, blood gases, and serum electrolytes.

Additional therapies in acute asthma attacks may include the use of IV magnesium sulfate, a potent muscle relaxant that decreases inflammation and improves pulmonary function and peak flow rate among patients with moderate to severe asthma when treated in the ED or ICU. Heliox (a mixture of 70% to 80% helium and 20% to 30% oxygen) may be administered to decrease airway resistance and thereby decrease the work of breathing; it can be delivered via a nonrebreathing face mask from premixed tanks, which may be blended in a standalone unit or within a ventilator. It may be used in acute exacerbations as an adjunct to β_2-agonist and IV corticosteroid therapy to improve pulmonary function until the two latter medications have time to take full effect in decreasing bronchospasm; the effects of heliox are usually seen within 20 minutes of administration, whereas other drugs may take longer to exert the desired effect. Ketamine, a dissociative anesthetic, is believed to cause smooth muscle relaxation and decrease airway resistance caused by severe bronchospasm in acute asthma; it may be administered as an adjunct to other therapies mentioned previously. Antibiotics should not be used to treat stable asthma except when a bacterial infection is present.

A child suspected of having status asthmaticus is usually seen in the ED and is often admitted to a pediatric ICU for close observation and continuous cardiorespiratory monitoring. A key component in the prevention of morbidity is helping the child, parents, teachers, coaches, and other adults recognize features of deteriorating respiratory status, use the correct rescue drugs effectively, and immediately place the child with deteriorating respiratory status into the care of health care professionals instead of waiting to see if the asthma gets better on its own. For the child going into early status asthmaticus, immediate medical care is required to prevent irreversible respiratory failure and possible death (see Next-Generation NCLEX® Examination-Style Unfolding Case Study).

Prognosis

Although deaths from asthma have been relatively uncommon since the 1980s, the rate of death from asthma increased steadily in the United States until it peaked in the mid-1990s and then slowly decreased over the next 10 years. In 2016, 209 children younger than 18 years old died from asthma (Centers for Disease Control and Prevention, 2018b). In 2011, 14% of all children in the United States were diagnosed with asthma, and 70% of these children had recurrent asthma (Liu et al., 2020). There has been a significant increase in asthma-related ED visits and hospitalizations. Mortality and morbidity rates for asthma are especially high among African American children, whose hospitalization and death rates are two to seven times higher than non–African American children (Fitzpatrick, Gillespie, Mauger, et al., 2019; Liu et al., 2020). Most asthma deaths in children occur in the home, school, or community before life-saving medical care can be administered.

Some children's asthma symptoms may improve at puberty, but up to two-thirds of children with asthma continue to have symptoms through puberty and into adulthood. The prognosis for control or disappearance of symptoms varies in children from those who have rare and infrequent attacks to those who are constantly wheezing or are subject to status asthmaticus. Risk factors that may predict the persistence of symptoms into childhood (from infancy) include atopy, male gender, exposure to environmental tobacco, and maternal history of asthma. Many children

NEXT-GENERATION NCLEX® EXAMINATION-STYLE UNFOLDING CASE STUDY

The Child With Acute Asthma Exacerbation

Day 1, 10:00 am

7. A 15-year-old male presents to the Emergency Department with a history of asthma and symptoms that are not resolving with his current rescue medications. His asthma symptoms have been controlled with use of a long-acting inhaler twice daily, but an increase in seasonal allergies and a recent upper respiratory infection (URI) have caused an exacerbation of his symptoms. The patient rarely uses his peak expiratory flow meter (PEFM); instead, he waits until his symptoms become severe before starting to use his rescue medications. The nurse completes a history and physical assessment and finds the following. **Highlight the assessment findings that require follow-up by the nurse.**
   A. Temperature = 98.6° F (37° C)
   B. Heart Rate = 114 beats/min
   C. Respirations = 28 breaths/min
   D. SpO_2 = 88% on room air
   E. Blood Pressure = 110/64 mmHg
   F. Wheezing auscultated in both lungs
   G. Unable to lie down on the stretcher
   H. Peak expiratory flow meter results are <50% of baseline

8. Based on these findings, what are the most important subjective and objective data that should be considered as the defining characteristics of an acute asthma exacerbation? **Select all that apply.**
   A. Dyspnea
   B. Moist cough
   C. Shortness of breath
   D. High blood pressure
   E. Increased respiratory rate
   F. Profuse thick secretions
   G. Chest tightness or chest pain
   H. Use of accessory muscles (retractions)
   I. Diminished breath sounds and/or adventitious breath sounds (wheezing)

Day 1, 10:15 am

9. A 15-year-old male with a history of asthma is in the Emergency Department for immediate treatment. The physician has examined the patient and written orders. Which nursing interventions are of **highest priority** for this adolescent with an asthma exacerbation? **Use an X to indicate whether the nursing actions listed below are Emergent (appropriate or immediately necessary) or Not Emergent (not appropriate or not immediately necessary) for the patient's care at this time.**

Nursing Action	Emergent	Not Emergent
Administer humidified oxygen to keep the oxygen saturation (SpO_2) above 90%.		
Administer methylprednisolone per the physician order.		
Administer albuterol per hospital protocol.		
Place the patient in a comfortable standing, sitting upright or learning forward position.		
Discuss possible allergens in the home that might have triggered the attack.		
Review how to use the metered dose inhaler.		

10. Indicate which nursing action number listed in the far-left column is most appropriate for each potential complication listed in the middle column. **Place the number in the far-right column. Note that not all actions will be used.**

Nursing Action	Potential Complication	Nursing Action to Prevent Complication
1. Allow patient to assume position of comfort.	To minimize drying of nasal mucous membranes	
2. Administer rescue medications (as prescribed) that can include inhalers, nebulization, and/or oral or intravenous (IV) steroids.	To prevent airway obstruction	
3. Administer humidified oxygen to maintain oxygen saturation (SaO_2) above 90%.	Decreased patient's awareness of factors that exacerbate asthma	
4. Assess patient's response to rescue medications.	To prevent constricted airways and decreased air exchange	
5. Assist patient in recognizing factors that trigger asthma symptoms.	Lack of awareness of need for more aggressive interventions	
6. Assure respirations will be easy and nonlabored at a rate within normal limits for age.		
7. Teach the patient how to use the peak expiratory flow meter (PEFM).		
8. Evaluate the use of the PEFM.		

Day 2, 11:00 am

11. A 15-year-old male with a history of asthma was admitted yesterday for acute asthmatic care. He has responded well to treatment and will be discharged. The nurse will be discussing discharge plans that are essentials aspects of asthma care and prevention. What would the nurse include in the teaching plan? **Select all that apply.**
   A. Avoiding smoke and other irritants
   B. Avoiding Tylenol containing products
   C. Encouraging daily albuterol use.
   D. Identifying early signs of an asthma exacerbation
   E. Identifying specific asthmatic triggers in the environment
   F. Reviewing home medications, dosing and precautions
   G. Recommending physical exercise and mental training
   H. Avoiding exposure to excessive cold, wind and other extremes of weather

Continued

NEXT-GENERATION NCLEX® EXAMINATION-STYLE UNFOLDING CASE STUDY—cont'd

Day 2, 2:00 pm

12. A 15-year-old male with a history of asthma who is in the Emergency Department for immediate treatment. He has responded well to treatment and no longer needs oxygen and plans are being discussed for discharge. Since there is a history of this adolescent not using the PEFM the nurse will meet with him and his mother to review how to use the PEFM. The nurse realizes that the adolescent and his mother must understand how to interpret the peak expiratory flow rates using the peak expiratory flow meter (PEFM). **Choose the most likely options for the information missing from the statements below by selecting from the lists of options provided.** The PEFR measures the maximum ____1____ that can be forcefully exhaled in ____2____. Asthma is under reasonably good control when the PEFR indicates ____3____ of the patient's personal best value is obtained. This value is established by obtaining a PEFR over a ____4____ period of time.

Options for 1	Options for 2	Options for 3	Options for 4
flow of air	5 seconds	80-100%	4-5 week
flow of oxygen	10 seconds	50-70%	2-3 week
flow of water	1 second	60-80%	1-2 day

who outgrow their exacerbations continue to have airway hyperresponsiveness and cough as adults. Furthermore, airway hyperresponsiveness in adults appears to be associated with decreased lung function.

The adolescent age-group appears to be the most vulnerable, with the greatest increase in mortality from the condition occurring in children 10 to 14 years of age. No reliable data exist to explain this increase. Factors that have been postulated include exposure of atopic persons to more allergens (particularly in large urban centers), change in severity of the disease, abuse of drug therapy (toxicity), failure of families and practitioners to recognize the severity of asthma, and psychologic factors, such as denial and refusal to accept the disease. Risk factors for asthma-related deaths include early onset, frequent attacks, difficult-to-manage disease, adolescence, history of respiratory failure, psychologic problems (refusal to take medications), dependency on or misuse of asthma drugs (high use), presence of physical stigmata (barrel chest, intercostal retractions), and abnormal PFTs.

Nursing Care Management

Acute Asthma Care

Children who are admitted to the hospital with acute asthma are ill, anxious, and uncomfortable. Continual observation and assessment are essential. Pediatric Quality Indicators for appropriate asthma medication implications are shown in Table 21.3.

When β_2-agonists, corticosteroids, and supplemental oxygen are given, the child is monitored closely and continuously for relief of respiratory distress and signs of side effects or toxicity (e.g., tachycardia, restlessness, irritability, hyperactivity). Pulse oximetry is monitored along with rate and depth of breathing, auscultation of air movement, adventitious sounds, and any signs of respiratory distress (e.g., nasal flaring, tachypnea, retractions). The child on supplemental oxygen requires intermittent or continuous oxygenation monitoring depending on severity of respiratory compromise and initial oxygenation status. The child in status asthmaticus should be placed on continuous cardiorespiratory (including blood pressure) and pulse oximetry monitoring. Oral fluid intake may be limited during the acute phase; IV fluid replacement may be required to provide adequate tissue hydration.

Children with acute asthma may be apprehensive and anxious. The calm, efficient presence of a nurse helps reassure children that they are safe and will be cared for during this stressful period. Assure children that they will not be left alone and that their parents can remain with them. Parents need reassurance and want to be informed of their child's condition and therapies. They may believe that they have in some way contributed to the child's condition or could have prevented the episode. Reassurance regarding their efforts expended on the child's behalf and their parenting capabilities can help alleviate their stress. Efforts to reduce parental apprehension will also reduce the child's distress. Anxiety is easily communicated to the child from parents and other family members.

Provide Long-Term Asthma Care

The nursing care of the child with asthma begins with a review of the child's health history; the home, school, and play environment; the parents' and child's attitudes about the child's condition; and a comprehensive physical assessment with focus on the respiratory system. Physical assessment of asthma involves the same observations and techniques described in Chapter 4. In addition, the nurse identifies and evaluates physical characteristics of chronic respiratory involvement, including chest configuration (e.g., barrel chest), posturing (tripod), and type of breathing. A history of the current and previous episodes and precipitating factors or events provides important information. An asthma scoring system may be used to determine severity of symptoms. The nursing assessment should include questions about nighttime waking related to symptoms, frequency of use of the quick-acting bronchodilator, ability to participate in school or other activities, PEFR scores, any medication side effects, and other visits to a provider related to asthma symptoms.

Nursing care of children with asthma involves both acute and long-term care. Nurses who are involved with children in the home, hospital, school, outpatient clinic, or practitioner's office play an important role in helping children and their families learn to live with the condition. The disease can be managed so that it does not require ED visits or hospitalization, or interfere with family life, physical activity, or school attendance. The nursing process in the care of the child with asthma is outlined in the Next-Generation NCLEX® Examination-Style Unfolding Case Study box.

Nurses may perform a variety of vital functions in asthma care, including asthma education in the primary care setting and in schools and other community settings and care of the child with asthma in the acute care setting, ambulatory care, and intensive care. Nurses also obtain information on how asthma affects the child's everyday

TABLE 21.3 Pediatric Quality Indicator[a]

Appropriate Medications for Asthma	
Measure	Asthma patients who were identified as having moderate to severe persistent asthma and had a ratio of controller medications to total asthma medications of 0.50 or greater during the measurement year.
Numerator	The number of patients who have a medication ratio of at least 0.50 during the measurement year who were identified as having moderate to severe persistent asthma.
Denominator	All patients during the measurement year who were identified as having moderate to severe persistent asthma.

[a]Endorsed by the National Quality Forum NQF #1800 and 2019 Core Set of Children's Health Care Quality Measures for Medicaid and CHIP, https://www.medicaid.gov/federal- policy-guidance/downloads/cib112018.pdf.

activities and self-concept, the child's and family's adherence to the prescribed therapy, and their personal treatment goals. Every effort is made to build a partnership between the child and family and the health care team, and effective communication is an essential part of this partnership. Assess the child and family's satisfaction with asthma control and with the quality of care, their perception of the severity of the disease, and their level of social support.

One of the major emphases of nursing care is outpatient management by the family. Parents are taught how to recognize and respond to symptoms of bronchospasm, to maintain health and prevent complications, and to promote normal activities. The child's asthma action plan should be reviewed periodically at least every 6 months in children with moderate to severe disease; precipitating factors, illness management, and medication use should be discussed. The nurse determines any cultural or ethnic beliefs or practices that influence self-management and may necessitate modifications in educational approaches to meet the family's needs.

Avoid Allergens

One goal of asthma management is avoidance of an exacerbation. Parents and children need to know how to avoid allergens that precipitate asthma episodes. The nurse educates the parent and child on how to modify the environment to reduce contact with the offending allergen(s). Caution parents to avoid exposing a sensitive child to extremes of weather (e.g., excessive cold, wind) and other irritants (e.g., smoke, sprays, scents). Foods known to provoke symptoms should be eliminated from the diet.

Approximately 2% to 6% of children with asthma are sensitive to aspirin; therefore nurses should caution parents to use other analgesic or antipyretic drugs for discomfort or fever and to read package labeling. Parents are taught to avoid administering aspirin to *any* child because of its association with Reye syndrome unless specifically recommended by and under the supervision of a health practitioner. Salicylate compounds are contained in other common medicines such as Pepto-Bismol, which should be avoided. Children with aspirin-induced asthma may also be sensitive to nonsteroidal antiinflammatory drugs (NSAIDs) and tartrazine (yellow dye number 5, a common food coloring).

> **! NURSING ALERT**
>
> Acetaminophen is the analgesic of choice for asthmatic children.

Relieve Bronchospasm

Teach parents and older children to recognize early signs and symptoms of an impending attack so that it can be controlled before symptoms become distressing. Most children can recognize prodromal symptoms well before an attack (about 6 hours) and implement preventive therapy. Objective signs that parents may observe include rhinorrhea, cough, low-grade fever, irritability, itching (especially in front of the neck and chest), apathy, anxiety, sleep disturbance, abdominal discomfort, and loss of appetite.

Children who use a nebulizer, MDI, Diskus, or Turbuhaler to deliver drugs need to learn how to use the device correctly (Fig. 21.8). The MDI device (Fig. 21.9) delivers medication directly to the airways; therefore the child needs to learn to breathe slowly and deeply for better distribution to narrowed airways (see Family-Centered Care box).

FAMILY-CENTERED CARE

Use of a Metered-Dose Inhaler[a]

Steps for Checking How Much Medicine Is in the Canister

1. If the canister is new, it is full.
2. Check product label to see how many inhalations should be in each canister.
3. The most accurate way to determine how many doses remain in a metered-dose inhaler (MDI) is to count and record each dose as it is used.
4. Many dry powder inhalers have a dose-counting device or dose indicator on the canister to specify when the canister is empty.
5. Placing dry powder inhalers or MDIs with hydrofluoroalkanes in water will destroy them.

Steps for Using the Inhaler With Mouthpiece

1. Remove the cap and hold inhaler upright
2. Shake the inhaler.
3. Attach spacer, as appropriate.
4. Tilt the head back slightly and breathe out slowly.
5. With the inhaler in an upright position, insert the mouthpiece about 3 to 4 cm (1 to 1½ inches) from the mouth or into the mouth, forming an airtight seal between the lips and mouthpiece.
6. At the end of a normal expiration, depress the top of the inhaler canister firmly to release the medication (into the mouth) and breathe in slowly (about 3 to 5 seconds). Relax the pressure on the top of the canister.
7. Hold the breath for at least 5 to 10 seconds to allow the aerosol medication to reach deeply into the lungs.
8. Remove the inhaler and breathe out slowly through the nose.
9. Wait 1 minute between puffs (if an additional puff is needed) when using a bronchodilator.
10. Replace the cap on the MDI.
11. If using a corticosteroid, rinse mouth or take a drink to remove residual medication (which can cause a yeast infection to develop).

Steps for Using the Inhaler With an AeroChamber (see Fig. 21.9)

1. Remove the cap and hold inhaler upright.
2. Shake the inhaler.
3. Attach AeroChamber
4. For AeroChamber with a mouthpiece, place the inhaler in an upright position, then insert the mouthpiece into the mouth, forming an airtight seal between the lips and mouthpiece.
5. For AeroChamber with a mask, apply AeroChamber mask to child's face and make sure that there is a good seal.
6. Have child breathe slow, regular breaths. Depress the top of the inhaler canister firmly to release the medication (into the AeroChamber) as the child breathes slowly in and out. Relax the pressure on the top of the canister.
7. Hold the AeroChamber in place over the child's face until six breaths have been taken. Give one puff at a time and wait 1 minute in between puffs when using a bronchodilator.
8. Remove the inhaler and AeroChamber. Apply to cap to the MDI. The AeroChamber should be washed weekly using soap and water.

Common Problems for Children Using Inhalers

- Child refuses or resists treatment.
- Inhalation is too rapid.
- Child is unable to coordinate the spray with inhalation.
- Breath is not held long enough after inhalation.

[a]Inhaled dry powder such as budesonide (Pulmicort) requires a different inhalation technique. To use a dry powder inhaler, the base of the device is turned until a click is heard. It is important to close the mouth tightly around the mouthpiece of the inhaler and inhale rapidly.

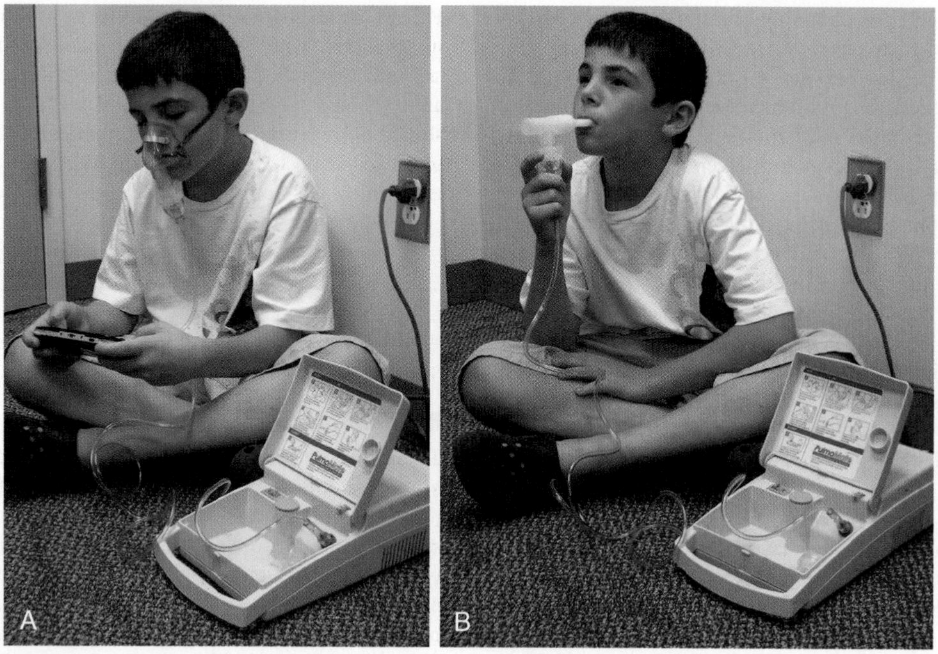

Fig. 21.8 Children with asthma may take a nebulized aerosol treatment with (A) a mask or (B) a mouthpiece. (Courtesy Texas Children's Hospital, Houston, TX.)

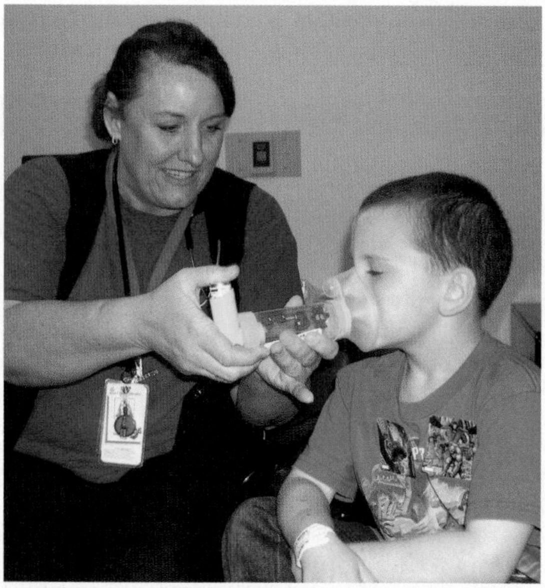

Fig. 21.9 Child using metered-dose inhaler (MDI) with spacer and face mask.

Young children and those who are unable to manipulate the MDI or hold their breath for 10 seconds should use a spacer. A spacer is a 4- to 8-inch tube that fits on the end of the MDI mouthpiece. These devices allow the parent or child to deliver the medication from the MDI into the spacer, from which the child then inhales the medication while taking slow, steady breaths at his or her own pace. Spacers also help prevent yeast infections in the mouth when corticosteroids are inhaled via an MDI.

! NURSING ALERT

Long-acting β_2-agonist (LABA) inhalers (salmeterol) should be used only as directed (usually every 12 hours) and not more frequently. They are not intended to relieve acute asthmatic symptoms.

The nurse also needs to caution the child and parents about the adverse effects of prescribed drugs and the dangers of overuse of β_2-agonists. They should know that it is important to use these drugs when needed but not indiscriminately or as a substitute for avoiding the symptom-provoking allergen. Caution parents against purchasing over-the-counter preparations because these medications can place the children at risk for increased dosage of a drug and toxicity. Educate parents on how to read labels on prepared foods and snacks to determine the presence of allergens.

The family should obtain a PEFM and learn to use this device to monitor the child's asthma. A written asthma action plan that includes the three peak flow meter zones and the child's asthma medications may be obtained from the child's primary care provider. A written asthma action plan can significantly reduce ED visits, hospital stay days, school absence days, and the risk of asthma death (Lakupoch, Manuyakorn, Preutthipan, et al, 2018; Liu et al., 2020). Medications used for asthma exacerbations are also included in the asthma plan. This action plan should be used to make decisions about asthma management at home and at school. The nurse may assist the child and family in preparing this plan, emphasizing that the child and family determine the success of the plan, not the health professionals.

The child should be protected from a respiratory tract infection that can trigger an attack or aggravate the asthmatic state, especially in young children whose airways are mechanically smaller and more reactive. Annual influenza vaccinations are recommended for all children older than 6 months of age. Pneumococcal conjugate vaccine (PCV13) regimen for protection against pneumococcal infection is part of the routine childhood vaccination schedule that is recommended for all children from 2 to 59 months of age. Also, an additional pneumococcal polysaccharide vaccine (PPSV23) is recommended for high-risk children, including asthmatic children on prolonged high-dose corticosteroids (American Academy of Pediatrics, Committee on Infectious Diseases, 2018). Equipment used for the child, such as nebulizers, must be kept absolutely clean to decrease the chances of contamination with bacteria and fungi.

Teach and encourage breathing exercises and controlled breathing for motivated children, and provide information on activities that promote diaphragmatic breathing, side expansion, and improved mobility of the chest wall. Play techniques that can be used for younger children to extend their expiratory time and increase expiratory pressure include blowing cotton balls or a ping-pong ball on a table, blowing a pinwheel, blowing bubbles, or preventing a tissue from falling by blowing it against the wall.

Self-care and asthma self-management programs are important in helping the child and family cope with asthma. Most asthma self-management programs for children convey several principles. First, asthma is a common disease that can be controlled with appropriate drug therapy, environmental control, education, and management skills. Second, it is much easier to prevent than to treat an asthma episode; adherence to a therapeutic program is necessary to prevent exacerbations. Third, children with asthma can live full and active lives. Although a visit to the ED or hospital due to an asthma exacerbation is undesirable, it also presents an opportunity to assess the child's and family's current knowledge about asthma, its triggers, prevention, and treatment to prevent future visits. The technique used for MDI or nebulizer administration should be observed and education provided when needed.

Asthma camps provide an opportunity for children with asthma to engage in physical activity while learning about their disease in a controlled environment with their peers and health professionals. Children who attend asthma camps often demonstrate improved asthma self-management skills.

Self-contained programs and brochures for patient education are available from the Asthma and Allergy Foundation of America[b] and the American Lung Association.[c] The National Heart, Lung, and Blood Institute[d] provides educational materials for asthma education in the school setting. Practice parameters and guidelines designed for health care practitioners are available from the American Academy of Allergy Asthma and Immunology website.[e]

Child and Family Support

The nurse working with children with asthma can provide support in a number of ways. Many children voice frustration because their exacerbations interfere with their daily activities and social lives. These children need reassurance from the health team that they can learn to control and cope with their asthma and live a normal life.

Children in disruptive family situations (e.g., divorce, separation, violence, custodial battles) may disregard their daily asthma medication regimen or be at higher risk as a result of neglect by adults who are in charge of their care. Adolescents struggling with a sense of identity and body image often regard asthma as a condition that will "go away," especially if there is a time lapse between symptoms, and may abandon the therapeutic regimen. Referral for counseling and guidance is appropriate where the child's or adolescent's life is potentially in danger and the therapeutic regimen for asthma is abandoned due to personal or family crises.

The short- and long-term adaptation of children with asthma often depends on the family's acceptance of the disorder. The task of living day to day with affected children undergoing periodic asthmatic crisis involves the entire family. Throughout the stressful crisis, encourage parents to promote as normal a life as possible for their children.

CYSTIC FIBROSIS

Cystic fibrosis (CF) is a condition characterized by exocrine (or mucus-producing) gland dysfunction that produces multisystem involvement, especially in the pulmonary and digestive systems. The affected child inherits the autosomal recessive defective gene from both parents, with an overall 25% risk with each pregnancy of acquiring the defective genes. The condition has a frequency of 1 in 3500 live births among mostly whites; the incidence in other ethnic groups varies, affecting African Americans in 1 in 15,000 live births and Hispanics in 1 in 9200 live births (Egan, Schecter, & Voynow, 2020). The mutated gene responsible for CF is located on the long arm of chromosome 7. This gene codes a protein of 1480 amino acids called the cystic fibrosis transmembrane conductance regulator (CFTR). The CFTR protein is related to a family of membrane-bound glycoproteins. The glycoproteins constitute a cAMP-activated chloride channel and regulate other chloride and sodium channels at the surfaces of the epithelial cells.

Pathophysiology

With the discovery of the CFTR gene, research is continuing to determine its multisystem effects on the body. Several clinical features characterize CF: increased viscosity of mucous gland secretions, a striking elevation of sweat electrolytes, an increase in several organic and enzymatic constituents of saliva, and abnormalities in autonomic nervous system function. Although both sodium and chloride are affected, the defect appears to be primarily a result of abnormal chloride movement; the CFTR appears to function as a chloride channel.

Children with CF demonstrate decreased pancreatic secretion of bicarbonate and chloride and an increase in sodium and chloride in both saliva and sweat. This last characteristic is the basis for the sweat chloride diagnostic test. The sweat electrolyte abnormality is present from birth, continues throughout life, and is unrelated to the severity of the disease or the extent to which other organs are involved. The sodium and chloride content of sweat in 98% to 99% of children with CF is two to five times greater than that of children without CF.

The primary factor, and the one responsible for many of the clinical manifestations of the disease, is mechanical obstruction caused by the increased viscosity of mucous gland secretions (Fig. 21.10). Instead of forming a thin, freely flowing secretion, the mucous glands produce a thick mucoprotein that accumulates and dilates them. Small passages in organs such as the pancreas and bronchioles become obstructed as secretions precipitate or coagulate to form concretions in glands and ducts.

In the pancreas of many patients, thick secretions block the ducts, leading to pancreatic fibrosis caused by cystic dilations of the acini (small lobes of the gland) that undergo degeneration and progressive diffuse fibrosis. The blockage prevents essential pancreatic enzymes from reaching the duodenum, which causes marked impairment in the digestion and absorption of nutrients, especially fats and proteins. The disturbed absorption is reflected in bulky stools that are frothy from undigested fat (steatorrhea) and foul smelling from putrefied protein (azotorrhea).

The incidence of diabetes mellitus (cystic fibrosis–related diabetes [CFRD]) is greater in children with CF than in the general population, which may be caused by changes in pancreatic architecture and diminished blood supply over time. CFRD is reported to be the most common complication associated with CF. Approximately 40% to 50% of people with CF will develop diabetes by age 30 years, which is associated with increased morbidity and mortality.

However, as age increases the likelihood of developing CFRD and survival improves, the proportion of CF adults with CFRD may exceed the current 40% to 50% estimate (Kayani, Mohammed, & Mohiaddin, 2018). Severe insulin deficiency occurs as a result of β-islet cell dysfunction, and insulin resistance may occur, especially during acute illness. Therefore CFRD has characteristics of both type 1 diabetes mellitus and type 2 diabetes mellitus. Adequate insulin appears to be a key factor in maintaining nutritional status that correlates with optimal lung function. Adult studies have shown that

[b]1235 South Clark Street, Suite 305, Arlington, VA 22202; 800-7-ASTHMA; http://www.aafa.org.
[c]55 W. Wacker Drive, Suite 1150, Chicago, IL 60601; 1-800-586-4872; http://www.lungusa.org.
[d]NHLBI Health Information Center, Building 31, 31 Center Drive, Bethesda, MD 20892; 301-496-5449; http://www.nhlbi.nih.gov.
[e]555 E. Wells St., Suite 1100, Milwaukee, WI 53202; 414-272-6071; http://aaaai.org.

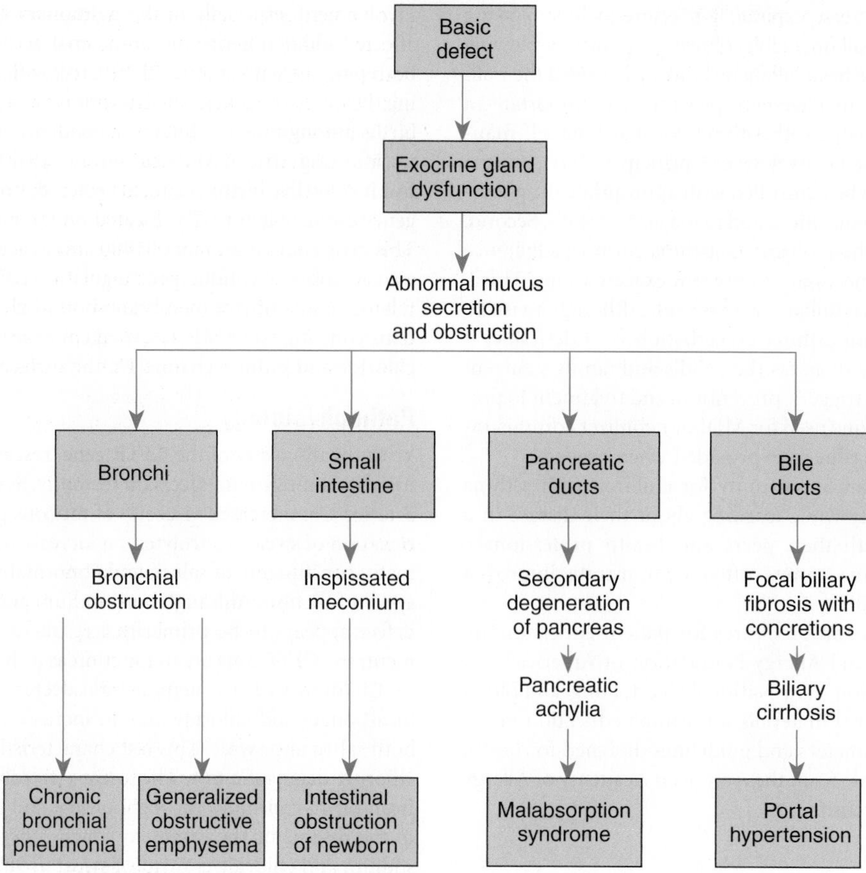

Fig. 21.10 Various effects of exocrine gland dysfunction in cystic fibrosis (CF).

reduced insulin (a potent anabolic hormone) contributes to a shift toward an inflammatory catabolic state, potentially compromising lung function (Kayani et al., 2018).

In the liver, focal biliary obstruction (e.g., cholelithiasis) and fibrosis are common and become more extensive with time, eventually giving rise to a distinctive type of multilobular biliary cirrhosis. Some children develop extensive liver involvement with fatty infiltration despite adequate nutrition.

Pulmonary complications are present in almost all children with CF, but the onset and extent of involvement are variable. Symptoms are produced by stagnation of mucus in the airways, with eventual bacterial colonization leading to destruction of lung tissue. The abnormally viscous and tenacious secretions are difficult to expectorate and gradually obstruct the bronchi and bronchioles, causing scattered areas of bronchiectasis, atelectasis, and hyperinflation. The stagnant mucus also offers a favorable environment for bacterial growth. Recurrent pulmonary infections in the child with CF result in greater and progressive damage to the airways. In severe, progressive lung involvement, compression of pulmonary blood vessels and progressive lung dysfunction frequently lead to pulmonary hypertension, cor pulmonale, respiratory failure, and death.

The most common pathogens responsible for pulmonary infections are *P. aeruginosa, Burkholderia cepacia,* methicillin-resistant *Staphylococcus aureus* (MRSA), *Burkholderia dolosa, S. aureus, H. influenzae, Escherichia coli,* and *Kiebsiella pneumoniae. P. aeruginosa* and *B. cepacia* are particularly pathogenic for children with CF, and infections with these organisms are difficult to eradicate. *P. aeruginosa* infection is not specific for CF but occurs much more frequently in CF than in other diseases characterized by chronic airway obstruction. Methicillin-sensitive *S. aureus* is the most common organism to colonize the respiratory tract and is likely to occur with coinfection of *P. aeruginosa, Aspergillus fumigatus,* or *H. influenzae* (Sobin, Kawai, Irace, et al., 2017). Children with CF who are chronically colonized with these organisms have poorer survival rates than children who are not colonized. Fungal colonization with *Candida* or *Aspergillus* organisms in the respiratory tract is also common in patients with CF.

The reproductive systems of both males and females with CF are adversely affected with CF. The glands of the uterine cervix are often filled with mucus, and copious amounts of mucus may block the cervical canal and prevent sperm entry. More than 95% of males with CF are sterile due to obliteration or atresia of the epididymis, vas deferens, and seminal vesicles, resulting in decreased or absent sperm production (Egan et al., 2020).

Growth and development are often affected in children with moderate to severe forms of CF. Physical growth may be restricted as a result of decreased absorption of nutrients, including vitamins and fat; increased oxygen demands for pulmonary function; and delayed bone growth. The usual pattern is one of growth failure (failure to thrive) with increased weight loss despite an increased appetite and gradual deterioration of the respiratory system. Clinical manifestations of CF are listed in Box 21.17.

Diagnostic Evaluation

Traditionally, the diagnosis of CF was based on a positive sweat chloride test, absence of pancreatic enzymes, radiography, chronic obstructive pulmonary disease, and family history. The addition of the positive newborn screen plus laboratory confirmation of an abnormality in the CFTR gene or protein makes it possible to diagnose CF in early infancy, so that therapies can be implemented to increase the child's overall survival and quality of life.

BOX 21.17 Clinical Manifestations of Cystic Fibrosis

Meconium Ileus[a]
Abdominal distention
Vomiting
Failure to pass stools
Rapid development of dehydration

Gastrointestinal Manifestations
Large, bulky, loose, frothy, extremely foul-smelling stools
Voracious appetite (early in disease)
Loss of appetite (later in disease)
Weight loss
Marked tissue wasting
Growth failure
Distended abdomen
Thin extremities
Sallow skin
Evidence of deficiency of fat-soluble vitamins A, D, E, and K
Anemia

Pulmonary Manifestations
Initial signs:
- Wheezy respirations
- Dry, nonproductive cough

Eventually:
- Increased dyspnea
- Paroxysmal cough
- Evidence of obstructive emphysema and patchy areas of atelectasis

Progressive involvement:
- Overinflated, barrel-shaped chest
- Cyanosis
- Clubbing of fingers and toes
- Repeated episodes of bronchitis and bronchopneumonia

[a]In about 10% of cases.

Universal newborn screening for CF is available in all 50 states in the United States. The newborn screening test consists of an immunoreactive trypsinogen (IRT) analysis performed on a dried spot of blood, which may be followed by direct analysis of DNA for the presence of the ΔF508 mutation or other mutations on the same dried blood spot. A positive screen indicates persistent hypertrypsinogenemia and does not diagnose CF but identifies infants at risk of CF. Further testing is needed to confirm or rule out CF. Benefits of newborn screening and detection include earlier nutritional intervention and preservation of lung function for identified infants. Perceived disadvantage of newborn screening is parental anxiety associated with a false-positive result. Children who were identified and treated early in infancy with aggressive nutritional support had improved height and weight well into adolescence (Egan et al., 2020). Although the technology is available to conduct carrier screening for the general population, this issue remains controversial, and widespread implementation of carrier screening programs is not recommended. An in-utero diagnosis of CF is also possible based on detection of two CF mutations in the fetus.

The consistent finding of abnormally high sodium and chloride concentrations in the sweat is a unique diagnostic characteristic of CF. Parents may report that their infant tastes "salty" when they kiss him or her. The quantitative sweat chloride test (pilocarpine iontophoresis) remains a diagnostic tool for CF and involves stimulating the production of sweat with a special device (involves stimulation with 3-mA electric current), collecting the sweat on filter paper, and measuring the sweat electrolytes. The quantitative analysis requires a sufficient volume of sweat (>75 mg). Two separate samples are collected to ensure the reliability of the test. Normally, sweat chloride content is less than 40 mEq/L, with a mean of 18 mEq/L. A chloride concentration greater than 60 mEq/L is diagnostic of CF; in infants younger than 3 months, a sweat chloride concentration greater than 40 mEq/L is highly suggestive of CF. In some situations, DNA testing may be substituted for the sweat test. The presence of a mutation known to cause CF on each CFTR gene predicts with a high degree of certainty that the individual has CF; however, multiple CFTR mutations may also be present and detected with DNA assay. More than 2000 mutations have now been identified in the CFTR gene, not all of which result in CF (Cystic Fibrosis Mutation Database, 2011).

Chest radiography reveals characteristic patchy atelectasis and obstructive emphysema. PFTs are sensitive indices of lung function, providing evidence of abnormal small airway function in CF. Radiographs, including contrast enema, are used for diagnosis of meconium ileus.

Other diagnostic tools that may aid in diagnosis include stool fat or enzyme analysis. Stool analysis requires a 72-hour sample with accurate recording of food intake during that time. In some cases, CF may go undiagnosed until the child is older and is seen with clinical manifestations that previously were not acute.

Therapeutic Management

Improved survival among patients with CF during the past 2 decades is attributable largely to antibiotic therapy and improved nutritional and respiratory management. Goals of CF therapy are to prevent or minimize pulmonary complications, ensure adequate nutrition for growth, encourage appropriate physical activity, and promote a reasonable quality of life for the child and the family. A multidisciplinary approach to treatment is needed to accomplish these goals.

Management of Pulmonary Problems

Management of pulmonary problems is directed toward prevention and treatment of pulmonary infection by improving ventilation, removing mucopurulent secretions, and administering antimicrobial agents. Many children develop respiratory symptoms by 3 years old. The large amounts and viscosity of respiratory secretions in children with CF contribute to the likelihood of respiratory tract infections. Recurrent pulmonary infections in children with CF result in greater damage to the airways; small airways are destroyed, causing bronchiectasis.

CPT has been the cornerstone of airway clearance therapy (ACT) in the prevention of pulmonary infection for many years. Several other ACT strategies are now available to assist with removal of secretions, including percussion and postural drainage, positive expiratory therapy (PEP), active cycle of breathing technique, autogenic drainage, oscillatory PEP, high-frequency chest compressions, and exercise. The decision of which technique to use is based on the child and the family. Several techniques may be used, and they are usually adapted over time. It is important to foster adherence to ACTs from a young age. They are usually performed on average twice daily (on rising and in the evening) and more frequently if needed, especially during pulmonary infection. Percussion and postural drainage are especially useful for infants and young children but are often not adequate for older children.

PEP is performed by breathing out with a moderate force through a device. This creates resistance and a positive pressure in the airways, helping keep them open. It allows airflow to get around the mucus and moves it toward the larger airways, where it can be expectorated. Three

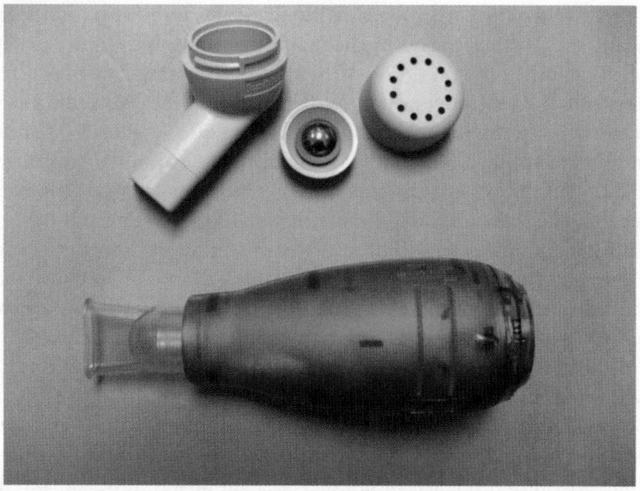

Fig. 21.11 *Top,* Flutter device components showing the pipe stem, cone with steel ball, and perforated top. *Bottom,* The acapella device. (From Marks, J. H. [2007]. Airway clearance devices in cystic fibrosis. *Paediatric Respiratory Reviews, 8*[1], 17–23.)

devices that help accomplish this are PEP valves, flutters, and acapellas. The PEP valve allows air to be inhaled through a one-way valve and blown out through a hole or resistance. The Flutter mucus clearance device is a small handheld plastic pipe with a stainless-steel ball on the inside that facilitates removal of mucus (Fig. 21.11). An acapella provides high-frequency oscillation as well as PEP.

The active cycle of breathing technique is a series of breathing techniques to help clear secretions. Examples include forced expiration, or "huffing," with the glottis partially closed; thoracic expansion exercises; and relaxation and breathing control. Young children can be taught games with breathing that can develop into these techniques as they get older.

Autogenic drainage involves a variety of breathing techniques that the older children can use to force mucus in lower lobes up into the airways so that it can be successfully expelled. Handheld percussors or electronic chest vibrators may be used to loosen secretions but may not be as effective as some of the other techniques described.

High-frequency chest compression (HFCC) is accomplished by use of a mechanical chest device that is worn for periodic treatments during the day. HFCC provides rapid entry and exit of air in the lungs and assists with mucus breakdown and clearance. It is a common ACT used in patients with CF. Nebulization therapies are generally administered during the vest therapy. Some studies have reported more effective mucus clearance with this treatment than with other conventional treatments.

Patients with CF have been found to regress when conventional ACT is discontinued. Although it is time consuming for the child and family, it is an essential part of care.

Physical exercise is an important adjunct to daily ACT. Exercise stimulates mucus excretion and provides a sense of well-being and increased self-esteem. Any aerobic exercise that the patient enjoys should be encouraged. The ultimate aim of exercise is to increase lung vital capacity, remove secretions, increase pulmonary blood flow, and maintain healthy lung tissue for effective ventilation.

Bronchodilator medication delivered in an aerosol opens bronchi for easier expectoration and is administered before or during ACTs when the patient exhibits evidence of reactive airway disease or wheezing. Another aerosolized medication is recombinant human deoxyribonuclease (DNase, known generically as dornase alfa [Pulmozyme]), which decreases the viscosity of mucus. It is well tolerated and has no major adverse effects; minor reactions are voice alterations and laryngitis. This medication, given once or twice daily via nebulization, generally has resulted in improvements in spirometry, PFTs, dyspnea scores, and perceptions of well-being and has reduced the viscosity of sputum (Yang, Chilvers, Montgomery, et al., 2016).

Nebulized hypertonic saline (6% to 7%) has shown some effectiveness in improving airway hydration and increases mucus clearance in patients with CF who are 6 years of age and older; this treatment, however, causes bronchospasm and may not be recommended for patients with severe disease (Goralski & Donaldson, 2014).

Pulmonary infections are treated as soon as they are recognized. In patients with CF, characteristic signs of pulmonary infection—fever, tachypnea, and chest pain—may be absent. Therefore a careful history and physical examination are essential. The presence of anorexia, weight loss, and decreased activity alerts the practitioner to pulmonary infection and the need for an antibiotic regimen. Aerosolized tobramycin is beneficial for patients with frequent pulmonary exacerbations (Egan et al., 2020). This medication is usually administered by jet or ultrasonic nebulizers after ACT is performed. This type of delivery system allows for direct antimicrobial application with little systemic absorption. It is not uncommon for the child with CF to be placed on as many as two or three antibiotics and one antifungal medication to treat coexisting pulmonary infections.

Colonization with *P. aeruginosa* and *B. cepacia* signals progressive involvement. Although the bacteria are impossible to eradicate, they can be successfully controlled. Patients with CF metabolize antibiotics more rapidly than normal; therefore drug dosage is often higher than would be expected. Depending on its sensitivity, *P. aeruginosa* is usually treated with piperacillin-tazobactam, ceftazidime, cefepime, imipenem-cilastin, meropenem or ticarcillin-clavulanate, ciprofloxacin, levofloxacin, tobramycin, or amikacin. Antibiotic treatment of *B. cepacia* and *S. aureus* should be based on susceptibility and synergy testing. The duration of therapy depends on the patient's response, which is measured by clinical indicators, including cough, fatigue, and exercise intolerance, in addition to tests such as PFTs, chest radiography, and oxygen measurements.

IV antibiotics may be administered at home as an alternative to hospitalization. The use of peripherally inserted central catheters (PICCs) for the administration of antibiotics in children with CF is a viable option with limited complications and fewer needle punctures to obtain blood specimens and to maintain often lengthy treatment with parenteral antibiotics. Alternatively, an implanted vascular access device offers the advantage of access for blood draws and antibiotic infusion. Patients may receive antibiotic therapy at home and continue daily activities with minimal disruptions. However, when pulmonary function does not improve with outpatient management, hospitalization may be recommended for continued antibiotic therapy and vigorous ACT. Oxygen administration is used for children with acute episodes but must be used cautiously because many children with CF have chronic carbon dioxide retention, and the unsupervised use of oxygen can be harmful (see Chapter 20, Oxygen Therapy). With repeated infection and inflammation, bronchial cysts and emphysema may develop. These cysts may rupture, resulting in a pneumothorax.

! NURSING ALERT

Signs of a pneumothorax are usually nonspecific and include tachypnea, tachycardia, dyspnea, pallor, and cyanosis. A subtle drop in oxygen saturation (measured by pulse oximetry) may be an early sign of pneumothorax.

Blood streaking of the sputum is usually associated with increased pulmonary infection or advanced lung disease. Hemoptysis greater than 250 ml/24 h for the older child (less for a younger child) indicates a potentially life-threatening event and needs to be treated immediately. Sometimes bleeding can be controlled with bed rest, IV antibiotics, replacement of acute blood loss, IV conjugated estrogens (Premarin) or vasopressin (Pitressin), and correction of any coagulation defects with vitamin K or fresh-frozen plasma. If hemoptysis persists, the site of bleeding should be localized via bronchoscopy and cauterized or embolized.

Nasal polyposis can develop in two-thirds of patients with CF and occur due to chronic inflammation. Treatment of nasal polyps includes intranasal corticosteroids, oral antihistamines, decongestants and sometimes prescribed nasal irrigations. If these measures are ineffective, surgical interventions may be necessary.

Because pulmonary damage in patients with CF is believed to be caused by the inflammatory process that occurs with frequent infections, the use of corticosteroids has been studied. However, treatment with corticosteroids for prolonged periods found only a modest efficacy and numerous side effects, including linear growth restriction, glucose tolerance abnormalities, and cataract formation. Antiinflammatory medications (NSAIDs) have been shown to slow the rate of decline in pulmonary function and to decrease the need for IV antibiotics in young patients with mild pulmonary involvement. Although this therapy is generally well tolerated, careful monitoring for adverse effects (GI bleeding) is essential.

Lung transplantation is a final therapeutic option for many CF patients with severe disease. Heart-lung and double-lung procedures have been performed successfully in children with advanced pulmonary vascular disease and hypoxia; however, whether such procedures significantly improve quality of life and survival rates in children with CF is debated in the current literature. Some experts state that infections such as *B. cepacia,* diabetes, and older age represent a negative factor for long-term survival after transplant (Egan et al., 2020).

Management of Gastrointestinal Problems

The principal treatment for pancreatic insufficiency is replacement of pancreatic enzymes, which are administered with meals and snacks to ensure that digestive enzymes are mixed with food in the duodenum. Enteric-coated products prevent the neutralization of enzymes by gastric acids, thus allowing activation to occur in the alkaline environment of the small bowel. The amount of enzyme depends on the severity of the insufficiency, the child's response to enzyme replacement, and published guidelines. A dosing schedule is based on grams of consumed fat or body weight. Usually one to five capsules are administered with a meal, and fewer are taken with snacks. To avoid overdosing, enzyme replacement should not exceed 2500 units lipase/kg/meal for children older than 12 months of age (Egan et al., 2020). Capsules can be swallowed whole or taken apart and the contents sprinkled on a small amount of food to be taken at the beginning of the meal. The amount of enzyme is adjusted to achieve normal growth and a decrease in the number of stools to one or two per day. Pancreatic enzymes should be taken within 30 minutes of eating. The enteric-coated beads should not be chewed or crushed because destroying the enteric coating can lead to inactivation of the enzymes and excoriation of oral mucosa. The powder form is used with infants and young children but should be used cautiously because inhalation of the powder may precipitate acute bronchospasm. The powder may also start to predigest the food, making it unpalatable. Enzymes are mixed into cereal or fruit such as applesauce for small children or into a small amount of breast milk or formula for infants. Enzyme dosing may need to be adjusted by the provider if abdominal side effects such as flatus, pain, loose stools, bloating, or steatorrhea occur.

Children with CF require a well-balanced, high-protein, high-caloric diet (because of their impaired intestinal absorption). In fact, a group of experts recommend that children and adolescents with CF who are 2 to 20 years of age should have an energy intake of 110% to 200% of standards for healthy persons (Turck, Braegger, Colombo, et al., 2016).

Regular nutritional monitoring should be a standard part of the medical care of the child with CF and should occur every month from birth to 6 months, then every 2 months until 12 months of age. During the second year of life, growth assessments should take place every 2 to 3 months, and between 2 and 18 years of age, they should take place every 3 months (Turck et al., 2016). The weight-for-length goal for growth in the first 2 years of life should be above the 50th percentile on World Health Organization standard growth charts, and in children 2 to 18 years of age a body mass index (BMI) above the 50th percentile should be the goal for growth (Turck et al., 2016). Breastfeeding with enzyme supplementation should be continued for as long as possible and, when necessary, supplemented with a higher-calorie-per-ounce (e.g., 24 kcal/oz) formula to achieve adequate growth. For formula-fed infants, commercial cow's milk–based formulas may be adequate to achieve desired growth. Because the uptake of fat-soluble vitamins is decreased, water-miscible forms of these vitamins (A, D, E, and K) are given along with multivitamins and the enzymes. When high-fat foods are eaten, the child is encouraged to add extra enzymes.

Growth failure despite adequate nutritional support may indicate deterioration of pulmonary status. Patients with CF may experience frequent anorexia as a result of the copious amounts of mucus produced and expectorated, persistent cough, effects of medications, fatigue, and sleep disruption. They may be placed on oral nutritional supplements, nighttime (or continuous) supplemental NG or gastrostomy feedings, or, rarely, parenteral alimentation in an effort to build up nutritional reserves if there has been a history of inability to maintain weight. An enzyme supplement is encouraged with enteric feedings; these may be given at the initiation of the infusion, at bedtime, and at the conclusion of the feeding infusion.

Meconium ileus and meconium ileus equivalent, or total or partial intestinal obstruction, can occur at any age. Constipation is often the result of a combination of malabsorption (either from inadequate pancreatic enzyme dosage or a failure to take the enzymes), decreased intestinal motility, and abnormally viscous intestinal secretions. These problems usually do not require surgical interventions and may be treated with Miralax or Colyte (osmotic solutions given orally or by NG tubes), other laxatives, stool softeners, or rectal administration of diatrizoate meglumine (Gastrografin).

Rectal prolapse occurs in a small number of infants with CF, due to steatorrhea, malnutrition, and repetitive coughing (Egan et al., 2020). The first episode of rectal prolapse is frightening to both the parents and child. Its reduction usually requires immediate intervention, which is managed by simply guiding the rectum back into place with a gloved, lubricated finger with the child in a side-lying position. Further management usually involves attempting to decrease the bulk of daily stools through enzyme replacement.

Children with CF often experience transient or chronic gastroesophageal reflux, which should be treated with the appropriate histamine-receptor antagonist and GI motility drug, dietary modifications, and an upright position after feedings or meals.

Management of Endocrine Problems

The management of CFRD is critical in the therapeutic treatment of the child with CF. CFRD presents a combination of insulin resistance and insulin deficiency, with unstable glucose homeostasis in the presence of acute lung infection and treatment. Children with CF may be at increased risk for glucose management problems as a result of decreased nutrient absorption, anorexia, and severity of pulmonary illness. Diagnosis of CFRD is made using an oral glucose tolerance test. Children with CFRD require close monitoring of blood glucose and administration of insulin, diet and exercise management, and quarterly glycosylated hemoglobin (A1c) measurements. The prevalence of CFRD increases with age, and there is increased morbidity and mortality among children with CFRD compared to those without (Castellani & Assael, 2017). Microvascular complications, such as retinopathy and nephropathy, may occur in children and adolescents with CFRD (O'Riordan, Dattani, & Hindmarsh, 2010). However, ketoacidosis is reported to be rare in individuals with CFRD (Egan et al., 2020).

Children with CFRD on an insulin regimen should perform blood glucose checks three times daily, preferably before meals. With mild CFRD, a single daily dose of long-acting insulin may be sufficient for glycemic control. During illness exacerbations, hyperglycemia may be prevalent.

Bone health is of concern in children and adults with CF. The pancreatic insufficiency of CF and chronic steroid use present potential risks for less than optimum bone growth in such children. Assessment of bone health by history and bone mass density evaluation should be considered in assessing the child's (≤8 years old) health status to detect and prevent osteoporosis and osteopenia.

The administration of recombinant human growth hormone is being used for children with CF who have growth delay to achieve optimum growth. A Cochrane review reported that human growth hormone benefits for children with CF are increased height, weight, and lean tissue mass and improved lung functioning (Thaker, Haagensen, Carter, et al., 2015). However, there is no evidence that it improves clinical status or health-related quality of life.

Prognosis

The median survival age for the patient with CF is 37 years (Egan et al., 2020). Despite considerable progress and a recent surge in new treatment modalities, CF remains a progressive and incurable disease. Lung, heart, pancreas, and liver transplantation have increased survival rates among some CF patients. Heart-lung and double-lung procedures have been successfully performed in children with advanced pulmonary vascular disease and hypoxia. The obstacles surrounding this technique are availability of donated organs; complications from surgery; pulmonary infections; and recurrence of obstructive bronchiolitis, which decreases transplanted lung function.

CFTR modulator therapies are available to patients who have specific mutations in the CFTR gene. The US Food and Drug Administration (2016) approved CFTR pharmacotherapy, namely ivacaftor (Kalydeco), which is available for children ages 2 years and older, and lumacaftor/ivacaftor (Orkambi), which is available for children ages 6 years and older. The medications last 12 hours, so twice-daily dosing is required (Bulloch, Hanna, & Giovane, 2017; Ren, Morgan, Oermann, et al., 2018). These medications regulate the flow of sodium and fluids in cell linings in the affected organs, reducing the likelihood of the development of sticky mucus in organs. Recommendations for the use of CFTR modulators in patients with CF were developed to help CF clinicians, patients, and their families in their decisions on the use of these medications (Ren et al., 2018).

Clinical trials are in progress to examine the effects of inhaled dry powder mannitol for improving mucociliary clearance in CF by rehydrating the airway. Initial reports showed significant improvement in lung function and sputum (De Boeck, Haarman, Hull, et al., 2017).

Current research and modern technologies are exploring methods to attack the genetic defect. For example, a number of clinical trials are underway to examine the feasibility of correcting the underlying genetic defect using gene therapy where patients inhale the CF gene monthly via a nebulizer.

With advances in technology, parents and adolescents are challenged to set future goals that may include college, careers, social relationships, and marriage. Concurrently, they are faced with increasing morbidity and higher rates of CF complications as they grow older.

Nursing Care Management

Assessment of the child with CF involves comprehensive assessment of all affected systems with special focus on the pulmonary and GI systems. Pulmonary assessment is the same as described for asthma, with special attention to lung sounds, observation of cough, and evidence of decreased activity or fatigue. Gastrointestinal assessment primarily involves observing the frequency and nature of the stools and abdominal distention. The nurse should be alert to evidence of growth failure or failure to thrive (e.g., weight loss, muscle wasting, pallor, anorexia, decreased activity [from baseline norm]). Family members are interviewed to determine the child's eating and elimination habits and confirm a history of frequent respiratory tract infections or bowel obstruction in infancy.

The nurse assesses the newborn for feeding and stooling patterns, which may indicate a potential problem, such as meconium ileus. The nurse also participates in diagnostic testing, such as the initial newborn screening, immunoreactive trypsinogen, DNA analysis, or sweat chloride test.

The uncertainty, fear, and initial shock associated with the diagnosis are overwhelming to parents. They must face the impact of the chronic, life-threatening nature of the disease and the prospect of intensive treatment, for which they must assume a major part of the responsibility and for which they may be ill prepared. They often fear that they will be unable to provide the care the child needs. They need careful explanations of the disease, how it might affect their family, and what they can do to provide the best possible care for their child. One of the most difficult aspects of the diagnosis is the implications inherent in its etiology (i.e., the recognition that each parent contributed the gene responsible for the defect).

Hospital Care

Most patients with CF require hospitalization for treatment of pulmonary infection (exacerbation of their pulmonary symptoms), uncontrolled diabetes, or a coexisting medical problem that cannot be treated on an outpatient basis. Patients with CF may require contact isolation for their own protection and should wear a mask in communal areas of the hospital.

When the child with CF is hospitalized for diagnosis or treatment of pulmonary complications, aerosol therapy, chest percussion therapy, and postural drainage are instituted or continued. Respiratory therapists often initiate, supervise, and provide these treatments; however, it is the nurse's responsibility to monitor the patient's tolerance to the procedure and evaluate the effectiveness of the procedure in relation to treatment goals. The nurse may at times administer aerosol therapy, perform chest percussion and postural drainage, assist with ACTs such as the mechanical vest, and teach breathing exercises. Planning ACT so that it does not coincide with meals is difficult in the hospital setting but is essential for the effectiveness of this treatment.

Nursing assessments, including observation of respiratory pattern, work of breathing, and lung auscultation, are vital. Noninvasive pulse oximetry provides valuable data about the patient's oxygenation status.

Supplemental oxygen therapy is administered to the child with mild or moderate respiratory distress.

One of the nursing challenges in the care of the child with CF is encouraging compliance with the therapeutic regimen, which often involves taking a significant number of medications, including pancreatic enzymes; vitamins A, D, E, and K; oral antifungals for *Candida* infection; antihistamines; antiinflammatory agents; and oral antibiotics. This may be overwhelming to the child. Factor in multiple inhaled bronchodilators, ACT and aerosol treatments, potential blood glucose monitoring and insulin administration, various other medications, and increased mucus production during the acute phase, and it is common for the child with CF to rebel and be uncooperative with the prescribed regimen. Gentle coaxing, positive reinforcement, and frank negotiation may be required to enlist cooperation for effective therapy compliance.

The diet for the child with CF represents another challenge; careful planning using a pediatric dietitian with the family and child's input may help decrease the loss of appetite and weight loss that are often part of the condition. With infection and increased lung involvement, the child's appetite tends to diminish, and eventually it can become a challenge to provide appropriate nutrition due to failing appetites. Age-appropriate nutrition education with specific nutritional goals for patients with CF may increase compliance with prescribed enzyme therapy and nutritional supplements.

When dietary intake fails to meet the child's needs for growth, enteral feedings or supplements may be considered. These feedings may be administered via an enteric tube during the night to minimize the disruption of daily activities, including school. A low-profile gastrostomy tube affords the child few activity restrictions and minimum disruption of body image in comparison to an NG tube or conventional gastrostomy tube. The child and parents are encouraged to perceive this therapy not as a last-ditch effort but as an adjunct therapy to maintain optimum growth and prevent excessive weight loss. In some cases, the nurse shows adolescents how to insert a NG tube for nighttime supplemental feedings; the tube may then be removed in the morning.

The child needs support during the many treatments and tests that are a part of the hospitalization. Vascular access (e.g., blood test, IV fluids and medications) are almost always a part of the acute care treatment, and the child soon associates hospitalization with these stress-provoking procedures. Depression, anxiety, and disturbed self-image may occur in children and adolescents with CF. Older adolescents and young adults are especially prone to depression due to the realization of the poor prognosis and unmet life expectations and goals.

Providing support to both the child and the family is essential. The progressive nature of the disease makes each illness requiring hospitalization a potentially life-threatening event. Skilled nursing care and sympathetic attention to the emotional needs of the child and family help them cope with the stresses associated with repeated respiratory tract infections and hospitalizations.

Home Care

Most children and adolescents with CF can be managed at home. The goals of care include normalization of daily activities, including school and peer involvement. The care plan should be flexible so that family activities are disrupted as little as possible. Parents may initially require assistance in finding and contacting durable medical equipment companies that will provide home care equipment. They also need opportunities to learn how to use the equipment and to solve problems they may encounter while delivering therapy at home (see Chapter 19).

Patients and family members need education about the preferred diet of nutritious meals with tolerated fat, increased protein and carbohydrate, and the administration of pancreatic enzymes and nutritional supplements. It is important to stress to parents that the enzymes, in the amount regulated to the child's needs, should be administered at the beginning of all meals and snacks. For enteral feeds administered overnight, enzymes are generally administered at the start and finish of the feeds.

One of the most important aspects of educating parents for home care is teaching ACTs. The success of a therapy program depends on conscientious performance of these treatments regularly as prescribed. The number of times these therapies are performed each day is determined on an individual basis, and often parents readily learn to adjust the number and intensity of the treatments to the child's needs. For pulmonary infection, home IV antibiotics may be prescribed. Home IV care may be preferred for willing and competent families; however, this option depends on a number of factors, including availability of an agency with adequate staff to perform multiple home antibiotic infusions, willingness of the family to assist with infusions, and adherence to therapy at home. With use of venous access devices such as PICC lines or vascular access devices, the parents and child learn the correct technique of direct administration into the IV line. Families also need information about medications and possible side effects.

The child diagnosed with CFRD should be educated on self–blood glucose monitoring, insulin therapy, diet control, and possible related complications. Follow-up with a pediatric endocrinologist is recommended.

Children and adolescents with CF should receive routine primary care with special attention to diet, growth and development, and immunizations. Primary care providers should be alert to any weight loss or flattening in the growth curve associated with loss of appetite, which could indicate a pulmonary exacerbation in children with CF. Anticipatory guidance concerning issues of discipline, how to incorporate aspects of the treatment regimen into the school environment, and delayed pubertal development is also an important consideration for the primary care provider. Home palliative care for the child or adolescent with CF who is in the terminal stages may be carried out with the assistance of hospice (see Chapter 17).

The nurse can assist the family in contacting resources that provide help to families with affected children. Various special child health services, many local clinics, private agencies, service clubs, and other community groups often offer equipment and medications either free or at reduced rates. The Cystic Fibrosis Foundation[f] has chapters throughout the United States that provide education and services to families and professionals.

Family Support

One of the most challenging aspects of providing care for a child or adolescent with CF is meeting the emotional needs of the child and family. The diagnosis, treatment, and prognosis for CF are often associated with many problems and frustrations. The diagnosis can evoke feelings of guilt and self-recrimination in parents.

The long-range problems for an infant, child, or adolescent with CF are those encountered in any chronic illness (see Chapter 17). Both the child and the family must make many adjustments, the success of which depends on their ability to cope and on the quality and quantity

[f]4550 Montgomery Avenue, Suite 1100N, Bethesda, MD 20814; 301-951-4422 or 800-344-4823; http://www.cff.org. In Canada: Canadian Cystic Fibrosis Foundation, 2323 Yonge St., Suite 800, Toronto, ON M4P 2C9; 800-378-2233 (toll-free in Canada only); http://www.cysticfibrosis.ca.

of support they receive from outside sources. The combined efforts of various health professionals are needed to provide the most comprehensive services to families. It is often the nurse who assesses the home situation, organizes and coordinates these services, and collects the data needed to evaluate the effectiveness of the services.

The persistent need for treatment several times a day places tremendous strain on the family. Children often balk at these treatments, and parents are placed in the position of insisting on adherence. The stress and anxiety related to this routine may produce feelings of resentment in both the child and the family members. When possible, occasional trusted respite care should be available to allow parents to leave the situation for short periods without undue anxiety about the child's welfare.

The affected child or adolescent may become resentful about the disease, its relentless routine of therapy, and the necessary curtailment it places on activities and relationships. The child's activities are interrupted or built around treatments, medications, and diet. This imposes hardships and influences the child's quality of life. The nurse should encourage the child to attend school and join age-appropriate peer groups to live as normally and productively as possible. Sports are often an important part of the child's and adolescent's life; interaction with peers includes valuable life experiences, especially for adolescents. The child or adolescent with CF should be encouraged to participate in sports activities in as much as physical and pulmonary health allows. Exercise is encouraged to increase pulmonary vital capacity, promote muscle development, and enhance cardiovascular function.

The nurse should monitor adolescents with CF for signs of eating disturbances. The need for high calorie consumption along with early satiety and a potential body image disorder leave adolescents vulnerable to eating disorders (Quick, Byrd-Bredbenner, & Neumark-Sztainer, 2013). In addition, depression in CF patients has been associated with worse health outcomes, less adherence, and decreased quality of life (Smith, Georgiopoulos, & Quittner, 2016). As the disease progresses, however, family stress should be expected, and the patient may become angry and noncompliant. It is important for the nurse to recognize the family's changing needs and the grief they may experience as the CF worsens. Families should be made aware of resources for counseling. Patients need to be guided toward activities that enable them to express anger, sorrow, and fear without guilt.

Transition to Adulthood

As life expectancy continues to rise for children and adolescents with CF, issues related to marriage, sexuality, childbearing, and career choice become more pressing. Males must be informed at some point that they will often be unable to produce offspring. It is important that the distinction be made between sterility and impotence. Normal sexual relationships can be expected. Female patients may be able to bear children but should be informed of the possible deleterious effects on the respiratory system created by the burden of pregnancy. Women with CF who become pregnant have an increased incidence of premature labor and delivery and low birth weight in the infant. However, favorable nutritional status and pulmonary function are positively correlated with favorable pregnancy outcomes, therefore adequate nutritional status and pulmonary status should be reinforced during pregnancy. Women with CF also need to know that their children will be carriers of the CF gene; therefore genetic counseling for those planning to have children is essential. Adolescent females may need counseling on the use of oral contraceptives and other contraceptive options.

Adolescents with CF are encouraged to take personal ownership and management of the illness to maximize their life's potential. Many adolescents and young persons with the illness enroll in college or vocational and technical training school and complete degrees either by distance learning or by attending a local school. Young people should set life goals and live normal lives to the extent that their illness allows.

Life as an independent adult should be encouraged for children with CF. From the time that children can take partial responsibility for their own care (e.g., ACT, taking pancreatic enzymes), independence and accountability should be fostered. Although the prognosis for these children has improved, many will need continued support as they cope with the demands of surviving with CF.

Anticipatory grieving and other aspects related to care of a child with a terminal illness are also part of nursing care. It is important to prepare the child and family members for end-of-life decisions and care when appropriate. Families may need information about specific interventions such as hospice (see Chapter 17).

OBSTRUCTIVE SLEEP-DISORDERED BREATHING

Pediatric obstructive sleep-disordered breathing reportedly affects approximately 600,000 children 5 to 19 years old in the United States (Weiss & Owens, 2018). Sleep-disordered breathing problems in this spectrum range from partial obstruction of the upper airway to continuous episodes of complete upper airway obstruction, with the most severe form being obstructive sleep apnea (OSA) (Owens, 2020).

Obstructive sleep apnea is defined by the American Thoracic Society (1996) as a disorder of breathing during sleep with prolonged partial upper airway obstruction and/or complete obstruction that disrupts normal respiration during sleep and normal sleep patterns. Adenotonsillar hypertrophy is a common cause of OSA, but tonsil size does not correlate with the degree of OSA (Owens, 2020). Other causes of OSA include allergies associated with chronic rhinitis or nasal obstruction, craniofacial abnormalities, gastroesophageal reflux, nasal septal deviation, and cleft palate repair (Owens, 2020).

Common OSA symptoms include nightly snoring, breathing pauses, choking or gasping on arousal, disturbed sleep patterns, secondary enuresis, daytime sleepiness, and daytime neurobehavioral problems (Owens, 2020). OSA is to be distinguished from primary snoring, which is snoring without obstructive apnea, or abnormalities in gas exchange. If left untreated, OSA may result in complications such as growth failure, cor pulmonale, hypertension, poor attention span, behavioral problems (impulsiveness, hyperactivity, rebelliousness, and aggression), attention-deficit/hyperactivity disorder, hypertension, cardiac ventricle dysfunction, and death.

The diagnosis of OSA is made by an overnight sleep study (polysomnography), which provides evidence of sleep disturbance, respiratory pauses, and changes in oxygenation. The six-channel polysomnography can be performed in children of all ages with videotaping or audiotaping. Polysomnography can distinguish between OSA and primary snoring (Owens, 2020).

Adenotonsillectomy is a common treatment for OSA in children with adenotonsillar hypertrophy (Owens, 2020). However, evidence indicates that this procedure may not be as successful in children with obesity as previously reported (Boudewyns, Abel, Alexopoulos, et al., 2017).

CPAP and BiPAP (cycles between high and low pressure) may be helpful in older children with OSA whose condition persists after surgical intervention or in children who are not good candidates for surgical intervention. These long-term therapies require frequent assessments to evaluate the required amount of pressure and the overall effectiveness of the intervention.

Nursing care of the child with OSA involves early detection by observation of the infant's or child's sleep patterns, active participation in the diagnostic polysomnography, observation of oxygenation and vital signs, application of CPAP when indicated, and monitoring the patient's response to diagnostic therapy. Counseling families of children with OSA may involve dietary counseling for exercise programs and weight management, use of the CPAP or BiPAP equipment, and direct postoperative care after the surgical intervention of tonsillectomy or adenoidectomy. Some children may resist wearing the CPAP or BiPAP devices. Gentle coaxing, patience, reassurance, and gradually building up the duration of time on the therapies may help the child's adjustment to these devices.

RESPIRATORY EMERGENCY

RESPIRATORY FAILURE

Effective pulmonary gas exchange requires clear airways, normal lungs and chest wall, and adequate pulmonary circulation. Anything that affects these functions or their relationships can compromise respiration. In general, the term respiratory insufficiency is applied to two conditions: when there is increased work of breathing, but gas exchange function remains near normal and when normal blood gas tensions cannot be maintained, and hypoxemia and acidosis develop secondary to carbon dioxide retention.

Respiratory failure is the inability of the respiratory system to maintain adequate gas exchange. This process involves pulmonary dysfunction that generally results in impaired alveolar-capillary gas exchange, which can lead to hypoxemia or hypercapnia. Respiratory arrest is the complete cessation of respiration. Respiratory failure is the most common cause of cardiopulmonary arrest in children.

Apnea is generally defined as cessation of breathing for more than 20 seconds or for a shorter period when associated with hypoxemia or bradycardia (Kline-Tilford, Sorce, Levin, et al., 2013; Krishnan, Raghunandhan, Kumar, et al., 2014). Apnea can be (1) central, in which both airflow and chest wall movement are absent; (2) obstructive, in which airflow is absent but chest wall motion is present; and (3) mixed, in which both central and obstructive components are present.

Respiratory dysfunction may have an abrupt or an insidious onset. Conditions that predispose to respiratory failure are obstructive lung disease (increase resistance to airflow), restrictive lung disease (impaired lung expansion), primary inefficient gas transfer (respiratory control dysfunction or diffusion defect), or a combination of these disorders. Respiratory failure can occur as an emergency or may be preceded by gradual and progressive deterioration of respiratory function. Most clinical manifestations are nonspecific and are affected by variations among individual patients and differences in the severity and duration of inadequate gas exchange.

Recognition of Respiratory Failure

Respiratory failure that occurs as a result of acute obstruction of a major airway or cardiac arrest is sudden and readily apparent. Gradual and more covert development of signs and symptoms is less easily recognized. Evaluation of respiratory adequacy is based on both clinical assessment and laboratory studies.

Unless respiratory arrest occurs suddenly, signs of hypoxemia and hypercapnia are usually subtle in their development, becoming more obvious as respiratory failure progresses. In clinical situations in which impaired ventilation can be anticipated or clinical manifestations indicate impending hypoxemia, serial measurements of blood gases should be obtained and monitored to detect impending respiratory failure, and therapy should be implemented before respiratory acidosis becomes extreme.

BOX 21.18 Clinical Manifestations of Respiratory Failure

Cardinal Signs
- Restlessness
- Tachypnea
- Tachycardia
- Diaphoresis

Early but Less Obvious Signs
- Mood changes, such as euphoria or depression
- Headache
- Altered depth and pattern of respirations
- Hypertension
- Exertional dyspnea
- Anorexia
- Increased cardiac output and renal output
- Central nervous system symptoms (e.g., decreased efficiency, impaired judgment, anxiety, confusion, restlessness, irritability, depressed level of consciousness)
- Nasal flaring
- Retractions
- Expiratory grunt
- Wheezing or prolonged expiration

Signs of More Severe Hypoxia
- Depressed respirations
- Hypotension or hypertension
- Altered vision
- Bradycardia
- Arrhythmias
- Somnolence
- Stupor
- Coma
- Dyspnea
- Cyanosis, peripheral or central

Nursing observation and judgment are vital to the recognition and successful management of respiratory failure. Nurses must be able to assess a situation and initiate appropriate action within moments. Clinical manifestations of respiratory failure are listed in Box 21.18.

Therapeutic Management

The interventions used in the management of respiratory failure are often dramatic, requiring special skills and emergency procedures. If respiratory arrest occurs, the primary objectives are to recognize the situation and immediately initiate resuscitative measures, such as opening the airway and positioning, administering supplemental oxygen and positive pressure ventilation, suctioning if needed, performing cardiopulmonary resuscitation (CPR), and intubating if the child's status continues to deteriorate.

When the situation is not an arrest, the suspicion of respiratory failure is confirmed by assessment, and the severity is defined by capillary or arterial blood gas analysis. Interventions such as opening the airway, administering supplemental oxygen, positioning, stimulation, suctioning, CPAP, BiPAP, or early intubation may avert an arrest. When the severity is established, an attempt is made to determine the underlying cause by thorough evaluation.

The principles of management are to (1) maintain ventilation and maximize oxygen delivery, (2) correct hypoxemia and hypercapnia, (3) treat the underlying cause, (4) minimize extrapulmonary organ failure, (5) apply specific and nonspecific therapy to control oxygen demands, and (6) anticipate complications. Monitoring the patient's condition closely is critical.

Nursing Care Management

Nursing observation and judgment are vital to successful management of respiratory failure. The nurse monitors the child to anticipate respiratory failure, determine a course of action, and assess the patient's response to treatment. Often the child is transferred to a pediatric ICU. The child is kept as comfortable as possible, and observation is geared toward general appearance, responsiveness, pulse oximetry, and vital signs. The child is positioned to allow maximum lung expansion and comfort, such as sitting upright or leaning forward (depending on respiratory status). The nurse closely monitors the child's cardiac and respiratory status by observation and by electronic means.

Children who are in respiratory distress often relax after an airway is established and their respiratory effort is assisted. However, they are anxious and frightened when they are unable to communicate; therefore it is important to effectively manage the child's anxiety. This may be accomplished initially with mild sedation until the child's ventilatory status has improved. Assistive communication devices should be offered as appropriate to age and development (e.g., electronic pads, paper and pen, picture boards).

Parents are often concerned about the life-threatening implications generated by the need for the breathing tube (endotracheal tube or tracheostomy) and the possible long-term residual effects on the brain and on the child's psychologic status. For families whose child has a respiratory arrest, support focuses on keeping the family informed of the child's status and helping them cope with a near-death experience or an actual death (see Chapter 17). Knowing that their child requires CPR is a frightening and often overwhelming experience for parents. Uncertainty about the outcome regarding morbidity and mortality is a primary concern.

Regardless of whether an institution permits parental presence during CPR, nurses must consider the needs, fears, and concerns of family members during this situation. If family presence is not permitted during CPR, nurses should arrange for someone to remain with the family. After the child's recovery or death, the family will continue to need support and thorough medical information regarding life-saving measures, the prognosis if the child survives, and the cause of death if the child dies.

CARDIOPULMONARY RESUSCITATION

Cardiac arrest in children occurs more frequently due to prolonged hypoxemia secondary to inadequate oxygenation, ventilation, and circulation (shock) than due to a cardiac condition. Some causes of cardiac arrest are injuries, suffocation (e.g., FB aspiration), smoke inhalation, anaphylaxis, apparent life-threatening event, or infection. Respiratory arrest is associated with a better survival rate than cardiac arrest. After cardiac arrest occurs, the outcome of resuscitative efforts is poor.

Apnea signals the need for rapid, vigorous action to prevent cardiac arrest. In such situations, nurses must initiate action immediately and notify emergency personnel. In the hospital, emergency equipment must be available and easily accessible in all patient care areas. The status of emergency equipment must be checked at least once daily.

Outside the hospital, the first action in an emergency is to quickly assess the extent of any injury and determine whether the child is unconscious. A child who is struggling to breathe but conscious should be transported immediately to an advanced life support (ALS) facility, with the child maintaining whatever position affords the most comfort. Transportation by an emergency medical service (EMS) is recommended, as the service can institute ALS immediately or en route to a medical facility.

An unconscious child is managed with care to prevent additional trauma if a head or spinal cord injury has been sustained (see Chapter 30, Spinal Cord Injuries).

Resuscitation Procedure

Historically, the sequence for CPR was A-B-C (airway, breathing or ventilation, and chest compressions [or circulation]), but the 2010 American Heart Association guidelines changed this recommended sequence to C-A-B to reduce the amount of time to the initiation of chest compressions (Fig. 21.12). Modifications were also made to the depth of compressions, which should be at least one-third of the anteroposterior diameter of the chest (4 cm in infants and 5 cm in older children). The American Heart Association stipulates that having rescuers stop to detect a pulse is not reliable and wastes time. Instead, rescuers should start CPR if the child is unresponsive and not breathing or not breathing normally or if they failed to detect a pulse within 10 seconds. The "look, listen, and feel for breathing" practice is no longer recommended. In 2015 the American Heart Association implemented a few changes in CPR guidelines. Chest compressions should be at a rate of 100 to 120 per minute and chest compression depth should be at least 2 inches (5 cm) but not more than 2.4 inches (6 cm). Each breath should be delivered at a rate of 1 breath every 6 seconds. The American Heart Association updated the recommendation for lay rescuer or bystander compression-only CPR to include chest compressions with rescue breaths for infants and children in cardiac arrest since most pediatric arrests have an asphyxial basis that necessitates ventilation. However, if bystanders are unwilling or unable to deliver rescue breaths, the recommendation is that rescuers provide chest compressions for infants and children (American Heart Association, 2017). The American Heart Association stipulates that a manual defibrillator is preferred to an automatic external defibrillator (AED) for defibrillation of infants. The AED is used as a part of the treatment of cardiorespiratory arrest in children older than 1 year of age. If a manual defibrillator is not available, an AED equipped with a pediatric dose attenuator is preferred. If neither is available, an AED without a pediatric dose attenuator may be used (American Heart Association, 2015; Travers, Rea, Bobrow, et al., 2010). There is still limited evidence to support the safety of AED use in infants, but it may be safe and effective in this group. Appropriate-size pediatric pads must be used for small children. Health care providers are advised to give children age 1 year and older a defibrillatory shock after providing approximately five cycles of CPR (≈2 minutes of cycles of 30 compressions and 2 ventilations by the lone rescuer), provided the AED is sensitive to pediatric rhythms, the device is capable of delivering a pediatric dose of 2 to 4 joules/kg, and a shockable rhythm (usually ventricular fibrillation) is present. In a hospital situation in which weight-based defibrillation dosing is possible, manual defibrillation is the mode of choice instead of AED. When using an AED, health care providers are advised to give adults and children older than 8 years of age a defibrillatory shock within 5 minutes of collapse outside the hospital and within 3 minutes in the hospital.

If two rescuers are present, one rescuer should begin CPR while the second rescuer activates the EMS system by calling 9-1-1 and obtaining an AED. Pediatric rescuers provide five cycles of basic life support (≈2 minutes) before activating EMS; each cycle consists of 30 chest compressions and 2 ventilations. Because pediatric arrests are most commonly caused by respiratory arrest, maintaining ventilation is key.

Component	RECOMMENDATIONS		
	Adults	Children	Infants
Recognition	Unresponsive (for all ages)		
	No breathing or no normal breathing (i.e., only gasping)	No breathing or only gasping	
	No pulse palpated within 10 seconds for all ages (HCP only)		
CPR sequence*	C-A-B		
Compression rate	100 to 120 per minute		
Compression depth	At least 2 inches (5 cm) but not more than 2.4 inches (6 cm)	At least ⅓ AP diameter About 2 inches (5 cm)	At least ⅓ AP diameter About 1½ inches (4 cm)
Chest wall recoil	Allow complete recoil between compressions HCPs rotate compressors every 2 minutes		
Compression interruptions	Minimize interruptions in chest compressions Attempt to limit interrruptions to <10 seconds		
Airway	Head tilt/chin lift (HCP suspected trauma: jaw thrust)		
Compression-to-ventilation ratio (until advanced airway placed)	30:2 1 or 2 rescuers	30:2 Single rescuer 15:2 2 HCP rescuers	
Ventilations: when rescuer untrained or trained and not proficient	Compressions only		
Ventilations with advanced airway (HCP)	1 breath every 6 seconds (10 breaths/min) Asynchronous with chest compressions About 1 second per breath Visible chest rise		
Defibrillation	Attach and use AED as soon as available. Minimize interruptions in chest compressions before and after shock; resume CPR beginning with compressions immediately after each shock.		

*Excluding the newly born, in whom the etiology of an arrest is nearly always asphyxial.
NOTE: Newborn/neonatal information not included.

Fig. 21.12 Summary of basic life support maneuvers for infants, children, and adults. *AED,* Automatic external defibrillator; *AP,* anterior-posterior; *C-A-B,* chest compressions (or circulation), airway, breathing or ventilation; *CPR,* cardiopulmonary resuscitation; *HCP,* health care provider. (Adapted from American Academy of Pediatrics, Committee on Infectious Diseases, Kimberlin, D. W., Brady, M. T., Jackson, M. A., & Long, S. S. [Eds.]. [2018]. *Red book: 2018 report of the Committee on Infectious Diseases* [31st ed.]. Itaca, IL: American Academy of Pediatrics)

Pulse Check

During an emergent situation, palpating the pulse can be a challenge. The patient should be reassessed for a pulse after every 2 minutes of CPR. The pulse should not be assessed for longer than 10 seconds. The carotid is the most central and accessible artery in children older than 1 year of age, but the femoral pulse may also be used. An infant's short and often fat neck makes the carotid pulse difficult to palpate. Therefore, in an infant, it is preferable to use the brachial pulse, located on the inner side of the upper arm midway between the elbow and the shoulder (Fig. 21.13). Absence of a carotid or brachial pulse is considered sufficient indication to begin external cardiac massage. Lay rescuers are not taught to check the pulse but are taught to look for signs of circulation (e.g., normal breathing, coughing, air movement) in response to rescue breaths.

Chest Compression

External chest compression consists of serial, rhythmic compressions of the chest to maintain circulation to vital organs until the child achieves spontaneous vital signs or ALS can be provided. Chest compressions are always interspersed with ventilation of the lungs; however, laypersons who witness an adult cardiac arrest should perform continuous chest compressions without ventilations (American Heart Association, 2015, 2017; Berg, Hemphill, Abella, et al., 2010). For optimal compressions, it is essential that the child's spine is supported on a firm surface during compressions of the sternum and that sternal pressure is forceful but not traumatic. The child's head is positioned for optimal airway opening using the head tilt/chin lift maneuver if the cervical spine is stable and no neck injuries are present. It is essential to prevent overextension of the head of small infants because this tends to close the flexible trachea.

The placement of the fingers for compression in infants is at a point on the lower sternum just below the intersection of the sternum and an imaginary line drawn between the nipples (Fig. 21.14). Compressions on the child 1 to 8 years old are applied to the lower half of the sternum (Fig. 21.15). Sternal compression to infants is applied with two fingers on the sternum, exerting a firm downward thrust; for children, pressure is applied with the heel of one hand or two hands, depending on the child's size. American Heart Association guidelines include the addition of the

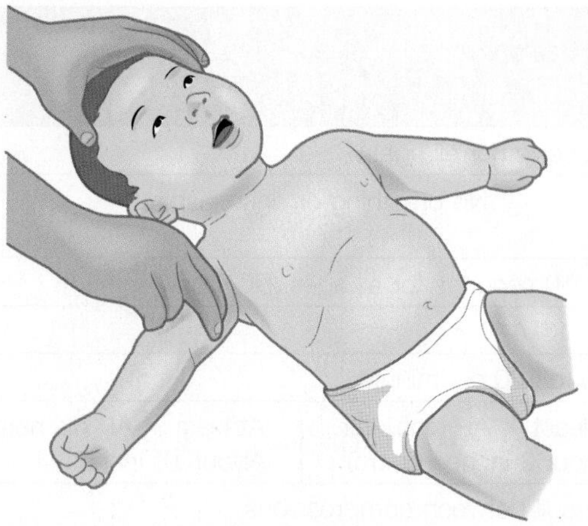

Fig. 21.13 Locating the brachial pulse in an infant. (From Proctor, B. D., Niedzwiecki, B., Pepper, J., Madero, P., & Garrels, M. [2017]. *Kinn's the medical assistant* [13th ed.]. St. Louis, MO: Elsevier.)

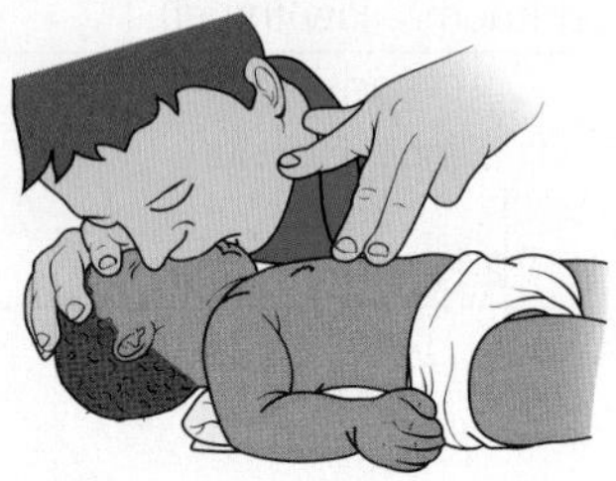

Fig. 21.14 Combining chest compressions with breathing in an infant.

two-thumb-encircling hands technique for chest compressions for infants when two health care providers are present (American Heart Association, 2015, 2017; Travers et al., 2010). In the two-thumb-encircling technique, one of the two rescuers places both thumbs side by side over the lower half of the infant's sternum; the remaining fingers encircle the infant's chest and support the back. The two-thumb-encircling technique is not taught to lay rescuers and is not practical for a health care provider working alone.

Lone-rescuer CPR is continued at the ratio of 2 breaths to 30 compressions for all ages until signs of recovery appear. These signs include palpable peripheral pulses, return of pupils to normal size, the disappearance of mottling and cyanosis, and possibly return of spontaneous respiration. When two rescuers are present, they should deliver 2 breaths to each 15 compressions.

Open the Airway

For effective CPR, the victim is placed on the back on a firm, flat surface using appropriate precautions. With loss of consciousness, the tongue, which is attached to the lower jaw, may relax and fall back, obstructing the airway. To open the airway, the head is positioned with a head tilt/chin lift maneuver (if stable cervical spine) by the lay rescuer. Health professionals should open the airway using either a head tilt/chin lift or a jaw thrust maneuver if an unstable cervical spine is suspected. A head tilt is accomplished by placing one hand on the victim's forehead and applying firm, backward pressure with the palm to tilt back the head. The fingers of the free hand are placed under the bony portion of the lower jaw near the chin to lift and bring the chin forward (chin lift). This supports the jaw and helps tilt the head back (Fig. 21.16).

The jaw thrust is accomplished by grasping the angles of the victim's lower jaw and lifting with both hands, one on each side, displacing the mandible upward and outward. The jaw thrust is recommended only for health care workers. In suspected neck injuries, the jaw thrust method should be used while the cervical spine is completely immobilized. After

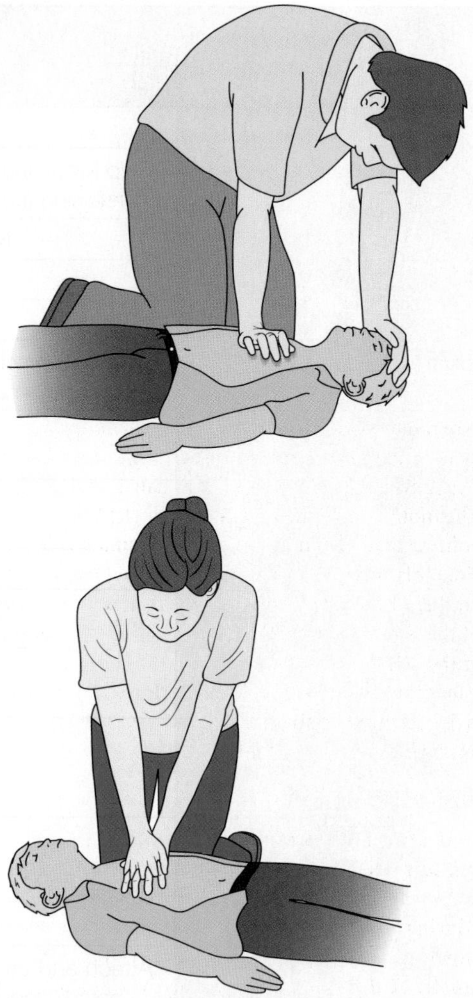

Fig. 21.15 Chest compressions in a child: **(A)** one hand for a smaller child and **(B)** two hands for a larger child.

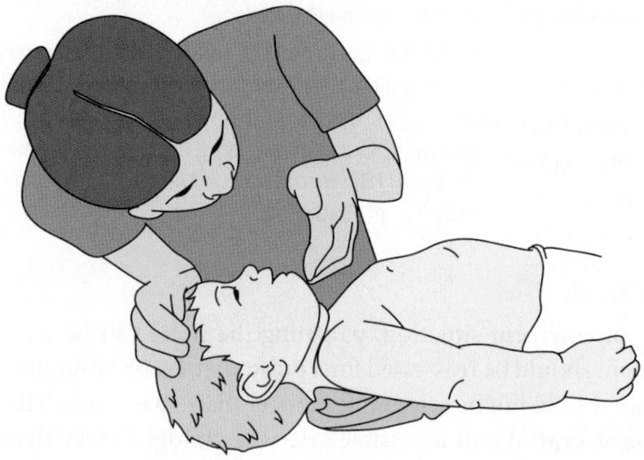

Fig. 21.16 Open the airway using the head tilt/chin lift maneuver, and check breathing.

a patent airway has been restored by removal of foreign material and secretions (if indicated) and if the child is not breathing, maintenance of the airway is continued, and rescue breathing is initiated.

Give Breaths

To ventilate the lungs in the infant (from birth to 1 year old), the bag valve mask (BVM) or operator's mouth is placed in such a way that both the mouth and the nostrils are covered (Fig. 21.17) using the E-C technique. With the BVM, the thumb and index finger of the nondominant

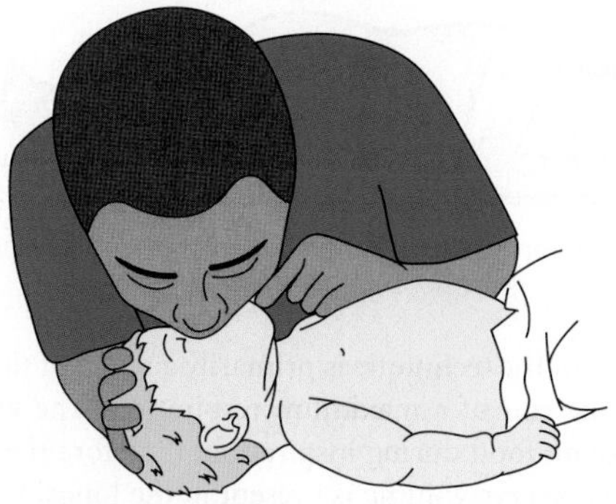

Fig. 21.17 Mouth-to-mouth and nose breathing for an infant.

hand secure the mask on the patient's face (forming a C), while the first three fingers of the same hand are used to lift the jaw (forming an E). If no BVM is available, children (older than 1 year old) are ventilated through the mouth while the nostrils are pinched for airtight contact.

The volume of air in an infant's lungs is small, and the air passages are considerably smaller, with resistance to flow potentially higher than in adults. The rescuer should deliver small puffs of air and assess the rise of the chest to ensure that overinflation does not occur. A gentle rise of the chest is a sufficient indicator of adequate inflation and indicates that the airway is clear. Breaths should be given over 1 second with sufficient volume to make the chest rise. If the chest does not rise, reposition the head or jaw and try again.

Medications

Medications are an important adjunct to CPR, especially with cardiac arrest, and are used during and after resuscitation in children. Medications are used to (1) correct hypoxemia, (2) increase perfusion pressure during chest compression, (3) stimulate spontaneous or more forceful myocardial contraction, (4) accelerate cardiac rate, (5) correct metabolic acidosis, and (6) suppress ventricular ectopy. In 2015 the American Heart Association changed the guidelines to report that bystanders may administer naloxone for suspected life-threatening opioid-associated emergencies.

Appropriate fluid therapy is initiated immediately in the hospital or by EMS personnel during transport (see Chapter 20, Parenteral Fluid Therapy, and Chapter 23, Shock). A complete supply of emergency medications is maintained in all EMS vehicles and on all hospital units. The supply is checked on a regular basis (usually once a day at minimum). When administering drugs during CPR (or a "code"), use a saline flush or other compatible flush solution between medications to prevent drug interactions. Document all drugs, dosages, and the time and route of administration.

AIRWAY OBSTRUCTION

Attempts at clearing the airway should be considered for (1) children in whom aspiration of an FB is witnessed or strongly suspected, and (2) unconscious, nonbreathing children whose airways remain obstructed despite the usual maneuvers to open them. When aspiration is strongly suspected, the child is encouraged to continue coughing for as long as the cough remains forceful. In a conscious choking child, attempt to relieve the obstruction only if:

- The child is unable to make any sounds.
- The cough becomes ineffective.
- There is increasing respiratory difficulty with stridor.

! NURSING ALERT

Blind finger sweeps are avoided in all infants and children.

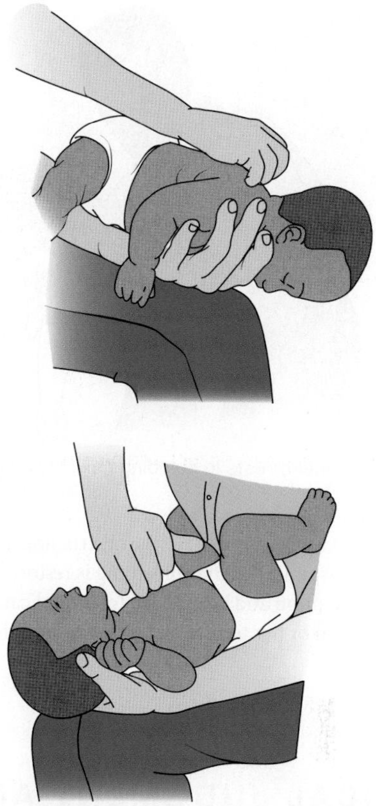

Fig. 21.18 Relief of foreign body (FB) obstruction in infant. A, Back blows. B, Chest thrusts.

Infants

A combination of back blows (over the spine between the shoulder blades) and chest thrusts (on the sternum, the same location as for chest compressions) is recommended to relieve an FB obstruction in infants (Fig. 21.18). A choking infant is placed face down over the rescuer's arm with the head lower than the trunk and the head supported. The rescuer should support the holding arm firmly against the thigh. Up to five quick, sharp back blows are delivered between the infant's shoulder blades with the heel of the rescuer's hand. Less force is required than would be applied to an adult. After delivery of the back blows, the rescuer's free hand is placed flat on the infant's back so that the infant is "sandwiched" between the two hands, making certain that the neck and chin are well supported. While the rescuer maintains support with the infant's head lower than the trunk, the infant is turned and placed supine on the rescuer's thigh, where up to five quick downward chest thrusts are applied in rapid succession in the same location as external chest compressions described for CPR. Back blows and chest thrusts are continued until the object is removed or the infant becomes unconscious. If the infant does lose consciousness, CPR should be initiated.

Children

A series of subdiaphragmatic abdominal thrusts (Heimlich maneuver) is recommended for children older than 1 year of age. The maneuver creates an artificial cough that forces air—and with it, the FB—out of the airway. The procedure is carried out with the child in a standing, sitting, or lying position (Fig. 21.19). In a conscious choking child, upward thrusts are delivered to the upper abdomen with the fisted hand at a point just below the rib cage. To prevent damage to the internal organs, the rescuer's hands should not touch the xiphoid process of the sternum or the lower margins of the ribs. Up to five thrusts are repeated in rapid succession until the FB is expelled.

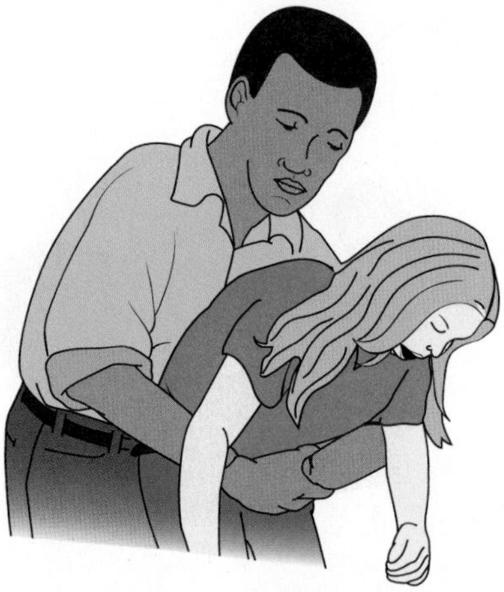

Fig. 21.19 Abdominal thrusts in standing child for relief of foreign body (FB) obstruction.

The child may vomit after relief of the obstruction and should be positioned to prevent aspiration. After breathing is restored, the child should receive medical attention and be assessed for complications. If the child is coughing, allow him or her to relieve the obstruction this way.

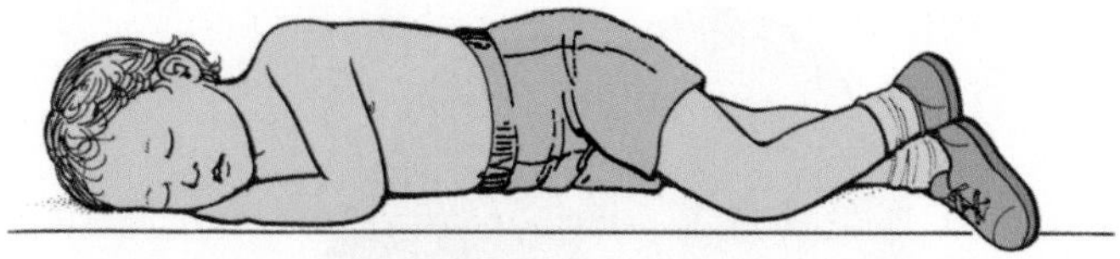

Fig. 21.20 Recovery position for a child after a respiratory emergency.

The success of the technique is primarily a result of the obstruction occurring at the end of a maximum respiration. The victim is most likely to choke on food during inspiration; therefore the tidal volume plus expiratory reserve volume is present in the lungs. When pressure is exerted on the diaphragm by the maneuver, the food bolus is ejected with considerable force by this trapped air.

If the victim is breathing or resumes effective breathing after emergency interventions, place him or her in the recovery position—move the head, shoulders, and torso simultaneously and turn onto the side. The leg not in contact with the ground may be bent and the knee moved forward to stabilize the victim (Fig. 21.20). The victim should not be moved in any way if trauma is suspected and should not be placed in the recovery position if rescue breathing or CPR is required.

CLINICAL JUDGMENT AND NEXT-GENERATION NCLEX® EXAMINATION-STYLE QUESTIONS

1. A 12-year-old boy is in the urgent care clinic with a complaint of fever, headache, and sore throat. The nurse performs a complete history and physical and obtains a throat swab for rapid antigen testing. A diagnosis of group A beta-hemolytic streptococcus (GABHS) pharyngitis is confirmed. The nurse's assessment findings are listed below. **Select the assessment findings that reflect the diagnosis of GABHS. Select all that apply.**
   - **A.** Tonsils are inflamed and covered with exudate
   - **B.** Temperature 100.4° F (38° C)
   - **C.** Headache for the past 2 days
   - **D.** Small, <.5cm cervical lymph nodes
   - **E.** Constipation for the past 3 days
   - **F.** Throat pan increased when swallowing
   - **G.** Abdomen painful to touch

2. A 5-year-old girl is recovering from a tonsillectomy and adenoidectomy and is being discharged home with her mother. She is taking oral fluids but says it still hurts to swallow. She has no fever. The nurse is preparing to discharge the patient. Home care instructions for the mother would include which of the following? **Select all that apply.**
   - **A.** Observe the child for ability to swallow.
   - **B.** Encourage the child to take sips of cool, clear liquids.
   - **C.** Administer codeine elixir as necessary for throat pain.
   - **D.** Administer an analgesic such as acetaminophen for pain.
   - **E.** Observe the child for restlessness or difficulty breathing.
   - **F.** Encourage the child to cough every 4 to 5 hours to prevent pneumonia.

3. A 4-year-old girl is seen in the urgent care clinic with the following history and symptoms: sudden onset of severe sore throat after going to bed, drooling and difficulty swallowing, axillary temperature of 102.2°F (39°C), clear breath sounds, and absence of cough. The child appears anxious and is flushed. Her pulse if 149 beats/min and respirations are 36 breaths/min. **Choose the most likely options for the information missing from the statements below by selecting from the lists of options provided.**

   Based on these symptoms and history, the nurse anticipates a diagnosis of:____1____ hat is most frequently caused by a ____2____ infection. When considering the diagnosis, examination of the throat with a ____3____ is contraindicated without experienced personnel and equipment available for immediate intubation or tracheostomy

Options for 1	Options for 2	Options for 3
Acute Laryngotracheo-bronchitis	Fungal	flashlight
Acute Tracheitis	Protozoic	tongue depressor
Acute Epiglottitis	Bacterial	microscope
Acute Spasmodic Laryngitis	Idiopathic	otoscope light

4. A 2-month-old, formerly healthy infant boy, born at term is seen in the urgent care clinic with intercostal retractions, respiratory rate of 62 breaths/min, heart rate of 128 beats/min, refusal to breastfeed, abundant nasal secretions, and a pulse oximeter reading of 88% in room air. The diagnosis of respiratory syncytial virus (RSV) is made, a bronchodilator is administered, and intravenous (IV) bolus of fluids is given. The infant's oxygen saturation (SpO_2) remains 95% on room air, and the respiratory rate is 54 breaths/min, with intercostal retractions; heart rate is 120 beats/min. After overnight observation the infant is being discharged home. The nurse provides which of the following home care instructions for this infant? **Select all that apply.**

   A. Continue breastfeeding infant.
   B. Keep the infant out of day care or nursery.
   C. Discontinue breastfeeding and administer Pedialyte for 24 hours.
   D. Observe infant for labored breathing or apnea (cessation of breathing).
   E. Instil normal saline drops in both nares and suction before feeding and before placing to sleep.
   F. Place infant to sleep on his side with the head of bed slightly elevated to facilitate breathing.

REFERENCES

Abdallah, C. (2012). Acute epiglottitis: Trends, diagnosis and management. *Saudi Journal of Anesthesia, 6*(3), 279–281.

Abrahams, S. W., & Labbok, M. H. (2011). Breastfeeding and otitis media: A review of recent evidence. *Current Allergy and Asthma Reports, 11*(6), 508–512.

American Academy of Otolaryngology- Head and Neck Surgery. (2011). Clinical practice guideline: Tonsillectomy in children. *Bulletin, 19*, 6.

American Academy of Pediatrics, Committee on Infectious Diseases. (2014). American Academy of Pediatrics Bronchiolitis Guidelines Committee: Updated guidance for palivizumab prophylaxis among infants and young children at increased risk of hospitalization for respiratory syncytial virus infection. *Pediatrics, 134*(2), 415–420.

American Academy of Pediatrics, Committee on Infectious Diseases. (2018). In D. W. Kimberlin, M. T. Brady, M. A. Jackson, & S. S. Long (Eds.), *Red book: 2018 report of the committee on infectious diseases* (31st ed.). Itaca, IL.

American Heart Association. (2015). Web-based integrated guidelines for cardiopulmonary resuscitation and emergency cardiovascular care-Part12: *Pediatric Advance life support*. ECC guidelines.heart.org.

American Heart Association. (2017). Web-based integrated guidelines for cardiopulmonary resuscitation and emergency cardiovascular care-Part11: *Pediatric basic life support and cardiopulmonary resuscitation quality*. ECC guidelines.heart.org.

American Thoracic Society. (1996). Standards and indications for cardiopulmonary sleep studies in children. *American Journal of Respiratory and Critical Care Medicine, 153*(2), 866–878.

Amrock, S. M., Lee, L., & Weitzman, M. (2016). Perceptions of e-cigarettes and noncigarette tobacco products among US youth. *Pediatrics, 138*(5), e20154306.

Antoon, A. Y. (2020). Burn injuries. In R. M. Kliegman, J. W. St. Geme, N. L. Blum, et al. (Eds.), *Nelson textbook of pediatrics* (21st ed.). Philadelphia: Saunders/Elsevier.

ARDS Definition Task Force, Ranieri, V. M., Rubenfeld, G. D., et al. (2012). Acute respiratory distress syndrome: The Berlin definition. *Journal of the American Medical Association, 307*(23), 2526–2533.

Barson, W. J. (2015). *Pneumonia in children: inpatient treatment*. Retrieved from http://www.uptodate.com/contents/pneumonia-in-children-inpatient-treatment.

Baugh, R. F., Archer, S. M., Mitchell, R. B., et al. (2011). Clinical practice guideline: Tonsillectomy in children. *Otolaryngology Head and Neck Surgery, 144*(Suppl. 1), S1–S30.

Bekmezian, A., Fee, C., & Weber, E. (2015). Clinical pathway improves pediatrics asthma management in the emergency department and reduces admissions. *The Journal of Asthma, 52*(8), 806–814.

Belongia, E. A., Karron, R. A., Reingold, A., et al. (2018). The advisory committee on immunization practices recommendation regarding the use of live influenza vaccine: A rejoinder. *Vaccine, 36*(3), 343–344.

Berg, R. A., Hemphill, R., Abella, B. S., et al. (2010). Part 5: Adult basic life support: 2010 American Heart Association guidelines for cardiopulmonary resuscitation and emergency cardiovascular care. *Circulation, 122*(18 Suppl. 3), S685–S705.

Bernard, G. R., Artigas, A., Brigham, K. L., et al. (1994). Report of the American-European consensus conference on ARDS: Definitions, mechanisms, relevant outcomes and clinical trial coordination. The Consensus Committee. *Intensive Care Medicine, 20*(3), 225–232.

Boudewyns, A., Abel, F., Alexopoulos, E., et al. (2017). Adenotonsillectomy to treat obstructive sleep apnea: Is it enough? *Pediatric Pulmonology, 52*(5), 699–709.

Bulloch, M. N., Hanna, C., & Giovane, R. (2017). Lumacaftor/ivacaftor, a novel agent for the treatment of cystic fibrosis patients who are homozygous for the F580del CFTR mutation. *Expert Review of Clinical Pharmacology, 10*(10), 1055–1072.

Burton, M. J., Glasziou, P. P., Chong, L. Y., et al. (2014). Tonsillectomy or adenotonsillectomy versus non-surgical treatment for chronic/recurrent acute tonsillitis. *Cochrane Database of Systematic Review* (11), CD001802.

Canistro, D., Vivarelli, F., Cirillo, S., et al. (2017). E-cigarettes induce toxicological effects that can raise the cancer risk. *Scientific Reports, 7*(1), 2028.

Castellani, C., & Assael, B. M. (2017). Cystic fibrosis: A clinical view. *Cellular and Molecular Life Sciences, 74*(1), 129–140.

Centers for Disease Control and Prevention. (2016). *Clinical signs and symptoms of influenza-Influenza prevention and control recommendations*. Retrieved from https://www.cdc.gov/flu/professionals/acip/clinical.htm.

Centers for Disease Control and Prevention. (2018a). *Key facts about influenza (Flu)*. Retrieved from https://www.cdc.gov/flu/about/keyfacts.htm.

Centers for Disease Control and Prevention. (2018b). *Most recent asthma data*. Retrieved from https://www.cdc.gov/asthma/most_recent_data.htm.

Cherry, J. D. (2016). Pertussis in young infants throughout the world. *Clinical Infectious Diseases, 63*(Suppl. 4), S119–S122.

Clarke, K. E. N. (2017). Can I give my 5-year-old over-the-counter cough medicine? *American Academy of Pediatrics*. Retrieved from https://www.healthychildren.org/English/tips-tools/ask-the-pediatrician/Pages/Can-I-give-my-5-year-old-cough-medicine.aspx.

Chun, L. F., Moazed, F., Calfee, C. S., et al. (2017). Pulmonary toxicity of e-cigarettes. *American Journal of Physiology. Lung Cellular and Molecular Physiology, 313*(2), L193–L206.

Cruz A, Zeichner S. (2020). COVID-19 in children: initial characterization of the pediatric disease. *Pediatrics*. https://doi.org/10.1542/peds.2020-0834.

Cystic Fibrosis Mutation Database. (2011). Retrieved from http://www.genet.sickkids.on.ca/cftr/StatisticsPage.html.

Davies, A. (2015). Management of gastroenteritis in children under five years. *Nursing Standard, 29*(27), 51–57.

De Boeck, K., Haarman, E., Hull, J., et al. (2017). Inhaled dry powder mannitol in children with cystic fibrosis: A randomised efficacy and safety trial. *Journal of Cystic Fibrosis, 16*(3), 380–387.

Drehmer, J. E., Walters, B. H., Nabi-Burza, et al. (2017). Guidance for clinical management of thirdhand smoke exposure in the child health care setting. *Journal of Clinical Outcomes Management, 24*(12), 551–559.

Egan, M., Schecter, M. S., & Voynow, J. A. (2020). Cystic fibrosis. In R. M. Kliegman, J. W. St. Geme, N. L. Blum, et al. (Eds.), *Nelson textbook of pediatrics* (21th ed.). Philadelphia: Saunders/Elsevier.

Falk, N. P., Hughes, S. W., & Rodgers, B. C. (2016). Medications for chronic asthma. *American Family Physician, 94*(6), 454–462.

Fan, E., Brodie, D., & Slutsky, A. (2018). Acute respiratory distress syndrome: Advances in diagnosis and treatment. *Journal of the American Medical Association, 319*(7), 698–710.

Fitzpatrick, A. M., Gillespie, S. E., Mauger, D. T., et al. (2019). Racial disparities in asthma-related health care use in the National Heart, Lung, and

Blood Institute's severe asthma research program. *Journal of Allergy and Clinical Immunology, S0091-6749*(18), 31732–31739.

Friedmann, I., Dahdouh, E. M., Kugler, P., et al. (2017). Maternal and obstetrical predictors of sudden infant death syndrome (SIDS). *The Journal of Maternal-fetal and Neonatal Medicine, 30*(19), 2315–2323.

Goralski, J. L., & Donaldson, S. H. (2014). Hypertonic saline for cystic fibrosis: Worth its salt? *Expert Review of Respiratory Medicine, 8*(3), 267–269.

Griffiths, B., Kew, K. M., & Normansell, R. (2016). Intravenous magnesium sulfate for treating children with acute asthma in the emergency department. *Paediatric Respiratory Reviews, 20*, 45–47.

Harju, M., Keski-Nisula, L., Georgiadis, L., et al. (2016). Parental smoking and cessation during pregnancy and risk of childhood asthma. *BMC Public Health, 16*, 428.

Howard, D., Finn Davis, K., Phillips, E., et al. (2014). Pain management for pediatric tonsillectomy: An integrative review through the perioperative and home experience. *Journal for Specialists in Pediatric Nursing, 19*(1), 5–16.

Ingram, D. G., & Friedman, N. R. (2015). Toward adenotonsillectomy in children: As review for the general pediatrician. *Journal of the American Medical Association pediatrics, 169*(12), 1155–1161.

Jacob, P., III, Benowitz, N. L., Destaillats, et al. (2017). Thirdhand smoke: New evidence, challenges and future directions. *Chemical Research in Toxicology, 30*(1), 270–294.

Jain, S., Williams, D. J., Arnold, S. R., et al. (2015). Community-acquired pneumonia requiring hospitalization among U.S. children. *The New England Journal of Medicine, 372*(9), 835–845.

Kanchongkittiphon, W., Mendell, M. J., Gaffin, J. M., et al. (2015). Indoor environmental exposures and exacerbation of asthma: An update to the 2000 review by the Institute of Medicine. *Environmental Health Perspectives, 123*(1), 6–20.

Kayani, K., Mohammed, R., & Mohiaddin, H. (2018). Cystic-Fibrosis-related diabetes. *Front Endocinol, 9*(20). https://doi.org/10.3389/fendo.2018.00020.

Kerschner, J. E., & Preciado, D. (2020). Otitis media. In R. M. Kliegman, J. W. St. Geme, N. L. Blum, et al. (Eds.), *Nelson textbook of pediatrics* (21st ed.). Philadelphia: Saunders/Elsevier.

Kline-Tilford, A. M., Sorce, L. R., Levin, D. L., et al. (2013). Pulmonary disorders. In M. F. Hazinski (Ed.), *Nursing care of the critically ill child* (3rd ed.). St Louis: Elsevier.

Knudson, C. J., & Varga, S. M. (2015). The relationship between respiratory syncytial virus and asthma. *Veterinary Pathology, 52*(1), 97–106.

Korvel-Hanquist, A., Djurhuus, B. D., & Homoe, P. (2017). The effect of breastfeeding on childhood otitis media. *Current Allergy and Asthma Reports* (7), 45.

Krishnan, P. V., Raghunandhan, S., Kumar, R. S., et al. (2014). A rational approach to the management of obstructive sleep apnea syndrome. *Indian Journal of Otolaryngology and Head and Neck Surgery, 66*(Suppl. 1), 138–146.

Lakupoch, K., Manuyakorn, W., Preutthipan, A., et al. (2018). The effectiveness of newly written asthma action plan in improvement of asthma outcome in children. *Asian Pac J Allergy Immunol, 36*, 88–92.

Liu, A. H., Spahn, J. D., & Sicherer, S. H. (2020). Childhood asthma. In R. M. Kliegman, J. W. St. Geme, N. L. Blum, et al. (Eds.), *Nelson textbook of pediatrics* (21st ed.). Philadelphia: Saunders/Elsevier.

Livingston, M. H., Colozza, S., Vogt, K. N., et al. (2016). Making the transition from video-assisted thoracoscopic surgery to chest tube with fibrinolytics for empyema in children: Any change in outcomes? *Canadian Journal of Surgery, 59*(3), 167–171.

Lonie, S., Baker, P., & Teixeira, R. (2016). Steam vaporizers: A danger for paediatric burns. *Burns: Journal of the International Society for Burn Injuries, 42*(8), 1850–1853.

Lopez-Fernandez, Y., Azagra, A. M., de la Oliva, P., et al. (2012). Pediatric acute lung injury epidemiology and natural history study: Incidence and outcome of the acute respiratory distress syndrome in children. *Critical Care Medicine, 40*(12), 3238–3245.

Lowry, J. A., & Leeder, J. S. (2015). Over-the-counter medications: Update on cough and cold preparations. *Pediatrics in Review, 36*(7), 286–297.

Makadia, L. D., Roper, P. F., Andrews, J. O., et al. (2017). Tobacco use and smoke exposure in children: New trends, harm, and strategies to improve health outcomes. *Current Allergy and Asthma Reports, 17*(8), 55.

Mejias, A., & Ramilo, O. (2015). New options in the treatment of respiratory syncytial virus disease. *The Journal of Infection, 71*(Suppl. 1), S80–S87.

Mitchell, R. B., Archer, S. M., Ishman, S. L., et al. (2019). Clinical practice guideline: Tonsillectomy in children (Update). *Otolaryngology-Head and Neck Surgery, 160*(Suppl. 1), S1–S42.

Mitselou, N., Hedlin, G., & Hederos, C. A. (2016). Spacers versus nebulizers in treatment of acute asthma – a prospective randomized study in preschool children. *The Journal of Asthma, 53*(10), 1059–1062.

Morad, A., Sathe, N. A., Francis, D. O., et al. (2017). Tonsillectomy versus watchful waiting for recurrent throat infection: A systematic review. *Pediatrics, 139*(2), e20163490.

Moualed, D., Masterson, L., Kumar, S., et al. (2016). Water precautions for prevention of infection in children with ventilation tubes (grommets). *Cochrane Database of Systematic Review*, CD010375.

Mussman, G. M., Parker, M. W., Statile, A., et al. (2013). Suctioning and length of stay in infants hospitalized with bronchiolitis. *Journal of the American Medical Association pediatrics, 167*(5), 414–421.

Nagarajan, S., Ahmad, S., Quinn, M., et al. (2018). Allergic sensitization and clinical outcomes in urban children with asthma. 2013-2016. *Allergy and Asthma Proceedings, 39*(4), 281–288.

National Asthma Education and Prevention Program. (2007). *Expert panel report: Guidelines for the diagnosis and management of asthma*. Bethesda, MD: National Heart Lung and Blood Institute, National Institutes of Health. Retrieved from https://www.nhlbi.nih.gov/health-topics/guidelines-for-diagnosis-management-of-asthma.

National Asthma Education and Prevention Program. (2012). *Asthma care quick reference diagnosing and managing asthma*. https://www.nhlbi.nih.gov/health-topics/all-publications-and-resources/asthma-care-quick-reference-diagnosing-and-managing.

National Heart, Lung, & Blood Institute. (2014). What is asthma? . Retrieved from https://www.nhlbi.nih.gov/health/health-topics/topics/asthma/.

Onell, A., Whiteman, A., Nordlund, B., et al. (2017). Allergy testing in children with persistent asthma: Comparison of four diagnostic methods. *Allergy, 72*, 590–597.

O'Riordan, S. M. P., Dattani, M. T., & Hindmarsh, P. C. (2010). Cystic fibrosis–related diabetes in childhood. *Hormone Research in Paediatrics, 73*(1), 15–24.

Owens, J. A. (2020). Sleep medicine. In R. M. Kliegman, J. W. St. Geme, N. L. Blum, et al. (Eds.), *Nelson textbook of pediatrics* (21st ed.). Philadelphia: Saunders/Elsevier.

Pediatric Acute Lung Injury Consensus Conference Group. (2015). Pediatric acute respiratory distress syndrome: Consensus recommendations from the Pediatric Acute Lung Injury Consensus Conference. *Pediatric Critical Care Medicine Journal, 16*(5), 428–439.

Petrocheilou, A., Tanou, K., Kalampouka, E., et al. (2014). Viral croup: Diagnosis and a treatment algorithm. *Pediatric Pulmonology, 49*, 421–429.

Pinfield, J., Gaskin, K., Bentley, J., et al. (2015). Recognition and management of asthma in children and young people. *Nursing Standard, 39*(3), 50–58.

Powell, J., Graham, D., O'Reilly, S., et al. (2016). Acute pulmonary oedema. *Nursing Standard, 39*(23), 51–59.

Quick, V. M., Byrd-Bredbenner, C., & Neumark-Sztainer, D. (2013). Chronic illness and disordered eating: A discussion of the literature. *Advances in Nutrition, 4*(3), 277–286.

Ren, C. L., Morgan, R. L., Oermann, C., et al. (2018). Cystic Fibrosis Foundation pulmonary guideline: Use of cystic fibrosis transmembrane conductance regulator. *Annals of the American Thoracic Society, 15*(3), 271–280.

Rodrigues, K. K., & Roosevelt, G. E. (2020). Acute inflammatory upper airway obstruction. In R. M. Kliegman, B. F. Stanton, J. W. St. Geme, et al. (Eds.), *Nelson textbook of pediatrics* (21st ed.). Philadelphia: Elsevier/Saunders.

Rosenfeld, R. M., Shin, J. J., Schwartz, S. R., et al. (2016). Clinical practice guideline: Otitis media with effusion (Update). *Journal of Otolaryngology and Head and Neck Surgery, 154*(Suppl. 1), S1–S41.

Samet, J. M., Chanson, D., & Wipfli, H. (2015). The challenges of limiting exposure to THS in vulnerable populations. *Current Environmental Health Reports, 2*(3), 215–225.

Santhi, N., Ramsey, D., Phillipson, G., et al. (2107). Efficacy of a topical aromatic rub (Vicks VapoRub) on effects on self-reported and actigraphically assessed aspects of sleep in common cold patients. *Open Journal of Respiratory Diseases, 7,* 83-101.

Schilder, A. G. M., Marom, T., Bhutta, M. F., et al. (2017). Otitis media: Treatment and complictions. *Otolaryngology-Head and Neck Surgery, 156*(4s), S88–S105.

Schuh, S., Sweeney, J., Freedman, S. B., et al. (2016). Magnesium nebulization utilization in management of pediatric asthma (MagNUM PA) trial: Study protocol for a randomized controlled trial. *Trials, 17*(1), 261.

Skaaby, T., Taylor, A. E., Jacobsen, R. K., et al. (2017). Investigating the causal of smoking on hayfever and asthma: A Mendelian randomization meta-analysis in the CARTA Consortium. *Scientific Reports, 7,* 2224.

Smith, B. A., Georgiopoulos, A. M., & Quittner, A. L. (2016). Maintaining mental health and function for the long run in cystic fibrosis. *Pediatric Pulmonology, 51*(S44), S71–S78.

Smith, D. K., Seales, S., & Budzik, C. (2017). Respiratory syncytial virus bronchiolitis in children. *American Family Physician, 95*(2), 94–99.

Sobin, L., Kawai, K., Irace, A. L., et al. (2017). Microbiology of the upper and lower airways in pediatric cystic fibrosis patients. Otolaryngology–Head and Neck Surgery. *Official Journal of American Academy of Otolaryngology-Head and Neck Surgery, 157*(2), 302–308.

Steele, D. W., Adam, G. P., Di, M., et al. (2017). Effectiveness of tympanostomy tubes for otitis media: a meta-analysis. *Pediatrics, 139*(6), e20170125.

Stewart, R. J., Tsang, C. A., Pratt, R. H., Price, S. F., & Langer, A. J. (2018). Tuberculosis — United States, 2017. *MMWR: Morbidity and Mortality Weekly Report, 67,* 317–323.

Thaker, V., Haagensen, A. L., Carter, B., et al. (2015). Recombinant growth hormone therapy for cystic fibrosis in children and young adults. *Cochrane Database of Systematic Review* (5), CD008901.

Thomson, N. C., & Chaudhuri, R. (2012). Omalizumab: Clinical use for the management of asthma. *Clinical medicine insights. Circulatory, Respiratory and Pulmonary Medicine, 6*(1), 27–40.

Travers, A. H., Rea, T. D., Bobrow, B. J., et al. (2010). Part 4: CPR overview: 2010 American Heart Association guidelines for cardiopulmonary resuscitation and emergency cardiovascular care. *Circulation, 122*(Suppl. 3), S676–S684.

Trent, C. A., Zimbro, K. S., & Rutledge, C. M. (2015). Barriers in asthma care for pediatric patients in primary care. *Journal of Pediatric Health Care, 29*(1), 70–79.

Turck, D., Braegger, C. P., Colombo, C., et al. (2016). ESPEN-ESP-GHAN-ECFS guidelines on nutrition care for infant, children, and adults with cystic fibrosis. *Clinical Nutrition: Official Journal of the European Society of Parenteral and Enteral Nutrition, 35*(3), 557–577.

US Food and Drug Administration. (2007). *Genentech adds black box warning to Xolair, US Food and drug administration news drug daily bulletin.* https://www.fdanews.com/articles/ 95475-genentech-adds-black-box-warning-to-xolair.

US Food and Drug Administration. (2016). *Allergenic products advisory committee: Clinical development of allergen immunotherapies for the treatment of Food Allergy.* Retrieved from https://www.fda.gov/media/95961/download.

van Loo, A., van Loo, E., Selvadurai, H., et al. (2014). Intrapleural urokinase versus surgical management of childhood empyema. *Journal of Paediatrics and Child Health, 50*(10), 823–826.

Venekamp, R. P., Damoiseaux, R. A., & Schilder, A. G. (2017). Acute otitis media in children. *American Family Physician, 95*(2), 109–110.

Verma, N., Lodha, R., & Kabra, S. K. (2013). Recent advances in management of bronchoiolitis. *Indian Pediatrics, 50*(10), 939–949.

Walter, H., Sadeque-Igbal, F., Ulysse, R., et al. (2015). The effectiveness of school-based family asthma educational programs on the quality of life and number of asthma exacerbations of children aged five to 18 years diagnosed with asthma: A systematic review protocol. *JBI Databased SystemReviews and Implementation Reports, 13*(10), 69–81.

Weiss, M., & Owens, J. (2018). Recognizing pediatric sleep apnea. *Nurse Pract, 39*(8), 43–49.

World Health Organization. (2018). *Global tuberculosis report 2018. World Health Organization.* https://apps.who.int/iris/handle/10665/274453.

Wong, J. J., Jit, M., Sultana, R., et al. (2017). Mortality in pediatric acute respiratory distress syndrome: A systematic review and meta-analysis. *Journal of Intensive Care Medicine, 34*(7), 563–571.

Woods, B. T., & Mazor, R. (2020). Pulmonary edema. In R. M. Kliegman, J. W. St. Geme, N. L. Blum, et al. (Eds.), *Nelson textbook of pediatrics* (21st ed.). Philadelphia: Saunders/Elsevier.

Yang, C., Chilvers, M., Montgomery, M., et al. (2016). Dornase alfa for cystic fibrosis. *Cochrane Database of Systematic Review* (4), CD001127.

22

The Child With Gastrointestinal Dysfunction

Micah Skeens, Marilyn J. Hockenberry

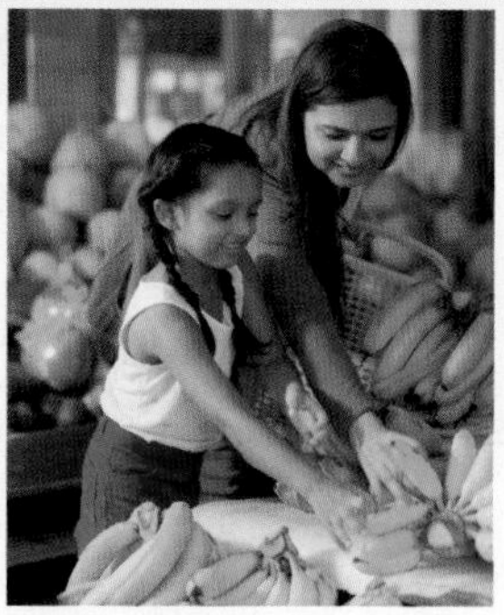

http://evolve.elsevier.com/wong/ncic

CONCEPTS

- Elimination
- Nutrition
- Fluid and Electrolyte Balance
- Inflammation
- Infection
- Tissue Integrity
- Patient Education

DISTRIBUTION OF BODY FLUIDS

The distribution of body fluids, or **total body water (TBW)**, involves the presence of **intracellular fluid (ICF)** and **extracellular fluid (ECF)**. Water is the major constituent of body tissues, and the TBW in an individual ranges from 45% (in late adolescence) to 75% (in term newborn) of total body weight.

The ICF refers to the fluid contained within the cells, whereas the ECF is the fluid outside the cells. The ECF is further broken down into several components: intravascular (contained within the blood vessels), interstitial (surrounding the cell; the location of most ECF), and transcellular (contained within specialized body cavities such as cerebrospinal, synovial, and pleural fluid). In the newborn, about 50% of the body fluid is contained within the ECF, whereas 30% of the toddler's body fluid is contained within the ECF.

Body water is important in body function not only because of its abundance but also because it is the medium in which body solutes are dissolved and all metabolic reactions take place. Because even small alterations in fluid composition affect these metabolic processes, precise regulation of the volume and composition of the fluid is essential. In healthy individuals, body water remains singularly constant, but marked alterations in either its volume or distribution, which occur in many disease states, can produce severely damaging physiologic consequences.

WATER BALANCE

Under normal conditions the amount of water ingested closely approximates the amount of urine excreted in a 24-hour period, and the water in food and from oxidation approximates the amount lost in feces and through evaporation. In this way, the body maintains equilibrium.

Mechanisms of Fluid Movement

Water is retained in the body in a relatively constant amount and, with few exceptions, is freely exchangeable among all body fluid compartments. The proximity of the extravascular compartment to the cells allows for continuous change in volume and distribution of fluids, largely determined by solutes (especially sodium) and physical forces. Transport mechanisms are the basis for all activity within the cells, and because the cells have limited ability to store materials, movement in and out of cells must be rapid. Internal control mechanisms are responsible for distribution and maintenance of fluid balance.

Maintaining Water Balance

Maintenance water requirement is the volume of water needed to replace obligatory fluid loss, such as that from insensible water loss (through the skin and respiratory tract), evaporative water loss, and losses through urine and stool formation. The amount and type of these losses may be altered by disease states such as fever (with increased sweating), diarrhea, gastric suction, and pooling of body fluids in a body space (often referred to as **third spacing**).

Nurses should be alert for altered fluid requirements in various conditions:

Increased requirements:

- Fever (add 12% per rise of 1°C)
- Vomiting, diarrhea
- High-output kidney failure
- Diabetes insipidus
- Diabetic ketoacidosis
- Burns
- Shock
- Tachypnea
- Radiant warmer (preterm infant)
- Phototherapy (infants)
- Postoperative bowel surgery (e.g., gastroschisis)

Decreased requirements:

- Heart failure
- Syndrome of inappropriate antidiuretic hormone
- Mechanical ventilation
- After surgery
- Oliguric renal failure
- Increased intracranial pressure

Basal maintenance calculations for required body water are based on the body's requirements for water in a normometabolic state, at rest; estimated fluid requirements are then increased or decreased from these parameters based on increased or decreased water losses, such as with elevated body temperature or congestive heart failure. Daily maintenance fluid requirements are listed in Table 22.1.

TABLE 22.1 Daily Maintenance Fluid Requirements[a]

Body Weight	Amount of Fluid per Day
1-10 kg	100 ml/kg
11-20 kg	1000 ml plus 50 ml/kg for each kg >10 kg
>20 kg	1500 ml plus 20 ml/kg for each kg >20 kg

[a]Not appropriate for neonatal use.

Maintenance fluids contain both water and electrolytes and can be estimated from the child's age, body weight, degree of activity, and body temperature. Basal metabolic rate (BMR) is derived from standard tables and adjusted for the child's activity, temperature, and disease state. For example, for afebrile patients at rest, the maintenance water requirement is approximately 100 ml for each 100 kcal expended. Children with fluid losses or other alterations require adjustment of these basic needs to accommodate abnormal losses of both water and electrolytes as a result of a disease state. For example, insensible losses increase when basal expenditure increases by fever or hypermetabolic states. Hypometabolic states, such as hypothyroidism and hypothermia, decrease the BMR.

CHANGES IN FLUID VOLUME RELATED TO GROWTH

The percentage of TBW varies among individuals, and in adults and older children it is related primarily to the amount of body fat. Consequently, females, who have more body fat than males, and obese persons tend to have less water content in relation to weight.

The fetus is composed primarily of water, with little tissue substance. As the organism grows and develops, a progressive decrease occurs in TBW, with the fastest rate of decline taking place during fetal life. The changes in water content and distribution that occur with age reflect the changes that take place in the relative amounts of bone, muscle, and fat making up the body. At maturity the percentage of TBW is somewhat higher in the male than in the female and is probably a result of the differences in body composition, particularly fat and muscle content.

Another important aspect of growth change as it corresponds to water distribution is related to the ICF and ECF compartments. In the fetus and prematurely born infant, the largest proportion of body water is contained in the ECF compartment. As growth and development proceed, the proportion within the ECF compartment decreases as the ICF and cell solids increase. The ECF diminishes rapidly from approximately 40% of body weight at birth to less than 30% at 1 year of age. The different effects on males and females become apparent at puberty.

Water Balance in Infants

Because of several characteristics, infants and young children have a greater need for water and are more vulnerable to alterations in fluid and electrolyte balance. Compared with older children and adults, they have a greater fluid intake and output relative to size. Water and electrolyte disturbances occur more frequently and more rapidly, and children adjust less promptly to these alterations.

The fluid compartments in the infant vary significantly from those in the adult, primarily because of an expanded extracellular compartment. The ECF compartment constitutes more than half of the TBW at birth and has a greater relative content of extracellular sodium and chloride. The infant loses a considerable amount of fluid in the first few days after birth and still maintains a larger amount of ECF than the adult until about 2 to 3 years of age. This contributes to greater and more rapid water loss during this age period.

Fluid losses create compartment deficits that reflect the duration of dehydration. In general, approximately 60% of fluid is lost from the ECF, and the remaining 40% comes from the ICF. The amount of fluid lost from the ECF increases with acute illness and decreases with chronic loss.

Fluid losses may be divided into insensible, urinary, and fecal losses and vary with the patient's age. Approximately two-thirds of insensible water loss occurs through the skin, and the remaining one-third is lost through the respiratory tract. Environmental heat and humidity, skin integrity, body temperature, and respiratory rate all influence insensible fluid loss. Infants and children have a much greater tendency to become highly febrile than do adults. Fever increases insensible water loss by approximately 7 ml/kg/24 h for each 1°F rise in temperature above 99°F (37.2°C). Fever and increased surface area relative to volume both contribute to greater insensible fluid losses in young patients.

Body Surface Area

The infant's relatively greater body surface area (BSA) allows larger quantities of fluid to be lost through the skin. It is estimated that the BSA of the premature neonate is five times more, and that of the newborn is two or three times more, than that of the older child or adult. The proportionately longer gastrointestinal (GI) tract in infancy is also a source of relatively greater fluid loss, especially from diarrhea.

Metabolic Rate

The rate of metabolism in infancy is significantly higher than in adulthood because of the larger BSA in relation to the mass of active tissue. Consequently, infants have a greater production of metabolic wastes that the kidneys must excrete. Any condition that increases metabolism causes greater heat production, with its concomitant insensible fluid loss and an increased need for water for excretion. The BMR in infants and children is higher to support cellular and tissue growth.

Kidney Function

The infant's kidneys are functionally immature at birth and are therefore inefficient in excreting waste products of metabolism. Of particular importance for fluid balance is the inability of the infant's kidneys to concentrate or dilute urine, to conserve or excrete sodium, or to acidify urine. Therefore the infant is less able to handle large quantities of solute-free water than is the older child and is more likely to become dehydrated when given concentrated formulas or overhydrated when given excessive free water or dilute formula.

Fluid Requirements

As a result of these characteristics, infants ingest and excrete a greater amount of fluid per kilogram of body weight than do older children. Because electrolytes are excreted with water and the infant has limited ability for conservation, maintenance requirements include both water and electrolytes. The daily exchange of ECF in the infant is much greater than that of older children, which leaves the infant little fluid volume reserve in dehydrated states. Fluid requirements depend on hydration status, size, environmental factors, and underlying disease.

DISTURBANCES OF FLUID AND ELECTROLYTE BALANCE

Disturbances of fluids and their solute concentration are closely interrelated. Alterations in fluid volume affect the electrolyte component, and changes in electrolyte concentration influence fluid movement. Because intracellular water and electrolytes move to and from the ECF compartment, any imbalance in the ICF is reflected by an imbalance in the ECF. Disturbances in the ECF involve either an excess or a deficit of fluid or electrolytes. Of these, fluid loss occurs more frequently.

Sodium is the chief solute in ECF and the primary determinant of ECF volume. It is considered a unique electrolyte in that water balance determines sodium concentration; when water is lost and sodium concentration becomes elevated, compensatory mechanisms in the kidney stop antidiuretic hormone (ADH) secretion so that water is retained. The thirst mechanism (not fully functional in infants) is also stimulated so that water is replaced, thus increasing the total body water content and returning sodium to a normal level (Greenbaum, 2020). Sodium depletion in diarrhea occurs in two ways: out of the body in stool and into the ICF compartment to replace potassium to maintain electrical equilibrium. Potassium is found primarily inside the cell (intracellular), but small amounts are also found in ECF.

Depletion of ECF, usually caused by gastroenteritis, is one of the most common problems encountered in infants and children. Until modern techniques for fluid replacement were perfected, gastroenteritis was one of the chief causes of infant mortality. Fluid and electrolyte problems related to specific diseases and their management are discussed throughout the book where appropriate. The major fluid disturbances, their usual causes, and clinical manifestations are listed in Table 22.2; the most common fluid disturbances, dehydration and edema, are discussed in the following sections. Problems of fluid and electrolyte disturbance always involve both water and electrolytes; therefore replacement includes administration of both, calculated based on ongoing processes and laboratory serum electrolyte values.

In conditions that involve alterations in the amount and composition of body fluid compartments, nurses consider many factors

TABLE 22.2 Disturbances of Select Fluid and Electrolyte Balance

Mechanisms and Situations	Manifestations	Management and Nursing Care
Water Depletion		
Failure to absorb or reabsorb water Complete or sudden cessation of intake or prolonged diminished intake: • Neglect of intake by self or caregiver—confused, psychotic, unconscious, or helpless • Loss from gastrointestinal tract—vomiting, diarrhea, nasogastric suction, fistula Disturbed body fluid chemistry: inappropriate ADH secretion Excessive renal excretion: glycosuria (diabetes) Loss through skin or lungs: • Excessive perspiration or evaporation—febrile states, hyperventilation, increased ambient temperature, increased activity (basal metabolic rate) • Impaired skin integrity—transudate from injuries • Hemorrhage Iatrogenic: • Overzealous use of diuretics • Improper perioperative fluid replacement • Use of radiant warmer or phototherapy	General symptoms dependent to some extent on proportion of electrolytes lost with water Thirst Variable temperature—increased (infection) Dry skin and mucous membranes Poor skin turgor Poor perfusion (decreased pulse, slowed capillary refill time) Weight loss Fatigue Diminished urinary output Irritability and lethargy Tachycardia Tachypnea Altered level of consciousness, disorientation Laboratory findings: • High urine specific gravity • Increased hematocrit • Variable serum electrolytes • Variable urine volume • Increased blood urea nitrogen • Increased serum osmolality	Provide replacement of fluid losses commensurate with volume depletion. Provide maintenance fluids and electrolytes. Determine and correct cause of water depletion. Measure fluid intake and output. Monitor vital signs. Monitor urine specific gravity. Monitor body weight. Monitor serum electrolytes.
Water Excess		
Water intake in excess of output: • Excessive oral intake • Hypotonic fluid overload • Plain water enemas Failure to excrete water in presence of normal intake: • Kidney disease • Congestive heart failure • Malnutrition	Edema: • Generalized • Pulmonary (moist rales or crackles) • Intracutaneous (noted especially in loose areolar tissue) Elevated central venous pressure Hepatomegaly Slow, bounding pulse Weight gain Lethargy Increased spinal fluid pressure Central nervous system manifestations (seizures, coma) Laboratory findings: • Low urine specific gravity • Decreased serum electrolytes • Decreased hematocrit • Variable urine volume	Limit fluid intake. Administer diuretics. Monitor vital signs. Monitor neurologic signs as necessary. Determine and treat cause of water excess. Analyze serum electrolytes frequently. Implement seizure precautions.

TABLE 22.2 Disturbances of Select Fluid and Electrolyte Balance—cont'd

Mechanisms and Situations	Manifestations	Management and Nursing Care
Sodium Depletion (Hyponatremia) Prolonged low-sodium diet Decreased sodium intake Fever Excess sweating Increased water intake without electrolytes Tachypnea (infants) Cystic fibrosis Burns and wounds Vomiting, diarrhea, nasogastric suction, fistulas Adrenal insufficiency Renal disease Diabetic ketoacidosis (DKA) Malnutrition	Associated with water loss: • Same as with water loss—dehydration, weakness, dizziness, nausea, abdominal cramps, apprehension • Mild—apathy, weakness, nausea, weak pulse • Moderate—decreased blood pressure, lethargy Laboratory findings: • Sodium concentration <130 mEq/L (may be normal if volume loss) • Urine specific gravity depends on water deficit or excess	Determine and treat cause of sodium deficit. Administer IV fluids with appropriate saline concentration. Monitor fluid intake and output.
Sodium Excess (Hypernatremia) High salt intake—enteral or IV Renal disease Fever Insufficient breast milk intake in neonate (dehydration hypernatremia) High insensible water loss: • Increased temperature • Increased humidity • Hyperventilation • Diabetes insipidus • Hyperglycemia	Intense thirst Dry, sticky mucous membranes Flushed skin Temperature possibly increased Hoarseness Oliguria Nausea and vomiting Possible progression to disorientation, convulsions, muscle twitching, nuchal rigidity, lethargy at rest, hyperirritability when aroused Laboratory findings: • Serum sodium concentration ≤150 mEq/L • High plasma volume • Alkalosis	Determine and treat cause of sodium excess. Administer IV fluids as prescribed. Measure fluid intake and output. Monitor laboratory data. Monitor neurologic status. Ensure adequate intake of breast milk and provide lactation assistance with new mother-baby pair before hospital discharge.
Potassium Depletion (Hypokalemia) Starvation Clinical conditions associated with poor food intake Malabsorption IV fluid without added potassium Gastrointestinal losses—diarrhea, vomiting, fistulas, nasogastric suction Diuresis Administration of diuretics Administration of corticosteroids Diuretic phase of nephrotic syndrome Healing stage of burns Potassium-losing nephritis Hyperglycemic diuresis (e.g., diabetes mellitus) Familial periodic paralysis IV administration of insulin in DKA Alkalosis	Muscle weakness, cramping, stiffness, paralysis, hyporeflexia Hypotension Cardiac arrhythmias, gallop rhythm Tachycardia or bradycardia Ileus Apathy, drowsiness Irritability Fatigue Laboratory findings: • Decreased serum potassium concentration ≥3.5 mEq/L • Abnormal ECG—notched or flattened T waves, decreased ST segment, premature ventricular contractions	Determine and treat cause of potassium deficit. Monitor vital signs, including ECG. Administer supplemental potassium. Assess for adequate renal output before administration. For IV replacement, administer potassium slowly. Always monitor ECG for IV bolus potassium replacement. For oral intake, offer high-potassium fluids and foods. Evaluate acid-base status.

Continued

TABLE 22.2 Disturbances of Select Fluid and Electrolyte Balance—cont'd

Mechanisms and Situations	Manifestations	Management and Nursing Care
Potassium Excess (Hyperkalemia)		
Renal disease Renal failure Adrenal insufficiency (Addison disease) Associated with metabolic acidosis Too-rapid administration of IV potassium chloride Transfusion with old donor blood Severe dehydration Crushing injuries Burns Hemolysis Dehydration Potassium-sparing diuretics Increased intake of potassium (e.g., salt substitutes)	Muscle weakness, flaccid paralysis Twitching Hyperreflexia Bradycardia Ventricular fibrillation and cardiac arrest Oliguria Apnea—respiratory arrest Laboratory findings: • High serum potassium concentration ≤5.5 mEq/L • Variable urine volume • Flat P wave on ECG, peaked T waves, widened QRS complex, increased PR interval	Determine and treat cause of potassium excess. Monitor vital signs, including ECG. Administer exchange resin, if prescribed. Administer IV fluids as prescribed. Administer IV insulin (if ordered) to facilitate movement of potassium into cells. Monitor potassium levels. Evaluate acid-base status.
Calcium Depletion (Hypocalcemia)		
Inadequate dietary calcium Vitamin D deficiency Rapid transit through gastrointestinal tract Advanced renal insufficiency Administration of diuretics Hypoparathyroidism Alkalosis Calcium trapped in diseased tissues Increased serum protein (albumin) Cow's milk—tetany of the newborn (inappropriate calcium/phosphorus ratio in whole milk for newborn) Exchange transfusion with citrated blood Inadequate parenteral administration in diseased status	Neuromuscular irritability Tingling of nose, ears, fingertips, toes Tetany Laryngospasm Generalized convulsions May be changes in clotting Positive Chvostek and Trousseau signs Hypotension Cardiac arrest Laboratory findings: • Decreased serum calcium concentration (8.8-10.8 mEq/L) or increased serum protein levels • Prolonged QT interval	Determine and treat cause of calcium deficit. Administer oral calcium supplements as prescribed; administer IV slowly and diluted. Monitor IV site; calcium may cause vascular irritation. Monitor serum calcium, vitamin D, and parathyroid levels. Monitor serum protein levels. Avoid cow's milk in infants younger than 12 months.
Calcium Excess (Hypercalcemia)		
Acidosis Prolonged immobilization Conditions associated with increased bone catabolism Hypoproteinemia Kidney disease Hypervitaminosis D Hyperparathyroidism Hyperthyroidism Excessive IV or oral administration	Constipation Weakness, fatigue Nausea, vomiting Anorexia Dry mouth (thirst) Muscle hypotonicity Bradycardia or cardiac arrest Increased calcium concentration in urine, causing formation of kidney stones Laboratory findings: • Increased serum calcium levels or decreased serum protein levels • Prolonged QRS complex or PR interval, shortened QT interval	Determine and treat cause of calcium excess. Monitor serum calcium levels. Monitor ECG.

ADH, Antidiuretic hormone; *ECG,* electrocardiogram; *IV,* intravenous.

when planning management. The following discussion is concerned with the general concepts of two common fluid volume disturbances, dehydration and edema, which are features of a variety of conditions.

DEHYDRATION

Dehydration is a common body fluid disturbance encountered in the nursing care of infants and young children; it occurs whenever the total output of fluid exceeds the total intake, regardless of the underlying cause. Dehydration is also commonly referred to as volume depletion. Although dehydration can result from lack of oral intake (especially in elevated environmental temperatures), more often it is a result of abnormal losses, such as those that occur in vomiting or diarrhea, when oral intake only partially compensates for the abnormal losses. Other significant causes of dehydration are diabetic ketoacidosis and extensive burns.

! NURSING ALERT

In a child with a history of fluid loss and potential or actual dehydration, direct nursing assessment toward the possibility of impending shock.

In early dehydration (during the first 2 days), fluid loss is derived from both the ECF and the ICF because the increased osmolality of the diminished ECF volume causes fluid from the ICF compartment to move into the ECF compartment. As dehydration becomes chronic, the cellular losses become greater.

Types of Dehydration

Because sodium is the primary osmotic force that controls fluid movement between the major fluid compartments, dehydration is often described according to plasma sodium concentrations (e.g., isonatremic, hyponatremic, or hypernatremic). Other osmotic forces, however, such as glucose in diabetic ketoacidosis and protein in nephrotic syndrome, may also play a dominant role. Consequently, dehydration is conventionally classified as isotonic, hypotonic, or hypertonic.

Isotonic (isosmotic or isonatremic) dehydration occurs in conditions in which electrolyte and water deficits are present in approximately balanced proportions. This is the primary form of dehydration occurring in children. The observable fluid losses are not necessarily isotonic, but losses from other avenues make adjustments so that the sum of all losses, or the net loss, is isotonic. Because no osmotic force is present to cause a redistribution of water between the ICF and ECF, the major loss is sustained from the ECF compartment. This significantly reduces the plasma volume and thus the circulating blood volume, with its effect on the skin, muscles, and kidneys. Shock is the greatest threat to life in isotonic dehydration, and the child with isotonic dehydration displays symptoms characteristic of hypovolemic shock. Plasma sodium remains within normal limits, between 130 and 150 mEq/L (Huether, 2019).

Hypotonic (hyposmotic or hyponatremic) dehydration occurs when the electrolyte deficit exceeds the water deficit. Because ICF is more concentrated than ECF in hypotonic dehydration, water transfers from the ECF to the ICF to establish osmotic equilibrium. This movement further increases the ECF volume loss, and shock is a frequent result. Because there is a greater proportional loss of ECF in hypotonic dehydration, the physical signs tend to be more severe with smaller fluid losses than in isotonic or hypertonic dehydration. Plasma sodium concentrations are typically less than 130 mEq/L (Huether, 2019).

Hypertonic (hyperosmotic or hypernatremic) dehydration results from water loss in excess of electrolyte loss and is usually caused by a proportionately larger loss of water or a larger intake of electrolytes. This type of dehydration is the most dangerous and requires much more specific fluid therapy. This sometimes occurs in infants with diarrhea who are given fluids by mouth that contain large amounts of solute or in children receiving high-protein nasogastric (NG) tube feedings that place an excessive solute load on the kidneys. In hypertonic dehydration, fluid shifts from the lesser concentration of the ICF to the ECF. Plasma sodium concentration is greater than 150 mEq/L (Huether, 2019).

Because the ECF volume is proportionately larger, hypertonic dehydration consists of a greater degree of water loss for the same intensity of physical signs. Shock is less apparent in hypotonic dehydration. However, neurologic disturbances, such as seizures, are more likely to occur. Cerebral changes are serious and may result in permanent damage. These include disturbance of consciousness, poor ability to focus attention, lethargy, increased muscle tone with hyperreflexia, and hyperirritability to stimuli (e.g., tactile, auditory, bright lights).

Degree of Dehydration

A determination of the type and degree of dehydration is necessary to develop an effective plan of therapy. The degree of dehydration has been described as a percentage of body weight dehydrated: mild—less than 3% in older children or less than 5% in infants; moderate—5% to 10% in infants and 3% to 6% in older children; and severe—more than 10% in infants and more than 6% in older children (Carson, Mudd, & Madati, 2017; Greenbaum, 2020). Water constitutes only 60% to 70% of the infant's weight. However, adipose tissue contains little water and is highly variable in individual infants and children. A more accurate means of describing dehydration is to reflect acute fluid loss (time frame of ≥48 hours) in milliliters per kilogram of body weight. For example, a loss of 50 ml/kg is considered to be a mild fluid loss, whereas a loss of 100 ml/kg produces severe dehydration.

Weight is the most important determinant of the percent of total body fluid loss in infants and younger children. However, often the pre-illness weight is unknown. Other predictors of fluid loss include a changing level of consciousness (irritability to lethargy), altered response to stimuli, decreased skin elasticity and turgor, prolonged capillary refill (>2 seconds), increased heart rate, and sunken eyes and fontanels.

Clinical signs provide clues to the extent of dehydration (Table 22.3). The earliest detectable sign is usually tachycardia, followed by dry skin and mucous membranes, sunken fontanels, signs of circulatory failure (coolness and mottling of extremities), loss of skin elasticity, and prolonged capillary filling time (see Table 22.4 for clinical manifestations of dehydration). There is evidence that the clinical signs of abnormal capillary refill, abnormal skin turgor, and abnormal respiratory pattern are the most useful in predicting dehydration of 5% or more in children (Carson, Mudd, & Madati, 2017).

Compensatory mechanisms attempt to maintain fluid volume by adjusting to these losses. Interstitial fluid moves into the vascular compartment to maintain the blood volume in response to hemoconcentration and hypovolemia, and vasoconstriction of peripheral arterioles helps maintain pumping pressure. When fluid losses exceed the body's ability to sustain blood volume and blood pressure, circulation is seriously compromised and the blood pressure falls. This results in tissue hypoxia with accumulation of lactic acid, pyruvate, and other acid metabolites, which contribute to the development of metabolic acidosis.

Renal compensation is impaired by reduced blood flow through the kidneys, and little urine is formed. Increased serum osmolality stimulates the secretion of **antidiuretic hormone (ADH)** to conserve fluid and initiates the renin-angiotensin mechanisms in the kidney, causing further vasoconstriction. Aldosterone is released to promote sodium retention and conserve water in the kidneys. If dehydration increases in severity, urine formation is greatly diminished and metabolites and hydrogen ions that are normally excreted by this route are retained.

Shock, a common manifestation of severe depletion of ECF volume, is preceded by tachycardia and signs of poor perfusion and tissue oxygenation (by pulse oximeter readings). Peripheral circulation is poor as a result of reduced blood volume; therefore the skin is cool and mottled with decreased capillary filling. Impaired kidney circulation often leads to **oliguria** and **azotemia**. Although low blood pressure may accompany other symptoms of shock, in infants and young children it is usually a late sign and may herald the onset of cardiovascular collapse (see Congestive Heart Failure in Chapter 23).

TABLE 22.3 Evaluating Extent of Dehydration

	LEVEL OF DEHYDRATION		
Clinical Signs	**Mild**	**Moderate**	**Severe**
Weight loss—infants	3%-5%	6%-9%	≤10%
Weight loss—children	3%-4%	6%-8%	10%
Pulse	Normal	Slightly increased	Very increased
Respiratory rate	Normal	Slight tachypnea (rapid)	Hyperpnea (deep and rapid)
Blood pressure	Normal	Normal to orthostatic (>10 mm Hg change)	Orthostatic to shock
Behavior	Normal	Irritable, more thirsty	Hyperirritable to lethargic
Thirst	Slight	Moderate	Intense
Mucous membranes[a]	Normal (moist)	Dry	Parched
Tears	Present	Decreased	Absent, sunken eyes
Anterior fontanel	Normal	Normal to sunken	Sunken
External jugular vein	Visible when supine	Not visible except with supraclavicular pressure	Not visible even with supraclavicular pressure
Skin[a]	Capillary refill >2 sec	Slowed capillary refill (2-4 sec [decreased turgor])	Very delayed capillary refill (>4 sec) and tenting; skin cool, acrocyanotic or mottled
Urine	Decreased	Oliguria	Oliguria or anuria

[a]These signs are less prominent in patients who have hypernatremia.
Data from Jospe, N., & Forbes, G. (1996). Fluids and electrolytes—Clinical aspects. *Pediatrics in Review, 17*(11), 395–403; and Steiner, M. J., DeWalt, D. A., & Byerly, J. S. (2004). Is this child dehydrated? *Journal of the American Medical Association, 291*(22), 2746–2754.

TABLE 22.4 Clinical Manifestations of Dehydration

Manifestation	Isotonic (Loss of Water and Salt)	Hypotonic (Loss of Salt in Excess of Water)	Hypertonic (Loss of Water in Excess of Salt)
Skin			
• Color	Gray	Gray	Gray
• Temperature	Cold	Cold	Cold or hot
• Turgor	Poor	Very poor	Fair
• Feel	Dry	Clammy	Thickened, doughy
Mucous membranes	Dry	Slightly moist	Parched
Tearing and salivation	Absent	Absent	Absent
Eyeball	Sunken	Sunken	Sunken
Fontanel	Sunken	Sunken	Sunken
Body temperature	Subnormal or elevated	Subnormal or elevated	Subnormal or elevated
Pulse	Rapid	Very rapid	Moderately rapid
Respirations	Rapid	Rapid	Rapid
Behavior	Irritable to lethargic	Lethargic or comatose; convulsions	Marked lethargy with extreme hyperirritability on stimulation

Diagnostic Evaluation

To initiate a therapeutic plan, several factors must be determined:

- The degree of dehydration based on physical assessment
- The type of dehydration based on the pathophysiology of the specific illness responsible for the dehydrated state
- Specific physical signs other than general signs
- Initial plasma sodium concentrations
- Serum bicarbonate concentration
- Any associated electrolyte (especially serum potassium) and acid-base imbalances (as indicated)

Initial and regular, ongoing evaluations assess the patient's progress toward equilibrium and the effectiveness of therapy.

In the examination of an infant or younger child, one of the most important determinants of the extent of dehydration is body weight because this can assist in determining the percentage of total body fluid lost; however, because the pre-illness weight is often unknown, clinical manifestations must be evaluated. Important clinical manifestations include changing sensorium (irritability to lethargy); decreased response to stimuli; integumentary changes (decreased elasticity and turgor); prolonged capillary refill; increased heart rate; sunken eyes; and, in infants, sunken fontanels. Using multiple predictors increases the sensitivity of assessing the fluid deficit, and studies have shown a reasonably high degree of agreement between experienced observers in assessment of the level

BOX 22.1 Model for Rehydration

- For mild to moderate dehydration, rehydration solution should consist of 50 mEq of sodium per liter. In infants who are breastfed, breastfeeding should continue.
- For mild to moderate dehydration, give 50 ml/kg of oral rehydration solution to children.
- For severe dehydration, give 30 ml/h of oral rehydration for infants, 60 ml/h for toddlers, and 90 ml/h for older children. There is a high likelihood for intravenous fluid when children cannot tolerate these oral intake requirements.
- Add 10 ml/kg of fluid for every loose stool or episode of vomiting.
- Reevaluate the need for further rehydration; initiate maintenance therapy using maintenance formulations.
- In children with diarrhea without significant dehydration, the maintenance phase may be initiated without the need for rehydration solution.
- As soon as adequate rehydration has been achieved, start a regular diet along with fluid therapy and wean intravenous fluids.

Modified from Churgay, C. A., & Aftab, A. (2012). Gastroenteritis in children: Part II, prevention and management. *American Family Physician, 85*(11), 1066–1070.

of dehydration. Objective signs of dehydration are present at a fluid deficit of less than 5%.

Therapeutic Management

Medical management is directed at correcting the fluid imbalance and treating the underlying cause. When the child is alert, awake, and not in danger, correction of dehydration may be attempted with oral fluid administration. Most cases of dehydration are mild and can be managed at home by this method. See Box 22.1 for a model for rehydration. Oral rehydration management consists of replacement of fluid loss over 4 to 6 hours, replacement of continuing losses, and provision for maintenance fluid requirements. In general, the mildly dehydrated child may be given 50 ml/kg of **oral rehydration solution (ORS)**, whereas the child with moderate dehydration may be given 100 ml/kg of ORS. The child with fluid losses from diarrhea may be given an additional 10 ml/kg for each stool (Greenbaum, 2020). Amounts and rates are determined from body weight and severity of dehydration and are increased if rehydration is incomplete or if excess losses continue, until the child is well hydrated and the basic problem is under control.

The child may not be thirsty even though dehydrated and may refuse oral fluids initially for fear of continued emesis (if occurring) or because of decreased strength, oral stomatitis, or thrush. In such children rehydration may proceed by administering 2 to 5 ml of ORS by a syringe or small medication cup every 2 to 3 minutes until the child is able to tolerate larger amounts; if the child has emesis, administering small amounts (5 ml) of ORS every 5 minutes or so may help overcome fluid deficit, and the emesis will often lessen over time (Hendrickson, Zaremba, Wey, et al., 2017). Evidence indicates that oral administration of ondansetron (Zofran) to children with acute gastroenteritis and vomiting reduces emesis and increases time to oral rehydration, thus preventing intravenous (IV) therapy (Carter & Fedorowicz, 2012; Hendrickson et al., 2017). Oral rehydration therapy (ORT) is effective for treating mild or moderate dehydration in children, is less expensive, and involves fewer complications than therapy (Carson et al., 2017; Kleinman & Greer, 2014). ORSs enhance and promote the reabsorption of sodium and water. These solutions greatly reduce vomiting and the need for IV infusions (Hendrickson et al., 2017). ORSs, including lower-osmolarity ORS (224 mmol/L), are available in the United States as commercially prepared solutions and are successful in treating the majority of infants with dehydration. See the Quality Patient Outcomes box.

QUALITY PATIENT OUTCOMES: Fluid Volume Deficit

- Moist mucous membranes
- Sodium and potassium within normal limits
- Voiding (>1 ml/kg/h)
- Capillary refill of 2 seconds or less
- Skin turgor brisk
- Fluid intake and output balanced

NURSING TIP: Enhance the flavor of an oral rehydration solution (ORS) such as Pedialyte (unflavored) by adding a teaspoon of unsweetened powder Kool-Aid to each 60 to 90 ml of ORS. Older children may take a small Popsicle orally instead of fluids that require drinking. Many commercially available Popsicles are relatively inexpensive, contain small amounts of sucrose, and contain approximately 40 to 50 ml of fluid. Frozen oral hydration may be accepted by some children when conventional ORS is rejected.

Parenteral Fluid Therapy

Parenteral fluid therapy is initiated whenever the child is unable to ingest sufficient amounts of fluid and electrolytes to meet ongoing daily physiologic losses, replace previous deficits, and replace ongoing abnormal losses. Patients who usually require IV fluids are those with severe dehydration, those with uncontrollable vomiting, those who are unable to drink for any reason (e.g., extreme fatigue, coma), or those with severe gastric distention.

Because dehydration (volume depletion) constitutes a great threat to life, the first priority is the restoration of circulation by rapid expansion of the ECF volume to treat or prevent shock. IV administration of fluid begins immediately, although the exact nature of the dehydration and the serum electrolyte values are not known. The solution selected is based on what is known regarding the probable type and cause of the dehydration. This usually involves an isotonic solution such as 0.9% sodium chloride or lactated Ringer, both of which are close to the body's serum osmolality of 285 to 300 mOsm/kg and do not contain dextrose (which is contraindicated in the early treatment stages of rehydration, but especially in diabetic ketoacidosis).

Parenteral rehydration therapy has three phases. The initial therapy is used to expand ECF volume quickly and to improve circulatory and renal function. During initial therapy, an isotonic electrolyte solution is used at a rate of 20 ml/kg, given as an IV bolus over 5 to 20 minutes, and repeated as necessary after assessment of the child's response to therapy. In a meta-analysis of 10 randomized clinical trials, isotonic fluids were found to be safer than hypotonic fluids in preventing severe hyponatremia following administration (Wang, Xu, & Xiao, 2014). Subsequent therapy is used to replace deficits, meet maintenance water and electrolyte requirements, and catch up with ongoing losses. Water and sodium requirements for the deficit, maintenance, and ongoing losses are calculated at 8-hour intervals, taking into consideration the amount of fluids given with the initial boluses and the amount administered during the first 24-hour period. With improved circulation during this phase, water and electrolyte deficits can be evaluated, and acid-base status can be corrected either directly through the administration of fluids or indirectly through improved renal function. Potassium is withheld until kidney function is restored and assessed and circulation has improved.

The final phase of therapy allows the patient to return to normal and begin oral feedings, with a gradual correction of total body deficits. The potassium loss in ICF is replaced slowly by way of the ECF. The body fat and protein stores are replaced through diet. If the child is unable to eat or if feeding aggravates a chronic condition, IV maintenance fluids are provided.

Although the initial phase of fluid replacement is rapid in both isotonic and hypotonic dehydration, it is contraindicated in hypertonic dehydration because of the risk of water intoxication, especially in the brain cells, specifically the central pontine cells. Central pontine myelinolysis may occur with an overcorrection of fluid deficit and an overly rapid correction of serum sodium concentration (Greenbaum, 2020). There is an apparent lag time for sodium to reach a steady state when diffusing in and out of brain cells, whereas water diffuses almost instantaneously. Consequently, rapid administration of fluid will cause equally rapid diffusion of water into the dehydrated brain cells, causing marked cerebral edema. Because ECF volume is maintained relatively well in hypertonic as opposed to the other types of dehydration, shock is not a usual manifestation.

WATER INTOXICATION

Water intoxication, or water overload, is observed less often than dehydration. However, it is important that nurses and others who care for children be alert to this possibility in certain situations. Children who ingest excessive amounts of electrolyte-free water develop a concurrent decrease in serum sodium accompanied by central nervous system (CNS) symptoms. There is a large urinary output, and because water moves into the brain more rapidly than sodium moves out, the child may also exhibit irritability, somnolence, headache, vomiting, diarrhea, or generalized seizures. The affected child usually appears well hydrated but may be edematous or even dehydrated.

Fluid intoxication can occur during acute IV water overloading, too-rapid dialysis, tap water enemas, feeding of incorrectly mixed infant formula, or excess water ingestion, or with too rapid reduction of glucose levels in diabetic ketoacidosis (Greenbaum, 2020). Patients with CNS infections occasionally retain excessive amounts of water. Administration of inappropriate hypotonic solutions (e.g., 0.45% sodium chloride) may cause a rapid reduction in sodium and result in symptoms of water overload.

Infants are especially vulnerable to fluid overload. Their thirst mechanism is not well developed; therefore they are unable to "turn off" fluid intake appropriately. A decreased glomerular filtration rate does not allow for repeated excretion of a water load, and ADH levels may not be maximally reduced. Consequently, infants are unable to excrete a water overload effectively.

Administration of inappropriately prepared formula is one of the more common causes of water intoxication in infants (Greenbaum, 2020). Families who cannot afford to buy enough formula may dilute the formula to increase the volume or even substitute water for the formula. A family may run out of formula and dilute the remaining amount to make it last until they are able to purchase more. In addition, water is sometimes used for pacification. Water intoxication can also occur in infants who receive overly vigorous hydration during a febrile illness.

A number of clinicians have reported water intoxication in infants after swimming lessons, in water births (Byard & Zuccollo, 2010), with excessive enema administration, and with gastric lavage (Manz, 2007). Although they hold their breath, some infants apparently swallow a large amount of water during repeated submersion. Anticipatory guidance to parents should include a discussion of swimming instruction and advice to stop a lesson if the child swallows unusual amounts of water or exhibits any symptoms of hyponatremia.

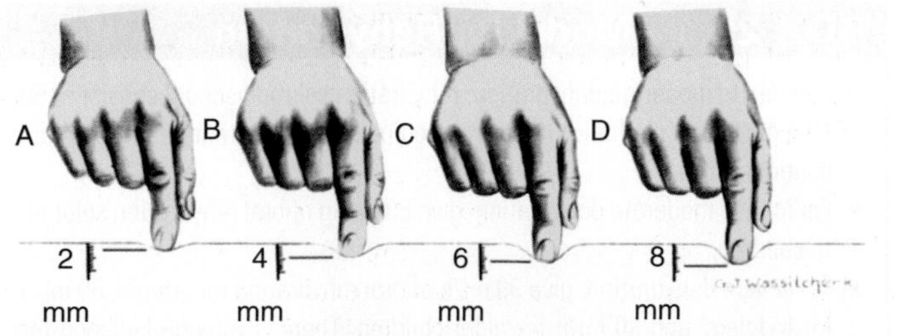

Fig. 22.1 Assessment of pitting edema. **A,** +1; **B,** +2; **C,** +3; **D,** +4.

EDEMA

Edema represents an abnormal accumulation of fluid within the interstitial tissue and subsequent tissue expansion and develops when a defect in the normal cardiovascular circulation or a failure in the lymphatic drainage to remove the increased amounts occurs. The processes responsible for fluid removal include venous hydrostatic pressure, oncotic pressure of intravascular and interstitial spaces, an intact semipermeable capillary wall, tissue tension, and lymphatic flow.

Assessment

Generalized edema resulting from any of the previously listed types is manifested by swelling in the extremities, face, perineum, and torso. Loss of normal skin creases may be assessed. Daily weights are more sensitive indicators of water gain or loss and should be obtained. Abdominal girth measurement changes may also be an indicator of edema in children. Pitting edema may occur and can be assessed by pressing the fingertip against a bony prominence for 5 seconds. If the tissue rebounds immediately on removing the finger, the patient does not have pitting edema. A quick way to determine the severity is to measure the degree of pitting edema (Fig. 22.1).

Therapeutic Management

The primary goal in the management of edema is treatment of the underlying disease process, which is discussed elsewhere in relation to the specific disorder. However, an essential aspect in the management of any fluid overload is early recognition, in which nurses play a vital role. The management of edema is discussed throughout the text with specific conditions. See the Quality Patient Outcomes box.

QUALITY PATIENT OUTCOMES: Fluid Volume Excess

- Fluid intake and output balanced
- No edema
- No weight gain
- No respiratory distress related to fluid volume excess

DISORDERS OF MOTILITY

DIARRHEA

Diarrhea is a symptom that results from disorders involving digestive, absorptive, and secretory functions. Diarrhea is caused by abnormal intestinal water and electrolyte transport. Worldwide, there are an estimated 1.7 billion episodes of diarrhea each year (Leung, Chisti, & Pavia, 2016). The incidence and morbidity of diarrhea are more prominent in low-income countries such as areas of Asia and Africa (Leung et al., 2016) and among children younger than 5 years of age (Leung et al., 2016).

The transport of fluid and electrolytes in the developing GI tract is related to the child's age. The intestinal mucosa of the young infant is more permeable to water than that of an older child. Therefore in young infants with increased intestinal luminal osmolality caused by diarrhea, more fluid and electrolytes are lost than in older children. Diarrhea results from several pathophysiologic processes.

Types of Diarrhea

Diarrheal disturbances involve the stomach and intestines (gastroenteritis), the small intestine (enteritis), the colon (colitis), or the colon and intestines (enterocolitis). Diarrhea is classified as acute or chronic.

Acute diarrhea is defined as a sudden increase in frequency and a change in consistency of stools, often caused by an infectious agent in the GI tract. It may be associated with upper respiratory or urinary tract infections, antibiotic therapy, or laxative use. Acute diarrhea is usually self-limited (14 days' duration) and subsides without specific treatment. Acute infectious diarrhea (infectious gastroenteritis) is caused by a variety of viral, bacterial, and parasitic pathogens (Table 22.5).

Chronic diarrhea is an increase in stool frequency and increased water content with duration of more than 14 days. It is often caused by chronic conditions such as malabsorption syndromes, inflammatory bowel disease (IBD), immunodeficiency, food allergy, lactose intolerance, or chronic nonspecific diarrhea, or as a result of inadequate management of acute diarrhea.

TABLE 22.5 Infectious Causes of Acute Diarrhea

Agents	Pathology	Characteristics	Comments
Viral			
Rotavirus Incubation—48 hours Diagnosis—EIA	Fecal-oral transmission 8 groups (A-H)—Most group A virus replicates in mature villus epithelial cells of small intestine; leads to (1) imbalance in ratio of intestinal fluid absorption to secretion and (2) malabsorption of complex carbohydrates	Mild to moderate fever Vomiting followed by onset of watery stools Fever and vomiting generally abate in approximately 2 days, but diarrhea persists 5-7 days	Most common cause of diarrhea in children <5 years old; infants 6-12 months old most vulnerable; affects all ages; usually milder in children >3 years old Immunocompromised children at greater risk for complications Peak occurrences in winter months Important cause of nosocomial infections
Norovirus Incubation—12-48 hours Diagnosis—PCR assays	Fecal-oral; contaminated water Pathology similar to that of rotavirus; affects villus epithelial cells of small intestine, leading to (1) imbalance in ratio of intestinal fluid absorption to secretion and (2) malabsorption of complex carbohydrates	Abdominal cramps, nausea, vomiting, malaise, low-grade fever, watery diarrhea without blood; duration 2-3 days; tends to resemble so-called food poisoning symptoms with nausea predominating	Affects all ages Multiple strains often named for the location of outbreak (e.g., Norwalk, Sapporo, Snow Mountain, Montgomery)
Bacterial			
Escherichia coli Incubation—3-4 days; variable depending on strain Diagnosis—Sorbitol MacConkey (SMAC) agar positive for blood, but fecal leukocytes absent or rare	*E. coli* strains produce diarrhea as result of enterotoxin production, adherence, or invasion (enterotoxigenic-producing *E. coli*, enterohemorrhagic *E. coli*, enteroaggregative *E. coli*)	Watery diarrhea 1-2 days, then severe abdominal cramping and bloody diarrhea Can progress to hemolytic uremic syndrome	Foodborne pathogen Traveler's diarrhea Cause of nursery epidemics Symptomatic treatment Antibiotics may worsen course Avoid antimotility agents and opioids
***Salmonella* groups** (nontyphoidal) Gram-negative rods, nonencapsulated, nonsporulating Incubation—6-72 hours Diagnosis—Gram stain, stool culture	Invasion of mucosa in the small and large intestine, edema of the lamina propria, focal acute inflammation with disruption of the mucosa and microabscesses	Nausea, vomiting, colicky, abdominal pain, bloody diarrhea, fever; symptoms variable (mild to severe) May have headache and cerebral manifestations (e.g., drowsiness, confusion, meningismus, seizures) Infants may be afebrile and nontoxic May result in life-threatening septicemia and meningitis Nausea and vomiting typically of short duration; diarrhea may persist as long as 2-3 weeks Typically shed virus for average of 5 weeks; cases reported up to 1 year	Incidence highest in summer months; foodborne outbreaks common Usually transmitted person to person but may transmit via undercooked meats or poultry; about half the cases caused by poultry and poultry products In children, related to pets (e.g., dogs, cats, hamsters, turtles) Communicable as long as organisms are excreted Antibiotics not recommended in uncomplicated cases Antimotility agents also not recommended—prolong transit time and carrier state

Continued

TABLE 22.5 Infectious Causes of Acute Diarrhea—cont'd

Agents	Pathology	Characteristics	Comments
Salmonella typhi Produces enteric fever—systemic syndrome Incubation—usually 7-14 days but could be 3-30 days, depending on size of inoculum Diagnosis—positive blood cultures; also sometimes positive stool and urine cultures Late stage—positive bone marrow culture	Bloodstream invasion; after ingestion, organism attaches to microvilli of ileal brush borders, and bacteria invade the intestinal epithelium via Peyer patches Next, organism is transported to intestinal lymph nodes and enters bloodstream via thoracic ducts, and circulating organism reaches reticuloendothelial cells, causing bacteremia	Manifestations dependent on age Abdominal pain, diarrhea, nausea, vomiting, high fever, lethargy Must be treated with antibiotics	Incidence much lower in developed countries; about 400 cases/year in United States; 65% of US cases acquired via international cases Ingestion of foods and water contaminated with human feces is most common mode of transmission Congenital and intrapartum transmission possible Two vaccines available
***Shigella* groups** Gram-negative nonmotile anaerobic bacilli Incubation—1-7 days Diagnosis—stool culture loaded with polymorphonuclear leukocytes	Enterotoxins—invade the epithelium with superficial mucosal ulcerations	Children appear sick Symptoms begin with fever, fatigue, anorexia Crampy abdominal pain preceding watery or bloody diarrhea Symptoms usually subside in 5-10 days	Most cases in children <9 years old, with about one-third of cases in children ages 1-4 weeks old Antibiotics shorten illness and lower mortality All patients at risk for dehydration Acute symptoms may persist for ≤1 week Antidiarrheal medications not recommended because they may predispose patient to toxic megacolon
***Yersinia* enterocolitis** Incubation—dose dependent, 1-3 weeks Diagnosis—stool culture, ELISA Patients have leukocytosis, elevated sedimentation rate	Pathology poorly understood; possibly caused by production of enterotoxin	Mucoid diarrhea, sometimes bloody; abdominal pain suggestive of appendicitis; fever, vomiting	Seen more frequently in the winter months Transmitted by pets and food Antibiotics usually do not alter the clinical course in uncomplicated cases; antibiotics used in complicated infections and compromised hosts
Campylobacter jejuni Microaerophilic, motile, gram-negative bacilli Incubation—1-7 days Ability to cause illness appears dose related Diagnosis—stool culture, sometimes blood culture Commonly found in GI tract of wild or domestic animals	Not fully understood, possibly (1) adherence to intestinal mucosa by toxin, (2) invasion of the mucosa in the terminal ileum and colon, (3) translocation in which the organisms penetrate the mucosa and replicate in the lamina propria	Fever, abdominal pain, diarrhea that can be bloody, vomiting Watery, profuse, foul-smelling diarrhea Clinically similar to infection by *Salmonella* or *Shigella* organisms Fecal-oral transmission	Most infections in humans relate to consumption of contaminated foods or water, such as undercooked meats, particularly chicken Also acquired from contaminated household pets (e.g., dogs, cats, hamsters) Bimodal peaks in infants <1 year old and again at ages 15-29 years old Antibiotics do not prolong the carriage of bacteria and may eliminate organism more quickly Erythromycin is the drug of choice Antimotility agents not recommended because they tend to prolong symptoms
Vibrio cholerae Gram-negative, motile, curved bacillus living in bodies of salt water Incubation—1-3 days Diagnosis—stool culture	Enters via oral route in contaminated food or water; if survives acid stomach environment, travels to the small intestine, adheres to the mucosa, and produces toxin	Onset abrupt; vomiting, watery diarrhea without cramping or tenesmus Dehydration can occur quickly	More prevalent in developing countries Rehydration most important treatment Antibiotics can shorten diarrhea Despite continued efforts, still no vaccine
Clostridium difficile Gram-positive anaerobic bacillus with the ability to produce spores Diagnosis—by detecting *C. difficile* toxin in stool culture	Produces two important toxins (A and B) Toxin binds to the enterocyte surface receptor, resulting in alteration permeability, protein synthesis, and direct cytotoxicity	Mostly mild watery diarrhea lasting a few days Some prolonged diarrhea and illness May cause pseudomembranous colitis Some individuals extremely ill with high fever, leukocytosis, hypoalbuminemia	Associated with alteration of normal intestinal flora by antibiotics Adults tend to have more severe symptoms than children Treatment with antibiotics (metronidazole) in mildly to moderately symptomatic patients; for nonresponders, give vancomycin Resistant strains have developed Relapse common

TABLE 22.5 Infectious Causes of Acute Diarrhea—cont'd

Agents	Pathology	Characteristics	Comments
Clostridium perfringens Anaerobic, gram-positive, spore-producing bacilli Incubation—8-24 hours	Toxins produced in the intestine after ingestion of organism	Acute onset—watery diarrhea, crampy abdominal pain Fever, nausea, and vomiting are rare Duration of illness usually 24 hours	Transmitted by contaminated food products, most often meats and poultry Usually self-limiting and medical intervention not needed Oral rehydration usually sufficient Antibiotics serve no purpose and should not be used
Clostridium botulinum Gram-positive anaerobic spore-producing bacilli Incubation—12-26 hours (range, 6 hours to 8 days) Diagnosis—To detect toxin, submit blood and stool culture to special laboratory (usually state health department)	Botulism caused by binding of toxin to the neuromuscular junction	Clinical presentation related to age and the strain of the botulism GI—abdominal pain, cramping, and diarrhea Other strains—respiratory compromise, CNS symptoms	Transmitted in contaminated food products Can be acquired via wound infection Treatment is supportive care and neutralization of the toxin
***Staphylococcus* organisms** Gram-positive nonmotile, aerobic or facultative anaerobic bacteria Incubation—generally short, 1-8 hours Diagnosis—identify organism in food, blood, pus, aspirate	Direct tissue invasion and production of toxin	Clinical presentation dependent on site of entry In food poisoning, profuse diarrhea, nausea, and vomiting	Transmitted in inadequately cooked or refrigerated foods Self-limiting Symptomatic treatment

CNS, Central nervous system; *EIA,* enzyme immunoassay; *ELISA,* enzyme-linked immunosorbent assay; *GI,* gastrointestinal; *PCR,* polymerase chain reaction.

Intractable diarrhea of infancy is a syndrome that occurs in the first few months of life, persists for longer than 2 weeks with no recognized pathogens, and is refractory to treatment. The most common cause is acute infectious diarrhea that was not managed adequately.

Chronic nonspecific diarrhea (CNSD), also known as *irritable colon of childhood* and *toddlers' diarrhea,* is a common cause of chronic diarrhea in children 6 to 54 months of age. These children have loose stools, often with undigested food particles, and diarrhea lasting longer than 2 weeks. Children with CNSD grow normally and have no evidence of malnutrition, no blood in their stool, and no enteric infection. Poor dietary habits and food sensitivities have been linked to chronic diarrhea. The excessive intake of juices and artificial sweeteners such as sorbitol, a substance found in many commercially prepared beverages and foods, may be a factor.

Etiology

Most pathogens that cause diarrhea are spread by the fecal-oral route through contaminated food or water or are spread from person to person where there is close contact (e.g., daycare centers). Lack of clean water, crowding, poor hygiene, nutritional deficiency, and poor sanitation are major risk factors, especially for bacterial or parasitic pathogens. Infants are often more susceptible to frequent and severe bouts of diarrhea because their immune system has not been exposed to many pathogens and has not acquired protective antibodies. Worldwide, the most common causes of acute gastroenteritis are infectious agents, viruses, bacteria, and parasites.

Rotavirus is the most important cause of serious gastroenteritis among children, with 28% of all cases causing fatality (Lamberti, Ashraf, Walker, et al., 2016). The virus is spread through the fecal-oral route or by person-to-person contact, and almost all children are infected with rotavirus at least once by the age of 5 years (Bass, 2020). Rotavirus is the most common cause of diarrhea-associated hospitalization, with an estimated 80,000 hospitalizations occurring annually in the United States in children less than 5 years of age (Bass, 2020).

Salmonella, Campylobacter, Yersinia, and *Shigella* organisms are the most frequently isolated bacterial pathogens in the United States (Kotloff, 2017). These organisms are gram-negative bacteria and can be contracted through raw or undercooked food, contaminated food or water, or the fecal-oral route. Among children and adults in the United States annually, *Salmonella* occurs in approximately 8172 people; *Campylobacter* occurs in 8547 people; *Shigella* occurs in 2913 people; and *Yersinia* occurs in 302 people (Marder, Cieslak, Cronquist, et al., 2017). (See also Chapter 6, Intestinal Parasitic Diseases.)

Antibiotic administration is frequently associated with diarrhea because antibiotics alter the normal intestinal flora, resulting in an overgrowth of other bacteria. *Clostridium difficile* is the most common bacterial overgrowth with a 12-fold increases in pediatric incidence from 1991 to 2009 (McFarland, Ozen, Dinleyici, et al., 2016). Children acquire most *C. difficile* infections in health care facilities, but 41% are acquired from the community, such as day care centers (McFarland, Ozen, Dinleyici, et al., 2016).

Pathophysiology

Invasion of the GI tract by pathogens results in increased intestinal secretion as a result of enterotoxins, cytotoxic mediators, or decreased intestinal absorption secondary to intestinal damage or inflammation. Enteric pathogens attach to the mucosal cells and form a cuplike pedestal on which the bacteria rest. The pathogenesis of the diarrhea depends on whether the organism remains attached to the cell surface, resulting in a secretory toxin (noninvasive, toxin-producing, noninflammatory-type diarrhea), or penetrates the mucosa (systemic diarrhea). Noninflammatory diarrhea is the most common diarrheal illness, resulting from the action of enterotoxin that is released after attachment to the mucosa. The most serious and immediate physiologic disturbances associated with severe diarrheal disease are dehydration, acid-base imbalance with acidosis, and shock that occurs when dehydration progresses to the point that circulatory status is seriously impaired.

TABLE 22.6 Treatment of Acute Diarrhea

Degree of Dehydration	Signs and Symptoms	Rehydration Therapy[a]	Replacement of Stool Losses	Maintenance Therapy
Mild (5%-6%)	Increased thirst Slightly dry buccal mucous membranes	ORS, 50 ml/kg within 4 hours	ORS, 10 ml/kg (for infants) or 150 to 250 ml at a time (for older children) for each diarrheal stool	Breastfeeding, if established, should continue; give regular infant formula if tolerated. If lactose intolerance suspected, give undiluted lactose-free formula (or half-strength lactose-containing formula for brief period only); infants and children who receive solid food should continue their usual diet.
Moderate (7%-9%)	Loss of skin turgor, dry buccal mucous membranes, sunken eyes, sunken fontanel	ORS, 100 ml/kg within 4 hours	Same as above	
Severe (>9%)	Signs of moderate dehydration plus one of following: rapid thready pulse, cyanosis, rapid breathing, lethargy, coma	Intravenous fluids (lactated Ringer solution), 40 ml/kg until pulse and state of consciousness return to normal; then 50-100 ml/kg or ORS	Same as above	

[a]If no signs of dehydration are present, rehydration therapy is not necessary. Proceed with maintenance therapy and replacement of stool losses.
ORS, Oral rehydration solution.

Diagnostic Evaluation

Evaluation of the child with acute gastroenteritis begins with a careful history that seeks to discover the possible cause of diarrhea, to assess the severity of symptoms and the risk of complications, and to elicit information about current symptoms indicating other treatable illnesses that could be causing the diarrhea. The history should include questions about recent travel, exposure to untreated drinking or washing water sources, contact with animals or birds, daycare center attendance, recent treatment with antibiotics, or recent diet changes. History questions should also explore the presence of other symptoms such as fever and vomiting, frequency and character of stools (e.g., watery, bloody), urinary output, dietary habits, and recent food intake.

Extensive laboratory evaluation is not indicated in children who have uncomplicated diarrhea and no evidence of dehydration because most diarrheal illnesses are self-limiting. Laboratory tests are indicated for children who are severely dehydrated and receiving IV therapy. Watery, explosive stools suggest glucose intolerance; foul-smelling, greasy, bulky stools suggest fat malabsorption. Diarrhea that develops after the introduction of cow's milk, fruits, or cereal may be related to enzyme deficiency or protein intolerance. Neutrophils or red blood cells in the stool indicate bacterial gastroenteritis or IBD. The presence of eosinophils suggests protein intolerance or parasitic infection. Stool cultures should be performed only when blood, mucus, or polymorphonuclear leukocytes are present in the stool; when symptoms are severe; when there is a history of travel to a developing country; and when a specific pathogen is suspected. Gross blood or occult blood may indicate pathogens such as *Shigella, Campylobacter,* or hemorrhagic *Escherichia coli* strains. Providers may use an enzyme-linked immunosorbent assay (ELISA) to confirm the presence of rotavirus or *Giardia* organisms. If there is a history of recent antibiotic use, test the stool for *C. difficile* toxin. When bacterial and viral cultures are negative and when diarrhea persists for more than a few days, examine stools for ova and parasites. A stool specimen with a pH of less than 6 and the presence of reducing substances may indicate carbohydrate malabsorption or secondary lactase deficiency. Stool electrolyte measurements may help identify children with secretory diarrhea.

Determine urine specific gravity if dehydration is suspected. Obtain a complete blood count (CBC), serum electrolytes, creatinine, and blood urea nitrogen (BUN) in the child who has moderate to severe dehydration or who requires hospitalization. The hemoglobin, hematocrit, creatinine, and BUN levels are usually elevated in acute diarrhea and should normalize with rehydration.

Therapeutic Management

The major goals in the management of acute diarrhea include assessment of fluid and electrolyte imbalance, rehydration, maintenance fluid therapy, and reintroduction of an adequate diet. Treat infants and children with acute diarrhea and dehydration first with **oral rehydration therapy (ORT)**. ORT is one of the major worldwide health care advances. It is more effective, safer, less painful, and less costly than IV rehydration. The American Academy of Pediatrics, World Health Organization, and Centers for Disease Control and Prevention all recommend ORT as the treatment of choice for most cases of dehydration caused by diarrhea. **Oral rehydration solutions (ORSs)** enhance and promote the reabsorption of sodium and water. These solutions greatly reduce vomiting, duration of illness, and the need for IV infusions (Dekate, Jayashree, & Singhi, 2013). ORSs, including reduced-osmolarity ORS, are available in the United States as commercially prepared solutions and are successful in treating the majority of infants with dehydration. Guidelines for rehydration recommended by the American Academy of Pediatrics are given in Table 22.6 (See Quality Patient Outcomes box.)

QUALITY PATIENT OUTCOMES: Diarrhea

- Adequate hydration maintained during illness
- Appropriate diagnostic tests performed
- Antibiotics given only if appropriate
- No repeat visits to the emergency department or pediatrician during the course of the illness
- No tissue breakdown
- Normal elimination returns

After rehydration, ORS may be used during maintenance fluid therapy by alternating the solution with a low-sodium fluid such as breast milk, lactose-free formula, or half-strength lactose-containing formula. In older children, ORS can be given and a regular diet continued. Ongoing stool losses should be replaced on a 1:1 basis with ORS. If the stool volume is not known, approximately 10 ml/kg (4 to 8 oz) of ORS should be given for each diarrheal stool.

Solutions for oral hydration are useful in most cases of dehydration, and vomiting is not a contraindication. Give a child who is vomiting an ORS at frequent intervals and in small amounts. For young children, the caregiver may give the fluid with a spoon or small syringe in 5- to 10-ml increments every 1 to 5 minutes. An ORS may also be given via NG or gastrostomy tube infusion. Infants without clinical signs of dehydration do not need ORT. They should, however, receive the same fluid recommended for infants with signs of dehydration in the maintenance phase and for ongoing stool losses. Probiotics when used in conjunction with ORS reduce the duration of antibiotic-associated diarrhea in children (Barnes & Yeh, 2015).

> **! NURSING ALERT**
>
> Encouraging intake of clear fluids by mouth, such as fruit juices, carbonated soft drinks, and gelatin, does not help diarrhea. These fluids usually have a high carbohydrate content, a very low electrolyte content, and a high osmolality. Have patients avoid caffeinated beverages because caffeine is a mild diuretic and may lead to increased loss of water and sodium. Chicken or beef broth is not given because it contains excessive sodium and inadequate carbohydrate. A BRAT diet (bananas, rice, applesauce, and toast or tea) is contraindicated for the child and especially for the infant with acute diarrhea because this diet has little nutritional value (low in energy and protein), is high in carbohydrates, and is low in electrolytes.

Early reintroduction of nutrients is desirable and has gained more widespread acceptance. Continued feeding or early reintroduction of a normal diet after rehydration has no adverse effects, lessens the severity and duration of the illness, and improves weight gain when compared with the gradual reintroduction of foods (Kotloff, 2020). Infants who are breastfeeding should continue to do so, and ORS should be used to replace ongoing losses in these infants. Formula-fed infants should resume their formula; if it is not tolerated, a lactose-free formula may be used for a few days. In toddlers there is no contraindication to continuing soft or pureed foods. In older children a regular diet, including milk, can generally be offered after rehydration has been achieved. In cases of severe dehydration and shock, IV fluids are initiated whenever the child is unable to ingest sufficient amounts of fluid and electrolytes to (1) meet ongoing daily physiologic losses, (2) replace previous deficits, and (3) replace ongoing abnormal losses. Patients who usually require IV fluids are those with severe dehydration, uncontrollable vomiting, inability to drink for any reason (e.g., extreme fatigue, coma), and severe gastric distention.

Select the IV solution on the basis of what is known regarding the probable type and cause of the dehydration. The type of fluid normally used is a saline solution containing 5% dextrose in water. Sodium bicarbonate may be added because acidosis is usually associated with severe dehydration. Although the initial phase of fluid replacement is rapid in both isotonic and hypotonic dehydration, rapid replacement is contraindicated in hypertonic dehydration because of the risk of water intoxication.

After the severe effects of dehydration are under control, begin specific diagnostic and therapeutic measures to detect and treat the cause of the diarrhea. Because of the self-limiting nature of vomiting and its tendency to improve when dehydration is corrected, the use of antiemetic agents is usually not needed; however, ondansetron has few side effects and may be administered if vomiting persists and interferes with ORT (Kotloff, 2020).

The use of antibiotic therapy in children with acute gastroenteritis is controversial. Antibiotics may shorten the course of some diarrheal illnesses (e.g., those caused by *Shigella* organisms). However, most bacterial diarrheas are self-limiting, and the diarrhea often resolves before the causative organism can be determined. Antibiotics may prolong the carrier period for bacteria such as *Salmonella*. Antibiotics may be considered, however, in patients who are younger than 3 months of age or on immunosuppressive medication, or who have clinical signs of shock, severe malnutrition, dysentery, suspected cholera, or suspected giardiasis (Wen, Best, & Nourse, 2017). (See Chapter 6, Intestinal Parasitic Diseases.)

Nursing Care Management

The management of most cases of acute diarrhea takes place in the home with education of the caregiver. Teach caregivers to monitor for signs of dehydration (especially the number of wet diapers or voidings) and the amount of fluids taken by mouth and to assess the frequency and amount of stool losses. Education relating to ORT, including the administration of maintenance fluids and replacement of ongoing losses, is important (see Critical Thinking Case Study box). ORS should be administered in small quantities at frequent intervals. Vomiting is not a contraindication to ORT unless it is severe. Information concerning the introduction of a normal diet is essential. Parents need to know that a slightly higher stool output initially occurs with continuation of a normal diet and with ongoing replacement of stool losses. The benefits of a better nutritional outcome with fewer complications and a shorter duration of illness outweigh the potential increase in stool frequency. Address parents' concerns to ensure adherence to the treatment plan.

CRITICAL THINKING CASE STUDY

Diarrhea

A mother brings her 8-month-old infant, Mary, to the primary care clinic. The mother reports that Mary has had a "cold" for about 2 days, and this morning she began to vomit and has had diarrhea for the past 8 hours. Mary's mother states that she is still breastfeeding, but Mary is not taking as much fluid as usual and she is having three times as many stools as usual (the stools are watery). When the nurse practitioner examines Mary, she notes that her temperature is 38°C (100.4°F), her pulse and blood pressure are in the normal range, her mucous membranes are slightly dry, but she has tears when she cries. The nurse practitioner also notes that Mary's weight has not changed from what it was when she was seen in the clinic 2 weeks ago for her well-child visit.

Initial Assessment. How would you classify the degree of dehydration that Mary is experiencing? Mild, moderate, or severe?

Clinical Reasoning. What interventions are appropriate for the degree of dehydration?

Teaching Points

- Infants or children with mild dehydration are managed with oral rehydration therapy (ORT) and early reintroduction of an adequate diet.
- Breastfeeding generally can be continued in mild dehydration.
- Antidiarrheal medications are not recommended for the treatment of acute infectious diarrhea. These medications have adverse effects such as slowed motility and can prolong the illness.

Critical Thinking Answers

Initial Assessment. Mary is experiencing mild dehydration based on the history and exam.

Clinical Reasoning. An appropriate nursing action is to continue oral rehydration at frequent intervals using small amounts. The mother should *not* administer any antidiarrheal medications.

If the child with acute diarrhea and dehydration is hospitalized, the nurse must obtain an accurate weight and carefully monitor intake and output. The child may be placed on parenteral fluid therapy with nothing by mouth (NPO) for 12 to 48 hours. Monitoring the IV infusion is an important nursing function. The nurse must ensure that the correct fluid and electrolyte concentration is infused, that the flow rate is adjusted to deliver the desired volume in a given time, and that the IV site is maintained.

Accurate measurement of output is essential to determine whether renal blood flow is sufficient to permit the addition of potassium to the IV fluids. The nurse is responsible for examination of stools and collection of specimens for laboratory examination. (See Chapter 20, Collection of Specimens.) Take care when obtaining and transporting stools to prevent possible spread of infection. Use a clean tongue depressor to obtain specimens for laboratory examination or as an applicator for transfer to a culture medium. Transport stool specimens to the laboratory in appropriate containers and media according to hospital policy.

Diarrheal stools are highly irritating to the skin, and extra care is necessary to protect the skin of the diaper region from excoriation. (See Chapter 31, Diaper Dermatitis.) Avoid taking temperatures rectally because they stimulate the bowel, increasing passage of stool.

Support for the child and family involves the same care and consideration given to all hospitalized children (see Chapter 19). Keep parents informed of the child's progress and instruct them in the use of frequent and proper hand washing and the disposal of soiled diapers, clothes, and bed linens. Everyone caring for the child must be aware of "clean" areas and "dirty" areas, especially in the hospital, where the sink in the child's room is used for many purposes. Discard soiled diapers and linens in receptacles close to the bedside.

Prevention

The best intervention for diarrhea is prevention. The fecal-oral route spreads most infections, and parents need information about preventive measures such as personal hygiene, protection of the water supply from contamination, and careful food preparation.

> **! NURSING ALERT**
>
> To reduce the risk of bacteria transmitted via food, encourage parents to do the following:
> - Quickly freeze or refrigerate all ground meat and other perishable foods.
> - Never thaw food on the counter or let it sit out of the refrigerator for more than 2 hours.
> - Wash hands, utensils, and work areas with hot, soapy water after contact with raw meat to keep bacteria from spreading.
> - Check ground meat with a fork to make certain no pink is showing before taking a bite.
> - Cook all dishes made with ground meat until brown or gray inside or to an internal temperature of 71°C (160°F).

Meticulous attention to perianal hygiene, disposal of soiled diapers, proper hand washing, and isolation of infected persons also minimize the transmission of infection. (See Chapter 20, Infection Control.)

Parents need information about preventing diarrhea while traveling. Caution them against giving their children adult medications that are used to prevent traveler's diarrhea. The best measure during travel to areas where water may be contaminated is to allow children to drink only bottled water and carbonated beverages (from the container through a straw supplied from home). Children should also avoid tap water, ice, unpasteurized dairy products, raw vegetables, unpeeled fruits, meats, and seafood.

Vaccines can protect children from some diarrhea-related diseases. The rotavirus vaccine was integrated into the national immunization program in the United States in 2006, and subsequently the rotavirus season was noted to be shorter, along with a 76% decline in diarrhea hospitalization rates among children younger than 5 years of age (Lamberti et al., 2016).

CONSTIPATION

Constipation is an alteration in the frequency, consistency, or ease of passing stool. It is defined as unsatisfactory defecation due to infrequent stools, difficult stool passage, or perceived incomplete defecation (Bruce, Bruce, Short, et al., 2016). The frequency of bowel movements varies by age, but children ages 4 years and older can be diagnosed with constipation if they have fewer than three stools per week (Poddar, 2016). Constipation is often associated with painful bowel movements, blood-streaked or retained stool, abdominal pain, lack of appetite, and stool incontinence (i.e., soiling) (Bruce et al., 2016). Having extremely long intervals between defecation is **obstipation**. Constipation with fecal soiling is **encopresis**.

Constipation may arise secondary to a variety of organic disorders or in association with a wide range of systemic disorders. Structural disorders of the intestine, such as strictures, ectopic anus, and Hirschsprung disease (HD), may be associated with constipation. Systemic disorders associated with constipation include hypothyroidism, hypercalcemia resulting from hyperparathyroidism or vitamin D excess, and chronic lead poisoning. Constipation is also associated with drugs such as antacids, diuretics, antiepileptics, antihistamines, opioids, and iron supplementation. Spinal cord lesions may be associated with loss of rectal tone and sensation. Affected children are prone to chronic fecal retention and overflow incontinence.

Most children have **idiopathic** or **functional constipation** because no underlying cause can be identified. Chronic constipation may occur as a result of environmental or psychosocial factors, or a combination of both. Transient illness, withholding and avoidance secondary to painful or negative experiences with stooling, and dietary intake with decreased fluid and fiber all play a role in the etiology of constipation.

Newborn Period

Normally, newborn infants pass a first meconium stool within 24 to 36 hours of birth. Any newborn that does not do so should be assessed for evidence of intestinal atresia or stenosis, HD, hypothyroidism, meconium plug, or meconium ileus. **Meconium plug** is caused by meconium that has reduced water content and is usually evacuated after digital examination but may require irrigations with a hypertonic solution or contrast medium. **Meconium ileus**, the initial manifestation of cystic fibrosis, is the luminal obstruction of the distal small intestine by abnormal meconium. Treatment is the same as for a meconium plug; early surgical intervention may be needed to evacuate the small intestine.

Infancy

The onset of constipation frequently occurs during infancy and may result from organic causes such as HD, hypothyroidism, and strictures. It is important to differentiate these conditions from functional constipation. Constipation in infancy is often related to dietary practices. It is less common in breastfed infants, who have softer stools than bottle-fed infants. Breastfed infants may also have decreased stools because of more complete use of breast milk with little residue. When constipation occurs with a change from human milk or modified cow's milk to whole cow's milk, simple measures such as adding or increasing the amount of vegetables and fruit in the infant's diet and increasing fluids such as sorbitol-rich juices usually correct the problem. When a bottle-fed infant passes a hard stool that results in an anal fissure, stool-withholding behaviors may develop in response to pain on defecation (see Critical Thinking Case Study box).

CRITICAL THINKING CASE STUDY

Constipation

Harry, an 8-month-old infant, is seen by the pediatric nurse practitioner for his well-child visit. Harry's mother states that he usually has one hard stool every 4 or 5 days, which causes discomfort when the stool is passed. He has also had one episode of diarrhea and two episodes of ribbonlike stools. Abdominal distention and vomiting have not accompanied the constipation, and Harry's growth has been appropriate for his age. Currently his diet consists of cow's milk–based formula only. Harry's mother reports that the infrequent passage of hard stools began approximately 6 weeks ago when she stopped breastfeeding.

Initial Assessment. What are the immediate concerns regarding Harry's symptoms?

Clinical Reasoning. What interventions are most appropriate for the degree of symptoms?

Teaching Points

- Functional constipation may occur with changes in the diet (e.g., the change from breastfeeding 6 weeks ago to bottle-feeding of cow's milk–based formula).
- Prune juice could be slowly introduced into Harry's diet.
- Offering fruits and vegetables each day may help prevent further constipation.
- Often, simple measures such as the introduction of solid foods or other dietary modifications help to remedy functional constipation.

Critical Thinking Answers

Initial Assessment. The immediate concern is constipation. The initial data seem to point to the conclusion that Harry has functional constipation. However, diarrhea and the passage of ribbonlike stools do not usually occur with functional constipation; therefore Harry should be monitored closely.

Clinical Reasoning. Constipation in infancy can be caused by medical conditions such as Hirschsprung disease, hypothyroidism, or strictures, or it can be simple functional constipation. In infancy, changes in dietary practices such as a change from human milk to cow's milk may precipitate functional constipation. Functional constipation is usually treated by dietary modifications such as increasing the amount of fluids, fruits, or vegetables in the infant's diet.

Childhood

Most constipation in early childhood is due to environmental changes or normal development when a child begins to attain control over bodily functions. A child who has experienced discomfort during bowel movements may deliberately try to withhold stool. Over time, the rectum accommodates to the accumulation of stool, and the urge to defecate passes. When the bowel contents are ultimately evacuated, the accumulated feces are passed with pain, thus reinforcing the desire to withhold stool.

Constipation in school-age children may represent an ongoing problem or a first-time event. The onset of constipation at this age is often the result of environmental changes, stresses, and changes in toileting patterns. A common cause of new-onset constipation at school entry is fear of using the school bathrooms, which are noted for their lack of privacy. Early and hurried departure for school immediately after breakfast may also impede bathroom use.

Therapeutic Management

Treatment of constipation depends on the cause and duration of symptoms. A complete history and physical examination are essential to determine appropriate management. It may be necessary to facilitate passage of the obstruction by irrigation with a hypertonic solution or water-soluble enema. If the constipation is due to HD, surgical treatment may include resection of the intestine and saline irrigations.

Management of the infant should include education of the parents concerning normal bowel habits. Short, transient periods of constipation usually require no intervention. Mild constipation usually resolves as solid food is introduced in the diet. Stool softeners such as malt extract or lactulose may be used for hard stools or anal fissures. The persistent use of rectal stimulation with thermometers or cotton-tipped applicators is discouraged because these methods often result in anal fissures and increased pain that may trigger stool withholding.

The management of simple constipation consists of a plan to promote regular bowel movements. Often this is as simple as changing the diet to provide more fiber and fluids, eliminating foods known to be constipating, and establishing a bowel routine that allows for regular passage of stool. Stool-softening agents such as docusate or lactulose may also be helpful. Polyethylene glycol (PEG) 3350 without electrolytes (MiraLax) is a chemically inert polymer that has been introduced as a new laxative in recent years. Children tolerate it well because it can be mixed in any beverage of choice. If other symptoms such as vomiting, abdominal distention, or pain and evidence of growth failure are associated with the constipation, investigate the condition further.

Management of chronic constipation requires an organized and ongoing approach. It is important for families to realize that it usually requires months or years to resolve, and relapse is common. The goals for management include restoring regular evacuation of stool, shrinking the distended rectum to its normal size, and promoting a regular toileting routine. This requires a combination of therapies and should include bowel cleansing, maintenance therapy to prevent stool retention, modification of diet, bowel habit training, and behavioral modification.

DRUG ALERT

Mineral Oil

Mineral oil must be given carefully to avoid the risk of aspiration. It should not be used in children younger than 1 year old (Poddar, 2016).

After the impaction is removed, maintenance therapy often lasting for 6 to 12 months is necessary to promote easy passage of stool and prevent stool retention. Maintenance therapy includes stool softeners and laxatives. Stool softeners are often ineffective for severe constipation; laxative therapy may be necessary to return the rectum to its normal size. Because of the minimal side effects, taste, and efficacy, PEG is a more favorable constipation intervention than lactulose (Poddar, 2016). PEG increases fluid in the colon. The additional volume of fluid stimulates the urge to defecate.

Changes in the diet may be helpful but are usually not effective alone. Encouraging the intake of fiber ultimately helps maintain regular elimination once the rectum returns to normal size and the laxatives are tapered. Recommended daily fiber intake is age in years plus 5 grams of fiber per day (Poddar, 2016). Effective counseling is an essential element of the treatment plan for children with chronic constipation. Explain normal bowel function, the purpose of interventions, and the need for persistence to the child and family.

Retraining therapy involves habit training, reinforcement for sitting on the toilet and defecating, and emotional support. Parents should establish a regular toilet time once or twice a day, preferably after a meal. A reasonable amount of time (5 to 10 minutes) should be spent attempting to defecate completely. Biofeedback may be indicated as a form of behavior modification and as a means to teach children to relax the anal sphincter during defecation.

Nursing Care Management

Unfortunately, constipation tends to be self-perpetuating. A child who has difficulty or discomfort when attempting to evacuate the bowels has a tendency to retain the bowel contents, and thus constipation becomes a chronic problem. Nursing assessment begins with a history of bowel habits; diet; events that may be associated with the onset of constipation; drugs or other substances that the child may be taking; and the consistency, color, frequency, and other characteristics of the stool. If there is no evidence of a pathologic condition that requires further investigation, the nurse's major task is to educate the parents regarding normal stool patterns and to participate in the education and treatment of the child.

Dietary modifications are helpful in preventing constipation. Fiber is an important part of the diet. Parents benefit from guidance about foods that are high in fiber and ways to promote healthy food choices in children. If bran is added to the diet, creative ways to disguise the consistency, such as adding it to cereal, peanut butter, mashed potatoes, fruit shakes, and baked goods, are helpful. Beans are often found in Mexican dishes children enjoy and can be added to soups, salads, and stews. Beyond the age when foreign body aspiration is a hazard, a good source of fiber is corn and popcorn.

VOMITING

Vomiting is the forceful ejection of gastric contents through the mouth. It is a well-defined, complex, coordinated process that is under CNS control and is often accompanied by nausea and retching. In contrast, regurgitation is a simpler, more passive, and effortless phenomenon. Vomiting has many causes, including acute infectious diseases, increased intracranial pressure, toxic ingestions, food intolerances and allergies, mechanical obstruction of the GI tract, adrenal insufficiency, nephrologic disease, pregnancy, and psychogenic problems (Maqbool & Liacouras, 2020c). Vomiting is common in childhood, is usually self-limiting, and requires no specific treatment. However, complications can occur in children, including acute fluid volume loss (dehydration) and electrolyte disturbances, malnutrition, aspiration, and Mallory-Weiss syndrome (small tears in the distal esophageal mucosa).

Etiology

The child's age, pattern of vomiting, and duration of symptoms help determine the cause. For example, chronic and intermittent episodes of vomiting may indicate malrotation, whereas vomiting on a specific day at the same time before school is not likely to be a result of organic disease. The color and consistency of the emesis vary according to the cause. Green, bilious vomiting suggests bowel obstruction. Curdled stomach contents, mucus, or fatty foods that are vomited several hours after ingestion suggest poor gastric emptying or high intestinal obstruction. Gastric irritation by certain medicines, foods, or toxic substances may cause vomiting. Forceful vomiting is associated with pyloric stenosis.

Associated symptoms also help identify the cause. Fever and diarrhea accompanying vomiting suggest an infection. Constipation associated with vomiting suggests an anatomic or functional obstruction. Localized abdominal pain and vomiting often occur with appendicitis, pancreatitis, or peptic ulcer disease. A change in the level of consciousness or a headache associated with vomiting indicates a central nervous system or metabolic disorder.

Pathophysiology

The act of vomiting, including nausea and retching, is under the control of the CNS. Two areas of the medulla are involved as the vomiting center. The medullary center is also activated by impulses from a second center, the chemoreceptor trigger zone, which is located in the floor of the fourth ventricle. **Nausea** is a sensation that may be induced by visceral, labyrinthine (inner ear), or emotional stimuli. It is characterized by the desire to vomit, with discomfort felt in the throat or abdomen. Nausea is often associated with autonomic symptoms such as salivation, pallor, sweating, and tachycardia. Retching may occur with or without vomiting. **Retching** involves a series of spasmodic movements during inspiration, creating a negative intrathoracic pressure, and contraction of the abdominal muscles. Projectile vomiting is preceded and accompanied by vigorous peristaltic waves.

Vomiting is a well-recognized response to psychologic stress. During stress, adrenaline levels rise and may stimulate the chemoreceptor trigger zone. Nausea and vomiting are likely a protective mechanism to remove toxins from the system. Vomiting may follow GI infection or toxic ingestion, or it can be a learned behavioral response.

Cyclic vomiting syndrome is a rare disorder, affecting approximately 2% of children in the United States, and is characterized by bouts of vomiting that can last from hours to several days (Maqbool & Liacouras, 2020c). The cause of this syndrome is unknown, although a family history of migraines is usually present in at least 80% of the patients (Maqbool & Liacouras, 2020c).

Diagnostic Evaluation

The diagnostic evaluation includes a thorough history and physical examination. The description of the vomitus; relationship to meals or specific foods; behavior; and presence of pain, constipation, diarrhea, or jaundice are important components of the history. Physical examination should include an assessment of the hydration status and an abdominal examination.

Further evaluation may include analysis of urine for protein or blood, serum electrolytes, and radiographic studies. A plain radiograph of the chest or abdomen or ultrasonography may reveal anatomic abnormalities. Brain scans are used when tumors are considered. Endoscopy of the upper GI tract may be a valuable diagnostic procedure if the provider suspects esophagitis. A psychiatric evaluation may be indicated if cyclic vomiting, anorexia nervosa, bulimia, or self-poisoning is present. Self-induced vomiting and rumination may be a self-stimulation or gratification activity.

Therapeutic Management

Management is directed toward detection and treatment of the cause of the vomiting and prevention of complications, such as dehydration and malnutrition. Vomiting is often a symptom of a common infectious illness that is self-limiting and resolves with no specific treatment.

Further investigation is indicated if there is dehydration, progressively severe vomiting, or persistent vomiting for more than 24 hours, or if the history and physical examination fail to suggest a diagnosis. If vomiting leads to dehydration, oral rehydration or parenteral fluids may be required.

Antiemetic drugs may be indicated when the child is not able to tolerate anything orally or in cases of postoperative vomiting, chemotherapy-induced vomiting, cyclic vomiting syndrome, or acute motion sickness (Maqbool & Liacouras, 2020c). Ondansetron (Zofran) is an antiemetic with limited adverse effects and is beneficial when the child is not able to tolerate anything orally or in the case of postoperative vomiting, chemotherapy-induced vomiting, cyclic vomiting syndrome, or acute motion sickness (Maqbool & Liacouras, 2020c). Adverse effects with earlier-generation antiemetics (such as promethazine and metoclopramide) include somnolence, nervousness, irritability, and dystonic reactions, and they should not be routinely administered to children. For children who are prone to motion sickness, it is often helpful to administer an appropriate dose of dimenhydrinate (Dramamine) before a trip (see Translating Evidence Into Practice box).

TRANSLATING EVIDENCE INTO PRACTICE

Use of Antiemetics in Children With Acute Gastroenteritis

Ask the Question

In children with acute gastroenteritis (AGE), should antiemetics be used?

Search for the Evidence

Search Strategies

Search criteria included English-language publications within the years 2011 to 2017, research-based articles (level 3 or higher) regarding antiemetic use among children with AGE.

Databases Used

PubMed/Medline; CINAHL; Cochrane; National Guideline Clearinghouse (Agency for Healthcare Research and Quality); American Academy of Pediatrics; National Institute of Health and Clinical Excellence; European Society for Paediatric Gastroenterology, Hepatology, and Nutrition; Joanna Briggs Institute.

Critically Analyze the Evidence

There is **moderate evidence** with a **strong recommendation** (Balshem, Hefland, Schunemann, et al., 2011).

A review of the literature revealed two systematic reviews and three randomized control trials from 2011 to 2017 that evaluated the use of antiemetics in the treatment of children with AGE.

- A Cochrane review in 2011 revealed 7 randomized controlled trials (1020 patients) evaluating the safety and efficacy of antiemetics to treat gastroenteritis-induced vomiting in children (Fedorowicz, Jagannath, & Carter, 2011). Ondansetron was found more effective than placebo in studies evaluating hospital admission rates, need for intravenous (IV) rehydration therapy, and resolution of vomiting. When comparing placebo, dimenhydrinate was found more effective in one study, and metoclopramide was more effective in another single study.
- A systematic review from 1980 to 2012 revealed 10 studies (1479 participants) evaluating the evidence of safety and effectiveness of antiemetics (dexamethasone, dimenhydrinate, granisetron, metoclopramide, and ondansetron) for gastroenteritis-induced vomiting in children and adolescents (Carter & Fedorowicz, 2012). There is clear evidence from nine studies that ondansetron is more effective than placebo in resolving vomiting, reducing the need for IV rehydration therapy, and reducing the hospital admission rate. A single study showed a reduction in mean vomiting days among children receiving dimenhydrinate versus placebo and among granisteron versus placebo. Studies of metoclopramide were underpowered, and a single study of dexamethasone versus placebo showed no statistically significant difference in vomiting.
- A group of 144 children diagnosed with AGE were randomized to receive dimenhydrinate or placebo in a pediatric emergency department (Gouin, Vo, Roy, et al., 2012). No statistically significant difference in the frequency of vomiting was noted between the two groups.
- A group of 76 children diagnosed with AGE were randomized to receive an orally disintegrating ondansetron tablet or domperidone suspension (dosing based on body weight), then evaluated for vomiting for the next 24 hours (Rerksuppaphol & Rerksuppaphol, 2013). Sixty-two percent of patients in the ondansetron group and 44% of patients in the domperidone group had no vomiting after treatment, although no statistically significant difference was noted ($P = 0.16$).
- Another study randomized 356 children who failed oral rehydration in an emergency department to receive ondansetron ($n = 119$) versus domperiodone ($n = 119$) versus placebo ($n = 118$) for treatment of AGE (Marchetti, Bonati, Maestro, et al., 2016). Fourteen children (12%) needed IV rehydration in the ondansetron group compared with 30 children (25%) in the domperidone and 34 children (29%) in the placebo group.

Apply the Evidence: Nursing Implications

Ondansetron reduces the duration of vomiting in children with AGE, and ondansetron and domperidone relieves the incidence of vomiting in children with AGE. There is limited evidence for dimenhydrinate and metoclopramide and no evidence for other antiemetics in children with AGE who are vomiting. The number of children requiring IV rehydration and hospital admission for AGE is reduced with administration of ondansetron.

References

Balshem, H., Hefland, M., Schunemann, H. J., et al. (2011). GRADE guidelines: Rating the quality of evidence. *Journal of Clinical Epidemiology, 64*(4), 401–406.

Carter, B., & Fedorowicz, Z. (2012). Antiemetic treatment for acute gastroenteritis in children: An updated Cochrane systematic review with meta-analysis and mixed treatment comparison in a Bayesian framework. *BMJ Open, 2*, 1–11.

Fedorowicz, Z., Jagannath, V. A., & Carter, B. (2011). Antiemetics for reducing vomiting related to acute gastroenteritis in children and adolescents. *Cochrane Database of Systematic Reviews, 9*, CD005506.

Gouin, S., Vo, T., Roy, M., et al. (2012). Oral dimenhydrinate versus placebo in children with gastroenteritis: A randomized controlled trial. *Pediatrics, 129*, 1050–1055.

Marchetti, F., Bonati, M., Maestro, A., et al. (2016). Oral ondansetron versus domperidone for acute gastroenteritis in pediatric emergency departments: Multicenter double blind randomized controlled trial. *PLoS ONE, 11*(11), e0165441.

Rerksuppaphol, S., & Rerksuppaphol, L. (2013). Randomized study of ondansetron versus domperidone in the treatment of children with acute gastroenteritis. *Journal of Clinical Medicine Research, 5*(6), 460–466.

Nursing Care Management

The major emphasis of nursing care of the vomiting infant or child is on observation and reporting of vomiting behavior and associated symptoms and on the implementation of measures to reduce the vomiting. Accurate assessment of the type of vomiting, appearance of the emesis, and the child's behavior in association with the vomiting greatly aids in establishing a diagnosis.

The cause of the vomiting determines the nursing intervention. When the vomiting is a manifestation of improper feeding methods, establishing proper techniques through teaching and example ordinarily corrects the situation. If the vomiting is a probable sign of GI obstruction, the nurse usually withholds food or implements special feeding techniques. The nurse should direct efforts toward maintaining hydration and preventing dehydration in a vomiting child.

The thirst mechanism is the most sensitive guide to fluid needs, and ad libitum administration of a glucose-electrolyte solution to an alert child restores water and electrolytes satisfactorily. It is important to include carbohydrates to spare body protein and to avoid ketosis resulting from exhaustion of glycogen stores. Small, frequent feedings of fluids or foods are preferable and more effective. Once vomiting has abated, offer more liberal amounts of fluids, followed by gradual resumption of the regular diet.

Position the infant or child who is vomiting upright to prevent aspiration and observe him or her for evidence of dehydration. Carefully monitor fluid and electrolyte status to avoid the possibility of electrolyte imbalance. It is important to emphasize the need for the child to brush the teeth or rinse the mouth after vomiting to dilute the hydrochloric acid that comes in contact with the teeth.

HIRSCHSPRUNG DISEASE (CONGENITAL AGANGLIONIC MEGACOLON)

Hirschsprung disease (HD) is a congenital anomaly that results in mechanical obstruction from inadequate motility of part of the intestine. It accounts for about one-fourth of all cases of neonatal intestinal obstruction. The incidence is 1 in 5000 live births (Maqbool & Liacouras, 2020a). It is four times more common in males than in females and follows a familial pattern in a small number of cases. Mutations in the *RET* proto-oncogene have been found in children with HD (Maqbool & Liacouras, 2020a).

Pathophysiology

The pathology of HD relates to the absence of ganglion cells in the affected areas of the intestine, resulting in a loss of the rectosphincteric reflex and an abnormal microenvironment of the cells of the affected intestine. The term *congenital aganglionic megacolon* describes the primary defect, which is the absence of ganglion cells in the myenteric plexus of Auerbach and the submucosal plexus of Meissner (Fig. 22.2).

The absence of ganglion cells in the affected bowel results in a lack of enteric nervous system stimulation, which decreases the internal sphincter's ability to relax. Unopposed sympathetic stimulation of the intestine results in increased intestinal tone. In addition to the contraction of the abnormal bowel and the resulting lack of peristalsis, there is a loss of the rectosphincteric reflex. Normally, when a stool bolus enters the rectum, the internal sphincter relaxes and the stool is evacuated. In HD, the internal sphincter does not relax. In about 80% of the cases, the aganglionic segment includes only the rectum and some portion of the distal colon, called *short-segment disease* (Maqbool & Liacouras, 2020a). However, the entire colon or part of the small intestine may be involved; this is considered *long-segment HD*. Occasionally, skip segments or total intestinal aganglionosis may occur. Approximately 15% have long-segment disease, and 5% have total intestinal aganglionosis (Maqbool & Liacouras, 2020a).

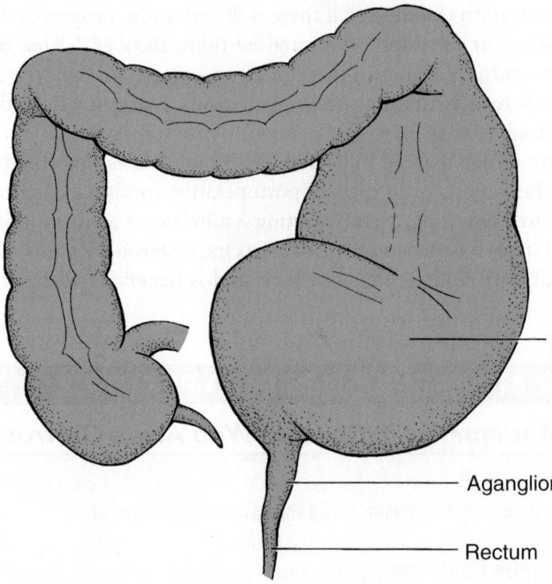

Fig. 22.2 Hirschsprung disease.

BOX 22.2 Clinical Manifestations of Hirschsprung Disease

Newborn Period
Failure to pass meconium within 24 to 48 hours after birth
Refusal to feed
Bilious vomiting
Abdominal distention

Infancy
Failure to thrive
Constipation
Abdominal distention
Episodes of diarrhea and vomiting
Signs of enterocolitis
- Explosive, watery diarrhea
- Fever
- Appears significantly ill

Childhood
Constipation
Ribbonlike, foul-smelling stools
Abdominal distention
Visible peristalsis
Easily palpable fecal mass
Undernourished, anemic appearance

Clinical Manifestations

Most children with HD are diagnosed in the first few months of life. Clinical manifestations vary according to the age when symptoms are recognized and the presence of complications, such as enterocolitis (Box 22.2). A neonate usually is seen with a distended abdomen, feeding intolerance with bilious vomiting, and a delay in the passage of meconium. Typically, 99% of term infants pass meconium in the first 48 hours of life, whereas few infants with HD do so (Maqbool & Liacouras, 2020a).

Diagnostic Evaluation

In the neonate the diagnosis is suspected on the basis of clinical signs of intestinal obstruction or failure to pass meconium. In infants and children the history is an important part of diagnosis and typically includes a chronic pattern of constipation. On examination the rectum is empty of feces, the internal sphincter is tight, and leakage of liquid stool and accumulated gas may occur if the aganglionic segment is short. A contrast enema often demonstrates the transition zone between the dilated proximal colon (megacolon) and the aganglionic distal segment. However, this typical megacolon and narrow distal segment may not develop until age 2 months or later.

To confirm the diagnosis, rectal biopsy is performed either surgically to obtain a full-thickness biopsy specimen or by suction biopsy for histologic evidence of the absence of ganglion cells. A noninvasive procedure that may be used is anorectal manometry, in which a catheter with a balloon attached is inserted into the rectum. The test records the reflex pressure response of the internal anal sphincter to distention of the balloon. A normal response is relaxation of the internal sphincter, followed by a contraction of the external sphincter. In HD the external sphincter contracts normally but the internal sphincter fails to relax.

Therapeutic Management

The majority of children with HD require surgery rather than medical therapy. One of three operative procedures is performed: a Soave pull-through, the Swenson procedure, and the Duhamel procedure (Maqbool & Liacouras, 2020a). Once the child is stabilized with fluid and electrolyte replacement and colonic cleansing with enemas, if needed, surgery is performed, usually with a high rate of success. Surgical management consists primarily of the removal of the aganglionic portion of the bowel to relieve obstruction, restore normal motility, and preserve the function of the external anal sphincter. The transanal Soave endorectal pull-through procedure consists of pulling the end of the normal bowel through the muscular sleeve of the rectum, from which the aganglionic mucosa has been removed. With earlier diagnosis the proximal bowel may not be extremely distended, thus allowing for a primary pull-through or one-stage procedure and eliminating the need for a temporary colostomy. Simpler operations, such as an anorectal myomectomy, may be indicated in very short-segment disease.

After the pull-through procedure, the majority of children achieve fecal continence. However, some children may experience anal stricture, recurrent enterocolitis, prolapse, or perianal abscess, and incontinence may occur and require further therapy, including dilations or bowel retraining therapy (Maqbool & Liacouras, 2020a).

Nursing Care Management

The nursing concerns depend on the child's age and the type of treatment. If the disorder is diagnosed during the neonatal period, the main objectives are to help the parents adjust to a congenital defect in their child, foster infant-parent bonding, prepare the parents for the medical-surgical intervention, and prepare the parents to assume the care of the child after surgery.

The child's preoperative care depends on the age and clinical condition. A child who is malnourished may not be able to withstand surgery until his or her physical status improves. Often this involves symptomatic treatment with enemas and a low-fiber, high-calorie, high-protein diet. Physical preoperative preparation includes the same measures that are common to any surgery. (See Chapter 20, Surgical Procedures.) In the newborn, whose bowel is presumed sterile, no additional preparation is necessary. However, in other children, preparation for the pull-through procedure involves emptying the bowel with repeated saline enemas and decreasing bacterial flora with oral or systemic antibiotics and colonic irrigations using antibiotic solution. Enterocolitis is the most serious complication of HD. Emergent preoperative care includes frequent monitoring of vital signs and blood pressure for signs of shock; monitoring fluid and electrolyte replacements, as well as plasma or other blood derivatives; and observing for symptoms of bowel perforation, such as fever, increasing abdominal distention, vomiting, increased tenderness, irritability, dyspnea, and cyanosis.

Because progressive distention of the abdomen is a serious sign, the nurse measures abdominal circumference with a paper tape measure, usually at the level of the umbilicus or at the widest part of the abdomen. The point of measurement is marked with a pen to ensure reliability of subsequent measurements. Abdominal measurement can be obtained with the vital sign measurements and is recorded in serial order so that any change is obvious. To reduce stress to the acutely ill child when frequent measurements of abdominal circumference are needed, the tape measure can be left in place beneath the child rather than removed each time.

Postoperative care is the same as that for any child or infant with abdominal surgery. (See Chapter 20, Surgical Procedures.) The nurse involves the parents in the care of the child, allowing them to help with feedings and observe for signs of wound infection or irregular passage of stool. After surgery, parents need instruction concerning the development of complications such as enterocolitis, fecal incontinence, and obstruction. Some children will require daily anal dilations in the postoperative period to avoid anastomotic strictures; parents are often taught to perform the procedure in the home and will need encouragement and detailed instructions to perform these dilations. Although less common, a diverting colostomy may be performed in some children with HD. Parents are taught how to care for the colostomy and how to provide meticulous skin care to prevent skin breakdown; the assistance of a wound and skin care specialist is essential for optimal follow-up and consistent skin care.

Parents may need to bring the child with an ostomy to an outpatient clinic for support, encouragement, and additional instructions on skin and ostomy care after the child is discharged. In general, the prognosis for the infant or child with HD is positive, and most live a normal life. In a few cases, problems with fecal incontinence may persist. A long-term study of children with HD for 1 to 19 years reported satisfying bowel control among 53% of the sample, soiling with 13%, constipation among 6%, and abdominal distention with 26% (Muller, Rossignol, Montalva, et al., 2016).

GASTROESOPHAGEAL REFLUX

Gastroesophageal reflux (GER) is defined as the transfer of gastric contents into the esophagus. This phenomenon is physiologic, occurring throughout the day, most frequently after meals and at night; therefore it is important to differentiate GER from **gastroesophageal reflux disease (GERD)**. GERD represents symptoms or tissue damage that results from GER. The peak incidence of GER occurs at 4 months of age, and GER generally resolves spontaneously in most infants by 1 year of age (Mousa & Hassan, 2017). GER becomes a disease when complications such as failure to thrive, respiratory problems, or dysphagia develop.

Certain conditions predispose children to a high prevalence of GERD, including neurologic impairment, chronic respiratory disorders, esophageal atresia, and obesity (Mousa & Hassan, 2017). Family clustering has also been identified; therefore a genetic predisposition to GERD is also likely (Khan & Matta, 2020a). Sandifer syndrome is an uncommon condition, usually occurring in young children, that is characterized by repetitive stretching and arching of the head and neck that

BOX 22.3 Clinical Manifestations and Complications of Gastroesophageal Reflux

Symptoms in Infants

Spitting up, regurgitation, recurrent vomiting (may be forceful)
Excessive crying, irritability, arching of the back, stiffening
Poor weight gain
Respiratory problems (e.g., cough, wheeze, stridor, gagging, choking with feedings)
Feeding refusal

Symptoms in Children

Heartburn
Abdominal pain
Chronic cough, hoarse voice
Dysphagia
Asthma
Recurrent vomiting

Complications

Esophagitis
Esophageal stricture
Laryngitis
Recurrent pneumonia
Anemia
Barrett esophagus

Adapted from Lightdale, J. R., Gremse, D. A., & Section on Gastroenterology, Hepatology, and Nutrition. (2013). Gastroesophageal reflux: Management guidance for the pediatrician. *Pediatrics, 131*(5), e1684–e1695.

can be mistaken for a seizure. This maneuver likely represents a physiologic neuromuscular response attempting to prevent acid refluxate from reaching the upper portion of the esophagus (Khan & Matta, 2020a).

Infants who are prone to develop GER include premature infants and infants with bronchopulmonary dysplasia. Children who have had tracheoesophageal or esophageal atresia repairs, neurologic disorders, scoliosis, asthma, cystic fibrosis, or cerebral palsy are also prone to develop GER.

Pathophysiology

Although the pathogenesis of GER is multifactorial, its primary causative mechanism likely involves inappropriate transient relaxation of the lower esophageal sphincter (LES). Factors that increase abdominal pressure (e.g., coughing and sneezing, scoliosis, overeating) may contribute to GER. Esophageal symptoms are caused by inflammation from the acid in the gastric refluxate, whereas reactive airway disease may result from stimulation of airway reflexes by the acid refluxate.

Clinical Manifestations

During infancy the most common clinical manifestation of GER is passive regurgitation. Regurgitation generally resolves spontaneously in most infants by 12 months of age and in almost all infants by 24 months of age (Khan & Matta, 2020a). Clinical manifestations of GER are listed in Box 22.3. GER is one of the causes of apparent life-threatening events and has also been associated with chronic respiratory disorders, including reactive airway disease, recurrent stridor, chronic cough, and recurrent pneumonia in infants. Esophagitis can also cause discomfort in the chest area, which may be manifested as unusual irritability or poor intake of nutrients. Poor weight gain and poor growth may occur in a child with an insufficient intake of nutrients or with a large amount of regurgitation.

In preschool children, GER may occur with intermittent vomiting. Older children tend to initially come to the physician with a more adult-like pattern of heartburn, regurgitation, and reswallowing. GERD may cause severe inflammation, chronic blood loss with anemia and hematemesis, hypoproteinemia, or melena. If the inflammation goes untreated, scarring and strictures may form. Barrett mucosa, another potential finding in the presence of chronic inflammation, is characterized by changes in the distal esophageal mucosa with metaplastic, potentially malignant epithelium.

GER is common in children with asthma, but recurrent pneumonia caused by GER is uncommon except in children with neurologic impairments. Hoarseness has also been associated with GER in children.

Diagnostic Evaluation

The history and physical examination are usually sufficiently reliable to establish the diagnosis of GER. Standardized questionnaires, such as the Infant Gastroesophageal Reflux Questionnaire, are commonly used to assist with the diagnosis (Khan & Matta, 2020a). An upper GI series is helpful in evaluating the presence of anatomic abnormalities (e.g., pyloric stenosis, malrotation, annular pancreas, hiatal hernia, esophageal stricture). The 24-hour intraesophageal pH monitoring study was the gold standard in the diagnosis of GER; however, this test is a poor detector of weakly acidic (pH 4 to 7) reflux, which is prevalent in infants and children (Mousa & Hassan, 2017). Endoscopy with biopsy may be helpful to assess the presence and severity of esophagitis, strictures, and Barrett esophagus and to exclude other disorders such as Crohn disease. Scintigraphy detects radioactive substances in the esophagus after a feeding of the compound and assesses gastric emptying. It can differentiate between aspiration of gastric contents from reflux and aspiration from poor oropharyngeal muscle coordination.

Therapeutic Management

Therapeutic management of GER depends on its severity. No therapy is needed for the infant who is thriving and has no respiratory complications. Avoidance of certain foods that exacerbate acid reflux (e.g., caffeine, citrus, tomatoes, alcohol, peppermint, spicy or fried foods) can improve mild GER symptoms. Lifestyle modifications in children (e.g., weight control if indicated; small, more frequent meals) and feeding maneuvers in infants (e.g., thickened feedings; upright positioning) can help as well.

Feedings thickened with 1 teaspoon to 1 tablespoon of rice cereal per ounce of formula may be recommended. This may benefit infants who are underweight as a result of GERD; however, the additional calories are not beneficial among infants who are overweight. These infants may benefit from prethickened formulas that are now commercially available. Constant NG feedings may be necessary for the infant with severe reflux and failure to thrive until surgery can be performed. Elevating the head of the bed and weight loss, if applicable, can reduce GER symptoms. Prone positioning of infants also decreases episodes of GER; however, due to the risk of sudden infant death syndrome, all infants should sleep in the supine position (Khan & Matta, 2020a). The American Academy of Pediatrics continues to recommend supine positioning for sleep (see Chapter 8).

Pharmacologic therapy may be used to treat infants and children with GERD. Both histamine (H_2)–receptor antagonists (ranitidine [Zantac] or famotidine [Pepcid]) and proton pump inhibitors (PPIs; esomeprazole [Nexium], lansoprazole [Prevacid], omeprazole [Prilosec], pantoprazole [Protonix], and rabeprazole [Aciphex]) reduce gastric hydrochloric acid secretion and may stimulate some increase in the lower esophageal sphincter tone. Use of metoclopramide for GERD in infants and children is no longer recommended

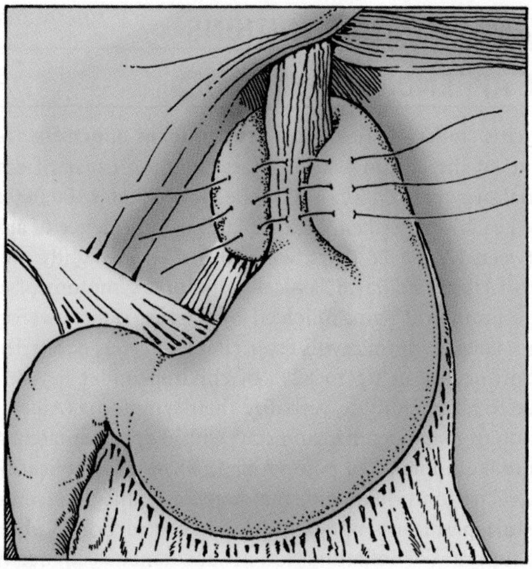

Fig. 22.3 Nissen fundoplication sutures passing through esophageal musculature. (Redrawn from Campbell, A., & Ferrara, B. [1993]. Toupet partial fundoplication. *AORN Journal, 57,* 671–679.)

due to the common incidence of side effects without significant benefit (Cohen, Bueno de Mesquita, & Mimouni, 2015).

Surgical management of GER is reserved for children with severe complications such as recurrent aspiration pneumonia, apnea, severe esophagitis, or failure to thrive and for children who have failed to respond to medical therapy. The **fundoplication** (Fig. 22.3) is a common surgical procedure for the treatment of GERD in children who have failed medical therapy or have life-threatening complications of GERD (Mousa & Hassan, 2017). This surgery involves passage of the gastric fundus behind the esophagus to encircle (i.e., wrap) the distal esophagus. Complications after fundoplication include a wrap that is too tight, causing dysphagia, small bowel obstruction, or gas-bloat; or a wrap that is too loose, causing continuation of symptoms (Khan & Matta, 2020a).

Prognosis

The majority of infants with GER have a mild problem that generally improves by 12 to 18 months of age and requires only conservative lifestyle changes or medical therapy. If GER is severe and remains unsuccessfully treated, multiple complications can occur. Esophageal strictures caused by persistent esophagitis with scarring are one of the most significant complications. Recurrent respiratory distress with aspiration pneumonia, another serious complication, is an indication for surgery. Failure to thrive caused by GER can often be managed with medical therapy and nutritional support. (See Quality Patient Outcomes box.)

QUALITY PATIENT OUTCOMES: Gastroesophageal Reflux

- Adequate weight gain
- Limited spitting up or vomiting
- Good sleep habits
- No recurrent pneumonias

Nursing Care Management

Nursing care is directed at identifying children with symptoms suggestive of GER; educating parents on home care, including feeding, positioning, and medications when indicated; and caring for the child undergoing surgical intervention. For the majority of infants, parental reassurance of the benign nature of the condition and its relationship to physiologic maturity is the most important intervention. To help parents cope with the inconvenience of dealing with a child who spits up or regurgitates frequently, simple tips such as using bibs and protective clothes during feeding and prone positioning when holding the infant after feeding are beneficial.

It is important to educate and reassure parents about positioning. In the past, recommendations encouraged upright positioning during sleeping for both infants and older children. The supine position for sleeping continues to be the recommended infant sleeping position. Parents should not place infants on their sides as an alternative to fully supine sleeping, and avoidance of soft bedding and soft objects in the bed is important. Rescheduling of the family's routine may be required to accommodate more frequent feeding times. If parents use thickened formula, they should also enlarge the nipple opening for easier sucking. Usually breastfeeding may continue, and the mother may provide more frequent feeding times or express the milk for thickening with rice cereal. Parents should avoid feeding the child spicy foods or any foods that they find aggravate symptoms in general and should avoid caffeine, chocolate, tobacco smoke, and alcohol when breastfeeding. Other practical advice includes advising the parents to avoid vigorous play after feedings and to avoid feeding just before bedtime.

When regurgitation is severe and growth is a problem, continuous NG tube feedings may decrease the amount of emesis and provide constant buffering of gastric acid. Special preparation of caregivers is required when this type of nutritional therapy is indicated.

The nurse can support the family by providing information about all aspects of treatment. Parents often require specific information about the medications given for GER. PPIs are most effective when administered 30 minutes before breakfast so that the peak plasma concentrations occur with mealtimes. If they are given twice a day, the second best time for administration is 30 minutes before the evening meal. Parents need to be reassured because it takes several days of administration to achieve a steady state of acid suppression. They may not see the results that they expect right away. A number of formulations available in PPIs allow for more efficient administration. Some preparations are available in dissolvable pills. There are powder and granule preparations as well. Many pharmacies will compound the medication in a liquid form for administration.

Postoperative nursing care after the Nissen fundoplication is similar to that for other types of abdominal surgery (see Chapter 20, Surgical Procedures). Gastric decompression by an NG tube or gastrostomy must be maintained to avoid distention in the immediate postoperative period. Usually the NG tube should not be replaced by the nurse if it is accidentally removed because of the risk of injury to the operative site. When postoperative ileus resolves, the NG tube is removed or the gastrostomy tube is elevated in preparation for feeding. If bolus feedings are initiated through the gastrostomy, the tube may need to remain vented for several days or longer to avoid gastric distention from swallowed air. Edema surrounding the surgical site and a tight gastric wrap may prohibit the infant from expelling air through the esophagus. Some infants benefit from clamping of the tube for increasingly longer intervals until they are able to tolerate continuous clamping between feedings. During this time, if the infant displays increasing irritability and evidence of cramping, some relief may be provided by venting the tube.

Preparation for Home Care

If medical management is prescribed or surgery is performed, nursing responsibilities include educating caregivers about administering drugs at home, special feeding regimens or formula preparation, gastrostomy care, and postoperative care (see Chapter 20). After surgery, reflux is completely controlled in most cases, with these children attaining normal health and growth. If a gastrostomy tube is inserted during surgery, it may be removed after several months unless nutritional supplementation is needed. In severe cases of bloating or dumping syndrome, continuous tube feedings may be better tolerated. Caregivers should be aware of potential postoperative problems, such as difficulty vomiting, bloating symptoms, or discomfort with large solid-food meals, and seek guidance from their health care provider as needed.

IRRITABLE BOWEL SYNDROME

Irritable bowel syndrome (IBS) is classified as a functional GI disorder. IBS occurs more frequently in adolescents than in children, 22% to 35% versus 6% to 14%, respectively (Giannetti, Maglione, Sciorio, et al., 2017). Children with IBS often have alternating diarrhea and constipation, flatulence, bloating or a feeling of abdominal distention, lower abdominal pain, a feeling of urgency when needing to defecate, and a feeling of incomplete evacuation of the bowel. Abdominal pain should be present for at least 4 days per month over the last 2 months, plus there should be a change in either frequency or appearance of stool (Chopra, Patel, Basude, et al., 2017). IBS has been identified as a cause of recurrent abdominal pain in 68% of children (Giannetti et al., 2017).

The cause of IBS is not clear, but it is believed to involve a combination of genetic and environmental factors. Strong predictors for the development of IBS in a child include having a mother, father, or twin with IBS (Kridler & Kamat, 2016). In addition, children with IBS have been noted to be less confident in their ability to deal with daily stress and have higher prevalence of anxiety, depression, introverted personalities, and difficulty sleeping (Kridler & Kamat, 2016). The intestinal microbiome is the focus of IBS research to evaluate whether inflammation may trigger nerves in the gut to cause IBS symptoms (Chopra et al., 2017; Kridler & Kamat, 2016).

Children with IBS are evaluated to rule out organic causes for their symptoms, such as IBD, lactose intolerance, and parasitic infections. A comprehensive history is obtained, including features and triggers of the symptoms, as well as associated symptoms such as headaches, recent infections, diet history, family history, and social history. Typically there are no abnormal physical findings on examination. Many children with symptoms appear active and healthy and have normal growth.

Therapeutic Management

There is no cure for IBS, so management involves controlling the child's symptoms. The long-range goal of treatment is development of regular bowel habits and relief of symptoms. Management depends on whether IBS is constipation or diarrhea predominant. Constipation-predominant IBS is managed by increasing fiber with diet changes and supplements, whereas diarrhea-predominant IBS is managed with diet changes, PPIs, and loperamide (Chopra et al., 2017; Kridler & Kamat, 2016). A recent Cochrane systematic review found evidence suggesting that probiotics are effective in relieving recurrent abdominal pain (Newlove-Delgado, Martin, Abbott, et al., 2017).

Psychosocial interventions, including cognitive-behavioral therapy and hypnotherapy, can decrease abdominal pain in children (Abbott, Martin, Newlove-Delgado, et al., 2017; Chopra et al., 2017). Cognitive-behavioral therapy provides stress management and coping skills that may lessen IBS symptoms.

Nursing Care Management

The primary nursing goal is family support and education. The disorder is stressful to children and parents. The nurse can help by providing support and reassurance that, although the symptoms are difficult to deal with, the disorder is not generally a threat to the child's health.

INFLAMMATORY CONDITIONS

ACUTE APPENDICITIS

Appendicitis, inflammation of the **vermiform appendix** (blind sac at the end of the cecum), is the most common cause of emergency abdominal surgery in childhood. In the United States 100,000 cases are diagnosed each year (Aiken, 2020a). The peak incidence of appendicitis is between 12 and 18 years, with boys affected slightly more often than girls (Aiken, 2020a). Classically, the first symptom of appendicitis is periumbilical pain, followed by nausea, right lower quadrant pain, and, later, vomiting with fever (Rentea, Peter, & Snyder, 2017). Perforation occurs in up to 82% of children under 5 years of age, likely due to an inability to verbalize their symptoms (Aiken, 2020a). Perforation of the appendix can occur within approximately 48 hours of the initial complaint of pain (Aiken, 2020a). Complications from appendiceal perforation include major abscess, phlegmon, enterocutaneous fistula, peritonitis, and partial bowel obstruction. A **phlegmon** is an acute suppurative inflammation of subcutaneous connective tissue that spreads.

Etiology

The cause of appendicitis is obstruction of the lumen of the appendix, usually by hardened fecal material (fecalith). Swollen lymphoid tissue, frequently occurring after a viral infection, can also obstruct the appendix. Another rare cause of obstruction is a parasite such as *Enterobius vermicularis,* or pinworms, which can obstruct the appendiceal lumen.

Pathophysiology

With acute obstruction, the outflow of mucus secretions is blocked and pressure builds within the lumen, resulting in compression of blood vessels. The resulting ischemia is followed by ulceration of the epithelial lining and bacterial invasion. Subsequent necrosis causes perforation or rupture with fecal and bacterial contamination of the peritoneal cavity. The resulting inflammation spreads rapidly throughout the abdomen (**peritonitis**), especially in young children, who are unable to localize infection. Progressive peritoneal inflammation results in functional intestinal obstruction of the small bowel (**ileus**) because intense GI reflexes severely inhibit bowel motility. Because the peritoneum represents a major portion of total body surface, the loss of ECF to the peritoneal cavity leads to electrolyte imbalance and hypovolemic shock.

Clinical Manifestations

The first symptom of appendicitis is usually colicky, cramping, abdominal pain located around the umbilicus (Box 22.4). **Referred pain** is the term used for this vague periumbilical localization. The midgut shares the same T10 dermatome, so pain is often perceived to be coming from this area. Generally, this pain progresses and becomes constant. The most important physical finding is focal abdominal tenderness. As the inflammation progresses to involve the serosa of the appendix and the peritoneum of the abdominal wall, the pain may shift to the right lower quadrant. The **McBurney point**, located two-thirds the distance along a line between the umbilicus and the anterosuperior iliac spine, is the most common point of tenderness. Localized peritoneal signs may occur with gentle percussion or maneuvers such as heel strike or shaking the bed. Other helpful findings are Rovsing sign, tenderness in the right lower quadrant that occurs during palpation or percussion of other abdominal quadrants; obturator sign, pain with flexion and internal rotation of the right hip; psoas sign, pain on the left side with right hip extension; and Dunphy sign, pain with coughing (Rentea et al., 2017). Rebound tenderness—pain on deep palpation

BOX 22.4 Clinical Manifestations of Appendicitis

- Right lower quadrant abdominal pain
- Fever
- Rigid abdomen
- Decreased or absent bowel sounds
- Vomiting (typically follows onset of pain)
- Constipation or diarrhea
- Anorexia
- Tachycardia
- Rapid, shallow breathing
- Pallor
- Lethargy
- Irritability
- Stooped posture

with sudden release—may be present, but it is not a finding specific to appendicitis (Aiken, 2020a). Nausea, vomiting, and anorexia typically occur after the pain starts. Diarrhea, as well as other common signs of childhood illness such as upper respiratory tract congestion, poor feeding, lethargy, or irritability, may accompany appendicitis.

The child may not be able to walk well and may complain of pain in the right hip caused by inflammation in the psoas or iliopsoas muscles. Low-grade fever (38°C [100.4°F]) may occur with the initial presentation; however, the absence of fever does not exclude appendicitis. Because of the great variability in the presentation and location of appendicitis, any child with focal tenderness, regardless of the location, should be considered to potentially have acute appendicitis (see Community Focus box).

COMMUNITY FOCUS

Acute Appendicitis

Abdominal pain is a common complaint among school-age children, but in some cases it may indicate acute appendicitis. School nurses and nurse practitioners in school-based clinics should become familiar with the "typical" pattern of symptoms in acute appendicitis and how to assess and evaluate an acute abdomen. School nurses also need to impress on teachers and coaches the importance of early referral to the health suite for further assessment. Early referral to the health suite and an alert school nurse or nurse practitioner may make the difference between an uncomplicated appendectomy and a delayed diagnosis of a perforated appendix with peritonitis.

! NURSING ALERT

Signs of peritonitis in addition to fever usually include sudden relief from pain after perforation; subsequent increase in pain, which is usually diffuse and accompanied by rigid guarding of the abdomen; progressive abdominal distention; tachycardia; rapid, shallow breathing as the child refrains from using abdominal muscles; pallor; chills; irritability; and restlessness.

Diagnostic Evaluation

Diagnosis is not always straightforward. Fever, vomiting, abdominal pain, and an elevated white blood cell count are associated with appendicitis but are also seen in IBD, pelvic inflammatory disease, gastroenteritis, urinary tract infection, right lower lobe pneumonia, mesenteric adenitis, Meckel diverticulum, and intussusception. Prolonged symptoms and delayed diagnosis often occur in younger children, in whom the risk of perforation is greatest because of their inability to verbalize their complaints.

The diagnosis is based primarily on the history and physical examination (see Box 22.4). Pain, the cardinal feature, is initially generalized (usually periumbilical). However, it usually descends to the lower right quadrant. The most intense site of pain may be at the McBurney point. Rebound tenderness is not a reliable sign and is extremely painful to the child. Referred pain, elicited by light percussion around the perimeter of the abdomen, indicates peritoneal irritation. Movement, such as riding over bumps in an automobile or gurney, aggravates the pain. In addition to pain, significant clinical manifestations include fever, a change in behavior, anorexia, and vomiting.

Laboratory studies usually include a CBC; urinalysis (to rule out a urinary tract infection); and, in adolescent females, serum human chorionic gonadotropin (to rule out an ectopic pregnancy). A white blood cell count greater than $10,000/mm^3$ and an elevated C-reactive protein (CRP) are common but not necessarily specific for appendicitis. An elevated percentage of bands (often referred to as "a left shift") may indicate an inflammatory process. CRP is an acute-phase reactant that rises within 12 hours of the onset of infection. A CRP level greater than 10 mg/mL is a sign of infection.

Ultrasound is the imaging technique of choice in diagnosing appendicitis, although a computed tomography (CT) scan may be used. Ultrasound is considered positive in the presence of enlarged appendiceal diameter; appendiceal wall thickening; and periappendiceal inflammatory changes, including fat streaks, phlegmon, fluid collection, and extraluminal gas (Aiken, 2020a). The accuracy of imaging for diagnosing appendicitis is 95% (Rentea et al., 2017).

Therapeutic Management

The treatment for appendicitis before perforation is surgical removal of the appendix (appendectomy). Usually antibiotics are administered preoperatively. IV fluids and electrolytes are often required before surgery, especially if the child is dehydrated as a result of the marked anorexia characteristic of appendicitis.

The operation is usually performed through a right lower quadrant incision (open appendectomy). Laparoscopic surgery is commonly used to treat nonperforated acute appendicitis in pediatric patients. Three cannulas are inserted in the abdomen: one in the umbilicus, one in the left lower abdominal quadrant, and one in the suprapubic area. A small telescope is inserted through the left lower quadrant cannula, and an endoscopic stapler is inserted through the umbilical cannula. The appendix is ligated with the stapler and removed through the umbilical cannula. Advantages of laparoscopic appendectomy include reduced time in surgery and under anesthesia and reduced risk of postoperative wound infection (Aiken, 2020a).

Ruptured Appendix

Management of the child diagnosed with peritonitis caused by a ruptured appendix often begins preoperatively with IV administration of fluid and electrolytes, systemic antibiotics, and NG suction. Postoperative management includes IV fluids, continued administration of antibiotics, and NG suction for abdominal decompression until intestinal activity returns. Sometimes surgeons close the wound after irrigation of the peritoneal cavity. Other times they leave the wound open (delayed closure) to prevent wound infection.

The treatment of a localized perforation with an appendiceal abscess is controversial. Some surgeons prefer to treat these children with antibiotics and IV fluids and allow the abscess to drain spontaneously. An elective appendectomy is then performed 2 to 3 months later.

Prognosis

Complications are uncommon after a simple appendectomy, and recovery is usually rapid and complete. The mortality rate from perforating appendicitis has improved from nearly certain death a century ago to less than 1% at the present time (Rentea et al., 2017). Complications, however, including wound infection and intra-abdominal abscess, are not uncommon. Early recognition of the illness is important to prevent complications.

! NURSING ALERT

In any instance in which severe abdominal pain is observed, the nurse must be aware of the danger of administering laxatives or enemas. Such measures stimulate bowel motility and increase the risk of perforation.

Nursing Care Management

Because successful treatment of appendicitis is based on prompt recognition of the disorder, an important nursing objective is to assist in establishing a diagnosis. Because abdominal pain is a common childhood complaint, the nurse needs to make some preliminary assessment of the severity of the pain (see Chapter 5). One of the most reliable estimates is the degree of change in behavior. A child who stays home from school and voluntarily lies down or refuses to play is much more likely to have considerable pain than a child who is absent from school but plays contentedly at home. Younger, nonverbal children will assume a rigid, side-lying position with the knees flexed and have decreased range of motion of the right hip.

For nurses involved in primary ambulatory care, the responsibility of recognizing a possible case of appendicitis and prompt medical or surgical referral is particularly important. The importance of a detailed history and thorough abdominal examination cannot be overemphasized. Palpating the abdomen should be delayed until all other assessments have been made. Instruct the child to point with one finger to the site of the abdominal pain. Rebound tenderness may be present but is not always a sufficiently reliable test in children. Light palpation will satisfactorily elicit pain without causing excessive trauma (see Atraumatic Care box). Ask the child with mild pain to lift the heels and drop them to the floor two or three times, to hop on one foot, or to "puff out" or "pull in" the abdomen to check for tenderness without more painful probing. Chapter 4 discusses other techniques for assessment of the abdomen.

ATRAUMATIC CARE

Palpating the Abdomen for Abdominal Pain

Because children associate the stethoscope with listening, use the bell piece for initial palpation of the abdomen for tenderness. Children usually endure pressure from the stethoscope that they would not tolerate from a probing hand. Follow with manual palpation, using a gentle touch without lifting the hand from the abdomen while observing the child's face for signs of discomfort, such as a grimace and watchful eyes on the examination of the abdomen.

Physical preparation of the child with appendicitis is similar to that for any child undergoing surgery (see Chapter 20, Surgical Procedures). In situations in which medical treatment is required to correct problems associated with peritonitis, the nurse must anticipate procedures and set up equipment as quickly as possible to avoid any delay in preparing the child for surgery. Psychologic preparation of the child and parents is similar to that used in other emergency situations (see Chapter 20).

Postoperative care for the nonperforated appendix is the same as for most abdominal operations. Care of the child with a ruptured appendix and peritonitis is more complex. The child may need to remain in the hospital for several days or may be discharged with home care services to provide IV antibiotics and dressing changes.

Postoperatively the child is maintained on IV fluids and antibiotics and is allowed nothing by mouth (NPO). The child also remains on low, intermittent gastric decompression until there is evidence of return of intestinal motility. Listening for bowel sounds and observing for other signs of bowel activity (such as passage of stool) are part of the routine assessment.

A drain may be placed in the wound during surgery, and frequent dressing changes with meticulous skin care are essential to prevent excoriation of the surgery area. If the wound is left open, moist dressings (usually saline-soaked gauze) and wound irrigations with antibacterial solution are used to provide an optimum healing environment.

Pain management is an essential part of the child's care. Not only is the incision painful, but the repeated dressing changes and irrigations also cause considerable distress. Because pain is continuous during the first few postoperative days, analgesics are given regularly to control pain. Procedures are performed when the analgesics are at peak effect. (See Chapter 5.)

Psychosocial care after surgery is also important. Sudden, acute illnesses cause unique stress because there is little time for preparation or planning. Parents and older children need an opportunity to express their feelings and concerns regarding the events surrounding the illness and hospitalization. The nurse can provide important education and psychosocial support to promote adequate coping, with alleviation of anxiety for both the child and the family (see Next-Generation NCLEX® Examination-Style Unfolding Case Study box).

MECKEL DIVERTICULUM

Meckel diverticulum is a remnant of the fetal omphalomesenteric duct, which connects the yolk sac with the primitive midgut during fetal life (Maqbool & Liacouras, 2020d). Normally the structure is obliterated between the fifth and seventh week of gestation, when the placenta replaces the yolk sac as the source of nutrition for the fetus. Failure of obliteration may result in an omphalomesenteric fistula (a fibrous band connecting the small intestine to the umbilicus), umbilical cyst, vitelline duct remnant, mesodiverticular bands, and Meckel diverticula (Bagade & Khanna, 2015).

Meckel diverticulum is a true diverticulum because it arises from the antimesenteric border of the small intestine and includes all layers of the intestinal wall. Meckel diverticulum is often referred to by the "rule of 2s" because it occurs in 2% of the population, has a 2:1 male-to-female ratio, is located within 2 feet of the ileocecal valve, is commonly 2 cm in diameter and 2 inches in length, contains 2 types of ectopic tissue (pancreatic and gastric), and is more common before age 2 years (Maqbool & Liacouras, 2020d).

Pathophysiology

Bleeding, obstruction, or inflammation causes the symptomatic complications of Meckel diverticulum (Lin, Huang, Bao, et al., 2017). Bleeding, which is the most common problem in children, is caused by peptic ulceration or perforation because of the unbuffered acidic secretion. Several mechanisms may cause obstruction, such as intussusception or entanglement of the small intestine.

NEXT-GENERATION NCLEX® EXAMINATION-STYLE UNFOLDING CASE STUDY

The Child With Appendicitis

Day 1, 11:00 am

1. A 10-year-old girl has a 2-day history of generalized periumbilical pain and anorexia. Today she developed a fever and vomiting, so her parents took her to the clinic. On review of the history, physical examination, and laboratory results, the nurse notes the findings below. Select findings that require follow-up by the nurse. **Select all that apply.**
   A. Weight 70lb (32kg)
   B. Hemoglobin = 13.8 g/dL
   C. Platelets = 252,000/mm^3
   D. C-reactive Protein (CRP) of 40 mg/dL
   E. Pain intensifies with any activity or deep breathing
   F. Oral temperature of 102° F (38.9° C)
   G. Pulse of 80 beats/min and blood pressure is 108/74 mm/Hg
   H. Abdominal pain midway between the anterior superior iliac crest and umbilicus
   I. White blood cell (WBC) count of 21,000/mm^3, 79% bands, 14% lymphocytes, 6% eosinophils
2. Based on the case presented in the question above, **choose the most likely options for the information missing from the statements below by selecting from the lists of options provided.** Based on the child's assessment data, the nurse determines that the laboratory findings reflect the probable presence of ____1____. The ____2____ is elevated and her periumbilical pain, along with other symptoms is most likely due to ____3____.

Options for 1	Options for 2	Options for 3
Anemia	Blood pressure of 108/74	Ruptured kidney
Pain	Pulse of 80	Acute abdomen
Bleeding	CRP	Influenza
Infection	Hemoglobin	Urinary Tract Infection
Heart failure	Platelets	Vomiting
Cancer	Serum sodium	Anxiety

Day 1, 11:30 am

Unfolding Case Continues: A 10-year-old girl who has a 2-day history of generalized periumbilical pain and anorexia. Today she developed a fever and vomiting, so her parents took her to her pediatrician. On review of the history, physical examination, and laboratory results, the nurse notes the following:

- Oral temperature of 102° F (38.9° C)
- Pulse of 80 beats/min and blood pressure is 108/74 mm/Hg
- Abdominal pain midway between the anterior superior iliac crest and umbilicus
- Pain intensifies with any activity or deep breathing
- White blood cell (WBC) count of 21,000/mm^3, 79% bands, 14% lymphocytes, 6% eosinophils
- C-reactive Protein (CRP) of 18 mg/dL
- Hemoglobin = 13.8 g/dL
- Platelets = 252,000/mm^3
- Weight 70lb (32kg)

3. The pediatrician examines the child and highly suspects appendicitis. A CT scan of the abdomen has been prescribed and the child is placed on NPO status. When planning care for this child, which **priority** symptoms would the nurse consider most immediate at this time? **Select all that apply.**
   A. Pain
   B. Anemia
   C. Infection
   D. Vomiting
   E. Weight loss
   F. Dehydration
   G. Constipation
   H. Hyperthermia
   I. Rupture of the appendix

Unfolding Case Continues: A 10-year-old girl who has a 2-day history of generalized periumbilical pain and anorexia. Today she developed a fever and vomiting, so her parents took her to her pediatrician. On review of the history, physical examination, and laboratory results, the nurse notes the following:

- Oral temperature of 102° F (38.9° C)
- Pulse of 80 beats/min and blood pressure is 108/74 mm/Hg
- Abdominal pain midway between the anterior superior iliac crest and umbilicus
- Pain intensifies with any activity or deep breathing
- White blood cell (WBC) count of 21,000/mm^3, 79% bands, 14% lymphocytes, 6% eosinophils
- C-reactive Protein (CRP) of 18 mg/dL
- Hemoglobin = 13.8 g/dL
- Platelets = 252,000/mm^3
- Weight 70lb (32kg)

Day 1, 12:00 noon

Results of the CT scan demonstrate a ruptured appendix. The child is being prepared for surgery. The nurse performing the assessment finds her temperature is 102° F (38.9° C). The child reports that the pain had initially resolved but now reports increasing pain (rated 9 out of 10 on a 1 to 10 pain intensity scale) and nausea.

Day 1, 2:00 pm

The child undergoes surgery for an appendectomy. She is transferred to the pediatric unit from the recovery room and the nurse plans care.

4. Indicate which nursing action listed in the far-left column is appropriate for the potential postoperative complication following appendectomy listed in the middle column. **Indicate the nursing action number in the far-right column. Note that ONLY one nursing action can be used for each potential postoperative complication and that NOT all nursing actions will be used.**

Nursing Action	Potential Postoperative Complication	Nursing Action for Postoperative Complication
1. Administer pain medications	Inflammation at the wound site	
2. Initiate IV fluids and assess intake and output (I&O)	Electrolyte imbalance	
3. Assess temperature and report elevation	Fluid deficit	
4. Administer antiemetics	Pain	
5. Administer IV sodium heparin	Nausea and vomiting	
6. Draw blood as scheduled and evaluate results	Infection	
7. Report changes in vital signs, behavior and level of consciousness	Fever	
8. Administer IV antibiotics		
9. Administer a blood transfusion		
10. Observe wound site		

Continued

NEXT-GENERATION NCLEX® EXAMINATION-STYLE UNFOLDING CASE STUDY—cont'd

Day 3, 9:00 am Unfolding Case Continues

5. The child is recovering well following surgery. The nurse performing the assessment finds her oral temperature is 98.6° F (37° C). The child reports that the pain is a 1 out of 10 on a 10 point pain intensity scale). She has no nausea or vomiting. **For each nursing action, use an X to indicate whether it was Effective (helped to meet expected quality patient outcomes), Ineffective (did not help to meet expected quality patient outcomes), or Unrelated (not related to the quality patient outcomes).**

Nursing Action	Effective	Ineffective	Unrelated
Observe no signs of infection.			
Pain is controlled.			
Referral is made to a physical therapist.			
No complaints of nausea or vomiting and a regular diet is tolerated.			
No complaints of headaches.			
Temperature remains in the normal range			
Child spending all of the time in bed.			

Day 5, 10:00 am Unfolding Case Continues

6. The child has recovered and is ready for discharge and the nurse is providing essential education to the parents and child for care at home. **Use an X for the health teaching statement below that is Indicated (appropriate or necessary), Contraindicated (could be harmful), or Non-Essential (makes no difference or not necessary).**

Health Teaching	Indicated	Contraindicated	Non-Essential
"Take your child's temperature if she feels warm and call the surgeon if she has a fever over 101° F"			
"Give ibuprofen every 6 hours for the next 5 days."			
"Sit beside her all day and watch her favorite movies."			
"Inspect the surgical incision every day for increased redness, heat, or drainage; if present call the surgeon immediately."			
Ask the parents, "What are your concerns regarding your daughter's care at home?"			
"Apply a topical antibiotic to the surgical wound for the next week."			

Clinical Manifestations

Signs and symptoms are based on the specific pathologic process, such as inflammation, bleeding, or intestinal obstruction (Box 22.5). The most common clinical presentation is rectal bleeding caused by ulceration at the junction of the ectopic gastric mucosa and normal ileal mucosa. The bleeding is usually painless and may be dramatic and occur as bright red or currant jelly–like stools, or it may occur intermittently and appear as tarry stools. The bleeding may be significant enough to cause hypotension. Volvulus and intussusception are common obstructive mechanisms in children with Meckel diverticulum, and these children present with symptoms of abdominal pain, distention, nausea, and vomiting (Maqbool & Liacouras, 2020d).

Diagnostic Evaluation

Diagnosis is usually based on the history, physical examination, and radiographic studies. Meckel diverticulum is often a diagnostic challenge. A technetium-99m pertechnetate scan (Meckel scan) is the most effective diagnostic testing, especially for a bleeding diverticulum, with sensitivity ranging from 80% to 90% and a specificity of 95% (Lin et al., 2017). Laboratory studies such as a CBC and a basic metabolic panel are usually part of the general workup to rule out any bleeding disorder and to evaluate for dehydration.

Therapeutic Management

The standard treatment for symptomatic Meckel diverticulum is surgical removal. In instances in which severe hemorrhage increases the

BOX 22.5 Clinical Manifestations of Meckel Diverticulum

Abdominal Pain
Similar to appendicitis
May be vague and recurrent

Bloody Stools[a]
Painless
Bright or dark red with mucus (currant jelly–like stool)
In infants, bleeding sometimes accompanied by pain

Occasional
Severe anemia
Shock

[a]Often a presenting sign.

surgical risk, medical intervention to correct hypovolemic shock (e.g., blood replacement, IV fluids, oxygen) may be necessary. Antibiotics may be used preoperatively to control infection. If intestinal obstruction has occurred, appropriate preoperative measures are used to correct fluid and electrolyte imbalances and prevent abdominal distention.

Prognosis

If symptomatic Meckel diverticulum is diagnosed and treated early, full recovery is likely. Because of the potential for surgical complications, resection of asymptomatic Meckel diverticulum remains controversial.

Nursing Care Management

Nursing objectives are the same as for any child undergoing surgery (see Chapter 20, Surgical Procedures). When intestinal bleeding is present, specific preoperative considerations include frequent monitoring of vital signs and blood pressure, keeping the child on bed rest, and recording the approximate amount of blood lost in stools.

Postoperatively the child requires IV fluids and an NG tube for decompression and evacuation of gastric secretions. Because the onset of illness is usually rapid, psychologic support is important, as in other acute conditions, such as appendicitis. It is important to remember that massive rectal bleeding is usually traumatic to both the child and the parents and may significantly affect their emotional reaction to hospitalization and surgery.

INFLAMMATORY BOWEL DISEASE

Inflammatory bowel disease (IBD) should not be confused with IBS. *IBD* is a term used to refer to three major forms of chronic intestinal inflammation: Crohn disease (CD), ulcerative colitis (UC), and inflammatory bowel disease unspecified (IBDU). CD and UC have similar epidemiologic, immunologic, and clinical features, but they are distinct disorders. The diagnosis of IBDU is used for patients with colonic disease, but whose features are not specific to UC or CD; it is very rare (Conrad & Rosh, 2017).

Approximately 70,000 children in the United States have IBD (Rosen, Dhawan, & Saeed, 2017). Over the past 30 years the incidence of CD has risen, whereas the incidence of UC in children has remained stable (Stein & Baldassano, 2020). Both CD and UC tend to be more aggressive if the onset occurs in childhood (Conrad & Rosh, 2017). Exacerbations and remissions without complete resolution of symptoms are also characteristics of IBD.

Etiology

Despite decades of research, the etiology of IBD is not completely understood, and there is no known cure. There is evidence to indicate a multifactorial etiology. Genetic, environmental, and microbial factors are associated with IBD, and research focuses on genetic associations and theories of defective immunoregulation of the inflammatory response to bacteria or viruses in the GI tract (Rosen et al., 2017). Genome-wide studies have confirmed at least 150 genes that increase the risk for IBD in individuals (Rosen et al., 2017). Furthermore, children who immigrate from developing countries to Western countries show an incidence of IBD similar to that of Western populations, confirming an environmental factor with the disease (Rosen et al., 2017). Finally, most individuals have 10 trillion bacteria and fungi in their intestinal microbiome, but children and adults with IBD have small diversity of intestinal bacterial species with an overrepresentation and underrepresentation of some species (Rosen et al., 2017).

Pathophysiology

The inflammation found with UC is limited to the colon and rectum, with the distal colon and rectum the most severely affected. Inflammation affects the mucosa and submucosa and involves continuous segments along the length of the bowel with varying degrees of ulceration, bleeding, and edema. Thickening of the bowel wall and fibrosis are unusual, but long-standing disease can result in shortening of the colon and strictures. Toxic megacolon is the most dangerous form of severe colitis.

The chronic inflammatory process of CD involves any part of the GI tract from the mouth to the anus but most often affects the terminal ileum. The disease involves all layers of the bowel wall (transmural) in a discontinuous fashion, meaning that between areas of intact mucosa there are areas of affected mucosa (skip lesions). The inflammation may result in ulcerations; fibrosis; adhesions; stiffening of the bowel wall; stricture formation; and fistulas to other loops of bowel, bladder, vagina, or skin.

Clinical Signs and Symptoms

Children with UC may experience mild, moderate, or severe symptoms, depending on the extent of mucosal inflammation and systemic symptoms. UC often manifests with the insidious onset of diarrhea, possibly with hematochezia, and usually without fever or weight loss. The course of the disease may remain mild with intermittent exacerbations. Some children and adolescents are seen with grossly bloody diarrhea, cramps, urgency with defecation, mild anemia, fever, anorexia, weight loss, and moderate signs of systemic illness. Severe UC is characterized by frequent bloody stools, abdominal pain, significant anemia, fever, and weight loss. Extraintestinal manifestations are not common in UC. Enlarged lymph nodes (lymphadenopathy), arthritis, and the skin lesions of erythema nodosum may be present.

Common presenting manifestations of CD include diarrhea, abdominal pain with cramps, fever, and weight loss. Extraintestinal manifestations, including aphthous ulcers, peripheral arthritis, erythema nodosum, digital clubbing, renal stones, and gallstones, are more common with CD than UC (Stein & Baldassano, 2020). Growth failure and delayed sexual maturation are often present for several years before overt GI symptoms are present (Conrad & Rosh, 2017). Both malabsorption and anorexia are factors that contribute to the growth problems that are prevalent in CD. Children with CD may have perianal disease, including tags, fissures, fistulas, or abscesses (Rosen et al., 2017). The effects of UC and CD are listed in Table 22.7, which provides a comparison of UC and CD.

Diagnostic Evaluation

The diagnosis of UC and CD comes from the history, physical examination, laboratory evaluation, and other diagnostic procedures.

TABLE 22.7 Comparison of Inflammatory Bowel Diseases

Characteristics	Ulcerative Colitis	Crohn Disease
Rectal bleeding	Common	Uncommon
Diarrhea	Often severe	Moderate to severe
Pain	Less frequent	Common
Anorexia	Mild or moderate	May be severe
Weight loss	Moderate	May be severe
Growth retardation	Usually mild	May be severe
Anal and perianal lesions	Rare	Common
Fistulas and strictures	Rare	Common
Rashes	Mild	Mild
Joint pain	Mild to moderate	Mild to moderate

Laboratory tests include a CBC to evaluate anemia and an erythrocyte sedimentation rate (ESR) or CRP to assess the systemic reaction to the inflammatory process. The ESR or CRP may be elevated, indicating a systemic response to an inflammatory process. Levels of total protein, albumin, iron, zinc, magnesium, vitamin B_{12}, and fat-soluble vitamins may be low in children with CD. Stools are examined for blood, leukocytes, and infectious organisms. A serologic panel is often used in combination with clinical findings to diagnose IBD and to differentiate between CD and UC.

In patients with CD, an upper GI series with small bowel follow-through assists in assessing the existence, location, and extent of disease. Upper endoscopy and colonoscopy with biopsies are an integral part of diagnosing IBD (Rosen et al., 2017). Endoscopy allows direct visualization of the surface of the GI tract so that the extent of inflammation and narrowing can be evaluated. CT and ultrasound also may be used to identify bowel wall inflammation, intra-abdominal abscesses, and fistulas. Colonoscopy can confirm the diagnosis and evaluate the extent of the disease. Discrete ulcers are commonly seen in patients with CD, whereas microulcers and diffuse abnormalities and inflammation are seen in patients with UC (Stein & Baldassano, 2020). CD lesions may pierce the walls of the small intestine and colon, creating tracts called *fistulas* between the intestine and adjacent structures such as the bladder, anus, vagina, or skin.

Therapeutic Management

The natural history of the disease continues to be unpredictable and characterized by recurrent flare-ups that can severely impair patients' physical and social functioning (Stein & Baldassano, 2020). The goals of therapy are to control the inflammatory process to reduce or eliminate the symptoms, obtain long-term remission, promote normal growth and development, and allow as normal a lifestyle as possible. Treatment is individualized and managed according to the type and the severity of the disease, its location, and the response to therapy. CD is more disabling, has more serious complications, and is often less amenable to medical and surgical treatment than is UC. Because UC is confined to the colon, a colectomy may cure UC.

Medical Treatment

The goal of any treatment regimen is first to induce remission of acute symptoms and then to maintain remission over time. 5-Aminosalicylates (5-ASAs) are effective in the induction and maintenance of remission in mild to moderate UC. Mesalamine, olsalazine, and balsalazide are preferred over sulfasalazine because of reduced side effects (e.g., headache, nausea, vomiting, neutropenia, oligospermia). Suppository and enema preparations of mesalamine are used to treat left-sided colitis. These drugs decrease inflammation by inhibiting prostaglandin synthesis. 5-ASAs can be used to induce remission in mild CD.

Corticosteroids, such as prednisone and prednisolone, are indicated in induction therapy in children with moderate to severe UC and CD. These drugs inhibit the production of adhesion molecules, cytokines, and leukotrienes. Although these drugs reduce the acute symptoms of IBD, they are not commonly used for maintenance therapy because of their long-term side effects, including growth suppression (adrenal suppression), weight gain, and decreased bone density (Rosen et al., 2017). High doses of IV corticosteroids may be administered in acute episodes and tapered according to clinical response. Budesonide, a synthetic corticosteroid, is designed for controlled release in the ileum and is indicated for ileal and right-sided colitis; budesonide has fewer side effects than prednisone and prednisolone but is also less effective (Rosen et al., 2017).

Immunomodulators, such as azathioprine and its metabolite 6-mercaptopurine (6-MP), are used to induce and maintain remission in children with IBD who are steroid resistant or steroid dependent and to treat chronic draining fistulas. They block the synthesis of purine, thus inhibiting the ability of deoxyribonucleic acid (DNA) and ribonucleic acid (RNA) to hinder lymphocyte function, especially that of T cells. Side effects include infection, pancreatitis, hepatitis, bone marrow toxicity, arthralgia, and malignancy. Methotrexate is also useful in inducing and maintaining remission in patients with CD who are unresponsive to standard therapies. Cyclosporine and tacrolimus have both been effective in inducing remission in severe steroid-dependent UC. 6-MP or azathioprine is then used to maintain remission. Patients on immunomodulating medications require regular monitoring of their CBC and differential to assess for changes that reflect suppression of the immune system because many of the side effects can be prevented or managed by dose reduction or discontinuation of medication.

Antibiotics, such as metronidazole and ciprofloxacin, may be used as an adjunctive therapy to treat complications such as perianal disease or small bowel bacterial overgrowth in CD. Side effects of these drugs are peripheral neuropathy, nausea, and a metallic taste.

Biologic therapies act to regulate inflammatory and antiinflammatory cytokines. The use of anti–tumor necrosis factor-alpha (anti-TNF-α) agents such as infliximab and adalimumab decrease active inflammation, are effective in healing the intestinal mucosal lining and perianal fistulas, and have even improved linear growth in children (Rosen et al., 2017; Stein & Baldassano, 2020). These agents are now being used as front-line therapy in children with CD who have severe deep mucosal ulcerations, perianal fistulas, or growth failure (Rosen et al., 2017).

Nutritional Support

Nutritional support is important in the treatment of IBD. Growth failure is a common serious complication, especially in CD. Growth failure is characterized by weight loss, alteration in body composition, retarded height, and delayed sexual maturation. Malnutrition causes the growth failure, and its etiology is multifactorial. Malnutrition occurs as a result of inadequate dietary intake, excessive GI losses, malabsorption, drug-nutrient interaction, and increased nutritional requirements. Inadequate dietary intake occurs with anorexia and episodes of increased disease activity. Excessive loss of nutrients (e.g., protein, blood, electrolytes, and minerals) occurs secondary to intestinal inflammation and diarrhea. Carbohydrate, lactose, fat, vitamin, and mineral malabsorption, as well as vitamin B_{12} and folic acid deficiencies, occur with disease episodes and with drug administration and when the terminal ileum is resected. Finally, nutritional requirements are increased with inflammation, fever, fistulas, and periods of rapid growth (e.g., adolescence).

The goals of nutritional support include correction of nutrient deficits and replacement of ongoing losses, provision of adequate energy and protein for healing, and provision of adequate nutrients to promote normal growth. Nutritional support includes both enteral and parenteral nutrition. A well-balanced, high-protein, high-calorie diet is recommended for children whose symptoms do not prohibit an adequate oral intake. There is little evidence that avoiding specific foods influences the severity of the disease. Supplementation with multivitamins, iron, and folic acid is recommended.

Special enteral formulas, given either by mouth or continuous NG infusion (often at night), may be required. Elemental formulas are completely absorbed in the small intestine with almost no residue. A diet consisting only of elemental formula not only improves nutritional status but also induces disease remission, either without steroids or with a diminished dosage of steroids required. An elemental diet is a safe and potentially effective primary therapy for patients with CD. Unfortunately, remission is not sustained when NG feedings are discontinued unless maintenance medications are added to the treatment regimen.

Total parenteral nutrition (TPN) has also improved nutritional status in patients with IBD. Short-term remissions have been achieved after TPN, although complete bowel rest has not reduced inflammation or added to the benefits of improved nutrition by TPN. Nutritional support is less likely to induce a remission in UC than in CD. However, improvement of nutritional status is important in preventing deterioration of the patient's health status and in preparing the patient for surgery.

Surgical Treatment

Surgery is indicated for UC when medical and nutritional therapies fail to prevent complications. Surgical options include a subtotal colectomy and ileostomy that leaves a rectal stump as a blind pouch. A reservoir pouch is created in the configuration of a J or an S to help improve continence postoperatively. An ileoanal pull-through preserves the normal pathway for defecation. Pouchitis, an inflammation of the surgically created pouch, is the most common late complication of this procedure. In many cases, UC can be cured with a total colectomy.

Surgery may be required in children with CD when complications cannot be controlled by medical and nutritional therapy. Segmental intestinal resections are performed for small bowel obstructions, strictures, or fistulas. Diversion of the fecal stream, such as a colostomy, allows the colon to be less active and causes the disease to become dormant, but on reconnection of the colon, disease often reoccurs (Stein & Baldassano, 2020).

Prognosis

IBD is a chronic disease. Relatively long periods of quiescent disease may follow exacerbations. The outcome is influenced by the regions and severity of involvement, as well as by appropriate therapeutic management. Malnutrition, growth failure, and bleeding are serious complications. The overall prognosis for UC is good.

The development of colorectal cancer (CRC) is a long-term complication of IBD. Because the risk for CRC occurs 8 to 10 years after diagnosis, surveillance colonoscopy with multiple biopsies should begin approximately 7 to 10 years after diagnosis of UC or CD (Rosen et al., 2017). In CD, surgical removal of the affected colon does not prevent cancer from developing elsewhere in the GI tract.

Nursing Care Management

The nursing considerations in the management of IBD extend beyond the immediate period of hospitalization. These interventions involve continued guidance of families in terms of (1) managing diet; (2) coping with factors that increase stress and emotional lability; (3) adjusting to a disease of remissions and exacerbations; and (4) when indicated, preparing the child and parents for the possibility of diversionary bowel surgery. (See Quality Patient Outcomes box.)

> **QUALITY PATIENT OUTCOMES: Inflammatory Bowel Disease**
> - Remission without symptoms of abdominal pain, bloating, diarrhea, and rectal bleeding
> - Optimum quality of life maintained by minimizing impairment of daily activities

Because nutritional support is an essential part of therapy, encouraging the anorexic child to consume sufficient quantities of food is often a challenge. Successful interventions include involving the child in meal planning; encouraging small, frequent meals or snacks rather than three large meals a day; serving meals around medication schedules when diarrhea, mouth pain, and intestinal spasm are controlled; and preparing high-protein, high-calorie foods such as eggnog, milkshakes, cream soups, puddings, or custard (if lactose is tolerated) (see Chapter 20, Feeding the Sick Child). Using bran or a high-fiber diet for active IBD is questionable. Bran, even in small amounts, has been shown to worsen the patient's condition. Occasionally the occurrence of aphthous stomatitis further complicates adherence to dietary management. Mouth care before eating and the selection of bland foods help relieve the discomfort of mouth sores.

When NG feedings or TPN is indicated, nurses play an important role in explaining the purpose and the expected outcomes of this therapy. The nurse should acknowledge the anxieties of the child and family members and give them adequate time to demonstrate the skills necessary to continue the therapy at home, if needed.

The importance of continued drug therapy despite remission of symptoms must be stressed to the child and family members. Failure to adhere to the pharmacologic regimen can result in exacerbation of the disease (see Chapter 20, Compliance). Unfortunately, exacerbation of IBD can occur even if the child and family are compliant with the treatment regimen; this is difficult for the child and family to cope with.

Emotional Support

The nurse should attend to the emotional components of the disease and assess any sources of stress. Frequently, the nurse can help children adjust to problems of growth retardation, delayed sexual maturation, dietary restrictions, feelings of being "different" or "sickly," inability to compete with peers, and necessary absence from school during exacerbations of the illness.

If a permanent colectomy-ileostomy is required, the nurse can teach the child and family how to care for the ileostomy. The nurse can also emphasize the positive aspects of the surgery, particularly accelerated growth and sexual development, permanent recovery, and the normality of life despite bowel diversion. Introducing the child and parents to other ostomy patients, especially those who are the same age, is effective in fostering eventual acceptance. Whenever possible, offer continent ostomies as options to the child, although they are not performed in all centers in the United States.

Because of the chronic and often lifelong nature of the disease, families benefit from the educational services provided by organizations such as the Crohn's and Colitis Foundation.[a] If diversionary bowel

[a]3733 Third Ave., Suite 510, New York, NY 10017; 888-694-8872; http://www.ccfa.org. In Canada: Crohn's and Colitis Canada, https://crohnsandcolitis.ca/.

surgery is indicated, United Ostomy Associations of America[b] and the Wound, Ostomy and Continence Nurses Society[c] are available to assist with ileostomy care and provide important psychologic support through their self-help groups. Adolescents often benefit by participating in peer-support groups, which are sponsored by the CCFA.

PEPTIC ULCER DISEASE

Peptic ulcer disease (PUD) is a chronic condition that affects the stomach or duodenum. Ulcers are described as gastric or duodenal and as primary or secondary. A **gastric ulcer** involves the mucosa of the stomach; a **duodenal ulcer** involves the pylorus or duodenum. Most **primary ulcers** are idiopathic or associated with *Helicobacter pylori* infection and tend to be chronic, occurring more frequently in the duodenum (Blanchard & Czinn, 2020). **Secondary ulcers** result from the stress of a severe underlying disease or injury (e.g., severe burns, sepsis, increased intracranial pressure, severe trauma, multisystem organ failure) and are more frequently gastric with an acute onset (Blanchard & Czinn, 2020).

Etiology

The exact cause of PUD is unknown, although infectious, genetic, and environmental factors are important. There is an increased familial incidence, likely due to *H. pylori,* which is known to cluster in families (Blanchard & Czinn, 2020). *H. pylori* is a microaerophilic, gram-negative, slow-growing, spiral-shaped, and flagellated bacterium known to colonize the gastric mucosa in about half of the population of the world (Blanchard & Czinn, 2020). *H. pylori* synthesizes the enzyme urease, which hydrolyzes urea to form ammonia and carbon dioxide. Ammonia then absorbs acid to form ammonium, thus raising the gastric pH. *H. pylori* may cause ulcers by weakening the gastric mucosal barrier and allowing acid to damage the mucosa. It is believed that it is acquired via the fecal-oral route, and this hypothesis is supported by finding viable *H. pylori* in feces.

In addition to ulcerogenic drugs, both alcohol and smoking contribute to ulcer formation. There is no conclusive evidence to implicate particular foods, such as caffeine-containing beverages or spicy foods, but polyunsaturated fats and fiber may play a role in ulcer formation. Psychologic factors may play a role in the development of PUD, and stressful life events, dependency, passiveness, and hostility have all been implicated as contributing factors.

Pathophysiology

Most likely, the pathology is due to an imbalance between the destructive (cytotoxic) factors and defensive (cytoprotective) factors in the GI tract. The toxic mechanisms include acid, pepsin, medications such as aspirin and nonsteroidal antiinflammatory drugs (NSAIDs), bile acids, and infection with *H. pylori.* The defensive factors include the mucus layer, local bicarbonate secretion, epithelial cell renewal, and mucosal blood flow. Prostaglandins play a role in mucosal defense because they stimulate both mucus and alkali secretion. The primary mechanism that prevents the development of peptic ulcer is the secretion of mucus by the epithelial and mucus glands throughout the stomach. The thick mucus layer acts to diffuse acid from the lumen to the gastric mucosal surface, thus protecting the gastric epithelium. The stomach and the duodenum produce bicarbonate, decreasing acidity on the epithelial cells and thereby minimizing the effects of the low pH. When abnormalities in the protective barrier exist, the mucosa is vulnerable to damage by acid and pepsin. Exogenous factors, such as aspirin and NSAIDs, cause gastric ulcers by inhibition of prostaglandin synthesis.

Zollinger-Ellison syndrome is rare but may occur in children who have multiple, large, or recurrent ulcers. This syndrome is characterized by hypersecretion of gastric acid, intractable ulcer disease, and intestinal malabsorption caused by a gastrin-secreting tumor of the pancreas.

BOX 22.6 Characteristics of Peptic Ulcers

Neonates

Usually gastric and secondary ulcers

Commonly a history of prematurity, respiratory distress, sepsis, hypoglycemia, or an intraventricular hemorrhage

Perforation possibly leading to massive bleeding

Infants to 2-Year-Old Children

Most likely to have a secondary ulcer located equally in the stomach or duodenum

Primary ulcers less common and usually located in stomach

Likely to be noticed in relation to illness, surgery, or trauma

Hematemesis, melena, or perforation

2- to 6-Year-Old Children

Primary or secondary ulcers

Located equally in stomach and duodenum

Perforation more likely in secondary ulcers

Periumbilical pain, poor eating, vomiting, irritability, nighttime wakening, hematemesis, melena

Children Over 6 Years

Usually primary and most often duodenal ulcers

More typical of adult type

Chance of recurrence greater

Often associated with *Helicobacter pylori*

Epigastric pain or vague abdominal pain

Nighttime wakening, hematemesis, melena, and anemia possible

Clinical Manifestations

The clinical manifestations of PUD vary according to the child's age and the ulcer's location. Common clinical manifestations include chronic abdominal pain, especially when the stomach is empty, such as during the night or early morning; recurrent vomiting; hematemesis; melena; chronic anemia; and abdominal tenderness (Box 22.6).

Diagnostic Evaluation

Diagnosis is based on the history of symptoms, physical examination, and diagnostic testing. The focus is on symptoms such as epigastric abdominal pain, nocturnal pain, oral regurgitation, heartburn, weight loss, hematemesis, and melena. History should include questions relating to the use of potentially causative substances such as NSAIDs, corticosteroids, alcohol, and tobacco. Frequently a history of epigastric and periumbilical pain accompanies PUD. However, children often find it difficult to describe the location of their pain and frequently indicate the location by moving their hand in a circular movement all around the stomach area. Asking the child to take one finger and point to the area where it hurts the most often helps identify the location of the pain. Pain may also be elicited during the examination with palpation.

---

[b]PO Box 525, Kennebunk, ME 04043-0525; 800-826-0826; http://www.ostomy.org. In Canada: Ostomy Canada Society, 5800 Ambler Drive, Suite 210, Mississauga, Ontario L4W 4J4; 1-888-969-9698; http://www.ostomycanada.ca.

[c]1120 Rt. 73, Suite 200, Mt. Laurel, NJ 08054; 888-224-9626; http://www.wocn.org.

Laboratory studies may include a CBC to detect anemia, stool analysis for occult blood, liver function tests (LFTs), ESR, or CRP to evaluate IBD; amylase and lipase to evaluate pancreatitis; and gastric acid measurements to identify hypersecretion. Stool analysis is performed to rule out infection. Polyclonal and monoclonal stool antigen tests are an accurate, noninvasive method both for the initial diagnosis of *H. pylori* and for the confirmation of its eradication after treatment (Yang, 2016). A C13 urea breath test measures bacterial colonization in the gastric mucosa and can be used as an additional noninvasive test to determine the presence of antibodies to *H. pylori*.

An upper GI series is the most reliable way to detect and diagnose PUD in children (Blanchard & Czinn, 2020). Direct visualization of the gastric and duodenal mucosa helps identify specific lesions, and biopsy specimens can determine the presence of *H. pylori*.

Therapeutic Management

The major goals of therapy for children with PUD are to relieve discomfort, promote healing, prevent complications, and prevent recurrence. Management is primarily medical and consists of administration of medications to treat the infection and to reduce or neutralize gastric acid secretion. Antacids are beneficial medications to neutralize gastric acid. H_2-receptor antagonists (antisecretory drugs) act to suppress gastric acid production. These medications have few side effects. PPIs, such as omeprazole, lansoprazole, pantoprazole, and esomeprazole, act to inhibit the hydrogen ion pump in the parietal cells, thus blocking the production of acid. Although these drugs have not been well studied in children, they are used in clinical practice to treat ulcers, GER, esophagitis, and gastritis, and appear to be well tolerated with infrequent side effects (e.g., headache, diarrhea, nausea) (Blanchard & Czinn, 2020).

Mucosal protective agents, such as sucralfate and bismuth-containing preparations, may be prescribed for PUD. Sucralfate is an aluminum-containing agent that forms a barrier over ulcerated mucosa to protect against acid and pepsin. Bismuth compounds are sometimes prescribed for the relief of ulcers, but they are used less frequently than PPIs. Although these compounds inhibit the growth of microorganisms, the mechanism of their activity is poorly understood. In combination with antibiotics, bismuth is effective against *H. pylori*. Although concern has been expressed about the use of bismuth salts in children because of potential side effects, none of these side effects has been reported when these compounds have been used in the treatment of *H. pylori* infection. These agents are available in both pill and liquid forms. Because they block the absorption of other medications, they should be given separately from other medications.

Triple-drug therapy is the standard first-line treatment regimen for *H. pylori* and has demonstrated 90% efficacy in the eradication of *H. pylori* (Kalach, Bontems, & Cadranel, 2015). Examples of drug combinations used in triple therapy are (1) bismuth, clarithromycin, and metronidazole; (2) lansoprazole, amoxicillin, and clarithromycin; and (3) metronidazole, clarithromycin, and omeprazole. Common side effects of medications include diarrhea, nausea, and vomiting.

Children with an acute ulcer who have developed complications, such as massive hemorrhage, require emergency care. The administration of IV fluids, blood, or plasma depends on the amount of blood loss. Replacement with whole blood or packed cells may be necessary for significant loss.

Surgical intervention may be required for complications such as hemorrhage, perforation, or gastric outlet obstruction. Ligation of the source of bleeding or closure of a perforation is performed. A vagotomy and pyloroplasty may be indicated in children with bleeding ulcers despite aggressive medical treatment (Patel, Bommayya, Choudhry, et al., 2015).

Prognosis

The long-term prognosis for PUD is variable. Many ulcers are successfully treated with medical therapy; however, primary duodenal peptic ulcers often recur. Complications such as GI bleeding can occur and extend into adult life. The effect of maintenance drug therapy on long-term morbidity remains to be established with further studies.

Nursing Care Management

The primary nursing goal is to promote healing of the ulcer through compliance with the medication regimen. If an analgesic-antipyretic is needed, acetaminophen, not aspirin or NSAIDs, is used. Critically ill neonates, infants, and children in intensive care units should receive H_2 blockers to prevent stress ulcers.

DRUG ALERT

H_2 Blockers

Critically ill children receiving intravenous (IV) histamine (H_2) blockers should have their gastric pH values checked at frequent intervals.

For nonhospitalized children with chronic illnesses, consider the role that stress plays. In children, many ulcers occur secondary to other conditions, and the nurse should be aware of family and environmental conditions that may aggravate or precipitate ulcers. Children may benefit from psychologic counseling and from learning how to cope constructively with stress.

OBSTRUCTIVE DISORDERS

Obstruction in the GI tract occurs when the passage of nutrients and secretions is impeded by a constricted or occluded lumen or when there is impaired motility (**paralytic ileus**). Obstructions may be congenital or acquired. Congenital obstructions, such as esophageal or intestinal atresias, imperforate anus, and meconium ileus, usually appear in the neonatal period. Other obstructions of congenital etiology (e.g., malrotation, HD, pyloric stenosis, volvulus, incarcerated hernia, Meckel diverticulum) appear after the first few weeks of life. Intestinal obstruction from acquired causes such as intussusception and tumors may occur in infancy or childhood.

Acute intestinal obstruction is commonly characterized by abdominal pain, nausea, vomiting, abdominal distention, and a change in stooling patterns. Pain is caused by intermittent muscular contractions proximal to the obstruction as the bowel attempts to move luminal contents along the normal path. It may also be due to severe abdominal distention, which results from accumulation of gas and fluid above the level of the obstruction. As abdominal distention progresses, the abdomen may become extremely tender, rigid, and firm.

When abdominal contents continue to accumulate, nausea and vomiting occur. Vomiting of gastric contents is often the first sign of a high obstruction, such as obstruction of the pylorus, and vomiting of bile-stained material is a sign of obstruction of the small intestine. Persistent vomiting can lead to dehydration and electrolyte disturbances. Constipation and obstipation (prolonged absence of defecation) are early signs of low obstructions and later signs of higher obstructions. In acute conditions such as intussusception, the clinical manifestations are apparent within a few hours of the onset of the disorder. In other conditions such as hypertrophic pyloric stenosis, the signs and symptoms may have a more gradual onset. Bowel sounds may initially be hyperactive, then diminish or cease. Respiratory distress may occur when the diaphragm is pushed up into the pleural cavity as a result of severe abdominal distention.

HYPERTROPHIC PYLORIC STENOSIS

Hypertrophic pyloric stenosis (HPS) occurs when the circumferential muscle of the pyloric sphincter becomes thickened, resulting in elongation and narrowing of the pyloric canal. This produces an outlet obstruction and compensatory dilation, hypertrophy, and hyperperistalsis of the stomach. This condition usually develops in the first few weeks of life, causing nonbilious vomiting, which occurs after a feeding; projectile vomiting may develop, and the infant is fussy and hungry after vomiting. If the condition is not diagnosed early, dehydration, metabolic alkalosis, and failure to thrive may occur. The precise etiology of HPS is not known. Boys are affected four to six times more frequently than girls (Maqbool & Liacouras, 2020b). It is more common in white infants and is seen less frequently in African American and Asian infants (Maqbool & Liacouras, 2020b).

Pathophysiology

The circular muscle of the pylorus thickens as a result of hypertrophy. This produces severe narrowing of the pyloric canal between the stomach and the duodenum. Consequently, the lumen at this point is partially obstructed. Over time, inflammation and edema further reduce the size of the opening, resulting in complete obstruction. The hypertrophied pylorus may be palpable as an olive-like mass in the upper abdomen (Fig. 22.4).

Pyloric stenosis is not a congenital disorder. It is believed that local innervation may be involved in the pathogenesis. In most cases, HPS is an isolated lesion; however, it may be associated with intestinal malrotation, esophageal and duodenal atresia, and anorectal anomalies.

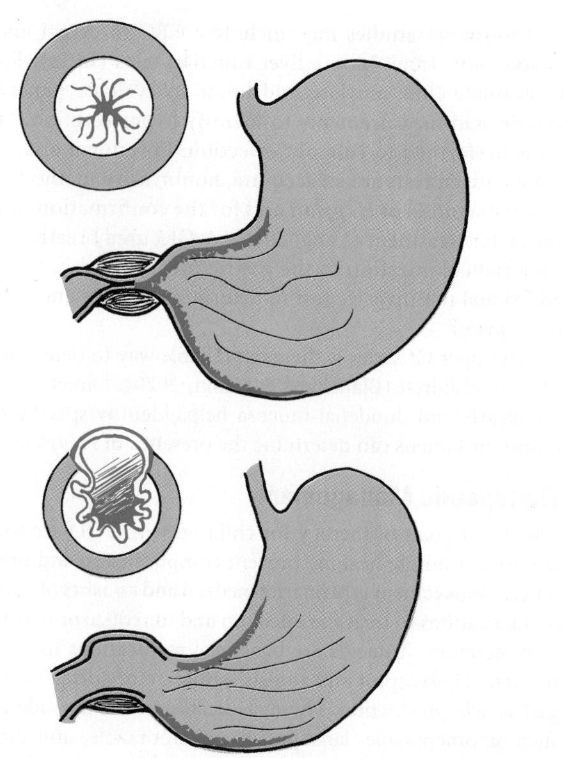

Fig. 22.4 Hypertrophic pyloric stenosis (HPS). **A,** Enlarged muscular area nearly obliterates the pyloric channel. **B,** Longitudinal surgical division of the muscle down to the submucosa establishes an adequate passageway.

Clinical Manifestations

Infants with HPS have nonbilious vomiting in the early stages (Box 22.7). Vomiting usually begins at 3 weeks of age but can start as early as 1 week and as late as 5 months. Vomiting usually occurs 30 to 60 minutes after feeding and becomes projectile as the obstruction progresses. Initially the infant is hungry and irritable, but prolonged vomiting may lead to dehydration, weight loss, and failure to thrive. Gastric peristalsis may be visible on examination, and the olive-shaped mass in the epigastrium just to the right of the umbilicus may be palpated (see Fig. 22.4A). Indirect (unconjugated) hyperbilirubinemia may be present in a small percentage of affected infants; this usually resolves with surgical correction and is reported to occur as a result of a decreased level of glucuronyl transferase (see also Chapter 8).

BOX 22.7 Clinical Manifestations of Hypertrophic Pyloric Stenosis

Projectile vomiting
- May be ejected 3 to 4 feet from the child when in a side-lying position, 1 foot or more when in a back-lying position
- Usually occurs shortly after a feeding but may not occur for several hours
- May follow each feeding or appear intermittently
- Nonbilious vomitus that may be blood tinged

Infant hungry, avid nurser; eagerly accepts a second feeding after vomiting episode
No evidence of pain or discomfort except that of chronic hunger
Poor weight gain
Signs of dehydration
Distended upper abdomen
Readily palpable olive-shaped tumor in the epigastrium just to the right of the umbilicus
Visible gastric peristaltic waves that move from left to right across the epigastrium

Diagnostic Evaluation

The diagnosis of HPS is often made after the history and physical examination. The olive-like mass is most easily palpated when the stomach is empty, the infant is quiet, and the abdominal muscles are relaxed. If the diagnosis is inconclusive from the history and physical examination, ultrasonography will demonstrate an elongated mass surrounding a long pyloric canal. If ultrasonography does not demonstrate a hypertrophied pylorus, upper GI radiography should be done to rule out other causes of vomiting.

If the condition is not diagnosed early, laboratory findings reflect the metabolic alterations created by moderate to severe depletion of both water and electrolytes from extensive and prolonged vomiting. There are decreased serum levels of both sodium and potassium, although these may be masked by the hemoconcentration from ECF depletion. Of greater diagnostic value are a decrease in serum chloride levels and increases in pH and bicarbonate (carbon dioxide content), indicative of metabolic alkalosis. The BUN will be elevated as evidence of dehydration. However, in those cases diagnosed early, laboratory findings may not be significant.

Therapeutic Management

Surgical relief of the pyloric obstruction by pyloromyotomy is the standard therapy for this disorder. Preoperatively the infant must be rehydrated and metabolic alkalosis corrected with parenteral fluid and electrolyte administration. Replacement fluid therapy usually delays surgery for 24 to 48 hours. The stomach is decompressed with an NG tube if the infant continues with vomiting. In infants with no evidence of fluid and electrolyte imbalance, surgery is performed without delay.

The surgical procedure is often performed by laparoscope and consists of a longitudinal incision through the circular muscle fibers of the pylorus down to, but not including, the submucosa (**pyloromyotomy**, or the Fredet-Ramstedt operation) (see Fig. 22.4B). The procedure has a high success rate. Laparoscopic surgery may result in a shorter surgical time, more rapid postoperative feeding, and shorter hospital stay (Maqbool & Liacouras, 2020b).

Feedings are usually begun 4 to 6 hours postoperatively, beginning with small, frequent feedings of water or electrolyte solution. If clear fluids are retained, formula is started in the same small increments about 24 hours after surgery. The amount and the interval between feedings are gradually increased until a full feeding schedule is reinstated, which usually takes about 48 hours.

Prognosis

The prognosis for infants and small children with HPS is excellent when the diagnosis is confirmed early, and the mortality rate is low (0% to 0.5%). A small percentage of children with HPS will have GER.

Nursing Care Management

Nursing care involves primarily observation for clinical features that help establish the diagnosis, careful regulation of fluid therapy, and reestablishment of normal feeding patterns. Nurses must be alert to signs of HPS in infants and refer them for medical evaluation. HPS should be considered a possibility in the very young infant who appears alert but fails to gain weight and has a history of vomiting after feedings. Assessment is based on observation of eating behaviors and evidence of other characteristic clinical manifestations, hydration, and nutritional status.

Preoperatively, the emphasis is on restoring hydration and electrolyte balance. The infant is kept NPO and given IV fluids with glucose and electrolytes based on serum electrolyte values and clinical appearance. Careful monitoring of the IV fluids and strict monitoring of intake and output are important. Record accurate description of any vomiting and the number and character of stools.

Observations include assessment of vital signs, particularly those that indicate fluid or electrolyte imbalances. These infants are especially prone to metabolic alkalosis from loss of hydrogen ions and depletion of potassium, sodium, and chloride, all of which are contained in gastric secretions. Assess the skin and mucous membranes for alterations in hydration status.

If stomach decompression and gastric lavage are part of preoperative management, the nurse is responsible for ensuring that the NG tube is patent and functioning properly and for measuring and recording the type and amount of drainage. Encourage parents to visit and become involved in the child's care. Most parents need support and reassurance that the condition is caused by a structural problem and is not a reflection of their parenting skills and capacities.

Postoperative vomiting is common, and most infants, even with successful surgery, exhibit some vomiting during the first 24 to 48 hours. IV fluids are administered until the infant is taking and retaining adequate amounts by mouth. Much of the same care that was instituted before surgery is continued postoperatively, including observation of vital signs, monitoring of IV fluids, and careful monitoring of intake and output. In addition, the infant is observed for responses to the stress of surgery and for evidence of pain. Appropriate analgesics should be given around the clock because pain is continuous. The surgical incision(s) is inspected for drainage or erythema, and any signs of infection are reported to the surgeon. A surgical adhesive may be used for incision closure, and parents are instructed regarding the care of the incision and any dressings before discharge.

Feedings are usually instituted within 12 to 24 hours postoperatively, beginning with clear liquids. They are offered in small quantities at frequent intervals. If the infant has been breastfed, breast milk expressed by the mother may be given by bottle when the infant is able to tolerate feedings, or the mother is instructed to limit nursing time and gradually increase the time to previous patterns. Observation and recording of feedings and the infant's responses to feedings are a vital part of postoperative care. Care of the operative site consists of observation for any drainage or signs of inflammation and care of the incision.

INTUSSUSCEPTION

Intussusception is the most common cause of intestinal obstruction in children between 3 months and 6 years old (Carroll, Kavanagh, Ni Leidhin, et al., 2017). Intussusception is more common in males than in females and is more common in children younger than 2 years old. Although specific intestinal lesions occur in a small percentage of the children, generally the cause is not known. Only 12.5% to 25% of intussusception cases have a pathologic lead point, such as a polyp, lymphoma, or Meckel diverticulum (Carroll et al., 2017). The idiopathic cases may be caused by hypertrophy of intestinal lymphoid tissue secondary to viral infection.

Pathophysiology

Intussusception occurs when a proximal segment of the bowel telescopes into a more distal segment, pulling the mesentery with it. The mesentery is compressed and angled, resulting in lymphatic and venous obstruction. As the edema from the obstruction increases, pressure within the area of intussusception increases. When the pressure equals the arterial pressure, arterial blood flow stops, resulting in ischemia and the pouring of mucus into the intestine. Venous engorgement also leads to leaking of blood and mucus into the intestinal lumen, forming the classic currant jelly–like stools. The most common site is the ileocecal valve (ileocolic), where the ileum invaginates into the cecum and then further into the colon (Fig. 22.5). Other forms include ileoileal (i.e., one part of the ileum invaginates into another section of the ileum) and colocolic (i.e., one part of the colon invaginates into another area of the colon) intussusceptions, usually in the area of the hepatic or splenic flexure or at some point along the transverse colon.

Clinical Manifestations

Intussusception usually manifests with the sudden onset of crampy abdominal pain, inconsolable crying, and a drawing up of the knees to the chest in an otherwise healthy child (Box 22.8). Between episodes the child appears normal. As the obstruction progresses, bilious vomiting may occur and lethargy increases. The classic triad of intussusception symptoms (abdominal pain, abdominal mass, bloody stools) is present in less than 30% of children (Maqbool & Liacouras, 2020d). A more chronic case, characterized by diarrhea, anorexia, weight loss, occasional vomiting, and periodic pain, may be presented. Because intussusception is potentially life threatening, be aware of such signs, and closely observe and refer these children for further medical evaluation. With atypical cases, lethargy may be the primary symptom. If the distal bowel remains distended, necrosis and perforation are possible.

Diagnostic Evaluation

Frequently, subjective findings lead to the diagnosis. However, definitive diagnosis is based on ultrasonography that reveals a characteristic heterogenous mass and a "bull's-eye." A rectal examination reveals mucus, blood, and occasionally a low intussusception itself.

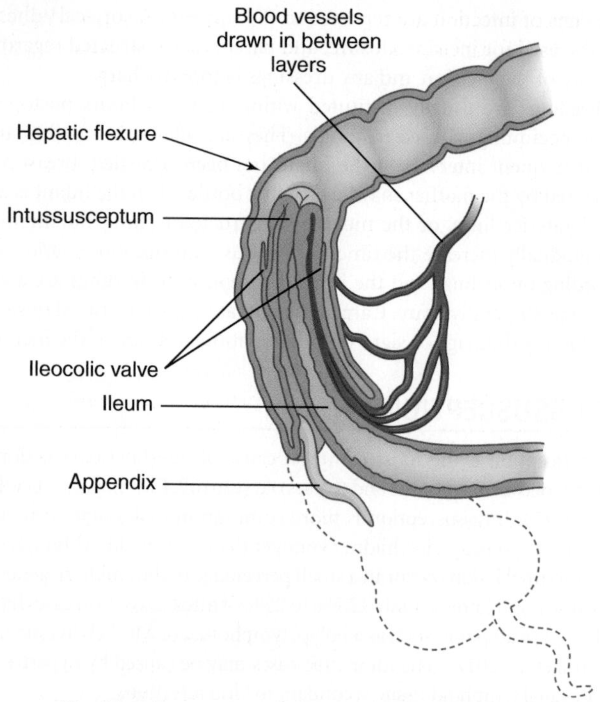

Fig. 22.5 Ileocecal valve (ileocolic) intussusception.

BOX 22.8 Clinical Manifestations of Intussusception

- Sudden acute abdominal pain
- Child screaming and drawing the knees onto the chest
- Child appearing normal and comfortable between episodes of pain
- Vomiting
- Lethargy
- Passage of red, currant jelly–like stools (stool mixed with blood and mucus)
- Tender, distended abdomen
- Palpable sausage-shaped mass in upper right quadrant
- Empty lower right quadrant (Dance sign)
- Eventual fever, prostration, and other signs of peritonitis

Therapeutic Management

Conservative treatment consists of radiologist-guided pneumoenema (gas enema) or ultrasound-guided hydrostatic enema, the advantage of the latter being that no ionizing radiation is needed (Maqbool & Liacouras, 2020e). Recurrence of intussusception after conservative treatment is rare; however, this procedure should not be attempted with prolonged intussusception, signs of shock, peritoneal irritation, or intestinal perforation (Maqbool & Liacouras, 2020e).

IV fluids, NG decompression, and antibiotic therapy may be used before hydrostatic reduction is attempted. If these procedures are not successful, the child may require surgical intervention. Surgery involves manually reducing the invagination and, when indicated, resecting any nonviable intestine.

Prognosis

Nonoperative reduction is successful in the majority of stable cases. Gas enema is slightly more successful with reduction compared to a hydrostatic enema (83% versus 70%, respectively) (Carroll et al., 2017). Surgery is required for patients in whom the reduction is unsuccessful or for patients who are unstable. With early diagnosis and treatment, serious complications and death are uncommon.

Nursing Care Management

The nurse can help establish a diagnosis by listening to the parents' description of the child's physical and behavioral symptoms. It is not unusual for parents to state that they thought something was seriously wrong before others shared their concerns. The description of the child's severe colicky abdominal pain combined with vomiting is a significant sign of intussusception.

As soon as a possible diagnosis of intussusception is made, the nurse prepares the parents for the immediate need for hospitalization, the nonsurgical technique of hydrostatic reduction, and the possibility of surgery. It is important to explain the basic defect of intussusception. The nurse can easily demonstrate this by creating a model of the defect. Use the example of a telescoping rod, or push the end of a finger on a rubber glove back into itself. Then demonstrate the principle of reduction by hydrostatic pressure by filling the glove with water, which pushes the "finger" into a fully extended position.

Physical care of the child does not differ from that for any child undergoing abdominal surgery. Even though nonsurgical intervention may be successful, the usual preoperative procedures, such as maintenance of NPO status, routine laboratory testing (CBC and urinalysis), signed parental consent, and preanesthetic sedation, are performed. Children with perforation will require IV fluids, systemic antibiotics, and bowel decompression before undergoing surgery. Fluid volume replacement and restoration of electrolytes may be required in such children before surgery. Before surgery the nurse monitors all stools.

! NURSING ALERT

Passage of a normal brown stool usually indicates that the intussusception has reduced itself. This is immediately reported to the practitioner, who may choose to alter the diagnostic and therapeutic care plan.

Postprocedural care includes observations of vital signs, blood pressure, intact sutures and dressing, and the return of bowel sounds. After spontaneous or hydrostatic reduction, the nurse observes for passage of water-soluble contrast material (if used) and stool patterns because the intussusception may recur. Children may be admitted to the hospital or monitored on an outpatient basis. A recurrence of intussusception is treated with the conservative reduction techniques described previously, but a laparotomy is considered for multiple recurrences.

MALROTATION AND VOLVULUS

Malrotation of the intestine is caused by the abnormal rotation of the intestine around the superior mesenteric artery during embryologic development. Malrotation may manifest in utero or at any age, but most patients (80%) present in the first month of life (Carroll et al., 2017). Infants may have intermittent bilious vomiting, recurrent abdominal pain, distention, or lower GI bleeding. Malrotation is the most serious type of intestinal obstruction because if the intestine undergoes complete volvulus (i.e., the intestine twisting around itself), compromise of the blood supply will result in intestinal necrosis, peritonitis, perforation, and death.

Diagnostic Evaluation

It is imperative that malrotation and volvulus be diagnosed promptly and surgical treatment instituted quickly. In addition to a history and physical, a plain abdominal radiograph and lateral decubitus view are obtained; bowel distention will be present proximal to the distention on plain radiograph, and a lateral view will demonstrate air-fluid levels in the distended bowel. An upper GI series is the most accurate imaging study (Carroll et al., 2017).

Therapeutic Management

Surgery is indicated to remove the affected area. Because of the extensive nature of some lesions, short bowel syndrome (SBS) is a postoperative complication.

Nursing Care Management

Preoperatively the nursing care is the same as that provided to an infant or child with intestinal obstruction. IV fluids, NG decompression, and systemic antibiotics are implemented. In the rapidly deteriorating infant, fluid volume resuscitation and vasopressors may be required for preoperative stabilization. Postoperatively, the nursing care is similar to that provided to the infant or child who has undergone abdominal surgery.

MALABSORPTION SYNDROMES

Chronic diarrhea and malabsorption of nutrients characterize malabsorption syndromes. An important complication of malabsorption syndromes in children is failure to thrive. Most cases are classified according to the location of the supposed anatomic or biochemical defect. The term celiac disease is often used to describe a symptom complex with four characteristics: (1) steatorrhea (fatty, foul, frothy, bulky stools), (2) general malnutrition, (3) abdominal distention, and (4) secondary vitamin deficiencies.

Digestive defects are conditions in which the enzymes necessary for digestion are diminished or absent, such as (1) cystic fibrosis, in which pancreatic enzymes are absent; (2) biliary or liver disease, in which bile flow is affected; or (3) lactase deficiency, in which there is congenital or secondary lactose intolerance.

Absorptive defects are conditions in which the intestinal mucosal transport system is impaired. This may occur because of a primary defect (e.g., celiac disease) or secondary to inflammatory disease of the bowel that results in impaired absorption because bowel motility is accelerated (e.g., ulcerative colitis). Obstructive disorders (e.g., Hirschsprung disease) also cause secondary malabsorption from enterocolitis.

Anatomic defects, such as extensive resection of the bowel or SBS, affect digestion by decreasing the transit time of substances and affect absorption by severely compromising the absorptive surface.

CELIAC DISEASE (GLUTEN-SENSITIVE ENTEROPATHY)

Celiac disease, also known as *gluten-induced enteropathy, gluten-sensitive enteropathy,* and *celiac sprue,* is an autoimmune disorder triggered by the ingestion of gluten in genetically susceptible individuals (Fok, Holland, Gil-Zaragozano, et al., 2016). The disorder results in permanent intestinal intolerance to dietary gluten, a protein present in wheat, barley, and rye that causes damage to the villi in the small intestine. Children with unexplained iron deficiency anemia, recurrent aphthous stomatitis, dental enamel defects, type 1 diabetes, Down syndrome, selective immunoglobulin A deficiency, autoimmune thyroid disease, Turner syndrome, or Williams syndrome are more susceptible to being diagnosed with the disease (Paul, McVeigh, Gil-Zaragozano, et al., 2016). The disease is seen more frequently in Europe and the United States in approximately 1% of these populations, and it is rarely reported in Asians or African Americans (Troncone & Shamir, 2020).

Pathophysiology

Celiac disease is characterized by villous atrophy in the small intestine in response to the protein gluten. When individuals are unable to digest the gliadin component of gluten, an accumulation of a toxic substance that is damaging to the mucosal cells occurs. Damage to the mucosa of the small intestine leads to villous atrophy, hyperplasia of the crypts, and infiltration of the epithelial cells with lymphocytes. Villous atrophy leads to malabsorption due to the reduced absorptive surface area.

Genetic predisposition is an essential factor in the development of celiac disease. Membrane receptors involved in preferential antigen presentation to $CD4^+$ T cells play a crucial role in the immune response characteristic of celiac disease. Children with genetic susceptibilities, namely *HLA-DQ2* or *HLA-DQ8,* are more susceptible to being diagnosed with celiac disease (Lebwohl, Sanders, & Green, 2017).

Clinical Manifestations

Symptoms of celiac disease appear when solid foods such as beans and pasta are introduced in the child's diet between the ages of 1 and 5 years (Box 22.9). There is usually an interval of several months between the introduction of gluten in the diet and the onset of symptoms. Intestinal symptoms are common in children diagnosed within the first 2 years of life. Other symptoms include failure to thrive, chronic diarrhea, abdominal distention and pain, muscle wasting, aphthous ulcers, and fatigue.

Diagnostic Evaluation

Gluten should not be excluded from the diet until the diagnostic evaluation is complete so that proper identification can occur. The first step is a serologic blood test for tissue transglutaminase and antiendomysial antibodies in children 18 months of age or older (Troncone & Shamir,

BOX 22.9 Clinical Manifestations of Celiac Disease

Impaired Fat Absorption
Steatorrhea (excessively large, pale, oily, frothy stools)
Exceedingly foul-smelling stools

Impaired Nutrient Absorption
Malnutrition
Muscle wasting (especially prominent in legs and buttocks)
Anemia
Anorexia
Abdominal distention

Behavioral Changes
Irritability
Uncooperativeness
Apathy

Celiac Crisis[a]
Acute, severe episodes of profuse watery diarrhea and vomiting
May be precipitated by:

- Infections (especially gastrointestinal)
- Prolonged fluid and electrolyte depletion
- Emotional disturbance

[a]In very young children.

2020). Positive serologic markers should be followed by an upper GI endoscopy with biopsy. The diagnosis of celiac disease is based on a biopsy of the small intestine demonstrating the characteristic changes of mucosal inflammation, crypt hyperplasia, and villous atrophy (Troncone & Shamir, 2020).

Therapeutic Management

Treatment of celiac disease consists primarily of dietary management. Although a gluten-free diet is prescribed, it is actually low in gluten because it is impossible to remove every source of this protein. Because gluten is found primarily in wheat and rye, but also in smaller quantities in barley and oats, these four foods are eliminated. Corn, rice, and millet are substitute grain foods.

Children with untreated celiac disease may have lactose intolerance, especially if their mucosal lesions are extensive. Lactose intolerance usually improves as the mucosa heals with gluten withdrawal. Specific nutritional deficiencies, such as iron, folic acid, and fat-soluble vitamin deficiencies, are treated with appropriate supplements.

Prognosis

Celiac disease is regarded as a chronic disease; its severity varies greatly among children. The most severe symptoms usually occur in early childhood and again in adult life. Most children who comply with dietary management are healthy and remain free of symptoms and complications; however, children should be evaluated annually for nutritional deficiencies, impaired growth, delayed puberty, and reduced bone mineral density (Fok et al., 2016).

Nursing Care Management

The main nursing consideration is helping the child adhere to the dietary regimen. Considerable time is involved in explaining the disease process to the child and parents, the specific role of gluten in aggravating the disorder, and those foods that must be restricted. It is difficult to maintain a diet indefinitely when the child has no symptoms and temporary transgressions result in no difficulties. However, the majority of individuals who relax their diet will experience a relapse of their disease.

Although the chief source of gluten is cereal and baked goods, grains are frequently added to processed foods as thickeners or fillers. To compound the difficulty, gluten is added to many foods as hydrolyzed vegetable protein, which is derived from cereal grains. The nurse must advise parents of the necessity of reading all label ingredients carefully to avoid hidden sources of gluten.

Many of children's favorite foods contain gluten, including bread, cake, cookies, crackers, donuts, pies, spaghetti, pizza, prepared soups, hot dogs, luncheon meats, and some prepared hamburgers. Many of these products can be eliminated from the infant's or young child's diet fairly easily, but monitoring the diet of the school-age child or adolescent is more difficult. Luncheon preparation away from home is particularly difficult because bread, luncheon meats, and instant soups are not allowed. For families on restricted food budgets, the diet adds another financial burden because many inexpensive or convenient foods cannot be used.

In addition to restricting gluten, other dietary alterations may be necessary. For example, in some children who have more severe mucosal damage, the digestion of disaccharides is impaired, especially in relation to lactose. Therefore these children often need a temporarily lactose-free diet, which necessitates eliminating all milk products. In general, dietary management includes a diet high in calories and proteins with simple carbohydrates such as fruits and vegetables, but low in fats. Because the bowel is inflamed as a result of the pathologic processes in absorption, the child must avoid high-fiber foods such as nuts, raisins, raw vegetables, and raw fruits with skin until inflammation has subsided.

It is important to stress long-range complications and to remind parents of the child's physical status before dietary treatment and the dramatic improvement after treatment. The nurse can be instrumental in allowing the child to express concerns and frustration while focusing on ways in which the child can still feel normal. Encourage the child and parents to find new recipes using suitable ingredients, such as Mexican or Chinese dishes that use corn or rice. Consult a registered dietitian to provide children and their families with detailed dietary instructions and education.

Several resources are available to assist children and parents in all aspects of coping with celiac disease. The National Celiac Association[d] provides support and guidance to families and supplies educational materials concerning a gluten-free diet, food sources, recipes, and travel information.

SHORT BOWEL SYNDROME

Short bowel syndrome (SBS) is a malabsorptive disorder that occurs as a result of decreased mucosal surface area, usually because of extensive resection of the small intestine. Malabsorption may be exacerbated by other factors, such as bacterial overgrowth and dysmotility. The most common congenital causes of SBS in children are multiple atresias, and gastroschisis; other causes resulting in bowel resection include necrotizing volvulus, meconium peritonitis, Crohn disease, and trauma (Avitzur & Shamir, 2020).

The definition of SBS includes two important findings: (1) decreased intestinal surface area for absorption of fluid, electrolytes, and nutrients; and (2) a need for parenteral nutrition (PN) (Martin, Ladd, Werts, et al., 2017). The prognosis for infants with SBS has improved dramatically, but the mortality rate within 5 years after diagnosis remains at 27% to 37% (Martin et al., 2017).

Therapeutic Management

The goals of therapy for infants and children with SBS include (1) preserving as much length of bowel as possible during surgery; (2) maintaining optimum nutritional status, growth, and development while intestinal adaptation occurs; (3) stimulating intestinal adaptation with enteral feeding; and (4) minimizing complications related to the disease process and therapy (Avitzur & Shamir, 2020).

Nutritional Support

Nutritional support is the long-term focus of care for children with SBS. The initial phase of therapy includes PN as the primary source of nutrition. The second phase is the introduction of enteral feeding, which usually begins as soon as possible after surgery. Elemental formulas containing glucose, sucrose and glucose polymers, hydrolyzed proteins, and medium-chain triglycerides facilitate absorption. Usually these formulas are given by continuous infusion through an NG or gastrostomy tube. As the enteral feedings are advanced, the PN solution is decreased in terms of calories, amount of fluid, and total hours of infusion per day. If enteral feedings are tolerated, oral feedings should be attempted to minimize oral aversion and preserve oral skills (Avitzur & Shamir, 2020).

[d]20 Pickering Street, Needham, MA 02492; 1-888-4CELIAC or 617-262-5422; http://www.nationalceliac.org. In Canada: Canadian Celiac Association, 1450 Meyerside Drive, Suite 503, Mississauga, Ontario L5T 2N5; 1-800-363-7296; http://www.celiac.ca.

The final phase of nutritional support occurs when growth and development are sustained. When PN is discontinued, there is a risk of nutritional deficiency secondary to malabsorption of fat-soluble vitamins (A, D, E, and K) and trace minerals (iron, selenium, zinc). Serum vitamin and mineral levels should be monitored closely and supplemented enterally, if needed. Pharmacologic agents have been used to reduce secretory losses. H_2 blockers, PPIs, and octreotide inhibit gastric or pancreatic secretion. Cholestyramine is often prescribed to improve diarrhea that is associated with bile salt malabsorption.

Numerous complications are associated with SBS and long-term PN. Infectious, metabolic, and technical complications can occur. Sepsis can occur after improper care of the catheter. The GI tract can also be a source of microbial seeding of the catheter. Bowel atrophy may foster increased intestinal permeability of bacteria. A lack of adequate sites for central lines may become a significant problem for the child in need of long-term PN. Hepatic dysfunction and cholestasis may also occur (Cohran, Prozialeck, & Cole, 2017).

Bacterial overgrowth is likely to occur when the ileocecal valve is absent or when stasis exists as a result of a partial obstruction or a dilated segment of bowel with poor motility. Alternating cycles of broad-spectrum antibiotics are used to reduce bacterial overgrowth. This treatment may also decrease the risk of bacterial translocation and subsequent central venous catheter infections. A high-fat and low-carbohydrate diet may be helpful in reducing bacterial overgrowth (Avitzur & Shamir, 2020). Other complications of bacterial overgrowth and malabsorption include metabolic acidosis and gastric hypersecretion.

Many surgical interventions, including intestinal valves, tapering enteroplasty or stricturoplasty, intestinal lengthening, and interposed segments, have been used to slow intestinal transit, reduce bacterial overgrowth, or increase mucosal surface area. Intestinal transplantation has been performed successfully in children. Children with a permanent dependence on PN or severe complications of long-term PN are candidates for transplantation.

Prognosis

The prognosis for infants with SBS has improved with advances in PN and with the understanding of the importance of intraluminal nutrition. Improved supportive care for the management of therapy-related problems and the development of more specific immunosuppressive medications for transplantation have all contributed to improved management. The prognosis depends in part on the length of the residual small intestine. An intact ileocecal valve also improves the prognosis. Infants and children with SBS die from PN-related problems, such as fulminant sepsis or severe PN cholestasis.

Nursing Care Management

The most important components of nursing care are administration and monitoring of nutritional therapy. During PN therapy, care must be taken to minimize the risk of complications related to the central venous access device (i.e., catheter infections, occlusions, dislodgment, or accidental removal). Care of the enteral feeding tubes and monitoring of enteral feeding tolerance are also important nursing responsibilities.

When hospitalization is prolonged, the child's developmental and emotional needs must be met. This often requires special planning to promote normal family adjustment and adaptation of the hospital routines. Family members require psychosocial support and education to cope successfully with SBS.

Many infants with SBS have an intestinal ostomy performed at the time of the initial bowel resection. Routine ostomy care is another important nursing responsibility. Because infants and children with SBS have chronic diarrhea, perineal skin irritation is often a problem after ostomy closure. Frequent diaper changes, gentle perineal cleansing, and protective skin ointments help prevent skin breakdown (see Chapter 31, Diaper Dermatitis).

Home Care

When long-term PN is required, preparation of the family for home care of the child is a major nursing responsibility. Preparation for home nutritional support begins as early as possible to prevent lengthy hospitalizations with subsequent problems such as developmental delays and family stresses. Many infants and children can be successfully cared for at home with enteral and parenteral nutrition if the family is thoroughly prepared and provided with adequate support services. Most families benefit from home nursing care to assist with and supervise therapy. Careful follow-up care by a multidisciplinary nutritional support service is essential. Most home health agencies now provide portable enteral and parenteral equipment, which enables the child and family to maintain a more normal and active lifestyle. The nurse plays an active and important role in the success of a home nutrition program. Home infusion companies provide portable equipment, which enables the child and family to maintain a more normal lifestyle.

HEPATIC DISORDERS

The liver is a vital organ whose functions can be divided into several groups: (1) vascular functions of storing and filtering blood; (2) secretory function of producing bile; (3) metabolism of carbohydrate, protein, and fat; (4) synthesis of blood-clotting components and storage of iron and vitamins (A, D, B_{12}, and K); and (5) detoxification and excretion of certain drugs and metabolic substances. Many disorders, including biliary atresia, hepatitis, and cirrhosis, can cause liver dysfunction in children.

ACUTE HEPATITIS

Hepatitis is an acute or chronic inflammation of the liver that can result from infectious or noninfectious reasons. Viruses such as hepatitis viruses, Epstein-Barr virus (EBV), and cytomegalovirus (CMV) are common causes of many types of hepatitis. Other causes of hepatitis are nonviral (e.g., abscess, amebiasis), autoimmune, metabolic, drug induced, anatomic (e.g., choledochal duct cyst and biliary atresia), hemodynamic (e.g., shock, congestive heart failure), and idiopathic (e.g., sclerosing cholangitis and Reye syndrome). Determining the cause of acute or chronic hepatitis is important in determining the treatment and prognosis for the child. Epidemiologic features and serologic testing are used to differentiate the causes. Table 22.8 compares the features of hepatitis A, B, and C viruses.

Hepatitis A Virus

Hepatitis A virus (HAV) incidence in the United States has declined since the introduction of a vaccine in 1995. There were approximately 1390 new cases in the United States in 2015 (Centers for Disease Control and Prevention, 2017). The virus is spread directly or indirectly by the fecal-oral route by ingestion of contaminated foods, direct exposure to infected fecal material, or close contact with an infected person. The virus is particularly prevalent in developing countries with poor living conditions, inadequate sanitation, crowding, and poor

TABLE 22.8 Comparison of Hepatitis Types A, B, and C

Characteristics	Type A	Type B	Type C
Incubation period	15-50 days, average 28 days	45-160 days, average 120 days	2-24 weeks, average 7-9 weeks
Period of communicability	Believed to be latter half of incubation period to first week after onset of clinical illness	Variable Virus in blood or other body fluids during late incubation period and acute stage of disease; may persist in carrier state for years to lifetime	Begins before onset of symptoms May persist in carrier state for years
Mode of transmission	Principal route—fecal-oral Rarely—parenteral	Principal route—parenteral Less frequent route—oral, sexual, any body fluid Perinatal transfer—transplacental blood (last trimester), at delivery, or during breastfeeding, especially if mother has cracked nipples	Principal route—parenteral Nonparenteral spread possible
Clinical features			
• Onset	Usually rapid, acute	More insidious	Usually insidious
• Fever	Common and early	Less frequent	Less frequent
• Anorexia	Common	Mild to moderate	Mild to moderate
• Nausea and vomiting	Common	Sometimes present	Mild to moderate
• Rash	Rare	Common	Sometimes present
• Arthralgia	Rare	Common	Rare
• Pruritus	Rare	Sometimes present	Sometimes present
• Jaundice	Present (many cases anicteric)	Present	Present
Immunity	Present after one attack; no crossover to type B or C	Present after one attack; no crossover to type A or C	Present after one attack; no crossover to type A or B
Carrier state	No	Yes	Yes
Chronic infection	No	Yes	Yes
Prophylaxis			
• Immune globulin (IG)	Passive immunity Successful, especially in early incubation period and preexposure prophylaxis	Passive immunity Inconsistent benefits; probably of no use	Not currently recommended by Centers for Disease Control and Prevention
• HAV vaccine	Two inactivated vaccines administered to all children ages 12-23 months old: Havrix and Vaqta; given in a 2-dose schedule (6 months between doses)		
• HBV immune globulin (HBIG)	No benefit	Postexposure protection possible if given immediately after definite exposure	No benefit
• HBV vaccine		Provides active immunity Universal vaccination recommended for all newborns	
Mortality rate	0.1%-0.2%	0.5%-2.0% in uncomplicated cases; may be higher in complicated cases	1%-2% in uncomplicated cases; may be higher in complicated cases

HAV, Hepatitis A virus; *HBV*, hepatitis B virus.

personal hygiene practices. The spread of HAV has been associated with improper food handling and high-risk areas such as households with infected persons, residential centers for the disabled, and day-care centers. The average incubation period is about 21 days (Jensen & Balistreri, 2020). Fecal shedding of the virus can occur for 2 weeks before and for 1 week after the onset of jaundice. During this time, although the individual is asymptomatic, the virus is most likely to be transmitted. Infants with HAV infection are likely to be asymptomatic (anicteric hepatitis). Children often have diarrhea, and their symptoms are frequently attributed to gastroenteritis. Younger children rarely develop jaundice; however, 70% of older children and adults infected with HAV develop clinical signs with icteric hepatitis that typically lasts 7 to 14 days (Jensen & Balistreri, 2020). The prognosis of HAV infection is usually good, and complications are rare.

Hepatitis B Virus

Although the incidence of hepatitis B virus (HBV) is declining after the introduction of a universal immunization program, approximately 1.25 million people in the United States are infected with HBV, with 400 million HBV cases worldwide (Jensen & Balistreri, 2020). HBV can be an acute or chronic infection, ranging from an asymptomatic, limited infection to fatal, fulminant (rapid and severe) hepatitis (Jensen & Balistreri, 2020). There are no environmental or animal reservoirs for HBV. Humans are the main source of infections. HBV may be transmitted parenterally, percutaneously, or transmucosally. Hepatitis B surface antigen (HBsAg) has been found in all body fluids, including feces, bile, breast milk, sweat, tears, vaginal secretions, and urine, but only blood, semen, and saliva have been found to contain infectious HBV particles. HBV infection from human bites has been documented, but transmission from feces has not. HBV has been acquired after blood transfusion, but the likelihood of this has been reduced through blood product–screening procedures. Adults whose occupations are associated with considerable exposure to blood or blood products, such as health care workers, are at an increased risk of contracting HBV.

Most HBV infections in children are acquired perinatally. Transmission from mother to infant during the perinatal period (i.e., blood exposure during delivery) results in chronic infection in up to 90% of infants if the mother is positive for HBsAg and HBeAg (Jensen & Balistreri, 2020). HBsAg has been inconsistently detected in breast milk, but no increased risk of transmission has been found, and breastfeeding is currently recommended after infant immunization (Jensen & Balistreri, 2020). Infants and children who are not infected during the perinatal period remain at high risk for acquiring person-to-person transmission from their mother.

HBV infection occurs in children and adolescents in the following specific high-risk groups: (1) individuals with hemophilia or other disorders who have received multiple transfusions, (2) children and adolescents involved in IV drug abuse, (3) institutionalized children, (4) preschool children in endemic areas, and (5) individuals engaged in sexual activity with an infected partner. The incubation period for HBV infection ranges from 45 to 160 days, with an average of 120 days (Jensen & Balistreri, 2020). HBV infection can cause a carrier state and lead to chronic hepatitis with eventual cirrhosis or hepatocellular carcinoma in adulthood.

Hepatitis C Virus

Hepatitis C virus (HCV) is the most common cause of chronic liver disease, with an estimated 4 million people in the United States and 170 million people worldwide infected (Jensen & Balistreri, 2020). HCV is transmitted parenterally through exposure to blood and blood products from HCV-infected persons, whereas perinatal transmission is the most common mode of transmission among children (Jensen & Balistreri, 2020). Recent improvements in donor screening and inactivation procedures for blood products, such as the factor concentrates used for hemophilia patients, have significantly reduced the risk of transmission through blood products. Currently the most common cause of HCV infection is illegal drug use with exposure to blood or blood products from an HCV-infected individual, and sexual transmission is the second most common cause of HCV infection (Jensen & Balistreri, 2020).

The clinical course is variable. The incubation period for HCV ranges from 2 to 24 weeks, with an average of 7 to 9 weeks (Jensen & Balistreri, 2020). The natural history of the disease in children is not well defined. Some children may be asymptomatic, but HCV can become a chronic condition and can cause cirrhosis and hepatocellular carcinoma. About 85% of individuals infected with HCV develop chronic disease (Jensen & Balistreri, 2020).

Hepatitis D Virus

Hepatitis D virus (HDV) rarely occurs in children and must occur in individuals already infected with HBV (Jensen & Balistreri, 2020). HDV is a defective RNA virus that requires the helper function of HBV. The incubation period is 2 to 8 weeks, but with coinfection of HBV the incubation period is similar to an HBV infection (Jensen & Balistreri, 2020). HDV infection occurs through blood and sexual contact, and commonly occurs among drug abusers, individuals with hemophilia, and persons immigrating from endemic areas.

Hepatitis E Virus

Hepatitis E virus (HEV) was formerly known as non-A, non-B hepatitis. Transmission may occur through the fecal-oral route or from contaminated water. The incubation period ranges from 15 to 60 days, with an average of 40 days (Jensen & Balistreri, 2020). This illness is uncommon in children, does not cause chronic liver disease, is not a chronic condition, and has no carrier state. However, it can be a devastating disease among pregnant women, with an unusually high fatality rate.

Pathophysiology

Pathologic changes occur primarily in the parenchymal cells of the liver and result in variable degrees of swelling; infiltration of liver cells by mononuclear cells; and subsequent degeneration, necrosis, and fibrosis. Structural changes within the hepatocyte account for altered liver functions, such as impaired bile excretion, elevated transaminase levels, and decreased albumin synthesis. The disorder may be self-limiting, with regeneration of liver cells without scarring, leading to a complete recovery. However, some forms of hepatitis do not result in complete return of liver function. These include fulminant hepatitis, which is characterized by a severe, acute course with massive destruction of the liver tissue causing liver failure and high mortality risk within 1 to 2 weeks, and subacute or chronic active hepatitis, which is characterized by progressive liver destruction, uncertain regeneration, scarring, and potential cirrhosis.

The progression of liver disease is characterized pathologically by four stages: (1) stage one is characterized by mononuclear inflammatory cells surrounding small bile ducts, (2) in stage two there is proliferation of small bile ductules, (3) stage three is characterized by fibrosis or scarring, and (4) stage four is cirrhosis.

Clinical Manifestations

The clinical manifestations and course of uncomplicated acute viral hepatitis are similar for most of the hepatitis viruses. Usually the prodromal, or anicteric, phase (absence of jaundice) lasts 5 to 7 days. Anorexia, malaise, lethargy, and easy fatigability are the most common symptoms. Fever may be present, especially in adolescents. Nausea, vomiting, and epigastric or right upper quadrant abdominal pain or tenderness may occur. Arthralgia and skin rashes may occur and are more likely in children with hepatitis B than those with hepatitis A. The transaminases, rather than the bilirubin, are often elevated in acute hepatitis, and hepatomegaly may be present. Some mild cases of acute viral hepatitis do not cause symptoms or can be mistaken for influenza.

In young children most of the prodromal symptoms disappear with the onset of jaundice, or the icteric phase. However, many children with acute viral hepatitis never develop jaundice. If jaundice occurs, it is often accompanied by dark urine and pale stools. Pruritus may accompany jaundice and can be bothersome for children.

Children with chronic active hepatitis may be asymptomatic but more commonly have nonspecific symptoms of malaise, fatigue, lethargy, weight loss, or vague abdominal pain. Hepatomegaly may be present, and the transaminases are often very high, with mild to severe hyperbilirubinemia.

Fulminant hepatitis is due primarily to HBV or HCV. Many children with fulminant hepatitis develop characteristic clinical symptoms and rapidly develop manifestations of liver failure, including encephalopathy, coagulation defects, ascites, deepening jaundice, and an increasing white blood cell count. Changes in mental status or personality indicate impending liver failure. Although children with acute hepatitis may have hepatomegaly, a rapid decrease in the size of the liver (indicating loss of tissue due to necrosis) is a serious sign of fulminant hepatitis. Complications of fulminant hepatitis include GI bleeding, sepsis, renal failure, and disseminated coagulopathy.

Diagnostic Evaluation

Diagnosis is based on the history, physical examination, and serologic markers for hepatitis A, B, and C. No LFT is specific for hepatitis, but serum aspartate aminotransferase (AST) and serum alanine aminotransferase (ALT) levels are markedly elevated. Serum bilirubin levels peak 5 to 10 days after clinical jaundice appears. Histologic evidence from liver biopsy may be required to establish the diagnosis and to assess the severity of the liver disease. Serologic markers indicate the antibodies or antigens formed in response to the specific virus and confirm the diagnosis. Serum immunologic tests are not available to detect HAV antigen, but there are two HAV antibody tests: anti-HAV immunoglobulin G (IgG) and immunoglobulin M (IgM). Anti-HAV antibodies are present at the onset of the disease and persist for life. A positive anti-HAV antibody test can indicate acute infection, immunity from past infection, passive antibody acquisition (e.g., from transfusion, serum immunoglobulin infusion), or immunization. To diagnose an acute or recent HAV infection, a positive anti-HAV IgM test that is present with the onset of the disease and that persists for only 2 or 3 days is required.

Diagnosis of hepatitis B is confirmed by the detection of various hepatitis virus antigens and the antibodies that are produced in response to the infection. These antibodies and antigens and their significance include the following:

HBsAg—Hepatitis B surface antigen (found on the surface of the virus), indicating ongoing infection or carrier state

Anti-HBs—Antibody to surface antigen HbsAg, indicating resolving or past infection

HBcAg—Hepatitis B core antigen (found on the inner core of the virus), detected only in the liver

Anti-HBc—Antibody to core antigen HbcAg, indicating ongoing or past infection

HBeAg—Hepatitis B antigen (another component of the HBV core), indicating active infection

Anti-HBe—Antibody to HbeAg, indicating resolving or past infection

IgM anti-HBc—IgM antibody to core antigen

Tests are available for detection of all the HBV antigens and antibodies except HBcAg. HBsAg is detectable during acute infection. Presence of HBsAg indicates that the individual has been infected with the hepatitis virus. If the infection is self-limiting, HBsAg disappears in most patients before serum anti-HBs can be detected (called the *window phase of infection*). IgM anti-HBc is highly specific in establishing the diagnosis of acute infection, as well as during the window phase in older children and adults. However, IgM anti-HBc usually is not present in perinatal HBV infection. Clinical improvement is usually associated with a decrease in or disappearance of these antigens, followed by the appearance of their antibodies. For example, anti-HBc of the IgM class often occurs early in the disease, followed by a rise in anti-HBc of the IgG class. Because the antibodies persist indefinitely, they are used to identify the carrier state (i.e., individuals with HBV who have no clinical disease but are able to transmit the organism). Persons with chronic HBV infection have circulating HBsAg and anti-HBc, and on rare occasions anti-HBsAg is present. Both anti-HBs and anti-HBc are detected in persons with resolved infection, but anti-HBs alone is present in individuals who have been immunized with the HBV vaccine.

HCV-RNA is the earliest serologic marker for HCV. HCV-RNA can be detected during the incubation period before symptoms of HCV disease are expressed. A positive HCV-RNA result indicates active infection, and persistence of HCV-RNA indicates chronic infection. A negative test correlates with resolution of the disease. HCV-RNA is also used to determine patient response to antiviral therapy for HCV.

The history of all patients should include questions to seek evidence of (1) contact with a person known to have hepatitis, especially a family member; (2) unsafe sanitation practices, such as contaminated drinking water; (3) ingestion of certain foods, such as clams or oysters (especially from polluted water); (4) multiple blood transfusions; (5) ingestion of hepatotoxic drugs, such as salicylates, sulfonamides, antineoplastic agents, acetaminophen, and anticonvulsants; and (6) parenteral administration of illicit drugs or sexual contact with a person who uses these drugs.

Therapeutic Management

The goals of management include early detection, support and monitoring of the disease, recognition of chronic liver disease, and prevention of spread of the disease. Special high-protein, high-carbohydrate, low-fat diets are generally not of value. The use of corticosteroids alone or with immunosuppressive drugs is not advocated in the treatment of chronic viral hepatitis. However, steroids have been used to treat chronic autoimmune hepatitis. Hospitalization is required in the event of coagulopathy or fulminant hepatitis.

Therapy for hepatitis depends on the severity of inflammation and the cause of the disorder. HAV is treated primarily with supportive care. The US Food and Drug Administration approved several medications for treatment of children with HBV and HCV. Human interferon-alpha is being used successfully in the treatment of chronic hepatitis B and C in children. Lamivudine is used for the treatment of HBV. It is well tolerated with no significant side effects and is approved for children older than 2 years of age (Jensen & Balistreri, 2020). Combined therapy with lamivudine and interferon-alpha does not improve response rates (Jensen & Balistreri, 2020). Adefovir is used to treat HBV in children older than 12 years of age. Entecavir and tenofovir have recently been approved for HBV treatment in adolescents ages 16 years or older (Jensen & Balistreri, 2020). Peginterferon alfa-2b has not been approved for use in children in the United States but has been used to treat HBV in people in other countries (Jensen & Balistreri, 2020).

Prevention

Proper hand washing and Standard Precautions prevent the spread of viral hepatitis. Prophylactic use of standard immune globulin is effective in preventing hepatitis A in situations of preexposure (such as anticipated travel to areas where HAV is prevalent) or within 2 weeks of exposure.

Hepatitis B immune globulin (HBIG) is effective in preventing HBV infection after one-time exposures such as accidental needle punctures or other contact of contaminated material with mucous membranes and should be given to newborns whose mothers are HbsAg positive. HBIG is prepared from plasma that contains high titers of antibodies against HBV. HBIG should be given within 72 hours of exposure.

Vaccines have been developed to prevent HAV and HBV infection (see Table 22.8). HBV vaccination is recommended for all newborns and for children who did not receive the vaccination as a newborn. (See Chapter 6, Immunizations.) Because HDV cannot be transmitted in the absence of HBV infection, it is possible to prevent HDV infection by preventing HBV infection. Routine serologic testing for anti-HCV of children older than 12 months of age who were born to women previously identified as being infected with HCV is also recommended (Jensen & Balistreri, 2020).

Prognosis

The prognosis for children with hepatitis is variable and depends on the type of virus and the child's age and immunocompetency. Hepatitis A and E are usually mild, brief illnesses with no carrier state. Hepatitis B can cause a wide spectrum of acute and chronic illness. Infants are more likely than older children to develop chronic hepatitis. Hepatocellular carcinoma during adulthood is a potentially fatal complication of chronic HBV infection. Hepatitis C frequently becomes chronic, and cirrhosis may develop in these children.

Nursing Care Management

Nursing objectives depend largely on the severity of the hepatitis, the medical treatment, and factors influencing the control and transmission of the disease. Because children with mild viral hepatitis are frequently cared for at home, it is often the nurse's responsibility to explain any medical therapies and infection control measures. When further assistance is needed for parents to comply with instructions, a public health nursing referral is necessary.

Encourage a well-balanced diet and a schedule of rest and activity adjusted to the child's condition. Because the child with HAV is not infectious within 1 week after the onset of jaundice, the child may feel well enough to resume school shortly thereafter. Caution parents about administering any medication to the child because normal doses of many drugs may become dangerous because of the liver's inability to detoxify and excrete them.

Standard Precautions are followed when children are hospitalized. However, these children are not usually isolated in a separate room unless they are fecally incontinent or their toys and other personal items are likely to become contaminated with feces. Discourage children from sharing their toys.

Hand washing is the single most effective measure in prevention and control of hepatitis in any setting. Parents and children need an explanation of the usual ways in which hepatitis is spread (fecal-oral route and parenteral route). Parents should also be aware of the recommendation for universal vaccination against HBV for newborns and adolescents (see Chapter 6).

In young people with HBV infection who have a known or suspected history of illicit drug use, the nurse has the responsibility of helping them realize the associated dangers of drug abuse, stressing the parenteral mode of transmission of hepatitis, and encouraging them to seek counseling through a drug program.

BILIARY ATRESIA

Biliary atresia (BA), or extrahepatic biliary atresia (EHBA), is a progressive inflammatory process that causes both intrahepatic and extrahepatic bile duct fibrosis, resulting in eventual ductal obstruction. The incidence of BA is approximately 1 in 10,000 to 15,000 live births (Hassan & Balistreri, 2020). Associated malformations include polysplenia and malrotation of the intestine. BA, if untreated, usually leads to cirrhosis, liver failure, and death.

Pathophysiology

The exact cause of BA is unknown, although immune- or infection-mediated mechanisms may be responsible for the progressive process that results in complete obliteration of the bile ducts. BA is not seen in the fetus or stillborn or newborn infant. This suggests that BA is acquired late in gestation or in the perinatal period and is manifested a few weeks after birth.

Congenital infections have been implicated as a cause of hepatocellular damage leading to BA, yet no specific agent is identified in every case. Immune-mediated bile duct injury from viral exposure and immaturity of the neonatal immune system may play a role in the destruction of bile ducts and development of EHBA. Other potential causes include an early first trimester insult to the developing bile ducts or a postnatal viral insult (Hassan & Balistreri, 2020). Early in the course of the disease, the intrahepatic ducts are patent from the interlobular ductules to the porta hepatis. The size of these structures is variable and is correlated with the infant's age and with bile excretion after surgical treatment. These structures are present in most affected infants under 2 months of age but gradually disappear over the next few months and by 4 months are completely replaced by fibrous tissue.

The degree of involvement of the extrahepatic biliary ducts is also variable. The majority of cases of BA (85%) have a complete obliteration of the extrahepatic biliary tree at or above the porta hepatis (Hassan & Balistreri, 2020). But some infants have a patent proximal portion of the extrahepatic duct or patency of the gallbladder, cystic duct, and common bile duct. Microscopic examination of the liver tissue reveals cholestasis with absent or diminished bile duct proliferation and fibrosis.

Clinical Manifestations

Many infants with BA are full term and appear healthy at birth. If **jaundice** persists beyond 2 weeks of age, especially if the direct (conjugated) serum bilirubin is elevated, the nurse should suspect BA. The urine may be dark, and the stools often become progressively acholic or gray, indicating absence of bile pigment. Hepatomegaly is present early in the course of the disease, and the liver is firm on palpation.

Diagnostic Evaluation

Early diagnosis is critical to the child with EHBA; the outcome in children surgically treated before 2 months of age is much better than in patients with delayed treatment. The diagnosis of BA is suspected on the basis of the history, physical findings, and laboratory studies. Laboratory tests include a CBC, bilirubin levels, and liver function studies. Additional laboratory analyses, including alpha-1 antitrypsin level, TORCH titers and other intrauterine infections (see Chapter 9), hepatitis serology, and urine cytomegalovirus, may be indicated to rule out other conditions that cause cholestasis and jaundice. An abdominal ultrasound is usually performed to identify potential causes of extrahepatic obstruction, such as a choledochal cyst. The patency of the extrahepatic biliary system is demonstrated by a nuclear scintiscan using technetium-99m iminodiacetic acid (^{99m}Tc IDA or HIDA; **HIDA scan**). If there is no evidence of radioactive material excreted into the duodenum, BA is the most probable diagnosis. Because the nuclear scan may take up to 5 days for the results, a percutaneous liver biopsy is probably the most useful method of diagnosing BA (Govindarajan, 2016). The definitive diagnosis of BA is further established during an exploratory laparotomy and an intraoperative cholangiogram that demonstrates complete obstruction at some level of the biliary tree.

Therapeutic Management

Medical management of BA is primarily supportive. It includes nutritional support with infant formulas that contain medium-chain triglycerides and essential fatty acids. Supplementation with fat-soluble vitamins (A, D, E, and K); a multivitamin; and minerals, including iron, zinc, and selenium, is usually required. Aggressive nutritional support in the form of continuous gastrostomy feedings or TPN may be indicated for moderate to severe growth failure; the enteral solution should be low in sodium. Phenobarbital may be prescribed after hepatic portoenterostomy to stimulate bile flow, and ursodeoxycholic acid may be used to decrease cholestasis and the intense pruritus from jaundice. In cases of advanced liver dysfunction, management is the same as in infants with cirrhosis.

The primary surgical treatment of BA is hepatic portoenterostomy (**Kasai procedure**), in which a segment of intestine is anastomosed to the resected porta hepatis to attempt bile drainage. A Roux-en-Y jejunal limb is then anastomosed to the porta hepatis (a Y-shaped anastomosis performed to provide bile drainage without reflux). Complications after portoenterostomy include ascending cholangitis, cirrhosis, portal hypertension, and GI bleeding. Prophylactic antibiotics are given after the Kasai procedure to minimize the risk of ascending cholangitis. After the Kasai procedure approximately one-third of infants become jaundice free and regain normal liver function. Another one-third of infants demonstrate liver damage; however, they may be supported by medical and nutritional interventions. A final third require liver transplantation. Liver transplantation is required for children who cannot regain bile flow and for those with end-stage liver disease or severe portal hypertension. Complications after liver transplantation include obstruction and bile leaks at the biliary anastomosis, portal hypertension, hemorrhage, infection, and rejection. Immunosuppressive drugs are required after transplantation.

Prognosis

Untreated BA results in progressive cirrhosis and death in most children by 3 years of age (Govindarajan, 2016). The Kasai procedure improves the prognosis but is not a cure. There is only 20% survival in patients 20 years after the Kasai procedure and only 10% survival in patients 30 years after the procedure (Govindarajan, 2016).

Biliary drainage can often be achieved if the surgery is performed before the intrahepatic bile ducts are destroyed; the success rate is much higher, up to 90%, if surgery is performed in an infant younger than 2 months of age (Hassan & Balistreri, 2020). Long-term survival rates of 64% to 92% have been noted in children after portoenterostomy (Govindarajan, 2016). However, even with successful bile drainage, many children ultimately develop liver failure and require liver transplantation.

The advances in surgical techniques for liver transplantation and the development of immunosuppressive and antifungal drugs have significantly improved the success of transplantation. Surgical techniques and immunosuppression have contributed to survival rates of 83% to 91% in children who underwent transplant (Yanagi, Matsuura, Hayashida, et al., 2017). The major obstacle remains the shortage of suitable infant donors.

Liver disease progresses in infants with delayed diagnosis or in children in whom surgery has failed to provide adequate bile drainage. Cirrhosis and splenomegaly occur with hypoalbuminemia, ascites, and coagulopathy. Malabsorption of fat and fat-soluble vitamins and malnutrition result in severe growth failure. Retained bile salts and cholesterol further contribute to **pruritus** (itching) and xanthomas, often requiring the administration of **ursodeoxycholic acid**. The severity of pruritus intensifies as the jaundice progresses as the result of disease advancement.

Nursing Care Management

There are many important nursing interventions for the child with BA. The nurse should educate family members on all aspects of the treatment plan and the rationale for therapy. Immediately after a hepatic portoenterostomy, nursing care is similar to that after any major abdominal surgery. If an interrupted jejunal conduit has been performed, the family needs to learn how to care for the two stomas and how to refeed the bile after feedings. Teaching includes the proper administration of medications. Administration of nutritional therapy, including special formulas, vitamin and mineral supplements, gastrostomy feedings, or parenteral nutrition, is an essential nursing responsibility. Growth failure in such infants is common, and increased metabolic needs combined with ascites, pruritus, and nutritional anorexia constitute a challenge for care. The nurse teaches caregivers how to monitor and administer nutritional therapy in the home. Pruritus may be a significant problem that is addressed by drug therapy or comfort measures such as baths in colloidal oatmeal compounds and trimming of fingernails. The risk of complications of BA, such as cholangitis, portal hypertension, GI bleeding, and ascites, should be explained to the caregivers.

These children and their families require special psychosocial support. The uncertain prognosis, discomfort, and waiting for transplantation can produce considerable stress (see Cirrhosis, next). In addition, extended hospitalizations, as well as pharmacologic and nutritional therapy, can impose significant financial burdens on the family, as with any chronic condition. The expertise of a multidisciplinary health care team, including surgeons, gastroenterologists, pediatricians, nurses, nutritionists, pharmacists, child life specialists, and social workers, is often necessary. Parent support groups can be beneficial as well. The Children's Liver Association for Support Services (C.L.A.S.S.)[e] and the American Liver Foundation[f] provide educational materials, programs, and support systems for parents of children with liver disease.

CIRRHOSIS

Cirrhosis occurs as an end stage of many chronic liver diseases, including BA and chronic hepatitis. Infectious, autoimmune, toxic injury, and chronic diseases such as hemophilia and cystic fibrosis can cause severe liver damage. A cirrhotic liver is irreversibly damaged.

Pathophysiology

Cirrhosis occurs as a result of hepatocyte injury with necrosis, fibrosis, regeneration, and eventual degeneration. The diminished parenchymal cell mass causes regeneration of tissue with nodular areas of proliferating hepatocytes that stretch the surrounding connective tissue. Hepatocytes respond to injury with deposition of collagen that forms fibrous connective tissue. This scar tissue and nodular areas of regeneration impair the intrahepatic blood flow. Ongoing necrosis and self-perpetuation of this pathologic process are the result of cirrhosis.

Failure of hepatocellular function and portal hypertension occur and often lead to complications, including ascites, severe cholestasis, encephalopathy (hepatic coma), and GI bleeding.

---

[e]P.O. Box 186, Monaca, PA 15061; (724) 581-5527; http://www.classkids.org.

[f]39 Broadway, Suite 2700, New York, NY 10006; 212-668-1000; http://www.liverfoundation.org.

Clinical Manifestations

Clinical manifestations of cirrhosis include jaundice, poor growth, anorexia, muscle weakness, and lethargy. Ascites, edema, GI bleeding, anemia, and abdominal pain may be present in children with impaired intrahepatic blood flow. Pulmonary function may be impaired because of pressure against the diaphragm due to hepatosplenomegaly and ascites. Dyspnea and cyanosis may occur, especially on exertion. Intrapulmonary arteriovenous shunts may develop, which can also cause hypoxemia. Spider angiomas and prominent blood vessels on the upper torso are often present.

Diagnostic Evaluation

The diagnosis of cirrhosis is based on (1) the history, especially in regard to prior liver disease, such as hepatitis; (2) physical examination, particularly hepatosplenomegaly; (3) laboratory evaluation, especially LFTs, such as bilirubin and transaminases, ammonia, albumin, cholesterol, and prothrombin time; and (4) liver biopsy for characteristic changes. Doppler ultrasonography of the liver and spleen is useful to confirm ascites, to evaluate the blood flow through the liver and spleen, and to determine the patency and size of the portal vein if liver transplantation is considered.

! NURSING ALERT

The most common complication from percutaneous liver biopsy is internal bleeding. Vital signs and laboratory values, especially hematocrit, should be monitored for evidence of hemorrhage and shock.

Therapeutic Management

Unfortunately, there is no successful treatment to arrest the progression of cirrhosis. The goals of management include monitoring liver function and managing specific complications such as esophageal varices and malnutrition. Assessment of the child's degree of liver dysfunction is important so that the child can be evaluated for transplantation at the appropriate time.

Liver transplantation has improved the prognosis substantially for many children with cirrhosis. Pediatric liver transplantation is one of the most successful solid organ transplants with a 1-year survival rate of 83% to 91%, depending on the age at transplant (Yanagi et al., 2017). The policy governing the allocation of livers for transplantation by the United Network for Organ Sharing allows pediatric patients younger than 12 years of age, those with acute fulminant liver failure, or those with chronic liver disease to be placed at the top of the network's transplantation lists (United Network for Organ Sharing, 2017). Although this change has benefited many pediatric patients, the shortage of available donors for children continues to dictate transplantation decisions, and many children continue to die while waiting for a suitable donor.

Nutritional support is an important therapy for children with cirrhosis and malnutrition. Supplements of fat-soluble vitamins are often required, and mineral supplements may be indicated. In some instances aggressive nutritional support in the form of enteral feeding or PN may be necessary.

Esophageal and gastric varices can be a life-threatening complication of portal hypertension. Acute hemorrhage is managed with IV fluids; blood products; vitamin K, if needed to correct coagulopathy; vasopressin or somatostatin; and gastric lavage. If acute hemorrhage persists, the most common secondary approach is endoscopic sclerotherapy or endoscopic banding ligation (Choudhary, Puri, Saigal, et al., 2016). Balloon tamponade with a Sengstaken-Blakemore tube may be indicated for the unstable patient with acute hemorrhage (Choudhary et al., 2016). Ascites is managed by sodium and fluid restrictions and diuretics. Severe ascites with respiratory compromise is managed with albumin infusions or by paracentesis.

Although the full mechanism of hepatic encephalopathy is unknown, failure of the damaged liver to remove endogenous toxins, such as ammonia, plays a role. Treatment is directed at limiting the ammonia formation and absorption that occur in the bowel, especially with the drugs neomycin and lactulose. Because ammonia is formed in the bowel by the action of bacteria on ingested protein, neomycin reduces the number of intestinal bacteria so that less ammonia is produced. The fermentation of lactulose by colonic bacteria produces short-chain fatty acids, which lower the colonic pH, thereby inhibiting bacterial metabolism. This decreases the formation of ammonia from bacterial metabolism of protein.

Prognosis

The success of liver transplantation has revolutionized the approach to liver cirrhosis. Liver failure and cirrhosis are indications for transplantation. Careful monitoring of the child's condition and quality of life is necessary to evaluate the need for and timing of transplantation.

Nursing Care Management

Several factors influence nursing care of the child with cirrhosis, including the cause of the cirrhosis, the severity of complications, and the prognosis. The prognosis is often poor unless successful liver transplantation occurs. Therefore nursing care of this child is similar to that for any child with a life-threatening illness (see Chapter 19). Hospitalization is required when complications such as hemorrhage, severe malnutrition, or hepatic failure occur. Nursing assessments are directed at monitoring the child's condition, and interventions are aimed at treatment of specific complications. If liver transplantation is an option, the family needs support and assistance to cope (see Family-Centered Care box).

FAMILY-CENTERED CARE

End-Stage Liver Disease

In many cases the child with liver disease and the family must cope with an uncertain progression of the disease. The only hope for long-term survival may be liver transplantation. Transplantation can be successful, but the waiting period may be long because there are many more children in need of organs than there are donors. The procedure is expensive and is performed only at designated medical centers, which are often far from the family's home. The nurse should recognize the unique stresses of coping with end-stage liver disease and waiting for transplantation and should offer support and assistance to the family in coping with these stressors. The assistance of social workers and support from other parents can also be beneficial.

STRUCTURAL DEFECTS

Congenital defects of the GI tract can involve any portion from the mouth to the anus. Most are apparent at birth or shortly thereafter and are anomalies in which normal growth ceased at a crucial stage of embryonic development, leaving the structure in an embryonic form or only partially completed. The result may be atresia, malposition, nonclosure, or any number of variations.

Atresia is absence of a normal opening or normally patent lumen. Atresia at any point along the length of the GI tract creates an obstruction to the normal progress of nutrients and secretions. The most common anomalies requiring surgical intervention are atresias of the esophagus, intestine, and anus. The congenital defects considered in this chapter include abnormalities of the lip, palate, trachea, esophagus, and anus.

ESOPHAGEAL ATRESIA AND TRACHEOESOPHAGEAL FISTULA

Congenital esophageal atresia (EA) and tracheoesophageal fistula (TEF) are rare malformations that represent a failure of the esophagus to develop as a continuous passage and a failure of the trachea and esophagus to separate into distinct structures. These defects may occur as separate entities or in combination, and without early diagnosis and treatment they pose a serious threat to the infant's well-being.

The incidence of EA is estimated to be approximately 1 in 3000 neonates (Wu, Kuang, Lv, et al., 2017). There appears to be a slightly higher incidence in males, and the birth weight of most affected infants is significantly lower than average, with an unusually high incidence of preterm birth in infants with EA and a subsequent increase in mortality. A history of maternal polyhydramnios is common.

Approximately 50% of the cases of EA or TEF are a component of VATER or VACTERL association, acronyms used to describe associated anomalies (VATER for *V*ertebral defects, imperforate *A*nus, *T*racheo*e*sophageal fistula, and *R*adial and *R*enal dysplasia; and VACTERL for *V*ertebral, *A*nal, *C*ardiac, *T*racheal, *E*sophageal, *R*enal, and *L*imb) (Khan & Matta, 2020b). Cardiac anomalies may also occur with EA or TEF; therefore all patients should undergo a workup for associated anomalies.

Pathophysiology

The esophagus develops from the first segment of the embryonic gut. During the fourth and fifth weeks of gestation, the foregut normally lengthens and separates longitudinally. Each longitudinal portion fuses to form two parallel channels (the esophagus and the trachea) that are joined only at the larynx. Anomalies involving the trachea and esophagus are caused by defective separation, incomplete fusion of the tracheal folds after this separation, or altered cellular growth during embryonic development.

The most commonly encountered form of EA and TEF (80% to 90% of cases) is one in which the proximal esophageal segment terminates in a blind pouch and the distal segment is connected to the trachea or primary bronchus by a short fistula at or near the tracheal bifurcation (Fig. 22.6C). The second most common type (7% to 8%) consists of a blind pouch at each end, widely separated and with no communication to the trachea (Fig. 22.6A). An H-type EA refers to an otherwise normal trachea and esophagus connected by a fistula (4% to 5%) (Fig. 22.6E). Extremely rare anomalies involve a fistula from the trachea to the upper esophageal segment (0.8%) (Fig. 22.6B) or to both the upper and lower segments (0.7% to 6%) (Fig. 22.6D).

Clinical Manifestations

The presence of EA is suspected in a newborn with frothy saliva in the mouth and nose, drooling, choking, and coughing. Respiratory distress may be mild or significant, depending on the type of defect and the infant's gestational age. If fed, the infant may swallow normally but suddenly cough and gag, with return of fluid through the nose and mouth. The infant may become cyanotic and apneic because of aspiration of breast milk or saliva.

In the infant who has EA with a distal TEF (type C), the stomach becomes distended with air, and thoracic and abdominal compressions (especially during crying) cause the gastric contents to be regurgitated through the fistula and into the trachea, producing a chemical pneumonitis. When the upper segment of the esophagus opens directly into the trachea (types B and D), the infant is in danger of aspirating any swallowed material. Cyanosis or choking during feeding may be the only symptom of type H fistula (see Fig. 22.6E). The child with this type of EA may not manifest symptoms until later in life when he or she shows signs of chronic respiratory problems, recurrent pneumonia, and signs of GER (Khan & Matta, 2020b).

Diagnostic Evaluation

Although the diagnosis is established on the basis of clinical signs and symptoms, the exact type of anomaly is determined by radiographic studies. A radiopaque catheter is inserted into the hypopharynx and advanced until it encounters an obstruction. Chest radiographs are taken to ascertain esophageal patency or the presence and level of a blind pouch. Films that show air in the stomach indicate a connection between the trachea and the distal esophagus in types C, D, and E. Complete absence of air in the stomach is seen in types A and B. Occasionally, fistulas are not patent, which makes their presence more difficult to diagnose. A careful bronchoscopic examination may be performed in an attempt to visualize the fistula.

The presence of **polyhydramnios** (accumulation of 2000 ml of amniotic fluid) prenatally is a clue to the possibility of EA in the unborn infant, especially with defect type A, B, or C. With these types of EA or TEF, amniotic fluid normally swallowed by the fetus is unable to reach the GI tract to be absorbed and excreted by the kidneys. The result is an abnormal accumulation of amniotic fluid, or polyhydramnios.

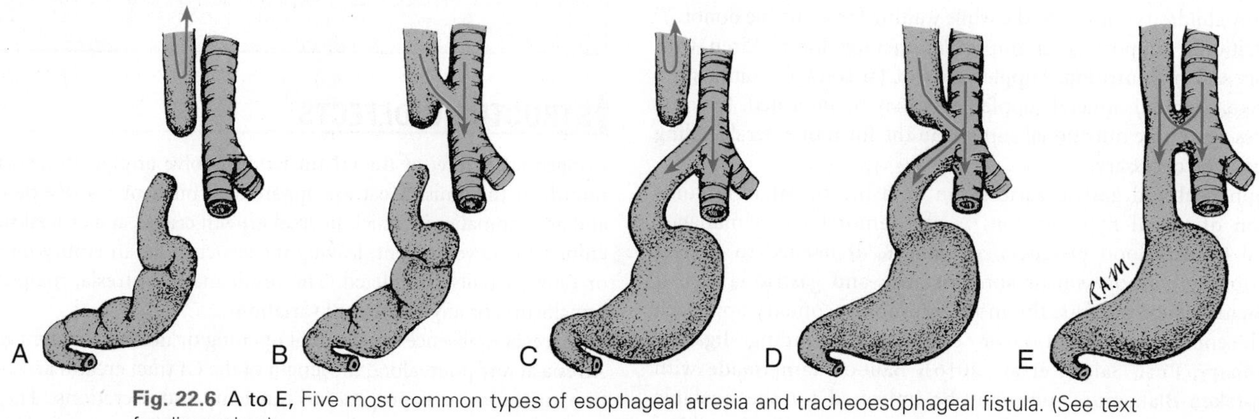

Fig. 22.6 A to E, Five most common types of esophageal atresia and tracheoesophageal fistula. (See text for discussion.)

Therapeutic Management

The treatment of EA and TEF includes maintenance of a patent airway, prevention of pneumonia, gastric or blind pouch decompression, supportive therapy, and surgical repair of the anomaly.

When EA with a TEF is suspected, the infant is immediately deprived of oral intake, IV fluids are initiated, and the infant is positioned to facilitate drainage of secretions and decrease the likelihood of aspiration. Accumulated secretions are suctioned frequently from the mouth and pharynx. A double-lumen catheter should be placed into the upper esophageal pouch and attached to intermittent or continuous low suction. The infant's head is kept upright to facilitate removal of fluid collected in the pouch and to prevent aspiration of gastric contents. Broad-spectrum antibiotic therapy is often instituted if there is a concern about aspiration of gastric contents.

Most malformations can be corrected surgically in one operation or in two or more staged procedures. The success depends on early diagnosis before complications occur and on the presence and severity of associated anomalies and illness factors, including preterm birth. With measures instituted to prevent aspiration pneumonia and to ensure adequate hydration and nutrition, surgery may be postponed to allow for more effective treatment of pneumonia and physiologic stabilization so that the infant can better withstand the complex surgery. The delay also offers an opportunity for further evaluation and assessment to rule out any associated anomalies and to optimize respiratory support.

Thoracoscopic repair of EA or TEF is being used successfully, thus negating the need for a thoracotomy and minimizing associated postoperative complications and morbidities (Khan & Matta, 2020b). The surgery consists of a thoracotomy with division and ligation of the TEF and an end-to-end or end-to-side anastomosis of the esophagus. A chest tube may be inserted to drain intrapleural air and fluid. For infants who are not stable enough to undergo definitive repair or those with a lengthy gap (>3 to 4 cm) between the proximal and distal esophagus, a staged operation is preferred that involves gastrostomy, ligation of the TEF, and constant drainage of the esophageal pouch (Khan & Matta, 2020b). A delayed esophageal anastomosis is usually attempted after several weeks to months.

A primary anastomosis may be impossible because of insufficient length of the two segments of esophagus. This occurs if the distance between the two segments is 3 to 4 cm (1.2 to 1.6 inches) (approximately three vertebral bodies) or greater; this is often referred to as *long-gap EA* (Khan & Matta, 2020b). In these cases an esophageal replacement procedure using a part of the colon or gastric tube interposition may be necessary to bridge the missing esophageal segment. Further surgical techniques may be performed later to facilitate esophageal lengthening.

Tracheomalacia may occur as a result of weakness in the tracheal wall that exists when a dilated proximal pouch compresses the trachea early in fetal life. It may also occur as a result of inadequate intratracheal pressure causing abnormal tracheal development. Clinical signs of tracheomalacia include barking cough, stridor, wheezing, recurrent respiratory tract infections, cyanosis, and sometimes apnea.

Prognosis

The survival rate is nearly 100% in otherwise healthy children. Most deaths are the result of extreme prematurity or other lethal associated anomalies.

Potential complications after the surgical repair of EA and TEF depend on the type of defect and surgical correction. Complications of repair include an anastomotic leak, strictures caused by tension or ischemia, esophageal motility disorders causing dysphagia, respiratory compromise, scoliosis, chest wall deformity, and GER. Anastomotic esophageal strictures may cause dysphagia, choking, and respiratory distress. The strictures are often treated with routine esophageal dilation. Feeding difficulties are often present for months or years after surgery, and the infant must be monitored closely to ensure adequate weight gain, growth, and development. In some cases laparoscopic fundoplication may be required. At times the infant must be fed via gastrostomy or jejunostomy to provide adequate caloric intake.

Nursing Care Management

Nursing responsibility for detection of this serious malformation begins immediately after birth. For the infant with the classic signs and symptoms of EA (see Nursing Alert) the major concern is the establishment of a patent airway and prevention of further respiratory compromise. Cyanosis is usually a result of laryngeal spasm caused by overflow of saliva into the larynx from the proximal esophageal pouch or aspiration; it normally resolves after removal of the secretions from the oropharynx by suctioning. The passage of a small-gauge orogastric (OG) feeding tube via the mouth into the stomach during the initial nursing physical assessment is helpful to determine the presence of EA or other obstructive defects.

! NURSING ALERT

Any infant who has an excessive amount of frothy saliva in the mouth or difficulty with secretions and unexplained episodes of apnea, cyanosis, or oxygen desaturation should be suspected of having an esophageal atresia (EA) or tracheoesophageal fistula (TEF) and referred immediately for medical evaluation.

Preoperative Care

The nurse carefully suctions the mouth and nasopharynx and places the infant in an optimum position to facilitate drainage and avoid aspiration. The most desirable position for a newborn who is suspected of having the typical EA with a TEF (e.g., type C) is supine (or sometimes prone) with the head elevated on an inclined plane of at least 30 degrees. This positioning minimizes the reflux of gastric secretions at the distal esophagus into the trachea and bronchi, especially when intra-abdominal pressure is elevated.

It is imperative to immediately remove any secretions that can be aspirated. Until surgery the blind pouch is kept empty by intermittent or continuous suction through an indwelling double-lumen catheter passed orally or nasally to the end of the pouch. In some cases a percutaneous gastrostomy tube is inserted and left open so that any air entering the stomach through the fistula can escape, thus minimizing the danger of gastric contents being regurgitated into the trachea. The gastrostomy tube is emptied by gravity drainage. Feedings through the gastrostomy tube and irrigations with fluid are contraindicated before surgery in the infant with a distal TEF.

Nursing interventions include respiratory assessment, airway management, thermoregulation, fluid and electrolyte management, and parenteral nutritional support.

Often the infant must be transferred to a hospital with a specialized care unit and pediatric surgical team. The nurse advises the parents of the infant's condition and provides them with necessary support and information.

Postoperative Care

Postoperative care for these infants is the same as for any high-risk newborn. Adequate thermoregulation is provided, the double-lumen NG catheter is attached to low-suction or gravity drainage, parenteral nutrition is provided, and the gastrostomy tube (if applicable) is returned to gravity drainage until feedings are tolerated. If a thoracotomy is performed and a chest tube is inserted, attention to the appropriate function of the closed drainage system is imperative. Pain management in the postoperative period is important even if only a thoracoscopic approach is used. In the first 24 to 36 hours the nurse should provide pain management for the neonate just as for an adult undergoing a similar procedure (see Chapter 5, Pain in Neonates). Tracheal suction should only be done using a premeasured catheter and with extreme caution to avoid injury to the suture line.

If tolerated, gastrostomy feedings may be initiated and continued until the esophageal anastomosis is healed. Before oral feedings are initiated and the chest tube (if applicable) is removed, a contrast study or esophagram will verify the integrity of the esophageal anastomosis.

The nurse must carefully observe the initial attempt at oral feeding to make certain the infant is able to swallow without choking. Oral feedings are begun with sterile water, followed by frequent small feedings of breast milk or formula. Until the infant is able to take a sufficient amount by mouth, oral intake may need to be supplemented by bolus or continuous gastrostomy feedings. Ordinarily infants are not discharged until they can take oral fluids well. The gastrostomy tube may be removed before discharge or maintained for supplemental feedings at home.

Special Problems

Upper respiratory tract complications are a threat to life in both the preoperative and the postoperative periods. In addition to pneumonia, the infants are in constant danger of respiratory distress resulting from atelectasis, pneumothorax, and laryngeal edema. Any persistent respiratory difficulty after removal of secretions must be reported to the surgeon immediately. The infant should be monitored for anastomotic leaks and signs of infection such as purulent chest tube drainage, an increased white blood cell count, and temperature instability.

For the infant who requires esophageal replacement, nonnutritive sucking should be provided with a pacifier. Infants who are on NPO status for an extended period and have not received oral stimulation frequently have difficulty eating by mouth after corrective surgery and may develop oral hypersensitivity and feeding aversion. They require patient, firm guidance in learning the techniques of taking food into the mouth and swallowing after repair. A referral to a multidisciplinary feeding behavior team may be necessary.

One of the difficulties in TEF is the immediate transfer of the sick infant to the intensive care unit and sometimes lengthy hospitalization. Parent-infant bonding is facilitated by encouraging parents to visit the infant, participate in his or her care when appropriate, and express their feelings regarding the infant's condition. The nurse in the intensive care unit should assume responsibility for ensuring that the parents are fully informed of the infant's progress.

Family Support, Discharge Planning, and Home Care

Some infants with EA or TEF may require periodic esophageal dilations on an outpatient basis. Discharge education should include instructions about feeding techniques in the child with a repaired esophagus, including a semiupright feeding position, small feedings, and observation for adequacy of swallowing (e.g., regurgitation, cyanosis, choking). Tracheomalacia is often a complication; parents are educated about the signs and symptoms of this condition, which include a barking cough, stridor, wheezing, recurrent respiratory tract infections, cyanosis, and sometimes apnea. GER may also occur when feedings resume and may contribute to reactive airway disease with wheezing and labored respirations as the prominent clinical manifestations. Problems with thriving and gaining weight may occur in the first 5 years of life in the child with EA or TEF, especially if the infant is born preterm. The nurse should be alert to the achievement of developmental milestones that indicate a need for early intervention and multidisciplinary referral.

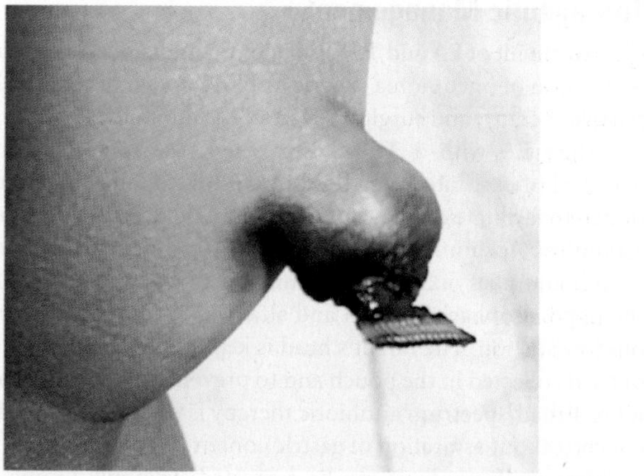

Fig. 22.7 Newborn with umbilical hernia. (From Zitelli, B. J., & Davis, H. W. [2007]. *Atlas of pediatric physical diagnosis* [5th ed.]. St. Louis, MO: Mosby.)

Preparing parents for discharge of their infant involves teaching the techniques that will be continued at home. The parents learn signs of respiratory difficulty and of esophageal stricture (e.g., poor feeding, choking, dysphagia, drooling, regurgitating undigested food) and GER.

Parents must be aware of feeding restrictions. Remind parents that it is particularly important to guard against the infant swallowing foreign objects. They should cut solid food into small pieces, teach the child to chew thoroughly, give frequent sips of liquid to help swallow food, and avoid foods such as whole hot dogs or large pieces of meat that may become lodged in the esophagus. (See Chapter 10.)

Discharge planning should include attainment of needed equipment and home nursing services to assist with ongoing assessment of the child and continuity of care.

HERNIAS

A **hernia** is a protrusion of a portion of an organ or organs through an abnormal opening. The danger of herniation arises when the protrusion is constricted, impairing circulation, or when the protrusion interferes with the function or development of other structures. The herniations discussed in this section are those that protrude through the diaphragm, the abdominal wall, or the inguinal canal.

Umbilical Hernia

The **umbilical hernia** is a common hernia observed in infants. It occurs when fusion of the umbilical ring is incomplete at the point where the umbilical vessels exit the abdominal wall. It affects low-birth-weight and preterm infants more often than full-term infants. An umbilical hernia usually is an isolated defect, but it may be associated with other congenital anomalies, such as Down syndrome (trisomy 21) and trisomies 13 and 18. The size of the defect is variable, and the protrusion is more prominent when the infant is crying (Fig. 22.7). **Incarceration**, in which the hernia is constricted and cannot be reduced manually, is rare. Hernias usually resolve spontaneously by 3 to 5 years of age. If the hernia persists beyond this age, it is usually surgically corrected on an elective basis.

Nursing Care Management

The appearance of an umbilical hernia may be disconcerting to parents. Therefore they need reassurance that the defect usually is not harmful. Taping or strapping the abdomen to flatten the protrusion does not aid in resolution and can produce skin irritation.

Nursing care of the child with an umbilical hernia repair is essentially the same as that for other minor GI surgery. The procedure may be performed on an outpatient basis. Observe the child for complications related to a hematoma or infection. The child may resume a normal diet and activity postoperatively; however, strenuous activity or play is restricted for 2 to 3 weeks.

Inguinal Hernia

Inguinal hernias account for approximately 80% of all childhood hernias and occur more frequently in boys than in girls (approximately 6:1). An incidence of 0.8% to 5% is reported in term newborns and of up to 30% is reported in low-birth-weight and preterm infants (Abdulhai, Glenn, & Ponsky, 2017).

Pathophysiology

Inguinal hernia comes from persistence of all or part of the processus vaginalis, the tube of peritoneum that precedes the testicle through the inguinal canal into the scrotum (in boys) or the round ligament into the labia (in girls), during the eighth month of gestation. After descent of the testicle, the proximal portion of the processus vaginalis normally atrophies and closes, whereas the distal portion forms the tunica vaginalis, which envelops the testicle in the scrotum. When the upper portion fails to atrophy, the abdominal fluid or an abdominal structure (e.g., bowel, ovary, fallopian tubes) can be forced into it, creating a palpable bulge or mass. The persistent sac may end at any point along the inguinal canal; it may stop at the inguinal ring or extend all the way into the scrotum or labia.

Clinical Manifestations

This common defect is usually asymptomatic unless the abdominal contents are forced into the patent sac. Most often it appears as a painless inguinal swelling that varies in size. It disappears during periods of rest or is reducible by gentle compression. It appears when the infant cries or strains or when the older child strains, coughs, or stands for a long time. The defect can be palpated as a thickening of the cord in the groin, and the silk glove sign can be elicited by rubbing together the sides of the empty hernial sac.

Sometimes the herniated loop of intestine becomes partially obstructed, producing variable symptoms that may include irritability, tenderness, anorexia, abdominal distention, and difficulty defecating. Occasionally the loop of bowel becomes **incarcerated** (irreducible) or strangulated (loss of blood supply), with symptoms of complete intestinal obstruction that, left untreated, will progress to strangulation and necrotic bowel. Incarceration occurs more often in infants younger than 12 months of age. The incidence of incarceration is reported to be 3% to 16% but as high as 30% in premature infants (Abdulhai et al., 2017).

Therapeutic Management

The treatment for hernias is prompt, elective surgical repair in the healthy child as soon as the defect is diagnosed. However, an incarcerated hernia requires emergent surgical care. Because there was believed to be a significant incidence of bilateral involvement, many surgeons advocated exploration of both sides; however, this practice has gained disfavor due to complications occurring with open exploration (Aiken, 2020b). Laparoscopic exploration of the contralateral side may be performed without risk of injury to the vas deferens (Aiken, 2020b).

Nursing Care Management

Prompt recognition of an inguinal hernia is imperative. The hernia may first be noticed when the infant is crying or straining to stool (Valsalva maneuver). Nursing care of the infant or child with an inguinal hernia involves preoperative preparation of the infant and appropriate explanation to the parents of the child's expected postoperative status. Most hernia repairs can be managed on an outpatient basis. The preterm infant usually has hernia repair several days before discharge. The former preterm infant diagnosed after discharge is admitted on the day of surgery and, after repair, is observed for 12 to 24 hours for apnea and bradycardia.

Postoperatively the incision is kept clean and dry, and the infant's pain is managed appropriately. In infants and small children who are not yet toilet trained, the wound may be covered with an occlusive dressing or left without a dressing. Changing diapers as soon as they become damp helps reduce the chance of irritation or infection of the incision.

No restrictions are placed on activity for the infant or toddler, but older children are cautioned against lifting, pushing, wrestling or fighting, bicycle riding, and participation in sporting events for about 3 weeks.

If surgery is postponed, parents need to learn the signs of incarcerated hernia, simple measures to reduce it (e.g., a warm bath, avoidance of upright positioning, and comfort measures to reduce crying), and where to call for assistance if relief is not obtained in a reasonably short time.

Femoral Hernia

Femoral hernias are rare in children, with a reported incidence of less than 1% (Abdulhai et al., 2017). The incidence is higher in girls than in boys. The hernia may manifest as a recurrent hernia after inguinal hernia repair. Initial symptoms are swelling in the groin area associated with severe abdominal pain and cramping. Treatment and management are the same as for inguinal hernia. Incarceration and strangulation are frequent complications.

ANORECTAL MALFORMATIONS

Anorectal malformations (ARMs) are among the more common congenital malformations caused by abnormal development, with an incidence of approximately 1 in 3000 births (Shanti, 2020). These malformations may range from simple imperforate anus to other associated complex anomalies of genitourinary (GU) and pelvic organs, which may require extensive treatment for fecal, urinary, and sexual function. Anorectal malformations may occur in isolation or as a part of the VACTERL association (see earlier in the chapter). These anomalies are classified according to the newborn's gender and abnormal anatomic features, including GU defects (Box 22.10). More than half of all ARMs are associated with other anomalies.

Rectal atresia and stenosis occur when the anal opening appears normal, there is a midline intergluteal groove, and usually no fistula exists between the rectum and urinary tract. **Rectal atresia** is a complete obstruction (inability to pass stool) and requires immediate surgical intervention. **Rectal stenosis** may not become apparent until later in infancy when the infant has a history of difficult stooling, abdominal distention, and ribbonlike stools. A **persistent cloaca** is a complex ARM in which the rectum, vagina, and urethra drain into a common channel opening into the perineum (Fig. 22.8A).

Imperforate anus includes several forms of malformation without an obvious opening (Fig. 22.8). Frequently a fistula (an abnormal communication) leads from the distal rectum to the perineum or GU system (see Fig. 22.8B and C). The fistula may be evidenced when meconium is evacuated through the vaginal opening, the perineum below the vagina, the male urethra, or the perineum under the scrotum. The presence of meconium on the perineum does not indicate anal patency. A fistula may not be apparent at birth, but as peristalsis increases, meconium is forced through the fistula into the urethra or onto the newborn's perineum.

Pathophysiology

During embryonic development the cloaca becomes the common channel for the developing urinary, genital, and rectal systems. The cloaca is divided at the sixth week of gestation into an anterior urogenital sinus and a posterior intestinal channel by the urorectal septum. After the lateral folds join the urorectal septum, separation of the urinary and rectal segments takes place. Further differentiation results in the anterior GU system and the posterior anorectal channel. An interruption of this development leads to incomplete migration of the rectum to its normal perineal position.

Diagnostic Evaluation

The diagnosis of an ARM is based on the physical finding of an absent anal opening. Other symptoms may include abdominal distention, vomiting, absence of meconium passage, or presence of meconium in the urine. Additional physical findings with an ARM are a flat perineum and the absence of a midline intergluteal groove. The appearance of the perineum alone does not accurately predict the extent of the defect and associated anomalies. GU and spinal-vertebral anomalies associated with ARMs should be considered when an anomaly is noted. EA with or without TEF, cardiac defects, and spinal or vertebral anomalies may occur in association with ARMs, and the infant should be carefully evaluated for the presence of these and other anomalies. Although rare, some ARMs may not be diagnosed until later in infancy or early childhood.

A perineal fistula (see Box 22.10) may be diagnosed by clinical observation. The presence of a prominent anal dimple and a band of skin tissue commonly known as a bucket handle is indicative of a perineal fistula. Abdominal and pelvic ultrasonography is performed to further evaluate the infant's anatomic malformation. An IV pyelogram and a voiding cystourethrogram are performed to evaluate associated anomalies involving the urinary tract. Other diagnostic examinations that may be performed include pelvic magnetic resonance imaging, radiography, ultrasound, and fluoroscopic examination of pelvic anatomic contents and lower spinal anatomy.

BOX 22.10 Classification of Anorectal Malformations

Male Defects

Perineal fistula
Rectourethral bulbar fistula
Rectourethral prostatic fistula
Rectovesicular (bladder neck) fistula
Imperforate anus without fistula
Rectal atresia

Female Defects

Perineal fistula
Rectovestibular fistula
Imperforate anus without fistula
Rectal atresia and stenosis
Cloaca

From Gangopadhyay, A. N., & Pandey, V. (2015). Anorectal malformations. *Journal of Indian Association of Pediatric Surgeons, 20*(1), 10–15.

Therapeutic Management

The primary management of ARMs is surgical. Once the defect is identified, take steps to rule out associated life-threatening defects, which need immediate surgical intervention. Provided no immediate life-threatening problems exist, the newborn is stabilized and kept NPO for further evaluation. IV fluids are provided to maintain glucose and fluid and electrolyte balance. Current recommendation is that surgery be delayed at least 24 hours to properly evaluate for the presence of a fistula and possibly other anomalies (Shanti, 2020).

The surgical treatment of ARMs varies according to the defect but usually involves one, or possibly a combination of several, of the following procedures: anoplasty, colostomy, **posterior sagittal anorectoplasty (PSARP)** or other pull-through with colostomy, and colostomy (take-down) closure. The Nursing Care Management discussion below outlines some aspects of preoperative and postoperative care.

A primary laparoscopic repair (without colostomy) of some ARMs is being used successfully for the treatment of ARMs. This minimizes surgical risks, associated morbidity, and postoperative pain management with no significant risk for rectal prolapse, anal stenosis, or anorectal manometry (Han, Xia, Guo, et al., 2017).

Prognosis

The long-term prognosis depends on such factors as the type of defect, anatomy of the sacrum and vertebrae, quality of muscles, and success of the surgery.

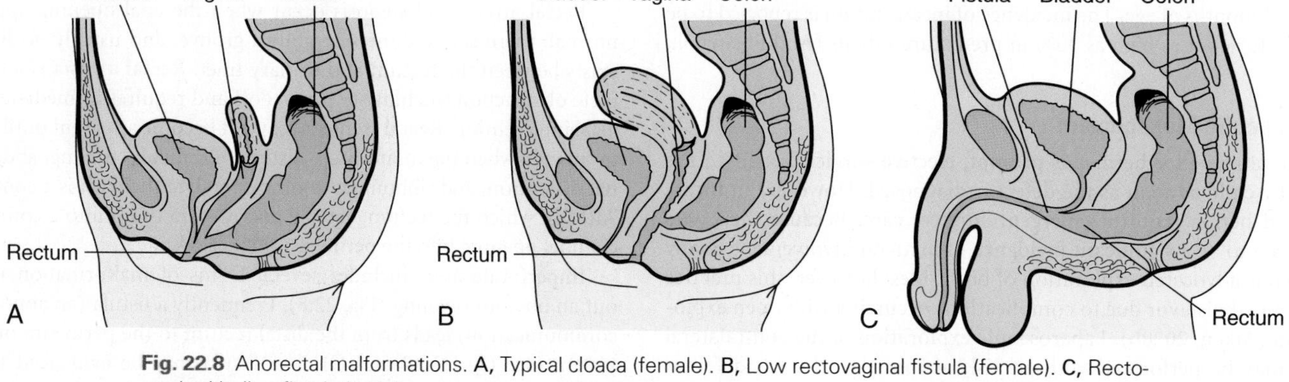

Fig. 22.8 Anorectal malformations. **A,** Typical cloaca (female). **B,** Low rectovaginal fistula (female). **C,** Rectourethral bulbar fistula (male).

The presence of a flat or "rocker" bottom and no midline groove usually carries a poor prognosis for bowel continence because of associated neurologic, muscular, and anatomic problems. When the internal anal sphincter is absent, incontinence is a common long-term problem. These children may achieve socially acceptable continence over time with the aid of a bowel management program. Other potential complications after surgical treatment of anorectal anomalies include strictures, recurrent rectourinary fistula, mucosal prolapse, and constipation. Long-term outcomes in adults with surgically treated ARM are reported to be positive, depending on the type and severity of the defect as well as associated anomalies (Gangopadhyay & Pandey, 2015). Constipation, fecal soiling, and fecal incontinence are problems that such children and adults must cope with on a regular basis, but the functional outcome is reported to be excellent (Gangopadhyay & Pandey, 2015).

Nursing Care Management

The first nursing responsibility is assisting in identification of ARMs. A newborn who does not pass stool within 24 hours after birth or has meconium that appears at a location other than the anal opening requires further assessment. Preoperative care includes diagnostic evaluation, GI decompression, bowel preparation, and IV fluids.

For the newborn with a perineal fistula, an **anoplasty** is performed, which involves moving the fistula opening to the center of the sphincter and enlarging the rectal opening. Postoperative nursing care after anoplasty is primarily directed toward healing the surgical site without other complications. A program of anal dilations is usually initiated when the child returns for the 2-week checkup. Feedings are started soon after surgical repair, and breastfeeding is encouraged because it causes less constipation.

In neonates with anomalies such as **cloaca** (female), rectourethral prostatic fistula (male), and vestibular fistula (female), a descending colostomy is performed to allow fecal elimination and avoid fecal contamination of the distal imperforate section and subsequent urinary tract infection in infants with urorectal fistulas. With a colostomy, postoperative nursing care is directed toward maintaining appropriate skin care at the stoma sites (both distal and proximal), managing postoperative pain, and administering IV fluids and antibiotics. Postoperative NG decompression may be required with laparotomy, and nursing care focuses on maintenance of appropriate drainage (see Chapter 20 for colostomy care).

The PSARP is a common surgical procedure for the repair of ARMs in infants approximately 1 to 2 months after the initial colostomy. Preoperative PSARP care often involves irrigation of the distal stoma to prevent fecal contamination of the operative site. During this time parents must be given accurate yet simple information regarding the infant's appearance postoperatively and expectations as to their level of involvement in the child's care.

In the PSARP procedure the repair is made via a posterior midline sacral approach to dissect the different muscle groups involved without damaging strategic innervation of pelvic structures so that optimum postoperative bowel continence is achieved. A laparotomy may be required if the rectum is unidentifiable by the posterior approach. Additional management after successful repair involves a program of anal dilations, colostomy closure, and a bowel management program.

Parents are instructed in perineal and wound care or care of the colostomy as needed. Anal dilations may be necessary for some infants. Parents should observe stooling patterns and observe for signs of anal stricture or complications. Information on dietary modifications and administration of medications is included in counseling. Nurses have a vital role in helping families of a child with ARMs provide optimum care so bowel management is successful and quality of life enhanced for the child and family.

Family Support, Discharge Planning, and Home Care

Long-term follow-up care is essential for children with complex malformations. When a colostomy is performed, parents need reassurance regarding the child's appearance and their ability to care for the child at home. With much patience and reassurance, parents learn how to provide optimum care of the skin and the appliance, while maintaining an appropriate bond with the child.

After the definitive pull-through procedure, toilet training may be delayed. Complete continence is seldom achieved at the usual age of 2 to 3 years. Bowel habit training, bowel management irrigation programs, diet modification, and administration of stool softeners or fiber help children improve bowel function and social continence. Some children never achieve bowel continence and must rely on daily bowel irrigations. Support and reassurance during the slow progression to normal, socially acceptable function are essential.

CLINICAL JUDGMENT AND NEXT-GENERATION NCLEX® EXAMINATION-STYLE QUESTIONS

1. A 16-month-old has a history of diarrhea for 3 days with poor oral intake. He received intravenous fluids, has tolerated some oral fluids in the emergency department, and is being discharged home. **For each home care instruction, use an X to indicate whether it was Indicated (appropriate or necessary), Contraindicated (could be harmful), or Non-Essential (makes no difference or not necessary).**

Home Care Instruction	Indicated	Contraindicated	Non-Essential
Keep on clear liquids and toast for 24 hours		X	
Offer a regular diet as child's appetite warrants	X		
Sterilize the infant's eating utensils before each meal			X
Give a BRAT diet (bananas, rice, applesauce, and toast) for 24 hours, then a soft diet as tolerated		X	
Find out what the infant's favorite food is			X
Give chicken or beef broth for 24 hours, then resume a soft diet		X	

2. A 3-year-old has a history of chronic diarrhea, lack of weight gain, and abdominal distension. He has a positive serological blood test and small intestine biopsy confirming Celiac Disease. **Choose the most likely options for the information missing from the statements below by selecting from the lists of options provided.**

Because children with celiac disease must limit their intake of products containing____1____ in many food items, one being____2____, they are at most risk for____3____ as well as a number of other deficiencies.

Options for 1	Options for 2	Options for 3
Sugar	Yogurt	Iron-deficiency anemia
Meat	Corn on the cob	Bleeding
Gluten	Lettuce and tomato salad	Asthma
Salt	Toast	Hepatitis
Milk	Baked chicken	Pyloric stenosis
Eggs	Carrot sticks	Hoarseness and difficulty swallowing

3. A preterm infant who had surgery for necrotizing enterocolitis is now 6 months old and has short bowel syndrome. He is unable to absorb most nutrients taken by mouth and is totally dependent on parenteral nutrition, which he receives via a central venous catheter. The clinic nurse following the care for this infant is aware that he should be closely observed for the development of which complications? **Select all that apply.**

A. Cholestasis
B. Constipation
C. Failure to thrive
D. Chronic diarrhea
E. Intestinal stricture
F. Intestinal failure
G. Hepatic dysfunction
H. Gastroesophageal reflux

4. A 3 month old infant who has not receive her immunizations is seen in the clinic following concerns that there was a Hepatitis outbreak in the day care where the infant was enrolled. The day care notified the mother that other children who were not immunized were also enrolled and that she should take her infant to the clinic. **Choose the most likely options for the information missing from the statements below by selecting from the list of options provided.**

The nurse recognizes that the principle mode of transmission for____1____ is by the____2____ route. The____3____, an inactivated vaccine, is approved for children 12-23 months of age and given in____4____ doses.

Options for 1	Options for 2	Options for 3	Options for 4
Hepatitis A	parenteral	HAV	Four
Hepatitis C	fecal-oral	HCV	Two
Hepatitis B	contaminated water	polio vaccine	Three
Hepatitis D	perinatal	HBV	One

REFERENCES

Abbott, R. A., Martin, A. E., Newlove-Delgado, T. V., et al. (2017). Psychosocial interventions for recurrent abdominal pain in childhood. *Cochrane Database of Systematic Review* (3), CD010973.

Abdulhai, S. A., Glenn, I. C., & Ponsky, T. A. (2017). Incarcerated pediatric hernias. *The Surgical Clinics of North America, 97*(1), 129–145.

Aiken, J. J. (2020a). Acute appendicitis. In R. M. Kliegman, J. W. St. Geme, N. J. Blum, et al. (Eds.), *Nelson textbook of pediatrics* (21st ed.). Philadelphia: Elsevier.

Aiken, J. J. (2020b). Inguinal hernias. In R. M. Kliegman, J. W. St. Geme, N. J. Blum, et al. (Eds.), *Nelson textbook of pediatrics* (21st ed.). Philadelphia: Elsevier.

Avitzur, Y., & Shamir, R. (2020). Short bowel syndrome. In R. M. Kliegman, J. W. St. Geme, N. J. Blum, et al. (Eds.), *Nelson textbook of pediatrics* (21st ed.). Philadelphia: Elsevier.

Bagade, S., & Khanna, G. (2015). Imaging of omphalomesenteric duct remnants and related pathologies in children. *Current Problems in Diagnostic Radiology, 44*(3), 246–255.

Barnes, D., & Yeh, A. M. (2015). Bugs and guts: Practical applications of probiotics for gastrointestinal disorders in children. *Nutrition in Clinical Practice, 30*(6), 747–759.

Bass, D. M. (2020). Rotaviruses, caliciviruses, and astroviruses. In R. M. Kliegman, J. W. St. Geme, N. J. Blum, et al. (Eds.), *Nelson textbook of pediatrics* (21st ed.). Philadelphia: Elsevier.

Blanchard, S. S., & Czinn, S. J. (2020). Peptic ulcer disease in children. In R. M. Kliegman, J. W. St. Geme, N. J. Blum, et al. (Eds.), *Nelson textbook of pediatrics* (21st ed.). Philadelphia: Elsevier.

Bruce, J. S., Bruce, C. S., Short, H., et al. (2016). Childhood constipation: Recognition, management and the role of the nurse. *British Journal of Nursing, 25*(22), 1231–1242.

Byard, R. W., & Zuccollo, J. M. (2010). Forensic issues in cases of water birth fatalities. *The American Journal of Forensic Medicine and Pathology, 31*(3), 258–260.

Carroll, A. G., Kavanagh, R. G., Ni Leidhin, C., et al. (2017). Comparative effectiveness of imaging modalities for the diagnosis and treatment of intussusception: A critically appraised topic. *Academic Radiology, 24*(5), 521–529.

Carson, R. A., Mudd, S. S., & Madati, J. (2017). Clinical practice guideline for the treatment of pediatric acute gastroenteritis in the outpatient setting. *Journal of Emergency Nursing*. http://www.jenonline.org.

Carter, B., & Fedorowicz, Z. (2012). Antiemetic treatment for acute gastroenteritis in children: An updated Cochrane systematic review with meta-analysis and mixed treatment comparison in a Bayesian framework. *BMJ Open, 2*, 1–11.

Centers for Disease Control and Prevention. (2017). *Surveillance for viral hepatitis – United States, 2015*. https://www.cdc.gov/hepatitis/statistics/2015surveillance/index.htm.

Chopra, J., Patel, N., Basude, D., et al. (2017). Abdominal pain-related functional gastrointestinal disorders in children. *British Journal of Nursing, 26*(11), 624–631.

Choudhary, N. S., Puri, R., Saigal, S., et al. (2016). Innovative approach of using esophageal stent for refractory post-band ligation esophageal ulcer bleed following liver donor liver transplantation. *Journal of Clinical and Experimental Hepatology, 6*(2), 149–150.

Cohen, S., Bueno de Mesquita, M., & Mimouni, F. B. (2015). Adverse effects reported in the use of gastroesophageal reflux disease treatments in children: A 10 years literature review. *British Journal of Clinical Pharmacology, 80*(2), 200–208.

Cohran, V. C., Prozialeck, J. D., & Cole, C. R. (2017). Redefining short bowel syndrome in the 21st century. *Pediatric Research, 81*(4), 540–549.

Conrad, M. A., & Rosh, J. R. (2017). Pediatric inflammatory bowel disease. *Pediatric Clinics of North America, 64*(3), 577–591.

Dekate, P., Jayashree, M., & Singhi, S. (2013). Management of acute diarrhea in emergency room. *Indian Journal of Pediatrics, 80*(3), 235–246.

Fok, C. Y., Holland, K. S., Gil-Zaragozano, E., et al. (2016). The role of nurses and dieticians in managing paediatric coeliac disease. *British Journal of Nursing, 25*(8), 449–455.

Gangopadhyay, A. N., & Pandey, V. (2015). Anorectal malformations. *Journal of Indian Association of Pediatric Surgeons, 20*(1), 10–15.

Giannetti, E., Maglione, M., Sciorio, E., et al. (2017). Do children just grow out of irritable bowel syndrome? *The Journal of Pediatrics, 183*, 122–126.

Govindarajan, K. K. (2016). Biliary atresia: Where do we stand now? *World Journal of Hepatology, 8*(36), 1593–1601.

Greenbaum, L. A. (2020). Acid-base balance. In R. M. Kliegman, J. W. St. Geme, N. J. Blum, et al. (Eds.), *Nelson textbook of pediatrics* (21st ed.). Philadelphia: Elsevier.

Han, Y., Xia, Z., Guo, S., et al. (2017). Laparoscopically assisted anorectal pull-through versus posterior sagittal anorectoplasy for high and intermediate anorectal malformations: A systematic review and meta-analysis. *PLoS ONE, 12*(1), e0170421.

Hassan, H. H., & Balistreri, W. F. (2020). Cholestasis. In R. M. Kliegman, J. W. St. Geme, N. J. Blum, et al. (Eds.), *Nelson textbook of pediatrics* (21st ed.). Philadelphia: Elsevier.

Hendrickson, M. A., Zaremba, J., Wey, A. R., et al. (2017). The use of a triage-based protocol for oral rehydration in a pediatric emergency department. *Pediatric Emergency Care*, pec-online.com.

Huether, S. E. (2019). The cellular environment: Fluids and electrolytes, acids and bases. In K. L. McCance, & S. E. Huether (Eds.), *Pathophysiology: The biologic basis for disease in adults and children* (8th ed.). St. Louis: Mosby.

Jensen, M. K., & Balistreri, W. F. (2020). Viral hepatitis. In R. M. Kliegman, J. W. St. Geme, N. J. Blum, et al. (Eds.), *Nelson textbook of pediatrics* (21st ed.). Philadelphia: Elsevier.

Kalach, N., Bontems, P., & Cadranel, S. (2015). Advances in the treatment of *Helicobacter pylori* infection in children. *Annals of Gastroenterology, 28*(1), 10–18.

Khan, S., & Matta, S. K. R. (2020a). Gastroesophageal reflux disease. In R. M. Kliegman, J. W. St. Geme, N. J. Blum, et al. (Eds.), *Nelson textbook of pediatrics* (21st ed.). Philadelphia: Elsevier.

Khan, S., & Matta, S. K. R. (2020b). Esophageal atresia and tracheoesophageal fistula. In R. M. Kliegman, J. W. St. Geme, N. J. Blum, et al. (Eds.), *Nelson textbook of pediatrics* (21st ed.). Philadelphia: Elsevier.

Kleinman, R. E., & Greer, F. R. (2014). *Pediatric nutrition* (7th ed.). Elk Grove Village, IL: American Academy of Pediatrics.

Kotloff, K. L. (2017). The burden and etiology of diarrheal illness in developing countries. *Pediatric Clinics of North America, 64*(4), 799–814.

Kotloff, K. L. (2020). Acute gastroenteritis in children. In R. M. Kliegman, J. W. St. Geme, N. J. Blum, et al. (Eds.), *Nelson textbook of pediatrics* (21st ed.). Philadelphia: Elsevier.

Kridler, J., & Kamat, D. (2016). Irritable bowel syndrome: A review for general pediatricians. *Pediatric Annals, 45*(1), e30–e33.

Lamberti, L. M., Ashraf, S., Walker, C. L., et al. (2016). A systematic review of the effect of rotavirus vaccination on diarrhea outcomes among children younger than 5 years. *The Pediatric Infectious Disease Journal, 35*(9), 992–998.

Lebwohl, B., Sanders, D. S., & Green, P. H. R. (2017). Coeliac disease. *Lancet, 391*(10115), 70–81.

Leung, D. T., Chisti, M. J., & Pavia, A. T. (2016). Prevention and control of childhood pneumonia and diarrhea. *Pediatric Clinics of North America, 63*(1), 67–79.

Lin, X. K., Huang, X. Z., Bao, X. Z., et al. (2017). Clinical characteristics of Meckel diverticulum in children: A retrospective review of a 15-year single-center experience. *Medicine, 96*(32), e7760.

Manz, F. (2007). Hydration in children. *Journal of the American College of Nutrition, 26*(Suppl. 5), S562–S569.

Maqbool, A., & Liacouras, C. A. (2020a). Congenital aganglionic megacolon (Hirschprung disease). In R. M. Kliegman, J. W. St. Geme, N. J. Blum, et al. (Eds.), *Nelson textbook of pediatrics* (21st ed.). Philadelphia: Elsevier.

Maqbool, A., & Liacouras, C. A. (2020b). Pyloric stenosis and other congenital anomalies of the stomach. In R. M. Kliegman, J. W. St. Geme, N. J. Blum, et al. (Eds.), *Nelson textbook of pediatrics* (21st ed.). Philadelphia: Elsevier.

Maqbool, A., & Liacouras, C. A. (2020c). Major symptoms and signs of digestive tract disorders. In R. M. Kliegman, J. W. St. Geme, N. J. Blum, et al. (Eds.), *Nelson textbook of pediatrics* (21st ed.). Philadelphia: Elsevier.

Maqbool, A., & Liacouras, C. A. (2020d). Intestinal duplications, Meckel diverticulum, and other remnants of the omphalomesenteric duct. In R. M. Kliegman, J. W. St. Geme, N. J. Blum, et al. (Eds.), *Nelson textbook of pediatrics* (21st ed.). Philadelphia: Elsevier.

Maqbool, A., & Liacouras, C. A. (2020e). Intussusception. In R. M. Kliegman, J. W. St. Geme, N. J. Blum, et al. (Eds.), *Nelson textbook of pediatrics* (21st ed.). Philadelphia: Elsevier.

Marder, E. P., Cieslak, P. R., Cronquist, A. B., et al. (2017). Incidence and trends of infections with pathogens transmitted commonly through food and the effect of increasing use of culture-independent diagnostic tests on surveillance – foodborne disease active surveillance network, 10 U.S. sites, 2013-2016. *MMWR. Morbidity and Mortality Weekly Report, 66*(15), 397–403.

Martin, L. Y., Ladd, M. R., Werts, A., et al. (2017). Tissue engineering for the treatment of short bowel syndrome in children. *Pediatric Research, 83*(1-2), 249–257.

McFarland, L. V., Ozen, M., Dinleyici, E. C., et al. (2016). Comparison of pediatric and adult antibiotic-associated diarrhea and *Clostridium dificile* infections. *World Journal of Gastroenterology: WJG, 22*(11), 3078–3104.

Mousa, H., & Hassan, M. (2017). Gastroesophageal reflux disease. *Pediatric Clinics of North America, 64*(3), 487–505.

Muller, C. O., Rossignol, G., Montalva, L., et al. (2016). Long-term outcome of laparoscopic Duhamel procedure for extended Hirschsprung's disease. *Journal of Laparoendoscopic and Advanced Surgical Techniques. Part A, 26*(12), 1032–1035.

Newlove-Delgado, T. V., Martin, A. E., Abbott, R. A., et al. (2017). Dietary interventions for recurrent abdominal pain in childhood. *Cochrane Database of Systematic Review* (3), CD010972.

Patel, R., Bommayya, N., Choudhry, M., et al. (2015). Bleeding duodenal ulcer in a healthy infant presenting with rectal bleeding and requiring surgical treatment. *Journal of Pediatric Surgical Special, 9*, 38–40.

Paul, S. P., McVeigh, L., Gil-Zaragozano, E., et al. (2016). Diagnosis and nursing management of coeliac disease in children. *Nursing Children and Young People, 28*(1), 18–24.

Poddar, U. (2016). Approach to constipation in children. *Indian Pediatrics, 53*(4), 319–327.

Rentea, R. M., Peter, D., & Snyder, C. L. (2017). Pediatric appendicitis: State of the art review. *Pediatric Surgery International, 33*(3), 269–283.

Rosen, M. J., Dhawan, A., & Saeed, S. A. (2017). Inflammatory bowel disease in children and adolescents. *JAMA Pediatrics, 169*(11), 1053–1060.

Shanti, C. M. (2020). Surgical conditions of the anus and rectum. In R. M. Kliegman, J. W. St. Geme, N. J. Blum, et al. (Eds.), *Nelson textbook of pediatrics* (21st ed.). Philadelphia: Elsevier.

Stein, R. E., & Baldassano, R. N. (2020). Chronic ulcerative colitis. In R. M. Kliegman, J. W. St. Geme, N. J. Blum, et al. (Eds.), *Nelson textbook of pediatrics* (21st ed.). Philadelphia: Elsevier.

Troncone, R., & Shamir, R. (2020). Celiac disease. In R. M. Kliegman, J. W. St. Geme, N. J. Blum, et al. (Eds.), *Nelson textbook of pediatrics* (21st ed.). Philadelphia: Elsevier.

United Network for Organ Sharing. (2017). *Questions and answers for transplant candidates about liver allocation*. https://www.unos.org/wp-content/uploads/unos/Liver_patient.pdf.

Wang, J., Xu, E., & Xiao, Y. (2014). Isotonic versus hypotonic maintenance IV fluids in hospitalized children: A meta-analysis. *Pediatrics, 133*(1), 105–113.

Wen, S. C., Best, E., & Nourse, C. (2017). Non-typhoidal Salmonella infections in children: Review of literature and recommendations for management. *Journal of Paediatrics and Child Health, 53*(10), 936–941.

Wu, Y., Kuang, H., Lv, T., et al. (2017). Comparison of clinical outcomes between open and thoracoscopic repairfor esophageal atresia with tracheoesophageal fistula: A systematic review and meta-analysis. *Pediatric Surgery International, 33*(11), 1147–1157.

Yanagi, Y., Matsuura, T., Hayashida, M., et al. (2017). Bowel perforation after liver transplantation for biliary atresia: A retrospective study of care in the transition from childhood to adulthood. *Pediatric Surgery International, 33*(2), 155–163.

Yang, H. R. (2016). Updates on the diagnosis of *Helicobacter pylori* infection in children: What are the differences between adults and children? *Pediatric Gastroenterology. Hepatology & Nutrition, 19*(2), 96–103.

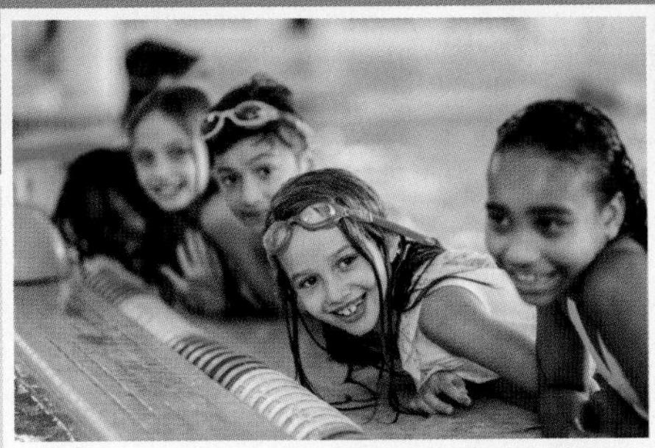

23

The Child With Cardiovascular Dysfunction

Margaret L. Schroeder, Annette L. Baker, Heather Bastardi, Patricia O'Brien

http://evolve.elsevier.com/wong/ncic

CONCEPTS

- Perfusion
- Hemodynamics

CARDIOVASCULAR DYSFUNCTION

Cardiovascular disorders in children are divided into two major groups: congenital heart disease and acquired heart disorders. Congenital heart disease (CHD) includes primarily anatomic abnormalities present at birth that result in abnormal cardiac function. The clinical consequences of congenital heart defects fall into two broad categories: heart failure (HF) and hypoxemia. Acquired cardiac disorders are disease processes or abnormalities that occur after birth and can be seen in the normal heart or in the presence of congenital heart defects. They result from various factors, including infection, autoimmune responses, environmental factors, and familial tendencies. The pathophysiology review found in Fig. 23.1 describes the flow of blood through the heart.

HISTORY AND PHYSICAL EXAMINATION

Taking an accurate health history is an important first step in assessing an infant or child for possible heart disease. Parents may have specific concerns, such as an infant with poor feeding or fast breathing, or a 7-year-old who can no longer keep up with friends on the soccer field. Others may not realize that their child has a medical problem because their baby has always been pale and fussy.

Asking details about the mother's health history, pregnancy, and birth history is important in assessing infants. Mothers with chronic health conditions, such as diabetes or lupus, are more likely to have infants with heart disease. Some medications, such as phenytoin (Dilantin), are teratogenic to fetuses. Maternal alcohol use or illicit drug use increases the risk of congenital heart defects. Exposures to infections, such as rubella, early in pregnancy may result in congenital anomalies. Infants with low birth weight resulting from intrauterine growth restriction are more likely to have congenital anomalies. High-birth-weight infants have an increased incidence of heart disease.

A detailed family history is also important. There is an increased incidence of congenital cardiac defects if either parent or a sibling has a heart defect. Some diseases, such as Marfan syndrome, and some cardiomyopathies are hereditary. A family history of frequent fetal loss, sudden infant death, and sudden death in adults may indicate heart disease. Congenital heart defects are seen in many syndromes such as Down and Turner syndromes.

The physical assessment of suspected cardiac disease begins with observation of general appearance and then proceeds with more specific observations. The following lists are supplementary to the general assessment techniques described for physical examination of the chest and heart in Chapter 4.

Inspection

Nutritional state: Failure to thrive or poor weight gain is associated with heart disease.

Color: Cyanosis is a common feature of CHD, and pallor is associated with poor perfusion.

Chest deformities: An enlarged heart sometimes distorts the chest configuration.

Unusual pulsations: Visible pulsations of the neck veins are seen in some patients.

Respiratory excursion: This refers to the ease or difficulty of respiration (e.g., tachypnea, dyspnea, expiratory grunt).

Clubbing of fingers: This is associated with cyanosis.

Palpation and Percussion

Chest: These maneuvers help discern heart size and other characteristics (e.g., thrills) associated with heart disease.

Abdomen: Hepatomegaly or splenomegaly may be evident.

Peripheral pulses: Rate, regularity, and amplitude (strength) may reveal discrepancies.

Auscultation

Heart rate and rhythm: Listen for fast heart rates (tachycardia), slow heart rates (bradycardia), and irregular rhythms.

Character of heart sounds: Listen for distinct or muffled sounds, murmurs, and additional heart sounds.

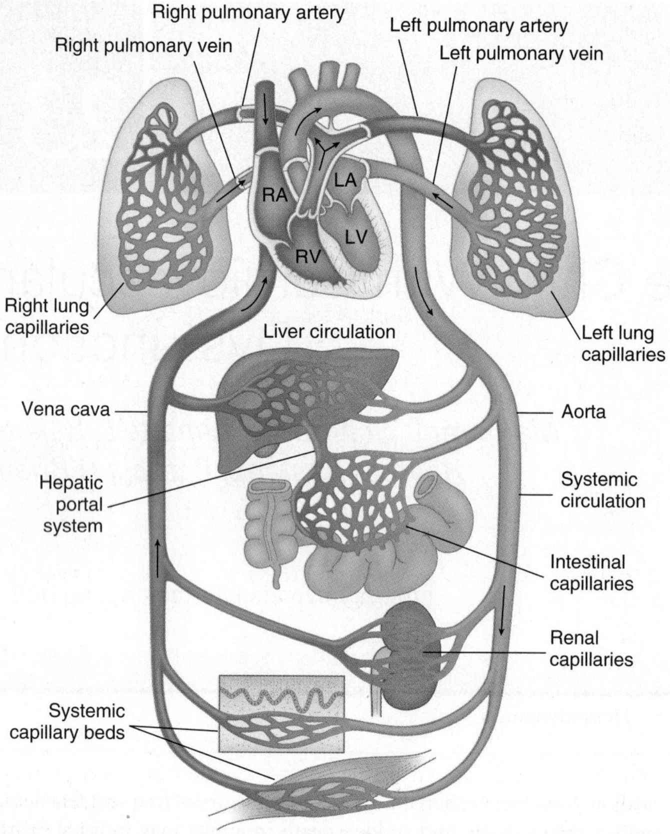

Fig. 23.1 Diagram showing serially connected pulmonary and systemic circulatory systems and how to trace the flow of blood. Right heart chambers propel unoxygenated blood through the pulmonary circulation, and the left side of the heart propels oxygenated blood through the systemic circulation. *LA*, Left atrium; *LV*, left ventricle; *RA*, right atrium; *RV*, right ventricle. (From McCance, K. L., & Huether, S. E. [2019]. *Pathophysiology: The biological basis for disease in adults and children* [8th ed.]. St. Louis, MO: Mosby.)

Diagnostic Evaluation

A variety of invasive and noninvasive tests may be used in the diagnosis of heart disease (Table 23.1). Some of the more common diagnostic tools that require nursing assessment and intervention are described in the following sections.

Electrocardiogram

Electrocardiography (ECG) measures the electrical activity of the heart; provides a graphic display; and supplies information on heart rate and rhythm, abnormal rhythms or conduction, ischemic changes, and other information. A standard ECG uses 12 leads to get different views of the heart. An ECG takes about 15 minutes to perform; infants and young children may be fussy with lead placement.

Bedside cardiac monitoring with a single lead of the ECG is commonly used in pediatrics, especially in the care of children with heart disease. An alarm can be set with parameters for individual patient requirements and will sound if the heart rate is above or below the set parameters. Gel foam electrodes are commonly used and placed on the right side of the chest (above the level of the heart) and on the left side of the chest, and a ground electrode is placed on the abdomen. Bedside monitors are an adjunct to patient care and should never be substituted for direct assessment and auscultation of heart sounds. The nurse should assess the patient, not the monitor.

TABLE 23.1 Procedures for Cardiac Diagnosis

Procedure	Description
Chest radiography (x-ray)	Provides information on heart size and pulmonary blood flow patterns
Electrocardiography (ECG)	Graphic measure of electrical activity of heart
Holter monitor	24-hour continuous ECG recording used to assess dysrhythmias
Echocardiography	Use of high-frequency sound waves obtained by a transducer to produce an image of cardiac structures
Transthoracic	Done with transducer on chest
M-mode	One-dimensional graphic view used to estimate ventricular size and function
Two-dimensional	Real-time, cross-sectional views of heart used to identify cardiac structures and cardiac anatomy
Doppler	Shows blood flow patterns and pressure gradients across structures
Fetal	Imaging fetal heart in utero
Transesophageal echocardiography (TEE)	Transducer placed in esophagus behind heart to obtain images of posterior heart structures or in patients with poor images from chest approach
Cardiac catheterization	Imaging study using radiopaque catheters placed in a peripheral blood vessel and advanced into heart to measure pressures and oxygen levels in heart chambers and visualize heart structures and blood flow patterns
Hemodynamics	Measurements of pressures and oxygen saturations in heart chambers
Angiography	Use of contrast material to illuminate heart structures and blood flow patterns
Biopsy	Use of special catheter to remove tiny samples of heart muscle for microscopic evaluation; used in assessing infection, inflammation, or muscle dysfunction disorders; also to evaluate for rejection after heart transplant
Electrophysiology study (EPS)	Special catheters with electrodes inserted to record electrical activity from within the heart; used to diagnose rhythm disturbances
Exercise stress test	Monitoring of heart rate, BP, ECG, and oxygen consumption at rest and during progressive exercise on a treadmill or bicycle
Cardiac MRI	Noninvasive imaging technique; used in evaluation of vascular anatomy outside of the heart (e.g., COA, vascular rings), estimates of ventricular mass and volume

BP, Blood pressure; *COA*, coarctation of the aorta; *MRI*, magnetic resonance imaging.

! NURSING ALERT

Electrodes for cardiac monitoring are often color coded: white for right, green (or red) for ground, and black for left. Always check to ensure that these colors are placed correctly.

Echocardiography

Echocardiography involves the use of ultra-high-frequency sound waves to produce an image of the heart's structure. A transducer placed directly on the chest wall delivers repetitive pulses of ultrasound and processes the returned signals (echoes). It is the most frequently used test for describing cardiac anatomy and detecting cardiac dysfunction in children. In many cases, a prenatal diagnosis of CHD can be made by fetal echocardiography.

Although the test is noninvasive, painless, and associated with no known side effects, it can be stressful for children. A full echocardiogram can take an hour, and the child must lie quietly in the standard echocardiographic positions. Therefore infants and young children may need conscious sedation or anesthesia, and older children benefit from preparation for the test. The distraction of a video or movie is often helpful.

Cardiac Magnetic Resonance Imaging

Cardiac magnetic resonance imaging (MRI) uses magnetic field and pulses of radio wave energy to produce real time three-dimensional (3D) images of the intracardiac and extracardiac vascular structures and assessments of ventricular function. It is often used in older children and adolescents when more quantitative information (i.e., volume of ventricular chambers, measurement of valve regurgitation) is needed that cannot be obtained by echocardiography or if echocardiography imaging windows have become limited. The use of MRI has rapidly expanded in the last decade. Although MRI is noninvasive, it can take an hour or more, and patients must lie still inside the scanner. Children under the age of 7 years, patients with claustrophobia, and those with developmental delays or other issues that limit cooperation will require anesthesia, deep sedation, or conscious sedation (depending on institutional preferences). Because the MRI is a magnet, patients with metal implants such as pacemakers, automatic implantable cardioverter defibrillators (AICDs), or cochlear implants cannot be scanned, and all patients are carefully screened for safety compatibility.

Cardiac Catheterization

Cardiac catheterization is an invasive diagnostic procedure in which a radiopaque catheter is introduced through a large-bore needle into a peripheral vessel (usually the femoral artery or vein in children) and then guided into the heart with the aid of fluoroscopy. After the tip of the catheter is within a heart chamber, measurements of pressures and saturations in the different cardiac chambers are obtained. Contrast material is injected, and images are taken of the circulation inside the heart (**angiography**). Types of cardiac catheterizations include:

Diagnostic catheterizations: These studies are used to diagnose congenital cardiac defects, particularly in symptomatic infants and before surgical repair. They can include right-sided catheterizations, in which the catheter is introduced through a vein (usually the femoral vein) and threaded to the right atrium, and left-sided catheterizations, in which the catheter is threaded through an artery into the aorta and into the heart.

Interventional catheterizations (therapeutic catheterizations): A balloon catheter or other device is used to alter the cardiac anatomy. Examples include dilating stenotic valves or vessels or closing abnormal connections (Table 23.2).

Electrophysiology studies: Catheters with tiny electrodes that record the impulses of the heart directly from the conduction system are used to evaluate dysrhythmias. Other catheters can destroy abnormal pathways that cause rapid rhythms (called ablation).

Nursing Care Management

Cardiac catheterization has become a routine procedure and may be done on an outpatient basis. Catheterization is not without risks, however, especially in neonates and seriously ill infants and children. Patients are exposed to radiation, general anesthesia for many cases, and contrast materials and medications that can cause allergic reactions or renal insufficiency. Possible complications include acute hemorrhage from the entry site requiring transfusion (more likely with interventional procedures because larger catheters are used), loss of a pulse due to vascular injury in the catheterized extremity (usually transient, resulting from a clot, hematoma, or intimal tear), and transient dysrhythmias (generally catheter induced). Serious complications such as valve damage, perforation of the heart, central nervous system (CNS) injury, stroke, or death is rare (Feltes, Bacha, Beekman, et al., 2011).

TABLE 23.2 Current Interventional Cardiac Catheterization Procedures in Children

Intervention	Diagnosis
Balloon atrial septostomy	Transposition of the great vessels Other complex defects
Balloon dilation	Valvar pulmonary stenosis Branch pulmonary artery stenosis Congenital valvar aortic stenosis Rheumatic mitral stenosis Recurrent coarctation of the aorta
Stent placement	Pulmonary artery stenosis Coarctation of the aorta in adolescents
Coil occlusion	Small patent ductus arteriosus Collateral vessels in single-ventricle patients
Transcatheter device closure	Some atrial septal defects (secundum type) Larger patent ductus arteriosus Fenestrations following Fontan procedures
Transcatheter pulmonary valve replacement	Incompetent pulmonary valves following surgery to repair right ventricular outflow tract
Radiofrequency (RF) ablation	Some tachydysrhythmias

Preprocedural Care

A complete nursing assessment is necessary to ensure a safe procedure with minimum complications. This assessment should include accurate height (essential for correct catheter selection) and weight. Obtaining a history of allergic reactions is important because some of the contrast agents are iodine based. Specific attention to signs and symptoms of infection is crucial. Severe diaper rash may be a reason to cancel the procedure if femoral access is required. Because assessment of pedal pulses is important after catheterization, the nurse should assess and mark the pulses (dorsalis pedis, posterior tibial) before the child goes to the catheterization room. Baseline oxygen saturation using pulse oximetry in children with cyanosis is also recorded.

Preparing the child and family for the procedure is the joint responsibility of the patient care team. School-age children and adolescents benefit from a description of the catheterization laboratory and a chronologic explanation of the procedure, emphasizing what they will see, feel, and hear. Older children and adolescents may bring earphones and favorite music so that they can listen to music during the catheterization procedure. Preparation materials such as picture books, videotapes, or tours of the catheterization laboratory may be helpful. Preparation should be geared to the child's developmental level. The child's caregivers often benefit from the same explanations. Additional information, such as the expected length of the catheterization, description of the child's appearance after catheterization, and usual postprocedure care, should be outlined (see also Prepare the

Child and Family for Invasive Procedures later in the chapter). Written informed consent is completed prior to the procedure.

Methods of sedation vary among institutions and may include oral or intravenous (IV) medications (see Chapter 20). The child's age, heart defect, clinical status, and type of catheterization procedure planned are considered when sedation is determined. General anesthesia is needed for most interventional procedures. Children are allowed nothing by mouth (NPO) for 6 to 8 hours or more before the procedure. Infants and patients with polycythemia may need IV fluids to prevent dehydration and hypoglycemia.

Postprocedural Care

Postcatheterization care may occur in a recovery unit, hospital room, or intensive care unit (ICU) depending on the patient's acuity and care needs. Some catheterizations may be done as outpatient procedures, but most patients having interventional procedures are observed overnight in the hospital. Patients are placed on a cardiac monitor and a pulse oximeter for the first few hours of recovery. The most important nursing responsibility is observation of the following for signs of complications:

- **Pulses,** especially below the catheterization site, for equality and symmetry (Pulse distal to the site may be weaker for the first few hours after catheterization but should gradually increase in strength.)
- **Temperature and color of the affected extremity** because coolness or blanching may indicate arterial obstruction
- **Vital signs,** which are taken as frequently as every 15 minutes, with special emphasis on heart rate, which is counted for 1 full minute for evidence of dysrhythmias or bradycardia
- **Blood pressure (BP),** especially for hypotension, which may indicate hemorrhage from cardiac perforation or bleeding at the site of initial catheterization
- **Dressing,** for evidence of bleeding or hematoma formation in the femoral or antecubital area
- **Fluid intake,** both IV and oral, to ensure adequate hydration (Blood loss in the catheterization laboratory, the child's NPO status, and diuretic actions of dyes used during the procedure put children at risk for hypovolemia and dehydration.)
- **Blood glucose levels** for hypoglycemia, especially in infants, who should receive IV fluids containing dextrose

! NURSING ALERT

If bleeding occurs, direct continuous pressure is applied 2.5 cm (1 inch) above the percutaneous skin site to localize pressure over the vessel puncture.

Depending on hospital policy, the child may be kept in bed with the affected extremity maintained straight for 4 to 6 hours after venous catheterization and 6 to 8 hours after arterial catheterization to facilitate healing of the cannulated vessel. If younger children have difficulty complying, they can be held in the parent's lap with the leg maintained in the correct position. The child's usual diet can be resumed as soon as tolerated, beginning with sips of clear liquids and advancing as the condition allows. The child is encouraged to void to clear the contrast material from the blood. Generally there is only slight discomfort at the percutaneous site. To prevent infection, the catheterization area is protected from possible contamination. If the child wears diapers, the dressing can be kept dry by covering it with a piece of plastic film and sealing the edges of the film to the skin with tape. However, the nurse must be careful to continue observing the site for any evidence of bleeding (see Family-Centered Care box and Critical Thinking Case Study).

FAMILY-CENTERED CARE

After Cardiac Catheterization

- Cover catheter insertion site with an adhesive bandage strip and change daily for 2 days.
- Keep site clean and dry. Avoid tub baths and swimming for several days; patient may shower or have a sponge bath.
- Observe site for redness, swelling, drainage, and bleeding. Monitor for fever. Notify practitioner if these occur.
- Encourage rest and quiet activities for the first 3 days and avoid strenuous exercise.
- Discuss returning to school and resuming other activities with the practitioner.
- Resume regular diet without restrictions.
- Use acetaminophen for pain.
- Keep follow-up appointments per practitioner's instruction.

CRITICAL THINKING CASE STUDY

Cardiac Catheterization

Tommy, a 3-year-old boy with tetralogy of Fallot, has just returned to his hospital room from the cardiac catheterization recovery room. His mother calls you to the bedside to tell you that he is vomiting and bleeding. You arrive to find Tommy anxious, pale, crying, and sitting in a puddle of blood.

Initial Assessment. What is the most likely explanation of what is going on?

Expected Nursing Action. What are the most appropriate immediate interventions?

Teaching Points

- Children must be kept in bed with the affected extremity maintained straight for 4 to 6 hours after venous catheterization and for 6 to 8 hours after arterial catheterization to facilitate healing of the cannulated vessel.
- Hematocrit and hemoglobin are usually checked 6 hours after catheterization but may be checked sooner if there are clinical signs of bleeding. If the level is low, a blood transfusion may be necessary.

Critical Thinking Answers

Initial Assessment. Tommy is experiencing bleeding at the catheterization site.

Expected Nursing Action. Lay Tommy flat and apply pressure. Tommy may also need his hemoglobin and hematocrit levels checked and a blood transfusion if these levels are low.

CONGENITAL HEART DISEASE

The incidence of CHD in children is approximately 1 in 110 live births in the United States (Reller, Strickland, Riehle-Colarusso, et al., 2008). Of these, approximately 25% of infants have a critical congenital heart defect and will require treatment within the first year of life (Botto, Correa, & Erickson, 2001). Nearly half (48%) of deaths due to CHD occur during the first year of life (Gilboa, Salemi, Nembhard, et al., 2010). Despite these statistics, mortality due to CHD has improved over the last few decades due to surgical and catheter interventions, early detection, and ongoing pharmaceutical advancements. In 2010 it was estimated that there were approximately 2.4 million people living with CHD in the United States, 1 million of whom were children (Gilboa, Devine, Kucik, et al., 2016).

The exact cause of most congenital cardiac diseases is unknown. Most are thought to be a result of multiple factors—a complex interaction of genetic and environmental influences. Some risk factors are known to be associated with increased incidence of congenital heart defects. Maternal risk factors include chronic illnesses such as diabetes or poorly controlled phenylketonuria, alcohol consumption, and exposure to environmental toxins and infections. Family history of a cardiac defect in a parent or sibling increases the likelihood of a cardiac anomaly. The risk of CHD increases if a first-degree relative (parent or sibling) is affected. The familial risk is higher with left-sided obstructive lesions.

Congenital heart anomalies are often associated with chromosomal abnormalities, specific syndromes, or congenital defects in other body systems. Down syndrome (trisomy 21) and trisomy 13 and 18 are highly correlated with congenital heart defects. Syndromes associated with heart defects include DiGeorge syndrome, also known as 22q11.2 deletion syndrome (heart defects, poor immune system function, a cleft palate, complications related to low levels of calcium in the blood, and delayed development with behavioral and emotional problems); Noonan syndrome (pulmonic valve anomalies and cardiomyopathy); Williams syndrome (aortic and pulmonic stenosis); and Holt-Oram syndrome (upper limb anomalies and atrial septal defect). Extracardiac defects such as tracheoesophageal fistula, renal abnormalities, and diaphragmatic hernia are seen in association with heart anomalies.

CIRCULATORY CHANGES AT BIRTH

Blood carrying oxygen and nutritive materials from the placenta enters the fetal system through the umbilicus via the large umbilical vein. The blood then travels to the liver, where it divides. Part of the blood enters the portal and hepatic circulation of the liver, and the remainder travels directly to the inferior vena cava (IVC) by way of the ductus venosus. Oxygenated blood enters the heart by way of the IVC. Because of the higher pressure of blood entering the right atrium, it is directed posteriorly in a straight pathway across the right atrium and through the **foramen ovale** to the left atrium. In this way, the better-oxygenated blood enters the left atrium and ventricle to be pumped through the aorta to the head and upper extremities. Blood from the head and upper extremities entering the right atrium from the superior vena cava is directed downward through the tricuspid valve into the right ventricle. From there it is pumped through the pulmonary artery, where the major portion is shunted to the descending aorta via the **ductus arteriosus**. Only a small amount flows to and from the nonfunctioning fetal lungs (Fig. 23.2A).

Before birth, the high pulmonary vascular resistance created by the collapsed fetal lung causes greater pressures in the right side of the heart and the pulmonary arteries. At the same time, the free-flowing placental circulation and the ductus arteriosus produce a low vascular resistance in the remainder of the fetal vascular system. With the cessation of placental blood flow from clamping of the umbilical cord and the expansion of the lungs at birth, the hemodynamics of the fetal vascular system undergo pronounced and abrupt changes (see Fig. 23.2B).

With the first breath, the lungs are expanded, and increased oxygen causes pulmonary vasodilation. Pulmonary pressures start to fall as systemic pressures, given the removal of the placenta, start to rise. Normally the foramen ovale closes as the pressure in the left atrium exceeds the pressure in the right atrium. The ductus arteriosus starts to close in the presence of increased oxygen concentration in the blood and other factors.

ALTERED HEMODYNAMICS

The physiology of heart defects is defined by pressure gradients, blood flow, and resistance within the circulation. As blood is pumped through the heart, it (1) flows from an area of high pressure to one of low pressure and (2) takes the path of least resistance. In general, the higher the pressure gradient, the faster the rate of flow; and the higher the resistance, the slower the rate of flow.

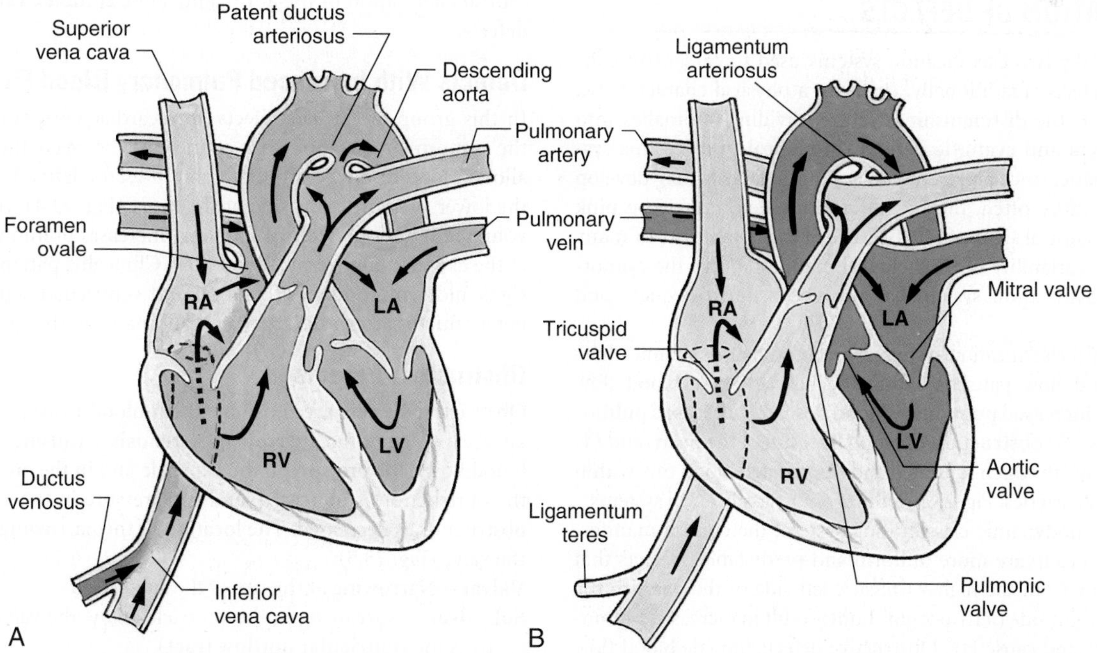

Fig. 23.2 Changes in circulation at birth. **A,** Prenatal circulation. **B,** Postnatal circulation. *Arrows* indicate direction of blood flow. Although four pulmonary veins enter the left atrium *(LA)*, for simplicity, this diagram shows only two. *LV,* Left ventricle; *RA,* right atrium; *RV,* right ventricle.

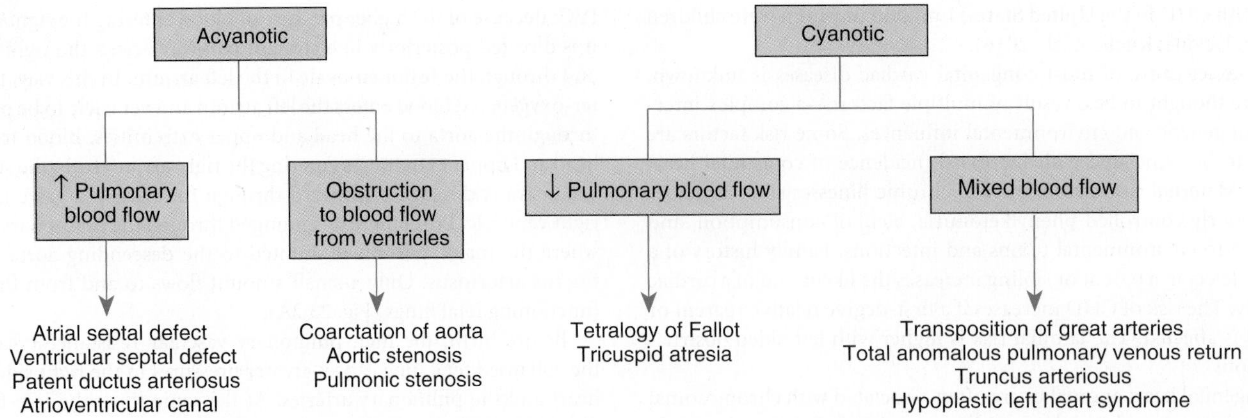

Fig. 23.3 Comparison of acyanotic-cyanotic and hemodynamic classification systems of congenital heart disease (CHD).

Normally, the pressure on the right side of the heart is lower than that on the left side, and the resistance in the pulmonary circulation is less than that in the systemic circulation. Likewise, vessels entering or exiting these chambers have corresponding pressures (e.g., lower pressure in the pulmonary artery and higher pressure in the aorta). Therefore if an abnormal connection exists between the heart chambers, such as a septal defect, blood flows from an area of higher pressure (left side) to one of lower pressure (right side). This directional flow of blood is termed a **left-to-right shunt**. If the opening is small, the amount of blood shunted to the atrium or ventricle may be minimal. Anomalies resulting in cyanosis may result from a change in pressure so that the blood is shunted from the right side to the left side of the heart (**right-to-left shunt**) because of either increased pulmonary vascular resistance or obstruction to blood flow through the pulmonic valve and artery. Cyanosis may also result from a defect that allows mixing of oxygenated and deoxygenated blood within the heart chambers or great arteries, such as occurs in truncus arteriosus.

CLASSIFICATION OF DEFECTS

There are typically two classification systems used to categorize congenital heart defects. Traditionally, cyanosis, a physical characteristic, has been used as the distinguishing feature, dividing anomalies into **acyanotic defects** and **cyanotic defects**. In clinical practice this system is problematic, since children with acyanotic defects may develop cyanosis. Also, more often, those with cyanotic defects may be pink and have more clinical signs of HF. Because of the complexity of many defects and the variability of their clinical manifestations, the cyanotic-acyanotic classification system has proven to be inadequate and misleading.

A more useful classification system is based on hemodynamic characteristics (blood flow patterns within the heart). These blood flow patterns are (1) **increased pulmonary blood flow**; (2) **decreased pulmonary blood flow**; (3) **obstruction to blood flow** out of the heart; and (4) **mixed blood flow**, in which saturated and desaturated blood mix within the heart or great arteries. Fig. 23.3 outlines both classification systems.

With the hemodynamic classification system, the clinical manifestations of each group are more uniform and predictable. Defects that allow blood flow from the higher pressure left side of the heart to the lower pressure right side (left-to-right shunt) result in increased pulmonary blood flow and cause HF. Obstructive defects impede blood flow out of the ventricles; obstruction on the left side of the heart results in HF, whereas severe obstruction on the right side causes cyanosis. Defects that cause decreased pulmonary blood flow result in cyanosis. Mixed lesions present a variable clinical picture based on the degree of mixing and amount of pulmonary blood flow; hypoxemia (with or without cyanosis) and HF usually occur together. Using this classification system, the clinical presentation and management of the most common defects are outlined in the following sections and in Boxes 23.1 to 23.4.

The outcomes of surgical treatment for patients with moderate to severe disease are variable. Patient risk factors for increased morbidity and mortality include prematurity or low birth weight, a genetic syndrome, multiple cardiac defects, a noncardiac congenital anomaly, and age at time of surgery (neonates are a higher risk group). The more common defects require no intervention or are treated with a single surgical intervention. Severe critical congenital heart defects often require multiple surgical and catheterization interventions and lifelong management by a cardiologist. Severe defects include all cyanotic heart disease and other complex defects such as hypoplastic left heart syndrome, atrioventricular (AV) canal, critical aortic stenosis, critical coarctation of the aorta, and some complex ventricular septal defects.

Defects With Increased Pulmonary Blood Flow

In this group of cardiac defects, intracardiac communications along the septum or an abnormal connection between the great arteries allows blood to flow from the higher pressure left side of the heart to the lower pressure right side of the heart (Fig. 23.4). Increased blood volume on the right side of the heart increases pulmonary blood flow at the expense of systemic blood flow. Clinically, patients demonstrate signs and symptoms of HF. Atrial and ventricular septal defects and patent ductus arteriosus are typical anomalies in this group (Box 23.1).

Obstructive Defects

Obstructive defects are those in which blood exiting the heart meets an area of anatomic narrowing (**stenosis**), causing obstruction to blood flow. The pressure in the ventricle and in the great artery before the obstruction is increased, and the pressure in the area beyond the obstruction is decreased. The location of the narrowing is usually near the valve (Fig. 23.5):

Valvar—Narrowing at the site of the valve itself
Subvalvar—Narrowing in the ventricle below the valve (also referred to as the **ventricular outflow tract**)
Supravalvar—Narrowing in the great artery above the valve

BOX 23.1 Defects With Increased Pulmonary Blood Flow

Atrial Septal Defect

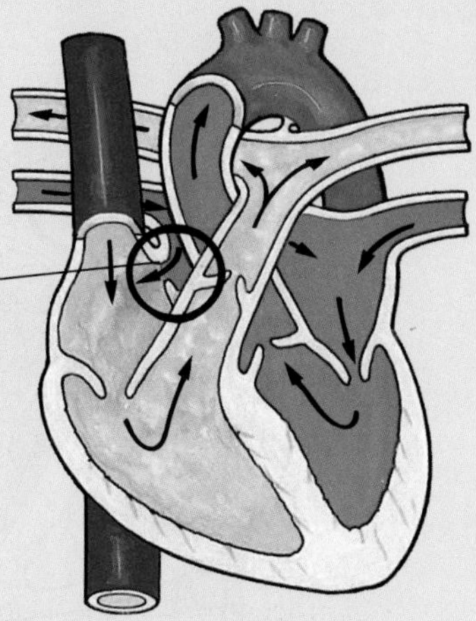

Description—Abnormal opening between the atria, allowing blood from the higher pressure left atrium to flow into the lower pressure right atrium. There are three types of atrial septal defect (ASD):

Ostium primum (ASD 1)—Opening at lower end of septum; may be associated with mitral valve abnormalities

Ostium secundum (ASD 2)—Opening near center of septum

Sinus venosus defect—Opening near junction of superior vena cava and right atrium; may be associated with partial anomalous pulmonary venous connection

Pathophysiology—Because left atrial pressure slightly exceeds right atrial pressure, blood flows from the left to the right atrium, causing an increased flow of oxygenated blood into the right side of the heart. Despite the low pressure difference, a high rate of flow can still occur because of low pulmonary vascular resistance and the greater distensibility of the right atrium, which further reduces flow resistance. This volume is well tolerated by the right ventricle because it is delivered under much lower pressure than with a ventricular septal defect. Although there is right atrial and ventricular enlargement, cardiac failure is unusual in an uncomplicated ASD. Pulmonary vascular changes usually occur only after several decades if the defect is left unrepaired.

Clinical manifestations—Patients may be asymptomatic. Spontaneous closure of ASDs are most likely to occur in younger patients and those with small defects (Vick & Bezold, 2018). They may develop heart failure (HF), particularly in the third or fourth decade of life if the ASD goes undiagnosed, as the pulmonary artery pressure then begins to rise. There is a characteristic murmur. Patients are at risk for atrial dysrhythmias (probably caused by atrial enlargement and stretching of conduction fibers) and pulmonary vascular obstructive disease and emboli formation later in life from chronically increased pulmonary blood flow.

Surgical closure—Surgical patch closure (pericardial patch or Dacron patch) is done for moderate to large defects. Open repair with cardiopulmonary bypass is usually performed before school age. In addition, the sinus venosus defect requires patch placement, so the anomalous right pulmonary venous return is directed to the left atrium with a baffle. The ASD 1 type may require mitral valve repair or, rarely, replacement of the mitral valve.

Transcatheter closure—ASD 2 closure with a device during cardiac catheterization is becoming commonplace and can be done as an outpatient procedure. The Amplatzer septal occluder is most commonly used. Smaller defects that have a rim around them for attachment of the device can be closed with a device; large, irregular defects without a rim require surgical closure. Successful closure in appropriately selected patients yields results similar to surgery but involves shorter hospital stays and fewer complications. Patients receive low-dose aspirin for 6 months (Moore, Hegde, El-Said, et al., 2013).

Prognosis—Outcomes for both treatment options are very good. Limited data also suggest that the rates of procedural success may be comparable to or possibly better with surgery versus transcatheter closure, but that there may be an increased rate of reintervention associated with percutaneous closure (Du, Hijazi, & Kleinman, 2002).

Ventricular Septal Defect

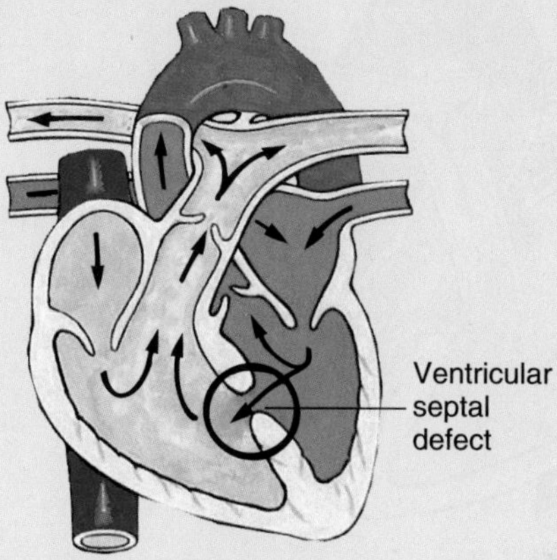

Description—Abnormal opening between the ventricles. May be classified according to location: membranous (accounting for 80%) or muscular. May vary in size from a small pinhole to absence of the septum, which results in a common ventricle. Ventricular septal defects (VSDs) are frequently associated with other defects, such as pulmonic stenosis, transposition of the great vessels, patent ductus arteriosus, atrial defects, and coarctation of the aorta. Many VSDs (20% to 60%) close spontaneously. Spontaneous closure is most likely to occur during the first year of life in children having small or moderate defects.

Pathophysiology—Because of the higher pressure within the left ventricle and because the systemic arterial circulation offers more resistance than the pulmonary circulation, blood flows through the defect into the pulmonary artery. The increased blood volume is pumped into the lungs, which may eventually result in increased pulmonary vascular resistance. Increased pressure in the right ventricle as a result of left-to-right shunting and pulmonary resistance causes the muscle to hypertrophy. If the right ventricle is unable to accommodate the increased workload, the right atrium may also enlarge as it attempts to overcome the resistance offered by incomplete right ventricular emptying.

Clinical manifestations—HF is common. There is a characteristic murmur.

Surgical treatment

Palliative—Pulmonary artery banding (placement of a band around the main pulmonary artery to decrease pulmonary blood flow) may be done in infants with multiple muscular VSDs or complex anatomy. Improvements in surgical techniques and postoperative care make complete repair in infancy the preferred approach.

Complete repair (procedure of choice)—Small defects are repaired with sutures. Large defects usually require sewing a knitted Dacron patch over the opening. Cardiopulmonary bypass is used for both procedures. The approach for the repair is generally through the right atrium and the tricuspid valve. Postoperative complications include residual VSD and conduction disturbances.

Transcatheter Closure

Description—Catheter closure of muscular, postoperative, or fenestrated defects is also widely used in centers nationwide. Device closures of VSDs carry more risk than with ASDs. The most common complication noted in one study was complete atrioventricular (AV) block requiring pacemaker placement in 5.7% of the subjects (Butera, Carminati, Chessa, et al., 2007).

Prognosis—Risks depend on the location of the defect, the number of defects, surgical versus transcatheter closure, and the presence of other associated cardiac defects. Single membranous defects are associated with low

Continued

BOX 23.1 Defects With Increased Pulmonary Blood Flow—cont'd

mortality (<2%); multiple muscular defects can carry a higher risk (Jacobs, Mavroudis, Jacobs, et al., 2004).

Atrioventricular Canal Defect

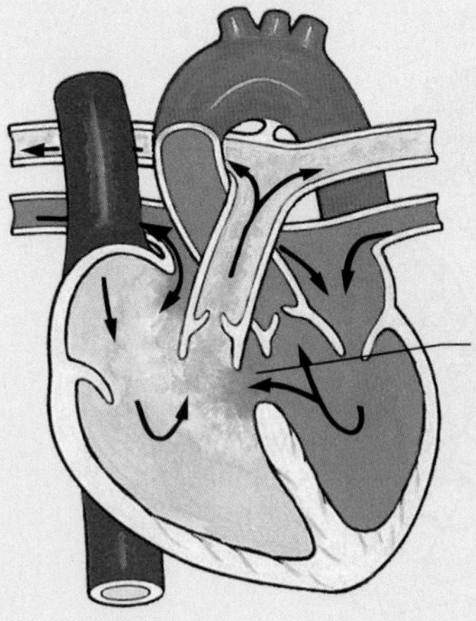

Description—Also referred to as *AV septal defects* or *endocardial cushion defects.* Incomplete fusion of the endocardial cushions. Consists of a low ASD that is continuous with a high VSD and clefts of the mitral and tricuspid valves, which creates a large central AV valve that allows blood to flow between all four chambers of the heart. The directions and pathways of flow are determined by pulmonary and systemic resistance, left and right ventricular pressures, and the compliance of each chamber, although flow is generally from left to right. It is the most common cardiac defect in children with Down syndrome.

Pathophysiology—The alterations in hemodynamics depend on the severity of the defect and the child's pulmonary vascular resistance. Immediately after birth, while the newborn's pulmonary vascular resistance is high, there is minimum shunting of blood through the defect. Once this resistance falls, left-to-right shunting occurs and pulmonary blood flow increases. The resultant pulmonary vascular engorgement predisposes the child to development of HF.

Clinical manifestations—Patients usually have moderate to severe HF. There is a characteristic murmur. There may be mild cyanosis that increases with crying. Patients are at high risk for developing pulmonary vascular obstructive disease.

Surgical treatment

Palliative—Pulmonary artery banding is occasionally done in small infants with severe symptoms. Single ventricle palliation is necessary for some infants who have a right or left ventricle dominant canal defect.

Complete repair—Surgical repair consists of patch closure of the septal defects and reconstruction of the AV valve tissue (either repair of the mitral valve cleft or fashioning of two AV valves). Postoperative complications include heart block, HF, mitral regurgitation, dysrhythmias, and pulmonary hypertension.

Prognosis—Operative mortality is generally low, with patients who are younger (>2.5 months) and smaller (<3.5 kg) having worse outcomes (Jacobs et al., 2004; St. Louis, Jodhka, Jacobs, et al., 2014). A potential later problem is mitral regurgitation, which may require valve replacement.

Patent Ductus Arteriosus

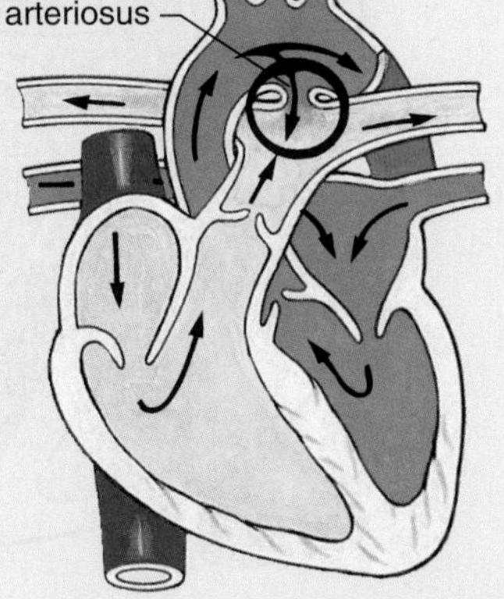

Description—Failure of the fetal ductus arteriosus (artery connecting the aorta and pulmonary artery) to close within the first weeks of life. The continued patency of this vessel allows blood to flow from the higher pressure aorta to the lower pressure pulmonary artery, which causes a left-to-right shunt.

Pathophysiology—The hemodynamic consequences of patent ductus arteriosus (PDA) depend on the size of the ductus and the pulmonary vascular resistance. At birth the resistance in the pulmonary and systemic circulations is almost identical, so the resistance in the aorta and pulmonary artery is equalized. As the systemic pressure comes to exceed the pulmonary pressure, blood begins to shunt from the aorta across the duct to the pulmonary artery (left-to-right shunt). The additional blood is recirculated through the lungs and returned to the left atrium and left ventricle. The effect of this altered circulation is increased workload on the left side of the heart, increased pulmonary vascular congestion and possibly resistance, and potentially increased right ventricular pressure and hypertrophy.

Clinical manifestations—The amount of shunting will determine the degree of clinical manifestations. There is a characteristic machinery-like murmur. Patients may be asymptomatic or show signs of HF. Moderate to large PDAs may present as left-sided volume overload or reversible pulmonary arterial hypertension.

Medical management—Administration of indomethacin (prostaglandin inhibitor) has proved successful in closing a patent ductus in premature infants and some newborns.

Surgical treatment—Surgical division or ligation of the patent vessel is performed via a left thoracotomy. In video-assisted thoracoscopic surgery, a thoracoscope and instruments are inserted through three small incisions on the left side of the chest to place a clip on the ductus. The surgical approach is dependent on the size and age of the patient.

Transcatheter treatment—Coils to occlude the PDA are placed in the catheterization laboratory in many centers. Premature or small infants (with small-diameter femoral arteries) and patients with large or unusual PDAs may require surgery.

Prognosis—Both surgical and nonsurgical procedures can be done at low risk with less than 1% mortality. PDA closure in very premature infants has a higher mortality rate because of the additional significant medical problems.

BOX 23.2 Obstructive Defects

Coarctation of the Aorta

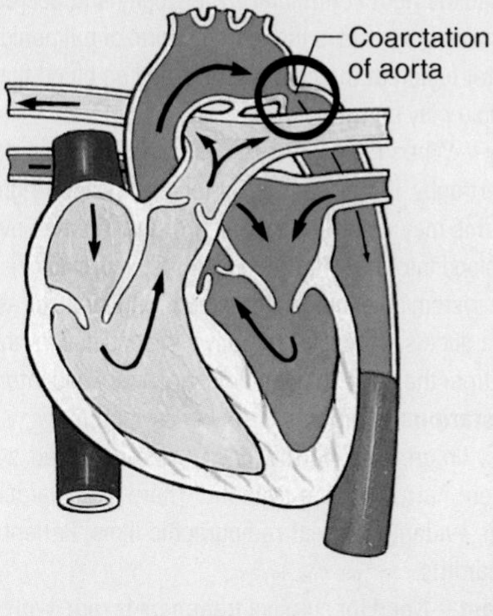

Description—Localized narrowing near the insertion of the ductus arteriosus, which results in increased pressure proximal to the defect (head and upper extremities) and decreased pressure distal to the obstruction (body and lower extremities).

Pathophysiology—The effect of a narrowing within the aorta is increased pressure proximal to the defect (upper extremities) and decreased pressure distal to it (lower extremities).

Clinical manifestations—There may be high blood pressure and bounding pulses in the arms, weak or absent femoral pulses, and cool lower extremities with lower blood pressure. There are signs of heart failure (HF) in infants. In infants with critical coarctation, the hemodynamic condition may deteriorate rapidly with severe acidosis and hypotension. Mechanical ventilation and inotropic support are often necessary before surgery. Older children may experience dizziness, headaches, fainting, and epistaxis resulting from hypertension. Patients are at risk for hypertension, ruptured aorta, aortic aneurysm, and stroke.

Surgical treatment—Surgical repair is the treatment of choice for infants younger than 6 months of age and for patients with long-segment stenosis or complex anatomy. Repair is by either (1) resection of the narrowed portion with an end-to-end anastomosis of the aorta or (2) enlargement of the section using a graft of prosthetic material or portion of the left subclavian artery. Because this defect is outside the heart and pericardium, cardiopulmonary bypass is not required, and a thoracotomy incision is used. Postoperative hypertension is treated with intravenous sodium nitroprusside, esmolol, or milrinone, followed by oral medications, such as angiotensin-converting enzyme inhibitors or beta-blockers. Residual permanent hypertension after repair of coarctation of the aorta (COA) seems to be related to age and time of repair. To prevent both hypertension at rest and exercise-provoked systemic hypertension after repair, elective surgery for COA is advised within the first 2 years of life. Percutaneous balloon angioplasty techniques have proved to be very effective in relieving residual postoperative coarctation gradients.

Transcatheter treatment—Balloon angioplasty is a primary intervention for COA in older infants and children. In adolescents, stents may be placed in the aorta to maintain patency. The goal of the procedure is to achieve a reduction in gradient to less than 10%, or more than 90% relief of obstruction angiographically. Dilation and/or stent implantation for native or recurrent coarctation seems to immediately relieve obstruction in more than 90% of cases (Holzer, Chisolm, Hill, et al., 2008).

Prognosis—There are low rates of morbidity, mortality, and reintervention for infants and children who underwent COA repair via a left thoracotomy (Mery, Guzmán-Pruneda, Trost, et al., 2015). Major long-term complications include recoarctation, aortic aneurysm, and systemic hypertension (Brown, Burkhart, Connolly, et al., 2013).

Aortic Stenosis

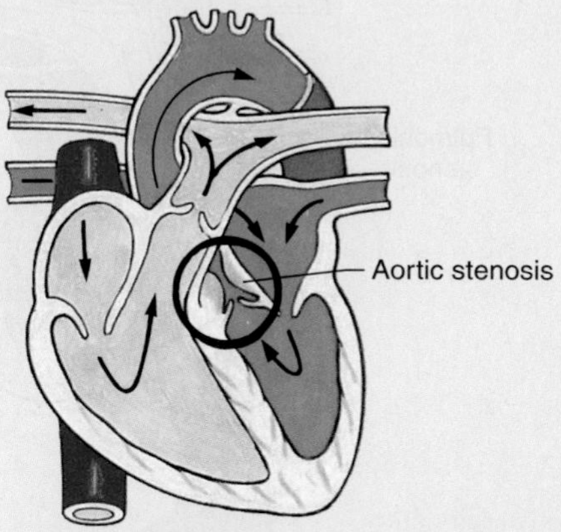

Description—Narrowing or stricture of the aortic valve, causing resistance to blood flow in the left ventricle, decreased cardiac output, left ventricular hypertrophy, and pulmonary vascular congestion. Valvular aortic stenosis (AS), the most common type, is usually caused by malformed cusps that result in a bicuspid rather than tricuspid valve or fusion of the cusps. Subvalvular stenosis is a stricture caused by a fibrous ring below a normal valve; supravalvular stenosis occurs infrequently. Valvular AS is a serious defect because (1) the obstruction tends to be progressive; (2) sudden episodes of myocardial ischemia, or low cardiac output, can result in sudden death; and (3) surgical repair rarely results in a normal valve. This is one of the rare instances in which strenuous physical activity may be curtailed because of the cardiac condition.

Pathophysiology—A stricture in the aortic outflow tract causes resistance to ejection of blood from the left ventricle. The extra workload on the left ventricle causes hypertrophy. If left ventricular failure develops, left atrial pressure will increase; this causes increased pressure in the pulmonary veins, which results in pulmonary vascular congestion (pulmonary edema).

Clinical manifestations—Newborns with critical AS demonstrate signs of decreased cardiac output with faint pulses, hypotension, tachycardia, and poor feeding. Children show signs of exercise intolerance, chest pain, and dizziness when standing for a long period. There is a characteristic murmur. Patients are at risk for infective endocarditis, coronary insufficiency, and ventricular dysfunction.

Valvular Aortic Stenosis

Surgical treatment—Aortic valvotomy is performed under inflow occlusion. Used rarely, since balloon dilation in the catheterization laboratory is the first-line procedure. Newborns with critical AS and small left-sided structures may undergo a stage 1 Norwood procedure (see Hypoplastic Left Heart Syndrome in Box 23.4).

Prognosis—Aortic valvotomy remains a palliative procedure, and the patient may require further surgery to repair or even replace the aortic valve. An aortic homograft with a valve may also be used (extended aortic root replacement), or the pulmonic valve may be moved to the aortic position and replaced with a homograft valve (Ross procedure). If the obstruction is at the subvalvular region and results from narrowing of the left ventricular outflow tract with a small aortic valve annulus, a patch may be required to enlarge the entire left ventricular outflow tract and annulus and replace the aortic valve, an approach known as the Konno procedure. Patients who have obstruction at both the valvular and the subvalvular regions may undergo a combination of these two procedures, also called a Ross-Konno procedure.

Nonsurgical treatment—The narrowed valve is dilated using balloon angioplasty in the catheterization laboratory. This procedure is usually the first intervention.

Prognosis—Complications include aortic insufficiency or valvular regurgitation, tearing of the valve leaflets, and loss of pulse in the catheterized limb.

Continued

BOX 23.2 Obstructive Defects—cont'd

Pulmonic Stenosis

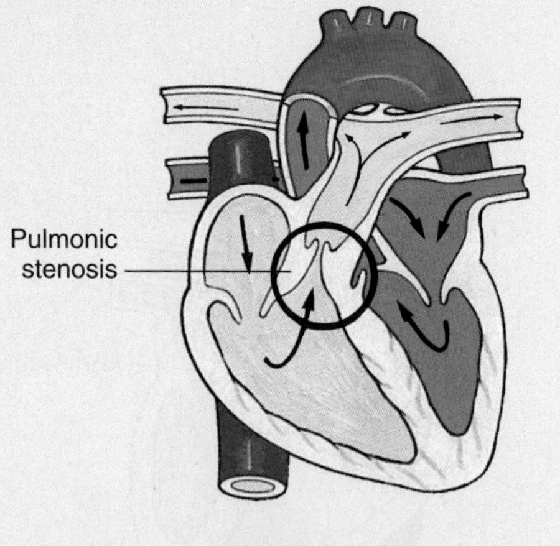

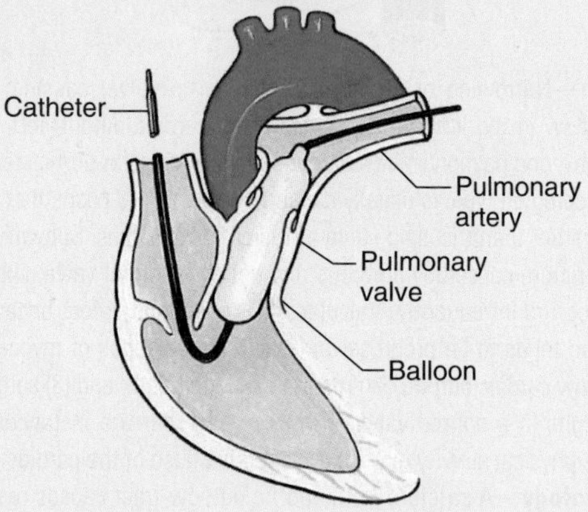

Description—Narrowing at the entrance to the pulmonary artery. Resistance to blood flow causes right ventricular hypertrophy and decreased pulmonary blood flow. Pulmonary atresia is the extreme form of pulmonic stenosis (PS) in that there is total fusion of the commissures and no blood flows to the lungs. The right ventricle may be hypoplastic.

Pathophysiology—When PS is present, resistance to blood flow causes right ventricular hypertrophy. If right ventricular failure develops, right atrial pressure increases, and this may result in reopening of the foramen ovale, shunting of deoxygenated blood into the left atrium, and systemic cyanosis. If PS is severe, HF occurs, and systemic venous engorgement is noted. An associated defect such as a patent ductus arteriosus partially compensates for the obstruction by shunting blood from the aorta to the pulmonary artery and into the lungs.

Clinical manifestations—Patients may be asymptomatic; some have mild cyanosis or HF. Progressive narrowing causes increased symptoms. Newborns with severe narrowing are cyanotic. There is a characteristic murmur. Cardiomegaly is evident on chest radiographic films. Patients are at risk for infective endocarditis.

Surgical treatment—Need for surgical treatment is rare, with widespread use of balloon angioplasty techniques, but in some cases pulmonary valvotomy with cardiopulmonary bypass is necessary.

Transcatheter treatment—Balloon angioplasty in the cardiac catheterization laboratory to dilate the valve. A catheter is inserted across the stenotic pulmonic valve into the pulmonary artery, and a balloon at the end of the catheter is inflated and rapidly passed through the narrowed opening. The procedure is associated with few complications and has proved to be highly effective. It is the treatment of choice for discrete PS in most centers and can be done safely in neonates.

Prognosis—Risk is low for both surgical and transcatheter procedures; mortality is low, slightly higher in neonates. Both balloon dilation and surgical valvotomy leave the pulmonary valve incompetent because they involve opening the fused valve leaflets; however, these patients are clinically asymptomatic. Long-term problems with restenosis or valve incompetence may occur.

BOX 23.3 Defects With Decreased Pulmonary Blood Flow

Tetralogy of Fallot

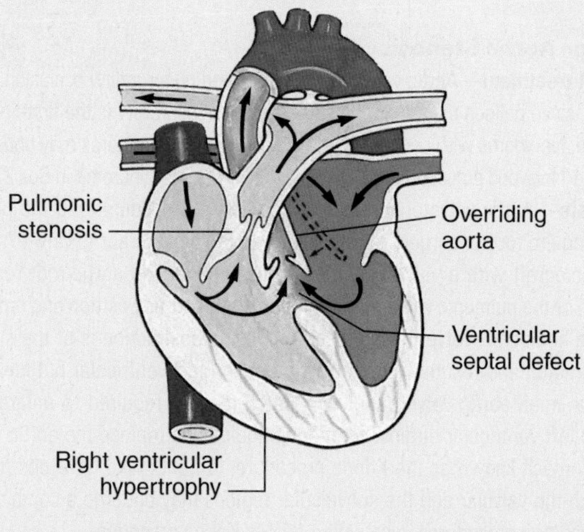

Description—The classic form includes four defects: (1) ventricular septal defect (VSD), (2) pulmonic stenosis, (3) overriding aorta, and (4) right ventricular hypertrophy.

Pathophysiology—The alteration in hemodynamics varies widely, depending primarily on the degree of pulmonary stenosis, but also on the size of the VSD and the pulmonary and systemic resistance to flow. Because the VSD is usually large, pressures may be equal in the right and left ventricles. Therefore the shunt direction depends on the difference between pulmonary and systemic vascular resistance. If pulmonary vascular resistance is higher than systemic resistance, the shunt is from right to left. If systemic resistance is higher than pulmonary resistance, the shunt is from left to right. Pulmonary stenosis decreases blood flow to the lungs and consequently the amount of oxygenated blood that returns to the left side of the heart. Depending on the position of the aorta, blood from both ventricles may be distributed systemically.

Clinical manifestations—Some infants may be acutely cyanotic at birth; others have mild cyanosis that progresses over the first year of life as the pulmonary stenosis worsens. There is a characteristic murmur. There may be acute episodes of cyanosis and hypoxia, called *blue spells* or *tet spells.* Anoxic spells occur when the infant's oxygen requirements exceed the blood supply, usually during crying or after feeding. Patients are at risk for emboli, seizures, and loss of consciousness or sudden death following an anoxic spell.

Surgical treatment—Elective repair is usually performed in the first year of life. Indications for repair include increasing cyanosis and the development of hypercyanotic spells. Complete repair involves closure of the VSD and resection of the

BOX 23.3 Defects With Decreased Pulmonary Blood Flow—cont'd

infundibular stenosis, with placement of a pericardial patch to enlarge the right ventricular outflow tract. In some repairs, the patch may extend across the pulmonic valve annulus (transannular patch), making the pulmonic valve incompetent. The procedure requires a median sternotomy and the use of cardiopulmonary bypass.

Prognosis—The operative mortality for total correction of tetralogy of Fallot is less than 3% (Jacobs et al., 2004). Long-term complications include chronic pulmonary regurgitation with right ventricular enlargement and decreased function requiring pulmonary valve replacement, residual right ventricular outflow tract obstruction, aortic root dilation and aortic valve insufficiency, arrhythmias, and sudden cardiac death. Pulmonary valve replacement is performed either surgically or in the catheterization lab using a transcatheter approach (Doyle, Kavanaugh-McHugh, & Fish, 2019).

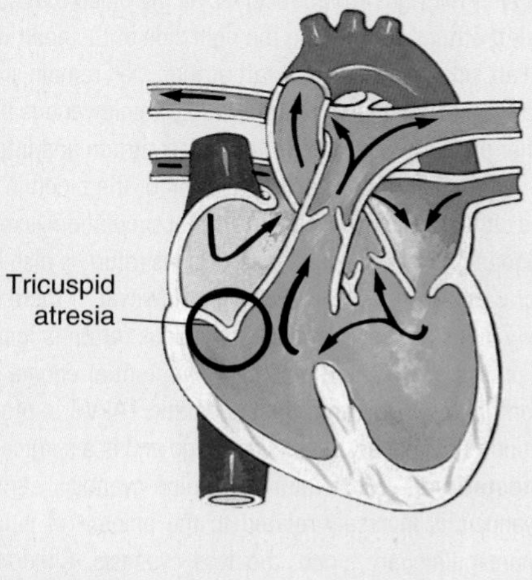

Tricuspid Atresia

Description—The tricuspid valve fails to develop; consequently, there is no communication from the right atrium to the right ventricle. Blood flows through an atrial septal defect (ASD) or a patent foramen ovale to the left side of the heart and through a VSD to the right ventricle and out to the lungs. The condition is often associated with pulmonary stenosis and transposition of the great arteries. There is complete mixing of deoxygenated and oxygenated blood in the left side of the heart, which results in systemic desaturation, and varying amounts of pulmonary obstruction, which causes decreased pulmonary blood flow.

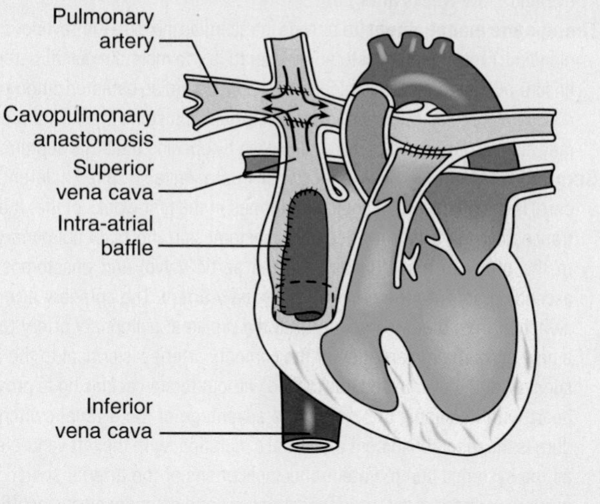

Pathophysiology—At birth the presence of a patent foramen ovale (or other atrial septal opening) is required to permit blood flow across the septum into the left atrium; the patent ductus arteriosus allows blood flow to the pulmonary artery into the lungs for oxygenation. A VSD allows a modest amount of blood to enter the right ventricle and pulmonary artery for oxygenation. Pulmonary blood flow is often diminished.

Clinical manifestations—Cyanosis is usually seen in the newborn period. There may be tachycardia and dyspnea. Older children have signs of chronic hypoxemia with clubbing.

Therapeutic management—For the neonate whose pulmonary blood flow depends on the patency of the ductus arteriosus, a continuous infusion of prostaglandin E1 is started at 0.1 mcg/kg/min until surgical intervention can be arranged.

Surgical treatment—Patients with tricuspid atresia follow the staged surgical approach for single ventricle anatomywith the left ventricle becoming the ventricular pump.

Prognosis—Surgical mortality is less than 5% (Jacobs et al., 2004); the rate increases when the anatomy is more complex and other risk factors are present. Postoperative complications include dysrhythmias, systemic venous hypertension, pleural and pericardial effusions, and ventricular dysfunction.

BOX 23.4 Mixed Defects

Transposition of the Great Arteries, or Transposition of the Great Vessels

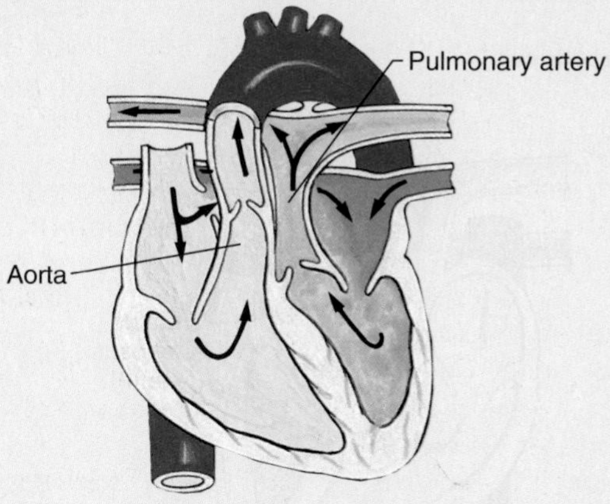

Description—The pulmonary artery leaves the left ventricle, and the aorta exits from the right ventricle, with no communication between the systemic and pulmonary circulations.

Pathophysiology—Associated defects such as septal defects or patent ductus arteriosus must be present to permit blood to enter the systemic circulation or the pulmonary circulation for mixing of saturated and desaturated blood. The most common defect associated with transposition of the great arteries (TGA) is a patent foramen ovale. At birth there is also a patent ductus arteriosus, although in most instances this closes after the neonatal period. Another associated defect may be a ventricular septal defect (VSD). The presence of a VSD increases the risk of heart failure (HF) because it permits blood to flow from the right to the left ventricle, into the pulmonary artery, and finally to the lungs. However, it also produces increased pulmonary blood flow under high pressure, which can result in high pulmonary vascular resistance.

Clinical manifestations—Vary according to the type and size of the associated defects. Newborns with minimum communication are severely cyanotic

Continued

and have depressed function at birth. Those with large septal defects or a patent ductus arteriosus may be less cyanotic but have symptoms of HF. Heart sounds vary according to the type of defect present. Cardiomegaly is usually evident a few weeks after birth.

Therapeutic management (to provide intracardiac mixing)—Intravenous prostaglandin E1 may be administered preoperatively to maintain ductal patency and ensure adequate systemic blood flow. During cardiac catheterization or under echocardiographic guidance, a balloon atrial septostomy (Rashkind procedure) may also be performed to increase mixing by opening the atrial septum.

Surgical treatment—An arterial switch operation (also called a Jatene procedure) is the procedure of choice performed in the first weeks of life. It involves transecting the great arteries and anastomosing the main pulmonary artery to the proximal aorta (just above the aortic valve) and anastomosing the ascending aorta to the proximal pulmonary artery. The coronary arteries are switched from the proximal aorta to the proximal pulmonary artery to create a new aorta. Reimplantation of the coronary arteries is critical to the infant's survival, and they must be reattached without torsion or kinking to provide the heart with its supply of oxygen. The advantage of the arterial switch procedure is the reestablishment of normal circulation, with the left ventricle acting as the systemic pump. Potential complications of the arterial switch include narrowing at the great artery anastomoses and coronary artery insufficiency.

Intra-atrial baffle repairs—Intra-atrial baffle repairs are rarely performed, although many adolescents and adults survive today with repairs that were done more than 15 years ago. An intra-atrial baffle is created to divert venous blood to the mitral valve and pulmonary venous blood to the tricuspid valve using the patient's atrial septum (Senning procedure) or a prosthetic material (Mustard procedure). A disadvantage is the continuing role of the right ventricle as the systemic pump and the late development of right ventricular failure and rhythm disturbances. Other potential postoperative complications include loss of normal sinus rhythm, baffle leaks, and ventricular dysfunction.

Rastelli procedure—This procedure is the operative choice in infants with TGA, VSD, and severe pulmonary stenosis. It involves closure of the VSD with a baffle so that left ventricular blood is directed through the VSD into the aorta. The pulmonary valve is then closed, and a conduit is placed from the right ventricle to the pulmonary artery to create a physiologically normal circulation. Unfortunately, this procedure requires multiple conduit replacements as the child grows.

Prognosis—Outcomes after the arterial switch operation are quite good. There are some long-term complications, including neoaortic, pulmonary, and coronary artery complications, but most patients maintain normal cardiovascular function and exercise capacity (Khairy, Clair, Fernandes, et al., 2013). Patients who undergo a Senning or Mustard procedure demonstrate diminished long-term survival rates and substantial morbidity (Cuypers, Eindhoven, Slager, et al., 2014).

Total Anomalous Pulmonary Venous Connection

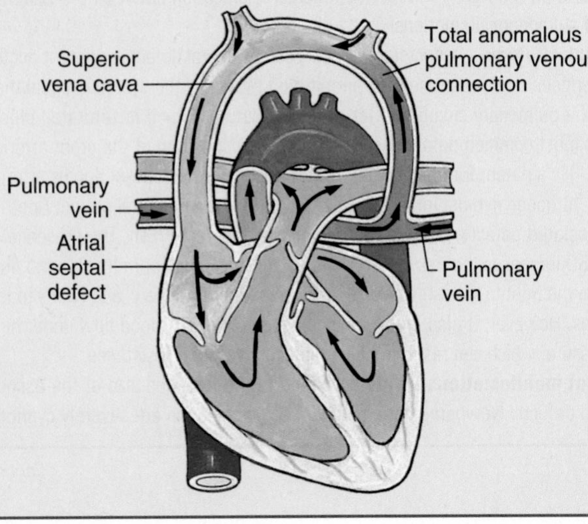

Description—Rare defect characterized by failure of the pulmonary veins to join the left atrium. Instead, the pulmonary veins are abnormally connected to the systemic venous circuit via the right atrium or various veins draining toward the right atrium, such as the superior vena cava. The abnormal attachment results in mixed blood being returned to the right atrium and shunted from the right to the left through an atrial septal defect (ASD). Total anomalous pulmonary venous connection (TAPVC; also called *total anomalous pulmonary venous return* or *total anomalous pulmonary venous drainage*) is classified according to the pulmonary venous point of attachment as follows:

Supracardiac—Attachment above the diaphragm, such as to the superior vena cava (most common form) but not directly to the heart (see accompanying figure).

Cardiac—Direct attachment to the heart, such as to the right atrium or coronary sinus

Infradiaphragmatic—Attachment below the diaphragm, such as to the inferior vena cava (most severe form)

Pathophysiology—The right atrium receives all the blood that normally would flow into the left atrium. As a result, the right side of the heart hypertrophies, whereas the left side, especially the left atrium, may remain small. An associated ASD or patent foramen ovale allows systemic venous blood to shunt from the higher pressure right atrium to the left atrium and into the left side of the heart. As a result, the oxygen saturation of the blood in both sides of the heart (and ultimately in the systemic arterial circulation) is the same. If the pulmonary blood flow is large, pulmonary venous return is also large, and the amount of saturated blood is relatively high. However, if there is obstruction to pulmonary venous drainage, pulmonary venous return is impeded, pulmonary venous pressure rises, and pulmonary interstitial edema develops and eventually contributes to HF. Infradiaphragmatic TAPVC is often associated with obstruction to pulmonary venous drainage and is a surgical emergency.

Clinical manifestations—Most infants develop cyanosis early in life. The degree of cyanosis is inversely related to the amount of pulmonary blood flow—the more pulmonary blood, the less cyanosis. Children with unobstructed TAPVC may be asymptomatic until pulmonary vascular resistance decreases during infancy, increasing pulmonary blood flow, with resulting signs of HF. Cyanosis becomes worse with pulmonary vein obstruction; once obstruction occurs, the infant's condition usually deteriorates rapidly. Without intervention, cardiac failure progresses to death.

Surgical treatment—Corrective repair is performed in early infancy. The surgical approach varies with the anatomic defect. In general, however, the common pulmonary vein is anastomosed to the back of the left atrium, the ASD is closed, and the anomalous pulmonary venous connection is ligated. The cardiac type is most easily repaired; the infradiaphragmatic type carries the highest morbidity and mortality because of the higher incidence of pulmonary vein obstruction. Potential postoperative complications include reobstruction; bleeding; dysrhythmias, particularly heart block; pulmonary artery hypertension; and persistent heart failure.

Prognosis—Mortality for all types is less than 10% (Jacobs et al., 2004) and is lowest for the cardiac type; morbidity increases with the presence of pulmonary vein obstruction.

Truncus Arteriosus

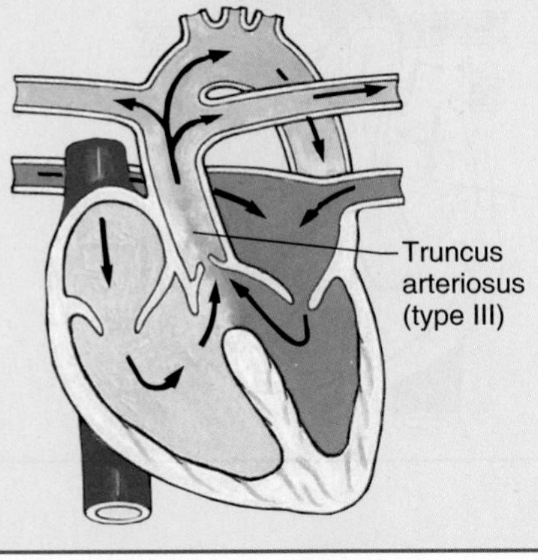

BOX 23.4 Mixed Defects—cont'd

Description—Failure of normal septation and division of the embryonic bulbar trunk into the pulmonary artery and the aorta, which results in development of a single vessel that overrides both ventricles. Blood from both ventricles mixes in the common great artery, which leads to desaturation and hypoxemia. Blood ejected from the heart flows preferentially to the lower pressure pulmonary arteries, so pulmonary blood flow is increased and systemic blood flow is reduced. There are three types:

Type I—A single pulmonary trunk arises near the base of the truncus and divides into the left and right pulmonary arteries.

Type II—The left and right pulmonary arteries arise separately but in close proximity and at the same level from the back of the truncus.

Type III—The pulmonary arteries arise independently from the sides of the truncus.

Pathophysiology—Blood ejected from the left and right ventricles enters the common trunk, so pulmonary and systemic circulations are mixed. Blood flow is distributed to the pulmonary and systemic circulations according to the relative resistances of each system. The amount of pulmonary blood flow depends on the size of the pulmonary arteries and the pulmonary vascular resistance. Generally, resistance to pulmonary blood flow is less than systemic vascular resistance, which results in preferential blood flow to the lungs. Pulmonary vascular disease develops at an early age in patients with truncus arteriosus.

Clinical manifestations—Most infants are symptomatic with moderate to severe HF and variable cyanosis, poor growth, and activity intolerance. There is a characteristic murmur. Thirty-five percent of patients have 22q11.2 deletions (Goldmuntz & Lin, 2008).

Surgical treatment—Early repair is performed in the first month of life. It involves closing the VSD so that the truncus arteriosus receives the outflow from the left ventricle, excising the pulmonary arteries from the aorta and attaching them to the right ventricle using a right ventricle to pulmonary artery conduit, and possible repair of the truncal valve. Postoperative complications include truncal valve insufficiency, persistent heart failure, bleeding, pulmonary artery hypertension, dysrhythmias, and residual VSD. Because conduits are not living tissue, they will not grow along with the child and may also become narrowed with calcifications. One or more conduit replacements will be needed in childhood.

Prognosis—Perioperative mortality is about 10%, with highest mortality in patients who required repair for both truncal valve and aortic arch interruption (Russell, Pasquali, Jacobs, et al., 2012). Long-term complications include truncal valve regurgitation and conduit stenosis.

Hypoplastic Left Heart Syndrome

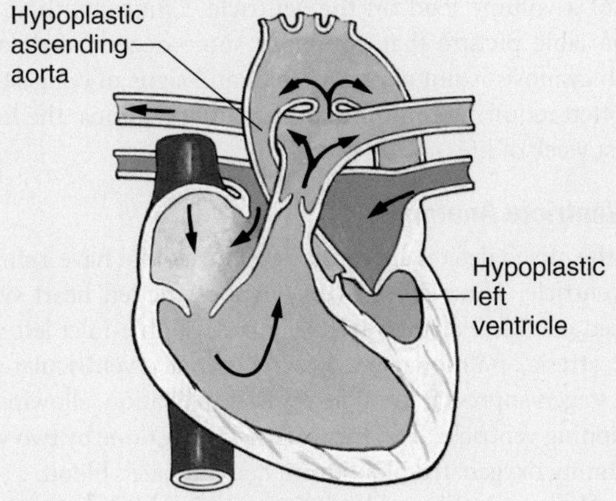

Description—Underdevelopment of the left side of the heart with significant hypoplasisa of the left ventricle including atresia, stenosis or hypoplasia of the aortic and/or mitral valves, and hypoplasia of the ascending arota and arch. Most blood from the left atrium flows across the patent foramen ovale to the right atrium, to the right ventricle, and out the pulmonary artery. The descending aorta receives blood from the patent ductus arteriosus supplying systemic blood flow.

Pathophysiology—An ASD or patent foramen ovale allows saturated blood from the left atrium to mix with desaturated blood from the right atrium and to flow through the right ventricle and out into the pulmonary artery. From the pulmonary artery, the blood flows both to the lungs and through the ductus arteriosus into the aorta and out to the body. The amount of blood flow to the pulmonary and systemic circulations depends on the relationship between the pulmonary and systemic vascular resistances. The coronary and cerebral vessels receive blood by retrograde flow through the hypoplastic ascending aorta.

Clinical manifestations—There is mild cyanosis and signs of HF until the patent ductus arteriosus closes, then progressive deterioration with cyanosis and decreased cardiac output, leading to cardiovascular collapse. The condition is usually fatal in the first months of life without intervention.

Therapeutic management—Neonates require stabilization with mechanical ventilation and inotropic support preoperatively. A prostaglandin E1 infusion is needed to maintain ductal patency and ensure adequate systemic blood flow until surgical intervention can occur.

Surgical treatment—Patients with hypoplastic left heart syndrome (HLHS) follow the staged surgical approach for single ventricle anatomy with the right ventricle becoming the ventricular pump. Postoperative complications include dysrhythmias, systemic venous hypertension, pleural and pericardial effusions, thrombotic events, and ventricular dysfunction.

Transplantation—Heart transplantation in the newborn period is another option for these infants. Problems include the shortage of newborn organ donors, risk of rejection, long-term problems with chronic immunosuppression, and infection.

Prognosis—Thirty years ago a diagnosis of HLHS was uniformly fatal. Today, for children who survive to the age of 12 months, long-term survival is approximately 90% (Alsoufi, Mori, Gillespie, et al., 2015; Siffel, Riehle-Colarusso, Oster, et al., 2015). Improved outcomes have been associated with early diagnosis and repair and increased monitoring in the hospital and at home, particularly between the first- and second-stage surgeries. Long-term problems include worsening ventricular function, tricuspid regurgitation, recurrent aortic arch narrowing, dysrhythmias, thrombotic complications, and developmental delays.

TABLE 23.3 Selected Shunt Procedures for Children With Cardiac Defects

Shunt Type	Comments
Modified Blalock-Taussig shunt—Subclavian artery to pulmonary artery using Gore-Tex or Impra tube graft	Shunt flow sometimes excessive, requiring use of diuretics Possibility of thrombosis; aspirin usually prescribed postoperatively Easy to ligate at time of definitive correction Shunt size fixed and may become too small as child grows
Sano modification—Right ventricular to pulmonary artery conduit using Gore-Tex graft	Prevents diastolic runoff of systemic blood into the pulmonary arteries Provides a higher diastolic blood pressure and seemingly better coronary perfusion Used in place of the modified Blalock-Taussig shunt in the Norwood procedure
Bidirectional Glenn shunt (cavopulmonary anastomosis)—Superior vena cava to side of right pulmonary artery; blood flows to both lungs	Done as a second shunt; often used as a staging step to a Fontan procedure Can be incorporated into eventual modified Fontan procedure Relieves severe cyanosis and decreases volume overload on ventricle Carries risk of embolic events (mixing defect); aspirin often prescribed Pulmonary arteriovenous fistulas may occur months or years later, causing desaturation (uncommon finding)
Central shunt—Ascending aorta to main pulmonary artery using Gore-Tex graft	Length of shunt acts to restrict blood flow; symptoms of heart failure may occur; diuretic therapy may be required Uncommon; used when modified Blalock-Taussig shunt cannot be used Easy to insert and remove at time of repair Possibility of thrombosis; aspirin usually prescribed postoperatively

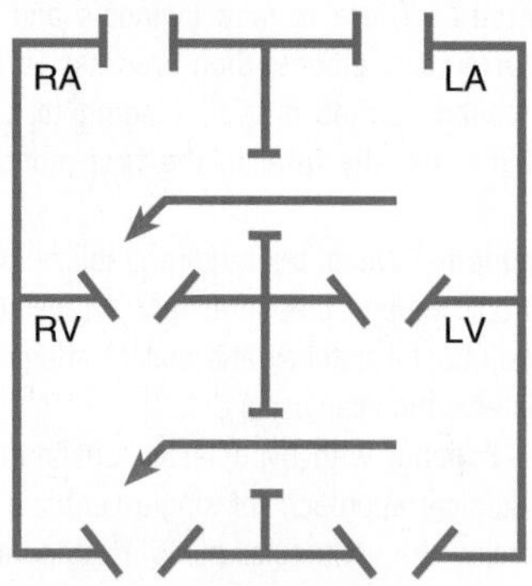

Fig. 23.4 Hemodynamics in defects with increased pulmonary blood flow. *LA,* Left atrium; *LV,* left ventricle; *RA,* right atrium; *RV,* right ventricle.

Coarctation of the aorta (narrowing of the aortic arch), aortic stenosis, and pulmonic stenosis are typical defects in this group (Box 23.2). Hemodynamically, there is a pressure load on the ventricle and decreased cardiac output. Clinically, infants and children exhibit signs of HF. Children with mild obstruction may be asymptomatic. Rarely, as in severe pulmonic stenosis, hypoxemia may occur.

Defects With Decreased Pulmonary Blood Flow

In this group of defects, there is obstruction of pulmonary blood flow and an anatomic defect (atrial septal defect or ventricular septal defect) between the right and left sides of the heart (Fig. 23.6). Because blood has difficulty exiting the right side of the heart via the pulmonary artery, pressure on the right side increases, exceeding left-sided pressure. This allows desaturated blood to shunt right to left, causing desaturation in the left side of the heart and in the systemic circulation. Clinically, these patients have hypoxemia and usually appear cyanotic. Tetralogy of Fallot and tricuspid atresia are the most common defects in this group (Box 23.3).

Mixed Defects

Many complex cardiac anomalies are classified together in the mixed category (Box 23.4), since survival in the postnatal period depends on mixing of blood from the pulmonary and systemic circulations within the heart chambers. Hemodynamically, fully saturated systemic blood flow mixes with the desaturated pulmonary blood flow, which causes

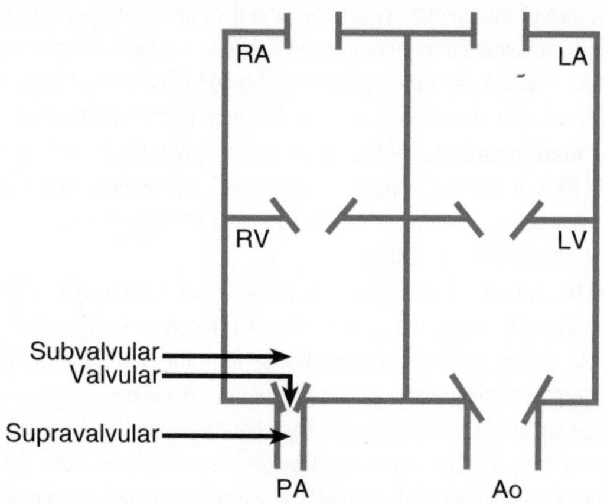

Fig. 23.5 Obstruction to ventricular ejection can occur at the valvular level (shown), below the valve (subvalvular), or above the valve (supravalvular). Pulmonic stenosis is shown here. *Ao,* Aorta; *LA,* left atrium; *LV,* left ventricle; *PA,* pulmonary artery; *RA,* right atrium; *RV,* right ventricle.

a relative desaturation of the systemic blood. Pulmonary congestion occurs because the differences in pulmonary artery pressure and aortic pressure favor pulmonary blood flow. Cardiac output decreases because of a volume load on the ventricle. Clinically, these patients have a variable picture that combines some degree of desaturation (although cyanosis is not always visible) and signs of congestive heart failure, often requiring multiple surgical interventions, the first being in the first week of life.

Single Ventricle Anatomy

Many of the mixed defects are cardiac anomalies that have a single functioning ventricle. These defects (e.g., hypoplastic left heart syndrome, unbalanced complete atrioventricular canal, double-inlet left ventricle, tricuspid atresia, pulmonary atresia with intact ventricular septum) require a staged approach to single ventricle palliation, allowing the single functioning ventricle to do the work normally done by two ventricles and separating oxygenated blood from deoxygenated blood.

Stage I or Norwood (first week of life)—(1) Establishes systemic blood flow by connecting the right ventricle to the aorta, (2) rebuilds a small aorta and connects it to the ventricle, and (3) creates pulmonary blood flow either through a modified Blalock-Taussig shunt

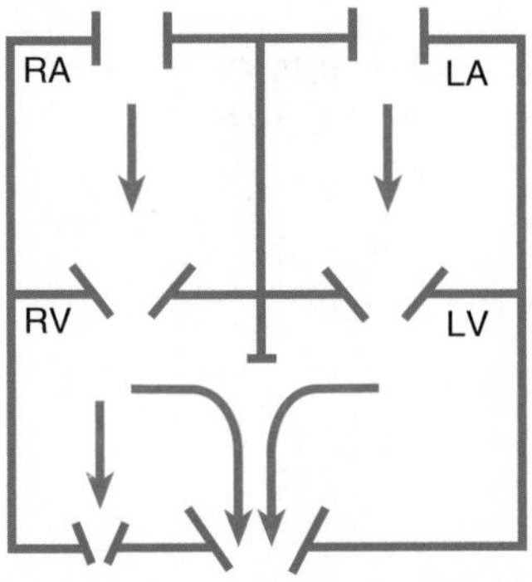

Fig. 23.6 Hemodynamic defects with decreased pulmonary blood flow. *LA,* Left atrium; *LV,* left ventricle; *RA,* right atrium; *RV,* right ventricle.

(3- to 4-mm Gore-Tex tube from the subclavian artery to the pulmonary artery) or a Sano modification (conduit from the right ventricle to the pulmonary artery) (Table 23.3).

Stage II or bidirectional Glenn (3 to 8 months of age)—Creates a direct connection between the superior vena cava and the pulmonary artery, allowing half of the systemic deoxygenated blood to return passively but directly to the lungs (see Table 23.3).

Stage III or Fontan (2 to 4 years of age)—Directs systemic venous return to the lungs without a ventricular pump through surgical connections between the right atrium and the pulmonary artery (Fig. 23.7). A fenestration (opening) is sometimes made in the right atrial baffle to relieve pressure. The patient must have normal ventricular function and a low pulmonary vascular resistance for the procedure to be successful. The modified Fontan procedure separates oxygenated and deoxygenated blood inside the heart and eliminates the excess volume load on the ventricle but does not restore normal anatomy or hemodynamics.

Between the first- and second-stage surgeries, the cardiac circulation is particularly fragile, and the infant requires extra care and careful monitoring at home (Ghanayem, Hoffman, Mussatto, et al., 2003; Petit, Fraser, Mattamal, et al., 2011). Long-term concerns for individuals who have completed single ventricle palliation and are living with Fontan physiology include the development of protein-losing enteropathy, atrial dysrhythmias, late ventricular dysfunction, and developmental delays. They will need lifelong care, including frequent follow-ups, procedures, and medications for most of their life.

CONGESTIVE HEART FAILURE

Congestive heart failure is the inability of the heart to pump an adequate amount of blood to the systemic circulation at normal filling pressures to meet the body's metabolic demands. It can be referred to as either congestive heart failure (CHF) or heart failure (HF). In children, HF occurs secondary to structural abnormalities (e.g., septal defects) that result in increased blood volume and pressure within the heart. It can also result from myocardial failure in which the contractility or relaxation of the ventricle is impaired. This can occur with cardiomyopathy, dysrhythmias, or severe electrolyte disturbances. HF can also occur because of excessive demands on a normal heart muscle, such as sepsis or severe anemia.

Pathophysiology

HF is often separated into two categories, right-sided and left-sided failure. In **right-sided failure**, the right ventricle is unable to pump blood effectively into the pulmonary artery, resulting in increased pressure in the right atrium and systemic venous circulation.

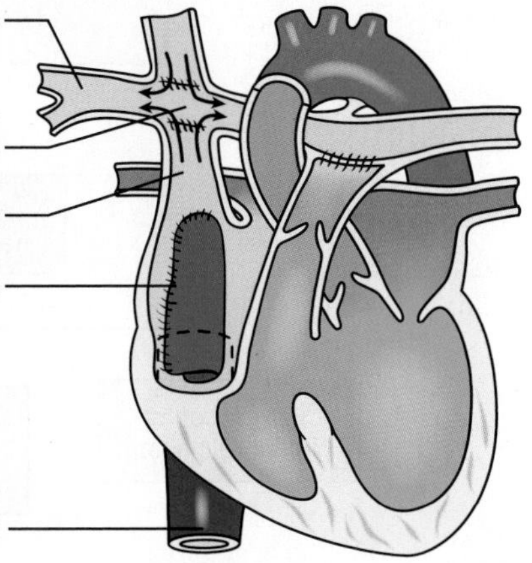

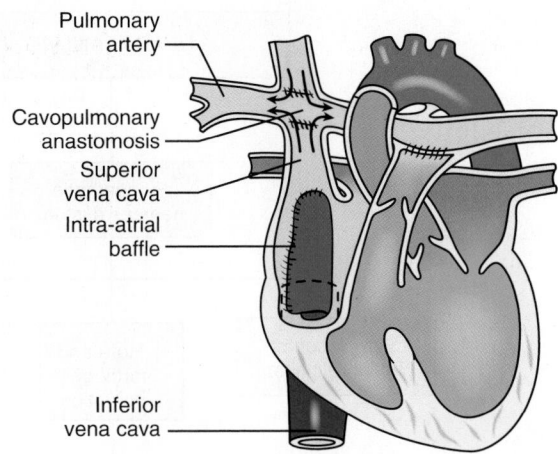

Fig. 23.7 Fontan procedure: third stage of single ventricle palliation.

Systemic venous hypertension causes hepatosplenomegaly and occasionally edema. In **left-sided failure**, the left ventricle is unable to pump blood into the systemic circulation, resulting in increased pressure in the left atrium and pulmonary veins. The lungs become congested with blood, causing elevated pulmonary pressures and pulmonary edema.

Although each type of HF produces different signs and symptoms, clinically it is unusual to observe solely right- or left-sided failure in children. Because each side of the heart depends on adequate function of the other side, failure of one chamber causes a reciprocal change in the opposite chamber.

If the abnormalities precipitating HF are not corrected, the heart muscle becomes damaged. Despite compensatory mechanisms, the heart is unable to maintain an adequate cardiac output. Decreased blood flow to the kidneys continues to stimulate sodium and water reabsorption, leading to fluid overload, increased workload on the heart, and congestion in the pulmonary and systemic circulations (Fig. 23.8).

Clinical Manifestations

The signs and symptoms of HF can be divided into three groups: (1) impaired myocardial function, (2) pulmonary congestion, and (3) systemic venous congestion (Box 23.5). Because these hemodynamic changes occur from different causes and at differing times, the clinical presentation may vary among children.

Diagnostic Evaluation

Diagnosis is made based on clinical symptoms, such as tachypnea and tachycardia at rest, dyspnea, retractions, activity intolerance (especially during feeding in infants), feeding intolerance, weight gain caused by fluid retention, and hepatomegaly. Chest radiography demonstrates cardiomegaly and increased pulmonary blood flow. Ventricular hypertrophy, abnormal rhythm, or decreased voltages appear on the ECG. An echocardiogram is done to determine the cause of HF, such as a congenital heart defect or poor ventricular function.

Therapeutic Management

The goals of treatment are to (1) improve cardiac function (increase contractility and decrease afterload), (2) remove accumulated fluid and sodium (decrease preload and minimize fluid overload), (3) decrease cardiac demands, and (4) improve tissue oxygenation and decrease oxygen consumption. For most infants diagnosed with HF, the cause is CHD. Infants are stabilized on medical therapy and then referred for surgical repair. Today many children are being surgically

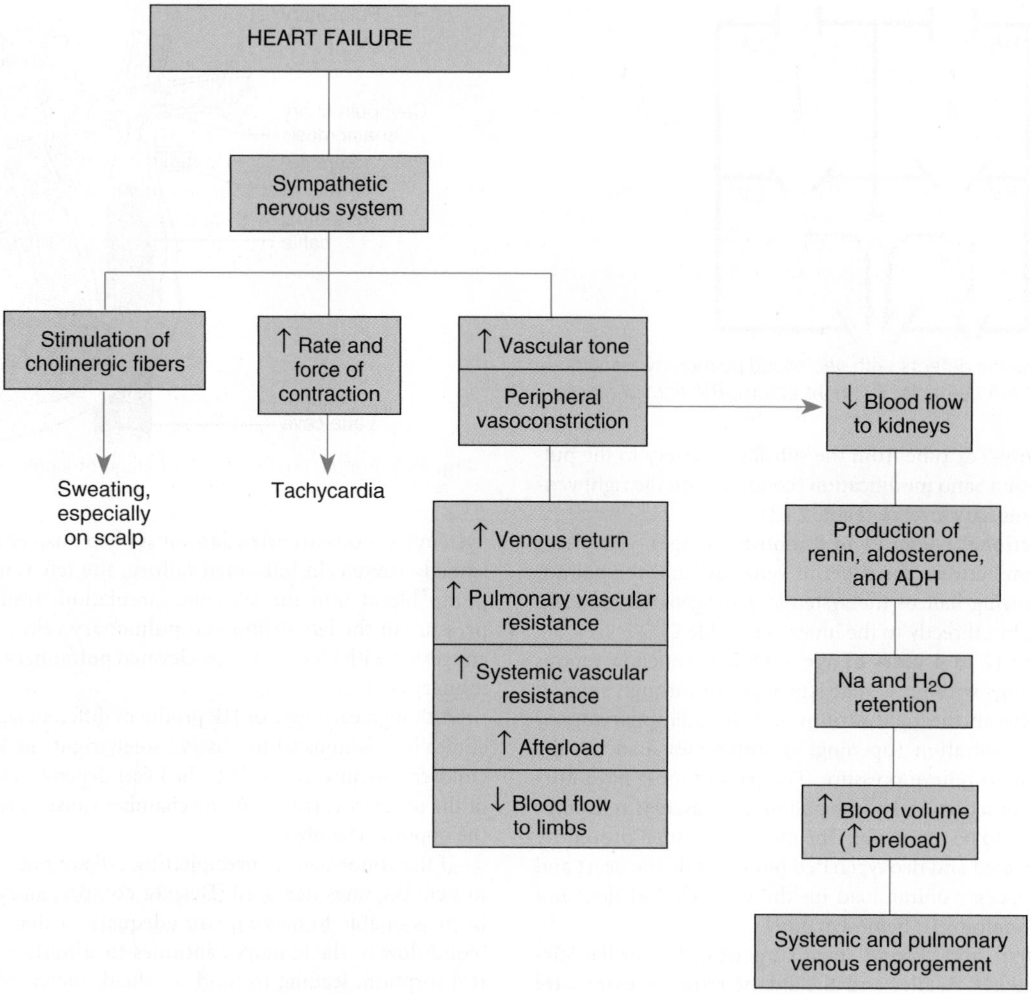

Fig. 23.8 Pathophysiology of heart failure. *ADH,* Antidiuretic hormone.

BOX 23.5 Clinical Manifestations of Heart Failure

Impaired Myocardial Function
- Tachycardia
- Sweating (inappropriate)
- Decreased urinary output
- Fatigue
- Weakness
- Restlessness
- Anorexia
- Pale, cool extremities
- Weak peripheral pulses
- Decreased blood pressure (BP)
- Gallop rhythm
- Cardiomegaly

Pulmonary Congestion
- Tachypnea
- Dyspnea
- Retractions (infants)
- Flaring nares
- Exercise intolerance
- Orthopnea
- Cough, hoarseness
- Cyanosis
- Wheezing
- Grunting

Systemic Venous Congestion
- Weight gain
- Hepatomegaly
- Peripheral edema, especially periorbital
- Ascites
- Neck vein distention (children)

repaired in the neonatal and early infancy stages before the onset of HF symptoms (Margossian, 2008). For children newly diagnosed with HF, the cause may be worsening ventricular function following a previous cardiac repair, cardiomyopathy, arrhythmia, or other conditions. In addition to management of HF, the underlying cause is treated if possible.

Improve Cardiac Function

Three groups of drugs are used to enhance myocardial function in HF: (1) digitalis glycosides (digoxin), which improve contractility, (2) angiotensin-converting enzyme (ACE) inhibitors, which reduce the afterload on the heart and thus make it easier for the heart to pump, and (3) beta-blockers. Myocardial efficiency is improved through administration of digitalis glycosides. The beneficial effects are increased cardiac output, decreased heart size, decreased venous pressure, and relief of edema. In children, digoxin (Lanoxin) is used almost exclusively because of its more rapid onset. Note that the dose is calculated in micrograms (1000 mcg = 1 mg). During initiation, the child is monitored by means of an ECG to observe for the desired effects (prolonged PR interval and reduced ventricular rate) and detect side effects, especially dysrhythmias.

! NURSING ALERT

A fall in the serum potassium level enhances the effects of digitalis, increasing the risk of digoxin toxicity. Increased serum potassium levels diminish digoxin's effect. Therefore serum potassium levels must be monitored carefully.

Digoxin is the only oral inotropic agent generally available for infants and children, although other oral inotropic agents are being used in clinical trials in adults. For patients with severe HF, IV inotropic agents such as dopamine or milrinone are used to improve contractility. They are generally given in the ICU setting.

Another group of drugs used in the treatment of HF, the ACE inhibitors, inhibit the normal function of the renin-angiotensin system in the kidney. The ACE inhibitors block the conversion of angiotensin I to angiotensin II so that, instead of vasoconstriction, vasodilation occurs. Vasodilation results in decreased pulmonary and systemic vascular resistance, decreased BP, and a reduction in afterload. It also reduces the secretion of aldosterone, which reduces preload by preventing volume expansion from fluid retention and decreases the risk of hypokalemia. Common medications used in children are captopril (Capoten), enalapril (Vasotec), and lisinopril. The principal side effects of ACE inhibitors are hypotension, cough, and renal dysfunction.

! NURSING ALERT

Because angiotensin-converting enzyme (ACE) inhibitors also block the action of aldosterone, the addition of potassium supplements or spironolactone (Aldactone) to the drug regimen of patients taking diuretics is usually not needed and may cause hyperkalemia.

Beta-blockers, specifically carvedilol (Coreg), are the newest medications to be added to the treatment of some children with chronic HF. The α- and β-adrenergic receptors are blocked, causing decreased heart rate, decreased BP, and vasodilation. These medications have been shown to decrease morbidity and mortality in some adults with HF and are being used selectively in children. Side effects included dizziness, headache, and hypotension.

Cardiac resynchronization therapy (CRT) using biventricular pacing is an effective treatment in adult patients with HF and is beginning to be applied in the pediatric population. With pharmacologic therapies described earlier, CRT has the potential to improve cardiac function in this group of patients, including those with a single ventricle (Cecchin, Frangini, Brown, et al., 2009; Dubin, Janousek, Rhee, et al., 2005).

Remove Accumulated Fluid and Sodium

Treatment consists of administration of diuretics, possible fluid restriction, and possible sodium restriction. Diuretics are the mainstay of therapy to eliminate excess water and salt to prevent reaccumulation. The most commonly used agents are listed in Table 23.4. Because furosemide (Lasix) and the thiazides cause potassium depletion, oral potassium supplements and rich dietary sources are often necessary.

Fluid restriction may be required in the acute stages of CHF and must be calculated carefully to avoid dehydrating the child, especially if cyanosis and significant polycythemia are present. Infants rarely need fluid restriction, since CHF makes feeding so difficult that they struggle to take maintenance fluids.

Sodium-restricted diets are used less often in children than in adults to control HF because of their potential negative effects on the child's appetite and ultimate growth. If salt intake is restricted, additional table salt and highly salted foods are avoided. Low-salt formulas are available but are used infrequently, since infants need a normal sodium source to offset the sodium depletion of chronic diuretic therapy.

Decrease Cardiac Demands

To lessen the workload on the heart, metabolic needs are minimized by (1) providing a neutral thermal environment to prevent cold stress in infants, (2) treating any existing infections, (3) reducing the effort of breathing (by placement in semi-Fowler position), (4) using medication to sedate an irritable child, and (5) providing for rest and decreasing environmental stimuli.

Improve Tissue Oxygenation

The preceding measures serve to increase tissue oxygenation, either by improving myocardial function or by lessening tissue oxygen demands. In addition, supplemental cool humidified oxygen may be administered to increase the amount of available oxygen during inspiration. Oxygen administration is especially helpful in patients with pulmonary edema, intercurrent respiratory tract infections, and increased pulmonary vascular resistance (oxygen is a vasodilator that decreases pulmonary vascular resistance).

! NURSING ALERT

Oxygen is a drug and is administered only with an appropriate order. There are some uncommon circumstances in patients with complex hemodynamics in which oxygen can be detrimental.

An oxygen hood, nasal cannula, or face tent is used to deliver oxygen. Nasal cannulas are ideal for long-term oxygen administration because the child can be ambulatory and can easily eat and drink. Cool humidification is necessary to counteract the drying effect of oxygen. The amount of cool humidity is carefully regulated to prevent chilling.

QUALITY PATIENT OUTCOMES: Heart Failure

- Adequate cardiac output
- Decreased cardiac demands
- Improved respiratory function
- No evidence of fluid excess
- Adequate support and education

Nursing Care Management

Infants or children with CHF may be acutely ill, and some may require intensive care until their symptoms improve. Expert nursing care is essential to reduce the cardiac demands that strain the failing heart muscle (see Next-Generation NCLEX® Examination-Style Unfolding Case Study box). During this time the child and family require emotional support; for some children, severe HF represents end-stage cardiac disease. Although the objectives of nursing care are the same, interventions for infants often differ from those for older children.

Assist in Measures to Improve Cardiac Function

Digoxin is used to improve cardiac function. Digoxin is a potentially dangerous drug because the margin of safety between therapeutic, toxic, and lethal doses is very narrow. Many toxic responses are extensions of its therapeutic effects. The nurse's responsibility in administering digoxin includes calculating and giving the correct dosage and observing for signs of toxicity. The child's apical pulse is always checked before administering digoxin. As a rule, the drug is not given

TABLE 23.4 Diuretics Used in Heart Failure

Actions	Comments	Nursing Care Management
Furosemide (Lasix)		
Blocks reabsorption of sodium and water in proximal renal tubule and interferes with reabsorption of sodium in the loop of Henle and in the most proximal portion of distal tubule	Drug of choice in severe heart failure Causes excretion of chloride and potassium (hypokalemia may precipitate digitalis toxicity)	Begin to record output as soon as drug is given. Observe for dehydration caused by profound diuresis. Observe for side effects (e.g., nausea and vomiting, diarrhea, ototoxicity, hypokalemia, dermatitis, postural hypotension). Encourage consumption of foods high in potassium and/or give potassium supplements. Monitor chloride and acid-base balance with long-term therapy. Observe for signs of digoxin toxicity.
Chlorothiazide (Diuril)		
Acts directly on distal tubules to decrease sodium, water, potassium, chloride, and bicarbonate absorption	Less frequently used drug Causes hypokalemia, acidosis in large doses	Observe for side effects (e.g., nausea, weakness, dizziness, paresthesia, muscle cramps, skin eruptions, hypokalemia, acidosis). Encourage consumption of foods high in potassium and/or give potassium supplements.
Spironolactone (Aldactone)		
Blocks action of aldosterone, which promotes retention of sodium and excretion of potassium	Weak diuretic Has potassium-sparing effect; frequently used with thiazides, furosemide Poorly absorbed from gastrointestinal tract Takes several days to achieve maximum actions	Observe for side effects (e.g., skin rash, drowsiness, ataxia, hyperkalemia). Do not administer potassium supplements.

NEXT-GENERATION NCLEX® EXAMINATION-STYLE UNFOLDING CASE STUDY

The Child With Coarctation of the Aorta

Day 1, 8:00 am Hospitalization

1. The nurse is caring for a 3-week-old male with congenital heart disease (CHD). At birth he initially showed no signs or symptoms, but within the second week of life he developed symptoms of heart failure (HF). He was found to have coarctation of the aorta and is now under the care of the cardiology team and scheduled for surgery. The infant is experiencing increased signs of HF and was hospitalized early this morning. His care is focused on preventing further symptoms before he goes to surgery. What are the most important signs of HF that the nurse would look for in this infant? **Select all that apply.**
   A. Edema
   B. Tachypnea
   C. Weight loss
   D. Tachycardia
   E. Hypotension
   F. Warm extremities
   G. Feeding difficulty
   H. Slow peripheral pulses
   I. Prolonged capillary refill, longer than 2 or 3 seconds
   J. Ineffective peripheral circulation, cool extremities
2. The nurse reviews the history of this 3-week old infant and reads that he is diagnosed with coarctation of the aorta. The nurse realizes that the symptoms experienced by the infant are caused by this congenital disorder. **Choose the most likely options for the information missing from the statements below by selecting from the lists of options provided.** Coarctation of the aorta is described as the _____1_____ of the aortic arch that results in _____2_____ cardiac output. A classic finding is _____3_____ pulses in the arms and _____4_____ femoral pulses.

Options for 1	Options for 2	Options for 3 and 4
widening	Increased	bounding = 3
absence	Decreased	Widening
narrowing	lack of	weak or absent = 4
crossing	Absent	Narrowing
absence	Complex	Unstable

Day 1, 2:00 pm Hospitalization

3. Surgery is planned for tomorrow. The infant's BP is 120/70mmHg, and the pulses in his arms are 220 beats/min and bounding. You find weak femoral pulses at 40 beats/min and his extremities are cool to touch. His breathing is at 36 breaths/min, and no nasal flaring or intercostal retractions are noted at this time. His color is pale without mottling. The infant is not on mechanical ventilation at this time. What are **priority** nursing actions? **Use an X to indicate which nursing actions listed below are <u>Emergent</u> (appropriate or immediately necessary) or <u>Not Emergent</u> (not appropriate or not immediately necessary) for the patient's care at this time.**

Nursing Action	Emergent	Not Emergent
Frequently assess and record heart rate, respiratory rate, blood pressure (BP), and any signs or symptoms of decreased cardiac output.		
Administer cardiac drugs on schedule. Assess and record any side effects or any signs and symptoms of toxicity. Follow hospital protocol for administration.		
Administer cool humidified oxygen to increase available oxygen during inspiration.		
Change the infant's position every 2 hours to prevent skin breakdown.		
Keep accurate record of intake and output.		
Weigh infant on same scale at same time of day.		
Maintain a 3-hour feeding schedule.		
Restrict fluids if the intake and output is unbalanced.		

NEXT-GENERATION NCLEX® EXAMINATION-STYLE UNFOLDING CASE STUDY—cont'd

The Child With Heart Failure

Day 1, 4:00 pm

4. The nurse continues to closely observe the infant since there are obvious signs of heart failure related to the congenital defect. **Indicate which nursing action listed in the far-left column is appropriate for each potential complication listed in the middle column. Indicate the nursing action number in the far-right column. Note that not all actions will be used.**

Nursing Action	Potential Complication	Nursing Action to Prevent Complication
1. Assess and record heart rate, respiratory rate, blood pressure (BP), and any signs or symptoms of altered cardiac output every 2 to 4 hours.	Decreased urinary output is a symptom of heart failure and could go unnoticed	
2. Administer cardiac drugs on schedule. Assess and record any side effects or any signs and symptoms of toxicity. Follow hospital protocol for administration.	Undetected changes in vital signs and infant's physical status that reflect altered cardiac output and high blood pressure	
3. Keep accurate record of intake and output.	Excess water and salt because fluid retention commonly occurs with heart failure	
4. Weigh infant on same scale at same time of day as previously. Document results and compare to previous weight.	Dangers inherent in failure to administer cardiac drugs as prescribed and to perform careful assessment before administration	
5. Administer diuretics on schedule. Assess and record effectiveness and any side effects noted.		
6. Offer small, frequent feedings to infant's tolerance.		
7. Organize nursing care to allow infant uninterrupted rest.		

Day 5 Hospitalization, 3 days post-surgery

5. The infant underwent surgery 3 days ago. Resection of the coarcted portion of the aorta was performed. Cardiopulmonary bypass was not required due to this defect being outside the heart and pericardium. The infant is in stable condition. The nurse is performing a change of shift assessment of the infant. What assessment findings demonstrate that the infant is stable at this time? **Select all that apply.**

A. Color pink
B. Lack of edema
C. Successful feeding
D. Heart rate 120 beats/min
E. Skin warm to touch
F. Weight gain (0.5kg/day)
G. Respiratory 48 breaths/min
H. Lack of distended neck veins
I. Strong and equal peripheral pulses
J. Brisk capillary refill within 5 seconds
K. Adequate urinary output (1 to 2 ml/kg/h)

Day of Discharge

6. The infant has recovered well from surgery with no complications. The nurse is preparing for discharge and notes that both parents are nervous and afraid of taking their infant home. What education would the nurse provide to the family at this time? **Use an X for the health teaching evaluation below that is Indicated (appropriate or necessary), Contraindicated (could be harmful), or Non-Essential (makes no difference or not necessary).**

Health Teaching	Indicated	Contraindicated	Non-Essential
Discuss the characteristics of COA and the surgery done to repair the obstructive defect.			
Review the infant's daily care including medication administration.			
Review signs and symptoms that could be of concern (fever, blue skin color, poor eating).			
Inform parents to purchase a pulse oximeter before taking the infant home so they can constantly monitor the oxygen level.			
Keep the infant supine at all times to assist with blood flow.			
Parents want to purchase another bed for the infant to keep her close to them at night.			
Give parents the opportunity to express their fears and concerns.			

BOX 23.6 Common Signs of Digoxin Toxicity in Children

Gastrointestinal	Cardiac
Nausea	Bradycardia
Vomiting	Dysrhythmias
Anorexia	

if the pulse is below 90 to 110 beats/min in infants and young children or below 70 beats/min in older children (the cutoff point for adults is 60 beats/min). The nurse should also use judgment in evaluating the pulse rate. If it is significantly lower than the previous recording, the dose should be withheld until the practitioner is notified.

The apical rate is measured because a pulse deficit (radial pulse rate lower than apical) may be present with decreased cardiac output. The pulse is auscultated for 1 full minute to evaluate alterations in rhythm. If the child is monitored by ECG, a rhythm strip is obtained and attached to the chart for rate and rhythm analysis, such as abnormal lengthening of the PR interval (>50% increase over the predigitalization interval) and dysrhythmias.

Digoxin is a potentially dangerous drug because of its narrow margin of safety of therapeutic, toxic, and lethal doses. Many toxic responses are extensions of its therapeutic effects. Therefore the nurse must maintain a high index of suspicion for signs of toxicity when administering digoxin (Box 23.6).

Because digoxin toxicity can occur from accidental overdose, great care must be taken in properly calculating and measuring the dosage. When converting milligrams to micrograms to milliliters, the nurse carefully checks the placement of the decimal point, because an error causes a significant change in dosage. For example, 0.1 mg is 10 times the dosage of 0.01 mg.

These same principles are taught to parents in preparation for the child's discharge, although the correct dose in milliliters is usually specified on the container, which reduces potential errors in calculation. The nurse watches the parent measure the elixir in the dropper and stresses the level mark as the meniscus of the fluid that is observed at eye level. Parents are also taught the signs of toxicity. According to the practitioner's preference, they may be taught to take the pulse before giving the drug, and a return demonstration of the procedure from the parents or another principal caregiver is included as part of the teaching plan.

Minimize Fluid Overload

Diuresis assists in decreasing preload and minimizing volume overload. When diuretics are given, the nurse records fluid intake and output and monitors body weight at the same time each day to evaluate the benefit of the drug. Because profound diuresis may cause dehydration and electrolyte imbalance (e.g., loss of sodium, potassium, chloride, bicarbonate), the nurse observes for signs indicating one of these complications, as well as signs and symptoms suggesting reactions to the drugs. Give diuretics early in the day to children who are toilet trained to avoid the need to urinate at night. If potassium-losing diuretics are given, the nurse encourages consumption of foods high in potassium, such as bananas, oranges, whole grains, legumes, and leafy vegetables, and administers prescribed supplements.

Fluid restriction is rarely necessary in infants because of their difficulty in feeding. With toddlers and preschoolers, it is psychologically advantageous to give small amounts of liquid in small cups so that the containers appear full. Older children's cooperation is gained by placing them in charge of recording their fluid intake.

Reduce Afterload

For patients receiving ACE inhibitors for afterload reduction, the nurse should carefully monitor BP before and after dose administration, observe for symptoms of hypotension, and notify the practitioner if BP is low. Numerous medications affecting the kidney can potentiate renal dysfunction, so children taking multiple diuretics and an ACE inhibitor require careful assessment of serum electrolytes and renal function.

Decrease Cardiac Demands

The infant requires rest and conservation of energy for feeding. Every effort is made to organize nursing activities to allow for uninterrupted periods of sleep. Whenever possible, parents are encouraged to stay with their infant to provide the holding, rocking, and cuddling that help children sleep more soundly. To minimize disturbing the infant, changing bed linens and complete bathing are done only when necessary. Feeding is planned to accommodate the infant's sleep and wake patterns. The child is fed at the first sign of hunger, such as when sucking on fists, rather than waiting until he or she cries for a bottle because the stress of crying exhausts the limited energy supply. Because infants with HF tire easily and may sleep through feedings, smaller feedings every 3 hours may be helpful. Gavage feedings may be instituted to provide adequate nutrition and allow the infant to rest.

Every effort is made to minimize unnecessary stress. Older children need an explanation of what is happening to them to decrease anxiety about their illness and necessary treatments, such as cardiac monitoring, oxygen administration, and medications. Outlining a plan for the day, preparing the child for tests and procedures, providing quiet activities, and providing adequate rest periods are all helpful interventions with older children. Some infants and children require sedation during the acute phase of illness to allow them to rest.

Temperature is carefully monitored because hyperthermia or hypothermia increases the need for oxygen. Febrile states are reported to the physician because infection must be promptly treated. Maintaining body temperature is important for children who are receiving cool, humidified oxygen and for children who tend to be diaphoretic, losing heat via evaporation.

Skin breakdown from edema is prevented with a change of position every 2 hours (from side to side while in semi-Fowler position) and use of a pressure-relieving mattress or bed. The skin, especially over the sacrum, is checked for evidence of redness from pressure.

Reduce Respiratory Distress

Careful assessment, positioning, and oxygen administration can reduce respiratory distress. Respirations are counted for 1 full minute during a resting state. Any evidence of increased respiratory distress is reported, because this may indicate worsening heart failure.

Infants are positioned to encourage maximum chest expansion, with the head of the bed elevated; they should sit up in an infant seat or be held at a 45-degree angle. Children may prefer to sleep on several pillows and remain in a semi-Fowler or high-Fowler position during waking hours.

The infant or child is often given humidified supplemental oxygen via oxygen hood or tent, nasal cannula, or mask. The child's response to oxygen therapy is carefully evaluated by noting respiratory rate, ease of respiration, color, and especially oxygen saturation as measured by oximetry.

Respiratory tract infections can exacerbate CHF and should be treated appropriately and prevented if possible. The child should be protected from persons with respiratory tract infections and have a noninfectious roommate. Good hand washing is practiced before and after caring for any hospitalized child. Antibiotics may be given to combat respiratory tract infection. The nurse ensures that the drug is given at equally divided times over a 24-hour schedule to maintain high blood levels of the antibiotic.

Maintain Nutritional Status

Meeting the nutritional needs of infants with CHF or serious cardiac defects is a nursing challenge. The metabolic rate of these infants is greater because of poor cardiac function and increased heart and respiratory rates. Their caloric needs are greater than those of the average infant because of their increased metabolic rate, yet fatigue limits their ability to take in adequate calories. For a fragile infant with serious CHD, feeding is similar to exercise in an adult, and the infant often does not have the energy or cardiac reserve to do extra work. The nurse seeks measures to enable the infant to feed easily without excess fatigue and to increase the caloric density of the formula.

The infant should be well rested before feeding and fed soon after awakening so as not to expend energy on crying. A 3-hour feeding schedule works well for many infants. (Feeding every 2 hours does not provide enough rest between feedings, and a 4-hour schedule requires an increased volume of feeding, which many infants are unable to take.) The feeding schedule should be individualized to the infant's needs. A feeding goal of 150 ml/kg/day and at least 120 kcal/kg/day is common for newborns with significant heart disease (Steltzer, Rudd, & Pick, 2005). Infants should be well supported and fed in a semi-upright position. The infant may need to rest frequently and may need to have the jaw and cheeks stroked to encourage sucking. Generally, giving an infant about a half-hour to complete a feeding is reasonable. Prolonging the feeding time can exhaust the infant and decrease the rest period between feedings.

Infants with feeding difficulties are often gavage fed using a nasogastric tube to supplement their oral intake and ensure adequate calories. Feeding team colleagues may be able to recommend bottle nipples and techniques to help the infant. If infants are very stressed and fatigued, in respiratory distress, or tachypneic to 80 to 100 breaths/min, oral feedings may be withheld and all nutrition given by gavage feedings. Gavage feedings are usually a temporary measure until the infant's medical status improves and nutritional needs can be met through oral feedings. Some infants with severe HF, neurologic deficits, or significant gastroesophageal reflux may need placement of a gastrostomy tube to allow adequate nutrition.

The caloric density of formulas is frequently increased by concentration and then adding Polycose, medium-chain triglyceride oil, or corn oil. Infant formulas provide 20 kcal/oz, and the use of additives can increase the calories to 30 kcal/oz or more. This allows the infant to obtain more calories despite a smaller volume intake of formula. The caloric density of the formula needs to be increased slowly (by 2 kcal/oz/day) to prevent diarrhea or formula intolerance. Breastfeeding mothers are encouraged to provide the infant with alternating feedings of breast milk and high-calorie formulas. Some lactating mothers prefer to feed the child expressed breast milk that has been fortified with Similac or Enfamil powder, Polycose, or corn oil to increase caloric intake. A diet plan specific to the individual infant's needs is calculated and prescribed by the nutritionist in collaboration with the other health personnel.

Support the Child and Family

Heart failure is a serious complication of heart disease. Parents and older children are usually acutely aware of the critical nature of the condition. Because stress places additional demands on cardiac function, the nurse should focus on reducing anxiety through anticipatory preparation, frequent communication with the parent regarding the child's progress, and constant reassurance that everything possible is being done.

Home care involves many of the same interventions discussed in Plan for Discharge and Home Care later in the chapter. The nurse teaches the family about the medications that need to be administered and alerts them to the signs of worsening HF that require medical attention, such as increased sweating, decreased urinary output (noted in fewer wet diapers or infrequent use of the toilet), or poor feeding. Every effort is made to improve the family's adherence to the medication schedule by adapting the schedule to their usual home routines, avoiding medications during the night, making it as simple as possible, and using charts or visual aids to remember when to give medications (see Chapter 20). If HF is the end stage of a severe heart defect, the nurse cares for this child as for any child who is terminally ill, using the principles discussed in Chapter 17.

HYPOXEMIA

Hypoxemia refers to an arterial oxygen tension (or pressure, PaO_2) that is lower than normal and can be identified by a decreased arterial saturation or a decreased PaO_2. **Hypoxia** is a reduction in tissue oxygenation that results from low oxygen saturations and PaO_2 and results in impaired cellular processes. **Cyanosis** is a blue discoloration in the mucous membranes, skin, and nail beds of the child with reduced oxygen saturation. It results from the presence of deoxygenated hemoglobin (hemoglobin not bound to oxygen) at a concentration of 5 g/dl of blood. Cyanosis is usually apparent when arterial oxygen saturation is 85% or lower. Determination of cyanosis is subjective. It can vary depending on skin pigment, quality of light, color of the room, or clothing worn by the child. The presence of cyanosis may not accurately reflect arterial hypoxemia because both oxygen saturation and the amount of circulating hemoglobin are involved. Children with severe anemia may not be cyanotic despite severe hypoxemia because the hemoglobin level may be too low to produce the characteristic blue color. Conversely, patients with polycythemia may appear cyanotic despite a near-normal PaO_2. Heart defects that cause hypoxemia and cyanosis result from desaturated venous blood (blue blood) entering the systemic circulation without passing through the lungs.

Clinical Manifestations

Over time, two physiologic changes occur in the body in response to chronic hypoxemia: polycythemia and clubbing. **Polycythemia**, an increased number of red blood cells, increases the oxygen-carrying capacity of the blood. However, anemia may result if iron is not readily available for the formation of hemoglobin. Polycythemia increases the viscosity of the blood and crowds out clotting factors. **Clubbing**, a thickening and flattening of the tips of the fingers and toes, is thought to occur because of chronic tissue hypoxemia and polycythemia (Fig. 23.9). Infants with mild hypoxemia may be asymptomatic except for cyanosis and exhibit near-normal growth and development. Those with more severe hypoxemia may exhibit fatigue with feeding, poor weight gain, tachypnea, and dyspnea. Severe hypoxemia resulting in tissue hypoxia is manifested by clinical deterioration and signs of poor perfusion.

Hypercyanotic spells, also referred to as **blue spells** or **tet spells** because they are often seen in infants with tetralogy of Fallot, may occur in any child whose heart defect includes obstruction to pulmonary blood flow and communication between the ventricles. The infant becomes acutely cyanotic and hyperpneic because sudden infundibular spasm decreases pulmonary blood flow and increases

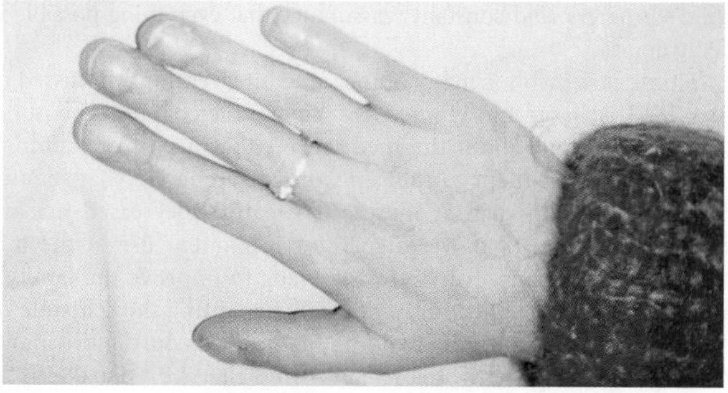

Fig. 23.9 Clubbing of the fingers.

right-to-left shunting (the proposed mechanism in tetralogy of Fallot). Spells, rarely seen before 2 months of age, occur most frequently in the first year of life. They occur more often in the morning and may be preceded by feeding, crying, defecation, or stressful procedures. Because profound hypoxemia causes cerebral hypoxia, hypercyanotic spells require prompt assessment and treatment to prevent brain damage or possibly death.

Persistent cyanosis as a result of cyanotic heart defects places the child at risk for significant neurologic complications. Cerebrovascular accident (CVA; stroke), brain abscess, and developmental delays (especially in motor and cognitive development) may result from chronic hypoxia.

Diagnostic Evaluation

Cyanosis in a newborn can be the result of cardiac, pulmonary, metabolic, or hematologic disease, although cardiac and pulmonary causes occur most often. To distinguish between the two, a hyperoxia test is helpful. The infant is placed in a 100% oxygen environment, and blood parameters are monitored. A PaO_2 of 100 mm Hg or higher suggests lung disease, and a PaO_2 lower than 100 mm Hg suggests cardiac disease (Park, 2014). An accurate history, a chest radiograph, and especially an echocardiogram contribute to the diagnosis of cyanotic heart disease.

Therapeutic Management

Newborns generally exhibit cyanosis within the first few days of life as the ductus arteriosus, which provided pulmonary blood flow, begins to close. Prostaglandin E1, which causes vasodilation and smooth muscle relaxation, thus increasing dilation and patency of the ductus arteriosus, is administered intravenously to reestablish pulmonary blood flow. The use of prostaglandins has been life-saving for infants with ductus-dependent cardiac defects. The increase in oxygenation allows the infant to be stabilized and have a complete diagnostic evaluation performed before further treatment is needed.

In the infant with tetralogy of Fallot, hypercyanotic spells occur suddenly, and prompt recognition and treatment are essential. In the hospital setting, spells are often seen during blood drawing or IV insertion, when the child is highly agitated, or after cardiac catheterization. Treatment of a hypercyanotic spell is outlined in the Nursing Care Guidelines box. Morphine, administered subcutaneously or through an existing IV line, helps reduce infundibular spasm. A spell indicates the need for prompt surgical treatment.

The cyanotic infant and child are well hydrated to keep the hematocrit and blood viscosity within acceptable limits to reduce the risk of CVAs. The infant is monitored closely for anemia because of the risk of CVAs and the reduced arterial oxygen-carrying capacity that

NURSING CARE GUIDELINES

Treating Hypercyanotic Spells

Place infant in knee-chest position (Fig. 23.10).
Use a calm, comforting approach.
Administer 100% "blow-by" oxygen.
Give morphine subcutaneously or through an existing intravenous (IV) line.
Begin IV fluid replacement and volume expansion if needed.
Repeat morphine administration.

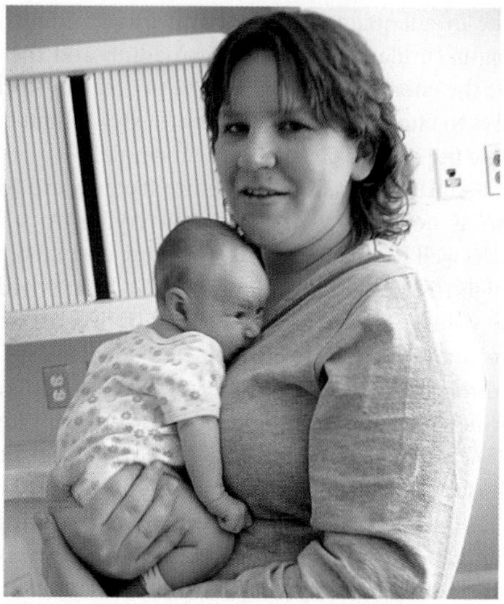

Fig. 23.10 Infant held in a knee-chest position.

occurs. Iron supplementation and possibly blood transfusion are used as needed.

Respiratory tract infections or reduced pulmonary function from any cause can worsen hypoxemia in the cyanotic child. Aggressive pulmonary hygiene, chest physical therapy, administration of antibiotics, and use of oxygen to improve arterial saturations are important interventions.

Surgical Intervention

Many cardiac causes of hypoxemia can be corrected surgically and are described in the discussion of particular cardiac defects (see Boxes 23.1 to 23.4). However, some severely hypoxemic newborns have cardiac defects, in particular those with single ventricle anatomy, which are not amenable to corrective repair and may undergo a three-stage surgical palliation. In the first surgery, the shunt serves the same purpose as the ductus arteriosus: to increase blood flow to the lungs through a systemic artery–to–pulmonary artery connection. The two most common connections are either (1) a modified Blalock-Taussig operation, in which a 3- to 3.5-mm tube graft is placed between the right or left subclavian artery and the pulmonary artery on the same side or (2) a Sano, in which a Gore-Tex tube is placed between the right ventricle and the pulmonary artery. Table 23.3 outlines the most commonly performed shunt procedures today.

Nursing Care Management

The general appearance of infants and children with significant cyanosis poses unique concerns. Blue lips and fingernails are obvious signs of their hidden cardiac defect. Clubbing and small, thin stature in older children further indicate severe heart disease. Adolescents are especially concerned about their body image; children with cyanosis are often teased about their appearance and singled out as different. Many children, when asked what surgery will do, reply, "Make me pink." Parents are often fearful of their child's bluish color because cyanosis is usually associated with lack of oxygen and severe illness. They also must deal with comments from relatives, friends, and strangers about their child's abnormal color. They need a simple explanation of hypoxemia and cyanosis, and reassurance that cyanosis does not imply a lack of oxygen to the brain. Their questions and fears need to be addressed in a calm, supportive manner, and positive aspects of their child's growth and development are emphasized.

Dehydration must be prevented in children with hypoxemia because it potentiates the risk of CVAs. Fluid status is carefully monitored, with accurate intake and output and daily weight measurements. Maintenance fluid therapy is the minimum requirement, supplemental fluids should be readily available, and gavage feeding or IV hydration is given to children unable to take adequate oral fluids. Fever, vomiting, and diarrhea can cause dehydration and require prompt treatment. Parents are instructed in the importance of adequate fluid intake and measures to prevent dehydration. An oral electrolyte solution should be available at home in the event that the infant is unable to tolerate the usual formula. The practitioner should be notified of fever, vomiting, diarrhea, or other problems.

Preventive measures and accurate assessment of respiratory infection are important nursing considerations. Any compromise in pulmonary function will increase the infant's hypoxemia. Good hand washing and protection from individuals with an obvious respiratory tract infection are important. Aggressive pulmonary hygiene, treatment with antibiotics or antiviral agents as indicated, and supplemental oxygen to decrease hypoxemia are necessary measures. Infants may need to be gavage fed or given parenteral hydration if respiratory distress prevents oral feeding.

! NURSING ALERT

Intracardiac shunting of blood from the right side (desaturated) to the left side of the heart allows air in the venous system to go directly to the brain, resulting in an air embolism. Therefore all IV lines should have filters in place to prevent air from entering the system, the entire tubing should be checked for air, all connections should be taped securely, and any air should be removed.

NURSING CARE OF THE FAMILY AND CHILD WITH CONGENITAL HEART DISEASE

When a child is born with a severe cardiac anomaly, parents face the immense psychologic and physical tasks of adjusting to the birth of a child with special needs. Family issues and nursing interventions to support the family are similar to those discussed in Chapters 10 and 19. The following discussion is primarily directed (1) toward the family of an infant who has a serious heart defect requiring home care before definitive repair and (2) toward preparation and care of the child and family when invasive procedures (catheterization and surgery) are performed. For nursing care related to the child with hypoxemia and HF, the reader should refer to earlier discussions of these topics.

Nursing care of the child with a congenital heart defect begins as soon as the diagnosis is suspected. Prenatal diagnosis of congenital heart defects is becoming increasingly frequent. New demands are being placed on nurses to counsel and support families as they prepare for the birth of these infants.

HELP THE FAMILY ADJUST TO THE DISORDER

When parents learn of the heart defect, they are often initially in a period of shock, followed by high anxiety and fear that their child may die. The family needs time to grieve before they can assimilate the meaning of the defect. Unfortunately, the demands for medical treatment may not allow this, instead necessitating that the parents immediately give informed consent for diagnostic-therapeutic procedures. The nurse can be instrumental in supporting parents in their loss, assessing their level of understanding, supplying information as needed, and helping other members of the health care team understand the parents' reactions (see Family-Centered Care box).

FAMILY-CENTERED CARE

Diagnosis of Heart Disease

Remember, we don't have your experience. We don't see children every day who have heart disease. We would have been upset finding out our child had to have his tonsils out. How could we ever be prepared for this? Please remember, we only know people who have trivial heart murmurs. How could we ever expect this to happen? And to us, this is the worst problem we've ever heard of.

We still fear most what we don't know and understand. Be honest with us. If you don't know either, tell us. But at least don't leave us wondering about what you know and we don't. Not knowing anything really can be worse than knowing something bad. Be honest but don't strip us of hope.

Please, remember we are trying to learn complex information in a moment of time. And trying to learn it in a context of great pain and emotional investment. This is our lives you're talking about. Please be thorough but keep it simple. Tell us again, maybe even again and again, when we can hear better.

From Schrey, C., & Schrey, M. A. (1994). Parent's perspective: Our needs and our message. *Critical Care Nursing Clinics of North America, 6*(1), 113–119.

Severely ill newborns usually remain in the hospital. Parent-infant attachment is supported by encouraging parents to hold, touch, and look at their child, and providing time and privacy for the parents to spend with their newborn. (See Chapter 8 for suggestions on promoting attachment between parents and their hospitalized newborn.)

The effect of a child with a serious heart defect on the family is complex. No member, regardless of the degree of positive adjustment, is unaffected. Mothers frequently feel inadequate in their mothering ability because of the complex care infants with congenital heart defects require. They often feel exhausted from the pressures of caring for these children and the other family members. Fathers and siblings may feel neglected and resentful, which is a reaction similar to the feelings toward family members with other chronic conditions (see Chapter 17). Parents may not feel confident leaving the child in another person's care. This often sets up a trap for parents, especially mothers, who become locked into the child's care with no relief. Although the fears are justified, they can be minimized by gradually teaching someone (a reliable relative or neighbor) how to care for the child.

The need to maintain discipline and set consistent limits can be difficult for parents. Using behavior modification techniques, in the form of either concrete awards (e.g., a favorite activity) or social reinforcement (e.g., approval), can be effective. To prevent later problems, it is necessary to begin discussions with parents while the child is in infancy regarding managing discipline as the child gets older.

The child also needs opportunities for normal social interaction with peers. These children do not need to be prevented from playing with other children because of concerns regarding overexertion. Children usually limit their activities if allowed to set their own pace.

A child with CHD may constitute a long-term family crisis. Frequently, the continuing unremitting stresses of care—physical exhaustion, financial costs, emotional upset, fear of death, and concern for the child's future—are not fully appreciated by those caring for the family. Even when the child's condition is stabilized or corrected, the family may need to make adjustments in their lifestyle.

EDUCATE THE FAMILY ABOUT THE DISORDER

When parents are ready to hear about the heart condition, they require a clear explanation based on their level of understanding. A review of the basic structure and function of the heart is helpful before describing the defect. A simple diagram, pictures, or a model of the heart can help parents visualize the heart and the congenital defect. Parents appreciate receiving written information about the specific condition. Health care professionals should take advantage of subsequent encounters to assess parental understanding of the condition and clarify information as needed.

Parents often use the Internet and social media to obtain information about their child's heart defect and support through contacts with other parents and parent groups.[a] Social media plays an important role for many families affected by congenital anomalies and offers a place for them to provide support, seek education, and make friends with other families sharing similar experiences (Jacobs, Boyd, Brennan, et al., 2016). It is important for parents to realize that not all websites offer medically accurate information and that information from other parents might not be applicable to their own situation. Some children with rare, complex heart defects require individualized treatment plans, and general information on the Internet or in books may not apply to these children. Parents should discuss information they have received from other sources with their health care team, in particular the cardiologist.

Information given to the child must be tailored to the child's developmental age. As the child matures, the level of information is revised to meet the child's new cognitive level. Preschoolers need basic information about what they will experience more than about what is occurring physiologically. School-age children benefit from a concrete explanation of the defect. Including the child at this age, early in their own health care and education about their condition, will improve self-care and their own accountability (Mickley, Burkhart, & Sigler, 2013). Preadolescents and adolescents often appreciate a more detailed description of how the defect affects their heart. Children of all ages need to express their feelings about the diagnosis.

HELP THE FAMILY MANAGE THE ILLNESS AT HOME

Parents are the child's principal caregivers and need to develop a positive, supportive working relationship with the health care team. Because most children spend most of their time at home with episodic trips to the hospital, parents manage their child's illness on a daily basis. They monitor for signs of illness, give medications and treatments, bring their child to appointments, work with a variety of caregivers, and alert the team about problems. Successful relationships are partnerships between parents and caregivers that are built on mutual trust and respect. Good communication among the family, the cardiology specialists, and the primary care practitioner is essential. As children reach adolescence, they begin to take a larger role in managing their illness and making decisions about their care.

Parents should be aware of the symptoms of their child's cardiac condition and signs of worsening clinical status. Parents of children who may develop HF should be familiar with the symptoms (see Box 23.5) and know when to contact the practitioner. Parents of children with cyanosis should be informed about fluid management and hypercyanotic spells. Parents should have an information sheet with their child's diagnosis, significant treatments such as surgical procedures, allergies, other health care problems, current medications, and health care providers' contact numbers available in case of emergencies and to share with other caregivers such as teachers, babysitters, and daycare providers.

The family also needs to be knowledgeable about the therapeutic management of the disorder and the role that surgery, other procedures, medications, and a healthy lifestyle play in maintaining good health. Medications play a critical role in managing some cardiac conditions, such as dysrhythmias, severe HF, anticoagulation for artificial valves, and antirejection medications after heart transplantation. Some patients must take multiple medications daily for their lifetime. Many medications can be dangerous if taken incorrectly and require close monitoring. Parents are taught the correct procedure for giving medications and cautioned to keep them in a safe area to prevent accidental ingestion.

Another area of parental concern is the child's level of physical activity. Most children do not need to restrict activity, and the best approach is to treat the child normally and allow self-limited activity. Exceptions to self-determined activity primarily involve strenuous recreational and competitive sports in children with specific cardiac problems. Activities and exercise restrictions should be discussed with the child's cardiologist. In 2013 the American Heart Association published guidelines for promotion of physical activity in children and adults with CHD. Regular exercise can assist the child with CHD in maintaining a healthy weight, foster normal development, help with self-esteem, and help with acceptance into peer groups (Longmuir, Brothers, de Ferranti, et al., 2013).

Infants and children with CHD require good nutrition. Breastfeeding is possible for many infants with CHD. Countering a common misconception that breastfeeding would not be possible for these infants because they would get tired or exhibit poor growth, Barbas and Kelleher (2004) found that breastfeeding could be successful with adequate support and education of the mother. Providing adequate nutrition to infants with HF or complex congenital defects is especially difficult due to their high caloric requirements and inability to suck effectively because of fatigue and tachypnea. Instructing parents in feeding methods that decrease the work of the infant and giving high-calorie formula are important interventions.

Infants with heart disease should be immunized according to the current guidelines. Immunization schedules may need to be modified around times of acute illness or surgical procedures (Smith, 2001). Infants and children younger than 2 years of age with unrepaired heart defects, cyanotic lesions, pulmonary hypertension, or a history of prematurity should receive the vaccine for respiratory syncytial virus (RSV) according to the American Academy of Pediatrics recommendations, which are updated annually. Use of the RSV vaccine palivizumab has been shown to reduce hospitalization due to RSV infection in infants and young children with hemodynamically significant CHD (Feltes, Cabalka, Meissner, et al., 2003) (see Chapter 6).

---

[a]American Heart Association, http://www.heart.org; National Association for Children's Heart Disorders, http://kidswithheart.org; Little Hearts, http://www.littlehearts.org; Congenital Heart Information Network, https://www.facebook.com/TCHIN.org?; Heart Rhythm Society (information on arrhythmias), http://www.hrsonline.org; Adult Congenital Heart Association, http://www.achaheart.org; National Pediatric Cardiology Quality Improvement Collaborative, https://npcqic.org; Children's Heart Foundation, http://www.childrensheartfoundation.org; Sisters by Heart, http://www.sistersbyheart.org.

Infants and children who have serious heart disease are at risk for developmental delays (Majnemer, Limperopoulous, Shevell, et al., 2009). There is growing interest in characterizing and mitigating these outcomes through early identification and initiation of integrated developmental services. Multiple factors can influence neurodevelopmental outcomes, including genetics (e.g., chromosomal abnormalities and microdeletions), family background (e.g., parental intelligence quotient [IQ] and socioeconomic status), preoperative factors (including prematurity, cyanosis, shock), intraoperative factors (e.g., use of cardiopulmonary bypass, deep hypothermic circulatory arrest), and postoperative factors (e.g., hemodynamic instability, hypoxia, acidosis, cardiac arrest, stroke, ischemic events). In 2012 the American Heart Association published guidelines for the evaluation and management of neurodevelopmental outcomes in children with CHD (Marino, Lipkin, Newburger, et al., 2012). The guidelines outline an algorithm for surveillance, screening, evaluation, reevaluation, and management of developmental disorder or disability to supplement the 2006 American Academy of Pediatrics statement on developmental surveillance and screening.

PREPARE THE CHILD AND FAMILY FOR INVASIVE PROCEDURES

Chapter 20 provides an extensive discussion of the principles for preparing children for invasive procedures. In 2003 the American Heart Association published a scientific statement, "Recommendations for Preparing Children and Adolescents for Invasive Cardiac Procedures" (LeRoy, Elixson, O'Brien, et al., 2003), that addresses issues specific to the child with heart disease. The reader is referred to these resources for a complete review of the topic. The following discussion highlights some important aspects of preparation for cardiac catheterization and cardiac surgery.

The expected outcomes for preprocedure preparation include reducing anxiety, improving patient cooperation with procedures, enhancing recovery, developing trust with caregivers, and improving long-term emotional and behavioral adjustments following procedures (LeRoy et al., 2003). Important factors to consider in planning preparation strategies are the child's cognitive development, previous hospital experiences, the child's temperament and coping style, the timing of preparation, and the involvement of parents. The most beneficial preparation strategies usually combine information giving and coping skills training, such as conscious breathing exercises, distraction techniques, guided imagery, and other behavioral interventions.

Outpatient preoperative and precatheterization workups are common for most elective procedures. Children are then admitted on the morning of the procedure. Preprocedure teaching is often done in the clinic setting or at home and may include a tour of the ICU and inpatient facilities. Children of different ages and developmental levels require different amounts of information and different approaches. Whereas young children should be prepared close in time to the event, older children and adolescents may benefit from teaching several weeks in advance. Parents should be included in the preparation session to support their child and learn about upcoming events.

Topics to include in preoperative or precatheterization preparation include information on the environment, equipment, and procedures that the child will encounter during and after the procedure. Many information-giving techniques can be used, such as verbal and written information, hospital tours, preoperative classes, picture books, or videos. Information about what the child will see, hear, and feel should be included, especially for older children and adolescents. Some of the sensory experiences of being in an ICU or catheterization laboratory include sights (monitors, many people, a lot of equipment), sounds (beeping noises, alarms, voices), and sensations (lines and dressings, tape, discomfort, thirst). Familiar aspects of the environment, such as BP cuffs, stethoscopes, or oximeter probes, are reviewed, and new equipment, such as monitors, IV lines, and oxygen masks, are described. Comforting aspects of the environment, such as play areas, chairs for parents, and televisions, are emphasized. Many patients who will be sedated during catheterization or receive narcotic pain relievers after surgery will have minimal recall of that period and will not need detailed information about the equipment or procedures used. Information should be specific to the planned procedure for each patient.

A discussion of ways the child can cope with the experience should be included. For a young child, bringing a familiar stuffed animal or comfort object will help relieve anxiety, and advising an older child to bring headphones and favorite music to the catheterization laboratory will help distract him or her during the procedure. Recovery topics after catheterization include lying still to prevent bleeding at the catheter site, advancing diet, controlling pain, and monitoring. After surgery, the nurse reviews the importance of ambulation, coughing, deep breathing, drinking, and eating, and describes pain management and monitoring routines. Simple coping strategies for use during painful procedures should be reviewed; these include distraction techniques such as counting, blowing, singing, and telling stories.

Children and their families should have a choice about an ICU tour. Exposure to the ICU environment can increase anxiety in some children, particularly young children, those with previous hospital experiences, and those who are highly anxious (LeRoy et al., 2003). Usually the day before the procedure is ample time to allow the child to ask questions and to prevent undue fantasizing about the experience. The child should be protected from the frightening sights in the unit; equipment not in view postoperatively, such as equipment located behind or below the bed, needs less attention. The child and parents are encouraged to ask questions or to explore further any equipment in the room, but they should not be pushed to assimilate more information than they are able.

Preoperative physical care differs little, if any, from that for any other surgery and is discussed in Chapter 20. The child should be assured that the parents will be there when the child wakes up; parents should be allowed to accompany their child as far as possible to the operating suite (see Chapter 20, Surgical Procedures). After all of the equipment and procedures have been explained, it is important to talk about "getting well" and going home.

PROVIDE POSTOPERATIVE CARE

Immediate postoperative care is usually provided by specially trained nurses in ICUs. Many of the procedures, such as arterial pressure and central venous pressure (CVP) monitoring, and the observations related to vital functions require advanced educational training (readers should refer to critical care texts for further information). However, nurses caring for the child before surgery and during the convalescent period need to be familiar with the major principles of care. Selected complications that may occur postoperatively are described in Box 23.7.

Observe Vital Signs

Vital signs and BP are recorded frequently until the child's condition is stable. Heart rate and respirations are counted for 1 full minute, compared with the ECG monitor, and recorded with activity. The heart rate is normally increased after surgery. The nurse observes cardiac rhythm and notifies the practitioner of any changes in regularity. Dysrhythmias may occur postoperatively secondary to anesthetics, acid-base and electrolyte imbalance, hypoxia, surgical intervention,

BOX 23.7 Selected Complications After Cardiac Surgery and Treatment Approaches

Cardiac

Heart failure: Digoxin, diuretics

Low cardiac output: Intravenous (IV) inotropes

Dysrhythmias: Identification, drug treatment, possible pacing, cardioversion

Tamponade (blood or fluid in the pericardial space constricting the heart): Prompt removal of fluid by pericardiocentesis

Respiratory

Atelectasis: Chest physical therapy, coughing, deep breathing, ambulation

Pulmonary edema: Diuretics

Pleural effusions: Diuretics, possible chest tube drainage

Pneumothorax: Possible chest tube drainage

Neurologic

Seizures: Assessment, antiepileptic drugs

Cerebrovascular accident (CVA; stroke), cerebral edema, neurologic deficits: Assessment and treatment

Infectious Disease

Infections (especially wound, pneumonia, otitis media, and sepsis): Antibiotics

Hematologic

Anemia: Iron supplementation, possible transfusion

Postoperative bleeding: Initially, clotting factors, blood products; may need repeat surgery to locate and ligate source of bleeding

Other

Postpericardiotomy syndrome (syndrome of fever, leukocytosis, friction rub, pericardial and pleural effusions, and lethargy seen about 7 to 21 days after cardiac surgery; possible viral or autoimmune etiologies): Antipyretics, diuretics, antiinflammatory medications

or trauma to conduction pathways. Cardiac arrest occurs at a higher rate in children with heart disease than in healthy children (Marino, Tabbutt, MacLaren, et al., 2018). Close monitoring in this postoperative period is essential to promote early recognition and treatment of decompensation to prevent cardiac arrest and support surgical recovery.

At least hourly, the lungs are auscultated for breath sounds. Diminished or absent sounds may indicate an area of atelectasis or a pleural effusion or pneumothorax, which necessitates further medical assessment. Temperature changes are typical during the early postoperative period. Hypothermia is expected immediately after surgery due to hypothermic procedures, effects of anesthesia, and loss of body heat to the cool environment. During this period, the child is kept warm to prevent additional heat loss. Infants may be placed under radiant heat warmers. During the next 24 to 48 hours the body temperature may rise to 37.7°C (100°F) or slightly higher as part of the inflammatory response to tissue trauma. After this period, an elevated temperature is most likely a sign of infection and warrants immediate investigation for probable cause.

Intra-arterial monitoring of BP is commonly done after open-heart surgery. A catheter is passed into the radial artery or other artery, and the other end is attached to an electronic monitoring system, which provides a continuous recording of the BP. The intra-arterial line is maintained with a low-rate, constant infusion of heparinized saline to prevent clotting.

Several IV lines are inserted preoperatively, including a peripheral IV to give fluids and medications and a central venous line, usually in a large vessel in the neck, to measure CVP. Additional, intracardiac monitoring lines are sometimes placed intraoperatively in the right atrium, left atrium, or pulmonary artery. Intracardiac lines allow assessment of pressures inside the cardiac chambers, providing vital information about volume status, cardiac output, and ventricular function. All lines must be cared for using strict aseptic technique, and patients must be carefully assessed for bleeding at the time of line removal.

Maintain Respiratory Status

Infants usually require mechanical ventilation in the immediate postoperative period. Early extubation in the operating room or early postoperative period is becoming more common. Children, especially those not requiring cardiopulmonary bypass, may be extubated in the operating room or in the first few postoperative hours. Suctioning is performed only as needed and performed carefully to avoid vagal stimulation (which can trigger cardiac dysrhythmias) and laryngospasm, especially in infants. Suctioning is intermittent and maintained for no more than 5 seconds at a time to avoid depleting the oxygen supply. Supplemental oxygen is administered with a manual resuscitation bag before and after the procedure to prevent hypoxia. The heart rate is monitored after suctioning to detect changes in rhythm or rate, especially bradycardia.

When ventilator weaning and extubation are completed, humidified oxygen is delivered by mask, hood, or nasal cannula to prevent drying of mucosa. The child is encouraged to turn and deep breathe at least hourly. Incentive spirometer use should be encouraged. Measures are used to enhance ventilation and decrease pain, such as splinting of the operative site and use of analgesics. Chest tubes are inserted into the pleural or mediastinal space during surgery or in the immediate postoperative period to remove drainage. This drainage is checked hourly for color and quantity. Immediately after surgery the drainage may be bright red, but afterwards it should be serous. The largest volume of drainage occurs in the first 12 to 24 hours and is greater in extensive heart surgery.

! NURSING ALERT

Chest tube drainage greater than 3 ml/kg/h for more than 3 consecutive hours or 5 to 10 ml/kg in any 1 hour is excessive and may indicate postoperative hemorrhage. The surgeon should be notified immediately because cardiac tamponade can develop rapidly and is life threatening.

Chest tubes are usually removed on the first to third postoperative day. Removal of chest tubes is an uncomfortable, frightening experience. Analgesics such as morphine sulfate, often combined with midazolam (Versed), should be given before the procedure. Older children are forewarned that they will feel a sharp, momentary pain. After the suture is cut, the tubes are quickly pulled out at the end of full inspiration in the extubated patient to prevent intake of air into the pleural cavity. (In the intubated patient, the tubes are pulled out on inspiration because the lungs are stented open with the positive pressure ventilation.) A purse-string suture (placed when the tubes were inserted) is pulled tight to close the opening. A petrolatum-covered gauze dressing is immediately applied over the wound and securely taped on all four sides to the skin so that an airtight seal is formed. It is left on for 1 or 2 days. Breath sounds are checked to assess for a pneumothorax, a possible complication of chest tube removal. A chest radiograph is usually obtained after removal to evaluate for possible pneumothorax or pleural effusion.

Monitor Fluids

Intake and output of all fluids must be accurately calculated. Intake is primarily IV fluids; however, a record of fluid used to flush the arterial and CVP lines or to dilute medications is also kept. Output includes hourly recordings of urine (usually a Foley catheter is inserted and attached to a closed collecting device), drainage from chest and nasogastric tubes, and blood drawn for analysis. Renal failure is a potential risk from a transient period of low cardiac output.

> **! NURSING ALERT**
>
> The signs of renal failure are decreased urinary output (<1 ml/kg/h) and elevated levels of blood urea nitrogen and serum creatinine.

Fluids are restricted during the immediate postoperative period to prevent hypervolemia, which places additional demands on the myocardium, predisposing the patient to cardiac failure. If the child is to be extubated within the first 24 to 48 hours, fluids are provided primarily intravenously. If the child is to be intubated longer, fluids may be given via a nasogastric or nasojejunal tube to optimize nutrition and gut motility. Approximately 4 hours after extubation, enteral fluids may be reinitiated in the setting of a stable hemodynamic and respiratory status. To monitor fluid retention, the child is weighed daily, and the same scale is used at approximately the same time each day to avoid errors in measurement. Fluid restriction may be imposed even when oral fluids are given. The nurse calculates the distribution over a 24-hour period based on the child's preoperative weight and drinking habits. The distribution should allow for most fluid to be given during the child's most wakeful and active periods.

Provide Rest and Progressive Activity

After heart surgery, rest should be provided to decrease the workload of the heart and promote healing. The simplest way to ensure individualized, efficient, high-quality care is to plan at the beginning of the shift the nursing procedures to be done, with periods of rest identified. The schedule should be shared with parents to allow them to visit at the most advantageous times, such as after a rest period when no special treatments are anticipated.

A progressive schedule of ambulation and activity is planned, based on the child's preoperative activity patterns and postoperative cardiovascular and pulmonary function. Ambulation is initiated early once the child is extubated. Activity progresses from sitting on the edge of the bed and dangling the legs to standing up and sitting in a chair. Heart rate and respirations are carefully monitored to assess the degree of cardiac demand imposed by each activity. Tachycardia, dyspnea, cyanosis, desaturation, progressive fatigue, and dysrhythmias indicate the need to limit further energy expenditure.

Provide Comfort and Emotional Support

Heart surgery is both painful and frightening for children, and comfort is a primary nursing concern. Several types of incisions are used by the cardiac surgeon. A median sternotomy is most common, following the sternum down the center of the chest. A mini-sternotomy opens the lower sternum. A thoracotomy incision is most uncomfortable because it goes through muscle tissue. It allows access to the side of the chest through an incision from under the arm around the back to the scapula.

Most patients need IV analgesics for pain control during the immediate postoperative period. Patient-controlled analgesia may be used with children old enough to understand the concept. Nonsteroidal antiinflammatory drugs (NSAIDs) such as ketorolac (Toradol) may be used intravenously. For patients with a thoracotomy, a nerve block placed at the time of surgery is helpful.

After extubation and removal of lines and tubes, pain can be satisfactorily controlled with oral medications such as ibuprofen, oxycodone, and acetaminophen. Acetaminophen alone provides adequate pain relief for most children at discharge. Sternotomy incisions are usually well tolerated, with some discomfort when walking and coughing. Thoracotomy incisions may require a more aggressive pain management plan with around-the-clock medications for several days to allow for adequate rest, ambulation, and pulmonary hygiene.

In addition to pharmacologic pain control, every effort is made to minimize the discomfort of procedures, such as using a firm pillow or favorite stuffed animal placed against the chest incision during movement and performing treatments after pain medication is given, preferably at a time that coincides with the drug's peak effect. Nonpharmacologic measures are used to lessen the perception of pain, and parents are encouraged to comfort their child as much as possible. (See also Chapter 5, Pain Assessment; Pain Management.)

Children may become depressed after surgery. This is thought to be caused by preoperative anxiety, postoperative psychologic and physiologic stress, and sensory overstimulation. Typically, the child's disposition improves on leaving the ICU.

Children may also be angry and uncooperative after surgery as a response to the physical pain and to the loss of control imposed by the surgery and treatments. They need an opportunity to express feelings, either verbally or through activity. Children often regress in their behavior during the stress of surgery and hospitalization. They also may express feelings of anger or rejection toward their parents. The nurse can support the parents by being available for information and explaining all procedures to them. The first few postoperative days are particularly difficult because parents see their child in pain and realize the potential risks from surgery. They often are overwhelmed by the physical environment of the ICU and feel useless because they can do so little for their child. The nurse can minimize such feelings by including parents in caregiving activities and comfort and play activities, providing information about the child's condition, and being sensitive to their emotional and physical needs. The importance of their presence in making the child feel more secure is stressed even if they do not provide physical care.

> **QUALITY PATIENT OUTCOMES: Congenital Heart Disease**
> - Improved cardiac function
> - Prevention of fluid and sodium overload
> - Decreased cardiac demands
> - Improved oxygenation
> - Reduced respiratory distress

PLAN FOR DISCHARGE AND HOME CARE

Ideally, discharge planning begins on admission for cardiac surgery and includes an assessment of the parents' adjustment to the child's altered state of health. Neonates need additional screening tests (e.g., newborn metabolic screen and hearing) and may need immunizations, as well as a car seat test before discharge. The family will need both verbal and written instructions on medication, nutrition, activity restrictions, return to school, wound care, and signs and symptoms of infection or complications (see Family-Centered Care box). Referrals to community agencies may be necessary to assist parents in the transition from the hospital to home and to reinforce the teaching.

FAMILY-CENTERED CARE

Topics to Include in Discharge Teaching After Cardiac Surgery

- Medication teaching
- Activity restrictions
- Diet and nutrition
- Wound care (including dressings, if any; suture removal; bathing)
- Bacterial (infective) endocarditis prophylaxis (see Box 23.9)
- Follow-up appointments (cardiologist, primary care provider)
- Community agencies as needed (visiting nurse service, early developmental intervention)
- When to call practitioner; signs and symptoms of postoperative problems
- Review of cardiac defect and surgical repair

The parents also need clear instructions on when to seek medical care for complications and how to contact the health care provider. Follow-up with the cardiologist and primary care provider is also arranged before discharge. Parents should have a summary, including their child's medical condition, medications, and health care providers available for emergencies. Appropriate identification, such as a MedicAlert device, is indicated for children with a pacemaker or a heart transplant and for those receiving anticoagulation therapy or antidysrhythmic medication.

Although surgical correction of heart defects has improved dramatically, it is still not possible to completely repair many of the complex anomalies. For many children, repeat procedures are required to replace conduits or grafts or to manage complications, such as re-stenosis. Consequently, the long-term prognosis is uncertain, and full recovery is not always possible. For these families, medical follow-up and continued emotional support are essential. The nurse can often serve as an important primary health professional and as a resource for referrals when needed.

ACQUIRED CARDIOVASCULAR DISORDERS

INFECTIVE ENDOCARDITIS

Infective endocarditis (IE) (also called bacterial endocarditis or subacute bacterial endocarditis [SBE] in the past) is an infection of the inner lining of the heart (endocardium), generally involving the valves. The incidence of IE is much less in children than adults but increasing in both groups (Gupta, Sakhuja, McGrath, et al., 2016). In the past, it was most often a result of bacteremia in children with acquired or congenital anomalies of the heart or great vessels. Now, the increased incidence is likely related to the increased use of indwelling lines in infants and children with many other illnesses.

Pathophysiology

Organisms may enter the bloodstream from any site of localized infection. Endocarditis may occur from routine exposure to bacteremia associated with usual daily activities such as brushing teeth, although it can also occur after procedures such as dental work; invasive procedures involving the gastrointestinal and genitourinary tracts; cardiac surgery, especially if synthetic material is used (valves, patches, conduits); or from long-term indwelling catheters. The most common causative agents are Staphylococcus aureus and viridans streptococci; other causative agents include gram-negative bacteria and fungi such as Candida albicans. The microorganisms grow on the endocardium, forming vegetations (verrucae), deposits of fibrin, and platelet thrombi. The lesion may invade adjacent tissues, such as the aortic and mitral valves, and may break off and embolize elsewhere, especially in the spleen, kidney, and CNS.

BOX 23.8 Clinical Manifestations of Infective Endocarditis

Onset usually insidious
Unexplained fever (low grade and intermittent)
Anorexia
Malaise
Weight loss
Characteristic findings caused by extracardiac emboli formation:
- Splinter hemorrhages (thin black lines) under the nails
- Osler nodes (red, painful intradermal nodes found on pads of phalanges)
- Janeway lesions (painless hemorrhagic areas on palms and soles)
- Petechiae on oral mucous membranes

May be present:
- Heart failure
- Cardiac dysrhythmias
- New murmur or change in previously existing one

Diagnostic Evaluation

The diagnosis of IE is suspected based on clinical manifestations (Box 23.8). The most commonly used diagnostic guidelines are the revised Duke criteria, which outline major and minor criteria consistent with IE (Li, Sexton, Mick, et al., 2000). Definitive diagnosis rests on growth and identification of the causative agent in the blood. At least three blood cultures are drawn at different times to aid in diagnosis. Vegetations on the valve and abnormal valve function can often be visualized by echocardiography. A diagnosis of culture-negative IE is made when the patient has echocardiographic or clinical evidence of IE but no organism can be cultured. Several laboratory findings, including anemia, elevated erythrocyte sedimentation rate [ESR], leukocytosis, and microscopic hematuria, may suggest IE.

Therapeutic Management

Treatment should be instituted immediately and consists of administration of high doses of appropriate antibiotics intravenously for 2 to 8 weeks. Blood cultures are taken periodically to evaluate the response to antibiotic therapy. Frequent echocardiograms are done to monitor for vegetations, valve function, and ventricular function. Heart surgery to repair or replace the affected valve may be necessary.

Prevention involves administration of prophylactic antibiotic therapy to high-risk patients prior to dental procedures that are associated with the risk of entry of organisms (Box 23.9). Drugs of choice for prophylaxis, given 1 hour prior to the procedure, include amoxicillin, ampicillin, and clindamycin in penicillin-allergic patients (Wilson, Taubert, Gewitz, et al., 2007).

QUALITY PATIENT OUTCOMES: Infective Endocarditis
- Prevention in high-risk patients with antibiotic prophylaxis
- Early recognition and treatment

Nursing Care Management

Nurses counsel parents of high-risk children concerning the signs and symptoms of endocarditis and the need for prophylactic antibiotic therapy before dental work. The family's dentist should be advised of the child's cardiac diagnosis as an added precaution to ensure preventive treatment. It is important that all children with congenital or acquired heart disease maintain the highest level of oral health to reduce the chance of bacteremia from oral infections.

BOX 23.9 Cardiac Conditions Associated With the Highest Risk of Adverse Outcome From Endocarditis

Prophylaxis with dental procedures recommended for[a]:

- Previous episode of infective endocarditis (IE)
- Prosthetic cardiac valve

Congenital heart disease (CHD), including only:

- Unrepaired cyanotic CHD, including palliative shunts and conduits
- Completely repaired congenital heart defect with prosthetic material or device, whether placed by surgery or by catheter intervention, during the first 6 months after the procedure

Repaired CHD with residual defects at the site or adjacent to the site of a prosthetic patch or prosthetic device (which inhibits endothelialization)

Cardiac transplantation recipients who develop cardiac valvulopathy

[a]Except for the conditions listed, antibiotic prophylaxis is no longer recommended for any other form of CHD.

Adapted from Wilson, W., Taubert, K. A., Gewitz, M., et al. (2007). Prevention of infective endocarditis: Guidelines from the American Heart Association. *Circulation, 116*(15), 1736–1754.

Parents should also have a high index of suspicion regarding potential infections. Without unduly alarming them, the nurse stresses that any unexplained fever, weight loss, or change in behavior (lethargy, malaise, anorexia) must be brought to the practitioner's attention. Children at risk (e.g., those with CHD) should have blood drawn for culture if they have a fever without an obvious source. Early diagnosis and treatment are important in preventing further cardiac damage, embolic complications, and growth of resistant organisms.

Treatment of endocarditis requires long-term parenteral drug therapy. In many cases, IV antibiotics may be administered at home with nursing supervision. Nursing goals during this period are (1) preparation of the child for IV infusion, usually with an intermittent infusion device and several venipunctures for blood cultures; (2) observation for side effects of antibiotics, especially inflammation along venipuncture sites; (3) observation for complications, including embolism and HF; and (4) education on the importance of follow-up visits for cardiac evaluation, echocardiographic monitoring, and blood cultures. Some children may need preparation for surgery and, later, postoperative care.

ACUTE RHEUMATIC FEVER AND RHEUMATIC HEART DISEASE

Acute rheumatic fever (ARF) is a result of an abnormal immune response to a group A strep (GAS) infection, usually pharyngitis, in a genetically susceptible host (Marijon, Mirabel, Celermajer, et al., 2012). It occurs most often in late school-age children and adolescents and is rare in adults. ARF is a self-limited illness that involves the joints, skin, brain, and heart, but cardiac valve damage, which is referred to as **rheumatic heart disease (RHD)**, the most significant complication of ARF, occurs in more than half of the cases. The mitral valve is most often affected. In developed countries, ARF and RHD have become uncommon. However, in developing countries, because of overcrowded living conditions and poor access to medical care, ARF and resulting RHD is the leading cause of HF in young people (Remenyi, Carapetis, Wyber, et al., 2013).

Etiology

Strong evidence supports a relationship between upper respiratory tract infection with GAS and subsequent development of ARF (usually within 2 to 6 weeks). Prevention or treatment of GAS infection prevents ARF. If the GAS infection is untreated, antibodies are produced to fight the infection, which can also act against the heart valves causing damage. If children have one strep infection, they are at greater risk for repeated infections, and recurrent infections cause the cumulative valve damage of RHD.

BOX 23.10 Clinical Manifestations of Acute Rheumatic Fever (Jones Criteria, 2015 Revision)

Major Manifestations

Carditis (seen in 50% to 70% of cases)
- New murmur of valve regurgitation (mitral valve most common)
- Echo Doppler evidence of cardiac involvement
- Tachycardia out of proportion to fever
- Pericardial friction rub
- Chest pain
- Muffled heart sounds
- Cardiomegaly on chest x-ray
- Prolonged PR interval on ECG

Polyarthritis (seen in 35% to 66%)
- Swollen, hot, red, very painful joint pain
- Migratory: affects one joint for 1 to 2 days, then another is affected
- Large joints: knees, elbows, hips, shoulders, wrists, chorea (seen in 10% to 30%) (also called Sydenham chorea or St. Vitus' dance)
- Sudden aimless, irregular movements of extremities, exacerbated by stress
- Profound muscle weakness
- Emotional lability
- Facial grimaces and speech disturbances
- More common in females

Subcutaneous nodules (0% to 10%)
- Nontender swelling over bony prominences
- May persist for many weeks and then resolve

Erythema marginatum (less than 6%)
- Pink rash with pale center and wavy, well-demarcated borders
- Seen on trunk and extremities
- More prominent with heat, blanches with pressure
- Nonpruritic

Minor Manifestations

Arthralgias

Fever (greater than 38.5°C)

ESR above 60 mm and/or CRP greater than 3 mg/dL

Prolonged PR interval

CRP, C-reactive protein; *ECG*, electrocardiogram; *ESR*, erythrocyte sedimentation rate.

Adapted from Gewitz, M. H., Baltimore, R. S., Tani, L. Y., et al. (2015). Revision of the Jones criteria for the diagnosis of acute rheumatic fever in the era of Doppler echocardiography: A scientific statement from the American Heart Association. *Circulation, 131*, 1806–1818.

Diagnostic Evaluation

The diagnosis is based on a set of diagnostic criteria first described by Dr. T. Duckett Jones in 1944 and known as the Jones criteria. Endorsed by the American Heart Association and the World Heart Federation, the most recent revision was completed in 2015 and added evidence supporting the use of Doppler echocardiogram in the diagnosis of carditis (Gewitz, Baltimore, Tani, et al., 2015). The revised Jones criteria are outlined in Box 23.10. The updated Jones criteria suggest that the presence of two major manifestations or one major and two minor manifestations, with supportive evidence of recent GAS infection, indicates a high probability of ARF (see Nursing Care Guidelines box). The most significant manifestation of ARF is carditis. Carditis is the only manifestation of ARF that leads to permanent damage.

Children suspected of having ARF are tested for streptococcal antibodies. The most reliable and best standardized test is an elevated or rising

NURSING CARE GUIDELINES

Diagnosis of Initial Attack of Rheumatic Fever (Jones Criteria, 1992 Update)[a]

Major Manifestations

Carditis

Tachycardia out of proportion to degree of fever
Cardiomegaly
New murmurs or change in preexisting murmurs
Muffled heart sounds
Pericardial friction rub
Chest pain
Changes in ECG (especially prolonged PR interval)

Polyarthritis

Swollen, hot, red, painful joint(s)
After 1 to 2 days, different joint(s) affected
Favors large joints: Knees, elbows, hips, shoulders, wrists

Erythema Marginatum

Erythematous macules with clear center and wavy, well-demarcated border
Transitory
Nonpruritic
Primarily affects trunk and extremities (inner surfaces)

Chorea (St. Vitus' Dance, Sydenham Chorea)

Sudden aimless, irregular movements of extremities
Involuntary facial grimaces
Speech disturbances
Emotional lability
Muscle weakness (can be profound)
Muscle movements exaggerated by anxiety and attempts at fine motor activity; relieved by rest

Subcutaneous Nodes

Nontender swelling
Located over bony prominences
May persist for some time and then gradually resolve

Minor Manifestations

Clinical Findings

Arthralgia
Fever

Laboratory Findings

Elevated acute-phase reactants

- ESR
- CRP
- Prolonged PR interval

Supporting Evidence of Antecedent Group A Streptococcal Infection

Positive throat culture or rapid streptococcal antigen test result
Elevated or rising streptococcal antibody titer

[a] If supported by evidence of preceding group A streptococcal infection, the presence of two major manifestations or of one major and two minor manifestations indicates a high probability of acute rheumatic fever.
CRP, C-reactive protein; *ECG,* electrocardiogram; *ESR,* erythrocyte sedimentation rate.
From Guidelines for the diagnosis of rheumatic fever, Jones criteria, 1992 update, Special Writing Group of the Committee on Rheumatic Fever, Endocarditis, and Kawasaki Disease of the Council on Cardiovascular Disease in the Young of the American Heart Association. (1992). *JAMA, 268*(15), 2069–2073.

antistreptolysin O (ASO or ASLO) titer, which occurs in 80% of children with ARF. Additional antistreptococcal antibody titers may be sent if ASO titers are negative. Acute-phase reactants, ESR, and C-reactive protein (CRP) are usually elevated as well. Echocardiograms play an important role in diagnosing RHD and monitoring deteriorating valve function.

Therapeutic Management

Primary prevention involves prompt diagnosis and treatment of strep throat infections so that ARF does not occur. Penicillin is the drug of choice or an alternative in penicillin-sensitive children (Gerber, Baltimore, Eaton, et al., 2009).

For children with ARF, treatment includes antibiotics, antiinflammatory therapy, and supportive care and management of HF in some. Antibiotics are given to treat the GAS infection and begin long-term prophylactic treatment to prevent future infections. Penicillin is the drug of choice. Salicylates are used to control the inflammatory process, especially in the joints, and reduce the fever and discomfort. The diagnosis must be confirmed before aspirin therapy is started so that clinical signs are not masked by the therapy. Aspirin up to 80-100 mg/kg/day has traditionally been given in four or five divided doses as initial therapy (Steer & Gibofsky, 2019). Newer nonsteroidal antiinflammatory agents such as Naproxen are now being used. Treatment continues until symptoms resolve which is usually within 2 weeks. Naproxen is dosed at 10 to 20 mg/kg/day in divided doses every 12 hours to a maximum of 1000 mg per day in children aged over two years (Steer & Gibofsky, 2019). Administration of prednisone may be indicated in patients with pericarditis or heart failure and in patients who do not respond to aspirin therapy. Neither salicylates nor prednisone has been shown to affect cardiac sequelae.

Supportive care involves initial bed rest during the acute illness and then quiet activities as symptoms subside. Good nutrition is important. Care for children with significant carditis includes HF therapies such as supplemental oxygen, diuretics, fluid and salt restriction, digoxin, or ACE inhibitors. Children with chorea with motor impairment must be protected from injury and eliminate physical and emotional stress, which can exacerbate their symptoms.

Children who have had ARF are susceptible to recurrent infections that are likely to result in RHD and further damage to the heart valves. Prophylactic treatment against recurrence of ARF (secondary prevention) is started after the acute therapy. The treatment of choice is intramuscular injections of benzathine penicillin G every 28 days because it is most effective. The duration of secondary prophylaxis is based on the presence of residual heart disease. If ARF occurs without carditis, prophylaxis is recommended for 5 years or until age 21 years, whichever is longer. In patients with carditis, 10 years is recommended or until 21 years old. Patients with RHD may need longer therapy (Steer & Gibofsky, 2019; Gerber et al., 2009).

Management of RHD may require surgical valve repair or replacement. Valve replacement with a mechanical valve requires lifelong anticoagulation with warfarin.

QUALITY PATIENT OUTCOMES: Acute Rheumatic Fever

- Group A strep (GAS) tonsillopharyngitis identified and treated
- Early recognition and treatment to prevent cardiac valve damage
- Recurrence prevented with prophylaxis compliance

Nursing Care Management

The objective of nursing care is, first, prevention. For the child with ARF, nursing care (1) encourages compliance with drug regimens, (2) facilitates recovery from the illness, and (3) provides emotional support. Nurses play an important role in prevention by educating parents about the complications of strep infections and working with patients and families to ensure follow-up with antibiotic prophylaxis. Because compliance is a major concern in long-term drug therapy, every effort is made to encourage adherence to the therapeutic plan (see Chapter 20, Compliance). When compliance is poor, monthly injections may be substituted for daily oral administration of antibiotics, and children need preparation for this often-dreaded procedure.

Interventions for ARF are primarily concerned with providing rest, adequate nutrition, and management of cardiac symptoms or chorea. One of the most disturbing manifestations of ARF is chorea. The onset is gradual and may occur weeks to months after the illness. Sometimes mistaken for nervousness, clumsiness, or inattentiveness, it is usually a source of great frustration to the child because the movements, incoordination, and weakness severely limit physical ability. It is important that parents and teachers are aware of the involuntary, sudden nature of the movements and that the movements are transitory and will eventually disappear.

Children with RHD will need lifelong follow-up, education, and management of HF, and monitoring for progressive valve disease. If surgery is required, preparation for the procedure is provided. An important aspect of postoperative care is education about anticoagulation medications and follow-up.

HYPERLIPIDEMIA (HYPERCHOLESTEROLEMIA)

Hyperlipidemia is a general term for excessive lipids (fat and fatlike substances); hypercholesterolemia refers to excessive cholesterol in the blood. Dyslipidemia is a term used to describe all abnormalities in lipid metabolism, including low levels of high-density lipoprotein (HDL) or "healthy" cholesterol, high low-density lipoprotein (LDL) or "lousy" cholesterol, or high triglycerides. Abnormal lipid or cholesterol levels play an important role in producing atherosclerosis (fatty plaque on the arteries), which eventually can lead to coronary artery disease, which is a primary cause of morbidity and mortality in the adult population. A presymptomatic phase of atherosclerosis begins in childhood or adolescence, providing the template for later clinical disease. Preventive cardiology focuses on the identification of high-risk patients and management of lipid levels in childhood or adolescence.

Cholesterol is part of the lipoprotein complex in plasma that is essential for cellular metabolism. Triglycerides, natural fats synthesized from carbohydrates, are used for energy. Both are major lipids transported on lipoproteins, a combination of lipids and proteins, which include:

Low-density lipoproteins (LDLs): LDL is the major carrier of cholesterol to the cells. Cells use cholesterol for synthesis of membranes and steroid production. Elevated circulating LDL is a strong risk factor in cardiovascular disease. In addition, particle size and density of LDL may affect overall risk, with small, dense particles associated with increased atherosclerosis.

High-density lipoproteins (HDLs): HDL cholesterol contains very low concentrations of triglycerides, relatively little cholesterol, and high levels of protein. They transport free cholesterol to the liver for excretion in the bile. High levels of HDL are thought to be protective against cardiovascular disease.

Very-low-density lipoproteins (VLDLs): VLDLs contain high concentration of triglycerides, some cholesterol, and a little protein. Triglycerides are the main storage form of fuel or energy for the body.

TABLE 23.5 Classification of Cholesterol Levels in Children

Category	Normal (mg/dl)	Borderline High (mg/dl)	Elevated (g/dl)
Total cholesterol	<170	170-199	≥200
Low-density lipoprotein (LDL)	<110	110-129	≥130
Non–high-density lipoprotein (HDL)	<120	120-144	≥145
High-density lipoprotein (HDL)[a]	>45	N/A	N/A

[a]Borderline low HDL, 40–45; low HDL, <40.

N/A, Not applicable.

Adapted from Expert Panel on Integrated Guidelines for Cardiovascular Health and Risk Reduction in Children and Adolescents & National Heart, Lung, and Blood Institute. (2011). Expert panel on integrated guidelines for cardiovascular health and risk reduction in children and adolescents: Summary report. *Pediatrics, 128*(Suppl 5), S213–S256.

Diagnostic Evaluation

Hyperlipidemia can have a genetic basis (familial homozygous or heterozygous hypercholesterolemia causing significantly elevated LDL and total cholesterol) and/or a lifestyle component or can be caused by secondary problems, such as hypothyroidism. Hyperlipidemia is diagnosed based on analysis of blood. A complete lipid profile should be drawn, ideally after a 12-hour fast. In children with elevated cholesterol levels, a screening thyroid-stimulating hormone is measured at diagnosis in order to rule out hypothyroidism as a cause of secondary hypercholesterolemia. Additional blood work is individualized based on other risk factors. Lipid values may be affected by recent high fevers, and therefore cholesterol values should not be drawn if a child has had a fever within the past 3 weeks. Diagnostic values for acceptable, borderline, and high total cholesterol and LDL cholesterol levels are listed in Table 23.5.

The National Heart, Lung, and Blood Institute published comprehensive guidelines for cardiovascular health and risk reduction in children and adolescents in 2011, recommending universal screening for all children between the ages of 9 and 11 years, and again between the ages of 17 and 21 years. In addition, earlier lipid screening continues to be recommended for children older than 2 years of age who have a family history of dyslipidemia or early heart disease in a first- or second-degree relative, as well as for those children who have individual coronary risk factors (Expert Panel on Integrated Guidelines for Cardiovascular Health and Risk Reduction in Children and Adolescents & National Heart, Lung, and Blood Institute, 2011) (see Translating Evidence Into Practice box). The goal of this approach is to identify children at risk, with the goal of decreasing coronary risk factors (Daniels, 2012; de Ferranti, Daniels, Gillman, et al., 2012; McCrindle, Kwiterovich, McBride, et al., 2012). In addition to abnormal cholesterol levels, known risk factors that correlate with the development of cardiovascular disease include:

- Positive family history of elevated cholesterol and/or early heart disease
- Cigarette smoking
- Obesity
- Sedentary lifestyle
- Nutritional factors
- Older age
- Male gender
- Hypertension
- Type 1 or type 2 diabetes

TRANSLATING EVIDENCE INTO PRACTICE

Rationale for Universal Cholesterol Screening for Children

Ask the Question

PICOT Question

Should cholesterol screening be performed in children?

Search for the Evidence

Search Strategies

The literature was searched to locate clinical research studies related to this issue. Selection criteria included English-language publications within the past 10 years, research-based articles (level 3 or lower), and infant and child populations.

Databases Used

PubMed, Cochrane Collaboration, MD Consult, Joanna Briggs Institute, National Guidelines Clearinghouse (Agency for Healthcare Research and Quality), TRIP Database Plus, PedsCCM, BestBETs.

Critically Analyze the Evidence

- In late 2011, an expert panel of the National Heart, Lung, and Blood Institute made a recommendation that lipid screening be performed on all children 9 to 11 years old; this recommendation was based on evidence that as many as 30% to 60% of children with dyslipidemia might be missed when screening is performed by family history alone (Expert Panel on Integrated Guidelines for Cardiovascular Health and Risk Reduction in Children and Adolescents & National Heart, Lung, and Blood Institute, 2011). The expert panel's guidelines also include comprehensive screening and treatment guidelines for children with cardiovascular disease risk factors.
- Diagnosis of obesity is paramount in enhancing care of pediatric patients who are obese. Current laboratory (cholesterol or glucose) screening rates (10%) are inadequate in the outpatient setting (Patel, Madsen, Maselli, et al., 2010).
- Testing for cardiovascular risk factors: HDL cholesterol, LDL cholesterol, fasting glucose, HgbA1c, BP, thyroid-stimulating hormone, and ALT should be considered in pediatric patients with increased waist circumference and even normal BMI (l'Allemand-Jander, 2010).
- In children who are obese, LDL cholesterol, HDL cholesterol, total cholesterol, and triglycerides are significantly different from those in subjects who are not obese (Simsek, Balta, Balta, et al., 2010).
- Serum triglyceride levels are a predictive risk factor of carotid intima-media thickness (Simsek et al., 2010).
- In children and adolescents (12 to 19 years old), fasting non-HDL cholesterol levels were strongly associated with metabolic syndrome. A non-HDL cholesterol threshold of 120 mg/dl indicated borderline risk for metabolic syndrome, and a threshold of 145 mg/dl indicated high metabolic syndrome risk (Li, Ford, McBride, et al., 2011).
- Cholesterol levels in childhood are a major population predictor for adult cholesterol levels (Daniels, Greer, & Committee on Nutrition, 2008).
- Precursors of atherosclerosis are present in young people. The atherosclerotic process begins early in life with early phases characterized by the development of fatty streaks in the vessels (PDAY study) (Enos, Holmes, & Beyer, 1953; Strong, Malcom, McMahan, et al., 1999).
- Atherosclerosis is related to the presence and degree of cardiovascular risk factors in adults (Berenson, Srinivasan, Bao, et al., 1998).
- Most severely affected children come from families with a high incidence of early heart disease. Children whose genetic family history is unknown should also be screened (Expert Panel on Integrated Guidelines for Cardiovascular Health and Risk Reduction in Children and Adolescents & National Heart, Lung, and Blood Institute, 2011).
- Universal cholesterol screening in children would identify all individuals with dyslipidemia. Using solely the family history to identify subjects for cholesterol screening missed individuals with moderate dyslipidemia and those with potentially genetic dyslipidemia (Ritchie, Murphy, Ice, et al., 2010).

Apply the Evidence: Nursing Implications

There are strong recommendations (Guyatt, Oxman, Vist, et al., 2008) that lipid screening should be performed on all children 9 to 11 years old and again between 17 and 21 years old. Selective screening is still recommended over the age of 2 years in children with affected first- or second-degree relatives or those with individual cardiac risk factors. The National Heart, Lung, and Blood Institute guidelines have been endorsed by the American Academy of Pediatrics (Expert Panel on Integrated Guidelines for Cardiovascular Health and Risk Reduction in Children and Adolescents & National Heart, Lung, and Blood Institute, 2011).

Quality and Safety Competencies: Evidence-Based Practice[a]

Knowledge

Differentiate clinical opinion from research and evidence-based summaries.

Describe use of cholesterol screening in children.

Skills

Base individualized care plan on patient values, clinical expertise, and evidence.

Integrate evidence into practice by using cholesterol screening in children.

Attitudes

Value the concept of evidence-based practice as integral to determining best clinical practice.

Appreciate strengths and weakness of evidence for using cholesterol screening in children.

Updated by Olga A. Taylor

References

Berenson, G. S., Srinivasan, S. R., Bao, W., et al. (1998). Association between multiple cardiovascular risk factors and atherosclerosis in children and young adults: The Bogalusa heart study. *New England Journal of Medicine, 338*(23), 1650–1656.

Daniels, S. R., Greer, F. R., & Committee on Nutrition. (2008). Lipid screening and cardiovascular health in childhood. *Pediatrics, 122*(1), 198–208.

Enos, W. F., Holmes, R. H., & Beyer, J. (1953). Coronary disease among United States soldiers killed in action in Korea: Preliminary report. *Journal of the American Medical Association, 152*(12), 1090–1093.

Expert Panel on Integrated Guidelines for Cardiovascular Health and Risk Reduction in Children and Adolescents & National Heart, Lung, and Blood Institute. (2011). Expert panel on integrated guidelines for cardiovascular health and risk reduction in children and adolescents: Summary report. *Pediatrics, 128*(Suppl. 5), S213–S256.

Guyatt, G. H., Oxman, A. D., Vist, G. E., et al. (2008). GRADE: An emerging consensus on rating quality of evidence and strength of recommendations. *British Medical Journal, 336*(7650), 924–926.

l'Allemand-Jander, D. (2010). Clinical diagnosis of metabolic and cardiovascular risk in overweight children: Early development of chronic diseases in the obese child. *International Journal of Obesity, 34*(Suppl. 2), S32–S36.

Li, C., Ford, E. S., McBride, P. E., et al. (2011). Non–high-density lipoprotein cholesterol concentration is associated with the metabolic syndrome among US youth aged 12–19 years. *Journal of Pediatrics, 158*(2), 201–207.

Patel, A. I., Madsen, K. A., Maselli, J. H., et al. (2010). Underdiagnosis of pediatric obesity during outpatient preventive care visits. *Journal of the Academic Pediatric, 10*(6), 405–409.

Ritchie, S. K., Murphy, E. C., Ice, C., et al. (2010). Universal versus targeted blood cholesterol screening among youth: The CARDIAC project. *Pediatrics, 126*(2), 260–265.

Simsek, E., Balta, H., Balta, Z., et al. (2010). Childhood obesity-related cardiovascular risk factors and carotid intima-media thickness. *Turkish Journal of Pediatrics, 52*(6), 602–611.

Strong, J. P., Malcom, G. T., McMahan, C. A., et al. (1999). Prevalence and extent of atherosclerosis in adolescents and young adults: Implications for prevention from the pathobiological determinants of atherosclerosis in youth study. *Journal of the American Medical Association, 281*(8), 727–735.

ALT, Alanine aminotransferase; *BMI,* body mass index; *BP,* blood pressure; *HDL,* high-density lipoprotein; *HgbA1c,* hemoglobin A1c test; *LDL,* low-density lipoprotein.

[a]Adapted from the Quality and Safety Education for Nurses website at http://www.qsen.org.

In addition to the risk factors noted earlier, the American Heart Association and National Heart, Lung, and Blood Institute have identified pediatric patients who are considered at higher risk for atherosclerosis because of coexisting health problems, including:

- Heterozygous or homozygous familial hyperlipidemia
- Chronic inflammatory diseases
  - Type 1 or 2 diabetes
  - Chronic kidney disease
- Cancer survivors
- Transplant patients
- CHD
- Kawasaki disease with current or history of coronary artery aneurysms (de Ferranti, Steinberger, Amerduri, et al., 2019)

Therapeutic Management

The first step in the treatment of high cholesterol is focused on lifestyle modification. The National Heart, Lung, and Blood Institute guidelines advocate the benefits of a heart-healthy diet for all children (Box 23.11). Children and adolescents with known dyslipidemia should have individual nutritional counseling, ideally by a dietitian with expertise in pediatric lipids.

BOX 23.11 Recommendations for Dietary and Lifestyle Management of Dyslipidemia for Children and Adolescents Older Than 2 Years of Age

For All Children and Adolescents

- Obtain 1 hour of moderate or vigorous physical activity at least 5 days a week
- Less than 2 hours per day of sedentary screen time
- Avoid firsthand and secondhand smoke exposure
- Eat a diverse diet rich in fruits, vegetables, whole grains, lean meats, and fish
- Refer to registered dietitian for individual nutritional counselling

Elevated Low-Density Lipoprotein Cholesterol

- 25% to 30% of calories from fat
- Less than 7% of calories from saturated fats (approximately 12 to 15 g/day)
- Avoid trans fats
- Favor monounsaturated fats
- Less than 200 mg/day of dietary cholesterol

Elevated Triglycerides or Non–High-Density Lipoprotein Cholesterol

- Decrease intake of simple sugars
  - Avoid white bread, white pasta, white potatoes, white rice, sugary cereals, cookies, cakes, candy
  - No sugar-sweetened beverages
  - Replace simple sugars with complex carbohydrates
- 25% to 30% of calories from fat
- Less than 7% of calories from saturated fat
- Favor monounsaturated fats (beneficial effects on high-density lipoprotein cholesterol)
  - Use olive oil, canola oil, avocados, nuts, and fish
- Avoid trans fats
- Increase dietary fish intake for omega-3 fatty acids

Adapted from Expert Panel on Integrated Guidelines for Cardiovascular Health and Risk Reduction in Children and Adolescents & National Heart, Lung, and Blood Institute. (2011). Expert panel on integrated guidelines for cardiovascular health and risk reduction in children and adolescents: Summary report. *Pediatrics, 128*(Suppl 5), S213–S256.

Research continues to support the benefit of diets low in saturated fats for patients with elevated LDL cholesterol. Current thinking favors a "Mediterranean"-type diet. Whole grains, fruits, and vegetables form the foundation of this diet. Patients who have elevated triglycerides, particularly those with an elevated body mass index (BMI), should also receive targeted counseling aimed at a low-glycemic diet. In both situations, monounsaturated fats are favored, as they have beneficial effects on HDL cholesterol. These fats include olive oil, canola oil, nuts, avocados, and fish. Regular aerobic exercise, at least 60 minutes a day 5 days a week, is recommended for all children and adolescents. In addition, patients and parents should be counseled regarding the negative effects of smoking (both firsthand and secondhand).

For some children, drug therapy may be necessary in addition to lifestyle modification, in order to achieve acceptable lipid values. After 6 months of lifestyle counselling, pharmacologic therapy is recommended for children older than 10 years of age who have LDL cholesterol values that are greater than 190 mg/dl without other risk factors or those with LDL values greater than 160 mg/dl in patients with additional risk factors and/or with a family history of early heart disease in a first-degree relative. In young people who are considered to have individual high-risk conditions (such as homozygous familial hypercholesterolemia, type 1 diabetes, chronic kidney disease, Kawasaki disease with aneurysms, or heart transplant recipients), the threshold for initiation of medication is lower and is considered when LDL values are greater than 130 mg/dl.

The use of medication in a child or adolescent needs to be a cooperative decision made with the patient and parents. Parents and patients should understand the available data related to statin use in young people, particularly because prospective, long-term evidence-based practice is not practical or available for this population. Options for lipid-lowering medications include bile acid–binding resins, 3-hydroxy-3-methylglutaryl coenzyme A (HMG-CoA) reductase inhibitors (statins), ezetimibe, and fibrates (for patients with severely elevated triglycerides). Nicotinic acid is generally not used in children and adolescents.

The most recent guidelines on lipid abnormalities in children recommend treatment with statins if pharmacologic therapy is indicated after lifestyle modification has been attempted (Expert Panel on Integrated Guidelines for Cardiovascular Health and Risk Reduction in Children and Adolescents & National Heart, Lung, and Blood Institute, 2011).

Statins are effective in lowering LDL cholesterol. To a lesser degree, they also help lower triglycerides levels and can raise HDL cholesterol somewhat. Statins work by inhibiting the enzyme necessary for cholesterol synthesis. Statins are started at the lowest possible dose in young people. Blood work should be followed closely in children and adolescents and usually includes a fasting lipid profile and an alanine aminotransferase (ALT) test repeated approximately 1 month after initiation and then monitored every 6 months to once a year as well as with any dosage changes.

Muscle symptoms should be assessed. Patients beginning therapy with a statin should be counseled regarding rare but potentially serious side effects (such as rhabdomyolysis) as well as more minor potential side effects. Patients should discontinue their medication and contact their practitioner if they develop dark urine or new muscle aches. Statin medications are not safe during pregnancy; therefore sexually active adolescents need to take adequate birth control measures. Very long–term studies are unlikely to be available over decades; however, in the shorter term studies that have been completed, statins seem to have a similar safety profile for children as they do for adults (McCrindle, Urbina, Dennison, et al., 2007). Ezetimibe is sometimes given in combination with statins to further reduce LDL cholesterol, which it accomplishes by decreasing reabsorption of cholesterol from the gut. Another class of lipid-lowering drugs is bile acid–binding resins. Bile acid–binding resins act by binding bile acids in the intestinal lumen. Because the intestine does not absorb them, resin binders do not produce systemic toxicity and are safe for children. Cholestyramine (Questran) and colestipol (Colestid) are both powders that are mixed with water or juice just before ingestion. Unfortunately, the vast majority of patients do not get adequate reduction in LDL cholesterol from bile acid–binding resins alone. Many cannot tolerate the medication because of the taste; gritty texture; and side effects, the most significant being constipation, abdominal pain, gastrointestinal bloating, flatulence, and nausea. Lastly, it is not common to use medications to lower triglyceride values unless they are significantly elevated (>500 mg/dl), in which case fibrates, which decrease the production of triglycerides, may be considered.

Nursing Care Management

Nurses play an important role in the screening, education, and support of children with lipid abnormalities and their families. When a child is referred to a preventive cardiology clinic, it is essential that the family be adequately prepared for the first visit. Generally, the parents will be asked to keep a dietary history of the child before this visit. Some clinics use questionnaires regarding the child's normal dietary habits. Families should be instructed to bring their child to the lab in the morning after fasting for at least 12 hours before blood work. In addition, parents should be aware that lipids should not be drawn within 3 weeks of a febrile illness because doing so can affect cholesterol values. It is important to schedule the blood test early in the morning and to arrange for nourishment immediately thereafter. At the visit, a full family history should be taken, including the health of both parents and all first- and second-degree relatives. Specific questions should be asked regarding early heart disease, hypertension, strokes (CVAs), sudden death, hyperlipidemia, diabetes, and endocrine abnormalities.

Patients and parents should be educated about cholesterol and lipid abnormalities. This should include a brief introduction of the different lipoprotein categories, including an explanation of the components of the lipid profile. In addition, lifestyle risk factors for heart disease, such as smoking, screen and sedentary time, exercise, and diet, should be reviewed in depth. For management to be effective, parents and patients need to understand the rationale for screening and treatment.

Ideally, a heart-healthy diet is reviewed by an experienced dietitian and should reflect national guidelines for healthy eating. Stringent dietary guidelines may become an issue of control and a source of great stress for many families. Rather, the positive aspects of healthy eating, regularly exercising, and avoiding smoking should be emphasized. Basic dietary changes should be encouraged for the whole family so that the affected child is not singled out. Cultural differences must be considered and recommendations individualized. Substitution rather than elimination needs to be emphasized. Visual aids (e.g., test tubes depicting the amount of fat in a hot dog or the number or packs of sugar in a glass of juice) are often helpful, especially for younger children. Diets should be flexible and individually tailored by a dietitian who is experienced in lipid disorders. Dietary recommendations need to meet the nutritional demands of growing children while providing benefit to the overall profile. Parents and patients are encouraged to participate in dietary and educational sessions, ask questions, and share ideas and experiences.

Parents often feel guilty about the hereditary component of hyperlipidemia. Many also believe that they have failed if the diet alone is not making a significant difference in their child's lipid profile. They need to be reassured that a dietary approach alone is often insufficient, especially for children with genetically elevated values.

Parents of children who require pharmacologic therapy need to understand the purpose, dosage, and possible side effects of the various drugs. Medication schedules should remain flexible and should not interfere with the child's daily activities. Follow-up phone calls by the nurse between visits allow parents to discuss their concerns and ask any questions that have arisen.

CARDIAC DYSRHYTHMIAS

Dysrhythmias, or abnormal heart rhythms, can occur in children with structurally normal hearts, as features of some congenital heart defects, and in patients following surgical repair of congenital heart defects. They are also seen in patients with cardiomyopathy and with cardiac tumors. They can occur secondary to metabolic and electrolyte imbalances. Childhood dysrhythmias can have a genetic or familial etiology. Dysrhythmias can be classified in several ways, such as by heart rate characteristics (bradycardia and tachycardia) or by the origin of the dysrhythmia in the atria or ventricles. Some dysrhythmias are well tolerated and self-limiting. Others may cause decreased cardiac output with associated symptoms. Some dysrhythmias can cause sudden death. Treatment depends on the cause of the dysrhythmia and its severity.

Many advances have been made in the diagnosis and treatment of pediatric dysrhythmias in the past decade. Improvements in technology have allowed better diagnosis, the development of ablation techniques, and the expansion of pacemaker capabilities. New antidysrhythmic medications have proven safe and effective in children. Radiofrequency ablation has offered a cure for some dysrhythmias. Pediatric electrophysiology has become a highly specialized field, and students should consult more detailed sources for an in-depth discussion. The following sections describe diagnostic studies and provide a general discussion of the most common tachycardia (supraventricular tachycardia) and the most common bradycardia (complete heart block) that require treatment in the pediatric population.

Diagnostic Evaluation

Nurses must be familiar with the standards of normal heart rate for the age-group. An initial nursing responsibility is recognition of an abnormal heartbeat, either in rate or in rhythm. When a dysrhythmia is suspected, the apical rate is counted for 1 full minute and compared with the radial rate, which may be lower because not all apical beats are felt. Consistently high or low heart rates should be regarded as suspicious. The patient should be placed on a cardiac monitor with recording capabilities. A 12-lead ECG yields more information than the monitor recording and should be done as soon as possible.

The basic diagnostic procedure is the ECG, including 24-hour Holter monitoring. Electrophysiologic cardiac catheterization allows for identification of the conduction disturbance and immediate investigation of drugs that may control the dysrhythmia. Another procedure that may be used is transesophageal recording. An electrode catheter is passed to the lower esophagus and, when in position at a point proximal to the heart, is used to stimulate and record dysrhythmias.

Dysrhythmias can be classified according to various criteria, such as effect on heart rate and rhythm, as follows:

Bradydysrhythmias: Abnormally slow rate
Tachydysrhythmias: Abnormally rapid rate
Conduction disturbances: Irregular heart rate

Bradydysrhythmias

Sinus bradycardia (slower than normal rate) in children can be attributed to the influence of the autonomic nervous system, as with hypervagal tone, or in response to hypoxia and hypotension. Sinus bradycardias are also known to develop after atrial repairs involving atrial suture lines, such as in the Fontan procedure.

Complete atrioventricular (AV) block is also referred to as **complete heart block**. This can be either congenital (occurring in children with structurally normal hearts) or acquired after surgery to repair cardiac defects. AV blocks are most often related to edema around the conduction system and resolve without treatment. Temporary epicardial wires are placed in most patients at surgery; if a rhythm disturbance occurs, temporary pacing can be used. Several days after surgery, the health practitioner removes the wires by pulling slowly and deliberately down on them from the site of insertion.

Some children may need a permanent pacemaker. The pacemaker takes over or assists in the heart's conduction function. Pacemaker functions have become more sophisticated, and some models can adjust the heart rate to activity demands or be programmed for overdrive pacing or cardioversion.

The implantation of a pacemaker, in the operating room or possibly the catheterization laboratory, is usually a low-risk procedure. The pacemaker is made up of two basic parts: the pulse generator and the lead. The pulse generator is composed of the battery and the electronic circuitry. The lead is an insulated, flexible wire that conducts the electrical impulse from the pulse generator to the heart. Two types of leads, transvenous and epicardial, are available. After the lead has been attached to the heart, a small incision is made, and a pocket is formed under the muscle to house and protect the generator. Continuous ECG monitoring is necessary during the recovery phase to assess pacemaker function. The nurse should be aware of the programmed rate and expected individual generator variations. The pacemaker insertion site is monitored for signs of infection. Analgesics are given for pain.

Discharge teaching includes information about the signs and symptoms of infection, general wound care, and activity restrictions. Parents, and patients if they are old enough, should be taught to take a pulse and know the settings of the pacemaker. If the patient's low rate is set at 80 beats/min and the heart rate is only 68 beats/min, there is a possible problem with the pacemaker that needs to be investigated. Instructions for telephone transmission of ECG readings are also given. Telephone transmission can be used to transmit ECG strips and to monitor battery life and pacemaker function. The pacemaker generator will have to be replaced periodically because of battery depletion. Children with pacemakers should wear a MedicAlert device, and their parents should have a paper identification card with specific pacer data in case of an emergency. Cardiopulmonary resuscitation (CPR) instruction is suggested for parents.

Tachydysrhythmias

Sinus tachycardia (an abnormally fast heart rate) secondary to fever, anxiety, pain, anemia, dehydration, or any other etiologic factor requiring increased cardiac output should be ruled out before diagnosing an increased heart rate as pathologic. Supraventricular tachycardia (SVT) is the most common tachydysrhythmia found in children and refers to a rapid regular heart rate of 200 to 300 beats/min. As many as 1 in 250 children experience SVT (Schlechte, Boramanand, & Funk, 2008). The onset of SVT is often sudden, the duration is variable, and the rhythm may end abruptly and convert back to a normal sinus rhythm. Clinical signs in infants and young children are poor feeding, extreme irritability, and pallor. Children may experience palpitations, dizziness, chest pain, and diaphoresis. If SVT is sustained, signs of HF may be seen.

The treatment of SVT depends on the degree of compromise imposed by the dysrhythmia. In some cases, vagal maneuvers, such as applying ice to the face, massaging the carotid artery (on one side of the neck only), or having an older child perform a Valsalva maneuver (e.g., exhaling against a closed glottis, blowing on a thumb as if it were a trumpet for 30 to 60 seconds), can terminate SVT. If vagal maneuvers fail or the child is hemodynamically unstable, adenosine (a drug that impairs AV conduction) may be used. Adenosine is given by rapid IV push with a saline bolus immediately after the drug because of its very short half-life. If this is unsuccessful or cardiac output is compromised, esophageal overdrive pacing or synchronized cardioversion (delivering an electrical shock to the heart) can be used in the intensive care setting. Sedation is needed for both procedures. Cardioversion should never be done in a conscious patient. Traditional first-line medical management of chronic SVT is a beta-blocker or digoxin. A primary focus of nursing care is education of the family regarding the symptoms of SVT and its treatment. If medication is prescribed, instructions on accurate dosage and the importance of administering the correct dose at specified intervals are stressed. SVT may occur again despite therapy. Parents should be taught to take a radial pulse for a full minute.

Radiofrequency ablation has become first-line therapy for some types of SVT. The procedure is done in the cardiac catheterization laboratory and begins with mapping of the conduction system to identify the dysrhythmia focus. A catheter delivering radiofrequency current is directed at the site, and the area is heated to destroy the tissue in the area. These are lengthy procedures, often lasting 6 to 8 hours, and sedation or general anesthesia is required. Preparation is similar to that for cardiac catheterization. Another procedure, cryoablation, is also used in treatment of SVT. For this kind of ablation, liquid nitrous oxide is used to cool a catheter to subfreezing temperatures, which then destroys the tissue of target by freezing.

PULMONARY HYPERTENSION

Pulmonary hypertension (PH) is a pulmonary vascular disease associated with diverse cardiac, lung, and systemic diseases as well as familial and idiopathic etiologies. The pulmonary arteries are described as having vascular narrowing due to decreased vascular growth and surface area and intraluminal obstruction, and they undergo structural remodeling of the vessel wall (Abman & Ivy, 2011). Pulmonary hypertension is defined by a mean pulmonary arterial pressure (mPAP) of 25 mm Hg or greater in children older than 3 months of age and is categorized based on a classification system created by the World Health Organization (Simonneau, Gatzoulis, Adatia, et al., 2013). In the pediatric population, there are three causes of PH: (1) increased pulmonary venous pressures (e.g., mitral stenosis, left ventricle noncompliance); (2) post-tricuspid cardiac shunts (e.g., large VSD, large patent ductus arteriosus [PDA]); and (3) small pulmonary arteries, that is, arteries that are too few or too narrow (e.g., idiopathic pulmonary arterial hypertension [IPAH], persistent pulmonary hypertension of the newborn [PPHN], connective tissue disorders, hypoxia, drugs, toxins). There is no cure for PH, and there is significant morbidity and mortality. However, advancements in therapeutic management in the last 10 to 15 years are helping to slow the progression of the disease and improve quality of life.

Clinical Manifestations

The clinical manifestations include dyspnea with exercise, chest pain, and syncope. Dyspnea is the most common symptom and is caused by impaired oxygen delivery. Chest pain is the result of coronary ischemia in the right ventricle from severe hypertrophy. Syncope reflects a limited cardiac output leading to decreased cerebral blood flow. Right-sided heart dysfunction is steadily progressive, and when symptoms of venous congestion and edema are present, the prognosis is poor.

Therapeutic Management

Pediatric PH guidelines from the American Heart Association and American Thoracic Society outline treatment recommendations for conditions specific to the pediatric population, including PPHN, congenital diaphragmatic hernia (CDH), bronchopulmonary dysplasia, and CHD (Abman, Hansmann, Archer, et al., 2015). The discussion here focuses on pharmacotherapy, supportive therapy, and, briefly, invasive interventions.

Three classes of drugs are used extensively in the treatment of pediatric PH: phosphodiesterase-5 (PDE5) inhibitors (sildenafil, tadalafil), endothelin receptor antagonists (ERAs; bosentan, ambrisentan), and prostanoids or prostacyclin (PGI_2) analogs (epoprostenol, treprostinil). Vasoconstriction is a primary component of PH, and these drugs work on different aspects to promote vasodilation and smooth muscle relaxation. For patients who are responsive to inhaled nitric oxide or vasodilator drug testing during cardiac catheterization, oral calcium channel blockers (nifedipine and diltiazem) have been successful and are the treatment of choice. Table 23.6 reviews the common PH drugs, dose form availability, adverse side effects, and comments on important aspects in the administration of these medications. Choice of treatment is determined by the severity of the disease, and all of these medications carry adverse effects.

In general, situations that may exacerbate the disease and cause hypoxia are avoided. Exercise prescriptions are specific to each patient. Patients should avoid high altitudes because of the relative hypoxia, and some patients have moved to sea level to slow the progress of the disease. Supplemental oxygen is commonly used to relieve hypoxia, especially at night while sleeping. Patients with pulmonary artery hypertension (PAH) are at risk for thromboembolic events. Anticoagulation therapy has been shown to increase survival in adults. Many patients are treated with warfarin to prevent pulmonary embolism, which can be fatal. Digoxin and diuretics are often used to treat right-sided heart failure.

Some patients fail to respond to medical management, and disease progression leads to severe right ventricle dysfunction. In these cases, two potential options are available. Creation of an atrial septostomy or communication between the two atria can be done in the catheterization lab. This often increases cardiac output and thus results in some improvement in function and quality of life. Lung transplantation may be another treatment option for children, primarily those with severe disease.

Nursing Care Management

The diagnosis of PH is devastating for the child and family. There is no known cure, and the treatments require significant lifestyle changes and commitment on the part of the patient and family to make them successful. Anxiety, depression, and fear of the future are common. Patients and families require extensive education about the disease and its management. They need emotional support to cope with a poor prognosis and make decisions about treatment options.

The medical treatment is complex and involves different medications and therapies. Families are often referred to a specialized center that has experience in the management of PH. This may involve travel far from home with associated emotional and financial hardships. The patient and family must cope with the symptoms of the disease and the side effects of the treatment. Dealing with a continuous IV infusion or continuous oxygen administration requires a major adjustment in lifestyle to accommodate the therapy. The prostacyclin infusion cannot be interrupted at any time, since symptoms can worsen and cause acute pulmonary hypertensive crisis, which can be fatal. Backup systems must be in place at all times. The patient and family must make a commitment to adhere to a complex regimen of preparing the infusion, maintaining the equipment, and maintaining sterility of the central line. Treatments are expensive, so insurance coverage and financial issues are critical. Nurses have an important role in educating and preparing families to perform these complex therapies. Discharge planning involves many team members and outside agencies. The nurse has a pivotal role in coordinating the child's care in the hospital and the transition to home.

CARDIOMYOPATHY

Cardiomyopathy refers to abnormalities of the myocardium in which the cardiac muscles' ability to contract is impaired. Cardiomyopathies are relatively rare in children. Possible etiologic factors include familial or genetic causes, infection, deficiency states, metabolic abnormalities, and collagen vascular diseases. Most cardiomyopathies in children are considered primary or idiopathic, in which the cause is unknown

TABLE 23.6 Pharmacologic Therapy for Pediatric Pulmonary Hypertension

Drug Class	Agent	Dose Form	Adverse Effects	Comments
Calcium channel blocker	Nifedipine, diltiazem	Oral	Bradycardia, decreased cardiac output, peripheral edema, rash, gum hyperplasia, constipation	Only effective for PH if patient is responsive to vasodilator testing in the cathetherization lab. Requires high (maximal) dosing to achieve desired vasodilation.
PDE5 inhibitor	Sildenafil, tadalafil	Oral	Flushing, hypotension, headache, priapism	
Endothelin receptor antagonist (ERA)	Bosentan, ambrisentan	Oral	Hepatotoxic, peripheral edema, teratogenic	Requires monthly LFTs; birth control important for adolescent and young women
Prostacyclin	Epoprostenol (Flolan), treprostinil (Remodulin)	IV/SC	Headache, flushing, hypotension, site pain (SC form), cellulitis, central line complications, jaw pain, nausea, or diarrhea	Flolan has an extremely short half-life (2-5 min), and PH crises occurs rapidly if infusion is stopped. Dosing is complex, and there is a high risk of error.
Prostacyclin	Treprostinil (Remodulin)	Oral	Headache, flushing, pain in extremities, jaw pain, nausea, or diarrhea (GI side effects can be greater than other dose forms)	Transition from IV/SC form occurs over days in the hospital. Timing of dosing is critical; if two doses are missed, need IV/SC form. Cannot be crushed, chewed, or compounded.
Prostacyclin	Treprostinil (Remodulin)	Inhaled	Headache, flushing, pain in extremities, jaw pain, nausea, or diarrhea	Must be inhaled 1-9 times every 6 hours. Can worsen reactive airway symptoms

GI, Gastrointestinal; *IV,* intravenous; *LFT,* liver function test; *PDE5,* phosphodiesterase-5; *PH,* pulmonary hypertension; *SC,* subcutaneous.
Adapted from Abman, S. H., Hansmann, G., Archer, S. L., et al. (2015). Pediatric pulmonary hypertension: Guidelines from the American Heart Association and American Thoracic Society. *Circulation, 132*(21), 2037–2099.

and the cardiac dysfunction is not associated with systemic disease. Some of the known causes of secondary cardiomyopathy are anthracycline toxicity (the antineoplastic agents, doxorubicin [Adriamycin] and daunomycin), hemochromatosis (from excessive iron storage), Duchenne muscular dystrophy, Kawasaki disease, collagen diseases, and thyroid dysfunction.

Cardiomyopathies can be divided into three broad clinical categories according to the type of abnormal structure and dysfunction present: (1) dilated cardiomyopathy, (2) hypertrophic cardiomyopathy, and (3) restrictive cardiomyopathy.

Dilated cardiomyopathy is characterized by ventricular dilation and greatly decreased contractility, resulting in symptoms of HF. This is the most common type of cardiomyopathy in children. Its cause is often unknown. The clinical findings are of HF with tachycardia, dyspnea, hepatosplenomegaly, fatigue, and poor growth. Dysrhythmias may be present and may be more difficult to control with worsening HF.

Hypertrophic cardiomyopathy is characterized by an increase in heart muscle mass without an increase in cavity size, usually occurring in the left ventricle and associated with abnormal diastolic filling. It is a familial autosomal dominant genetic abnormality in most cases and is probably the most common genetically transmitted cardiovascular disease (Gajarski, Naftel, Pahl, et al., 2009). The expression of clinical disease varies greatly among patients. Clinical symptoms usually appear in the school-age period or adolescence and may include anginal chest pain, dysrhythmias, and syncope. One recent study confirmed that unexplained syncope in the childhood age-group (younger than 18 years old) with known hypertrophic cardiomyopathy had a 60% cumulative risk of sudden death within 5 years of the syncopal event (Spirito, Autore, Rapezzi, et al., 2009). Presentation in infancy includes signs of HF and has a poor prognosis. The ECG demonstrates left ventricular hypertrophy, often with ST-T changes. The echocardiogram is most helpful and demonstrates asymmetric septal hypertrophy and an increase in left ventricular wall thickness, with a small left ventricle cavity.

Restrictive cardiomyopathy, which is rare in children, describes a restriction to ventricular filling caused by endocardial or myocardial disease or both. It is characterized by diastolic dysfunction and absence of ventricular dilation or hypertrophy. Symptoms are similar to those of HF (see discussion earlier in the chapter).

Therapeutic Management

Treatment is directed toward correcting the underlying cause whenever feasible. However, in most affected children, this is not possible, and treatment is aimed at managing HF (see discussion earlier in the chapter) and dysrhythmias. Digoxin, diuretics, and aggressive use of afterload reduction agents have been found to be helpful in managing symptoms in those with dilated cardiomyopathy. Practice guidelines for the management of HF in children have been outlined and provide an in-depth review of available therapies (Kirk, Dipchand, Rosenthal, et al., 2014; Rossano & Shaddy, 2014). Digoxin and inotropic agents usually are not helpful in the other forms of cardiomyopathy because increasing the force of contraction may exacerbate the muscular obstruction and actually impair ventricular ejection. Beta-blockers (such as carvedilol) and calcium channel blockers (such as verapamil) have been used to reduce left ventricular outflow obstruction and improve diastolic filling in those with hypertrophic cardiomyopathy.

Careful monitoring and treatment of dysrhythmias are essential. The placement of an AICD should be considered for patients at high risk of sudden death because of ventricular dysrhythmias. Anticoagulants may be given to reduce the risk of thromboemboli, a complication of the sluggish circulation through the heart. For worsening HF and signs of poor perfusion, IV inotropic or vasodilating drugs may be needed. Severely ill children may require mechanical ventilation, oxygen administration, IV medications, and placement of ventricular assist devices. Heart transplantation may be a treatment option for patients who have worsening symptoms despite maximum medical therapy.

Nursing Care Management

Because of the poor prognosis in many children with cardiomyopathy, nursing care is consistent with that for any child with a life-threatening disorder (see Chapter 17). One of the most difficult adjustments for the child may be the realization of failing health and the need for restricted activity. The child should be included in decisions regarding activity and allowed to discuss feelings, particularly if the disease follows a progressively fatal course. After symptoms of HF or dysrhythmias develop, the same nursing interventions discussed earlier in the chapter are implemented. If heart transplantation is considered, the needs of the child and family are great in terms of psychologic preparation and postoperative care. The nurse plays an important role in assessing the family's understanding of the procedure and long-term consequences. Children of school age and older should be fully informed to give their assent to the procedure (see Chapter 20, Informed Consent).

HEART TRANSPLANTATION

Heart transplantation has become a treatment option for infants and children with worsening HF and a limited life expectancy despite maximum medical and surgical management. Indications for heart transplantation in children are cardiomyopathy and end-stage CHD. It is also an option for patients with some forms of complex congenital cardiac defects, such as hypoplastic left heart syndrome (HLHS), for whom conventional surgical approaches have a high mortality rate.

The heart transplant procedure may be orthotopic or heterotopic. Orthotopic heart transplantation refers to removing the recipient's own heart and implanting a new heart from a donor who has had brain death but a healthy heart. The donor and recipient are matched by weight and blood type. Heterotopic heart transplantation refers to leaving the recipient's own heart in place and implanting a new heart to act as an additional pump, or "piggyback" heart; this type of transplant is rarely done in children.

Before transplantation, potential recipients undergo a careful cardiac evaluation to determine if there are any other medical or surgical options to improve the patient's cardiac status. Other organ systems are assessed to identify problems that might increase the risk of or preclude transplantation. A psychosocial evaluation of the patient and family is done to assess family function, support systems, and ability to comply with the complex medical regimen after the transplant. Support services to help the family successfully care for their child are provided when possible. Parents and older adolescents need extensive education about the risks and benefits of transplantation so that they can make an informed decision. Patients are listed on a national computer network organized by the United Network for Organ Sharing to match donors and recipients (see also Chapter 17, Organ or Tissue Donation and Autopsy).

The annual number of pediatric heart transplants has increased from 274 in 1998 to 684 in 2015 (Dipchand, Rossano, Edwards, et al., 2015). Primary diagnosis for most candidates older than 1 year of age at listing continues to be cardiomyopathy, and most (>85%) candidates are status 1A at the time of transplant (Scientific Registry of Transplant Recipients, 2015). The 1-year graft survival rate for pediatric heart transplants in the current era is 90% (Scientific Registry of Transplant Recipients, 2015).

Waiting list mortality remains high, particularly in the smallest children. Recent progress in suitable ventricular assist devices for use in children as a bridge to transplantation has made outcomes to survival for cardiac transplantation more successful (Blume, Naftel, Bastardi, et al., 2006). A multicenter study using the US Scientific Registry of Transplant Recipients to identify the vulnerable population was conducted (Almond, Thiagarajian, Piercy, et al., 2009). Among 3098 children listed for a heart transplant between 1999 and 2006, the median age was 2 years. Sixty percent of patients were listed as a top status (30% ventilated and 18% on supportive measures), and of those children, 17% died, 63% received transplants, 8% recovered, and 12% remained listed. These numbers concluded that US waiting time remains high in the current era, and high-risk groups in these categories could benefit from emerging cardiac assist devices, such as extracorporeal membrane oxygenation and ventricular assist devices. In response, donor centers and transplant centers are identifying strategies to increase donor supply, optimize donor management, and facilitate changes in the organ allocation system (Zafar, Castleberry, Khan, et al., 2015).

The posttransplant course is complex. Although heart function is greatly improved or normal after transplantation, the risk of rejection is serious. The leading cause of death in the first 3 years after heart transplantation is rejection, with the greatest risk in the first 6 months (Everitt, Pahl, Schechtman, et al., 2011). Rejection of the heart is diagnosed primarily by endomyocardial biopsy in older children. Serial echocardiograms are often used in infants and young children to reduce the need for invasive biopsies. Immunosuppressants must be taken for life and have many systemic side effects. Triple-drug therapy for immunosuppression with a calcineurin inhibitor (cyclosporine or tacrolimus), steroids, and mycophenolate mofetil or azathioprine is most commonly used in pediatric patients. Steroids are weaned in the first year and may be discontinued in some patients; many pediatric centers are avoiding long-term steroids by using induction therapy protocols of high-dose steroids and thymoglobulin at the time of transplant (Thrush & Hoffman, 2014).

Infection is always a risk. Potential long-term problems that may limit survival include chronic rejection, causing coronary artery disease; renal dysfunction and hypertension resulting from cyclosporine administration; lymphoma; and infection. Coronary artery disease is the leading cause of death among late survivors of heart transplantation (Boucek, Aurora, Edwards, et al., 2007). In the short term, after successful transplantation, children can return to full participation in age-appropriate activities and appear to adapt well to their new lifestyle. Transplantation is not a cure because patients must live with the lifetime consequences of chronic immunosuppression.

NURSING CARE MANAGEMENT

Successfully caring for a child after a heart transplant requires the expertise and dedication of many members of the health care team. Nurses play vital roles in assessment, coordination of care, psychosocial support, and patient and family education. The heart transplant recipient must be carefully monitored for signs of rejection, infection, and the side effects of the immunosuppressant medications. The patient's and family's psychosocial well-being also needs to be assessed to identify issues such as increased family stress, depression, substance abuse, and school problems. Noncompliance with an intense medication regimen, especially during adolescence, can lead to serious medical problems and can be fatal. Immunosuppressants and nursing implications are discussed in Chapter 26 in relation to renal transplantation. Care of the immunosuppressed child is reviewed in Chapter 25. Psychosocial concerns and appropriate interventions for the child with a life-threatening disorder are presented in Chapter 17.

The first 6 months to 1 year after the transplant are most intense because the risk of complications is greatest and the patient and family are adjusting to a new lifestyle. Patients are monitored closely by the health care team, with frequent visits and laboratory tests. Care is usually shared between local health care providers and the transplant center. Many patients can return to school and other age-appropriate activities within 2 to 3 months after the transplant.

VASCULAR DYSFUNCTION

SYSTEMIC HYPERTENSION

Hypertension is defined as the consistent elevation of BP beyond values considered to be the upper limits of normal. The two major categories of hypertension are **essential hypertension** (no identifiable cause) and **secondary hypertension** (subsequent to an identifiable cause). Whether essential or attributable to a secondary cause, hypertension is a major contributor to cardiovascular disease in the adult population. Recently published Clinical Practice Guidelines streamline the recommendations for the evaluation of BP and outline the parameters for testing and treatment of young people with high BP (Flynn, Kaelber, Baker-Smith, et al., 2017). These guidelines are endorsed in another American Heart Association Scientific Statement that is aimed at risk reduction in patients considered to be at high risk (de Ferranti et al., 2019). It is important to note that new normative BP tables are based only on children of normal weight, those below the 95th percentile BMI (as opposed to all children). The new guidelines rely on percentiles (based on age, sex, and height) to define norms only for children younger than 13 years old, whereas the definition of abnormal BP in adolescents older than 13 years of age is now defined using numeric cut points, designed to interface with adult hypertension guidelines (Whelton, Carey, Aranow, et al., 2018). The previous category of prehypertension has been relabeled as elevated blood pressure.

Abnormal BP categories are now defined as follows: (1) elevated blood pressure, (2) stage 1 hypertension, or (3) stage 2 hypertension (see https://pediatrics.aappublications.org/content/140/3/e20171904 for additional information). All BP normal values are based on auscultated blood pressures, the preferred method of measurement. The goal of treatment is decreasing systolic and diastolic BP values to below the 90th percentile in children younger than 13 years old and less than 130/80 mm Hg in adolescents older than 13 years of age (Flynn et al., 2017).

ETIOLOGY

Most instances of hypertension in very young children occur secondary to a structural abnormality or an underlying pathologic process, although this is being challenged by screening programs of relatively healthy children. The most common cause of secondary hypertension is renal disease followed by cardiovascular, endocrine, and some neurologic disorders. As a rule, the younger the child and the more severe the hypertension, the more likely it is to be secondary (Mattoo, 2019).

The causes of essential hypertension are undetermined, but evidence indicates that both genetic and environmental factors may play a role. The incidence of hypertension has been shown to be higher in children whose parents are hypertensive. African Americans have a higher incidence of hypertension than whites, and in African Americans hypertension develops earlier, is frequently more severe, and results in death at an earlier age. Environmental factors that contribute to the risk of developing hypertension include obesity, salt ingestion, smoking, and stress.

DIAGNOSTIC EVALUATION

BP assessment is recommended as a routine part of annual assessment in healthy children older than 3 years of age. BP readings should be taken in children younger than 3 years old if they have individual risk factors, including CHD, kidney disease, malignancy, transplant, certain neurologic problems, or systemic illnesses known to cause hypertension, or high-risk family history. Assessing for symptoms of BP elevation such as frequent headaches, dizziness, and visual changes should be part of the health history. In infants and very young children who cannot communicate symptoms, observation of behaviors such as head banging/rubbing or irritability may provide clues, although many behavioral changes are nonspecific.

Before a diagnosis of hypertension is made, BP should be measured on at least three separate occasions at healthy visits only. An ambulatory BP monitor may be helpful to assess for "white-coat hypertension" or for those patients who have had elevated BPs for a year or more as well as patients whose BPs fall in the range of stage 1 hypertension over three clinic visits. Appropriate cuff size should be specified. These monitors are useful in that they provide BP readings over a 24-hour period. There are different normative values for ambulatory BP readings (Flynn, Daniels, Hayman, et al., 2014).

A careful medical history and family history should be obtained to screen for other relatives with hypertension and other cardiovascular risk factors. In children with suspected hypertension, initial laboratory data include a urinalysis, renal function studies (such as creatinine and blood urea nitrogen), a lipid profile, and electrolytes. For obese patients, hemoglobin A1c (HgbA1c), aspartate aminotransferase (AST), ALT and fasting lipid values are recommended. Additional testing is determined based on the individual's age, history, degree of BP elevation, and physical examination and may include additional laboratory work (thyroid-stimulating hormone [TSH], complete blood count [CBC], drug screen, retinal examination, sleep study). Renal ultrasonography is now recommended only in children younger than 6 years old unless there are laboratory abnormalities or clinical reasons to prompt kidney imaging. If a renal ultrasound is indicated, it should include Doppler flow as well as kidney size. ECGs are no longer recommended as a routine part of the workup in children and adolescents. Echocardiograms are not recommended as part of the initial screening but should be obtained prior to initiating pharmacologic therapy in order to help evaluate the presence of end-organ involvement, such as left ventricular hypertrophy and effects on ejection fraction. The frequency of repeat surveillance echocardiograms depends on the presence or absence of left ventricular hypertrophy as well as the individual response to BP treatment. A more extensive workup for a secondary cause of hypertension may be indicated in children with significant hypertension in the setting of normal initial screening results (Flynn et al., 2017).

Therapeutic Management

Therapy for secondary hypertension involves the diagnosis and treatment of the underlying cause. Children and adolescents with consistently elevated BP readings from no known cause or those with secondary hypertension not amenable to surgical correction are treated with a combination of lifestyle and pharmacologic interventions. Dietary practices and lifestyle changes are important in the control of hypertension both for children and for adults. Nonpharmacologic measures, such as weight control in overweight patients, increased exercise, limited salt intake (such as recommended in the Dietary Approaches to Stop Hypertension [DASH] diet), and avoidance of stress and smoking, carry no risk and should be instituted as first-line therapy except in severe cases in which pharmacologic therapy may be indicated as well.

Drug therapy is instituted with caution in children but may be necessary to treat significant elevations of BP despite lifestyle modification. Pharmacologic treatment begins with one drug, with other drugs added if adequate control is not obtained. The classes of oral antihypertensive drugs now recommended for use in young people include ACE inhibitors, angiotensin-receptor blockers, long-acting calcium channel blockers, and thiazide diuretics. Beta-blockers are no longer recommended in children due to their side effects and the availability of other medications. The goal of treatment is to achieve a normotensive state without accompanying drug side effects.

Nursing Care Management

BP measurement should be a part of the routine assessment of children older than 3 years of age and patients younger than 3 years old who are considered to be at high risk for hypertension. To obtain an accurate reading, care is taken to quiet the child or relax the adolescent while the measurement is recorded to avoid false readings caused by excitement. BP should be measured in the sitting position with the arm at the level of the heart. Initial evaluation should also include four extremity pressures (in the supine position) to rule out COA. The chief cause of falsely elevated BP readings is the use of improperly fitting, narrow cuffs. Therefore attention to correct measurement technique is essential (see Chapter 4, Blood Pressure).

Education aimed at understanding hypertension and its implication over the life span is essential in promoting patient and family compliance with both nonpharmacologic and pharmacologic therapies (see Chapter 20, Compliance).

Ambulatory or home BP measurements can facilitate surveillance in youngsters being assessed for hypertension or can document the effectiveness of therapy for those being treated for chronic hypertension. In addition, a family member can be instructed on how to take and record accurate BP measurements, thus decreasing the number of trips to a health care facility. This individual needs to have parameters, above which they should contact the practitioner. In addition, the school nurse can often be a valuable resource in monitoring BP. The nurse plays an important role in assessing individual families and providing targeted information regarding nonpharmacologic modes of intervention, such as diet, weight loss, smoking cessation, and exercise programs. A DASH diet—low in sodium, red meats, and sugar and high in fruits, vegetables, whole grains, beans, nuts, low-fat dairy, fish, and poultry—is recommended for children and adolescents with elevated BP or hypertension. The child should be referred to a registered dietitian with expertise in working with children and adolescents with hypertension. Exercise regimens should be individualized but should emphasize the benefits of regular aerobic exercise (ideally 300 minutes of aerobic exercise weekly). School-age children and young adolescents generally prefer team sports to individual training, which they may view as a burden rather than an enjoyable activity. If peers and family members can be encouraged to participate in any of the management strategies, the child's compliance is likely to be greater.

If drug therapy is prescribed, the nurse needs to provide information to the family on the reasons for it, how the drug works, and possible side effects. General instructions for antihypertensive drugs include:

- Rise slowly from a horizontal position and avoid sudden position changes.
- Take drugs as prescribed.
- Maintain adequate hydration.
- Notify the practitioner if side effects occur but do not discontinue the drug.

- Avoid alcohol and stay on the prescribed diet (generally the DASH diet).

The need for regular follow-up is stressed, especially because antihypertensive therapy can sometimes be safely discontinued if BP remains under control over time.

KAWASAKI DISEASE

Kawasaki disease is an acute systemic vasculitis of unknown cause. It is seen in every racial group, with 76% of the cases occurring in children younger than 5 years old. The peak incidence is in the toddler age-group. The acute disease is self-limited; however, without treatment approximately 20% to 25% of children develop coronary artery dilation or aneurysm formation (coronary artery anomaly [CAA]). Infants younger than 1 year old are at the greatest risk for heart involvement, although an increased incidence has also been reported in older children, perhaps because of later diagnosis in many.

The etiology of Kawasaki disease is unknown. The illness is not spread by person-to-person contact; however, several factors support an infectious etiologic trigger, possibly in a genetically susceptible host. This theory is supported by a higher prevalence in Asian children and in siblings and children of patients with Kawasaki disease. Kawasaki disease is often seen in geographic and seasonal outbreaks, with an increased incidence reported in late winter and early spring (McCrindle, Rowley, Newburger, et al., 2017; Newburger, de Ferranti, & Fulton, 2017).

Pathophysiology

The principal area of concern in Kawasaki disease is the cardiovascular system. During the initial stage of the illness, extensive inflammation of the arterioles, venules, and capillaries is evident, resulting in many of the clinical symptoms. In addition, segmental damage to the medium-size muscular arteries, mainly the coronary arteries, can occur, resulting in the formation of coronary artery aneurysms in some children. Death is very rare in Kawasaki disease (<0.1% of cases) and is usually the result of myocardial ischemia from coronary thrombosis during the first few months of illness or years later from severe scar formation and stenosis in coronary aneurysms (Wilder, Palinkas, Kao, et al., 2007).

Clinical Manifestations

Because no specific diagnostic test exists for Kawasaki disease, the diagnosis is established based on clinical findings and associated laboratory results (Box 23.12). These criteria should be used as guidelines. It is important to note that many children with Kawasaki disease do not fulfill standard diagnostic criteria, and infants in particular often have an incomplete presentation. It is therefore important to consider Kawasaki disease as a possible diagnosis in any infant or child with prolonged fever that is unresponsive to antibiotics and is not attributable to another cause.

Kawasaki disease manifests in three phases: acute, subacute, and convalescent. The **acute phase** begins with abrupt onset of a high fever that is unresponsive to antibiotics and antipyretics. The remaining diagnostic symptoms evolve over the next week or so. Symptoms may come and go and do not need to be present simultaneously for diagnosis, although the fever is generally persistent throughout. During this stage, the child is typically very irritable. Laboratory tests may demonstrate an elevated white blood cell count, elevated liver function tests, and elevated markers of inflammation (ESR and CRP). Of note, the platelet count is initially normal, rising in the second week of illness. Patients may also present with sterile pyuria, hydrops of the gallbladder, and/or aseptic meningitis. The **subacute phase** begins with resolution of the fever and lasts until all clinical signs of Kawasaki disease have disappeared. During this phase, coronary artery aneurysms may become evident, and previously dilated vessels may continue to increase in size. Irritability persists during this phase. Lab work shows a normochromic, normocytic anemia as well as thrombocytosis. Inflammatory markers start to resolve (after intravenous immunoglobulin [IVIG] treatment, ESR is no longer an accurate marker of inflammation, as it is raised by IVIG, and therefore CRP is favored). In the **convalescent phase**, all clinical signs of Kawasaki disease have resolved, and laboratory values are returning to normal. The entire illness lasts 6 to 8 weeks until the child has regained his or her usual temperament, energy, and appetite and all blood tests are back to normal.

BOX 23.12 Diagnostic Criteria for Kawasaki Disease

Classic Kawasaki disease criteria include fever for 5 calendar days along with four of five clinical criteria[a] (diagnosis may be made on day 4 of fever by an experienced clinician in children with fever and more than four clinical criteria):

1. Changes in the extremities: In the acute phase, edema or erythema of the palms and soles; in the subacute phase, periungual desquamation (peeling) of the hands and feet
2. Bilateral conjunctival injection (inflammation) without exudation
3. Changes in the oral mucous membranes, such as erythema, cracking of the lips, oropharyngeal reddening; or "strawberry tongue" (large papillae are exposed)
4. Rash: Maculopapular, diffuse erythroderma, or erythema multiforme-like
5. Cervical lymphadenopathy (typically unilateral >1.5 cm)

[a]Incomplete Kawasaki disease should be considered in situations of prolonged fever (see algorithm for incomplete Kawasaki disease from American Heart Association guidelines). Kawasaki disease can be diagnosed with fewer clinical criteria when coronary artery changes are noted.

Adapted from McCrindle, B. W., Rowley, A. H., Newburger, J. W., et al. (2017). Diagnosis, treatment, and long-term management of Kawasaki disease: A scientific statement for health professionals from the American Heart Association. *Circulation, 135*(17), e927–e999.

Cardiac Involvement

Long-term complications of Kawasaki disease include the development of coronary artery aneurysms, potentially disrupting blood flow to the heart. Children with large (giant) aneurysms have a risk of myocardial infarction, resulting from thrombotic occlusion of a coronary aneurysm or late-stenosis and occlusion of the affected vessel.

Affected coronary arteries may dilate progressively over the initial few weeks of illness, reaching their maximal diameter approximately 4 to 6 weeks from the onset of fever. Over years, as the damaged vessel tries to heal, stenosis of the aneurysm may develop and may lead to myocardial ischemia. The vast majority of the morbidity in Kawasaki disease occurs in children affected with the largest aneurysms (giant aneurysms >8 mm or z-score >10). The actual mortality is low (<0.1% in Japan). Symptoms of acute myocardial infarction in young children can be confusing and may include abdominal pain, vomiting, restlessness, inconsolable crying, pallor, and shock, as well as chest pain or pressure (noted more often in older children). Cardiac involvement in the initial phase of the illness may also include effects related to inflammation of the myocardium, including myocarditis, valvulitis, or arrhythmias.

Echocardiograms are used to assess coronary artery dilation, monitoring coronary artery dimensions during the initial illness as well as myocardial and valvar function. A baseline echocardiogram should be obtained at the time of diagnosis and is then used for comparison with future studies. Follow-up echocardiograms should be obtained approximately 1 week after the initial diagnosis and again 4 to 6 weeks later in uncomplicated patients. Additional echocardiograms should be done (often as frequently as twice a week) in situations where a child has coronary artery dilation or obvious aneurysm formation or when response to treatment is incomplete.

Therapeutic Management

The current treatment of children with Kawasaki disease includes the administration of high-dose IVIG along with salicylate therapy. IVIG has been demonstrated to be effective at reducing the incidence of coronary artery abnormalities when given within the first 10 days of the illness and ideally in the first 7 days of illness. A single infusion of IVIG, 2 g/kg over 10 to 12 hours, is recommended. Retreatment with IVIG and/or other antiinflammatory drugs should be given to patients who have an incomplete response to the initial IVIG (those with continued or recrudescent fever 36 hours after the end of the initial IVIG infusion) or those with coronary artery dilation (McCrindle et al., 2017).

Aspirin has been used historically to control fever and symptoms of inflammation. Initial doses of aspirin have ranged from moderate to high dose (30 to 50 mg/kg/day in divided doses every 6 hours up to 80 to 100 mg/kg/day in divided doses every 6 hours). The use of aspirin is not associated with a decrease in the incidence of coronary aneurysms. After the patient is afebrile for 48 to 72 hours, aspirin can be reduced to an antiplatelet dose (3 to 5 mg/kg/day). Low-dose aspirin is continued in patients without echocardiographic evidence of coronary abnormalities until the platelet count has returned to normal (6 to 8 weeks) (McCrindle et al., 2017). If the child develops coronary abnormalities, salicylate therapy is continued indefinitely. Additional antithrombotic medications (e.g., clopidogrel [Plavix], enoxaparin [Lovenox], or warfarin) are added for children with coronary artery aneurysms depending on the size of the CAA.

Prognosis

Most children with Kawasaki disease recover fully after treatment. However, when cardiovascular complications occur, serious morbidity may result. The prognosis for patients is strongly related to the extent of coronary damage, with patients who have giant aneurysms being at the highest risk for complications and those with normal coronary dimensions having an excellent long-term prognosis.

QUALITY PATIENT OUTCOMES: Kawasaki Disease
- Early diagnosis and treatment
- Prevention of cardiovascular complications

Nursing Care Management

In the initial phase, the nurse must monitor the child's cardiac status carefully. Intake and output and daily weight measurements are recorded. Fluids are administered with care because of the usual finding of myocarditis. The child should be assessed frequently for signs of HF, including decreased urinary output, gallop rhythm (an additional heart sound), tachycardia, and respiratory distress.

Administration of IVIG should follow the same guidelines as for any blood product, with frequent monitoring of vital signs. Generally, IVIG rates are titrated up per individual hospital protocols. During the infusion and in the few days after, patients must be watched for reactions to this medication, which may include fever, headache, and nausea. Cardiac status must be monitored because of the large volume being administered to patients who may have diminished left ventricular function.

The majority of nursing care in the hospital focuses on symptomatic relief. To minimize skin discomfort, cool cloths; unscented lotions; and soft, loose clothing are helpful. During the acute phase, mouth care, including lubricating ointment to the lips, is important for mucosal inflammation. Clear liquids and soft foods can be offered.

Patient irritability and mood swings are pervasive in KD. During hospitalization, these children need a quiet environment that promotes adequate rest. Their parents need to be supported in their efforts to comfort an often inconsolable child. They may need time away from their child, and nurses can often provide respite care for the family. Parents need to understand that irritability is a hallmark of Kawasaki disease and that it will resolve. They need not feel guilty or embarrassed about their child's behavior.

Discharge Teaching

Parents need accurate information about the course of the illness, including the importance of follow-up monitoring and when they should contact their practitioner. Irritability may persist for up to 2 months after the onset of symptoms. Periungual desquamation (peeling of the hands and feet) begins in the second and third weeks. Usually the fingertips peel first, followed by the toes and feet. The peeling is painless, but the new skin may be tender. A temporary arthritis may occur in Kawasaki disease, involving the small joints initially but possibly also affecting the larger weight-bearing joints. Affected children are typically most stiff in the mornings, during cold weather, and after naps. Passive range-of-motion exercises in the bathtub are often helpful in increasing flexibility. Any live immunizations (e.g., measles, mumps, and rubella; varicella) should be deferred for 11 months after the administration of IVIG because the body might not produce the appropriate amount of antibodies to provide lifelong immunity. Daily temperatures should be recorded in the first week or two after discharge, and the occurrence of fever should be communicated to the health care provider, as continuing fever warrants evaluation and further treatment.

Parents of children with large or giant aneurysms should be educated on the unlikely but real possibility of myocardial infarction, as well as the signs and symptoms of cardiac ischemia in a child. CPR should be taught to parents of children with coronary artery aneurysms.

Long-Term Follow-Up

The frequency and type of follow-up are based on the presence or absence of coronary damage. The long-term outlook for children without aneurysms is excellent, and therefore long-term cardiology follow-up is no longer indicated in this group of patients (McCrindle et al., 2017). These patients should have a cholesterol screen performed at routine physical examinations as per the general population; routine BP monitoring; and education recommending a heart-healthy lifestyle, including exercise, a heart-healthy diet, and avoidance of smoking.

In patients with aneurysms, cardiology follow-up is necessary. The frequency of cardiology follow-up as well as the use of long-term antithrombotic therapy is based on the largest abnormal coronary dimension with patients classified according to the American Heart Association risk levels (McCrindle et al., 2017). Noninvasive coronary imaging (e.g., echocardiography, ECGs, and stress testing to assess for reversible ischemia) is used as much as possible, with other forms of imaging, such as low-radiation cardiac computed tomography, cardiac MRI, and cardiac angiography, recommended based on individual symptoms as well as the classification of risk according to the American Heart Association (McCrindle et al., 2017).

In addition to regular monitoring, patients with coronary aneurysms may require long-term antiplatelet or anticoagulation and possibly beta-blocker therapy or other therapies, depending on the severity of coronary involvement.

MULTISYSTEM INFLAMMATORY SYNDROME

Multisystem Inflammatory Syndrome in children (MIS-C) is associated with coronavirus disease (COVID-19) and causes different body systems to become inflamed, including the heart, lungs, kidneys, brain, skin, eyes, or gastrointestinal organs (Dufort, Koumans, Chow, et al., 2020). Many children have fever and mucocutaneous lesions similar to Kawasaki's disease; however, MIS-C is associated with more cardiovascular involvement.

Pathophysiology

Little is known about the pathophysiology of MIS-C. It is felt that MIS-C is a consequence of immune-mediated injury triggered by COVID-19 (Feldstein, Rose, Horwitz, et al., 2020).

Clinical Manifestations

The Centers for Disease Control (2020) describes MIS-C in children less than 21 years of age using the following criteria:

- Fever ≥38.0° C for ≥24 hours or report of subjective fever lasting ≥24 hours
- Laboratory evidence of inflammation including, but not limited to, one or more of the following: an elevated C-reactive protein (CRP), erythrocyte sedimentation rate (ESR), fibrinogen, procalcitonin, d-dimer, ferritin, lactic acid dehydrogenase (LDH), or interleukin 6 (IL-6), elevated neutrophils, reduced lymphocytes and low albumin
- Evidence of clinically severe illness requiring hospitalization, with multisystem (≥2) organ involvement (cardiac, renal, respiratory, hematologic, gastrointestinal, dermatologic or neurological)
- No alternative plausible diagnoses
- Positive for current or recent COVID-19 infection documented by reverse-transcriptase polymerase chain reaction (RT-PCR), serology, or antigen test; or COVID-19 exposure within the 4 weeks prior to the onset of symptoms

Therapeutic Management

Since MIS-C is a new syndrome in children numerous treatment options are being investigated. Some aspects of MIS-C management are similar to the therapeutic management of Kawasaki disease (see p....). Intravenous immune globulin and systemic glucocorticoids are given (Whittaker, Bamford, Kenny, et al., 2020). Antiviral agents are being explored during the acute stage of the illness. Many children with MIS-C require mechanical ventilation and some receive extracorporeal membrane oxygenation (ECMO) support (Feldstein, Rose, Horwitz, et al., 2020).

Until more is known about long-term cardiac sequelae of MIS-C, providers should consider following Kawasaki's disease guidelines for follow-up. Long-term monitoring for other potential sequelae of MIS-C will also be critical (Whittaker, Bamford, Kenny, et al., 2020).

Nursing Care Management

Caring for a child with MIS-C is similar to the care of a critically ill child with Kawasaki's disease (see p. 764).

SHOCK

Shock, or **circulatory failure**, is a complex clinical syndrome characterized by inadequate tissue perfusion to meet the metabolic demands of the body, resulting in cellular dysfunction and eventual organ failure. Although the causes are different, the physiologic consequences are the same and include hypotension, tissue hypoxia, and metabolic acidosis. Circulatory failure in children is a result of hypovolemia, altered peripheral vascular resistance, or pump failure. Types of shock and their clinical signs are listed in Table 23.7.

Pathophysiology

A healthy child's circulatory system is able to transport oxygen and metabolic substrates to body tissues, which require a constant source for these essential needs. The cardiac output and distribution to the various body tissues can change rapidly in response to intrinsic (myocardial and intravascular) or extrinsic (neuronal) control mechanisms. In shock states, these mechanisms are altered or challenged.

Reduced blood flow, as in hypovolemic shock, causes diminished venous return to the heart, low CVP, low cardiac output, and hypotension. Vasomotor centers in the medulla are signaled, causing a compensatory increase in the force and rate of cardiac contraction and constriction of arterioles and veins, thereby increasing peripheral vascular resistance. Simultaneously, the lowered blood volume leads to the release of large amounts of catecholamines, antidiuretic hormone, adrenocorticosteroids, and aldosterone in an effort to conserve body fluids. This causes reduced blood flow to the skin, kidneys, muscles, and viscera to shunt the available blood to the brain and heart. Consequently, the skin feels cold and clammy, there is poor capillary filling, and glomerular filtration rate and urinary output are significantly reduced.

As a result of impaired perfusion, oxygen is depleted in the tissue cells, causing them to revert to anaerobic metabolism, producing lactic acidosis. The acidosis places an extra burden on the lungs as

TABLE 23.7 Clinical Signs of Shock

Clinical Signs	Hypovolemic Shock	Distributive Shock	Cardiogenic Shock	Obstructive Shock
Respiratory rate	Normal to increased	Normal to increased	Labored	Labored
Breath sounds	Normal	Normal (crackles may or may not be present)	Crackles, grunting	Crackles, grunting
Systolic blood pressure	Compensated-normal	Compensated-normal	Hypotensive-low	Hypotensive-low
Pulse pressure	Narrow	Variable	Narrow	Narrow
Heart rate	Tachycardia	Tachycardia	Tachycardia	
Peripheral pulses	Weak	Bounding or weak	Weak	
Skin	Pale, cool	Warm or cool	Pale, cool	
Capillary refill	Delayed (>2 sec)	Variable	Delayed (>2 sec)	
Urine output	Decreased (<1 ml/kg/h [<30 kg; 66 pounds]; <30-50 ml/kg/h [>30 kg, 66 pounds])			
Level of consciousness	Irritable early	Late, lethargic		

Adapted from American Heart Association. (2016). Pediatric advanced life support (PALS) provider manual. Dallas, TX: American Heart Association.

they attempt to compensate for the metabolic acidosis by increasing the respiratory rate to remove excess carbon dioxide. Prolonged vasoconstriction results in fatigue and atony of the peripheral arterioles, which leads to vessel dilation. Venules, which are less sensitive to vasodilator substances, remain constricted for a time, causing massive pooling in the capillary and venular beds, which further depletes blood volume.

Complications of shock create further hazards. CNS hypoperfusion eventually may lead to cerebral edema, cortical infarction, or intraventricular hemorrhage. Renal hypoperfusion causes renal ischemia with possible tubular or glomerular necrosis and renal vein thrombosis. Reduced blood flow to the lungs can interfere with surfactant secretion and result in acute respiratory distress syndrome, which is characterized by sudden pulmonary congestion and atelectasis with formation of a hyaline membrane. Gastrointestinal tract bleeding and perforation are always possibilities after splanchnic ischemia and necrosis of intestinal mucosa. Metabolic complications of shock may include hypoglycemia, hypocalcemia, and other electrolyte disturbances.

Clinical Manifestations

Shock can be regarded as a form of compensation for circulatory failure and, because of its progressive nature, can be divided into two stages or phases: **compensated** and **hypotensive** (previously referred to as decompensated). Cardiac arrest represents irreversible shock. At all stages the principal differentiating signs are the degree of tachycardia and perfusion to extremities, the level of consciousness, and BP. Additional signs or modifications of these more universal signs may be present, depending on the type and cause of the shock. Initially, the child's ability to compensate is effective; therefore early signs are subtle. As the shock state advances, signs are more obvious and indicate early decompensation (Box 23.13).

BOX 23.13 Clinical Manifestations of Shock

Compensated
Apprehensiveness
Irritability
Unexplained tachycardia
Normal blood pressure (BP)
Narrowing pulse pressure
Thirst
Pallor
Diminished urinary output
Reduced perfusion of extremities

Hypotensive
Confusion and somnolence
Tachypnea
Moderate metabolic acidosis
Oliguria
Cool, pale extremities
Decreased skin turgor
Poor capillary filling

Irreversible
Thready, weak pulse
Hypotension
Periodic breathing or apnea
Anuria
Stupor or coma

Compensated Shock

When vital organ function is maintained by intrinsic mechanisms and the child's ability to compensate is effective, cardiac output and systemic arterial BP are usually normal or increased. However, blood flow is generally uneven or maldistributed in the microcirculation. Early clinical signs are subtle and include apprehension, irritability, normal BP, narrowing pulse pressure, thirst, pallor, and diminished urinary output.

> **! NURSING ALERT**
>
> Unexplained mild tachycardia and a decrease in perfusion of the hands and feet are differentiating features of compensated shock.

Hypotensive (Decompensated) Shock

As shock progresses, perfusion in the microcirculation becomes marginal despite compensatory adjustments, and the signs are more obvious and indicate early decompensation. These signs are tachypnea; moderate metabolic acidosis; oliguria; and cool, pale extremities with decreased skin turgor and poor capillary filling. Hypotensive shock may be differentiated from compensated shock by evaluating BP; the child in hypotensive shock will have a low BP, but hypotension is a late finding. Another clinical sign of hypotensive shock is a change in level of consciousness as brain perfusion declines. The outcomes of circulatory failure that progress beyond the limits of compensation are tissue hypoxia, metabolic acidosis, and eventual dysfunction of all organ systems

> **! NURSING ALERT**
>
> In hypotensive shock, tachycardia is pronounced and pulse pressure (difference between systolic and diastolic blood pressure) becomes narrowed. There is poor capillary filling, and the child exhibits confusion, sleepiness, and decreased responsiveness.

As hypotensive shock progresses along a physiologic continuum, clinical signs indicate a progression of circulatory damage. With the progression of shock, there is damage to vital organs (e.g., the heart or brain) of such magnitude that the entire system is disrupted regardless of therapeutic intervention. There is pronounced systemic vasoconstriction and hypoxia of visceral and cutaneous circulations with hypotension, acidosis, lethargy or coma, and oliguria or anuria. The child is totally obtunded. A thready and weak pulse, hypotension, periodic breathing or apnea, anuria, and stupor or coma are signs of impending cardiac arrest. Death occurs even if cardiovascular measurements return to normal levels with therapy.

> **! NURSING ALERT**
>
> Hypotension is a late and poor prognostic sign of shock, so signs of shock must be recognized and appropriate interventions implemented before hypotension is evident.

At all stages, the principal differentiating signs are observed in the (1) degree of tachycardia and perfusion to the extremities, (2) level of consciousness, and (3) BP. Additional signs or modifications of these more universal signs may be present depending on the type and cause of the shock. Initially, the child's ability to compensate is effective; therefore early signs are subtle. As the shock state advances, signs are more obvious and indicate early decompensation.

Additional signs may be present, depending on the type and cause of the shock. In early septic shock, there are chills, fever, and vasodilation, with increased cardiac output that results in warm, flushed skin (hyperdynamic, or "warm" shock). A later and ominous development is disseminated intravascular coagulation (DIC) (see Chapter 24), the major hematologic complication of septic shock. Anaphylactic shock is frequently accompanied by urticaria and angioneurotic edema, which is life threatening when it involves the respiratory passages (see Anaphylaxis later in the chapter).

Laboratory tests that assist in assessment are blood gas measurements, pH, and sometimes liver function tests. Coagulation tests are evaluated when there is evidence of bleeding, such as oozing from a venipuncture site, bleeding from any orifice, or petechiae. Cultures of blood and other sites are indicated when there is a high suspicion of sepsis. Renal function tests are performed when impaired renal function is evident.

Therapeutic Management

Treatment of shock consists of three major interventions: (1) oxygenation and ventilation, (2) fluid administration, and (3) improvement of the pumping action of the heart (vasopressor support). The priority is to establish an airway and administer oxygen. After the airway is ensured, circulatory stabilization is the major concern. Establishment of adequate IV access, ideally with multilumen central lines, is essential to deliver fluids and medications.

Oxygenation and Ventilatory Support

The lung is the organ most sensitive to shock. Decreased distribution or redistribution of blood flow to respiratory muscles plus the increased work of breathing can rapidly lead to respiratory failure. Supplemental oxygen is always given as soon as possible. Critically ill patients are unable to maintain an adequate airway. To place the lung at rest and improve ventilation, endotracheal intubation is initiated early with positive-pressure ventilation and oxygen. Blood gases, oxygen saturation (using pulse oximetry), and pH are monitored frequently.

Increased extravascular lung water caused by edema contributes to the development of respiratory complications. Therapy is directed toward maintaining normal arterial blood gas measurements, normal acid-base balance, and circulation. Efforts are made to remove fluid and prevent its accumulation with the use of diuretics.

Cardiovascular Support

In many cases, rapid restoration of blood volume is the main therapy needed in the resuscitation of the child in shock. An isotonic crystalloid solution (0.9% normal saline or lactated Ringer solution) is usually the first choice for fluid replacement. Crystalloid is given in IV boluses of 20 ml/kg over 5 to 20 minutes and repeated as necessary. Blood products may also be given if acute blood loss is the cause of hypovolemia. The child's response is assessed after each bolus. An increase in BP and a decrease in heart rate indicate successful resuscitation. An increased cardiac output results in improved capillary circulation and skin color. Colloids (protein-containing fluids) are often administered to children in shock; albumin is the most common. Because albumin is a protein solution, it remains in the vascular space much longer than crystalloid fluids.

For the critically ill child with shock and multisystem organ dysfunction, more aggressive monitoring is necessary. CVP measurements of right atrial pressure help guide fluid therapy, and urinary output measurement is an important indicator of adequacy of circulation. Correction of acidosis, hypoxemia, hypoglycemia, hypothermia, and any metabolic derangements is mandatory.

Temporary pharmacologic support may be required to enhance myocardial contractility, reverse metabolic or respiratory acidosis, and maintain arterial pressure. The principal agents used to improve cardiac output and circulation are catecholamines, such as dopamine (Intropin) and epinephrine (Adrenalin). Dopamine is the preferred drug in most situations because it also improves renal perfusion. Metabolic acidosis is usually corrected with adequate tissue perfusion and improved renal function. This is accomplished with adequate ventilatory support, including oxygen, and restoration of blood volume and peripheral circulation

QUALITY PATIENT OUTCOMES: Shock

- Oxygen content of blood optimized
- Cardiac output improved
- Oxygen demand reduced
- Metabolic abnormalities corrected
- Type of shock identified and treated

Nursing Care Management

The child who is in shock requires intensive observation and care. The initial action is to ensure adequate tissue oxygenation. The nurse should be prepared to administer oxygen by the appropriate route and to assist with any intubation and ventilatory procedures indicated. Other procedures and activities that require immediate attention are establishing an IV line, weighing the child, obtaining baseline vital signs, placing an indwelling catheter, obtaining blood gases and other measurements, and administering fluids and medications as indicated. The child is best positioned flat with the legs elevated.

! NURSING ALERT

Early clinical signs of shock include apprehension, irritability, normal blood pressure (BP), narrowing pulse pressure (difference between diastolic and systolic BP), thirst, pallor, diminished urinary output, unexplained mild tachycardia, and decreased perfusion of the hands and feet.

The nurse's responsibilities are to monitor the IV infusion, intake and output, vital signs (including CVP), and general systems assessments on a routine basis. IV medications are titrated according to patient responses, and vital signs are taken every 15 minutes during the critical periods and thereafter as needed. Urinary output is measured hourly; blood gases, hematocrit, pH, and electrolytes are monitored frequently to assess the child's status and the efficacy of therapy. An apnea and cardiac monitor and pulse oximeter is attached and monitored continuously. In the initial stages of acute shock, more than one nurse is often needed to manage the necessary activities that must be carried out simultaneously (see Emergency Treatment box).

EMERGENCY TREATMENT

Shock

Ventilation

Establish airway; be prepared for intubation.
Administer 100% oxygen.

Fluid Administration

Restore fluid volume as ordered via intravenous (IV) lines.

Cardiovascular Support

Administer inotropes and vasopressors as ordered.

General Support

Keep child flat with legs raised above level of heart.
Keep child warm and calm.

Throughout the intense activity, support for the family must not be overlooked. Someone should contact family members at frequent intervals to inform them of what is being done and whether there is any progress. Ideally, someone should remain with the parents to serve as a liaison between them and the intensive care team. However, this is not always feasible in such a critical situation. As soon as possible, the family should be allowed to see the child. A member of the clergy or a social worker may be called to help provide comfort and support.

ANAPHYLAXIS

Anaphylaxis is the acute clinical syndrome resulting from the interaction of an allergen and a patient who is hypersensitive to that allergen. When the antigen enters the circulatory system, a generalized reaction rapidly takes place, and chemical substances, primarily histamine, are released from mast cells and cause vasodilation, bronchoconstriction, and increased capillary permeability.

Severe reactions are immediate in onset; are often life threatening; and frequently involve multiple systems, primarily the cardiovascular, respiratory, gastrointestinal, and integumentary systems. Exposure to the antigen can be by ingestion, inhalation, skin contact, or injection. Examples of common allergens associated with anaphylaxis include drugs (e.g., antibiotics, chemotherapeutic agents, radiologic contrast media), latex, foods, venom from bees or snakes, and biologic agents (antisera, enzymes, hormones, blood products).

> **! NURSING ALERT**
>
> Penicillin allergy is associated with immediate onset (within 1 hour of administration) or accelerated onset (1 to 72 hours after administration) of skin eruption, especially an urticarial rash, or more serious symptoms such as laryngeal edema or anaphylactic shock.

Clinical Manifestations

The onset of clinical symptoms usually occurs within seconds or minutes of exposure to the antigen, and the rapidity of the reaction is directly related to its intensity: the sooner the onset, the more severe the reaction. The reaction may be preceded by symptoms of uneasiness, restlessness, irritability, severe anxiety, headache, dizziness, paresthesia, and disorientation. The patient may lose consciousness. Cutaneous signs of flushing and urticaria are common early signs followed by angioedema, most notable in the eyelids, lips, tongue, hands, feet, and genitalia.

Bronchiolar constriction may follow, causing narrowing of the airway; pulmonary edema and hemorrhage also may occur. Laryngeal edema with severe acute upper airway obstruction may be life threatening and requires rapid intervention. Shock occurs as a result of mediator-induced vasodilation, which causes capillary permeability and loss of intravascular fluid into the interstitial space. Sudden hypotension and impaired cardiac output with poor perfusion are seen.

Therapeutic Management

Successful outcome of anaphylactic reactions depends on rapid recognition and institution of treatment. The goals of treatment are to provide ventilation, restore adequate circulation, and prevent further exposure by identifying and removing the cause when possible.

A mild reaction with no evidence of respiratory distress or cardiovascular compromise can be managed with subcutaneous administration of antihistamines, such as diphenhydramine (Benadryl) and epinephrine.

Moderate or severe distress presents a potentially life-threatening emergency. Establishing an airway is the first concern, as with all shock states. Epinephrine is given subcutaneously or intravenously as an antihistamine and to support the cardiovascular system and increase BP. Other routes for giving epinephrine are intramuscular and via the airway, either nebulized or injected through an endotracheal tube. In severe anaphylaxis, epinephrine by any route is better than none. Fluids are given to restore blood volume. Additional vasopressors may be given to improve cardiac output. A **biphasic reaction** may occur within 4 hours after symptoms have originally subsided, so it is important to monitor the child closely for this reaction (Sampson, Wang, & Sicherer, 2020).

Prevention of a reaction is preferable. Preventing exposure is more easily accomplished in children known to be at risk, including those with (1) a history of previous allergic reaction to a specific antigen; (2) a history of atopy; (3) a history of severe reactions in immediate family members; and (4) a reaction to a skin test, although skin tests are not available for all allergens. Desensitization may be recommended in certain cases.

> **QUALITY PATIENT OUTCOMES: Anaphylaxis**
>
> - Early recognition of symptoms
> - Airway patency maintained
> - Adequate circulation restored and maintained
> - Further exposure to allergic agent prevented

Nursing Care Management

Major nursing responsibilities in anaphylaxis include anticipating which children are likely to develop a reaction, recognizing the early signs, and intervening appropriately. When an anaphylactic reaction is suspected, nursing responsibilities include immediate intervention and preparation for medical therapy. If emergency supplies such as epinephrine are not immediately available, emergency medical services should be accessed. Ventilation is ensured by placing the child in a head-elevated position, unless contraindicated by hypotension, to facilitate breathing and administer oxygen. If the child is not breathing, CPR is initiated and emergency medical services are summoned.

If the cause can be determined, measures are implemented to slow the spread of the offending substance. An IV infusion is established immediately. Emergency medications are given intravenously whenever possible; however, epinephrine may be given intramuscularly (see Drug Alert box). Vital signs and urinary output are monitored frequently. Medications are administered as prescribed, with regular assessment to monitor effectiveness and to detect signs of side effects of medication and fluid overload.

> **DRUG ALERT**
>
> ***Epinephrine***
>
> Intramuscular administration of epinephrine (0.01 mg/kg up to 0.3 mg) is the first line of therapy, and administration should never be delayed. Two premixed preparations are available: EpiPen Jr (0.15 mg) for children 8 to 25 kg (3.5 to 11.25 pounds) and EpiPen (0.3 mg) for children over 25 kg (11.25 pounds). As in any shock state, the airway is the first concern, followed by assessment of breathing and then circulation (ABCs).

To prevent an anaphylactic reaction, parents are always asked about possible allergic responses to foods, latex, medications, and environmental conditions. These are displayed prominently on the patient's chart. The specific allergen is noted, as are the type and severity of the reaction. Parents are excellent historians, especially when the child has displayed a pronounced reaction to a substance. Drugs, including related drugs (e.g., penicillin, nafcillin), and other items, such as latex, that have produced a reaction previously are never used. If the child is allergic to insect venom, the family is instructed to purchase an emergency kit to keep with the child at all times. Both the family and the child, if the child is old enough, are taught how to use the equipment. The patient should carry medical identification at all times.

SEPTIC SHOCK

Sepsis and septic shock are caused by infectious organisms. Normally, an infection triggers an inflammatory response in a local area, which results in vasodilation, increased capillary permeability, and eventually elimination of the infectious agent. The widespread activation and systemic release of inflammatory mediators is called the **systemic inflammatory response syndrome (SIRS)**. Box 23.14 provides the exact definitions for SIRS, infection, sepsis, and severe sepsis (Weiss, Peters, Alhazzani, et al., 2020). SIRS can occur in response to both infectious and noninfectious (e.g., trauma, burns) causes. When caused by infection, it is called **sepsis**. Septic shock is defined as sepsis with organ dysfunction and hypotension.

Most of the physiologic effects of shock occur because the exaggerated immune response triggers more than 30 different mediators that result in diffuse vasodilation, increased capillary permeability, and maldistribution of blood flow. This impairs oxygen and nutrient delivery to the cells, resulting in cellular dysfunction. If the process continues, multiple-organ dysfunction occurs and may result in death. Although the incidence of shock continues to be on the increase, survival rate due to early detection and treatment improves (Martin, 2012).

Three stages have been identified in septic shock. In early septic shock, the patient has chills, fever, and vasodilation with increased cardiac output, which results in warm, flushed skin that reflects vascular tone abnormalities and hyperdynamic, warm, or hyperdynamic-compensated responses. BP and urinary output are normal. The patient has the best chance for survival in this stage. The second stage—the normodynamic, cool, or hyperdynamic-decompensated stage—lasts only a few hours. The skin is cool, but pulses and BP are still normal. Urinary output diminishes, and the mental state becomes depressed. With advancing disease, certain signs of circulatory decompensation that deteriorate to signs of circulatory collapse are indistinguishable from late shock of any cause. In the hypodynamic, or cold, stage of shock, cardiovascular function progressively deteriorates even with aggressive therapy. The patient has hypothermia, cold extremities, weak pulses, hypotension, and oliguria or anuria. Patients are severely lethargic or comatose. Multiorgan failure is common. This is the most dangerous stage of shock.

Management of septic shock involves measures to provide hemodynamic stability and adequate oxygenation to the tissues and the use of antimicrobials to treat the infectious organism. As with other forms of shock, hemodynamic stability is achieved with fluid volume resuscitation and inotropic agents as needed. Providing adequate oxygenation often requires intubation and mechanical ventilation, supplemental oxygen, sedation, and paralysis to decrease the work of breathing. Septic shock involves activation of complement proteins that promote clumping of the granulocytes in the lung. The granulocytes can release chemicals that can cause direct lung injury to the pulmonary capillary endothelium. This causes a fluid leak into the alveoli, which causes stiff, noncompliant lungs. DIC and multiorgan dysfunction may also occur and require prompt assessment and management.

BOX 23.14 Definitions of Systemic Inflammatory Response Syndrome, Infection, and Septic Shock

Systemic inflammatory response syndrome (SIRS): The presence of at least two of the following four criteria, one of which must be abnormal temperature or leukocyte count:

1. Core temperature of more than 38.5°C (101.3°F) or less than 36°C (96.8°F)
2. Tachycardia, defined as a mean heart rate more than two standard deviations above normal for age in the absence of external stimulus, chronic drugs, or painful stimuli; or otherwise unexplained persistent elevation over a 0.5- to 4-hour period; or, for children younger than 1 year old, bradycardia, defined as a mean heart rate below the 10th percentile for age in the absence of external vagal stimulus, beta-blocker drugs, or CHD; or otherwise unexplained persistent depression over a 0.5-hour period
3. Mean respiratory rate more than two standard deviations above normal for age or mechanical ventilation for an acute process not related to underlying neuromuscular disease or the receipt of general anesthesia
4. Leukocyte count elevated or depressed for age (not secondary to chemotherapy-induced leukopenia) or more than 10% immature neutrophils

Infection: A suspected or proven (by positive culture, tissue stain, or PCR test) infection caused by any pathogen; or a clinical syndrome associated with a high probability of infection. Evidence of infection includes positive findings on clinical examination, imaging, or laboratory tests (e.g., white blood cells in a normally sterile body fluid, perforated viscus, chest radiograph consistent with pneumonia, petechial or purpuric rash, or purpura fulminans).

Septic Shock: Severe infection leading to cardiovascular dysfunction (including hypotension, need for treatment with a vasoactive medication, or impaired perfusion) and organ dysfunction in children as severe infection leading to cardiovascular and/or noncardiovascular organ dysfunction.

CHD, Congenital heart disease; *PCR,* polymerase chain reaction.
Adapted from Weiss, S.L., Peters, M.J., Alhazzani, W., et al. (2020). Surviving Sepsis Campaign International Guidelines for the Management of Septic Shock and Sepsis-Associated Organ Dysfunction in Children. *Pediatric Critical Care Medicine, 21*(2); e53-e106; Goldstein, B., Giroir, B., Randolph, A., et al. (2005). International Pediatric Sepsis Consensus Conference: Definitions for sepsis and organ dysfunction in pediatrics. *Pediatric Critical Care Medicine, 6*(1), 2–8.

Newer therapies are being developed to modify the host immune response by attempting to block various mediators, thereby interrupting the inflammatory cascade. Evidence-based management protocols for the management of adult and pediatric septic shock have recently been published (de Caen, Berg, Chameides, et al., 2015; Weiss, Peters, Alhazzani, et al., 2020).

Early identification of the symptoms of septic shock and starting antimicrobial therapy as soon as possible (within 1 hour of recognition) is critical to patient survival (Weiss, Peters, Alhazzani, et al., 2020). A high index of suspicion is required in all critically ill patients who are at greater risk for sepsis because of multiple invasive lines and devices, poor nutrition, and impaired immune function. Subtle alterations in tissue perfusion and unexplained tachypnea and tachycardia often are early warning signs. Identification of the infectious agent and prompt treatment are also critical to patient survival. Broad-spectrum antibiotics should be given, and the site of infection should be removed if possible (e.g., drain abscesses, remove indwelling lines). Patients should be managed in an ICU in which continuous monitoring and sophisticated cardiac and respiratory support are available. Multidisciplinary collaboration is essential in managing these critically ill patients.

BOX 23.15 Criteria for Definition of *Staphylococcus aureus* Toxic Shock Syndrome

Fever of 38.9°C (102°F) or higher
Presence of diffuse macular erythroderma
Desquamation, particularly of palms and soles, 1 to 2 weeks after onset of illness
Hypotension, defined as a systolic blood pressure of 90 mm Hg or less for adults, and below the 5th percentile for children younger than 16 years old; or an orthostatic drop in diastolic blood pressure of 15 mm Hg or more with a change from lying to sitting; or orthostatic syncope; or orthostatic dizziness
Involvement of three or more of the following organ systems: GI, muscular, mucous membrane, renal, hepatic, hematologic, or CNS
Toxic shock syndrome is probable when four of the five major criteria are fulfilled. In addition, if blood and cerebrospinal fluid cultures are obtained, they must be negative for any organisms other than *S. aureus*. Serologic tests for Rocky Mountain spotted fever, leptospirosis, and measles also must be negative.

CNS, Central nervous system; *GI*, gastrointestinal.
Adapted from Wharton, M., Chorba, T. L., Vogt, R. L., et al. (1990). Case definitions for public health surveillance. *MMWR Recommendations and Reports, 39*(RR-13), 1–43.

TOXIC SHOCK SYNDROME

Toxic shock syndrome (TSS) is a relatively rare condition caused by the toxins produced by the Staphylococcus bacteria. First described in 1978, TSS can cause acute multisystem organ failure and a clinical picture that resembles septic shock. TSS became well known in 1980 because of the striking relationship between the disease and tampon use. An aggressive health education campaign about the dangers of prolonged tampon use and a change in the chemical composition of tampons have markedly reduced the incidence of TSS in menstruating women. Cases of TSS have also been reported in men, older women, and children.

Diagnostic Evaluation

Diagnosis is made based on the criteria established by the Centers for Disease Control and Prevention's toxic case definition (Box 23.15). A history of tampon use contributes to the diagnosis. Additional laboratory tests include cultures from blood, the vagina, the cervix, and any discharge. Other laboratory tests are those that facilitate the management of shock.

Therapeutic Management

The management of patients with TSS is the same as management of shock of any cause and may range from supportive care in mild cases to hospitalization and intensive care in severe cases. Appropriate parenteral antibiotics are usually administered after cultures are obtained.

Nursing Care Management

Because the disease is relatively rare, the major efforts of nursing are directed toward prevention. The association between the disease and the use of tampons provides some direction for education. Avoiding the use of tampons offers the most certain preventive measure, although this approach is probably unacceptable to most adolescent girls, who prefer the freedom, comfort, and inconspicuousness that tampons afford.

Adolescent girls who use tampons can be taught general hygiene measures, such as good hand washing and careful insertion to avoid vaginal abrasion. It is wise to modify their use, alternating with sanitary napkins—perhaps using the napkins during the night, when at home during the day, and when flow is slight. Young girls are advised not to use super-absorbent tampons and not to leave any tampon in the body for more than 4 to 6 hours.

CLINICAL JUDGMENT AND NEXT-GENERATION NCLEX® EXAMINATION-STYLE QUESTIONS

1. A nurse is working with a new graduate on the pediatric unit, and the patient is returning from the cardiac catheterization lab. The patient is a 3-year-old with a congenital heart disease who is having more symptoms related to heart failure. The nurse determines that the graduate understands the important nursing interventions when she makes which statements? **Select all that apply.**
   A. "Check pulses, especially below the catheterization site, for equality and symmetry."
   B. "Check vital signs, which may be taken as frequently as every 30 to 45 minutes, with special emphasis on the heart rate, which is counted for 1 full minute for evidence of dysrhythmias or bradycardia."
   C. "Special attention needs to be given to the BP, especially for hypertension, which may indicate hemorrhage or bleeding from the catheterization site."
   D. "Check the dressing for evidence of bleeding or hematoma formation in the femoral or antecubital area."
   E. "Allow the child to ambulate because this will prevent skin breakdown from lying so long in one place."

2. A nurse recently accepted a position in the congenital heart disease clinic at a major children's hospital. It is important for her to understand the different types of heart defects in children. In the table below, which heart defect and hemodynamic change pairing is correct? **Choose the most likely options for the information missing from the table below by selecting from the lists of options provided.**

Diagnosis	Hemodynamic change	Defect
Ventricular Septal Defect (VSD)	Higher pressure in the left ventricle pumps more blood into the lungs causing increased pulmonary vascular resistance	3
Aortic Stenosis	2	Narrowing of the aortic valve
Tricuspid Atresia	Increased pulmonary blood flow	4
1	Structures on the left side of the heart (the side which receives oxygen-rich blood from the lungs and pumps it out to the body) are severely underdeveloped	Underdeveloped left side of the heart.

Select from these options.

1	2	3 and 4
Atrial Septal Defect (ASD)	Decreased pulmonary blood flow	Abnormal opening between right and left ventricles = 3
Coarctation of the Aorta	Resistance of blood flow in the left ventricle causing decreased cardiac output	Four defects of the heart disrupt blood flow
Heart Failure	Increased pressure proximal to the defect and decreased pressure distal to the obstruction	Valve fails to develop leaving no communication from the right atrium to the right ventricle = 4
Hypoplastic Left Heart Syndrome	Blood flows from the left to right atrium causing increased flow of blood to the right side of the heart	Local narrowing near the insertion of the ductus arteriosus

3. A nurse is discharging a 5-week-old infant male with a congenital heart defect who will be going home on digoxin. The child was born prematurely, and the medication has shown beneficial effects in increasing cardiac output. The nurse is preparing the family for discharge and has spent time teaching both parents how to give digoxin to the infant. Which of the following answers by the father indicate the need for more teaching? **Select all that apply.**
   A. "If more than two doses have been missed, I should call the doctor."
   B. "If I miss a dose, I don't give an extra dose, but I give the next dose as ordered."
   C. "If the baby vomits, I should give a second dose of 10mg of the medication."
   D. I know I should give the drug carefully by slowly directing it to the side and back of the mouth."
   E. "I give the medication every 8 hours, and I can place it in a bit of formula so that I know the baby will take it."

4. A 5-year-old boy presents with symptoms that are suspicious of the acute phase of Kawasaki disease. He was playing last week with a cousin who was staying with the family. The nurse completes a history and physical assessment, and the findings are listed below. Which history and assessment findings reflect the diagnosis of Kawasaki disease? **Select all that apply.**
   A. Irritability
   B. Loud pansystolic murmur
   C. Tender, swollen abdomen
   D. Cervical lymphadenopathy
   E. Erythema of the palms and soles
   F. Bilateral conjunctival inflammation
   G. Loss of ambulation and weakened muscles
   H. Temperature over 100° F (37.8° C) for the last 5 days
   I. Inflammation of the pharynx with red, cracked lips and a "strawberry tongue"

REFERENCES

Abman, S. H., Hansmann, G., Archer, S. L., et al. (2015). Pediatric pulmonary hypertension: Guidelines from the American Heart Association and American Thoracic Society. Circulation, 132(21), 2037–2099.

Abman, S. H., & Ivy, D. D. (2011). Recent progress in understanding pediatric pulmonary hypertension. Current Opinion in Pediatrics, 23(3), 298–304.

Almond, C., Thiagarajian, R. R., Piercy, G. E., et al. (2009). Waiting list mortality among children listed for heart transplantation in the United States. Circulation, 119(5), 717–727.

Alsoufi, B., Mori, M., Gillespie, S., et al. (2015). Impact of patient characteristics and anatomy on results of Norwood operation for hypoplastic left heart syndrome. The Annals of Thoracic Surgery, 100(2), 591–598.

Barbas, K. H., & Kelleher, D. K. (2004). Breastfeeding success among infants with congenital heart disease. Pediatric Nurses, 30, 285–289.

Blume, E. D., Naftel, D. C., Bastardi, H. J., et al. (2006). Outcomes of children bridged to heart transplantation with ventricular assist devices: A multi-institutional study. Circulation, 113(19), 2313–2319.

Botto, L. D., Correa, A., & Erickson, J. D. (2001). Racial and temporal variations in the prevalence of heart defects. Pediatrics, 107(3), E32.

Boucek, M. M., Aurora, P., Edwards, L. B., et al. (2007). The registry of the International Society for Heart and Lung Transplantation: Tenth official pediatric heart transplantation report—2007. Journal of Heart and Lung Transplantation, 26(8), 796–807.

Brown, M. L., Burkhart, H. M., Connolly, H. M., et al. (2013). Coarctation of the aorta: Lifelong surveillance is mandatory following surgical repair. Journal of the American College of Cardiology, 62(11), 1020–1025.

Butera, G., Carminati, M., Chessa, M., et al. (2007). Transcatheter closure of perimembranous ventricular septal defects: Early and long-term results. Journal of the American College of Cardiology, 50(12), 1189–1195.

Cecchin, F., Frangini, P. A., Brown, D. W., et al. (2009). Cardiac resynchronization therapy (and multisite pacing) in pediatrics and congenital heart disease: Five years' experience in a single institution. Journal of Cardiovascular Electrophysiology, 20(1), 58–65.

Center for Disease Control and Prevention. (n.d.). Coronavirus Disease 2019 (Covid-19). Retrieved from https://www.cdc.gov/coronavirus/2019-ncov/. Retrieved 24 June 2020.

Cuypers, J. A., Eindhoven, J. A., Slager, M. A., et al. (2014). The natural and unnatural history of the Mustard procedure: Long-term outcome up to 40 years. European Heart Journal, 35(25), 1666–1674.

Daniels, S. R. (2012). Management of hyperlipidemia in pediatrics. Current Opinion in Cardiology, 27(2), 92–97.

de Caen, A. R., Berg, M. D., Chameides, L., et al. (2015). Part 12: Pediatric advanced life support 2015 American Heart Association guidelines update for cardiopulmonary resuscitation and emergency cardiovascular care. Circulation, 132(suppl. 2), S526–S542.

de Ferranti, S. D., Daniels, S. R., Gillman, M., et al. (2012). NHLBI Integrated guidelines on cardiovascular disease risk reduction: Can we clarify the controversy about cholesterol screening and treatment in childhood? Clinical Chemistry, 58(12), 1626–1630.

de Ferranti, S. D., Steinberger, J., Amerduri, R., et al. (2019). Cardiovascular risk reduction in high-risk pediatric patients. A scientific statement from the American Heart Association. Circulation, 139(13), e603–e634.

Dipchand, A. I., Rossano, J. W., Edwards, L. B., et al. (2015). The Registry of the International Society for Heart and Lung Transplantation: Eighteenth official pediatric heart transplantation report--2015; Focus theme: Early graft failure. Journal of Heart and Lung Transplantation, 34(10), 1233–1243.

Doyle, T., Kavanaugh-McHugh, A., & Fish, F. A. (2019). Management and outcome of tetralogy of Fallot, 2018. UpToDate. Retrieved https://www.uptodate.com/contents/management-and-outcome-of-tetralogy-of-fallot. Retrieved 13 February 2019.

Du, Z. D., Hijazi, Z. M., Kleinman, C. S., et al. (2002). Comparison between transcatheter and surgical closure of secundum atrial septal defect in children and adults: Results of a multicenter nonrandomized trial. Journal of the American College of Cardiology, 39(11), 1836–1844.

Dubin, A. M., Janousek, J., Rhee, E., et al. (2005). Resynchronization therapy in pediatric and congenital heart disease patients. Journal of the American College of Cardiology, 46(12), 2277–2283.

Dufort, E. M., Koumans, E. H., Chow, E. J., et al. (2020). Multisystem Inflammatory Syndrome in Children in New York State. The New England Journal of Medicine, 383(4), 347–358.

Everitt, M. D., Pahl, E., Schechtman, K. B., et al. (2011). Rejection with hemodynamic compromise in the current era of pediatric heart transplantation: A multi-institutional study. Journal of Heart and Lung Transplantation, 30(3), 282–288.

Expert Panel on Integrated Guidelines for Cardiovascular Health and Risk Reduction in Children and Adolescents; National Heart, Lung, and Blood Institute. (2011). Expert panel on integrated guidelines for cardiovascular health and risk reduction in children and adolescents: Summary report. Pediatrics, 128(Suppl. 5), S213–S256.

Feldstein, L. R., Rose, E. B., Horwitz, S. M., et al. (2020). Multisystem Inflammatory Syndrome in U.S. Children and Adolescents. The New England Journal of Medicine, 383(4), 334–346.

Feltes, T. F., Bacha, E., Beekman, R. H., et al. (2011). Indications for cardiac catheterization and intervention in pediatric heart disease: A scientific statement from the American Heart Association. Circulation, 123(22), 2607–2652.

Feltes, T. F., Cabalka, A. K., Meissner, H. C., et al. (2003). Palivizumab prophylaxis reduces hospitalization due to respiratory syncytial virus in young children with hemodynamically significant congenital heart disease. Journal of Pediatrics, 143, 532–540.

Flynn, J. T., Daniels, S. R., Hayman, L. L., et al. (2014). On behalf of the American Heart Association atherosclerosis, hypertension and obesity in youth committee of the council on cardiovascular disease in the young. Update: Ambulatory blood pressure monitoring in children and adolescents: A scientific statement from the American Heart Association. Hypertension, 63(5), 1116–1135.

Flynn, J. T., Kaelber, D. C., Baker-Smith, C. M., et al. (2017). Clinical practice guideline for screening and management of high blood pressure in children and adolescents. Pediatrics, 140(3), e20171904.

Gajarski, R., Naftel, D. C., Pahl, E., et al. (2009). Outcomes of pediatric patients with hypertrophic cardiomyopathy listed for transplant. Journal of Heart and Lung Transplantation, 28(12), 1329–1334.

Gerber, M. A., Baltimore, R. S., Eaton, C. B., et al. (2009). Prevention of rheumatic fever and diagnosis and treatment of acute streptococcal pharyngitis: A scientific statement from the American Heart Association. Circulation, 119, 1541–1551.

Gewitz, M. H., Baltimore, R. S., Tani, L. Y., et al. (2015). Revision of the Jones criteria for the diagnosis of acute rheumatic fever in the era of Doppler echocardiography: A scientific statement from the American Heart Association. Circulation, 131, 1806–1818.

Ghanayem, N. S., Hoffman, G. M., Mussatto, K. A., et al. (2003). Home surveillance program prevents interstage mortality after the Norwood procedure. Journal of Thoracic and Cardiovascular Surgery, 126, 1367–1377.

Gilboa, S. M., Devine, O. J., Kucik, J. E., et al. (2016). Congenital heart defects in the United States: Estimating the magnitude of the affected population in 2010. Circulation, 134, 101–109.

Gilboa, S. M., Salemi, J. L., Nembhard, W. N., et al. (2010). Mortality resulting from congenital heart disease among children and adults in the United States, 1999 to 2006. Circulation, 122, 2254–2263.

Goldmuntz, E., & Lin, A. (2008). Genetics of congenital heart defects. In H. D. Allen, D. J. Driscoll, R. E. Shaddy, et al. (Eds.), Moss and Adams' heart disease in infants, children, and adolescents (7th ed.). Philadelphia, PA: Lippincott Williams & Wilkins.

Gupta, S., Sakhuja, A., McGrath, E., et al. (2016). Trends, microbiology, and outcomes of infective endocarditis in children during 2000-2010 in the United States. Congenital Heart Disease, 12(2), 196–201.

Holzer, R. J., Chisolm, J. L., Hill, S. L., et al. (2008). Stenting complex aortic arch obstructions. Catheterization and Cardiovascular Interventions, 71(3), 375–382.

Jacobs, J. P., Mavroudis, C., Jacobs, M. L., et al. (2004). Lessons learned from the data analysis of the second harvest (1998-2001) of the Society of Thoracic Surgeons (STS) congenital heart surgery database. European Journal of Cardio-throacic Surgery, 26(1), 18–37.

Jacobs, R., Boyd, L., Brennan, K., et al. (2016). The importance of social media for patients and families affected by congenital anomalies: A Facebook cross-sectional analysis and user survey. Journal of Pediatric Surgery, 51, 1766–1771.

Khairy, P., Clair, M., Fernandes, S. M., et al. (2013). Cardiovascular outcomes after the arterial switch operation for D-transposition of the great arteries. Circulation, 127(3), 331–339.

Kirk, R., Dipchand, A. I., Rosenthal, D. N., et al. (2014). The International Society for Heart and Lung Transplantation guidelines for the management of pediatric heart failure: Executive summary. [Corrected]. Journal of Heart and Lung Transplantation, 33(9), 888–909.

LeRoy, S. S., Elixson, E. M., O'Brien, P., et al. (2003). Recommendations for preparing children and adolescents for invasive cardiac procedures: A statement from the American Heart Association pediatric nursing subcommittee of the council on cardiovascular nursing in collaboration with the council on cardiovascular diseases of the young. Circulation, 108, 2550–2564.

Li, J. S., Sexton, D. J., Mick, N., et al. (2000). Proposed modifications to the Duke criteria for the diagnosis of infective endocarditis. Clinical Infectious Diseases, 30(4), 633–638.

Longmuir, P. E., Brothers, J. A., de Ferranti, S. D., et al. (2013). Promotion of physical activity for children and adults with congenital heart disease: A scientific statement from the American Heart Association. Circulation, 127(21), 2147–2159.

Majnemer, A., Limperopoulos, C., Shevell, M. I., et al. (2009). A new look at outcomes of infants with congenital heart disease. Pediatric Neurology, 40, 197–204.

Margossian, R. (2008). Contemporary management of pediatric heart failure. Expert Review of Cardiovascular Therapy, 6(2), 187–197.

Marijon, E., Mirabel, M., Celermajer, D. S., et al. (2012). Rheumatic heart disease. Lancet, 379, 953–964.

Marino, B. S., Lipkin, P. H., Newburger, J. W., et al. (2012). Neurodevelopmental outcomes in children with congenital heart disease: Evaluation and management: A scientific statement from the American Heart Association. Circulation, 126, 1143–1172.

Marino, B. S., Tabbutt, S., MacLaren, G., et al. (2018). Cardiopulmonary resuscitation in infants and children with cardiac disease. Circulation, 137, e691–e782.

Martin, G. S. (2012). Sepsis, severe sepsis and septic shock: Changes in incidence, pathogens, and outcomes. Expert Review of Anti-infective Therapy, 10(6), 701–706.

Mattoo, T. K. (2019). Evaluation and treatment of hypertension in children/adolescents, 2018. UpToDate. Retrieved https://www.uptodate.com/contents/evaluation-of-hypertension-in-children-and-adolescents. Retrieved 4 March 2019.

McCrindle, B. W., Kwiterovich, P. O., McBride, P. E., et al. (2012). Guidelines for lipid screening in children and adolescents: Bringing evidence to the debate. Pediatrics, 130(2), 353–356.

McCrindle, B. W., Rowley, A. H., Newburger, J. W., et al. (2017). Diagnosis, treatment, and long-term management of Kawasaki disease: A scientific statement for health professionals from the American Heart Association. Circulation, 135(17), e927–e999.

McCrindle, B. W., Urbina, E. M., Dennison, B. A., et al. (2007). Drug therapy of high-risk lipid abnormalities in children and adolescents: A scientific statement from the American Heart Association atherosclerosis, hypertension, and obesity in youth committee, council of cardiovascular disease in the young, with the council on cardiovascular nursing. Circulation, 115(14), 1948–1967.

Mery, C. M., Guzmán-Pruneda, F. A., Trost, J. G., et al. (2015). Contemporary results of aortic coarctation repair through left thoracotomy. The Annals of Thoracic Surgery, 100(3), 1039–1046.

Mickley, K. L., Burkhart, P. V., & Sigler, A. N. (2013). Promoting normal development and self-efficacy in the school-age children managing chronic conditions. Nursing Clinics of North America, 48(2), 319–328.

Moore, J., Hegde, S., El-Said, H., Beekman, R., Benson, L., Bergersen, L., et al. (2013). Transcatheter device closure of atrial septal defects: A safety review. JACC Cardiovascular Interventions, 6(5), 433–442.

Newburger, J. W., de Ferranti, S. D., & Fulton, D. R. (2017). Cardiovascular sequelae of Kawasaki disease, 2017. UpToDate. Retrieved http://www.uptodate.com/contents/cardiovascular-sequelae-of-kawasaki-disease. Retrieved 4 March 2019.

Park, M. K. (2014). Pediatric Cardiology for Practitioners (6th ed.). Philadelphia, PA: Elsevier/Saunders.

Petit, C. J., Fraser, C. D., Mattamal, R., et al. (2011). The impact of a dedicated single-ventricle home-monitoring program on interstage somatic growth, interstage attrition, and 1-year survival. Journal of Thoracic and Cardiovascular Surgery, 142, 1358–1366.

Reller, M. D., Strickland, M. J., Riehle-Colarusso, T., et al. (2008). Prevalence of congenital heart defects in metropolitan Atlanta, 1998-2005. Journal of Pediatrics, 153(6), 807–813.

Remenyi, B., Carapetis, J., Wyber, R., et al. (2013). Position statement of the World Heart Federation on the prevention and control of rheumatic heart disease. Nature Reviews Cardiology, 10(5), 284–292.

Rossano, J. W., & Shaddy, R. E. (2014). Heart failure in children: Etiology and treatment. Journal of Pediatrics, 165(2), 228–233.

Russell, H. M., Pasquali, S. K., Jacobs, J. P., et al. (2012). Outcomes of repair of common arterial trunk with truncal valve surgery: A review of the Society of Thoracic Surgeons congenital heart surgery database. The Annals of Thoracic Surgery, 93(1), 164–169.

Sampson, H. A., Wang, J., & Sicherer, S. H. (2020). Anaphylaxis. In R. M Kliegman, B. F Stanton, J. W. St. Geme., et al. (Eds.), Nelson textbook of pediatrics (21st ed.). Philadelphia, PA: Saunders.

Schlechte, E. A., Boramanand, N., & Funk, M. (2008). Supraventricular tachycardia in the pediatric primary care setting: Age-related presentation, diagnosis, and management. Journal of Pediatric Health Care, 22(5), 289–299.

Scientific Registry of Transplant Recipients. (2015). OPTN/SRTR 2015 annual data report. Rockville, MD: Department of Health and Human Services, Health Resources and Services Administration, Healthcare Systems Bureau, Division of Transplantation.

Siffel, C., Riehle-Colarusso, T., Oster, M. E., et al. (2015). Survival of children with hypoplastic left heart syndrome. Pediatrics, 136(4), e864–e870.

Simonneau, G., Gatzoulis, M. A., Adatia, I., et al. (2013). Updated clinical classification of pulmonary hypertension. Journal of the American College of Cardiology, 62(Suppl. 25), D34–41.

Smith, P. A. (2001). Primary care in children with congenital heart disease. Journal of Pediatric Nursing, 16, 308–319.

Spirito, P., Autore, C., Rapezzi, C., et al. (2009). Syncope and risk of sudden death in hypertrophic cardiomyopathy. Circulation, 119(13), 1703–1710.

Steer, A., & Gibofsky, A. (2019). Acute rheumatic fever: Treatment and prevention. UpToDate. Retrieved from https://www.uptodate.com/contents/acute-rheumatic-fever-treatment-and-prevention/print.

Steltzer, M., Rudd, N., & Pick, B. (2005). Nutrition care for newborns with congenital heart disease. Clinics in Perinatology, 32(4), 1017–1030.

St Louis, J. D., Jodhka, U., Jacobs, J. P., et al. (2014). Contemporary outcomes of complete atrioventricular septal defect repair: Analysis of the Society of Thoracic Surgeons congenital heart surgery database. The Journal of Thoracic and Cardiovascular Surgery, 148(6), 2526–2531.

Thrush, P. T., & Hoffman, T. M. (2014). Pediatric heart transplantation—indications and outcomes in the current era. Journal of Thoracic Disease, 6(8), 1080–1096.

Vick, G. W., & Bezold, L. I. (2018). Isolated atrial septal defects (ASDs) in children: Classification, clinical features, and diagnosis, 2018. UpToDate. Retrieved https://www.uptodate.com/contents/isolated-atrial-septal-defects-asds-in-children-classification-clinical-features-and-diagnosis. Retrieved 13 February 2019.

Weiss, S. L., Peters, M. J., Alhazzani, W., et al. (2020). Surviving Sepsis Campaign International Guidelines for the Management of Septic Shock and Sepsis-Associated Organ Dysfunction in Children. Pediatric Critical Care Medicine, 21(2), e53–e106.

Whelton, P. K., Carey, R. M., Aranow, W. S., et al. (2018). 2017 ACC/AHA/AAPA/ABC /ACPM/AGS/APhA/ASH/ASPC/NMA/PCNA Guideline for the prevention, detection, evaluation, and management of high blood pressure in adults: A report of the American College of Cardiology/American Heart Association task force on clinical practice guidelines. Circulation, 138(17), e426–e483.

Whittaker, E., Bamford, A., Kenny, J., et al. (2020). Clinical Characteristics of 58 Children With a Pediatric Inflammatory Multisystem Syndrome Temporally Associated With SARS-CoV-2. The Journal of the American Medical Association, 324(3), 259–269.

Wilder, M. S., Palinkas, L. A., Kao, A. S., et al. (2007). Delayed diagnosis by physicians contributes to the development of coronary artery aneurysms in children with Kawasaki syndrome. Pediatric Infectious Disease, 26(3), 256–260.

Wilson, W., Taubert, K. A., Gewitz, M., et al. (2007). Prevention of infective endocarditis: Guidelines from the American Heart Association. Circulation, 116(15), 1736–1754.

Zafar, F., Castleberry, C., Khan, M. S., et al. (2015). Pediatric heart transplant waiting list mortality in the era of ventricular assist devices. Journal of Heart and Lung Transplantation, 34, 82–88.

24

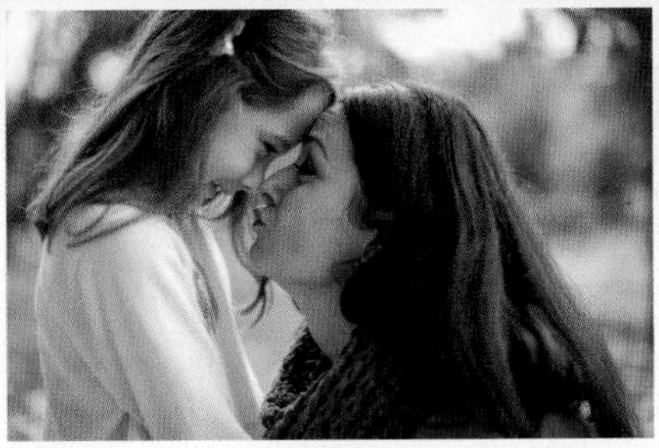

The Child With Hematologic or Immunologic Dysfunction

Rosalind Bryant

http://evolve.elsevier.com/wong/essentials

CONCEPTS

- Perfusion
- Clotting

HEMATOLOGIC AND IMMUNOLOGIC DYSFUNCTION

Several tests can be performed to assess hematologic function, including additional procedures to identify the cause of the dysfunction. The following discussion is limited to a description of the most common and one of the most valuable tests, the **complete blood count (CBC)**. Other procedures, such as those related to iron, coagulation, and immune status, are discussed throughout the chapter as appropriate. The nurse should be familiar with the significance of the findings from the CBC (Table 24.1).

As with any disorder, the history and physical examination are essential to identify hematologic dysfunction, and the nurse is often the first person to suspect a problem based on information from these sources. Comments by the parent regarding the child's lack of energy, food diary of poor sources of iron, frequent infections, and bleeding that is difficult to control offer clues to the more common disorders affecting the blood. A careful physical appraisal, especially of the skin, can reveal findings (e.g., pallor, petechiae, bruising) that may indicate minor or serious hematologic conditions. Nurses need to be aware of the clinical manifestations of blood diseases to assist in recognizing symptoms and establishing a diagnosis.

> **NURSING TIP:** A common term used in describing an abnormal complete blood count (CBC) is **shift to the left**, which refers to the presence of immature neutrophils in the peripheral blood from hyperfunction of the bone marrow, as seen during a bacterial infection.

RED BLOOD CELL DISORDERS

ANEMIA

Anemia is a reduction in red blood cell (RBC) mass per volume and/or hemoglobin (Hgb or Hb) concentration compared with normal values for age (Brugnara, Oski, & Nathan, 2015; Thornburg, 2020). This diminishes the oxygen-carrying capacity of the blood, causing a reduction in the oxygen available to the tissues. The anemias are the most common hematologic disorder of infancy and childhood and are not diseases but an indication or manifestation of an underlying pathologic process.

Classification

Anemias can be classified using two basic approaches: **etiology** or **physiology**, manifested by erythrocyte or Hgb depletion, and **morphology**, the characteristic changes in RBC size, shape, or color (Box 24.1). Although the morphologic classification is useful in terms of laboratory evaluation of anemia, the etiology provides direction for planning nursing care. For example, anemia with reduced Hgb concentration may be caused by a dietary depletion of iron, and the principal intervention is replenishing iron stores. The classification of anemias is found in Fig. 24.1.

Consequences of Anemia

The basic physiologic defect caused by anemia is a decrease in the oxygen-carrying capacity of blood and consequently a reduction in the amount of oxygen available to the body cells. When the anemia has developed slowly, the child usually adapts to the declining Hgb level.

The effects of anemia on the circulatory system can be profound. Because the viscosity of blood depends almost entirely on the concentration of RBCs, the resulting hemodilution of severe anemia decreases peripheral resistance, causing greater quantities of blood to return to the heart. The increased circulation and turbulence within the heart may produce a murmur. Because the cardiac workload is greatly increased, especially during exercise, infection, or emotional stress, cardiac failure may ensue.

Children seem to have a remarkable ability to function well despite low levels of Hgb. **Cyanosis**, which results from an increased quantity of deoxygenated Hgb in arterial blood, is typically not evident. Growth retardation, resulting from decreased cellular metabolism, and coexisting anorexia is a common finding in chronic severe anemia. It is frequently accompanied by delayed sexual maturation in the older child.

Diagnostic Evaluation

In general, anemia may be suspected based on history and physical examination findings, such as a lack of energy, easy fatigability, and pallor. Laboratory tests are another clue to the disorder, with possible alterations in the CBC, such as decreased RBCs, and decreased Hgb and hematocrit (Hct) levels (see Fig. 24.1). Although anemia is sometimes defined as decreased Hgb level, it important to be aware that normal Hgb levels vary with age (see Table 24.1).

Other tests specific to a particular type of anemia are used to determine the underlying cause of anemia. These are discussed in relation to the particular disorder.

TABLE 24.1 Tests Performed as Part of a Complete Blood Count

Test (Average Value)	Description, Comments
RBC count (4.5-5.5 million/mm^3)	Number of RBCs/mm^3 of blood Indirectly estimates Hgb content of blood Reflects function of bone marrow
Hgb determination (11.5-15.5 g/dl)	Amount of Hgb (g)/dl of whole blood Total blood Hgb primarily depends on number of circulating RBCs but also on amount of Hgb in each cell
Hct (35%-45%)	Percent volume of packed RBCs in whole blood Indirectly measures Hgb content Is approximately three times Hgb content
RBC indices	
MCV (77-95 fl)	Average or mean volume (size) of a single RBC MCV value is expressed as femtoliter (fl) or cubic micron (mm^3)
MCH (25 to 33 pg/cell)	Average or mean quantity (weight) of Hgb in a single RBC MCH value is expressed as picogram (pg) or micromicrogram (mmcg) Whereas MCV and MCH depend on accurate counts of RBCs, MCHC does not; therefore MCHC is often more reliable All indices depend on average cell measurements and do not show individual RBC variations (anisocytosis)
MCHC (31%-37% Hgb [g]/dl RBC)	Average concentration of Hgb in a single RBC MCHC values are expressed as percent Hgb (g)/cell or Hgb (g)/dl RBC
RBC volume distribution width (13.4% ± 1.2%)	Average size of RBCs Differentiates some types of anemia
Reticulocyte count (0.5%-1.5% erythrocytes)	Percent reticulocytes in RBCs Index of production of mature RBCs by bone marrow Decreased count indicates depressed bone marrow function Increased count indicates erythrogenesis in response to some stimulus When reticulocyte count is extremely high, other forms of immature RBCs (normoblasts, even erythroblasts) may be present Indirectly estimates hypochromic anemia Usually elevated in patients with chronic hemolytic anemia
WBC count (4.5-13.5 × 10^3 cells/mm^3)	Number of WBCs/mm^3 of blood Total number of WBCs less important than differential count
Differential WBC count	Inspection and quantification of WBC types present in peripheral blood Values are expressed as percentages; to obtain absolute number of any type of WBC, multiply its respective percentage by total number of WBCs
Neutrophils (polys) (54%-62%) (3-5.8 × 10^3 cells/mm^3)	Primary defense in bacterial infection; capable of phagocytizing and killing bacteria
Bands (3%-5%) (0.15-0.4 × 10^3 cells/mm^3)	Immature neutrophil Increased numbers in bacterial infection Also capable of phagocytosis and killing
Eosinophils (1%-3%) (0.05-0.25 × 10^3 cells/mm^3)	Named for their staining characteristics with eosin dye Increased in allergic disorders, parasitic diseases, certain neoplasms, and other diseases
Basophils (0.075%) (0.015-0.030 × 10^3 cells/mm^3)	Named for their characteristic basophilic stippling Contain histamine, heparin, and serotonin; believed to cause increased blood flow to injured tissues while preventing excessive clotting
Lymphocytes (25%-33%) (1.5-3.0 × 10^3 cells/mm^3)	Involved in development of antibody and delayed hypersensitivity
Monocytes (3%-7%)	Large phagocytic cells that are involved in early stage of inflammatory reaction
ANC (>1000/mm^3)	Percent neutrophils/bands times WBC count Indicates body's capability to handle bacterial infections
Platelet count (150-400 × 10^3/mm^3)	Number of platelets/mm^3 of blood Cellular fragments that are necessary for clotting to occur
Stained peripheral blood smear	Visual estimation of amount of Hgb in RBCs and overall size, shape, and structure of RBCs Various staining properties of RBC structures may be evidence of immature forms of erythrocytes Shows variation in size and shape of RBCs: microcytic, macrocytic, poikilocytic (variable shapes)

ANC, Absolute neutrophil count; *Hct,* hematocrit; *Hgb,* hemoglobin; *MCH,* mean corpuscular hemoglobin; *MCHC,* mean corpuscular hemoglobin concentration; *MCV,* mean corpuscular volume; *RBC,* red blood cell; *WBC,* white blood cell.

Therapeutic Management

The objective of medical management is to reverse the anemia by treating the underlying cause. In nutritional anemias, the specific deficiency is replaced. In blood loss from acute hemorrhage, RBC transfusion may be given. In patients with severe anemia, supportive medical care may include oxygen therapy, bed rest, and replacement of intravascular volume with intravenous (IV) fluids. In addition to these general measures, the nurse may implement more specific interventions, depending on the cause. The next sections will discuss these interventions.

Nursing Care Management

The assessment of anemia includes the basic techniques that are applicable to any condition. The age of the infant or child provides some clues regarding the possible etiology of the anemia. For example, iron-deficiency anemia occurs more frequently in toddlers between 12 and 36 months old and during the growth spurt of adolescence.

BOX 24.1 Red Blood Cell Morphology

Size (Cell Size)

Variation in red blood cell (RBC) sizes (anisocytosis)

- Normocytes (normal cell size)
- Microcytes (smaller than normal cell size)
- Macrocytes (larger than normal cell size)

Shape (Cell Shape)

Variation in RBC shapes (poikilocytosis)

- Spherocytes (globular cells)
- Drepanocytes (sickle-shaped cells)
- Numerous other irregularly shaped cells

Color (Cell Staining Characteristics)

Variation in hemoglobin concentration in the RBC

- Normochromic (sufficient or normal amount of hemoglobin per RBC)
- Hypochromic (reduced amount of hemoglobin per RBC)
- Hyperchromic (increased amount of hemoglobin per RBC)

In interviewing the family, the nurse assesses the following areas: (1) nutrition, especially if the child is lactose intolerant or has inadequate intake of iron; (2) history of chronic, recurrent infection; (3) eating habits, particularly pica (consumption of nonnutritive substances such as dirt, starch, lead-based paint chips, paper); (4) bowel habits and presence of frank blood in stools or black, tarry stools as a result of chronic blood loss; and (5) familial history of hereditary diseases, such as sickle cell disease (SCD) or thalassemia.

The nurse should also obtain pertinent information that may aid in identifying the cause of the anemia. For example, a statement such as "My child drinks a lot of milk" is a frequent finding in toddlers with iron-deficiency anemia.

The stool examination using the Hemoccult test for occult (microscopic) blood can identify chronic intestinal bleeding that results from a primary or secondary lactase deficiency. It is also important to understand the significance of various blood tests (see Table 24.1).

Prepare the Child and Family for Laboratory Tests

Several blood tests are generally ordered sequentially. Therefore the child may undergo multiple finger or heel punctures or venipunctures. These invasive procedures may be better tolerated (see Chapter 20, Blood Specimens) with the topical anesthetic known as eutectic mixture of lidocaine and prilocaine (EMLA) or lidocaine (ELA-Max or LMX) cream applied prior to needle punctures (see Chapter 5, Pain Management). Therefore the nurse is responsible for preparing the child and family for the tests by:

- Explaining the significance of each test, particularly why the tests are not all done at one time
- Encouraging parents or another supportive person to be with the child during the procedure
- Allowing the child to play with the equipment on a doll or participate in the actual procedure (e.g., by holding the Band-Aid)

Older children may appreciate the opportunity to observe the blood cells under a microscope or in photographs. This experience is especially important if a serious blood disorder, such as aplastic anemia, is suspected because it serves as a foundation for explaining the pathophysiology of the disorder.

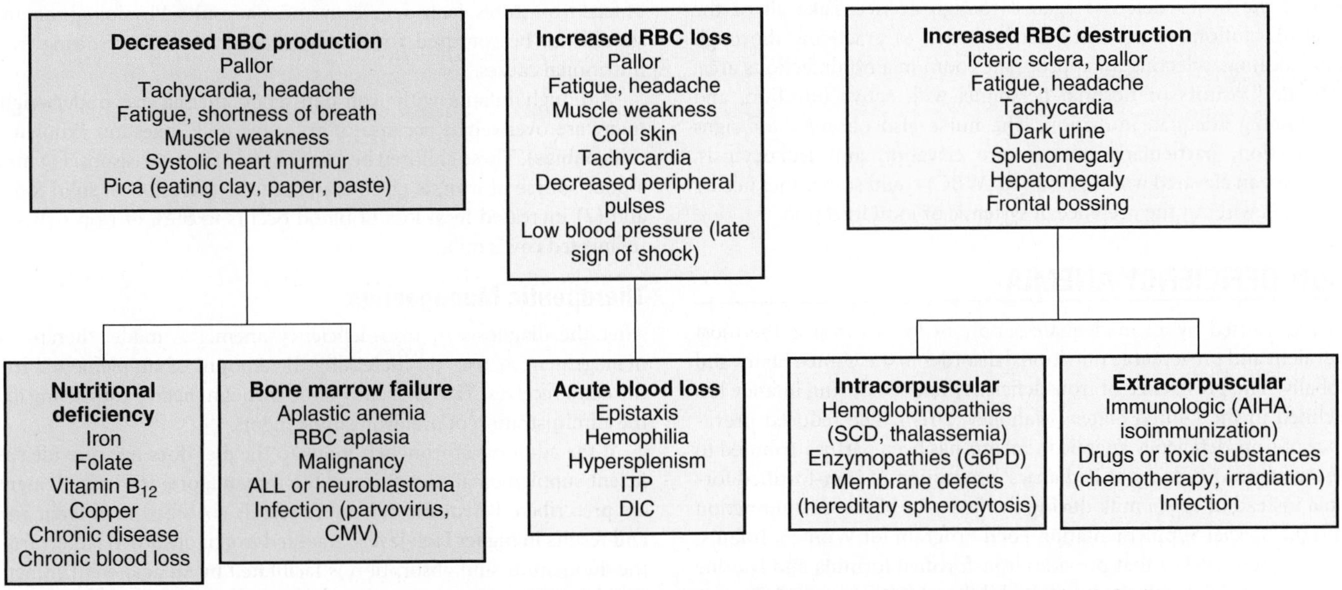

Fig. 24.1 Classifications of anemias. *AIHA,* Autoimmune hemolytic anemia; *ALL,* acute lymphoblastic leukemia; *CMV,* cytomegalovirus; *DIC,* disseminated intravascular coagulation; *G6PD,* glucose-6-phosphate dehydrogenase; *ITP,* idiopathic thrombocytopenic purpura; *RBC,* red blood cell; *SCD,* sickle cell disease.

Bone marrow aspiration is not a routine hematologic test but is essential for definitive diagnosis of certain anemias, such as severe aplastic anemia.

NURSING TIP: Suggested explanations for teaching children about blood components are:

Red blood cells: Carry the oxygen you breathe from your lungs to all parts of your body

White blood cells: Help keep germs from causing infection

Platelets: Small parts of cells that help make bleeding stop by forming a clot (scab) over the hurt area

Plasma: The liquid portion of blood; has clotting factors that help make bleeding stop

Decrease Tissue Oxygen Needs

Because the basic pathologic process in anemia is a decrease in oxygen-carrying capacity of the RBCs, an important nursing responsibility is to minimize tissue oxygen needs by continual assessment of the child's energy level. Assess the child's level of tolerance for activities of daily living and play, and make adjustments to allow as much self-care as possible without undue exertion. During periods of rest, the nurse measures vital signs and observes behavior to establish a baseline of nonexertion energy expenditure. During periods of activity, the nurse repeats these measurements and observations to compare them with resting values.

NURSING TIP: Signs of exertion include tachycardia, palpitations, tachypnea, dyspnea, shortness of breath, hyperpnea, dizziness, lightheadedness, diaphoresis, and change in skin color. The child looks fatigued (e.g., sagging, limp posture; slow, strained movements; inability to tolerate additional activity; difficulty sucking in infants).

Prevent Complications

Children with anemia are prone to infection because tissue hypoxia causes cellular dysfunction, and the disturbed metabolic processes weaken the host's defenses against foreign agents. Take all of the usual precautions to prevent infection, such as practicing thorough hand washing, selecting an appropriate room in a noninfectious area, restricting visitors or hospital personnel with active infection, and maintaining adequate nutrition. The nurse also observes for signs of infection, particularly temperature elevation and leukocytosis. However, an elevated white blood cell (WBC) count sometimes occurs in anemia without the presence of systemic or local infection.

IRON-DEFICIENCY ANEMIA

Anemia caused by an inadequate supply or loss of iron is the most prevalent and preventable nutritional disorder in the United States and globally. The prevalence of iron-deficiency anemia during infancy has declined in the United States (Mahoney, 2017). The reduced prevalence of iron-deficiency anemia in infants has been partly attributed to the American Academy of Pediatrics' promotion of iron-fortified formula instead of cow's milk during the first year of life in conjunction with the Special Supplementation Food Program for Women, Infants, and Children (WIC) that provides iron-fortified formula and routine screening of Hgb levels during early childhood (Fleming, 2015; Powers & Buchanan, 2014). The promotion of iron supplement in the exclusively breastfed infant, introduction of iron-fortified infant formula and cereal, weaning from the bottle by 1 year of age, limiting intake of cow's milk to 16 to 24 oz/day, and delayed introduction of cow's milk into the diet have also contributed to the decreased incidence of iron-deficiency anemia in infants and young children (Fleming, 2015). Preterm infants are especially at risk because of their reduced fetal iron supply. Children 12 to 36 months old are at risk for anemia as a result of excessive cow's milk consumption, not eating an adequate amount of iron-containing food, and possible blood loss from milk protein colitis (Eussen, Alles, Uijterschout, et al., 2015; Paoletti, Bogen, & Ritchey, 2014; Rothman, 2020). Adolescents are also at risk for iron deficiency because of their rapid growth rate combined with poor eating habits, menses, obesity, or strenuous activities. However, iron deficiency both with and without anemia remains a relatively common health problem, especially among at-risk children and pregnant women (Fleming, 2015; Juul, Derman, & Auerbach, 2019; Mahoney, 2017; Miller, 2013).

Pathophysiology

Iron-deficiency anemia can be caused by any number of factors that decrease the supply of iron, impair its absorption, increase the body's need for iron, or affect the synthesis of Hgb. Although the clinical manifestations and diagnostic evaluation are similar regardless of the cause, the therapeutic and nursing care management depends on the specific reason for the iron deficiency. The following discussion is limited to iron-deficiency anemia resulting from inadequate iron in the diet.

During the last trimester of pregnancy, iron is transferred from the mother to the fetus at the rate of 4 mg/day. Most of the iron is stored in the circulating erythrocytes of the fetus, with the remainder stored in the fetal liver, spleen, and bone marrow. When iron stores are deficient, the production of hemoglobin is reduced. Consequently, the main effect of iron deficiency is decreased Hgb level and reduced oxygen-carrying capacity of the blood.

Along with maternal iron supplements, delayed umbilical clamping for 1 to 3 minutes can improve iron status and reduce the risk of iron deficiency in the newborn (Anderson, Domeliof, Anderson, et al., 2014; Mercer, Erickson-Owens, Collins, et al., 2017; Miller, 2013; Rothman, 2020). Maternally derived iron stores are usually adequate for the first 5 to 6 months in a full-term infant but for only 2 to 3 months in preterm infants and multiple births. If dietary sources of iron are not supplied to meet the infant's growth demands after the depletion of fetal iron stores, iron-deficiency anemia results. Physiologic anemia should not be confused with iron-deficiency anemia resulting from nutritional causes.

Although infants with iron-deficiency anemia are underweight, many are overweight because of excessive milk ingestion (known as **milk babies**). These children become anemic for two reasons: (1) milk, a poor source of iron, is given almost to the exclusion of solid foods; and (2) increased fecal loss of blood occurs in 50% of iron-deficient infants fed cow's milk.

Therapeutic Management

After the diagnosis of iron-deficiency anemia is made, therapeutic management focuses on increasing the amount of supplemental iron the child receives. This is usually done through dietary counseling and the administration of oral iron supplements.

If the addition of iron-rich foods to the diet does not provide sufficient supplemental quantities of the mineral, oral iron supplements are prescribed. Ferrous iron is more readily absorbed than ferric iron and results in higher Hgb levels. Ingested iron is absorbed largely from the duodenum, and absorption is facilitated by an acid environment. Children normally absorb an average of 10% to 20% of the iron in oral supplements, but during periods of iron deficiency they absorb an additional 5% to 10%. Oral iron supplementation is prescribed as

3 to 6 mg of elemental iron per kilogram per day. Side effects of oral iron therapy may include nausea, gastric irritation, diarrhea or constipation, and anorexia. If the iron produces vomiting and diarrhea, it should be administered with meals. Lower dosages of iron are associated with fewer side effects.

Ideally, the daily dose of iron should be given in two or three divided doses between meals. Ascorbic acid (vitamin C) appears to facilitate absorption of iron and may be given as vitamin C–enriched foods and juices with the iron preparation. The administration of oral iron with vitamin C supplementation was supported in a recent cohort study. The oral iron with vitamin C was given over a period of 10 weeks and had a complete response in majority (6/7 = 86%) with greater than 2 g/dl rise in Hgb along with significant improvement of other iron-related indices (Sourabh, Bhatia, & Jain, 2019).

The response to oral iron therapy is reflected in a peak increase in the reticulocyte count by the fifth to tenth day of administration. Following the reticulocyte rise, the Hgb and Hct levels and RBC count increase. The Hgb level rises from 0.1 to 0.4 g/dl/24 h depending on anemia severity; therefore a substantial increase should occur by the end of 1 month (Rothman, 2020).

If the Hgb level fails to rise after 1 month of oral therapy, it is important to assess for persistent bleeding, iron malabsorption, noncompliance, improper iron administration, or other causes of the anemia. Parenteral (IV or intramuscular [IM]) iron administration is safe and effective but is expensive, and occasionally is associated with regional lymphadenopathy, transient arthralgias, or serious allergic reaction (Bregman & Goodnough, 2014; Fleming, 2015). Therefore parenteral iron is reserved for children who have iron malabsorption, chronic hemoglobinuria, or intolerance to oral preparations. The deep IM injection route for iron administration is discouraged because it is painful; requires multiple injections; may leak into the subcutaneous tissue, causing skin discoloration at the injection site; and is associated with gluteal sarcoma (Juul, Derman, & Auerbach, 2019). Careful observation with IV iron administration is required because of the risk of anaphylaxis, so a test dose is recommended before use. Several IV iron preparations (e.g., ferumoxytol, ferric carboxymaltose, iron sucrose complex, iron isomaltoside) show promise in complete replacement of iron with little toxicity (Auerbach, James, Nicoletti, et al., 2017; DeLoughery, 2014; Mantadakis, 2018; Smith, 2012). Transfusions are indicated for the most severe anemia and in cases of serious infection, cardiac dysfunction, or surgical emergency when anesthesia is required. Packed RBCs (2 to 3 ml/kg), not whole blood, are used to minimize the chance of circulatory overload. Supplemental oxygen is administered when tissue hypoxia is severe.

Prognosis

The prognosis for a child with iron-deficiency anemia is very good. There is evidence that if the anemia is severe and long-standing, then diminished cognitive function, behavioral changes, delayed infant growth and development, decreased exercise tolerance, and impaired immune function may develop (Angulo-Barroso, Li, Santos, et al., 2016; Fleming, 2015; Jauregui-Lobera, 2014; Pivina, Semenova, Dosa, et al., 2019). However, there is lack of convincing evidence that iron treatment of young children with iron-deficiency anemia or nonanemic iron deficiency has an effect on psychomotor development or cognitive function (Abdullah, Thorpe, Mamak, et al., 2015; McDonagh, Blazina, Dana, et al., 2015; Thompson, Biggs, & Pasricha, 2013; Wang, Zhan, Gong, et al., 2013). Therefore there is a need for further large, long-term follow-up, randomized interventional studies.

QUALITY PATIENT OUTCOMES: Iron-Deficiency Anemia

- Early recognition of signs and symptoms of iron-deficiency anemia
- Appropriate quantity of milk, use of iron-fortified infant formula, and introduction of solid foods
- Adherence to oral iron supplement with appropriate administration
- Hemoglobin increase within 1 month and anemia resolved within 6 months

Nursing Care Management

An essential nursing responsibility is instructing parents in the administration of iron. Oral iron should be given as prescribed in two divided doses between meals, when the presence of free hydrochloric acid is greatest, because more iron is absorbed in the acidic environment of the upper gastrointestinal (GI) tract. A citrus fruit or juice taken with the medication aids in absorption.

DRUG ALERT

Cow's milk contains substances that bind the iron and interfere with absorption. Iron supplements should not be administered with milk or milk products (Powers & Buchanan, 2014; Walczyk, Muthayya, Wegmuller, et al., 2014).

An adequate dosage of oral iron turns the stools a tarry green or black color. The nurse advises parents of this normally expected change and inquires about its occurrence on follow-up visits. Absence of the greenish black stool may be a clue to poor compliance (e.g., in schedule, in dosage, in administration, in side effects). If compliance is an issue, make every effort to institute strategies to improve adherence to the medication regimen, such as changing the schedule to more convenient times.

DRUG ALERT

Liquid preparations of iron may temporarily stain the teeth. If possible, the medication should be taken through a straw or given through a syringe or medicine dropper placed toward the back of the mouth. Brushing the teeth after administration of the drug lessens the discoloration.

NURSING ALERT

Because iron ingestion in excessive quantities is toxic or even fatal, parents should be instructed to keep no more than a month's supply in the home and store it safely away from the reach of children.

Diet

A primary nursing objective is to prevent nutritional anemia through family education. The nurse must reinforce the importance of administering iron supplementation to exclusively breastfed infants by 4 months of age because breast milk is a low iron source (American Academy of Pediatrics, 2016; Centers for Disease Control and Prevention, 2018a; Lokeshwar, Mehta, Mehta, et al., 2011; Ziegler, Nelson, & Jeter, 2011). The American Academy of Pediatrics recommends that preterm infants, marginally low– and low-birth-weight infants, or infants with inadequate iron stores at birth receive iron supplements at approximately 2 months old (Berglund, Westrup, & Domellof, 2010).

In formula-fed infants, the most convenient and best sources of supplemental iron are iron-fortified commercial formula and iron-fortified infant cereal (National Institutes of Health, Office of Dietary Supplements, 2018). Iron-fortified formula provides a relatively constant and predictable amount of iron and is not associated with an increased incidence of GI symptoms, such as colic, diarrhea, or constipation. Infants younger than 12 months old should *not* be given fresh cow's milk because it may increase the risk of GI blood loss occurring from exposure to a heat-labile protein in cow's milk or cow's milk–induced GI mucosal damage resulting from a lack of cytochrome iron (heme protein) (Subramaniam & Girish, 2015). If GI bleeding is suspected, several stool analyses for occult blood known as *guaiac tests* are performed to identify any intermittent blood loss.

Since the best first solid-food source of iron is commercial iron-fortified cereals, it may be difficult initially to teach the infant to accept foods other than milk. Predominantly milk-fed infants tend to rebel against solid foods, and parents are cautioned about this and the need to be firm in not relinquishing control to the child. It may require intense problem solving on the part of both the family and the nurse to overcome the child's resistance.

A difficulty encountered in discouraging the parents from feeding milk to the exclusion of other foods is dispelling the popular myth that milk is a "perfect food." Many parents believe that milk is best for infants and equate weight gain with "healthiness." Although milk is an excellent food, it is deficient in iron, vitamin C, zinc, and fluoride. Sources of each of these nutrients and the role they play in preventing deficiencies need to be discussed with the family, especially the persons responsible for feeding the infant. Also stress that overweight is not synonymous with good health. The same principles are applied as those for introducing new foods (see Chapter 7, Provide Optimal Nutrition), especially feeding the solid food prior to milk intake.

Counseling families whose children are anemic is often a difficult and challenging task. Meal planning must be based on the family's budget, cultural pattern, and food preferences. Diet education of teenagers is difficult, especially because teenage girls are particularly prone to following weight-reduction diets. Stressing the physical and behavioral improvements and effect that the improved diet will have on all family members may encourage parents and teens to adhere to the treatment plan.

SICKLE CELL ANEMIA

Sickle cell anemia (SCA) is one of a group of diseases collectively called **hemoglobinopathies** in which normal adult Hgb (Hgb A or HbA) is partly or completely replaced by abnormal sickle Hgb (HbS). **Sickle cell disease (SCD)** refers to a group of hereditary disorders, all of which are related to the presence of HbS. Although the term *SCD* is sometimes used to refer to SCA, this use is incorrect. The correct terms for SCA are homozygous sickle cell disease (HgbSS) and **homozygous SCD**.

The following are the most common forms of SCD in the United States:

- **SCA,** the homozygous form of the disease (HbgSS), in which valine, an amino acid, is substituted for glutamic acid at the sixth position of the beta chain
- **Sickle cell–C disease,** a heterozygous variant of SCD (HgbSC), is characterized by the presence of both HgbS and HgbC, in which lysine is substituted for glutamic acid at the sixth position of the beta chain
- **Sickle thalassemia disease,** a combination of sickle cell trait and beta thalassemia trait (Sβthal). In the β^+ (beta plus) form, some normal HbA can be produced. In the β^0 (beta zero) form, there is no ability to produce HbA.

Of the SCDs, SCA is the most common form in African Americans, followed by sickle cell–C disease and sickle thalassemia disease. Numerous other sickle syndromes exist in which HbS is paired with other mutant globin.

SCD is one of the most common genetic diseases worldwide, affecting approximately 100,000 Americans and including other nationalities, such as Africans, Hispanics, Italians, Greeks, Iranians, Turks, and individuals of Arab, Caribbean, Asian Indian descent, and other ethnic groups. The incidence of the disease varies in different geographic locations. Among African Americans, the incidence of sickle cell trait is about 8%, whereas among inhabitants of West Africa, the incidence is reported to be as high as 40%. The high incidence of sickle cell trait in West Africans is believed to be the result of selective protection afforded trait carriers against malaria caused by endemic *Plasmodium falciparum* infection (Nussbaum, McInnes, & Willard, 2016).

The gene that determines the production of HbS is situated on an autosome and, when present, is always detectable. Heterozygous persons who have both normal HbA and abnormal HbS are said to have **sickle cell trait**. Persons who are homozygous have predominantly HbS and have SCA. The inheritance pattern is essentially that of an autosomal recessive disorder. Therefore when both parents have sickle cell trait, there is a 25% chance with each pregnancy of producing an offspring with SCA.

Although the defect is inherited, the sickling phenomenon is usually not apparent until later in infancy because of the presence of fetal Hgb (HbF). As long as the child has predominantly HbF, sickling does not occur because there is less HbS. Newborns with SCA are generally asymptomatic because of the protective effect of HbF (60% to 80% HbF), but this rapidly decreases during the first year, so these children are at risk for sickle cell–related complications (Heeney & Ware, 2015; Piel, Steinberg, & Rees, 2017).

Pathophysiology

The clinical manifestations of SCA are primarily the result of (1) obstruction caused by the sickled RBCs with other cells, (2) vascular inflammation, and (3) increased RBC destruction (Fig. 24.2). The abnormal adhesion, entanglement, and enmeshing of rigid sickle-shaped cells accompanied by the inflammatory process intermittently blocks the microcirculation causing vasoocclusion (Fig. 24.3). The resultant absence of blood flow to adjacent tissues causes local hypoxia, leading to tissue ischemia and infarction (cellular death). Most of the complications seen in SCA can be traced to this process and its impact on various organs of the body (Box 24.2).

The clinical manifestations of SCA vary greatly in severity and frequency. The most acute symptoms of the disease occur during periods of exacerbation called **crises**. There are several types of episodic crises, including vasoocclusive, acute splenic sequestration, aplastic, hyperhemolytic, cerebrovascular accident (CVA), acute chest syndrome, and infection. The crises may occur individually or concomitantly with one or more other crises. The **vasoocclusive crisis (VOC)**, preferably called a "painful episode," is characterized by ischemia causing mild to severe pain that may last from minutes to days or longer. Dactylitis (swelling in hands and feet) is often the first painful manifestation of VOC in children, usually occurring from 6 months to 2 years old. **Sequestration crisis** is a pooling of a large amount of blood, usually in the spleen and infrequently in the liver, that causes a decreased blood volume and may ultimately cause shock. **Aplastic crisis** is diminished RBC production, usually triggered by viral infection that may result in profound anemia. **Hyperhemolytic crisis** is an accelerated rate of RBC destruction characterized by anemia, jaundice, and reticulocytosis.

Another serious complication is **acute chest syndrome (ACS)**, which is clinically similar to pneumonia. It is the presence of a new

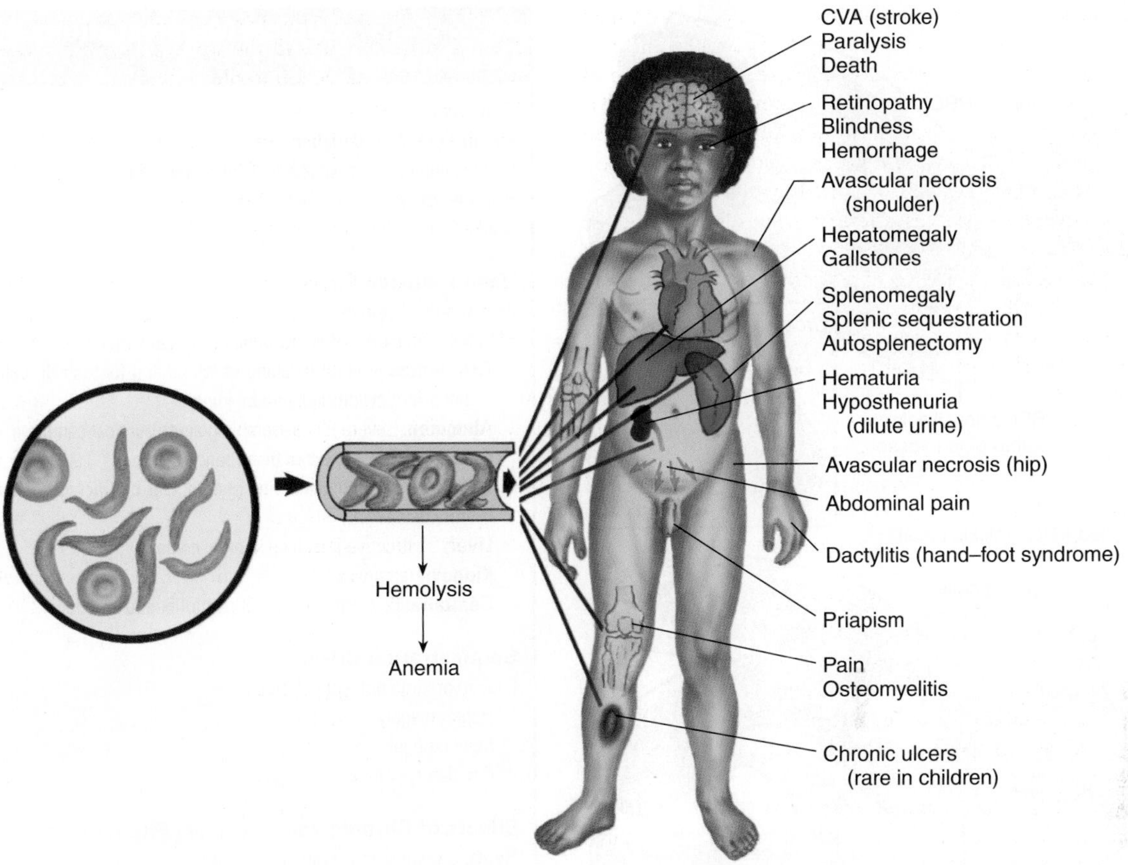

Fig. 24.2 Clinical features of sickle cell anemia (SCA) from red blood cell (RBC) obstruction and destruction. *CVA,* Cerebrovascular accident.

pulmonary infiltrate and may be associated with chest pain, fever, cough, tachypnea, wheezing, and hypoxia.

A **cerebrovascular accident (CVA, stroke)** is a major complication, often primarily vascular as sickled cells block the blood vessels in the brain, resulting in cerebral infarction, which causes variable degrees of neurologic impairment. Before the development of transcranial Doppler ultrasonography (TCD; described later in the chapter) to screen for stroke risk among children with sickle cell anemia, approximately 11% experienced an overt stroke and 20% a silent stroke before age 18 years (Estcourt, Fortin, Hopewell, et al., 2017; Smith-Whitley & Kwiatkowski, 2020). A functional definition of overt stroke is the presence of a focal neurologic deficit lasting for more than 24 hours and/or abnormal neuroimaging of the brain indicating a cerebral infarct on magnetic resonance imaging (MRI) corresponding to the focal neurologic deficit, whereas a silent cerebral infarct lacks focal neurologic findings lasting more than 24 hours and is diagnosed as an abnormality on MRI (Smith-Whitley & Kwiatkowski, 2020). Any number of neurologic symptoms, such as headache, aphasia, weakness, convulsions, visual disturbances, or unilateral hemiplegia, can indicate a minor cerebral insult. Cognitive impairment (e.g., developmental delays, poor or declining school performance) from SCA without any other overt signs tends to be associated with silent cerebral infarct (Choudhury, DeBaun, Rodeghier, et al., 2018; DeBaun, Armstrong, McKinstry, et al., 2012; Kawadler, Clayden, Clark, et al., 2016; Yawn, Buchanan, Afenyi-Annan, et al., 2014).

Diagnostic Evaluation

Universal screening of newborns for SCD has become standard in all US states and territories (McGann, Nero, & Ware, 2013; Meier & Miller, 2012). The global newborn screening program varies by country and is not a common practice in most countries where SCD is a public health concern, but such programs are being developed in India and some African countries (Huttle, Maestre, Lantigua, et al., 2015; Piel et al., 2017). The screening provides early identification of these children before complications develop. At birth, infants have up to 80% of HbF, which does not carry the defect. Because levels of HbS are low at birth, Hgb electrophoresis or other tests that measure Hgb concentrations are indicated.

Although SCD is usually reported during the prenatal or neonatal periods, it may not be recognized until the toddler and preschool periods during a crisis precipitated by an acute respiratory tract or GI infection. Early diagnosis (before the age of 2 months) facilitates parental education on the importance of maintaining hydration, current immunizations, administering prophylaxtic antibiotics, detecting splenomegaly, recognizing early signs of infection and other SCD complications, and seeking prompt medical attention as indicated.

Several specific tests detect abnormal Hgb in the homozygous or heterozygous form of SCD. For screening purposes, the sickle-turbidity test (Sickledex) is used because it can be performed on blood from a finger or heel stick and yields accurate results in 3 minutes, yet it is not able to distinguish between the sickle cell trait and SCD. If the test result is positive, Hgb electrophoresis is necessary to distinguish between children with the trait and those with the disease. **Hemoglobin electrophoresis,** referred to as "fingerprinting" of the protein, is a specially prepared blood test that separates various hemoglobins by high voltage. The blood test is accurate, rapid, and specific for detecting the homozygous and heterozygous forms of the disease, as well as the percentages of the various types of Hgb. The hemoglobin electrophoresis increasingly is used as the initial screening test in centers within the United States.

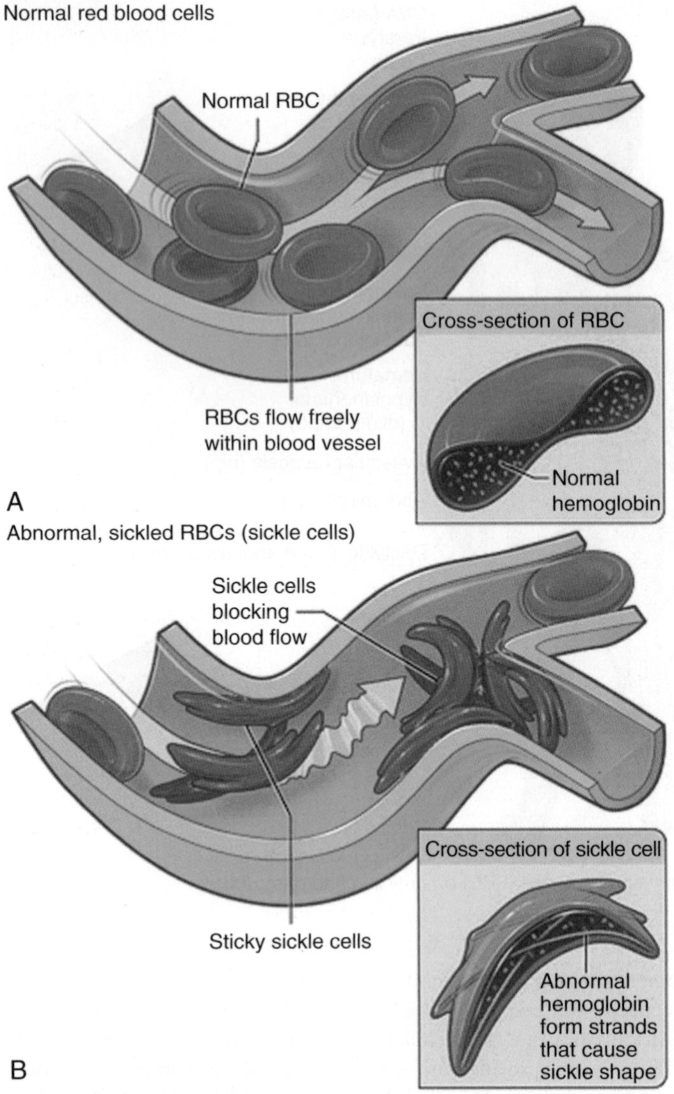

Fig. 24.3 **A,** Normal red blood cells *(RBCs)* flowing freely in a blood vessel. The *inset* shows a cross-section of a normal RBC with normal hemoglobin. **B,** Abnormal, sickled RBCs clumping and blocking blood flow in a blood vessel. (Other cells also may play a role in this clumping process.) The *inset* shows a cross-section of a sickle cell with abnormal hemoglobin. (From National Heart, Lung, and Blood Institute. [2016]. *What is sickle cell anemia?* Bethesda, MD: National Institutes of Health.)

BOX 24.2 Clinical Manifestations of Sickle Cell Anemia

General

Possible growth retardation
Chronic anemia (hemoglobin level of 6 to 9 g/dl)
Possible delayed sexual maturation
Marked susceptibility to sepsis

Vasoocclusive Crisis

Pain in area(s) of involvement
Manifestations related to ischemia of involved areas

- **Extremities:** Painful swelling of hands and feet (sickle cell dactylitis, or hand-foot syndrome), painful joints
- **Abdomen:** Severe pain resembling acute surgical condition
- **Cerebrum:** Stroke, visual disturbances
- **Chest:** Symptoms resembling pneumonia, protracted episodes of pulmonary disease
- **Liver:** Obstructive jaundice, hepatic coma
- **Kidney:** Hematuria
- **Genitalia:** Priapism (persistent painful penile erection)

Sequestration Crisis

Pooling of large amounts of blood

- Hepatomegaly
- Splenomegaly
- Circulatory collapse

Effects of Chronic Vasoocclusive Phenomena

Heart: Cardiomegaly, systolic murmurs
Lungs: Altered pulmonary function, susceptibility to infections, pulmonary insufficiency
Kidneys: Inability to concentrate urine, enuresis, progressive renal failure
Liver: Hepatomegaly, cirrhosis, intrahepatic cholestasis
Spleen: Splenomegaly, susceptibility to infection, functional reduction in splenic activity progressing to autosplenectomy
Eyes: Intraocular abnormalities with visual disturbances; sometimes progressive retinal detachment and blindness
Extremities: Avascular necrosis of hip or shoulder; skeletal deformities, especially lordosis and kyphosis; chronic leg ulcers; susceptibility to osteomyelitis
Central nervous system (CNS): Hemiparesis, seizures

Therapeutic Management

The aims of therapy are to prevent the sickling phenomena, which are responsible for the pathologic sequelae, and treat the medical emergencies of sickle cell crisis. The successful achievement of these aims depends on prompt nursing interventions, medical therapies, patient and family preventive measures, and use of innovative treatments.

Medical management of a crisis is usually directed toward supportive, symptomatic, and specific treatments. The main objectives are to provide (1) rest to minimize energy expenditure and to improve oxygen use; (2) hydration through oral and IV therapy; (3) electrolyte replacement because hypoxia results in metabolic acidosis, which also promotes sickling; (4) analgesia for the severe pain from vasoocclusion; (5) blood replacement to treat progressing severe anemia; and (6) antibiotic therapy to treat any existing infection.

Administration of pneumococcal, *Haemophilus influenzae,* and meningococcal vaccines is recommended for these children because of their susceptibility to infection as a result of functional asplenia. In addition to routine immunizations, children with SCD should receive a yearly influenza vaccination (see Chapter 6, Immunizations). Oral penicillin prophylaxis is recommended by 2 months old to reduce the chance of pneumococcal sepsis (see Translating Evidence Into Practice box).

Oxygen therapy is of little therapeutic value unless the patient has hypoxia (Heeney & Ware, 2015). Severe hypoxia must be prevented because it causes massive systemic sickling that can be fatal. Oxygen administration is usually not effective in reversing sickling or reducing pain because the oxygen is unable to reach the enmeshed sickled erythrocytes through the clogged vessels. In addition, prolonged administration of oxygen can depress bone marrow, further aggravating the anemia.

Another important component of care is the use of blood transfusions. Exchange RBC transfusion (erythrocytapheresis) is the replacement of sickle cells with normal RBCs. Exchange transfusion is a successful, rapid method of reducing the number of circulating sickle cells and therefore slowing down the vicious cycle of hypoxia,

TRANSLATING EVIDENCE INTO PRACTICE

Sickle Cell Anemia and Penicillin Prophylaxis

Ask the Question

PICOT Question

In children with sickle cell anemia (SCA), does prophylaxis with penicillin reduce the risk of pneumococcal infection?

Search for the Evidence

Search Strategies

Search selection criteria included English-language publications within the past 27 years, research-based articles (level 3 or lower), and child populations.

Databases Used

PubMed, Cochrane Collaboration, MD Consult.

Critically Analyze the Evidence

- Rankine-Mullings and Owusu-Ofori (2017) conducted an update of a Cochrane review first published in 2002 and previously updated in 2014. Five randomized or quasi-randomized control trials were identified by the searches, of which three trials (880 children randomized) met the inclusion criteria. All of the included trials showed a reduced incidence of infection in children with SCD (HgbSS or HgbSβ0Thal) receiving prophylactic penicillin. The evidence examined suggests that prophylactic penicillin significantly reduces risk of pneumococcal infection in children with HgbSS and is associated with minimal adverse reactions.
- Hirst and Owusu-Ofori (2014) conducted an updated systematic Cochrane review of three trials that showed a reduced rate of infection in children with homozygous sickle cell disease (HgbSS or HgbSβ0Thal) receiving prophylactic penicillin. Two trials looked at whether treatment was effective. The third trial followed from one of the early trials and looked at when it was safe to stop treatment. Adverse drug effects were rare and minor. Penicillin given prophylactically significantly reduces the risk of pneumococcal infection in children with SCD younger than 5 years old and is associated with minimal adverse reactions. Support for the same conclusion that there is strong evidence that daily oral penicillin prophylaxis greatly reduces the risk of pneumococcal infection in children with SCA younger than 3 years old was reported in a systematic review (Gwaram & Gwaram, 2014).
- Researchers combined the clinical experiences of three sickle cell programs in the eastern United States in an attempt to determine the age and disease-specific risk of *Streptococcus pneumoniae* bacteremia and meningitis in children with SCD at a time when penicillin prophylaxis was routine. Forty-seven pneumococcal infections (44 bacteremia, 3 meningitis) among 40 patients with SCD were observed. Most children in whom infections developed were taking prophylactic penicillin and received Pneumovax at 24 months old. The observed severe pneumococcal infection rate in children with HgbSS younger than 5 years old was less than that reported before penicillin prophylaxis in this specific population (Hord, Byrd, Stowe, et al., 2002).
- Administration of oral prophylactic penicillin was compared with the 14-valent pneumococcal vaccine in preventing pneumococcal infection in 242 children with HgbSS between the ages of 6 months and 3 years. In the first 5 years of the trial, there were 11 pneumococcal infections in the pneumococcal vaccine group and higher infection rates in those given the vaccine before 1 year of age. No pneumococcal isolates were found in the group receiving penicillin, although four pneumococcal isolates were found in this group within 1 year of stopping the penicillin prophylaxis at 3 years old. This study supported the use of penicillin prophylaxis to prevent pneumococcal infection in children younger than 3 years old (John, Ramlal, Jackson, et al., 1984).
- In a multicenter, randomized, double-blind, placebo-controlled clinical trial, 105 children received penicillin twice daily; a control group of 110 children received a placebo twice daily. The trial was terminated 8 months early when an 84% reduction in the incidence of pneumococcal infections was observed in the group treated with penicillin compared with the placebo group. There were no deaths in the penicillin group, but three deaths from infection occurred in the placebo group. Researchers stressed the importance of screening children during the neonatal period and prescribing prophylactic penicillin to decrease the morbidity and mortality associated with pneumococcal infection (Gaston, Verter, Woods, et al., 1986).
- Zarkowsky and colleagues (1986) conducted a retrospective analysis of 178 episodes of bacteremia in children with sickle hemoglobinopathies that occurred during 13,771 patient-years of follow-up ($n = 3451$). The predominant pathogen in patients younger than 6 years old was *S. pneumoniae* (66%), and gram-negative organisms were responsible for 50% of the bacteremias in patients 6 years of age and older. The incidence of pneumococcal bacteremia in children with SCA younger than 3 years old was 6.1 events per 100 patient-years. The results of this study supported prophylactic administration of penicillin for prevention of pneumococcal bacteremia in children younger than 3 years old.
- A cohort study of 315 patients with HgbSS who lived in Jamaica was conducted between June 1973 and December 1981. The patients were divided into three groups to determine whether interventions such as penicillin prophylaxis, parental education on early diagnosis of acute splenic sequestration, and close monitoring in a sickle cell clinic improved survival. A significant decline in deaths from acute splenic sequestration and pneumococcal septicemia and meningitis was found. The research indicated that early detection of SCD and prophylactic measures could significantly reduce deaths associated with HgbSS (Lee, Thomas, Cupidore, et al., 1995).
- Riddington and Owusu-Ofori (2002) conducted a systematic review of randomized controlled trials evaluating the effectiveness of prophylactic antibiotic administration in preventing pneumococcal infection in children with SCD. The review of published research found that penicillin prophylaxis significantly reduced the risk of pneumococcal infection in children with HgbSS with minimal adverse reactions.
- McCavit, Gilbert, and Buchanan (2013) conducted a cross-sectional electronic survey of 106 pediatric hematologists with expertise in SCD regarding their practices related to penicillin prophylaxis in children with SCD older than 5 years of age. Eighty-four percent of pediatric hematologists from 76 centers completed the survey, and 76% routinely recommended cessation of penicillin prophylaxis after 5 years of age.

Apply the Evidence: Nursing Implications

There is **good evidence** with a **strong recommendation** (Guyatt, Oxman, Vist, et al., 2008) that penicillin prophylaxis significantly reduces the risk of pneumococcal infection in children with SCA. The epidemiologic studies strongly suggest that all children with SCA should be started on prophylactic penicillin at 2 months old. Parents and children with SCA should be instructed on the importance of taking the prophylactic penicillin twice daily and seeking medical attention immediately for acute illness, especially if the temperature exceeds 38.3°C (101°F), regardless of the use of prophylaxis. Most pediatric hematologists with SCD expertise recommend cessation of prophylactic penicillin after 5 years of age.

Quality and Safety Competencies: Evidence-Based Practice[a]

Knowledge

Differentiate clinical opinion from research and evidence-based summaries.

Summarize the epidemiologic studies that strongly suggest that children with SCA should be started on prophylactic penicillin. A survey of pediatric experts recommends stopping prophylactic penicillin after 5 years of age.

Continued

TRANSLATING EVIDENCE INTO PRACTICE—cont'd

Skills

Base individualized care plan on patient values, clinical expertise, and evidence.

Integrate evidence into practice by making sure infants with SCD are started on penicillin at 2 months old. Most pediatric SCD experts recommend stopping prophylactic penicillin in children with SCD after 5 years of age.

Attitudes

Value the concept of evidence-based practice as integral to determining best clinical practice.

Appreciate the strength and weakness of evidence for preventing pneumococcal infection in children with SCD.

References

Gaston, M. H., Verter, J. I., Woods, G., et al. (1986). Prophylaxis with oral penicillin in children with sickle cell anemia: A randomized trial. *New England Journal of Medicine, 314*(25), 1593–1599.

Guyatt, G. H., Oxman, A. D., Vist, G. E., et al. (2008). GRADE: An emerging consensus on rating quality of evidence and strength of recommendations. *BMJ, 336*(7650), 924–926.

Gwaram, H. A., & Gwaram, B. A. (2014). A systematic review of effectiveness of daily oral penicillin v prophylaxis in the prevention of pneumococcal infection in children with sickle cell anaemia. *Nigerian Journal of Medicine, 23*(2), 118–129.

Hirst, C., & Owusu-Ofori, S. (2014). Prophylactic antibiotics for preventing pneumococcal infection in children with sickle cell disease. *Cochrane Database of Systematic Reviews, 11*, CD003427.

Hord, J., Byrd, R., Stowe, L., et al. (2002). Streptococcus pneumoniae sepsis and meningitis during the penicillin prophylaxis era in children with sickle cell disease. *Journal of Pediatric Hematology/Oncology, 24*(6), 470–472.

John, A. B., Ramlal, A., Jackson, H., et al. (1984). Prevention of pneumococcal infection in children with homozygous sickle cell disease. *BMJ, 288*(6430), 1567–1570.

Lee, A., Thomas, P., Cupidore, L., et al. (1995). Improved survival in homozygous sickle cell disease: Lessons from cohort study. *BMJ, 311*(7020), 1600–1602.

McCavit, T. L., Gilbert, M., & Buchanan, G. R. (2013). Prophylactic penicillin after 5 years of age in patients with sickle cell disease: A survey of sickle cell disease experts. *Pediatric Blood & Cancer, 60*(6), 935–939.

Rankine-Mullings, A. E., & Owusu-Ofori, S. (2017). Prophylactic antibiotics for preventing pneumococcal infection in children with sickle cell disease. *Cochrane Database of Systematic Reviews, 10*, CD003427.

Riddington, C., & Owusu-Ofori, S. (2002). Prophylactic antibiotics for preventing pneumococcal infection in children with sickle cell disease. *Cochrane Database of Systematic Reviews* (3), CD003427.

Zarkowsky, H. S., Gallagher, D., Gill, F. M., et al. (1986). Bacteremia in sickle hemoglobinopathies. *Journal of Pediatrics, 109*(4), 579–585.

[a] Adapted from the Quality and Safety Education for Nurses website at http://www.qsen.org.
HgbSβ0Thal, Sickle Beta 0 Thalassemia; *HgbSS,* homozygous sickle cell disease; *SCD,* sickle cell disease.

thrombosis, tissue ischemia, and injury. Therapy including simple and exchange transfusions is used in life-threatening ACS and also after acute overt stroke to prevent reoccurrence and further tissue damage (Azar & Wong, 2017; Fortin, Hopewell, & Estcourt, 2018; Hirtz & Kirkham, 2019; Rees, Robinson, & Howard, 2018; Wang & Dwan, 2013).

Children with HgbSS disease and sickle beta thalassemia have the highest risk of stroke and should be monitored with annual TCD (Heeney & Ware, 2015). TCD is a cost-effective, noninvasive ultrasound technique that screens for stroke risk in children who have SCD. TCD is performed on children with SCD from 2 to 16 years of age and measures the average velocity of intracranial vascular flow within the large cerebral arteries (Smith-Whitley & Kwiatkowski, 2020; Yawn et al., 2014; Yawn & John-Sowah, 2015). The recommended treatment for children with confirmed abnormal TCD is chronic transfusion therapy (Armstrong-Wells, Grimes, Sidney, et al., 2009; Fortin et al., 2018; Hirtz & Kirkham, 2019; Kwiatkowski, Yim, Miller, et al., 2011; Smith-Whitley & Kwiatkowski, 2020; Wang & Dwan, 2013). The duration of transfusion is indefinite, although studies are addressing whether patients may be transitioned safely from red cell transfusions and chelation to hydroxyurea and phlebotomy to prevent stroke and decrease iron concentration (Estcourt et al., 2017). Hydroxyurea and phlebotomy were found to be an acceptable alternative to standard treatment (transfusion/chelation therapy) for primary stroke prevention in children with abnormal TCD velocities without evidence of severe vasculopathy on brain MRI or magnetic resonance angiography (MRA) (Helton, Adams, Kesler, et al., 2014).

After a CVA, blood transfusions are usually given every 3 to 4 weeks to help prevent a repeat stroke. Multiple transfusions carry the risk of transmission of viral infection, hyperviscosity, transfusion reactions, alloimmunization, hemosiderosis, and transfusion-related acute lung injury (Heeney & Ware, 2015; Pahuja, Puri, Mahajan, et al., 2017; Rees et al., 2018; Secher, Stensballe, & Afshari, 2013; Yawn et al., 2014). To reduce iron overload from chronic transfusion therapy, chelation therapy may be started (see later in the chapter).

In children with recurrent life-threatening splenic sequestration, splenectomy may be a life-saving measure. However, the spleen usually atrophies on its own through progressive fibrotic changes (**functional asplenia**) by 6 years of age in children with SCA. Prophylactic penicillin and pneumococcal vaccines have decreased the incidence of pneumococcal sepsis in children with SCD. Packed RBC transfusions are recommended for treatment of not only splenic sequestration but also stroke and are used preoperatively accompanied by maintenance IV hydration for major surgical procedures in children with SCD.

Painful VOC, the most common acute SCD complication, is considered the clinical hallmark of SCD that is usually accompanied by increasing health care cost because of prolonged hospitalization (Bou-Maroun, Meta, Hanba, et al., 2018; Meier & Rampersad, 2017; Raphael, Mei, Mueller, et al., 2012; Yawn et al., 2014). The chronic nature of this pain can greatly affect the child's development. A multidisciplinary team (e.g., physician, psychologist, child life specialist, family, nurse, social worker) approach is best for vasoocclusive pain management that includes pharmacologic treatments, hydration, physical therapy, and nonpharmacologic and complementary treatment (e.g., prayer, spiritual healing, massage, heating pads, herbs, relaxation, breathing exercises, distraction, music, guided imagery, exercise, self-motivation, acupuncture, biofeedback) (Brown, Weisberg, Balf-Soran, et al., 2015; Campelo, Oliveira, Magalhaes, et al., 2018; Meier & Rampersad, 2017; Williams & Tanabe, 2016). When mild to moderate VOC is reported, nonsteroidal antiinflammatory medication (e.g., ibuprofen, ketorolac) or nonopioids (e.g., acetaminophen) are used initially. If these drugs are not effective alone, an opioid may be added. The dosages of both drugs are titrated (adjusted) to a therapeutic level. Opioids such as immediate- and sustained-release morphine, oxycodone, hydrocodone, hydromorphone (Dilaudid), and methadone are administered intravenously or orally for severe pain and are given around the clock. In conjunction with the opioid, IV ketorolac for a maximum 5-day course is commonly used to enhance the pain management effect. Patient-controlled analgesia (PCA) has been used successfully for sickle cell–related pain. PCA reinforces the patient's role and responsibility in managing the pain and provides flexibility in dealing with pain, which may vary in severity over time (see Chapter 5, Pain Management).

DRUG ALERT

Meperidine (Demerol) is not recommended. Normeperidine, a metabolite of meperidine, is a central nervous system (CNS) stimulant that produces anxiety, tremors, myoclonus, and generalized seizures when it accumulates with repetitive dosing. Patients with sickle cell disease (SCD) are particularly at risk for normeperidine-induced seizures (National Institutes of Health, National Heart, Lung, and Blood Institute, Division of Blood Disease and Resources, 2014).

Prognosis

The prognosis varies, but most patients live into the fifth decade. The greatest risk is usually in children younger than 5 years old, and most deaths in these children are caused by overwhelming infection. Consequently, SCA is a chronic illness with a potentially terminal outcome. Physical and sexual maturation are delayed in adolescents with SCA. Although adults achieve normal height, typically below normal weight, and normal sexual function, the delay may present problems to the adolescent (Heeney & Ware, 2015). A recent retrospective study of children with SCA reported the effect of disease-modifying therapies (hydroxyurea, transfusion) on growth and puberty patterns compared to no therapy, with transfusion therapy demonstrating an earlier height velocity as compared to either hydroxyurea or no therapy (Nagalapuram, Kulkami, Leach, et al., 2019).

Individuals with SCD who have higher levels of HbF tend to have a milder disease with fewer complications than those with lower levels of HbF (Meier & Miller, 2012; Meier & Rampersad, 2017). Hydroxyurea is a US Food and Drug Administration–approved medication that increases the production of HbF, reduces endothelial adhesion of sickle cells, improves the sickle cell hydration and cell size, increases nitric oxide production (a vasodilator), and lowers leukocyte and reticulocyte counts (National Institutes of Health, National Heart, Lung, and Blood Institute, Division of Blood Disease and Resources, 2014; Nevitt, Jones, & Howard, 2017; Yawn et al., 2014). Long-term follow-up of patients taking hydroxyurea alone revealed at least a 40% reduction in mortality and decreased frequency of VOC, ACS, hospital admissions, and need for transfusions, thus making SCD crises milder (DeBaun & Kirkham, 2016; Ghafuri, Chaturvedi, Rodeghier, et al., 2016; Nevitt et al., 2017; Quarmyne, Dong, Theodore, et al., 2017; Smith-Whitley & Kwiatkowski, 2020; Thomas, Dulman, Lewis, et al., 2019). Pediatric studies have shown that hydroxyurea can be safely used in children (Estepp, Smeltzer, Kang, et al., 2017; Rodriguez, Duez, Dedeken, et al., 2018; Thomas et al., 2019; Wang, Ware, Miller, et al., 2011). The 2014 National Heart, Lung, and Blood Institute evidence-based management guidelines for sickle cell disease recommends that all infants 9 months of age and older with SCA be offered hydroxyurea as treatment, regardless of the frequency or severity of disease complications (National Institutes of Health, National Heart, Lung, and Blood Institute, Division of Blood Disease and Resources, 2014; Yawn et al., 2014).

Despite the positive effects of hydroxyurea, new therapeutic agents are being investigated that focus on preventing sickle red cell dehydration, reducing endothelial adhesion, and using antioxidant treatments (Matte, Zorzi, Mazzi, et al., 2019). Since there has not been any long-term use of these agents, further clinical studies are required.

Hematopoietic stem cell transplantation (HSCT) from a human leukocyte antigen (HLA)–matched sibling or unrelated donor is the only potential cure for SCD, with a high risk of neurologic complications (Azar & Wong, 2017; Heeney & Ware, 2015; Locatelli & Pagliara, 2012). Allogeneic HSCT offers a curative treatment for children with SCD, with overall survival of 92% to 95% and event-free survival of 82% to 86% (Hsieh, Fitzhugh, Weitzel, et al., 2014; Krishnamurti, Neuberg, Sullivan, et al., 2019; Locatelli & Pagliara, 2012). Children and adolescents younger than 16 years of age who have severe complications (e.g., stroke, recurrent ACS, refractory pain, abnormal TCD) and have an HLA-matched donor available may be offered HSCT as a treatment modality (Haining, Duncan, El-haddad, et al., 2015; Lucarelli, Isgro, Sodani, et al., 2012; Smith-Whitley & Kwiatkowski, 2020). Substantial risks such as graft rejection, infections, prolonged immunosuppression, graft-versus-host disease, and disease relapse are associated with HSCT and limit its broad acceptance in SCD patients (Khemani, Katoch, & Krishnamurti, 2019; National Institutes of Health, National Heart, Lung, and Blood Institute, Division of Blood Disease and Resources, 2014). Eventually, improved survival with other HSCT modalities, such as umbilical cord blood transplantation, haploidentical transplants, and nonmyeloablative conditioning regimens, may augment sibling donor protocols and widen the availability of HSCT as a potential cure to SCD patients (Khemani et al., 2019; Lucarelli et al., 2012).

Since SCD is an autosomal recessive disorder, investigative strategies for correction, replacement, addition, or modulation of the globin gene continue to evolve in the basic and clinical research settings (Bourzac, 2017; Matte et al., 2019; Negre, Eggimann, Beuzard, et al., 2016; Sii-Felice, Giorgi, Leboulch, et al., 2018). With fewer than 20% of people with SCD having a matched sibling donor for HSCT, gene therapy may be an attractive curative option (Matte et al., 2019; Meier & Rampersad, 2017; Rubin, 2019).

QUALITY PATIENT OUTCOMES: Sickle Cell Disease

- Early recognition of signs and symptoms of sickle cell anemia (SCA)
- Tissue deoxygenation minimized
- Sickle cell crisis prevented or quickly managed
- Pain appropriately managed
- Stroke prevented
- Prophylactic penicillin regimen followed
- Hypoxia prevented when surgery is necessary
- Pneumococcal, *Haemophilus influenzae* type b, and meningococcal vaccines administered

Nursing Care Management

Educate the Family and Child

Family education begins with an explanation of the disease and its consequences (see Nursing Care Plan and Case Study box). After this explanation, the most important issues to teach the family are to (1) seek early intervention for problems, such as fever of 38.5°C (101.3°F) or greater; (2) give penicillin as ordered; (3) recognize signs and symptoms of stroke, splenic sequestration, as well as respiratory problems that can lead to hypoxia; and (4) treat the child normally.

The nurse emphasizes the importance of adequate hydration to prevent sickling and delay the vasoocclusion and hypoxia-ischemia cycle. It is not sufficient to advise parents to "force fluids" or "encourage drinking." They need specific instructions on how many daily glasses or bottles of fluid are required. Many foods are also a source of fluid, particularly soups, flavored ice pops, ice cream, sherbet, gelatin, and puddings.

NEXT-GENERATION NCLEX® EXAMINATION-STYLE UNFOLDING CASE STUDY

The Child With Sickle Cell Anemia

Day 1, 9:00 am

1. A 12-year-old male with sickle cell anemia (homozygous sickle cell disease [HgbSS]) is being seen in the emergency department (ED) for increasing pain over the past 2 days. The mother is giving him the pain medications as prescribed by the hematology team, but she feels that his pain is getting worse. Which assessment findings require follow-up by the nurse? **Select all that apply.**
   A. Pulse oximetry 96%
   B. Hematocrit = 34%
   C. Pulse = 112 beats/min
   D. Hemoglobin = 10.6 g/dL
   E. Respiration = 24 breaths/min
   F. Abdomen tender to palpation
   G. 8/10 on the number pain scale
   H. Blood pressure = 102/50 mm Hg
   I. Total serum bilirubin = 0.3 mg/dL
   J. Oral temperature = 100.4° F (38° C) K. Weight = 40 kg
2. **Review the case study above. Choose the most likely options for the information missing from the statements below by selecting from the lists of options provided.** As a result of this child's diagnosis of sickle cell disease, the nurse is aware, based on the assessment findings, that the child may be experiencing_____1_____. This is caused by_____2_____

Options for 1	Options for 2
Aplastic crisis	High blood pressure
Sequestration crisis	Ischemia
Acute chest syndrome	Bleeding
Vasoocclusive crisis	Infection
Hyper hemolytic crisis	Diminished red blood cell production
Cerebral vascular accident	Decreased serum sodium

Day 1, 9:30 am

3. The hematologist arrives to examine the child. At this time the child has findings that are consistent with a vasoocclusive crisis (VOC). When planning care for this child, which **priority** interventions would the nurse consider at this time? **Select all that apply.**
   A. Hydration
   B. Antibiotics
   C. Strict bedrest
   D. Pain medication
   E. Pain assessment
   F. Blood transfusion
   G. Oxygen therapy

Day 1, 10:00 am

4. In the last hour an IV dose of morphine (0.1 mg/kg) was given every 10 minutes for three doses. The numeric pain score of 7/10 is assessed after these initial doses. A decision is made to start both morphine and ketorolac since the pain was not relieved after three doses of IV morphine. The morphine is changed to patient-controlled analgesia (PCA). Ketorolac 1 mg/kg for the first dose, then 0.5 mg/kg/dose (maximum of 30 mg/dose) IV every 6 hours also is started. IV fluids at 1½ maintenance rate are administered. What are the **most appropriate** nursing interventions for this child with SCD experiencing pain who is now receiving morphine by PCA and IV Ketorolac? **Indicate which nursing action listed in the far-left column is appropriate for each potential complication listed in the middle column. Indicate the nursing action number in the far-right column. <u>Note that ONLY one nursing action can be used for each potential complication and that NOT all nursing actions will be used.</u>**

Nursing Action	Potential Complication	Nursing Action for Complication
1. Discuss schedule of medication around the clock with parents.	Uncontrolled pain	
2. Encourage high level of fluid intake.	Breakthrough pain	
3. Recognize that various analgesics, including opioids and medication schedules, may need to be tried.	To avoid needless suffering because of unfounded fears	
4. Reassure child and family that analgesics, including opioids, are medically indicated; that high doses may be needed; and that children rarely become addicted.	To prevent vasoconstriction that may enhance sickling with cold applications	
5. Apply heat application or massage to affected area. Avoid applying cold compresses.	Dehydration	
6. Provide protein shake with each meal.		
7. Weigh the child each morning with the same scale.		

NEXT-GENERATION NCLEX® EXAMINATION-STYLE UNFOLDING CASE STUDY—cont'd

Day 1, 2:00 pm

5. The patient is now resting comfortably having been admitted to the pediatric unit. His mother is at the bedside and the last numeric pain assessment reveals his level of pain a 3/10. These are the PCA doses used: Loading dose of 0.1 mg/kg (maximum 8 mg); basal rate of 0.01 mg/kg and intermittent dose 0.035 mg/kg (maximum 8 mg) with the interval lockout at approximately 10 minutes. A 4-hour limit of 0.5 mg/kg is set. His weight is 40 kg. **Based on these PCA loading doses above, choose the most likely options for the information missing from the table by selecting from the list of options provided.**

Loading Dose	Basal Rate	Intermittent Dose	Interval Lockout
1	2	3	4

Options for 1	Options for 2	Options for 3	Options for 4
6	0.4	2.2	5 min
4	0.2	1.8	6 min
8	0.8	1.4	8 min
2	0.9	1.2	10 min

Day 1, 7:00 pm

6. A 12-year-old male with sickle cell anemia (homozygous sickle cell disease [HgbSS]) was seen this morning in the emergency department (ED) for increasing pain over the past 2 days. He is admitted for pain management and is on IV Morphine and Ketorolac. His pain assessment is 2/10 on the numeric scale. Assessment findings at the nurse's change of shift at 7pm reveal:

- Oral temperature = 99.0° F (37.2° C)
- Pulse = 60 beats/min
- Respiration = 16 breaths/min
- Blood pressure = 100/48 mm Hg
- Weight = 89 lbs (40kg)
- Abdomen slightly tender to palpation
- 2/10 on the number pain scale
- Pulse oximetry 98%

The patient is resting comfortably and the nurse at the end of her shift is assessing important nursing actions for the care of this child. **For each nursing action, use an X to indicate whether it was Effective (helped to meet expected quality patient outcomes), Ineffective (did not help to meet expected quality patient outcomes), or Unrelated (not related to the quality patient outcomes).**

Nursing Action	Effective	Ineffective	Unrelated
Administer morphine and ketorolac safely.			
Monitor for side effects of morphine; assess respiratory status closely and prevent constipation.			
Monitor for side effects of ketorolac; assess for bleeding (gastrointestinal [GI] or renal) closely.			
Educate parents on the safety and effectiveness of IV morphine and ketorolac when using them at home.			
Reassess the child's pain level once a shift after administering morphine and ketorolac.			
Read a children's book to the child while he is asleep.			
Recognize that various analgesics and doses may need to be tried.			

NURSING TIP: One simple yet graphic way to demonstrate the effect of sickling is to roll rounded objects, such as marbles or beads, through a tube to simulate normal circulation and then roll pointed objects, such as screws or jacks, through the tube. The effect of sickling and clumping of the pointed objects is especially noticeable at a bend or slight narrowing of the tube.

Increased fluids combined with impaired kidney function result in the problem of **enuresis**. Parents who are unaware of this fact frequently use the usual measures to discourage bedwetting, such as limiting fluids at night, and may resort to punishment and shame to force bladder control. The nurse should discuss this problem with the parents, stressing that the child's ability to concentrate urine is impaired. Reminding the child to urinate frequently during the day and prior to bedtime may be helpful, as may be waking the child during the night if the child's sleep pattern is not disturbed. Enuresis is treated as a complication of the disease, such as joint pain or some other symptom, to alleviate parental pressure on the child.

Promote Supportive Therapies During Crises

The success of many of the medical therapies relies heavily on nursing implementation. Management of pain is an especially difficult problem and often involves experimenting with various analgesics, including opioids, and schedules before relief is achieved. Unfortunately, these children tend to be undermedicated, which results in "clock watching" and demands for additional doses sooner than might be expected. Often this incorrectly raises suspicions of drug addiction, when in fact the problem is one of improper dosage (see Family-Centered Care box). In choosing and scheduling analgesics, the goal should be *prevention* of pain.

FAMILY-CENTERED CARE

Fear of Addiction

Although the pain during a sickle cell crisis is usually severe and opioids are needed, many families fear that their child will become addicted to the narcotic. Unfortunately, misinformed health professionals may foster this unfounded fear, which results in needless suffering. Extremely few children who receive opioids for severe pain become behaviorally addicted to the drug (American Pain Society, 2015). Opioid dependency in children with sickle cell disease is rare and should never be used as a reason to withhold pain medication (Smith-Whitley & Kwaitkowski, 2020). Families and older children, especially adolescents, need to be reassured that opioids are medically indicated, high doses may be needed, and children rarely become addicted.

NURSING TIP: Advise parents to be particularly alert to situations in which dehydration may be a possibility (e.g., hot weather, playing sports) and to recognize early signs of reduced fluid intake, such as decreased urinary output (e.g., fewer wet diapers) and increased thirst.

Any pain program should be combined with psychologic support to help the child deal with the depression, anxiety, and fear that may accompany the disease. This includes regular visits with the child to discuss any concerns during the hospitalization and positive reinforcement of coping skills, such as successful methods of dealing with the pain and compliance with treatment prescriptions. To reduce the negative connotation associated with the term *crisis,* it is best to say *pain episode.*

If blood transfusions or exchange transfusions are given, the nurse has the responsibility of observing for signs of transfusion reaction (see Table 24.3 later in the chapter). Because hypervolemia from too-rapid transfusion can increase the workload of the heart, the nurse also must be alert to signs of cardiac failure.

In splenic sequestration, gently measure the size of the spleen, because increasing splenomegaly is an ominous sign (see Chapter 4, Abdomen). A decrease in spleen size denotes response to therapy. The nurse also closely monitors vital signs and blood pressure to detect impending shock. Anemia is typically not a presenting complication in VOC but is a critical problem in other types of crises. The nurse monitors for evidence of increasing anemia and institutes appropriate nursing interventions (see earlier in the chapter). Oxygen therapy does not reverse sickled RBCs, and if used in a nonhypoxic patient, it will decrease erythropoiesis (Vichinsky & Styles, 1996). Because prolonged use of oxygen can aggravate the anemia, report any signs of lack of therapeutic benefit, such as restlessness, increased pallor, and continued pain.

Record intake, especially of IV fluids, and output. The child's weight should be taken on admission, because it serves as a baseline for evaluating hydration. Because diuresis can result in electrolyte loss, the nurse observes for signs of hypokalemia and should be familiar with normal serum electrolyte values to report changes.

Recognize Other Complications

Nurses also need to be aware of the signs of ACS and CVA, which are both potentially fatal complications.

! NURSING ALERT

Report signs of the following immediately:

Acute chest syndrome (ACS):

- Severe chest, back, or abdominal pain
- Fever of 38.5°C (101.3°F) or higher
- Cough
- Dyspnea, tachypnea
- Retractions
- Declining oxygen saturation (oximetry)

Cerebrovascular accident (CVA):

- Severe, unrelieved headaches
- Severe vomiting
- Jerking or twitching of the face, legs, or arms
- Seizures
- Strange, abnormal behavior
- Inability to move an arm or leg
- Stagger or an unsteady walk
- Stutter or slurred speech
- Weakness in extremities
- Changes in vision

Support the Family

Families need the opportunity to discuss their feelings regarding transmitting a potentially fatal, chronic illness to their child. Because of the widely publicized prognosis for children with SCA, many parents express their fear of the child's death. The prognosis varies; with early diagnosis and treatment, these children are living longer. Previously identified predictors of a severe course of SCA included low hemoglobin level (approximately 7 g/dl), dactylitis or painful episode, and elevated WBC count exhibited before the age of 24 months (Miller, Sleeper, Pegelow, et al., 2000). However, a systematic review identified that the only predictive tests consistently associated with severe SCA outcome are elevated TCD velocities and increased reticulocyte count (Meier, Fasano, & Levett, 2017). All other prognostic predictors had mixed results that were attributed to improved supportive care with reduction in infectious deaths and stroke rate (Meier et al., 2017). The nurse should care for the family as for any family with a child who has a chronic and life-threatening illness and consider the siblings' reactions, the stress on the marital relationship, and the childrearing attitudes displayed toward the child (see Chapter 17). Several resources are available to families with a sickling disorder.[a]

The nurse advises parents to inform all treating personnel of the child's condition. The use of medical identification, such as a bracelet, is another way to ensure awareness of the disease.

If family members have the SCD trait or SCA, genetic counseling is necessary. A primary consideration in genetic counseling is informing parents of the 25% chance with each pregnancy of having a child with the disease when both parents carry the trait.

BETA THALASSEMIA (COOLEY ANEMIA)

Thalassemia is a common genetic disorder, affecting millions globally, that occurs in approximately 4.4 of every 10,000 live births throughout the world (Smith, 2018; Yaish, 2015). In the United States, an estimated 2000 persons have beta thalassemia major (Centers for Disease Control and Prevention, 2019a; Smith-Whitley & Kwiatkowski, 2020). The term **thalassemia**, which is derived from the Greek word *thalassa,* meaning "sea," is applied to various inherited blood disorders characterized by deficiencies in the rate of production of specific globin chains in Hgb. The name appropriately refers to people living near the Mediterranean Sea, namely Italians, Greeks, Syrians, Asians, Africans, and their descendants. Evidence suggests that the high incidence of the disorders among these groups is a result of the selective advantage the trait has in protecting against malaria, as is postulated in SCD. The disorder has a wide geographic distribution, probably as a result of genetic migration through intermarriage or possibly as a result of spontaneous mutation. However, in the past few decades there has been an influx of migrants from these high-prevalence countries, mainly into North America and Central and North Europe, with rapid increase in the thalassemia population.

Beta thalassemia is the most common of the thalassemias and classified in the following forms:

- Two heterozygous forms, **thalassemia minor**, an asymptomatic silent carrier, and **thalassemia trait**, which produces a mild microcytic anemia
- **Thalassemia intermedia**, which may involve either homozygous or heterozygous abnormalities and is manifested as splenomegaly and moderate to severe anemia
- A homozygous form, **thalassemia major** (also known as **Cooley anemia**), which results in a severe anemia that that is not compatible with life without transfusion support

Mode of Transmission

Thalassemia is an autosomal recessive disorder. Both parents must be carriers of the thalassemia trait to produce a child with beta thalassemia major. The typical mode of transmission is between parents who both carry the trait and therefore have a 25% chance with each pregnancy that their child will be born with thalassemia.

BOX 24.3 Clinical Manifestations of Beta Thalassemia

Anemia (Before Diagnosis)

Pallor
Unexplained fever
Poor feeding
Enlarged spleen or liver

Progressive Anemia

Signs of chronic hypoxia
- Headache
- Precordial and bone pain
- Decreased exercise tolerance
- Listlessness
- Anorexia

Other Features

Small stature
Delayed sexual maturation
Bronzed, freckled complexion (if not receiving chelation therapy)

Bone Changes (Older Children If Untreated)

Enlarged head
Prominent frontal and parietal bossing
Prominent malar eminences
Flat or depressed bridge of the nose
Enlarged maxilla
Protrusion of the lip and upper central incisors and eventual malocclusion
Generalized osteoporosis

Pathophysiology

Normal postnatal HbA is composed of two α- and two β-polypeptide chains. In beta thalassemia, there is a partial or complete deficiency in the synthesis of the β-chains of the Hgb molecule. Consequently, there is a compensatory increase in the synthesis of the α-chains, and γ-chain production remains activated, resulting in defective Hgb formation. This unbalanced polypeptide unit is very unstable; when it disintegrates, it damages RBCs, causing severe anemia.

To compensate for the hemolytic process, an overabundance of erythrocytes is formed unless the bone marrow is suppressed by transfusion therapy. Excess iron from packed RBC transfusions and from the rapid destruction of defective cells is stored in various organs (**hemosiderosis**).

Diagnostic Evaluation

The onset of clinical manifestations in thalassemia major may be insidious and not recognized until late infancy or early toddlerhood. The clinical effects of thalassemia major are primarily attributable to defective synthesis of HbA, structurally impaired RBCs, and shortened life span of erythrocytes (Box 24.3).

Hematologic studies reveal the characteristic changes in RBCs (e.g., microcytosis, hypochromia, anisocytosis, poikilocytosis, target cells, basophilic stippling of various stages). Low Hgb and Hct levels are seen in severe anemia, although they are typically lower than the reduction in RBC count because of the proliferation of immature erythrocytes. Hgb electrophoresis confirms the diagnosis and is helpful in distinguishing the type of thalassemia because it analyzes the quantity and kind of Hgb variants found in the blood.

[a]Sickle Cell Disease Association of America, Inc., 231 E. Baltimore St., Suite 800, Baltimore, MD 21202; 410-528-1555, 800-421-8453; fax: 410-528-1495; email: scdaa@sicklecelldisease.org; http://www.sicklecelldisease.org; http://www.facebook.com/sicklecellcampaign; Sickle Cell Information Center, PO Box 109, Grady Memorial Hospital, 80 Jesse Hill Jr Drive SE, Atlanta, GA 30303; 404-616-3572; fax: 404-616-5998; email: aplatt@emory.edu; http://scinfo.org; National Heart, Lung, and Blood Institute Health Information Center, PO Box 30105, Bethesda, MD 20824-0105; 301-592-8573; fax: 301-592-8563; http://www.nhlbi.nih.gov; http://www.ahcpr.gov.

Therapeutic Management

The objectives of supportive therapy are to maintain sufficient Hgb levels to prevent bone marrow expansion and bony deformities and to provide sufficient RBCs to support normal growth and normal physical activity. Transfusions are the foundation of medical management, with the goal of maintaining the Hgb level at approximately 9.5 g/dl, an aim that may require transfusions as often as every 2 to 5 weeks. The advantages of this therapy include (1) improved physical and psychologic well-being because of the ability to participate in normal activities, (2) decreased cardiomegaly and hepatosplenomegaly, (3) fewer bone changes, (4) normal or near-normal growth and development until puberty, and (5) fewer infections.

One of the potential complications of frequent blood transfusions is iron overload (hemosiderosis). Because the body has no effective means of eliminating the excess iron, the mineral is deposited in body tissues. To minimize the development of hemosiderosis and hemochromatosis in patients with thalassemia major, there are three approved iron-chelating agents: deferoxamine, deferasirox, and deferiprone (Khandros & Kwaitkowski, 2019; Origa, 2017; Smith-Whitley & Kwiatkowski, 2020).

In some children with severe splenomegaly who require repeated transfusions, a splenectomy may be necessary to decrease the disabling effects of abdominal pressure and to increase the life span of supplemental RBCs. Over time, the spleen may accelerate the rate of RBC destruction and thus increase transfusion requirements. After a splenectomy, children generally require fewer transfusions, although the basic defect in Hgb synthesis remains unaffected. A major postsplenectomy complication is severe and overwhelming infection. Therefore these children are often on prophylactic antibiotics with close medical supervision for many years and should receive the pneumococcal and meningococcal vaccines in addition to the regularly scheduled immunizations (see Chapter 6, Immunizations).

> **NURSING TIP:** Ensure that the family and patient understand the need to notify the health professional of all fevers of 38.5°C (101.3°F) or greater because of the risk of sepsis in a child with asplenia.

Prognosis

Most children treated with blood transfusions and early chelation therapy have a remarkably improved survival and quality of life as they survive well into adulthood (Cappellini, Porter, Viprakasit, et al., 2018; Sankaran, Nathan, & Orkin, 2015). The most common causes of death are heart disease, liver damage with cirrhosis, postsplenectomy sepsis, and multiorgan failure secondary to hemochromatosis (Choudhry, 2017; Sankaran et al., 2015; Yaish, 2015). The three adverse prognostic factors for event-free survival are presence of hepatomegaly, iron overload, and portal fibrosis (Choudhry, 2017). Children without these adverse prognostic factors have greater than 97% event-free survival (Choudhry, 2017). A curative treatment for some children is HSCT. Children younger than 14 years of age without excessive iron stores and hepatomegaly who undergo allogeneic HSCT have a high rate of complication-free survival; approximately 80% to 97% of these children are cured (Issaragrisil & Kunacheewa, 2016; Origa, 2017; Smith-Whitley & Kwiatkowski, 2020). Also, related cord-blood transplantation has a disease-free survival of about 90% (Higgs, Engel, & Stamatoyannopoulos, 2012; Issaragrisil & Kunacheewa, 2016). Children without a matched donor may benefit from haploidentical family member transplant, which has shown encouraging results (Locatelli, Merli, & Strocchio, 2016; Lucarelli et al., 2012). New approaches for correction of thalassemia through the introduction of gene therapy strategies, including the use of lentiviral vectors, generation of pluripotent stem cells, gene targeting, and gene editing, are ongoing but continue to have concerns (Arlet, Dussiot, Moura, et al., 2016; El-Beshlawy & El-Ghamrawy, 2019; Makis, Hatzimichael, Papassotiriou, et al., 2016; Sankaran et al., 2015; Xu, Luk, Yao, et al., 2019).

Nursing Care Management

The objectives of nursing care are to (1) promote compliance with transfusion and chelation therapy, (2) assist the child in coping with the anxiety-provoking treatments and the effects of the illness, (3) foster the child's and family's adjustment to a chronic illness, and (4) observe for complications of multiple blood transfusions. Basic to each of these goals is explaining to parents and older children the defect responsible for the disorder, its effect on RBCs, and the potential effects of untreated iron overload (e.g., delayed growth and maturation, heart disease). Because this condition is prevalent among families of Mediterranean descent, the nurse also inquiries about the family's previous knowledge about thalassemia. All families with a child with thalassemia should be tested for the trait and referred for genetic counseling.

As with any chronic illness, the family's needs must be met for optimal adjustment to the stresses imposed by the disorder (see Chapter 17). Sources of information for the family include the Cooley's Anemia Foundation[b] and the Northern California Comprehensive Thalassemia Center. Genetic counseling for the parents and fertile offspring is mandatory, and both prenatal diagnosis using amniocentesis or fetal blood sampling and screening for thalassemia trait are available.

APLASTIC ANEMIA

Aplastic anemia (AA) is a rare and life-threatening disorder that affects approximately 2 to 6 in 1 million children and adults each year (Fargo & Hord, 2020; Korthof, Bekassy, & Hussein, 2013). AA refers to a bone marrow failure condition in which the formed elements of the blood are simultaneously depressed. The peripheral blood smear demonstrates cytopenia with at least two of the following present: profound anemia, leukopenia, and thrombocytopenia. In contrast, **hypoplastic anemia** is characterized by a profound depression of RBCs but normal or slightly decreased WBCs and platelets.

Etiology

AA can be primary (**congenital**, or present at birth) or secondary (**acquired**). The best-known congenital disorder of which AA is an outstanding feature is **Fanconi syndrome**, a rare hereditary disorder characterized by pancytopenia, hypoplasia of the bone marrow, and patchy brown discoloration of the skin resulting from the deposit of melanin. It is associated with multiple congenital anomalies of the musculoskeletal and genitourinary systems. The syndrome appears to be inherited as an autosomal recessive trait with varying penetrance; therefore affected siblings may demonstrate several different combinations of defects.

Several etiologic factors contribute to the development of acquired AA; however, most cases are considered idiopathic (Box 24.4). The following discussion focuses on severe acquired AA, which carries a poorer prognosis and follows a more rapidly fatal course than the primary types.

Diagnostic Evaluation

The onset of clinical manifestations, which include anemia, leukopenia, and decreased platelet count, is usually insidious. Definitive diagnosis is

[b]330 Seventh Ave., No. 200, New York, NY 10001; 800-522-7222; fax: 212-279-5999; email: info@cooleysanemia.org; http://www.thalassemia.org; www.facebook.com/pages/Thalassemia-org/162500870481012.

BOX 24.4 Common Causes of Acquired Aplastic Anemia

- Human parvovirus infection, hepatitis, or overwhelming infection
- Irradiation
- Immune disorders, such as eosinophilic fasciitis and hypoimmunoglobulinemia
- Drugs, such as certain chemotherapeutic agents, anticonvulsants, and antibiotics
- Industrial and household chemicals, including benzene and its derivatives, which are found in petroleum products, dyes, paint remover, shellac, and lacquers
- Infiltration and replacement of myeloid elements, such as in leukemia or the lymphomas
- Idiopathic (In most cases, no identifiable precipitating cause can be found.)

determined from bone marrow examination, which demonstrates the conversion of red bone marrow to yellow, fatty bone marrow. Severe AA is based on Camitta criteria, which include less than 25% bone marrow cellularity with at least two of the following findings: absolute granulocyte count less than 500/mm^3, platelet count less than 20,000/mm^3, and absolute reticulocyte count less than 40,000/mm^3 (Miano & Dufour, 2015; Passweg & Marsh, 2010). Moderate AA is defined as less than 50% bone marrow cellularity with presence of mild to moderate cytopenia (Shimamura & Williams, 2015).

Therapeutic Management

The objectives of treatment are based on the recognition that the underlying disease process is failure of the bone marrow to carry out its hematopoietic functions. Therefore therapy is directed at restoring function to the marrow and involves two main approaches: (1) immunosuppressive therapy (IST) to remove the presumed immunologic functions that prolong aplasia or (2) replacement of the bone marrow through transplantation. Bone marrow transplantation is the treatment of choice for severe AA when a suitable donor exists (see later in the chapter).

Antilymphocyte globulin (ALG) or **antithymocyte globulin (ATG)** is the principal drug treatment used for AA. The rationale for using ATG is based on the theory that AA may be a result of autoimmunity. IST is a combination of ATG and cyclosporine that suppress T cell–dependent autoimmune responses by recognizing human lymphocyte cell surface antigen and decreasing the lymphocytes without causing bone marrow suppression (Peinemann & Labeit, 2014; Young, 2018). ATG usually is administrated intravenously over 12 to 16 hours for 4 days after a test dose to check for hypersensitivity. Cyclosporine is administered orally for several months to a year after ATG therapy until achievement of stable maximally improved blood counts, then is slowly tapered over the course of approximately a year (Fargo & Hord, 2020; Peslak, Olson, & Babushok, 2017). Response to IST is typically delayed, and responses generally do not start before 3 to 4 months with a median time of 6 months (Fargo & Hord, 2020; Samarasinghe & Webb, 2012; Shimamura & Williams, 2015). An IST course may be repeated, depending on the reduction in circulating lymphocytes and the patient's response. Because of the hypersensitivity response associated with ATG (i.e., fever, chills, myalgias), methylprednisolone is given intravenously to prevent these side effects. Granulocyte colony-stimulating factor (G-CSF) is usually ineffective, with no clear evidence of improving the overall survival when added to IST, therefore routine G-CSF used outside febrile neutropenic episodes is controversial (Fargo & Hord, 2020; Tichelli, Schrezenmeier, Socie, et al., 2011; Young, 2018). However, studies reported the use of another growth factor with encouraging preliminary results when eltrombopag (thrombopoietic growth factor) was added to IST in treatment of refractory severe AA (Desmond, Townsley, Dumitriu, et al., 2014; Townsley, Scheinberg, Winkler, et al., 2017). Androgens may be used with ATG to stimulate erythropoiesis if the AA is unresponsive to initial therapies.

HSCT should be considered early in the course of the disease if a compatible donor can be found. Transplantation is more successful when performed before multiple transfusions have sensitized the child to leukocyte and **human leukocyte antigens (HLAs)**. HSCT is associated with an approximately 90% survival rate in patients who receive a bone marrow transplant from an HLA-identical sibling, but the risk of graft failure, graft-versus-host disease, and infectious complications should also be taken into account (Fargo & Hord, 2020; Halkes, de Wreede, Knol-Bout, et al., 2019; Scheinberg, 2012). Recently, survival outcomes from unrelated HLA-matched bone marrow transplantation have been approaching the success seen with HLA-identical sibling bone marrow transplant (Georges & Storb, 2016).

Nursing Care Management

The care of the child with AA is similar to that of the child with leukemia (see Chapter 25) and includes preparing the child and family for the diagnostic and therapeutic procedures, preventing complications from the severe pancytopenia, and emotionally supporting them in the face of a potentially fatal outcome. Information and support are available from the Aplastic Anemia and MDS International Foundation.[c]

The drug ATG is usually administered by way of a central vein. If not, vigilant care must be directed to the IV infusion to prevent extravasation. Meticulous care of the venous access is essential because of the child's susceptibility to infection. Chemotherapeutic agents have been used in the treatment of relapsed patients with AA after unresponsive IST. Many of the side effects associated with chemotherapy, such as nausea and vomiting, alopecia, and mucositis, are experienced by children receiving treatment for AA. Specialized care is required for children with AA who have HSCT (discussed in Chapter 25).

DEFECTS IN HEMOSTASIS

Hemostasis is the process that stops bleeding when a blood vessel is injured. Vascular and plasma clotting factors, as well as platelets, are required. A complex system of clotting, anticlotting, and clot breakdown (**fibrinolysis**) mechanisms exists in equilibrium to ensure clot formation only in the presence of blood vessel injury and to limit the clotting process to the site of vessel wall injury. Dysfunction in these systems leads to bleeding or abnormal clotting. Although the coagulation process is complex, clotting depends on three factors: (1) vascular influence, (2) platelet role, and (3) clotting factors.

HEMOPHILIA

The term **hemophilia** refers to a group of bleeding disorders resulting from congenital deficiency or dysfunction, or absence of specific coagulation proteins or factors (Di Paola, Montgomery, Gill, et al., 2015; Sharathkumar & Pipe, 2008). Although the symptomatology is similar regardless of which clotting factor is deficient, the identification of specific factor deficiencies allows definitive treatment with replacement agents.

In about 80% of all cases of hemophilia, the inheritance pattern is demonstrated as X-linked recessive. The two most common forms of the disorder are **factor VIII deficiency** (hemophilia A, or classic hemophilia) and **factor IX deficiency** (hemophilia B, or Christmas disease) with prevalence of approximately 1 in 5000 and 1 in 20,000 to 30,000 live births, respectively (Centers for Disease Control and Prevention,

[c]100 Park Avenue, Suite 108, Rockville, MD 20850; 800-747-2820, 301-279-7202; fax: 301-279-7205; email: help@aamds.org; http://www.aamds.org; http://www.facebook.com/aamds.

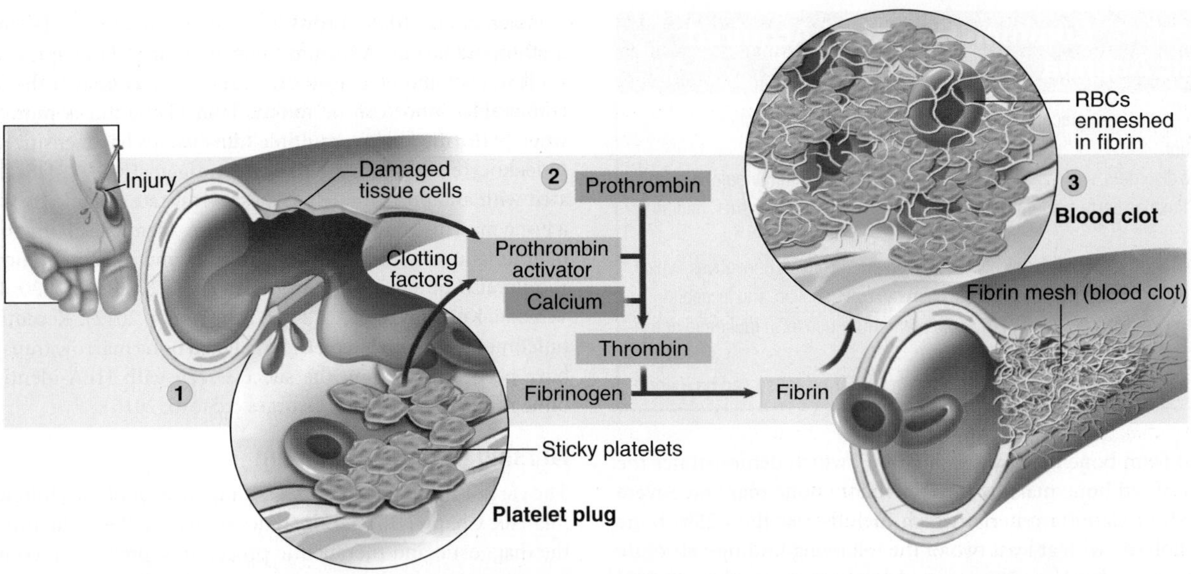

Fig. 24.4 Blood clotting. The extremely complex clotting mechanism can be distilled into three basic steps: (1) release of clotting factors from both injured tissue cells and sticky platelets at the injury site (which form a temporary platelet plug); (2) a series of chemical reactions that eventually result in the formation of thrombin; and (3) formation of fibrin and trapping of red blood cells *(RBCs)* to form a clot. (From Thibodeau, G. A. [2010]. *The human body in health and disease* [5th ed.]. St Louis, MO: Mosby.)

2018b; Scott & Flood, 2020a; Sharathkumar & Carcao, 2011). There are about 20,000 people of all races and ethnic groups affected with hemophilia in the United States (National Hemophilia Foundation, 2019). Von Willebrand disease (vWD) is another hereditary bleeding disorder characterized by a deficiency, abnormality, or absence of the protein called *von Willebrand factor (vWF)*. The following discussion is primarily concerned with factor VIII deficiency, which accounts for 80% to 85% of all hemophilia cases.

Pathophysiology

The basic defect of hemophilia A is a deficiency of factor VIII (antihemophilic factor [AHF]). Factor VIII is produced by the liver and is necessary for the formation of thromboplastin in phase I of blood coagulation (Fig. 24.4). The less factor VIII that is found in the blood, the more severe the disease. Individuals with hemophilia have two of the three factors required for coagulation: vascular influence and platelets. Therefore they may bleed for longer periods but not at a faster rate.

A major feature of hemophilia is that its expression varies markedly regarding the degree of bleeding severity. Hemophilia is generally classified into three groups (severe, moderate, mild) according to the severity of the factor deficiency; 60% to 70% of children with hemophilia demonstrate the severe form of the disorder. With severe factor deficiencies, hemorrhage can occur spontaneously or as a result of minor trauma, such as after circumcision. In children with less severe deficiencies (moderate, mild), however, the bleeding tendency may not be noted until the onset of walking.

Subcutaneous and IM hemorrhages are common. Hemarthrosis, which refers to bleeding into joint cavities, especially the knees, elbows, and ankles, is the most frequent form of internal bleeding. Bony changes and crippling deformities occur after repeated bleeding episodes over several years. Early signs of hemarthrosis are a feeling of stiffness, tingling, or achiness in the affected joint, followed by decrease in joint movement. Obvious affected joint signs and symptoms are increased warmth, redness, and swelling and severe pain with loss of movement. Bleeding in the neck, mouth, or thorax is serious because the airway can become obstructed. Intracranial hemorrhage can have fatal consequences and is one of the major causes of death. Hemorrhage anywhere along the GI tract can lead to anemia, and bleeding into the retroperitoneal cavity is especially hazardous because of the large space for blood to accumulate. Hematomas in the spinal cord can cause paralysis.

Diagnostic Evaluation

The diagnosis is usually made from a history of bleeding episodes, evidence of X-linked inheritance (only one-third of the cases are new mutations), and laboratory findings. To understand the significance of various tests of hemostasis, it is helpful to recall the usual mechanism to control bleeding (e.g., the function of platelets and clotting factors). The test specific for hemophilia plasma includes factor VIII and factor IX assay, procedures normally performed in specialized laboratories. Other tests are those that depend on specific factors for a reaction to occur, especially the partial thromboplastin time (PTT). Carrier detection is possible in classic hemophilia using deoxyribonucleic acid (DNA) testing and is an important consideration in families in which female offspring may have inherited the trait.

Therapeutic Management

The primary therapy for hemophilia is replacement of the missing clotting factor. The products available are factor VIII concentrates, either produced through genetic engineering (recombinant form) or derived from pooled plasma, which are reconstituted with sterile water immediately before use. A synthetic form of vasopressin, 1-deamino-8-d-arginine vasopressin (DDAVP), increases plasma factor VIII activity and is the treatment of choice in mild hemophilia and vWD types I and IIA only if the child shows an appropriate response. After DDAVP administration, a threefold to fourfold rise in factor VIII level activity should occur. It is not effective in the treatment of severe hemophilia A, severe vWD, or any form of hemophilia B. Aggressive factor concentrate replacement therapy is initiated to prevent chronic crippling effects from joint bleeding.

Other drugs may be included in the therapy plan, depending on the source of the hemorrhage. Corticosteroids are given for hematuria, acute hemarthrosis, and chronic synovitis. It is recommended that patients with hemophilia avoid aspirin and traditional nonsteroidal antiinflammatory drugs (NSAIDs) such as ibuprofen because they inhibit platelet function associated with GI bleeding (Scott & Flood, 2020a; World Federation of Hemophilia, 2012). However, cyclooxygenase-2 (COX-2) inhibitors, selective NSAIDs that have comparable analgesic effect to traditional NSAIDs with less chance of GI bleeding, have been recommended as a suitable option for hemophilic arthropathy (Arachchillage & Markis, 2016; World Federation of Hemophilia, 2012). Oral administration of ε-aminocaproic acid (Amicar) prevents clot destruction. Its use is limited to mouth trauma or surgery, with a dose of factor concentrate given first.

A regular program of exercise and physical therapy is an important aspect of management. Physical activity within reasonable limits strengthens muscles around joints and may decrease the number of spontaneous bleeding episodes.

Treatment without delay results in more rapid recovery and a decreased likelihood of complications; therefore most children are treated at home. The family is taught the technique of venipuncture and to administer the AHF to children older than 2 to 3 years old. The child learns the procedure for self-administration at 8 to 12 years old. Home treatment is highly successful, and the rewards, in addition to the immediacy, are less disruption of family life, fewer school or work days missed, and enhancement of the child's self-esteem and independence.

Prophylactic therapy is periodic factor replacement for children with severe hemophilia to prevent bleeding complications, including arthropathy and spontaneous life-threatening bleeding events (Di Paola et al., 2015; Scott & Flood 2020a; von der Lippe, Frich, Harris, et al., 2017). Primary prophylaxis involves the infusion of factor VIII concentrate on a regular basis before the onset of joint damage. Secondary prophylaxis involves the infusion of factor VIII concentrate on a regular basis after the child experiences his or her first joint bleed. The administration of infusions differs among treatment centers and may range from every other day to three times a week for several weeks to promote healing. On-demand factor replacement may be a cost-effective alternative to primary prophylaxis, but prophylaxis decreases the development of joint disease and preserves joint function compared with on-demand factor replacement treatment (Chozie, Primacakti, Gatot, et al., 2019; Iorio, Marchesini, Marcucci, et al., 2011; Nugent, O'Mahony, Dolan, et al., 2018). Prompt appropriate treatment of hemorrhage and prophylactic therapy are key to excellent care and prevention of long-term morbidity in patients with hemophilia (Di Paola et al., 2015; Hanley, McKernan, Creagh, et al., 2017; Lillicrap, 2013; Nugent et al., 2018).

Prognosis

Although there is no cure for hemophilia, its symptoms can be controlled and its potentially crippling deformities greatly reduced or even avoided. Today, many children with hemophilia function with minimal or no joint damage. They have an average life expectancy and are normal in every respect but one—they have a tendency to bleed, which is a significant inconvenience but not necessarily a life-threatening event.

Unfortunately, those individuals with hemophilia who were treated before the development of current purification techniques for factor VIII concentrate (between 1979 and 1985) may have been exposed to human immunodeficiency virus (HIV). It is estimated that 90% of severe hemophiliacs seroconverted to HIV-positive status (National Hemophilia Foundation, 2019). Individuals with hemophilia diagnosed since the 1990s and treated with recombinant factor products are at virtually no risk for developing HIV infection from treatment. Recombinant factor VIII and factor IX products that are devoid of human protein materials have become the treatment of choice for children and previously untreated hemophilia patients (Di Paola et al., 2015).

Gene therapy may prove to be a treatment option in the future. Techniques are under development to introduce factor VIII and factor IX genes into hepatocytes, fibroblast, and endothelial cells using adeno-associated viral vectors and other novel ideas for genetic correction (Branchford, Monahan, & Di Paola, 2013; Nienhuis, Nathwani, & Davidoff, 2017; Walsh & Batt, 2013). Efforts are underway to improve viral vector strategies, including selection of both appropriate vectors and the appropriate cell in which to express the gene, and to obtain a better understanding of the immune consequences of gene transfer (Di Paola et al., 2015; Doshi & Arruda, 2018; Lytle, Brown, Paik, et al., 2016; Nienhuis et al., 2017).

QUALITY PATIENT OUTCOMES: Hemophilia

- Early recognition of signs and symptoms of hemophilia
- Bleeding episodes prevented
- Bleeding episodes treated early with factor replacement
- Adherence to prophylactic factor replacement program when indicated
- Hemarthrosis prevented when possible with limited joint damage
- Exercise program and physical therapy ongoing

Nursing Care Management

The earlier a bleeding episode is recognized, the more effectively it can be treated. Signs that indicate internal bleeding are especially important to recognize. Children are aware of internal bleeding and are reliable in telling the examiner the location of an internal bleed. In addition to the manifestations described (Box 24.5), the nurse maintains a high level of suspicion when a child with hemophilia shows signs such as headache; slurred speech; loss of consciousness (from cerebral bleeding); and black, tarry stools (from GI bleeding).

Prevent Bleeding

The goal of prevention of bleeding episodes is directed toward decreasing the risk of injury. Prevention of bleeding episodes is geared mostly toward appropriate exercises to strengthen muscles and joints and to allow age-appropriate activity. During infancy and toddlerhood, the normal acquisition of motor skills creates innumerable opportunities for falls, bruises, and minor wounds. Restraining the child from mastering motor development can bring more serious long-term problems than allowing the behavior. However, the environment should be made as safe as possible, with close supervision during playtime to minimize incidental injuries.

For older children, the family usually needs assistance in preparing for school. A nurse who knows the family can be instrumental in discussing the situation with the school nurse and in jointly planning an appropriate activity schedule. Because almost all individuals with hemophilia are boys, the physical limitations regarding active sports may be a difficult adjustment, and activity restrictions must be

BOX 24.5 Clinical Manifestations of Hemophilia

- Prolonged bleeding anywhere from or in the body
- Hemorrhage from any trauma: Loss of deciduous teeth, circumcision, cuts, epistaxis, injections
- Excessive bruising, even from a slight injury, such as a fall
- Subcutaneous and intramuscular (IM) hemorrhages
- Hemarthrosis (bleeding into the joint cavities), especially the knees, ankles, and elbows
- Hematomas: Pain, swelling, and limited motion
- Spontaneous hematuria

tempered with sensitivity to the child's emotional and physical needs. Use of protective equipment, such as helmets, face masks, shin/wrist/forearm guards, kneepads, and other equipment appropriate for the type of athletic activity, is encouraged to prevent injury. Children and adolescents with severe hemophilia may participate in noncontact sports with a low injury risk, such as aerobic exercise, stretching exercises, swimming, yoga, archery, walking, jogging, tennis, golf, fishing, and bowling (Anderson & Forsyth, 2017; World Federation of Hemophilia, 2012). Athletic participation is recommended after careful consideration of different activities with proper prophylaxis, precautions, and surveillance by caregivers and physicians (Howell, Scott, & Patel, 2017; National Hemophilia Foundation, 2019)

To prevent oral bleeding, some readjustment in terms of dental hygiene may be needed to minimize trauma to the gums, such as use of a water irrigating device, softening the toothbrush in warm water before brushing, or using a sponge-tipped disposable toothbrush. A regular toothbrush should be soft bristled and small. Adolescents also need to be advised of the dangers of using safety razors with blades and should use an electric shaver.

Because any trauma can lead to a bleeding episode, all persons caring for these children must be aware of their disorder. These children should wear medical identification, and older children should be encouraged to recognize situations in which disclosing their condition is important, such as during dental extraction or injections. Health personnel need to take special precautions to prevent the use of procedures that may cause bleeding, such as IM injections. The subcutaneous route is substituted for IM injections whenever possible. Venipunctures for blood samples are usually preferred for these children. There is usually less bleeding after the venipuncture than after finger or heel punctures. Neither aspirin nor any aspirin-containing compound should be used. Acetaminophen is a suitable aspirin substitute, especially for controlling pain at home.

Recognize and Control Bleeding

As noted, the earlier a bleeding episode is recognized, the more effectively it can be treated. Factor replacement therapy should be instituted according to established medical protocol, and supportive measures may be implemented, such as **RICE**, which stands for *r*est, *i*ce, *c*ompression, and *e*levation. When parents and older children are taught such measures beforehand, they can be prepared to initiate immediate treatment. Plastic bags of ice or cold packs should be kept in the freezer for such emergencies. However, such measures do not take the place of factor replacement.

Prevent Crippling Effects of Bleeding

As a result of repeated episodes of hemarthrosis, incompletely absorbed blood in the joints, and limitation of motion, bone and muscle changes occur that result in flexion contractures and joint fixation. During bleeding episodes, the joint is elevated and immobilized. Active range-of-motion exercises are usually instituted after the acute phase. This allows the child to control the degree of exercise according to the level of discomfort. If an exercise program is instituted in the home, a physical therapist or public health nurse may need to supervise compliance with the regimen. Rarely, orthopedic intervention (such as casting, application of traction, or aspiration of blood) may be necessary to preserve joint function. Diet is also an important consideration because excessive body weight can increase the strain on affected joints, especially the knees, and predispose the child to hemarthrosis. Consequently, calories need to be supplied in accordance with energy requirements.

Support the Family and Prepare for Home Care

Genetic counseling is essential as soon as possible after diagnosis. Unlike many other disorders in which both parents carry the trait, the feeling of responsibility for this condition usually rests with the mother. Unless she has an opportunity to discuss her feelings, the couple's relationship can suffer. Technology is available to identify classic hemophilia carriers using DNA testing and may reduce the anxiety regarding childbearing in women who may be at risk of carrying the defective gene. Factor concentrates have greatly changed the outlook for these children by minimizing bleeding and allowing the child to live a normal, unrestricted life. Children are taught to take responsibility for their disease at an early age. They learn their limitations, preventive measures, and self-administration of the prophylactic AHF.

The needs of families who have children with hemophilia are best met through a comprehensive team approach of physicians (pediatrician, hematologist, orthopedist), nurse practitioner, nurse, social worker, and physical and psychologic therapists. Parent-group discussions are beneficial in meeting the needs that are often best met by similarly affected families. For example, with the improved prognosis for these children, parents and adolescents with hemophilia face vocational and financial problems in addition to concern over future childbearing. This can be disastrous in terms of the cost of treatment, which can exceed $100,000 a year. Financial support is particularly important. The National Hemophilia Foundation[d] and the Canadian Hemophilia Society[e] provide numerous services and publications for both health providers and families.

Children who have become infected with HIV through transfusions and factor replacement products are faced with the consequences of this dreaded disease. Consequently, they need the support of health professionals, especially in the areas of safe sexual practices to avoid disease transmission and public education regarding acquired immune deficiency syndrome (AIDS) and ways to deal with public reactions to persons who have AIDS.

IMMUNE THROMBOCYTOPENIA (IDIOPATHIC THROMBOCYTOPENIC PURPURA)

Idiopathic thrombocytopenic purpura (ITP), the term formerly used because purpura is an infrequent sign at presentation, is now referred to as *immune thrombocytopenia* (Rodeghiero, Stasi, Gernsheimer, et al., 2009). ITP is an acquired hemorrhagic disorder characterized by (1) **thrombocytopenia**, (2) absence or minimal signs of bleeding (easy bruising, mucosal bleeding, petechiae) in most childhood cases, and (3) normal bone marrow with a normal or increased number of immature platelets (**megakaryocytes**) and **eosinophils**. Although the causes are not known, it is understood that ITP involves the evolution of antibodies against multiple platelet antigens and cytotoxic T cells that cause platelet destruction in blood and spleen and/or inhibition of platelet production in the bone marrow (Consolini, 2011; Scott & Flood, 2020b; Wilson, 2015). ITP is the most common thrombocytopenia of childhood that typically presents 1 to 4 weeks after a viral illness, and the majority of cases are in children younger than 10 years old, with the peak incidence between 1 to 6 years old (Consolini, 2011; Cooper, 2017; Scott & Flood, 2020b; Wilson, 2015).

The disease occurs in one of the following forms: (1) as newly diagnosed acute ITP that is less than 3 months from diagnosis, (2) as persistent

[d]116 W. 32nd St., 11th Floor, New York, NY 10001; 800-42-HANDI, 212-328-3700; email: handi@hemophilia.org; http://www.hemophilia.org; http://www.facebook.com/NationalHemophiliaFoundation.

[e]400–1255 University St., Montreal, Quebec, Canada H3B 3B6; 800-668-2686, 514-848-0503; fax: 514-848-9661; email: chs@hemophilia.ca; http://www.hemophilia.ca; http://www.facebook.com/CanadianHemophiliaSociety.

BOX 24.6 Clinical Manifestations of Immune Thrombocytopenia (Idiopathic Thrombocytopenic Purpura)

Easy Bruising
- Petechiae
- Ecchymoses
- Most often over bony prominences

Bleeding From Mucous Membranes
- Epistaxis
- Bleeding gums
- Internal hemorrhage evidenced by the following:
    - Hematuria
    - Hematemesis
    - Melena
    - Hemarthrosis
    - Menorrhagia
    - Hematomas over lower extremities

ITP that occurs from 3 months to 1 year, or (3) as a chronic condition lasting more than 12 months' duration (Cooper, 2017; Onisai, Vladareanu, Spinu, et al., 2019). The acute form occurs most commonly after upper respiratory tract infections; after the childhood diseases measles, rubella, mumps, and chickenpox; or after infection with human parvovirus.

Diagnostic Evaluation

The diagnosis is suspected based on clinical manifestations (Box 24.6). In ITP, the platelet count is reduced to less than 20,000/mm^3; therefore tests that depend on platelet function, such as the tourniquet test, bleeding time, and clot retraction, are abnormal. There is no definitive test that establishes a diagnosis of ITP; several tests are usually performed to rule out other disorders in which thrombocytopenia is a manifestation, such as systemic lupus erythematosus, lymphoma, or leukemia.

Therapeutic Management

Management of ITP is primarily supportive because the disease is self-limiting in most cases. Activity is restricted at the onset while the platelet count is low and while active bleeding or progression of lesions is occurring. Treatment for acute presentation is symptomatic and has included prednisone, intravenous immunoglobulin (IVIG), and anti-D antibody. These are not curative therapies. Experts suggest that no therapy is necessary for asymptomatic patients because there is no difference in the recovery time of platelet counts with and without treatment (Cooper, 2017; Kuhne & Imbach, 2013; Scott & Flood, 2020b; Wilson, 2015). **Anti-D antibody** is a plasma-derived immunoglobulin that causes a transient hemolytic anemia in Rh (D)-positive patients with ITP. With the clearance of antibody-coated RBCs, there is prolonged survival of platelets resulting from the blockade of the Fc receptors of the reticuloendothelial cells. The platelet count usually increases approximately 48 hours after an infusion of anti-D antibody; therefore it is not appropriate therapy for patients who are actively bleeding. The benefits of choosing anti-D antibody IV therapy over prednisone or IVIG are that anti-D antibody can be given in one dose over 5 to 10 minutes and is significantly less expensive than IVIG. Before receiving the initial dose of anti-D antibody, patients must meet certain criteria (Box 24.7). Premedication with acetaminophen 5 to 10 minutes before the infusion is recommended. Bone marrow examination is not recommended in patients with typical ITP, particularly in patients who respond well to treatment, but bone marrow examination may be done in patients with refractory disease (Cooper, 2017; Onisai et al., 2019).

BOX 24.7 Criteria for Anti-D Antibody Therapy

- Age between 1 and 19 years; Rh (D)–positive blood type
- Normal WBC count and hemoglobin level for age; platelet count of 20,000/mm^3
- No active mucosal bleeding
- No history of reaction to plasma products
- No known immunoglobulin A deficiency
- No concurrent infection
- Absence of Evans syndrome (characterized by the combination of ITP and autoimmune hemolytic anemia)
- No suspicion of lupus erythematosus or other collagen vascular disorder
- No splenectomy

ITP, Idiopathic thrombocytopenic purpura; *WBC*, white blood cell.

NURSING TIP: After administration of anti-D antibody, observe the child for a minimum of 1 hour and maintain a patent intravenous (IV) line. Obtain baseline vital sign measurements before the infusion and again 5, 20, and 60 minutes after beginning the infusion. If fever, chills, and headache occur during or shortly after the infusion, the nurse should administer acetaminophen, diphenhydramine (Benadryl), and/or hydrocortisone (Solu-Cortef) as ordered and observe the patient for an additional hour after the reaction.

Splenectomy is for patients who have chronic ITP that is not responsive to pharmacologic management and have increased risk of severe hemorrhage. It is an option associated with long-term remission for these children and reduces the risk of hemorrhage but increases the risk of lifelong postsplenectomy infection (Onisai et al., 2019; Scott & Flood, 2020b; Wilson, 2015). Before splenectomy is considered, it is recommended to wait until the child is older than 5 years of age because of the increased risk of bacterial infection. Administration of pneumococcal, meningococcal, and *H. influenzae* vaccines is recommended before splenectomy (see Chapter 6, Immunizations). The child also receives penicillin prophylaxis after splenectomy. The length of prophylactic therapy is controversial, but in general a minimum of 3 years of therapy is recommended.

Prognosis

Most children have a self-limited course without major complications. Some children may develop chronic ITP and require ongoing therapies such as rituximab, azathioprine, or agents (romiplostim, eltrombopag) that stimulate thrombopoiesis (Cooper, 2017; Scott & Flood, 2020b). A splenectomy may modify the disease process, and the child may be asymptomatic.

QUALITY PATIENT OUTCOMES: Idiopathic Thrombocytopenic Purpura
- Serious bleeding episode prevented
- Activities that increase risk for serious bleeding avoided
- Treatment administered without serious side effects

Nursing Care Management

Nursing care is largely supportive and should include teaching on the possible side effects of therapy and restriction of contact sports while the child's platelet count is less than 50,000/mm^3 (Consolini, 2011; Kumar, Lambert, Breakey, et al., 2015). Restricted physical activities or contact sports should include football, rugby, bike riding, skateboarding, in-line skating, gymnastics, climbing, and running. Parents may engage their children in physical activities such as swimming (no diving), golf, walking, fishing, and aim to prevent any injuries, especially to the child's head. Instruct the parents to obtain prompt medical evaluation if the child sustains head or abdominal trauma. As in any condition with an uncertain outcome, the family needs emotional support.

DISSEMINATED INTRAVASCULAR COAGULATION

Disseminated intravascular coagulation (DIC), also known as **consumption coagulopathy**, is characterized by diffuse fibrin deposition in the microvasculature, consumption of coagulation factors, and endogenous generation of thrombin and plasmin. DIC is a secondary disorder of coagulation that occurs as a complication of a number of pathologic processes, such as hypoxia, acidosis, shock, endothelial damage (e.g., burns), and many severe systemic diseases (e.g., congenital heart disease, necrotizing enterocolitis, gram-negative bacterial sepsis, rickettsial infections, some severe viral infections). The hallmarks of this disorder are bleeding and clotting that occurs simultaneously.

Pathophysiology

DIC occurs when the first stage of the coagulation process is abnormally stimulated. Although no well-defined sequence of events occurs, two distinct phases can be identified. First, when the clotting mechanism is triggered in the circulation, thrombin is generated in greater amounts than can be neutralized by the body. Consequently, there is rapid conversion of fibrinogen to fibrin, with aggregation and destruction of platelets. Local and widespread fibrin deposition occurs in blood vessels, which causes obstruction of blood flow with eventual necrosis of tissues. Concurrently, the fibrinolytic mechanism is activated, which causes extensive destruction of clotting factors. With a deficiency of clotting factors, the child is vulnerable to uncontrollable hemorrhage into vital organs. An additional complication is damage and hemolysis of RBCs.

Diagnostic Evaluation

DIC is suspected when the patient has an increased tendency to bleed (Box 24.8). Hematologic findings include prolonged prothrombin time, PTT, thrombin time, and increased D-dimer antigen (byproduct of fibrinolytic process). There is a profoundly depressed platelet count, fragmented RBCs, and depleted fibrinogen.

Therapeutic Management

Treatment of DIC is directed toward control of the underlying or initiating cause, which in most instances stops the coagulation problem spontaneously. Platelets and fresh-frozen plasma may be needed to replace lost plasma components, especially in children whose underlying disease remains uncontrolled. Extremely ill newborn infants may require exchange transfusion with fresh blood. The administration of IV heparin to inhibit thrombin formation is most often restricted to patients who have no response to treatment of the underlying disease or replacement of coagulation factors and platelets.

Nursing Care Management

The goals of nursing care are to be aware of the possibility of DIC in severely ill children and to recognize signs that might indicate its presence. The skills needed to monitor IV infusion and blood transfusions and to administer heparin are the same as for any child receiving these therapies. (See Chapter 17 for care of children with life-threatening illnesses.)

BOX 24.8 Clinical Manifestations of Disseminated Intravascular Coagulation

Petechiae
Purpura
Bleeding from openings in the skin
- Venipuncture site
- Surgical incision

Bleeding from umbilicus, trachea (newborn)
Evidence of gastrointestinal (GI) bleeding
Hypotension
Organ dysfunction from infarction and ischemia

EPISTAXIS (NOSEBLEEDING)

Isolated and transient episodes of epistaxis, or nosebleeding, are common in childhood. The nose, especially the septum, is a highly vascular structure, and bleeding usually results from direct trauma, including blows to the nose, foreign bodies, and nose picking, or from mucosal inflammation associated with allergic rhinitis and upper respiratory tract infections. The bleeding usually stops with minimal pressure and requires no medical evaluation or therapy.

Recurrent epistaxis and severe bleeding may indicate an underlying disease, particularly vascular abnormalities, leukemia, thrombocytopenia, and clotting factor deficiency diseases (e.g., hemophilia, vWD). Nosebleeds are sometimes associated with administration of aspirin, even in normal amounts. Persistent episodes of epistaxis require medical evaluation.

Nursing Care Management

In the event of a nosebleed, an essential intervention is to remain calm. Otherwise, the child will become more agitated, the blood pressure will increase, and the child may not cooperate. Although in most instances a nosebleed is not serious, it can be upsetting to family members as well. They need reassurance that the loss of blood is not serious and that the bleeding usually stops in less than 10 minutes with nasal pressure.

To control the bleeding, the child is instructed to sit up and lean forward (not to lie down or hold the head backwards) to avoid aspiration of blood. Most of the nosebleeding originates in the anterior part of the nasal septum and can be controlled by applying pressure to the soft lower portion of the nose with the thumb and forefinger (see Emergency Treatment box). During this time, the child breathes through the mouth.

If hemorrhage continues, the child should be evaluated by a practitioner, who may pack the nose with epinephrine-soaked gauze. After a nosebleed, a water-soluble jelly can be inserted into each nostril

EMERGENCY TREATMENT

Epistaxis

- Have child sit up and lean forward (not lie down or tilt head backwards).
- Apply continuous pressure to tip of nose with thumb and forefinger for at least 10 minutes.
- Do not insert cotton or wadded tissue into each nostril, as it may reopen wound when removed.
- Discourage nose blowing or picking or rubbing nose, as this may dislodge the clot.
- Apply ice pack or cold cloth to bridge of nose if bleeding persists.
- Keep child calm and quiet.

to prevent crusting of old blood and to lessen the likelihood of the child's picking at the nose and restarting the hemorrhage. If a child has numerous nosebleeds, factors believed to increase the likelihood of bleeds are eliminated, such as discouraging nose picking or altering the household humidity by placing a cool-mist humidifier in the child's room. Repeated bleeding episodes lasting longer than 30 minutes may be an indication to refer the child for evaluation for the possibility of a bleeding disorder.

IMMUNOLOGIC DEFICIENCY DISORDERS

A number of disorders can cause profound, often life-threatening alterations within the body's immune system. The most serious are those conditions that completely depress immunity, such as severe combined immunodeficiency disease (SCID). However, the one disorder that generates the most anxiety in both the family and the community is HIV infection and the subsequent development of AIDS.

Several classifications of immune dysfunction exist. AIDS, SCID, and **Wiskott-Aldrich syndrome (WAS)** are disorders wherein the body is unable to mount an immune response. The immune response can also be misdirected. In **autoimmune disorders**, antibodies, macrophages, and lymphocytes attack healthy cells.

HUMAN IMMUNODEFICIENCY VIRUS INFECTION AND ACQUIRED IMMUNE DEFICIENCY SYNDROME

HIV infection and AIDS is a persistent global problem that has generated intense medical investigation and constitutes one of world's most serious medical, public health, and social challenges of our time (Centers for Disease Control and Prevention, 2019b; Grace, 2015; United Nations AIDS, 2016). Research has led to early diagnosis and improved medical treatments for HIV infection, changing this disease from a rapidly fatal one to a chronic disease.

Epidemiology

The first AIDS cases in the pediatric population in the United States were identified in children born to HIV-infected mothers and in children who received blood products. More than 90% of these children acquired the disease perinatally from their mothers. Smaller numbers of children were infected through the transfusion of contaminated blood or blood products before blood products were routinely screened for HIV. Currently, the principal modes of HIV transmission to the pediatric population are mother-to-child transmission and adolescent and young adult (13 to 24 years of age) risky behaviors, such as unprotected sexual activity and IV drug use (Centers for Disease Control and Prevention, 2019b; Hayes, 2020; Siberry, 2014; UN Joint Programme on HIV/AIDS [UNAIDS], 2019).

New cases of perinatally acquired HIV have declined approximately 70% with the use of preventive measures such as HIV counseling; voluntary testing practices; antiretroviral therapy (ART) during pregnancy, intrapartum, and neonatal periods; elective cesarean delivery; avoidance of breastfeeding; and avoidance of premastication of food by a caregiver with HIV (Centers for Disease Control and Prevention, 2017a; Hayes, 2020; Nesheim, Fitzharris, Gray, et al., 2019). ART is typically a combination of three or more antiretroviral drugs, with each drug inhibiting a specific stage of the HIV cycle. Two nucleoside analog reverse transcriptase inhibitors in combination with either a nonnucleoside reverse transcriptase inhibitor protease inhibitor or an integrase inhibitor is the current standard in the United States for the treatment of HIV-infected pregnant women and has significantly reduced the transmission of HIV to babies more than 90% of the time (Centers for Disease Control and Prevention, 2019b; Givens, Dotters-Katz, Stringer, et al., 2018; Siberry, 2014). Routine HIV counseling and voluntary testing using the opt-in (must agree) or opt-out (right of refusal) approach is the recommended standard of care for pregnant women in the United States (American Academy of Pediatrics Committee on Pediatric AIDS, 2008; Centers for Disease Control and Prevention, 2017a, 2019b; Siberry, 2014).

BOX 24.9 Common Clinical Manifestations of Human Immunodeficiency Virus Infection in Children

- Lymphadenopathy
- Hepatosplenomegaly
- Oral candidiasis
- Chronic or recurrent diarrhea
- Failure to thrive
- Developmental delay
- Parotitis

Etiology

HIV is a retrovirus that is the primary cause of AIDS. It is found in the blood, semen, vaginal secretions, rectal fluids, and breast milk. It has an incubation or latency period of months to years (Hayes, 2020). There are different strains of HIV. Whereas HIV-2 is prevalent in Africa, HIV-1 is the dominant strain in the United States and elsewhere. **Horizontal transmission** of HIV occurs through intimate sexual contact or parenteral exposure to blood or body fluids containing visible blood. **Perinatal (vertical) transmission** occurs when an HIV-infected pregnant woman passes the infection to her infant. There is no evidence that *casual* contact between infected and uninfected individuals can spread the virus.

Pathophysiology

The HIV virus primarily infects a specific subset of T lymphocytes, the $CD4^+$ T cells, but it can also invade cells of the monocyte-macrophage lineage. The virus takes over the machinery of the $CD4^+$ lymphocyte, using it to replicate itself, rendering the $CD4^+$ cell dysfunctional. The $CD4^+$ lymphocyte count gradually decreases over time; at some point, physical symptoms appear. The count eventually reaches a critical level at which there is substantial risk of opportunistic illnesses, followed by risk of death.

Clinical Manifestations

Common clinical manifestations of HIV infection in children vary (Box 24.9). The diagnosis of AIDS is associated with certain illnesses or conditions. The most common AIDS-defining conditions observed among American children are listed in Box 24.10. Other problems in these children may include short stature, malnutrition, and cardiomyopathy. CNS abnormalities resulting from HIV infection may include neuropsychologic deficits; developmental disabilities; and deficits in motor skills, communication, and behavioral functioning.

Diagnostic Evaluation

For children 18 months of age and older, the HIV enzyme-linked immunosorbent assay (ELISA) and Western blot immunoassay are performed to determine HIV infection. In infants born to HIV-infected mothers, results of these assays are positive because of the presence of maternal antibodies derived transplacentally. Since maternal antibodies may persist in the infant up to 18 to 24 months of age, other diagnostic tests are used—most commonly the HIV polymerase chain reaction (PCR) for detection of proviral DNA (US Department of Health and Human Services, 2018a).

Currently, several rapid HIV inexpensive tests are available with sensitivity and specificity better than those of the standard enzyme immunoassay, with only a single step that allows test results to be reported within 30 minutes (Hayes, 2020). A positive rapid test is either confirmed by Western blot testing or two different positive rapid tests (testing different HIV-associated antibodies). Viral diagnostic assays, such as HIV DNA or ribonucleic acid (RNA) PCR or HIV culture, are considerably more useful in young infants, allowing a definitive diagnosis in most infected infants by 1 to 4 months of age (Hayes, 2020; US Department of Health and Human Services, 2018b). In the United States, HIV testing approved by the Food and Drug Administration includes (1) combination tests that detect both HIV antigen and antibody and (2) tests that accurately differentiate HIV-1 from HIV-2 antibodies (Centers for Disease Control and Prevention, 2019b; US Department of Health and Human Services, 2018b). With the identification of HIV antigen, individuals may be diagnosed with HIV infection prior to development of symptoms.

The Centers for Disease Control and Prevention (1994, 2006, 2008, 2014) has developed a revised classification system to describe the spectrum of HIV disease in children (Selik, Mokotoff, Branson, et al., 2014) (Table 24.2). The system indicates the degree of immunosuppression and the severity of clinical signs and symptoms. The immune categories are based on $CD4^+$ lymphocyte counts and percentages that are divided into the following categories: 0 = previous negative or indeterminate test (not included on table), 1 = no evidence of immune suppression, 2 = moderate suppression, and 3 = severe suppression (Selik et al., 2014; Weinberg, 2018) (see Table 24.2). Age adjustment of the category numbers is necessary because normal counts, which are relatively high in infants, decline steadily until 6 years of age, when they reach adult norms.

The clinical categories are defined by the presence or absence of certain opportunistic infections or cancers (e.g., non-Hodgkin lymphoma, leiomyosarcoma, Kaposi sarcoma) (Weinberg, 2018). The nonsymptomatic category includes either no signs and symptoms or one of the conditions listed in the mildly symptomatic category. The mildly symptomatic category includes signs and symptoms such as lymphadenopathy, parotitis, hepatosplenomegaly, dermatitis, and recurrent or persistent sinusitis or otitis media. The moderately symptomatic category includes signs and symptoms such as lymphoid interstitial pneumonitis (LIP) and a variety of organ-specific dysfunctions or infections. The severely symptomatic category includes signs and symptoms such as AIDS-defining illnesses, with the exception of LIP. Children with LIP have a better prognosis than those with other AIDS-defining illnesses.

The immunologic and clinical categories are becoming less relevant in the era of combination ART. When ART is taken as prescribed, it almost invariably increases $CD4^+$ T-cell counts and decreases the symptoms. Therefore the categories are useful for clinical research and for describing the severity of illness at time of diagnosis in children younger than 13 years old (Selik et al., 2014; Weinberg, 2018) (see Table 24.2). For adolescents older than 13 years of age and adults, classification systems use $CD4^+$ T-cell count as the major staging unless AID-defining conditions (opportunistic infections) are present (Selik et al., 2014; Weinberg, 2018) (see Table 24.2).

BOX 24.10 Common Defining Conditions for Acquired Immune Deficiency Syndrome in Children

- *Pneumocystis carinii* pneumonia (PCP)
- Lymphoid interstitial pneumonitis (LIP)
- Recurrent bacterial infections
- Wasting syndrome
- Candidal esophagitis
- Human immunodeficiency virus (HIV) encephalopathy
- Cytomegalovirus disease
- *Mycobacterium avium-intracellulare* complex infection
- Pulmonary candidiasis
- Herpes simplex disease
- Cryptosporidiosis

Therapeutic Management

The goals of therapy for HIV infection include slowing the growth of the virus, preventing and treating opportunistic infections, and providing nutritional support and symptomatic treatment. **Antiretroviral drugs** work at various stages of the HIV life cycle to prevent reproduction of functional new virus particles. Although antiretroviral drugs are not a cure, they can delay progression of the disease (Centers for Disease Control and Prevention, 2016; Hayes, 2020). Classes of antiretroviral agents include nucleoside reverse transcriptase inhibitors (e.g., zidovudine, didanosine, stavudine, lamivudine, abacavir), nonnucleoside reverse transcriptase inhibitors (e.g., nevirapine, delavirdine, efavirenz), nucleotide reverse transcriptase inhibitors (e.g., adefovir), protease inhibitors (e.g., indinavir, saquinavir, ritonavir, nelfinavir,

TABLE 24.2 Human Immunodeficiency Virus Infection Stage[a] Based on Age-Specific $CD4^+$ T-Lymphocte or $CD4^+$ T-Lymphocyte Percentage of Total Lymphocytes

	AGE ON DATE OF $CD4^+$ T LYMPHOCYTE TEST		
Stage	**<1 Year (cells/µL, %)**	**1-6 Years (cells/µL, %)**	**>6 Years (cells/µL, %)**
1	>1500, >34	>1000, >30	>500, >26
2	750-1499, 26-33	500-999, 22-29	200-499, <14-25
3	<750	<500, <22	<200, <14

[a]The stage is based primarily on the $CD4^+$ T-lymphocyte count; the $CD4^+$ T-lymphocyte count takes precedence over the CD4 T-lymphocyte percentage, and the percentage is considered only if the count is missing. There are three situations in which the stage is not based on this table: (1) if the criteria for stage 0 are met, the stage is 0 regardless of criteria for other stages (CD4 T-lymphocyte test results and opportunistic illness diagnoses); (2) if the criteria for stage 0 are not met and a stage 3–defining opportunistic illness has been diagnosed, the stage is 3 regardless of CD4 T-lymphocyte test results; and (3) if the criteria for stage 0 are not met and information on the above criteria for other stages is missing, the stage is classified as unknown.

Modified from Centers for Disease Control and Prevention. (1994). 1994 Revised classification system for human immunodeficiency virus infection in children less than 13 years of age. *MMWR Recommendations and Reports, 43*(RR-12), 1–10; and Selik, R. M., Mokotoff, E. D., Branson, B., et al. (2014). Revised surveillance case definition for HIV infection—United States. *Morbidity and Mortality Weekly Report, 63*(RR-3), 1–10.

amprenavir), and fusion inhibitors (e.g., enfuvirtide) (Givens et al., 2018). Combinations of antiretroviral drugs are used to stall the emergence of drug resistance, including the addition of other drug classes approved by the US Food and Drug Administration (e.g., entry inhibitors, integrase inhibitors, pharmacokinetic enhancers) (Huang, Chen, Dolan, et al., 2017; US Department of Health and Human Services, 2019). Antiretroviral therapy regimens and guidelines are continually evolving. Therapy is lifelong, making adherence difficult. Laboratory markers ($CD4^+$ lymphocyte count, viral load) assist in monitoring both disease progression and response to therapy. If people with HIV take ART as prescribed, their viral load can become undetectable (Centers for Disease Control and Prevention, 2019b).

Pneumocystis carinii pneumonia (PCP) is the most common opportunistic infection of children infected with HIV. It occurs most frequently between 3 and 6 months old. All infants born to HIV-infected women should receive prophylaxis until HIV infection is reasonably excluded (Hayes, 2020; Siberry, 2014; Simpkins, Siberry, & Hutton, 2009). Trimethoprim/sulfamethoxazole (TMP-SMZ) is the agent of choice. If adverse effects are experienced with TMP-SMZ, dapsone, atovaquone, or pentamidine can be used.

Prophylaxis is often given for other opportunistic infections, such as disseminated *Mycobacterium avium-intracellulare* complex, candidiasis, or herpes simplex. Intravenous gamma globulin (IVGG) has been helpful in preventing recurrent or serious bacterial infections in some HIV-infected children.

Immunization against common childhood illnesses, including the pneumococcal and influenza vaccines, is recommended for all children exposed to and infected with HIV (Bamford, Manno, Mellado, et al., 2016; Leggat, Iyer, Ohtola, et al., 2015; Simpkins et al., 2009). Varicella (chickenpox) vaccine and measles, mumps, and rubella (MMR) vaccine can be administered if there is no evidence of severe immunocompromise (Hayes, 2020; Weinberg, 2018). Because antibody production to vaccines may be poor or decrease over time, immediate prophylaxis after exposure to several vaccine-preventable diseases (e.g., measles, varicella) is warranted. It should be recognized that children receiving IVGG prophylaxis may not respond to the MMR vaccine if it is given in close proximity to the IVGG dose (McLean, Fiebelkorn, Temte, et al., 2013).

HIV infection often leads to marked failure to thrive and multiple nutritional deficiencies. Nutritional management may be difficult because of recurrent illness, diarrhea, and other physical problems. The nurse should implement intensive nutritional interventions if the child's growth begins to slow or weight begins to decrease.

Prognosis

Early recognition and improved medical care have changed HIV disease from a rapidly fatal illness to a chronic disease. After the introduction of combination ART, the numbers of new AIDS cases and deaths declined substantially. In the United States, from 2009 to 2013, the annual estimated number and rate of deaths of HIV-infected children younger than 13 years old has remained stable (Centers for Disease Control and Prevention, 2015; Simpkins et al., 2009). In contrast, adolescents and young adults (13 to 24 years old) with AIDS represent a minority of cases in the United States yet constitute one of the fastest-growing groups of newly infected persons in the country, most likely because they are unaware of the infection (Centers for Disease Control and Prevention, 2019b; Hayes, 2020; Simpkins et al., 2009). During the 20th International AIDS Conference in Melbourne, Australia, in 2014, the 90–90–90 targets were launched as a global quest with a December 2020 deadline (UN Joint Programme on HIV/AIDS [UNAIDS], 2017). Targets were aimed at maximizing viral suppression among people living with HIV, with a focus on 90% of people living with HIV knowing their status, 90% of those who know their status being on treatment, and 90% of those on treatment being virally suppressed (UN Joint Programme on HIV/AIDS [UNAIDS], 2017).

> **QUALITY PATIENT OUTCOMES: Human Immunodeficiency Virus**
> - Early recognition of human immunodeficiency virus (HIV) infection
> - HIV infection slowed or maintained
> - Growth and development promoted
> - No infectious complications or cancer development
> - Adherence to antiretroviral therapy
> - Prolonged survival
> - Quality of life supported

Nursing Care Management

Education on transmission and control of infectious diseases, including HIV infection, is essential for children with HIV infection and anyone involved in their care. The basic tenets of Standard Precautions should be presented in an age-appropriate manner, with careful consideration of the educational levels of the individuals (see Chapter 20, Infection Control). Safety issues, including appropriate storage of special medications and equipment (e.g., needles, syringes), are emphasized.

Unfortunately, relatives, friends, and others in the general public may be fearful of contracting HIV infection, and criticism and ostracism of the child and family may occur. In an effort to protect the child and deal with fears of the community, the family may limit the child's activities outside the home. Although certain precautions are justified in limiting exposure to sources of infections, they must be tempered with concern for the child's normal developmental needs. Both the family and the community need ongoing education about HIV to dispel many of the myths that have been perpetuated by uninformed persons.[f]

Prevention is a key component of HIV education. Educating adolescents about HIV is essential in preventing HIV infection in this age-group. Education should include the routes of transmission, the hazards of IV and other recreational drug use, and the value of sexual abstinence and safe sex practices (Hayes, 2020; United Nations AIDS, 2016). Such education should be a part of anticipatory guidance provided to all adolescent patients. Nurses should also encourage adolescents at risk to undergo HIV counseling and testing. In addition to identifying infected teenagers and getting them into care, such counseling affords adolescents an opportunity to learn about, and possibly change, their risky behaviors.

Because approximately 1 in 7 individuals living with HIV infection are unaware of their positive status, the Centers for Disease Control and Prevention recommends that clinicians screen for HIV infection in all persons 13 to 64 years old at least once during routine health care and in all those individuals who are at increased risk regardless of age (Centers for Disease Control and Prevention, 2019b; Moyer and US Preventive Services Task Force, 2013). Early detection of HIV-infected individuals and linking them to medical care and counseling through screening programs in the health care setting provides effective treatment and decreases the transmission of HIV (Suthar, Ford, Bachanas, et al., 2013; Weinberg, 2018).

[f]Additional information is available from the National HIV/AIDS Hotline: 800-342-AIDS (2437) or 800-HIV-0440 (448-0440); TTY/TDD: 800-243-7889 or 888-480-3739; outside of the United States: 301-315-2816; contactus@aidsinfo.nih.gov; http://aidsinfo.nih.gov.

The multiple complications associated with HIV disease are potentially painful. Aggressive pain management is essential for these children to have an acceptable quality of life. Their pain may be caused by infections (e.g., otitis media, dental abscess), encephalopathy (e.g., spasticity), adverse effects of medications (e.g., peripheral neuropathy), or an unknown source (e.g., deep musculoskeletal pain). Common psychosocial concerns include disclosing the diagnosis to the child, making custody plans when the parent is infected, and anticipating the loss of a family member. Other stressors may include financial difficulties, HIV-associated stigma, attempts to keep the diagnosis secret, infection of other family members, and any losses associated with HIV. Most mothers of these children are single mothers who are also HIV infected. As primary caretakers, they often attend to the needs of their child first, neglecting their own health in the process. The nurse should encourage the mother to receive regular health care. As an integral part of the multidisciplinary team, the nurse is necessary for the successful management of the complex medical and social problems of these families.

Children with HIV infection attend daycare centers and schools. It is well established that the risk of HIV transmission in these settings is minimal. These institutions are required to follow Centers for Disease Control and Prevention and Occupational Safety and Health Administration guidelines for infection control measures. Standard Precautions describing proper management of blood and body fluids should also be followed. It is recommended that school personnel receive current HIV information and include it in the health education curriculum for kindergarten through twelfth grade (Nacken, Rehfuess, Paul, et al., 2018; Naidoo & Rule, 2016; National Association of School Psychologists, 2012). School nurses play a vital role in educating the school staff, students, and parents. They are also invaluable in monitoring the needs of known affected children.

Confidentiality is another major issue in daycare or school attendance. Parents and legal guardians have the right to decide whether they inform the daycare or school of their child's HIV diagnosis. Unfortunately, myths about HIV infection continue to exist, and the family often wishes to avoid any potential criticism or ostracism of the child.

SEVERE COMBINED IMMUNODEFICIENCY DISEASE

SCID is a defect characterized by absence of both humoral and cell-mediated immunity. The terms **Swiss-type lymphopenic agammaglobulinemia,** which refers to the autosomal recessive form of the disease, and **X-linked lymphopenic agammaglobulinemia** have been used to describe this disorder, which, as the names imply, can follow either mode of inheritance.

The most common manifestation is susceptibility to infection early in life, most often in the first month. The disorder in children is characterized by chronic infections, failure to recover completely from infections, frequent reinfection, and infection with unusual agents. Failure to thrive is a consequence of the persistent illnesses.

Diagnosis is usually based on a history of recurrent, severe infections from early infancy; a familial history of the disorder; and specific laboratory findings, which include lymphopenia, lack of lymphocyte response to antigens, and absence of plasma cells in the bone marrow. Documentation of immunoglobulin deficiency is difficult during infancy because of the normally delayed response of infants in producing their own immunoglobulins and material transfer of immunoglobulin G (IgG). Currently, newborn screening for SCID can be performed by quantifying levels of T-cell receptor (TCR) excision circles (TRECs) in dried blood spots collected at birth (Centers for Disease Control and Prevention, 2017b; Cross, 2013; Dorsey, Dvorak, Cowan, et al., 2017; King & Hammarstrom, 2018). TRECs are a byproduct of rearrangement of TCR genes during intrathymic T-cell development, and the TREC levels are extremely low or absent in patients with SCID. Since newborn screening for SCID, most states as well as the District of Columbia and Puerto Rico have identified several cases of SCID at birth in otherwise healthy-looking newborns (Centers for Disease Control and Prevention, 2019c; Dorsey et al., 2017; King & Hammarstrom, 2018). Quantification of TRECs represents an important yet nonspecific indicator of a possible severe T-cell immunodeficiency, the diagnosis of which must be confirmed by appropriate immunophenotypic, functional, and molecular tests (Bonilla & Notarangelo, 2015). Advances in SCID newborn screening have profoundly improved outcomes of children born in the United States, with identification of an increased number of expected cases from approximately 40 to 69 annually, equating to an additional 29 cases each year managed with potentially curative treatment (Dorsey & Puck, 2017; King & Hammarstrom, 2018).

Therapeutic Management

The definitive treatment for SCID is HSCT. If the condition is diagnosed at birth or within the first 3 months of life, more than 95% of cases can be treated successfully with HLA-identical or T-cell depleted haploidentical donor (usually a parent) or a matched unrelated donor bone marrow stem cells transplant or umbilical cord donor (Bonilla & Notarangelo, 2015; Sullivan & Buckley, 2020). Before newborn screening for SCID became a reality, most patients were infected when initially diagnosed and required immediate aggressive interventions (Bonilla & Notarangelo, 2015). Approaches to manage SCID patients include providing passive immunity with IVIG and maintaining the child in a sterile environment. The latter is effective only if the measure is instituted before any infectious process takes hold in the infant, and it represents an extreme effort to prevent life-threatening infections. Investigators using research protocols reported tremendous advances with gene therapy, offering hope that gene therapy may eventually be the treatment of choice for cases of SCID (Bonilla & Notarangelo, 2015; Booth, Romano, Roncarolo, et al., 2019; Dorsey & Puck, 2017; Sullivan & Buckley, 2020).

Nursing Care Management

Nursing care focuses on preventing infection and supporting the child and family. The care is consistent with that needed for HSCT for any condition (see earlier in the chapter). Because the prognosis for SCID is very poor if a compatible bone marrow donor is not available, nursing care is directed at supporting the family in caring for a child with a life-threatening illness (see Chapter 17). Genetic counseling is essential because of the modes of transmission in either form of the disorder.

WISKOTT-ALDRICH SYNDROME

WAS is a congenital X-linked recessive disorder characterized by a triad of abnormalities: thrombocytopenia, eczema, and immunodeficiency of selective functions of B and T lymphocytes. An abnormal gene has been identified on the proximal arm of the X chromosome and designated the WAS protein (Bonilla & Notarangelo, 2015). Today, it is well recognized that the syndrome has a wide clinical spectrum ranging from mild, isolated thrombocytopenia to the severe classic presentation that can be complicated by life-threatening hemorrhages, immunodeficiency, atopy, autoimmunity, and cancer (Candotti, 2018). However, it is important to keep in mind that patients with initial mild form can transition to severe condition with the development of chronic or life-threatening clinical problems (Candotti, 2018). At birth, the presenting feature may be prolonged bleeding at the circumcision site or bloody diarrhea as a result of thrombocytopenia. As the child grows older, recurrent infection and eczema become more severe, and the bleeding becomes less frequent.

Eczema is typical of the allergic type and readily becomes superinfected. Chronic infection with herpes simplex is a frequent problem and may lead to chronic keratitis of the eye with loss of vision. Chronic pulmonary disease, sinusitis, and otitis media result from repeated infections. In children who survive the bleeding episodes and overwhelming infections, malignancy presents an additional risk to survival.

Since medical and supportive care is tailored toward the degree of severity and specific clinical manifestations, it primarily involves counteracting the bleeding tendencies with platelet transfusions, promoting appropriate nutrition, giving IVIG to provide passive immunity, using G-CSF to correct neutropenia and prevent infections, administering prophylactic antibiotics to prevent and control infection, and providing aggressive local therapy for the eczema (Bonilla & Notarangelo, 2015; Candotti, 2018; Dale, 2017; Sullivan & Buckley, 2020). Splenectomy may improve the platelet count, although the risk of asplenic sepsis in these infants is extremely high. These children require the same prophylactic antibiotics and appropriate immunizations as any child with asplenia. Despite their immunodeficiency, they can mount an adequate immunologic response to the inactivated vaccines. When an HLA-matched donor exists, WAS is usually cured with HSCT, which should be performed as early as possible (Albert, Notarangelo, & Ochs, 2011; Mahlaoui, Pellier, Mignot, et al., 2013; Sullivan & Buckley, 2020). However, further research is needed to determine optimal conditioning for WAS to minimize the HSCT-related complications (Iguchi, Cho, Hiromasa, et al., 2019).

More recently, transplantation of autologous gene-corrected hematopoietic stem or progenitor cells (gene therapy) has become an alternative, albeit still investigational, option (Booth et al., 2019; Candotti, 2018). Therefore gene therapy provides a valuable treatment for patients with severe WAS, particularly those who do not have a suitable HSCT donor. The efficiency, efficacy, and long-term safety are yet largely untested in humans, but there is likely to be rapid evolution of the technology with autologous somatic gene modification that may become a standard of care within 5 to 10 years (Booth et al., 2019; Ferrua, Cicalese, Galimberti, et al., 2019).

Nursing Care Management

Because of the poor prognosis for children with WAS, the main nursing consideration is supporting the family in the care of a fatally ill child (see Chapter 17). Physical care should be directed at controlling the problems imposed by the disorder. The measures used to control bleeding are similar to those for hemophilia and vWD (see discussions earlier in the chapter). Another major goal is prevention or control of infection. Because eczema is a troublesome problem, nursing measures specific to this condition are especially important. The genetic implications of this X-linked recessive disorder differ little from those of any other X-linked disease. Since the multiplicity of defects tends to affect emotional adjustment and physical care, the nurse must be especially supportive by providing short-term goals during periods of hospitalization and by focusing on long-range needs through coordinated efforts with a public health nurse.

TECHNOLOGIC MANAGEMENT OF HEMATOLOGIC AND IMMUNOLOGIC DISORDERS

BLOOD TRANSFUSION THERAPY

Technologic advances in blood banking and transfusion medicine enable the administration of only the blood component needed by the child, such as packed RBCs in anemia or platelets for bleeding disorders. Regardless of the blood component administered, the nurse must be aware of the possible transfusion reactions. Table 24.3 summarizes the major complications of transfusions, the signs and symptoms typically associated with each, and nursing responsibilities. General guidelines that apply to all transfusions include:

TABLE 24.3 Nursing Care of the Child Receiving Blood Transfusions

Complication	Signs and Symptoms	Precautions and Nursing Responsibilities
Immediate Reactions		
Hemolytic reactions Most severe type but rare Incompatible blood Incompatibility in multiple transfusions	Sudden, severe headache Chills Shaking Fever Pain at needle site and along venous tract Nausea and vomiting Sensation of tightness in chest Red or black urine Flank pain Progressive signs of shock or renal failure	Identify donor and recipient blood types and groups before transfusion is begun; verify with another nurse or practitioner. Transfuse blood slowly for the first 15-20 min or initial 20% of blood volume; remain with patient. Stop transfusion immediately in the event signs or symptoms occur, maintain patent IV line, and notify practitioner. Save donor blood to recrossmatch with patient's blood. Monitor for evidence of shock. Insert urinary catheter and monitor hourly outputs. Send samples of patient's blood and urine to laboratory for presence of hemoglobin (indicates intravascular hemolysis). Observe for signs of hemorrhage resulting from DIC. Support medical therapies to reverse shock.
Febrile reactions Leukocyte or platelet antibodies Plasma protein antibodies	Fever Chills	May give acetaminophen for prophylaxis. Leukocyte-poor RBCs are less likely to cause reaction. Stop transfusion immediately; report to practitioner for evaluation.

Continued

TABLE 24.3 Nursing Care of the Child Receiving Blood Transfusions—cont'd

Complication	Signs and Symptoms	Precautions and Nursing Responsibilities
Allergic reactions Recipient reaction to allergens in donor's blood	Urticaria Pruritus Flushing Asthmatic wheezing Laryngeal edema	Give antihistamines for prophylaxis to children with tendency to allergic reactions. Stop transfusion immediately. Administer epinephrine for wheezing or anaphylactic reaction.
Circulatory overload Too rapid transfusion (even a small quantity) Transfusion of excessive quantity of blood (even slowly)	Precordial pain Dyspnea Rales Cyanosis Dry cough Distended neck veins Hypertension	Transfuse blood slowly. Prevent overload by using packed RBCs or administering divided amounts of blood. Use infusion pump to regulate and maintain flow rate. Stop transfusion immediately if there are signs of overload. Place child upright with feet in dependent position to increase venous resistance.
Air emboli May occur when blood is transfused under pressure	Sudden difficulty in breathing Sharp pain in chest Apprehension	Normalize pressure before container is empty when infusing blood under pressure. Clear tubing of air by aspirating air with syringe at nearest Y connector if air is observed in tubing; disconnect tubing and allow blood to flow until air has escaped only if a Y connector is not available.
Hypothermia	Chills Low temperature Irregular heart rate Possible cardiac arrest	Allow blood to warm at room temperature (<1 h). Use approved mechanical blood warmer or electric warming coil to warm blood rapidly; never use microwave oven. Take temperature if patient complains of chills; if subnormal, stop transfusion.
Electrolyte disturbances Hyperkalemia (in massive transfusions or in patients with renal problems)	Nausea, diarrhea Muscular weakness Flaccid paralysis Paresthesia of extremities Bradycardia Apprehension Cardiac arrest	Use washed RBCs or fresh blood if patient is at risk.
Delayed Reactions		
Transmission of infection Hepatitis HIV infection Malaria Syphilis Other bacterial or viral infection	Signs of infection (e.g., jaundice) Toxic reaction: High fever, severe headache or substernal pain, hypotension, intense flushing, vomiting, or diarrhea	Blood is tested for antibodies to HIV, hepatitis C virus, and hepatitis B core antigen; in addition, blood is tested for hepatitis B surface antigen and alanine aminotransferase, and a serologic test is performed for syphilis. Units that test positive are destroyed. Individuals at risk for carrying certain viruses are deterred from donation. Report any sign of infection, and if it occurs during transfusion, stop transfusion immediately, send sample for culture and sensitivity testing, and notify practitioner.
Alloimmunization Antibody formation Occurs in patients receiving multiple transfusions	Increased risk of hemolytic, febrile, and allergic reactions	Use limited number of donors. Observe carefully for signs of reactions.
Delayed hemolytic reaction	Destruction of RBCs and fever 5-10 days after transfusion	Observe for posttransfusion anemia and decreasing benefit from successive transfusion.

DIC, Disseminated intravascular coagulation; *HIV,* human immunodeficiency virus; *IV,* intravenous; *RBC,* red blood cell.

- Take vital signs, including blood pressure, *before* administering blood to establish baseline data for pretransfusion and posttransfusion comparison; 15 minutes after initiation; hourly while blood is infusing; and on completion of transfusion.
- Check the identification of the recipient and the blood type and group of the recipient against the donor's, regardless of the blood product being used.
- Administer the first 50 ml of blood or initial 20% of the volume (whichever is smaller) *slowly* and stay with the child.

- Administer with normal saline on a piggyback setup or have normal saline available.
- Administer blood through an appropriate filter to eliminate particles in the blood and prevent the precipitation of formed elements; gently shake the container frequently.
- Use blood within 30 minutes of its arrival from the blood bank; if it is not used, return it to the blood bank—do not store it in the regular unit refrigerator.
- Infuse a unit of blood (or the specified amount) within 4 hours. If the infusion will exceed this time, the blood should be divided into appropriate-size quantities by the blood bank and the unused portion refrigerated under controlled conditions.
- If a reaction of any type is suspected, stop the transfusion, take vital signs, maintain a patent IV line with normal saline and new tubing, notify the practitioner, and do not restart the transfusion until the child's condition has been medically evaluated.

Although hemolytic reactions are rare, ABO incompatibility remains the most common cause of death from blood transfusion, and human error is usually responsible (e.g., administration of the wrong type to the patient or mislabeling of the blood product) (Josephson & Strauss, 2020; Pahuja et al., 2017). Hemolysis can also cause the release of large quantities of phospholipids, which are capable of stimulating DIC. Acute kidney shutdown and eventual renal failure are a result of renal vasoconstriction from antigen–antibody complexes derived from the RBC surface.

Blood is usually administered to children by infusion pump; therefore the usual precautions and management related to pumps apply. When the blood infusion begins with a standard transfusion set, the filter chamber is filled to allow the total filter to be used. The drip chamber is partially filled with blood to permit counting of the drops. In adjusting the flow rate, it is important to remember that blood administration sets do not use microdrops (60 drops/ml) but regular drops (usually 10 to 15 drops/ml). The nurse must consider this when calculating the flow rate.

APHERESIS

Apheresis is the removal of blood from an individual, separation of the blood into its components, retention of one or more of these components, and reinfusion of the remainder of the blood into the individual. These transfusion components have greatly prolonged the survival of patients with hematologic and oncologic diseases.

CLINICAL JUDGMENT AND NEXT-GENERATION NCLEX® EXAMINATION-STYLE QUESTIONS

1. A 10-month-old boy is scheduled for a follow-up clinic visit. His mother reports that her son is anemic and needs further evaluation. What assessment findings below would the nurse expect to find to confirm iron deficiency anemia? **Select all that apply.**
   A. MCV = 67 fl
   B. Hematocrit = 30%
   C. Poor intake of solid food
   D. Pulse oximetry 98%
   E. Hemoglobin = 10.2 g/dL
   F. Respirations- 14 breaths/min
   G. Blood pressure = 102/50 mm Hg
   H. Serum iron concentration- 12 mcg/dL
   I. Total iron-binding capacity = 450 mcl/dL
   J. History of 28-32 oz/day of cow's milk intake

2. The nurse is working with a 4-year-old girl who is newly diagnosed with beta thalassemia. Hemoglobin electrophoresis confirms the diagnosis of β-thalassemia. In preparing for discharge teaching with the parents and patient, which statements below would be discussed? **Use an X for the health teaching statement below that is Indicated (appropriate or necessary), Contraindicated (could be harmful), or Non-Essential (makes no difference or not necessary).**

Health Teaching	Indicated	Contraindicated	Non-Essential
"We need to check your iron level to make sure you are not anemic."			
"I believe your disease is most common in those of Hispanic descent, although you are Mediterranean."			
"I would like to talk to you about the diagnosis and provide you with some information about β-thalassemia."			
"You look much younger than I would expect. I guess you are a late bloomer."			
"I think a transfusion will be ordered because your hemoglobin level is 9.5."			

3. A 9-year-old girl has been diagnosed with severe aplastic anemia. She presented with a two-week history of nosebleeds and developed a fever to 102 F the past few days. She complains of fatigue and notices bruising of her arms and legs. Her peripheral blood counts show marked reduction in the red blood cells, white blood cells and platelets. A bone marrow aspiration and biopsy were performed and demonstrated conversion of the red bone marrow to yellow, fatty bone marrow with a bone marrow cellularity of 20%. Based on her diagnosis, what are the **most appropriate** nursing actions at this time? **Select all the apply.**
   A. Advise the family what to do if fever develops.
   B. Recommend eating fruits and vegetables each day.
   C. Review the importance of the spleen and how it works.
   D. Discuss the diagnosis with the child in an age appropriate manner.
   E. Review how to use an epinephrine pen at home if anaphylaxis should occur.
   F. Provide opportunities for the child and family to ask questions and express feelings.
   G. Discuss how blood cells work and what side-effects to look for due to low blood cell counts.

4. The nurse is discharging a 5-year-old patient newly diagnosed with hemophilia. He was hospitalized because of a severe joint bleed following a fall. Which of the following responses are appropriate for the nurse to discuss with the parents? **Use an X for the health teaching statement below that is Indicated (appropriate or necessary), Contraindicated (could be harmful), or Non-Essential (makes no difference or not necessary).**

Health Teaching	Indicated	Contraindicated	Non-Essential
"Your child should remain active to decrease joint problems, and most children with hemophilia can participate in the same activities as their peers."			
"Care should be taken to avoid bleeding of gums; soften the toothbrush in warm water before brushing or using a sponge-tipped disposable toothbrush may be helpful."			
"Signs of internal bleeding should be recognized, such as headache, slurred speech, loss of consciousness (from cerebral bleeding), and black, tarry stools (from gastrointestinal bleeding)."			
"If there is bleeding in a joint, elevation, ice, and rest should prevent the need for factor VIII replacement."			
"All of your son's teachers need to be aware of what to do if he gets a bloody nose."			
"Your child should drink a lot of fluids to decrease the possibility of dehydration."			

REFERENCES

Abdullah, K., Thorpe, K. E., Mamak, E., et al. (2015). Optimizing early child development for young children with non-anemic iron deficiency in primary care practice setting (OptEC): Study protocol for a randomized controlled trial. *Trials, 16*, 132.

Albert, M. H., Notarangelo, L. D., & Ochs, H. D. (2011). Clinical spectrum, pathophysiology and treatment of Wiskott-Aldrich syndrome. *Current Opinion in Hematology, 18*(1), 42–48.

American Academy of Pediatrics. (2016). *Vitamin D and iron supplements for babies: AAP recommendations.* Accessed April 10, 2019 from https://www.healthychildren.org/English/ ages-stages/baby/feeding-nutrition/Pages/Vitamin-Iron-Supplements.aspx.

American Academy of Pediatrics Committee on Pediatric AIDS. (2008). HIV testing and prophylaxis to prevent mother-to-child transmission in the United States. *Pediatrics, 122*(5), 1127–1134.

American Pain Society. (2015). *Guidelines for the management of acute and chronic pain in sickle-cell disease.* Glenview, IL: Author.

Anderson, A., & Forsyth, A. (2017). *Playing it safe: Bleeding disorders, sports and exercise.* The National Hemophilia Foundation. Retrieved from https://www.hemophilia.org/node/4041.

Anderson, O., Domeliof, M., Anderson, D., et al. (2014). Effect of delayed vs early umbilical cord clamping on iron status and neurodevelopment at age 12 months: A randomized clinical trial. *Journal of the American Medical Association Pediatrics, 168*(6), 547–554.

Angulo-Barroso, R. M., Li, M., Santos, D. C. C., et al. (2016). Iron supplementation in pregnancy or infancy and motor development: A randomized controlled trial. *Pediatrics, 137*(4), e20153547.

Arachchillage, D. R., & Markis, M. (2016). Choosing and using non-steroidal anti-inflammatory drugs in haemophilia. *Haemophilia, 22*(2), 179–187.

Arlet, J., Dussiot, M., Moura, I. C., et al. (2016). Novel players [beta]-thalassemia dyserythropoiesis and new therapeutic strategies. *Current Opinion in Hematology, 23*(3), 181–188.

Armstrong-Wells, J., Grimes, B., Sidney, S., et al. (2009). Utilization of TCD screening for primary stroke prevention in children with sickle cell disease. *Neurology, 72*(15), 1316–1321.

Auerbach, M., James, S. E., Nicoletti, M., et al. (2017). Results of first American prospective study of intravenous iron in oral iron-intolerant iron deficient gravidas. *American Journal of Medical Sciences*, *130*(12), 1402–1407.

Azar, S., & Wong, T. E. (2017). Sickle cell disease: A brief update. *The Medical Clinics of North America*, *101*(2), 375–393.

Bamford, A., Manno, E. C., Mellado, M. J., et al. (2016). Immunisation practices in centres for children perinatally acquired HIV: A call for harmonization. *Vaccine*, *34*(46), 5587–5594.

Berglund, S., Westrup, B., & Domellof, M. (2010). Iron supplements reduce the risk of iron deficiency anemia in marginally low birth weight infants. *Pediatrics*, *126*(4), e874–e883.

Bonilla, F. A., & Notarangelo, L. D. (2015). Primary immunodeficiency diseases. In S. H. Orkin, D. E. Fisher, D. Ginsburg, et al. (Eds.), *Nathan and Oski's hematology of infancy and childhood* (8th ed.). Philadelphia: Saunders.

Booth, C., Romano, R., Roncarolo, M., et al. (2019). Gene therapy for primary immunodeficiency. *Human Molecular Genetics* (Epub ahead or print).

Bou-Maroun, L. M., Meta, F., Hanba, C., et al. (2018). An analysis of inpatient pediatric sickle cell disease: Incidence, cost, and outcomes. *Pediatric Blood & Cancer*, *65*(1), e26758.

Bourzac, K. (2017). Gene therapy: Erasing sickle-cell disease. *Nature*, *549*(7673), s28–s30.

Branchford, B. R., Monahan, P. E., & Di Paola, J. (2013). New developments in the treatment of pediatric hemophilia and bleeding disorders. *Current Opinion in Pediatrics*, *25*(1), 23–30.

Bregman, D. B., & Goodnough, L. T. (2014). Experience with intravenous ferric carboxymaltose in patients with iron deficiency anemia. *Therapeutic Advances in Hematology*, *5*(2), 48–60.

Brown, S. E., Weisberg, D. F., Balf-Soran, G., et al. (2015). Sickle cell disease patients with and without extremely high hospital use: Pain, opiods, and coping. *Journal of Pain and Symptom Management*, *49*(3), 539–547.

Brugnara, C., Oski, F. A., & Nathan, D. G. (2015). Diagnostic approach to the anemic patient. In S. H. Orkin, D. E. Fisher, D. Ginsburg, et al. (Eds.), *Nathan and Oski's hematology of infancy and childhood* (8th ed.). Philadelphia: Saunders.

Campelo, L. M. N., Oliveira, N. F., Magalhaes, J. M., et al. (2018). The pain of children with sickle cell disease: The nursing approach. *Revista Brasileira de Enfermagem*, *71*(Suppl. 3), 1381–1387.

Candotti, F. (2018). Clinical manifestations and pathophysiological mechanisms of the Wiskott-Aldrich syndrome. *The Journal of Allergy and Clinical Immunology*, *38*(1), 13–27.

Cappellini, M. D., Porter, J. B., Viprakasit, V., et al. (2018). A paradigm shift on beta-thalassemia treatment: How will we manage this old disease with new therapies? *Blood Reviews*, *32*(4), 300–311.

Centers for Disease Control and Prevention. (1994). 1994 revised classified system for human immunodeficiency virus infection in children less than 13 years of age. *MMWR Recommendations and Reports*, *43*(RR–12), 1–10.

Centers for Disease Control and Prevention. (2006). Revised recommendations for HIV testing of adults, adolescents, and pregnant women in health-care settings. *MMWR Recommendations and Reports*, *55*(RR–14), 1–17.

Centers for Disease Control and Prevention. (2008). Revised surveillance case definitions for HIV infection among adults, adolescents, and children aged <18 months and for HIV infection and AIDS among children aged 18 months to <13 years — United States, 2008. *MMWR Recommendations and Reports*, *57*(10), 1–12.

Centers for Disease Control and Prevention. (2014). National HIV Testing Day and new testing recommendations. *Morbidity and Mortality Weekly Report*, *63*(25), 537.

Centers for Disease Control and Prevention. (2015). *HIV surveillance report, 2013*. vol 25. Published February 2015, https://www.cdc.gov/hiv/pdf/library/reports/surveillance/cdc-hiv-surveillance-report-2013-vol-25.pdf.

Centers for Disease Control and Prevention. (2016). HIV in the United States: At a glance, 2016. Accessed May 29, 2017 from https://www.cdc.gov/hiv/statistics/overview/ataglance.html.

Centers for Disease Control and Prevention. (2017a). HIV and pregnant women, infants and children. Accessed May 29, 2017 from https://www.cdc.gov/hiv/group/gender/pregnantwomen/index.html.

Centers for Disease Control and Prevention. (2017b). Newborn screening for severe combined immunodeficiency (SCID) saves lives and money: A cost-effective public health policy. Accessed on July 19, 2019 from https://blogs.cdc.gov/genomics/2016/03/15/scid/.

Centers for Disease Control and Prevention. (2018a). Breastfeeding and special circumstances. Accessed August 10, 2019 from https://www.cdc.gov/breastfeeding/breastfeeding-special-circumstances/index.html.

Centers for Disease Control and Prevention. (2018b). Hemophilia Facts—United States. Accessed June 29, 2018 from www.cdc.gov/ncbddd/hemophilia/facts.html.

Centers for Disease Control and Prevention. (2019a). *Thalassemia awareness, National Center on Birth Defects and Developmental Disabilities, Division of Blood Disorders*. https://www.cdc.gov/features/international-thalassemia/index.html.

Centers for Disease Control and Prevention (CDC). (2019b). Division of HIV/AIDS Prevention, National Center, National Center for HIV/AIDS, Viral Hepatitis, STD and TB Prevention-Basic statistics. Accessed July 10, 2019 from https://www.cdc.gov/hiv/basics/transmission.html.

Centers for Disease Control and Prevention. (2019c). Newborn screening and molecular biology branch: Severe combined immunodeficiency (SCID). Accessed on July 19, 2019 from https://www.cdc.gov/nceh/dis/nsmbb.html.

Choudhry, V. P. (2017). Thalassemia minor and major: Current management. *Indian Journal of Pediatrics*, *84*(8), 607–611.

Choudhury, N. A., DeBaun, M. R., Rodeghier, M., et al. (2018). Silent cerebral infarct definitions and full-scale IQ loss in children with sickle cell anemia. *Neurology*, *90*(3), e239–e246.

Chozie, N. A., Primacakti, F., Gatot, D., et al. (2019). Comparison of the efficacy and safety of 12 month low-dose factor VIII prophylaxis vs. on-demand treatment in severe haemophilia A children. *Haemophilia*, *25*(4), 633–639.

Consolini, D. M. (2011). Thrombocytopenia in infants and children. *Pediatrics in Review*, *32*(4), 135–151.

Cooper, N. (2017). State of the art-how I manage immune thrombocytopenia. *British Journal of Haematology*, *177*(1), 39–54.

Cross, C. (2013). Ontario newborns now screened for SCID. *Canadian Medical Association Journal*, *185*(13), E616.

Dale, D. C. (2017). How to manage children with neutropenia. *British Journal of Haematology*, *178*(3), 351–363.

DeBaun, M. R., Armstrong, F. D., McKinstry, R. C., et al. (2012). Silent cerebral infarcts: A review on a prevalent and progressive cause of neurologic injury in sickle cell anemia. *Blood*, *119*(20), 4587–4596.

DeBaun, M. R., & Kirkham, F. J. (2016). Central nervous system complications and management in sickle cell disease. *Blood*, *127*(7), 829–838.

DeLoughery, T. G. (2014). Microcytic anemia. *The New England Journal of Medicine*, *371*, 1324–1331.

Desmond, R., Townsley, D., Dumitriu, B., et al. (2014). Eltrombopag restores trilineage hematopoiesis in refactory severe aplastic anemia that can be sustained on discontinuation of drug. *Blood*, *123*, 1818–1825.

Di Paola, J., Montgomery, R. R., Gill, J. C., et al. (2015). Hemophilia and von Willebrand disease. In S. H. Orkin, D. E. Fisher, D. Ginsburg, et al. (Eds.), *Nathan and Oski's hematology of infancy and childhood* (8th ed). Philadelphia: Elsevier Saunders.

Dorsey, M. J., Dvorak, C. C., Cowan, M. J., et al. (2017). Treatment of infants identified as having severe combined immunodeficiency by means of newborn screening. *The Journal of Allergy and Clinical Immunology*, *139*, 733–742.

Dorsey, M. J., & Puck, J. (2017). Newborn screening for severe combined immunodeficiency in U.S.: Current status and approach to management. *International Journal of Neonatal Screening*, *3*(2), 15.

Doshi, B. S., & Arruda, V. R. (2018). Gene therapy for hemophilia:What does the future hold? *Therapeutic Advances in Hematology*, *9*(9), 273–293.

El-Beshlawy, A., & El-Ghamrawy, M. (2019). Recent trends in treatment of thalassemia. *Blood Cells, Molecules & Diseases*, *76*, 53–58.

Estcourt, L. J., Fortin, P. M., Hopewell, S., et al. (2017). Blood transfusion for preventing primary and secondary stroke in people with sickle cell disease. *Cochrane Database of Systematic Reviews*, *1*, CD003146.

Estepp, J. H., Smeltzer, M. P., Kang, G., et al. A clinically meaningful fetal hemoglobin threshold for children with sickle cell anemia during hydroxyurea therapy. *American Journal of Hematology*, 92(12), 1333–1339.

Eussen, S., Alles, M., Uijterschout, L., et al. (2015). Iron intake and status of children aged 6-36 months in Europe: A systematic review. *Annals of Nutrition and Metabolism*, *66*(2–3), 80–92.

Fargo, G. H., & Hord, J. D. (2020). The acquired pancytopenia. In R. M. Kliegman, J. W. St. Geme, N. J. Blum, et al. (Eds.), *Nelson textbook of pediatrics* (21st ed). Philadelphia: Elsevier.

Ferrua, F., Cicalese, M. P., Galimberti, S., et al. (2019). Lentiviral haemopoietic stem/progenitor of Wiskott-Aldrich syndrome: Interim results of a non-randomized, open-label, phase1/2 clinical study. *The Lancet Haematology, 6*, e239–e253.

Fleming, M. D. (2015). Disorders of iron and copper metabolism, the sideroblastic anemias and lead toxicity. In S. H. Orkin, D. E. Fisher, D. Ginsburg, et al. (Eds.), *Nathan and Oski's hematology of infancy and childhood* (8th ed.). Philadelphia: Saunders.

Fortin, P. M., Hopewell, S., & Estcourt, L. J. (2018). Red blood cell transfusion to treat or prevent complications in sickle cell disease: An overview of Cochrane reviews. *Cochrane Database of Systematic Reviews, 8*, CD012082.

Georges, G. E., & Storb, R. (2016). Hematopoietic stem cell transplantation for acquired aplastic anemia. *Current Opinion in Hematology, 23*(6), 495–500.

Ghafuri, D. L., Chaturvedi, S., Rodeghier, M., et al. (2016). Secondary benefit of maintaining normal transcranial Doppler velocities when using hydroxyurea for prevention of severe sickle cell anemia. *Pediatric Blood & Cancer, 64*(7).

Givens, M., Dotters-Katz, S. K., Stringer, E., et al. (2018). Minimizing risk perinatal HIV Transmission. *Obstetrical and Gynecological Survey, 73*(7), 423–432.

Grace, R. F. (2015). Hematologic manifestations of systemic diseases. In S. H. Orkin, D. E. Fisher, D. Ginsburg, et al. (Eds.), *Nathan and Oski's hematology of infancy and childhood* (8th ed.). Philadelphia: Saunders.

Haining, W. N., Duncan, C., El-haddad, et al. (2015). Principles of bone marrow and stem cell transplantation. In S. H. Orkin, D. E. Fisher, D. Ginsburg, et al. (Eds.), *Nathan and Oski's hematology of infancy and childhood* (8th ed.). Philadelphia: Saunders.

Halkes, C., de Wreede, L. C., Knol-Bout, J. P., et al. (2019). Allogeneic stem cell transplantation for acquired pure red cell aplasia. *American Journal of Hematology*. Epub ahead of print.

Hanley, J., McKernan, A., Creagh, M. D., et al. (2017). Guildelines for the management of acute joint bleeds and chronic synovitis in haemophilia. *Haemophilia, 23*, 511–520.

Hayes, E. V. (2020). Human immunodeficiency virus and acquired immunodeficiency syndrome. In R. M. Kliegman, J. W. St. Geme, N. J. Blum, et al. (Eds.), *Nelson textbook of pediatrics* (21st ed.). Philadelphia: Elsevier.

Heeney, M., & Ware, R. (2015). Sickle cell disease. In S. H. Orkin, D. E. Fisher, D. Ginsburg, et al. (Eds.), *Nathan and Oski's hematology of infancy and childhood* (8th ed.). Philadelphia: Saunders.

Helton, K. J., Adams, R. J., Kesler, K. L., et al. (2014). Magnetic resonance imaging/ angiography and transcranial Doppler velocities in sickle cell anemia: Results from the SWITCH trial. *Blood, 124*(6), 891–898.

Higgs, D. R., Engel, J. D., & Stamatoyannopoulos, G. (2012). Thalassaemia. *Lancet, 379*, 373–383.

Hirtz, D., & Kirkham, F. J. (2019). Sickle cell disease and stroke. *Pediatric Neurology, 95*, 34–41.

Howell, C., Scott, K., & Patel, D. (2017). Sports participation recommendations for patients with bleeding disorders. *Translational Pediatrics, 6*(3), 174–180.

Hsieh, M. M., Fitzhugh, C. D., Weitzel, R. P., et al. (2014). Nonmyeloablative HLA-matched sibling allogeneic hematopoietic stem cell transplantation for severe sickle cell phenotype. *Journal of the American Medical Association, 312*(1), 48–56.

Huang, R., Chen, Z., Dolan, S., et al. (2017). The dual modulatory effects of efavirenz on GABAa receptors are mediated via two distinct sites*. *Neuropharmacology, 121*, 167–178.

Huttle, A., Maestre, G. E., Lantigua, R., et al. (2015). Sickle cell in Latin America and the United States. *Pediatric Blood & Cancer, 62*(7), 1131–1136.

Iguchi, A., Cho, Y., Hiromasa, Y., et al. (2019). Long-term outcome and chimerism in patients with Wiskott-Aldrich syndrome treated by hematopoietic cell transplantation: A retrospective nationwide survey. *International Journal of Hematology, 110*(3), 364–369.

Iorio, A., Marchesini, E., Marcucci, M., et al. (2011). Clotting factor concentrates given to prevent bleeding and bleeding-related complications in people with hemophilia A or B. *The Cochrane Database of Systematic Reviews* (9), CD003429.

Issaragrisil, S., & Kunacheewa, C. (2016). Matched sibling donor hematopoietic stem cell transplantation for thalassemia. *Current Opinion in Hematology, 23*(6), 506–514.

Jauregui-Lobera, I. (2014). Iron deficiency and cognitive functions. *Neuropsychiatric Disease and Treatment, 10*, 2087–2095.

Josephson, C. D., & Strauss, R. G. (2020). Risk of blood transfusions. In R. M. Kliegman, J. W. St. Geme, N. J. Blum, et al. (Eds.), *Nelson textbook of pediatrics* (21th ed.). Philadelphia: Elsevier.

Juul, S. E., Derman, R. J., & Auerbach, M. (2019). Perinatal iron deficiency: Implications for mothers and infants. *Neonatology, 115*, 269–274.

Kawadler, J. M., Clayden, J. D., Clark, C. A., et al. (2016). Intelligence quotient in paediatric sickle cell disease: A systematic review and meta-analysis. *Developmental Medicine and Child Neurology, 58*(7), 672–679.

Khandros, E., Kwaitkowski, J. L. Beta-thalassemia: Monitoring and new treatment approaches. *Hematology/Oncology Clinics of North America, 33*(3), 339–353.

Khemani, K., Katoch, D., & Krishnamurti, L. (2019). Curative therapies for sickle cell disease. *Oshsner Journal, 19*, 131–137.

King, J. R., & Hammarstrom, L. (2018). Newborn screening for primary immunodeficiency diseases: History, current and future practice. *The Journal of Allergy and Clinical Immunology, 38*(1), 56–66.

Korthof, E. T., Bekassy, A. N., & Hussein, A. A. (2013). Management of acquired aplastic anemia in children. *Bone Marrow Transplant, 48*(2), 191–195.

Krishnamurti, L., Neuberg, D. S., Sullivan, K. M., et al. (2019). Bone marrow transplantation for adolescents and young adults with sickle cell disease: Results of a prospective multicenter pilot study. *The American Journal of Hematology, 94*(9), 446–454.

Kuhne, T., & Imbach, P. (2013). Management of children and adolescents with primary immune thrombocytopenia: Controversies and solutions. *Vox Sanguinis, 104*(1), 55–66.

Kumar, M., Lambert, M. P., Breakey, V., et al. (2015). Sports participation in children and adolescents with immune thrombocytopenia (ITP). *Pediatr Blood Cancer, 62*, 2223–2225.

Kwiatkowski, J. L., Yim, E., Miller, S., et al. (2011). Effect of transfusion therapy on transcranial Doppler ultrasonography velocities in children with sickle cell disease. *Pediatric Blood & Cancer, 56*(5), 777–782.

Leggat, D. J., Iyer, A. S., Ohtola, J. A., et al. (2015). Response to pneumococcal polysaccharide vaccination in newly diagnosed HIV-positive individuals. *Journal of AIDS & Clinical Research, 6*(2).

Lillicrap, D. (2013). The future of hemostasis management. *Pediatric Blood & Cancer, 60*(Suppl. 1), S44–S47.

Locatelli, F., Merli, P., & Strocchio, L. (2016). Transplantation for thalassemia major: Alternative donors. *Current Opinion in Hematology, 23*(6), 515–523.

Locatelli, F., & Pagliara, D. (2012). Allogeneic hematopoietic stem cell transplantation in children with sickle cell disease. *Pediatric Blood & Cancer, 59*(2), 372–376.

Lokeshwar, H. R., Mehta, M., Mehta, N., et al. (2011). Prevention of iron deficiency anemia (IDA): How far have we reached? *Indian Journal of Pediatrics, 78*(5), 593–602.

Lucarelli, G., Isgro, A., Sodani, P., et al. (2012). Hematopoietic stem cell transplantation in thalassemia and sickle cell anemia. *Cold Spring Harbor Perspectives in Medicine, 2*(5), a011825.

Lytle, A. M., Brown, H. C., Paik, N. Y., et al. (2016). Effects of FVIII immunity on hepatocyte and hematopoietic stem cell-directed gene therapy of murine hemophilia A, molecular therapy-methods and clinical development. *Molecular Therapy. Methods & Clinical Development, 10*(3), 15056.

Mahlaoui, N., Pellier, I., Mignot, C., et al. (2013). Characteristics and outcome of early-onset, severe forms of Wiskott-Aldrich syndrome. *Blood, 121*(9), 1510–1516.

Mahoney, D. H. (2017). Iron deficiency in infants and young children: Screening, prevention, clinical manifestations, and diagnosis. UpToDate. Accessed June 20, 2017 from https://www.uptodate.com/contents/iron-deficiency-in-infants-and-children-less-than12-years-screening-prevention-clinical-manifestations-and-diagnosis.

Makis, A., Hatzimichael, E., Papassotiriou, I., et al. (2016). Clinical trials update in new treatments of β-thalassemia. *American Journal of Hematology, 91*(11), 1135–1145.

Mantadakis, E. (2018). Intravenous iron: Safe and underutilized in children. *Pediatric Blood & Cancer, 65*(6), e27016.

Matte, A., Zorzi, F., Mazzi, F., et al. (2019). New therapeutic options for the treatment of sickle cell disease. *Mediterranean Journal of Hematology and Infectious Diseases, 11*(1), e2019002.

McDonagh, M. S., Blazina, I., Dana, T., et al. (2015). Screening and routine supplementation for iron deficiency anemia: A systematic review. *Pediatrics, 135*(4), 723–733.

McGann, P. T., Nero, A. C., & Ware, R. E. (2013). Current management of sickle cell anemia. *Cold Spring Harbor Perspectives in Medicine, 3*(8), a011817.

McLean, H. Q., Fiebelkorn, A. P., Temte, J. L., et al. (2013). Prevention of measles, rubella, congenital rubella syndrome, and mumps, 2013: Summary recommendations of the Advisory Committee on Immunization Practices (ACIP). *MMWR Recommendations and Reports, 62*(RR–04), 1–34.

Meier, E. M., Fasano, R. M., & Levett, P. R. (2017). A systematic review of the literature for severity predictors in children with sickle cell anemia. *Blood Cells, Molecules & Diseases, 65*, 86–94.

Meier, E. R., & Miller, J. L. (2012). Sickle cell disease in children. *Drugs, 72*(7), 895–906.

Meier, E. R., & Rampersad, A. (2017). Pediatric sickle cell disease: Past successes and future challenges. *Pediatric Research, 81*(1), 249–258.

Mercer, J. S., Erickson-Owens, D. A., Collins, J., et al. (2017). Effects of delayed cord clamping on residual placental blood volume, hemoglobin and bilirubin levels in term infants: A randomized controlled trial. *Journal of Perinatology, 37*(3), 260–264.

Miano, M., & Dufour, C. (2015). The diagnosis and treatment of aplastic anemia: A review. *International Journal of Hematology, 101*(6), 527–535.

Miller, J. L. (2013). Iron deficiency anemia: A common and curable disease. *Cold Spring Harbor Perspectives in Medicine, 3*(7), a011866.

Miller, S. T., Sleeper, L. A., Pegelow, C. H., et al. (2000). Prediction of adverse outcomes in children with sickle cell disease. *The New England Journal of Medicine, 342*(2), 83–89.

Moyer, V. A., & US Preventive Services Task Force. (2013). Screening for HIV: US Preventive Services Task Force recommendation statement. *Annals of Internal Medicine, 159*(1), 51–60.

Nacken, A., Rehfuess, E. A., Paul, I., et al. (2018). Teachers' competence, school policy and social context-HIV prevention needs of primary schools in Kagera, Tanzania. *Health Education Reseach, 33*(6), 505–521.

Nagalapuram, V., Kulkami, V., Leach, J., et al. (2019). Effect of sickle cell anemia therapies on the natural history of growth and puberty patterns. *Journal of Pediatric Hematology and Oncology*, (Epub ahead of print).

Naidoo, J., & Rule, P. (2016). Teachers' subjectivities and emotionality in HIV/AIDS teaching. *African Journal of AIDS Research, 15*(3), 233–241.

National Association of School Psychologists. (2012). *Supporting students with HIV/AIDS (position statement)*. Bethesda, MD: Author.

National Hemophilia Foundation. 2019. Accessed June 19, 2019 from https://www.hemophilia.org/

National Institutes of Health; National Heart, Lung, and Blood Institute, & Division of Blood Disease and Resources. (2014). Evidence-based management of sickle cell disease, Expert Panel Report, 2014. Retrieved from https://www.nhlbi.nih.gov/health-topics/evidence-based-management-sickle-cell-disease.

National Institutes of Health, Office of Dietary Supplements. (2018). Iron dietary supplement fact sheet for health professionals. Accessed April 15, 2019 from https://ods.od.nih.gov/factsheets/Iron-HealthProfessional/.

Negre, O., Eggimann, A. V., Beuzard, Y., et al. (2016). Gene therapy of the β-hemoglobinopathies by lentiviral transfer of the βA(T87Q)-globin gene. *Human Gene Therapy, 27*(2), 148–165.

Nesheim, S. R., Fitzharris, L. F., Gray, K. M., et al. (2019). Epidemiology of perinatal HIV transmission in United States in the era of its elimination. *Pediatric Infectious Disease Journal, 38*, 611–616.

Nevitt, S. J., Jones, A. P., & Howard, J. (2017). Hydroxyurea (hydroxycarbamide) for sickle cell disease. *Cochrane Database of Systemic Reviews, 4*, CD002202.

Nienhuis, A. W., Nathwani, A. C., & Davidoff, A. M. (2017). Gene therapy for hemophilia. *Molecular Therapy, 25*(5), 1163–1167.

Nugent, D., O'Mahony, B., Dolan, G., et al. (2018). Value of prophylaxis vs. on demand treatment: Application of a value framework in hemophilia. *Haemophilia, 24*(5), 755–765.

Nussbaum, R. L., McInnes, R. R., & Willard, H. F. (2016). Genetic variation in populations. In R. L. Nussbaum, R. R. McInnes, & H. F. Willard (Eds.), *Thompson and Thompson genetics in medicine* (8th ed.). Philadelphia, PA: Elsevier Inc.

Onisai, M., Vladareanu, A., Spinu, A., et al. (2019). Idiopathic thrombocytopenic purpura (ITP)-new era for old disease. *Romanian Journal of Internal Medicine* Epub ahead of print.

Origa, R. (2017). β-Thalassemia. *Genetics in Medicine, 19*, 609–619.

Pahuja, S., Puri, V., Mahajan, G., et al. (2017). Reporting adverse transfusion reactions: A retrospective study from tertiary care hospital from New Delhi, India. *Asian Journal of Transfusion Science, 11*(1), 6–12.

Paoletti, G., Bogen, D. L., & Ritchey, A. K. (2014). Severe iron-deficiency anemia still an issue in toddlers. *Clinical Pediatrics (Phila), 53*(14), 1352–1358.

Passweg, J. R., & Marsh, J. C. (2010). Aplastic anemia: First-line treatment by immunosuppression and sibling marrow transplantation. *American Society of Hematology Education Program book*, 2010, 36–42.

Peinemann, F., & Labeit, A. M. (2014). Stem cell transplantation of matched sibling donors compared with immunosuppressive therapy for acquired severe aplastic anaemia: A Cochrane systematic review. *British Medical Journal Open, 4*(7), e005039.

Peslak, S. A., Olson, T., & Babushok, D. V. (2017). Diagnosis and treatment of aplastic anemia. *Current Treatment Options in Oncology, 18*(12), 70.

Piel, F. B., Steinberg, M. H., & Rees, D. C. (2017). Sickle cell disease. *The New England Journal of Medicine, 376*, 1561–1573.

Pivina, L., Semenova, Y., Dosa, M. D., et al. (2019). Iron deficiency, cognitive functions and neurobehavioral disorders in children. *Journal of Molecular Neuroscience, 68*(1), 1–10.

Powers, J. M., & Buchanan, G. R. (2014). Diagnosis and management of iron deficiency anemia. *Hematology/Oncology Clinics of North America, 28*(4), 729–745.

Quarmyne, M. D., Dong, W., Theodore, R., et al. (2107). Hydroxyurea effectiveness in children and adolescents with sickle cell anemia: A large retrospective, population-based cohort. *American Journal of Hematology, 92*(1), 77–81.

Raphael, J. L., Mei, M., Mueller, B. U., et al. (2012). High resource hospitalizations among children with vaso-occlusive crises in sickle cell disease. *Pediatric Blood & Cancer, 58*(4), 584–590.

Rees, D. C., Robinson, S., & Howard, J. (2018). How I manage red cell transfusions in patients with sickle cell disease. *British Journal of Haematology, 180*, 607–617.

Rodeghiero, F., Stasi, R., Gernsheimer, T., et al. (2009). Standardization of terminology, definitions, and outcome criteria in immune thrombocytopenic purpura of adults and children: Report from an international working group. *Blood, 113*(11), 2386–2393.

Rodriguez, A., Duez, P., Dedeken, L., et al. (2018). Hydroxyurea (hydroxycarbamide) genotoxicity in pediatric patients with sickle cell disease. *Pediatric Blood & Cancer, 65*, e27022.

Rothman, J. A. (2020). Iron-deficiency anemia. In R. M. Kliegman, J. W. St. Geme, N. J. Blum, et al. (Eds.), *Nelson textbook of pediatrics* (21st ed.). Philadelphia: Elsevier.

Rubin, R. (2019). Gene therapy for sickle cell disease shows promise. *Journal of the American Medical Association, e321*(4), 334.

Samarasinghe, S., & Webb, D. K. (2012). How I manage aplastic anaemia in children. *British Journal of Haematology, 157*(1), 26–40.

Sankaran, V. G., Nathan, D. G., & Orkin, S. H. (2015). The thalassemias. In S. H. Orkin, D. E. Fisher, D. Ginsburg, et al. (Eds.), *Nathan and Oski's hematology of infancy and childhood* (8th ed.). Philadelphia: Saunders.

Scheinberg, P. (2012). Aplastic anemia: Therapeutic updates in immunosuppressive and transplantation. *Hematology American Society of Hematology Education Program book*, 2012(1), 292–300.

Scott, J. P., & Flood, V. H. (2020a). Hereditary clotting factor deficiencies (bleeding disorders). In R. M. Kliegman, J. W. St.Geme, N. J. Blum, et al. (Eds.), *Nelson textbook of pediatrics* (21st ed.). Philadelphia: Elsevier.

Scott, J. P., & Flood, V. H. (2020b). Platelet and blood vessel disorders. In R. M. Kliegman, J. W. St.Geme, N. J. Blum, et al. (Eds.), *Nelson textbook of pediatrics* (21st ed.). Philadelphia: Elsevier.

Secher, E. L., Stensballe, J., & Afshari, A. (2013). Transfusion in critically ill children: An ongoing dilemma. *Acta Anaesthesiologica Scandinavica, 57*(6), 684–691.

Selik, R. M., Mokotoff, E. D., Branson, B., et al. (2014). Revised surveillance case definition for HIV infection-United States. *MMWR. Morbidity and Mortality Weekly Report, 63*(No. RR-3), 1–10.

Sharathkumar, A. A., & Carcao, M. (2011). Clinical advances in hemophilia management. *Pediatric Blood & Cancer, 57*(6), 910–920.

Sharathkumar, A. A., & Pipe, S. W. (2008). Post-thrombotic syndrome in children: A single center experience. *Journal of Pediatric Hematology and Oncology, 30*(4), 261–266.

Shimamura, A., & Williams, D. A. (2015). Aquired aplastic anemia and pure red cell aplasia. In S. H. Orkin, D. E. Fisher, D. Ginsburg, et al. (Eds.), *Nathan and Oski's hematology of infancy and childhood* (8th ed.). Philadelphia: Saunders.

Siberry, G. K. (2014). Preventing and managing HIV infection in infants, children, and adolescents in the United States. *Pediatrics in Review, 35*(7), 268–286.

Sii-Felice, K., Giorgi, M., Leboulch, P., et al. (2018). Hemoglobin disorders: Lentiviral gene therapy in the starting blocks to enter clinical practice. *Experimental Hematology, 64*, 12–32.

Simpkins, E. P., Siberry, G. K., & Hutton, N. (2009). Thinking about HIV infection. *Pediatrics in Review, 30*(9), 337–349.

Smith, A. (2012). Guide to evaluation and treatment of anaemia in general practice. *Prescriber, 23*(21), 25–42.

Smith-Whitley, K., & Kwiatkowski, J. L. (2020). Hemoglobinopathies. In R. M. Kliegman, J. W. St. Geme, N. J. Blum, et al. (Eds.), *Nelson textbook of pediatrics* (21st ed.). Philadelphia: Elsevier.

Smith, Y. (2018). Thalassemia prevalence. News-Medical, 2018. Accessed on June 16, 2019 from https://www.news-medical.net/health/Thalassemia-Prevalence.aspx.

Sourabh, S., Bhatia, P., & Jain, R. (2019). Favourable improvement in haematological parameters in response to oral iron and vitamin C combination in children with iron refractory iron deficiency anemia (IRIDA) phenotype. *Blood Cells, Molecules & Diseases, 75*, 26–29.

Subramaniam, G., & Girish, M. (2015). Iron deficiency anemia in children. *Indian Journal of Pediatrics, 82*(6), 558–564.

Sullivan, K. E., & Buckley, R. H. (2020). Severe combined immunodeficiency. In R. M. Kliegman, J. W. St. Geme, N. J. Blum, et al. (Eds.), *Nelson textbook of pediatrics* (21st ed.). Philadelphia: Elsevier.

Suthar, A. B., Ford, N., Bachanas, P. J., et al. (2013). Towards universal voluntary HIV testing and counseling: A systematic review and meta-analysis of community-based approaches. *PLoS Medicine, 10*(8), e1001496.

Thomas, R., Dulman, R., Lewis, A., et al. (2019). Prospective longitudinal follow-up of children with sickle cell disease treated with hydroxyurea since infancy. *Pediatric Blood & Cancer, 66*(9), e27816.

Thompson, J., Biggs, B. A., & Pasricha, S. R. (2013). Effects of daily iron supplementation in 2- to 5-year-old children: Systematic review and meta-analysis. *Pediatrics, 131*(4), 739–753.

Thornburg, C. D. (2020). The anemias. In R. M. Kliegman, J. W. St. Geme, N. J. Blum, et al. (Eds.), *Nelson textbook of pediatrics* (21st ed.). Philadelphia: Elsevier.

Tichelli, A., Schrezenmeier, H., Socie, G., et al. (2011). A ramdomized controlled study in patients with newly diagnosed severe aplastic anemia receiving antithymocyte globulin (ATG), cyclosporine, with or without GCSF: A study of the SAA Working Party of the European Group for Blood and Marrow Transplatation. *Blood, 117*(17), 4434–4441.

Townsley, D. M., Scheinberg, P., Winkler, T., et al. (2017). Eltrombopag added to standard immunosuppression for aplastic anemia. *The New England Journal of Medicine, 376*(16), 1540–1550.

United Nations AIDS. (2016). Global AIDS update, 2016. Accessed May 30, 2017 from www.unaids.org/en/resources/documents/2016/Global-AIDS-update-2016.

UN Joint Programme on HIV/AIDS (UNAIDS), *Ending AIDS: Progress towards the 90–90– 90 targets*, 20 July 2017. Accessed July 15, 2019 from https://www.unaids.org/en/resources/documents/2017/20170720_Global_AIDS_update_2017.

UN Joint Programme on HIV/AIDS (UNAIDS). (2019). Accessed July 15, 2019 from https://www.unaids.org/en/keywords/unaids-joint-united-nations-programme-hivaids.

US Department of Health and Human Services. (2018a). *Guidelines for the prevention and treatment of opportunistic infections in HIV-exposed and HIV-infected children. AIDSinfo*. Accessed July 15, 2019 from http://AIDSinfo.nih.gov.

US Department of Health and Human Services. (2018b). *Guidelines for use of antiretroviral agents in pediatric HIV infection. AIDSinfo*. Accessed July 15, 2019 from http://AIDSinfo.nih.gov.

US Department of Health and Human Services. (2019). Panel on antiretroviral therapy and medical management of children living with HIV. Guidelines for use of antiretroviral agents in pediatric HIV infection. AIDS info. Accessed July 15, 2019 from https://aidsinfo.nih.gov/guidelines/html/2/pediatric-arv/45/whats-new-in-the-guidelines.

Vichinsky, E., & Styles, L. (1996). Pulmonary complications. *Hematology/Oncology Clinics of North America, 10*(6), 1275–1286.

von der Lippe, C., Frich, J. C., Harris, A., et al. (2017). Treatment of hemophilia: A qualitative study of mothers' perspectives. *Pediatric Blood & Cancer, 64*, 121–127.

Walczyk, T., Muthayya, S., Wegmuller, R., et al. (2014). Inhibition of iron absorption by calcium is modest in iron-fortified, casein and whey-based drink in Indian children and is easily compensated by the addition of ascorbic acid. *Journal of Nutrition, 44*(1), 1703–1709.

Walsh, C. E., & Batt, K. M. (2013). Hemophilia clinical gene therapy: Brief review. *Translational Research, 161*(4), 307–312.

Wang, B., Zhan, S., Gong, T., et al. (2013). Iron therapy for improving psychomotor development and cognitive function in children under the age of three with iron deficiency anemia. *The Cochrane Database of Systematic Reviews* (6), CD001444.

Wang, W. C., & Dwan, K. (2013). Blood transfusion for preventing primary and secondary stroke in people with sickle cell disease. *The Cochrane Database of Systematic Reviews, 11*, CD003146.

Wang, W. C., Ware, R. E., Miller, S. T., et al. (2011). Hydroxycarbamide in very young children with sickle-cell anaemia: A multicenter, randomized, controlled trial (BABY HUG). *Lancet, 377*(9778), 1663–1672.

Weinberg, G. A. (2018). *Human immunodeficiency virus (HIV) infection in infants and children, Merck Manual Professional Version*. Kenilworth, NJ: Merck Sharp and Dohme Corp. A subsidiary of Merck and Co., Inc.

Williams, H., & Tanabe, P. (2016). Sickle cell disease: A review of nonpharmacological approaches for pain. *Journal of Pain and Symptom Management, 51*(2), 163–177.

Wilson, D. B. (2015). Acquired platelet defects. In S. H. Orkin, D. E. Fisher, D. Ginsburg, et al. (Eds.), *Nathan and Oski's hematology of infancy and childhood* (8th ed.). Philadelphia: Saunders.

World Federation of Hemophilia. (2012). *About bleeding disorders*. Accessed July 20, 2019 from https://www.wfh.org.

Xu, S., Luk, K., Yao, Q., et al. (2019). Editing aberrant splice sites efficiently restores β-globin expression in β-thalassemia. *Blood, 133*, 2255–2262.

Yaish, H. M. (2015). *Pediatric thalassemia*. Retrieved from http://emedicine.medscape.com/article/958850-overview.

Yawn, B. P., Buchanan, G. R., Afenyi-Annan, A. N., et al. (2014). Management of sickle cell disease summary of the 2014 evidence-based report by expert panel members. *Journal of the American Medical Association, 312*(10), 1033–1048.

Yawn, B. P., & John-Sowah, J. (2015). Management of sickle cell disease: Recommendations from the 2014 expert panel report. *American Family Physician, 92*(12), 1069–1076.

Young, N. S. (2018). Aplastic anemia. *N Engl J Med, 379*(17), 1643–1656.

Ziegler, E. E., Nelson, S. E., & Jeter, J. M. (2011). Iron supplementation of breastfed infants. *Nutrition Reviews, 69*(Suppl. 1), S71–S77.

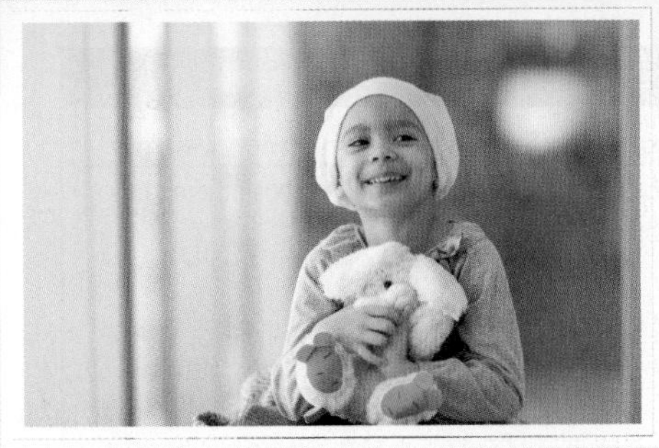

25

The Child With Cancer

Kathleen S. Ruccione

http://evolve.elsevier.com/wong/essentials

CONCEPTS

- Cellular Regulation
- Family Dynamics
- Patient/Family Education
- Nutrition
- Infection

CANCER IN CHILDREN

Few situations in nursing exceed the challenges of caring for a child with cancer. Despite dramatic improvements in prognosis, cancer remains a life-threatening, life-altering illness that has a major impact on family life and places significant demands on family strengths in coping with informational and support needs. Nurses should base support of patients and their families on the premise that with clear communication and compassionate care, fear diminishes, hope emerges, and the cancer journey feels less overwhelming. Effective communication, including nurse listening behaviors, also promotes understanding that aids treatment adherence.

This chapter summarizes clinical overviews and nursing care issues for the most common types of pediatric cancer. Chapter 17 discusses situations when the disease is imminently life threatening, as well as the general psychologic needs of these children and their families in terms of chronic illness.

EPIDEMIOLOGY: INCIDENCE RATES

Childhood cancer is rare; approximately 16,400 cases are diagnosed in children younger than 20 years of age in the United States each year (Scheurer, Lupo, & Bondy, 2016). Approximately 1700 children die of the disease in the United States annually, making cancer the leading cause of death from disease after infancy in this age-group (Scheurer et al., 2016). Worldwide, it is estimated that 300,000 new cases are diagnosed annually and that there are an estimated 80,000 deaths per year; in addition, survival rates in low-income countries are lower than in high-income countries (American Childhood Cancer Organization, 2016).

The incidence of specific types of childhood cancer varies according to demographic risk factors such as age, sex, and race or ethnicity. Cancer incidence is higher in children from infancy to 4 years of age and in adolescents ages 15 to 19 years; however, the types of cancers occurring among these two groups are distinct, with neuroblastoma and retinoblastoma more common in young children and lymphoma and sarcoma more common in adolescents (Scheurer et al., 2016). Males have a higher overall incidence of cancer compared to females, with a ratio of 1.1:1 (Scheurer et al., 2016). This difference reflects the higher incidence of acute lymphoblastic leukemia (ALL), non-Hodgkin lymphoma (NHL), and central nervous system (CNS) tumors—the most common types of childhood cancer—in young boys. White children have an overall higher incidence of cancer compared with African American children. This is accounted for by the higher incidence of ALL, Ewing sarcoma, and melanoma in white children.

Childhood cancer survival has dramatically increased over the past 5 decades with improved treatment and supportive care. In the 1960s, the overall (all cancer types combined) survival rate for childhood cancer was 28% compared with 3-year survival rates that now exceed 80% (Scheurer et al., 2016). Improvement in survival among adolescents has lagged behind younger age-groups, although that is changing. Survival rates remain low for some types of cancer, such as a brain tumor called diffuse intrinsic pontine glioma (DIPG), and for some age-groups, such as older children with a kidney tumor called Wilms tumor. ALL and NHL have demonstrated the greatest improvement in survival rates. Recent estimates indicate that there are now more than 400,000 survivors of childhood and adolescent cancer in the United States. A general definition of "cure" includes completion of all therapy, no clinical and radiologic evidence of disease, and a period of 5 years since diagnosis.

ETIOLOGY

Often the first questions asked by parents of children newly diagnosed with cancer are "How did my child get this, and could it have been prevented?" Lifestyle-related behaviors are the main factors that increase the risk of cancer in adults, but as far as is now known, they have little to no effect on cancer incidence in children. Apart from exposure to high-dose radiation and prior chemotherapy, there is relatively little evidence to support a major external or environmental role in the development of childhood cancer (Spector, Pankratz, & Marcote, 2015). Thus, given current understanding, it is unlikely that parents could have done anything to prevent their child's cancer.

On the other hand, characteristics such as birth weight, advanced parental age, and congenital anomalies have been found to be risk factors for childhood cancer (Spector et al., 2015). In addition, a small percentage of cancer occurs in children with cancer predisposition syndromes. The intrinsic risk factors, the association of germline

TABLE 25.1 Risk Factors Associated With Childhood Cancers

Cancer Type	Risk Factors	Selected Examples of Genomic Lesions
Acute lymphoblastic leukemia	• Ionizing radiation (primarily of historical importance) • Race (i.e., White) • Genetic conditions (i.e., Down syndrome, Bloom syndrome, and others) • Birth weight more than 400 g	• *ABL* family genes activated by translocation in a subset of cases
Acute myeloid leukemia (NIH, 2019d)	• Chemotherapeutic agents (i.e., alkylating agents and epipodophyllotoxins) • Genetic conditions (i.e., Down syndrome and neurofibromatosis 1)	
Brain tumors	• Therapeutic radiation to the head • Genetic conditions (i.e., neurofibromatosis 1, tuberous sclerosis, and others)	• BRAF and other kinase genomic mutations associated with subsets of pediatric glioma cases • Hedgehog pathway mutations associated with a subset of medulloblastoma cases
Hodgkin disease	• Family history (i.e., monozygotic twins) • Infections (i.e., Epstein-Barr virus)	
Non-Hodgkin lymphoma	• Immunodeficiency (i.e., acquired and congenital immunodeficiency, immunosuppressive therapy) • Infections (i.e., Epstein-Barr virus associated with Burkitt lymphoma in African countries)	
Osteosarcoma	• Ionizing radiation (i.e., cancer radiation therapy and high radium exposure) • Chemotherapy (i.e., alkylating agents) • Genetic conditions (i.e., Li-Fraumeni syndrome, hereditary retinoblastoma)	
Ewing sarcoma	• Race (White)	
Neuroblastoma	• None known	• *ALK* point mutations in a subset of neuroblastoma cases
Retinoblastoma	• No known nonhereditary risk factors	
Wilms tumor	• Congenital anomalies (i.e., aniridia, Beckwith-Wiedemann syndrome, other congenital and genetic conditions) • Race (White and Black)	
Rhabdomyosarcoma	• Congenital anomalies and genetic conditions (i.e., Li-Fraumeni syndrome and neurofibromatosis 1)	
Hepatoblastoma	• Genetic conditions (i.e., Beckwith-Wiedemann syndrome, hemihypertrophy, Gardner syndrome, family history of adenomatous polyposis)	
Malignant germ cell tumors	• Cryptorchidism associated with testicular germ cell tumors	

From Scheurer, M. E., Lupo, P. J., & Bondy, M. L. (2016). Epidemiology of childhood cancer. In P. A. Pizzo & D. G. Poplack (Eds.), *Principles and practice of pediatric oncology* (7th ed.). Philadelphia, PA: Lippincott. Also from https://www.cancer.gov/types/childhood-cancers/pediatric-genomics-hp-pdq

mutations (passed from parents to children) with certain malignancies such as retinoblastoma, and the existence of familial cancer predisposition syndromes point to the importance of genetic mechanisms in childhood cancer etiology.

Genomic technology, including the ability to analyze vast amounts of data and data sharing across institutions and organizations, is rapidly advancing understanding of the biology of childhood cancer. A working definition of genomics is the study of a person's complete set of genes, their functions, and their interrelationships (World Health Organization, 2019). Genome-wide association studies (GWASs) compare the genomes of people who have a disease such as cancer with people who do not have it. Scientists look for genetic variations and/or mutations that may be involved in the development of the disease. These changes could be small, such as substitution, deletion, or addition of a single base pair, or large, such as deletion of thousands of bases. The value of this research is the ability to identify subsets of patients whose prognosis is associated with a particular genetic change; these subsets could be studied separately in the future to find the most effective and least toxic treatment specifically for them. Genomic research also offers the opportunity for developing new treatment approaches that are precisely tailored to the particular cancer's molecular abnormality. This is the promise of precision medicine. Risk factors associated with childhood cancer, including genetic mutations, are summarized in Table 25.1.

Prevention

Knowledge of the risk factors that increase the likelihood of cancer holds the promise of prevention. However, there are no generally recognized preventive measures for childhood cancer.

Nevertheless, pediatric health professionals have another role in cancer prevention, namely educating parents and children about the hazards of known carcinogens associated with adult-type cancers. This is particularly true for the effects of cigarette smoking (and exposure to secondhand smoke) and excessive exposure to ultraviolet radiation (e.g., exposure to sunlight and tanning) because lung cancer is the leading cause of death from cancer in adults, and malignant melanoma is the leading cause of death from diseases of the skin. Children at higher risk for skin cancer are those with sun or tanning bed exposure; light-colored eyes, complexion, and hair; a history of sunburn; skin that burns, freckles, and reddens easily; and certain types of moles (Centers for Disease Control and Prevention, 2019). Not only these children but all children should be protected from overexposure to the sun and to tanning beds.

To provide early detection of other types of cancer, clinicians have historically recommended that males learn testicular self-examination and that females learn breast self-examination. However, teaching breast self-examination and testicular self-examination is no longer supported by the US Preventive Services Task Force (2016, 2018). Some clinicians endorse being breast "self-aware," meaning that females should know what is normal for their own breasts. All children and teens should have periodic health examinations by a health care professional, including a Papanicolaou smear for females and testicular examination for males when developmentally appropriate. In addition, to prevent human papillomavirus (HPV)–associated malignancies, HPV vaccine is recommended for routine vaccination at age 11 or 12 years (Centers for Disease Control and Prevention, 2018).

DIAGNOSTIC EVALUATION

The evaluation of a child suspected of having cancer may take several days to complete. The essential components of a comprehensive evaluation include complete history and review of symptoms, physical examination, laboratory tests, diagnostic imaging, diagnostic procedures (e.g., lumbar puncture [LP], bone marrow aspirate, biopsy), and surgical pathology depending on whether biopsy or surgical resection is performed.

Laboratory Tests

Several laboratory tests must be performed to accurately diagnose and treat children with cancer. Most patients have a complete blood count (CBC), serum chemistries, liver function tests, coagulation studies, and urinalysis done on initial presentation. For example, the CBC for patients with leukemia often reveals low hemoglobin; low platelet count; and low, normal, or high white blood cell (WBC) counts. In addition, these patients may have elevated lactate dehydrogenase, creatinine, and uric acid, which require close monitoring when therapy is initiated. Frequent CBCs are necessary to monitor effects of therapy and, in some hematologic malignancies, response to therapy.

Blood chemistry yields important information with regard to kidney, liver, and bone function and electrolyte balance. These tests are important to help detect the extent of disease and also to monitor for side effects during therapy. For example, a patient with bone metastasis may have elevated alkaline phosphatase. Elevations in blood urea nitrogen and creatinine may reflect kidney damage from chemotherapy agents. Consequently, regular blood chemistries and urinalysis are standard procedures throughout the course of the disease and its treatment.

Diagnostic Procedures

An LP is a routine test used in leukemia, brain tumors, and other cancers that may metastasize to the CNS. An LP also is used to administer intrathecal drugs in patients with various malignancies, such as leukemia.

A bone marrow test is performed by aspirating marrow with a large- or fine-bore needle. A bone marrow biopsy is performed by obtaining a piece of bone through a special type of needle. These tests are performed to determine the presence or absence of cancer cells or response to therapy in the bone marrow. For example, the type of leukemia can be identified by examination of the patient's bone marrow and core biopsy. Also, patients with other solid tumors, such as neuroblastoma, may have spread of disease to the bone marrow, which can be determined by these procedures.

Diagnostic Imaging

Modern diagnostic imaging has greatly improved the ability to accurately diagnose childhood cancers. The most commonly used modes of imaging include x-rays, computed tomography (CT), magnetic resonance imaging (MRI), and positron emission tomography (PET); in addition, metaiodobenzylguanidine (MIBG) scan is used in certain pediatric malignancies such as neuroblastoma and soft tissue tumors. Interventional radiology uses imaging to guide diagnostic and treatment procedures in the diagnosis and management of pediatric malignancies. The nurse should be aware of the Image Gently campaign to improve safe and effective imaging care of children. Parents who have heard of this effort may have questions about radiation exposure in the imaging of their children (Image Gently, 2014).

Pathologic and Molecular Evaluation

For most solid tumors, a biopsy is necessary to establish the diagnosis. Besides determining what type of cancer the patient has, this tissue sample can also be sent for various biologic or molecular studies that help define the patient's risk of relapse or recurrence and allow the health care team to plan risk-adapted therapy. For example, a bone marrow biopsy determines whether the patient has acute lymphoblastic leukemia or acute myeloid leukemia and indicates the specific leukemia subtype that is the basis for how aggressively it should be treated (NIH, 2019d). Similarly, patients with neuroblastoma undergo a biopsy of the tumor to establish the diagnosis and to evaluate the tumor for amplification of an oncogene, *MYCN,* which is a prognostic factor considered in treatment planning. Increasingly, the diagnostic evaluation includes molecular genetic testing (e.g., deoxyribonucleic acid [DNA] sequencing, reverse transcription polymerase chain reaction [RT-PCR], fluorescence in situ hybridization [FISH]) to find biologic abnormalities of the cancer cells. As more is learned about these cell changes in cancer, it is becoming possible to design therapies that target these abnormalities or block their effects; this is called **targeted therapy**, which is the basis of precision medicine.

TREATMENT MODALITIES

Survival of children with cancer has greatly improved through the use of (1) multimodal therapy consisting of surgery, chemotherapy or biotherapy, blood or marrow transplant (now referred to as hematopoietic stem cell transplant [HSCT]), and radiation therapy; (2) enrollment of large numbers of children in cooperative group clinical trials or protocols; and (3) improvements in supportive care. Current efforts are aimed at increasing the survival of patients with high-risk malignancies, decreasing the acute and long-term side effects of treatment, and studying the biology and genomics of the diseases to better identify

TABLE 25.2 Early Side Effects of Radiation Therapy

Site	Effects	Nursing Interventions
Gastrointestinal tract	Nausea and vomiting	Give antiemetic on schedule around the clock. Measure amount of emesis to assess for dehydration.
	Anorexia	Encourage fluids and foods best tolerated, usually light, soft, small, and frequent meals. Monitor weight.
	Mucosal ulceration	Use frequent mouth rinses and oral hygiene to prevent mucositis.
	Diarrhea	Control with antispasmodics and kaolin pectin preparations. Observe for signs of dehydration.
Skin	Alopecia (occurs within 2 weeks; hair may regrow by 3-6 months)	Introduce idea of wig. Stress necessity of scalp hygiene and need for head covering in sun and cold weather.
	Dry or moist desquamation	Do not refer to skin change as a "burn" (implies use of too much radiation). Avoid lotions and other creams to skin. Wash daily, using mild soap (e.g., Dove) sparingly. Do not remove skin marking for radiation fields. Avoid exposure to sun. For desquamation, consult radiation therapy practitioner for skin hygiene and care.
Head	Nausea and vomiting (from stimulation of vomiting center in brain)	Same as for gastrointestinal tract.
	Alopecia	Same as for skin.
	Mucositis	Encourage regular dental care, fluoride treatments.
	Potential effects: • Parotitis • Sore throat • Loss of taste • Xerostomia (dry mouth)	Provide analgesics as needed to relieve discomfort Combat severe dryness of mouth with oral hygiene and liquid diet.
Urinary bladder	Radiation cystitis (rarely)	Encourage liberal fluid intake and frequent voiding. Monitor for hematuria.
Bone marrow	Myelosuppression	Observe for fever (temperature >101°F [38.3°C]). Initiate workup for sepsis as ordered. Administer antibiotics as prescribed. Avoid use of suppositories, rectal temperatures. Institute bleeding precautions. Observe for signs of anemia.

patients who are at different risk levels for disease recurrence and can therefore benefit from risk-adapted and targeted therapies.

Surgery

The main goal of surgery, besides obtaining biopsies, is to remove the tumor and restore normal body functioning to the greatest extent possible. Surgery is most successful when the tumor is encapsulated and localized (confined to the site of origin). Surgery may be used for palliation when the cancer is regional (metastasized to an area adjacent to the original site) or advanced (widespread throughout the body). Generally, the best prognosis is directly related to early detection of the tumor because that facilitates surgical removal.

Because the majority of pediatric cancers respond well to chemotherapy, more conservative surgical excision is increasingly used in a variety of tumors in an attempt to preserve function and cosmesis. For example, in some types of bone cancer, such as osteosarcoma, patients are successfully treated with resection of the diseased portion of the bone rather than amputation.

Radiation Therapy

Radiation therapy is frequently used in the treatment of childhood cancer, usually in conjunction with chemotherapy or surgery. It can be used for curative purposes and for palliation to relieve symptoms by shrinking the size of the tumor. Recent advances in radiation therapy that allow the beam to be aimed precisely have optimized its beneficial effects and minimized many of the undesirable side effects by sparing normal tissue.

Ionizing radiation is cytotoxic in at least three different ways: (1) damaging the pyrimidine bases cytosine, thymine, and uracil needed for the synthesis of nucleic acids; (2) causing single-strand breaks in the DNA or ribonucleic acid (RNA) molecule; or (3) causing double helical-strand breaks in these molecules. Disturbing cellular metabolic and reproductive functions causes lethal or sublethal damage. *Lethal damage* refers to the death of the cell. *Sublethal damage* refers to injured cells that may subsequently be repaired. Many acute side effects are the result of lethal damage to radiosensitive tissue, particularly proliferating cells such as those of the bone marrow, gastrointestinal tract, and hair follicles. Late effects (late-occurring or long-term effects) are usually the result of cell death.

The acute untoward reactions from radiation therapy depend on the area being irradiated. Total body irradiation is associated with the most severe reactions and is used to prepare the immune system for HSCT. Table 25.2 summarizes the acute effects of radiation therapy and nursing interventions that may be helpful in mitigating or preventing them.

In some areas of the United States, proton beam radiation is available. Protons are positively charged subatomic particles. Protons deposit energy differently than x-ray beams. There is no "exit dose" beyond the tumor involved in proton radiation therapy; therefore local control of the tumor is a major benefit with no long-term effects to organs surrounding the target area (Hill-Kayser, Tochner, Both, et al., 2013). For example, some brain tumor patients receive radiation to the spine. With traditional forms of radiation therapy, lasting damage to nearby vital organs such as the heart and lungs is possible; however, with proton therapy the heart and lungs would not be affected, avoiding long-term cardiac and pulmonary damage.

Chemotherapy

Chemotherapy may be the primary form of treatment, or it may be an adjunct to surgery, radiation therapy, or HSCT. The majority of traditional chemotherapy agents work by interfering with the function or production of nucleic acids, DNA, or RNA. Although several drugs have been effective in treating different forms of cancer as single agents, the remarkable increase in survival rates has been the result of improved combination drug regimens. Combining drugs allows for optimum cell cycle destruction with minimum toxic effects and decreased resistance by the cancer cells to the agent. For example, a treatment regimen called VAC (vincristine [Oncovin], doxorubicin [Adriamycin], and cyclophosphamide [Cytoxan]) combines complementary cytotoxic effects with distinct side effects. Doxorubicin and cyclophosphamide are myelosuppressive, whereas vincristine is neurotoxic.

In addition to more effective combinations of drugs, several advances in the administration of chemotherapy have permitted continuous or intermittent intravenous (IV) administration without multiple venipunctures. The use of venous access devices (e.g., catheters, implantable infusion ports) has greatly facilitated safe and effective drug administration with minimum discomfort for the child (see Chapter 20). Continuous infusions over an extended period using syringe pumps have made possible the administration of certain drugs, such as cytosine arabinoside, in higher doses with less toxicity than when the drug is administered intermittently.

An understanding of the actions and side effects of these drugs is essential to nursing care of children with cancer. Unfortunately, almost all standard chemotherapy drugs are not selectively cytotoxic for malignant cells, and other cells with a high rate of proliferation, such as the bone marrow elements, hair, skin, and epithelial cells of the gastrointestinal tract, are also affected. Frequently the problems related to the destruction of these normal cells require more nursing care than those related to the disease itself.

Precautions in Administering and Handling Chemotherapeutic Agents

Many chemotherapeutic agents are **vesicants** (sclerosing agents) that can cause severe cellular damage if even minute amounts of the drug infiltrate surrounding tissue. Only nurses experienced with chemotherapeutic agents should administer vesicants (Fig. 25.1). Standards are available[a] and must be followed meticulously to prevent tissue damage to patients. Interventions for extravasation vary, but each nurse should be aware of the institution's policies before giving any vesicant and implement them at once if indicated.

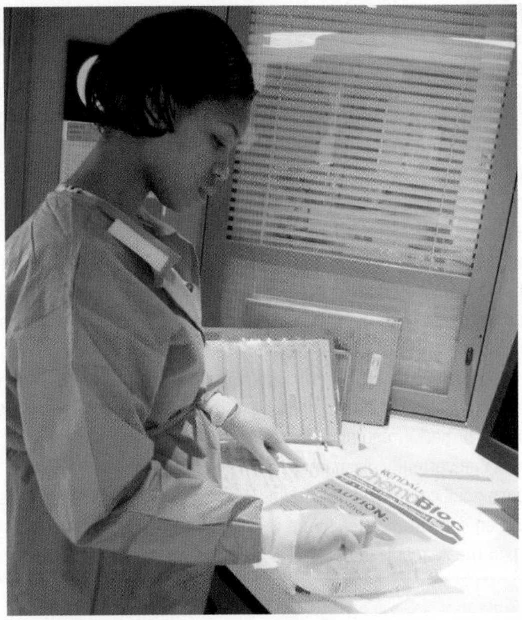

Fig. 25.1 Nurses caring for children with cancer require expertise in the safe administration of chemotherapy.

> **! NURSING ALERT**
>
> Chemotherapeutic drugs must be given through a free-flowing intravenous (IV) line. The infusion is stopped immediately if any sign of infiltration (e.g., pain, stinging, swelling, redness at needle site) occurs.

> **! NURSING ALERT**
>
> When chemotherapy or immunotherapy agents with known anaphylactic potential are given, it is standard practice to observe the child for 1 hour after the infusion for signs of anaphylaxis (e.g., rash, urticaria, hypotension, wheezing, nausea, vomiting). Emergency equipment (especially blood pressure monitor, bag valve mask, and suction) and emergency drugs (especially oxygen, epinephrine, antihistamine, aminophylline, corticosteroids, and vasopressors) must be readily available.

In addition to the many patient-focused responsibilities during chemotherapy administration, nurses must also use safeguards to protect themselves. Handling chemotherapeutic agents may present risks to handlers and to their offspring, although the exact degree of risk is not known. The Oncology Nursing Society has published comprehensive guidelines for safe practice issues related to administration of chemotherapy.[b] The Oncology Nursing Society also has established safe management procedures for chemotherapy administered in the home.[b] Basic nursing guidelines are in the Nursing Care Guidelines box.

---

[a] *2016 Updated American Society of Clinical Oncology/Oncology Nursing Society Chemotherapy Administration Safety Standards, Including Standards for Pediatric Oncology* is available from the Oncology Nursing Society, 125 Enterprise Drive, Pittsburgh, PA 15275; 412-859-6100; http://www.ons.org.

[b] *Chemotherapy and Biotherapy Guidelines and Recommendations for Practice* (4th edition) can be obtained from the Oncology Nursing Society, 125 Enterprise Drive, Pittsburgh, PA 15275; 866-257-4667, 412-859-6100; http://www.ons.org.

NURSING CARE GUIDELINES

Handling Chemotherapeutic Agents

- Use great care and strict aseptic technique in handling chemotherapeutic agents to prevent any physical contact with the substance.
- Drugs are prepared in a properly ventilated room (which incorporates a protective front panel and vertical laminar airflow to reduce potential for inhalation during preparation).
- Wear disposable gloves and protective clothing and discard in a special container after each use.
- Wear face and eye protection when splashing is possible and wear a respirator when the risk of inhalation is possible.
- Use a sterile gauze pad when priming intravenous (IV) tubing, connecting and disconnecting tubing, inserting syringes into vials, breaking glass ampules, or performing any other procedure in which antineoplastic drugs may be inadvertently discharged.
- Dispose of all contaminated needles, syringes, IV tubing, and other contaminated equipment in a leakproof and puncture-resistant container; do not recap or break needles.

Biologic Therapy

Biologic therapy, also called biotherapy, uses substances made from living organisms, derived from living organisms, or laboratory-produced versions of these substances to treat cancer (Ceppi, Beck-Popovic, Bourquin, et al., 2017). Biotherapies can be grouped into three main types: (1) those that do not target cancer cells directly but stimulate the body's immune system to act against cancer cells and that are collectively referred to as immunotherapy or biologic response modifier therapy; (2) those that use antibodies or segments of genetic material to target cancer cells directly; and (3) therapies that interfere with specific molecules involved in tumor growth and progression and that are referred to as targeted therapies (Ceppi et al., 2017).

Immunotherapy works by stimulating the activity of the immune system against cancer cells or by counteracting signals produced by cancer cells that suppress immune responses (US Food and Drug Administration, 2016). Immunotherapy includes the use of monoclonal antibodies that attach to proteins on cancer cells so that the immune system can find and destroy the cells. Other antibodies block pathways that allow cancer cells to escape the immune system; these are called checkpoint inhibitors. Nonspecific immunotherapies include two types of cytokines: interferons and interleukins. Other immunotherapies include oncolytic virus therapy and chimeric antigen receptor (CAR) T-cell therapy. CAR T-cell therapy is being studied in childhood acute leukemia that does not respond to traditional chemotherapy. Surveillance for and management of side effects of immunotherapy are critical nursing responsibilities. Side effects may range from mild to severe. For example, with CAR T-cell therapy, adverse events may include cytokine release syndrome, neurologic symptoms, tumor lysis syndrome, and graft-versus-host disease (Becze, 2017).

Targeted therapies are substances that interfere with specific molecules involved in cancer. They are different from standard chemotherapy in two ways (National Institutes of Health, 2019a): (1) they act on molecular targets rather than affecting all rapidly dividing normal and malignant cells; and (2) they are selected or designed to affect their target, compared with chemotherapy drugs that were identified because they kill cells. Previously, targeted therapies have had limited use in pediatric patients, but they are now being evaluated in clinical trials. Careful monitoring of side effects is essential because the profile of adverse events may be different than that seen in adults and because these agents may affect the process of growth and development in pediatric patients in unexpected ways (Gore, DeGregori, & Porter, 2013).

Hematopoietic Stem Cell Transplant

Another approach to the treatment of childhood cancer is transplantation of hematopoietic (blood-forming) stem cells. HSCT restores stem cells in children who have diseases that require high doses of chemotherapy or radiation therapy and/or replacement of dysfunctional bone marrow. Blood-forming stem cells from bone marrow, peripheral blood, or cord blood can be sources for HSCT. The main types of HSCT are **allogeneic**, where cells are obtained from a family member or volunteer donor, and **autologous**, where cells previously stored from the patient are given back to the patient by IV infusion. In either type of HSCT, if it is successful, the newly transfused cells begin to produce functioning nonmalignant blood cells. In essence, the recipient accepts a new blood-forming organ.

Children receiving an allogeneic HSCT undergo a pretransplant conditioning regimen consisting of radiation therapy and/or high-dose chemotherapy to rid the body of malignant cells and suppress the immune system to prevent rejection of the transplanted marrow (see Family-Centered Care box).

FAMILY-CENTERED CARE

Decision for Transplant

A family's decision for a child to undergo a hematopoietic stem cell transplant (HSCT) is fraught with uncertainties. Often the child faces certain death from the malignancy without the HSCT. The preparation of the child for the transplant also places the patient at great medical risk.

Once the preparatory regimen begins and the child's immune system is destroyed, there is no turning back. Unlike kidney transplantation, HSCT does not have a "rescue" procedure, such as dialysis, for supportive therapy. If the donor is a sibling, the expectation that his or her marrow will "save" the brother or sister can be a concern, especially if the transplant is not successful. Parents often must leave home to stay at the transplant center and encounter additional stressors such as arranging child care, taking leave from work, and managing finances. If old enough to understand the risks, the patient faces the greatest stress, such as fear of HSCT failure or life-threatening complications.

The selection process for a suitable donor and the potential complications in allogeneic transplantation are related to the human leukocyte antigen (HLA) system complex. Some of the major HLA antigens are A, B, C, D, DR, and DQ. There is wide diversity for each of these HLA loci. For example, more than 20 different HLA-A antigens and more than 40 different HLA-B antigens can be inherited. The genes are inherited as a single unit, or haplotype. A child inherits one unit from each parent; thus a child and each parent have one identical and one nonidentical haplotype. Because the possible haplotype combinations among siblings follow the laws of Mendelian genetics, there is a 1 in 4 chance that two siblings have identical haplotypes and are perfectly matched at the HLA loci.

The importance of HLA matching is to prevent the serious complication of graft-versus-host disease (GVHD) after allogeneic transplant. Because the child's immune system is essentially rendered nonfunctional, the recipient is unlikely to reject the bone marrow. However, the donor's marrow may contain antigens not matched to the recipient's antigens, which begin attacking body cells. The more closely the HLA systems match, the less likely GVHD is to develop. However, GVHD can occur even with a perfect HLA match because of unidentified and thus unmatched histocompatibility antigens (Gottschalk, Naik, Hegde, et al., 2016).

Umbilical cord blood or haploidentical family donors (i.e., parents) are additional sources of hematopoietic stem cells for use in children with cancer (Gottschalk, Naik, Hegde, et al., 2016). The benefit of using umbilical cord blood is the blood's relative immunodeficiency at birth, allowing for partially matched, unrelated cord blood transplants to be successful, with a lower risk of GVHD-related problems (Sarvaria, Jawdat, Madrigal, et al., 2017). A benefit of using a haploidentical family member is the likely immediate availability of the donor, which is especially important when children urgently need HSCT.

Autologous Transplantation

Autologous transplants use the patient's own marrow that was collected from disease-free tissue, frozen, and may have been treated to remove malignant cells. Peripheral blood stem cell transplant (PBSCT) is also used in children with cancer. This type of transplant differs in the way stem cells are collected. Most commonly, colony-stimulating factor (CSF) is first given to stimulate the production of many stem cells (Karakukcu & Unal, 2015). Once the WBC count is high enough, the stem cells are collected by an apheresis machine. This machine filters out peripheral stem cells from whole blood and returns the remainder of the blood cells and plasma to the child. Stem cells have been collected without problems in even very small children weighing 20 kg (44 pounds) or less (Gottschalk et al., 2016). The peripheral stem cells are then frozen until the patient is ready for the PBSCT. Children with solid tumors such as neuroblastoma, Hodgkin lymphoma, NHL, rhabdomyosarcoma, Ewing sarcoma, and Wilms tumor have been treated with autologous transplants.

COMPLICATIONS OF THERAPY

Although great advances have been achieved through current modes of cancer therapy, the successes are not without consequences. Numerous acute side effects are commonly expected with chemotherapy or biotherapy and radiation therapy. Several complications that are less frequent but generally more serious are described here.

Pediatric Oncologic Emergencies

Tumor Lysis Syndrome

Life-threatening conditions may develop in children with cancer as a result of the malignancy and/or aggressive treatment modalities. Acute tumor lysis syndrome has hallmark metabolic abnormalities that are the direct result of rapid release of intracellular contents during the lysis of malignant cells. This typically occurs in patients with acute lymphoblastic leukemia or Burkitt lymphoma during the initial treatment period but may occur spontaneously before onset of therapy. The metabolic abnormalities of tumor lysis syndrome include hyperuricemia, hypocalcemia, hyperphosphatemia, and hyperkalemia. The crystallization of uric acid that can occur with hyperuricemia can lead to acute renal failure (Freedman, Rheingold, & Fisher, 2016).

Risk factors for development of tumor lysis syndrome include high WBC count at diagnosis, large tumor burden, cancer cell sensitivity to chemotherapy, and high proliferative rate. In addition to the described metabolic abnormalities, children may develop a spectrum of clinical symptoms, including flank pain, lethargy, nausea and vomiting, muscle cramps, pruritus, tetany, and seizures.

Management of tumor lysis syndrome consists of early identification of patients at risk, prophylactic measures, and early interventions. Patients at risk for tumor lysis syndrome should have serum chemistries and urine pH monitored frequently, strict recording of intake and output, and aggressive administration of IV fluids. Medications, such as allopurinol, that reduce uric acid formation and promote excretion of byproducts of purine metabolism are often used. If tumor lysis syndrome occurs, IV hydration continues and the specific metabolic abnormalities are treated. Hyperuricemia is now effectively treated with recombinant urate oxidase, or rasburicase. This medication converts uric acid to allantoin, which is more soluble in urine. Exchange transfusions are sometimes necessary to reduce the metabolic consequences of massive tumor lysis, especially in children with a high tumor burden.

Hyperleukocytosis

Hyperleukocytosis, defined as a peripheral WBC count greater than 100,000/mm^3, can lead to capillary obstruction, microinfarction, and organ dysfunction. Children often experience respiratory distress and cyanosis. They also experience neurologic changes, including altered level of consciousness, visual disturbances, agitation, confusion, ataxia, and delirium. Management consists of rapid cytoreduction by chemotherapy, hydration, urinary alkalinization, and allopurinol. Leukapheresis or exchange transfusion may be necessary.

Superior Vena Cava Syndrome

Space-occupying lesions located in the chest, especially from Hodgkin disease and NHL, may cause superior vena cava syndrome (SVCS), leading to airway compromise and potentially to respiratory failure. The second leading cause of SVCS is thrombotic complications of implantable IV devices, such as central venous catheters and port catheters (Freedman et al., 2016).

Children are initially seen with cyanosis of the face, neck, and upper chest; facial and upper extremity edema; and distended neck and chest veins. They may be anxious and have dyspnea, wheezing, or a frequent cough from airway obstruction. Management consists of airway protection and alleviation of respiratory distress. Rapid treatment is initiated, and symptoms typically improve as the disease is effectively treated.

Spinal Cord Compression

Malignancies can invade or impinge on the spinal cord, causing acute symptoms of cord compression. Primary CNS tumors can originate or spread to the spinal cord. Other solid tumors, such as neuroblastoma or rhabdomyosarcoma, can metastasize to the spinal cord and cause compression. Back pain is a common initial manifestation, but other symptoms can include sensation change, extremity weakness, loss of bowel and bladder function, and respiratory insufficiency. Careful physical examination is essential in early detection of symptoms, and MRI is the gold standard for diagnosis (Freedman et al., 2016). Treatment may include high-dose steroids to reduce associated edema and alleviate symptoms and rapid initiation of treatment such as emergent radiation or laminectomy if indicated.

Disseminated Intravascular Coagulation

Overwhelming infections in the immunocompromised child constitute an emergency situation. Sepsis from bacteria or fungus can result in numerous complications, including disseminated intravascular coagulation (DIC). Children with DIC form excessive microthrombi throughout the vascular system due to hyperactivation of the clotting cascade, downregulation of anticoagulants, and impaired fibrinolysis, which leaves the child susceptible to hemorrhage. Life-threatening hemorrhage can occur from DIC with thrombocytopenia (platelet count of less than 20,000/mm^3) (Andrews, Galel, Wong, et al., 2016).

Treatment is focused on identifying and treating the underlying cause, along with infusing heparin to minimize microthrombi and cryoprecipitate to replace fibrinogen.

GENERAL NURSING CARE MANAGEMENT

This section presents an overview of general nursing concepts that apply to most childhood cancers. Specific nursing care for children with a particular type of cancer is discussed under each disease section later in the chapter. This discussion focuses on the physical aspects of care. In addition, refer to Chapter 19 for family-centered care and Chapter 17 for end-of-life care (see Quality Patient Outcomes box).

QUALITY PATIENT OUTCOMES: The Child With Cancer

- Child and family educated about disease and treatment
- Child and family safely perform self-care as appropriate
- Treatment administered on schedule with appropriate drug doses
- Side effects of treatment managed
- Treatment complications prevented
- Child and family strengths and coping skills supported
- Quality of life during treatment maintained
- Child and family adjusted to chronic illness
- Growth and development maintained during treatment

SIGNS AND SYMPTOMS OF CANCER IN CHILDREN

Early detection is critical to starting treatment with the best prospect for eventual cure. Cancers in children are often difficult to recognize. Therefore being alert to the persistence of possible signs and symptoms is essential (Box 25.1). This section discusses some of the more significant clues leading to a diagnosis of pediatric cancer.

Pain may be an early or late initial sign of cancer and requires a careful history of its onset, characteristics, location, intensity, and alleviating factors. Pain may be generalized or present at a specific location. For example, bone pain occurs in approximately 20% of children with leukemia. Pain, swelling, and tenderness at the tumor site may be initial signs in solid tumors. In addition, a mass is a typical finding in children with solid tumors. An abdominal mass in a child must be evaluated for a malignancy, such as Wilms tumor or neuroblastoma.

Fever is a frequent occurrence during childhood and is caused by numerous illnesses, including cancer. The cause of fever in cancer patients is infection or the malignant process itself. The latter is often referred to as tumor-associated fever. The exact mechanism by which the malignancy causes a fever is not completely understood. Cytokines (e.g., interleukin, tumor necrosis factor) are known to be involved and are thought to be released either directly from tumor cells or from macrophages responding to tumor (Foggo & Cavenagh, 2015).

A careful skin assessment will reveal signs of a low platelet count. Ecchymosis and petechiae are most commonly found on the child's extremities and under constricting parts of clothing like waistbands. Spontaneous gum or nose bleeding may occur when the platelet count falls below 20,000/mm^3.

The child with malignant invasion of the bone marrow often appears pale, with symptoms of lethargy, weight loss, and malaise. These symptoms may be attributed to anemia caused by the replacement of normal cells with malignant cells in the bone marrow. The nurse should assess for signs and symptoms of anemia (see Chapter 24).

Swollen lymph nodes are another common finding in children. However, enlarged, firm lymph nodes in a child with fever for more than 1 week; a recent history of weight loss; or an abnormal chest x-ray film may indicate a serious disease and should be evaluated further.

BOX 25.1 Possible Signs and Symptoms of Childhood Cancer

- Unusual mass or swelling
- Unexplained paleness and loss of energy
- Easy bruising
- Persistent, localized pain or limping
- Prolonged, unexplained fever or illness
- Frequent headaches, often with vomiting
- Sudden eye or vision changes
- Unexplained, rapid weight loss

Data from American Cancer Society. (2016). Finding cancer in children. Retrieved from https://www.cancer.org/cancer/cancer-in-children/finding-childhood-cancers-early.html

Recognizing one sign is facilitated by the widespread use of cell phone photography. Leukocoria or white eye reflex can be seen as a yellow "glow" in the pupil, as opposed to the normal red pupillary reflex, in photographs. It can be a sign of retinoblastoma that needs prompt medical attention. Squinting, strabismus, or swelling can indicate other solid tumors of the eye.

The child with a brain tumor develops signs and symptoms related to the area of the brain involved. The nurse's thorough physical assessment can indicate the likely area of tumor involvement.

MANAGING COMMON ACUTE SIDE EFFECTS OF TREATMENT

Cancer care encompasses more than treatments aimed at eliminating the malignant cells. Because of the delicate balance between killing malignant cells and preserving functional cells, supportive therapy usually is needed during those times that serious damage occurs to normal body tissues. A major concern for the child receiving treatment for cancer is the risk for the development of complications secondary to the treatment.

Infection

The nurse caring for the child with fever must be aware of the signs and symptoms of septic shock, as discussed in Chapter 23. The child with fever who has an absolute neutrophil count (ANC) lower than 500/mm^3 is at risk for the following (see Nursing Care Guidelines box):

- Overwhelming infection
- Malaise
- Dehydration
- Seizures (young infants and children)
- Invasion of organisms producing secondary infections

NURSING CARE GUIDELINES

Calculating the Absolute Neutrophil Count (ANC)

1. Determine the total percentage of neutrophils ("polys, or segs" and "bands").
2. Multiply white blood cell (WBC) count by percentage of neutrophils.

Example

WBC = 1000/mm^3, neutrophils = 7%, nonsegmented neutrophils (bands) = 7%
Step 1: 7% + 7% = 14%
Step 2: 0.14 × 1000 = 140/mm^3 ANC

The child with fever is evaluated for potential sites of infection, such as from a needle puncture, mucosal ulceration, minor abrasion, or skin tears (e.g., a hangnail). Although the body may not be able to produce an adequate inflammatory response to the infection and the usual clinical signs of infection may be partially expressed or absent, fever will occur. Therefore the child's temperature is monitored closely. To identify the source of infection, the health care team takes blood, stool, urine, and nasopharyngeal cultures and chest x-rays.

Once infection is suspected, broad-spectrum IV antibiotic therapy is begun before the organism is identified and may be continued for 7 to 10 days. If the child does not have a venous access device, a heparin lock peripheral IV should be inserted to prevent the inconvenience and discomfort of multiple venipunctures in administering antibiotic therapy.

The organisms most lethal to these children are (1) viruses, particularly varicella (chickenpox), herpes zoster, herpes simplex, respiratory syncytial virus, influenza, and cytomegalovirus; (2) protozoan, *Toxoplasma gondii;* (3) fungi, especially *Pneumocystis jirovecii* (formally known as *Pneumocystis carinii*) and *Candida albicans;* (4) gram-negative bacteria, such as *Pseudomonas aeruginosa, Escherichia coli,* and *Klebsiella* organisms; and (5) gram-positive bacteria, especially *Staphylococcus* and *Enterococcus* species (Ardura & Koh, 2016).

Prophylaxis against *Pneumocystis* pneumonia, such as trimethoprim-sulfamethoxazole, is routinely given to most children during treatment for cancer (Ardura & Koh, 2016). Colony-stimulating factors (CSFs), a family of glycoprotein hormones that regulate the reproduction, maturation, and function of blood cells, are now routinely used as supportive measures to prevent the side effects caused by low blood counts. CSFs promote stem cell proliferation and stimulate a more rapid maturation of the cells, allowing them to enter the bloodstream earlier. Granulocyte colony-stimulating factor (G-CSF; filgrastim [Neupogen], pegfilgrastim [Neulasta]) directs granulocyte development and can decrease the duration of neutropenia. This reduces the incidence and duration of infection in children receiving treatment for cancer. G-CSF is also being used to decrease the bone marrow recovery time after HSCT (Ardura & Koh, 2016). G-CSF is usually administered intravenously or subcutaneously 24 hours after chemotherapy is discontinued and is given for 10 to 14 days. G-CSF is discontinued when the ANC surpasses 10,000/mm^3. The pegylated or long-acting form of G-CSF, pegfilgrastim, is given only once after completion of therapy and typically has its peak efficacy (highest WBC count) about 8 to 10 days after administration. During G-CSF therapy, children may experience bone pain, fever, rash, malaise, and headaches.

Prevention of infection continues as a priority after discharge from the hospital. Some institutions allow the child to return to school when the ANC is above 500/mm^3. Other institutions place no restrictions on the child, regardless of the blood count. If the ANC falls below 500/mm^3, cautious isolation from crowded areas, such as shopping centers or subways, is advisable. At all times, family members should be encouraged to practice good hand washing to avoid introducing pathogens into the home, and they should know how to take a temperature and who to call in the event of fever (see the Next-Generation NCLEX® Examination-Style Unfolding Case Study).

Hemorrhage

Before the use of transfused platelets, hemorrhage was a leading cause of death in children with some types of cancer. Now most bleeding episodes can be prevented or controlled with judicious administration of platelet concentrates or platelet-rich plasma. The incidence of severe spontaneous internal hemorrhage varies but usually does not occur until the platelet count is 20,000/mm^3 or less (Hockenberry, Kline, & Rodgers, 2016).

Because infection increases the tendency toward hemorrhage and because bleeding sites become more easily infected, special care should be taken to avoid performing skin punctures whenever possible. When performing finger sticks, venipunctures, intramuscular injections, and bone marrow tests, use aseptic technique with continued observation for bleeding. Meticulous mouth care is essential because gingival bleeding with resultant mucositis is a frequent problem. Because the rectal area is prone to ulceration from various drugs, hygiene is essential. To prevent additional trauma, avoid rectal temperatures and suppositories. Frequent turning and the use of a pressure-reducing mattress under bony prominences prevent development of pressure sores and decubital ulcers.

Platelet transfusions are generally reserved for active bleeding episodes that do not respond to local treatment and that may occur during induction or relapse therapy. Epistaxis and gingival bleeding are the most common. The nurse teaches parents and children measures to control nose bleeding. Applying pressure at the site without disturbing clot formation is the general rule. Platelet concentrates normally do not have to be cross-matched for blood group or type. However, because platelets contain specific antigen components similar to blood group factors, children who receive multiple transfusions may become sensitized to a platelet group other than their own. Therefore platelets are cross-matched with the donor's blood components whenever possible.

Transfused platelets generally survive in the body for 1 to 3 days. The peak effect is reached in about 1 hour and decreased by half in 24 hours. After a transfusion, the nurse observes and records the approximate time when hemostasis of bleeding sites occurs. Delayed hemostasis is evidence of platelet destruction. For long-term patients, multiple transfusion therapy becomes progressively less effective.

During bleeding episodes the parents and child need much emotional support. The sight of oozing blood is upsetting. Often parents request a platelet transfusion, unaware of the necessity of trying local measures first. The nurse can help calm their anxiety by explaining the reason for delaying a platelet transfusion until absolutely necessary. Because compatible donors decrease the risk of antigen formation in the recipient, the nurse should encourage parents to locate suitable donors for eventual blood use.

Children at home who have low platelet counts (usually <100,000/mm^3) should avoid activities that might cause injury or bleeding, such as riding bicycles or skateboards, skating, climbing trees or playground equipment, and contact sports such as football or soccer. Once the platelet count rises, these restrictions are not necessary. In addition, aspirin and aspirin-containing products are not used; for mild pain or significantly elevated temperature, acetaminophen is substituted.

Anemia

Initially anemia may be profound if there is complete replacement of the bone marrow by cancer cells. During induction therapy, blood transfusions with packed red blood cells may be necessary to raise the hemoglobin to levels approaching 10 g/dl. The usual precautions in caring for the child are instituted (see Chapter 24).

Anemia is also a consequence of drug-induced myelosuppression. Although not as severely affected as the WBCs, erythrocyte production may be delayed. Because children have an amazing capacity to withstand low hemoglobin levels, the best approach is to allow the child to regulate activity with reasonable adult supervision. It may be necessary for the parents to alert the schoolteacher to the child's physical limitations, particularly in terms of strenuous activity.

Nausea and Vomiting

The nausea and vomiting that occur shortly after administration of several of the drugs and as a result of cranial or abdominal irradiation can be profound and debilitating. The advent of serotonin receptor blockers (5-hydroxytryptamine-3 or 5-HT3 receptor antagonists) has greatly improved management of nausea and vomiting caused by chemotherapy and radiation therapy. The advantage of these agents over conventional drugs is that they produce no extrapyramidal side effects, such as difficulty speaking or swallowing, shuffle walk, slow movements, trembling, stiffness of the arms and legs, or loss of balance. Published guidelines recommend 5-HT3 antagonists and corticosteroids for children receiving highly or moderately emetogenic chemotherapy (Patel, Robinson, Thackray, et al., 2017).

For mild to moderate vomiting, phenothiazine-type drugs remain the mainstay of therapy. Promethazine (Phenergan), prochlorperazine (Compazine), or trimethobenzamide (Tigan) may be effective agents. Metoclopramide is a more effective antiemetic for acute nausea or vomiting. Unfortunately, the drug causes a number of side effects in children, particularly extrapyramidal reactions, such as muscle tremors or twitching, agitation, grimacing, dysarthria, and oculogyric crisis (fixation of eyes in one position for minutes or hours). Prophylaxis with diphenhydramine (Benadryl) is recommended to reduce the incidence of extrapyramidal symptoms when metoclopramide is given (Krane, Casillas, & Zeltzer, 2016).

There is increasing interest in the use of cannabis and its components, cannabinoids, for symptom relief in pediatric patients, including antiemetic effects, appetite stimulation, pain relief, and improved sleep (National Institutes of Health, 2019b). Although cannabis has been approved by a number of states for medical use, some have limited approval to only one ingredient (e.g., cannabidiol, or CBD). It remains illegal by federal law in the United States (except in approved research settings), is not approved by the US Food and Drug Administration, and is not endorsed by the American Academy of Pediatrics because of concerns about brain development (National Institutes of Health, 2019b). These constraints have limited clinical trials and thus the evidence for practice. Commercially available synthetic cannabinoids (e.g., dronabinol, nabilone) are approved drugs for chemotherapy-induced nausea and vomiting (CINV) and have shown evidence of effectiveness for relief of CINV (Wong & Wilens, 2017).

The most beneficial regimen for antiemetic control has been the administration of the antiemetic before chemotherapy begins (30 minutes to 1 hour before) and regular (not as-needed) administration for at least 24 hours after chemotherapy. The goal is to prevent the child from ever experiencing nausea or vomiting in order to prevent the development of anticipatory symptoms (the conditioned response of developing nausea and vomiting before receiving the drug). Other nonpharmacologic interventions (similar to those discussed for pain management in Chapter 5) can be useful in controlling posttherapy and anticipatory nausea and vomiting. Giving the antineoplastic drug with a mild sedative at bedtime is also helpful for some children, and there is evidence that nighttime administration of drugs such as methotrexate and 6-mercaptopurine may be more effective than morning administration.

More detailed information about preventing and treating CINV is available in the Children's Oncology Group's COG Supportive Care Endorsed Guidelines (https://childrensoncologygroup.org/downloads/COG_SC_Guideline_Document.pdf). This resource lists the strength of each recommendation and the quality of the evidence wherever possible.

Altered Nutrition

Altered nutrition is a common side effect of treatment. Continued assessment of the child's nutritional status, child's intake, and energy expenditure must occur throughout treatment. The child's height, weight, and head circumference (for children younger than 3 years old) must be measured routinely during visits to the hospital or clinic. Energy reserves should be evaluated with routine skinfold measurements. Biochemical assays such as serum prealbumin, transferrin, and albumin may be helpful to evaluate nutritional status in some children, but a single assay should not be used alone for a nutritional evaluation (Lawson, Daley, Sams, et al., 2013). There are no specific criteria that mandate nutritional interventions in children undergoing cancer treatment. Instead, each child should have an individualized nutritional care plan based on routine assessments. Most pediatric cancer treatment centers have a nutritionist who can be consulted to develop the nutritional care plan and revise it as needed. Nutritional status is important to maintain because a compromised nutritional status can contribute to reduced tolerance to treatment, altered metabolism of chemotherapy drugs, prolonged episodes of neutropenia, and increased risk for infection.

> **! NURSING ALERT**
>
> Some children develop conditioned aversions to certain foods if they are eaten during a period of chemotherapy. It is best to refrain from offering the child's favorite foods while the child is receiving chemotherapy.

Supportive nutrition measures include oral supplements with high-protein and high-calorie foods. Ways to increase calories include using whole milk; adding tofu (high in protein) to most meals; and serving full-fat yogurt, ice cream, and milk instead of nonfat or low-fat items. Cooking with butter; putting sugar on cereal; and making high-calorie snacks such as trail mix, peanut butter, or dried fruit readily available for the child are other ways to increase calories. Enteral feeding may be necessary when children are unable to maintain the necessary calories to prevent weight loss. Parenteral hyperalimentation is used most frequently for children who have digestive problems, after surgery, or with HSCT. Chapter 22 discusses these interventions in more detail.

Despite such approaches, some children still do not eat. Theories to explain persistent anorexia include the following: (1) a nonspecific physical effect related to the cancer and/or substances it secretes or evokes from the immune system; (2) a conditioned aversion to food from nausea and vomiting during treatment; (3) a response to stress in the environment related to eating or to the child's condition; (4) a result of depression; and (5) a control mechanism when so much else has been imposed on the child. When loss of appetite and weight loss persist, the nurse should investigate the family situation to determine whether any of these variables are contributing to the problem and discuss with the treatment team.

Mucosal Ulceration

One of the most distressing side effects of several drugs is gastrointestinal mucosal cell damage, which results in ulcers anywhere along the alimentary tract. Oral ulcers (stomatitis) are red, eroded, painful areas in the mouth or pharynx (see Chapter 6, Stomatitis). Similar lesions may extend along the esophagus and occur in the rectal area. Mucositis greatly compounds anorexia because eating becomes extremely uncomfortable.

! NURSING ALERT

Viscous lidocaine is not recommended for young children. If applied to the pharynx, it may depress the gag reflex, increasing the risk of aspiration. Seizures have also been associated with the use of oral viscous lidocaine, most likely as a result of the rapid absorption into the bloodstream via the oral lesions (Lutwak, Howland, Gambetta, et al., 2013).

Some helpful interventions when oral ulcers develop are feeding a bland, moist, soft diet; using a soft sponge toothbrush (Toothette) instead of a toothbrush; frequently rinsing the mouth with chlorhexidine mouthwash or sodium bicarbonate and salt mouth rinses (using a solution of 1 tsp of baking soda and ½ tsp of table salt in 1 quart of water); using sucralfate; and administering local anesthetics without alcohol, such as a solution of diphenhydramine and Maalox (aluminum and magnesium hydroxide) or UlcerEase (Chaveli-Lopez & Bagan-Sebastian, 2016). Although local anesthetics are effective in temporarily relieving the pain, many children dislike the taste and numb feeling they produce.

More detailed information about preventing and treating mucositis is available in the Children's Oncology Group's COG Supportive Care Endorsed Guidelines (https://childrensoncologygroup.org/downloads/COG_SC_Guideline_Document.pdf). This resource lists the strength of each recommendation and the quality of the evidence wherever possible.

! NURSING ALERT

Avoid agents such as lemon glycerin swabs and hydrogen peroxide because of their drying effects on the mucosa. In addition, the acidity of lemon may be very irritating, especially on eroded tissue.

Administering mouth care is particularly difficult in infants and toddlers. A satisfactory method of cleaning the gums is to wrap a piece of gauze around a finger; soak it in saline or plain water; and swab the gums, palate, and inner cheek surfaces with the finger. Mouth care should be performed routinely before and after any feeding and as often as every 2 to 4 hours to rid mucosal surfaces of debris, which becomes an excellent medium for bacterial and fungal growth if left undisturbed.

Dental hygiene can become a serious problem if the child wears an orthodontic appliance. The accumulated debris on braces is difficult to remove without vigorous brushing, and the appliance itself traumatizes the gums. For this reason, sometimes braces are removed before starting chemotherapy treatment.

Difficulty eating is a major problem with stomatitis and may warrant hospitalization if the child refuses fluids. The child usually chooses the foods that are best tolerated. Surprisingly, some children prefer salty foods to bland ones. Drinking can usually be encouraged if a straw is used to bypass the ulcerated oral mucosa. The nurse should encourage parents to relax any eating pressures because the anorexia accompanying stomatitis is well justified. In addition, because it is a temporary condition, the child can resume good food habits once the ulcers heal. Ordinarily, severe mucosal ulceration indicates a need for reduced chemotherapy until complete healing takes place, usually within a week. Analgesics, including opioids, may be needed when treatment cannot be altered, such as during HSCT.

If rectal ulcers develop, meticulous toilet hygiene, warm sitz baths after each bowel movement, and an occlusive ointment applied to the ulcerated area promote healing; the use of stool softeners is necessary to prevent further discomfort. The child may avoid defecation to prevent discomfort; for this reason, parents should record bowel movements to keep track. Rectal temperatures and suppositories are always avoided because they may traumatize the area.

Neurologic Problems

Vincristine, and to a lesser extent vinblastine, can cause various neurotoxic effects. One of the more common neurotoxic effects is severe constipation caused by decreased bowel innervation. Administration of opioids can further aggravate constipation. The nurse advises parents to record bowel movements and to notify the practitioner of a change in stool habits. Physical activity and stool softeners are helpful in preventing the problem, but laxatives, such as polyethylene glycol, are often necessary to stimulate evacuation. Dietary changes such as increased fiber may not be effective because the increased bulk tends to increase fecal distention and discomfort without producing the necessary mechanical stimulation.

Footdrop and weakness and numbness of the extremities may cause difficulty in walking or fine hand movement. The nurse should observe for these problems and warn parents of these side effects, which are reversible once the drug is stopped. Wearing high-top tennis shoes or using a footboard in bed may help preserve proper alignment. If weakness occurs while the child is attending school, temporary alteration of activity may be necessary. Parents should inform the teacher of the situation to avoid unrealistic expectations of the child's abilities.

Another neurotoxic effect is severe jaw pain. Analgesics may help relieve the discomfort. Children may avoid movement by not talking or chewing, although continuous chewing, such as with gum, may actually help reduce the pain.

A neurologic syndrome, postirradiation somnolence, may develop 5 to 8 weeks after CNS irradiation and last for 4 to 15 days. It is characterized by somnolence with or without fever, anorexia, and nausea and vomiting. Parents should be warned of the possibility of such symptoms and be encouraged to seek medical evaluation because somnolence may be an early indicator of long-term neurologic sequelae after cranial irradiation.

Hemorrhagic Cystitis

Sterile hemorrhagic cystitis is a side effect of chemical irritation to the bladder from chemotherapy. It can be prevented by (1) a liberal oral or parenteral fluid intake (at least 1.5 times the recommended daily fluid requirement [2 L/m^2/day]); (2) frequent voiding immediately after feeling the urge, including immediately before bed, one nighttime void, and on arising; (3) administration of chemotherapy early in the day to allow for sufficient fluids and frequent voiding; and (4) administration of mesna, a drug that inhibits the urotoxicity of cyclophosphamide and ifosfamide (Freedman et al., 2016).

! NURSING ALERT

If signs of cystitis such as burning on urination occur, prompt medical evaluation is needed. Hemorrhagic cystitis warrants a full workup and timely intervention.

In most cases IV fluids are given before, during, and after the drug to ensure adequate hydration, thereby eliminating the need for the child to drink large amounts of fluid. If oral home administration is prescribed, the family needs specific instructions on exactly how much fluid the child must have.

Alopecia

Hair loss is a side effect of several chemotherapeutic drugs and cranial irradiation. Not all children lose their hair during chemotherapy, and some children may experience thinning of the hair rather than baldness. However, retaining hair is the exception rather than the rule. It is better to warn children and parents of this side effect to allow them some time to adapt to hair loss.

The family should know that the hair falls out in clumps, causing patchy baldness. To lessen the trauma of seeing large amounts of hair on bed linens or clothing, the child can wear a disposable surgical cap to collect the shed hair during the period of greatest hair loss, or the hair can be cut short or the head shaved. Families should also be aware that wigs are a tax deductible expense. Hair typically regrows in 3 to 6 months, and it is often a different color and texture than before cancer treatment.

NURSING TIP: Encouraging children to choose a wig similar to their own hairstyle and color before the hair falls out is helpful in fostering later adjustment to hair loss.

If the child chooses not to wear a wig, attention to some type of head covering is important, especially in cold or sunny climates. Scalp hygiene is also important. The scalp should be washed regularly as with any other body part.

Steroid Effects

Short-term steroid therapy produces physical changes and alterations in body image, which although not clinically significant, can be extremely distressing to older children. One of these is Cushingoid appearance. The child's face becomes rounded and puffy (see Fig. 28.2). Unlike hair loss, little can be done to camouflage this obvious change, although careful avoidance of salt and salt-containing foods can help reduce fluid accumulation. It is not unusual for other children to tease the child. It is helpful to reassure the child that, after the drug is stopped, the facial contours will return to normal. The use of loose-fitting clothes can help camouflage changes in weight.

The moon face, red cheeks, supraclavicular fat pads, protuberant abdomen, and fluid retention in children receiving steroid therapy indicate weight gain. However, the actual weight gain resulting from increased muscle mass and subcutaneous tissue may be small. Therefore the nurse should evaluate weight gain by observing the extremities and measuring skinfold thickness and arm circumference during steroid therapy to determine whether the weight gain is a result of increased dietary intake.

Shortly after beginning steroid therapy, children may experience mood changes, which range from feelings of well-being and euphoria to depression and irritability. If parents are unaware of these drug-induced changes, they may become unduly concerned. Therefore the nurse should warn them of the reactions and encourage them to discuss the behavioral changes with each other and the child.

NURSING CARE DURING HEMATOPOIETIC STEM CELL TRANSPLANTATION

Because of the aggressive preconditioning therapy used to remove the marrow and the potential for complications while waiting for engraftment of transplanted stem cells, children undergoing HSCT are usually hospitalized for several weeks. HSCT patients must have numerous procedures performed, such as the insertion of a venous access device, administration of intensive chemotherapy and irradiation, and strict infection precautions. During the period after transplantation and before the new marrow begins adequately replacing granulocytes, the child is extremely susceptible to infection, and any infection can be life threatening. In addition, many of the side effects previously discussed occur in the child undergoing HSCT.

The most common complication in allogeneic transplants is acute GVHD, which can affect the skin, gastrointestinal tract, and liver. The characteristics and severity of the manifestations vary according to the severity and area affected. Emphasis is now placed on the prevention of GVHD, using various agents such as a calcineurin inhibitor in conjunction with mycophenolate mofetil, methotrexate, or sirolimus (Gottschalk et al., 2016). Treatment involves the use of steroids or other immunosuppressive medications. However, this treatment further increases the risk of infection in the already susceptible patient. All blood products are irradiated to minimize the introduction of additional antigens.

Skin breakdown and delayed wound healing frequently occur in the patient undergoing HSCT. Preventive interventions to minimize pressure on dependent areas of the skin include the use of pressure-relieving or pressure-reducing beds or mattresses and frequent movement. Measures to promote healing when breakdown occurs include frequent sitz baths to the perianal area and protective skin barriers, such as hydrocolloid dressings or occlusive ointments.

Throughout this long ordeal the family is worried about successful engraftment and possible fatal complications. An unfortunate post-transplant possibility is recurrence of the disease after engraftment. Consequently, nurses need to provide sensitive care and maintain a supportive attitude during the many crises that may arise. If the procedure is not successful, the care needed by these families is consistent with that required by the family of any child with a life-threatening disorder (see Chapter 17).

PREPARATION FOR PROCEDURES

Children in particular need psychologic preparation for the various treatment interventions, which often involve surgery, IV injections, bone marrow aspirations, and LPs. The diagnostic procedures initially used to confirm the diagnosis and those that are repeated to monitor treatment can be a source of discomfort and stress to the child and family. Even noninvasive procedures such as imaging and radiologic tests are frightening to a young child and may be stressful at any age. Some of these tests require the child to lie motionless for a prolonged time in a confined space with little or no communication. Consequently, infants and young children are usually sedated, and older children need an explanation of what to expect and reminders during the test of how much longer they must remain still. The same principles for preparing children for procedures that are discussed in Chapter 20 apply here, including the option of having parents stay with the child whenever possible. Children who undergo repeated tests need additional preparation and emotional support to manage their stress.

Two procedures, bone marrow studies and LPs, are so commonly performed in many types of childhood cancer that they deserve special consideration (Fig. 25.2). Both tests can be frightening because they are done behind the child's field of vision. Professionals caring for children with cancer recommend the use of developmentally appropriate support using both pharmacologic and nonpharmacologic approaches and sedation if required (see Chapter 20).

Topical anesthetics such as eutectic mixture of local anesthetics (EMLA) and LMX4 creams are used as a local anesthetic before intrusive procedures, including venipunctures, implanted port access, LPs, and subcutaneous or intramuscular injections (Hockenberry et al., 2016). Local intradermal anesthesia with lidocaine is frequently used for LP and bone marrow examination. To reduce the stinging sensation from lidocaine, sodium bicarbonate should be added (see Chapter 5, Pain Management). Deeper infiltration of the muscle and periosteum of the bone with buffered lidocaine further reduces the

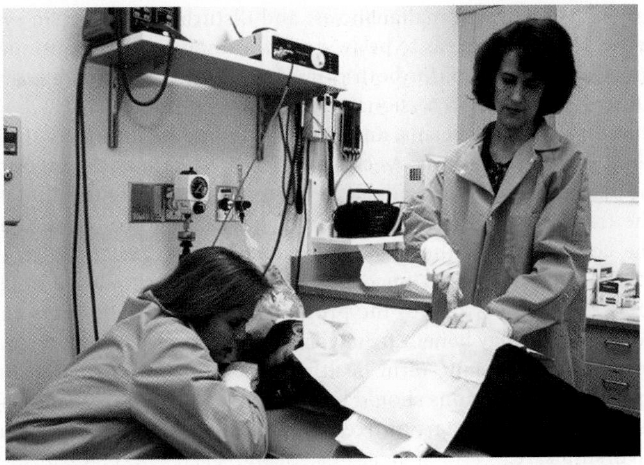

Fig. 25.2 Child with leukemia undergoing bone marrow aspiration.

pain from the large-bore aspiration or biopsy needle entering the bone.

For bone marrow studies, LPs, and other procedures, children of preschool age and older should be prepared beforehand. Physical care after the procedures is minimal. A small pressure bandage is applied to the bone marrow puncture site, and an adhesive bandage is applied to the LP site. No activity restriction is necessary after the bone marrow test, although the site is usually sore and the child may prefer to remain quiet. Recommendations after LP vary, and nurses should know their institutional practice. If medication was instilled, the child may be placed in a slight Trendelenburg position to facilitate circulation of the medicated spinal fluid.

PAIN MANAGEMENT

Nurses must be knowledgeable about the basic pathophysiology of cancer pain and treatment-related side effects. The World Health Organization's three-step analgesic pain ladder should be incorporated into the approach to pain management for every child with cancer (Ullrich, Sourkes, & Wolfe, 2016). Nurses must acquire extensive knowledge of nonopioid and opioid analgesics, as well as nonpharmacologic approaches used in pediatric pain management (see Chapter 5). Interdisciplinary pain management teams are used in many pediatric cancer centers. These teams serve as consultants and provide expertise in the assessment and management of pain. The nurse often serves as the coordinator of care, playing a key role in cancer pain management and implementing the pain team's plan of care.

Pharmacologic management of disease-related pain involves a variety of methods. It may take more than one trial of one type of medication to find the appropriate agent to manage a patient's pain. The route of administration must be considered as well. Providing "pain relief" by administering painful intramuscular injections as an alternative to the IV route is not appropriate therapy because many oral preparations are now available with comparable efficacy. Furthermore, children may refuse needed pain medication if it involves an injection. Nonsteroidal antiinflammatory drugs (NSAIDs), acetaminophen with codeine, oxycodone, and morphine are commonly used in the management of disease-related pain (Fielding, Sanford, & Davis, 2013). All are available in the oral form, and morphine and the NSAID ketorolac (Toradol) are available as IV preparations. Appropriate dosing is imperative. Doses are titrated to increase the amount of analgesia and minimize side effects. If opioids are prescribed, families will need guidance from the treatment team regarding pharmacy and regulatory practices enacted in the context of the opioid epidemic, such as barriers and restrictions to accessing adequate pain control (Page & Blanchard, 2019).

HEALTH PROMOTION

Children with cancer require the same basic health supervision as do any children. Sometimes the overwhelming needs and demands placed on the family, coupled with the singular concern focused on the cancer by both family and health care professionals, result in a lack of attention to typical health care needs. Nurses should monitor the type of primary care the child receives, using guidelines for recommended medical supervision (American Academy of Pediatrics, 2019). Areas of particular concern are (1) dental care because of potential side effects from treatment, and (2) immunizations because of concerns with live virus vaccines and immunosuppression.

Dental Care

Irradiation to the head and neck can cause a number of late complications (Landier, Armenian, Meadows, et al., 2016). Some are irreversible, such as facial asymmetry, but those affecting the teeth and gums (e.g., caries, periodontal disease) benefit from excellent oral hygiene, including regular use of systemic and topical fluoride and regular dental examinations and cleaning (see Chapter 12, Dental Health). Delayed or absent development of the permanent teeth can occur (Effinger, Migliorati, Hudson, et al., 2014). Depending on the child's age, this can be a source of acute psychologic distress, especially during early school-age years, when "losing a tooth" is a status symbol. Children need to be aware of this possibility and need help to explain the delay to peers.

Daily toothbrushing and flossing are encouraged in children with granulocyte counts in excess of $500/mm^3$ and platelet counts above $40,000/mm^3$. Fluoride rinses are used as discussed in Chapter 12. Oral hygiene for children whose counts are below these parameters is limited to wiping the teeth with moistened gauze sponges or Toothettes.

Immunizations and Communicable Disease Exposure

Viral replication after the administration of live vaccine for polio, measles, rubella, and mumps can cause serious disease in immunocompromised children. The child receiving chemotherapy for cancer should not receive live, attenuated vaccines. Inactivated vaccines can be given to immunosuppressed children. Siblings and other family members can receive the live measles, mumps, and rubella vaccine and the varicella vaccine without risk to the child who is immunosuppressed. Guidelines for immunization of children receiving chemotherapy and HSCT patients have been published (Ardura & Koh, 2016).

An important indication for isolation is an outbreak of childhood communicable disease, such as rubella and varicella. Ideally, the school nurse should work with the treating practitioner to decide the optimum time for school attendance. Parents should be taught to work with the school or daycare staff to be sure they understand the risk to the child being treated for cancer and that they notify the parents immediately of any exposure. If the child has been exposed to the varicella virus, varicella-zoster immune globulin given within 96 hours may favorably alter the course of the disease. Antiviral agents, such as acyclovir, should be given if the child develops varicella. Without treatment, death from disseminated varicella can occur due to disease in the liver, lung, and CNS (Ardura & Koh, 2016) (see also Chapter 6, Immunizations).

! NURSING ALERT

Children who were vaccinated 2 weeks before or during chemotherapy should be considered unimmunized and should be revaccinated or receive live virus vaccines 6 months after chemotherapy has stopped (American Academy of Pediatrics, 2018). Most institutions have individual guidelines regarding vaccinations in a child undergoing immunosuppressive therapy. The nurse should be aware of these guidelines and educate patients and families about the need for and timing of immunizations.

PATIENT AND FAMILY EDUCATION

Nurses working with children being treated for cancer have a significant role in helping the family understand the treatment plan, preventing or managing side effects, and transitioning to off-treatment and adult-focused health care. Little data to support evidence-based practices for patient and family education exist. Most children with cancer are enrolled in clinical trials through the Children's Oncology Group. The Children's Oncology Group Nursing Discipline has conducted several activities focusing on patient and family education during the new diagnosis period. They identified five broad principles with expert consensus recommendations: (1) patient and family education is family centered; (2) a diagnosis of childhood cancer is overwhelming, and the family needs time to process the diagnosis and develop a plan for managing ongoing life demands before they can successfully learn to care for the child; (3) patient and family education should be an interprofessional endeavor with three key areas of focus: (a) diagnosis and treatment, (b) psychosocial coping, and (c) care of the child; (4) patient and family education should occur across the continuum of care; and (5) a supportive environment is necessary to optimize learning (Landier, Ahern, Barakat, et al., 2016). According to the authors, "Dissemination and implementation of these recommendations will set the stage for future studies that aim to develop evidence to inform best practices, and ultimately to establish the standard of care for effective patient/family education in pediatric oncology" (Landier et al., 2016). In current practice, several excellent resources for teaching and learning are available. The National Cancer Institute (https://www.cancer.gov/) and the Children's Oncology Group (https://www.childrensoncologygroup.org/) websites are reliable sources of regularly updated information on childhood cancer research and care. The Association of Pediatric Hematology/Oncology Nurses[c] has developed a portfolio of educational materials for family education. The American Childhood Cancer Organization[d] is an international organization providing support, education, and advocacy programs for children with cancer and their families. Similarly, the Coalition Against Childhood Cancer (https://cac2.org/) is composed of numerous foundations that provide advocacy and resources focused on childhood cancer; it also hosts the HOPE Portal, an online guide to available information and support resources (https://cac2.org/family-resources/).

COMPLETION OF THERAPY

Care does not end when the child completes therapy. With the increasing awareness of late effects, nurses have an important role in the assessment of the child for problems such as delayed growth, subsequent malignancies, and disturbances in organ systems. The family needs to be aware of the importance of continued medical supervision, for both primary care and survivorship care. Other health care professionals caring for the child, such as school nurses, family physicians, and dentists, should be informed of the child's cancer diagnosis. As children reach young adulthood, transition services may be available in the treatment center to help ease the transfer of primary care to adult health care professionals in the community. If there is a survivorship program at the treating hospital or nearby, oncology follow-up care should be transferred there according to the program's criteria. Adolescents and young adults may benefit from genetic or genomic counseling that may affect their long-term health. If the possibility of infertility exists, fertility options should be discussed for pubertal males and females before the start of treatment and readdressed during survivorship care.

The Children's Oncology Group has developed guidelines for long-term follow-up care for pediatric cancer survivors.[e] Nurses involved with care of these children should be familiar with these guidelines and use all opportunities to help patients and families access needed survivorship and transition care.

CANCERS OF BLOOD AND LYMPH SYSTEMS

ACUTE LEUKEMIAS

Leukemia is a broad term given to a group of malignant diseases of the bone marrow, blood, and lymphatic system. In healthy children, the bone marrow makes blood stem cells that mature to become lymphoid or myeloid stem cells. Myeloid cells differentiate into red blood cells, platelets, and WBCs. Lymphoid stem cells become lymphoblasts that differentiate into B lymphocytes, T lymphocytes, and natural killer cells (National Institutes of Health, 2019c). In acute leukemias, immature cells that cannot function effectively predominate. Two types of leukemia are seen most often in children: acute lymphoblastic leukemia (ALL) and acute myeloid leukemia (AML).

ACUTE LYMPHOBLASTIC LEUKEMIA

Older synonyms for ALL include acute lymphatic, lymphocytic, and lymphoid leukemia. ALL is the most common form of childhood cancer, with an annual incidence of approximately 4900 new cases annually in the United States (Rabin, Gramatges, Margolin, et al., 2016). It occurs more often in boys than in girls, and it is 20% more common in Hispanics than non-Hispanic whites; it is more common in whites than in African Americans (Rabin et al., 2016; Wiemels, Walsh, deSmith, et al., 2018). The peak age of onset is between 2 and 3 years old. Risk factors for ALL include prenatal exposure to x-rays, previous treatment with chemotherapy, and certain genetic conditions (e.g., Down syndrome, Bloom syndrome, Fanconi anemia, Li-Fraumeni syndrome) (National Institutes of Health, 2019c). Genetic predisposition also includes a number of germline polymorphisms (genetic variations) in common alleles found by GWAS, as well as rare germline variants (e.g., *PAX5*, *ETV6*, *TP53*). There is evidence to suggest that some ALL begins prenatally.

---

[c]8735 W. Higgins Road, Suite 300, Chicago, IL 60631; 847-375-4724; fax: 847-375-6478; http://www.aphon.org.

[d]PO Box 498, Kensington, MD 20895; 855-858-2226 or 301-962-3520; fax: 301-962-3521; http://www.acco.org.

[e]Long-Term Follow-up Guidelines for Survivors of Childhood, Adolescent, and Young Adult Cancers (Version 5.0). Retrieved from http://www.survivorshipguidelines.org/.

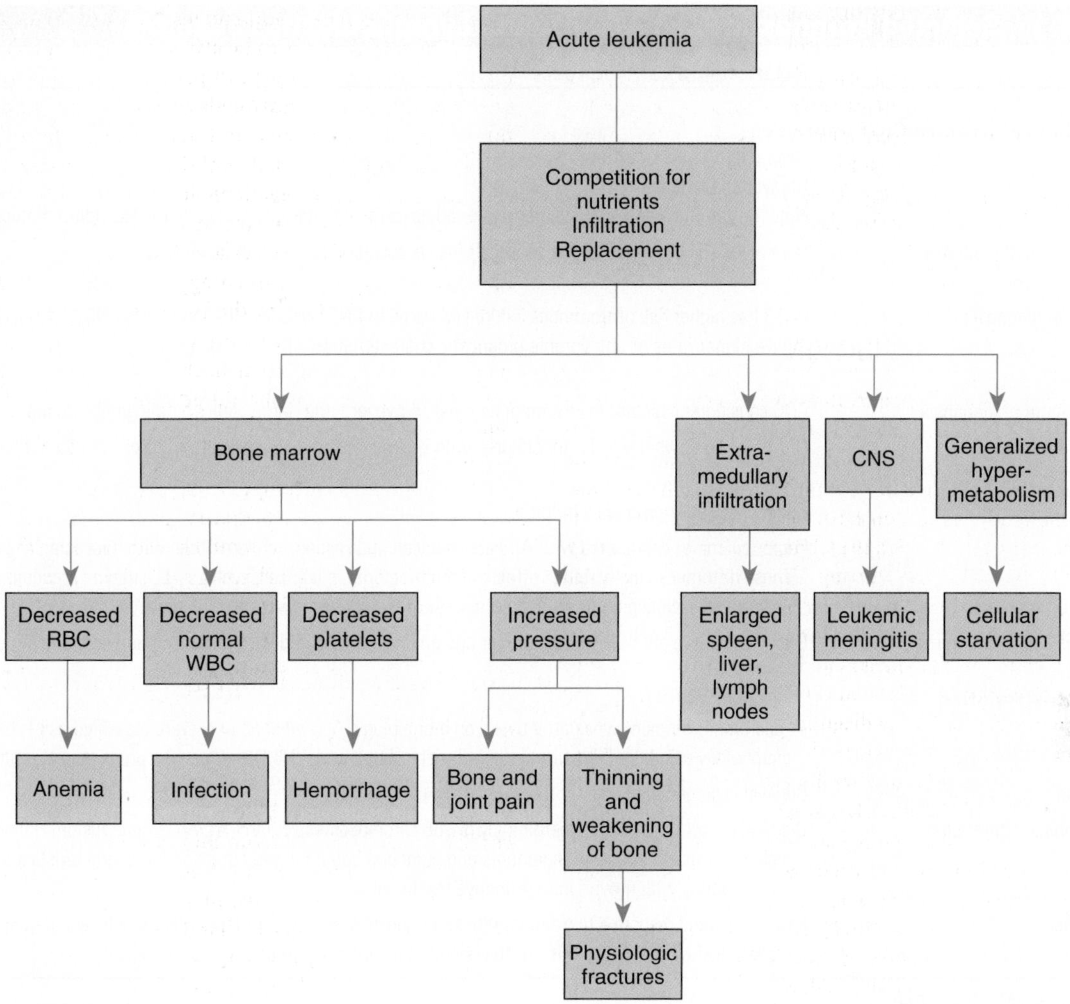

Fig. 25.3 Principal sites of tissue involvement in leukemia. *CNS,* Central nervous system; *RBC,* red blood cell; *WBC,* white blood cell.

Clinical Manifestations

The onset of leukemia varies from acute to insidious. In most instances the child displays remarkably few symptoms. For example, leukemia may be diagnosed when a minor infection, such as a cold, fails to disappear completely. The child continues to be pale, listless, irritable, febrile, and anorexic. Parents often suspect some underlying problem when they observe the child's weight loss, petechiae, bruising without cause, and continued complaints of bone and joint pain. At other times there may be an extended history of signs and symptoms mimicking such conditions as rheumatoid arthritis or mononucleosis. Sometimes leukemia is an incidental finding on a routine physical examination or during treatment for an injury. Fig. 25.3 displays the sites for tissue involvement in leukemia.

Signs and symptoms of ALL reflect infiltration of the bone marrow by nonfunctional leukemic cells ("blasts"). The three main consequences of bone marrow infiltration are (1) anemia from decreased erythrocytes, (2) infection from neutropenia, and (3) bleeding from decreased platelet production. Approximately half of patients have an elevated WBC count at presentation (>10,000/mm^3). Other signs and symptoms indicate leukemic cell infiltration of various organs; highly vascular organs, such as the spleen and liver, are most severely affected. Commonly seen are hepatosplenomegaly (68% of patients), splenomegaly (63%), fever (61%), lymphadenopathy (50%), bleeding (e.g., petechiae or purpura, 48%), and bone pain (23%) (Rabin et al., 2016).

Two important sites of extramedullary (outside the bone marrow) disease are the CNS and testes because they can serve as "sanctuaries" for leukemic cells; these sites require specific therapy.

Diagnostic Evaluation

Leukemia is usually suspected from the history, physical manifestations, and a peripheral blood smear that contains leukemic blasts, frequently in combination with low blood counts. The diagnostic evaluation includes a thorough history and physical examination, laboratory tests (CBC with differential, blood chemistries), and bone marrow aspiration or biopsy (cytogenetic analysis, immunophenotyping). A chest x-ray may be performed to determine whether there is a mass of leukemic cells in the chest. Definitive diagnosis is based on analysis of the bone marrow sample. Typically the bone marrow of a child with ALL shows a monotonous infiltrate of blast cells. Once the diagnosis is confirmed, an LP is performed to determine whether there is any CNS involvement. Only a small number of children have CNS involvement at diagnosis, and they are usually asymptomatic.

Clinical Staging and Prognosis

In the past, the standard ways to classify ALL were with the French-American-British (FAB) morphologic system and cytochemical stains. Now the standard accepted method is immunophenotyping, in which panels of monoclonal antibodies are used to determine

TABLE 25.3 Selected Prognostic Factors for Acute Lymphoblastic Leukemia

Factor	Relationship to Prognosis
Patient and Clinical Disease Characteristics	
Age at diagnosis	Favorable: >1 year or ≤10 years. Unfavorable: infants Note: Better outcomes are documented for adolescents when treated on pediatric (vs. adult) protocols.
White blood cell count at diagnosis	Favorable: ≤50,000/mm³ (precursor B-cell ALL; association not seen in T-cell ALL).
CNS involvement at diagnosis	CNS3 has higher risk of treatment failure compared to CNS1 or CNS2. Patients with CNS2, CNS3, or traumatic LP have higher rates of unfavorable prognostic characteristics.
Testicular involvement at diagnosis	COG considers testicular involvement high risk; however, other large clinical trials groups do not.
Down syndrome (trisomy 21)	Outcomes somewhat inferior for children with Down syndrome compared to children who do not have Down syndrome.
Sex	Somewhat better prognosis for girls.
Race and ethnicity	Poorer outcomes associated with African American and Hispanic children than with Caucasian and Asian children. These differences likely reflect effects of multifactorial influences, such as ALL subtype predominance, treatment adherence, socioeconomic status, access to care, and ancestry-related genomic variations.
Weight at diagnosis and during treatment	Both obesity (weight >95th percentile for age and height) and underweight have been studied with variable results.
Leukemic Characteristics	
Morphology	At one time, treatment was partly based on morphology. ALL lymphoblasts were classified as L1, L2, or L3 morphology using the French-American-British (FAB) criteria. No longer used in prognostic classification.
Immunophenotype	Survival is somewhat better in B-cell ALL than in T-cell ALL.
Cytogenetics/genomic alterations	B-cell ALL: Favorable: high hyperdiploidy (51-65 chromosomes); *ETV6-RUNX1* gene fusion. Unfavorable: includes various gene rearrangements and numbers. Some formerly unfavorable characteristics are losing their unfavorability with newer, more effective treatment.
Treatment response	Favorable: rapid response to treatment (best prognosis associated with undetectable levels of minimal residual disease (MRD) or at least $<10^{-4}$ at the end of standard induction).

ALL, Acute lymphoblastic leukemia.
Adapted from Rabin, K. R., Gramatges, M. M., Margolin, J. F., & Poplack, D. G. (2016). Acute lymphoblastic leukemia. In P. A. Pizzo & D. G. Poplack (Eds.), *Principles and practice of pediatric oncology* (7th ed.). Philadelphia, PA: Lippincott; National Institutes of Health, National Cancer Institute. (2017). Childhood acute lymphoblastic leukemia treatment. Retrieved from https://www.cancer.gov/types/leukemia/hp/child-all-treatment-pdq.

T-lineage, B-lineage, and myeloid antigens (Rabin et al., 2016). In addition, chromosomal number (ploidy) and structural rearrangements are evaluated using molecular genetic analyses. In 2016 the World Health Organization revised the classification of ALL into B-lymphoblastic leukemia subgroups characterized by specific chromosomal abnormalities, T-lymphoblastic leukemia, and acute leukemias of ambiguous lineage (having characteristics of both ALL and AML).

The most important prognostic factors in determining assignment to risk-based treatment for children with ALL (Table 25.3) include the child's age and WBC count at diagnosis, CNS involvement as indicated by cerebrospinal fluid sample (CNS1 = negative for blasts; CNS2 = fewer than 5 WBC/μL and positive for blasts; CNS3 = 5 or more WBC/μL and positive for blasts), testicular involvement, Down syndrome, sex, race and ethnicity, and nutritional status; leukemic cell characteristics, including immunophenotype and cytogenetics or genomic alterations such as ploidy and structural rearrangements; response to initial treatment; and minimal residual disease (MRD) determination (National Institutes of Health, 2019c).

Therapeutic Management

ALL has demonstrated dramatic improvements in survival rates such that current long-term disease-free survival rates for children with ALL approach 90% in major pediatric cancer treatment centers. Treatment is based on assignment to risk groups. Children with a higher risk of relapse or recurrence are treated with the most intensive therapy. Different research groups have similar but varying criteria for risk groups. Children's Oncology Group risk groups include age, WBC count at diagnosis, immunophenotype, cytogenetics or genomic alterations, presence of extramedullary disease, Down syndrome, and steroid pretreatment. With advances in treatment, refinement of risk groups is constantly under study.

Although specifics for various risk groups vary, treatment is generally divided into three phases: remission induction, consolidation/intensification, and maintenance (also called continuation). Four types of standard treatment are used: chemotherapy, radiation therapy, chemotherapy with stem cell transplant, and targeted therapy. Targeted therapy includes tyrosine kinase inhibitors (TKIs), monoclonal antibodies, and proteasome inhibitor therapy.

Almost immediately after confirmation of the diagnosis, induction therapy begins and lasts for 4 to 5 weeks (Rabin et al., 2016). The principal drugs are the corticosteroids (dexamethasone or prednisone), vincristine, and L-asparaginase or PEG-asparaginase, with or without an anthracycline. A complete remission (CR) is determined by the presence of less than 5% blast cells in the bone marrow and no detectable leukemia in extramedullary sites.

Because many of the drugs also cause myelosuppression of normal blood elements, the period immediately after a remission can be critical. The body is defenseless against invading organisms (especially normal bacterial flora) and susceptible to spontaneous hemorrhage. Consequently, supportive therapy during this time is essential. Supportive care consists of transfusion support and use of antibacterial and antifungal agents.

With achievement of CR, systemic treatment plus CNS-directed therapy begins. CNS-directed therapy is based on the understanding that leukemic cells could be present in the CNS where they are protected from many systemic chemotherapy drugs by the blood-brain barrier. For this reason, all children receive CNS prophylactic therapy. The combination of intrathecal chemotherapy (either methotrexate alone or in combination with cytarabine and hydrocortisone) plus CNS-directed systemic chemotherapy (dexamethasone, L-asparaginase, and high-dose methotrexate with leucovorin rescue) is standard; cranial radiation may be used for children at highest risk for CNS relapse (National Institutes of Health, 2019c).

Past clinical trials have shown that postinduction therapy is needed to maintain remission. Treatment regimens vary, but all patients receive consolidation/intensification after achieving CR. Most commonly used is the Berlin-Frankfurt-Münster (BFM) "backbone" (a very intensive chemotherapy regimen from the International BFM Study Group that greatly increases ALL survival). This backbone includes consolidation with cyclophosphamide, cytarabine, and mercaptopurine given initially, followed by interim maintenance with high-dose methotrexate with or without leucovorin rescue. Next, delayed intensification is given using drugs and schedules similar to those used in the induction and consolidation phases.

This is followed by maintenance therapy with daily mercaptopurine and weekly low-dose methotrexate; vincristine and a corticosteroid may be given, as well as continued intrathecal therapy (National Institutes of Health, 2019c; Rabin et al., 2016). A critical challenge during maintenance therapy is medication adherence because it has been shown that anything less than 95% adherence increases the risk of relapse (Bhatia, Landier, Shangguan, et al., 2012).

Nursing Care

Nursing care of the child with acute leukemia is directly related to the regimen of therapy. Myelosuppression, drug toxicity, and leukemic infiltration cause secondary complications that necessitate supportive physical care. This discussion focuses on supportive interventions for the child with leukemia and the family. General aspects of care appropriate for the child with leukemia are discussed earlier under General Nursing Care Management.

Prepare the Family for Diagnostic and Therapeutic Procedures

From the time before diagnosis to cessation of therapy, children must undergo several tests, the most traumatic of which are bone marrow aspiration or biopsy and LP. Finger sticks and venipunctures for blood analysis and drug infusion are common occurrences for several years after the diagnosis. Therefore children need an explanation of the rationale for each procedure, what can be expected, and what they can do to help (see Chapter 20, Preparation for Diagnostic and Therapeutic Procedures).

Depending on the child's age, one way of beginning diagnostic preparation is to explain the tests, procedures, and treatment plan. Using a drawing or letting the child look at a drop of blood under a microscope not only teaches but also fosters trust between the nurse and the child. It also allows the nurse to assess the child's level of understanding. An error many health professionals make is to overestimate children's knowledge about their bodies. For example, a bone marrow aspiration makes sense only when it is clarified that the center of a bone contains the cells that later become "working" blood cells or leukemic cells.

Provide Continued Emotional Support

Nursing care of the child with leukemia is based on typical problems the family confronts during the treatment phases and afterwards. Therefore the nurse's role is one of continual support, guidance, clarification, and clinical judgment. Parents need to know how to recognize symptoms that demand medical attention. Although some of the reactions discussed are expected, parents should still report them to their practitioner. Warning parents of their possible occurrence beforehand also allows parents to prepare themselves. At the same time, it reassures them that these reactions are not caused by a return of leukemic cells.

The nurse must also use judgment in recognizing which side effects are typical reactions and which indicate toxicity. Frequently it is the office or clinic nurse who screens such telephone calls and gives advice, when appropriate. Usually nausea and vomiting are not indications for drug cessation. However, severe vomiting or diarrhea may require immediate intervention to prevent dehydration. Signs of infection, mucosal ulceration, hemorrhagic cystitis, peripheral neuropathy, and constipation require medical evaluation.

Another aspect of continued emotional support involves prognosis. Leukemia is not invariably fatal, but present statistics must be interpreted correctly. Although almost 80% of children with ALL live for 5 years or longer, these are average estimates that apply to those children treated with the most successful protocols since diagnosis. For the high-risk child with ALL or the child with AML, the prognosis may be significantly poorer. Of those who do survive after completing therapy, some will experience recurrence of the leukemia.

LYMPHOMAS

The lymphomas, a group of malignant diseases that arise from the lymphoid and hematopoietic systems, are divided into Hodgkin lymphoma (HL) and NHL. These diseases are further subdivided according to tissue type and extent of disease. In children, NHL is more common than HL.

Hodgkin Lymphoma

Hodgkin lymphoma affects about 29 in 1 million children (National Institutes of Health, 2019e). Its incidence is age related. In the United States there is a striking increased incidence in adolescents 15 to 19 years of age. The Epstein-Barr virus (EBV) is thought to have a role in the causation of HL. Age cohorts vary in the predominant HL subtypes and in the association with EBV. The risk of HL is increased among individuals with immunodeficiency and those with a history of HL among immediate family members. Exposure to infections in early childhood may decrease HL risk (National Institutes of Health, 2019e).

Hodgkin lymphoma originates in the lymphoid system and primarily involves the lymph nodes. It predictably metastasizes to nonnodal or extralymphatic sites, especially the spleen, liver, bone marrow, lungs, and mediastinum (i.e., mass of tissues and organs separating the lungs, including the heart and its vessels, trachea, esophagus, thymus, and lymph nodes), although no tissue is exempt from involvement (Fig. 25.4).

Clinical Staging and Prognosis

Accurate clinical staging of the extent of disease is essential for assignment to treatment protocols based on expected prognosis. The four stages in the Ann Arbor Staging Classification are shown in Box 25.2.

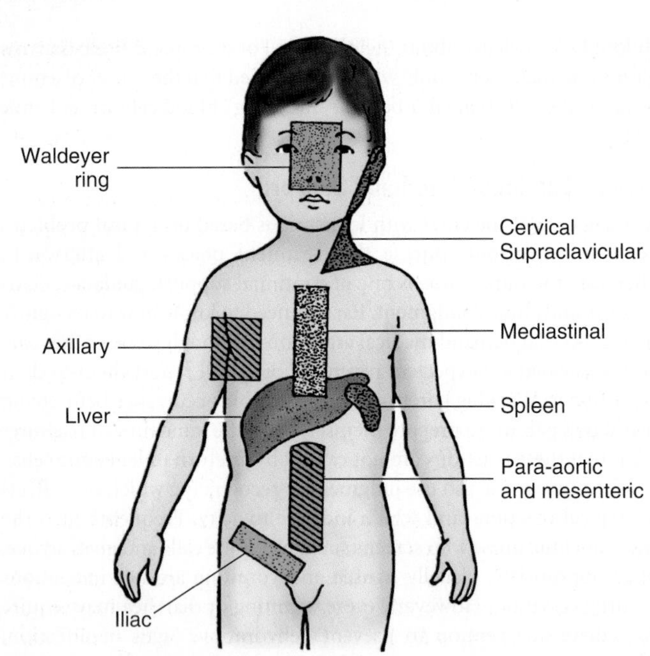

Fig. 25.4 Main areas of lymphadenopathy and organ involvement in Hodgkin disease.

BOX 25.2 Ann Arbor Staging of Hodgkin Disease

Stage I: Lesions are limited to one lymph node area or only one additional extralymphatic site (I_E), such as the liver, lungs, kidney, or intestines.
Stage II: Two or more lymph node regions on the same side of the diaphragm or one additional extralymphatic site or organ (II_E) on the same side of the diaphragm is involved.
Stage III: Lymph node regions on both sides of the diaphragm are involved with spread to one extralymphatic site (III_E), spleen (III_S), or both (III_{SE}).
Stage IV: Diffuse spread throughout the body to one or more extralymphatic sites with or without involvement of associated lymph nodes.

Each stage is further subdivided into A, B, E, or S. Stage A denotes absence of symptoms. Stage B indicates presence of symptoms, such as drenching night sweats, fever (100.4°F [38°C]), or weight loss of 10% or more during the preceding 6 months. Stage E represents involvement of a single extranodal site contiguous or proximal to the known nodal site. Stage S indicates splenic involvement.

The prognosis for patients with HL has improved dramatically, largely as a result of systematic staging, risk group stratification, and improved treatment protocols. The prognosis is excellent in children with localized disease. Overall survival rates for patients with HL are as high as 95%; however, survival rates vary with tumor histology and staging (Frew, Lewis, & Lucraft, 2013). Even in those with disseminated disease, long-term remissions are possible in more than half of patients. For relapses, CR may occur in 30% to 60% of patients undergoing autologous HSCT (Metzger, Krasin, Choi, et al., 2016).

Clinical Manifestations

Hodgkin lymphoma is characterized by painless enlargement of lymph nodes. The most common finding is enlarged, firm, nontender, movable nodes in the supraclavicular or cervical area. Other signs and symptoms depend on the extent and location of involvement. Mediastinal lymphadenopathy may cause a persistent, nonproductive cough. Enlarged retroperitoneal nodes may produce otherwise unexplained abdominal pain. Systemic symptoms include low-grade or intermittent fever, anorexia, nausea, weight loss, night sweats, and pruritus. Generally, such symptoms indicate advanced lymph node and extralymphatic involvement.

Diagnostic Evaluation

The history and physical examination often yield important clues to the disease, such as a history of systemic symptoms, presence of a mediastinal mass, and enlargement of lymph nodes, spleen, or liver. Enlarged nodes should be measured as baseline for later evaluation of treatment response. Because multiple organs can become involved, the diagnostic evaluation requires several tests to confirm the diagnosis and assess the extent of involvement for accurate staging. Laboratory tests include CBC and chemistry panel with albumin, erythrocyte sedimentation rate, and C-reactive protein. Imaging tests include chest x-ray; anatomic imaging with CT or MRI of neck, chest, abdomen, and pelvis; and functional imaging with PET scan (National Institutes of Health, 2019e).

Biopsy of one or more peripheral lymph nodes is used to establish histologic diagnosis. The presence of Hodgkin and Reed-Sternberg cells is considered diagnostic of Hodgkin disease because it is absent in the other lymphomas; however, it may occur in infectious mononucleosis. Hodgkin lymphoma is classified into one of four histologic types: (1) lymphocytic-rich HL, (2) nodular sclerosing HL, (3) mixed cellularity HL, and (4) lymphocytic-depleted HL. For some patients, the histologic subtype may determine therapy. A bone marrow aspiration or biopsy also may be performed.

Therapeutic Management

The primary treatment modalities for HL are chemotherapy and radiation. The length and intensity of therapy are based on disease-related factors (e.g., stage, number of involved nodal regions, tumor bulk, B symptoms, and early response); other factors that may be considered are age, sex, and histology (National Institutes of Health, 2019e). For treatment planning, patients are classified into favorable and unfavorable risk groups, indicating their risk of relapse or lack of response to treatment. Favorable clinical features include localized nodal involvement and no B symptoms or bulky disease. Unfavorable features include presence of B symptoms, bulky lymphadenopathy, extranodal extension, and advanced disease (stages IIIB to IV). Other features may be included in risk stratification (e.g., presence of a pleural effusion), depending on the treatment group or protocol.

The goal of treatment is cure; however, aggressive therapy increases the chances of complications that can seriously compromise quality of life. One of the major concerns with combined radiation and chemotherapy is the risk of serious late effects in children with an excellent prognosis. Consequently, treatment that is risk adapted and response based aims to minimize long-term complications. Because of the diversity of approaches to treatment, the following is an overview of general principles that may not apply to all children.

Most newly diagnosed children are treated with risk-adapted chemotherapy alone or in combination with radiation therapy. Radiation may entail involved field radiation or extended field radiation (involved areas plus adjacent nodes) depending on the extent of involvement. Combination chemotherapy, abbreviated as ABVE-PC, is used: doxorubicin (Adriamycin), bleomycin, vincristine (Oncovin), etoposide, prednisone, and cyclophosphamide. Monoclonal antibodies and other new agents/approaches are being studied in clinical trials for refractory/relapsed HL.

Nursing Care Management

Nursing care involves preparation for diagnostic and operative procedures, explanation of treatment side effects, and child and family support. When HL is suspected, a battery of diagnostic tests is ordered. The family and child need an explanation of why each test is performed because many of them, such as bone marrow aspiration and lymph node biopsy, are invasive procedures (see Chapter 20).

Explanations of chemotherapeutic reactions are based on the specific drug regimen. The most common side effects, such as nausea and vomiting, body image changes, neuropathy, and mucosal ulceration, are discussed in the General Nursing Care Management section. Involved-field radiation results in few side effects, sometimes consisting only of a mild skin reaction. With extended-field radiation to the chest and abdomen, nausea and vomiting, weight loss, and mucosal ulceration (esophagitis, gastric ulcers) are common. The usual measures for providing relief are discussed earlier in the chapter and outlined in Table 25.2.

The most common side effect of extensive irradiation is fatigue, which may result from damage to the thyroid gland, causing hypothyroidism. Lack of energy is particularly difficult for adolescents because it prevents them from keeping up with their peers. Sometimes adolescents push themselves to the point of physical exhaustion rather than admit fatigue and give in to their decreased activity tolerance. Parents should observe for such behavior, such as extreme fatigue at the end of the day, falling asleep at the dinner table, inability to concentrate on homework, or an increased susceptibility to infection. Regular bedtimes and periodic rest times are important, especially during chemotherapy, when myelosuppression increases the risk of infection and debilitation. Before discharge (if the child has been hospitalized), the nurse should discuss a feasible school schedule with the parents and child; home schooling or tutoring may be an option. If alterations are necessary, such as elimination of strenuous physical education, they are discussed with the teacher, school nurse, and principal. If a central venous access device is in place, no gym or contact sports are permitted. Follow-up care is essential to diagnose hypothyroidism early and institute thyroid replacement.

An area of concern for adolescents is the risk of infertility from irradiation and chemotherapy. Both irradiation to the gonads and drugs, particularly procarbazine and alkylating agents, may lead to infertility. Younger females with a greater complement of oocytes are more likely to retain ovarian function. Adolescents should be informed of these side effects and offered options for fertility preservation early in the course of diagnosis and treatment. Although sexual function is not altered, the appearance of secondary sexual characteristics and menstruation may be delayed in the pubescent child. Delayed sexual maturation may be an extremely sensitive and painful area for children (see Chapter 16).

Non-Hodgkin Lymphoma

Approximately 800 new cases of NHL are diagnosed each year in the United States, with an incidence of 10 children per 1 million under the age of 20 years (Allen, Kamdar, Bollard, et al., 2016). Risk factors include infection with EBV, inherited or acquired immunodeficiency, DNA repair syndromes (e.g., ataxia-telangiectasia), and previous cancer (National Institutes of Health, 2019f).

Staging and Prognosis

NHL exhibits various morphologic, cytochemical, and immunologic features. The World Health Organization's histopathologic classification is based on immunophenotype, molecular biology, and clinical response to treatment. Most cases are categorized into one of three groups: mature B-cell NHL (including Burkitt lymphoma), lymphoblastic lymphoma, and anaplastic large cell lymphoma (National Institutes of Health, 2019f).

BOX 25.3 St. Jude Staging of Non-Hodgkin Lymphoma

Stage I: Disease limited to one lymph node area or only one additional extralymphatic site (excluding thoracic or abdomen).

Stage II: Single tumor with regional lymph node involvement; two or more lymph node regions on the same side of the diaphragm; two single tumors with or without regional involvement on the same side of the diaphragm; or primary resectable gastrointestinal tumor with or without involvement of adjacent mesenteric nodes.

Stage III: Two single tumors on opposite sides of the diaphragm; two nodal areas above or below the diaphragm; primary intrathoracic tumor or extensive intra-abdominal disease; or paraspinal or epidural tumors.

Stage IV: Tumor has spread into central nervous system and/or bone marrow

Prognostic staging is shown in Box 25.3. The St. Jude Children's Research Hospital Murphy Staging System is widely used for childhood NHL. A favorable prognosis is defined by young age, low stage without mediastinal involvement, low tumor burden, and good response to initial therapy (Allen et al., 2016). The use of aggressive combination chemotherapy has had a major impact on NHL survival rates in children. The most effective treatment regimens result in cure in 85% to 95% of children with limited disease involvement, and 70% to 90% of children with extensive disease are cured (Allen et al., 2016).

Clinical Manifestations

Many of the signs and symptoms seen in HL may be present in NHL, although it is rare for a single symptom to lead to the diagnosis. Rather, metastasis to the bone marrow or CNS may produce signs and symptoms typical of leukemia. Lymphoid tumors compressing various organs may cause intestinal or airway obstruction, cranial nerve palsies, or spinal paralysis. A large mediastinal mass and tumor lysis syndrome are medical emergencies requiring urgent attention because they may be life threatening.

The exception to the usual presentation of NHL is Burkitt lymphoma, a type of cancer that is rare in the United States but endemic in parts of Africa. It is a rapidly growing neoplasm that is most commonly seen as a mass in the jaw, abdomen, or orbit. However, no anatomic site appears exempt from involvement. Peripheral lymphadenopathy, hepatosplenomegaly, or signs of conversion to leukemia are rarely seen.

Diagnostic Evaluation

Current recommendations for diagnostic evaluation and staging include history and physical examination; blood chemistries; total body imaging (CT, PET, MRI); LP; bone marrow aspiration; and biopsy. Cancer cells are examined by immunophenotyping (immunohistochemistry, flow cytometry), cytogenetics, and/or FISH (National Institutes of Health, 2019f).

Therapeutic Management

Because NHL is generally considered to be widespread at diagnosis, most children are treated with combination chemotherapy. The role of radiation is limited, although it may be used in emergency situations at diagnosis, such as deviated trachea with impingement on the airway with associated respiratory compromise (National Institutes of Health, 2019f).

Treatment for NHL is based on histologic subtype. Lymphoblastic lymphoma therapy is similar to leukemia therapy; the protocols include induction, consolidation, and maintenance phases, some with intrathecal chemotherapy with or without cranial-spinal radiation therapy. The most commonly used chemotherapy regimens for

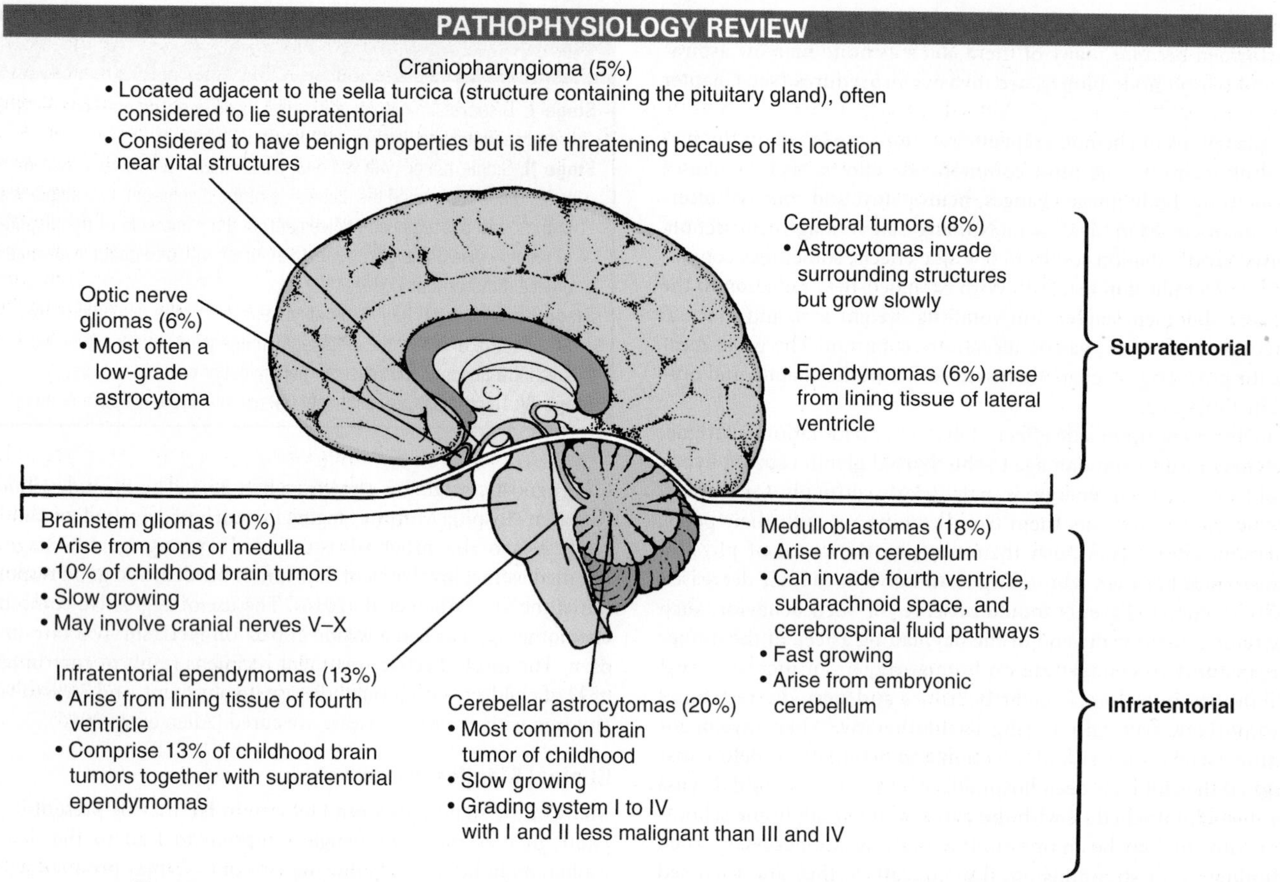

Fig. 25.5 Location of brain tumors in children. (From McCance KL, Huether SE. [2014]. *Pathophysiology: The biological basis for disease in adults and children* [7th ed.]. St. Louis, MO: Elsevier.)

newly diagnosed lymphoblastic lymphoma include prednisone, dexamethasone, vincristine, daunorubicin, doxorubicin, L-asparaginase, cyclophosphamide, cytarabine, methotrexate, 6-mercaptopurine, 6-thioguanine, and intrathecal treatments during maintenance. Newly diagnosed children with diffuse mature B-cell lymphoma are treated with surgery (stage I and II only) and chemotherapy with or without a monoclonal antibody; those with lymphoblastic lymphoma receive chemotherapy (plus cranial radiation for overt CNS disease); and patients with anaplastic large cell lymphoma are treated with surgery (stage I) and chemotherapy. These multiagent regimens are administered for 6 to 24 months.

Nursing Care Management

Nursing care of the child with NHL is similar to the care discussed under General Nursing Care Management. With intensive chemotherapy, nursing care is primarily directed toward managing the side effects of these agents.

NERVOUS SYSTEM TUMORS

BRAIN TUMORS

Primary tumors of the CNS, when grouped together, are the most common solid tumor in children and account for about 25% of all childhood cancers, with an annual incidence of 5 per 100,000 children younger than 20 years of age in the United States (Crawford, 2013). Brain tumors may be benign or malignant, although what matters the most is location, given the vital functions the brain controls. About 60% of the tumors are **infratentorial** (below the tentorium cerebelli), which means they occur in the posterior part of the brain, primarily in the cerebellum or brainstem. This anatomic distribution accounts for the frequency of symptoms resulting from increased intracranial pressure (ICP). The other tumors are **supratentorial** or lie within the midbrain structures. Fig. 25.5 shows the major brain tumors of childhood.

Because brain tumors can arise from any cell within the cranium, it is possible to have tumors originating from the glial cells, nerve cells, neuroepithelium, cranial nerves, blood vessels, pineal gland, and pituitary. Within each of these structures, specific cells may be involved that provide a histologic classification. For example, astrocytes, cells that form most of the supportive tissue for the neurons, may form astrocytomas, the most common glial tumor. Germline mutations are being increasingly recognized as cancer predisposing in childhood brain tumors (up to 8%); examples include Li-Fraumeni syndrome and neurofibromatosis. Other known risk factors include cranial irradiation and immunosuppression (Parsons, Pollack, Hass-Kogan, et al., 2016). Molecular or genomic studies of brain tumors are an active area of research and are changing traditional concepts of histology-based risk classification.

Clinical Manifestations

The signs and symptoms of brain tumors are directly related to their anatomic location, tumor size, rate of tumor growth, and the child's chronological and developmental age. For instance, in infants whose sutures are still open, a bulging fontanel indicates hydrocephalus. Head circumference measurements allow for detection of increased head size. Even in older children, clinical manifestations may be nonspecific.

However, the most common symptoms of infratentorial brain tumors are headache, especially on awakening, and vomiting that is not related to feeding. Tumors in this area of the brain often obstruct the flow of cerebrospinal fluid, causing increased ICP and the symptoms mentioned earlier. In addition, patients may have symptoms related to the specific structure involved. Tumors of the cerebellum often cause nystagmus, ataxia, dysarthria, and dysmetria. Supratentorial tumor symptoms more commonly include seizures, personality or behavioral changes, visual disturbances, and hemiparesis. Tumors involving the structures of the midbrain, including the hypothalamus and pituitary gland, may cause endocrinopathies such as diabetes insipidus, delayed or precocious puberty, and growth failure. Table 25.4 shows common presenting symptoms of brain tumors.

Diagnostic Evaluation

Diagnosis of a brain tumor is initially based on presenting clinical signs and diagnostic imaging. Because the signs and symptoms may be vague and easily overlooked, early diagnosis requires a high index of suspicion during history taking. A number of tests may be used in the neurologic evaluation, but the gold standard diagnostic procedure is MRI, which permits early diagnosis of brain tumors and assessment of tumor growth during or after treatment. Diffusion-weighted imaging, spectroscopy, and perfusion imaging are other MRI tools used to investigate and diagnose tumor types (Poussaint, Panigrahy, & Huisman, 2015). The CT scan permits direct visualization of the brain parenchyma, ventricles, and surrounding subarachnoid space, and it is commonly used in urgent cases of suspected tumors when MRI is not available. Other tests may include an MRI of the spine and electroencephalography. In the presence of increased ICP, LP is avoided due to the danger of possible brainstem herniation after sudden release of pressure.

Definitive diagnosis is based on tissue specimens obtained during surgery. Classification of pediatric brain tumors is evolving, and it is important that the diagnostic tissue be examined by a neuropathologist with special expertise in this area (National Institutes of Health, 2019g). Occasionally, special techniques are required for determining the cell type. The location of some brain tumors, such as brainstem tumors, may mean biopsy is avoided and the diagnosis is made by imaging findings alone; however, this is changing with recognition that postoperative complications of biopsy are mostly transient.

Therapeutic Management

Treatment depends on the type of brain tumor and may involve the use of surgery, radiation therapy, and chemotherapy (as well as targeted therapy). All three may or may not be used, depending on the type of tumor. The treatment of choice is total removal of the tumor without residual neurologic damage. Patients with the most complete tumor removal have the greatest chance of survival. Several surgical advances have allowed the biopsy and removal of tumors in areas previously considered too dangerous for traditional operative techniques. Stereotactic surgery involves the use of CT and MRI in conjunction with other special computer techniques to reconstruct the tumor in three dimensions. With computer-assisted instruments, total resection of the tumor is sometimes possible. Stereotactic biopsy is performed with CT or MRI computer guidance for inserting the biopsy needle. This procedure has the benefit of a shorter hospital stay and a lower morbidity and mortality rate in comparison with an open craniotomy (Parsons et al., 2016). Other procedures include the use of lasers to vaporize tumor tissue and brain mapping to determine the precise location of critical brain areas to avoid during surgery.

Radiation therapy is used to treat most tumors and to shrink the size of the tumor before attempting surgical removal. The use of chemotherapy has had an increasingly important role, either in combination with surgery and/or radiation or alone. All three modes of therapy are associated with serious late effects. Surgery can cause injury to important areas of the brain, especially when the surgeon is attempting to remove invasive tumors. The long-term consequences of radiation therapy include tissue necrosis, subsequent malignancies, endocrine dysfunction, and behavioral or intellectual deficits. For these reasons, the use of irradiation is deferred for as long as possible in young children. Chemotherapy may allow a delay or reduction in radiation therapy. Targeted therapy is being used in some types of brain tumors. Proton beam radiation therapy, available at some sites, is being studied to learn whether it offers greater efficacy and less long-term toxicity (Parsons et al., 2016).

Nursing Care

Nursing care of the child with a brain tumor is similar regardless of the type of intracranial lesion. Because a brain tumor is potentially fatal, the reader is urged to incorporate the psychologic interventions discussed in Chapter 19 with those elaborated on in this section. However, it is important to remember that many brain tumors are curable. Medulloblastoma, for instance, has a survival rate of approximately 80% in those patients without metastatic disease. Despite the grave nature of some brain tumors, new and emerging therapies are bringing hope to the families of many pediatric patients with brain tumor.

Assess for Signs and Symptoms

A child admitted to the hospital with neurologic dysfunction is often suspected of having a brain tumor, even though the actual diagnosis is not yet confirmed. Establishing baseline data for comparing preoperative and postoperative changes is an essential step toward planning physical care and preventing complications. It also allows the nurse to assess the degree of physical incapacity and the family's emotional response to the diagnosis. For example, children with cerebellar astrocytoma may have displayed vague cerebellar symptoms for several years before a tumor is suspected. For these parents the revelation of a neoplasm may be as shocking as for those who witnessed a rapid deterioration in their child's abilities. Table 25.4 summarizes common presenting signs and assessment procedures to document significant changes in the child's condition.

Prepare the Family for Diagnostic and Operative Procedures

The suspected diagnosis of a brain tumor is always a crisis. Although some tumors are removed with excellent results, the physician can rarely give definitive answers regarding prognosis until after surgery. Therefore parents, the child, and other family members require excellent emotional support to face the diagnostic procedures and a craniotomy.

How the child is prepared for the diagnostic tests depends on the child's age and experience. Chapter 20 discusses preparing children for an MRI or a CT scan. Once surgery is scheduled, the child needs an explanation of what to expect. By the time most children are late preschoolers, they know that the head and brain are important parts of their body. It may be helpful to have children draw their concept of the brain to clarify misconceptions and base the explanation on their level of understanding. Although it may be tempting to justify the surgery by stating that removing the tumor will take away various symptoms, the nurse should refrain from emphasizing this point too strenuously. Postsurgical headaches and cerebellar symptoms, such as ataxia, may be aggravated rather than improved. Surgery may not improve vision. With optic gliomas, the child will be blind in one eye even if the tumor is fully resected. Finally, surgical removal of the mass may

TABLE 25.4 Clinical Manifestations and Assessment of Brain Tumors

Signs and Symptoms	Assessment
Headache Recurrent and progressive In frontal or occipital areas Usually dull and throbbing Worse on arising, less during day Intensified by lowering head and straining, such as during bowel movement, coughing, sneezing	Record description of pain, location, severity, and duration. Use pain rating scale to assess severity of pain (see Chapter 5). Note changes in relation to time of day and activity. Observe changes in behavior in infants (e.g., persistent irritability, crying, head rolling).
Vomiting With or without nausea or feeding Progressively more projectile More severe in morning on arising Relieved by moving about and changing position	Record time, amount, and relationship to feeding, nausea, and activity.
Neuromuscular Changes Incoordination or clumsiness Loss of balance (e.g., use of wide-based stance, falling, tripping, banging into objects) Poor fine motor control Weakness Hyporeflexia or hyperreflexia Positive Babinski sign Spasticity Paralysis	Test muscle strength, gait, coordination, and reflexes (see Chapter 4).
Behavioral Changes Irritability Decreased appetite Failure to thrive Fatigue (frequent naps) Lethargy Coma Bizarre behavior (e.g., staring, automatic movements)	Observe behavior regularly. Compare observations with parental reports of normal behavioral patterns. Monitor growth and food intake. Monitor activity and sleep.
Cranial Nerve Neuropathy Cranial nerve involvement varied according to tumor location Most common signs: • Head tilt • Visual defects (e.g., nystagmus, diplopia, strabismus, episodic "graying out" of vision, visual field defect)	Assess cranial nerves especially VII (facial), IX (glossopharyngeal), X (vagus), V (trigeminal sensory roots), and VI (abducens see Chapter 4). Assess visual acuity binocularity and peripheral vision (see Chapter 4).
Vital Sign Disturbances Decreased pulse and respiration Increased blood pressure Decreased pulse pressure Hypothermia or hyperthermia	Measure vital signs frequently. Monitor pulse and respirations for 1 full minute. Record pulse pressure (difference between systolic and diastolic blood pressure).
Other Signs Seizures Cranial enlargement[a] Tense, bulging fontanel at rest[a] Nuchal rigidity Papilledema (edema of optic nerve)	Record seizure activity (see Chapter 27). Measure head circumference daily (infant and child). Perform funduscopic examination if skilled in procedure.

[a]Present only in infants and young children.

be impossible, and after surgery functioning may temporarily deteriorate or result in permanent damage. Being honest before surgery most often makes honesty after the procedure easier because no false hopes were created.

The hair is usually shaved in the operating room just before surgery or sometimes in the child's room, typically on the night before surgery. When shaving is done with the child awake, the procedure is approached in a sensitive, positive way. If the child's hair is long, braid it so that the long swatch can be saved. Showing children how they look at different stages of the process helps them prepare for their changed appearance.

Once the hair is clipped short or shaved, give the child a cap or scarf to camouflage the baldness. Take every precaution to provide privacy during the procedure and to protect the child from teasing or ridicule by other children before surgery. Also emphasize that the hair will regrow shortly after surgery. Depending on the child's immediate adjustment to the hair loss, the nurse may introduce the idea of wearing a wig until the hair grows in, particularly if additional irradiation or chemotherapy is anticipated.

Also tell children about the size of the dressing. Usually the entire scalp is covered to maintain tight wound closure, even if a small incision is made. Infratentorial head dressings may be attached to the upper back and extend forward to the neck to maintain slight extension and alignment as a precaution against wound rupture. Applying a similar dressing or "special hat" to a doll is often a less traumatic way of demonstrating the physical appearance.

Children also need a brief explanation of how they will feel after surgery and where they will be. Ordinarily they will return to a special intensive care unit, which they may visit beforehand, depending on hospital policy. They should be aware that they may be sleepy for some time after surgery and that a headache is likely and may last for a few days.

Parents need similar explanations before surgery, especially in terms of special equipment used in the intensive care unit, dressings, and their child's behavior. For example, they should know that it is not unusual for the child to be lethargic for a few days after surgery. The nurse may wish to encourage less frequent visiting during this period so that parents can rest and be able to support their child when the child is awake. The nurse should participate in preoperative conferences with the physician and parents. The nurse needs to know what information the parents have been given in order to provide further explanations or emotional support as needed.

! NURSING ALERT

Report sluggish, dilated, or unequal pupils immediately because they may indicate increased intracranial pressure (ICP) and potential brainstem herniation—a medical emergency.

Prevent Postoperative Complications

After surgery the surgeon prescribes specific orders for taking vital signs, positioning, regulating fluids, and administering medication. These vary somewhat, depending on the location of the craniotomy. The following are general principles of care for patients undergoing infratentorial or supratentorial surgery. Chapter 27 discusses additional aspects of care, such as care of the child with seizures and care of the unconscious child in terms of respiratory status and neurologic assessment.

Assessment

Vital signs are taken as often as every 15 to 30 minutes until the patient is stable. Temperature measurement is particularly important because of hyperthermia resulting from surgical intervention in the hypothalamus or brainstem and from some types of general anesthesia. To prepare for this reaction, a cooling blanket may be placed on the bed before the child returns to the unit, or it may be used when needed. Because the temperature control centers are affected and hypothermia can occur suddenly, the nurse monitors body temperature often when any cooling measures are used.

! NURSING ALERT

To keep an accurate account of drainage, circle the soiled area with a pen and monitor for signs of continuous bleeding. The presence of colorless drainage is reported immediately because it most likely is cerebrospinal fluid leaking from the incisional area. A foul odor from the dressing may indicate an infection. Such a finding is reported, and a culture is taken.

The most likely types of infection are meningitis and respiratory tract infection. The probable cause of meningitis is wound contamination. The risk of respiratory tract infections is high because of the imposed immobility, danger of aspiration, and possible respiratory depression from the brainstem. The usual precautions of deep breathing and turning as allowed are instituted. Regular pulmonary assessments are performed to identify adventitious sounds or any areas of diminished or absent breath sounds. Blood pressure is also taken at frequent intervals. The deflated cuff is left on the arm between readings to allow for the least movement and disturbance of the child. Ocular signs are recorded at least every hour.

As soon as possible, the nurse should begin testing reflexes, hand grip, and functioning of the cranial nerves. Muscle strength is usually reduced after surgery because of general weakness but should improve daily. Ataxia may be significantly worse with cerebellar intervention, but it slowly improves. Edema near the cranial nerves may depress important functions such as the gag, blink, or swallowing reflex.

Neurologic checks are an essential aspect of care and include pupillary reaction to light, level of consciousness, sleep patterns, and response to stimuli. Although children may be comatose for a few days, once they regain consciousness there should be a steady increase in alertness. Regression to a lethargic, irritable state indicates increasing pressure, possibly caused by meningitis, hemorrhage, or edema.

Dressings are observed for evidence of drainage. If soiled, the dressing is not removed but reinforced with dry sterile gauze. The approximate amount of drainage is estimated and recorded.

Once the younger child is alert, the arms may need to be restrained to preserve the dressing. Even a child who has been cooperative before surgery must be closely supervised during the initial stages of regaining consciousness, when disorientation and restlessness are common. Elbow restraints are satisfactory to prevent the hands from reaching the head, although additional restraint may be necessary to preserve an infusion line and maintain a specific position.

Positioning

Correct positioning after surgery is critical to prevent pressure against the operative site, reduce ICP, and avoid the danger of aspiration. If a large tumor was removed, the child is not placed on the operative side because the brain may suddenly shift to that cavity, causing trauma to the blood vessels, linings, and the brain itself. The nurse confers with the surgeon to be certain of the correct position, including the degree of neck flexion. The first 24 to 48 hours after brain surgery are critical.

If positioning is restricted, notice of this is posted above the head of the bed. When the child is turned, every precaution is used to prevent jarring or misalignment to prevent undue strain on the sutures. Two nurses, one supporting the head and the other supporting the body, are needed. The use of a turning sheet may facilitate turning a heavy child.

! NURSING ALERT

The Trendelenburg position is contraindicated in both infratentorial and supratentorial surgeries because it increases intracranial pressure (ICP) and the risk of hemorrhage. If shock is impending, the practitioner is notified immediately, before the head is lowered.

The child with an infratentorial craniotomy is usually positioned flat and on either side. Pillows should be placed against the child's back, not head, to maintain the desired position. Ordinarily the head and neck are kept in midline with the body and slightly extended. After a supratentorial craniotomy the head is usually elevated above the heart to facilitate cerebrospinal fluid drainage and decrease excessive blood flow to the brain to prevent hemorrhage.

Fluid Regulation

With an infratentorial craniotomy the child is allowed nothing by mouth for at least 24 hours or longer if the gag and swallowing reflexes are depressed or the child is comatose. With a supratentorial procedure, feeding may be resumed soon after the child is alert, sometimes within 24 hours. Clear water is always started first because of the danger of aspiration. If the child vomits, stop oral liquids. Vomiting not only predisposes the child to aspiration but also increases ICP and the risk for incisional rupture.

IV fluids are continued until fluids are well tolerated by mouth. Because of cerebral edema postoperatively and the danger of increased ICP, fluids are carefully monitored and usually infused less than the maintenance rate. If drugs such as prophylactic antibiotics are given intravenously, the medication amount is calculated as part of the IV fluid. For example, if the child is to receive 20 ml/h and the diluted drug is 5 ml, the IV solution is reduced to 15 ml for that hour.

A hypertonic solution such as mannitol may be necessary to remove excess fluid. These drugs cause rapid diuresis. After surgery the child may have a Foley catheter in place. Urinary output is monitored after administration of these drugs to evaluate their effectiveness.

When able to take fluids, the child should be fed to conserve strength and minimize movement. If there is any sign of facial paralysis, the child is fed slowly to prevent choking or aspiration. Scrupulous mouth care is essential to prevent oral infection. Sometimes gavage feeding is necessary when body functions are too depressed to permit safe oral feedings or the child refuses to eat or drink. In the latter instance the nurse should use every measure to encourage acceptance of fluids or solids (see Chapter 20 for nursing interventions).

Comfort Measures

Headache may be severe and is largely the result of cerebral edema. Measures to relieve some of the discomfort include providing a quiet, dimly lit environment; restricting visitors; preventing any sudden jarring movement, such as banging into the bed; and preventing an increase in ICP. The last is most effectively achieved by proper positioning and prevention of straining, such as during coughing, vomiting, or defecating. The use of opioids, such as morphine, to relieve pain has been controversial because it is thought that they may mask signs of altered consciousness or depress respirations. However, opioids are considered safe because naloxone can be used to reverse opioid effects, such as sedation or respiratory depression. Acetaminophen and codeine are also effective analgesics. Regardless of the drugs used, adequate dosage and regular administration are essential to provide optimum pain relief (see Chapter 5, Pain Assessment and Pain Management).

Monitor bowel movements to prevent constipation. Stool softeners may be given as soon as liquids are tolerated to facilitate easy passage of stool.

Brain edema may severely depress the gag reflex, necessitating suctioning of oral secretions. Facial edema may also be present, necessitating eye care if the lids remain partially open. Ice compresses applied to the eyes for short periods help relieve the edema. A depressed blink reflex also predisposes the corneas to ulceration. Irrigating the eyes with saline drops and covering them with eye dressings are important steps in preventing this complication.

Support the Family

The family's informational and support needs are great when the diagnosis is a brain tumor and are influenced by the extent of surgery, any neurologic deficits, the prognosis, and additional therapy. Because few definitive answers can be given before surgery, the surgeon's report is a significant finding that can vary from a completely benign, resected neoplasm to a highly malignant, invasive, and only partially removed tumor. Although parents try to prepare themselves for a potentially fatal diagnosis, it is understandably a shock for them.

Ideally, a nurse who will be involved in the continuing care of this child should be with the family when the physician discusses the prognosis and plan of therapy. Although parents may absorb only a fraction of what they are told, they can begin to put the future into perspective. Regardless of the future prospects, direct the parents' thinking toward helping the child recover and resume a normal life to his or her fullest potential. Providing the opportunity for the family to share their concerns and questions with other families who have a child with a brain tumor may help the family cope, and the nurse can direct them to resources.[f]

It is also a time to encourage parents to verbalize their feelings about the diagnosis. Often they express guilt for attributing the insidious onset of symptoms, such as ataxia, visual difficulty, or headache, to minor "complaints" by the child. Parents may have punished their child for clumsiness, mistaking it for carelessness, or for their declining performance in school. The nurse listens to such statements and emphasizes the normality of the parents' reactions. Sometimes it may be helpful to start a discussion with a statement such as "It is difficult to know when a child's complaints are significant because so often they are caused by minor ailments and you would never have imagined they were the result of a brain tumor." The nurse avoids any comments that insinuate the parents should have sought medical advice sooner because such remarks only add to the parents' feelings of guilt.

During this period the nurse should also discuss with parents what they plan to tell the child. If the child was prepared honestly, as described previously, the diagnosis can be expressed in a similar manner, such as "The surgeon removed most of the tumor, and the rest will be treated with special drugs and x-ray treatments." During recovery the child needs additional explanation about the treatment and the reason for residual neurologic effects, such as ataxia or blindness.

[f]Information about support groups is available from the National Brain Tumor Society, 22 Battery St., Suite 612, San Francisco, CA 94111; 800-934-CURE; email: info@braintumor.org; http://www.braintumor.org; and the Pediatric Brain Tumor Foundation, 302 Ridgefield Court, Asheville, NC 28806; 800-253-6530; email: info@curethekids.org; http://www.curethekids.org.

Hair loss is a normal concern for the child, and hair regrowth will be delayed, depending on the length of therapy. This is an appropriate time to reintroduce the idea of a wig, scarf, or hat.

Promote Return to Optimum Functioning

The ultimate goal is a cured child who has optimum functioning. As soon as possible, the child should resume usual activities within tolerable limits, especially returning to school.[g] Until the skull is completely healed, the child may need to wear a helmet when engaging in any active sport. This decision is made by the child's neurosurgeon. The school nurse and teacher should confer with the parents on activity restrictions, such as physical education, as well as the reactions of schoolmates to the child's appearance.

After discharge the family needs continuing medical and emotional support from health personnel. Children who are long-term survivors after treatment for a brain tumor require ongoing follow-up due to residual disabilities, such as short stature, cranial nerve palsies, sensory defects, motor abnormalities (especially ataxia), intellectual deficits, dysphagia, dysgraphia, and behavioral problems (Parsons et al., 2016).

The realm of all possible consequences after the diagnosis of a brain tumor is not discussed here. The reader is referred to other sections of the text that deal with possible outcomes, such as the paralyzed, visually impaired, or unconscious child or the child with a ventricular shunt, seizure disorder, or meningitis. Numerous physical problems can occur with progression of the tumor, and these may necessitate additional procedures. For example, frequent vomiting, anorexia, and nausea may require nonoral routes of feeding, such as gastrostomy or parenteral alimentation. Trials with chemotherapy may necessitate the use of central venous access devices. Whenever these procedures are instituted, the nurse may be responsible for teaching the family appropriate home care to allow the child the highest quality of life for the longest time (see discussion of discharge planning and home care in Chapter 19).

NEUROBLASTOMA

With approximately 650 new cases of neuroblastoma diagnosed every year in the United States, neuroblastoma is the most common extracranial childhood solid tumor (National Institutes of Health, 2019h). It is a disease of infancy and early childhood, with a median age at diagnosis of about 19 months (Brodeur, Hogarty, Bagatell, et al., 2016). Neuroblastoma sometimes occurs in a hereditary form, although this is rare. Three genes or mutations that play a part in hereditary neuroblastoma have been identified (*ALK* and *PHOX2B*, deletion at 1p36 or 11q14-23 locus). Also, several syndromes contribute to neuroblastoma predisposition, including Costello and Noonan syndromes, and neurofibromatosis (Brodeur et al., 2016). Genomic studies (GWAS) are an active area of research. Within the tumor cells, a hallmark is amplification of an oncogene, *MYCN*, a variation seen in 16% to 25% of neuroblastoma tumors and mainly associated with high-risk disease.

Neuroblastomas originate from embryonic neural crest cells (neuroblasts) that normally give rise to the adrenal medulla and the sympathetic nervous system. Consequently, the majority of the tumors arise from the adrenal gland or in the neck, chest, or spinal cord.

Clinical Manifestations

The signs and symptoms of neuroblastoma depend on the location and extent of disease (National Institutes of Health, 2019h). The most common primary site is within the abdomen; other sites include the head and neck region, chest, and pelvis. With abdominal tumors, the most common presenting sign is a firm, nontender, irregular mass in the abdomen that crosses the midline (in contrast to Wilms tumor, which is usually confined to one side). Other signs related to abdominal location include pain or discomfort, vomiting, anorexia, and respiratory compromise; compression of the kidney, ureter, or bladder may cause urinary frequency or retention. Tumors in the thoracic or cervical region can involve dyspnea, Horner syndrome (ptosis, miosis, anhidrosis), neck mass, stridor, and dysphagia. Spinal cord and brain sites can present with neurologic deficits, difficulty breathing, bladder and bowel dysfunction, paraparesis, paraplegia, or seizures. Neuroblastoma that infiltrates the bone marrow can produce anemia, thrombocytopenia, and neutropenia. Tumors in the orbit or optic nerves can produce exophthalmos, periorbital ecchymosis, and impaired vision. Tumors in bone can result in pain or limping. Metastases to the skin can appear as subcutaneous skin nodules, described as "blueberry muffin lesions" due to their color; this is usually only seen in infants.

Diagnostic Evaluation

Diagnostic evaluation is aimed at determining the primary site and extent of disease. Physical exam and history, blood chemistry studies, and neurologic exam are performed. Tumor imaging by CT or MRI is used to locate the primary tumor in neck, chest, abdomen, and pelvis. Evaluation for metastases includes examination of the bone marrow with bilateral aspirates and biopsies and of the bony skeleton with MIBG scanning.

Neuroblastomas, particularly those arising on the adrenal glands or from a sympathetic chain, excrete the catecholamines epinephrine and norepinephrine. Urinary excretion of catecholamine metabolites (vanillylmandelic acid [VMA] and homovanillic acid [HVA]) is measured before therapy; these markers can be used to monitor response to therapy and detection of relapse after therapy (National Institutes of Health, 2019h).

Diagnosis is based on the presence of tumor cells in a biopsy of tumor tissue (biopsy also provides tissue for determining *MYCN* copy number [amplification] and other chromosomal or genetic tests) or the presence of tumor cells in bone marrow plus increased urinary catecholamine metabolites (National Institutes of Health, 2019h).

Staging and Prognosis

Neuroblastoma is a "silent" tumor. In more than 70% of cases, diagnosis is made after metastasis occurs, with the first signs caused by involvement in a nonprimary site, usually the lymph nodes, bone marrow, skeletal system, or liver. Accurate clinical staging is important for establishing initial treatment. The International Neuroblastoma Risk Group staging system is used to classify neuroblastoma patients to a pretreatment risk group based on International Neuroblastoma Risk Group image-defined risk factors, age, histologic category, grade of tumor differentiation, *MYCN* amplification, 11q aberration, and ploidy (National Institutes of Health, 2019h). Future versions of the International Neuroblastoma Risk Group staging system are expected to include more tumor genomic criteria as new biomarkers that affect outcomes are identified. The International Neuroblastoma Risk Group staging system is shown in Box 25.4.

Therapeutic Management

For patients considered to be low risk, treatment may include surgery followed by observation or chemotherapy (carboplatin, cyclophosphamide, doxorubicin, etoposide) with or without surgery for those with

[g]The American Brain Tumor Association has information on returning to school: 8550 W. Bryn Mawr Ave. Suite 550, Chicago, IL 60631; 1-800-886-2282; email: info@abta.org; http://www.abta.org/returning-to-school/.

BOX 25.4 Staging of Neuroblastoma by International Neuroblastoma Risk Group

Stage L1: Localized tumor not involving vital structures as defined by the list of image-defined risk factors and confined to one body compartment

Stage L2: Local-regional tumor with presence of one or more image-defined risk factors

Stage M: Distant metastatic disease (except stage MS)

Stage MS: Metastatic disease in children younger than 18 months with metastases confined to skin, liver, and/or bone marrow

Note: Patients with multifocal primary disease should be staged according to the greatest extent of disease. Image-defined risk factors are grouped by anatomic location and include multiple body compartments, neck, cervicothoracic junction, thorax, thoracoabdominal junction, abdomen and pelvis, and intraspinal tumor extension.

Data from Monclair, T., Brodeur, G. M., Ambros, P., et al. (2009). The International Neuroblastoma Risk Group (INRG) staging system: An INRG task force report. Journal of Clinical Oncology, 27(2), 298–303; and Chen, A. M., Trout, A. T., & Towbin, A. J. (2018). A review of image-defined risk factors on magnetic resonance imaging. Pediatric Radiology, 48, 1337–1347.

symptomatic disease or unresectable disease after surgery. For certain low-risk patients, observation without biopsy is being studied.

For intermediate-risk patients, treatment may include chemotherapy (carboplatin, cyclophosphamide, doxorubicin, etoposide) with or without surgery, surgery, and observation (infants). Radiation therapy is used for patients with progressive disease during chemotherapy or progressive unresectable disease after chemotherapy.

Patients with high-risk neuroblastoma are treated with chemotherapy (cisplatin, etoposide, vincristine, cyclophosphamide, doxorubicin, topotecan), surgery, tandem cycles of myeloablative therapy and HSCT, radiation therapy, immunotherapy, and retinoid therapy. This treatment is usually divided into three phases. Induction includes chemotherapy and surgery; consolidation includes tandem cycles of myeloablative therapy and HSCT; and postconsolidation includes radiation to the primary tumor site and residual metastatic sites, immunotherapy, and retinoid therapy. Treatment plans are actively being studied in order to improve response rates and reduce long-term complications.

Nursing Care

Nursing care is similar to that discussed under General Nursing Care Management, including psychologic and physical preparation for diagnostic and operative procedures; prevention of postoperative surgical complications; and explanation of chemotherapy, immunotherapy, HSCT, and radiation therapy, as well as their side effects as appropriate for the patient.

Because this tumor carries a poor prognosis for many children, the nurse evaluates and addresses the needs of the family in terms of coping with a life-threatening illness (see Chapter 17). Because of the high frequency of metastasis at the time of diagnosis, many parents suffer guilt for not having recognized signs earlier. Parents need skilled support in dealing with these feelings and expressing them to the appropriate members of the health care team. In addition, many neuroblastoma patients will go home with tube feedings, and the family will need relevant education and skills training.

BONE TUMORS

Osteosarcoma (OS) and Ewing sarcoma (EWS) are the primary bone tumors that occur most often in young people. Although both are bone tumors, they are different in many ways. OS is the most common bone tumor in adolescents and young adults, with approximately 400 new cases annually in the United States (National Institutes of Health, 2019i). EWS is less common, with about 200 cases diagnosed annually among children under the age of 20 years in the United States (Hawkins, Brennan, Bolling, et al., 2016). EWS occurs predominantly in whites, and more than half of affected patients are adolescents (National Institutes of Health, 2019j). Risk factors for OS include ionizing radiation exposure, genetic predisposition syndromes, and a history of retinoblastoma, particularly the hereditary form (Gorlick, Janeway, & Marina, 2016).

CLINICAL MANIFESTATIONS

Most malignant bone tumors produce localized pain in the affected site, which may be severe or dull and may be attributed to trauma or the vague complaint of "growing pains." The pain is often relieved by a flexed position, which relaxes the muscles overlying the stretched periosteum. Frequently a bone tumor draws attention when the child limps, curtails physical activity, or is unable to hold heavy objects. A palpable mass is also a common manifestation of bone tumors. Systemic symptoms (such as fever) and other clinical symptoms (such as spinal cord compression and respiratory distress) are more frequent in patients with Ewing sarcoma.

DIAGNOSTIC EVALUATION

Diagnosis begins with a thorough history and physical examination. A primary objective is to rule out causes such as trauma or infection. Careful questioning regarding pain is essential in attempting to determine the duration and rate of tumor growth. Physical assessment focuses on functional status of the affected area; signs of inflammation; size of the mass; and any systemic indication of generalized malignancy, such as anemia, weight loss, and frequent infection.

Definitive diagnosis is based on imaging studies, such as plain films and CT or MRI scan of the primary site, CT scan of the chest, and PET scan to evaluate metastasis. Because EWS may be found in bone marrow, a bone marrow examination is performed; this is not the case in patients with OS. A needle or surgical biopsy is necessary to establish the diagnosis. EWS most commonly involves the pelvis, long bones of the lower extremities, and chest wall; imaging reveals involvement of the diaphysis with detachment of the periosteum from the bone (Codman triangle). In OS, lesions are most commonly located in the metaphyseal region of the bone, often involving the long bones. Radial ossification in the soft tissue gives the tumor a "sunburst" appearance on plain radiograph. It should be noted that the particular radiology findings associated with bone tumors are not themselves diagnostic of either OS or EWS.

PROGNOSIS

A better understanding of the biology of neoplastic growth has resulted in more aggressive treatment and improved prognosis. The natural history of OS and EWS suggests that multiple submicroscopic foci of metastatic disease are present at the time of diagnosis despite clinical evidence indicating only localized involvement. The lungs, distant bones, and bone marrow are the most common sites for metastatic bone tumor disease. With current therapies that include surgery and chemotherapy for OS and surgery, radiation therapy, and chemotherapy for EWS, the majority of patients with localized disease can be cured.

Pretreatment factors that influence OS outcome include primary tumor site and initial treatment, size of the primary tumor, and presence of clinically detectable metastatic disease; postchemotherapy treatment factors that influence outcome include surgical resectability of the tumor and degree of tumor necrosis assessed by the pathologist. Greater tumor necrosis has been associated with better prognosis in OS (National Institutes of Health, 2019i). Older adolescents and young adults with OS tend to have a worse prognosis than do younger patients.

For patients with EWS, the pretreatment factors that are associated with better prognosis are distal site of tumor, extraskeletal primary tumor, smaller tumor size or volume (larger tumors tend to occur in unfavorable sites), younger age, female sex, lactic acid dehydrogenase (LDH) levels not increased, and absence of metastases. Adverse prognostic factors include pathologic fracture, previous cancer treatment, certain chromosomal abnormalities, and other biologic factors (National Institutes of Health, 2019j). A key feature of EWS (in 85% of cases) is the translocation between chromosomes 11 and 22, fusing the *EWS* gene of chromosome 22 to the *FLLI1* gene of chromosome 11.

OSTEOSARCOMA

Osteosarcoma occurs most often in adolescents and young adults, coinciding with the period of rapid bone growth (Gorlick et al., 2016; National Institutes of Health, 2019i). It presumably arises from bone-forming mesenchyme, which gives rise to malignant osteoid tissue. Most primary tumor sites are in the diametaphyseal region (wider part of the shaft, adjacent to the epiphyseal growth plate) of long bones, especially in the lower extremities. More than half occur in the femur, particularly the distal portion, with the rest involving the humerus, tibia, pelvis, jaw, and phalanges.

Therapeutic Management

Optimum treatment of OS includes surgery and chemotherapy. The surgical approach consists of surgical biopsy followed by either limb salvage or amputation. Biopsy and surgery should be performed by an orthopedic oncology surgeon. To ensure local control, all gross and microscopic tumors must be resected. A limb salvage procedure has become the standard approach to surgical intervention and involves resection of the primary tumor with prosthetic replacement of the involved bone (Gorlick et al., 2016). For example, with OS of the distal femur, a total femur and joint replacement is performed. Frequently children undergoing a limb salvage procedure receive preoperative chemotherapy in an attempt to decrease the tumor size and make surgery more manageable (Gorlick et al., 2016).

Treatment for OS with few exceptions is preoperative chemotherapy, local control, and postoperative chemotherapy. The standard of care for localized OS is three-drug treatment with cisplatin, doxorubicin, and methotrexate with citrovorum. These combined-modality approaches have significantly improved the prognosis in OS to approximately 70% for patients with nonmetastatic disease (Gorlick et al., 2016). OS is not a very radiation-sensitive tumor. Thus radiation is used only in palliative situations for unresectable tumors of the axial skeleton.

Nursing Care

Nursing care depends on the type of surgical approach. The family may or may not have more difficulty adjusting to an amputation than a limb salvage procedure. In either instance, preparation of the child and family is critical. Straightforward honesty is essential in gaining the child's cooperation and trust. The emphasis is on early preparation and planning with the child and family. This is done with the multidisciplinary treating team, including the oncologist, surgeon, advanced practice registered nurse (APRN), physical therapist, psychologist, and social worker, as well as the staff nurse. It is a process, not a one-time discussion, in order to allow time to think about the diagnosis and consequent treatment and to ask questions.

Sometimes children have many questions about the prosthesis, limitations on physical ability, and prognosis in terms of cure. At other times they react with silence or with a calm manner that belies their concern and fear. Either response must be accepted because it is part of grieving the loss of an aspect of their physical appearance and function. For those who desire information, it may be helpful to introduce them to another amputee or survivor with a limb salvage procedure before surgery or to show them pictures of the prosthesis.[h] However, the nurse must be careful not to overwhelm children with information. A sound approach is to answer questions without offering additional information. For those who do not pursue additional information, the nurse expresses a willingness to talk.

Children are informed of the need for chemotherapy from the beginning of the treatment process through surgery and beyond. Children have a variety of responses to side effects of chemotherapy. The nurse should be aware of expected side effects, normalize the patient's responses, and be aware of resources within the hospital and outside the hospital for patients.

If an amputation is performed, the child may be fitted with a temporary prosthesis immediately after surgery, which permits early functioning and fosters psychologic adjustment. Stump care is provided the same as for any amputee. A permanent prosthesis is typically fitted within 6 to 8 weeks. During hospitalization the child begins physical therapy to become proficient in the use and care of the device. Wound healing is a significant issue for patients with OS, and they may have a significant delay in getting their prosthesis if they do not have complete surgical incisional healing. This can be frustrating and difficult for patients who are actively receiving chemotherapy and likely to have delayed healing.

Phantom limb pain may develop in 60% to 80% of patients after amputation. The exact pathophysiology is still unclear but may include a combination of physical and psychologic factors that need to be further clarified by research (Luo & Anderson, 2016). This symptom is characterized by sensations such as tingling, itching, and, more frequently, pain felt in the amputated limb. The child and family need to know that the sensations are real, not imagined. Although various pharmacologic and nonpharmacologic techniques have been used for phantom limb pain, none provides complete relief or is curative (Luo & Anderson, 2016). A study of pediatric patients with cancer-related amputation found that 76% had phantom limb pain during the first year after amputation, but only 10% still had phantom limb pain more than 1 year after amputation (Burgoyne, Billups, Jirón, et al., 2012). The nurse works with the institution's pain team to address the problem of phantom limb pain.

Discharge planning begins early in the postoperative period. Once the child has begun physical therapy, the nurse consults with the therapist and oncology team to evaluate the child's physical and emotional readiness to reenter school. However, patients with OS often do not attend school until their intense chemotherapy is complete and efforts are made to maintain school work until the end of treatment. Every effort is made to promote normality and gradual resumption of realistic presurgery activities. Role playing in anticipation of such

[h]Information about prostheses can be obtained from the National Amputation Foundation, 40 Church St., Malverne, NY 11565; 516-887-3600; http://www.nationalamputation.org.

experiences is beneficial in preparing the child for inevitable confrontations by others. Environmental barriers, such as stairs, are assessed in terms of accessibility in the school and home, especially because the child may need to use crutches or a wheelchair before complete healing and prosthetic competency are achieved. Information about special programs for children with amputations is available from the American Childhood Cancer Organization (see footnote earlier in the chapter).

The nurse encourages the child to select from among the many options available for personalization of prosthetics and sleeves. Well-fitted prostheses are so natural looking that girls usually can wear sheer stockings without revealing the device if that is their desire. The key is that the child can personalize the prosthetic device and apparel according to personal preference.

The family and child need much support in adjusting not only to a life-threatening diagnosis but also to alteration in body form and function. Because loss of a limb entails a grieving process, those caring for the child need to recognize that reactions of anger and depression are normal and necessary. Often parents view anger as a direct affront to them for allowing the amputation to occur, or they see the depression as rejection. These are not personal attacks but the child's attempts to cope with a loss. Psychosocial support programs (or members of the health care team such as psychologists, social workers, and child life specialists) at the institution may be particularly helpful in supporting the patient's and family's strengths in coping.

EWING SARCOMA (PRIMITIVE NEUROECTODERMAL TUMOR OF THE BONE)

Ewing sarcomas, or the EWS family of tumors, which includes primitive neuroectodermal tumor of the bone, are the second most common malignant bone tumor (after OS) in childhood (Hawkins et al., 2016). EWS arises in the marrow spaces of the bone rather than from osseous tissue. The tumor originates in the shaft of long and trunk bones, most often affecting the pelvis, femur, tibia, fibula, humerus, ulna, vertebra, scapula, ribs, and skull (Hawkins et al., 2016).

Therapeutic Management

Surgery is the main local therapy for EWS. However, radiation may be used for patients with unresectable disease or for patients who would have functional compromise by surgery (National Institutes of Health, 2019j). Limb salvage procedures may be feasible in extremity lesions, although amputation may be considered if the results of radiation therapy would render the extremity useless or deformed (e.g., from growth retardation in young children). Patients with EWS are encouraged to have surgical resection when possible, however, because it is associated with a slight survival advantage and fewer long-term morbidities.

The treatment of choice for most localized lesions is involved-field radiation therapy and chemotherapy. The standard chemotherapy protocol includes vincristine, doxorubicin, ifosfamide, and etoposide; cyclophosphamide and dactinomycin may also be used. High-dose chemotherapy with stem cell rescue may be used for patients at high risk of relapse.

Approximately two-thirds of patients with localized EWS can expect to be cured (Hawkins et al., 2016). Improving survival, especially for patients with metastatic or recurrent disease, is a focus of ongoing research.

Nursing Care Management

Ewing sarcoma differs from OS because preservation of the affected limb is more likely. Families may accept the diagnosis with some relief in knowing that this type of bone cancer does not necessitate amputation. They need preparation for the various diagnostic tests, including bone marrow aspiration and surgical biopsy, and adequate explanation of the treatment regimen.

High-dose radiation therapy often causes a skin reaction of dry or moist desquamation followed by hyperpigmentation. The child should wear loose-fitting clothes over the irradiated area to minimize additional skin irritation. Because of increased sensitivity, the area should be protected from sunlight and sudden changes in temperature, such as from heating pads or ice packs. Encourage the child to use the extremity as tolerated. The physical therapist may plan an active exercise program to preserve maximum function.

The child needs the same considerations for adjusting to the effects of chemotherapy as any other patient with cancer. The drug regimen usually results in hair loss, severe nausea and vomiting, peripheral neuropathy, and possible cardiotoxicity. Make every effort to outline a treatment plan that allows the child maximum resumption of a normal lifestyle and activities.

OTHER SOLID TUMORS

In addition to the cancers already discussed, several other types of solid tumors may occur in children. This section covers Wilms tumor, rhabdomyosarcoma, and retinoblastoma. These tumors tend to be diagnosed early, typically before 5 years of age. Wilms tumor and retinoblastoma are unusual in that they are among the few types of cancer that may occur in both hereditary and nonhereditary forms.

WILMS TUMOR

Of the many types of childhood kidney tumors, Wilms tumor (nephroblastoma) is the most common, with approximately 650 new cases per year in the United States (National Institutes of Health, 2019k). The average age at diagnosis is 44 months in children with tumor in one kidney but younger (31 months) in those with tumor in both kidneys. Although the specific cause is unknown, certain genetic syndromes or conditions increase the risk of Wilms tumor, such as WAGR (**W**ilms tumor, **a**niridia, **g**enitourinary anomalies, and cognitive impairment [mental **r**etardation]), Denys-Drash, and Beckwith-Wiedemann syndromes (hemihypertrophy, macroglossia, omphalocele, and visceromegaly) (National Institutes of Health, 2019k). Approximately 10% of children with Wilms tumor have congenital anomalies, such as cryptorchidism or hypospadias.

A number of genes and chromosomal alterations have been implicated in the biology of Wilms tumor, including *WT1, CTNNB1, WTX* on the X chromosome, imprinting cluster regions on chromosome 11p15 (*WT2),* and other genes or chromosomal alterations (National Institutes of Health, 2019k). Families of children at significantly increased risk of developing Wilms tumor are referred for genetic or genomic testing and counseling. In addition, children at increased risk are usually screened with ultrasound every 3 months until they are 8 years of age (National Institutes of Health, 2019k).

Clinical Manifestations

The most common presenting sign is swelling or mass within the abdomen; pain is present in about 40% of patients (Fernandez, Geller, Ehrlich, et al., 2016). The mass is characteristically firm, nontender, confined to one side, and deep within the flank. If it is on the right side, it may be difficult to distinguish from the liver, although unlike that organ, it does not move with respiration. The mass is typically discovered during routine bathing or dressing of the child.

Other clinical manifestations may result from compression by the tumor mass, metabolic alterations secondary to the tumor, or metastases. Hematuria occurs in less than one-fourth of children with Wilms tumor. Anemia, usually secondary to hemorrhage within the tumor, results in pallor, anorexia, and lethargy. Hypertension, probably caused by secretion of excess amounts of renin by the tumor, occurs in about 25% of children. Other effects of malignancy include anorexia, weight loss, and fever (10%). If pulmonary metastasis has occurred, symptoms of lung involvement, such as dyspnea, cough, shortness of breath, and pain in the chest, may be evident.

Diagnostic Evaluation

In a child suspected of having Wilms tumor, special emphasis is placed on the history and physical examination for the presence of congenital anomalies (e.g., aniridia, developmental delay, hypospadias, cryptorchidism); a family history of cancer; and clinical signs of Wilms tumor. The diagnostic workup includes abdominal imaging studies (abdominal x-ray, ultrasound, CT or MRI of the abdomen); chest x-ray; CT of the chest to look for lung metastases; and von Willebrand disease workup. Laboratory studies should include a CBC (polycythemia is sometimes present if the tumor secretes excess erythropoietin), biochemical studies, and urinalysis. Studies to assess intravascular extension of the tumor and tumor rupture also are performed.

Staging and Prognosis

There are two main staging systems for Wilms tumor, one used by the Children's Oncology Group and the other used by the European group SIOP. In the Children's Oncology Group system, disease staging (ranging from stage I to V) is determined by results of imaging studies and pathologic findings at nephrectomy (Box 25.5), with stage I being localized to one kidney and stage V indicating bilateral involvement by tumor (National Institutes of Health, 2019k). The histology of the tumor cells is classified into two groups: favorable histology (FH) and anaplastic (unfavorable) histology; the anaplastic group is further subdivided into diffuse and focal (Fernandez et al., 2016).

Prognosis depends on histology of the tumor (FH versus anaplastic), stage of disease at diagnosis, molecular features of the tumor, and age. Five-year survival rates for Wilms tumor with FH are above 90%. Anaplastic histology, disseminated disease, 1q gain, and older age confer a worse prognosis (National Institutes of Health, 2019k).

Therapeutic Management

The standard of care is combined treatment with surgery and chemotherapy; radiation therapy may be used, based on clinical stage and tumor histology. In unilateral disease, nephrectomy and lymph node sampling are performed; a transabdominal or thoracoabdominal incision is used for greatest visibility of the kidney. Great care is taken to keep the encapsulated tumor intact because intraoperative spill can seed cancer cells throughout the abdomen, lymph channel, and bloodstream. If imaging studies do not indicate bilateral kidney involvement, exploration of the contralateral kidney is not necessary during the operative procedure (National Institutes of Health, 2019k).

In the United States, the standard approach to treatment is immediate surgery followed by postoperative chemotherapy, except for selected cases who do not receive chemotherapy; in advanced stages, radiation therapy is used in a risk-adapted approach. Standard chemotherapy regimens for Wilms tumor include some or all of the following: vincristine, dactinomycin, doxorubicin, cyclophosphamide, and etoposide. Postoperative radiation therapy is indicated for children with tumors classified as stage II focal or diffuse anaplastic histology, stage III, and stage IV (National Institutes of Health, 2019k). Options for stage V tumors may include preoperative chemotherapy and surgery and/or renal transplantation.

The child may be treated with chemotherapy preoperatively under some circumstances (e.g., tumor is bilateral or child has a single kidney) after biopsy confirmation of the diagnosis. The rationale is that preoperative chemotherapy reduces the size and vascular supply of the tumor, thereby making tumor removal easier (National Institutes of Health, 2019k).

BOX 25.5 Children's Oncology Group Staging of Wilms Tumor

Stage I: Tumor is limited to one kidney and completely resected without rupture or previous biopsy. All sampled lymph nodes negative for tumor.

Stage II: Tumor extends beyond kidney but is completely resected; lymph nodes do not contain tumor cells.

Stage III: There is postoperative residual tumor confined to abdomen. Lymph nodes in abdomen or pelvis contain tumor cells.

Stage IV: Hematogenous metastases with disease spread to the lung, liver, bone, brain, or distant lymph nodes.

Stage V: Bilateral renal involvement is present at diagnosis.

Nursing Care

The nursing care of the child with Wilms tumor is similar to that of other cancers treated with surgery and chemotherapy and possibly radiation therapy. However, some significant differences are discussed for each phase of nursing intervention.

Preoperative Care

As with most cancers, the diagnosis of Wilms tumor is a shock for the family. Frequently the child has no physical indication of the seriousness of the disorder other than a palpable abdominal mass. The nurse needs to take particular account the parents' feelings, since parents are often the ones who discover the mass. Whereas some parents are grateful for detecting the tumor so that it can be treated, others feel guilty for not finding it sooner or feel angry toward the health care professional, believing it was missed on earlier examinations.

The preoperative period is one of swift diagnostic workup. Typically, surgery is scheduled within 24 to 48 hours of admission. The nurse is faced with the challenge of preparing the child and parents for all laboratory and operative procedures. Explanations should be simple and repeated, with attention to what the child will experience. In addition to usual preoperative observations, blood pressure is monitored because hypertension from excess renin production is possible.

There are several special preoperative concerns, the most important of which is not to palpate the tumor unless absolutely necessary because manipulation of the mass may cause dissemination of cancer cells to adjacent and distant sites.

! NURSING ALERT

To reinforce the need for caution, it may be necessary to post a sign on the bed that reads "Do not palpate abdomen." Careful bathing and handling are also important in preventing trauma to the tumor site.

Because chemotherapy and radiation therapy (if used) are usually begun immediately after surgery, parents need an explanation of what to expect, such as major benefits and side effects, although the timing of the information should be considered to avoid overwhelming the family. Ideally the nurse should be present during physician-parent conferences to answer questions as they arise afterwards.

Postoperative Care

Despite the extensive surgical intervention necessary in many children with Wilms tumor, the recovery period is usually rapid. The major nursing responsibilities are those after any abdominal surgery. Because of the risk for intestinal obstruction from vincristine-induced adynamic ileus, radiation-induced edema, and postsurgical adhesion formation, the nurse monitors gastrointestinal activity, such as bowel movements, bowel sounds, distention, and vomiting. Other considerations are frequent evaluation of blood pressure and observation for signs of infection, especially during chemotherapy.

Support the Family

The postoperative period may be difficult for parents. The shock of seeing their child immediately after surgery may be the first realization of the seriousness of the diagnosis. From surgery, the stage and pathology of the tumor are determined. The physician discusses this information with the parents. The nurse's presence during this conversation is important to provide additional support and assess the parents' understanding of the information.

Children need an opportunity to deal with their feelings concerning the many procedures to which they have been subjected in rapid succession. Therapeutic play can be beneficial in helping children understand what they have undergone and express their feelings.

RHABDOMYOSARCOMA

Sarcomas, including rhabdomyosarcoma (*rhabdo* means striated), are tumors arising from mesenchymal cells, which normally develop into muscle and other tissues (Wexler, Skapek, & Helman, 2016). Approximately 400 new cases are diagnosed in the United States each year, with almost two-thirds occurring in children younger than 10 years of age; a smaller peak in incidence occurs in early to middle adolescence (Wexler et al., 2016).

Rhabdomyosarcomas originate from undifferentiated mesenchymal cells in muscles, tendons, bursae, and fascia or in fibrous, connective, lymphatic, or vascular tissue. The most common primary sites are the head and neck (especially the orbit), the genitourinary tract, and the extremities, but these tumors can occur in other sites as well.

Rhabdomyosarcoma is classified into histologic subtypes (Box 25.6): embryonal, alveolar, and pleomorphic. More than half are embryonal. Risk factors for rhabdomyosarcoma include high birth weight (embryonal rhabdomyosarcoma) and several genetic conditions, including Li-Fraumeni syndrome, neurofibromatosis type 1, Costello syndrome, and Beckwith-Wiedemann syndrome. At the molecular level, embryonal and alveolar histologies are associated with characteristic genetic abnormalities. As one example, translocations between the *FOXO1* gene on chromosome 13 and either the *PAX3* gene on chromosome 2 or the *PAX7* gene on chromosome 1 are seen in 70% to 80% of alveolar tumors (National Institutes of Health, 2019l).

Clinical Manifestations

The initial signs and symptoms are related to the site of the tumor and compression of adjacent organs (Table 25.5). Some tumor locations, such as the orbit, manifest early in the course of the illness. Other tumors, such as those of the retroperitoneal area, produce symptoms only when they are large enough to cause organ compression. Unfortunately, many of the signs and symptoms attributable to rhabdomyosarcoma are vague and frequently suggest a common childhood illness, such as "earache" or "runny nose." Often it is not possible to identify the site of the primary tumor.

BOX 25.6 Subtypes of Rhabdomyosarcoma

Embryonal—Most common type; most frequently found in the head, neck, abdomen, and genitourinary tract
Alveolar—Second most common type; most often seen in deep tissues of the extremities and trunk
Pleomorphic—Rare in children (adult form); most often occurs in soft parts of extremities and trunk

TABLE 25.5 Clinical Manifestations of Rhabdomyosarcoma According to Tumor Site

Location	Signs and Symptoms
Orbit	Rapidly developing unilateral proptosis Ecchymosis of conjunctiva Loss of extraocular movements (strabismus)
Nasopharynx	Stuffy nose (earliest sign) Nasal obstruction—dysphagia, nasal voice (obstruction of posterior nasal conches), serous otitis media (obstruction of eustachian tube) Pain (sore throat and ear) Epistaxis Palpable neck nodes Visible mass in oropharynx (late sign)
Paranasal sinuses	Nasal obstruction Local pain Discharge Sinusitis Swelling
Middle ear	Signs of chronic serous otitis media Pain Sanguinopurulent drainage Facial nerve palsy
Retroperitoneal area (usually a "silent" tumor)	Abdominal mass Pain Signs of intestinal or genitourinary obstruction
Perineum	Visible superficial mass Bowel or bladder dysfunction (from tumor compression)

Diagnostic Evaluation

Diagnosis begins with a careful history and physical examination, imaging studies, and baseline laboratory studies. An extensive evaluation is then performed to determine the extent of disease. Metastatic evaluation includes chest x-ray and CT scan, CT or MRI for abdominal or pelvic tumors, MRI of the skull and brain for parameningeal tumors, imaging of regional lymph nodes, bilateral bone marrow aspirates and biopsies, and bone scan for selected patients. An excisional biopsy or surgical resection of the tumor, when possible, is done to confirm the diagnosis.

Staging and Prognosis

Careful staging is extremely important for planning treatment and determining the prognosis. Two staging systems are used in

BOX 25.7 Surgicopathologic Staging of Rhabdomyosarcoma

Group I: Localized disease; tumor completely resected and regional nodes not involved
Group II: Localized disease; tumor completely removed; microscopic residual that may have spread into nearby lymph nodes
Group III: Incomplete resection with gross residual disease
Group IV: Metastatic disease present at diagnosis

combination: a surgicopathologic staging system (Box 25.7) and a modified tumor, node, metastasis (TNM) pretreatment staging system. A stage is assigned, based on primary site, tumor size, and whether there is regional lymph node involvement or distant metastasis. A group is assigned based on the status of the surgical resection or biopsy, pathologic assessment of the tumor margin, and lymph node involvement before therapy. Then a risk group is assigned, based on stage, group, and histology (National Institutes of Health, 2019l). Risk refers to the risk of disease recurrence.

Prognosis is related to age, with children ages 1 to 9 years having the best prognosis; primary tumor site, size, and resectability; whether there is lymph node involvement or metastasis at diagnosis; and histologic subtype. The alveolar histologic subtype is associated with worse outcomes. Most rhabdomyosarcomas are curable with the use of contemporary multimodal therapy. More than 70% of patients with localized disease are expected to survive (Wexler et al., 2016). However, if relapse occurs, the prognosis for long-term survival is poor.

Therapeutic Management

Rhabdomyosarcoma is treated with multimodality therapy that includes chemotherapy plus surgery or radiation therapy, or both modalities. The intensity and duration of chemotherapy are based on risk group. Some or all of the following chemotherapeutic drugs are used: vincristine, dactinomycin, cyclophosphamide, ifosfamide, irinotecan, vinorelbine, and doxorubicin. Complete resection of the primary tumor before chemotherapy is advocated whenever possible, if it will not result in disfigurement, functional compromise, or organ dysfunction (National Institutes of Health, 2019l). Otherwise, only an initial biopsy is performed. Radiation therapy is based on risk group and tailored to the primary site and the sites of metastatic disease.

Nursing Care

The nursing responsibilities in caring for a child with rhabdomyosarcoma are similar to those for other types of cancer, especially the other solid tumors for which surgery is used. Specific objectives include careful assessment for signs of tumor, especially during well-child examinations; preparation of the child and family for the multiple diagnostic tests; and supportive care during each stage of multimodal therapy. The reader is urged to review the General Nursing Care Management section earlier in the chapter and Chapter 17 for emotional support of the family in the event of a poor prognosis.

RETINOBLASTOMA

Retinoblastoma, so named because it arises from the retina, is the most common intraocular malignancy of childhood, with approximately 300 new cases diagnosed annually in the United States (Hurwitz, Shields, Shields, et al., 2016). Retinoblastoma can be present at birth, can have single or multiple foci in one or both eyes, and occurs in a heritable form. Of all cases of retinoblastoma, 60% are unilateral and nonhereditary (also called sporadic), 25% are bilateral and hereditary, and 15% are unilateral and hereditary (Hurwitz et al., 2016). Retinoblastoma occurs predominantly in very young children; most cases are diagnosed before 2 years of age (National Institutes of Health, 2019m).

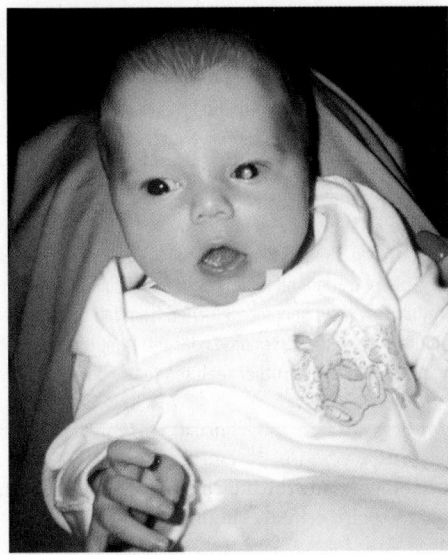
Fig. 25.6 Cat's eye reflex. Whitish appearance of lens is produced as light falls on tumor mass in left eye.

Children with hereditary retinoblastoma tend to be diagnosed at a younger age. In the hereditary form of retinoblastoma, germline mutation of the *RB1* gene is present. The mutation may have been inherited, occurred in a germ cell before conception, or occurred in utero during embryogenesis (Hurwitz et al., 2016). The "two-hit model" was developed to explain hereditary and sporadic retinoblastoma. According to the model, as few as two mutation events can lead to tumor formation; in the hereditary form, the "first hit" occurs in the germline, whereas both hits occur somatically in the sporadic form.

Clinical Manifestations

Retinoblastoma has few grossly obvious signs. Typically parents or relatives are the ones who first observe a whitish "glow" in the pupil, known as the **cat's eye reflex**, or **leukocoria** (Fig. 25.6), which prompts ophthalmoscopic examination. The reflex represents visualization of the tumor as light momentarily falls on the mass. When a tumor arises in the macular region (area directly at the back of the retina when the eye is focused straight ahead), a white reflex may be visible when the tumor is small. It is best observed when a bright light is shining toward the child as the child looks forward, which is why it may be discovered when a flash photograph is taken.

When the tumor arises in the periphery of the retina, it must grow to a considerable size before light can strike it sufficiently to produce the cat's eye reflex. In this situation it is visible only when the child looks sideways or if the observer stands at an oblique angle to the child's face as the child looks straight ahead. The fleeting nature of the reflex often results in a delayed diagnosis because health care professionals fail to appreciate the ominous significance of the parents' observation.

The next most common sign is strabismus resulting from poor fixation of the visually impaired eye, particularly if the tumor develops in the macula, the area of sharpest visual acuity. Blindness is usually a late sign, but it may not be obvious unless the parent or other caregiver consciously observes for behaviors indicating loss of sight, such as bumping into objects, slowed motor development, or turning of

BOX 25.8 International Classification of Retinoblastoma

Group A: Small (3 mm or less) intraretinal tumors away from the optic disc and foveola
Group B: All remaining tumors that are larger than 3 mm and/or close to the optic disc or foveola but remain confined to the retina
Group C: Discrete local disease with minimal disease under the retina (subretinal seeding) or in the gelatinous material of the eye (vitreous seeding)
Group D: Large or poorly defined tumors with significant vitreous or subretinal seeding; retina may have become detached from the back of the eye
Group E: Tumor is very large, extending near the front of the eye; is bleeding or causing glaucoma; or has other features that indicate it is not possible to save the eye

the head to see objects lateral to the affected eye. Other late signs and symptoms include pain, orbital cellulitis, and glaucoma.

Diagnostic Evaluation

A detailed family history and recording of eye signs and symptoms are essential. Children suspected of having retinoblastoma are referred to an ophthalmologist; the diagnosis usually is based on indirect ophthalmoscopy (under anesthesia), ultrasound, CT, and MRI scans. Blood and tumor samples can be tested for *RB1* gene mutations.

Metastatic disease at the time of retinoblastoma diagnosis is rare. For patients with suspected metastatic disease, bone marrow aspirates and biopsies, bone scan, and LP may be performed.

Staging and Prognosis

Staging of retinoblastomas is done under indirect ophthalmoscopy before surgery to accurately determine the tumor size (measured in disc diameter [DD]) and location (according to an imaginary line called the equator drawn on the midplane of the eye) (Hurwitz et al., 2016).

Various classification systems have been used to stage or group retinoblastomas. The Reese-Ellsworth system classifies tumors according to five groups and is used to compare therapeutic results in patients treated with methods other than enucleation (i.e., radiation therapy). A revised classification system, the International Classification of Retinoblastoma, is based on the extent and location of the intraocular tumor; it better predicts globe salvage using contemporary treatments (Box 25.8). The overall 10-year survival rate is nearly 90% for unilateral and bilateral tumors (Hurwitz et al., 2016). Like neuroblastoma, retinoblastoma may spontaneously regress.

A major concern for long-term survivors is the development of SNs. Children with bilateral disease (hereditary form) are more likely to develop subsequent cancers than are children with unilateral disease, and radiation therapy increases their risk.

Therapeutic Management

Treatment of retinoblastoma is complex. Enucleation may be used to treat advanced disease with optic nerve invasion in which vision cannot be salvaged. Radiation therapy can be used when there is vitreous seeding. Chemotherapy has been used to decrease the tumor size to allow treatment with local therapies such as plaque brachytherapy (surgical implantation of an iodine-125 applicator on the sclera until the maximum radiation dose has been delivered to the tumor), photocoagulation (use of a laser beam to destroy retinal blood vessels that supply nutrition to the tumor), and cryotherapy (freezing of the tumor, which destroys the microcirculation to the tumor and the cells themselves through microcrystal formation). Chemotherapy, along with radiation

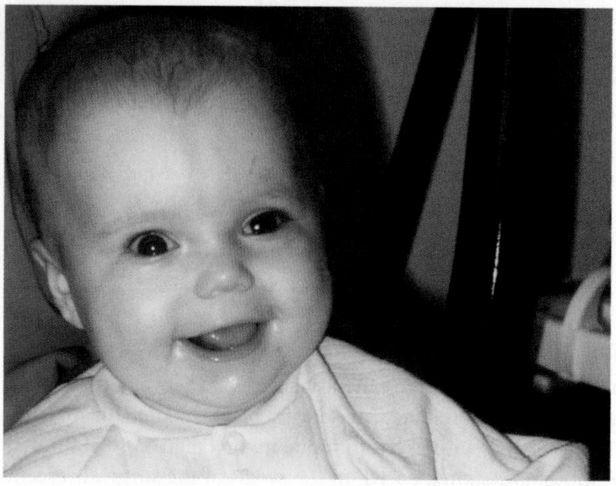

Fig. 25.7 Infant with left prosthetic eye.

or high-dose chemotherapy with autologous stem cell rescue, is used to treat metastatic disease (Hurwitz et al., 2016).

Nursing Care

Prepare the Family for Diagnostic and Therapeutic Procedures and Home Care

Because the tumor is usually diagnosed in infants or very young children, most of the preparation for diagnostic tests and treatment involves parents. Once the disease is staged, the treating team confers with the parents regarding the plan of care. In most cases, enucleation can be avoided. If enucleation is performed, the procedure and the benefits of a prosthesis are explained. Showing parents pictures of another child with an artificial eye may help with adjustment to the procedure (Fig. 25.7). Although the loss of vision is distressing, acknowledging the significance of the loss and emphasizing that the unaffected eye retains normal vision and that the affected eye is probably already blind may be helpful in promoting acceptance of the imposed impairment.

After surgery the parents need to be prepared for the child's facial appearance. An eye patch is in place, and the child's face may be edematous and ecchymotic. Parents often fear seeing the surgical site because they imagine a cavity in the skull. On the contrary, the lids are usually closed, and the area does not appear sunken because a surgically implanted sphere maintains the shape of the eyeball. The implant is covered with conjunctiva, and when the lids are open, the exposed area resembles the mucosal lining of the mouth. Once the child is fitted for a prosthesis, usually within 3 weeks, the facial appearance returns to normal.

After an uneventful recovery from enucleation, plans can be made for discharge from the hospital, usually within 3 to 4 days postoperatively. Parents need instruction on care of the surgical site and preparation for any additional therapy. They should be given the opportunity to see the socket as soon after surgery as possible. A good time to do this without unduly pressuring them is during dressing changes. They should then be encouraged to participate in the dressing changes.

Care of the socket is minimal and easily accomplished. The wound itself is clean and has little or no drainage. If an antibiotic ointment is prescribed, it is applied in a thin line on the surface of the tissues of the socket. The dressing consists of an eye pad changed daily. Once the socket has healed completely, a dressing is no longer necessary, although there are several reasons for having the child continue to wear an eye patch. Infants and toddlers explore their environment with their hands, and without an eye patch in place, the socket is available to exploring fingers. Although there is little danger of the child injuring the socket, parents may feel more secure with the socket covered. This also helps prevent infection.

The ocularist, who fits and manufactures the prosthesis, gives initial instructions for care of the device. Once in place, the prosthesis need not be removed unless cleaning is necessary, in which case it is taken out by gently pulling down on the lower lid, which frees the lower edge of the prosthesis, and applying pressure to the upper lid. The prosthesis is cleaned by placing it in hot water and soaking it for several minutes. Reinsertion is easier if the prosthesis remains wet. To reinsert the prosthesis, the lids are separated, and with the prosthesis held in the correct position (it should be marked to indicate the nasal side), it is pushed up under the upper lid, allowing the lower lid to cover its lower edge.

Safety is a major concern to prevent damage to the unaffected eye. Safety measures should be practiced at all times, and children should avoid rough contact sports or wear protective eyewear.

Support the Family

The diagnosis of retinoblastoma presents some special concerns in addition to those raised by cancer in general. Families with a history of retinoblastoma may feel guilt for transmitting the mutation to their offspring, especially if they knowingly "played the odds" in conceiving an affected child. Conversely, when parents are aware of the probability and have an affected child, early treatment results in such favorable outcomes that parental adjustment may be rapid. In families with no history of retinoblastoma, the diagnosis is a shock, frequently complicated by guilt for not having discovered it sooner. Because parents often are the first to observe the cat's eye reflex, they may be angry at themselves or others, especially health care professionals, if a more thorough examination was delayed. The nurse should consider each of these variables while offering supportive care to the family. Active listening is helpful.

Other concerns also relate to the hereditary aspects of the disease. Of great importance to parents is the risk of retinoblastoma in their subsequent offspring and in the offspring of the surviving affected child. With improving prognoses for these children, genetic counseling is assuming greater importance (see Chapter 3 for a discussion of the nurse's role in genetic counseling).

Encourage these families to seek regular follow-up care for the affected child for early identification of possible SNs. Offspring of unaffected parents and survivors should undergo regular ophthalmoscopy to detect retinoblastoma at its earliest stage.

GERM CELL TUMORS

Germ cell tumors (GCTs) account for approximately 3% of cancers in children younger than 15 years and 14% of cancers in adolescents 15 to 19 years (National Institutes of Health, 2019n). They can arise in gonadal and extragonadal sites and are broadly classified as teratomas (mature and immature) or malignant germ cell tumors (National Institutes of Health, 2019n). GCTs can appear in various body sites, including the testicles (e.g., yolk sac tumor, teratoma), ovaries (e.g., teratoma, germinoma, yolk sac tumor), sacrococcyx, mediastinum, and retroperitoneum (Frazier, Olson, Schneider, et al., 2016; National Institutes of Health, 2019n). In general, most children with teratomas and localized gonadal tumors that are surgically resected can be observed without the need for further therapy. For patients with more advanced disease, chemotherapy has produced excellent results.

LIVER TUMORS

Primary liver tumors are rare in childhood; they are divided into two main histologic subtypes, hepatoblastoma (infants and young children) and hepatocellular carcinoma (individuals ages 5 to 15 years), with hepatoblastoma being most common (National Institutes of Health, 2019o). Surgical resection is the treatment of choice for liver tumors, usually performed after the administration of platinum-based chemotherapy to increase the likelihood of complete resection (Meyers, Trobaugh-Lotrario, Malogolowkin, et al., 2016). Liver transplant should be used for unresectable tumors. Survival rates for patients with hepatoblastoma can be as high as 90% with current therapies (Aronson & Meyers, 2016).

THE CHILDHOOD CANCER SURVIVOR

Survival rates for children with cancer have greatly improved over the past decades, so that long-term survival is expected for more than 80% of children with access to contemporary therapy for cancer (National Institutes of Health, 2019p). Curative therapy can also produce adverse health outcomes, referred to as late effects, which may become apparent months to years after cancer treatment is completed. Survivorship research has demonstrated that 60% to 90% of adult survivors of childhood cancer develop chronic health conditions; of these, 20% to 80% experience severe or life-threatening complications (Landier et al., 2016). Late effects are related to therapeutic exposures (chemotherapy, surgery, radiation therapy, HSCT) and are also influenced by host factors such as genetic predisposition, age at diagnosis or treatment, comorbid health conditions, and health habits (National Institutes of Health, 2019p).

All survivors should have risk-based medical follow-up that includes a survivorship care plan for lifelong screening, surveillance, and health promotion. Because nurses in pediatric and adult primary care settings may encounter childhood cancer survivors, they should be aware of the risk-based, exposure-based guidelines developed by the Children's Oncology Group (2013) and endorsed by the American Academy of Pediatrics (2009). The Children's Oncology Group long-term follow-up guidelines include patient education materials ("Health Links") on guideline-specific topics that can be downloaded for use (Landier et al., 2016). The current fifth edition can be retrieved from http://www.survivorshipguidelines.org/.

Childhood cancer survivors have an elevated risk for disease and treatment-related morbidity and mortality that persists long after disease cure (Landier et al., 2016). Survivorship research has contributed to better characterization of late effects, as well as to modification of treatment regimens to minimize the risk of late effects. As therapeutic options evolve, nurses will need to stay current with ongoing research to determine best practices for continued improvement in both the duration and the quality of survival after childhood cancer.

NEXT-GENERATION NCLEX® EXAMINATION-STYLE UNFOLDING CASE STUDY

The Child With Acute Lymphoblastic Leukemia

Tadala Mulemba

Day 1, 8:00 am

1. A 7-year-old male developed bilateral neck swelling 1 month ago and is being seen in the Emergency Department. His mother had taken him to a nearby health center twice because the swelling is increasing in size; oral antibiotics were prescribed. Two-weeks later, he now has hoarseness when speaking and his mother also reports that he is sleeping most of the time. On presentation to the hospital this morning, the complete blood count revealed a hemoglobin of 6.0 g/dl, white blood cell (WBC) of 85,000/mm^3 and a platelet count of 60,000/mm^3. On examination, the child has bilateral parotid gland enlargement, submental nodes and axillary nodes, and hepatomegaly approximately 6cm below the right subcostal margin. Leukemia is suspected and the child is admitted for further evaluation. Based on the list below, what are the most common signs and symptoms of leukemia the nurse would look for? **Select all that apply.**
   A. Fever
   B. Seizure
   C. Fatigue
   D. Infection
   E. Bone pain
   F. Short stature
   G. Shortness of breath
   H. Lymphadenopathy
   I. Hepatosplenomegaly
   J. Bruising and bleeding

Day 1, 8:00 am Continued

2. It is important for the nurse to be aware of the pathophysiology associated with the signs and symptoms of childhood leukemia. Symptoms are caused by bone marrow dysfunction that cause the rapidly proliferating leukemia cells to depress bone marrow production of the formed elements of the blood. **Choose the most likely options for the information missing from the table below by selecting from the lists of options provided.**

Symptom	Pathophysiology	Assessment Finding
Anemia	2	Pale, tired, listless
Infection	Decreased production of WBCs	3
1	Decreased production of platelets	Nosebleed, bruising
Bone pain	Increased pressure	Unable to bear weight on legs

Option 1	Option 2	Option 3
Seizure	Decreased production of RBCs	Lack of appetite and weight loss
Blindness	Increased production of plasma cells	Headache and seizure
Hemorrhage	Decreased production of CNS fluid	Enlarged spleen
Hearing loss	Increased production of bilirubin	Fever and infection

Day 1, 4:00 pm

3. This afternoon a diagnostic work-up was completed and the child underwent a bone marrow aspiration and biopsy. Flow cytometry revealed 70% B-cell leukemia blast cells and the diagnosis of acute lymphoblastic leukemia (ALL) is confirmed. He is to start chemotherapy tomorrow as part of the initial therapy for ALL. The child's WBC is extremely high, 85,000/mm^3 this morning and he is at risk for tumor lysis syndrome. **Choose the most likely options for the information missing from the statements below by selecting from the lists of options provided.**
   Children who present with a high WBC caused by leukemia are at risk for ____1____ abnormalities that are a direct result of the ____2____ release of intracellular contents during the ____3____ of malignant cells, in this child's case- leukemia cells.

Options for 1	Options for 2	Options for 3
cardiac	rapid	production
cellular	slow	growth
metabolic	intermittent	lysis
neurologic	prolonged	mitosis

Day 1, 5:00 pm

4. A 7-year-old male was diagnosed with acute lymphocytic leukemia and has done well overnight. He continues on IV fluids and medication to reduce uric acid formation and prevent tumor lysis syndrome. He is due to start chemotherapy today and will undergo a lumbar puncture with intrathecal chemotherapy administered to prevent invasion of leukemia cells into the CNS. The nurse is preparing the child and family for the lumbar puncture procedure. **For each nursing action, use an X to indicate whether it was Effective (helped to meet expected quality patient outcomes), Ineffective (did not help to meet expected quality patient outcomes), or Unrelated (not related to the quality patient outcomes).**

Nursing Action	Effective	Ineffective	Unrelated
Explain the procedure to the patient and family and obtain informed consent.			
Monitor vital signs during the procedure (pulse rate, oxygen saturation, respirations, blood pressure).			
Administer a bolus of IV fluids before the procedure begins.			
Administer sedation during the procedure to provide optimal comfort and minimize pain.			
Provide comfort and reassure the patient and family throughout the procedure.			
Allow the child to watch a favorite show before the procedure.			
Watch for signs of bleeding from the puncture site.			

NEXT-GENERATION NCLEX® EXAMINATION-STYLE UNFOLDING CASE STUDY—cont'd

The Child With Acute Lymphoblastic Leukemia

Day 2, 8:00 am

25.5. A 7-year-old male was diagnosed today with Acute Lymphocytic Leukemia confirmed by bone marrow examination and a complete diagnostic work up. He will begin chemotherapy tomorrow. Orders are written for preventing tumor lysis syndrome since his WBC is 85,000mm^3. Which of the following actions would the nurse take? **Select all that apply.**

A. Restrict IV fluids
B. Monitor WBC
C. Check urine pH with each void
D. Administer aggressive IV fluids
E. Monitor serum chemistries frequently
F. Maintain strict record of intake and output
G. Administer medication to prevent heart failure
H. Administer medication to reduce uric acid formation

Day 5, 8:00 am

6. A 7-year-old male was diagnosed with acute lymphocytic leukemia five days ago and has no complications from starting chemotherapy. He remains afebrile and the blood count today reveals a hemoglobin of 8.0 g/dl, white blood cell (WBC) of 10,000/mm^3 and a platelet count of 65,000/mm^3. Packed red blood cells were given on day 3 due to decreasing hemoglobin. The WBC count has decreased dramatically from 85,000/mm^3 to 10,000/mm^3. Chemistries are without evidence of tumor lysis syndrome. Plans are for the child to be discharged in the next 2 days if he does not develop fever and there are no signs of tumor lysis. The nurse begins preparing the child and family for discharge. **Indicate which nursing action listed in the far-left column is appropriate for potential complications following the start of leukemia treatment listed in the middle column, indicate the nursing action number in the far-right column.**

<u>Note that ONLY one nursing action can be used for each potential complication and that NOT all nursing actions will be used.</u>

Nursing Action	Potential Complication	Nursing Action to prevent Complication
1. Explain the disease course of treatment and adverse effects to the family.	Skin as an entry point for infection	
2. Teach the patient and family ways to prevent infection through hand washing, bathing frequently, and not using cups and utensils used by another person.	Lack of recognition of infection	
3. Teach the family how to recognize symptoms of infection such as fever, chills, cough, and sore throat and report these to the health care worker immediately.	Lack of understanding of leukemia treatment	
4. Provide skin care to patient by keeping the skin and perianal area clean and apply mild lotion.	Mouth ulceration	
5. Provide a high-protein and high-calorie diet.	Lack of knowledge on how to prevent infection in the home	
6. Provide adequate hydration and encourage a high-fiber diet and stool softeners.	Bleeding	
7. Educate family and patient on how to recognize and report abnormal bleeding through bruising and petechiae.		
8. Provide frequent mouth care and saline rinses and check for ulcers in the mouth and gum swelling.		
9. Instruct patient and family to avoid contact sports.		

CLINICAL JUDGMENT AND NEXT-GENERATION NCLEX® EXAMINATION-STYLE QUESTIONS

1. A new nurse is in orientation on the pediatric cancer ward. She is working with her preceptor to administer chemotherapy to a newly diagnosed child with leukemia. The child is to receive intravenous Vincristine today. Which nursing actions are appropriate for the nurse to perform? **Select all that apply.**
   A. Wear disposable gloves and protective clothing
   B. Make sure drugs are prepared in a properly ventilated room
   C. Use strict aseptic technique when administering chemotherapy agents
   D. Use a sterile gauze pad when connecting the syringe to the IV tubing
   E. Make sure air is out of the chemotherapy syringe by slowly injecting into the air
   F. Dispose of all contaminated materials in a leak-proof and puncture-resistant contained
   G. Wear face and eye protection that includes a respirator at all times when handling the agent

2. A 5-year-old boy with cancer is experiencing mucositis from receiving methotrexate a week ago. He had a fever and since his blood count shows the WBCs are less than 1,000,/mm ^{3} he is admitted for antibiotics and observation. The nurse is to provide mouth care this morning. Which of the following principles would be followed when providing oral care for a child with mucositis? **Use an X for the nursing action statement below that is Indicated (appropriate or necessary), Contraindicated (could be harmful), or Non-Essential (makes no difference or not necessary).**

Nursing Action	Indicated	Contraindicated	Non-Essential
Viscous lidocaine should be used to swish the mouth three times per day			
Perform mouth care routinely before and after feeding			
Lemon glycerin swabs are helpful because they remind children of lemon drops.			
Allowing the child to sleep 8 hours will help recovery			
Using a soft sponge–type toothbrush will decrease the tendency of gums to bleed.			
Sodium bicarbonate and saltwater rinses can be used			

3. Infection prevention is a major goal during treatment for childhood cancer. The nurse is caring for a family who has a newly diagnosed child with lymphoma. The doctor has told them that their child's blood counts will be extremely low after receiving chemotherapy. Their child is a 6-year-old boy who just finished his first treatment cycle. When considering the need for the family to understand the importance of the white blood cell count, complete the following statements. **Choose the most likely options for the information missing from the statements below by selecting from the lists of options provided.**
   Children receiving treatment for cancer experience low white blood cell counts and for this reason, they are closely monitored. The ____1____ cell count reflects the risk for infection and is determined by ____2____ the white blood cell count by percentage of ____3____.

Options for 1	Options for 2	Options for 3
absolute red blood	subtracting	platelets
absolute platelet	multiplying	monocytes
absolute neutrophil	dividing	neutrophils
absolute white blood	adding	eosinophils

4. The parents of a child with a possible cancer diagnosis ask how the physician will know what type of cancer their child has. Their son is 14 years of age and presented with an enlarged subclavian lymph node. He completed the diagnostic evaluation and the diagnosis is confirmed as Hodgkin lymphoma. What teaching would the nurse present at this time on Hodgkin lymphoma to answer the parent's question? **Select all that apply.**
   A. Radiographic tests are used to determine the extent of disease.
   B. A lymph node biopsy is essential to establish the histologic diagnosis.
   C. Hodgkin lymphoma is staged to determine the extent of spread throughout the body.
   D. The presence of lymphoblastic cells is considered diagnostic of Hodgkin lymphoma.
   E. Hodgkin lymphoma often presents with an enlarged, firm, nontender, movable nodes in the supraclavicular or cervical area.
   F. Tests used to confirm the diagnosis include a complete blood count, prothrombin time and
   G. glucose-6-phosphate dehydrogenase (G6PD), erythropoietin, and sedimentation rate.
   H. The presence of a white reflection as opposed to the normal red pupillary reflex in the pupil of a child's eye is a classic sign.

REFERENCES

Allen, C. E., Kamdar, K. Y., Bollard, C. M., et al. (2016). Non-Hodgkin lymphomas in children. In P. A. Pizzo, & D. G. Poplack (Eds.), *Principles and practices of pediatric oncology* (7th ed.). Philadelphia: Lippincott.

American Academy of Pediatrics (AAP). (2009). Long-term follow-up care for pediatric cancer survivors. *Pediatrics, 123*, 906–915.

American Academy of Pediatrics (AAP). (2018). Committee on Infectious Diseases. In D. W. Kimberlin, M. T. Brady, & M. A. Jackson (Eds.), *2015 Red book: Report of the committee on infectious diseases* (31st ed.). Elk Grove Village, IL: AAP.

American Academy of Pediatrics (AAP). (2019). 2019 Recommendations for Preventive Pediatric Health Care. *Pediatrics, 143*(3). Retrieved from https://pediatrics.aappublications.org/content/143/3/e20183971.

American Childhood Cancer Organization. (2016). *International statistics (summary of IARC Report)*. Retrieved from https://www.acco.org/global-childhood-cancer-statistics/.

Andrews, J., Galel, S. A., Wong, W., et al. (2016). Hematologic supportive care for children with cancer. In P. A. Pizzo, & D. G. Poplack (Eds.), *Principles and practice of pediatric oncology* (7th ed.). Philadelphia: Lippincott.

Ardura, M. I., & Koh, A. Y. (2016). Infectious complications in pediatric cancer patients. In P. A. Pizzo, & D. G. Poplack (Eds.), *Principles and practice of pediatric oncology* (7th ed.). Philadelphia: Lippincott.

Aronson, D. C., & Meyers, R. L. (2016). Malignant tumors of the liver in children. *Seminars in Pediatric Surgery, 25*(5), 265–275.

Becze, E. (2017). Nursing considerations for adverse events from CAR T-cell therapy. ONS Voice. May 9. Retrieved from https://voice.ons.org/news-and-views/nursing-considerations-for-adverse-events-from-car-t-cell-therapy.

Bhatia, S., Landier, W., Shangguan, M., et al. (2012). Nonadherence to oral mercaptopurine and risk of relapse in Hispanic and non-Hispanic white children with acute lymphoblastic leukemia: A report from the Children's Oncology Group. *Journal of Clinical Oncology: Official Journal of the American Society of Clinical Oncology, 30*(17), 2094–2101.

Brodeur, G. M., Hogarty, M. D., Bagatell, R., et al. (2016). Neuroblastoma. In P. A. Pizzo, & D. G. Poplack (Eds.), *Principles and practice of pediatric oncology* (7th ed.). Philadelphia: Lippincott.

Burgoyne, L. L., Billups, C. A., Jirón, J. L., Jr., et al. (2012). Phantom limb pain in young cancer related amputees: Recent experience at St Jude Children's Research Hospital. *Clinical Journal of Pain, 28*, 222–225.

Centers for Disease Control and Prevention (CDC), & U.S. Department of Health & Human Services. (2018). *HPV vaccine recommendations*. Retrieved from https://www.cdc.gov/vaccines/vpd/hpv/hcp/recommendations.html.

Centers for Disease Control and Prevention (CDC), & U.S. Department of Health & Human Services. (2019). *What are the risk factors for skin cancer*. Retrieved from https://www.cdc.gov/cancer/skin/basic_info/risk_factors.htm.

Ceppi, F., Beck-Popovic, M., Bourquin, J. P., et al. (2017). Opportunities and challenges in the immunological therapy of pediatric malignancy: A concise snapshot. *European Journal of Pediatrics*.

Chaveli-Lopez, B., & Bagan-Sebastian, J. V. (2016). Treatment of oral mucositis due to chemotherapy. *J Clin Exp Denta, 8*(2), e201–e209.

Children's Oncology Group. (2013). *Long-term follow-up guidelines for survivors of childhood, adolescent and young adult cancers*. Retreived from http://www.survivorshipguidelines.org.

Crawford, J. (2013). Childhood brain tumors. *Pediatrics in Review, 34*(2), 63–78.

Effinger, K. E., Migliorati, C. A., Hudson, M. M., et al. (2014). Oral and dental late effects in survivors of childhood cancer: A Children's Oncology Group report. *Supportive Care in Cancer, 22*(7), 2009–2019.

Fernandez, C. V., Geller, J. I., Ehrlich, P. F., et al. (2016). Renal tumors. In P. A. Pizzo, & D. G. Poplack (Eds.), *Principles and practice of pediatric oncology* (7th ed.). Philadelphia.

Fielding, F., Sanford, T. M., & Davis, M. P. (2013). Achieving effective control in cancer pain: A review of current guidelines. *International Journal of Palliative Nursing, 19*, 584–591.

Foggo, V., & Cavenagh, J. (2015). Malignant causes of fever of unknown origin. *Clin Med (Lond), 15*, 252–294.

Frazier, A. L., Olson, T. A., Schneider, D. R., et al. (2016). Germ cell tumors. In P. A. Pizzo, & D. G. Poplack (Eds.), *Principles and practice of pediatric oncology* (7th ed.). Philadelphia: Lippincott.

Freedman, J. L., Rheingold, S. R., & Fisher, M. J. (2016). Oncologic emergencies. In P. A. Pizzo, & D. G. Poplack (Eds.), *Principles and practice of pediatric oncology* (7th ed.). Philadelphia: Lippincott.

Frew, J. A., Lewis, J., & Lucraft, H. H. (2013). The management of children with lymphomas. *Clinical Oncology, 25*, 11–18.

Gore, L., DeGregori, J., & Porter, C. C. (2013). Targeting developmental pathways in children with cancer: What price success? *The Lancet Oncology, 14*(2), e70–e78.

Gorlick, R., Janeway, K., & Marina, N. (2016). Osteosarcoma. In P. A. Pizzo, & D. G. Poplack (Eds.), *Principles and practice of pediatric oncology* (7th ed.). Philadelphia: Lippincott.

Gottschalk, S., Naik, S., Hegde, M., et al. (2016). Hematopoietic stem cell transplantation in pediatric oncology. In P. A. Pizzo, & D. G. Poplack (Eds.), *Principles and practice of pediatric oncology* (7th ed.). Philadelphia: Lippincott.

Hawkins, D. S., Bolling, T., Brennan, B. M. D., et al. (2016). Ewing sarcoma. In P. A. Pizzo, & D. G. Poplack (Eds.), *Principles and practice of pediatric oncology* (7th ed.). Philadelphia: Lippincott.

Hill-Kayser, C., Tochner, Z., Both, S., et al. (2013). Proton versus photon radiation therapy for patients with high-risk neuroblastoma: The need for a customized approach. *Pediatric Blood and Cancer, 60*(10), 1606–1611.

Hockenberry, M. J., Kline, N. E., & Rodgers, C. (2016). Nursing support of the child with cancer. In P. A. Pizzo, & D. G. Poplack (Eds.), *Principles and practice of pediatric oncology* (7th ed.). Philadelphia: Lippincott.

Hurwitz, R. L., Shields, C. L., Shields, J. A., et al. (2016). Retinoblastoma. In P. A. Pizzo, & D. G. Poplack (Eds.), *Principles and practice of pediatric oncology* (7th ed.). Philadelphia: Lippincott.

Image Gently®. (2014). *Mission statement update*. Retrieved from http://www.imagegently.org/.

Karakukcu, M., & Unal, E. (2015). Stem cell mobilization and collection from pediatric patients and healthy children. *Transfusion and Apheresis Science, 53*, 17–22.

Krane, E. J., Casillas, J., & Zeltzer, L. K. (2016). Pain and symptom management. In P. A. Pizzo, & D. G. Poplack (Eds.), *Principles and practice of pediatric oncology* (7th ed.). Philadelphia: Lippincott.

Landier, W., Ahern, J., Barakat, L. P., et al. (2016). Patient/family education for newly diagnosed pediatric oncology patients. *Journal of Pediatric Oncology Nursing, 33*(6), 422–431.

Landier, W., Armenian, S. H., Meadows, A. T., et al. (2016). Late effects of childhood cancer and its treatment. In P. A. Pizzo, & D. G. Poplack (Eds.), *Principles and practice of pediatric oncology* (7th ed.). Philadelphia: Lippincott.

Lawson, C. M., Daley, B. J., Sams, V. G., et al. (2013). Factors that impact patient outcome: Nutrition assessment. *Journal of Parenteral and Enteral Nutrition, 37*(Suppl. 5), 30S–38S.

Luo, Y., & Anderson, T. A. (2016). Phantom limb pain: A review. *International Anesthesiol Clinics, 54*, 121–139.

Lutwak, N., Howland, M. A., Gambetta, R., et al. (2013). Even "safe" medications need to be administered with care. *BMJ Case Reports*.

Metzger, M., Krasin, M. J., Choi, J. K., et al. (2016). Hodgkin lymphoma. In P. A. Pizzo, & D. G. Poplack (Eds.), *Principles and practices of pediatric oncology* (7th ed.). Philadelphia: Lippincott.

Meyers, R. L., Trobough-Lotrario, A. D., Malogolowkin, M. H., et al. (2016). Pediatric liver tumors. In P. A. Pizzo, & D. G. Poplack (Eds.), *Principles and practice of pediatric oncology* (7th ed.). Philadelphia: Lippincott.

National Institutes of Health (NIH), & National Cancer Institute. (2019a). *Targeted cancer therapies*. Retrieved from https://www.cancer.gov/about-cancer/treatment/types/targeted-therapies/targeted-therapies-fact-sheet.

National Institutes of Health (NIH), & National Cancer Institute. (2019b). *Cannabis and cannabinoids (PDQ)*. Retrieved from https://www.cancer.gov/about-cancer/treatment/cam/hp/cannabis-pdq#cit/section_2.4.

National Institutes of Health (NIH), & National Cancer Institute. (2019c). *Childhood acute lymphoblastic leukemia treatment*. Retrieved from https://www.cancer.gov/types/leukemia/hp/child-all-treatment-pdq.

National Institutes of Health (NIH), & National Cancer Institute. (2019d). *Childhood acute myeloid malignancies treatment*. Retrieved from https://www.cancer.gov/types/leukemia/hp/child-aml-treatment-pdq.

National Institutes of Health (NIH), & National Cancer Institute. (2019e). *Childhood Hodgkin lymphoma treatment*. Retrieved from https://www.cancer.gov/types/lymphoma/hp/child-hodgkin-treatment-pdq.

National Institutes of Health (NIH), & National Cancer Institute. (2019f). *Childhood Non-Hodgkin lymphoma treatment*. Retrieved from https://www.cancer.gov/types/lymphoma/patient/child-nhl-treatment-pdq.

National Institutes of Health (NIH), & National Cancer Institute. (2019g). *Childhood astrocytomas treatment*. Retrieved from https://www.cancer.gov/types/brain/hp/child-astrocytoma-treament-pdq.

National Institutes of Health (NIH), & National Cancer Institute. (2019h). *Neuroblastoma treatment*. Retrieved from https://www.cancer.gov/types/neuroblastoma/hp/neuroblastoma-treatment-pdq.

National Institutes of Health (NIH), & National Cancer Institute. (2019i). *Osteosarcoma and malignant fibrous histiocytoma of bone treatment*. Retrieved from https://www.cancer.gov/types/bone/hp/osteosarcoma-treatment-pdq.

National Institutes of Health (NIH), & National Cancer Institute. (2019j). *Ewing sarcoma treatment*. Retrieved from https://www.cancer.gov/types/bone/hp/ewing-treatment-pdq.

National Institutes of Health (NIH), & National Cancer Institute. (2019k). *Wilms tumor treatment*. Retrieved from https://www.cancer.gov/types/kidney/hp/wilms-treatment-pdq.

National Institutes of Health (NIH), & National Cancer Institute. (2019l). *Childhood rhabdomyosarcoma treatment*. Retrieved from https://www.ncbi.nlm.nih.gov/pubmedhealth/PMH0032852/.

National Institutes of Health (NIH), & National Cancer Institute. (2019m). *Retinoblastoma treatment*. Retrieved from https://www.ncbi.nlm.nih.gov/pubmedhealth/PMH0032680/.

National Institutes of Health (NIH), & National Cancer Institute. (2019n). *Childhood extracranial germ cell tumors treatment*. Retrieved from https://www.cancer.gov/types/extracranial-germ-cell/hp/germ-cell-treatment-pdq.

National Institutes of Health (NIH), & National Cancer Institute. (2019o). *Childhood liver cancer treatment*. Retrieved from https://www.ncbi.nlm.nih.gov/pubmedhealth/PMH0032595/.

National Institutes of Health (NIH), & National Cancer Institute. (2019p). *Late effects of treatment for childhood cancer*. Retrieved from https://www.cancer.gov/types/childhood-cancers/late-effects-hp-pdq.

Page, R., & Blanchard, E. (2019). Opioids and cancer pain: Patients' needs and access challenges. *Journal of Oncology Practice, 15*(5), 229–232.

Parsons, D. W., Pollack, I. F., Hass-Kogan, D. A., et al. (2016). Gliomas, ependymomas, and other nonembryonal tumors of the central nervous system. In P. A. Pizzo, & D. G. Poplack (Eds.), *Principles and practice of pediatric oncology* (7th ed.). Philadelphia: Lippincott.

Patel, P., Robinson, P. D., Thackray, J., et al. (2017). Guideline for the prevention of acute chemotherapy-induced nausea and vomiting in pediatric cancer patients: A focused update. *Pediatric Blood and Cancer,* epub ahead of print.

Poussaint, T. Y., Panigrahy, A., & Huisman, T. A. (2015). Pediatric brain tumors. *Pediatric Radiology, 45*(Suppl. 3), S443–S453.

Rabin, K. R., Gramatges, M. M., Margolin, J. F., et al. (2016). Acute lymphoblastic leukemia. In P. A. Pizzo, & D. G. Poplack (Eds.), *Principles and practice of pediatric oncology* (7th ed.). Philadelphia: Lippincott.

Sarvaria, A., Jawdat, D., Madrigal, J. A., et al. (2017). Umbilical cord blood natural killer cells, their characteristics, and potential clinical applications. *Frontiers in Immunology, 23*(8), 329.

Scheurer, M. E., Lupo, P. J., & Bondy, M. L. (2016). Epidemiology of childhood cancer. In P. A. Pizzo, & D. G. Poplack (Eds.), *Principles and practice of pediatric oncology* (7th ed.). Philadelphia: Lippincott.

Spector, L. G., Pankratz, N., & Marcotte, E. L. (2015). Genetic and nongenetic risk factors for childhood cancer. *Pediatr Clin North Am, 62*(1), 11–25.

Ullrich, C. K., Sourkes, B. M., & Wolfe, J. (2016). Palliative care for the child with cancer. In P. A. Pizzo, & D. G. Poplack (Eds.), *Principles and practice of pediatric oncology* (7th ed.). Philadelphia: Lippincott.

US Food and Drug Administration (FDA). (2016). *Information about chemotherapy, biological therapy and immunotherapy*, November 10. Retrieved from https://www.fda.gov/forpatients/illness/cancer/ucm412505.htm.

US Preventive Services Task Force (USPSTF). (2016). *Final Update Summary: Testicular Cancer: Screening, September*. Retrieved from https://www.uspreventiveservicestaskforce.org/Page/Document/UpdateSummaryFinal/testicular-cancer-screening.

US Preventive Services Task Force (USPSTF). (2018). *Final Update Summary: Breast cancer: Screening, February*. Retrieved from https://www.uspreventiveservicestaskforce.org/Page/Document/UpdateSummaryFinal/breast-cancer-screening1.

Wexler, L. H., Skapek, S. X., & Helman, L. J. (2016). Rhabdomyosarcoma. In P. A. Pizzo, & D. G. Poplack (Eds.), *Principles and practice of pediatric oncology* (7th ed.). Philadelphia: Lippincott.

Wiemels, J. L., Walsh, K. M., deSmith, A. J., et al. (2018). GWAS in childhood acute lymphoblastic leukemia reveals novel genetic associations at chromosomes 17q12 and 8q24.21. *Nature Communications, 9*(1), 1–8.

Wong, S. S., & Wilens, T. E. (2017). Medical cannabinoids in children and adolescents: A systematic review. *Pediatrics, 140*(5), e20171818.

World Health Organization (WHO). (2019). *WHO definitions of genetics and genomics*. Retrieved from https://www.who.int/genomics/geneticsVSgenomics/en/.

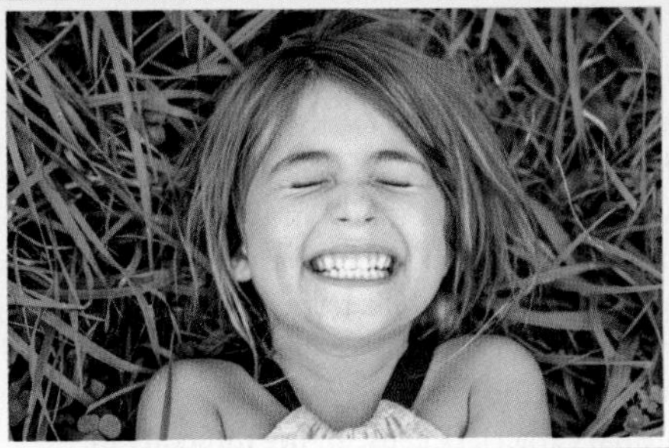

26

The Child With Genitourinary Dysfunction

Maryellen S. Kelly

http://evolve.elsevier.com/wong/essentials

CONCEPTS

- Infection
- Acid-Base Balance
- Fluid Reflection

GENITOURINARY DYSFUNCTION

Assessment of kidney and urinary tract integrity and diagnosis of renal or urinary tract disease are based on several evaluative tools. Physical examination, history taking, and observation of symptoms are the initial procedures. In suspected urinary tract diseases or disorders, further assessment by laboratory, radiologic, and other evaluative methods is carried out. Fig. 26.1 provides a review of the kidney and nephron structures.

CLINICAL MANIFESTATIONS

As in most disorders of childhood, the incidence and type of kidney or urinary tract dysfunction will change with the age and maturation of the child. In addition, the presenting complaints and the significance of these complaints vary with age. For example, a complaint of enuresis has greater significance at 8 years old than at 4 years old. In newborns, renal abnormalities may be associated with a number of other malformations—for example, obvious neural tube defects to the subtle abnormal shape or position of the outer ear. Failure to thrive in children may be a sign of impaired renal function.

Many of the clinical manifestations of renal disease are common to a variety of childhood disorders, but their presence is an indication to obtain further information from the child's history, family history, and laboratory studies as part of a complete physical examination. Suspected renal disease can be further evaluated by means of radiographic studies and renal biopsy (Table 26.1).

LABORATORY TESTS

Both urine and blood studies contribute vital information for detection of renal problems. The single most important test is probably routine urinalysis. Specific urine and blood tests provide additional information. Because nurses are usually the individuals who collect the specimens for examination and who often perform many of the screening tests, they should be familiar with the test, its function, and factors that can alter or distort the results of the test. The major urine and blood tests are outlined in Tables 26.2 and 26.3.

NURSING CARE MANAGEMENT

Nursing responsibilities in the assessment of genitourinary disorders or diseases begin with observation of the child for any manifestations that might indicate dysfunction. Many conditions have specific characteristics that distinguish them from other disorders. These are discussed as appropriate throughout the chapter.

The nurse is generally responsible for preparing infants, children, and parents for tests and for collection of urine and (sometimes) blood specimens for observation and laboratory analysis (see Chapter 20, Preparation for Diagnostic and Therapeutic Procedures and Collection of Specimens). An important nursing responsibility is to maintain careful intake and output measurements and blood pressure for most children with genitourinary dysfunction and those who might be at risk for developing renal complications (e.g., children in shock, postoperative patients). For example, any significant degree of renal disease can diminish the glomerular filtration rate (GFR), a measure of the amount of plasma from which a given substance is totally cleared in 1 minute. A number of substances can be used, but the most useful clinical estimation of glomerular filtration is the clearance of **creatinine**, an end product of protein metabolism in muscle and a substance that is freely filtered by the glomerulus and secreted by renal tubular cells. The nurse's responsibility in this test is collection of urine, usually a 12- or 24-hour specimen.

GENITOURINARY TRACT DISORDERS AND DEFECTS

Urinary Tract Infection

Urinary tract infection (UTI) is a common and potentially serious problem in children. The overall prevalence is approximately 7% in infants and young children, although there is some variability based on age,

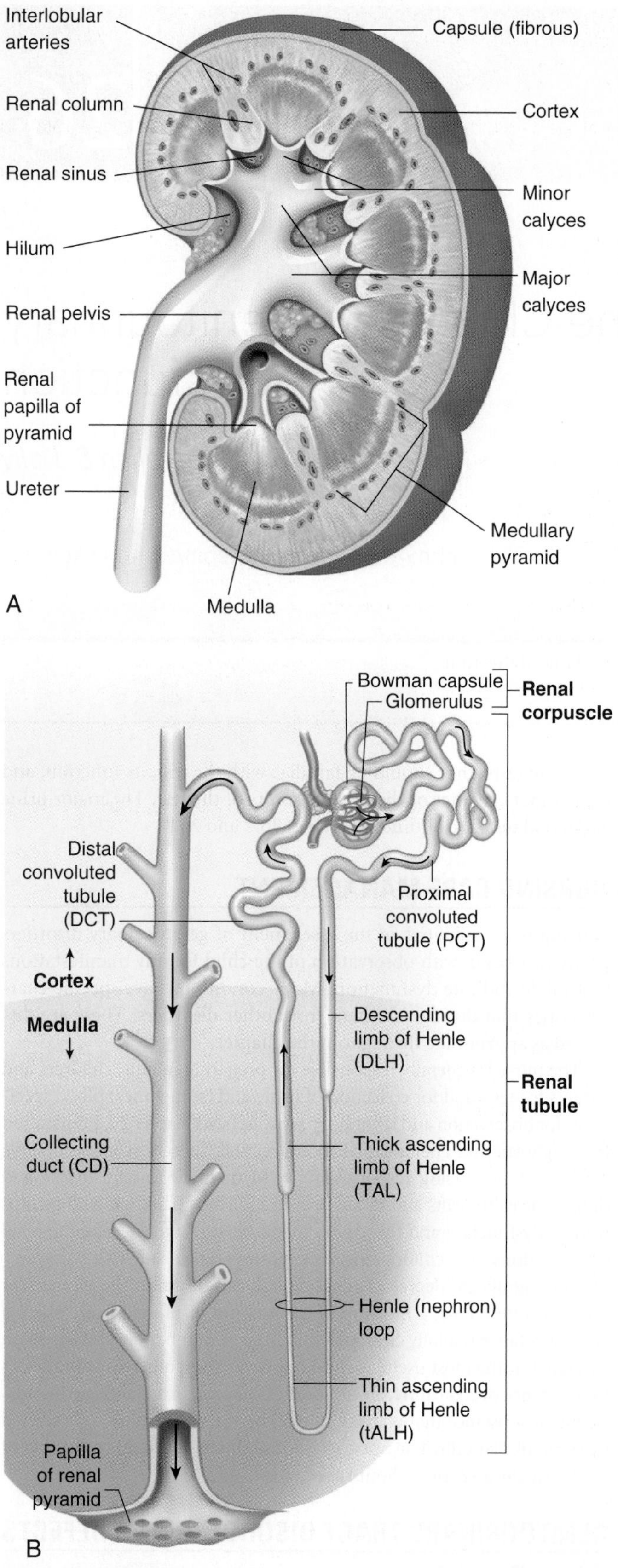

Fig. 26.1 **A,** Kidney structure. **B,** Components of the nephron. (From Patton, K. T., & Thibodeau, G. A. [2010]. *Anatomy and physiology* [7th ed.]. St. Louis, MO: Mosby.)

gender, race, and circumcision status (Shaikh, Morone, Bost, et al., 2008). Whites, females, and uncircumcised boys have the highest rates. Specifically, girls have a twofold to fourfold higher prevalence than do circumcised boys. Uncircumcised males younger than 3 months old and females younger than 12 months old have the highest baseline prevalence of UTI (Shaikh et al., 2008). UTI is an umbrella term for infections of either the upper or the lower urinary tract. UTIs may involve the urethra and bladder (lower urinary tract) or the ureters, renal pelvis, calyces, and renal parenchyma (upper urinary tract). Because of the difficulty in distinguishing upper from lower tract infection, particularly in young children, UTI is often broadly defined. Lower UTIs are often characterized by symptoms of irritation to the bladder, such as hesitancy to void, dysuria, frequency of voiding, and urine incontinence. Upper UTIs or kidney infections (pyelonephritis) tend to present with fever and may lead to renal scarring that may be associated with decreased kidney function, hypertension, and renal disease over time. Upper UTIs may also present with additional symptoms of flank pain, nausea, or vomiting. Diagnosis of UTI is made based on the presence of both pyuria and at least 50,000 colonies/ml of a single uropathic organism in an appropriately collected specimen (Roberts, 2011).

Classification

Infection of the urinary tract may be present with or without clinical symptoms. As a result, the site of infection is often difficult to pinpoint with any degree of accuracy. Various terms used to describe urinary tract disorders include:

Bacteriuria: Presence of bacteria in the urine
Pyuria: Presence of white blood cells in the urine
Asymptomatic bacteriuria: Significant bacteriuria (usually defined as >100,000 colony-forming units [CFUs]) with no clinical symptoms
Symptomatic bacteriuria: Bacteriuria accompanied by physical signs of UTI (dysuria, suprapubic discomfort, hematuria, fever)
Recurrent UTI: Repeated episode of bacteriuria or symptomatic UTI with the same strain of bacteria
Frequent UTI: More than three UTIs within a 6-month period; they do not have to be infections characterized by the same strain of bacteria
Persistent UTI: Persistence of bacteriuria despite antibiotic treatment
Febrile UTI: Bacteriuria accompanied by fever and other physical signs of UTI; presence of a fever typically implies pyelonephritis
Cystitis: Inflammation of the bladder
Urethritis: Inflammation of the urethra
Pyelonephritis: Inflammation of the upper urinary tract and kidneys; kidney infection, usually characterized by presence of bacteriuria and clinical symptoms that include fever
Urosepsis: Febrile UTI coexisting with systemic signs of bacterial illness; blood culture reveals presence of urinary pathogen

Etiology

A variety of organisms can be responsible for UTI. *Escherichia coli* remains the most common uropathogen overall, but the prevalence is higher in females (83%) than males (50%) (Edlin, Shapiro, Hersh, et al., 2013). Other gram-negative organisms associated with UTI include *Proteus mirabilis, Pseudomonas aeruginosa, Klebsiella,* and *Enterobacter.* Gram-positive bacterial pathogens include *Enterococcus, Staphylococcus saprophyticus,* and, rarely, *Staphylococcus aureus.* Viruses and fungi are uncommon causes of UTI in children. Most uropathogens originate in the gastrointestinal tract, migrate to the periurethral area, and ascend to the bladder. Organ cross-talk between the bladder and the colon can also contribute to pathologic changes that may increase risks for UTI (Malykhina, Wyndaele, Andersson, et al., 2012). A number of factors contribute to the development of UTI, including anatomic, physical, and chemical conditions or properties of the host's urinary tract.

TABLE 26.1 Radiologic and Other Tests of Urinary System Function

Test	Procedure	Purpose	Comments and Nursing Responsibilities
Urine culture and sensitivity	Collection of sterile specimen	Determines presence of pathogens and the drugs to which they are sensitive	Send specimen to laboratory immediately after collection Catheterization, clean-catch, or suprapubic specimen
Renal and bladder ultrasonography	Transmission of ultrasonic waves through renal parenchyma, along ureteral course, and over bladder	Allows visualization of renal parenchyma and renal pelvis without exposure to external-beam radiation or radioactive isotopes Visualization of dilated ureters and bladder wall also possible Can show renal cysts and stones, though less sensitive than CT Doppler ultrasonography can be used to evaluate renal vascular flow	Noninvasive procedure
Testicular (scrotal) ultrasonography	Transmission of ultrasonic waves through scrotal contents and testis	Allows visualization of scrotal contents, including testis Testicular ultrasonography is used to identify masses, and Doppler-enhanced ultrasonography is used to differentiate hyperemia of epididymo-orchitis from ischemia or torsion	Noninvasive procedure
Plain film of the abdomen	Flat plate radiograph of abdomen and pelvis for KUB	Can identify certain types of stones that are calcium containing as well as calculi or opaque foreign bodies in bladder (diagnostic test of choice for nephrolithiasis is noncontrast helical CT)	Prepare as for routine x-ray film
Voiding cystourethrography	Contrast medium injected into bladder through urethral catheter until bladder is full; films taken before, during, and after voiding	Visualizes bladder outline and urethra, reveals VUR Provides information on bladder emptying and is also used to diagnosis PUV	Prepare child for catheterization Should not be done at time of active UTI
Radionuclide (nuclear) cystogram	Radionuclide-containing fluid injected through urethral catheter until bladder is full; images generated before, during, and after voiding	Alternative to voiding cystourethrography to evaluate reflux, although visualization of anatomic details is relatively poor Used in some institutions for follow-up due to less radiation	Prepare child for catheterization
Radioisotope imaging studies (renal scans)	Contrast medium injected intravenously; computer analysis to measure uptake or washout (excretion) for analysis of organ function	DMSA radioisotope used to visualize renal scars and differential renal function; does not visualize ureters and bladder MAG3 radioisotope assesses obstruction and differential function between the two kidneys DTPA is an alternative to MAG3, but imaging is limited because it is only filtered at the glomerulus	Insert or assist with insertion of IV infusion Monitor IV infusion Urethral catheterization may accompany MAG3 scan; prepare child for catheterization when indicated
MRI	Uses strong magnetic fields and radio waves to form images	MRI of kidneys used to evaluate renal mass Magnetic resonance angiography used to evaluate renovascular hypertension and has reduced need for renal angiography Magnetic resonance urogram used to detect specific urologic abnormalities, such as ectopic ureter	MRI often requires sedation in infants and children due to need to stay still, typically in an enclosed space; follow NPO guidelines depending on timing of study Assist with IV access if indicated Magnetic devices or implants may be unsafe for MRI, including cochlear implants and permanent pacemakers
CT	Narrow-beam x-rays and computer analysis provide precise reconstruction of area	Visualizes vertical or horizontal cross-section of kidney Especially valuable to distinguish tumors, cysts, and stones Noncontrast helical CT is gold standard for radiologic diagnosis of renal stone disease Renal CT angiogram used to evaluate blood flow in hypertensive patients and is now used more commonly than renal arteriography	Noncontrast scan is noninvasive Contrast-enhanced CT scan preparation may require child be NPO for a few hours With speed of newer scans, the need for sedation is decreased but if required will also require NPO Assist with IV access if needed *Used selectively due to higher radiation exposure*

Continued

TABLE 26.1 Radiologic and Other Tests of Urinary System Function—cont'd

Test	Procedure	Purpose	Comments and Nursing Responsibilities
Cystoscopy	Direct visualization of bladder and lower urinary tract through small scope inserted via urethra	Investigation of bladder and lower tract lesions; visualizes ureteral openings, bladder wall, trigone, and urethra	NPO orders per protocol, typically no solid food after midnight, liquids until 4-6 h before procedure Carry out preoperative preparations; cystoscopy is done under anesthesia in children
Renal biopsy	Removal of kidney tissue by open or percutaneous technique for study by light, electron, or immunofluorescent microscopy	Yields histologic and microscopic information about glomeruli and tubules; helps distinguish among types of nephritic syndromes Distinguishes other renal disorders	Nothing orally 4-6 h before test Premedicate as ordered Prepare setup for procedure Assist with procedure Take vital signs Apply pressure to area with pressure dressing and, if feasible, a sandbag Bed rest for 24 h Observe for abdominal pain, tenderness Monitor input and output Surgical incision may be required in infants
Urodynamics	Set of tests designed to measure bladder filling, storage, and evacuation functions: **Uroflowmetry:** Test to determine efficiency of urination **Cystometrography:** Graphic comparison of bladder pressure as a function of volume **Voiding pressure study:** Comparison of detrusor contraction pressure, sphincter electromyelogram, and urinary flow	Determine characteristic of voiding dysfunction Used to identify type (cause) of incontinence or urinary retention Especially valuable for voiding dysfunction complicated by urinary infection, urinary retention, or neurogenic bladder dysfunction	Prepare child for urinary catheterization The bladder will be filled with contrast, sterile water, or saline solution, and filling pressures will be recorded; the child may experience fullness, coolness from the fluid, and urine leakage during the study Insertion of needles may be required for sphincter EMG (institution specific, often use electrode patches)

CT, Computed tomography; *DMSA,* dimercaptosuccinic acid; *DTPA,* diethylenetriamine pentaacetic acid; *EMG,* electromyography; *IV,* intravenous; *KUB,* kidney, ureters, and bladder; *MAG3,* mercaptoacetyltriglycine; *MRI,* magnetic resonance imaging; *NPO,* nothing by mouth; *PUV,* posterior urethral valve; *UTI,* urinary tract infection; *VUR,* vesicoureteral reflux.

TABLE 26.2 Urine Tests of Renal Function

Test	Normal Range	Deviations	Significance of Deviations
Physical Tests			
Volume	Age related Newborn: 30-60 ml Children: Bladder capacity (oz) = Age (years) + 2	Polyuria Oliguria	Osmotic factors (urinary glucose level in diabetes mellitus) Retention caused by obstructive disease Inadequate bladder emptying caused by neurogenic bladder or obstructive disorder
		Anuria	Obstruction of urinary tract; AKI
Specific gravity	With normal fluid intake: 1.016-1.022 Newborn: 1.001-1.020 Others: 1.001-1.030	High	Dehydration Presence of protein or glucose Presence of radiopaque contrast medium after radiologic examinations
		Low	Excessive fluid intake Distal tubular dysfunction Insufficient ADH Diuresis

TABLE 26.2 Urine Tests of Renal Function—cont'd

Test	Normal Range	Deviations	Significance of Deviations
Osmolality	Newborn: 50-600 mOsm/L	Fixed at 1.010	Chronic glomerular disease
	Thereafter: 50-1400 mOsm/L	High or low	Same as for specific gravity More sensitive index than specific gravity
Appearance	Clear pale yellow to deep gold	Cloudy Cloudy reddish-pink to reddish-brown Light Dark Red	Contains sediment Blood from trauma or disease Myoglobin after severe muscle destruction Dilute Concentrated Trauma
Chemical Tests			
pH	Newborn: 5-7 Thereafter: 4.8-7.8 Average: 6	Weak acid or neutral Alkaline	If associated with metabolic acidosis, suggests tubular acidosis If associated with metabolic alkalosis, suggests potassium deficiency Urinary infection Metabolic alkalosis
Protein level	Absent	Present	Abnormal glomerular permeability (e.g., glomerular disease, changes in blood pressure) Most kidney disease Orthostatic in some individuals
Glucose level	Absent	Present	Diabetes mellitus Infusion of concentrated glucose-containing fluids Glomerulonephritis Impaired tubular reabsorption
Ketone levels	Absent	Present	Conditions of acute metabolic demand (stress) Diabetic ketoacidosis
Leukocyte esterase	Absent	Present	Can identify both lysed and intact WBCs via enzyme detection
Nitrites	Absent	Present	Most species of bacteria convert nitrates to nitrites in the urine
Microscopic Tests			
WBC count	<1 or 2	>5 polymorphonuclear leukocytes/field	Urinary tract inflammatory process
		Lymphocytes	Allograft rejection Malignancy
RBC count	<1 or 2	4-6/field in centrifuged specimen	Trauma Stones Glomerular injury Infection Neoplasms
Presence of bacteria	Absent to a few	>100,000 organisms/ml in centrifuged specimen	UTI
Presence of casts	Occasional	Granular casts Cellular casts WBC RBC Hyaline casts	Tubular or glomerular disorders Degenerative process in advanced renal disease Pyelonephritis Glomerulonephritis Proteinuria; usually transient

ADH, Antidiuretic hormone; *AKI*, acute kidney injury; *RBC*, red blood cell; *UTI*, urinary tract infection; *WBC*, white blood cell.

Anatomic and Physical Factors

The structure of the lower urinary tract has traditionally been thought to account for the increased incidence of bacteriuria in females. The short urethra, which measures about 2 cm in young girls and 4 cm in women, provides a ready pathway for invasion of organisms. In addition, the closure of the urethra at the end of micturition may return contaminated bacteria to the bladder. The longer male urethra (as long as 20 cm in an adult male) and the antibacterial properties of prostatic secretions inhibit the entry and growth of pathogens. The importance of the length of the urethra in the pathogenesis of UTI has been questioned because of the high incidence of UTI in male neonates. The presence or absence of the foreskin has been shown to be a significant factor, with prevalence of UTI in infant males younger than 3 months old being 2.4% in circumcised and 20.1% in uncircumcised males (Shaikh et al., 2008). The presence of a foreskin is associated with a preputial colonization of uropathic bacteria that

TABLE 26.3 Blood Tests of Renal Function

Test	Normal Range (mg/dl)	Deviations	Significance of Deviations
BUN	Newborn: 4-18 Infant, child: 5-18	Elevated	Renal disease: Acute or chronic (the higher the BUN, the more severe the disease) Increased protein catabolism Dehydration Hemorrhage High protein intake Corticosteroid therapy
Uric acid	Child: 2.0-5.5	Increased	Severe renal disease
Creatinine	Infant: 0.2-0.4 Child: 0.3-0.7 Adolescent: 0.5-1.0	Increased	Renal impairment

BUN, Blood urea nitrogen.

can ascend the urethra easily (Balat, Karakok, Guler, et al., 2008). Virulence factors are important in the pathogenesis, and these, coupled with the propensity of bacteria to adhere to the female periurethral mucosa, may explain the increased incidence of UTI in females.

NURSING TIP: Considerable evidence shows significant reductions in the risk of urinary tract infection (UTI) in the first year of life in circumcised male infants. Current evidence indicates that the health benefits of circumcision outweigh the risks and that the benefits of the procedure justify access for families who choose it but are not sufficient to recommend routine circumcision for all male newborns (American Academy of Pediatrics Task Force on Circumcision, 2012).

The single most important host factor influencing the occurrence of UTI is **urinary stasis**. Under normal conditions, the act of completely and repeatedly emptying the bladder flushes away any uropathogens before they have an opportunity to multiply and invade surrounding tissue. However, urine that remains in the bladder after voiding allows uropathogens to rapidly establish in bladder tissue and cause symptoms. Incomplete bladder emptying (stasis) may result from **reflux** (see Vesicoureteral Reflux later in the chapter), anatomic abnormalities, neurogenic bladder, voiding dysfunction, or extrinsic ureteral or bladder compression that may be caused by constipation. Overdistention of the bladder may increase risk of infection by decreasing host resistance, probably as a result of decreased blood flow to the mucosa. This occurs more often in a neurogenic bladder with increased bladder pressure, but it can be the result of voluntary urine holding (Vasudeva & Madersbacher, 2014).

Altered Urine and Bladder Chemistry

Increased fluid intake promotes flushing of the normal bladder and lowers the concentration of organisms in the infected bladder, thereby decreasing risk of UTI. Children with UTIs should be encouraged to have adequate water intake (generally accepted as one 8-oz cup of water per year of age until age 8) to aid in prevention of further infections. Diuresis also seems to enhance the antibacterial properties of the renal medulla.

Most pathogens favor an alkaline medium. Normally, urine is slightly acidic with a median pH of 6. A urine pH of 5 hampers but does not eliminate bacterial multiplication. Much has been reported about the use of cranberry products for prevention of UTI. Initially it was thought to alter the urine acidity, but studies have not shown that ingestion results in a lower pH; instead it appears to decrease the adherence of certain bacteria *(E. coli)* to the bladder wall. Recent review of the literature showed that cranberry products did not significantly reduce the occurrence of symptomatic UTI overall or in any of the subgroups, including children. Because the benefit is small, cranberry juice cannot currently be recommended for prevention of UTIs. Other cranberry preparations need to be quantified using standardized methods to ensure their potency before being evaluated in clinical studies or recommended for use (Jepson, Williams, & Craig, 2012; Ranfaing, Dunyach-Remy, Lavigne, et al., 2018; Sihra, Goodman, Zakri, et al., 2018).

Diagnostic Evaluation

The clinical manifestations of UTI depend on the child's age (Box 26.1). Diagnosis of UTI is confirmed by detection of bacteria in urine culture, but urine collection is often difficult, especially in infants and very small children. Several factors may alter a urine specimen, and contamination of a specimen by organisms from sources other than the urine, such as perineal and perianal flora in bag specimens or clean-catch specimens, is the most frequent cause of false-positive results. Unless the specimen is a first morning sample, a recent high fluid intake may indicate a falsely low organism count. Therefore children should not be encouraged to drink large volumes of water in an attempt to obtain a specimen quickly.

! NURSING ALERT

A child who exhibits the following should be evaluated for urinary tract infection (UTI):

- Incontinence in a toilet-trained child
- Frequency or urgency of voiding
- Dysuria
- Gross hematuria

The most accurate tests of bacterial content are **suprapubic aspiration** (for children younger than 2 years old) and properly performed **bladder catheterization** (as long as the first few milliliters are excluded from collection). The specimen must be fresh (<1 hour with storage at room temperature or <4 hours with refrigeration) to ensure sensitivity and specificity of the urinalysis and to prevent growth of organisms (Roberts, 2011). Clean catch and specimens collected by urine bags are prone to contamination, given the difficulty of obtaining a true midstream specimen with wiping of the meatus and retraction of the labia or foreskin or cleaning the perineum. In these instances, a negative specimen excludes infection and a positive culture is not necessarily diagnostic.

Predictive tests are used to direct therapy when UTI is suspected. Urine dipsticks indicate the presence of leukocyte esterase and nitrites and are quick and inexpensive. Leukocyte esterase is a surrogate marker for pyuria, and nitrite is converted from dietary nitrates in the presence of most gram-negative enteric bacteria in the urine. Because the conversion takes 4 hours in the bladder, it is not a sensitive marker for infants or children who empty their bladder frequently. Also, not all urinary pathogens reduce nitrate to nitrite (Roberts, 2011). Use of a microscopic urinalysis for pyuria should be used for confirmation and diagnosis.

Further radiographic evaluation, such as ultrasonography, voiding cystourethrogram (VCUG), and renal scans such as a dimercaptosuccinic acid (DMSA) scan, may be performed after the infection subsides to identify anatomic abnormalities contributing to the development of infection and existing kidney changes from recurrent infection.

Therapeutic Management

The objectives of treatment of children with UTI are to (1) eliminate current infection, (2) identify contributing factors to reduce the risk of recurrence, (3) prevent systemic spread of the infection, and (4) preserve renal function. Antibiotic therapy should be initiated on the

BOX 26.1 Clinical Manifestations of Urinary Tract Disorders or Disease

Neonatal Period (Birth to 1 Month Old)
Poor feeding
Vomiting
Failure to gain weight
Rapid respiration (acidosis)
Respiratory distress
Spontaneous pneumothorax or pneumomediastinum
Frequent urination
Screaming on urination
Poor urine stream
Jaundice
Seizures
Dehydration
Other anomalies or stigmata
Enlarged kidneys or bladder

Infancy (1 to 24 Months Old)
Poor feeding
Vomiting
Failure to gain weight
Excessive thirst
Frequent urination
Straining or screaming on urination
Foul-smelling urine
Pallor
Fever
Persistent diaper rash
Seizures (with or without fever)
Dehydration
Enlarged kidneys or bladder

Childhood (2 to 14 Years Old)
Poor appetite
Vomiting
Growth failure
Excessive thirst
Enuresis, incontinence, frequent urination
Painful urination
Swelling of face
Seizures
Pallor
Fatigue
Blood in urine
Abdominal or back pain
Edema
Hypertension
Tetany

basis of identification of the pathogen, the child's history of antibiotic use, and the location of the infection. Several antimicrobial drugs are available for treating UTI, but all of them can occasionally be ineffective because of resistance of organisms. Common anti-infective agents used for UTI include the penicillins, sulfonamide (including trimethoprim-sulfamethoxazole), the cephalosporins, and nitrofurantoin (not to be used if pyelonephritis is suspected or confirmed).

If anatomic defects such as primary reflux or bladder neck obstruction are present, surgical correction or urinary prophylaxis may be necessary to prevent further infections. The aim of therapy and careful follow-up is to reduce the chance of renal scarring.

Vesicoureteral Reflux

Vesicoureteral reflux (VUR) refers to the retrograde flow of urine from the bladder into the upper urinary tract. **Primary reflux** results from congenitally abnormal insertion of ureters into the bladder; **secondary reflux** occurs as a result of an acquired condition.

VUR does not cause UTIs but does increase the risk that a lower UTI will become an episode of pyelonephritis. When bladder pressure is high enough, refluxing urine can fill the ureter and the renal pelvis. The International Reflux Study Group developed a classification system that describes the degree of VUR, ranging from Grade I to V, which is important because higher grades are associated with increased renal abnormalities and renal damage. In addition, higher grades are less likely to spontaneously resolve than lower grades. Children with pyelonephritis are often very symptomatic with high fevers, vomiting, and chills. In most cases, conservative therapy is sufficient, with a high rate of spontaneous resolution of VUR over time: 51% at a mean duration of 2 years for all grades of VUR (Estrada, Passerotti, Graham, et al., 2009). Prevention of infection has been the goal with use of continuous antibiotic prophylaxis (CAP) common practice until resolution or correction of VUR. This practice was reviewed in a recent multisite trial and found to be associated with a substantially decreased risk of recurrence of UTI but not of renal scarring, leaving the use of CAP controversial (Hoberman & Chesney, 2014). Urine cultures are not recommended routinely for children with VUR but should be obtained if there are symptoms or unexplained fevers present, because breakthrough infections can occur despite CAP.

Surgical management of VUR corrects the anatomy at the insertion of the refluxing ureter into the bladder and consists of open or laparoscopic and robotic techniques or endoscopic correction. Surgical intervention is indicted in patients who are unlikely to resolve their VUR and are at risk for renal scarring, including those with Grade V reflux with scarring, those with Grade V reflux over 6 years of age, and children who fail medical therapy (have breakthrough infections).

Prognosis

With prompt and adequate treatment at the time of diagnosis, the long-term prognosis for UTI is usually excellent. However, the risk of progressive renal injury due to scarring from a first UTI has been found to be highest in children with an abnormal renal bladder ultrasound or with a combination of high fever (≥39°C) and an etiologic organism other than *E. coli* (Shaikh, Craig, Rovers, et al., 2014). The presence of VUR, particularly high grade (IV to V), is an important risk factor for the development of renal scarring.

QUALITY PATIENT OUTCOMES: Urinary Tract Infections
- Treatment based on culture and sensitivity
- Renal function maintained
- Appropriate diagnosis of renal abnormalities

Nursing Care Management

Nurses should instruct parents of those with VUR to observe for signs and symptoms suggestive of UTI. These are not always obvious, particularly in an infant, young child, or developmentally delayed child. A high fever without obvious cause should be a signal to check the urine. Because infants and young children often are unable to express their feelings and sensations verbally, it is difficult to detect discomfort they may be experiencing from dysuria. A careful history regarding voiding habits, stooling pattern, feeding tolerance, and episodes of unexplained irritability may assist in detecting less obvious cases of UTI.

NURSING TIP: Another strategy for obtaining a daily urine protein is to place cotton balls in the diaper at night before bedtime and then squeeze them out in the morning. This should not be used if looking for urinary tract infections (UTIs).

When infection is suspected, collecting an appropriate specimen is essential. It is the nurse's responsibility to take every precaution to obtain acceptable clean-voided specimens in a child who is able to void volitionally, taking care to cleanse the meatus and retract the foreskin in uncircumcised males or keep the labia separated in females. Having a young girl sit backwards on the toilet can facilitate this process, particularly the ability to obtain urine midstream, decreasing the risk of contamination. Because of the unreliability of a specimen obtained via a urine collection bag, sterile catheterization should be done in infants and young children whose illness warrants immediate antibiotic therapy, such as with high fever, vomiting, and lethargy.

Frequently, additional tests are performed to detect anatomic defects. Children are prepared for these tests as appropriate for their age. This includes an explanation of the procedure, its purpose, and what the children will experience (see Chapter 20, Preparation for Diagnostic and Therapeutic Procedures). Sometimes a simple description of the urinary system is helpful. For children younger than 3 to 4 years old, the procedure can be explained on a doll. For those who are older, a simple drawing of the bladder, urethra, ureters, and kidneys makes the procedure more understandable.

Handling actual equipment when feasible can be helpful in allaying anxiety in children of all ages. Anticipatory instruction on distraction techniques such as deep breathing, storytelling, and imagery may help the child relax and be more cooperative during the actual procedures.

Because antibacterial drugs are indicated in UTI, the nurse advises parents of proper dosage and administration. When used in low dose for prevention of UTI, parents need an explanation of the drug's continued necessity when no signs of infection are present. For all children, adequate fluid intake is encouraged.

Prevention

Prevention is the most important goal in both primary and recurrent infection, and many preventive measures are simple hygienic habits that should be a routine part of daily care (see Nursing Care Guidelines box). For example, parents are taught to cleanse their infant's genital areas from front to back to avoid contaminating the urethral area with fecal organisms. Girls are taught to wipe from front to back after voiding and defecating. Children should void as soon as they feel the urge and should not be encouraged to hold their urine for prolonged periods.

NURSING CARE GUIDELINES

Prevention of Urinary Tract Infection

Factors Predisposing to Development

Short female urethra close to vagina and anus
Incomplete emptying and overdistention of bladder
Concentrated urine
Constipation

Measures of Prevention

Practice perineal hygiene; wipe from front to back in females.
Avoid tight clothing or diapers; wear cotton panties rather than nylon.
Avoid "holding" urine; encourage child to void frequently.
Take time to empty bladder completely. This may be helped by relaxed toilet posture for girls, with feet supported on a stool and knees apart. Some children benefit from "double voiding" (void, wait a few minutes, and void again).
Avoid constipation.
Encourage adequate fluid intake.

Sexually active female adolescents are advised to urinate as soon as possible after they have intercourse to flush out any bacteria introduced. Children who have recurrent UTIs or neurogenic bladder are sometimes maintained on daily low-dose antibiotics. Giving the dose at bedtime in children who stay dry through the night allows the drug to remain in the bladder longer. The nurse should reinforce the importance of compliance to parents and older children.

Obstructive Uropathy

Structural or functional abnormalities of the urinary system that obstruct the normal flow of urine can result in renal dysfunction. The area above the obstruction may demonstrate increased pressure, dilation, and urinary stasis. If the blockage is low in the urinary tract, both ureters and kidneys may be affected; if one kidney or ureter is affected, the other may be normal. The renal pelvis and calyces typically show dilation called **hydronephrosis** from obstruction, although a kidney may have hydronephrosis and not be obstructed.

Obstruction may be congenital or acquired, unilateral or bilateral, and complete or incomplete with acute or chronic manifestations. The obstruction can occur at any level of the upper or lower urinary tract (Fig. 26.2). Partial obstruction may not be symptomatic, and changes caused may be partially or completely reversible if there is early intervention. Boys are affected more frequently than girls, and malformations should be suspected when patients have associated congenital defects (e.g., prune belly syndrome, chromosomal anomalies, anorectal malformations, neural tube defects). Prenatal diagnosis with ultrasonography has been a factor leading to early diagnosis and intervention with subsequent decrease in renal impairment.

Causes of obstructive uropathy include congenital problems, such as posterior urethral valves (PUVs), ureteropelvic junction (UPJ) and ureterovesical junction (UVJ) obstruction, and ureterocele. Acquired causes include renal or bladder stones, tumor, and trauma. PUVs are obstructing membranous folds within the lumen of the posterior urethra and are the most common cause of obstruction of the urinary

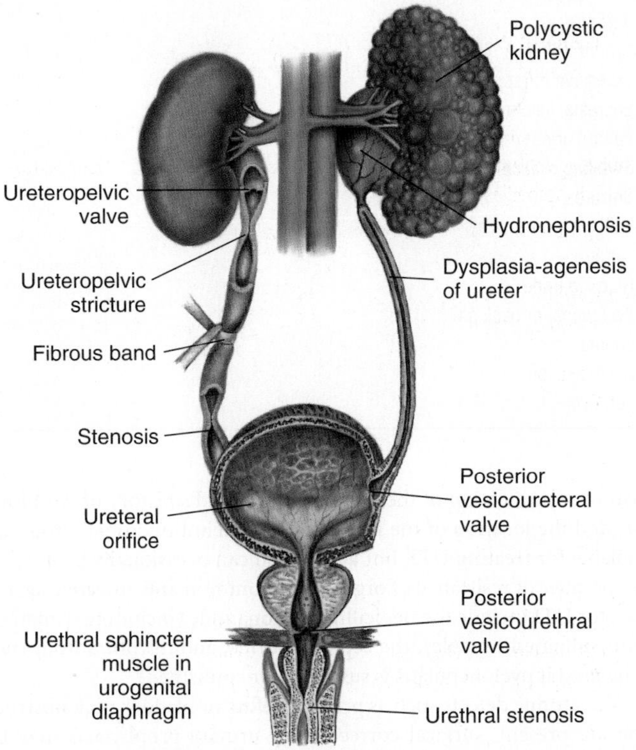

Fig. 26.2 Major sites of urinary tract obstruction.

tract in newborn males, as well as the most common cause of chronic renal injury from obstructive uropathy. Because the obstruction occurs in the urethra, the bladder and upper urinary tract are affected. Damage to distal nephrons in chronic uropathy may cause decreased glomerular filtration, which can lead to renal insufficiency (Chevalier, 2015). Damage to smooth muscle of the bladder and upper urinary tract also may occur with obstruction and can contribute to bladder dysfunction. Because stasis of urine serves as a medium for bacterial growth, infection can magnify destructive changes of obstruction and cause increased renal damage as well as increased morbidity.

Early diagnosis and surgical correction or procedures that divert the flow of urine to bypass the obstruction may prevent progressive renal damage. Medical complications of acute or chronic renal failure (CRF) or infection are managed as described for those disorders.

Nursing Care Management

Nursing goals in urinary tract obstruction include helping to identify cases, assisting with diagnostic procedures, and caring for children with complications (described elsewhere). Preparing parents and children for procedures is a major nursing responsibility (see Chapter 20, Preparation for Diagnostic and Therapeutic Procedures).

Parents and children need emotional support and counseling during the potentially lengthy management of these disorders. Children may be discharged with urinary drainage systems that require nursing education of the parents and older child to provide care and to recognize problems, such as obstruction of urine flow or infection. Drainage tubes should be observed for obstruction resulting from sediment, small blood clots, or kinking. If indicated, instructions on site care and drainage tube irrigation need to be provided, including observation for signs of infection or dislodgement.

Children with external diversional systems need psychologic support and guidance, especially as they reach adolescence and body image concerns assume more prominence. Those with progressive renal deterioration may face the prospect of dialysis or transplantation and the physical and psychologic challenges that accompany these procedures.

EXTERNAL DEFECTS OF THE GENITOURINARY TRACT

Defects of the external genitourinary tract have the potential to cause distortions of body image. Satisfactory surgical repair is successful for the more common disorders and is carried out or initiated as early as possible. The major anomalies of the lower genitourinary tract, their description, and their management are outlined in Table 26.4.

PHIMOSIS

Phimosis is a narrowing or stenosis of the preputial opening of the foreskin that prevents retraction of the foreskin over the glans penis.

TABLE 26.4 Defects of the Genitourinary Tract

Defect	Therapeutic Management
Inguinal hernia: Protrusion of abdominal contents through inguinal canal into scrotum	Detected as painless inguinal swelling of variable size Surgical closure of inguinal defect
Hydrocele: Fluid in scrotum	Surgical repair may be indicated if persists past 1 year old and symptomatic
Phimosis: Narrowing or stenosis of preputial opening of foreskin	**Mild cases:** May not require therapy if urine flow not obstructed; steroid cream may be prescribed, typically twice a day for 1 month **Severe cases:** Circumcision or dorsal slit in severe, rare cases
Hypospadias: Urethral opening located behind glans penis or anywhere along ventral surface of penile shaft	Objectives of surgical correction: • Enable child to void in standing position and direct stream voluntarily in usual manner • Improve physical appearance of genitalia • Produce a sexually adequate organ
Chordee: Ventral curvature of penis, often associated with hypospadias	Surgical release of fibrous band causing the deformity
Epispadias: Meatal opening located on dorsal surface of penis	Surgical correction, usually including penile and urethral lengthening and bladder neck reconstruction (if necessary)
Cryptorchidism: Failure of one or both testes to descend normally through inguinal canal	Detected by inability to palpate testes within scrotum **Medical:** Administration of hormonal therapy has historically been used in some centers to induce testicular descent but is controversial and not currently recommended **Surgical:** Orchiopexy Objectives of therapy: Place and fix viable undescended testes in a normal scrotal position or remove nonviable testicular remnants Allows for easier examination of the testis because there is an increased risk of testicular cancer in undescended testes; early surgical correction may reduce the risk of cancer as well as infertility Decrease risk of trauma and torsion Decrease risk of inguinal hernia by closing the inguinal canal Potential improved body satisfaction
Exstrophy of bladder: Eversion of posterior bladder through anterior bladder wall and lower abdominal wall; associated with open pubic arch (a severe defect)	Potential objectives of surgical correction: • Preserve renal function • Attain urinary control • Provide adequate reconstructive repair • Improve sexual function

It is a normal finding in infants and young boys and usually resolves as the child grows and the distal prepuce dilates. Occasionally the narrowing obstructs the flow of urine, resulting in a dribbling stream or even ballooning of the foreskin with accumulated urine during voiding. Phimosis causing urinary obstruction is often treated effectively by application of steroid cream twice a day for 1 month, with the option for surgical treatment with circumcision in severe cases.

Balanitis is an inflammation or infection of the phimotic foreskin, which occurs occasionally and is managed as any other inflammation or infection.

Nursing Care Management

Proper hygiene of the phimotic foreskin in infants and young boys consists of external cleansing during routine bathing. The foreskin should not be forcibly retracted because this may create scarring that can prevent future retraction. Furthermore, retraction of the tight foreskin can result in paraphimosis, a condition in which the retracted foreskin cannot be replaced in its normal position over the glans. This causes edema and venous congestion created by constriction by the tight band of foreskin—a urologic emergency that requires immediate evaluation.

HYDROCELE

A **hydrocele** is the presence of peritoneal fluid in the scrotum between the parietal and visceral layers of the tunica vaginalis and is the most common cause of painless scrotal swelling in children and adolescents, along with nonincarcerated inguinal hernia. Hydroceles may be communicating or noncommunicating. A communicating hydrocele usually develops when the processus vaginalis does not close during development, allowing for communication with the peritoneum. Noncommunicating hydroceles have no connection to the peritoneum, with fluid coming from the mesothelial lining of the tunica vaginalis. Hydroceles are common in newborns and often resolve spontaneously, usually by 1 to 3 years of age. In older children, noncommunicating hydroceles may be idiopathic or a result of trauma, epididymitis, orchitis, testicular torsion, torsion of the appendix testis or appendix epididymis, or tumor.

Communicating hydroceles may change in size during the day or with straining, whereas noncommunicating hydroceles are not reducible and so do not change size with crying or straining. Surgical repair is indicated for communicating hydroceles persisting past 1 year old because there is a risk for development of incarcerated inguinal hernia. Idiopathic hydroceles are repaired if symptomatic, and reactive hydroceles usually resolve with treatment of underlying cause, such as epididymitis.

Nursing Care Management

Surgical correction is an outpatient procedure. Advise parents that there may be temporary swelling and discoloration of the scrotum that resolves spontaneously. Straddle toys are avoided for 2 to 4 weeks, and strenuous activities in older boys may be avoided for 1 month. If a dressing is used, it is removed in 2 to 3 days, and typically the child can bathe in 3 days.

CRYPTORCHIDISM (CRYPTORCHISM)

Cryptorchidism, commonly referred to as undescended testicle(s), is failure of one or both testes to descend normally through the inguinal canal into the scrotum. It is the most common disorder of sexual development in boys. Absence of testes within the scrotum can be a result of undescended (cryptorchid) testes, retractile testes, or anorchism (absence of testes). Undescended testes can be categorized further according to location:

Abdominal: Proximal to the internal inguinal ring
Canalicular: Between the internal and external inguinal rings
Ectopic: Outside the normal pathways of descent between the abdominal cavity and the scrotum

The incidence of cryptorchidism is reported to be as high as 45% in preterm boys and less than 5% in full-term boys; by 1 year old, the incidence decreases to less than 2% and does not change thereafter (Sijstermans, Hack, Meijer, et al., 2008). Guidelines from the American Urological Association recommend that boys with cryptorchidism be referred to a surgeon by 6 months of age (Kolon, Herndon, Baker, et al., 2014).

Pathophysiology

Cryptorchidism occurs when one or both testes fail to descend through the inguinal canal and into the scrotum. Several processes may slow or arrest testicular descent, including endocrinologic abnormalities affecting the hypothalamic-pituitary-testicular axis, denervation of the genitofemoral nerve, traction of the gubernaculum, abnormal development of the epididymis, or preterm birth. Congenital hernias and abnormal testes often accompany cryptorchid testes, and they are at risk for subsequent torsion.

Anorchism is the complete absence of a testis. Anorchism is suspected whenever one or both testes cannot be palpated in the patient with apparent cryptorchidism. In some cases, bilateral anorchism is associated with disorders of sex development with genotypic and phenotypic abnormalities, specifically congenital adrenal hyperplasia (CAH). Although it is commonly associated with a normal karyotype (46, XY) and normal genital development, it is critical to rule out the possibility of CAH in the newborn because of the potential for serious harm due to inability to regulate electrolyte levels (Kolon et al., 2014). An absent testis may be due to atrophy from prenatal testicular torsion, also known as *vanishing testes* or *testicular regression syndrome.*

The cryptorchid or ectopic testis must be differentiated from anorchism because of the risk for malignant degeneration and subfertility when the testis is left in an extrascrotal location. This differentiation requires laparoscopic or direct surgical exploration (Kolon et al., 2014).

Retractile testes can be found at any level within the path of testicular descent, but they are most commonly identified in the groin. Fortunately, they are not truly cryptorchid. Instead, they are introverted to an inguinal or abdominal position because of an overactive cremasteric reflex. The cremasteric reflex, observed as withdrawal of the testis above the scrotum and into the inguinal canal in response to various stimuli, including exposure to cool temperatures, is active during infancy and peaks around 4 to 5 years old. Unlike the cryptorchid testis, the retractile testis can be gently moved into the scrotum without residual tension and does not require treatment. Retractile testes can become ascending testes and require annual monitoring. Retractile testicles do not require surgical intervention unless they do become ascended testicles that can no longer be brought into the scrotum.

Clinical Manifestations

A nonpalpable testis is typically observed by the parent or detected during routine physical examination by a nurse practitioner, physician assistant, or physician. If one testis is not palpable, the affected hemiscrotum will appear smaller than the other. With bilateral nonpalpable testes, both hemiscrota appear small. In the case of retractile testes, the parents may report intermittently observing the testes in the scrotum, interspersed with periods when they cannot be visualized or palpated. Frequently, the retractile testis will be observed in the scrotum when the child is being bathed in warm water.

Diagnostic Evaluation

It is important to differentiate the true undescended testis from the more common retractile testis. Retractile testes can be "milked" or pushed back into the scrotum, but truly undescended ones cannot. For examination, the nurse can obviate the cremasteric reflex by placing the child in a squatting or cross-legged sitting position prior to checking the position of the testes.

Therapeutic Management

Although primary hormonal therapy with luteinizing hormone–releasing hormone (nasal spray) and human chorionic gonadotropin (injection) has been used more commonly in Europe, it is no longer recommended to induce testicular descent (Kolon et al., 2014). Evidence shows low response rates and lack of long-term efficacy (Kolon et al., 2014). Orchiopexy, or surgical repositioning of the testis, is performed on palpable testes. Exploratory surgery may be required if the testis is not palpable. The goal of surgery is to place and fix viable undescended testes to a normal scrotal position or to remove nonviable testicular remnants. Scrotal positioning reduces the risk of torsion and trauma and permits easier examination of the testis because there is an increased risk of testicular cancer despite treatment of undescended testes. In the routine surgical procedure for undescended testes, the testes are brought down into the scrotum and secured in that position without tension or torsion. A simple orchiopexy for a palpable testis can usually be performed in an outpatient setting. If exploratory surgery is needed to determine whether a testis is present, an examination under anesthesia is the initial step. Depending on findings, a diagnostic laparoscopic procedure or an open inguinal approach may be performed. If an intra-abdominal testis is identified, this permits planning for a definitive procedure, which may be open or laparoscopic; some boys will require a planned two-stage surgical repair to bring an intra-abdominal testis into the scrotum. Approximately 10% of boys with nonpalpable testes are found to have an absent testicle at the time of surgery.

Nursing Care Management

Postoperative nursing care is directed toward preventing infection and instructing parents in home care of the child, including pain control. Observation of the wound for complications and activity restrictions are discussed. The child should avoid vigorous sports activities and use of toys that are straddled for 2 to 4 weeks postoperatively. General care is similar to that described for hydrocele repair.

Parents may be concerned about the child's future fertility, and recent studies show some decreased fertility in bilateral cryptorchidism, but in unilateral patients the fertility rate approximates that found in the general population. The risk of testicular cancer is a concern that is decreased if surgery is done before puberty, but all boys with cryptorchidism should be taught testicular self-examination at puberty to potentially facilitate early detection (Kolon et al., 2014). Surgical treatment is indicated as soon as possible after 6 months of age and definitely should be completed by 2 years old, because spontaneous descent rarely occurs after 6 months and treatment by 1 to 2 years old is associated with improved fertility and testicular growth (Kolon et al., 2014).

HYPOSPADIAS

Hypospadias is a congenital anomaly of the male urethra that results in abnormal ventral placement of the urethral opening on the underside of the penis, ranging from the glans to the perineum (Fig. 26.3). It is one of the most common congenital anomalies with an incidence report varied around the world, with 10% to 15% having a first-degree male relative (sibling or father) with the same condition (Gray, 2009; Springer, van den Heijkant, & Baumann, 2016). Both genetic and environmental factors have been associated with hypospadias. Severity of hypospadias is based on the position of the urethral opening and the degree of chordee, or ventral curvature of the penis. The more distant the opening from the normal position at the tip of the glans and the more marked curvature increases the severity and the need for more extensive surgical correction. In mild cases, the meatus is just below

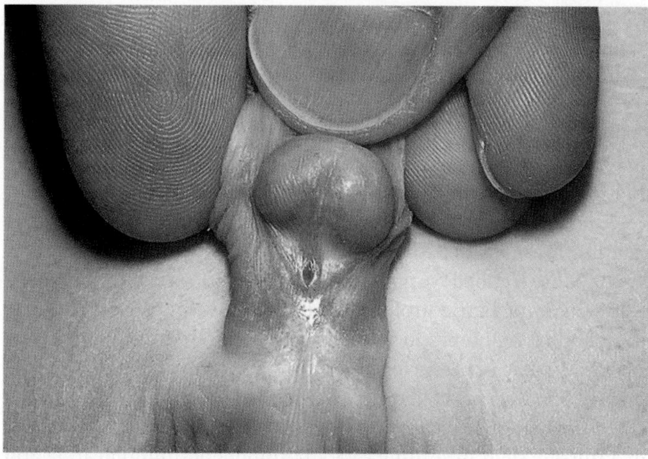

Fig. 26.3 Hypospadias. (Courtesy H. Gil Rushton, MD, Children's National Medical Center, Washington, DC.)

the tip of the penis. In the most severe malformation, the meatus is on the perineum between the halves of the bifid scrotum. In addition, the foreskin is usually absent ventrally and, when combined with chordee, gives the organ a hooded and crooked appearance. In severe cases the altered appearance may leave the infant's gender in doubt at birth because of the perineal position of the meatus and small penis. In any case of ambiguous genitalia, additional evaluation is essential. Cryptorchidism is present in about 10% of infants with hypospadias and increases with more proximal hypospadias with the meatus at the scrotum or perineum. There is an increased risk of disorders of sex development in patients with severe hypospadias, both with and without cryptorchidism.

Surgical Correction

The principal objectives of surgical correction are (1) to enhance the child's ability to void in the standing position with a straight stream, (2) to improve the physical appearance of the genitalia for psychologic reasons, and (3) to preserve a sexually adequate organ. The choice of surgical procedure is affected primarily by the severity of the defect and the presence of associated anomalies. Numerous techniques are used in repair of hypospadias and are performed under general anesthesia and typically as an outpatient procedure.

Hypospadias repair may be done by primary tubularization for milder forms in which a new urethra is made by rolling a ventral strip of penile shaft skin that normally would have formed the urethra. For more severe hypospadias, an onlay island flap is used to create the urethra, transferring a strip of inner foreskin onto the ventral urethral plate. In severe forms of hypospadias, including those with significant chordee, a two-stage repair is used to straighten the penis and create a new urethra. These are typically performed at least 6 months apart. There is no consensus on the best surgical approach for correcting severe hypospadias, and complication rates—specifically, development of urethrocutaneous fistula, urethral stricture or meatal stenosis, and urethral diverticulum—are high.

The preferred time for surgical repair is 6 to 12 months old, before the child has developed body image. Occasionally a short course of testosterone is administered preoperatively to achieve additional penile size to facilitate the surgery. If preoperative testosterone is used it does not have an effect on the eventual adult size of the phallus.

Nursing Care Management

Neonatal circumcision should be avoided in hypospadias where there is incomplete foreskin, because this is not conductive to a safe clamp or Plastibell circumcision. In severe cases, the foreskin may be used in reconstruction. In mild hypospadias, the foreskin may not be incomplete and the abnormality may not be noted until after a circumcision is complete. This does not affect future successful reconstruction if it is needed. In most cases, the appearance after reconstruction will be of a circumcised normal penis. Preparation of parents for the type of procedure to be done and the expected cosmetic result helps avert problems.

Frequently parents are informed of what is to be surgically corrected but are not advised of what to expect as a reasonable consequence. More refined surgical techniques performed by surgeons specializing in pediatric urologic conditions have improved cosmetic and functional outcomes in these boys. If children are old enough to understand what is occurring, the nurse also prepares them for the operation and the expected outcome.

Hypospadias repair may require some type of urinary diversion with a silicone stent or feeding tube to promote optimum healing and to maintain the position and patency of the newly formed urethra. This is left in the bladder to drain urine for 5 to 10 days. In most infants and children who are not toilet trained, the catheter drains directly into the diaper. In older children, the catheter is connected to a leg bag or a larger bedside bag at night. Drainage bags should always be positioned below the bladder level for proper drainage. Tub baths are avoided until the catheter is removed. Most children will have a caudal or penile nerve block in addition to general anesthesia, which lasts 6 to 8 hours. Appropriate administration of prescribed pain medication for 48 to 72 hours after surgery will help control discomfort. When a catheter is left in place, bladder spasms are common and are very uncomfortable. Anticholinergic medications, such as oxybutynin, are typically used to prevent spasms. Parents should be advised of the possibility of bladder spasms, which are usually brief and intense and during which the child may arch his back and bring his knees up to his chest and urine may leak around the catheter. Oxybutynin is given every 8 hours typically and may require dosing adjustment, such as increasing frequency to every 6 hours to control spasms. Once the catheter is removed, the medication is no longer needed. Often a prophylactic antibiotic is given until shortly after catheter removal. Anticholinergic medication is constipating, and this is a problem that is common in the postoperative period and may be avoided with preventative measures, such as giving adequate fluid and a stool softener or laxative if needed. Preparing parents for these potential problems is an important nursing responsibility. Patients usually go home with a dressing that often comes off in 1 to 2 days and typically is removed in the bath in 3 days if there is no stent in place. If the dressing is soiled, it can be cleaned gently and removed once the parent is prepared that the appearance of the penis is often swollen, discolored, and/or bruised and that this is expected and will resolve with time. While healing, applying petroleum jelly or KY jelly to the diaper to prevent the penis from sticking can help prevent bleeding and increase comfort.

EXSTROPHY-EPISPADIAS COMPLEX

Bladder exstrophy is a severe defect involving the musculoskeletal system and the urinary, reproductive, and intestinal tracts. It is one of three anomalies that define the exstrophy-epispadias complex (EEC). **Epispadias** is an exposed or open dorsal urethra. Bladder exstrophy is a more severe defect characterized by an open, inside-out bladder with the inner surface exposed and the dorsal urethra on the lower abdominal wall (Figs. 26.4 and 26.5). The third disorder, **cloacal exstrophy**, is the most severe, and includes bladder exstrophy as well as exstrophy of the large intestine (hindgut) through an abdominal wall defect. In addition, there is anal atresia, omphalocele, hypoplasia of the colon, anomalous genitalia, and often spinal dysraphism. Fortunately,

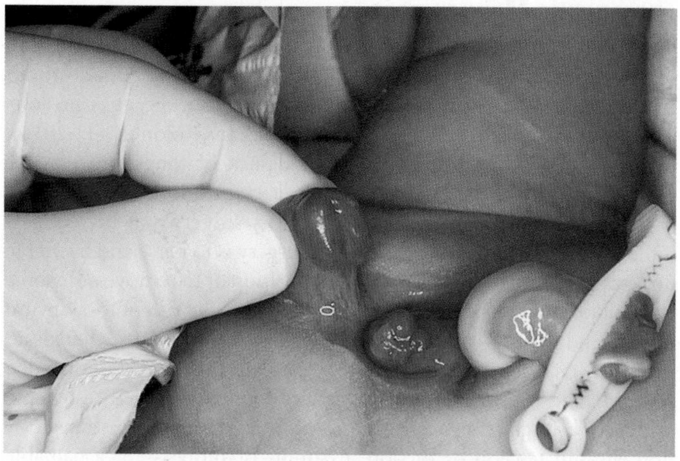

Fig. 26.4 Newborn with bladder exstrophy and epispadias. (Courtesy Tim Yankee, St. Francis Hospital, Tulsa, OK.)

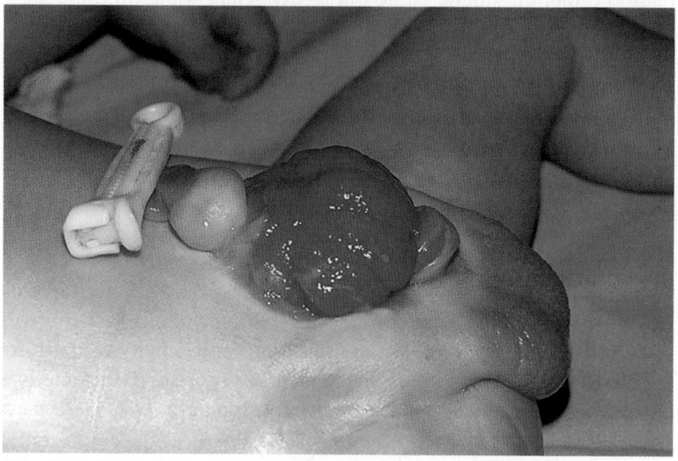

Fig. 26.5 Exstrophy of bladder. (Courtesy H. Gil Rushton, MD, Children's National Medical Center, Washington, DC.)

incidence of cloacal exstrophy is low—less than 1 per 100,000 live births (Feldkamp, Botto, Amar, et al., 2011). Classic bladder exstrophy typically includes findings of diastasis (separation) of the symphysis pubis (pelvic bone), low-set umbilicus, anteriorly displaced anus, defects of the genitalia, and inguinal hernia. The incidence of bladder exstrophy ranges from 3.3 to 5 per 100,000 live births and is more common in males than females (Jayachandran, Bythell, Platt, et al., 2011).

Pathophysiology

Exstrophy results from failure of the abdominal wall and underlying structures, including the ventral wall of the bladder, to fuse in utero. As a result, the lower urinary tract is exposed, and the everted bladder appears bright red through the abdominal opening. This is accompanied by a constant seepage of urine from the exposed ureteral orifices, making the area malodorous and susceptible to infection. The constant accumulation of urine on the surrounding skin produces tissue ulceration and further infection. Progressive renal damage from infection and obstruction may cause renal failure if left untreated.

In males with bladder exstrophy, the defect of the genitalia includes epispadias and upward curvature of a shortened penis and may include other problems, such as undescended testes and inguinal hernias. In females, there is epispadias, a bifid clitoris, and small labia minora. The vagina is shortened compared with normal, and vaginal dilation may be needed to allow for sexual intercourse. In patients with cloacal exstrophy, there are often more severe anomalies, such as bifid or duplicated uterus, split clitoris, completely separated labia, and a duplicate or absent vagina in females. Males may have a split penis and scrotum or a short, flat penis with hypospadias. In either sex, separation of the pubic bones is generally corrected by pelvic osteotomy, particularly if there is extreme diastasis to increase the likelihood of successful bladder closure. In patients with bladder exstrophy, the upper urinary tract is usually normal. Fertility is possible in females but decreased in males, possibly because of semen abnormalities, abnormal ejaculation, or both. Assisted reproductive techniques remain a viable option for patients with infertility. Recent studies indicate good long-term outcomes on erectile and general sexual function in both men and women with epispadias and bladder exstrophy (Suominen, Santtila, & Taskinen, 2015).

Therapeutic Management

The objectives of treatment are (1) preservation of renal function, (2) attainment of urinary control, (3) adequate reconstructive repair for acceptable appearance, (4) prevention of UTIs, and (5) preservation of optimum external genitalia with continence and sexual function. Two surgical approaches currently are used to correct bladder exstrophy. One is called *modern staged repair of exstrophy (MSRE),* typically involving three surgeries beginning with closure of the bladder and abdominal wall. Complete primary repair of bladder exstrophy (CPRE) is a single-stage surgical closure combining closure of the bladder and abdominal wall, partial tightening of the bladder neck, and bilateral ureteral reimplantation to correct reflux. Often pelvic osteotomies are performed at the time of primary closure to deepen the flattened pelvis, close the pubic diastasis, and release tension on the abdominal wall to improve success of primary closure (Inouye, Massanyi, Di Carlo, et al., 2013; Inouye, Tourchi, Di Carlo, et al., 2014; Kasprenski, Benz, Maruf, et al., 2018).

For the child with bladder exstrophy, CPRE may be performed within the first 72 hours of life or as a delayed procedure at about 2 months old. For the child with cloacal exstrophy, pelvic osteotomies are needed because of the wide pelvic diastasis, and surgery is done within 48 to 72 hours of life to close the bladder and omphalocele and perform intestinal diversion (Inouye et al., 2013, 2014; Kasprenski et al., 2018).

In some children, reconstruction (tightening) of the bladder neck may not provide sufficient resistance to achieve urinary continence. In these cases, suburethral collagen injections or implantation of an artificial urinary sphincter may be performed. Occasionally the bladder fails to achieve an adequate functional capacity, and augmentation enterocystoplasty is required. This procedure is typically combined with the creation of a Mitrofanoff appendiceal stoma, because catheterization is difficult after reconstruction of the proximal urethra. Abnormalities of the genitalia are addressed to ensure optimal sexual function. In boys, the testes are typically cryptorchid, and bilateral orchiopexy is combined with reconstruction of the bifid scrotum to preserve testicular function. In girls, surgical enlargement of the vaginal introitus may be needed to permit intercourse. In both genders, plastic surgery to reduce scarring of the genital area or to create an umbilicus may significantly improve the child's body image and emerging sexual identity.

Nursing Care Management

It is important to limit trauma to the exposed bladder mucosa, and the bladder is covered with a nonadherent film of plastic wrap or transparent dressing that will not stick to the bladder but can adhere to the surrounding skin. After bladder closure, the neonate is monitored for urinary output and for signs of urinary tract or wound infection. At the time of closure, the pelvic diastasis may be corrected with an osteotomy, but even if that is not performed, these patients typically require immobilization of the pelvis with traction for 2 to 4 weeks. A common form of traction for newborns is modified Bryant's traction, but spica casting and other alternatives are used. Monitoring of skin condition and circulation is critical, as is monitoring the incision for wound dehiscence. The focus of nursing care is pain management and maintenance of immobilization. Pain management may be achieved with continuous epidural therapy or patient-, parent-, or nurse-controlled intravenous analgesia and may involve the acute pain service working with the bedside nurse to provide optimal pain control (Kozlowski, 2008). Postoperative nursing care also includes monitoring of hemodynamic stability, maintaining patency and stability of tubes and drains, provision of intravenous (IV) fluids and nutrition, and inclusion of the family in care.

Postoperative nursing care after bladder neck reconstruction and antireflux surgery (ureteral reimplantation) includes routine wound care and careful monitoring of urinary output from the bladder and ureteral drainage tubes. Care after a penile lengthening, chordee release, and urethral reconstruction is similar to care after hypospadias repair.

Children who fail to attain urinary continence after bladder neck reconstruction are offered a continent diversion. In addition to routine postoperative care, nursing care after a continent diversion includes wound care, observation of nasogastric (NG) suction (surgery requires bowel resection), and measurement and observation of urinary output. Clean intermittent catheterization (CIC) is used to regularly empty the urinary reservoir. Most children are able to learn self-catheterization by 6 or 7 years old. Adult supervision is needed to ensure that the child is compliant.

Family Support and Home Care

Bladder exstrophy and the other disorders of the EEC are significant congenital abnormalities that require lifelong care by a team of specialists. Improvement in surgical techniques has helped achieve better outcomes, specifically that of the goal of continence. Parental stress is significant, and support services may be helpful for positive adaptation. Patients may also benefit from psychologic support, as adjustment problems are common, particularly in adolescents. Parents should receive teaching and practice on care of the infant or child at home and have access to resources to call if there are questions. Allowing time for the parent to voice concerns can facilitate evaluation of their understanding and help direct discharge needs. When the infant is discharged with an unrepaired defect, plastic wrap is placed over the defect, and diapers are changed frequently to prevent infection, ulceration, and odor. Parents are taught to recognize the signs of UTI and to report a suspected infection to the practitioner. General infant care remains unchanged—except for sponge baths rather than immersion in water.

DISORDERS OF SEX DEVELOPMENT

Infants born with a discrepancy between external genitalia, gonadal, and chromosomal sex are now referred to as having a **disorder of sex development (DSD)** (Lee, Nordenstrom, Houk, et al., 2016). The presentation at birth may be a genital appearance that does not permit gender declaration, and this is called **ambiguous genitalia**. These may include bilateral cryptorchidism, perineal hypospadias with bifid scrotum, clitoromegaly, posterior labial fusion, phenotypic female appearance with a palpable gonad, and hypospadias and unilateral nonpalpable gonad. Also included in the DSD category are infants with discordant genitalia and sex chromosomes. Turner syndrome (45, XO) and Klinefelter syndrome (47, XXY) are also DSDs that do not present with ambiguous genitalia.

Pathophysiology

Normal sexual differentiation starts at 7 weeks' gestation when fetuses with a Y chromosome begin developing testes. Early on, both female (XX) and male (XY) fetuses have a similar reproductive structure. Multiple genes contribute to this process, and mutations in these genes can lead to various DSDs. Congenital malformation of the genitalia are most frequently because of androgen deficiency in XY individuals and androgen excess in XX patients, though in many cases no endocrine etiology can be found (Grinspon & Rey, 2014).

Initial evaluation includes karyotype and assessment of adrenal and gonadal function, and this information can be used to categorize the infant into one of three categories:

- Virilized XX (XX DSD)
- Undervirilized XY (XY DSD)
- Mixed sex chromosome pattern

Therapeutic Management

The most common cause of ambiguous genitalia is **congenital adrenal hyperplasia (CAH)**, which can lead to life-threatening salt-wasting adrenal insufficiency in the first weeks of life. Though now a part of neonatal screening in the United States, any infant with genital ambiguity should be evaluated urgently. Laboratory testing includes a measurement of 17-hydroxyprogesterone in addition to karyotype with immediate probe for SRY (sex-determining region on the Y chromosome). Serum electrolytes are monitored, as signs and symptoms of adrenal insufficiency may include hypoglycemia, hypovolemia, hyponatremia, hyperkalemia, vomiting, and diarrhea. Fluids and electrolytes need to be replaced urgently, and the nurse plays a key role in assessing the infant and providing prescribed therapy. Additional laboratory testing may be indicated, as may be pelvic and abdominal ultrasonography to evaluate for gonads, uterus, and vagina.

Family Support

The birth of a child with ambiguous genitalia has been called a *psychosocial emergency for the family.* They require support because the answer to a seemingly simple question as to the sex of their child requires evaluation and time. Involvement in a multidisciplinary team that may include endocrinology, urology, genetics, surgeons, nurses, and social workers can make clear communication challenging, and the nurse may be instrumental in coordinating family meetings with the team.

The infant and child with DSD poses very complex and controversial management questions, including sex assignment and potential genital surgery. Traditional approaches are being questioned and continue to evolve. Referral to a specialized center for children with DSD is recommended.

Psychological Problems Related to Genital Surgery

Improved understanding of the psychologic implications of genitourinary surgery in children, improvements in technical aspects of surgery, and advances in pediatric anesthesia have resulted in modifications of the surgical approach to children requiring genitourinary surgery. Some of the problems of hospitalization, separation, and anxiety can be eased by hospital practices that are sensitive to the child's needs (see Chapter 19).

A child's body image is largely derived as a result of feedback from primary caregivers and peers, and parental anxiety regarding an acceptable physical appearance is readily communicated to an affected child. This subtle communication increases the risk of development of a distorted body image, and early repair may facilitate a positive body image. Sexual body image is another area that has been thought to be largely a function of socialization. In terms of disorders of sex development, this becomes a much more complex and multifaceted area.

The child's reaction to surgery is related to emotional and cognitive development. Separation of parent and child is important to minimize, particularly in the first 1 to 2 years of life. From about 3 to 6 years old, children are frightened of what they perceive to be threats to their body and bodily function. They are egocentric in their view of the world and may perceive surgery as punishment for real or imagined wrongdoing and require reassurance that they are not to blame. By age 7 years, they have more ability to understand but may still associate surgery with punishment. Surgical repair is ideally performed before these fears and anxieties develop. In terms of anesthesia risk, elective procedures are generally performed after 6 months of age. It is thought that children do not have memory of procedures performed by 18 to 24 months old. Age 24 to 36 months may be a time when trauma of surgery is relatively less, but in the case of an external defect this prolongs correction. The American Academy of Pediatrics Action Committee on Surgery first published recommendations on timing of elective surgery on the genitalia of male children as a review in 1996.

Nursing Care Management

Preparing children and their families for diagnostic and surgical procedures (see Chapter 20, Preparation for Diagnostic and Therapeutic Procedures) and for home care is a major nursing function. Most postoperative care involves care of the surgical site. Tub baths may be discouraged for a few days or longer, depending on procedure (if a stent or catheter is left in place) and surgeon preference. It is common practice to leave a urethral stent or catheter in place to drain directly into the diaper after some reconstructive procedures, such as hypospadias repair. The surgical site is kept clean and is inspected for signs of infection or bleeding. More complex surgeries require additional care and observation, such as drainage tube care and irrigation, dressing changes, and monitoring of collection devices.

Postoperative activity restrictions vary with age and type of surgery. Activity of infants and toddlers is not typically limited, with the exception of avoiding straddle toys following penile or scrotal surgery. Older children may need more restriction from strenuous activity for 1 month after these types of procedures. In the case of more extensive abdominal surgery, there may be restrictions on lifting and strenuous activity for a longer period. Swimming may be restricted, especially when any drains are still in place or until incisions are healed. Precise restrictions depend on the specific type of surgery and surgeon preference.

In most cases, the results of surgery are satisfactory. However, in some of the more severe defects, such as exstrophy and severe hypospadias, additional psychologic support may be needed to help adjust to concerns about penis size, appearance of the genitalia, potential ability to procreate, and rejection by peers (especially the opposite sex). Ongoing open discussion and support groups for parents and children are useful in promoting optimum emotional adjustment, particularly during adolescence.

GLOMERULAR DISEASE

NEPHROTIC SYNDROME

Nephrotic syndrome is a clinical state that includes massive proteinuria, hypoalbuminemia, hyperlipidemia, and edema. The disorder can occur as (1) a primary disease known as **idiopathic nephrosis, childhood nephrosis,** or **minimal-change nephrotic syndrome (MCNS)**; (2) a secondary disorder that occurs as a clinical manifestation after or in association with glomerular damage that has a known or presumed cause; or (3) a congenital form inherited as an autosomal recessive disorder. The disorder is characterized by increased glomerular permeability to plasma protein, which results in massive urinary protein loss. This discussion is devoted to MCNS because it constitutes 80% of nephrotic syndrome cases.

Pathophysiology

The onset of MCNS can occur at any age but predominantly occurs in children between 2 and 7 years old. It is rare in children younger than 6 months old, uncommon in infants younger than 1 year old, and unusual after 8 years old. Patients with MCNS are twice as likely to be male.

The pathogenesis of MCNS is not fully understood. There may be a metabolic, biochemical, physiochemical, or immune-mediated disturbance that causes the basement membrane of the glomeruli to become increasingly permeable to protein, but the cause and mechanisms are only speculative.

The glomerular membrane, normally impermeable to albumin and other proteins, becomes permeable to proteins, especially albumin, that leak through the membrane and are lost in urine (**hyperalbuminuria**). This reduces the serum albumin level (**hypoalbuminemia**), decreasing the colloidal osmotic pressure in the capillaries. As a result, the vascular hydrostatic pressure exceeds the pull of the colloidal osmotic pressure, causing fluid to accumulate in the interstitial spaces (**edema**) and body cavities, particularly in the abdominal cavity (**ascites**). The shift of fluid from the plasma to the interstitial spaces reduces the vascular fluid volume (**hypovolemia**), which in turn stimulates the renin-angiotensin system and the secretion of antidiuretic hormone and aldosterone. Tubular reabsorption of sodium and water is increased in an attempt to increase intravascular volume. The elevation of serum lipids is not fully understood. The sequence of events in nephrotic syndrome is diagrammed in Fig. 26.6.

Diagnostic Evaluation

The disease is suspected based on clinical manifestations (Box 26.2). The generalized edema may develop rapidly or gradually but eventually prompts the family to seek medical attention. Parents usually give a history of the child being well but steadily gaining weight; appearing edematous; and then becoming anorexic, irritable, and less active.

The diagnosis of MCNS is suspected on the basis of the history and clinical manifestations (edema, proteinuria, hypoalbuminemia, and hypercholesterolemia in the absence of hematuria and hypertension) in children between 2 and 8 years old. The hallmark of MCNS is massive proteinuria (higher than 2+ on urine dipstick). Hyaline casts, oval fat bodies, and a few red blood cells (RBCs) can be found in the urine of some affected children, although there is seldom gross hematuria. The GFR is usually normal or high. Kidney function must be monitored, however, because acute kidney injury (AKI) may occur due to intravascular volume depletion, interstitial nephritis, acute tubular necrosis, or other factors (Rheault, Wei, Hains, et al., 2014).

Total serum protein concentration is low, with the serum albumin significantly reduced and plasma lipids elevated. Hemoglobin and hematocrit are usually normal or elevated as a result of hemoconcentration. The platelet count may be elevated. Serum sodium concentration may be low. If the patient does not respond to an 8-week course of daily steroids, a renal biopsy may be needed to distinguish among other types of nephrotic syndrome. The biopsy results of children with MCNS are remarkable for effacement of the foot processes of the epithelial cells lining the basement membrane, but otherwise the kidney tissue is normal.

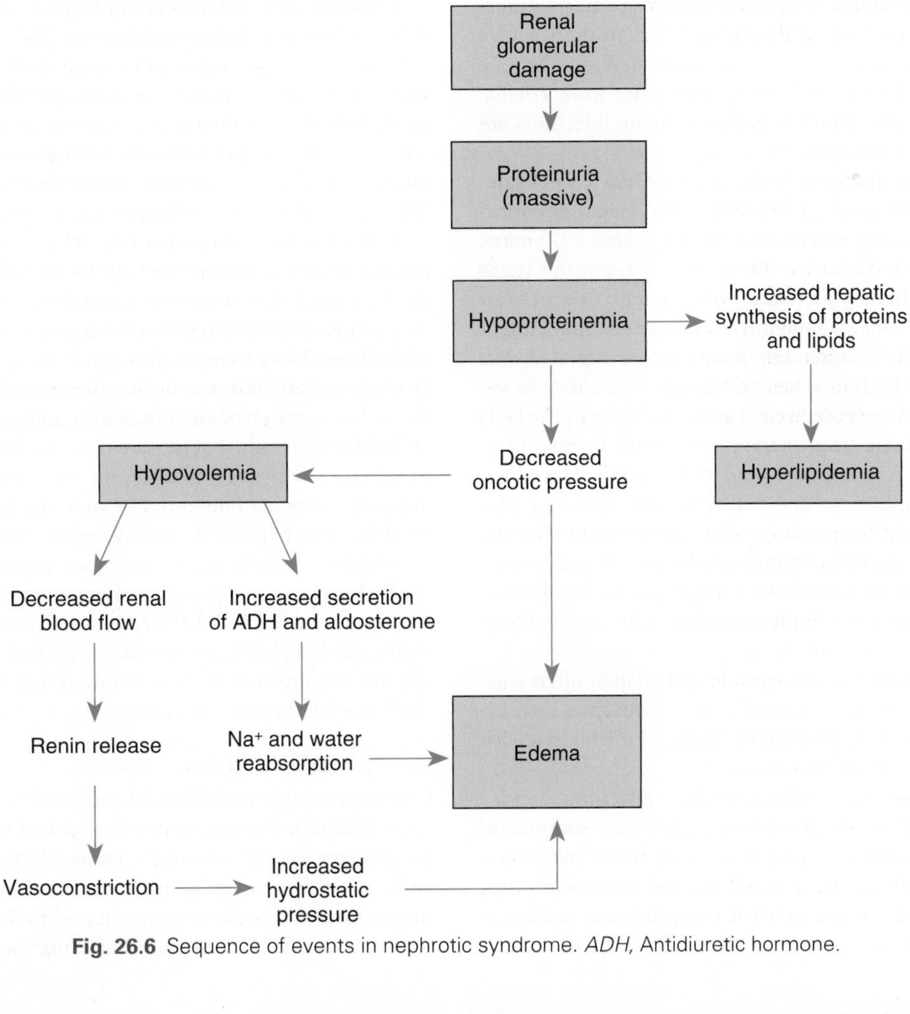

Fig. 26.6 Sequence of events in nephrotic syndrome. *ADH*, Antidiuretic hormone.

BOX 26.2 Clinical Manifestations of Nephrotic Syndrome

Weight gain
Puffiness of face (facial edema):
- Especially around the eyes
- Apparent on arising in the morning
- Subsides during the day

Abdominal swelling (ascites)
Pleural effusion
Labial or scrotal swelling
Edema of intestinal mucosal, possibly causing:
- Diarrhea
- Anorexia
- Poor intestinal absorption

Ankle or leg swelling
Irritability
Easily fatigued
Lethargic
Blood pressure normal or slightly decreased
Susceptibility to infection
Urine alterations:
- Decreased volume
- Frothy

Therapeutic Management

Objectives of therapeutic management include (1) reducing excretion of urinary protein, (2) reducing fluid retention in the tissues, (3) preventing infection, and (4) minimizing complications related to therapies. Dietary restrictions include a low-salt diet and, in more severe cases, fluid restriction. If complications of edema develop, diuretic therapy may be initiated to provide temporary relief from edema. Sometimes infusions of 25% albumin are used. Acute infections are treated with appropriate antibiotics.

Corticosteroids are the first line of therapy for MCNS. The starting dosage for prednisone is usually 2 mg/kg body weight/day for 6 weeks followed by 1.5 mg/kg every other day for 6 weeks (Lombel, Gipson, & Hodson, 2013). About two-thirds of children with MCNS have a relapse, heralded first by increased urine protein. Relapses can be diagnosed early if parents are taught routine home monitoring of urine protein by dipstick. Relapses are treated with a repeated, but usually shorter, course of high-dose steroid therapy. Side effects of the steroids include increased appetite, weight gain, rounding of the face, and behavior changes. Long-term therapy may result in hirsutism, growth retardation, cataracts, hypertension, gastrointestinal bleeding, bone demineralization, infection, and hyperglycemia. Children who do not respond to steroid therapy, those who have frequent relapses, and those in whom the side effects threaten their growth and general health may be considered for a course of therapy using other immunosuppressant medications (cyclophosphamide, chlorambucil, or cyclosporine).

Episodes of MCNS, both the first episode and relapse, often happen in conjunction with a viral or bacterial infection. Relapses can also be triggered by allergies and immunizations. Relapses in children with MCNS may continue over many years.

Complications of nephrotic syndrome include infection, circulatory insufficiency secondary to hypovolemia, and thromboembolism. Infections that may be seen in children with nephrotic syndrome include peritonitis, cellulitis, and pneumonia and require prompt recognition and vigorous treatment with appropriate antibiotic therapy.

Prognosis

The prognosis for ultimate recovery in most cases is good. In children who respond to steroid therapy, the tendency to relapse decreases with time. With early detection and prompt implementation of therapy to eradicate proteinuria, progressive basement membrane damage is minimized so that when the tendency to relapse is past, renal function is usually normal or near normal. It is estimated that approximately 80% of affected children have this favorable prognosis.

QUALITY PATIENT OUTCOMES: Nephrotic Syndrome
- Protein-free urine
- Acute infections prevented
- Edema absent or minimal
- Nutrition maintained
- Metabolic abnormalities controlled

Nursing Care Management

Continuous monitoring of fluid retention or excretion is an important nursing function. Strict intake and output records are essential but may be difficult to obtain from very young children. Application of collection bags is irritating to edematous skin that is readily subject to breakdown. Applying diapers or weighing wet pads may be necessary.

Other methods of monitoring progress include urine examination for albumin, daily weight, and measurement of abdominal girth. Assessment of edema (e.g., increased or decreased swelling around the eyes and dependent areas), the degree of pitting, and the color and texture of skin are part of nursing care. Vital signs are monitored to detect any early signs of complications, such as shock or an infective process.

Infection is a constant source of danger to edematous children and those receiving corticosteroid therapy. These children are particularly vulnerable to upper respiratory tract infection; therefore they must be kept warm and dry, active, and protected from contact with infected individuals (e.g., roommates, visitors, personnel). The Centers for Disease Control and Prevention recommend the pneumococcal conjugate vaccine (13-valent) and pneumococcal polysaccharide vaccine (PPSV, 23-valent) for children with nephrotic syndrome.

Loss of appetite accompanying relapse creates a perplexing problem for nurses. The combined efforts of nurse, dietitian, parents, and child are needed to formulate a nutritionally adequate and attractive diet. Salt is restricted (but not eliminated) during the edema phase and while the child is on steroid therapy. Fluid restriction (if prescribed) is limited to short-term use during massive edema. Every effort should be made to serve attractive meals with preferred foods and a minimum of fuss, but it usually requires considerable ingenuity to entice the child to eat (see Chapter 20, Feeding the Sick Child). Once the child feels better, the appetite (enhanced by steroids) returns. At this point, care must be taken to prevent excessive caloric intake and weight gain.

Children usually adjust activities according to their tolerance level. However, they may require guidance in selecting play activities. Suitable recreational and diversional activities are an important part of their care. Irritability and mood swings that accompany steroid therapy are not unusual in these children and may create an additional challenge for the nurse and family.

Family Support and Home Care

Continuous support of the child and family is one of the major nursing considerations. Parents are taught to detect signs of relapse and to call for changes in treatment at the earliest indication. Unless the edema and proteinuria are severe or the parents, for some reason, are unable to care for the ill child, *home care is preferred.* Parents are instructed in testing urine for albumin, administering medications, and providing general care. Parents are also instructed on avoiding contact with infected playmates, but the child should attend school.

The prolonged course of the relapsing form of nephrotic syndrome is taxing to both the child and the family. The up-and-down course of remissions and exacerbations with periodic disruption of family life by hospitalization places a severe strain on the child and the family, both psychologically and financially. Reassurance regarding this characteristic of the course of the disease, with emphasis on the importance of long-term care, needs to be provided to parents and children. A satisfactory response is more likely when relapses are detected and therapy is instituted early, and remissions are prolonged when instructions are carried out faithfully. Continuous support of the child and family is one of the major nursing considerations (see Chapter 17).

ACUTE GLOMERULONEPHRITIS

Acute glomerulonephritis (AGN) may be a primary event or a manifestation of a systemic disorder that can range from minimal to severe. Common features include oliguria, edema, hypertension and circulatory congestion, hematuria, and proteinuria. Most cases are postinfectious and have been associated with pneumococcal, streptococcal, and viral infections. Acute poststreptococcal glomerulonephritis (APSGN) is the most common of the postinfectious renal diseases in childhood and the one for which a cause can be established in most cases. APSGN can occur at any age but affects primarily early school-age children, with a peak age of onset of 6 to 7 years old. It is uncommon in children younger than 2 years old, and boys outnumber girls 2 to 1.

Etiology

APSGN is an immune-complex disease that occurs after an antecedent streptococcal infection with certain strains of the group A beta-hemolytic streptococci (GABHS). Most streptococcal infections *do not* cause APSGN. A latent period of 10 to 21 days occurs between the streptococcal infection and the onset of clinical manifestations. Disease secondary to streptococcal pharyngitis is more common in the winter or spring, but when APSGN is associated with pyoderma (principally impetigo), it may be more prevalent in late summer or early fall, especially in warmer climates. Second episodes of APSGN are rare.

Pathophysiology

The pathophysiology of APSGN is still uncertain. Immune complexes are deposited in the glomerular basement membrane. The glomeruli become edematous and infiltrated with polymorphonuclear leukocytes, which occlude the capillary lumen. The resulting decrease in plasma filtration results in an excessive accumulation of water and retention of sodium that expands plasma and interstitial fluid volumes, leading to circulatory congestion and edema. The cause of the hypertension associated with AGN cannot be completely explained by fluid retention. Excess renin may also be produced.

Diagnostic Evaluation

Typically, affected children are in good health until they experience a streptococcal infection. In some instances, they have a history of only a mild cold or no previous infection at all. The onset of nephritis appears after an average latency period of about 1 to 3 weeks (Box 26.3). Because the child appears to be well during the latency period, parents may not recognize the association. The edema is usually relatively moderate and may not be appreciated by someone unfamiliar with the child's normal appearance.

BOX 26.3 Clinical Manifestations of Acute Poststreptococcal Glomerulonephritis

Edema:
- Especially periorbital
- Facial edema more prominent in the morning
- Spreads during the day to involve extremities, genitalia, and abdomen

Anorexia
Urine:
- Cloudy, smoky brown (resembles tea or cola)
- Severely reduced volume

Pallor
Irritability
Lethargy
Child appearing ill
Child seldom expresses specific complaints
Older children complaining of:
- Headaches
- Abdominal discomfort
- Dysuria

Vomiting possible
Mild to severely elevated blood pressure

Urinalysis during the acute phase characteristically shows hematuria and proteinuria. Proteinuria generally parallels the hematuria and may be 3+ or 4+ in the presence of gross hematuria. Gross discoloration of the urine reflects RBC and hemoglobin content. Microscopic examination of the sediment shows many RBCs, leukocytes, epithelial cells, and granular and RBC casts. Bacteria are not seen.

Azotemia that results from impaired glomerular filtration is reflected in elevated blood urea nitrogen (BUN) and creatinine levels in at least 50% of cases. Occasionally, proteinuria is excessive, and the patient may have nephrotic syndrome (i.e., hypoproteinemia and hyperlipidemia).

Cultures of the pharynx are rarely positive for streptococci because the renal disease occurs weeks after the infection.

Some serologic tests are necessary to make the diagnosis of APSGN. Circulating serum antibodies to streptococci indicate the presence of a previous infection. The antistreptolysin O (ASO) titer is the most familiar and readily available test for streptococcal infection. Other antibodies that may aid in diagnosis are elevated antihyaluronidase (AHase), anti-deoxyribonuclease B (ADNase-B), and streptozyme. All patients with APSGN have reduced serum complement 3 (C3) activity in the early stages of the disease. Rising C3 levels are used as a guide to indicate improvement of the disease and should be normal in almost all patients 8 weeks after the disease onset.

Studies that may be useful include chest x-ray examination, which generally shows cardiac enlargement, pulmonary congestion, or pleural effusion during the edematous phase of acute disease. Renal biopsy for diagnostic purposes is seldom required but may be useful in the diagnosis of atypical cases.

Therapeutic Management

Management consists of general supportive measures and early recognition and treatment of complications. Children who have normal blood pressure and a satisfactory urinary output can generally be treated at home. Those with substantial edema, hypertension, gross hematuria, or significant oliguria should be hospitalized because of the unpredictability of complications.

Dietary restrictions depend on the stage and severity of the disease, especially the extent of edema. Moderate sodium restriction and even fluid restriction may be instituted for children with hypertension and edema. Foods with substantial amounts of potassium are generally restricted during the period of oliguria.

Regular measurement of vital signs, body weight, and intake and output is essential to monitor the progress of the disease and to detect complications that may appear at any time during the course of the disease. A record of daily weight is the most useful means for assessing fluid balance. Rarely, children with APSGN will develop AKI with oliguria that significantly alters the fluid and electrolyte balance (resulting in hyperkalemia, acidosis, hypocalcemia, or hyperphosphatemia). These children require careful management. Peritoneal dialysis or hemodialysis is seldom needed.

Acute, sometimes severe, hypertension must be anticipated and identified early. Blood pressure measurements are taken every 4 to 6 hours. A variety of antihypertensive medications and diuretics are used to control hypertension. Antibiotic therapy is indicated only for children with evidence of persistent streptococcal infections. It is used to prevent transmission of nephritogenic streptococci to other family members.

Prognosis

Almost all children correctly diagnosed as having APSGN recover completely, and specific immunity is conferred, so subsequent recurrences are uncommon. Less than 1% of children will go on to develop **end-stage renal disease (ESRD)**, although abnormal urinalysis and renal function may persist for decades (Nast, 2012).

Nursing Care Management

Nursing care of the child with glomerulonephritis involves careful assessment of the disease status, with regular monitoring of vital signs (including frequent measurement of blood pressure), fluid balance, and behavior.

Vital signs provide clues to the severity of the disease and early signs of complications. They are carefully measured, and any deviations are reported and recorded. The volume and character of urine are noted, and the child is weighed daily. Children with restricted fluid intake, especially those who are not severely edematous or those who have lost weight, are observed for signs of dehydration.

Assessment of the child for signs of cerebral complications is an important nursing function, because the severity of the acute phase is variable and unpredictable. The child with edema, hypertension, and gross hematuria may be subject to complications, and anticipatory preparations such as seizure precautions and IV equipment are included in the unfolding case study (see the Next-Generation NCLEX® Examination-Style Unfolding Case Study box later in the chapter).

For most children, a regular diet is allowed, but it should contain no added salt. Foods high in sodium and salted treats are eliminated, and parents and friends are advised not to bring snacks, such as potato chips or pretzels. Fluid restriction, if prescribed, is more difficult, and the amount permitted should be evenly divided throughout the waking hours. Meal preparation and service require special attention because the child is indifferent to meals during the acute phase. Again, collaboration with parents and the dietitian and special consideration for food preferences facilitate meal planning.

During the acute phase, children are generally content to lie in bed. As they begin to feel better and their symptoms subside, they will want to be up and about. Activities should be planned to allow for frequent rest periods and avoidance of fatigue. Children who have mild edema and no hypertension, as well as convalescent children who are being treated at home, need follow-up care. Parent education and support in preparation for discharge and home care include education in home management, dietary restrictions, infection prevention, and the need for follow-up care and health supervision. Health supervision is continued with weekly and then monthly visits for evaluation and urinalysis.

MISCELLANEOUS RENAL DISORDERS

HEMOLYTIC UREMIC SYNDROME

Hemolytic uremic syndrome (HUS) is an uncommon, acute renal disease that occurs primarily in infants and small children between 6 months and 5 years old. HUS is one of the most frequent causes of acquired AKI in children (Walsh & Johnson, 2018). The clinical features of the disease include acquired hemolytic anemia, thrombocytopenia, renal injury, and central nervous system (CNS) symptoms. The etiology of HUS is thought to be associated with bacterial toxins, chemicals, and viruses. The appearance of the disease has been associated with *Rickettsia* organisms, viruses (especially coxsackievirus, echovirus, and adenovirus), *E. coli,* pneumococci, shigellae, and salmonellae and may represent an unusual response to these infections. Multiple cases of HUS caused by enteric infection of the *E. coli* O157:H7 serotype have been traced to undercooked meat, especially ground beef. Other sources are unpasteurized milk or fruit juice, especially apple; alfalfa sprouts; lettuce; and salami. Drinking or swimming in sewage-contaminated water can also cause infection. The clinical presentation is usually a history of a prodromal illness (most often gastroenteritis or an upper respiratory tract infection) followed by the sudden onset of hemolysis and renal failure.

Pathophysiology

The primary site of injury appears to be the endothelial lining of the small glomerular arterioles, which become swollen and occluded with deposits of platelets and fibrin clots (intravascular coagulation). RBCs are damaged as they attempt to move through the partially occluded blood vessels. These damaged cells are removed by the spleen, causing acute hemolytic anemia. The platelet aggregation within the damaged blood vessels or the damage and removal of platelets produce the characteristic thrombocytopenia.

Diagnostic Evaluation

The triad of anemia, thrombocytopenia, and renal failure is sufficient for diagnosis (Box 26.4). Renal involvement is evidenced by proteinuria, hematuria, and urinary casts; BUN and serum creatinine levels are elevated. A low hemoglobin and hematocrit and a high reticulocyte count confirm the hemolytic nature of the anemia.

BOX 26.4 Clinical Manifestations of Hemolytic Uremic Syndrome

Vomiting
Irritability
Lethargy
Marked pallor
Hemorrhagic manifestations:
- Bruising
- Petechiae
- Jaundice
- Bloody diarrhea

Oliguria or anuria
Central nervous system (CNS) involvement:
- Seizures
- Stupor or coma

Signs of acute heart failure (sometimes).

Therapeutic Management

The goals of therapy are early diagnosis and aggressive, supportive care of the AKI and hemolytic anemia. Hemodialysis or peritoneal dialysis is instituted in any child who has been anuric for 24 hours or who demonstrates oliguria with uremia or hypertension and seizures. Other treatments include use of pharmacologic agents, fresh-frozen plasma, and plasmapheresis. Blood transfusions with fresh, washed packed cells are administered for severe anemia but are used with caution to prevent circulatory overload from added volume.

Prognosis

With prompt treatment, the recovery rate is about 95%, but residual renal impairment ranges from 10% to 50%. Long-term complications include chronic kidney disease (CKD), hypertension, and CNS disorders. Death is usually caused by residual renal impairment or CNS injury.

Nursing Care Management

Nursing care is the same as that provided in AKI and, for children with continued impairment, includes management of chronic disease. Because of the sudden and life-threatening nature of the disorder in a previously well child, parents are often ill prepared for the impact of hospitalization and treatment. Therefore support and understanding are especially important aspects of care.

RENAL FAILURE

Renal failure is the inability of the kidneys to excrete waste material, concentrate urine, and conserve electrolytes. It can occur suddenly (e.g., AKI) in response to inadequate perfusion, kidney disease, or urinary tract obstruction, or it can develop slowly (e.g., CKD) as a result of long-standing kidney disease or an anomaly.

Azotemia and *uremia* are terms often used in relation to renal failure. **Azotemia** is the accumulation of nitrogenous waste within the blood. **Uremia** is a more advanced condition in which retention of nitrogenous products produces toxic symptoms. Whereas azotemia is not life threatening, uremia is a serious condition that often involves other body systems.

ACUTE KIDNEY INJURY

AKI is said to exist when the kidneys suddenly are unable to regulate the volume and composition of urine appropriately in response to food and fluid intake and the needs of the organism. The principal feature of AKI is oliguria[a] associated with azotemia, metabolic acidosis, and diverse electrolyte disturbances. AKI is not common in childhood, and the outcome depends on the cause, associated findings, and prompt recognition and treatment.

The pathologic conditions that produce AKI caused by glomerulonephritis and HUS are discussed in relation to those disorders. AKI can also develop as a result of a large number of related or unrelated clinical conditions: poor renal perfusion; urinary tract obstruction; acute renal injury; cardiac surgery (Susantitaphong, Cruz, Cerda, et al., 2013); or the final expression of chronic, irreversible renal disease. The most common cause in children is transient renal failure resulting from severe dehydration or other causes of poor perfusion that may respond to restoration of fluid volume.

[a]The definition of oliguria varies extensively in the literature, from 1.8 to 4 dl/m² every 24 hours.

BOX 26.5 Clinical Manifestations of Acute Kidney Injury

Specific:
- Oliguria
- Anuria uncommon (except in obstructive disorders)

Nonspecific (may develop):
- Nausea
- Vomiting
- Drowsiness
- Edema
- Hypertension

Manifestations of underlying disorder or pathologic condition

Pathophysiology

AKI is usually reversible, but the deviations of physiologic function can be extreme, and mortality in the pediatric age-group remains high. There is severe reduction in the GFR, an elevated BUN level, and a significant reduction in renal blood flow.

The clinical course is variable and depends on the cause. In reversible AKI, there is a period of severe oliguria, or a low-output phase, followed by an abrupt onset of diuresis, or a high-output phase, and then a gradual return to (or toward) normal urine volumes.

In many instances of AKI, the infant or child is already critically ill with the precipitating disorder, and the explanation for development of oliguria may or may not be readily apparent (Box 26.5). When a previously well child develops AKI without an obvious cause, a careful history is taken to reveal symptoms that may be related to glomerulonephritis, obstructive uropathy, or exposure to chemicals (e.g., ingestion of heavy metals; inhalation of organic solvents; medications such as vancomycin, aminoglycosides, or nonsteroidal antiinflammatory drugs) known to be toxic to the kidneys (Goldstein, 2016). Significant laboratory measurements during renal failure that serve as a guide for therapy are BUN, serum creatinine, pH, sodium, potassium, and calcium.

Diminished urinary output and lethargy in a child who is dehydrated, is in shock, or has recently undergone surgery should be evaluated for possible AKI.

! NURSING ALERT

Any of the following signs of hyperkalemia constitute an emergency and are reported immediately:
- Serum potassium concentrations in excess of 7 mEq/L
- Presence of electrocardiographic abnormalities, such as prolonged QRS complex, depressed ST segment, high peaked T waves, bradycardia, or heart block

Therapeutic Management

Treatment of AKI is directed toward (1) treatment of the underlying cause, (2) management of the complications of renal failure, and (3) provision of supportive therapy within the constraints imposed by the renal failure.

Treatment of poor perfusion resulting from dehydration consists of volume restoration, as described in Chapter 22, in treatment of dehydration. If oliguria persists after restoration of fluid volume or if the renal failure is caused by intrinsic renal damage, the physiologic and biochemical abnormalities that have resulted from kidney dysfunction must be corrected or controlled. Initially, a Foley catheter is inserted to rule out urine retention, to collect available urine for analysis, and to monitor results of diuretic administration. The catheter may or may not be removed during the oliguric phase.

The amount of exogenous water provided should not exceed the amount needed to maintain zero water balance. It is calculated on the basis of estimated endogenous water formation and losses from sensible (primarily gastrointestinal) and insensible sources. No allotment is calculated for urine as long as oliguria persists.

When the output begins to increase, either spontaneously or in response to diuretic therapy, the intake of fluid, potassium, and sodium must be monitored and adequate replacement provided to prevent depletion and its consequences. Some patients pass enormous amounts of electrolyte-rich urine.

Complications

The child with AKI has a tendency to develop water intoxication and hyponatremia, which makes it difficult to provide calories in sufficient amounts to meet the child's needs and reduce tissue catabolism, metabolic acidosis, hyperkalemia, and uremia. If the child is able to tolerate oral foods, food sources high in concentrated carbohydrate and fat but low in protein, potassium, and sodium may be provided. However, many children have functional disturbances of the gastrointestinal tract, such as nausea and vomiting; therefore the IV route is generally preferred and usually consists of essential amino acids or a combination of essential and nonessential amino acids administered by the central venous route.

Control of water balance in these patients requires careful monitoring of feedback information, such as accurate intake and output, body weight, and electrolyte measurements. In general, during the oliguric phase, no sodium, chloride, or potassium is given unless there are other large, ongoing losses. Regular measurement of plasma electrolyte, pH, BUN, and creatinine levels is required to assess the adequacy of fluid therapy and to anticipate complications that require specific treatment.

Hyperkalemia is the most immediate threat to the life of the child with AKI. Hyperkalemia can be minimized and sometimes avoided by eliminating potassium from all food and fluid, reducing tissue catabolism, and correcting acidosis. Measures used for the reduction of serum potassium levels are oral or rectal administration of an ion-exchange resin, such as sodium polystyrene sulfonate (Kayexalate) and peritoneal dialysis or hemodialysis (see later in the chapter). The resin produces its effect by exchange of its sodium for the potassium, thus binding potassium for removal from the body. This increased sodium concentration may contribute to fluid overload, hypertension, and cardiac failure. Dialysis removes potassium and other waste products from the serum by diffusion through a semipermeable membrane.

Hypertension is a frequent and serious complication of AKI, and to detect it early, blood pressure measurements are made every 4 to 6 hours. The most common cause of hypertension in AKI is overexpansion of extracellular fluid and plasma volume together with activation of the renin-angiotensin system. Hypertension is controlled with antihypertensive drugs. Other measures that may be used include limiting fluids and salt.

Anemia is frequently associated with AKI, but transfusion is not recommended unless the hemoglobin drops below 6 g/dl. Transfusions, if used, consist of fresh, packed RBCs given slowly to reduce the likelihood of increasing blood volume, hypertension, and hyperkalemia.

Seizures may occur when renal failure progresses to uremia and are also related to hypertension, hyponatremia, and hypocalcemia. Treatment is directed to the specific cause when known. More obscure causes are managed with antiepileptic drugs.

Cardiac failure with pulmonary edema is almost always associated with hypervolemia. Treatment is directed toward reduction of fluid volume, with water and sodium restriction and administration of diuretics.

Prognosis

The prognosis of AKI depends largely on the nature and severity of the causative factor or precipitating event and the promptness and competence of management. The outcome is least favorable in children with rapidly progressive nephritis and cortical necrosis. Children in whom AKI is a result of HUS or AGN may recover completely, but residual renal impairment or hypertension is more often seen. Complete recovery is usually expected in children whose renal failure is a result of dehydration, nephrotoxins, or ischemia. AKI after cardiac surgery is less favorable. It is often impossible to assess the extent of recovery for several months.

QUALITY PATIENT OUTCOMES: Acute Kidney Injury

- Underlying cause of acute kidney injury (AKI) identified and treated
- Water balance maintained
- Hypertension controlled
- Electrolyte balance maintained
- Diet maintains calories while minimizing tissue catabolism, metabolic acidosis, hyperkalemia, and uremia

Nursing Care Management

Meticulous attention to fluid intake and output is mandatory and includes all of the physical measurements discussed previously in relation to problems of fluid balance. Monitoring fluid balance and vital signs is a continuous process, and observers are constantly on the alert for signs of complications so that appropriate interventions can be implemented. Because these children require intensive observation and often specialized treatment (such as dialysis), they are usually admitted to an intensive care unit in which needed equipment and trained personnel are available (see the Next-Generation NCLEX® Examination-Style Unfolding Case Study box later in the chapter).

Limiting fluid intake requires ingenuity on the part of caregivers to cope with the child who is thirsty. Rationing the daily intake in small amounts of fluid served in containers that give the impression of larger volumes is one strategy. Older children who understand the rationale of fluid limits can help determine how their daily ration should be distributed.

Meeting nutritional needs is sometimes a problem; the child may be nauseated, and encouraging concentrated foods without fluids may be difficult. When nourishment is provided by the IV route, careful monitoring is essential to prevent fluid overload. In addition, nursing measures such as maintaining an optimal thermal environment, reducing any elevation of body temperature, and reducing restlessness and anxiety are used to decrease the rate of tissue catabolism.

The nurse must be continually alert for changes in behavior that indicate the onset of complications. Infection from reduced resistance, anemia, and general morbidity is a constant threat. Fluid overload and electrolyte disturbances can precipitate cardiovascular complications, such as hypertension and cardiac failure. Fluid and electrolyte imbalances, acidosis, and accumulation of nitrogenous waste products can produce neurologic involvement manifested by coma, seizures, or alterations in sensorium.

Although children with AKI are usually quite ill and voluntarily diminish their activity, infants may become restless and irritable, and children are often anxious and frightened. Frequent, painful, and stress-producing treatments and tests must be performed. A supportive, empathetic nurse can provide comfort and stability in a threatening and unnatural environment.

Family Support

Providing support and reassurance to parents is among the major nursing responsibilities. The seriousness of AKI and its emergency nature are stressful to parents, and most feel some degree of guilt regarding the child's condition, especially when the illness is a result of ingestion of a toxic substance, dehydration, or a genetic disease. They also need to be kept informed of the child's progress and provided explanations regarding the therapeutic regimen. The equipment and the child's behavior are sometimes frightening and anxiety provoking. Nurses can do much to help parents comprehend and deal with the stresses of the situation.

CHRONIC KIDNEY DISEASE

The kidneys are able to maintain the chemical composition of fluids within normal limits until more than 50% of functional renal capacity is destroyed by disease or injury. Chronic renal insufficiency or failure begins when the diseased kidneys can no longer maintain the normal chemical structure of body fluids under normal conditions. Progressive deterioration over months or years produces a variety of clinical and biochemical disturbances that eventually culminate in the clinical syndrome known as **uremia**.

A variety of diseases and disorders can result in CKD. The most frequent causes are congenital renal and urinary tract malformations, VUR associated with recurrent UTI, chronic pyelonephritis, hereditary disorders, chronic glomerulonephritis, and glomerulonephropathy associated with systemic diseases, such as anaphylactoid purpura and lupus erythematosus (see the Next-Generation NCLEX® Examination-Style Unfolding Case Study)

Pathophysiology

Early in the course of progressive renal failure, the child remains asymptomatic with only minimal biochemical abnormalities. Unless the presence of CKD is detected in the process of routine assessment, signs and symptoms that indicate advanced renal damage frequently emerge only late in the course of the disease. Midway in the disease process, as increasing numbers of nephrons are totally destroyed and most others are damaged to varying degrees, the few that remain intact

NEXT-GENERATION NCLEX® EXAMINATION-STYLE UNFOLDING CASE STUDY

The Child With Chronic Kidney Disease

Day 1 9:00 am

1. A 9-year-old girl who has a history of chronic pyelonephritis has increased symptoms. Over the past several months, she has experienced increased fatigue and lack of appetite, is unable to participate in physical activities, and appears pale and listless. Her parents took her to the pediatrician, who on examination found signs and symptoms of weight loss, facial puffiness, bone and joint pain, and dryness of the skin. She told the pediatrician she was having headaches. With the child's history of chronic pyelonephritis, she was immediately referred to a pediatric nephrologist. The nurse in the pediatric nephrology clinic performs a complete history and physical examination and finds the following data. Select the history and physical assessment findings that require follow-up by the nurse. **Select all that apply.**
   A. Nausea
   B. Pallor
   C. Headache
   D. Facial edema
   E. Increased fatigue
   F. Pulse 90 beats/min
   G. Muscle cramps
   H. Height=128 cm (25% for height)
   I. BP= 128/90 mmHg
   J. Weight=55 lbs (24.9 kg)
   K. Respirations= 20 breaths/min
   L. Temperature 98.4F (36.9C)
   M. Dryness and itchiness of the skin

Day 1, 10:00 am

2. Chronic kidney disease (CKD) occurs when the diseased kidneys can no longer maintain the normal chemical structure of blood fluids and chronic pyelonephritis can cause CKD. The pediatric nephrologist confirms that this young girl has CKD. What are the most appropriate nursing actions for a child with chronic kidney disease (CKD)? **Indicate which nursing action listed in the far-left column is appropriate to prevent the potential complication of chronic kidney disease listed in the middle column. Indicate the nursing action number in the far-right column.**
   <u>Note that ONLY one nursing action can be used for each potential postoperative complication and that NOT all nursing actions will be used.</u>

Nursing Action	Potential Complication	Nursing Action to Prevent Complication
1. Close monitoring of the patient's status. Follow clinical and laboratory findings. Blood studies included complete blood count (CBC), electrolytes, and kidney status.	waste products accumulate	
2. Observe for evidence of accumulated waste products.	increased excretory kidney demands	
3. Provide dietary instructions for foods that reduce excretory demands on kidneys and provide sufficient calories and protein for growth.	changes in kidney status go unrecognized	
4. Limit phosphorus, salt, and potassium as prescribed.	growth failure unrecognized	
5. Monitor growth closely since short stature is a significant side effect.	accumulation of minerals	
6. Monitor cardiovascular status, including blood pressure measurement.	renal bone disease	
7. Minimize renal bone disease by maintaining optimal calcium, phosphorus, and intact parathyroid hormone levels, and acid-base balance.		
8. Monitor for anemia. Child may require school accommodations and rest periods due to fatigue.		
9. Identify patient and family stressors that may accompany a diagnosis of CKD.		

Continued

NEXT-GENERATION NCLEX® EXAMINATION-STYLE UNFOLDING CASE STUDY—cont'd

The Child With Chronic Kidney Disease

30. days later, 9:00 am

3. A 9-year-old girl diagnosed with CKD is now being followed by a nephrology specialty team and has returned to the clinic for her monthly evaluation. The nurse performing the assessment finds Susie's blood pressure elevated and notices the child's skin is pale and sallow in appearance. The child tells the nurse that she has been really tired lately and her headaches have returned. She also says her feet are more swollen than usual. Which **immediate** steps would be taken to further evaluate the kidney status? **Select all that apply.**
   A. Check CBC.
   B. Check electrolyte status.
   C. Check kidney function.
   D. Check liver function.
   E. Perform lumbar puncture.
   F. Document weight, height and blood pressure.
   G. Compare vital signs and weight to previous visit.
   H. Evaluate patient adherence to medication and dietary recommendations.
4. The laboratory tests are ordered, and results are found below. Which findings require immediate follow-up? **Select all that apply.**
   A. hematocrit, 29%
   B. hemoglobin, 9.8 gm/dl
   C. platelets, 150,000/mm^3
   D. potassium, 4.9 mmol/L
   E. sodium, 139 mmol/L
   F. phosphorus 5.4 mmol/L
   G. serum creatinine, 1.9 mg/dL
   H. white blood count (WBC), 8,500/mm^3
   I. blood urea nitrogen (bun), 25 mg/dL
   J. urinalysis, elevated protein and hematuria
   K. glomerular function rate (GFR), 45 ml/min/1.73 m^2

30. Days later, 11:00 am

5. A 9-year-old girl diagnosed with CKD is now being followed by a nephrology specialty team. There is concern that the kidney status may be deteriorating based on the history and physical examination. Based on the abnormal history, physical and laboratory findings, what are the most appropriate dietary management strategies at this time? **Select all that apply.**
   A. Restrict sodium intake.
   B. Restrict foods high in sugar.
   C. Reduce foods high in calories.
   D. Limit protein to the reference daily intake for age.
   E. Reduce milk intake to correct sodium-glucose imbalance.
   F. Give oral medications to decrease creatinine gastrointestinal absorption.
   G. Provide sufficient calories and protein for growth while limiting excretory demands on the kidneys.

30. Days later, 1:00 pm

6. The nurse is meeting with the child and family to discuss CKD and what to observe for at home. The mother confides she is extremely scared that she will miss something, and symptoms will worsen without her recognizing them. She states, "I did not even realize her blood pressure was up and her kidneys were worse. How will I know when they are abnormal at home?" The nurse spends time reviewing the most important concerns to look for at home. The mother and child also meet with the dietician to review important things to remember about the diet. Which statements by the mother indicate that the health teaching was effective? **Select all that apply.**
   A. "My child will need to restrict her total calories each day to under 1,500 a day."
   B. "Her kidneys do not work to extract wastes from my child's body and we have to be careful about her diet."
   C. "Her protein intake will be limited to the reference daily intake for her age and outlined by the dietician."
   D. "I will need to call the health care team if I notice more swelling in her arms and feet and if she develops frequent headaches at home."
   E. "Frequent rest periods can help my child have more energy since she is anemic."
   F. "Since her blood pressure is elevated, I will follow the guidelines for medication administration and sodium restriction discussed with me by the dietician."

are hypertrophied but functional. These few normal nephrons are able to make sufficient adjustments to stresses to maintain reasonable degrees of fluid and electrolyte balance. Definitive biochemical examination at this time will reveal restricted tolerance to excesses or restrictions. As the disease progresses to the end stage, because of a severe reduction in the number of functioning nephrons, the kidneys are no longer able to maintain fluid and electrolyte balance, and the features of uremic syndrome appear.

The accumulation of various biochemical substances in the blood resulting from diminished renal function produces complications such as the following:

Retention of waste products, especially BUN and creatinine

Water and sodium retention, which contributes to edema and vascular congestion

Hyperkalemia of dangerous levels

Metabolic acidosis of a sustained nature because of continual hydrogen ion retention and bicarbonate loss

Calcium and phosphorus disturbances, resulting in altered bone metabolism, which in turn causes growth arrest or retardation, bone pain, and deformities known as **renal osteodystrophy**

Anemia caused by hematologic dysfunction, including a shortened life span of RBCs, impaired RBC production related to decreased production of erythropoietin, prolonged bleeding time, and nutritional anemia

Growth disturbance, probably caused by such factors as renal osteodystrophy, poor nutrition associated with dietary restrictions and loss of appetite, and biochemical abnormalities

Children with CKD seem to be more susceptible to infection, especially pneumonia, UTI, and septicemia, although the reason for this is unclear. These children become extraordinarily sensitive to changes in vascular volume that may cause pulmonary overload, CNS symptoms, hypertension, and cardiac failure.

Diagnostic Evaluation

The diagnosis of CKD is usually suspected on the basis of any number of clinical manifestations, a history of prior renal disease, or biochemical findings. The onset is usually gradual, and the initial signs and symptoms are vague and nonspecific (Box 26.6).

Laboratory and other diagnostic tools and tests are of value in assessing the extent of renal damage, biochemical disturbances, and related physical dysfunction (see Tables 26.1 to 26.3). Often they can help establish the nature of the underlying disease and differentiate among other disease processes and the pathologic consequences of renal dysfunction.

Therapeutic Management

In irreversible renal failure, the goals of medical management are to (1) promote maximum renal function, (2) maintain body fluid and electrolyte balance within safe biochemical limits, (3) treat systemic

BOX 26.6 Clinical Manifestations of Chronic Renal Failure

Early signs:
- Loss of normal energy
- Increased fatigue on exertion
- Pallor, subtle (may not be noticed)
- Elevated blood pressure (sometimes)

As the disease progresses:
- Decreased appetite (especially at breakfast)
- Less interest in normal activities
- Increased or decreased urinary output with compensatory intake of fluid
- Pallor more evident
- Sallow, muddy appearance of skin

Child may complain of:
- Headache
- Muscle cramps
- Nausea

Other signs and symptoms:
- Weight loss
- Facial edema
- Malaise
- Bone or joint pain
- Growth retardation
- Dryness or itching of the skin
- Bruised skin
- Sensory or motor loss (sometimes)
- Amenorrhea (common in adolescent girls)

Uremic syndrome (untreated):
- Gastrointestinal symptoms
  - Anorexia
  - Nausea and vomiting
- Bleeding tendencies
  - Bruises
  - Bloody diarrheal stools
  - Bleeding from lips and mouth
- Stomatitis
- Intractable itching
- Uremic frost (deposits of urea crystals on skin)
- Unpleasant "uremic" breath odor
- Deep respirations
- Hypertension
- Congestive heart failure
- Pulmonary edema
- Neurologic involvement
  - Progressive confusion
  - Dulled sensorium
  - Coma (ultimately)
  - Tremors
  - Muscular twitching
  - Seizures

complications, and (4) promote as active and normal a life as possible for the child for as long as possible. The child is allowed unrestricted activity and is allowed to set his or her own limits regarding rest and extent of exertion. School attendance is encouraged as long as the child is able. When the effort is too great, home tutoring is arranged.

Diet regulation is the most effective means, short of dialysis, of reducing the quantity of materials that require renal excretion. The goals of diet management in renal failure are to provide sufficient calories and protein for growth while limiting the excretory demands made on the kidneys, to minimize metabolic bone disease (**osteodystrophy**), and to minimize fluid and electrolyte disturbances. Dietary protein intake is limited only to the reference daily intake (Recommended Dietary Allowance [RDA]) for the child's age. Restriction of protein intake below the RDA is believed to negatively affect growth and neurodevelopment. Malnutrition due to factors including anorexia, dietary restrictions, metabolic acidosis, and increased energy expenditure is common in these children (Carrero, Stenvinkel, Cuppari, et al., 2013).

Sodium and water are not usually limited unless there is evidence of edema or hypertension, and potassium is not usually restricted. However, restrictions of any or all three may be imposed in later stages or at any time that abnormal serum concentrations are evident.

Dietary phosphorus is controlled through reduction of protein and milk intake to prevent or correct the calcium-phosphorus imbalance. Phosphorus levels can be further reduced by oral administration of calcium carbonate preparations or other phosphate-binding agents that combine with the phosphorus to decrease gastrointestinal absorption and thus the serum levels of phosphate. Treatment with (inactive) 25-OH vitamin D and/or (active) 1,25-dihydroxy vitamin D is begun to increase calcium absorption and suppress elevated parathyroid hormone levels (Wesseling-Perry & Salusky, 2013).

Metabolic acidosis is alleviated through administration of alkalizing agents, such as sodium bicarbonate or a combination of sodium and potassium citrate.

Growth failure is one major consequence of CKD, especially in preadolescents. These children grow poorly both before and after the initiation of hemodialysis. The use of recombinant human growth hormone to accelerate growth in children with growth retardation secondary to CKD has been successful (Gupta & Lee, 2012). **Osseous deformities** that result from renal osteodystrophy, especially those related to ambulation, are troublesome and require correction if they occur. Dental defects are common in children with CKD, and the earlier the onset of the disease, the more severe are the dental manifestations (including hypoplasia, hypomineralization, tooth discoloration, alteration in size and shape of teeth, malocclusion, and ulcerative stomatitis). Therefore regular dental care is important in these children.

Anemia in children with CKD is related to decreased production of erythropoietin. Recombinant human erythropoietin (rHuEPO) is being offered to these children as thrice-weekly or weekly subcutaneous injections and is replacing the need for frequent blood transfusions. The drug corrects the anemia, which in turn increases appetite, activity, and general well-being in the children who receive it.

Hypertension may be managed initially by cautious use of a low-sodium diet, fluid restriction, and perhaps diuretics, such as hydrochlorothiazide or furosemide. Severe hypertension requires the use of other antihypertensive agents, singly or in combination.

Intercurrent infections are treated with appropriate antimicrobials at the first sign of infection; however, any drug eliminated through the kidneys is administered with caution. Other complications are treated symptomatically (e.g., central-acting antiemetics for nausea, antiepileptics for seizures, and diphenhydramine [Benadryl] for pruritus).

When the child reaches end-stage renal failure, death will eventually occur unless waste products and toxins are removed from body fluids by dialysis or kidney transplantation. These techniques have been adapted for infants and small children and are implemented in most cases of renal failure after conservative management is no longer effective (see Technologic Management of Renal Failure later in the chapter).

Prognosis

Dialysis and transplantation are the only treatments currently available for children with ESRD. Although children may survive on dialysis, it is not an ideal long-term modality. Complications include infection of access sites, growth failure, and disruption of normal socialization. Many pediatric centers encourage families of children with ESRD to consider kidney transplantation. The North American Pediatric Renal Trials and Collaborative Studies' annual transplant report documents graft survival of 96% at 1 year and 84% at 5 years for living donor kidneys and of 95% at 1 year and 78% at 5 years for deceased donor kidneys (Smith, Martz, & Blydt-Hansen, 2013).

Posttransplant complications include infection, hypertension, steroid toxicity, hyperlipidemia, aseptic necrosis, malignancy, and growth retardation (Verghese, 2017). Long-term graft survival is not guaranteed, and many children require a second or third transplant. Successful kidney transplantation does improve rehabilitation of children with CKD, both educationally and psychologically. Increasing use of primary or preemptive kidney transplants is becoming the optimal form of renal replacement therapy, leading to substantial improvement in quality of life (Goldstein, Rosburg, Warady, et al., 2009).

QUALITY PATIENT OUTCOMES: Chronic Kidney Disease

- Sufficient calories and protein for growth maintained
- Excretory demands made on the kidney are limited
- Metabolic bone disease (osteodystrophy) minimal
- Fluid and electrolyte disturbances managed
- Hypertension managed
- Growth retardation treated

Nursing Care Management

The multiple complications of ESRD are managed according to medical protocols, such as the National Kidney Foundation Kidney Disease Outcomes Quality Initiative's evidence-based clinical practice guidelines (https://www.kidney.org/professionals/guidelines). However, progressive disease places a number of stresses on the child and family, including those of a potentially fatal illness (see Chapter 17). There is a continuing need for repeated examinations that often entail painful procedures, side effects, and frequent hospitalizations. Diet therapy becomes progressively more restricted and intense, and the child is required to take a variety of medications. Ever present in all aspects of the treatment regimen is the realization that without treatment, death is inevitable.

Some specific stresses related to ESRD and its treatment are predictable. When it first becomes apparent that ESRD is inevitable, both parents and child experience depression and anxiety. Acceptance is particularly difficult if renal failure progresses rapidly after diagnosis. Denial and disbelief are usually pronounced. After renal failure is established and symptoms become progressively more distressing, the initiation of dialysis is usually perceived as a positive experience, and after experiencing initial concerns regarding the treatment, the child begins to feel better, and parental anxiety is relieved for a time.

For children, however, initiating a dialysis regimen is a traumatic and anxiety-provoking experience, because it involves surgery for implantation of a graft, fistula, or peritoneal catheter. The initial experience with the dialysis procedure is frightening to most children. They need reassurance about the nature of the preparations for dialysis and the conduct of the treatment.

Adolescents, with their increased need for independence and their urge for rebellion, usually adapt less well than younger children. They resent the control and enforced dependence imposed by the rigorous and unrelenting therapy program. They resent being dependent on hemodialysis technology, their parents, and the professional staff. Depression or hostility is common in adolescents undergoing hemodialysis.

Both the graft and the fistula require needle insertions at each dialysis. The goal is to perform pain-free venipuncture. Using buffered lidocaine with a small-gauge needle (30-gauge) to anesthetize the area before venipuncture of the graft or fistula is one method. Using an anesthetizing topical preparation, such as eutectic mixture of local anesthetics (EMLA; lidocaine and prilocaine) 1 hour before venipuncture is another approach (see Chapter 5, Pain Management). External dual-lumen venous access devices eliminate the need for needles but are more prone to infection and other central line complications.

The availability of home peritoneal dialysis has offered a greater degree of freedom for persons undergoing long-term dialysis. The nurse is responsible for teaching the family about (1) the disease, its implications, and the therapeutic plan; (2) the possible psychologic effects of the disease and the treatment; and (3) the technical aspects of the procedure. The family learns to manage the various aspects of the dialysis procedure, how to maintain accurate records, and how to observe for signs of complications that need to be reported to the proper persons.

Body changes related to the disease process (such as pale or ashen skin color, growth retardation, and lack of sexual maturation) are stress provoking. Dietary restrictions are particularly burdensome for both children and parents. Children feel deprived when they are unable to eat foods previously enjoyed and that are unrestricted for other family members. Consequently, they may fail to cooperate. Diet restrictions may be interpreted as punishment. Some children, unable to understand fully the purpose of restrictions, will sneak forbidden food items at every opportunity. Allowing children, especially adolescents, maximum participation in and responsibility for their own treatment program is helpful.

After months or years of dialysis, the parents and child feel anxiety associated with the prognosis and continued pressures of the treatment. The continuous need for treatment interferes with family plans. The time spent in transportation to and from the dialysis unit and the time spent undergoing dialysis treatments cut into time for outside activities, including school. Graft and fistula problems, as well as peritoneal catheter exit site infections, may develop and present a common source of aggravation.

The possibility of kidney transplantation often provides hope for relief from the rigors of hemodialysis and peritoneal dialysis. Most children and families respond well to a kidney transplant, and most children can be successfully rehabilitated.

The National Kidney Foundation[b] and other agencies provide a number of services and information for families of children with renal disease.

TECHNOLOGIC MANAGEMENT OF RENAL FAILURE

DIALYSIS

Dialysis is the process of separating colloids and crystalline substances in solution by the difference in their rate of diffusion through a semipermeable membrane. Methods of dialysis currently available for

[b]30 E. 33rd St., New York, NY 10016; 212-889-2210, 800-622-9010; http://www.kidney.org. In Canada: Kidney Foundation of Canada, 310–5160 Decarie Blvd., Montreal, QC H3X 2H9; 514-369-4806, 800-361-7494; http://www.kidney.ca.

clinical management of renal failure are **peritoneal dialysis**, wherein the abdominal cavity acts as a semipermeable membrane through which water and solutes of small molecular size move by osmosis and diffusion according to their respective concentrations on either side of the membrane, and **hemodialysis**, in which blood is circulated outside the body through artificial membranes that permit a similar passage of water and solutes. A third type of dialysis is **hemofiltration**, in which blood filtrate is circulated outside the body by hydrostatic pressure exerted across a semipermeable membrane with simultaneous infusion of a replacement solution. Types of hemofiltration include continuous venovenous hemofiltration and continuous venovenous hemodialysis. These continuous renal replacement therapies are used in AKI, severe fluid overload, and inborn errors of metabolism or after bone marrow transplant.

Peritoneal dialysis is the preferred form of dialysis for infants, children, and parents who wish to remain independent, families who live a long distance from the medical center, and children who prefer fewer dietary restrictions and a gentler form of dialysis. Chronic peritoneal dialysis is most often performed at home. The two types of peritoneal dialysis are **continuous ambulatory peritoneal dialysis** and **continuous cycling peritoneal dialysis**. In both methods, commercially available sterile dialysis solution is instilled into the peritoneal cavity through a surgically implanted indwelling catheter tunneled subcutaneously and sutured into place. The warmed solution is allowed to enter the peritoneal cavity by gravity and remains for a variable length of time according to the rate of solute removal and glucose absorption in individual patients. The care and management of the procedure are the responsibility of the parents of young children. Some centers have initiated use of home health nurses to give parents respite from care. Older children and adolescents can carry out the procedure themselves, which provides them with some control and less dependency. This is especially important for adolescents.

Hemodialysis requires the creation of a vascular access and the use of special dialysis equipment—the hemodialyzer, or so-called artificial kidney. Vascular access may be one of three types: fistulas, grafts, or external vascular access devices. An **arteriovenous fistula** is an access in which a vein and artery are connected surgically. The preferred site is the radial artery and a forearm vein that produces dilation and thickening of the superficial vessels of the forearm to provide easy access for repeated venipuncture. An alternative is the creation of a subcutaneous (internal) **arteriovenous graft** by anastomosing artery and vein, with a synthetic prosthetic graft for circulatory access. The most commonly used material is expanded polytetrafluoroethylene (ePTFE). Both the graft and the fistula require needle insertions with each dialysis treatment.

For external vascular access devices, percutaneous catheters are inserted in the femoral, subclavian, or internal jugular veins, even in very small children. A more permanent form of external access is available via a central catheter inserted surgically into the internal jugular vein. This catheter has a dual lumen, which allows a larger volume of blood flow with minimum recirculation. Catheters eliminate the need for skin punctures but require some home care.

Hemodialysis is best suited to children who do not have someone in the family who is able to perform home peritoneal dialysis and to those who live close to a dialysis center. The procedure is usually performed three times per week for 4 to 6 hours, depending on the child's size. Studies suggest that intensified hemodialysis (shorter sessions done 5 to 7 days weekly or longer sessions done overnight three to seven times weekly) may improve outcomes (Thumfart, Pommer, Querfeld, et al., 2014). Hemodialysis achieves rapid correction of fluid and electrolyte abnormalities but can cause problems in association with this rapid change, such as muscle cramping and hypotension. Disadvantages include school absence during dialysis and strict fluid and dietary restrictions between dialysis sessions. Boredom for the child and family is often a problem during dialysis, and planned activities should be introduced (Fig. 26.7).

> **! NURSING ALERT**
>
> Observe for changes in the color of the dialysate draining from the child. The spent solution should be clear. If the color is cloudy, notify the practitioner immediately.

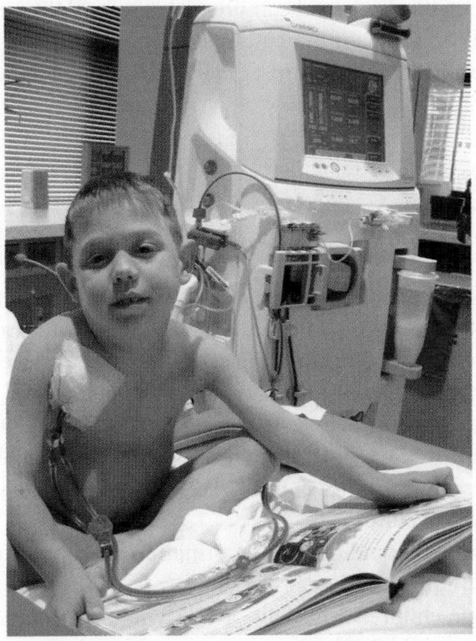

Fig. 26.7 Diversional activities help lessen the boredom children can experience during hemodialysis.

Most children show rapid clinical improvement with the implementation of dialysis, although this is directly related to the duration of uremia before dialysis and good nutrition. Growth rate and skeletal maturation improve, but recovery of normal growth is infrequent. In many cases, sexual development, although delayed, progresses to completion.

TRANSPLANTATION

Kidney transplantation is an acceptable and effective means of therapy in the pediatric age-group. Although peritoneal dialysis and hemodialysis are life preserving, both require major alterations in lifestyle. Transplantation offers the opportunity for a relatively normal life and is the preferred form of treatment for children with ESRD.

Kidneys for transplant are available from two sources: a **living related donor**, usually a parent or a sibling, or a **cadaver donor**, wherein the family of a dead or brain-dead patient consents to donation of a healthy kidney. Retransplantation may be required if rejection occurs.

The primary goal in transplantation is the long-term survival of grafted tissue by securing tissue that is antigenically similar to that of the recipient and by suppressing the recipient's immune mechanism. The immunosuppressant therapy of choice has been corticosteroids (prednisone) in conjunction with cyclosporine or tacrolimus and mycophenolate mofetil. Other therapies include antilymphoblast globulin or monoclonal antibodies. New immunosuppressant medications and early withdrawal of steroids or steroid-free protocols are rapidly coming into clinical trials and use in large transplant centers (Kim, Webster, & Craig, 2013). It is important for the nurse to learn about the medications used in the antirejection protocols and their side effects.

Because the immunosuppressant medications are taken indefinitely, transplant patients experience many side effects of the drugs, including hypertension, growth retardation, cataracts, risk of infection, obesity, characteristics of Cushing syndrome, and hirsutism.

Rejection of the transplanted kidney is the most common cause of transplant failure. Rejection is treated aggressively with immunosuppressant medications and can often be reversed. Some patients do not respond to treatment of acute rejection or develop chronic rejection and must eventually return to dialysis or undergo another kidney transplant.

! NURSING ALERT

The child with a kidney transplant who exhibits any of the following should be evaluated immediately for possible rejection:

- Fever
- Swelling and tenderness over graft area
- Diminished urinary output
- Elevated blood pressure
- Elevated serum creatinine

CLINICAL JUDGMENT AND NEXT-GENERATION NCLEX® EXAMINATION-STYLE QUESTIONS

1. The nurse is caring for a 4-year-old girl with a history of frequent urinary tract infections (UTIs). The child presents with strong-smelling urine, frequency and pain on urination. A urinalysis is needed for diagnostic evaluation and the nurse is preparing the child and mother for a clean voided urine specimen for evaluation. What does the nurse need to be aware of before obtaining the urine sample? **Select all that apply.**
   A. Children who are toilet trained can provide a clean voided urine sample for culture.
   B. The nurse should obtain the urine specimen through suprapubic aspiration.
   C. Because children who have a UTI will have painful urination, have the child drink a large amount of fluid before obtaining the sample.
   D. The specimen should be sent to the laboratory less than 8 hours after voiding with storage at room temperature or less than 8 hours after voiding with refrigeration.
   E. The child should be told to urinate in the toilet and that midway through urination a small amount of urine should be collected in a sterile container.
   F. Because the child is febrile, the nurse should immediately start an antimicrobial and then obtain a urine culture.

2. A 7-year-old girl with periorbital edema, hypertension, decreased urine output, pallor, and fatigue is admitted to the pediatric unit. She had a cold and sore throat 2 weeks ago that resolved. Her brother and younger sister also had these symptoms. She is active in school and plays soccer. **Choose the most likely options for the information missing from the statements below by selecting from the lists of options provided.**
   Children who present with ____1____ glomerulonephritis may have a history of a ____2____ infection. ____3____ tests during the acute phase shows hematuria and proteinuria.

Options for 1	Options for 2	Options for 3
post staphylococcal	Group A beta-hemolytic streptococci	Blood
post meningitis	Group B beta-hemolytic streptococci	Urine
post streptococcal	Group A beta-hemolytic staphylococcus	Radiographic
post pneumococcal	Group B beta-hemolytic staphylococcus	Ultrasound

3. A three-year-old girl has a urinary tract infection (UTI) and is seen for follow-up in the pediatric office. The nurse after completing a history and physical examination is meeting with the mother to discuss important ways to prevent another urinary tract infection. Which of the topics listed below would be included in the health teaching for the parent before leaving the clinic? **Select all that apply.**
   A. Give prophylactic antibiotics.
   B. Encourage adequate fluid intake.
   C. Make sure the child is not constipated.
   D. How to cleanse the genital areas from front to back.
   E. Encourage the child to hold urine as long as possible.
   F. Make sure mother is aware of the signs and symptoms of UTI.
   G. Make sure the child empties the bladder completely and frequently.

4. A 4-month-old child has had surgical correction for hypospadias. The nurse is meeting with the mother to give discharge instructions for home care. The mother is young and recently divorced. This is her first child. The infant will have a stent in place to drain urine for the next 5-10 days. The nurse recognizes a **need for additional teaching** when the mother says which of the following? **Select all that apply.**
   A. "I know that the catheter will drain into the diaper for 5-10 days."
   B. "I will give pain medication around the clock for 14 days after surgery."
   C. "My child can take a tub bath when we arrive home because it will soothe the area."
   D. "My child will be on an antibiotic to prevent infection until the catheter is removed."
   E. "I realize that bladder spasms may occur and my child may arch his back and bring his knees up to his chest during the spasm."

REFERENCES

American Academy of Pediatrics Task Force on Circumcision. (2012). Circumcision policy statement. *Pediatrics, 130*(3), 585–586.

Balat, A., Karakok, M., Guler, E., Ucaner, N., & Kibar, Y. (2008). Local defense systems in the prepuce. *Scandinavian Journal of Urology and Nephrology, 42*(1), 63–65.

Carrero, J. J., Stenvinkel, P., Cuppari, L., Ikizler, T. A., Kalantar-Zadeh, K., Kaysen, G., et al. (2013). Etiology of the protein-energy wasting syndrome in chronic kidney disease: A consensus statement from the International Society of Renal Nutrition and Metabolism (ISRNM). *The Journal of Renal Nutrition, 23*(2), 77–90.

Chevalier, R. L. (2015). Congenital urinary tract obstruction: The long view. *Advances in Chronic Kidney Disease, 22*(4), 312–319.

Edlin, R. S., Shapiro, D. J., Hersh, A. L., & Copp, H. L. (2013). Antibiotic resistance patterns of outpatient pediatric urinary tract infections. *Journal of Urology, 190*(1), 222–227.

Estrada, C. R., Jr., Passerotti, C. C., Graham, D. A., Peters, C. A., Bauer, S. B., Diamond, D. A., et al. (2009). Nomograms for predicting annual resolution rate of primary vesicoureteral reflux: Results from 2,462 children. *Journal of Urology, 182*(4), 1535–1541.

Feldkamp, M. L., Botto, L. D., Amar, E., Bakker, M. K., Bermejo-Sanchez, E., Bianca, S., et al. (2011). Cloacal exstrophy: An epidemiologic study from the International Clearinghouse for Birth Defects Surveillance and Research. *American Journal of Medical Genetics Part C: Seminars in Medical Genetics, 157c*(4), 333–343.

Goldstein, S. L. (2016). Medication-induced acute kidney injury. *Current Opinion in Critical Care, 22*(6), 542–545.

Goldstein, S. L., Rosburg, N. M., Warady, B. A., Seikaly, M., McDonald, R., Limbers, C., et al. (2009). Pediatric end stage renal disease health-related quality of life differs by modality: A PedsQL ESRD analysis. *Pediatric Nephrology, 24*(8), 1553–1560.

Gray, M., & Moore, K. N. (Eds.). (2009). *Urologic disorders: Adult and pediatric care*. St Louis. MO: Mosby/Elsevier.

Grinspon, R. P., & Rey, R. A. (2014). When hormone defects cannot explain it: Malformative disorders of sex development. *Birth Defects Research Part C: Embryo Today, 102*(4), 359–373.

Gupta, V., & Lee, M. (2012). Growth hormone in chronic renal disease. *Indian Journal of Endocrinology and Metabolism, 16*(2), 195–203.

Hoberman, A., & Chesney, R. W. (2014). Antimicrobial prophylaxis for children with vesicoureteral reflux. *The New England Journal of Medicine, 371*(11), 1072–1073. https://doi.org/10.1056/NEJMc1408559.

Inouye, B. M., Massanyi, E. Z., Di Carlo, H., Shah, B. B., & Gearhart, J. P. (2013). Modern management of bladder exstrophy repair. *Current Urology Reports, 14*(4), 359–365.

Inouye, B. M., Tourchi, A., Di Carlo, H. N., Young, E. E., & Gearhart, J. P. (2014). Modern management of the exstrophy-epispadias complex. *Surgery Research and Practice, 2014*, 587064.

Jayachandran, D., Bythell, M., Platt, M. W., & Rankin, J. (2011). Register based study of bladder exstrophy-epispadias complex: Prevalence, associated anomalies, prenatal diagnosis and survival. *Journal of Urology, 186*(5), 2056–2060.

Jepson, R. G., Williams, G., & Craig, J. C. (2012). Cranberries for preventing urinary tract infections. *The Cochrane Database of Systematic Reviews, 10*, CD001321.

Kasprenski, M., Benz, K., Maruf, M., Jayman, J., Di Carlo, H., & Gearhart, J. (2018). Modern management of the failed bladder exstrophy closure: A 50-yr experience. *European Urology Focus*. https://doi.org/10.1016/j.euf.2018.09.008.

Kim, S., Webster, A. C., & Craig, J. C. (2013). Current trends in immunosuppression following organ transplantation in children. *Current Opinion in Organ Transplantation, 18*(5), 537–542.

Kolon, T. F., Herndon, C. D., Baker, L. A., Baskin, L. S., Baxter, C. G., Cheng, E. Y., et al. (2014). Evaluation and treatment of cryptorchidism: AUA guideline. *Journal of Urology, 192*(2), 337–345.

Kozlowski, L. J. (2008). The acute pain service nurse practitioner: A case study in the postoperative care of the child with bladder exstrophy. *The Journal of Pediatric Health Care, 22*(6), 351–359.

Lee, P. A., Nordenstrom, A., Houk, C. P., Ahmed, S. F., Auchus, R., Baratz, A., et al. (2016). Global disorders of sex development update since 2006: perceptions, approach and care. *Hormone Research in Paediatrics, 85*(3), 158–180.

Lombel, R. M., Gipson, D. S., & Hodson, E. M. (2013). Treatment of steroid-sensitive nephrotic syndrome: New guidelines from KDIGO. *Pediatric Nephrology, 28*(3), 415–426.

Malykhina, A. P., Wyndaele, J. J., Andersson, K. E., De Wachter, S., & Dmochowski, R. R. (2012). Do the urinary bladder and large bowel interact, in sickness or in health? ICI-RS 2011. *Neurourology and Urodynamics, 31*(3), 352–358.

Nast, C. C. (2012). Infection-related glomerulonephritis: Changing demographics and outcomes. *Advances in Chronic Kidney Disease, 19*(2), 68–75.

Ranfaing, J., Dunyach-Remy, C., Lavigne, J. P., & Sotto, A. (2018). Propolis potentiates the effect of cranberry (Vaccinium macrocarpon) in reducing the motility and the biofilm formation of uropathogenic Escherichia coli. *PLoS One, 13*(8), e0202609.

Rheault, M. N., Wei, C. C., Hains, D. S., Wang, W., Kerlin, B. A., & Smoyer, W. E. (2014). Increasing frequency of acute kidney injury amongst children hospitalized with nephrotic syndrome. *Pediatric Nephrology, 29*(1), 139–147.

Roberts, K. B. (2011). Urinary tract infection: Clinical practice guideline for the diagnosis and management of the initial UTI in febrile infants and children 2 to 24 months. *Pediatrics, 128*(3), 595–610.

Shaikh, N., Craig, J. C., Rovers, M. M., Da Dalt, L., Gardikis, S., Hoberman, A., et al. (2014). Identification of children and adolescents at risk for renal scarring after a first urinary tract infection: A meta-analysis with individual patient data. *JAMA Pediatrics, 168*(10), 893–900.

Shaikh, N., Morone, N. E., Bost, J. E., & Farrell, M. H. (2008). Prevalence of urinary tract infection in childhood: A meta-analysis. *The Pediatric Infectious Disease Journal, 27*(4), 302–308.

Sihra, N., Goodman, A., Zakri, R., Sahai, A., & Malde, S. (2018). Nonantibiotic prevention and management of recurrent urinary tract infection. *Nature Reviews Urology, 15*(12), 750–776.

Sijstermans, K., Hack, W. W., Meijer, R. W., & van der Voort-Doedens, L. M. (2008). The frequency of undescended testis from birth to adulthood: A review. *International Journal of Andrology, 31*(1), 1–11.

Smith, J. M., Martz, K., & Blydt-Hansen, T. D. (2013). Pediatric kidney transplant practice patterns and outcome benchmarks, 1987-2010: A report of the north american pediatric renal trials and collaborative studies. *Pediatric Transplant, 17*(2), 149–157.

Springer, A., van den Heijkant, M., & Baumann, S. (2016). Worldwide prevalence of hypospadias. *Journal of Pediatric Urology, 12*(3), 152.e151-e157.

Suominen, J. S., Santtila, P., & Taskinen, S. (2015). Sexual function in patients operated on for bladder exstrophy and epispadias. *Journal of Urology, 194*(1), 195–199.

Susantitaphong, P., Cruz, D. N., Cerda, J., Abulfaraj, M., Alqahtani, F., Koulouridis, I., et al. (2013). World incidence of AKI: A meta-analysis. *Clinical Journal of the American Society of Nephrology, 8*(9), 1482–1493.

Thumfart, J., Pommer, W., Querfeld, U., & Muller, D. (2014). Intensified hemodialysis in adults, and in children and adolescents. *Deutsches Ärzteblatt International, 111*(14), 237–243.

Vasudeva, P., & Madersbacher, H. (2014). Factors implicated in pathogenesis of urinary tract infections in neurogenic bladders: Some revered, few forgotten, others ignored. *Neurourology and Urodynamics, 33*(1), 95–100.

Verghese, P. S. (2017). Pediatric kidney transplantation: A historical review. *Pediatric Research, 81*(1-2), 259–264.

Walsh, P. R., & Johnson, S. (2018). Treatment and management of children with haemolytic uraemic syndrome. *Archives of Disease in Childhood, 103*(3), 285–291.

Wesseling-Perry, K., & Salusky, I. B. (2013). Phosphate binders, vitamin D and calcimimetics in the management of chronic kidney disease-mineral bone disorders (CKD-MBD) in children. *Pediatric Nephrology, 28*(4), 617–625.

27

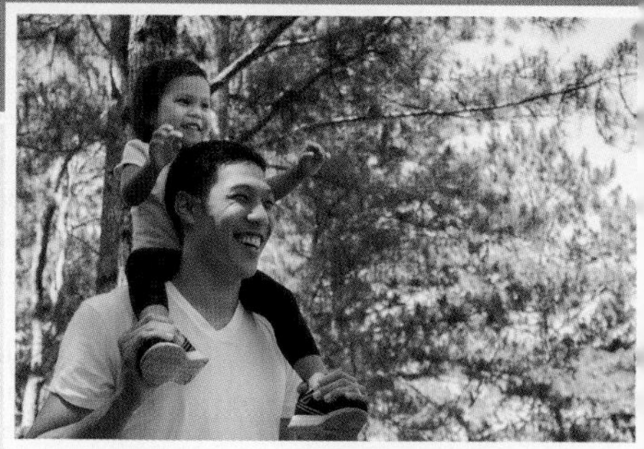

The Child With Cerebral Dysfunction

Marilyn J. Hockenberry

http://evolve.elsevier.com/wong/essentials

CONCEPTS

- Intracranial Regulation
- Sensory Perception
- Infection
- Safety

THE BRAIN AND INCREASED INTRACRANIAL PRESSURE

The brain, tightly enclosed in the solid bony cranium, is well protected but highly vulnerable to pressure that may accumulate within the enclosure (Fig. 27.1). Its total volume—brain (80%), cerebrospinal fluid (CSF; 10%), and blood (10%)—must remain approximately the same at all times. A change in the proportional volume of one of these components (e.g., increase or decrease in intracranial blood) must be accompanied by a compensatory change in another (e.g., decrease or increase in CSF). In this way the volume and pressure normally remain constant. Examples of compensatory changes are reduction in blood volume, decrease in production of CSF, increase in CSF absorption, or shrinkage of brain mass by displacement of intracellular and extracellular fluid.

Children with open fontanels compensate for increased volume by skull expansion and widened sutures. However, at any age the capacity for spatial compensation is limited. An increase in intracranial pressure (ICP) may be caused by tumors or other space-occupying lesions, accumulation of fluid within the ventricular system, bleeding, or edema of cerebral tissues. Once compensation is exhausted, any further increase in volume results in a rapid rise in ICP.

The early signs and symptoms of increased ICP, such as headache, vomiting, personality changes, irritability, and fatigue, are often subtle (Box 27.1). In older children, subjective symptoms are headache, especially when arising after lying flat (e.g., on awakening in the morning) or when coughing, sneezing, or bending over, and nausea and vomiting. The child may complain of double vision or blurred vision with movement of the head. Seizures may occur. In children whose cranial sutures have not closed, there is an increase in head circumference and tense or bulging fontanels. Cranial sutures may widen. Head circumference can enlarge until the child is 5 years of age if the condition progresses slowly. As pressure increases, the pupils become progressively sluggish in reaction and eventually become fixed and dilated. The level of consciousness progressively deteriorates from drowsiness to eventual coma. Problems related to increased ICP are discussed later in the chapter in relation to head injury and hydrocephalus (see Chapter 25, Brain Tumors).

Physiologic and biochemical changes within the cerebral vasculature serve to complicate the primary causes of increased ICP. Especially in cases of trauma, blood flow often initially increases as a result of venous congestion or vasomotor paralysis. If cerebral hypoxia is associated with the cerebral dysfunction, the compensatory vasodilation caused by oxygen deficiency will tend to increase the cerebral flow. However, blood flow is reduced as ICP progressively increases, with diminished blood supply to the brain tissues. The classic responses observed in adults (widening pulse pressure, increased blood pressure) rarely occur in children or are very late signs. Periodic or irregular breathing is an ominous sign of brainstem (especially medullary) dysfunction that often precedes apnea.

EVALUATION OF NEUROLOGIC STATUS

Earlier chapters discuss methods to evaluate neurologic function in relation to numerous aspects of child care. The neurologic examination is an integral part of the health assessment (see Chapter 4) and newborn assessment (see Chapter 7). Chapter 30 discusses some of the tests used to differentiate neuromuscular disorders. The assessment tools and examinations in this chapter are primarily those used to assess intracranial integrity.

ASSESSMENT: GENERAL ASPECTS

Children younger than 2 years of age require special evaluation because they are unable to respond to directions designed to elicit specific neurologic responses. Early neurologic responses in infants are primarily reflexive; these responses are gradually replaced by meaningful movement in the characteristic cephalocaudal direction of development. This evidence of progressive maturation reflects more extensive myelinization and changes in neurochemical and electrophysiologic properties.

Most information about infants and small children comes from observation of spontaneous and elicited reflex responses. As they develop increasingly complex gross and fine motor skills and communication skills, more sophisticated techniques are used to assess acquisition of developmental milestones. Delay or deviation from expected milestones helps identify high-risk children. Persistence or reappearance of primitive reflexes indicates a pathologic condition. In evaluating the infant or young child, it is important to obtain the history of the pregnancy, delivery, respiratory status at birth, and neonatal health, including any need for intensive care hospitalization to determine the possible impact of intrauterine and extrauterine environmental influences known to affect the orderly maturation of the central nervous system (CNS). These influences include maternal infections, chemical exposure, trauma, medication, illicit drug use, and metabolic insults.

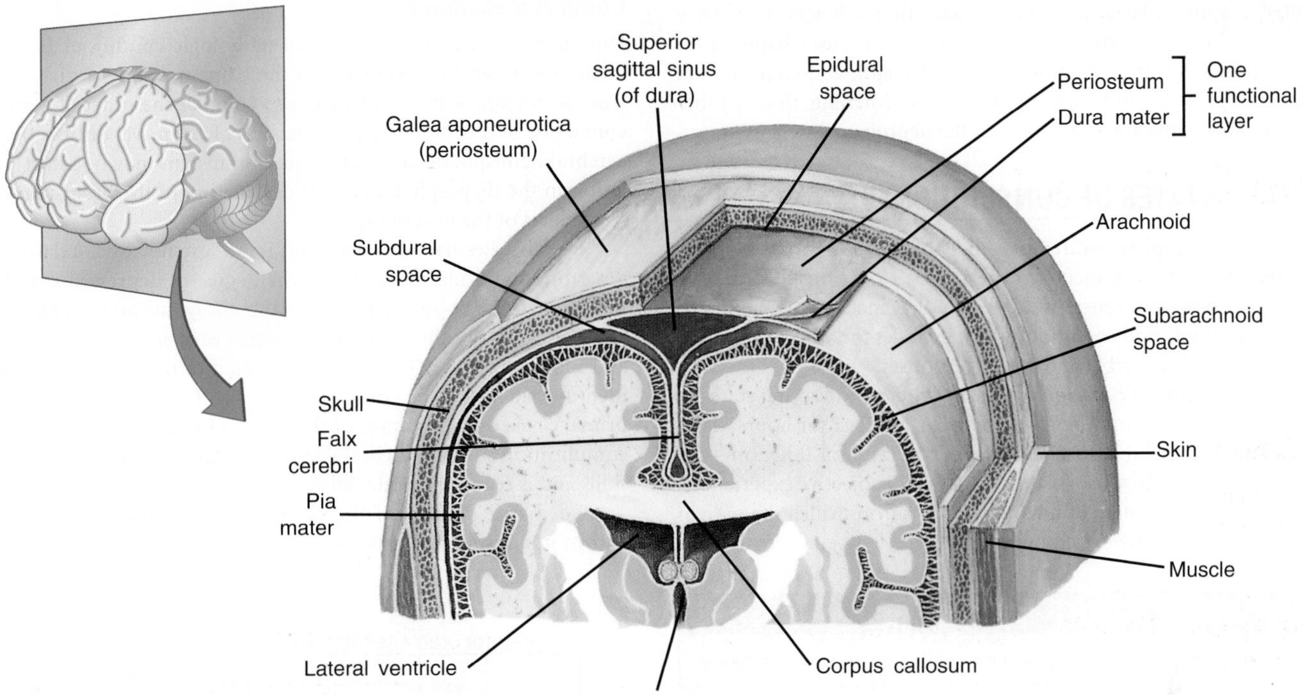

Fig. 27.1 Coronal section of top of head showing meningeal layers. (From Patton, K. T., & Thibodeau, G. A. [2010]. *Anatomy and physiology* [7th ed.]. St. Louis, MO: Mosby.)

BOX 27.1 Clinical Manifestations of Increased Intracranial Pressure in Infants and Children

Infants
- Tense, bulging fontanel
- Separated cranial sutures
- Macewen (cracked-pot) sign
- Irritability and restlessness
- Drowsiness
- Increased sleeping
- High-pitched cry
- Increased frontooccipital circumference
- Distended scalp veins
- Poor feeding
- Crying when disturbed
- Setting-sun sign

Children
- Headache
- Nausea
- Forceful vomiting
- Diplopia, blurred vision
- Seizures
- Indifference, drowsiness
- Decline in school performance
- Diminished physical activity and motor performance
- Increased sleeping
- Inability to follow simple commands
- Lethargy

Late Signs in Infants and Children
- Bradycardia
- Decreased motor response to command
- Decreased sensory response to painful stimuli
- Alterations in pupil size and reactivity
- Extension or flexion posturing
- Cheyne-Stokes respirations
- Papilledema
- Decreased consciousness
- Coma

History

A family history can sometimes offer clues regarding possible genetic disorders with neurologic manifestations. A review of family members often identifies conditions that might otherwise be overlooked, especially increased number of miscarriages or siblings or relatives who died at an early age. The nurse asks questions regarding specific neurologic problems, such as intellectual and developmental disabilities, deafness, epilepsy, blindness, unusual movements, weakness, ataxia, stroke, and progressive mental deterioration. History of consanguinity is also important.

A health history provides valuable clues regarding the cause of neurologic dysfunction. A history is assessed for injury with loss of consciousness, febrile illness, an encounter with an animal or insect, ingestion of neurotoxic substances, inhalation of chemicals, past illness, and known diabetes mellitus or sickle cell disease. Sudden or progressive alterations in movement or mental abilities may provide clues for investigation. It is also important to ascertain the chronologic course of the illness.

Physical Examination

Physical examination includes observation of the size and shape of the head (particularly in the infant and young child), spontaneous activity and postural reflex activity, and sensory responses. Note whether the patient is lethargic, drowsy, stuporous, alert, active, or irritable. The nurse also observes the overall tone, noting whether there is a normal flexed posture or one of extreme extension, opisthotonos, or hypotonia. Symmetry of movement is also assessed.

Facial features may suggest a specific syndrome. A high-pitched, piercing cry in an infant is often associated with CNS disorders. An abnormal respiratory cycle, such as prolonged apnea, ataxic breathing, paradoxic chest movement, and hyperventilation, may be the result of a neurologic problem.

Older children can be evaluated by the usual methods used in a neurologic examination. In addition, an estimation of the level of development provides essential information about neurologic function. This assessment is discussed throughout the book in relation to evaluation for specific disorders such as intellectual and developmental disabilities, failure to thrive, attention-deficit/hyperactivity disorder, cerebral palsy, cerebral tumors, and other physical or behavioral problems. Developmental screening tests can assess developmental progress in the young child.

Muscular activity and coordination, including ocular movements and gait, are valuable sources of information. Ocular movements, pupillary response, facial movements, and mouth functions provide clues regarding CNS involvement or impingement (see Chapter 4 for CNS and reflex testing). Testing reflexes, strength, and coordination and for the presence and location of tremors, twitching, tics, or other unusual movements are also aspects of the neurologic assessment.

ALTERED STATES OF CONSCIOUSNESS

Consciousness implies awareness—the ability to respond to sensory stimuli and have subjective experiences. Consciousness has two aspects: alertness, an arousal-waking state that includes the ability to respond to stimuli, and cognition, which includes the ability to process stimuli and produce verbal and motor responses.

An *altered state of consciousness* usually refers to varying states of unconsciousness that may be momentary or may last for hours, days, or indefinitely. Unconsciousness is depressed cerebral function—the inability to respond to sensory stimuli and have subjective experiences. Coma is defined as a state of unconsciousness from which the patient cannot be aroused, even with powerful stimuli.

! NURSING ALERT

Lack of response to painful stimuli is abnormal and must be reported immediately.

Etiology

An altered state of consciousness may be the outcome of several processes that affect the CNS. Impaired neurologic function can result from a direct or indirect cause. Some altered states, such as the diffuse changes observed in encephalitis, are directly related to cerebral insult. Others are the result of dysfunction in other organs or processes. For example, biochemical changes can impair neurologic function without morphologic findings, as in hypoglycemia.

Level of Consciousness

Assessment of level of consciousness (LOC) remains the earliest indicator of improvement or deterioration in neurologic status. LOC is determined by observations of the child's responses to the environment. Other diagnostic tests, such as motor activity, reflexes, and vital signs, are more variable and do not necessarily directly parallel the depth of the comatose state. The most consistently used terms are described in Box 27.2.

BOX 27.2 Levels of Consciousness

Full consciousness—Awake and alert, orientated to time, place, and person; behavior appropriate for age.

Confusion—Impaired decision making.

Disorientation—Confusion regarding time, place, and/or person; decreased level of consciousness.

Lethargy—Limited spontaneous movement, sluggish speech, drowsiness.

Obtundation—Arousable with stimulation.

Stupor—Remaining in a deep sleep, responsive only to vigorous and repeated stimulation.

Coma—No motor or verbal response to noxious (painful) stimuli.

Persistent vegetative state (PVS)—Permanently lost function of the cerebral cortex. Eyes follow objects only by reflex or when attracted to the direction of loud sounds; all four limbs are spastic but can withdraw from painful stimuli; hands show reflexive grasping and groping; the face can grimace, some food may be swallowed, and the child may groan or cry but utter no words.

Modified from Ball, J. W., Dains, J. E., Flynn, J. A., et al. (Eds.). (2019). *Seidel's guide to physical examination* (9th ed.). St. Louis, MO: Elsevier.

Coma Assessment

Diminished alertness as a result of pathologic conditions occurs on a continuum and is designated as the comatose state, which extends from somnolence at one end to deep coma at the other. To produce coma, one of the following must occur: (1) extensive, diffuse, bilateral cerebral hemispheric destruction (the brainstem may be intact); (2) a lesion in the diencephalon; or (3) destruction of the brainstem down to the level of the lower pons.

Several scales have been devised in an attempt to standardize the description and interpretation of the degree of depressed consciousness. The most popular of these is the *Glasgow Coma Scale (GCS)*, which consists of a three-part assessment: eye opening, verbal response, and motor response. The GCS was created to meet a clinical need to identify criteria for the consciousness level. For clinical purposes, the primary role of observation of the LOC is to detect a life-threatening complication such as cerebral edema. The GCS requires observational skills and is readily reproducible between observers.

A pediatric version of the GCS recognizes that expected verbal and motor responses must be related to the child's age (Fig. 27.2).

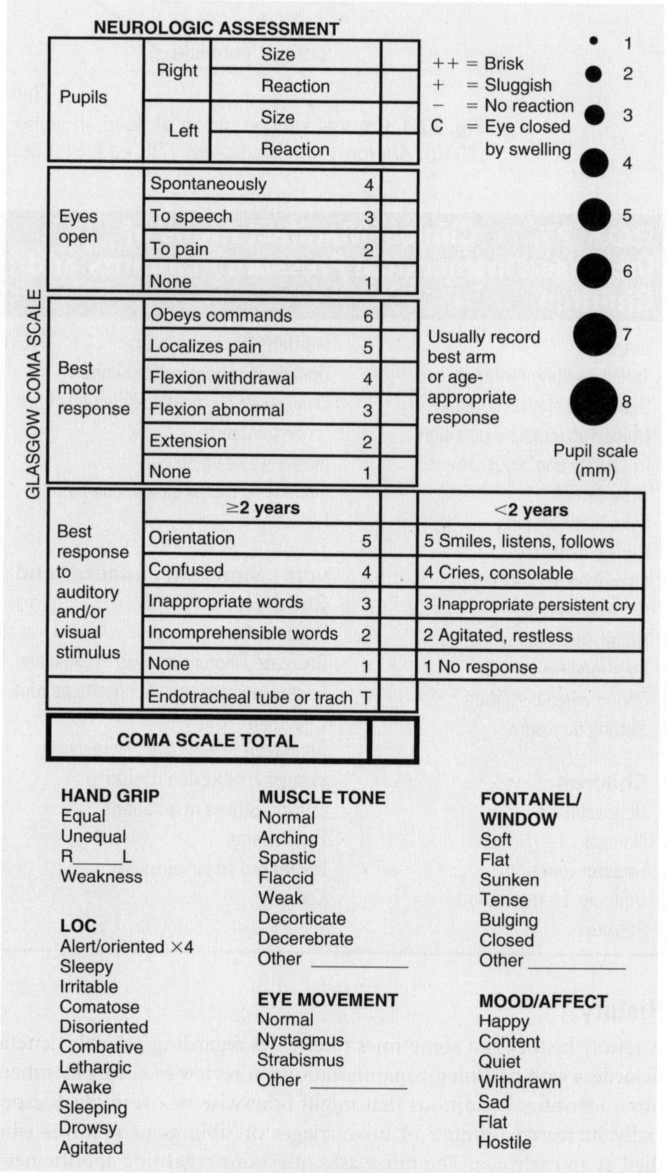

Fig. 27.2 Pediatric coma scale.

The pediatric coma scale does not assess verbal responses as such but records smiling, crying, and interaction. It uses a 6-point motor scale that is inappropriate for children younger than 6 months of age. In children younger than 5 years of age, speech is understood to be any sound at all, even crying. Young children demonstrate orientation by identifying their parents correctly or giving their own names. When assessing LOC in young children, the nurse may find it helpful to have a parent present to help elicit a desired response. An infant or child may not respond in an unfamiliar environment or to unfamiliar voices.

Numeric values are assigned to the levels of response in each category. The sum of these numeric values provides an objective measurement of the patient's LOC. The lower the score, the deeper the coma. A person with an unaltered LOC would score the highest, 15; a score of 8 or below is generally accepted as a definition of coma; the lowest score, 3, indicates deep coma or death.

The GCS in itself is not sufficient to determine depressed consciousness in all children. For example, because a child with quadriplegia cannot respond to commands physically, the child's GCS can be very low but the child may be cognitively intact. Nevertheless, the GCS provides a more objective method for evaluating the state of consciousness in most cases. Severely injured children (GCS ≤8) may have a consistent grading of motor response, verbal response, and eye opening.

The GCS score performed during preadmission (i.e., assessment in the field), in the emergency department, and throughout the inpatient admission is universally accepted as one criterion to determine the patient's prognosis (Braine & Cook, 2017). GCS scores of 5 or less are associated with poor outcome (Murphy, Thomas, Gertz, et al., 2017).

Clinical Death

There is no precise diagnosis for clinical death. Different tissues undergo permanent damage after varying periods of exposure to an ongoing insult; the brain (especially the cerebrum) has become the tissue of most importance in determining the time of death. The current concept of dying is a process that takes place over a finite interval of time rather than an event that occurs spontaneously. ***Brain death*** is a clinical diagnosis based on the total cessation of brainstem and cortical brain function that causes irreversible widespread brain injury and coma. In children the most common causes are trauma, anoxic encephalopathy, infections, and cerebral neoplasms. The pronouncement of brain death requires two conditions: (1) complete cessation of clinical evidence of brain function and (2) irreversibility of the condition. It is essential to establish the absence of a reversible condition, especially a toxic and metabolic disorder, sedative-hypnotic drugs, paralytic agents, hypothermia, hypotension, and surgically remediable conditions (Nakagawa, Ashwal, Mathur, et al., 2012).

Organ transplantation has created a need to separate the process of death from the retrieval of viable tissues at a time when the brain is already dead. The clinical criteria for brain death must be met so that there is no error. Although the legal status of the concept of death varies among individual states and communities in the United States, the Task Force for the Determination of Brain Death in Children has established guidelines for the determination of brain death in children (see Nursing Care Guidelines box and Chapter 17, Organ or Tissue Donation and Autopsy). At least two different attending physicians should participate in diagnosing brain death in children (Nakagawa et al., 2012).

NURSING CARE GUIDELINES

Establishing Brain Death in Children

Coma and apnea must coexist. Child must exhibit complete loss of consciousness, vocalization, and volitional activity.

Brainstem function must be absent, as defined by the following:

- Midposition or fully dilated pupils in both eyes that do not respond to light.
- Absence of spontaneous eye movements and those induced by oculocephalic and caloric (oculovestibular) testing.
- Absence of movement of bulbar musculature, including facial and oropharyngeal muscles.
- Absence of the corneal, gag, cough, sucking, and rooting reflexes.
- Absence of respiratory movements when child is removed from respirator. Apnea testing using standardized methods can be performed but is done after other criteria are met.

Child must not be significantly hypothermic or hypotensive for age.

Flaccid tone and absence of spontaneous or induced movements, including spinal cord events such as reflex withdrawal or spinal myoclonus, should exist.

Examination should remain consistent with brain death throughout the observation and testing period.

Observation periods according to age:

- Term newborn 37 weeks of gestational age and up to 30 days of age—Two separate examinations separated by at least 24 hours
- 31 days to 18 years old—Two separate examinations separated by at least 12 hours

Ancillary testing with electroencephalogram or cerebral blood flow testing should be considered if there is concern about the validity of the examination.

Data from Nakagawa, T. A., Ashwal, S., Mathur, M., et al. (2012). Guidelines for the determination of brain death in infants and children: An update of the 1987 task force recommendations—Executive summary. *Annals of Neurology, 71*(4), 573–585.

NEUROLOGIC EXAMINATION

The purpose of the neurologic examination is to establish an accurate, objective baseline of neurologic function. Therefore it is essential that the neurologic examination be documented in a descriptive and detailed fashion, thereby enhancing the ability to detect subtle changes in neurologic status over time. Descriptions of behaviors should be simple, objective, and easily interpreted—for example, "Drowsy but awake and conversationally rational/oriented" or "Sleepy but arousable with vigorous physical stimuli; pressure to nail base of right hand results in upper extremity flexion/lower extremity extension."

Vital Signs

Pulse, respiration, and blood pressure provide information on the adequacy of circulation and the possible underlying cause of altered consciousness. Autonomic activity is most intensively disturbed in deep coma and in brainstem lesions. Body temperature is often elevated; sometimes the elevation is extreme. High temperature is most often a sign of an acute infectious process or heatstroke, but it may be caused by ingestion of some drugs (especially salicylates, alcohol, and barbiturates) or by intracranial bleeding, especially subarachnoid hemorrhage. Hypothalamic involvement may cause elevated or decreased temperature. Serious infection may produce hypothermia.

The pulse is variable and may be rapid, slow and bounding, or feeble. Blood pressure may be normal, elevated, or very low. The Cushing reflex, or pressor response that causes a slowing of the pulse and an increase in blood pressure, is uncommon in children; when it does occur, it is a very late sign of increased ICP. Medications can also affect vital signs. For assessment purposes, actual changes in pulse and blood pressure are more important than the direction of the change.

Respirations are more often slow, deep, and irregular. Slow and deep breathing often occurs in the heavy sleep caused by sedatives, after seizures, or in cerebral infections. Slow, shallow breathing may result from sedatives or opioids. Hyperventilation (deep and rapid respirations) is usually the result of metabolic acidosis or abnormal stimulation of the respiratory center in the medulla caused by salicylate poisoning, hepatic coma, or Reye syndrome. A pattern of alternating hyperventilation and breath holding during wakefulness is common in Rett syndrome.

Breathing patterns have been described with a number of terms (e.g., *apneustic, cluster, ataxic, Cheyne-Stokes*). However, it is better to describe what is being observed rather than placing a label on it because the terms are often used and interpreted incorrectly. Periodic or irregular breathing is a sign of brainstem (especially medullary) dysfunction. This is an ominous sign that often precedes complete apnea. The odor of the breath may provide additional clues (e.g., the fruity and acetone odor of ketosis, the foul odor of uremia, the fetid odor of hepatic failure, or the odor of alcohol).

Skin

The skin may offer clues to the cause of unconsciousness. The body surface should be examined for injury, needle marks, petechiae, bites, and ticks. Evidence of toxic substances may be found on the hands, face, mouth, and clothing—especially in small children.

Eyes

Assess pupil size and reactivity (Fig. 27.3). Pupils either do or do not react to light. Pinpoint pupils are commonly observed in poisoning (e.g., opiate or barbiturate poisoning) or in brainstem dysfunction. Widely dilated and reactive pupils are often seen after seizures and may involve only one side. Widely dilated and fixed pupils suggest paralysis of CN III (oculomotor nerve) secondary to pressure from herniation of the brain through the tentorium. A unilateral fixed pupil usually suggests a lesion on the same side. Bilateral fixed pupils, if present for more than 5 minutes, usually imply brainstem damage. Dilated and nonreactive pupils also occur in hypothermia, anoxia, ischemia, poisoning with atropine-like substances, or prior instillation of mydriatic drugs. Some of the therapies used (e.g., barbiturates) can alter pupil size and reaction.

The description of eye movements should indicate whether one or both eyes are involved and how the reaction was elicited. Ask the parents if the child has strabismus, which may cause the eyes to appear misaligned.

! NURSING ALERT

The sudden appearance of a fixed and dilated pupil is a neurosurgical emergency.

Blinking observed at rest or in response to a sudden loud noise or bright light implies that the pontine reticular formation is intact. The corneal reflex, blinking of the eyelids when the cornea is touched with a wisp of cotton, can test the integrity of the ophthalmic division of CN V (trigeminal nerve). Posttraumatic strabismus indicates CN VI (abducens nerve) damage.

Eye movements are assessed by the doll's head maneuver, in which the child's head is rotated quickly to one side and then to the other. When the brainstem centers for eye movement are intact, there is conjugate (paired or working together) movement of the eyes in the direction opposite the head rotation. Absence of this response suggests dysfunction of the brainstem or CN III. Downward or lateral deviation is often observed in association with pupillary dilation in dysfunction of CN III.

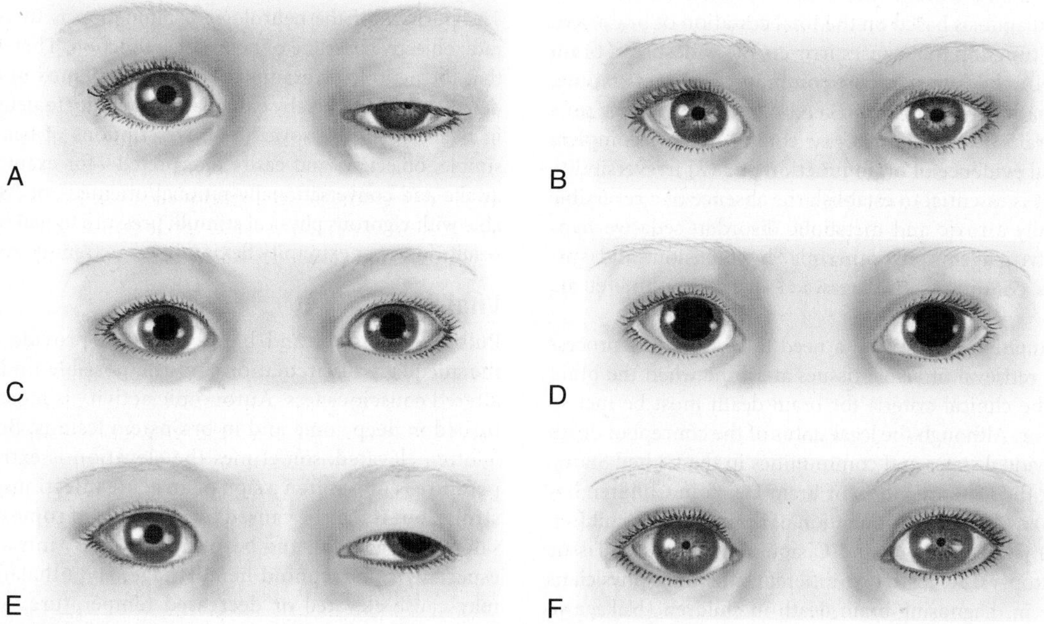

Fig. 27.3 Variations in pupil size with altered states of consciousness. **A,** Ipsilateral pupillary constriction with slight ptosis. **B,** Bilateral small pupils. **C,** Midposition, light fixed to all stimuli. **D,** Bilateral dilated and fixed pupils. **E,** Dilated pupils, left eye abducted with ptosis. **F,** Pinpoint pupils.

! NURSING ALERT

Any tests that require head movement are not attempted until after cervical spine injury has been ruled out.

The caloric test, or oculovestibular response, is elicited by irrigating the external auditory canal with 10 ml of ice water over a period of approximately 20 seconds (with the head of bed elevated at a 30-degree angle). This test normally causes movement of the eyes toward the side of stimulation. This response is lost when the pontine centers are impaired and thus provides important information in assessment of the comatose patient.

! NURSING ALERT

The ice water caloric test is painful and is never performed if the child is awake or the tympanic membranes are ruptured.

Funduscopic examination reveals additional clues. Because it takes 24 to 48 hours to develop, papilledema (e.g., optic disc swelling, indistinct margins, hemorrhages, tortuosity of vessels, absence of venous pulsations), if it develops at all, will not be evident early in the course of unconsciousness. The presence of retinal hemorrhages in children is usually the result of accidental or inflicted trauma with intracranial bleeding (usually subarachnoid or subdural hemorrhage) but is sometimes caused by infection (Minns, Jones, Tandon, et al., 2017).

Motor Function

Observation of spontaneous activity, posture, and response to painful stimuli provides clues to the location and extent of cerebral dysfunction. Asymmetric movements of the limbs or the absence of movement suggests paralysis. In hemiplegia the affected limb lies in external rotation and falls uncontrollably when lifted and allowed to drop. Observations should be described rather than labeled.

In the deeper comatose states, the child has little or no spontaneous movement, and the musculature tends to be flaccid. There is considerable variability in motor behavior in lesser degrees of coma. For example, the child may be relatively immobile or restless and hyperkinetic; muscle tone may be increased or decreased. Tremors, twitching, and spasms of muscles are common observations. The patient may display purposeless plucking or tossing movements. Combative or negativistic behavior is not uncommon. Hyperactivity is more common in acute febrile and toxic states than in cases of increased ICP. Seizures are common in children and may be present in coma as a result of any cause. Any repetitive movements and movements during seizures are described.

Posturing

Primitive postural reflexes emerge as cortical control over motor function is lost in brain dysfunction. These reflexes are evident in posturing and motor movements directly related to the area of the brain involved. Posturing reflects a balance between the lower exciting and the higher inhibiting influences. Strong muscles overcome weaker ones. Flexion posturing (Fig. 27.4A) occurs with severe dysfunction of the cerebral cortex or with lesions to corticospinal tracts above the brainstem. Typical flexion posturing includes rigid flexion, with arms held tightly to the body; flexed elbows, wrists, and fingers; plantar flexed feet; legs extended and internally rotated; and possibly fine tremors or intense stiffness. Extension posturing (see Fig. 27.4B) is a sign of dysfunction at the level of the midbrain or lesions to the brainstem. It is characterized by rigid extension and pronation of the arms and legs, flexed wrists and fingers, clenched jaw, extended neck, and possibly an arched back. Unilateral extension posturing is often caused by tentorial herniation.

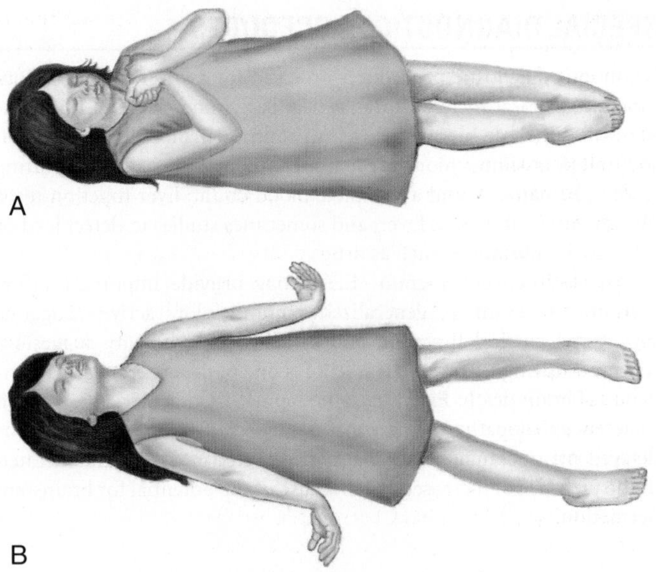

Fig. 27.4 A, Flexion posturing. B, Extension posturing.

Posturing may not be evident when the child is quiet but can usually be elicited by applying painful stimuli such as a blunt object pressed on the base of the nail. Nurses should avoid applying thumb pressure to the supraorbital region of the frontal bone (risk of orbital damage). Noxious stimuli (e.g., suctioning), turning, or touching will elicit a response. When the nurse is describing posturing, the stimulus needed to provoke the response is as important as the reaction.

Reflexes

Testing of certain reflexes, such as those present in an intact spinal cord, may be of limited value (see Chapter 4). In general, the corneal, pupillary, muscle-stretch, superficial, and plantar reflexes tend to be absent in deep coma. The state of reflexes is variable in lighter grades of unconsciousness and depends on the underlying pathologic process and the location of the lesion. The doll's eye reflex maneuver, described previously, reflects paralysis of CN III. The absence of corneal reflexes (CN V) and the presence of a tonic neck reflex are associated with severe brain damage. The Babinski reflex, in which the lateral portion of the bottom of the foot is stroked and causes the big toe to go up, may be of value if it is found to be present consistently in children older than 1 year. A positive Babinski reflex is significant in the assessment of pyramidal tract lesions when it is unilateral and associated with other pyramidal signs. A fluctuating Babinski reflex is often observed after seizures (see Fig. 7.8B).

NURSING TIP: Three key reflexes that demonstrate neurologic health in young infants are the Moro, tonic neck, and withdrawal reflexes.

SPECIAL DIAGNOSTIC PROCEDURES

Numerous diagnostic procedures are used for assessment of cerebral function. Laboratory tests that may help determine the cause of unconsciousness include blood glucose, urea nitrogen, and electrolyte (pH, sodium, potassium, chloride, calcium, and bicarbonate) tests; clotting studies, hematocrit, and a complete blood count; liver function tests; blood cultures if there is fever; and sometimes studies to detect lead or other toxic substances, such as drugs.

An electroencephalogram (EEG) may provide important information. For example, generalized random, slow activity suggests suppressed cortical function, and localized slow activity suggests a space-occupying lesion. A flat tracing is one of the criteria used as evidence of brain death. Examination of spinal fluid is carried out when toxic encephalopathy or infection is suspected. Lumbar puncture is delayed if intracranial hemorrhage is suspected and is contraindicated in the presence of increased ICP because of the potential for brainstem herniation.

Auditory and visual evoked potentials are sometimes used in neurologic evaluation of very young children. Brainstem auditory evoked potentials are useful for evaluating the continuity of brainstem auditory tracts and are particularly useful for detecting demyelinating disease and neoplasms of the brainstem and for distinguishing between brainstem and cortical lesions. For example, a normal evoked potential in a comatose patient suggests involvement of the cerebral hemispheres.

Highly sophisticated tests are carried out with specialized equipment. Two imaging techniques, computed tomography (CT) and magnetic resonance imaging (MRI), assist in diagnosis by scanning both soft tissues and solid matter. Most of these tests are listed in Table 27.1. Because these tests can be threatening to children, the nurse needs to prepare patients and their parents or guardians for the tests and provide support and reassurance during the tests. Consultation with a child life specialist can also be helpful (see Chapter 20, Preparation for Diagnostic and Therapeutic Procedures).

TABLE 27.1 Neurologic Diagnostic Procedures

Test	Description	Purpose	Comments
Lumbar puncture (LP)	Spinal needle is inserted between L3 and L4 or L4 and L5 vertebral spaces into subarachnoid space; cerebrospinal fluid (CSF) pressure is measured, and sample is collected for examination.	Measures spinal fluid pressure Obtains CSF for laboratory analysis Injection of medication	Contraindicated in patients with increased intracranial pressure (ICP) or infected skin over puncture site.
Subdural tap	Needle is inserted into anterior fontanel or coronal suture (midline to pupil).	Helps rule out subdural effusions Removes CSF to relieve pressure	Place infant in semierect position after subdural tap to minimize leakage from site; prevent child from crying if possible. Check site frequently for evidence of leakage.
Ventricular puncture	Needle is inserted into lateral ventricle via coronal suture (midline to pupil).	Removes CSF to relieve pressure	Risk of intracerebral or ventricular hemorrhage.
Electroencephalography (EEG)	EEG records changes in electrical potential of brain. Electrodes are placed at various points to assess electrical function in a particular area. Impulses are recorded by electromagnetic pen or digitally.	Detects spikes, or bursts of electrical activity, that indicate the potential for seizures Used to determine brain death	Patient should remain quiet during procedure; may require sedation. Minimize external stimuli during procedure.
Nuclear brain scan	Radioisotope is injected intravenously, then counted and recorded after fixed time intervals. Radioisotope accumulates in areas where blood-brain barrier is defective.	Identifies focal brain lesions (e.g., tumors, abscesses) Positive uptake of material with encephalitis and subdural hematoma Visualizes CSF pathways	Requires intravenous (IV) access; patient may require sedation. In normal children or noncommunicating hydrocephalus, no retrograde filling of ventricles occurs. Areas of concentrated uptake of material are termed *hot spots.*
Endocephalography	Pulses of ultrasonic waves are beamed through head; echoes from reflecting surfaces are recorded graphically.	Identifies shifts in midline structures from their normal positions as a result of intracranial lesions May show ventricular dilation	Simple, safe, rapid procedure.
Real-time ultrasonography (RTUS)	RTUS is similar to CT but uses ultrasound instead of ionizing radiation.	Allows high-resolution anatomic visualization in variety of imaging planes	Produces images similar to CT scan. Especially useful in neonatal central nervous system problems.

TABLE 27.1 Neurologic Diagnostic Procedures—cont'd

Test	Description	Purpose	Comments
Radiography	Skull films are taken from different views—lateral, posterolateral, axial (submentoventricular), half-axial.	Shows fractures, dislocations, spreading suture lines, craniostenosis Shows degenerative changes, bone erosion, calcifications	Simple, noninvasive procedure.
Computed tomography (CT) scan	Pinpoint x-ray beam is directed on horizontal or vertical plane to provide series of images that are fed into computer and assembled in image displayed on video screen. CT uses ionizing radiation.	Visualizes horizontal and vertical cross-section of brain in three planes (axial, coronal, sagittal) Distinguishes density of various intracranial tissues and structures—congenital abnormalities, hemorrhage, tumors, demyelinating and inflammatory processes, calcification	Requires IV access if contrast agent is used. Patient may require sedation.
Magnetic resonance imaging (MRI)	MRI produces radiofrequency emissions from elements (e.g., hydrogen, phosphorus), which are converted to visual images by computer.	Permits visualization of morphologic feature of target structures Permits tissue discrimination unavailable with many techniques	MRI is noninvasive procedure except when IV contrast agent is used. No exposure to radiation occurs. Patient may require sedation. Parent or attendant can remain in room with child. MRI does not visualize bone detail or calcifications. No metal can be present in scanner.
Positron emission tomography (PET)	PET involves IV injection of positron-emitting radionucleotide; local concentrations are detected and transformed into visual display by computer.	Detects and measures blood volume and flow in brain, metabolic activity, biochemical changes within tissue	Requires lengthy period of immobility. Minimum exposure to radiation occurs. Patient may require sedation.
Digital subtraction angiography (DSA)	Contrast dye is injected intravenously; computer "subtracts" all tissues without contrast medium, leaving clear image of contrast medium in vessels studied.	Visualizes vasculature of target tissue Visualizes finite vascular abnormalities	Safe alternative to angiography. Patient must remain still during procedure; may require sedation.
Single-photon emission computed tomography (SPECT)	SPECT involves IV injection of photon-emitting radionuclide; radionuclides are absorbed by healthy tissue at different rate than diseased or necrotic tissue; data are transferred to computer that converts image to film.	Provides information regarding blood flow to tissues; analyzing blood flow to organ may help determine how well it is functioning	Requires lengthy period of immobility. Minimum exposure to radiation occurs. Patient may require sedation.

Children who are old enough to understand require careful explanation of the procedure, why it is being done, what they will experience, and how they can help. School-age children usually appreciate a more detailed description of why contrast material is injected. Because children are often frightened of needles, they and their families need to be informed of any medication or contrast medium that will be administered intravenously. Special anxiety reduction strategies may be necessary for children who have blood-injury-injection (needle) phobia (McMurtry, Taddio, Noel, et al., 2016). This phobia is the most inheritable of all phobias. The nurse should talk with parents to find out if they also have this phobia and will need help with anxiety management.

The importance of lying still for tests needs to be stressed. Children unfamiliar with the machines can be shown a picture beforehand. Although radiographic examinations are not painful, the machinery often appears so frightening that the child protests because of anxiety. This is especially true of CT and MRI, both of which require that the child's head be placed within a special immobilizing device. Chin and cheek pads are sometimes used to prevent the slightest head movement, and straps are applied to the body to prevent a slight change in body position. The nurse can explain these events to a frightened child by comparing them to an astronaut's preparation for a space flight. It is important to emphasize to the child that at no time is the procedure painful.

It is helpful for nurses to become acquainted with the equipment and the general environment in which the test will take place so that they can better explain the procedure to children and their families at their level of understanding. Written material describing the procedure should be available for parents and may be appropriate to share with children. Equipment is often strange and ominous to children. They need constant reassurance from a trusted companion. The nurse should not expect cooperation from a young child. Sedation may be required. Many different agents are currently used for sedation of children undergoing neurologic diagnostic procedures (see Chapter 5, Pain Management).

Physical preparation for the diagnostic test may involve administration of a sedative. If so, children should be helped through the preparation and administration and assured that someone will remain with them (if this is possible). Children need continual support and reinforcement during procedures in which they remain conscious. Vital signs and physiologic responses to the procedure are monitored throughout. Many diagnostic procedures performed on an outpatient basis require sedation, and children need recovery time and observation. The nurse should review written instructions with parents if the child is discharged after a procedure. Children who have undergone a procedure with a general anesthetic require postanesthesia care, including positioning to prevent aspiration of secretions and frequent assessment of vital signs, oxygen saturation, and LOC. In addition, other neurologic functions such as pupillary responses, motor strength, and movement are tested at regular intervals. Any surgical wound resulting from the test is checked for bleeding, CSF leakage, and other complications. Children who undergo repeated subdural taps should have their hematocrit monitored to detect excessive blood loss from the procedure.

THE CHILD WITH CEREBRAL COMPROMISE

NURSING CARE OF THE UNCONSCIOUS CHILD

The unconscious child requires nursing attendance with observation, recording, and evaluation of changes in objective signs. These observations provide valuable information regarding the patient's progress and often serve as a guide to diagnosis and treatment. Careful and detailed observations are essential for the child's welfare. In addition, vital functions must be maintained and complications prevented through conscientious and meticulous nursing care. The outcome of unconsciousness is variable and ranges from early and complete recovery to death within a few hours or days, or persistent and permanent unconsciousness, or recovery with varying degrees of residual mental or physical disability. The outcome and recovery of the unconscious child may depend on the level of nursing care and observational skills.

Direct emergency measures toward ensuring circulation, airway, and breathing (CAB); stabilizing the spine when indicated; treating shock; and reducing ICP (if present). Delayed treatment often leads to increased damage. Therapies for specific causes of unconsciousness begin as soon as emergency measures have been implemented; in many cases they occur concurrently. Because nursing care is closely related to the medical management, both are considered here.

Continual observation of the LOC, pupillary reaction, and vital signs is essential to management of CNS disorders. Regular assessment of neurologic status and vital signs is an integral part of the nursing care of unconscious children. The frequency depends on the cause of unconsciousness, the LOC, and the progression of cerebral involvement. Intervals between observations may be as short as every 15 minutes or as long as every 2 hours. Significant alterations are reported immediately.

The temperature is measured every 2 to 4 hours, depending on the child's condition. An elevated temperature may occur in children with CNS dysfunction; therefore a light covering may be sufficient. Vigorous efforts, such as tepid sponge baths or application of a hypothermia blanket, are needed to prevent brain damage if the rectal temperature exceeds 104°F (40°C).

The LOC is assessed periodically, including pupillary size, equality, and reaction to light. Signs of meningeal irritation, such as nuchal rigidity, need to be assessed. Assessment of LOC also includes response to vocal commands, spontaneous behavior, resistance to care, and response to painful stimuli. Note any abnormal movements, changes in muscle tone or strength, and body position. If a seizure occurs, describe the seizure, including the body areas involved from the beginning to the end of the seizure, and the duration of seizure (see Box 27.8 and Critical Thinking Case Study later in the chapter).

Pain management for the unconscious child requires astute nursing observation and management. Signs of pain include changes in behavior (e.g., increased agitation and rigidity) and alterations in vital signs and perfusion (usually an increased heart rate, respiratory rate, and blood pressure and decreased oxygen saturation). Because these findings are not specific for pain, the nurse should be alert for their appearance during times of induced or suspected pain and for their disappearance after the inciting procedure or the administration of analgesia. A pain assessment record is used to document indications of pain and the effectiveness of interventions (see Chapter 5, Pain Assessment). The use of opioids, such as morphine, to relieve pain is controversial because these drugs can mask signs of altered consciousness or depress respirations. However, unrelieved pain activates the stress response, which can elevate ICP. To block the stress response, some authorities advocate the use of analgesics, sedatives, and, in some cases such as head injury, paralyzing agents via continuous intravenous (IV) infusion. A commonly used combination is fentanyl, midazolam, and vecuronium (Norcuron). If there are concerns about assessing the LOC or respiratory depression, naloxone can be used to reverse the opioid effects. Regardless of the drugs used, adequate dosage and regular administration are essential to provide optimum pain relief.

> **! NURSING ALERT**
>
> When opioids are used, bowel elimination must be closely monitored because of the potential constipating effect. A stool softener should be given regularly with laxatives as needed to prevent constipation.

Other measures to relieve discomfort include providing a quiet, dimly lit environment; limiting visitors; preventing any sudden, jarring movement, such as banging into the bed; and preventing an increase in ICP. The latter is most effectively achieved by proper positioning and prevention of straining, such as during coughing, vomiting, or defecating (see Chapter 5, Pain Management). Antiepileptic drugs, such as fosphenytoin (Cerebyx) or phenobarbital, may be ordered for control of seizure activity.

Respiratory Management

Respiratory effectiveness is the primary concern in the care of the unconscious child, and establishment of an adequate airway is always the first priority. Carbon dioxide has a potent vasodilating effect and will increase cerebral blood flow (CBF) and ICP. Cerebral hypoxia at normal body temperature that lasts longer than 4 minutes often causes irreversible brain damage.

> **! NURSING ALERT**
>
> Respiratory obstruction and subsequent compromise lead to cardiac arrest. Always maintain an adequate, patent airway.

Children in lighter stages of coma may be able to cough and swallow, but those in deeper states of coma are unable to manage secretions, which tend to pool in the throat and pharynx. Dysfunction of CNs IX and X (glossopharyngeal and vagus nerves) places the child at risk of aspiration and cardiac arrest. Therefore position the child with the head and body to the side to prevent aspiration of secretions and empty the stomach to reduce the likelihood of vomiting. In infants, the blockage of air passages from secretions can happen in seconds. In addition, upper airway obstruction from laryngospasm is a common complication in comatose children.

An oral airway can be used for the child who is suffering a temporary loss of consciousness, such as after a contusion, seizure, or anesthesia. For children who remain unconscious for a longer time, a nasotracheal or orotracheal tube is inserted to maintain the open airway and facilitate removal of secretions. A tracheostomy is performed in cases where laryngoscopy for introduction of an endotracheal tube would be difficult or dangerous or for a child who needs long-term ventilatory support. Suctioning is used only as needed to clear the airway, exerting care to prevent increasing ICP. Respiratory status is observed and evaluated regularly. Signs of respiratory distress may indicate a need for ventilator assistance.

Mechanical ventilation is usually indicated when the respiratory center is involved. Blood gas analysis is performed regularly, and oxygen is administered when indicated. Moderately severe hypoxia and respiratory acidosis are often present, but they are not always evident from clinical manifestations. Hypoventilation often accompanies unconsciousness and may lead to respiratory alkalosis, or it may represent the body's attempt to compensate for metabolic acidosis. Blood gas and pH determinations are essential guides for electrolyte therapy. Chest physiotherapy is carried out on a regular basis, and the child's position is changed at least every 2 hours to prevent pulmonary complications. Regular oral hygiene is recommended to reduce the risk of ventilator-associated pneumonia (VAP) (Hua, Xie, Worthington, et al., 2016).

Intracranial Pressure Monitoring

The role of ICP monitoring after traumatic brain injury (TBI) is controversial. Placement of the ICP monitor often occurs in the emergency department and where older in age (Kannan, Quistberg, Wang, et al., 2017). Early placement of ICP monitors may guide assessment management of patients with intracranial hypertension or those at higher risk for developing intracranial hypertension. ICP monitoring also may assist with decision making regarding transfer to the operating room or pediatric intensive care unit (PICU). However, in a large study using two national databases of 3084 children with severe TBI, no evidence was found of a benefit from ICP monitoring on functional survival of children with severe TBI (Bennett, DeWitt, Greene, et al., 2017). Development of noninvasive ICP sensors has the potential of decreasing the need for invasive interventions in pediatric patients in the future (Harary, Dolmans, & Gormley, 2018).

Direct ventricular pressure measurement remains the gold standard of ICP monitoring. The catheter method involves introduction of a catheter into the lateral ventricle on the nondominant side, if known, or placement in the subdural space. The catheter has the advantage of providing a means of extraventricular (or continuous) drainage of CSF to reduce pressure. A drainage bag attached to the system is kept at the level of the ventricles and can be lowered to decrease ICP. This device requires full penetration of the brain, requires skill and experience with placement, and carries the risk of infection. Infection risks can be lowered by always using aseptic technique when handling the external ventricular drainage (EVD) system, manipulating the EVD as little as possible, and sterile dressing changes only weekly or when the dressing is compromised, whichever occurs first (Hepburn-Smith, Dynkevich, Spektor, et al., 2016).

! NURSING ALERT

If the external ventricular drain is unclamped for cerebrospinal fluid (CSF) drainage, carefully monitor the level of the collection container. If the container is positioned too low, improper CSF decompression could lower intracranial pressure (ICP) too rapidly, causing bleeding and pain.

With the bolt method, the end of the bolt is placed into the subarachnoid space. The bolt cannot be adequately secured in a small child's pliant skull, although special modifications have been developed for children younger than 6 years of age. The placement of the bolt is not adjusted by anyone except the neurosurgeon who placed the device. The neurosurgeon is notified if a satisfactory waveform is not observed.

! NURSING ALERT

With the bolt method, the bolt is stabilized with dressings, but these are not changed or disturbed—not even to check the site.

An epidural sensor can be placed between the dura and the skull through a burr hole and connected to a stopcock assembly and a transducer, which provides a readout of the pressure. Although less invasive, the epidural sensor may have inconsistent correlation of pressure readings. In infants, a fontanel transducer can be used to detect impulses from a pressure sensor and convert them to electrical energy. The electrical energy is then converted to visible waves or numeric readings on an oscilloscope. ICP measurement from the anterior fontanel is noninvasive but may prove to be inaccurate if the equipment is poorly placed or inconsistently recalibrated. Intraparenchymal pressure monitoring devices (e.g., Camino) use fiberoptic technology and perform reliably.

ICP can be increased by direct instillation of solutions; antibiotics are administered systemically if a positive CSF culture is obtained. However, ICP monitoring rarely causes infection. CSF is a body fluid; implement Standard Precautions according to hospital policy (see Chapter 20, Infection Control).

Nurses caring for patients with intracranial monitoring devices must be acquainted with the system, assist with insertion, interpret the monitor readings, and be able to distinguish between danger signals and mechanical dysfunction. Because systemic blood pressure, ICP, and therefore cerebral perfusion pressure (CPP) are normally lower in children, the child's age must be taken into account when deciding what constitutes abnormally high ICP or abnormally low CPP.

Several medical measures are available to treat increased ICP resulting from cerebral edema. These include sedation, CSF drainage, and osmotic diuretics. Osmotic diuretics may provide rapid relief of ICP in emergency situations. Although their effect is transient, lasting only about 6 hours, they can be life-saving in emergencies. These substances are rapidly excreted by the kidneys and carry with them large quantities of sodium and water. Mannitol (or sometimes urea) administered intravenously is the drug most commonly used for rapid reduction of ICP. The infusion is generally given slowly but may be pushed rapidly if there is herniation or impending herniation. Because of the profound diuretic effect of the drug, an indwelling catheter is inserted to ensure bladder emptying. Arterial carbon dioxide ($PaCO_2$) should be maintained at approximately 30 mm Hg to produce vasoconstriction, which reduces CBF, thereby decreasing ICP. Recording and analyzing the child's volume state, plasma sodium concentration, and serum osmolarity can avert potential fluid and electrolyte problems. Administration of adrenocorticosteroids is not recommended for cerebral edema secondary to head trauma.

Nursing Activities

In cases of high levels of increased ICP, nursing procedures tend to trigger reactive pressure waves in many children. For example, increased intrathoracic or abdominal pressure will be transmitted to the cranium. The goals of monitoring a child who is neurologically compromised include maintaining CPP; controlling ICP, cerebral edema, and factors that increase cerebral metabolism (e.g., fever, seizures); and maintaining hemodynamic stability. Take particular care in positioning these patients to avoid neck vein compression that may further increase ICP by interfering with venous return.

! NURSING ALERT

Elevate the head of the bed 15 to 30 degrees and position the child so that the head is maintained in midline to facilitate venous drainage and avoid jugular compression. Turning side to side is contraindicated because of the risk of jugular compression.

Sandbags or other support devices can help maintain correct head position. The child can be propped to one side or the other, and the use of a pressure-relieving or pressure-decreasing mattress decreases the chance of prolonged pressure to vulnerable skin areas. Frequent clinical assessment of the child cannot be replaced by an ICP monitoring device.

It is important to avoid activities that may increase ICP by causing pain or emotional stress. Clustering nursing activities together and minimizing environmental stimuli by decreasing noxious procedures help control ICP. Range-of-motion exercises can be carried out gently but should not be performed vigorously. Any necessary disturbing procedures should be scheduled to take advantage of therapies that reduce ICP, such as osmotherapy and sedation. Make efforts to minimize or eliminate environmental noise, including managing the number of visitors. Assessment and intervention to relieve pain are important nursing functions to decrease ICP.

Suctioning and percussion are poorly tolerated; these procedures are contraindicated unless the child has concurrent respiratory problems. Hypoxia and the Valsalva maneuver associated with cough acutely elevate ICP. Vibration, which does not increase ICP, accomplishes excellent results and should be tried first if treatment is needed. If suctioning is necessary, it should be used judiciously and preceded by hyperventilation with 100% oxygen, which can be monitored during suctioning with a pulse oxygen sensor reading to determine oxygen saturation.

Nutrition and Hydration

In the unconscious child, fluids and calories are supplied initially by the IV route. The type of fluid administered depends on the patient's general condition. Children on the ketogenic diet and with certain metabolic disorders, such as pyruvate dehydrogenase deficiency, should receive normal saline rather than fluids containing dextrose, which can cause seizures and worsen their condition. Fluid therapy requires careful monitoring and adjustment based on neurologic signs and electrolyte determinations. Often unconscious children cannot tolerate the same amounts of fluid as when they are healthy. Overhydration must be avoided to prevent fatal cerebral edema. When cerebral edema is a threat, fluids may be restricted to reduce the chance of fluid overload. Examine skin and mucous membranes for signs of dehydration. Adjustments to fluid administration are based on urinary output, serum electrolytes and osmolarity, blood pressure, and arterial filling pressure. Observation for signs of altered fluid balance related to abnormal pituitary secretions is a part of nursing care.

Provide long-term nutrition in a balanced formula given by nasogastric or gastrostomy tube. The nasogastric tube is usually taped in place, with care taken to prevent pressure on the nares. Most children have continuous feedings. When bolus feedings are used, the tube is rinsed with water after each feeding. Tubes are replaced according to institutional policy. Irritation of the nasal mucosa is prevented by alternating nares each time the nasogastric tube is replaced.

Avoid overfeeding to prevent vomiting and the associated risk of aspiration. Stomach contents are aspirated with a syringe and measured before feeding to ascertain the amount remaining in the stomach. The removed contents may be refed. If the residual volume is excessive (depending on the child's size), consult the dietitian and physician regarding the composition and amount to determine whether changes are required to provide calories and nutrients in a smaller volume.

Altered Pituitary Secretion

An altered ability to handle fluid loads is attributed in part to the syndrome of inappropriate antidiuretic hormone secretion (SIADH) and diabetes insipidus (DI) resulting from hypothalamic dysfunction (see Chapter 28). SIADH often accompanies CNS conditions such as head injury, meningitis, encephalitis, brain abscess, brain tumor, and subarachnoid hemorrhage. In the child with SIADH, scant quantities of urine are excreted, electrolyte analysis reveals hyponatremia and hypoosmolality, and manifestations of overhydration are evident. It is important to evaluate all parameters because the reduced urinary output might be erroneously interpreted as a sign of dehydration. The treatment of SIADH consists of fluid restriction until serum electrolytes and osmolality return to normal levels. If fluid restriction is not completely ineffective, medications such as sodium chloride and diuretics may be used.

DI may occur after intracranial trauma. In DI there is increased urinary volume and the accompanying danger of dehydration. Adequate replacement of fluids is essential, and observation of electrolyte balance is necessary to detect signs of hypernatremia and hyperosmolality. Exogenous vasopressin may be administered.

Medications

The cause of unconsciousness determines specific drug therapies. Children with infectious processes are given antibiotics appropriate to the disease and the infecting organism. Corticosteroids are prescribed for inflammatory conditions and edema. Cerebral edema is an indication for osmotic diuretics. Antiepileptic medications are prescribed for seizure activity. Sedation in the combative child provides amnesic and anxiolytic properties in conjunction with a paralytic agent. This combination decreases ICP and allows treatment of cerebral edema. Usual drugs include morphine and midazolam. Midazolam is attractive because of its short half-life.

Deep coma induced by the administration of barbiturates is controversial in the management of ICP. Barbiturates are currently reserved for the reduction of increased ICP when all else has failed. Barbiturates decrease the cerebral metabolic rate for oxygen and protect the brain during times of reduced CPP. Barbiturate coma requires extensive monitoring. EEG monitoring can assess depth of coma, record EEG background abnormalities that can help predict outcome, and evaluate any seizure activity. Cardiovascular and respiratory support and ICP monitoring are needed to assess response to therapy. Paralyzing agents such as vecronium may be needed to aid in performing diagnostic tests, improving effectiveness of therapy, and reducing the risks of secondary complications. Elevation of ICP or heart rate in patients who are being given paralyzing agents or are under sedation may indicate the need for another dose of either or both medications or the need for pain medication.

Thermoregulation

Hyperthermia often accompanies cerebral dysfunction; if it is present, the nurse implements measures to reduce the temperature to prevent brain damage from hyperthermia and to reduce metabolic demands generated by the increased body temperature. Antipyretics are the method of choice for fever reduction; cooling devices are used for hyperthermia (see Chapter 20, Controlling Elevated Temperatures). Laboratory tests and other methods help determine the cause, if any, of the hyperthermia. Treatment with hypothermia and barbiturates increases the risk of iatrogenic complications.

Elimination

A urinary catheter is usually inserted in the acute phase, but diapers may be used and weighed to record urinary output. The child who previously had bowel and bladder control is generally incontinent. If the child remains comatose for a long period, the indwelling catheter may be removed and periodic bladder emptying accomplished by intermittent catheterization. Stool softeners are usually sufficient to maintain bowel function, but suppositories or enemas may be needed occasionally for adequate elimination and to prevent fecal impaction. The passage of liquid stool after a period of no bowel activity is usually a sign of impaction. To avoid this preventable problem, daily recording of bowel activity is essential.

Hygienic Care

Routine measures for cleansing and maintaining skin integrity are an integral part of nursing care of the unconscious child. Skinfolds require special attention to prevent excoriation. The child who is unable to move is prone to develop tissue breakdown and necrosis; the child is placed on a resilient appliance (e.g., alternating-pressure or water-filled mattress) to prevent pressure on prominent areas of the body. The goal is prevention by regular change of position and inspection of vulnerable areas (e.g., the ankle, heels, trochanter, sacrum, and shoulder). Unconscious children undergo numerous invasive procedures, and the skin sites used for these procedures require special assessment and intervention to promote healing and prevent infection. Keep bed linens and any clothing dry and free of wrinkles. Rubbing the back and extremities with lotion stimulates circulation and helps prevent drying of the skin. However, to prevent further tissue damage, do not massage reddened and nonblanching skin (see Chapter 20, Maintaining Healthy Skin). If the child requires surgery or radiography, the nurse checks all dressings, bony sites, catheters, and IV access lines before and after the procedure.

Oral care is performed at least twice daily because the mouth tends to become dry or coated with mucus. The teeth are carefully brushed with a soft toothbrush or cleaned with gauze saturated with saline. Commercially prepared cleansing devices, such as Toothettes, are convenient for cleansing the mouth and teeth. Lips are coated with ointment to protect them from drying, cracking, or blistering.

The unconscious child is also prone to eye irritation. The corneal reflexes are absent; therefore the eyes are easily irritated or damaged by linens, dust, or other substances that may come in contact with them. Excessive dryness results from incomplete closure of the lids and/or decreased secretions, especially if the child is undergoing osmotherapy to reduce or prevent brain edema.

! NURSING ALERT

The eyes are examined regularly and carefully for early signs of irritation or inflammation. Artificial tears (methylcellulose) are placed in the eyes every 1 to 2 hours. Eye patches may be required to protect the eyes from possible damage.

Keep the child's hair combed and secure to prevent tangling. Keep the scalp clean with dry or wet shampoos as needed. The child's head may need to be shaved for tests or surgical procedures. The family may want the hair saved.

Positioning and Exercise

The unconscious child is positioned to minimize ICP and to prevent aspiration of saliva, nasogastric secretions, and vomitus. The head of the bed is elevated, and the child is placed in a side-lying or semiprone position. A small, firm pillow is placed under the head, and the uppermost limbs are flexed and supported with pillows. The weight of the body should not rest on the dependent arm. In the semiprone position the child lies with the dependent arm at the side behind the body; the opposite side is supported on pillows, and the uppermost arm and leg are flexed and resting on the pillows. This position prevents undue pressure on the dependent extremities. The dependent position of the face encourages drainage of secretions and prevents the flaccid tongue from obstructing the airway.

Normal range-of-motion exercises help maintain function and prevent contractures of joints. Perform exercises gently to minimize increasing ICP and with full range of motion. Place a small rolled pad in the palms to help maintain proper positioning of fingers. Splinting may be needed to prevent severe contractures of the wrists, knees, or ankles.

Stimulation

Sensory stimulation is as important in the care of the unconscious child as it is in the care of the alert child. For the temporarily unconscious or semiconscious child, sensory stimulation helps arouse the child to the conscious state and orient the child in terms of time and place. Auditory and tactile stimulation are especially valuable. Tactile stimulation is not appropriate for a child in whom it may elicit an undesirable response. However, for other children tactile contact often has a relaxing and calming effect. When the child's condition permits, holding or rocking the child is soothing and provides the body contact needed by young children.

Hearing is often intact in a state of coma. Hearing is the last sense to be lost and the first one to be regained; speak to the child as any other child. Conversation around the child should not include thoughtless or derogatory remarks. Soft music is often used to provide auditory stimulation. Singing the child's favorite songs or reading a favorite story is a strategy used to maintain the child's contact with a familiar world. Playing songs or favorite stories recorded in the parents' voices can provide a continuous source of familiar stimulation.

Family Support

Helping the parents of an unconscious child cope with the situation is especially difficult. They may demonstrate all of the guilt, fear, hostility, and anxiety of any parent of a seriously ill child (see Chapter 19). In addition, these parents face the uncertain outcome of the cerebral dysfunction. The fear of death, cognitive impairment, or permanent physical disability is present. Nursing intervention with parents depends on the nature of the pathologic condition, the parents' coping skills, and the parent-child relationship before injury or illness.

Awakening from a coma is a gradual process; however, some children regain consciousness within a short time. If there is little or no residual effect, the child is discharged home fairly soon. The parents need the most intensive nursing intervention during the period of crisis and uncertainty. During the recovery phase the nurse gives them information, clarifies it as needed, and encourages them to become involved in the child's care. Often the child's hospitalization is brief; however, some children require extended hospitalization for intensive therapy and rehabilitation. The parents of children who die require support and guidance to cope with the reality of the death and to resolve their grief (see Chapter 17).

Probably the most difficult situations are those that involve children who never regain consciousness. Unlike losing a child through death, these children lack finality, which often leaves the parents in a state of suspended grief. Like parents of dying children, parents of comatose children search for any signs of hope. Well-meaning friends and relatives relate instances of miraculous recoveries. The parents seek confirmation and support for such possibilities and assign erroneous meanings to any sign in the child that might be interpreted as evidence of recovery (e.g., reflexive muscle contractions).

At these times nurses need to respond with compassion and honesty. They can acknowledge that miraculous recoveries do occur but are rare. The important message is to maintain open communication with the family.

Like parents who lose a child through death, the parents of a child who is unconscious attempt to construct a representation of the child. They bring items that belong to the child, such as favorite toys or music. This may be interpreted as an attempt to provide stimulation for the child in the hope of eliciting a response, to let the hospital staff know the child as the unique individual he or she was, and to reconstitute an image of the child "lost" to them and for whom they mourn. The nurses' recognition and understanding of these behaviors and coping mechanisms is important to support the parents in their grief process.

In addition to the process of grieving for the "lost" child, the parents may face difficult decisions. When the child's brain is so severely damaged that vital functions must be maintained by artificial means, the parents must make the final decision whether to remove the life support systems and allow a natural death. After parents are provided with information about what allowing a natural death and removal from life support mean, the parents may turn to both the provider and the nurses with their questions and concerns. Nurses play a critical role in assisting families in participating in their child's care to the greatest extent possible and in planning the child's death when that is the inevitable outcome of the neurologic disorder (Bloomer, Endacott, Copnell, et al., 2016).

HEAD INJURY

Head injury is a pathologic process involving the scalp, skull, meninges, or brain as a result of mechanical force. Unintentional injuries are the number-one health risk for children and the leading cause of death in children older than 1 year of age (Chen, Shi, Stanley, et al., 2017). However, children younger than 1 year of age have a significantly higher rate of severe head injury (Chen et al., 2017). In 2013 approximately 660,000 children 0 to 14 years old experienced a TBI and 17,900 of those children were hospitalized; 1484 children died as a result of their brain injury (Taylor, Bell, Breiding, et al., 2017).

Etiology

The most common causes of head injury in children are falls, being struck by or striking an object with one's head, and motor vehicle accidents, in that order (Centers for Disease Control and Prevention, 2017a). Assaults are the leading cause of death from TBI in children 4 years of age or younger (Taylor et al., 2017). Neurologic injury accounts for the highest mortality rate, with boys usually affected twice as often as girls. There are a number of head trauma strategies, including safety gates on stairs, restricting sleeping in the top bunk to children older than 6 years of age, seat belts and car seat use, and helmets during recreational activities such as biking and skiing. Furthermore, preventing child abuse is necessary and possible.

Pathophysiology

The pathology of brain injury is directly related to the force of impact. Intracranial contents (brain, blood, CSF) are damaged because the force is too great to be absorbed by the skull and musculoligamentous support of the head. Although nervous tissue is delicate, it usually requires a severe blow to cause significant damage.

A child's response to head injury is different from that of adults. The larger head size in proportion to body size and insufficient musculoskeletal support render the very young child particularly vulnerable to acceleration-deceleration injuries.

Primary head injuries are those that occur at the time of trauma and include skull fractures, contusions, intracranial hematomas, and diffuse injuries. Subsequent complications include hypoxic brain injury, increased ICP, and cerebral edema. The predominant feature of a child's brain injury is the diffuse amount of swelling that occurs. Hypoxia and hypercapnia threaten the energy requirements of the brain and increase CBF. The added volume across the blood-brain barrier along with the loss of autoregulation exacerbates cerebral edema. Pressure inside the skull that is greater than arterial pressure results in inadequate perfusion. Because the cranium of very young children has the ability to expand and the thin skull is more compliant, they may tolerate increases in ICP better than older children and adults.

Physical forces act on the head through acceleration, deceleration, or deformation. Acceleration or deceleration is more descriptive of the circumstances responsible for most head injuries. When the stationary head receives a blow, the sudden acceleration causes deformation of the skull and mass movement of the brain. Continued movement of the intracranial contents allows the brain to strike parts of the skull (e.g., the sharp edges of the sphenoid or the irregular surface of the anterior fossa) or the edges of the tentorium.

Although the brain volume remains unchanged, significant distortion and cavitation occur as the brain changes shape in response to the force transmitted from the impact to the skull. This deformation can cause bruising at the point of impact (coup) or at a distance as the brain collides with the unyielding surfaces opposite or far removed from the point of impact (contrecoup) (Fig. 27.5). Thus a blow to the occipital region can cause severe injury to the frontal and temporal areas of the brain.

When a moving head strikes a stationary surface, such as during a fall, sudden deceleration occurs and causes the greatest cerebral injury

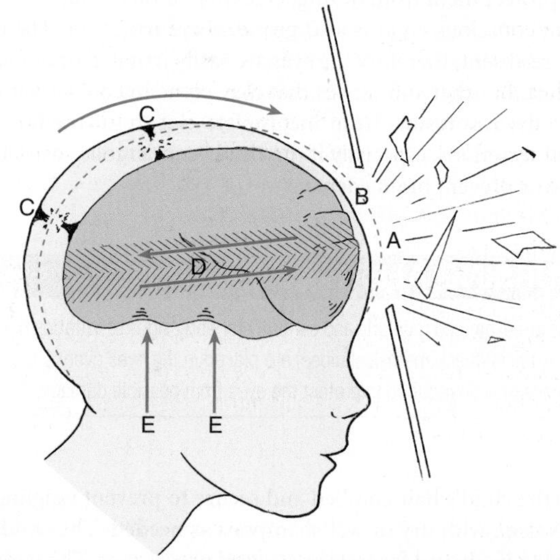

Fig. 27.5 Mechanical distortion of cranium during closed head injury. *A,* Preinjury contour of skull. *B,* Immediate postinjury contour of skull. *C,* Torn subdural vessels. *D,* Shearing forces. *E,* Trauma from contact with floor of cranium. (Redrawn from Grubb, R. L., & Coxe, W. S. [1974]. Central nervous system trauma: Cranial. In S. G. Eliasson, A. L. Presky, & W. B. Hardin [Eds.], *Neurological pathophysiology.* New York, NY: Oxford University Press.)

at the point of impact. Deceleration is responsible for most severe brainstem injuries.

Children with an acceleration-deceleration injury demonstrate diffuse generalized cerebral swelling produced by increased blood volume or by a redistribution of cerebral blood volume (cerebral hyperemia) rather than by the increased water content (edema).

Another effect of brain movement is shearing forces, which are caused by unequal movement or different rates of acceleration at various levels of the brain. A shearing force may tear small arteries that travel from the cerebral surfaces through the meninges to the dural sinuses and cause subdural hemorrhages. Shearing or stretching effects can also be transmitted to nerve fibers. Maximum stress from the shearing force occurs at the interface between structures of different density so that the gray matter (cell body) rapidly accelerates, whereas the white matter (axons) tends to lag behind. Although maximum shearing forces are at the cerebral surface and extend toward the center of rotation within the brain, the most serious effects are often in the area of the brainstem. Severe compression of the skull can cause the brain to be forced through the tentorial opening and produce irreparable damage to the brainstem.

A GCS value of 8 or less in pediatric patients indicates severe injury and requires aggressive therapeutic management (Hartman & Cheifetz, 2020). Three out of four children with a score of 3 or 4 will be severely disabled, be in a persistent vegetative state, or die within a year of their injury (Fulkerson, White, Rees, et al., 2015). A number of studies indicate that the Simplified Motor Scale (SMS) is equivalent to the GCS in predictive power but that the GCS is better for prognosticating death (Singh, Murad, Prokop, et al., 2013).

Concussion

The most common and mildest TBI is ***concussion***, an alteration in mental status with or without loss of consciousness that occurs immediately after a head injury (McCrea, Nelson, & Guskiewicz, 2017). Direct head trauma and "whiplash" seen with rapid acceleration and deceleration of the head are the most frequent causes in children. Sports-related activities are responsible for the majority of concussions (Mullally, 2017).

The hallmarks of a concussion are confusion and amnesia. These are often not preceded by loss of consciousness and may occur immediately after the injury or several minutes later. The belief that loss of consciousness is the hallmark of concussion is a common misconception. A study of 182 adolescent athletes who sustained a concussion found that only 22% lost consciousness, whereas 34% experienced amnesia (Meehan, Mannix, Stracciolini, et al., 2013).

The pathogenesis of concussion is still unclear, but it may be a result of shearing forces that cause stretching, compression, and tearing of nerve fibers, particularly in the area of the central brainstem, the seat of the reticular activating system. It has also been suggested that the anatomic alterations of nerve fibers cause the release of large quantities of acetylcholine into the CSF and a reduction in oxygen consumption with increased lactate production.

Contusion and Laceration

The terms *contusion* and *laceration* are used to describe visible bruising and tearing of cerebral tissue. Contusions represent petechial hemorrhages or localized bruising along the superficial aspects of the brain at the site of impact (coup injury) or a lesion remote from the site of direct trauma (contrecoup injury). In serious accidents there may be multiple sites of injury.

The major areas of the brain susceptible to contusion or laceration are the occipital, frontal, and temporal lobes. In addition, the irregular surfaces of the anterior and middle fossae at the base of the skull are capable of producing bruises or lacerations on forceful impact. Contusions may cause focal disturbances in strength, sensation, or visual awareness. The degree of brain damage in the contused areas varies according to the extent of vascular injury. Signs vary from mild, transient weakness of a limb to prolonged unconsciousness and paralysis. However, the signs and symptoms may be clinically indistinguishable from those of concussion.

Infants who are roughly shaken, referred to as shaken baby syndrome or abusive head trauma, can sustain profound neurologic impairment, seizures, retinal hemorrhages (usually bilateral), and intracranial subarachnoid or subdural hemorrhages (Joyce & Huecker, 2019).

Cerebral lacerations are generally associated with penetrating or depressed skull fractures. However, they may occur without fracture in small children. When brain tissue is actually torn, with bleeding into and around the tear, more severe and prolonged unconsciousness and paralysis usually occur, leaving permanent scarring and some degree of disability.

Fractures

Skull fractures result from a direct blow or injury to the skull and are often associated with intracranial injury. Many of the falls that resulted in a skull fracture in children younger than 2 years of age involved short distances of less than 3 feet, such as falls from a caregiver's arms (Burrows, Trefan, Houston, et al., 2015).

The types of skull fractures that occur are linear, comminuted, depressed, open, basilar, and growing fractures. As a rule, the faster the blow, the greater the likelihood of a depressed fracture; a low-velocity impact tends to produce a linear fracture.

Linear skull fractures are a single fracture line that starts at the point of maximum impact and spreads; however, they do not cross suture lines. Linear skull fractures constitute the majority of childhood skull fractures and typically occur in the parietal bone. Most linear skull fractures are associated with an overlying scalp hematoma, particularly in infants younger than 2 years of age and in the parietal or temporal region (Burns, Grool, Klassen, et al., 2016). Scalp hematomas, in turn, are associated with the presence of intracranial injury whether there is a linear fracture or not (Burns et al., 2016).

Comminuted fractures consist of multiple associated linear fractures. They usually result from intense impact, often from repeated blows against an object or ejection from a car at a high rate of speed. They may suggest child abuse.

Depressed fractures are those in which the bone is locally broken, usually into several irregular fragments that are pushed inward. The greater the depression, the higher the risk of a tear in the dura or cortical laceration. Depressed skull fractures may be associated with direct underlying parenchymal damage and should be suspected when a child's head appears misshapen. Surgery may be needed to elevate the depressed bone fragment if there is an associated intracranial hematoma and if the depression is greater than 1 cm (0.4 inch).

Basilar fractures involve the bones at the base of the skull in either the posterior or the anterior region. The bones involved are the ethmoid, sphenoid, temporal, or occipital bones. These fractures usually result in a dural tear. Because of the proximity of the fracture line to structures surrounding the brainstem, a basal skull fracture is a serious head injury. Basilar fractures often involve frontal bone fractures. This can result in clinical features such as leakage of CSF from the nose (CSF rhinorrhea) or ear (CSF otorrhea), blood behind the tympanic membrane (hemotympanum), subcutaneous bleeding over the mastoid process that is located posterior to the ear, and subcutaneous bleeding around the orbit (Bonfield, Naran, Adetayo, et al., 2014). Meningitis, although rare, is always a potential risk with CSF leakage.

> **! NURSING ALERT**
>
> Suspect posttraumatic meningitis in children with increasing drowsiness and fever who also have basilar skull fractures.

Open fractures result in a communication between the skull and the scalp or the mucosa of the upper respiratory tract. The risk of CNS infection is increased with open fractures. Compound fractures consist of a skin laceration overlying the bone fracture. Open fractures that involve the paranasal sinuses or middle ear may lead to leakage of CSF (rhinorrhea or otorrhea). Prophylactic antibiotics are recommended to prevent osteomyelitis.

Growing skull fracture is an unusual complication of head trauma. The fracture is accompanied by an underlying tear in the dura or brain injury that fails to heal properly. A leptomeningeal cyst, dilated ventricles, or herniated brain may result and cause growth of the original fracture. Most growing skull fractures occur before 30 months of age and occur in the parietal bone (Vezina, Al-Halabi, Shash, et al., 2017). Physical examination usually shows a swelling scalp and skull defect. Clinical neurologic symptoms may be delayed for months to years after the initial skull fracture and include headache, seizures, hemiparesis, and learning and intellectual disabilities (Vezina et al., 2017).

Complications

The major complications of trauma to the head are hemorrhage, infection, edema, and herniation through the brainstem. Infection is always a hazard in open injuries. Edema is related to tissue trauma. Vascular rupture may occur even in minor head injuries, causing hemorrhage between the skull and cerebral surfaces. Compression of the underlying brain produces effects that can be rapidly fatal or insidiously progressive.

Epidural Hematoma

Epidural (extradural) hematoma is a hemorrhage into the space between the dura and the skull. As the hematoma enlarges, the dura is stripped from the skull; this accumulation of blood results in a mass effect on the brain, forcing the underlying brain contents downward as it expands (Fig. 27.6A). Because bleeding is generally arterial, brain compression occurs rapidly. The lower incidence of epidural hematoma in childhood is attributed to the fact that the middle meningeal artery is not embedded in the skull's bone surface until approximately 2 years old. Therefore a temporal bone fracture is less likely to lacerate the artery. Neuroimaging studies in 210 infants and young children with isolated mild TBI showed skull fractures with extra-axial hemorrhage/no midline shift (30%), nondisplaced skull fractures (28%), and intracranial hemorrhage without fractures/midline shift (19%) (Noje, Jackson, Nasr, et al., 2019).

Child abuse accounts for a significant number of cases of epidural hematomas in infants and children, whereas motor vehicle accidents account for most epidural hematomas in adolescents.

Because bleeding is generally arterial, brain compression occurs rapidly. Most often the expanding hematoma is located in the parietal and temporal regions (Teichert, Rosales, Lopes, et al., 2012), which forces the medial portion of the temporal lobe under the edge of the tentorium, where it places pressure on nerves and blood vessels. Pressure on the arterial supply and venous return to the reticular formation causes loss of consciousness; pressure on CN III produces dilation and (later)

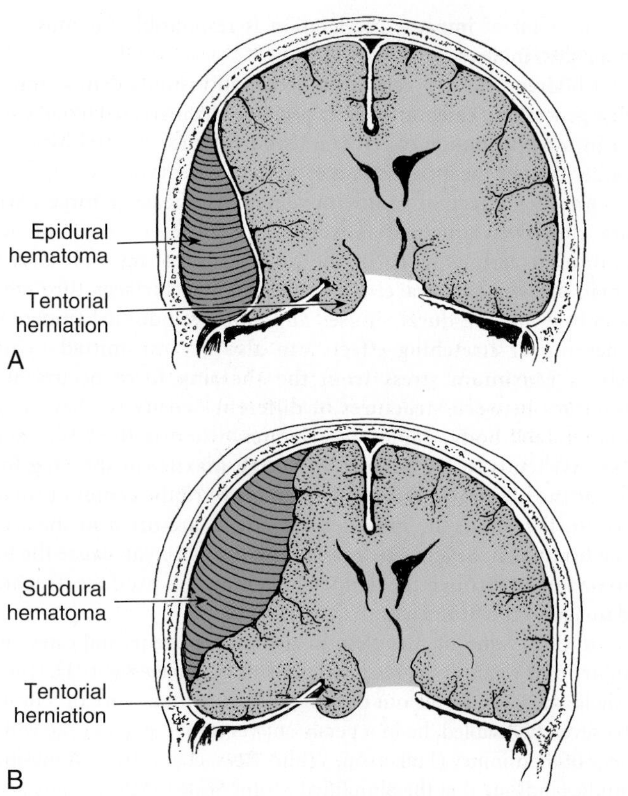

Fig. 27.6 **A,** Epidural (extradural) hematoma and compression of temporal lobe through tentorial herniation. **B,** Subdural hematoma.

fixation of the ipsilateral pupil. Pressure on the fibers of the pyramidal tract is evidenced by contralateral weakness or paralysis and increased deep tendon reflexes. Extreme pressure may cause brain herniation and death. Expanding epidural hemorrhages may be better tolerated in young children with open sutures that allow for expansion of the skull. In addition, young children have larger subarachnoid and extracellular spaces, which provide space for the expanding hematoma without compression on the brain parenchyma.

The classic clinical picture of an epidural hemorrhage is a lucid interval of minutes to hours followed by rapidly altered mental status, then loss of consciousness or coma due to blood accumulation in the epidural space and compression of the brain. The child may be seen with varying degrees of impaired consciousness, depending on the severity of the traumatic injury. Common symptoms in a child with no neurologic deficit are irritability, headache, and vomiting. In infants younger than 24 months of age, common symptoms are scalp swelling, irritability, and lethargy. They may also have seizures, reduced oral intake, and increasing head circumference (Sellin, Moreno, Ryan, et al., 2017).

An epidural hematoma can be detected by an initial CT scan. If the severity of the child's symptoms is not recognized, herniation and death will result. ***Cushing triad*** (systemic hypertension, bradycardia, and respiratory depression) is a late sign of impending brainstem herniation.

> **! NURSING ALERT**
>
> Children with a subdural hematoma and retinal hemorrhages should be evaluated for the possibility of child abuse, especially shaken baby syndrome.

Subdural Hematoma

A subdural hematoma is a hemorrhage between the dura and the arachnoid membrane that overlies the brain and the subarachnoid space. The hemorrhage may be from two sources: (1) tearing of the veins that bridge the subdural space and (2) hemorrhage from the cortex of the brain caused by direct brain trauma (see Fig. 27.6B). Subdural hematomas are much more common than epidural hematomas in infants and children.

Unlike epidural hemorrhage, which develops inwardly against the less resistant brain tissue, subdural hemorrhage tends to develop more slowly and spreads thinly and widely, crossing cranial sutures, until it is limited by the dural barriers: the falx and the tentorium. The small subdural space and the dura, which is firmly attached to the skull in this area, are highly vulnerable to increased ICP.

Subdural hematoma is fairly common in infants. Most often it is the result of assaults or violent shaking. The caregiver's response to infant crying, often perceived as inconsolable, is an important risk factor (Barr, 2014). In neonates, subdural hematoma can be a consequence of labor and delivery. Subdural hemorrhage can cause either acute or chronic subdural hematoma. Acute subdural hematoma may be associated with contusions or lacerations and develops within minutes or hours of injury. Chronic subdural hematoma is more common. The clinical course and manifestations vary depending on the damage sustained by the brain and the child's age.

Presenting signs of acute hematoma include irritability, vomiting, increased head circumference, bulging anterior fontanel (in the infant), lethargy, coma, or seizures. In infants with open fontanels, large amounts of intracranial blood may accumulate, causing hemorrhagic shock or fever before there are any changes in the neurologic examination. Retinal hemorrhages and skull and skeletal fractures are suggestive of physical abuse. An infant who has an altered LOC and in whom the CT scan shows subarachnoid hemorrhage or subdural hematoma may have been physically abused. A child with a GCS of 12 or less or a decrease in GCS score by 2 or more points requires emergency consultation with the neurosurgeon (Huang, Bi, Abd-El-Barr, et al., 2016).

Closely observe older children for signs of neurologic deterioration, including altered mental status, vomiting, lethargy, and signs of increased ICP. Hemiparesis, hemiplegia, and anisocoria (unequal pupils) are signs of brainstem compression and require emergency treatment targeted at decreasing ICP. The surgical management of subdural hematomas depends on the physical examination, size of the hematoma, and presence of other abnormalities on the CT scan. Not all children require surgery or are candidates for surgery. Various surgical options to treat subdural hematomas include transfontanel percutaneous aspiration, subdural drains, placement of burr hole, or craniotomy (Huang et al., 2016).

Other Hemorrhagic Lesions

A subarachnoid hemorrhage is bleeding within the subarachnoid space, which is normally filled with CSF. Nontraumatic intracranial hemorrhages are rare in children. The most common causes of spontaneous intracranial hemorrhage in children are arteriovenous malformations and fistulas and brain tumors (Ding, Starke, Kano, et al., 2017). Sudden onset of a severe headache, headaches occurring out of sleep, first-time seizure, and abnormal neurologic examination are symptoms that require evaluation including neuroimaging (Blume, 2017).

Cerebral Edema

Some degree of brain edema is expected after craniocerebral trauma and often accompanies any of the previously mentioned disorders. Cerebral edema peaks at 24 to 72 hours after injury and may account for changes in a child's neurologic status. Cerebral edema associated with traumatic brain injury may be a result of two different mechanisms: cytotoxic edema or vasogenic edema. Cytotoxic edema is a result of direct cell injury and is caused by intracellular swelling. In many cases the brain cells are irreversibly damaged. Vasogenic edema is due to increased permeability of capillary endothelial cells, resulting in increased intracellular fluid. In vasogenic edema the nerve cells are not primarily injured. Either mechanism can result in increased ICP as a result of increased intracranial volume and changes in CBF as a result of loss of autoregulation and/or hypercapnia or hypoxia. Children at risk for deterioration can be identified by abnormalities seen on noncontrast CT scans.

Sequelae of Traumatic Brain Injury

Postconcussion syndrome is a sequela to brain injury with or without loss of consciousness. Concussions usually resolve in 1 to 3 weeks without complications. Up to a third of children may have ongoing somatic, behavioral, cognitive, and psychologic symptoms, including headaches, visual and balance problems, difficulty concentrating, irritability, and changes in their sleep patterns (Morgan, Zuckerman, Lee, et al., 2015). The pathophysiology of these symptoms is unclear. When these symptoms continue for more than 4 weeks after the concussion, the term *postconcussion syndrome* (PCS) is used (Zemek, Barrowman, Freedman, et al., 2016). Risk factors for PCS in youth athletes include a personal or family history of mood disorders and other psychiatric illnesses and migraines (Morgan et al., 2015). Previously, concussion treatment guidelines recommended cognitive and physical rest as a path to recovery. Recent studies, though, have found that early participation in physical activity is significantly likely to prevent the development of PCS (Grool, Aglipay, Momoli, et al., 2016).

Posttraumatic headaches, one of the most common symptoms after mild TBI, may occur within 1 week to 3 months after a mild TBI. They occur in 25% to 75% of individuals and are most commonly classified as migraines (Kuczynski, Crawford, Bodell, et al., 2013). Posttraumatic headaches are treated based on the primary headache type: migraine or tension/chronic headache (Kacperski & Arthur, 2016).

Posttraumatic seizures occur in a number of children who survive a head injury, often within 24 hours, but they also can occur sometime after the injury (Rumalla, Smith, Letchuman, et al., 2018). Risk factors for seizures include preexisting comorbidities, shaken infant syndrome, subdural hematoma, closed-type injury, and changes in LOC (Rumalla et al., 2018).

Hydrocephalus may develop after subarachnoid hemorrhage or infection. Normal pressure hydrocephalus can be a complication of TBI. In infants, signs and symptoms include rapidly increasing head circumference, irritability, refusal to feed, and sleepiness. The clinical signs and symptoms in children include changes in personality, developmental regression, ataxia, and incontinence. These signs are also seen during posttraumatic amnesia, making early recognition of this syndrome difficult. Focal deficits, including optic atrophy, cranaial nerve (CN) palsies, motor deficits, DI, or aphasia, may be seen. The type of residual effect depends on the location and nature of the trauma.

Diagnostic Evaluation

A detailed health history, both past and present, is essential in evaluating the child with head trauma. Certain disorders such as drug allergies, hemophilia, diabetes mellitus, or epilepsy may produce similar symptoms. Even a minor traumatic injury can aggravate a preexisting

BOX 27.3 Clinical Manifestations of Acute Head Injury

Minor Injury
May or may not lose consciousness
Transient period of confusion
Somnolence
Listlessness
Irritability
Pallor
Vomiting (one or more episodes)

Signs of Progression
Altered mental status (e.g., difficulty arousing child)
Mounting agitation
Development of focal lateral neurologic signs
Marked changes in vital signs

Severe Injury
Signs of increased intracranial pressure (see Box 27.1)
Bulging fontanel (infant)
Retinal hemorrhages
Extraocular palsies (especially cranial nerve III)
Hemiparesis
Quadriplegia
Elevated temperature
Unsteady gait (older child)
Papilledema (older child)
Retinal hemorrhages

Associated Signs
Scalp trauma
Other injuries (e.g., to extremities)

disease process, thereby producing neurologic signs out of proportion to the injury.

After a minor injury, initial unconsciousness (if present) is brief. The child ordinarily exhibits a transient period of confusion, somnolence, and listlessness; this period is most often accompanied by irritability, pallor, and one episode of vomiting. A severe head injury requires immediate evaluation and treatment. Because head injuries are often accompanied by injuries in other areas (e.g., spine, viscera, extremities), the examination is performed with care to avoid further damage. Box 27.3 lists manifestations of head injury.

NURSING ALERT

Stabilize the spine after head injury until spinal cord injury is ruled out.

Initial Assessment

Priorities in the initial phase in the care of a child with a head injury include assessment of the CAB (circulation, airway, breathing); neurologic examination focusing on mental status, papillary responses, and motor responses; and assessment for spinal cord injury. The assessment is carried out quickly in relation to vital signs (see Emergency Treatment box).

EMERGENCY TREATMENT

Head Injury

1. Assess child:
   - C—Circulation
   - A—Airway
   - B—Breathing
   - Neurologic and thermoregulatory status
2. Stabilize neck and spine immediately. Use jaw thrust, not chin lift, to open airway.
3. Clean any abrasions with soap and water.
   - Apply clean dressing.
   - If child is bleeding, apply ice to relieve pain and swelling.
4. Keep child NPO (nothing by mouth) until instructed otherwise.
5. Assess pain but give no analgesics or sedatives.
6. Check level of consciousness and pupillary reaction every 4 hours (including twice during night) for 48 hours.
7. Seek medical attention for any of the following:
   - Injury sustained at high speed (e.g., automobile)
   - Fall from a significant distance (height greater than that of the child)
   - Injury sustained from great force (e.g., baseball bat)
   - Injury sustained under suspicious circumstances
   - Loss of consciousness
   - Amnesia
   - Discomfort (crying) more than 10 minutes after injury
   - Headache that is severe, worsens, interferes with sleep, or lasts more than 24 hours
   - Vomiting three or more times or vomiting that begins or continues 4 to 6 hours after injury
   - Swelling in front of or above earlobe or swelling that increases in size
   - Fluid leak from ears or nose; blackened eyes
   - Confusion or abnormal behavior
   - Difficulty arousing child from sleep
   - Difficulty speaking
   - Blurring of vision or diplopia
   - Unsteady gait
   - Difficulty using extremities; weakness or incoordination
   - Neck pain or stiffness
   - Pupils dilated, fixed, or unequal
   - Infant with bulging fontanel
   - Seizures

NURSING ALERT

Deep, rapid, periodic, or intermittent and gasping respirations; wide fluctuations or noticeable slowing of the pulse; and widening pulse pressure or extreme fluctuations in blood pressure are signs of brainstem involvement. Marked hypotension may represent internal injuries.

Ocular signs such as fixed, dilated, and unequal pupils; fixed and constricted pupils; and pupils that are poorly reactive or unreactive to light and accommodation indicate increased ICP or brainstem involvement. It is important to remain with the patient who demonstrates fixed and dilated pupils because these are ominous signs often associated with impending respiratory arrest. Dilated, nonpulsating blood vessels indicate increased ICP before the appearance of papilledema. Retinal hemorrhages often occur with acute head injuries, specifically with shaken baby syndrome.

! NURSING ALERT

Observation of asymmetric pupils or one dilated, unreactive pupil in a comatose child is a neurologic emergency.

Funduscopic examination should be performed routinely to detect retinal hemorrhages in a child with CNS trauma. Vestibulo-ocular symptoms such as diplopia, dizziness, motion sensitivity, eye-tracking and eye-focusing problems, photosensitivity, and visual inattention may develop (Ellis, Cordingley, Vis, et al., 2015). Transient vision loss may occur after mild head trauma but may not be obvious in children unless this diagnosis is evaluated. Theories of possible causes are vasospasm or localized cerebral edema.

Less urgent but important assessments include examination of the scalp for lacerations, widely separated sutures, and the size and tension of fontanels, which indicate intracranial hemorrhage or rapidly developing cerebral edema. Scalp lacerations may require surgical intervention. A significant amount of blood loss can occur from scalp lacerations. CT scan may be necessary to evaluate possible skull fractures and acute intracranial hemorrhage (Ryan, Jaju, Ciolino, et al., 2016).

! NURSING ALERT

Bleeding from the nose or ears needs further evaluation, and a watery discharge from the nose (rhinorrhea) that is positive for glucose (as tested with reagent strips [e.g., Dextrostix]) suggests leaking of cerebrospinal fluid (CSF) from a skull fracture.

A documented accurate assessment of clinical signs provides baseline information. Serial evaluations, preferably by a single observer, help detect changes in neurologic status. Alterations in mental status, evidenced by increased difficulty in rousing the child, mounting agitation, development of focal neurologic signs, or marked changes in vital signs, usually indicate extension or progression of the basic pathologic process.

Evaluation of reflexes provides information about cerebral and pyramidal involvement, although transient abnormalities of the primitive reflexes and Babinski sign may be present in children with mild head trauma. Conscious, cooperative children are examined for cerebellar signs such as ataxia and dysmetria. Children may display unsteadiness, clumsiness, or tremor with intentional movement after head injury. Temperature may be moderately elevated for 1 or 2 days after an initial mild hypothermia after injury. A persistent fever may indicate subarachnoid hemorrhage or infection.

Special Tests

After a thorough clinical examination, a variety of diagnostic tests are helpful in providing a more definitive diagnosis of the type and extent of the trauma. A hematocrit and urinalysis are typically done. Serum electrolytes and glucose may also be measured in children with severe head injuries; hyperglycemia and disseminated intravascular coagulation are associated with a poor prognosis. The severity of a head injury may not be apparent on clinical examination of the child but detectable on a CT scan. Whenever the child has a history consistent with a serious head injury (as with an unrestrained occupant in a severe motor vehicle accident or a fall from higher than their own height), it is important to perform a scan even if the child initially appears alert and oriented. All children with head injuries who have any alteration of consciousness, headache, vomiting, skull fracture, seizure, or predisposing medical condition should undergo a diagnostic evaluation that includes CT scanning.

MRI may be done to further assess cerebral edema or other structural brain abnormalities. A neurodevelopmental assessment after early head injury may be useful in documenting cognitive impairment. Skull radiographs are of little benefit in diagnosing skull fractures. Other radiographic tests may be indicated, depending on the severity or cause of the trauma. Electroencephalography is not helpful for diagnosis of a head injury but is useful for defining seizures and looking for subclinical seizures, which can impair consciousness (Gainza-Lein, Sanchez-Fernandez, & Loddenkemper, 2017). Lumbar puncture is rarely used for craniocerebral trauma and is contraindicated in the presence of increased ICP because of the possibility of herniation.

Therapeutic Management

Most children with mild TBI who have not lost consciousness can be cared for and observed at home after careful examination reveals no serious intracranial injury. The nurse should give parents both verbal and written instructions of signs and symptoms that warrant concern and the need for reevaluation. These include persistent or worsening headaches, vomiting, change in mental status or behavior, unsteady gait, or seizure. The child should have a physical examination 1 or 2 days after the injury. The manifestations of epidural hematoma in children do not generally appear until 24 hours or more after injury.

Maintaining contact with parents for continued observation and reevaluation of the child, when indicated, facilitates early diagnosis and treatment of possible complications from head injury, such as hematoma, cerebral edema, and posttraumatic seizures. Children are generally hospitalized for 24 to 48 hours of observation if their family lives far from medical facilities or lacks transportation or a telephone, which would provide access to immediate help. Other circumstances, such as language or other communication barriers or even emotional trauma, may hinder learning and make it difficult for families to feel confident caring for their child at home.

! NURSING ALERT

If a child loses consciousness or develops a severe headache after a head injury, medical attention should be sought.

Children with severe injuries, those who have lost consciousness for more than a few minutes, and those with prolonged and continued seizures or other focal or diffuse neurologic signs must be hospitalized until their condition is stable and their neurologic signs have diminished. The child is maintained on nothing-by-mouth (NPO) status or restricted to clear liquids (if able to take fluids by mouth) until it is determined that vomiting will not occur. IV fluids are indicated in the child who is comatose, displays dulled sensorium, or is persistently vomiting.

The volume of IV fluid is carefully monitored to minimize the possibility of overhydration in case of SIADH and cerebral edema. However, damage to the hypothalamus or pituitary gland may produce DI, with its accompanying hypertonicity and dehydration. Fluid balance is closely monitored by daily weight, strict intake and output measurement, and serum osmolality (to detect early signs of water retention).

Sedating drugs are usually withheld in the acute phase. Headache is usually controlled with acetaminophen, although opioids may be needed. Antiepileptics are used for seizure control. Antibiotics are administered if there are lacerations or penetrating injuries. Prophylactic tetanus toxoid is given as appropriate (see Chapter 6). Cerebral edema is managed as described for the unconscious child. Hyperthermia is controlled with tepid sponges or a hypothermia blanket.

Surgical Therapy

Approximately 10% to 30% of pediatric head traumas will result in skull fractures. Because of the greater capacity of a child's skull fracture to heal, conservative nonsurgical management is often adequate. Children hit in the head or who have TBI as a result of a motor vehicle accident are more likely to require surgical intervention, especially if the frontal bones have been fractured (Bonfield et al., 2014).

Scalp lacerations are sutured after careful examination of underlying bone. The use of topical lidocaine, adrenaline, and tetracaine (LAT) or lidocaine, epinephrine, and tetracaine (LET) provides noninvasive, effective anesthesia for suturing, particularly when combined with consultation from and the bedside presence of a child life specialist (Martin, 2017).

Depressed fractures require surgical reduction and removal of bone fragments. Torn dura is also sutured. A skull fracture depressed more than the thickness of the skull or an intracranial hematoma that causes more than a 5-mm (0.2-inch) midline shift is an indication for surgery. Direct pressure should never be applied to a depressed skull fracture. Parents should be advised that painful hardware and wound infections may need further surgical intervention. Parents and other caregivers must be taught the importance of meticulous hand washing after surgical repair of a skull fracture.

Prognosis

The outcome of craniocerebral trauma depends on the extent of injury and complications. Neurologic, cognitive, emotional, and behavioral symptoms can result in significant impairment. They may not present until the child is older and preparing to reach certain developmental milestones (Babikian, Merkley, Savage, et al., 2015). These symptoms can become chronic and include epilepsy, attention-deficit/hyperactivity disorder, and learning or psychiatric disorders. Children with learning and behavior problems before their head trauma are more likely to suffer these consequences (Beauchamp & Anderson, 2013). More than 90% of children with concussions or simple linear fractures recover without symptoms after the initial period.

Children may be more vulnerable than adults to long-term cognitive and behavioral dysfunction after diffuse brain injury. Contrary to what was previously thought about "brain plasticity," evidence now indicates that children's brains may be especially vulnerable to early injury due to their ongoing maturation processes, which can be disrupted by head trauma (Babikian et al., 2015). Parents of children who have suffered TBI should be advised to seek evaluation and treatment sooner rather than later if any of these symptoms present. TBI is recognized as a disability that may qualify a child for special education services under the Individuals with Disabilities Education Act (IDEA) of 1990.

True coma (i.e., not obeying commands, eyes closed, and not speaking) usually does not last for more than 2 weeks. A child's eventual outcome can range from brain death to a persistent vegetative state to complete recovery. However, even the best recovery may be associated with personality changes, including mood lability and loss of confidence, impaired short-term memory, headaches, and subtle cognitive impairments. In general, 90% of the long-term neurologic outcome has been achieved within 6 months to 1 year after the injury.

Nursing Care Management

The hospitalized child requires careful neurologic assessment and evaluation repeated as frequently as every 15 minutes to establish a correct diagnosis, identify signs and symptoms of increased ICP, determine clinical management, and prevent many complications. The goals of nursing management of the child with a head injury are to maintain adequate ventilation, oxygenation, and circulation; to monitor and treat increased ICP; to minimize cerebral oxygen requirements; and to support the child and family during recovery (see Quality Patient Outcomes box).

> **QUALITY PATIENT OUTCOMES: Acute Head Injury**
> - Early recognition of signs and symptoms of increased intracranial pressure
> - Adequate ventilation, oxygenation, and circulation maintained
> - Cerebral oxygen requirements minimized
> - Sedation and analgesia provided while allowing for neurologic assessment

The child is placed on bed rest, usually with the head of the bed elevated slightly and the head in midline position. Appropriate safety measures, such as side rails kept up and seizure precautions, are implemented. If the child is extremely restless, hard surfaces may be padded and restraints used to prevent further injury. Individualize care according to the child's specific needs.

A key nursing role is to provide sedation and analgesia for the child. The conflict between the need to promote the child's comfort and relieve anxiety versus the need to assess for neurologic changes presents a dilemma. Both goals can be achieved with close observation of the child's LOC and response to analgesics (using a pain assessment record) and effective communication with the provider. Decreasing restlessness after administration of an analgesic most likely reflects pain control rather than a decreasing LOC (see Chapter 5, Pain Assessment and Pain Management).

Children may be restless and irritable, but more often their reaction is to fall asleep when left undisturbed. A quiet environment can help reduce restlessness and irritability. Bright lights are irritating. This often makes checking the ocular responses more difficult and aggravating to the child.

Frequent examinations of vital signs, neurologic signs, and LOC are extremely important nursing observations. When possible, they should be performed by a single observer to better detect subtle changes that may indicate worsening of neurologic status. Pupils are checked for size, symmetry, reaction to light, and accommodation. Unless there is brainstem involvement, vital signs generally return to normal after the initial changes seen after injury.

The most important nursing observation is assessment of the child's LOC. In the progression of an injury, alterations in consciousness appear earlier than alterations in vital signs or focal neurologic signs (see evaluation of responsiveness later in the chapter). Frequent examinations of alertness are fatiguing to the child; the child often desires to fall asleep, which may be confused with depressed consciousness. It is not uncommon to observe ocular divergence through the partially closed eyelids.

Observations of position and movement provide additional information. Note any abnormal posturing and whether it occurs continuously or intermittently. Questions nurses might ask include the following:

- Are the child's hand grips strong and equal in strength?
- Are there any signs of extension or flexion posturing?
- What is the child's response to auditory and physical stimulation?
- Is movement purposeful, random, or absent?
- Are movement and sensation equal on both sides or restricted to one side only?

The child may report a headache or other discomfort. The child who is too young to describe a headache may be fussy and resist being handled. The child who suffers from vertigo often vigorously resists being moved from a position of comfort. Forcible movement causes the child to vomit and display spontaneous nystagmus. Seizures are relatively common in children at the time of head injury and may be of any type. Carefully observe any seizure activity and describe it in detail. Children in postictal states are more lethargic, with sluggish pupils.

Document drainage from any orifice. Bleeding from the ear suggests the possibility of a basal skull fracture. Clear nasal drainage is suggestive of an anterior basal skull fracture. Observe the amount and characteristics of the drainage.

! NURSING ALERT

Suctioning through the nares is contraindicated because there is a risk of the catheter entering the brain through a fracture in the skull.

Head trauma is often accompanied by other undetected injuries; therefore any bruises, lacerations, or evidence of internal injuries or fractures of the extremities are noted and reported. Associated injuries are evaluated and treated appropriately.

The child with a normal LOC is usually allowed clear liquids unless fluid is restricted. If the child has an IV infusion, it is maintained as prescribed. The diet is advanced to that appropriate for the child's age as soon as the condition permits. Intake and output are measured and recorded with attention to the development of constipation. Any incontinence of bowel or bladder is noted for the child who has been toilet trained.

Assessment for unusual behavior can be made only in relation to the child's typical behavior. For example, urinary incontinence during sleep would be of no consequence in a child who routinely wets the bed but would be highly significant for one who is always dry. Parents are invaluable resources in evaluating objective behaviors of their children. Information obtained from parents at or shortly after admission is essential in evaluating the child's behavior (e.g., the ease with which the child is roused normally, the usual sleeping position, how much the child sleeps during the day, the child's motor activities [rolling over, sitting up, climbing], hearing and visual acuity, appetite, and manner of eating [spoon, bottle, cup]). Documentation of the child's baseline developmental and behavioral level is crucial. There is less concern about a child who falls asleep several times during the day if this is consistent with the child's usual behavior.

When the child is discharged, advise the parents of probable posttraumatic symptoms they may observe, such as behavioral changes, sleep disturbances, phobias, and seizures. Parents should be taught seizure first aid. They should understand observations they need to make and when and how to contact the provider or health facility in case the child develops any unusual signs or symptoms. Emphasize the importance of follow-up evaluation.

Family Support

The emotional and educational support of the family presents a challenge. Witnessing the parents' grief and helplessness on seeing their child in an intensive care unit connected to monitoring equipment and in an altered state evokes empathy. The nurse can encourage the family to be involved in the child's care, to bring in familiar belongings, or to make a recording of familiar voices and sounds. Parents may need a demonstration on how to touch or cuddle their child and may want to talk about their grief. The nurse listens attentively, reinforces what is being done to assist the child, and directs parents toward signs and symptoms of recovery to instill hope without promises. Honesty and kindness, along with consistent and competent care, help families through this difficult time.

Rehabilitation

Rehabilitation and management of the child with permanent brain injury are essential aspects of care. Rehabilitation begins as soon as possible and usually involves the family and a rehabilitation team. The nurse makes a careful assessment of the child's capabilities and limitations and implements appropriate interventions to maximize the residual capacities. The Brain Injury Association of America[a] provides information and listings of rehabilitation services and support groups throughout the country.

The child with a disability resulting from head trauma requires functional assessment of his or her physical, cognitive, emotional, and social levels. The child has experienced separation, pain, sensory deprivation and overload, changes in circadian cycle, and fear of the unknown. Recovery and transition require new coping strategies at the same time that regressive and acting-out behaviors may start. Parents and children need honest communication for decision making.

Rehabilitation is recommended when the child is making progress and no longer requires acute care hospitalization but continues to require daily therapies to return to his or her premorbid functional level. Children are more likely to continue in outpatient rehabilitation if they have had an inpatient assessment of their rehabilitation needs (Jimenez, Symons, Wang, et al., 2016). The Rancho Los Amigos Scale provides a systematic assessment of the progress that a child with a severe head injury may achieve.

Pediatric rehabilitation focuses on the child's strengths and needs. The rehabilitation team should include physical medicine; rehabilitation nursing; nutritional counseling; physical, occupational, and speech therapy; special education; and psychologic, neuropsychologic, child life, and social services support. Before the child's transfer, the hospital team should provide a detailed care plan of the child's needs and abilities, especially communication skills, and a description of the child's usual schedule, nursing care interventions, and the family's concerns and needs. To augment the care plan, a video introducing the child and family and showing any unique aspects of their care can be sent to the rehabilitation center.

Prevention

Preventive strategies are underused in almost all cases of accidental childhood injury. Head injuries occur in the most serious accidents—especially motor vehicle accidents, sports, and falls.

Strides are being made in the prevention of secondary brain tissue damage after the initial head injury in children. This secondary injury is caused by altered cerebral blood flow that results in ischemia, hypoxia, and eventually the death of brain cells (Popernack, Gray, & Reuter-Rice, 2015). Studies are ongoing in both humans and animals using therapeutic hypothermia, glucagon, blood pressure medications, and antioxidants (Toth, Szarka, Farkas, et al., 2016). The roles of calcium, oxyradicals, and prostaglandins are being investigated.

However, the greatest benefit lies in prevention of head injuries. Nurses can exert a valuable influence on behalf of children through education. Accidents that are preventable occur because unnecessary risks go unchecked. Inadequate supervision combined with a child's natural sense of curiosity and exploration can lead to lethal results. Nurses are in the unique position of influencing caregivers in terms of growth and development. The use of car seats; seat belts in strollers and feeding chairs; and helmets for biking, skateboarding, and other sports

[a]1608 Spring Hill Road, Suite 110, Vienna, VA 22182; 703-761-0750; fax: 703-761-0755; http://www.biausa.org.

has been shown to reduce both the number and the severity of head injuries in children (Gaw, Chounthirath, & Smith, 2017).

Studies of ways to prevent abusive head trauma are ongoing. Promising interventions include teaching parents about infant crying and ways to cope with it (Lopes & Williams, 2016). Infants who have been hospitalized after birth have an increased risk of being abused after discharge. Neonatal nurses have an important role to play in teaching parents of these children about child abuse prevention.

Public education coupled with legislative support can aid in the prevention of childhood injuries. Research has shown that increased household income can prevent abusive head trauma (Klevens, Schmidt, Luo, et al., 2017). For extensive discussions of childhood injuries, see the information on injury prevention in Chapters 10, 12, 13, and 15.

SUBMERSION INJURY

Drowning is one of the major causes of unintentional injury-related death in children ages 1 to 19 years. In children ages 1 to 4 years it is the leading cause of unintentional injury-related death (Gilchrist & Parker, 2014). The term *near-drowning* is no longer used; instead, the term *submersion injury* should be used until the time of drowning-related death.

Most cases of submersion injury are accidental, usually involving children who are helpless in water, such as inadequately attended children in or near swimming pools or infants in bathtubs; small children who fall into ponds, streams, and flooded excavations, usually near home; occupants of pleasure boats who fail to wear life preservers; children who have diving accidents; and children who are able to swim but overestimate their endurance. Accidental submersion injury occurs predominantly in males, toddlers, and African Americans (Gilchrist & Parker, 2014).

Submersion injury can take place in any body of water. Children less than 1 year of age are most likely to have a submersion injury in a bathtub, whereas top-heavy toddlers fall headfirst into a pail of water and are unable to free themselves (Xu, 2014). Preschoolers are at risk for injury in swimming pools, and school-age children and adolescents are most commonly at risk in natural bodies of water such as lakes, ponds, and rivers (Xu, 2014). The suction created at the outlet of pools, hot tubs, or whirlpool spas is strong enough to trap even larger children underwater. Submersion injury as a form of fatal child abuse also occurs. Homicidal submersion injuries are not witnessed, usually occurring in the home, and the victims are either infants or toddlers.

Pathophysiology

Physiologically, most organ systems are affected, especially the pulmonary, cardiovascular, and neurologic systems. The major pulmonary changes that occur in submersion injury are directly related to the length of submersion (regardless of the type and amount of fluid aspirated), the victim's physiologic response, and the development and degree of immersion hypothermia. Cerebral hypoxia is a major component of morbidity and mortality in these individuals. Therefore early and aggressive resuscitation is imperative.

Physiologic factors in submersion injuries are hypothermia, aspiration, and hypoxia. The temperature of the liquid plays an important role. Cold water decreases metabolic demands and activates the diving reflex, which causes blood to be shunted away from the periphery to vital organs (i.e., the brain and heart). Hypothermia occurs rapidly in infants and children, partly because of their large surface area relative to size and partly as a result of the cold water itself. Profound hypothermia is usually evidence of lengthy submersion. Prolonged submersion in cold liquids can impair cognition, coordination, and muscle strength that ultimately results in loss of consciousness, decreased cardiac output, and cardiac arrest (Thomas & Caglar, 2020). Submersion in cold water had previously been thought to be somewhat neuroprotective, but it is not (Quan, Mack, & Schiff, 2014).

Submerged children struggle initially to stay above water, and often breath-holding leads to air hunger. Reflex inspiration eventually occurs, which leads to aspiration (Thomas & Caglar, 2020). Fluid is quickly absorbed in the pulmonary circulation, resulting in pulmonary edema, atelectasis, and airway spasm. Hypoxia is the primary problem because it results in global cell damage, with different cells tolerating variable lengths of anoxia. Neurons, especially cerebral cells, sustain irreversible damage after 4 to 6 minutes of submersion. The heart and lungs can survive up to 30 minutes. Regardless of the amount of water aspirated, the victim suffers arterial hypoxemia (resulting from atelectasis and shunting of blood through the nonventilated alveoli), combined respiratory acidosis (resulting from retained carbon dioxide), and metabolic acidosis (caused by buildup of acid metabolites because of anaerobic metabolism). Although electrolyte imbalances are contributing factors, they are not the major causes of morbidity and mortality. The pathologic events are directly related to the duration of submersion. Approximately 10% of submersion injury victims die without aspirating fluid but succumb from acute asphyxia as a result of prolonged reflex laryngospasm.

! NURSING ALERT

All children who have a submersion injury should be admitted to the hospital for observation. Although many patients do not appear to have suffered adverse effects from the event, complications (e.g., respiratory compromise, cerebral edema) may occur 24 hours after the incident.

Aspiration of fluid occurs in most submersion injuries. The aspirated fluid results in pulmonary edema, atelectasis, airway spasm, and pneumonitis, which aggravates hypoxia. Submersion in salt water is associated with better outcomes than submersion in fresh water, although duration of the submersion is the main factor that predicts outcome (Quan, Bierens, Lis, et al., 2016).

Clinical Manifestations

Clinical manifestations are directly related to the duration of loss of consciousness and neurologic status after rescue and resuscitation.

Therapeutic Management

With rapid treatment, some children can be saved. Resuscitative measures should begin at the scene, and the victim should be transported to the hospital with maximum ventilatory and circulatory support. In the hospital, intensive pulmonary care is implemented and continued according to the patient's needs.

In general, management of the victim with a submersion injury is based on the degree of cerebral insult. The first priority is to restore oxygen delivery to the cells and prevent further hypoxic damage. A spontaneously breathing child does well in an oxygen-enriched atmosphere; the more severely affected child requires endotracheal intubation and mechanical ventilation. Blood gases and pH are monitored at frequent intervals as a guide to oxygen, fluid, and electrolyte therapies. Rewarming the hypothermic patient is initiated. Seizures may occur due to hypoxia and cerebral edema. Seizures result in increased cerebral oxygen consumption. Therefore it is imperative to aggressively control seizure activity. In addition, blood glucose should be monitored; both hypoglycemia and hyperglycemia are harmful to the brain.

All children who have a submersion injury should be hospitalized for observation. Although some children do not appear to have sustained adverse effects from the event, respiratory compromise or cerebral edema may occur within 24 hours after the incident. In the acute recovery period, fever should be prevented, although prophylactic antibiotics are not recommended. Aspiration pneumonia is a common complication that occurs approximately 48 to 72 hours after the episode. Bronchospasm, alveolar-capillary membrane damage, atelectasis, abscess formation, and acute respiratory distress syndrome are other complications that occur after aspiration of fluid.

Prognosis

Children who have submersion injuries usually have a good outcome with no or mild neurologic sequelae, no severe neurologic disabilities, and rarely morbidity (Thomas & Caglar, 2020). The best predictors of a good outcome are length of submersion less than 5 minutes and the presence of sinus rhythm, reactive pupils, and neurologic responsiveness at the scene. The worst outcomes are for children submerged for more than 10 minutes and unresponsive to advanced life support within 25 minutes. All children without spontaneous, purposeful movement and normal brainstem function 24 hours after sustaining a submersion injury suffered severe neurologic deficits or death (Thomas & Caglar, 2020).

Nursing Care Management

Nursing care depends on the child's condition. A child who survives may need intensive respiratory nursing care with attention to vital signs, mechanical ventilation or tracheostomy, blood gas determination, chest physiotherapy, and IV infusion. Often the child has sustained a hypoxic insult and requires the same care as an unconscious child.

A difficult aspect in the care of the child who sustained a submersion injury is helping the parents cope with the grief, guilt, and anger reactions. Given the magnitude of the event, parents need repeated assurance that everything possible is being done to treat their child.

Nurses often have difficulty relating to the parents if obvious neglect has precipitated the accident and subsequent problems; it is important for those who care for these children and their families to assess their own feelings about the situation, in addition to assessing the family's coping abilities and resources. Caring for victims of a submersion injury and their families requires the nurse to be sensitive to the needs of the child and the family and to recognize his or her own reactions and emotions.

Prevention

Most submersion injuries are preventable. The most common cause of submersion injury in infants and young children is inadequate adult supervision, including a momentary lapse of supervision. Parents are often unaware that they must be within arm's reach and constantly supervising without being distracted (Thomas & Caglar, 2020). Children with known risk factors such as epilepsy and autism require eyes-on surveillance. In general, children are not developmentally ready for formal swimming lessons until their fourth birthday. All parents and swimming pool owners should be familiar with basic cardiopulmonary resuscitation (CPR) because rapid, basic CPR is one of the keys to improving outcomes (Tobin, Ramos, Pu, et al., 2017). Water safety and survival training should be required for all school-age children. Pool covers and fencing on all sides and the presence of lifeguards can prevent accidents.

Nurses can be active advocates in their communities. Nurses are also in a position to emphasize the importance of adequate adult supervision when children are around any body of water and should include the necessity of the adult not engaging in distracting activities.

INTRACRANIAL INFECTIONS

The nervous system is subject to infection by the same organisms that affect other organs of the body. However, the nervous system is limited in the ways in which it responds to injury. Laboratory studies are needed to identify the causative agent. The inflammatory process can affect the meninges (meningitis) or brain (encephalitis).

Meningitis can be caused by a variety of organisms, but the three main types are (1) bacterial, or pyogenic, caused by pus-forming bacteria, especially meningococci and pneumococci organisms; (2) viral, or aseptic, caused by a wide variety of viral agents; and (3) tuberculous, caused by the tuberculin bacillus. The majority of children with acute febrile encephalopathy have either bacterial meningitis or viral meningitis as the underlying cause.

BACTERIAL MENINGITIS

Bacterial meningitis is an acute inflammation of the meninges and CSF. The advent of antimicrobial therapy has had a marked effect on the course and prognosis. The introduction of conjugate vaccines against *Haemophilus influenzae* type b (Hib vaccine) in 1990 and *Streptococcus pneumoniae* (pneumococcus) in 2000 has led to dramatic changes in the epidemiology of bacterial meningitis (see Translating Evidence Into Practice box). Today, Hib infection has been virtually eradicated among young children in areas where the Hib vaccine is administered routinely. By 2013 there were fewer than 40 cases of Hib disease in children younger than 5 years old (Centers for Disease Control and Prevention, 2016). Before the vaccine, Hib was responsible for almost half of all cases of bacterial meningitis, but now it is the least likely pathogen to cause meningitis (Castelblanco, Lee, & Hasbun, 2014). Since the introduction of widespread vaccination for *S. pneumoniae,* the incidence of pneumococcal meningitis in children in the United States has decreased, but it remains the most common cause of meningitis in children ages 3 months to 11 years (Castelblancoet al., 2014). It is also the most likely to result in death (Heckenberg, Brouwer, & Van de Beek, 2014).

Etiology

A variety of bacterial agents can cause bacterial meningitis. Since the introduction of vaccinations against most common causes of community-acquired pathogens, the incidence of bacterial meningitis has declined precipitously. The leading causes of neonatal meningitis are group B streptococcus (GBS) and *Escherichia coli* (Ku, Boggess, & Cohen-Wolkowiez, 2015).

Meningococcal meningitis is the only type readily transmitted by droplet infection from nasopharyngeal secretions and so has the potential to occur in outbreaks (Vetter, Baxter, Denizer, et al., 2016). Before the development of a vaccine it occurred predominantly in school-age children and adolescents; now it is most common in children under 12 months old, with a secondary peak in incidence in 16- to 23-year-olds (Centers for Disease Control and Prevention, 2017b). Meningitis caused by pneumococcal and meningococcal infections can occur at any time but is more common in late winter and early spring.

Maternal factors, such as premature rupture of fetal membranes and maternal infection during the last week of pregnancy, are major causes of neonatal meningitis. It is a devastating disease with significant morbidity and mortality. Vaccination of pregnant women is being explored as a way to protect infants from meningitis (Jones, Munoz, Spiegel, et al., 2016). Children who survive neonatal meningitis are 10 times more likely to have moderate to severe disabilities than those who have not had meningitis (Ku et al., 2015). The incidence of early-onset GBS meningitis has been reduced by more than 70% with the adoption of antenatal screening and administration of intrapartum prophylactic antibiotics (Ku et al., 2015).

TRANSLATING EVIDENCE INTO PRACTICE

Children With Bacterial Meningitis and Preventive Vaccines

Ask the Question

In children and adolescents with bacterial meningitis, has the administration of *Haemophilus influenzae* type b (Hib), pneumococcal, and meningococcal preventive vaccines reduced the incidence and mortality rates associated with bacterial meningitis?

Search for the Evidence

Search Strategies

Search selection criteria included English-language publications within the past 10 years, research-based articles, children and adult populations.

Databases Used

PubMed and Cochrane Collaboration.

Critically Analyze the Evidence

GRADE criteria: Evidence quality high; recommendation strong (Balshem, Hefland, Schunemann, et al., 2011). A review of the literature revealed two literature reviews, one Cochrane review, and one population-based observational study.

- Watt and colleagues (2009) performed a literature review with studies evaluating Hib disease incidence, fatality ratios, and the effect of the Hib vaccine. In 2000 there were 173,000 cases of Hib meningitis and 78,300 deaths among children under the age of 5 years worldwide. Expanded use of the Hib vaccine can reduce the incidence and mortality rates of Hib-related disease.
- A Cochrane review determined the effect, duration of protection, and age-specific effects of polysaccharide serogroup A vaccine (SgAV) to prevent meningococcal meningitis in children. The vaccine had a 95% protective effect during the first year in children older than 5 years of age, but its efficacy after the first year could not be determined. Children ages 1 to 5 years in low-income countries also experienced protective effects from the SgAV, but the exact efficacy could not be determined (Patel & Lee, 2010).
- A literature review assessed the impact of the 7-valent pneumococcal conjugate vaccination on morbidity and mortality rates from invasive pneumococcal diseases. The six studies from North America consistently reported a decline in invasive pneumococcal disease mortality rate after the introduction of the pneumococcal vaccine, with reductions ranging from 57% to 62% among children and 37% to 76% among all age-groups (Myint, Madhava, Balmer, et al., 2013).
- A population-based observational study evaluated the incidence of bacterial meningitis from 1997 to 2010, after conjugate vaccination introduction. The incidence of *Streptococcus pneumoniae* decreased from 0.8 to 0.3 per 100,000 people; the incidence of *Neisseria* meningitis decreased from 0.721 to 0.123 per 100,000 people; and the mortality rate from pneumococcal meningitis decreased from 0.073 to 0.024 per 100,000 people (Castelblanco, Lee, & Hasbun, 2014).

Apply the Evidence: Nursing Implications

The evidence strongly suggests that all children should be immunized against the most common organisms responsible for bacterial meningitis (i.e., Hib, *S. pneumoniae,* and *Neisseria meningitidis*) as prevention to decrease the incidence of bacterial meningitis. Nurses should stress to the parents, children, adolescents, and young adults the importance of adhering to the immunization schedule to protect against serious childhood diseases.

References

Balshem, H., Hefland, M., Schunemann, H. J., et al. (2011). GRADE guidelines: Rating the quality of evidence. *Journal of Clinical Epidemiology, 64,* 401–406.

Castelblanco, R. L., Lee, M., & Hasbun, R. (2014). Epidemiology of bacterial meningitis in the USA from 1997 to 2010: A population-based observational study. *The Lancet Infectious Diseases, 14*(9), 813–819.

Myint, T., Madhava, H., Balmer, P., et al. (2013). The impact of 7-valent pneumococcal conjugate vaccine on invasive pneumococcal disease: A literature review. *Advances in Therapy, 30*(2), 127–151.

Patel, M., & Lee, C. K. (2010). Polysaccharide vaccines for preventing serogroup A meningococcal meningitis. *Cochrane Database of Systematic Reviews* (1), CD001093.

Watt, J. P., Wolfson, L. J., O'Brien, K. L., et al. (2009). Burden of disease caused by *Haemophilus influenzae* type b in children younger than 5 years. *Lancet, 374,* 903–911.

Risk factors for children developing meningitis include lack of immunization to the specific pathogen; recent exposure to someone with invasive *Neisseria meningitidis* or Hib disease; penetrating head trauma; cochlear implant devices; and anatomic defects such as midline facial defects, inner ear fistulas, or recent placement of a ventricular shunt (Swanson, 2015).

Pathophysiology

The most common route of infection is vascular dissemination from a focus of infection elsewhere. For example, organisms from the nasopharynx invade the underlying blood vessels, cross the blood-brain barrier, and multiply in the CSF. Invasion by direct extension from infections in the paranasal and mastoid sinuses is less common. Organisms also gain entry by direct implantation after penetrating wounds, skull fractures that provide an opening into the skin or sinuses, lumbar puncture or surgical procedures, anatomic abnormalities such as spina bifida, or foreign bodies such as an internal ventricular shunt or an external ventricular device. Once implanted, the organisms spread into the CSF, by which the infection spreads throughout the subarachnoid space.

The infective process is like that seen in any bacterial infection: inflammation, exudation, white blood cell accumulation, and varying degrees of tissue damage. The brain becomes hyperemic and edematous, and the entire surface of the brain is covered by a layer of purulent exudate that varies with the type of organism. For example, meningococcal exudate is most marked over the parietal, occipital, and cerebellar regions; the thick, fibrinous exudate of pneumococcal infection is confined chiefly to the surface of the brain, particularly the anterior lobes; and the exudate of streptococcal infections is similar to that of pneumococcal infections but thinner. As infection extends to the ventricles, thick pus, fibrin, or adhesions may occlude the narrow passages and obstruct the flow of CSF.

Clinical Manifestations

The clinical manifestations of acute bacterial meningitis depend to a large extent on the child's age. The type of organism, the effectiveness of therapy for antecedent illness, and whether it occurs as an isolated entity or as a complication of another illness or injury also influence the clinical manifestation (Box 27.4).

Children and Adolescents

The onset of illness may be abrupt and rapid, or develop progressively over one or several days, and may be preceded by a febrile illness. Most children with meningitis are seen with fever, chills, headache, and vomiting that are associated with or quickly followed by alterations in sensorium; however, some may present only with lethargy and irritability (Weinberg & Thompson-Stone, 2018). The child is extremely irritable and agitated and may develop seizures, photophobia, confusion, hallucinations, aggressive behavior, drowsiness, stupor, or coma.

BOX 27.4 Clinical Manifestations of Bacterial Meningitis

Children and Adolescents
Usually abrupt onset
Fever
Chills
Headache
Vomiting
Alterations in sensorium
Seizures (often the initial sign)
Irritability
Agitation
May develop the following:
- Photophobia
- Delirium
- Hallucinations
- Aggressive behavior
- Drowsiness
- Stupor
- Coma

Nuchal rigidity; may progress to opisthotonos
Positive Kernig and Brudzinski signs
Hyperactivity but variable reflex responses
Signs and symptoms peculiar to individual organisms:
- Petechial or purpuric rashes (meningococcal infection), especially when associated with a shock-like state
- Joint involvement (meningococcal or *Haemophilus influenzae* infection)
- Chronically draining ear (pneumococcal meningitis)

Infants and Young Children
Classic picture (above) rarely seen in children between 3 months and 2 years of age
Fever
Poor feeding
Vomiting
Marked irritability
Frequent seizures (often accompanied by a high-pitched cry)
Bulging fontanel
Nuchal rigidity possible
Brudzinski and Kernig signs not helpful in diagnosis
Difficult to elicit and evaluate in this age-group
Subdural empyema (*H. influenzae* infection)

Neonates
Specific Signs
Child well at birth but within a few days begins to look and behave poorly
Refuses feedings
Poor sucking ability
Vomiting or diarrhea
Poor tone
Lack of movement
Weak cry
Full, tense, and bulging fontanel may appear late in course of illness
Neck usually supple

Nonspecific Signs That May Be Present
Hypothermia or fever (depending on the infant's maturity)
Jaundice
Irritability
Drowsiness
Seizures
Respiratory irregularities or apnea
Cyanosis
Weight loss

The child resists flexion of the neck (nuchal rigidity). Kernig and Brudzinski signs are positive. Reflex responses are variable, although they show hyperactivity (see Chapter 4, Reflexes). The skin may be cold and cyanotic with poor peripheral perfusion.

Other signs and symptoms that are specific to individual organisms may appear. Petechial or purpuric rashes occur in 50% of cases and indicate a meningococcal infection (meningococcemia), especially when the eruption is associated with a septic shock–like state. Joint involvement is seen in meningococcal and *H. influenzae* infection. A chronically draining ear commonly accompanies pneumococcal meningitis. *E. coli* infection may be associated with a congenital dermal sinus that communicates with the subarachnoid space.

Infants and Young Children

Between 3 months and 2 years of age, the illness is characterized by fever or hypothermia, poor feeding, vomiting, marked irritability, restlessness, seizures, and a bulging or tense fontanel, which are often accompanied by a high-pitched cry.

Neonates

Meningitis in newborn and premature infants is extremely difficult to diagnose. The vague and nonspecific manifestations, which are characteristic of all neonatal sepsis, bear little resemblance to the findings in older children. These infants are usually well at birth but within a few days begin to appear ill. They refuse feedings, have poor sucking ability, and may vomit or have diarrhea. They display poor muscle tone and lack of movement and have a poor cry. Other nonspecific signs that may be present include hypothermia or fever (depending on the infant's maturity), jaundice, irritability, drowsiness, seizures, respiratory irregularities or apnea, cyanosis, and weight loss. The full, tense, and bulging fontanel may or may not be present until late in the course of the illness, and the neck is usually supple. Untreated, the infant's condition will decline to cardiovascular collapse, seizures, and apnea. Even with improved antibiotics and more rapid diagnosis, the prognosis of neonatal meningitis has not improved in decades, likely due to the virulence of the infectious pathogen (Gordon, Srinivasan, & Harris, 2017).

Complications

The incidence of complications from acute bacterial meningitis has been significantly reduced with early diagnosis and vigorous antimicrobial therapy. If infection extends to the ventricles, thick pus, fibrin, or adhesions may occlude the narrow passages, thereby obstructing the flow of CSF and causing obstructive hydrocephalus. Subdural effusions often occur, and thrombosis may occur in meningeal veins or venous sinuses. Destructive changes may take place in the cerebral cortex, and brain abscesses may form by direct extension of the infection or by vascular dissemination. Extension of the infection to the areas of the cranial nerves or compression necrosis from increased pressure may cause deafness, blindness, or weakness or paralysis of facial or other muscles of the head and neck.

One of the most dramatic and serious complications usually associated with meningococcal infections is meningococcal sepsis, or meningococcemia. When the onset is severe, sudden, and rapid, it is known as the Waterhouse-Friderichsen syndrome. The syndrome is characterized by overwhelming septic shock, disseminated intravascular coagulation, massive bilateral adrenal hemorrhage, and purpura. Meningococcemia requires immediate emergency treatment, hospitalization, and intensive care because of the serious sequelae that can quickly develop (Weinberg & Thompson-Stone, 2018).

! NURSING ALERT

Any child who is ill and develops a petechial or purpural rash may have meningococcemia and must receive immediate medical attention.

Other acute complications of meningitis include SIADH (see Chapter 28), subdural effusions, seizures, cerebral edema and herniation, and hydrocephalus. Obstruction to the flow of CSF occurs during the acute phase of illness by clumping of purulent material in the drainage channels and during the chronic phase of illness by adhesive arachnoiditis or fibrotic obstruction through any of the ventricular foramina. Postmeningitic complications in neonates include ventriculitis, which results in cystic, walled-off areas of the brain with fluid accumulation and pressure.

Extension of the inflammation to cranial nerves or compression and destruction of the nerves from ICP can produce permanent impairment of vision or hearing and other nerve palsies. CN VIII damage is usually followed by permanent deafness, the most common permanent neurologic sequela of bacterial meningitis (Weinberg & Thompson-Stone, 2018). Other long-term complications include cerebral palsy, cognitive impairments, learning disorders, attention-deficit/hyperactivity disorder, and seizures.

Hemiparesis and quadriparesis may result from damage caused by arteritis or thrombosis or other mechanisms. Behavioral changes occur in some children. Evidence indicates that psychometric and behavioral defects may be a significant concomitant sign of meningitis in childhood, although it is difficult to determine the degree to which meningitis affects the intelligence of young children. Meningitis in the neonatal period is more likely to cause lifelong impairments, including moderate to severe developmental delay, blindness, deafness, and epilepsy (Swanson, 2015).

Diagnostic Evaluation

A lumbar puncture is the definitive diagnostic test. The fluid pressure is measured, and samples are obtained for culture, Gram stain, blood cell count, and determination of glucose and protein levels. The findings are usually diagnostic. Culture and sensitivity are needed to identify the causative organism. Spinal fluid pressure is usually elevated, but interpretation is often difficult when the child is crying. Sedation with fentanyl and midazolam can alleviate the child's pain and fear associated with this procedure (see Atraumatic Care box). If there is evidence or suspicion of increased ICP, a CT scan of the head may be warranted before the procedure (Weinberg & Thompson-Stone, 2018).

ATRAUMATIC CARE

Lumbar Puncture

If time permits, LMX (4% lidocaine) or EMLA cream (a eutectic mixture of lidocaine and prilocaine), both topical anesthetics, should be applied to the skin overlying L3 to L5 to reduce pain before lumbar puncture. For maximum effect, apply EMLA cream at least 1 hour or LMX 30 minutes before the procedure.

The patient generally has an elevated white blood cell count, often predominantly polymorphonuclear leukocytes. The glucose level is reduced, generally in proportion to the duration and severity of the infection. The relationship between the CSF glucose and serum glucose levels is important in evaluating the glucose content of CSF; therefore a serum glucose sample is drawn approximately a half-hour before the lumbar puncture. Protein concentration is usually increased.

Blood culture is advisable for all children suspected of having meningitis if antibiotics are started before obtaining CSF. Blood culture will occasionally be positive when CSF culture is negative. Nose and throat cultures may provide helpful information in some cases.

Therapeutic Management

Acute bacterial meningitis is a medical emergency that requires early recognition and immediate therapy to prevent death and avoid residual disabilities. The initial therapeutic management includes the following:

- Isolation precautions
- Initiation of antimicrobial therapy
- Maintenance of hydration
- Maintenance of ventilation
- Reduction of increased ICP
- Management of systemic shock
- Control of seizures
- Control of temperature
- Treatment of complications

The child is usually moved to an intensive care unit for close observation. An IV infusion is started to facilitate administration of antimicrobial agents, fluids, antiepileptic drugs, and blood, if needed. The child is placed in respiratory isolation.

Drugs

Until the causative organism is identified, empiric therapy is administered. After identification of the organism, antimicrobial agents are adjusted accordingly. Signs of gastrointestinal hemorrhage or secondary infection may complicate steroid administration. Antibiotic treatment with cephalosporins demonstrates superiority for promptly sterilizing the CSF and reducing the incidence of severe hearing impairment. With increasing prevalence of antibiotic-resistant *S. pneumoniae,* vancomycin should be given until antibiotic susceptibility test results are available.

Nonspecific Measures

Maintaining hydration is a prime concern. The patient's condition determines whether IV fluids are needed and the type and amount of fluid. The optimum hydration involves correction of any fluid deficits and electrolyte abnormalities, followed by fluid restriction until normal serum sodium levels and no signs of increased ICP are present. If needed, measures to decrease ICP are implemented (see earlier in the chapter); however, long-term fluid restriction is not the standard of care because a lack of fluid volume can reduce blood pressure and CPP, causing CNS ischemia (Janowski & Hunstad, 2020c).

Complications, such as subdural effusion in infants and disseminated intravascular coagulation syndrome, are treated appropriately. Shock is managed by restoration of circulating blood volume and maintenance of electrolyte balance. Seizures can occur during the first few days of treatment. These are controlled with the appropriate antiepileptic drug.

Hearing loss is common. The patient should undergo auditory evaluation shortly after discharge so that audiology and speech and communication therapies can begin as soon as possible.

Lumbar puncture is carried out as needed to determine the effectiveness of therapy. The patient is evaluated neurologically during the convalescent period.

Prognosis

Less than 10% of cases of bacterial meningitis are fatal; the highest mortality rate is seen in pneumococcal meningitis and in infants under the age of 6 months (Janowski & Hunstad, 2020c). Prognosis is dependent in large part on the length of time between onset of illness and initiation of antibiotic therapy, rapidity of diagnosis after onset, type of organism, prolonged or complicated seizures, low CSF glucose concentration, and adequacy of therapy. Up to half of those who recover from meningitis will have some neurodevelopmental sequelae ranging from mild behavioral and learning problems to profound hearing impairment, intractable epilepsy, and significant intellectual disability (Janowski & Hunstad, 2020c).

DRUG ALERT

Antibiotic Use in Meningitis

A major priority of nursing care of a child suspected of having meningitis is to administer antibiotics as soon as they are ordered. The child is placed on respiratory isolation for at least 24 hours after initiation of antimicrobial therapy.

The sequelae of bacterial meningitis occur most often when the disease occurs in the first 2 months of life and least often in children with meningococcal meningitis. The residual deficits in infants are primarily a result of communicating hydrocephalus and the greater effects of cerebritis on the immature brain. In older children the residual effects are related to the inflammatory process itself or result from vasculitis associated with the disease. Bacterial meningitis continues to cause substantial morbidity in infants and children.

Prevention

Vaccination is the foundation of prevention of CNS infections. Vaccines are available for pneumococci; types A, C, Y, and W-135 meningococci; and Hib. Routine meningococcal conjugate vaccination of children is recommended at age 11 to 12 years, with a booster at 16 years, but can be given to children 2 months to 10 years of age if they are considered at high risk (e.g., asplenia, foreign travel to high-risk areas, or present during outbreaks). Routine vaccinations for Hib and pneumococcal conjugate vaccines are recommended for all children beginning at 2 months of age (see Chapter 6, Immunizations).

Nursing Care Management

Nurses should take the necessary precautions to protect themselves and others from possible infection. Teach parents proper hand washing technique and remind them as needed.

Keep the room as quiet as possible and environmental stimuli at a minimum, as most children with meningitis are sensitive to noise, bright lights, and other external stimuli. Help the family limit the number and frequency of visitors until the child is and feels better. Most children are more comfortable without a pillow under their head but with the head of the bed slightly elevated. Use pillows alongside a child in a side-lying position and between the child's knees for comfort in cases of nuchal rigidity. Avoid actions that cause pain or increase discomfort, such as lifting the child's head. Evaluating the child for pain and implementing appropriate relief measures are important ongoing interventions. Measures are used to ensure safety because the child is often restless, disoriented, and subject to seizures. Prevention of falls is essential.

The nursing care of the child with meningitis is determined by the child's symptoms and treatment (see Box 27.4). Observation of vital signs, neurologic signs, LOC, urinary output, and other pertinent data is carried out at frequent intervals. The child who is unconscious is managed as described previously, and all children are observed carefully for signs of the complications just described, especially increased ICP, shock, and respiratory distress. Frequent assessment of the open fontanels is needed in the infant because subdural effusions and obstructive hydrocephalus can develop as a complication of meningitis.

Administration of fluids and nourishment is determined by the child's status. The child who is not alert and oriented is given nothing by mouth. Other children are allowed clear liquids initially and, if tolerated, progress to a diet suitable for their age. Careful monitoring and recording of intake and output are needed to determine deviations that might indicate impending shock or increasing fluid accumulation, such as cerebral edema or subdural effusion.

One of the most challenging issues in the nursing care of children with meningitis is maintaining IV infusion for the length of time needed to provide adequate antimicrobial therapy (usually 10 days). Because continuous IV fluids are usually not necessary, an intermittent infusion device is used. In some cases children who are recovering uneventfully are sent home with the device, and the parents are taught IV drug administration (see Quality Patient Outcomes box).

QUALITY PATIENT OUTCOMES: Bacterial Meningitis

- Early recognition of signs and symptoms of meningitis
- Antibiotics administered as soon as diagnosis is established
- Cerebral edema prevented
- Exposure prevented by early isolation
- Side effects managed
- Neurologic sequelae prevented

Family Support

The sudden nature of the illness makes emotional support of the child and parents extremely important (see Family-Centered Care box). Parents are upset and concerned about their child's condition and often feel guilty for not having suspected the seriousness of the illness sooner. They need reassurance that the natural onset of meningitis is sudden and that they acted responsibly in seeking medical assistance when they did. The nurse encourages the parents to openly discuss their feelings to minimize blame and guilt. Some parents will benefit from referral to a hospital chaplain, social worker, psychologist, or psychiatrist. The nurse keeps parents informed of the child's progress and of all procedures, results, and treatments. In the event that the child's condition worsens, the parents need the same psychologic care as other parents facing the possible death of their child (see Chapter 17).

FAMILY-CENTERED CARE

Preventing Bacterial Meningitis

With immunization schedules calling for administration of *Haemophilus influenzae* type b vaccine and pneumococcal conjugate vaccine to infants at 2 months of age, encourage parents to bring their child to a health facility so that the full series of inoculations is completed. Given the 10% mortality rate associated with bacterial meningitis, early immunization can help families avoid the tragic death or permanent disability of a child. Nurses play a significant role in educating families on preventive measures, such as having children immunized on schedule.

NONBACTERIAL (ASEPTIC) MENINGITIS

The term *aseptic meningitis* refers to the onset of meningeal symptoms, fever, and pleocytosis without bacterial growth from CSF cultures. Aseptic meningitis is caused by many different viruses, including arbovirus, enterovirus, herpes simplex virus, cytomegalovirus, and human immunodeficiency virus. Enterovirus is the most common cause of aseptic meningitis (Janowski & Hunstad, 2020b).The onset may be abrupt or gradual, and many of the presenting signs and symptoms are the same as for bacterial meningitis, including headache, fever, photophobia, and nuchal rigidity.

Diagnosis is based on clinical features and CSF findings. Table 27.2 lists variations in CSF values in bacterial and viral meningitis. It is important to differentiate this usually self-limiting disorder from the more serious forms of meningitis.

Treatment is primarily symptomatic, such as acetaminophen for headache and muscle pain, maintenance of hydration, and positioning for comfort. Until a definitive diagnosis is made, antimicrobial agents may be administered and isolation enforced as a precaution against the possibility that the disease might be of bacterial origin. Nursing care is similar to the care of the child with bacterial meningitis. The course of aseptic meningitis is usually much shorter and typically without significant complications.

TUBERCULOUS MENINGITIS

Tuberculous meningitis must be considered in children who have traveled to or lived in developing countries or who live with or are immigrants from developing countries. In 2015 the incidence of tuberculous meningitis in the United States increased for the first time in more than 2 decades (Smith, Pratt, Trieu, et al., 2017). Tuberculous meningitis is more likely to be disseminated (including CNS involvement) in very young or immunosuppressed children.

Ischemic infarction can occur with tuberculous meningitis. The most common clinical findings are meningeal signs, fever, altered consciousness, CN involvement, seizures, and focal neurologic deficit.

Early diagnosis of tuberculous meningitis in the child can significantly reduce the disability caused by hydrocephalus, a common complication of this type of meningitis. Nursing care is similar to the care of the child with bacterial meningitis and involves administration of medications, support of the child, control of pain, and neurologic monitoring.

BRAIN ABSCESS

Intracerebral abscesses form when pyogenic organisms gain access to neural tissue by way of the bloodstream from foci of infection or from direct inoculation of organisms from infections, penetrating trauma, or surgical procedures. Chronic ear infection, mastoiditis, sinusitis, and congenital heart disease are the most common predisposing factors for children with brain abscesses. The majority (70%) of brain abscesses are caused by aerobic and anaerobic streptococci (Janowski & Hunstad, 2020a). In neonates, *Citrobacter* is most common, and fungi are more common in immunocompromised children (Janowski & Hunstad, 2020a).

The most common sites of intracerebral abscesses are the parietal, temporal, and frontal lobes. Early signs of the disease are vague; however, the most common symptom is a severe headache. As the inflammatory process proceeds, symptoms intensify and include vomiting, lethargy, fever, seizures, papilledema, focal neurologic signs (hemiparesis), and progression to coma (Janowski & Hunstad, 2020a). Because mortality rates from brain abscesses may exceed 20%, prompt diagnosis and treatment are critical (Janowski & Hunstad, 2020a). Successful management consists of surgical drainage and antibiotic therapy. Surgical drainage is necessary if the mass is greater than 2 cm in diameter or there are signs of increased ICP. Where possible, the source of the infection is eradicated. Children may experience epilepsy, hemiparesis, cranial nerve abnormalities, and behavior or learning problems as long-term complications (Janowski & Hunstad, 2020a).

ENCEPHALITIS

Encephalitis is an inflammatory process of the CNS that is caused by a variety of organisms, including bacteria, spirochetes, fungi, protozoa, helminths, and viruses. Most infections are associated with viruses, and this discussion is limited to those agents.

Etiology

Encephalitis can occur as a result of direct invasion of the CNS by a virus or postinfectious involvement of the CNS after a viral disease. Enteroviruses are the most common etiology (Janowski & Hunstad, 2020b); however, the specific type of encephalitis often may not be identified. The cause of more than half of the cases reported in the United States is unknown.

Autoimmune encephalitis syndromes are a recently recognized cause of new-onset neurologic deficits in children (Longoni, Levy, & Yeh, 2016). In some children, antibodies are identified, and there is a small group (<20%) whose etiology is a tumor, particularly ovarian teratoma, but the majority of children will not have either of these conditions (Dubey, Sawhney, Greenberg, et al., 2015). Diagnosis is usually based on clinical symptoms, which can be neurologic, psychiatric, or both (Scheer & John, 2016). Neurologic symptoms include seizures, encephalopathy, and movement disorders (Dale, Gorman, & Lim, 2017). Behavioral changes, hallucinations, anxiety, and aggression are some of the more commonly seen psychiatric manifestations (Scheer & John, 2016).

TABLE 27.2 Variation of Cerebrospinal Fluid Analysis in Bacterial and Viral Meningitis

Manifestations	Bacterial[a]	Viral
White blood cell count	Elevated; increased neutrophils	Slightly elevated; increased lymphocytes
Protein content	Elevated	Normal or slightly increased
Glucose content	Decreased	Normal
Gram stain; bacteria culture	Positive	Negative
Color	Turbid or cloudy	Clear or slightly cloudy
Opening pressure	Elevated	Normal

[a]Results may vary in the neonate.

Herpes simplex encephalitis is an uncommon disease, but 30% of cases involve children. The initial clinical findings are nonspecific (e.g., fever, altered mental status), but most cases evolve to demonstrate focal neurologic signs and symptoms. Children may experience focal seizures. The CSF is abnormal in most cases. Because of a rise in the number of children with herpes simplex encephalitis, suspected cases require prompt attention, especially because the diagnosis can be difficult. CSF polymerase chain reaction (PCR) testing can confirm the clinical diagnosis rapidly. The early use of IV acyclovir reduces mortality and morbidity rates. Empiric therapy with acyclovir is given before precise virologic diagnosis has been established.

The multiple causes of viral encephalitis make diagnosis difficult. Most are those involved with arthropod vectors (e.g., togaviruses, bunyaviruses) and those associated with hemorrhagic fevers (e.g., arenaviruses, filoviruses, hantaviruses). In the United States, the vector reservoir for most agents pathogenic for humans is the mosquito (St. Louis or West Nile encephalitis); therefore most cases of encephalitis appear during the hot summer months and subside during the autumn.

Clinical Manifestations

The clinical features of encephalitis are similar regardless of the agent involved. Manifestations can range from a mild benign form that resembles aseptic meningitis, lasts a few days, and is followed by rapid and complete recovery, to a rapidly progressing encephalitis with severe CNS involvement. The onset may be sudden or may be gradual with malaise, fever, headache, dizziness, apathy, nuchal rigidity, nausea and vomiting, ataxia, tremors, hyperactivity, and speech difficulties (Box 27.5). In severe cases the patient has high fever, stupor, seizures, disorientation, spasticity, and coma that may proceed to death. Ocular palsies and paralysis also may occur.

Diagnostic Evaluation

The diagnosis is made based on clinical findings and, where possible, identification of the specific virus. Early in the course of encephalitis, CT scan results may be normal. Later, hemorrhagic areas in the frontotemporal region may be seen. Arboviruses are rarely detected in the blood or spinal fluid, but viruses of herpes, mumps, measles, and enteroviruses may be found in the CSF. Serologic testing may be required. The first blood sample should be drawn as soon as possible after onset, with the second sample drawn 2 or 3 weeks later.

Therapeutic Management

Patients suspected of having encephalitis are hospitalized promptly for observation, including ICP monitoring. In autoimmune encephalitis rapid initiation of immunotherapy, including corticosteroids, plasmapheresis, and IV immunoglobulin, improves outcomes. Herpes simplex virus encephalitis is the only viral encephalitis that has specific treatment available. In other cases, treatment is primarily supportive and includes conscientious nursing care, control of cerebral manifestations, and adequate nutrition and hydration, with observations and management as for other cerebral disorders.

Prognosis

Viral encephalitis can cause devastating neurologic injury. The prognosis for the child with encephalitis depends on the child's age, the type of encephalitis, and residual neurologic damage. Very young children (younger than 2 years of age) with viral encephalitis have an increased risk of neurologic disability, including learning difficulties and epilepsy. About 80% of patients with autoimmune encephalitis make a full or nearly full recovery (Longoni et al., 2016).

Follow-up care with periodic reevaluation and rehabilitation is important for patients who develop residual effects of encephalitis.

BOX 27.5 Clinical Manifestations of Encephalitis

Onset: Sudden or Gradual

Malaise
Fever
Headache
Dizziness
Apathy
Lethargy
Nuchal rigidity
Ataxia
Tremors
Hyperactivity
Speech difficulties: mutism
Altered mental status

Severe Cases

High fever
Stupor
Seizures
Disorientation
Spasticity
Coma (may proceed to death)
Ocular palsies
Paralysis

Nursing Care Management

Nursing care of the child with encephalitis is the same as for any unconscious child and for the child with meningitis. Additional nursing interventions include observation for deterioration in consciousness. Isolation of the child is not necessary; however, always use good hand washing technique. A main focus of nursing management is the control of rapidly rising ICP. Neurologic monitoring, administration of medications, and support of the child and parents are the major aspects of care (see Quality Patient Outcomes box).

QUALITY PATIENT OUTCOMES: Encephalitis

- Early recognition of signs and symptoms
- Cerebral edema prevented
- Side effects managed
- Neurologic sequelae prevented

RABIES

Rabies is an acute infection of the nervous system caused by a virus that is almost invariably fatal if left untreated. It is transmitted to humans by the saliva of an infected mammal introduced through a bite or skin abrasion. After entry into a new host, the virus multiplies in muscle cells and is spread through neural pathways without stimulating a protective host immune response.

Through dog vaccination, rabies from dog bites has been eliminated in the United States (World Health Organization, 2017). Carnivorous wild animals (e.g., raccoons, skunks, bats, foxes) are the animals most often infected with rabies and the cause of most indigenous cases of human rabies in the United States (Singh, Singh, Cherian, et al., 2017).

The circumstances of a biting incident are important. An unprovoked attack is more likely than a provoked attack to indicate a rabid animal. Bites inflicted on a child attempting to feed or handle an apparently healthy animal can generally be regarded as provoked. Any child bitten by a wild animal is assumed to be exposed to rabies.

! NURSING ALERT

Unusual behavior in an animal is cause for suspicion; children should be warned to beware of wild animals that appear to be friendly.

Although rabies is common among wildlife species, human rabies is rarely acquired. The highest incidence of rabies occurs in children under age 15 years. The incubation period usually ranges from 1 to 3 months but may be as short as 5 days or longer than 6 months (Willoughby, 2020). Modern-day prophylaxis is nearly 100% successful. Only 10% to 15% of persons bitten develop the disease, but once symptoms are present, rabies progresses to a fatal outcome. In the United States, human fatalities associated with rabies occur in people who fail to seek medical attention, usually because they are unaware of their exposure.

The disease is characterized by a period of nonspecific flulike symptoms, including general malaise, anorexia, fever, and sore throat, followed by a phase of excitement that features hypersensitivity and increased reaction to external stimuli, seizures, hallucinations, hypersalivation, and choking. Attempts at swallowing may cause spasms of respiratory muscles so severe that they produce apnea, cyanosis, and anoxia—the characteristics from which the term *hydrophobia* was derived.

Diagnosis is made on the basis of history and clinical features. Hydrophobia is a cardinal sign of rabies. The diagnosis is confirmed by skin biopsy. Antibodies maybe detected 7 to 8 days after the onset of clinical symptoms (Crowcroft & Thampi, 2015).

Therapeutic Management

Treatment is of little avail once symptoms appear, but the long incubation period allows time for the induction of active and passive immunity before the onset of illness. Two types of immunizing products are available for use in humans: (1) the inactivated rabies vaccines, which induce an active immune response; and (2) the globulins, which contain preformed antibodies. The two types of products should be used concurrently for rabies postexposure treatment when prophylaxis is indicated.

The current therapy for a rabid animal bite consists of three steps: (1) thorough cleansing of the wound with soap and water (suturing should be avoided whenever possible); (2) administration of rabies vaccine; and (3) administration of rabies immunoglobulin. The rabies vaccine and immunoglobulin should be initiated as soon as possible after exposure. The rabies vaccine consists of four doses administered intramuscularly at days 0, 3, 7, and 14 but can be stopped if the animal remains healthy throughout the 10-day observation period or is proved to be negative for rabies by a reliable laboratory (Crowcroft & Thampi, 2015). Rabies immunoglobulin is administered locally at the wound and provides passive antibodies at the site of exposure. Rabies immunoglobulin is given once within 7 days after the first vaccine dose before the child develops an active immune response (Crowcroft & Thampi, 2015).

Nursing Care Management

Parents and children are frightened by the urgency and seriousness of the situation. They need anticipatory guidance for the therapy and support and reassurance regarding the efficacy of the preventive measures for this dreaded disease. The vaccine is well tolerated by children, although they need preparation for the series of injections. Mass immunization is unnecessary and unlikely to be implemented. In areas in which rabies is rare, the schedule given is sufficient. However, certain circumstances may warrant preexposure vaccination, such as when a child is being taken to an area of the world where rabies in stray dogs is still a problem.

REYE SYNDROME

Reye syndrome (RS) is a disorder defined as a metabolic encephalopathy associated with other characteristic organ involvement. It is characterized by fever, profoundly impaired consciousness, and disordered hepatic function.

The etiology of RS is not well understood, but most cases follow a common viral illness, typically influenza or varicella. RS is a condition characterized pathologically by cerebral edema and fatty changes of the liver. The onset of RS is notable for profuse effortless vomiting and lethargy that quickly progresses to neurologic impairment, including delirium, seizures, and coma, and can ultimately lead to increased ICP, herniation, and death (Ibrahim & Balistreri, 2016). The cause of RS is a mitochondrial insult induced by various viruses, drugs, exogenous toxins, and genetic factors. Elevated serum ammonia levels tend to correlate with the clinical manifestations and prognosis.

Definitive diagnosis is established by liver biopsy. The staging criteria for RS are based on liver dysfunction and on neurologic signs that range from lethargy to coma. As a result of improved diagnostic techniques, children who in the past would have been diagnosed with RS are now diagnosed with other illnesses such as viral or inborn metabolic errors affecting organic acid, ammonia, and carbohydrate metabolism. Cases of unrecognized, drug-induced encephalopathy by antiemetics given to children during viral illnesses have symptoms similar to those of RS.

The potential association between aspirin therapy for the treatment of fever in children with varicella or influenza and the development of RS precludes its use in these patients. However, by the time the Food and Drug Administration required aspirin product labeling in 1986, most of the decline in RS incidence had already occurred.

Nursing Care Management

The most important aspect of successful management of the child with RS is early diagnosis and aggressive therapy. Rapid progression to coma and high peak ammonia concentrations are associated with a more serious prognosis. Cerebral edema with increased ICP represents the most immediate threat to life.

Care and observations are implemented as for any child with an altered state of consciousness (see earlier in the chapter) and increasing ICP. Accurate and frequent monitoring of intake and output is essential for adjusting fluid volumes to prevent both dehydration and cerebral edema. Because of related liver dysfunction, monitor laboratory studies to determine impaired coagulation, such as prolonged bleeding time.

Keep the parents of children with RS informed of the child's progress and explain diagnostic procedures and therapeutic management. Recovery from RS is rapid and usually without sequelae if the diagnosis is determined early and therapy is initiated promptly. Patients who survive have full liver function recovery (Ibrahim & Balistreri, 2020).

DRUG ALERT

Salicylates

Families need to be aware that salicylates, the alleged offending ingredient in aspirin, are contained in other products (e.g., Pepto-Bismol). They should refrain from administering any product for influenza-like symptoms without first checking the label for "hidden" salicylates.

SEIZURES AND EPILEPSY

A seizure is a "transient occurrence of signs and/or symptoms due to abnormal excessive and synchronous neuronal activity in the brain" (Fisher, Acevedo, Arzimanoglou, et al., 2014). Seizures are the most common pediatric neurologic disorder. About 4% to 10% of children will have at least one seizure in the first 16 years of life (Mikati & Tchapyjnikov, 2020). The manifestation of seizures depends on the region of the brain in which they originate and may include unconsciousness or altered consciousness; involuntary movements; and changes in perception, behaviors, sensations, and/or posture. Seizures are a symptom of an underlying disease process. They are individual events. Potential causes include infections, intracranial lesions or hemorrhage, metabolic disorders, trauma, brain malformations, genetic disorders, or toxic ingestion (see Nursing Care Guidelines box).

NURSING CARE GUIDELINES

Terminology for Seizures

Many words are used synonymously with the terms *seizure, epilepsy,* and *seizure disorder.* Epilepsy used to belong to the medical discipline of psychiatry, and therefore words such as *attacks* and *fits* are sometimes used to describe seizure events. These words, however, still create images of medieval superstitions, evil spirits, and the horrors of mental institutions. Parents are often hesitant to inform caregivers and the school that their child has a seizure disorder or epilepsy for fear of prejudice and misunderstandings. When working with families, health professionals should consider the words they use to discuss epilepsy and seizures. Correct terminology can help lessen the stigma and fear often associated with epilepsy and seizures.

The words *convulsion, convulsive disorder,* and *anticonvulsive drugs* are often used to cover all seizure types and antiepileptic drugs. However, the word *convulsion* conjures up images of a raving, wild person who is out of control and possibly dangerous. Therefore referring to all seizures as convulsions is questionable because most seizures are not convulsive in nature. In this chapter the word *event, episode,* or *experience* is used to describe a seizure; likewise, medications are referred to as *antiepileptic drugs.*

Epilepsy is defined as two or more unprovoked seizures more than 24 hours apart and can be caused by a variety of pathologic processes in the brain. A single seizure is not classified as epilepsy and is generally not treated with long-term antiepileptic drugs. Some seizures may result from an acute medical or neurologic illness and cease after the illness is treated. In other cases, children may have one or more seizures without the cause ever being found.

When a child has had a seizure, it is important to classify the seizure according to the International Classification of Epileptic Seizures. Optimal treatment and prognosis require an accurate diagnosis and a determination of the cause whenever possible.

EPILEPSY

The clinical definition of epilepsy was recently updated by the International League Against Epilepsy (ILAE). "Epilepsy is a disease of the brain defined by the following conditions: (1) at least two unprovoked seizures occurring more than 24 hours apart OR (2) one unprovoked seizure and a probability of further seizures similar to the general recurrence risk (at least 60%) after two unprovoked seizures occurring over the next 10 years" (Fisher et al., 2014). Seizures are a symptom of an underlying disease process. A single seizure event should be classified as epilepsy only if it meets criteria in number 2. Single seizures in children are generally not treated with long-term antiepileptic drugs. Some seizures may result from an acute medical or neurologic illness and cease once the illness is treated. In other cases, children may have a single seizure without the cause ever being known.

Etiology

Seizures in children have many different causes (Box 27.6). Seizures had been classified according to type and etiology. The ILAE 2017 classification of seizures focuses on location of onset rather than etiology: focal

BOX 27.6 Etiology of Seizures in Children

Nonrecurrent (Acute)

Febrile episodes
Intracranial infection
Intracranial hemorrhage
Space-occupying lesions (cyst, tumor)
Acute cerebral edema
Anoxia
Toxins
Drugs
Tetanus
Lead encephalopathy
Shigella and *Salmonella* organisms
Metabolic alterations:
- Hypocalcemia
- Hypoglycemia
- Hyponatremia or hypernatremia
- Hypomagnesemia
- Alkalosis
- Disorders of amino acid metabolism
- Deficiency states
- Hyperbilirubinemia

Recurrent (Chronic)

Idiopathic epilepsy
Epilepsy secondary to the following:
- Trauma
- Hemorrhage
- Anoxia
- Infections
- Toxins
- Degenerative phenomena
- Congenital defects
- Parasitic brain disease
- Hypoglycemia injury

Epilepsy—sensory stimulus
Epilepsy-stimulating states
- Narcolepsy and catalepsy
- Psychogenic
- Tetany from hypocalcemia, alkalosis

Hypoglycemic states
- Hyperinsulinism
- Hypopituitarism
- Adrenocortical insufficiency
- Hepatic disorders

Uremia
Allergy
Cardiovascular dysfunction or syncopal episodes
Migraine

(formerly known as partial), generalized, or unknown and unclassified (Fisher, Cross, French, et al., 2017). Focal seizures are divided into those with preserved awareness and those with impaired awareness and those with or without motor manifestations. Generalized onset seizures are also divided by their motor symptoms: tonic for the stiffening movements and clonic for the rhythmic jerking that may accompany tonic stiffening, and absence of nonmotor seizures. Unknown onset seizures are classified using the same motor criteria as generalized seizures.

The causes of seizures in children are many. Acute reactive seizures are caused by an acute condition such as electrolyte imbalance, acute stroke, head trauma, meningitis, or encephalitis. These seizures may continue and become epilepsy depending on the ability to treat the underlying condition. New-onset seizures may be the initial presentation of a child with a brain malformation. More than 100 genes have been found to cause epilepsy syndromes in children (Mikati & Tchapyjnikov, 2020). Many, but not all, of these genetic orders cause intellectual disability in addition to epilepsy. The proportion of seizures and epilepsy for which we have no identifiable cause becomes smaller each year as neuroimaging and genetic testing improve. Those children who do not have an identifiable cause for their seizures and epilepsy have a better prognosis for eventual resolution of their epilepsy.

Incidence

Epilepsy and seizures affect about 3 million Americans; it is the most common neurologic condition of children. The prevalence of epilepsy in children is consistently higher than the incidence and ranges from 3.2 to 5.5 in 1000 (Camfield & Camfield, 2015). The onset of epilepsy in children is highest during the first few months of life. The causative factors associated with childhood seizures are often linked to the child's age. In infants the most common causes are congenital brain malformations and genetic disorders, including metabolic disorders. Infections and epilepsy of unknown etiology are common causes of seizures in childhood. Children with intellectual disability, cerebral palsy, and/or autism spectrum disorder are more likely to have epilepsy than their typically developing peers.

Pathophysiology

Regardless of the etiologic factor or type of seizure, the basic mechanism is the same. Abnormal electrical discharges (1) may arise from the simultaneous activation of neurons in both hemispheres of the brain (generalized seizures); (2) may be restricted to one area of the cerebral cortex, producing manifestations characteristic of that particular anatomic focus; or (3) may begin in a localized area of the cortex as a focal seizure and spread to other portions of the brain and, if sufficiently extensive, produce generalized seizure activity.

A seizure occurs when there is sudden excessive excitation and loss of inhibition within neuronal circuits, allowing the circuits to amplify their discharges simultaneously. These discharges occur in response to the activity of sodium, potassium, calcium, and chloride ion channels. Normally these discharges are restrained by inhibitory mechanisms. In response to physiologic stimuli, such as brain injury or infection, genetic abnormalities, severe hypoglycemia, electrolyte imbalance, sleep deprivation, and toxic exposures, these abnormal neuronal discharges can spread to nearby cortex and subcortical structures. Primary generalized seizures begin with abnormal discharges in both hemispheres, which can involve connections between the thalamus and neocortex. On the basis of these characteristic neuronal discharges (manifested as stereotypical symptoms observed and reported during seizures and/or as recorded by the EEG), seizures are designated as focal, generalized, and unclassified epileptic seizures.

Seizure Classification and Clinical Manifestations

There are many different types of seizures, and each has unique clinical manifestations (Box 27.7). Seizures are classified into two major categories: (1) focal seizures (previously referred to as partial seizures), which have a local onset and involve a relatively small location in the brain; and (2) generalized seizures, which involve both hemispheres of the brain and are without local onset.

Focal Seizures (Formerly Known as Partial Seizures)

Focal seizures may arise from any area of the cerebral cortex, but the frontal, temporal, and parietal lobes are most often affected and are characterized by localized motor symptoms; somatosensory, psychic, or autonomic symptoms; or a combination of these. The abnormal EEG discharges begin unilaterally and are evident as focal spikes or sharp waves. Focal seizures are subdivided into three types:

Focal seizures without impaired awareness (formerly simple partial seizures)—Sensory symptoms that occur in one part of the brain and cause no alteration of consciousness, often referred to as aura. Sometimes accompanied by motor movements.

Focal seizures with impaired awareness (formerly complex partial seizures)—Sensory and/or motor symptoms that result in a change or loss of consciousness.

Focal to bilateral tonic-clonic seizures (formerly simple or complex seizures secondarily generalized)—Focal seizures with or without awareness that evolve into generalized seizures, usually a tonic-clonic event.

Focal seizures exhibit manifestations related to where they occur in the brain. A clear description of the seizure (***ictal state***) by an eyewitness is a valuable aid in localizing the brain area involved. Asking the child if he or she could hear, remember, and respond during the event is also helpful for localization. The initial event may provide the best clue for assessing the type of seizure and its localization. Correctly localizing the area of the brain involved with the seizure event is crucial for diagnostic and therapeutic reasons because many antiepileptic drugs are specific for each type of seizure.

In addition to the initial event, the circumstances that precipitated the episode are important. Identifying and eliminating triggering factors may be the only treatment needed. The ***postictal state*** (the period after a seizure) may be varied. The child may be drowsy, be uncoordinated, have transient aphasia or confusion, and display some sensory or motor impairment. Document neurologic changes. Weakness, hypotonia, or inactivity of a body part may indicate an epileptogenic focus in the corresponding contralateral cortical region.

Focal seizures without impaired awareness. Focal seizures with motor signs originate from the primary motor cortex, located in the temporal lobe, which is the area of the brain that controls muscle movement. They are the most frequent type of focal seizure. The simplest form of focal seizures with motor signs is ***clonus***, the rhythmic alternating contraction and relaxation of muscle groups.

Eye movements provide clues to the focus or origin of the seizure. Discharge in the cortex of one hemisphere tends to cause the eyes to deviate to the opposite side. Bilateral discharges tend to cause the eyes to move upward or straight ahead. While deviated, the eyes may rhythmically twitch.

Focal seizures with sensory symptoms are usually described as numbness, tingling, or pins and needles. This may be the only symptom of a seizure, or it may spread to involve an adjacent sensory cortex or motor cortex. Auditory seizures may manifest as sounds becoming painfully loud, humming, buzzing, or hissing. Visual seizures typically manifest as micropsia, macropsia, or flashes of light or colors. Focal seizures with autonomic symptoms may consist of feelings of nausea or epigastric rising. Flushing or pallor, sweating, or pupil dilation can

BOX 27.7 Classification and Clinical Manifestations of Partial and Generalized Seizures

Partial Seizures

Simple Partial Seizures With Motor Signs

Characterized by the following:

- Localized motor symptoms
- Somatosensory, psychic, autonomic symptoms
- Abnormal discharges remaining unilateral

Manifestations:

- Aversive seizure (most common motor seizure in children)—Eye or eyes and head turn away from the side of the focus; awareness of movement or loss of consciousness
- Rolandic (Sylvan) seizure—Tonic-clonic movements involving the face, salivation, arrested speech; most common during sleep
- Jacksonian march (rare in children)—Orderly, sequential progression of clonic movements beginning in a foot, hand, or face and moving, or "marching," to adjacent body parts

Simple Partial Seizures With Sensory Signs

Characterized by various sensations, including:

- Numbness, tingling, prickling, paresthesia, or pain originating in one area (e.g., face or extremities) and spreading to other parts of the body
- Visual sensations or formed images
- Motor phenomena such as posturing or hypertonia

Focal Seizures With Impaired Awareness

Observed more often in children from 3 years of age through adolescence

Characterized by the following:

- Period of altered behavior
- Amnesia for event (no recollection of behavior)
- Inability to respond to environment
- Impaired consciousness during event
- Drowsiness or sleep usually following seizure
- Confusion and amnesia possibly prolonged
- Complex sensory phenomena (aura)—Most frequent sensation is strange feeling in the pit of the stomach that rises toward the throat and is often accompanied by odd or unpleasant odors or tastes, complex auditory or visual hallucinations, ill-defined feelings of elation or strangeness (e.g., déjà vu, a feeling of familiarity in a strange environment), strong feelings of fear and anxiety, distorted sense of time and self, and in small children emission of a cry or attempt to run for help

Patterns of motor behavior:

- Stereotypic
- Similar with each subsequent seizure
- May suddenly cease activity, appear dazed, stare into space, become confused and apathetic, and become limp or stiff or display some form of posturing
- May be confused
- May perform purposeless, complicated activities in a repetitive manner (automatisms), such as walking, running, kicking, laughing, or speaking incoherently, most often followed by postictal confusion or sleep; may exhibit oropharyngeal activities, such as smacking, chewing, drooling, swallowing, and nausea or abdominal pain followed by stiffness, a fall, and postictal sleep; rarely manifests actions such as rage or temper tantrums; aggressive acts uncommon during seizure

Generalized Seizures

Tonic-Clonic Seizures (Formerly Known as Grand Mal)

Most common and most dramatic of all seizure manifestations

Occur without warning

Tonic phase lasts approximately 10 to 20 seconds

Manifestations:

- Eyes roll upward
- Immediate loss of consciousness
- If standing, falls to floor or ground
- Stiffens in generalized, symmetric tonic contraction of entire body musculature
- Arms usually flexed
- Legs, head, and neck extended
- May utter a peculiar piercing cry
- Apneic, may become cyanotic
- Increased salivation and loss of swallowing reflex

Clonic phase: lasts about 30 seconds but can vary from only a few seconds to a half-hour or longer

Manifestations:

- Violent jerking movements as the trunk and extremities undergo rhythmic contraction and relaxation
- May foam at the mouth
- May be incontinent of urine and feces

As event ends, movements less intense, occurring at longer intervals, then ceasing entirely

Status epilepticus—Series of seizures at intervals too brief to allow the child to regain consciousness between the time one event ends and the next begins:

- Requires emergency intervention
- Can lead to exhaustion, respiratory failure, and death

Postictal state:

- Appears to relax
- May remain semiconscious and difficult to arouse
- May awaken in a few minutes
- Remains confused for several hours
- Poor coordination
- Mild impairment of fine motor movements
- May have visual and speech difficulties
- May vomit or complain of severe headache
- When left alone, usually sleeps for several hours
- On awakening is fully conscious
- Usually feels tired and complains of sore muscles and headache
- No recollection of entire event

Absence Seizures (Formerly Called Petit Mal)

Characterized by the following:

- Onset usually between 4 and 12 years of age
- More common in girls than in boys
- Usually cease at puberty
- Brief loss of consciousness
- Minimum or no alteration in muscle tone
- May go unrecognized because of little change in child's behavior
- Abrupt onset; suddenly develops 20 or more attacks daily
- Event often mistaken for inattentiveness or daydreaming
- Events possibly precipitated by hyperventilation, hypoglycemia, stresses (emotional and physiologic), fatigue, or sleeplessness

Manifestations:

- Brief loss of consciousness
- Appear without warning or aura
- Usually last about 5 to 10 seconds
- Slight loss of muscle tone may cause child to drop objects
- Ability to maintain postural control; seldom falls
- Minor movements such as lip smacking, twitching of eyelids or face, or slight hand movements
- Not accompanied by incontinence
- Amnesia for episode
- May need to reorient self to previous activity

Continued

BOX 27.7 Classification and Clinical Manifestations of Partial and Generalized Seizures—cont'd

Atonic and Akinetic Seizures (Also Known as Drop Attacks)

Characterized by the following:

- Onset usually between 2 and 5 years of age
- Sudden, momentary loss of muscle tone and postural control
- Events recurring frequently during the day, particularly in the morning hours and shortly after awakening

Manifestations:

- Loss of tone causing child to fall to the floor violently; unable to break fall by putting out hand; may incur a serious injury to the face, head, or shoulder
- Loss of consciousness only momentary

Myoclonic Seizures

May be isolated as benign essential myoclonus

Characterized by the following:

- Sudden, brief contractures of a muscle or group of muscles
- Occur singly or repetitively
- No postictal state
- May or may not be symmetric
- May or may not include loss of consciousness

be observed. Focal seizures with psychic symptoms may include speech arrest or vocalizations, the sensation that an experience has occurred before (déjà vu), fear, displeasure, anger, or irritability. The affective symptoms associated with focal seizures last only a few minutes and are unprovoked.

Focal seizures with impaired awareness. During the period of impaired consciousness the child may look vacant, dazed, or frightened and be unable to respond when spoken to or to follow instructions and will not react when touched. Focal seizures with impaired awareness are the most common type of seizures. Focal seizures are observed in children of all ages and are the most common type in infants. These seizures may begin with an *aura*—a sensation or sensory phenomenon that precedes the seizure activity. Common sensations include a strange feeling at the bottom of the stomach that rises toward the throat, odd or unpleasant odors or taste, complex auditory or visual hallucinations, or ill-defined feelings of strangeness (e.g., déjà vu). Small children may emit a cry as a manifestation of an aura. Strong feelings of fear and anxiety and a disturbed sense of time can be associated with an aura. The aura is part of the seizure event and is associated with EEG changes.

Another feature of a focal seizures may be *automatisms* (repetitive involuntary activities without purpose, carried out in a dreamy state). The predominant observations may be oropharyngeal activities such as lip smacking, chewing, drooling, swallowing, or picking at clothing or bed linens; ambulatory activities such as wandering or running; and verbal manifestations such as repeating words ("please, please," or "help, help"). These automatisms may appear to be antisocial behaviors, such as removing clothes in public or attempting to open the door of a moving car. The child may begin walking or running and unknowingly run out into traffic or into obstacles. It is important to realize that the child's consciousness is impaired and that these actions are not deliberate. It is sometimes difficult to determine whether such behavior is related to the seizure activity or to a behavioral deviation. If the behavior results from seizure activity, all attempts to control such behavior by physical restraint, with counseling, or with behavior plans will be ineffective. The child may suddenly cease activity, appear dazed, stare into space, become confused or apathetic, become limp or stiff, or display some form of posturing. Because the seizure starts in the same part of the brain each time, the child will do the same thing during every event. The term *psychomotor seizure* was formerly used because of the frequent association of psychic symptoms and motor automatisms with focal seizures.

If the seizure involves areas of the brain that control motor function, the child exhibits movements such as jerking of the hands and arms. Focal seizures generally last only a few minutes. After the seizure the postictal period occurs, with signs of confusion and lack of recollection of the ictal period. Depending on the area of the brain involved during the episode, the child may sleep for a time (see Table 27.3 for a comparison of focal seizures without and with impaired awareness).

Focal seizures that generalize. Focal seizures may spread and become generalized, usually into a tonic-clonic seizure. In such cases the focal seizure is considered the primary seizure event, and the generalized seizure is considered the secondary one. It would be stated that the tonic-clonic seizure was not generalized at the onset but was a focal seizure that became a bilateral tonic-clonic or secondarily generalized seizure.

Generalized Seizures

Generalized seizures without a focal onset indicate that the initial involvement is from both hemispheres. Loss of consciousness and impairment of motor function occur from the outset. Unlike focal seizures that become generalized, there is no aura. Seizures can occur at any time, day or night. The interval between events may be minutes, hours, weeks, or even years.

Tonic-clonic seizures. The generalized tonic-clonic seizure, formerly known as *grand mal,* is the most dramatic of all seizure manifestations of childhood. The seizure usually occurs without warning and consists of two distinct phases: tonic and clonic. In the tonic phase the child stiffens, the eyes roll upward, and the child loses consciousness. If standing, the child falls to the ground. The musculature stiffens in a generalized and symmetric tonic contraction of the entire body. The arms usually flex, and the legs, head, and neck extend. The mouth snaps shut, and the tongue may be bitten. The thoracic and abdominal muscles contract and sometimes produce a "tonic cry" as air is forced over the vocal cords. Parents often misinterpret this as an expression of pain. The average tonic phase lasts 10 to 30 seconds, during which the child's respirations become slow and shallow and the child may become cyanotic. Autonomic phenomena that may be observed include increased blood pressure, increased heart rate, flushing, and increased salivation.

In the clonic phase the tonic rigidity is replaced by intense jerking movements as the trunk and extremities undergo rhythmic contraction and relaxation. During this time the child cannot control oral secretions and may be incontinent of urine and feces. As the seizure ends, the movements become less intense and occur at less frequent intervals until they cease entirely. The average clonic phase lasts 30 to 50 seconds.

In the postictal phase the child may remain semiconscious and difficult to arouse. The postictal phase can last 30 minutes to several hours (Mikati & Tchapyjnikov, 2020). The child may remain confused or sleep. He or she may have mild impairment of fine motor movements, have visual and speech difficulties, and may vomit or complain

TABLE 27.3 Comparison of Focal and Absence Seizures

Clinical Manifestations	Focal Seizures Without Impaired Awareness	Focal Seizures With Impaired Awareness	Absence Seizures
Frequency (per day)	Variable	Rarely over 1-2 times	Multiple
Duration	Usually <30 sec	Usually >60 sec, rarely <10 sec	Usually <10 sec, rarely >30 sec
Aura	May be sole manifestation of seizure	Frequent	Never
Impaired consciousness	Never	Always	Always, brief loss of consciousness
Automatisms	No	Frequent	Frequent
Clonic movements	Frequent	Occasional	Occasional
Postictal impairment	Rare	Frequent	Never
Mental disorientation	Rare	Common	Unusual

of headache. On awakening, he or she is fully conscious but usually feels tired and may complain of sore muscles and a headache. The child has no recollection of the event.

Absence seizures. Absence seizures, formerly called *petit mal,* are generalized seizures. They have a sudden onset and are characterized by a brief loss of awareness, a blank stare, and automatisms. Absence seizures are divided into typical and atypical. These seizures almost always first appear during childhood, usually between the ages of 5 to 8 years, and often stop spontaneously in the teenage years (Mikati & Tchapyjnikov, 2020).

The onset of typical absence seizures is abrupt, with the child suddenly experiencing 20 or more events daily. Characteristically the brief loss of consciousness appears without warning and usually lasts 5 to 10 seconds. The child has a motionless blank stare that may be confused with inattentiveness or daydreaming. Slight loss of muscle tone may cause the child to drop objects, but he or she seldom falls. There may be automatisms such as lip smacking, twitching of the eyelids or face, or fumbling with the clothes. The sudden arrest of activity and consciousness is not accompanied by incontinence. Although the child will not recall the episode, when the seizure ends, the child may be aware and able to report that he or she has missed things that happened. There is no postictal sleepiness. Most children can immediately resume previous activities but may be momentarily confused. Atypical absence seizures are accompanied by head nods and sudden myoclonic jerks. Atypical absence seizures, unlike typical absence seizures, can be difficult to treat (Mikati & Tchapyjnikov, 2020).

Hyperventilation and photic stimulation are potent precipitators of absence seizures (Mikati & Tchapyjnikov, 2020). If the child is involved in a group activity, such as classroom reading or discussion, he or she may need help to catch up with the group after the seizure. Frequent episodes can result in slowed intellectual processes and deterioration in schoolwork and behavior. This is often the first indication of the problem. Absence seizures can be distinguished from daydreaming and attention-deficit/hyperactivity disorder by attempting to physically interrupt the episode by touching the face and eyelashes. Children who are daydreaming will respond to touch, whereas those who are having an absence seizure cannot. The abnormal EEG pattern in absence epilepsy is diagnostic and distinguishes absence seizures from focal seizures.

Atonic seizures. Atonic seizures are a sudden, momentary, and total loss of muscle tone. The onset is usually between 2 and 5 years of age. During a mild seizure the child may simply experience several sudden brief head drops. During a more severe episode the child suddenly falls to the ground, loses consciousness briefly, and after a few seconds gets up as if nothing happened. Because of the sudden loss of tone, the child is unable to break the fall by putting out a hand and can suffer injuries to the head, teeth, and face. Therefore if a child has frequent atonic seizures, wearing a helmet with a face guard when the child is up and walking around should be considered.

Myoclonic seizures. Myoclonic seizures are characterized by sudden, brief, shocklike movements of a muscle or group of muscles (Holmes, 2018). The seizures may involve only the face and trunk or one or more extremities. They may occur singly or repetitively. The seizures may or may not be symmetric. Myoclonic seizures often occur in combination with other seizure types. Myoclonic seizures should not be confused with myoclonic jerks that can occur normally in the course of falling asleep.

The myoclonic seizure can be confused with the exaggerated startle reflex often seen in children with severe developmental delays. The startle reflex occurs immediately after a stimulus such as a loud noise. The child will stiffly and rapidly extend all four extremities, sometimes with a cry, and then quickly return to his or her usual posture. An EEG with video recording can distinguish between the two events.

Tonic seizures. Tonic seizures are characterized by a sudden onset of increased tone. The child falls if standing. The child may involuntarily cry out because of contraction of the respiratory and abdominal muscles. Tonic seizures are longer than myoclonic seizures, with an average duration of 10 seconds. Postictal confusion, tiredness, and headache are common.

Clonic seizures. Clonic seizures are characterized by loss of consciousness and decreased tone followed by jerking movements of the extremities. These movements may be more predominant in one extremity. The duration is typically from 1 to several minutes and may be followed by a rapid recovery or may have a period of postictal confusion.

Unknown Onset Epileptic Seizures

Unknown onset epileptic seizures are seizures that lack sufficient information to classify. For example, the location of the onset of epileptic spasms, a type of seizure found predominantly in children younger than 2 years old, is often unknown. In addition to the seizures listed in the International Classification of Epileptic Seizures, several types of epileptic syndromes display a group of signs and symptoms that collectively characterize or indicate a particular condition. Several syndromes associated with epilepsy occur in infants and children. Two of these are West syndrome and Lennox-Gastaut syndrome (LGS).

Infantile Spasms (West syndrome). Infantile spasms are the most common epilepsy of infancy and are also known as West syndrome. It has a peak onset between 4 and 8 months of age and rarely occurs after 2 years of age (Singhal, Harini, & Sullivan, 2018). The etiology can be genetic, metabolic, or structural but is unknown in about one-third of affected children. The pathophysiology is poorly understood. An abnormal EEG with hypsarrhythmia is pathognomonic. Nearly all children with infantile spasms have some degree of cognitive impairment (Singhal et al., 2018).

Flexor spasms consist of brief contractions of the neck, trunk, arms, and legs. The arms may either adduct or abduct, with the arms flexed at the elbow. Extensor spasms consist predominantly of extensor contractions resulting in abrupt extension of the neck and trunk with extensor adduction or abduction of the arms and legs. Eye deviation or nystagmus often occurs with infantile spasms. Infantile spasms may occur as a single event or in clusters, with as many as 150 seizures within a cluster. The infant often cries or is irritable during or after a cluster of spasms.

Adrenocorticotropic hormone (ACTH), an injectable hormonal treatment, is the first-line treatment recommended for infantile spasms. ACTH is more likely to provide short-term resolution of infantile spasms, but longer-term resolution is no different when prednisolone (oral hormonal treatment) is used (Jones, Snead, Boyd, et al., 2015). Due to the cost and difficulty obtaining ACTH, prednisone is considered to be a reasonable option by many epileptologists.

Vigabatrin is usually the choice of treatment for infantile spasms in tuberous sclerosis (Hancock, Osborne, & Edwards, 2013). There is evidence that it works as well as hormonal treatment in the rare children with infantile spasms and normal development (Jones, Go, Boyd, et al., 2015). Long-term use can damage the retinas, causing clinically asymptomatic peripheral visual field cuts. The risk of this visual field cut must be balanced with the benefit of controlling infantile spasms. New evidence suggests that combining vigabatrin with hormonal treatment is more effective than either treatment alone (O'Callaghan, Edwards, Alber, et al., 2017).

A Cochrane review of 18 randomized controlled studies found that no single treatment proved to be more efficacious than any other in the treatment of infantile spasms; hormonal treatments resolve spasms more often than vigabatrin, but the hormonal treatments may cause more long-term side effects (Hancock et al., 2013). Use of the ketogenic diet and other antiepileptic drugs as adjunctive therapy is increasing.

Lennox-Gastaut syndrome. Between 20% and 50% of infants who have infantile spasms eventually develop LGS (Germain & Maria, 2018). LGS is diagnosed on three criteria: (1) the presence of multiple seizure types (atonic, myoclonic, tonic, and atypical absence); (2) intellectual disability; and (3) slow spike wave discharges on EEG (Tenney & Glauser, 2018). Onset of LGS is between 1 and 8 years of age. Children with LGS typically have multiple seizures daily. Tonic seizures are the most common. There are many causes of LGS; about one-third of children with LGS have no known cause. Causes include brain malformations and injury, neurocutaneous disorders, brain infections, and genetic disorders. In addition to cognitive impairments, many of these children develop other problems, including hyperactivity, aggressive behavior, or autism spectrum disorder.

Treatment is challenging. Most children require more than one antiepileptic drug and even then many will continue to have some seizures. In addition, the ketogenic diet or implantation of a vagus nerve stimulator may be efficacious for some of these children. The prognosis of LGS is typically poor. Additional family support is often required to maintain the child at home.

Diagnostic Evaluation

Establishing a diagnosis is critical for establishing a prognosis and planning appropriate treatment. The process of diagnosis in a child suspected of having epilepsy includes first determining whether the events thought to be seizures are epileptic seizures or nonepileptic events and then identifying the underlying cause, if possible. The assessment and diagnosis rely heavily on a thorough history, skilled observation, and several diagnostic tests.

It is especially important to differentiate seizures from other brief alterations in consciousness or behavior. Clinical entities that mimic seizures include staring, migraine headaches, toxic effects of drugs, syncope (fainting), breath-holding spells in infants and young children, movement disorders (tics, tremor, chorea), prolonged QT syndrome and other cardiac arrhythmias, sleep disturbances (sleepwalking, night terrors), psychogenic seizures, rage attacks, and transient ischemic attacks (rare in children). The toxic effects of maternal drug use and withdrawal from these drugs should be considered in the differential diagnosis of new-onset seizure activity in a newborn.

A detailed description of the seizure should be obtained from the caregiver(s) who witnessed it. Ask questions about the child's behavior during the event, especially at the onset, and the time at which the seizure occurred (e.g., early morning, while awake, during sleep). Any factors that may have precipitated the seizure are important, including fever, infection, head trauma, anxiety, fatigue, sleep deprivation, menstrual cycle, alcohol, and activity (e.g., hyperventilation or exposure to strong stimuli such as bright flashing light or loud noises). Record any sensory phenomena that the child can describe and if the child was able to hear during the seizure. The duration and progression of the seizure (if any) and the postictal feelings and behavior (e.g., confusion, inability to speak, amnesia, headache, sleep) should also be noted. For children who have epilepsy, document how often they have seizures: daily, weekly, or monthly. Knowing the age at which the child had his or her first seizure is important. It is important to determine whether more than one seizure type exists. It is often more informative to ask the parents to show you what the seizure looked like rather than to rely on their verbal description. Demonstrating a seizure often reveals features, such as head turning, that would otherwise go unrecognized. Some seizures are overlooked by parents. For example, some parents may not identify brief head nods or brief single jerks as seizures unless specifically asked if their child has these symptoms.

A thorough medical history must be obtained, beginning with conception. Questions to consider include the following: Was the mother's pregnancy complicated by illness and drug use, either prescription or recreational? How old was the baby when discharged from the hospital after birth? Has the child had any overnight hospitalizations or surgeries? A complete history is designed to uncover possible risk factors for the development of seizures or epilepsy.

The family history should include whether other family members ever had a seizure of any kind, cognitive impairments, cerebral palsy, autism, or other neurologic disorders. Ask if there is a family history of sudden, unexpected deaths. A family history can offer clues to other paroxysmal disorders, such as migraine headaches, breath-holding spells, febrile seizures, or neurologic diseases.

A complete physical and neurologic examination, including developmental assessment of language, learning, behavior, and motor abilities, may provide clues to the cause of the seizures. A number of laboratory and neuroimaging tests may be ordered depending on the child's age, whether it is a new-onset seizure, characteristics of the seizure, and the history. Laboratory studies that may prove valuable include a white blood cell count (for signs of infection) and blood glucose measurements that may indicate hypoglycemic episodes. Serum electrolytes, blood urea nitrogen, calcium, serum amino acids, lactate, ammonia, and urine organic acids may indicate metabolic disturbances. Blood for chromosomal analysis may also be tested if a genetic etiology is suspected. A toxicology screen should be performed if alcohol or drug ingestion or withdrawal is suspected. Lumbar puncture can confirm a suspected diagnosis of meningitis. CT may be done to detect a cerebral hemorrhage, infarctions, brain tumors, and gross malformations. MRI provides greater anatomic detail and is used to detect developmental malformations, tumors, and cortical dysplasias.

Most children with seizures will have an EEG. The EEG is the most useful tool for evaluating the child's risk of recurrent seizures, helping determine the type of seizure the child had, and diagnosing the type of epilepsy. The EEG confirms the presence of abnormal electrical discharges and provides information on the seizure type and the location of onset. The EEG is carried out under varying conditions: with the child asleep, awake, awake with provocative stimulation (flashing lights, noise), and hyperventilation. Stimulation may elicit abnormal electrical activity that is recorded on the EEG. Various seizure types produce characteristic EEG patterns; for example, a three-per-second spike and wave pattern is observed in absence epilepsy, and a slow spike and wave pattern is observed in LGS.

A normal EEG does not rule out seizures. The EEG is only a surface recording, lasts approximately 1 hour, and therefore may show normal interictal activity. If there is concern about whether a child has seizures or if the seizure type cannot be determined, a long-term video EEG may be done to record the child during wakefulness and sleep. The full-body image is recorded on video, with selected EEG channels displayed on the same screen for simultaneous recording and viewing. Amplitude-integrated electroencephalography (aEEG) monitoring is increasingly available in neonatal and pediatric intensive care units. This is a method of continuous monitoring of brain activity using recordings from a handful of leads compared with the 24 leads of standard EEGs. aEEG is useful for diagnosing seizures when standard EEG or a neurophysiologist to interpret it is unavailable. Although the EEG is valuable, it should not be used alone to determine the type of seizure. Rather, the EEG interpretation with a thorough clinical description of the child's behavior during the seizure will inform the correct classification of the seizure and the appropriate treatment choice.

Therapeutic Management

The goal of treatment of seizure disorders is to control the seizures or to reduce their frequency and severity, discover and correct the cause when possible, and help the child live as normal a life as possible. Discovering and, when possible, correcting the underlying cause of the seizures can lead to complete control of all seizures. If the seizure activity is a manifestation of an infectious, traumatic, or metabolic process, seizure therapy is instituted as part of the general therapeutic regimen. Management of epilepsy has four treatment options: drug therapy, the ketogenic diet, vagus nerve stimulation, and epilepsy surgery.

Drug Therapy

It is known that persons predisposed to epilepsy have seizures when their basal level of neuronal excitability exceeds a critical point; no event occurs if the excitability is maintained below this threshold. The administration of antiepileptic drugs serves to raise this threshold and prevent seizures. Consequently, the primary therapy for epilepsy is the administration of the appropriate antiepileptic drug or combination of drugs in a dosage that provides the desired effect without causing adverse side effects or toxicity. Antiepileptic drugs are believed to exert their effect primarily by reducing the responsiveness of neurons to the sudden, high-frequency nerve impulses that arise in the epileptogenic focus. Thus the seizure is effectively suppressed; however, the abnormal brain waves may or may not be altered. The chance of total control of seizures depends on the underlying cause of the seizures. Children with epilepsy without any underlying pathology such as brain malformations or genetic disorders and with normal development have the best prognosis.

The initiation of anticonvulsant therapy is based on several factors, including the child's age, type of seizure, risk of recurrence, and other comorbid or predisposing medical issues. For children who develop recurrent seizures or epilepsy, treatment is begun with a single drug known to be effective for the child's seizure type and have the lowest risk of adverse side effects. The dosage is gradually increased until the seizures are controlled. If a child develops intolerable side effects, the medication is stopped and another one tried. If the drug at maximum doses reduces but does not stop all seizures, a second drug is added in gradually increasing doses. When seizures are controlled, the first drug may be tapered to reduce the potential adverse effects and drug interactions of polytherapy. Monotherapy remains the treatment of choice for epilepsy, but a combination of medications may be a viable alternative for children who do not have total seizure control with only one medication (Mikati & Tchapyjnikov, 2020).

If complete seizure control is maintained on an antiepileptic drug for 2 years, it may be safe to slowly discontinue the drug for patients with no risk factors. Risk factors for recurrence of seizures include history of status epilepticus, older age at onset, duration of treatment before seizure control is achieved, presence of a neurologic dysfunction (e.g., motor or cognitive impairment), and abnormal EEG findings when the medication is stopped (Lee, Li, & Chen, 2017). Recurrence occurs most often within the first year of discontinuation (Braun & Schmidt, 2014). When seizure medications are discontinued, the dosage is decreased gradually over weeks or months. Sudden withdrawal of a drug is not recommended because it can cause seizures, which may be longer and more intense than previously, to recur.

Potential complications of drug therapy. The side effects of continued use of antiepileptic medications are often distressing to the child and family. Most side effects are transient and dose related, but drug reactions warrant immediate attention. A serious potential adverse side effect of antiepileptic medication is allergic drug rash. The rash can start with hives and is usually very pruritic. Allergic drug rashes from antiepileptic drugs can spread quickly and become severe, life-threatening events. The drug should be stopped with any signs of a rash. A physician or nurse practitioner should evaluate the child within 24 hours or sooner if the child develops edema or respiratory problems. Treatment includes antihistamines, epinephrine, glucocorticosteroids, anabolic steroids, and/or airway management, depending on the severity of the reaction (Blaszczyk, Lasoń, & Czuczwar, 2015).

Sleepiness, changes in mood or behavior, vision changes, and ataxia are some of the potential side effects of antiepileptic medications. These are very distressing to both children and families. They often disappear over time or when drug dosages are reduced. Blood cell counts, urinalysis, and liver function tests are obtained at regular intervals in children receiving some older antiepileptic medications that can affect organ function.

Knowledge of drug-to-drug interactions, including other medications such as antibiotics, is critical in caring for the child with epilepsy. Knowledge of potential adverse effects is also imperative. Severe, potentially life-threatening side effects can occur with specific antiepileptic medications. For example, carbamazepine, phenytoin, and lamotrigine may cause a severe, life-threatening rash. Valproic acid may cause liver toxicity, particularly in a child less than 2 years of age. To avoid possible complications of tissue damage and difficulties with administration of IV phenytoin, fosphenytoin should be used. Therefore critical thinking and careful monitoring are necessary in providing optimum care to the child with epilepsy.

DRUG ALERT

Fosphenytoin

Fosphenytoin is often used to treat seizures instead of intravenous (IV) phenytoin because of possible complications and drug interactions associated with IV phenytoin. If IV phenytoin is used, it should be administered via slow IV push and at a rate that does not exceed 50 mg/min. Because phenytoin precipitates when mixed with glucose, only normal saline is used to flush the tubing or catheter. Fosphenytoin may be given in saline or glucose solutions at a rate of up to 150 mg PE (phenytoin equivalent)/min, and it may be given intramuscularly if necessary.

Chronic treatment with phenytoin may cause gum hypertrophy. Surgical removal of the excess tissue may be needed in severe cases. Enlargement of the tonsillar and adenoidal tissue can cause partial airway obstruction, which produces snoring during sleep. Chronic treatment with antiepileptic medications, particularly enzyme-inducing medications, has been associated with decreased bone mineral density that worsened with prolonged use of antiepileptic medications (Ahmad, Petty, Gorelik, et al., 2017). Prophylactic administration of calcium and vitamin D supplements is recommended for all patients receiving antiepileptic medications, and bone mineral density testing is recommended for patients on long-term antiepileptic medications (Ahmad et al., 2017).

Children whose mothers took antiepileptic medications in the first trimester of pregnancy have a twofold increased risk of being born with congenital malformations compared with children not exposed in utero to these drugs (Ban, Fleming, Doyle, et al., 2015). Folic acid can prevent birth defects, but women taking antiepileptic medications tend to have low levels of serum folic acid. The Centers for Disease Control and Prevention and the American Academy of Neurology recommend that all females capable of childbearing take 400 to 800 mcg of folic acid daily prior to conception.

Ketogenic Diet

The ***ketogenic diet*** is a high-fat, very-low-carbohydrate, and adequate-protein diet that has shown effectiveness for treatment of epilepsy (Martin, Jackson, Levy, et al., 2016). It is also the first-line treatment for certain metabolic disorders, including pyruvate dehydrogenase deficiency, glucose transporter type I deficiency, and glutaric aciduria type I. Consumption of the ketogenic diet forces the body to shift from using glucose as the primary energy source to using fat, and the individual develops a state of ketosis. The diet is rigorous. All foods and liquids the child consumes must be carefully weighed and measured. A liquid formula is available for children who cannot take solid food. The diet is deficient in vitamins and minerals; therefore vitamin and mineral supplementation is necessary. Potential adverse side effects of the diet include constipation, hypoglycemia during initiation of the diet, acidosis, and lethargy. Less common but more serious side effects include urinary tract infections, kidney stones, and insufficient weight gain (Luat, Coyle, & Kamat, 2016).

The ketogenic diet (and its variations) has been shown to be an effective and tolerable treatment for medically refractory epilepsy with seizure control comparable to or better than that obtained with antiepileptic medications in some children (Martin et al., 2016).

Vagus Nerve Stimulation

Vagus nerve stimulation (VNS) was developed as palliative treatment for patients with seizures not controlled by drugs and who are not candidates for diet or surgical therapy (Moshe, Perucca, Ryvlin, et al., 2015). The results in children have been mixed, with a usually modest reduction in seizures (Dhamne, Kaye, & Rotenberg, 2018). A programmable signal generator is implanted subcutaneously in the chest. Electrodes tunneled underneath the skin deliver electrical impulses to the left vagus nerve (CN X). The device is programmed noninvasively to deliver a precise pattern of stimulation to the left vagus nerve. The patient or caregiver can activate the device using a magnet at the onset of a seizure. No long-term adverse effects have been reported with VNS, but dysphonia, throat or neck pain, and cough can occur during stimulation.

Surgical Therapy

When seizures are caused by a hematoma, vascular malformation, tumor, or other cerebral lesion, surgical removal is usually recommended. Epilepsy surgery is the most effective treatment for children with medically refractory epilepsy due to focal cortical dysplasia and mesial temporal sclerosis. About 80% of these patients will be seizure free 4 years after surgery (Moosa & Gupta, 2014).

Epilepsy surgery does not always eliminate the need for antiepileptic drug therapy. The goal is to improve seizure control without worsening or producing serious deficits. Some children will see improvements in their cognition, behavior, and quality of life (Ryvlin, Cross, & Rheims, 2014). Types of surgeries include focal resection of the epileptogenic focus, functional hemispherectomy, and corpus callosotomy, which severs the connection between the hemispheres.

Status Epilepticus

Status epilepticus is a continuous seizure that lasts more than 30 minutes or a series of seizures from which the child does not regain a premorbid level of consciousness (Fernandez, Abend, & Loddenkemper, 2018). The term *impending status epilepticus* is used for a continuous seizure or series of seizures lasting between 5 and 30 minutes with the designation that treatment should begin within 5 minutes (Fernandez et al., 2018).

The initial treatment is directed toward support of vital functions (i.e., the CAB of life support), measuring blood glucose, administrating oxygen, and gaining IV access, immediately followed by IV administration of antiepileptic agents. Simultaneously with life support measures and emergency medications, the underlying cause of the status epilepticus is identified and corrected (Fernandez et al., 2018).

Buccal or intranasal midazolam and rectal diazepam are simple, effective, and safe treatments for home or prehospital management of prolonged seizures and impending status epilepticus (Brigo, Nardone, Tezzon, et al., 2015). Time to cessation of the seizure with midazolam was 4 minutes shorter than with rectal diazepam (Brigo et al., 2015). Respiratory depression is a potential side effect of these medications when more than two doses are given (Abend & Loddenkemper, 2014); however, respiratory depression is not a side effect of rectal diazepam when it is administered as recommended. Intranasal midazolam is safe and effective for stopping seizures but also is easier to administer than rectal diazepam (Glauser, Shinnar, Gloss, et al., 2016).

For in-hospital management of status epilepticus, IV diazepam or lorazepam (Ativan) is the first-line drug of choice (Glauser et al., 2016). If IV access has not been established, rectal diazepam or intramuscular, intranasal, or buccal midazolam should be given. It appears that the exact medication chosen is less important than choosing the one that can be administered fastest (Fernandez et al., 2018). The child must be closely monitored during administration to detect early alterations in vital signs that may indicate impending respiratory depression. When a benzodiazepine (diazepam or lorazepam) is ineffective, IV phenytoin or fosphenytoin followed by phenobarbital is given as the next line of treatment. Fosphenytoin is preferred over phenytoin because of better tolerability (Glauser et al., 2016). This combination of therapy places the child at high risk for apnea, and therefore respiratory support is generally necessary. Children may also receive other antiepileptic medications, including IV valproate or levetiracetam.

Children who continue to have seizures despite drug treatment may require general anesthesia with a continuous infusion of midazolam, propofol, or pentobarbital (Fernandez et al., 2018). In this situation the patient may need to be intubated, and continuous EEG monitoring is typically done to monitor for and treat electrographic seizures (Fernandez et al., 2018).

DRUG ALERT

Diazepam

Diazepam is incompatible with many drugs. To give intravenously, inject slowly and directly into the vein or through tubing as close as possible to the vein insertion site.

Nursing care of a child with status epilepticus includes, in addition to the CAB of life support, monitoring blood pressure and body temperature. During the first 30 to 45 minutes of the seizure, the blood pressure may be elevated. Thereafter the blood pressure typically returns to normal but may be decreased depending on the medications being administered for seizure control. Hyperthermia requiring treatment may occur as a result of increased motor activity.

Status epilepticus is a medical emergency that requires immediate intervention to prevent possible brain injury or death. Diagnosis and correction of the underlying cause of the status epilepticus is essential.

Prognosis

Only about half of children who experience a first seizure will have additional seizures (El-Radhi, 2015). Children who have cognitive impairments and/or cerebral palsy are at highest risk for developing epilepsy. Prognosis for eventual remission of childhood epilepsy depends on the etiology and epilepsy syndrome diagnosis. Some syndromes almost always remit, whereas others almost never do (Camfield & Camfield, 2015). ***Intractable seizures*** are defined as failure to control seizures after two appropriately selected antiepileptic medications are trialed (Wassenaar, Leijten, Egberts, et al., 2013). ***Refractory seizures*** are usually defined as the persistence of seizures despite adequate trials of three antiepileptic medications, alone or in combination (Téllez-Zenteno, Hernández-Ronquillo, Buckley, et al., 2014).

Most deaths in children with epilepsy are due to factors associated with a child's coexisting neurologic conditions and poorly controlled seizures (Berg & Rychlik, 2015). Deaths from epilepsy in children who have no other neurologic conditions occur at the same rate as childhood deaths from other causes, with the exception of drowning

BOX 27.8 General Observations of the Child During a Seizure

Observations During Seizure

General Description

Order of events (before, during, and after)

Duration of seizure

- Tonic-clonic—from first signs of event until jerking stops
- Absence—from loss of consciousness until consciousness is regained
- Focal seizures with impaired awareness—from first sign of unresponsiveness, motor activity, automatisms until there are signs of responsiveness to environment

Onset

Time of onset

Significant precipitating events—missed medication dosage, illness, stress, sleep deprivation, menses

Behavior

Change in facial expression

Cry or other sound

Stereotypic or automatous movements

Random activity (wandering)

Position of eyes, head, body, extremities

Unilateral or bilateral posturing of one or more extremities

Movement

Change of position, if any

Site of commencement—hand, thumb, mouth, generalized

Tonic phase—length, parts of body involved

Clonic phase—twitching or jerking movements, parts of body involved, sequence of parts involved, generalized, change in character of movements

Lack of movement or muscle tone of body part or entire body

Face

Color change—pallor, cyanosis, flushing

Perspiration

Mouth—position, deviating to one side, teeth clenched, tongue bitten, frothing at mouth

Lack of expression

Asymmetric expression

Eyes

Position—straight ahead, deviation upward or outward, conjugate or divergent gaze

Pupils—change in size, equality, reaction to light

Respiratory Effort

Presence and length of apnea

Other

Incontinence

Postictal Observations

Duration of postictal period

State of consciousness

Orientation

Arousability

Motor ability

- Any change in motor function
- Ability to move all extremities
- Paresis or weakness

Speech

Sensations

- Complaint of discomfort or pain
- Any sensory impairment
- Recollection of preseizure sensations or aura

(Franklin, Pearn, & Peden, 2017). The phenomenon of sudden unexpected death in epilepsy (SUDEP) is drawing increasing attention in child neurology and epilepsy clinics. It is an extremely rare condition in children with a risk of between 1.1 and 3.4 per 10,000 patient-years (Morse & Kothare, 2016). The major risk factor for SUDEP is uncontrolled generalized tonic-clonic seizures, particularly in sleep (Harden, Tomson, Gloss, et al., 2017).

Nursing Care Management

An important nursing responsibility is to observe the seizure episode and accurately document the events. Record and note any alterations in behavior preceding the seizure and the characteristics of the episode, such as sensory-hallucinatory phenomena (e.g., an aura), motor effects (e.g., eye movements, muscular contractions), alterations in consciousness, and postictal state (Box 27.8). The nurse should describe only what is observed rather than try to label a seizure type. Note the time that the seizure began and the duration of the seizure.

Generalized seizures and other types with clear manifestations are easy to detect, but absence seizures may present more difficulties. They are easily misinterpreted as inattention. Any unusual behavior, even seemingly inconsequential, such as a momentary interruption of activity, staring, or mental blankness, should be described. The more detailed these descriptions, the more valuable they are for assessment (see the Next-Generation NCLEX® Examination-Style Unfolding Case Study and Quality Patient Outcomes boxes).

NEXT-GENERATION NCLEX® EXAMINATION-STYLE UNFOLDING CASE STUDY

The Child With Seizures

Day 1, 10:00 am

1. A 7-year-old boy who was playing during physical education class at school when he suddenly stopped his activity, stared into space, repetitively moved his left arm up and down, and smacked his lips. After approximately 1 minute, he stopped the behavior and was drowsy but responsive to his environment. He had no memory of the event. He was accompanied by his teacher to the school nurse for further assessment. While waiting for the parents to arrive, what are the most important subjective and objective data that the nurse would document? **Select all that apply.**

From the boy:

A. Aura
B. Sensory phenomena that the child can describe during the event (i.e., ability to hear)
C. Postictal feelings (i.e., confusion, inability to speak, amnesia, headache, sleepiness)

From the person who observed the seizure:

A. Duration of seizure
B. Time of onset of seizure
C. Other students who have the same symptoms
D. Change in level of consciousness (LOC) before, during, and after the seizure
E. Movements (ask for demonstration of the seizure rather than relying on verbal description)

Day 1, 11:30 am

2. The child is seen in the Emergency Department after the mother picked him up from school. The physician wants to observe the child while tests results are pending. Blood work and an electroencephalogram (EEG) was done. **Indicate which nursing action listed in the far-left column is appropriate to prevent the potential complication following a seizure listed in the middle column. Indicate the nursing action number in the far-right column. <u>Note that ONLY one nursing action can be used for each potential complication and that NOT all nursing actions will be used</u>.**

Nursing Action	Potential Complication	Nursing Action to Prevent Complication
1. Monitor time (onset and duration), movements, and LOC during seizure.	Child experiences anxiety and fear	
2. If child is at risk of falling, ease child to floor. Prevent child from hitting head on objects. Do not attempt to restrain child or use force.	An accurate description of the seizure is not obtained	
3. During seizure, place child in a side-lying position on a flat surface such as floor. Do not put anything in child's mouth.	Parents unable to cope with the diagnosis and management of their son	
4. Stay with the child and reassure the child when awakening from seizure.	Physical harm occurs	
5. Involve child and parents in discussion of fears, anxieties, and resources and support options available to patient and family.	Aspiration can occur	
	Lack of description of the postictal state	
	Further seizures occur	

NEXT-GENERATION NCLEX® EXAMINATION-STYLE UNFOLDING CASE STUDY—cont'd

1 week later, 11:00 am

3. A 7-year-old boy who was playing during physical education class at school a week ago had a seizure. The work-up revealed an abnormal EEG and the physical examination and clinical history supported the decision to begin anticonvulsant therapy with a single medication. This morning he has another seizure while playing with his siblings in the backyard. His brother ran inside to get help and his mother ran outside to see him staring into space with his head turned to the side and his left arm moving rhythmically up and down. This activity stopped for a few seconds and then started again. His mother called for emergency assistance (911), and he was transported to the hospital. Which of the signs and symptoms experienced by this 7-year-old child would the nurse expect to find with a focal seizure? **Select all that apply.**
   A. Automatisms
   B. Aura experienced
   C. Mental disorientation
   D. Postictal impairment
   E. Lasted less than a minute
   F. Occurs multiple times a day
   G. Seizure lasted for 45 minutes

1 week later, 11:30 am

4. The child was transferred by ambulance to the hospital. He had not regained consciousness during the transport. **Choose the most likely options for the information missing from the statements below by selecting from the lists of options provided.**
   Since the child is not regaining a premorbid level of consciousness (LOC) between seizures is concerning and meets criteria for a diagnosis of____1____. The child's ____2____ should be monitored closely, and supportive measures (i.e., cardiopulmonary resuscitation) should be initiated as indicated. Simple, effective, and safe treatments for home or prehospital management of prolonged seizures and impending status epilepticus include ____3____ midazolam and rectal diazepam.

Options for 1	Options for 2	Options for 3
simple partial seizure	blood pressure	intrathecal
complex partial seizure	seizure activity	intravenous
status epilepticus	circulation, airway, and breathing (CAB)	rectal
absence seizure	blood levels	buccal

1 week later, 1:00 pm

5. The child is admitted to the hospital after the seizure was stopped in the Emergency Department by administering intravenous lorazepam. The child has gained consciousness and is being monitored closely with his parents at the bedside. He is undergoing a comprehensive neurological examination with neuroimaging studies. The child had no history of signs of infection or head trauma. **For each nursing action, use an X to indicate whether it was Effective (helped to meet expected patient outcomes), Ineffective (did not help to meet expected patient outcomes), or Unrelated (not related to the patient outcomes).**

Nursing Action	Effective	Ineffective	Unrelated
Monitor circulation, airway, and breathing closely.			
Ensure antiepileptic drugs are being administered as directed.			
Monitor and record characteristics, onset, and duration of any new seizures, including motor effects, alterations in consciousness, and postictal state.			
Attempt to stop the seizure if one occurs again; keep the child upright.			
Do not place anything in child's mouth during the seizure.			
Place child in a side-lying position; suction the oral cavity and posterior oropharynx as needed.			
Closely monitor hemoglobin and platelet count.			
Observe for hyperthermia, hypertension and respiratory depression.			

Three days later, 11:00 am

6. The child is stabilized and has completed the comprehensive neurological evaluation. The evaluation revealed no definitive etiology for the seizures. However, the EEG remains abnormal and the MRI study was also abnormal. He will remain on seizure medications at home and be followed by the neurology team. The child's parents are anxious and upset and concerned about taking their son home. The nurse caring for him is to begin discharge teaching today. What are the most important aspects of home care to discuss with his parents at this time? **Select all that apply.**
   A. Have the child wear a helmet to school.
   B. Have child wear medical identification.
   C. Arrange for a class presentation to all students to help with observation while at school.
   D. Educate family about characteristics of seizures, including aura, seizure activity, and postictal state.
   E. Educate family about safety precautions before and during a seizure, including side-lying positioning, padding area if needed, and not placing items in mouth or attempting to stop the seizure.
   F. Educate family about medication administration, including scheduled and as necessary (prn) medications and potential side effects of medications.
   G. Arrange for social worker to meet with family to assess emotional and financial needs.
   H. Consider consultation with child life specialist to assist with education of school personnel and classmates.
   I. Have eyes-on supervision when swimming in pools and an adult within arm's reach in natural bodies of water.
   J. Use protective helmet and padding during bicycle riding, skateboarding, and in-line skating.

QUALITY PATIENT OUTCOMES: Seizures

- Etiology of seizure determined
- Seizures controlled or reduced in frequency and severity
- Family and child receive education to manage seizures
- Child adhering to treatment
- Side effects of treatment minimized

The child must be protected from injury during the seizure. Nursing observations made during the event provide valuable information for diagnosis and management of the disorder (see Emergency Treatment box).

It is impossible to physically stop a seizure once it has begun, and no attempt should be made to do so. The nurse must remain calm, stay with the child, and prevent the child from injury during the seizure. If possible, isolate the child from the view of others by closing a door or curtain. A seizure can be upsetting to the child, other visitors, and their families. If other persons are present, reassure them that everything is being done for the child. After the seizure, they can be given a simple explanation about the event as needed.

If the nurse is able to reach the child in time, a child who is standing or seated in a chair is eased to the floor immediately. Do not remove a child from a wheelchair. During (and sometimes after) a tonic-clonic seizure, the swallowing reflex is lost, salivation increases, and the tongue is hypotonic. Therefore the child is at risk for aspiration and airway occlusion. Placing the child on the side facilitates drainage and helps maintain a patent airway. Suctioning of the oral cavity and posterior oropharynx may be necessary. Take vital signs and allow the child to rest. When feasible, the child is integrated into the environment as soon as possible. Sending a child with a chronic seizure disorder home from school is not necessary unless requested by the parents.

! NURSING ALERT

Do not move or forcefully restrain the child during a tonic-clonic seizure, and do not place a solid object between the child's teeth.

Seizure precautions are required for children who are known to have seizures or who are under observation for seizures. The extent of these measures depends on the type and frequency of the seizure (Box 27.9).

Long-Term Care

Care of the child with epilepsy involves physical care and instruction on the importance of adherence to the treatment plan. Probably more significant is support and education on the potential for the development of psychosocial, educational, and emotional problems in children with epilepsy and their families. Few diseases generate as much anxiety among family, friends, and school personnel as epilepsy (Jones & Reilly, 2016). Fears and misconceptions about the disease and its treatment are common. Nursing care is directed toward educating the child and family about epilepsy and helping them develop strategies to cope with the psychologic and sociologic problems related to epilepsy.

EMERGENCY TREATMENT

Seizures

Tonic-Clonic Seizure

During the Seizure

Remain calm.
Time seizure episode.
If child is standing or seated, ease child to the floor.
Place pillow or folded blanket under child's head.
Loosen restrictive clothing.
Remove eyeglasses.
Clear area of any hazards or hard objects.
Allow seizure to end without interference.
If vomiting occurs, turn child to one side.
Do *not:*

- Attempt to restrain child or use force.
- Put anything in child's mouth.
- Give any food or liquids.

After the Seizure

Time postictal period.
Check for breathing. Check position of head and tongue.
Reposition if head is hyperextended.
If breathing is not present, give rescue breathing and call emergency medical service (EMS).
Keep child on side.
Remain with child.
Do not give food or liquids until child is fully alert and swallowing reflex has returned.
Look for medical identification, and determine what factors occurred before onset of seizure that may have been triggering factors.
Check head and body for possible injuries.
Check inside of mouth to see if tongue or lips have been bitten.

Focal Seizure With Impaired Consciousness

During the Seizure

Do not restrain the child's movements.
Remove harmful objects from area.
Redirect to safe area.
Do not agitate; instead, talk in calm, reassuring manner.
Do not expect child to follow instructions.
Watch to see if seizure generalizes.

After the Seizure

Stay with child and reassure until fully conscious.

Call EMS If

Child stops breathing.
There is evidence of injury or child is diabetic or pregnant.
Seizure lasts for more than 5 minutes (unless seizures typically last longer than 5 minutes) and written medical order is present.
Status epilepticus occurs.
Pupils are not equal after seizure.
Child vomits continuously 30 minutes after seizure has ended (sign of possible acute problem).
Child cannot be awakened and is unresponsive to pain after seizure has ended.
Seizure occurs in water.
This is child's first seizure.

Data from Epilepsy Foundation. (2017). *Seizure first aid,* Retrieved from http://www.epilepsyfoundation.org/aboutepilepsy/firstaid/index.cfm.

BOX 27.9 Seizure Precautions

The extent of precautions depends on type, severity, and frequency of seizures. Precautions may include the following:

- Side rails raised when child is sleeping or resting
- Side rails and other hard objects padded
- Waterproof mattress or pad on bed or crib

Appropriate precautions during potentially hazardous activities may include the following:

- Swimming with a companion
- Showers preferred; bathing only with close supervision
- Use of protective helmet and padding during bicycle riding, skateboarding, and skating
- Supervision during use of hazardous machinery or equipment

Have child carry or wear medical identification.

Alert other caregivers to need for any special precautions.

Child may not drive or operate hazardous machinery or equipment unless seizure free for designated period (varies by state).

Children with epilepsy are prescribed antiepileptic medications, which are administered at regular intervals to maintain adequate levels in the blood. The nurse can help the parents plan the administration of the medication at convenient times, usually breakfast and dinner or bedtime, to make taking the medication as easy as possible. It is important to talk with the family about the importance of giving the antiepileptic medication as scheduled to prevent recurrent seizures. Using a pill box can prevent accidentally missing doses. The seizure threshold may be lowered during any illness but particularly with fever. Therefore parents should be aware that if their child has an illness he or she may be at increased risk for seizures. Parents should contact their health professional if their child misses medications due to vomiting.

Rectal preparations of some antiepileptic medications are highly effective when a child is unable to take oral medications because of repeated vomiting, surgery, or status epilepticus. Parents can learn to administer rectal antiepileptic medication for home treatment. Buccal and intranasal midazolam and rectal diazepam are useful adjunctive home treatments for children at risk for prolonged seizures or clusters of seizures and can minimize the need for hospitalization while enhancing parental confidence.

Usually antiepileptic medications are continued until the child has been seizure free for 2 years (Lee et al., 2017). The medication is then slowly tapered over a period of weeks to decrease the chances of precipitating a seizure.

DRUG ALERT

Vitamin D and Folic Acid Deficiency

Children taking phenobarbital or phenytoin should receive adequate vitamin D and folic acid because deficiencies of both have been associated with these drugs. Phenytoin should not be taken with milk.

Nurses should educate the child and parents about the possible adverse reactions to the medications used to treat seizures. Parents must understand the rare but potentially serious side effect of allergic reaction to the medication. They must immediately report rashes to the child's health care provider. More common but less serious potential side effects include excessive sleepiness, changes in appetite, and worsening behavior and mood. Parents should be encouraged to share their observations with their child's health care provider. Parents should understand that the child needs periodic physical assessment. Depending on the medication prescribed, some children will need regular testing of their complete blood count and liver functions. Possible adverse effects on the hematopoietic system, liver, and kidneys may be reflected in symptoms such as fever, sore throat, enlarged lymph nodes, jaundice, and bleeding (e.g., abnormally easy bruising, petechiae, ecchymosis, and epistaxis). The most common cause of status epilepticus in children taking antiepileptic medications is missed medication.

Children with epilepsy are not at increased risk for injury with the exception of head injury (Baca, Vickrey, Vassar, et al., 2013). The degree to which activities are restricted is individualized for each child and depends on the type, frequency, and severity of the seizures; the child's response to therapy; and the length of time the seizures have been controlled. To prevent head injuries, children should always wear helmets and other safety devices when participating in sports, such as biking, skiing, skateboarding, horseback riding, and skating. Only children with frequent seizures must avoid these activities. Children with epilepsy should avoid activities involving heights, such as climbing on play structures taller than they are. Submersion injuries are a serious risk for children with a history of seizures. Children should never be left alone in the bathtub, even for a few seconds. Older children and adolescents should be encouraged to use a shower and reminded not to lock the bathroom door when showering. They must have eyes-on supervision at all times when swimming.

Because the child is encouraged to attend school, camp, and other normal activities, the school nurse and teachers should be made aware of the child's condition and therapy. They can help ensure regularity of medication administration and provision of any special care the child might need. Teachers, child care providers, camp counselors, youth organization leaders, coaches, and other adults who assume responsibility for children should be instructed on care of the child during a seizure so that they can react calmly, provide for the child's safety, and influence the attitude of the child's peers.

DRUG ALERT

Rectal Antiepileptic Medications

Rectal preparations of some antiepileptic medications are highly effective when a child is unable to take oral medications because of repeated vomiting, gastrointestinal surgery, or status epilepticus. Parents can learn to administer rectal antiepileptic medication for home treatment. Rectal diazepam is a useful adjunctive home treatment for children at risk for prolonged seizures or clusters of seizures. It also minimizes hospitalization and enhances parental confidence.

Triggering Factors

Careful and detailed documentation of seizures over time may indicate a pattern of seizures. About half of people age 12 years and older with epilepsy can recognize at least one trigger for their seizures (Wassenaar, Kasteleijn-Nolst Trenite, de Haan, et al., 2014). When this occurs, the child, nurse, or responsible adult can intervene to make changes in the lifestyle or environment that may prevent seizures or decrease their frequency. Often the necessary changes are simple but can make an enormous difference in the lives of the child and family.

The most precipitating factors for seizures in children include physical and psychologic stress, sleep deprivation, fever, and illness (Novakova, Harris, Ponnusamy, et al., 2013). Other precipitating factors include flickering lights, menstrual cycle, stimulant recreational drugs, and alcohol (Wassenaar et al., 2014). Some individuals have pattern-sensitive or photosensitive epilepsy, that is, seizures precipitated by changes in dark-light patterns, such as those that occur with a flash on a camera, automobile headlights, reflections of light on snow or water, sunlight filtered through leafy trees, or rotating blades on a fan. Most of these individuals have absence, myoclonic, or generalized tonic-clonic seizures. A small minority of children have seizures while playing video games. Only these children need to be restricted from playing video games (see Critical Thinking Case Study).

CRITICAL THINKING CASE STUDY

Seizures

Jane is a 14-year-old girl with focal epilepsy with focal seizures with impaired awareness. Her seizures have been well controlled for the past 6 years on monotherapy, with only an occasional breakthrough seizure every 3 or 4 months, often in association with a concurrent illness. Six months ago she entered high school. She is active with cheerleading and practices for 2 hours after school each day. In addition, she is taking honors English and math classes, both of which have daily homework. Jane typically does homework until midnight and gets up at 6 AM for school. For the past 3 months she has had an increasing number of seizures and is now having at least one seizure per week. She has not had any recent illnesses. Her physical and neurologic examination is normal.

Initial Assessment. Should there be concern for the increase in seizures? What could be causing this?

Clinical Reasoning. What interventions should be explored and how will you include Jane in the plans?

Teaching Points

- Precipitating factors for seizures include physical and psychologic stress, sleep deprivation, fever, and illness.
- Careful and detailed documentation of seizures over time may indicate a pattern of seizures.
- Adolescents can often identify the triggers that cause their seizures.

Critical Thinking Answers

Initial Assessment. Changes with starting high school could be a precipitating factor for the increased number of seizures Jane is experiencing. Exploring this further with her will be important, and working together to establish ways to decrease her stress is important. Her sleep pattern has changed, and strategies to improve sleep hygiene should be explored.

Clinical Reasoning. Common precipitating factors for seizures in children and adolescents include physical and psychologic stress. Jane is now in high school with many new experiences that could be new stressors for her.

Family Support

Parental attitudes and management of a child with a seizure disorder vary. Whether the seizures result from illness, injury, or unknown cause, the parents may feel guilt, anxiety, and even humiliation. They want to know if the seizures will affect their child's ability to learn and develop. Many persons erroneously associate epilepsy with mental deficiency. Seizures commonly accompany other manifestations of severe brain damage from disease or injury, but children with seizures, like any population of healthy children, display a wide range of intelligence.

Parents also wonder how the illness will affect their child's future. The answer to this question depends on the cause of the seizures and other comorbid conditions. In many cases parents can be reassured that the illness will not shorten their child's life and that their child can attend school, marry, and have children. The child may need vocational guidance. Parents need to become familiar with the laws in their state regarding any limitations imposed on people with epilepsy. For children who are severely impaired, the family needs to become familiar with local early childhood programs. The nurse should emphasize that the seizures can be controlled or greatly reduced in the large majority of affected children.

Encourage a healthy attitude toward the child and the condition and help the parents feel competent in their ability to meet their responsibilities to their child. The child should be reared in the same manner as any normal child, with natural concern tempered by understanding of the need not to overprotect. Many parents refrain from correcting or punishing their child, especially if the child has had a seizure after being disciplined. The child must not be made to feel different in any way. Encourage parents to be honest and open about the disorder with their child and with others. Some parents try to conceal the nature of their child's illness because of their belief that the disorder is shameful or a disgrace to the family.

Educational materials and support groups may prove beneficial for families. The Epilepsy Foundation[b] is a national organization that works for the welfare of persons with epilepsy and their families; helps with employment and legal problems; and provides education to patients, families, and communities.

Febrile Seizures

A febrile seizure is a seizure associated with a febrile illness in the absence of a CNS infection. By definition, children who have a febrile seizure cannot have a history of afebrile seizures, must have a temperature of at least 38°C (100.4°F), and must be between the age of 6 and 60 months (Mikati & Tchapyjnikov, 2020). Febrile seizures are the most common type of seizure, affecting 2% to 4% of children (Weiss, Masur, Shinnar, et al., 2016).

There is evidence for both genetic and environmental causes of febrile seizures. Children with a family history of febrile seizures are at increased risk for both a single febrile seizure (10% to 46%) and recurrent febrile seizures (Saghazadeh, Matrangelo, & Rezaei, 2014). In some families the predisposition to febrile seizures is inherited as an autosomal dominant trait. In most families, though, the predisposition involves multiple genes that have not yet been found (Mikati & Tchapyjnikov, 2020). Environmental factors include viral illness and age under 18 months (Mewasingh, 2014).

! NURSING ALERT

If a febrile seizure lasts more than 5 minutes, parents should seek medical attention immediately. Instruct parents to call for emergency assistance (911) and not to place the child who is actively having a seizure in the car.

Most febrile seizures have stopped by the time the child is taken to a medical facility and require no treatment. There is no benefit of antiepileptic prophylaxis in these children; patients who were started on medication are exposed to several potential adverse side effects (Offringa, Newton, Cozijnsen, et al., 2017). Parents may be given a prescription to take home for a benzodiazepine for as-needed acute treatment of prolonged recurrent febrile seizures. If the child has recurrent febrile seizures that last more than 5 minutes, acute treatment

[b]8301 Professional Place, Landover, MD 20785; 800-332-1000; http://www.epilepsyfoundation.org/. In Canada: Epilepsy Canada, 2255B Queen St. E., Suite 336, Toronto, Ontario, Canada M4E 1G3; 877-734-0873; http://www.epilepsy.ca.

with rectal diazepam, buccal lorazepam, or intranasal midazolam is recommended (Silverman, Sporer, Lemieux, et al., 2017). The child whose seizure does not stop within 10 minutes of administration of acute treatment will need treatment for febrile status epilepticus with IV administration of both short-acting and long-acting antiepileptic medications.

Antipyretic therapy during febrile illness offers symptomatic relief for fever-associated symptoms but appears to be ineffective in preventing seizures (Patel, Ram, Swiderska, et al., 2015). Parental education and emotional support are important interventions. Parents need reassurance regarding the benign nature of febrile seizures. Several large studies show no difference in intelligence, memory, behavior, or academic performance in children with febrile seizures compared with either population or sibling controls (Weiss et al., 2016).

Parents need education on what to do during a seizure, that is, turn the child on his or her side, never put anything in the child's mouth, and time the seizure. Attempts to lower the temperature will not prevent a seizure. Tepid sponge baths are not recommended for several reasons: they are ineffective in significantly lowering the temperature, the shivering effect further increases metabolic output, and cooling causes discomfort to the child. Parental education and emotional support are important interventions, and information may need to be repeated, depending on the parents' anxiety and education level.

Long-term antiepileptic therapy is usually not required for children with simple febrile seizures. Children whose initial simple febrile seizure becomes febrile status epilepticus have an increased risk of subsequent febrile status epilepticus. Risk of recurrence of a simple febrile seizure is about 30% (Hesdorffer, Shinnar, Lax, et al., 2016). The risk of developing epilepsy after having simple febrile seizures is less than 3%, whereas the risk increases to 12% to 22% if the child has had prolonged febrile seizures and febrile status epilepticus. The risk of developing epilepsy for children with simple febrile seizures is increased if they have a family history of seizures (Seinfeld, Pellock, Kjeldsen, et al., 2016).

HEADACHE

Headaches are a common complaint of children. They can be either primary or secondary. Primary headaches are classified as migraine, tension-type headache, trigeminal autonomic cephalalgias, and other primary headache disorders by the International Headache Society (2018). A secondary headache is caused from another condition and should resolve once the underlying cause is treated. Headaches can be the result of a variety of conditions, including TBI, brain tumor, brain infections, cerebrovascular disorders, withdrawal from or exposure to substances, vision problems, hunger, psychiatric disorders, and medication overuse.

ASSESSMENT

It is important to determine the pattern of the headache—acute, acute recurrent, chronic progressive, or chronic nonprogressive (Langdon & DiSabella, 2017). Other assessment information includes the presence of seizures, ataxia, lethargy, weakness, nausea or vomiting, or any personality changes. Factors related to early development and past illnesses and a family history of headaches may also be pertinent. A "headache diary," which includes time of onset and termination of headaches, intensity, associated events, and actions taken and their effects, can be helpful for the patient and provider.

Clues to etiology may be found in the family history, including information about the home or social situation (e.g., divorce, separation, alcoholism, school avoidance). Thorough physical and neurologic examinations are performed. An abnormal neurologic examination or unusual neurologic symptoms indicate the need for further diagnostic tests (e.g., CT, MRI, EEG) (Hershey, Kabbouche, O'Brien, et al., 2020).

> **! NURSING ALERT**
>
> During the health history and neurologic assessment, the following abnormal signs require immediate follow-up for children:
> - The headache progresses in frequency and severity over a brief period (2 to 3 weeks).
> - It awakens the child from sleep (may also be migraine).
> - It occurs in early morning.
> - It is worse on arising.
> - It is characterized by persistent, occipital, or frontal pain.
> - It is accompanied by unexplained vomiting.
> - It is associated with a change in gait, personality, or behavior.
> - It is exacerbated by Valsalva maneuver (intensified by lowering head and straining, such as during a bowel movement, coughing, or sneezing).

Tension-type headaches are common in children. They are typically frontal, the pain is described as a pressing or tightness and nonthrobbing in character, and they are not typically accompanied by nausea or vomiting.

Management of tension-type headaches begins with headache hygiene or prevention (Gofshteyn & Stephenson, 2016). This includes adequate sleep, appropriate hydration, and regular meals and exercise. If headaches continue after the child is following a headache hygiene plan, ibuprofen is usually the most effective pharmacologic intervention. To prevent medication overuse headache, children with headaches should take no more than three doses of these medications per week (Kacperski, Kabbouche, O'Brien, et al., 2016). Biofeedback, cognitive-behavioral therapy, and relaxation techniques may be useful nonpharmacologic interventions in children with recurrent tension-type headaches (Langdon & DiSabella, 2017).

MIGRAINE HEADACHE

Migraine is in the top five common childhood diseases. Migraines can have their onset in very young children, including infants where they may manifest as colic. The onset tends to be earlier in boys than girls until puberty, when girls have a twofold increase over boys in migraines. This is thought to be due to the effects of estrogen (Langdon & DiSabella, 2017).

The exact pathophysiology of migraines is not completely known. Genetics, neurotransmitters, and neurophysiologic mechanisms appear to be involved to varying degrees (Puledda, Messina, & Goadsby, 2017). Familial hemiplegic migraine has an identified autosomal dominant genetic cause. A number of other genes have been identified in diseases that that are often accompanied by migraine (Sutherland & Griffiths, 2017). Previously, it was thought that migraine headaches were caused by dilation of cerebral blood vessels; however, this is no longer thought to be correct. There is much attention on the specific vulnerability factors of the individual that leads to neuron dysfunction and the generation of the acute attack.

Revisions in the classification of migraine headaches introduced some new terms and eliminated, renamed, or reclassified others. Migraine headaches are now classified as migraine without aura and migraine with aura; the latter category includes the following subtypes: auras and prodrome, familial hemiplegic migraine, sporadic hemiplegic migraine, and basilar-type migraine (International Headache Society, 2018).

Migraines are paroxysmal. The symptoms vary depending on age. Typical symptoms include nausea, vomiting, and abdominal pain, which are relieved by sleep. Toddlers may be seen with episodic pallor, decreased activity, and vomiting. In children the onset may be bifrontal, temporal, and bilateral or unilateral. As children and adolescents advance in age, many will develop phonophobia and/or photophobia. Compared with adults, migraine headaches in children are generally shorter in duration. If the child falls asleep during the headache, the amount of time the child is asleep is counted as part of the duration (Hershey et al., 2020). A family history of migraine is elicited in up to 90% of children with migraine; 28% of all children who have migraines experience a headache before age 15 years (Hershey et al., 2020).

Like tension-type headaches, migraine management begins with headache hygiene. Keeping a headache diary can help with identifying triggers so that they can be avoided. If these measures fail to prevent migraines, both abortive and prophylactic treatment may be needed. At the onset of the headache, the child should rest or sleep in a quiet, dark room when feasible. Migraine therapy, if administered early in the course of the headache, may provide rapid relief. Ibuprofen appears to be the safest and most effective treatment if given early (Patniyot & Gelfand, 2016). Prophylactic mediation can be considered if a child is having a migraine or more per week. Riboflavin and magnesium have helped some children (Merison & Jacobs, 2016). Topiramate, an antiepileptic drug, has been approved by the US Food and Drug Administration for use in children to prevent migraine (Kacperski et al., 2016).

DRUG ALERT

Triptans

Triptans are serotonin agonists and are effective in the abortive treatment of migraines. Almotriptan, zolmitriptan, and sumatriptan are approved by the US Food and Drug Administration for use in children ages 12 to 17 years, and rizatriptan is approved for children ages 6 years and older (Patniyot & Gelfand, 2016).

The outlook for a child with migraine is good, but the child and parents should be informed that predisposition to the headaches may be lifelong. Severe headaches can adversely affect the child's routine activities of daily living, including family relations and school. Many children and families will benefit from psychotherapy.

THE CHILD WITH CEREBRAL MALFORMATION

HYDROCEPHALUS

Hydrocephalus is a condition caused by an imbalance in the production and absorption of CSF in the ventricular system. The causes of hydrocephalus are varied and include either congenital (e.g., myelomeningocele, intrauterine viral infection [cytomegalovirus, toxoplasmosis], aqueduct stenosis) or acquired conditions (e.g., intraventricular hemorrhage, tumor, CSF infection, head injury). The result is either (1) impaired absorption of CSF fluid within the subarachnoid space, obliteration of the subarachnoid cisterns, or malfunction of the arachnoid villi (nonobstructive or communicating hydrocephalus); or (2) obstruction to the flow of CSF through the ventricular system (obstructive or noncommunicating hydrocephalus) (Kinsman & Johnston, 2020).

Any imbalance of secretion and absorption causes an increased accumulation of CSF in the ventricles, which become dilated (ventriculomegaly) and compress the brain tissue against the surrounding rigid bony cranium. When this occurs before fusion of the cranial sutures, it causes enlargement of the skull and dilation of the ventricles. In children younger than 12 years old, previously closed sutures, especially the sagittal suture, may become diastatic or opened. After 12 years old, the sutures are fused and will not open.

Pathophysiology

To appreciate the condition, an understanding of the dynamics of CSF, and the relationship between the various structures that make up the ventricular and subarachnoid spaces is necessary. The two mechanisms by which CSF is formed are secretion by the choroid plexuses and lymphatic-like drainage by the extracellular fluid of the brain. CSF circulates throughout the ventricular system and is then absorbed within the subarachnoid spaces by a mechanism that is not entirely clear.

Ventricular Circulation

The fluid flows from the lateral ventricles through the foramen of Monro to the third ventricle, where it combines with fluid secreted into the third ventricle. From there CSF flows through the aqueduct of Sylvius into the fourth ventricle, where more fluid is formed; it then leaves the fourth ventricle by way of the lateral foramen of Luschka and the midline foramen of Magendie and flows into the cisterna magna. From the cisterna magna, CSF flows to the cerebral and cerebellar subarachnoid spaces where it is absorbed. A large portion is absorbed through the arachnoid villi, but the sinuses, veins, brain substance, and dura also participate in absorption.

The terms *communicating* and *noncommunicating hydrocephalus* traditionally referred to obstructive and nonobstructive types of hydrocephalus. Because other diagnostic methods are now used, the terms may be used only as a reference point in the diagnosis. Hydrocephalus can also be classified according to the cause as either congenital or acquired hydrocephalus.

Etiology

Rarely, a tumor of the choroid plexus causes increased CSF secretion. Most cases of hydrocephalus are a result of developmental malformations. Although the defect usually is apparent in early infancy, it may become evident at any time from the prenatal period to late childhood or early adulthood. Other causes include neoplasms, CNS infections (e.g., meningitis, encephalitis), and trauma (e.g., shaken baby syndrome). An obstruction to the normal flow can occur at any point in the CSF pathway to produce increased pressure and dilation of the pathways proximal to the site of obstruction.

Developmental defects (e.g., Chiari malformation [see following discussion], aqueductal stenosis, aqueductal gliosis, atresia of the foramina of Luschka and Magendie [Dandy-Walker malformation]) account for most cases of hydrocephalus from birth to 2 years of age. Dandy-Walker malformation involves dilation of the fourth ventricle, partial or complete absence of the cerebellar vermis, and enlargement of the posterior fossa resulting in hydrocephalus in about 80% of children with Dandy-Walker (Shankar, Zamora, & Castillo, 2016).

Hydrocephalus is so often associated with myelomeningocele that all such infants should be observed for its development. In the remaining cases there is a history of intrauterine infection (e.g., toxoplasmosis, cytomegalovirus), hemorrhage (e.g., posthemorrhagic hydrocephalus in preterm infants), and neonatal meningoencephalitis (bacterial or viral). In older children hydrocephalus is most often a result of intracranial masses (e.g., vascular anomalies, cysts, tumors), preexisting developmental defects, intracranial infections, trauma, or hemorrhage.

Chiari I and II Malformations

Chiari malformations are structural defects in the base of the skull and cerebellum. They occur when the lower cerebellum extends below the foramen magnum and into the upper spinal canal (Chiari I) or when the lower cerebellum and brain stem protrude into the spinal canal through an enlarged foramen magnum (Chiari II). Chiari I malformation does not usually cause hydrocephalus. It is usually asymptomatic until adolescence, when it can cause headaches, neck pain, frequent urination, and lower limb progressive spasticity (Kinsman & Johnston, 2020). Type II Chiari malformation is seen almost exclusively with myelomeningocele and results in obstruction of CSF flow causing the hydrocephalus.

Clinical Manifestations

The three factors that influence the clinical picture in hydrocephalus are the acuity of onset, timing of onset, and associated structural malformations. In infancy, before closure of the cranial sutures, head enlargement (increasing occipitofrontal circumference [OFC]) is the predominant sign. The signs and symptoms in early to late childhood are caused by increased ICP. Specific manifestations are related to the location of the lesion.

Infancy

In infants with hydrocephalus, the head grows at an abnormal rate, although the first signs may be bulging fontanels with or without head enlargement (Fig. 27.7). The anterior fontanel is tense, often bulging, and nonpulsatile. Scalp veins are dilated, especially when the infant cries. With the increase in intracranial volume, the bones of the skull become thin and the sutures become palpably separated to produce the cracked-pot sound (***Macewen sign***) on percussion of the skull. In severe cases there may be frontal protrusion, or ***frontal bossing***, with depressed eyes, and the eyes may be rotated downward, producing a ***setting-sun sign***, in which the sclera may be visible above the iris. Pupils are sluggish, with unequal response to light.

The infant is irritable and lethargic, feeds poorly, and may display changes in LOC, opisthotonos (often extreme), and lower extremity spasticity. The infant cries when picked up or rocked and quiets when allowed to lie still. Early infantile reflexes may persist, and normally expected responses may not appear, indicating failure in the development of normal cortical inhibition.

Infants with Chiari malformations may exhibit behaviors that reflect cranial nerve dysfunction as a result of brainstem compression, including swallowing difficulties, stridor, apnea, aspiration, respiratory difficulties, and arm weakness.

The preterm infant with posthemorrhagic hydrocephalus may not exhibit any clinical signs and symptoms other than a gradual increase in head circumference. Alternatively, the nurse may note subtle seizure activity and alternating levels of consciousness. Ventricular size can be assessed by ultrasonography or CT scanning in preterm infants at high risk for intraventricular hemorrhage.

If hydrocephalus is allowed to progress, development of lower brainstem functions is disrupted, as manifested by difficulty in sucking and feeding and a shrill, brief, high-pitched cry. Eventually the skull becomes enlarged, and the cortex is destroyed. If the hydrocephalus is rapidly progressive, symptoms may include emesis, somnolence, seizures, and cardiopulmonary distress.

Childhood

The signs and symptoms in early to late childhood are caused by increased ICP, and specific manifestations are related to the location of the focal lesion. Most commonly resulting from posterior fossa neoplasms and aqueduct stenosis, the clinical manifestations are primarily those associated with space-occupying lesions (i.e., headache on awakening with improvement after emesis, papilledema, strabismus, extrapyramidal tract signs such as ataxia). As with infants, the child is irritable, lethargic, apathetic, confused, and often incoherent. In one of the congenital defects with later onset (by age 3 months), Dandy-Walker syndrome, characteristic manifestations are a bulging occiput, nystagmus, ataxia, and cranial nerve palsies.

Manifestations of Chiari malformation in children older than 3 years of age are related to spinal cord dysfunction rather than brainstem compression as observed in infants. Scoliosis proximal to the level of the myelomeningocele (usually associated with Chiari malformation) and development of upper extremity spasticity, which may progress to weakness and atrophy, are common. Cranial nerve deficits are rare.

Diagnostic Evaluation

Antenatal diagnosis of fetal ventriculomegaly, which is associated with postnatal hydrocephalus, is possible with fetal ultrasonography as early as 14 to 15 weeks of gestation, often followed by fetal MRI (Pisapia, Sinha, Zarnow, et al., 2017). There are ongoing trials in carefully selected pregnant women of fetal surgery for prevention of in utero brain damage from in utero hydrocephalus. Initial results were not

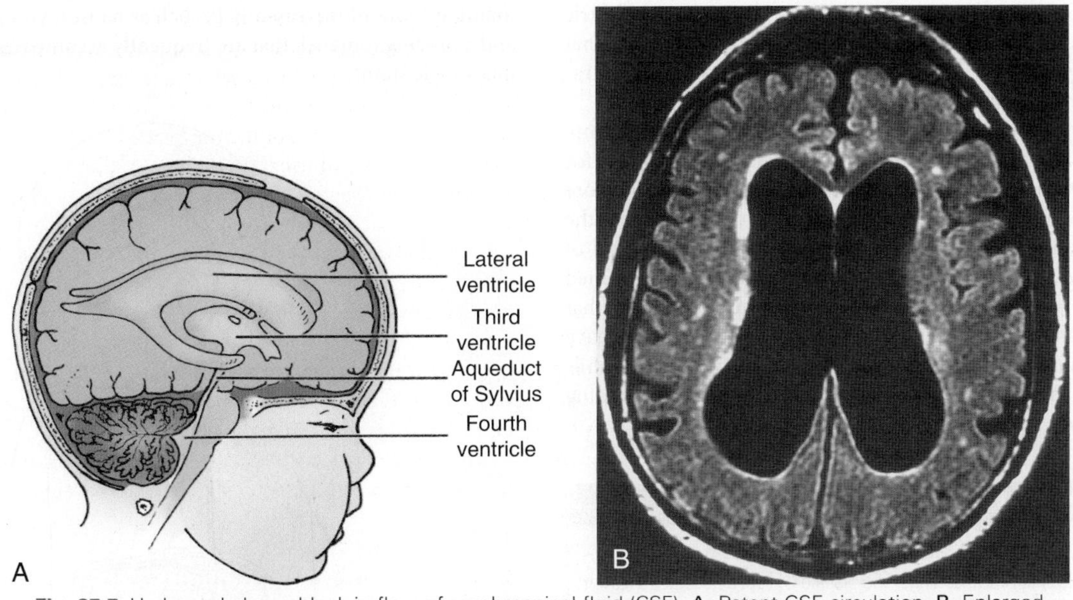

Fig. 27.7 Hydrocephalus: a block in flow of cerebrospinal fluid (CSF). **A**, Patent CSF circulation. **B**, Enlarged lateral and third ventricles caused by obstruction of circulation—stenosis of aqueduct of Sylvius.

promising, but recently outcomes have improved (Elbabaa, Gildehaus, Pierson, et al., 2017). Delivery is not currently recommended until fetal lung maturity has been achieved.

In infancy the diagnosis of hydrocephalus is based on head circumference that crosses one or more percentile lines on the head measurement chart within a period of 2 to 4 weeks and on associated neurologic signs that are progressive. However, other diagnostic studies are needed to localize the site of CSF obstruction. Routine daily head circumference measurements are carried out in infants with myelomeningocele, hemorrhage, or intrauterine viral or CNS infections. In evaluation of a preterm infant, specially adapted head circumference charts are consulted to distinguish abnormal head growth from rapid but normal head growth.

The primary diagnostic tools for detecting hydrocephalus in older infants and children are CT and MRI. Mild sedation or general anesthesia is usually required for children under age 8 years or with neurodevelopmental disabilities because the child must remain absolutely still for an accurate study. Diagnostic evaluation of children who have symptoms of hydrocephalus after infancy is similar to that used in those with a suspected intracranial tumor. In the neonate, echoencephalography is useful in comparing the ratio of lateral ventricle to cortex.

Problems in differential diagnosis are related to the child whose head circumference is greater than the 95th percentile but whose head growth parallels the normal growth curve. It is sometimes valuable to measure the parental OFC to detect a possible normal familial characteristic (benign familial megalencephaly) (see Table 27.1 for diagnostic tests for neurologic evaluation).

Therapeutic Management

The treatment of hydrocephalus is directed toward relief of ventricular pressure, treatment of the cause of the ventriculomegaly, treatment of associated complications, and management of problems related to the effect of the disorder on psychomotor development. The treatment is, with few exceptions, surgical.

Surgical Treatment

Improved neurosurgical techniques have established surgical treatment as the therapy of choice in almost all cases of hydrocephalus. This is accomplished by direct removal of an obstruction, such as resection of a neoplasm, cyst, or hematoma, or, in rare instances of fluid overproduction, by choroid plexus extirpation (plexectomy or electric coagulation). However, most children require a shunt procedure that provides primary drainage of the CSF from the ventricles to an extracranial compartment, usually the peritoneum.

Most shunt systems consist of a ventricular catheter, a flush pump, a unidirectional flow valve, and a distal catheter. All are radiopaque for easy visualization after placement, and all are tested for accuracy before insertion. A reservoir is frequently added to allow direct access to the ventricular system for administration of medications and removal of fluid. In all models the valves are designed to open at a predetermined intraventricular pressure and close when the pressure falls below that level, thus preventing backflow of fluid. Most shunts now in use have differential pressure and adjustable programmable valves with capability for changing the pressures with an external magnet, thus avoiding additional surgery.

! NURSING ALERT

Tablet computers, such as iPads, and magnetic toys may interfere with magnetically programmable shunt valve settings. They should be kept at least 2.5 cm from the shunt's valve (Strahle, Selzer, Muraszko, et al., 2012)

The standard procedure for many years has been the ***ventriculoperitoneal (VP) shunt***, especially in neonates and young infants (Fig. 27.8). There is greater allowance for excess tubing, which minimizes the number of revisions needed as the child grows. Because it requires repeated lengthening, the ventriculoatrial (VA) shunt (ventricle to right atrium) is reserved for older children who have attained most of their somatic growth and children with abdominal pathologic conditions. The VA shunt is contraindicated in children with cardiopulmonary disease or elevated CSF protein.

The initial shunt is placed when indicated based on individual assessment. The timing of revisions varies widely. In most instances, revisions are performed when physical signs indicate shunt malfunction (i.e., signs of elevated ICP). Sometimes revisions are planned for specific times during development. The initial success rate is relatively high. However, shunts are associated with complications that interfere with continued shunt function or that threaten the child's life.

Endoscopic third ventriculostomy (ETV) is a procedure that has potential for allowing greater independence from VA or VP shunting in children with obstructive hydrocephalus. ETV involves creating a small opening in the floor of the third ventricle, allowing CSF to flow freely through the previously blocked ventricle. Studies to date have not demonstrated improved short-term outcomes with ETV compared with VP shunting (Kulkarni, Sgouros, Constantini, et al., 2016). Long-term outcomes need to be studied. VP shunts have a risk of infection and shunt failure, whereas ETV does not; however, for the foreseeable future, placement of a VP shunt for treatment of hydrocephalus remains a frequent neurosurgical procedure (Venable, Rossi, Morgan Jones, et al., 2016).

Complications

The major complications of VP shunts are infection and malfunction. All shunts are subject to mechanical difficulties, such as kinking, plugging, or separation and migration of tubing. Malfunction is most often caused by mechanical obstruction either within the ventricles from particulate matter (tissue or exudate) or at the distal end from thrombosis or displacement as a result of growth. Functional obstruction of a shunt's antisiphon device remains a common complication. About 22% of shunt failures are reported within the first 90 days, the majority of these within the first month (Venable et al., 2016). The child with a shunt obstruction often is seen in an emergency visit with clinical manifestations of increased ICP, such as nausea, vomiting, irritability, and a bulging fontanel, that are frequently accompanied by worsening neurologic status.

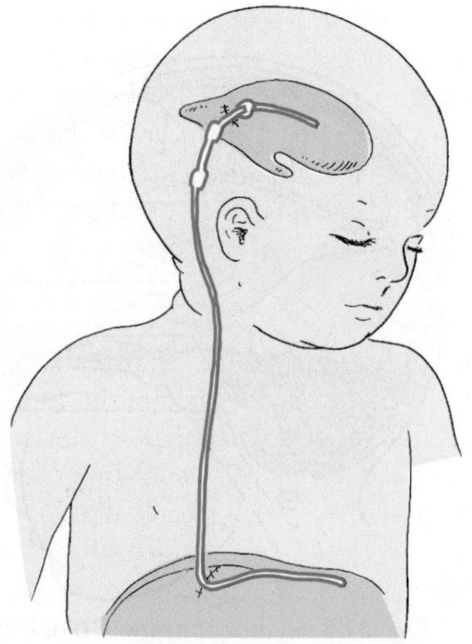

Fig. 27.8 Ventriculoperitoneal shunt. Catheter is threaded beneath skin.

One of the most common and serious complications, shunt infection, can occur at any time, but the period of greatest risk is within the first month after placement (Månsson, Johansson, Ziebell, et al., 2017). Within 2 years, shunt infection rates are reported to be approximately 5% to 10% (Månsson et al., 2017). Infections include sepsis, bacterial endocarditis, wound infection, shunt nephritis, meningitis, and ventriculitis, and may be a result of intercurrent infections at the time of shunt placement. Brain abscess associated with colonic perforation and infection with a gram-negative enteric organism suggests an ascending shunt infection in a child who has a VP shunt. Meningitis and ventriculitis are of greatest concern because any complicating CNS infection is a significant predictor of future intellectual disability. Infection is treated with antibiotics administered intravenously or intrathecally for a minimum of 7 to 10 days. The use of perioperative antibiotic prophylaxis or antibiotic-impregnated shunts has significantly decreased shunt infection rates, particularly acute infections, among all age ranges of patients and all types of shunts (Månsson et al., 2017). In addition, measures to reduce the number of people in the operating room and strictly enforced hand washing can help. A persistent infection may require removal of the shunt until the infection is controlled, and an EVD is used until CSF is sterile. EVD allows removal of CSF from a tube placed in the child's ventricle that flows by gravity into a collection device.

The primary reasons for inserting an EVD include unstable status, increased ICP that is difficult to stabilize, or infection from an existing VP shunt. The EVD may drain CSF intermittently or continuously according to need. The EVD is a closed system made up of transparent pliable tubing that should be labeled, a collection bag, and at times a drip chamber between the tubing and the collection bag. The EVD is placed at the level of the child's external auditory meatus with the head at a 20- to 30-degree elevation, depending on physician preference. Elevating the EVD above this level decreases the flow of CSF, and placing the device below the level of the external meatus increases the flow. Ambulation or sitting up in bed or a chair usually requires that the tubing be clamped to prevent imbalance in CSF drainage. In addition, the EVD is a closed sterile system. Aseptic technique should be used during any manipulation or maintenance of the EVD system, such as in relation to emptying the device or changing the scalp dressing (Hepburn-Smith et al., 2016). Accurate and frequent documentation of the incision site; amount, color, and consistency of drainage into the device; and the child's vital and neurologic signs are an important part of the nursing care.

Another serious shunt-related complication is subdural hematoma caused by too-rapid reduction of ICP and, in some cases, tentorial herniation as a result of imbalance in CSF drainage. These complications can be averted by careful assessment of ICP before insertion of the shunt and use of correct valvular pressure. Other complications that may occur include peritonitis, abdominal abscesses, perforation of abdominal organs by catheter or trocar (at the time of insertion), fistulas, hernias, and ileus. Some children require shunt lengthening as body growth occurs. This procedure usually involves replacing the distal catheter below the valve.

Prognosis

The prognosis of children with treated hydrocephalus depends largely on the cause of the dilated ventricles before shunt placement and the amount of irreversible brain damage before shunting (Kinsman & Johnston, 2020). Those children with isolated aqueductal stenosis usually function cognitively like their typically developing peers (Kahle, Kulkarni, Limbrick, et al., 2016). The neurologic disorders seen in children after shunting for hydrocephalus are most often due to the underlying cause of the hydrocephalus rather than the hydrocephalus itself (Paulsen, Lundar, & Lindegaard, 2015).

Survivors have a high incidence of intellectual disability and learning disorders, including challenges with memory, processing, and visual-spatial skills requiring special education services. Tumors, meningitis, and intraventricular hemorrhage are the conditions most closely associated with hydrocephalus accompanied by intellectual disability (Paulsen et al., 2015). Children with myelomeningocele or intraventricular hemorrhage often have motor disabilities. As with all pediatric neurologic conditions, social and behavior problems are common, including attention-deficit/hyperactivity disorder. Up to a third of children with hydrocephalus will have epilepsy (Kahle et al., 2016).

Surgically treated hydrocephalus in patients with little or no evidence of irreversible brain damage has a survival rate of about 80%, with most deaths occurring within the first year of treatment (Paulsen et al., 2015). Those with poor outcomes included children shunted for posthemorrhagic hydrocephalus or meningitis. Most children who require shunting must depend on the shunt for the remainder of their life.

Nursing Care Management

The infant with suspected or confirmed hydrocephalus is observed carefully for signs of increasing ventricular size and increasing ICP. In infants the head is measured daily at the point of largest measurement—the OFC (see Chapter 4 for technique). To avoid the likelihood of wide discrepancies, the point at which the measurements are taken is indicated on the head with a marking pen. Fontanels and suture lines are palpated for size, signs of bulging, tenseness, and separation. Irritability, lethargy, seizure activity, and altered vital signs and feeding behavior may indicate an advancing pathologic condition.

In older children, who are usually admitted to the hospital for elective or emergency shunt revision, the most valuable indicators of increasing ICP are an alteration in the child's LOC, complaint of headache, and changes in interaction with the environment. Changes are identified by observing and comparing present behavior with customary behavior, sleep patterns, developmental capabilities, and habits obtained through a detailed history and a baseline assessment. This baseline information serves as a guide for postoperative assessment and evaluation of shunt function.

The nurse is responsible for preparing the child for diagnostic tests such as MRI or a CT scan and for assisting with procedures such as a ventricular tap, which is often performed to relieve excessive pressure and to obtain CSF during the preoperative period. Sedation is required because the child must remain absolutely still during diagnostic testing. A variety of drugs are available for sedation (see Chapter 22 for preparing children for procedures). If surgery is anticipated, IV infusions should not be placed in a scalp vein.

Postoperative Care

In addition to routine postoperative care and observation, the infant or child is positioned carefully on the unoperated side to prevent pressure on the shunt valve. The child remains flat to help avert complications resulting from too-rapid reduction of intracranial fluid. The surgeon indicates the position to be maintained and the extent of activity allowed.

The nurse continues observation for signs of increased ICP that indicate obstruction of the shunt. Neurologic assessment includes pupil dilation (pressure causes compression or stretching of the oculomotor nerve, producing dilation on the same side as the pressure) and blood pressure (hypoxia to the brainstem causes variability in these vital signs). The nurse also observes for abdominal distention and constipation because CSF may cause peritonitis or a postoperative ileus as a complication of distal catheter placement.

Because infection is the greatest hazard of the postoperative period, nurses are continually on the alert for the usual manifestations of CSF infection, including elevated temperature, poor feeding, vomiting, decreased responsiveness, and seizure activity. There may be signs of local inflammation at the operative sites and along the shunt tract. Antibiotics are administered by the IV route as ordered, and the nurse may need to assist with intraventricular instillation. Inspect the incision site for leakage, and test any suspected drainage for glucose, an indication of CSF.

Family Support

Specific needs and concerns of parents during periods of hospitalization are related to the reason for the child's hospitalization (e.g., shunt revision, infection, diagnosis) and the diagnostic and surgical procedures to which the child must be subjected. Parents may have little understanding of anatomy; therefore they need further explanation and reinforcement of information that was given to them by the physician, neurosurgeon, and nurse practitioners, including information about what to expect. They are especially frightened of any procedure that involves the brain. The fear of disability or brain damage is real and pervasive. Nurses can calm their anxiety with explanations of the rationale underlying the various nursing and medical activities such as positioning or testing and by simply being available and willing to listen to their concerns.

To prepare for the child's discharge and home care, instruct the parents on how to recognize signs that indicate shunt malfunction or infection. Active children may have injuries, such as a fall, that can damage the shunt, and the tubing may pull out of the distal insertion site or become disconnected during normal growth. Contact sports such as football, rugby, boxing, and wrestling are usually prohibited if a person has a VP shunt; other sports such as swimming, soccer, and track are acceptable and even encouraged for the child's physical and emotional health. Families should consult with their child's neurosurgeon or neurosurgery nurse practitioner about activities after discharge, as providers vary in their recommendations. Helmets must be worn for skating, skiing, biking, and skateboarding. It is also important for the nurse to encourage families to enroll infants and toddlers with hydrocephalus into an early childhood development program to monitor their development and quickly address any signs that they are not keeping up with their typically developing peers.

The management of hydrocephalus in a child is a demanding task for both the family and health professionals. Helping the family cope with the child's difficulties is an important nursing responsibility. Children with hydrocephalus have lifelong special health care needs. The nurse can provide optimum primary health care, including teaching families hand hygiene and hand washing, advice on immunizations, treatments for common infectious conditions, or child care and school precautions. The overall aim is to establish realistic goals and an appropriate educational program that will assist the child in achieving the maximum potential. Families can be referred to community agencies for support and guidance. The National Hydrocephalus Foundation[c] and the Hydrocephalus Association[d] in the United States and the Spina Bifida and Hydrocephalus Association of Canada[e] provide information on the condition for families; the National Hydrocephalus Foundation also assists interested groups in establishing local organizations.

Anticipatory guidance will prepare parents for possible problems and help them avoid being overprotective of the child. Few restrictions need be placed on the child's activities (mainly contact sports), and the child is encouraged to live as would any other youngster of the same age and abilities. Parents need support and encouragement in coping with the child and problems the child may encounter in relationships with peers and others. Reactions of other children when the child has a noticeably enlarged head or requires special restrictions are stressful for both the child and the parents (see Chapter 19 for problems and coping with a child with a disability).

[c]12413 Centralia Road, Lakewood, CA 90715-1653; 888-857-3434; http://www.nhfonline.org.
[d]4340 East West Highway, Suite 905, Bethesda, MD 20814; 888-598-3789; http://www.hydroassoc.org.
[e]Suite 647–167 av. Lombard Avenue, Winnipeg MB, Canada R3B 0V3; 800-565-9488; http://www.sbhac.ca.

CLINICAL JUDGMENT AND NEXT-GENERATION NCLEX® EXAMINATION-STYLE QUESTIONS

1. A nurse is assigned to complete the initial assessment for a 5-year-old child with a basilar skull fracture from a fall this morning. He was taken by ambulance to the Emergency Department after his older brother found him; he had tried to climb a tree in their yard and fell backwards onto the ground. When he arrived at the Emergency Department, he was awake and knew his name. Because of the severity of this type of fracture the nurse completes a comprehensive history and assessment, and findings are found below. Which are clinical manifestations of severe acute head injury and need **immediate** intervention? **Select all that apply.**
   - **A.** Retinal hemorrhages
   - **B.** Bleeding from the ear
   - **C.** Respiration = 16 breaths/min
   - **D.** Pulse oximetry 96% room air
   - **E.** Clear fluid leaking from the nose
   - **F.** Oral temperature = 100.4 F (38 C)
   - **G.** Unsteady gait when moving from wheelchair to stretcher

2. A 7-year-old child is hospitalized with fever, chills, headache and vomiting the past 2 days. She is irritable when awake but sleeps most of the time and is extremely sensitive to the light in the room. On examination she exhibits nuchal rigidity with + Kernig and Brudzinski signs. A lumbar puncture was performed to confirm the diagnosis. **Choose the most likely options for the information missing from the statements below by selecting from the lists of options provided.** This child's diagnosis most likely is ____1____. Because of this diagnosis initial therapeutic management includes____2____. There are routine vaccinations available to prevent bacterial meningitis and includes the ____3____ vaccine for all children beginning at 2 months of age.

Options for 1	Options for 2	Options for 3
Aplastic crisis	Intubation	meningococcal
Bacterial meningitis	Suctioning	pneumococcal
Acute chest syndrome	Isolation	polio
Reye syndrome	Vaccination	tetanus
COVID 19	blood transfusion	pertussis

3. You are working with a pediatric nurse who has just transferred to the pediatric clinic from adult surgery. You are role-playing phone triage with a mother of a 10-month-old infant with a head injury. The infant was seen in the emergency center yesterday and sent home after observation. You ascertain that the nurse needs more teaching based on what response? **Select all that apply.**
   A. "Another physical examination should take place in 1 or 2 days."
   B. "After initial physical examination, if there was no loss of consciousness with the head injury the infant is observed at home."
   C. "If there is a language barrier, written instructions can be given, followed by discharge."
   D. "Parents should call the doctor if their child has any of these signs: blurred vision, walking unsteadily, or is hard to awaken."
   E. "An ultrasound of the head is needed to provide important follow-up to determine if your child had bleeding into the head."
   F. "Parents should give only clear liquids to the infant for the next 24 hours."

4. The nurse is caring for an infant with hydrocephalus who is postoperative day 1 from a shunt revision. A complete assessment is performed by the nurse and findings are below. Which history and assessment findings require **immediate** follow-up for this infant. **Select all that apply.**
   A. Pupil dilation
   B. Abdominal distention
   C. Easily awakened and cries
   D. Sleeping quietly
   E. Temperature of 38.2°C (100.8°F)
   F. Decrease in heart rate over the last hour

REFERENCES

Abend, N. S., & Loddenkemper, T. (2014). Pediatric status epilepticus management. *Current Opinion in Pediatrics, 26*(6), 668–674.

Ahmad, B. S., Petty, S. J., Gorelik, A., et al. (2017). Bone loss with antiepileptic drug therapy: A twin and sibling study. *Osteoporosis International, 28*(9), 2591–2600.

Babikian, T., Merkley, T., Savage, R. C., et al. (2015). Chronic aspects of pediatric traumatic brain injury: Review of the literature. *Journal of Neurotrauma, 32*(23), 1849–1860.

Baca, C. B., Vickrey, B. G., Vassar, S. D., et al. (2013). Injuries in adolescents with childhood-onset epilepsy compared with sibling controls. *The Journal of Pediatrics, 163*(6), 1684–1691.

Ban, L., Fleming, K. M., Doyle, P., et al. (2015). Congenital anomalies in children of mothers taking antiepileptic drugs with and without periconceptional high dose folic acid use: A population-based cohort study. *PLoS ONE, 10*(7), e0131130.

Barr, R. G. (2014). Crying as a trigger for abusive head trauma: A key to prevention. *Pediatric Radiology, 44*(suppl. 4), S559–S564.

Beauchamp, M. H., & Anderson, V. (2013). Cognitive and psychopathological sequelae of pediatric traumatic brain injury. *Handbook of Clinical Neurology, 112*, 913–920.

Bennett, T. D., DeWitt, P. E., Greene, T. H., et al. (2017). Function outcome after intracranial pressure monitoring for children with severe traumatic brain injury. *JAMA pediatrics, 171*(10), 965–972.

Berg, A. T., & Rychlik, K. (2015). The course of childhood-onset epilepsy over the first two decades: A prospective, longitudinal study. *Epilepsia, 56*(1), 40–48.

Blaszczyk, B., Lasoń, W., & Czuczwar, S. J. (2015). Antiepileptic drugs and adverse skin reactions: An update. *Pharmacological Reports, 67*(3), 426–434.

Bloomer, M. J., Endacott, R., Copnell, B., et al. (2016). 'Something normal in a very, very abnormal environment' – Nursing work to honour the life of dying infants and children in neonatal and paediatric intensive care in Australia. *Intensive and Critical Care Nursing, 33*, 5–11.

Blume, H. K. (2017). Childhood headache: A brief review. *Pediatric Annals, 46*(4), e155–e165.

Bonfield, C. M., Naran, S., Adetayo, O. A., et al. (2014). Pediatric skull fractures: The need for surgical intervention, characteristics, complications, and outcomes. *Journal of Neurosurgery. Pediatrics, 14*(2), 205–211.

Braine, M. E., & Cook, N. (2017). The Glasgow Coma Scale and evidence-informed practice: A critical review of where we are and where we need to be. *Journal of Clinical Nursing, 26*(1–2), 280–293.

Braun, K. P., & Schmidt, D. (2014). Stopping antiepileptic drugs in seizure-free patients. *Current Opinion in Neurology, 27*(2), 219–226.

Brigo, F., Nardone, R., Tezzon, F., et al. (2015). Nonintravenous midazolam versus intravenous or rectal diazepam for the treatment of early status epilepticus: A systematic review with meta-analysis. *Epilepsy and Behavior: E&B, 49*, 325–336.

Burns, E., Grool, A. M., Klassen, T. P., et al. (2016). Scalp hematoma characteristics associated with intracranial injury in pediatric minor head injury. Academic Emergency Medicine. *Official Journal of the Society for Academic Emergency Medicine, 23*(5), 576–583.

Burrows, P., Trefan, L., Houston, R., et al. (2015). Head injury from falls in children younger than 6 years of age. *Archives of Disease in Childhood, 100*(11), 1032–1037.

Camfield, P., & Camfield, C. (2015). Incidence, prevalence and aetiology of seizures and epilepsy in children. Epileptic Disorders. *International Epilepsy Journal With Videotape, 17*(2), 117–123.

Castelblanco, R. L., Lee, M., & Hasbun, R. (2014a). Epidemiology of bacterial meningitis in the USA from 1997 to 2010: A population-based observational study.. *The Lancet. Infectious Diseases, 14*(9), 813–819.

Centers for Disease Control and Prevention. (2016). Unintentional drowning: Get the facts. Available at https://www.cdc.gov/homeandrecreationalsafety/water-safety/waterinjuries-factsheet.html. [Accessed 22 July 2017].

Centers for Disease Control and Prevention. (2017a). *TBI: Get the facts.* Retrieved from https://www.cdc.gov/traumaticbraininjury/get_the_facts.html.

Centers for Disease Control and Prevention. (2017b). *Meningococcal disease surveillance.* Retrieved from https://www.cdc.gov/meningococcal/surveillance/index.html.

Chen, C., Shi, J., Stanley, R. M., et al. (2017). US trends of ED visits for pediatric traumatic brain injuries: Implications for clinical trials. *International Journal of Environmental Research and Public Health, 14*(4), 414.

Crowcroft, N. S., & Thampi, N. (2015). The prevention and management of rabies. *British Medical Journal (Clinical Research Ed.), 350*, g7827.

Dale, R. C., Gorman, M. P., & Lim, M. (2017). Autoimmune encephalitis in children: Clinical phenomenology, therapeutics, and emerging challenges. *Current Opinion in Neurology, 30*(3), 334–344.

Dhamne, S. C., Kaye, H. L., & Rotenberg, A. (2018). Neuromodulation in epilepsy. In K. F. Swaiman, S. Ashwal, D. M. Ferriero, et al. (Eds.), *Swaiman's pediatric neurology: Principles and practice* (6th ed.). Philadelphia, PA: Elsevier.

Ding, D., Starke, R. M., Kano, H., et al. (2017). International multicenter cohort study of pediatric brain arteriovenous malformations. Part 1: Predictors of hemorrhagic presentation. *Journal of Neurosurgery. Pediatrics, 19*(2), 127–135.

Dubey, D., Sawhney, A., Greenberg, B., et al. (2015). The spectrum of autoimmune encephalopathies. *Journal of Neuroimmunology, 287*, 93–97.

Elbabaa, S. K., Gildehaus, A. M., Pierson, M. J., et al. (2017). First 60 fetal in-utero myelomeningocele repairs at Saint Louis Fetal Care Institute in the post-MOMS trial era: Hydrocephalus treatment outcomes (endoscopic third ventriculostomy versus ventriculo-peritoneal shunt). *Child's Nervous System, 33*(7), 1157–1168.

Ellis, M. J., Cordingley, D., Vis, S., et al. (2015). Vestibulo-ocular dysfunction in pediatric sports-related concussion. *Journal of Neurosurgery. Pediatrics, 16*(3), 248–255.

El-Radhi, A. S. (2015). Management of seizures in children. *The British Journal of Nursing, 24*(3), 152–155.

Fernandez, I. S., Abend, N. S., & Loddenkemper, T. (2018). Status epilepticus. In K. F. Swaiman, S. Ashwal, D. M. Ferriero, et al. (Eds.), *Swaiman's pediatric neurology: Principles and practice* (6th ed.). Philadelphia, PA: Elsevier.

Fisher, R. S., Acevedo, C., Arzimanoglou, A., et al. (2014). ILAE official report: A practical clinical definition of epilepsy. *Epilepsia, 55*(4), 475–482.

Fisher, R. S., Cross, J. H., French, J. A., et al. (2017). Operational classification of seizure types by the international league against epilepsy: Position paper of the ILAE commission for classification and terminology. *Epilepsia, 58*(4), 522–530.

Franklin, R. C., Pearn, J. H., & Peden, A. E. (2017). Drowning fatalities in childhood: The role of pre-existing medical conditions. *Archives of Disease in Childhood, 102*(10), 888–893.

Fulkerson, D. H., White, I. K., Rees, J. M., et al. (2015). Analysis of long-term (median 10.5 years) outcomes in children presenting with traumatic brain injury and an initial Glasgow Coma Scale score of 3 or 4. *Journal of Neurosurgery. Pediatrics, 16*(4), 410–419.

Gainza-Lein, M., Sanchez-Fernández, I., & Loddenkemper, T. (2017). Use of EEG in critically ill children and neonates in the United States of America. *Journal of Neurology, 264*(6), 1165–1173.

Gaw, C. E., Chounthirath, T., & Smith, G. A. (2017). Nursery product-related injuries treated in United States emergency departments. *Pediatrics, 139*(4), e20162503.

Germain, B., & Maria, B. L. (2018). Epileptic encephalopathies: Clinical aspects, molecular features and pathogenesis, therapeutic targets and translational opportunities, and future research directions. *Journal of Child Neurology, 33*(1), 7–40.

Gilchrist, J., & Parker, E. M. (2014). Racial/ethnic disparities in fatal unintentional drowning among persons aged≤ 29 years – United States, 1999–2010. *MMWR. Morbidity and Mortality Weekly Report, 63*(19), 421–426.

Glauser, T., Shinnar, S., Gloss, D., et al. (2016). Evidence-based guideline: Treatment of convulsive status epilepticus in children and adults: Report of the guideline committee of the American Epilepsy Society. *Epilepsy Currents, 16*(1), 48–61.

Gofshteyn, J. S., & Stephenson, D. J. (2016). Diagnosis and management of childhood headache. *Current Problems in Pediatric and Adolescent Health Care, 46*(2), 36–51.

Gordon, S. M., Srinivasan, L., & Harris, M. C. (2017). Neonatal meningitis: Overcoming challenges in diagnosis, prognosis, and treatment with omics. *Frontiers in Pediatrics, 5*, 139.

Grool, A. M., Aglipay, M., Momoli, F., et al. (2016). Association between early participation in physical activity following acute concussion and persistent postconcussive symptoms in children and adolescents. *JAMA: The Journal of the American Medical Association, 316*(23), 2504–2514.

Hancock, E. C., Osborne, J. P., & Edwards, S. W. (2013). Treatment of infantile spasms. *Cochrane Database of Systematic Review* (6), CD001770.

Harary, M., Dolmans, R. G. F., & Gormley, W. B. (2018). Intracranial pressure monitoring- Review and avenues for development. *Sensors, 18*(465), 1–15.

Harden, C., Tomson, T., Gloss, D., et al. (2017). Practice guideline summary: Sudden unexpected death in epilepsy incidence rates and risk factors report of the guideline development, dissemination, and implementation subcommittee of the American Academy of Neurology and the American Epilepsy Society. *Neurology, 88*(17), 1674–1680.

Hartman, M. E., & Cheifetz, I. M. (2020). Pediatric emergencies and resuscitation. In R. Kliegman, J. W. St. Geme, N. J. Blum, et al. (Eds.), *Nelson textbook of pediatrics* (21st ed.). Philadelphia PA: Elsevier.

Heckenberg, S. G., Brouwer, M. C., & van de Beek, D. (2014). Bacterial meningitis. *Handbook of Clinical Neurology, 121*, 1361–1375.

Hepburn-Smith, M., Dynkevich, I., Spektor, M., et al. (2016). Establishment of an external ventricular drain best practice guideline: The quest for a comprehensive, universal standard for external ventricular drain care. *The Journal of Neuroscience Nursing: Journal of the American Association of Neuroscience Nurses, 48*(1), 54–65.

Hershey, A. D., Kabbouche, M. A., O'Brien, H. L., et al. (2020). Headaches. In R. Kliegman, J. W. St. Geme, N. J. Blum, et al. (Eds.), *Nelson textbook of pediatrics* (21st ed.). Philadelphia PA: Elsevier.

Hesdorffer, D. C., Shinnar, S., Lax, D. N., et al. (2016). Risk factors for subsequent febrile seizures in the FEBSTAT study. *Epilepsia, 57*(7), 1042–1047.

Holmes, G. L. (2018). Generalized seizures. In K. F. Swaiman, S. Ashwal, D. M. Ferriero, et al. (Eds.), *Swaiman's pediatric neurology: Principles and practice* (6th ed.). Philadelphia, PA: Elsevier.

Hua, F., Xie, H., Worthington, H. V., et al. (2016). Oral hygiene care for critically ill patients to prevent ventilator-associated pneumonia. *Cochrane Database of Systematic Review* (10), CD008367.

Huang, K. T., Bi, W. L., Abd-El-Barr, M., et al. (2016). The neurocritical and neurosurgical care of subdural hematomas. *Neurocritical Care, 24*(2), 294–307.

Ibrahim, S. H., & Balestreri, W. F. (2020). Mitonchondrial hepatopathies. In R. M. Kliegman, J. W. St. Geme, N. J. Blum, et al. (Eds.), *Nelson textbook of pediatrics* (21st ed.). Philadelphia PA: Elsevier.

International Headache Society. (2018). *The International Classification of Headache Disorders* (3rd ed). Available at: https://www.ichd-3.org/. [Accessed 18 May 2018].

Janowski, A. B., & Hunstad, D. A. (2020a). Brain abscess. In R. M. Kliegman, J. W. St. Geme, N. J. Blum, et al. (Eds.), *Nelson textbook of pediatrics* (21st ed.). Philadelphia PA: Elsevier.

Janowski, A. B., & Hunstad, D. A. (2020b). Central nervous system infections. In R. M. Kliegman, J. W. St. Geme, N. J. Blum, et al. (Eds.), *Nelson textbook of pediatrics* (21st ed.). Philadelphia PA: Elsevier.

Janowski, A. B., & Hunstad, D. A. (2020c). Acute bacterial meningitis. In R. M. Kliegman, J. W. St. Geme, N. J. Blum, et al. (Eds.), *Nelson textbook of pediatrics* (21st ed.). Philadelphia PA: Elsevier.

Jimenez, N., Symons, R. G., Wang, J., et al. (2016). Outpatient rehabilitation for Medicaid-insured children hospitalized with traumatic brain injury. *Pediatrics, 137*(6), e20153500.

Jones, C. E., Munoz, F. M., & Spiegel, H. M. (2016). Guideline for collection, analysis and presentation of safety data in clinical trials of vaccines in pregnant women. *Vaccine, 34*(49), 5998–6006.

Jones, C., & Reilly, C. (2016). Parental anxiety in childhood epilepsy: A systematic review. *Epilepsia, 57*(4), 529–537.

Jones, K., Go, C., Boyd, J., et al. (2015). Vigabatrin as first-line treatment for infantile spasms not related to tuberous sclerosis complex. *Pediatric Neurology, 53*(2), 141–145.

Jones, K., Snead, O. C., III, Boyd, J., et al. (2015a). Adrenocorticotropic hormone versus prednisolone in the treatment of infantile spasms post vigabatrin failure. *Journal of Child Neurology, 30*(5), 595–600.

Joyce, T., & Huecker, M. R. (2019). *Pediatric abusive head trauma (Shaken Baby Syndrome).*

Kacperski, J., & Arthur, T. (2016). Management of post-traumatic headaches in children and adolescents. *Headache, 56*(1), 36–48.

Kacperski, J., Kabbouche, M. A., O'Brien, H. L., et al. (2016). The optimal management of headaches in children and adolescents. *Therapeutic Advances in Neurological Disorders, 9*(1), 53–68.

Kahle, K. T., Kulkarni, A. V., Limbrick, D. D., et al. (2016). Hydrocephalus in children. *Lancet, 387*(10020), 788–799.

Kannan, N., Quistberg, A., Wang, J., et al. (2017). Frequency of and factors associated with emergency department intracranial pressure monitor placement in severe pediatric traumatic brain injury. *Brain Inj, 31*(13–14), 1745–1752.

Kinsman, S. L., & Johnston, M. V. (2020). Hydrocephalus. In R. M. Kliegman, J. W. St. Geme, N. J. Blum, et al. (Eds.), *Nelson Textbook of Pediatrics* (21st ed.). Philadelphia PA: Elsevier.

Klevens, J., Schmidt, B., Luo, F., et al. (2017). Effect of the earned income tax credit on hospital admissions for pediatric abusive head trauma, 1995-2013. *Public Health Reports, 132*(4), 505–511.

Ku, L. C., Boggess, K. A., & Cohen-Wolkowiez, M. (2015). Bacterial meningitis in infants. *Clinics in Perinatology, 42*(1), 29–45.

Kuczynski, A., Crawford, S., Bodell, L., et al. (2013). Characteristics of post-traumatic headaches in children following mild traumatic brain injury and their response to treatment: A prospective cohort. *Developmental Medicine and Child Neurology, 55*(7), 636–641.

Kulkarni, A. V., Sgouros, S., Constantini, S., et al. (2016). International infant hydrocephalus study: Initial results of a prospective, multicenter comparison of endoscopic third ventriculostomy (ETV) and shunt for infant hydrocephalus. *Child's Nervous System, 32*(6), 1039–1048.

Langdon, R., & DiSabella, M. T. (2017). Pediatric headache: An overview. *Current Problems in Pediatric and Adolescent Health Care, 47*(3), 44–56.

Lee, I. C., Li, S. Y., & Chen, Y. J. (2017). Seizure recurrence in children after stopping antiepileptic medication: 5-year follow-up. *Pediatrics and Neonatology, 58*(4), 338–343.

Longoni, G., Levy, D. M., & Yeh, E. A. (2016). The changing landscape of childhood inflammatory central nervous system disorders. *The Journal of Pediatrics, 179*, 24–32.

Lopes, N. R., & Williams, L. C. (epub ahead of print, 2016). Pediatric abusive head trauma prevention initiatives: A literature review. Trauma, Violence and Abuse.

Luat, A. F., Coyle, L., & Kamat, D. (2016). The ketogenic diet: A practical guide for pediatricians. *Pediatric Annals, 45*(12), e446–e450.

Månsson, P. K., Johansson, S., Ziebell, M., et al. (2017). Forty years of shunt surgery at Rigshospitalet, Denmark: A retrospective study comparing past and present rates and causes of revision and infection. *British Medical Journal Open, 7*(1), e013389.

Martin, H. A. (2017). The power of lidocaine, epinephrine, and tetracaine (LET) and a child life specialist when suturing lacerations in children. *Journal of Emergency Nursing, 43*(2), 169–170.

Martin, K., Jackson, C. F., Levy, R. G., et al. (2016). Ketogenic diet and other dietary treatments for epilepsy. *Cochrane Database of Systematic Review* (2), CD001903.

McCrea, M. A., Nelson, L. D., & Guskiewicz, K. (2017). Diagnosis and management of acute concussion. *Physical Medicine and Rehabilitation Clinics of North America, 28*(2), 271–286.

McMurtry, C. M., Taddio, A., Noel, M., et al. (2016). Exposure-based interventions for the management of individuals with high levels of needle fear across the lifespan: A clinical practice guideline and call for further research. *Cognitive Behaviour Therapy, 45*(3), 217–235.

Meehan, W. P., Mannix, R. C., Stracciolini, A., et al. (2013). Symptom severity predicts prolonged recovery after sport-related concussion, but age and amnesia do not. *The Journal of Pediatrics, 163*(3), 721–725.

Merison, K., & Jacobs, H. (2016). Diagnosis and treatment of childhood migraine. *Current Treatment Options in Neurology, 18*(11), 48.

Mewasingh, L. D. (2014). Febrile seizures. *BMJ Clinical Evidence, 2014*, 0324.

Mikati, M. A., & Tchapyjnikov, D. (2020). Seizures in childhood. In R. M. Kliegman, J. W. St. Geme, N. J. Blum, et al. (Eds.), *Nelson Textbook of Pediatrics* (21st ed.). Philadelphia PA: Elsevier.

Minns, R. A., Jones, P. A., Tandon, A., et al. (2017). Raised intracranial pressure and retinal haemorrhages in childhood encephalopathies. *Developmental Medicine and Child Neurology, 59*(6), 597–604.

Moosa, A. N., & Gupta, A. (2014). Outcome after epilepsy surgery for cortical dysplasia in children. *Child's Nervous System, 20*(11), 1905–1911.

Morgan, C. D., Zuckerman, S. L., Lee, Y. M., et al. (2015). Predictors of postconcussion syndrome after sports-related concussion in young athletes: A matched case-control study. *Journal of Neurosurgery. Pediatrics, 15*(6), 589–598.

Morse, A. M., & Kothare, S. V. (2016). Pediatric sudden unexpected death in epilepsy. *Pediatric Neurology, 57*, 7–16.

Moshe, S. L., Perucca, E., Ryvlin, P., et al. (2015). Epilepsy: New advances. *Lancet, 385*(9971), 884–898.

Mullally, W. J. (2017). Concussion. *The American Journal of Medicine.*

Murphy, S., Thomas, N. J., Gertz, S. J., et al. (epub ahead of print, 2017). Tripartite stratification of the Glasgow Coma Scale in children with severe traumatic brain injury and mortality: An analysis from a multi-center comparative effectiveness study. *Journal of Neurotrauma.*

Nakagawa, T. A., Ashwal, S., Mathur, M., et al. (2012). Guidelines for the determination of brain death in infants and children: An update of the 1987 task force recommendations. *Annals of Neurology, 71*(4), 573–585.

Noje, C., Jackson, E. M., Nasr, I. W., et al. (2019). Trauma bay disposition of infants and young children with mild traumatic brain injury and positive head imaging. *Operative Neurosurgery* [Epub ahead of print].

Novakova, B., Harris, P. R., Ponnusamy, A., et al. (2013). The role of stress as a trigger for epileptic seizures: A narrative review of evidence from human and animal studies. *Epilepsia, 54*(11), 1866–1876.

O'Callaghan, F. J., Edwards, S. W., Alber, F. D., et al. (2017). Safety and effectiveness of hormonal treatment versus hormonal treatment with vigabatrin for infantile spasms (ICISS): A randomised, multicentre, open-label trial. *The Lancet. Neurology, 16*(1), 33–42.

Offringa, M., Newton, R., Cozijnsen, M. A., et al. (2017). Prophylactic drug management for febrile seizures in children. *Cochrane Database of Systematic Review* (2), CD003031.

Patel, N., Ram, D., Swiderska, N., et al. (2015). Febrile seizures. *British Medical Journal (Clinical Research Ed.), 351*, 1–7.

Patniyot, I. R., & Gelfand, A. A. (2016). Acute treatment therapies for pediatric migraine: A qualitative systematic review. *Headache, 56*(1), 49–70.

Paulsen, A. H., Lundar, T., & Lindegaard, K. F. (2015). Pediatric hydrocephalus: 40-year outcomes in 128 hydrocephalic patients treated with shunts during childhood. Assessment of surgical outcome, work participation, and health-related quality of life. *Journal of Neurosurgery. Pediatrics, 16*(6), 633–641.

Pisapia, J. M., Sinha, S., Zarnow, D. M., et al. (2017). Fetal ventriculomegaly: Diagnosis, treatment, and future directions. *Child's Nervous System, 33*(7), 1113–1123.

Popernack, M. L., Gray, N., & Reuter-Rice, K. (2015). Moderate-to-severe traumatic brain injury in children: Complications and rehabilitation strategies. *Journal of Pediatric Health Care, 29*(3), e1–e7.

Puledda, F., Messina, R., & Goadsby, P. J. (2017). An update on migraine: Current understanding and future directions. *Journal of Neurology, 264*(9), 2031–2039.

Quan, L., Bierens, J. J., Lis, R., et al. (2016). Predicting outcome of drowning at the scene: A systematic review and meta-analyses. *Resuscitation, 104*, 63–75.

Quan, L., Mack, C. D., & Schiff, M. A. (2014). Association of water temperature and submersion duration and drowning outcome. *Resuscitation, 85*(6), 790–794.

Rumalla, K., Smith, K. A., Letchuman, V., et al. (2018). Nationwide incidence and risk factors for posttraumatic seizures in children with traumatic brain injury. *J Neurosurg Pediatr, 22*(6), 684–693.

Ryan, M. E., Jaju, A., Ciolino, J. D., et al. (2016). Rapid MRI evaluation of acute intracranial hemorrhage in pediatric head trauma. *Neuroradiology, 58*(8), 793–799.

Ryvlin, P., Cross, J. H., & Rheims, S. (2014). Epilepsy surgery in children and adults. *The Lancet. Neurology, 13*(11), 1114–1126.

Saghazadeh, A., Mastrangelo, M., & Rezaei, N. (2014). Genetic background of febrile seizures. *Reviews in the Neurosciences, 25*(1), 129–161.

Scheer, S., & John, R. M. (2016). Anti–N-Methyl-D-Aspartate receptor encephalitis in children and adolescents. *Journal of Pediatric Health Care, 30*(4), 347–358.

Seinfeld, S. A., Pellock, J. M., Kjeldsen, M. J., et al. (2016). Epilepsy after febrile seizures: Twins suggest genetic influence. *Pediatric Neurology, 55*, 14–16.

Sellin, J. N., Moreno, A., Ryan, S. L., et al. (2017). Children presenting in delayed fashion after minor head trauma with scalp swelling: Do they require further workup? *Child's Nervous System, 33*(4), 647–652.

Shankar, P., Zamora, C., & Castillo, M. (2016). Congenital malformations of the brain and spine. *Handbook of Clinical Neurology, 136*, 1121–1137.

Singh, B., Murad, M. H., Prokop, L. J., et al. (2013). Meta-analysis of Glasgow Coma Scale and simplified motor score in predicting traumatic brain injury outcomes. *Brain Injury: [BI], 27*(3), 293–300.

Singh, R., Singh, K. P., Cherian, S., et al. (2017). Rabies–epidemiology, pathogenesis, public health concerns and advances in diagnosis and control: A comprehensive review. *Veterinary Quarterly, 37*(1), 212–251.

Singhal, N. S., Harini, C., & Sullivan, J. (2018). Epileptic spasms and myoclonic seizures. In K. F. Swaiman, S. Ashwal, D. M. Ferriero, et al. (Eds.), *Swaiman's Pediatric Neurology: Principles and Practice* (6th ed.). Philadelphia, PA: Elsevier.

Smith, S. E., Pratt, R., Trieu, L., et al. (2017). Epidemiology of pediatric multidrug-resistant tuberculosis in the United States, 1993-2014. *Clinical Infectious Diseases, 65*(9), 1437–1443.

Strahle, J., Selzer, B. J., Muraszko, K. M., et al. (2012). Programmable shunt valve affected by exposure to a tablet computer. *Journal of Neurosurgery. Pediatrics, 10*(2), 118–120.

Sutherland, H. G., & Griffiths, L. R. (2017). Genetics of migraine: Insights into the molecular basis of migraine disorders. *Headache, 57*(4), 537–569.

Swanson, D. (2015). Meningitis. *Pediatrics in Review, 36*(12), 514–524.

Taylor, C. A., Bell, J. M., Breiding, M., et al. (2017). Traumatic brain injury–related emergency department visits, hospitalizations, and deaths—United States, 2007 and 2013. *MMWR. Surveillance Summaries: Morbidity and Mortality Weekly Report. Surveillance Summaries, 66*(9), 1–16.

Teichert, J. H., Rosales, P. R., Jr., Lopes, P. B., et al. (2012). Extradural hematoma in children: Case series of 33 patients. *Pediatric Neurosurgery, 48*(4), 216–220.

Téllez-Zenteno, J. F., Hernández-Ronquillo, L., Buckley, S., et al. (2014). A validation of the new definition of drug-resistant epilepsy by the International League Against Epilepsy. *Epilepsia, 55*(6), 829–834.

Tenney, J. R., & Glauser, T. (2018). Electroclinical syndromes: Childhood onset. In K. F. Swaiman, S. Ashwal, D. M. Ferriero, et al. (Eds.), *Swaiman's pediatric neurology: Principles and practice* (6th ed.). Philadelphia, PA: Elsevier.

Thomas, A. A., & Caglar, D. (2020). Drowning and submersion injury. In R. M. Kliegman, J. W. St. Geme, N. J. Blum, et al. (Eds.), *Nelson textbook of pediatrics* (21st ed.). Philadelphia PA: Elsevier.

Tobin, J. M., Ramos, W. D., Pu, Y., et al. (2017). Bystander CPR is associated with improved neurologically favourable survival in cardiac arrest following drowning. *Resuscitation, 115*, 39–43.

Toth, P., Szarka, N., Farkas, E., et al. (2016). Traumatic brain injury-induced autoregulatory dysfunction and spreading depression-related neurovascular uncoupling: Pathomechanisms, perspectives, and therapeutic implications. *American Journal of Physiology, Heart and Circulatory Physiology, 311*(5), H1118–H1131.

Venable, G. T., Rossi, N. B., Morgan Jones, G., et al. (2016). The preventable shunt revision pate: A potential quality metric for pediatric shunt surgery. *Journal of Neurosurgery. Pediatrics, 18*(1), 7–15.

Vetter, V., Baxter, R., Denizer, G., et al. (2016). Routinely vaccinating adolescents against meningococcus: Targeting transmission & disease. *Expert Review of Vaccines, 15*(5), 641–658.

Vezina, N., Al-Halabi, B., Shash, H., et al. (2017). A review of techniques used in the management of growing skull fractures. *The Journal of Craniofacial Surgery, 28*(3), 604–609.

Wassenaar, M., Kasteleijn-Nolst Trenite, D. G., de Haan, G. J., et al. (2014). Seizure precipitants in a community-based epilepsy cohort. *Journal of Neurology, 261*(4), 717–724.

Wassenaar, M., Leijten, F. S., Egberts, T. C., et al. (2013). Prognostic factors for medically intractable epilepsy: A systematic review. *Epilepsy Research, 106*(3), 301–310.

Weinberg, G. A., & Thompson-Stone, R. (2018). Bacterial infections of the nervous system. In K. F. Swaiman, S. Ashwal, D. M. Ferriero, et al. (Eds.), *Swaiman's pediatric neurology: Principles and practice* (6th ed.). Philadelphia, PA: Elsevier.

Weiss, E. F., Masur, D., Shinnar, S., et al. (2016). Cognitive functioning one month and one year following febrile status epilepticus. *Epilepsy & Behavior, 64*, 283–288.

Willoughby, R. E., Jr. (2020). Rabies. In R. M. Kliegman, J. W. St. Geme, N. J. Blum, et al. (Eds.), *Nelson textbook of pediatrics* (21st ed.). Philadelphia PA: Elsevier.

World Health Organization. (2017). Human rabies: 2016 updates and call for data. *Weekly Epidemiological Record, 92*(7), 77–86.

Xu, J. (2014). Unintentional drowning deaths in the United States 1999–2010. *NCHS Data Brief, 149*, 1–8.

Zemek, R., Barrowman, N., Freedman, S. B., et al. (2016). Clinical risk score for persistent postconcussion symptoms among children with acute concussion in the. *JAMA: The Journal of the American Medical Association, 315*(10), 1014–1025.

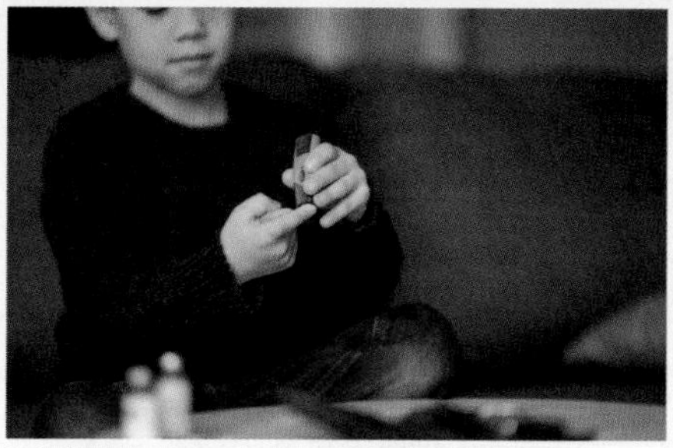

28

The Child With Endocrine Dysfunction

Amy Barry, Erin Connelly

http://evolve.elsevier.com/wong/essentials

CONCEPTS

- Cellular Regulation
- Glucose Regulation
- Patient Education
- Health Promotion

THE ENDOCRINE SYSTEM

The endocrine system controls and regulates metabolism; this includes energy production, growth, fluid and electrolyte balance, response to stress, and sexual development (Gardner & Shoback, 2011). This system has three components: (1) the cell that sends a chemical message using a hormone; (2) the target cells or organs, which receive the chemical message; and (3) the environment through which the chemical is transported from the site of synthesis to the site of cellular action (e.g., blood, lymph, extracellular fluids). The endocrine glands, which are distributed throughout the body, are listed in Table 28.1; also listed are several additional structures sometimes considered endocrine glands, although they are not usually included. The pathophysiology review in Fig. 28.1 provides a summary of the principle pituitary hormones and their target organs.

HORMONES

A hormone is a complex chemical substance produced and secreted into body fluids by a cell or group of cells that exerts a physiologic controlling effect on other cells (Garibaldi & Chemaitilly, 2016). These effects may be local or distant and may affect either most cells of the body or specific "target" tissues. Most hormones are released by the endocrine glands into the bloodstream, and production is regulated by a feedback mechanism (see Table 28.1). The master gland of the endocrine system is the anterior pituitary. The pituitary is responsible for stimulation and inhibition of tropic hormones. Other hormones, such as insulin, are not regulated by the pituitary gland.

DISORDERS OF PITUITARY FUNCTION

The pituitary gland is divided into two lobes: the anterior pituitary (adenohypophysis) and the posterior pituitary (neurohypophysis). It is controlled by hormones secreted from the hypothalamus. Each lobe of the pituitary is responsible for secreting different hormones. The cause of pituitary dysfunction may be organic or idiopathic and may involve one hormone or a combination of hormones. The clinical manifestations of pituitary dysfunction depend on the hormones involved and the age of the patient. Combined pituitary hormone deficiency (CPHD) is defined as the loss of more than one anterior pituitary hormone function (Gangat & Radovick, 2017). *Panhypopituitarism* is defined clinically as the loss of all anterior pituitary hormone function, leaving only posterior function intact (Toogood & Stewart, 2008).

> **! NURSING ALERT**
>
> Children with panhypopituitarism should wear medical identification, such as a bracelet.

HYPOPITUITARISM

Hypopituitarism or CPHD is the diminished secretion of one or more anterior pituitary hormones. The consequences of this condition depend on the degree of dysfunction and are often associated with increased risk of morbidity and mortality (Gangat & Radovick, 2017).

- Gonadotropin deficiency (decrease in luteinizing hormone [LH] or follicle-stimulating hormone [FSH]) where children show an absence or regression in secondary sex characteristics
- Growth hormone (GH) deficiency in which children display stunted somatic growth
- Thyroid-stimulating hormone (TSH) deficiency, which causes hypothyroidism
- Adrenocorticotropic hormone (ACTH) deficiency, which results in adrenal hypofunction

Hypopituitarism can result from any of the conditions listed in Box 28.1. The most common organic cause of pituitary undersecretion is a tumor in the pituitary or hypothalamic region. Craniopharyngiomas are tumors well known to invade these regions of the brain and cause panhypopituitarism. Clinical manifestations of panhypopituitarism are listed in Box 28.1. Children with panhypopituitarism should be advised to wear medical identification at all times.

Congenital hypopituitarism can be seen in newborn infants and can run in families, suggesting a genetic cause; however the majority of cases have no genetic association (Gangat & Radovick, 2017). Neonates may have symptoms of hypoglycemia and seizure activity (Schoenmaker, Alatzoglou, Chatterjee, et al., 2015). A child with combined GH deficiency and hypothyroidism should be screened for congenital pituitary defects and genetic mutations (Pine-Twaddell, Romero, & Radovick, 2013).

Idiopathic hypopituitarism, or idiopathic pituitary growth failure, is usually related to GH deficiency, which inhibits somatic growth in all cells of the body (Amin, Mushtaq, & Alvi, 2015). Isolated GH deficiency is seen in children, but these patients should be closely monitored for

TABLE 28.1 **Hormones and Their Function**

Hormone	Effect	Hypofunction	Hyperfunction
Adenohypophysis (Anterior Pituitary)[a]			
STH or GH (somatotropin) *Target tissue:* Bones	Promotes growth of bone and soft tissues Has main effect on linear growth Maintains a normal rate of protein synthesis Conserves carbohydrate use and promotes fat mobilization Is essential for proliferation of cartilage cells at epiphyseal plate Is ineffective for linear growth after epiphyseal closure Has hyperglycemic effect (anti-insulin action)	Epiphyseal fusion with cessation of growth Prepubertal dwarfism Pituitary cachexia (Simmonds disease) Generalized growth retardation Hypoglycemia	Prepubertal gigantism Acromegaly (after full growth is attained) DM Postpubertal hypoproteinemia
Thyrotropin (TSH) *Target tissue:* Thyroid gland	Promotes and maintains growth and development of thyroid gland Stimulates TH secretion	Hypothyroidism Marked delay of puberty Juvenile myxedema	Hyperthyroidism Thyrotoxicosis Graves disease
ACTH *Target tissue:* Adrenal cortex	Promotes and maintains growth and development of adrenal cortex Stimulates adrenal cortex to secrete glucocorticoids and androgens	Acute adrenocortical insufficiency (Addison disease) Hypoglycemia Increased skin pigmentation	Cushing syndrome
Gonadotropins *Target tissue:* Gonads	Stimulate gonads to mature and produce sex hormones and germ cells	Absent or incomplete spontaneous puberty	Precocious puberty Early epiphyseal closure
FSH *Target tissue:* Ovaries, testes	*Male:* Stimulates development of seminiferous tubules; initiates spermatogenesis *Female:* Stimulates Graafian follicles to mature and secrete estrogen	Hypogonadism Sterility Absence or loss of secondary sex characteristics Amenorrhea	Precocious puberty Primary gonadal failure Hirsutism Polycystic ovary Early epiphyseal closure
LH[b] *Target tissue:* Ovaries, testes	*Male:* Stimulates differentiation of Leydig cells, which secrete androgens, principally testosterone *Female:* Produces rupture of follicle with discharge of mature ovum; stimulates secretion of progesterone by corpus luteum	Hypogonadism Sterility Impotence Absence or loss of secondary sex characteristics Ovarian failure Eunuchism	Precocious puberty Primary gonadal failure Hirsutism Polycystic ovary Early epiphyseal closure
Prolactin (luteotropic hormone) *Target tissue:* Ovaries, breasts	Stimulates milk secretion Maintains corpus luteum and progesterone secretion during pregnancy	Inability to lactate Amenorrhea	Galactorrhea Functional hypogonadism
MSH *Target tissue:* Skin	Promotes pigmentation of skin	Diminished or absent skin pigmentation	Increased skin pigmentation
Neurohypophysis (Posterior Pituitary)			
ADH (vasopressin) *Target tissue:* Renal tubules	Acts on distal and collecting tubules, making them more permeable to water, thus increasing reabsorption and decreasing excretion of urine	DI	SIADH Fluid retention Hyponatremia
Oxytocin *Target tissue:* Uterus, breasts	Stimulates powerful contractions of uterus Causes ejection of milk from alveoli into breast ducts (letdown reflex)		
Thyroid			
THs: T_4 and T_3	Regulate metabolic rate; control rate of growth of body cells Especially important for growth of bones, teeth, and brain Promote mobilization of fats and gluconeogenesis	Hypothyroidism Myxedema Hashimoto thyroiditis General growth greatly reduced; extent dependent on age at which deficiency occurs Intellectual disability in infant	Exophthalmic goiter (Graves disease) Accelerated linear growth Early epiphyseal closure
Thyrocalcitonin	Regulates calcium and phosphorus metabolism Influences ossification and development of bone		
Parathyroid Glands			
PTH	Promotes calcium reabsorption from blood, bone, and intestines Promotes excretion of phosphorus in kidney tubules	Hypocalcemia (tetany)	Hypercalcemia (bone demineralization) Hypophosphatemia

TABLE 28.1 Hormones and Their Function—cont'd

Hormone	Effect	Hypofunction	Hyperfunction
Adrenal Cortex			
Mineralocorticoids Aldosterone	Stimulate renal tubules to reabsorb sodium, thus promoting water retention but potassium loss	Adrenocortical insufficiency	Electrolyte imbalance Hyperaldosteronism
Sex hormones: Androgens, estrogens, progesterone	Influence development of bone, reproductive organs, and secondary sex characteristics	Male feminization	Adrenogenital syndrome
Glucocorticoids Cortisol (hydrocortisone and compound F) Corticosterone (compound B)	Promote normal fat, protein, and carbohydrate metabolism Mobilize body defenses during periods of stress Suppress inflammatory reaction	Addison disease Acute adrenocortical insufficiency Impaired growth and sexual function	Cushing syndrome Severe impairment of growth with slowing in skeletal maturation In excess, tend to accelerate gluconeogenesis and protein and fat catabolism
Adrenal Medulla			
Epinephrine (adrenaline), norepinephrine (noradrenaline)	Produce vasoconstriction of heart and smooth muscles (raise blood pressure) Increase blood glucose via glycolysis Inhibit GI activity Activate sweat glands		Hyperfunction caused by: • Pheochromocytoma • Neuroblastoma • Ganglioneuroma
Islets of Langerhans of Pancreas			
Insulin (β cells)	Promotes glucose transport into the cells Increases glucose use, glycogenesis, and glycolysis Promotes fatty acid transport into cells and lipogenesis Promotes amino acid transport into cells and protein synthesis	DM	Hyperinsulinism
Glucagon (α cells)	Acts as antagonist to insulin, thereby increasing blood glucose concentration by accelerating glycogenolysis Able to inhibit secretion of both insulin and glycogen		Hyperglycemia May be instrumental in genesis of DKA in DM
Somatostatin (δ cells)	Able to inhibit secretion of both insulin and glycogen		
Ovaries			
Estrogen	Accelerates growth of epithelial cells, especially in uterus after menses Promotes protein anabolism Promotes epiphyseal closure of bones Promotes breast development during puberty and pregnancy Plays role in sexual function Stimulates water and sodium reabsorption in renal tubules Stimulates ripening of ova	Lack of or repression of sexual development	Precocious puberty, early epiphyseal closure
Progesterone	Prepares uterus for nidation of fertilized ovum and aids in maintenance of pregnancy Aids in development of alveolar system of breasts during pregnancy Inhibits myometrial contractions Has effect on protein catabolism Promotes salt and water retention, especially in endometrium		
Testes			
Testosterone	Accelerates protein anabolism for growth Promotes epiphyseal closure Promotes development of secondary sex characteristics Plays role in sexual function Stimulates testes to produce spermatozoa	Delayed sexual development or eunuchoidism	Precocious puberty, early epiphyseal closure

ACTH, Adrenocorticotropic hormone; *ADH,* antidiuretic hormone; *DI,* diabetes insipidus; *DKA,* diabetic ketoacidosis; *DM,* diabetes mellitus; *FSH,* follicle-stimulating hormone; *GH,* growth hormone; *GI,* gastrointestinal; *LH,* luteinizing hormone; *MSH,* melanocyte-stimulating hormone; *PTH,* parathyroid hormone; *SIADH,* syndrome of inappropriate antidiuretic hormone secretion; *STH,* somatotropin hormone; T_3, triiodothyronine; T_4, thyroxine; *TH,* thyroid hormone; *TSH,* thyroid-stimulating hormone.

[a]For each anterior pituitary hormone there is a corresponding hypothalamic-releasing factor. A deficiency in these factors caused by inhibiting anterior pituitary hormone synthesis produces the same effects. (See text for more detailed information.)

[b]In males, LH is sometimes known as interstitial cell–stimulating hormone (ICSH).

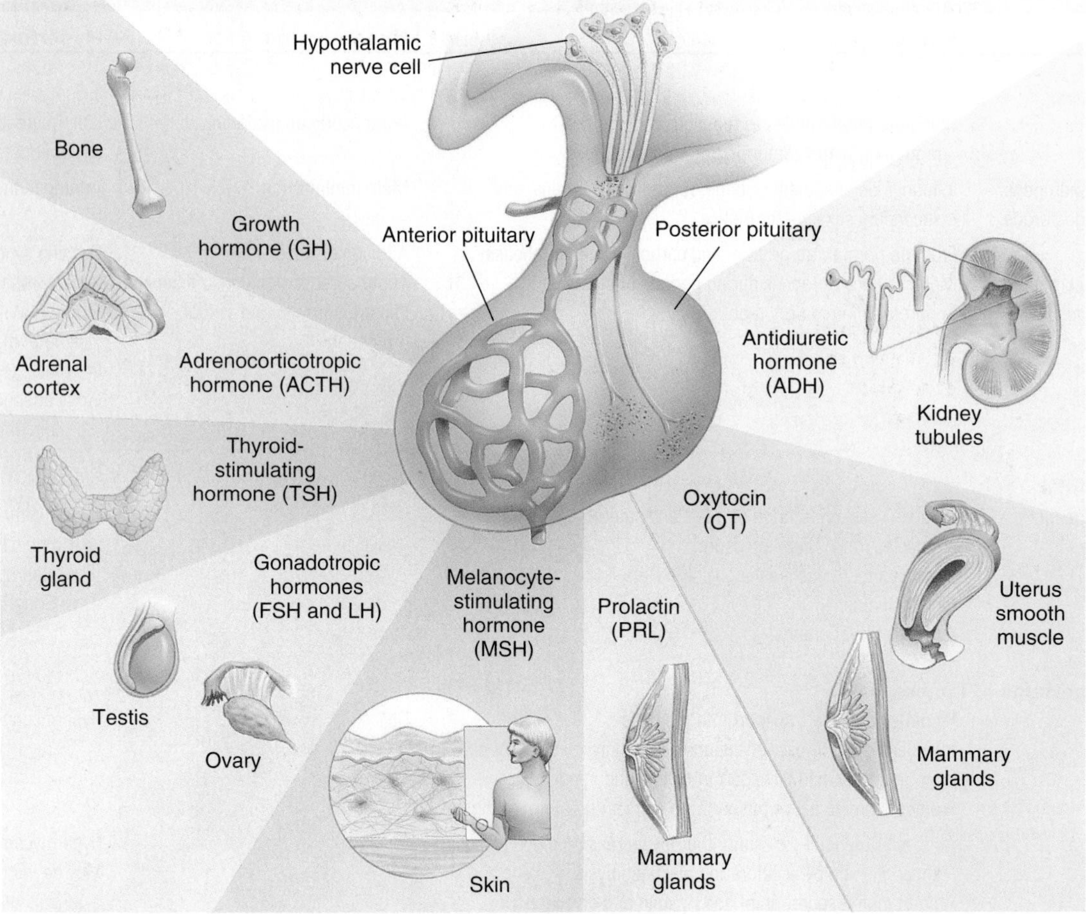

Fig. 28.1 Principal anterior and posterior pituitary hormones and their target organs. *FSH,* Follicle-stimulating hormone; *LH,* luteinizing hormone. (From Patton, K. T., & Thibodeau, G. A. [2013]. *Anatomy and physiology* [8th ed.]. St. Louis, MO: Mosby/Elsevier.)

BOX 28.1 Clinical Manifestations of Panhypopituitarism

Growth Hormone

Short stature but proportional height and weight
Delayed epiphyseal closure
Retarded bone age proportional to height
Premature aging common in later life
Increased insulin sensitivity

Thyroid-Stimulating Hormone

Short stature with infantile proportions
Dry, coarse skin; yellow discoloration, pallor
Cold intolerance
Constipation
Somnolence
Bradycardia
Dyspnea on exertion
Delayed dentition, loss of teeth

Gonadotropins

Absence of sexual maturation or loss of secondary sexual characteristics
Atrophy of genitalia, prostate gland, breasts
Amenorrhea without menopausal symptoms
Decreased spermatogenesis

Adrenocorticotropic Hormone

Severe anorexia, weight loss
Hypoglycemia
Hypotension
Hyponatremia, hyperkalemia
Adrenal apoplexy, especially in response to stress
Circulatory collapse

Antidiuretic Hormone

Polyuria
Polydipsia
Dehydration

Melanocyte-Stimulating Hormone

Decreased pigmentation

the development of other pituitary hormone deficiencies (Cerbone & Datanni, 2017). Growth failure is defined as an absolute height of less than −2 standard deviation (SD) for age or a linear growth velocity consistently less than −1 SD for age. When this occurs without the presence of hypothyroidism, systemic disease, or malnutrition, an abnormality of the GH–insulin-like growth factor (IGF-I) axis should be considered (Grimberg, Divall, Polychronakos, et al., 2016).

However, not all children with short stature have GH deficiency. In most instances, the cause is considered idiopathic. Most children with idiopathic short stature (ISS) have either familial short stature or constitutional growth delay. **Familial short stature** refers to otherwise healthy children who have ancestors with adult height in the lower percentiles. **Constitutional delay of growth and puberty** refers to individuals (usually boys) with delayed linear growth, with skeletal and sexual maturation that is behind that of age-mates (Amin et al., 2015). GH therapy in children with ISS continues to be debated frequently by pediatric endocrinologists (Murray, Dattani, & Clayton, 2016). New guidelines recommend the clinical management of children with growth failure related to GH deficiency and ISS. They now include recombinant IGF-1 therapy for primary IGF-1 deficiency (Grimberg et al., 2016).

Clinical Manifestations

Children with GH deficiency generally grow normally during the first year and then follow a slowed growth curve that is below the 3rd percentile. These children may appear overweight or obese due to stunted height in combination with good nutrition. A nourished appearance is an important diagnostic clue that may differentiate patients with GH deficiency from patients with failure to thrive. Sexual development is usually delayed but is otherwise normal unless the gonadotropin hormones are deficient. Growth may extend into the third or fourth decade of life, but permanent height is usually diminished if the disorder is left untreated. Because of an underdeveloped jaw, teeth may be crowded or malpositioned.

Diagnostic Evaluation

Only a small number of children with delayed growth or short stature have hypopituitary dysfunction. Diagnostic evaluation is aimed at isolating organic causes, which, in addition to GH deficiency, may include tumor growth, hypothyroidism, oversecretion of cortisol, gonadal aplasia, chronic illness, nutritional inadequacy, Russell-Silver dwarfism, or hypochondroplasia. A detailed family history, growth history and previous health status, physical examination, and psychosocial evaluation are important. Specific radiographic imaging, including magnetic resonance imaging (MRI), endocrine studies, and genetic testing, may be warranted (Stanley, 2012). Accurate measurement of height and weight and comparison of these measures with standard growth charts are essential. Multiple height measures reflect a more accurate assessment of abnormal growth patterns (Box 28.2). Parental height and familial patterns of growth are important clues to diagnosis. A skeletal survey in children younger than 3 years old and radiographic examination of the hand and wrist for centers of ossification (bone age) (Box 28.3) in older children are important in evaluating growth.

A definitive diagnosis of GH deficiency is based on absent or subnormal reserves of pituitary GH. Because GH levels are variable in children, GH stimulation testing is usually required for diagnosis. It is recommended that GH stimulation tests be reserved for children with low serum IGF-I and insulin-like growth factor binding protein 3 (IGFBP3) levels and poor growth who do not have other causes for short stature (Hokken-Koelega, 2011). GH stimulation testing involves the use of pharmacologic agents such as levodopa, clonidine, arginine, insulin, propranolol, or glucagon, followed by the measurement of GH blood levels (Patterson & Felner, 2020). Children with poor linear growth, delayed bone age, and abnormal GH stimulation tests are considered GH deficient. New reference standards that decrease the lower limit of normal GH levels have been proposed and continue to be debated (Murray et al., 2016).

Therapeutic Management

Treatment of GH deficiency caused by organic lesions is directed toward correction of the underlying disease process (e.g., surgical removal or irradiation of a tumor). The definitive treatment of GH deficiency is replacement of GH, which is successful in 80% of affected

BOX 28.2 Evaluating the Growth Curve

Ensure reliability of measurements: Accurately obtain and plot height and weight measurements.

Determine absolute height: The child's absolute height bears some relationship to the likelihood of a pathologic condition. However, most children who have a height below the lowest percentile (either the 3rd or 5th percentile on the height curve) do not have a pathologic growth problem.

Assess height velocity: The most important aspect of a growth evaluation is the observation of a child's height over time, or height velocity. Accurate determination of height velocity requires at least 4 and preferably 6 months of observation. A substantial deceleration in height velocity (crossing several percentiles) between 3 and 12 or 13 years of age indicates a pathologic condition until proven otherwise.

Determine weight-to-height relationship: Determination of the weight-to-height ratio has some diagnostic value in ascertaining the cause of growth retardation in a short child.

Project target height: The height of a child can be judged inappropriately short only in the context of his or her genetic potential. Determine the target height of the child with the formula:

[Father's height (cm) + Mother's height (cm) + 13] / 2 for boys

or

[Father's height (cm) + Mother's height (cm) − 13] / 2 for girls

Most children achieve an adult stature within approximately 10 cm (4 inches) of the target height.

Modified from Vogiatzi, M. G., & Copeland, K. C. (1998). The short child. *Pediatrics in Review, 19*(3), 92–99.

BOX 28.3 Bone Age for Evaluating Growth Disorders

Bone age refers to a method of assessing skeletal maturity by comparing the appearance of representative epiphyseal centers obtained on x-ray examination with age-appropriate published standards.

Most conditions that cause poor linear growth also cause a delay in skeletal maturation and a retarded bone age. Observation of even a profoundly delayed bone age is never diagnostic or even indicative of a specific diagnosis. A delayed bone age merely indicates that the associated short stature is to some extent "partially reversible" because linear growth will continue until epiphyseal fusion is complete. In comparison, a bone age that is not delayed in a short child is of much greater concern and may, in fact, be of some diagnostic value under certain circumstances.

Modified from Vogiatzi, M. G., & Copeland, K. C. (1998). The short child. *Pediatrics in Review, 19*(3), 92–99.

children. Biosynthetic GH is administered subcutaneously on a daily basis. Growth velocity increases in the first year of treatment and then declines in subsequent years (Patterson & Felner, 2020). Final height is likely to remain less than normal (Bryant, Baxter, Cave, et al., 2007; Deodati & Cianfarani, 2011), and early diagnosis and intervention are essential.

The decision to stop GH therapy is made jointly by the child, family, and health care team. Growth rates of less than 1 inch per year and a bone age of more than 14 years in girls and more than 16 years in boys are often used as criteria to stop GH therapy (Patterson & Felner, 2020).

Nursing Care Management

The principal nursing consideration is identifying children with growth problems. Even though the majority of growth problems are not a result of organic causes, any delay in normal growth and sexual development may pose special emotional adjustments for these children.

The nurse may be a key person in helping establish a diagnosis. For example, if serial height and weight records are not available, the nurse can question parents about the child's growth compared with that of siblings, peers, or relatives. Preparation of the child and family for diagnostic testing is especially important if a number of tests are being performed, and the child requires particular attention during testing. Blood samples are usually taken every 30 minutes for a 3-hour period. Children also have difficulty overcoming hypoglycemia generated by tests with insulin, so they must be observed carefully for signs of hypoglycemia. Those receiving glucagon are at risk of nausea and vomiting. Clonidine may cause hypotension, requiring administration of intravenous (IV) fluids.

Child and Family Support

Children undergoing hormone replacement require additional support. The nurse should provide education for patient self-management during the school-age years. Nursing functions include family education concerning medication preparation and storage, injection sites, injection technique, and syringe disposal (see Chapter 20). Administration of GH is facilitated by family routines that include a specific time of day for the injection.

> **NURSING TIP:** Optimum dosing is often achieved when growth hormone (GH) is administered at bedtime. The pituitary release of GH occurs during the first 45 to 90 minutes after the onset of sleep.

Even when hormone replacement is successful, these children attain their eventual adult height at a slower rate than their peers; therefore they need assistance in setting realistic expectations regarding improvement. Because these children appear younger than their chronologic age, others may relate to them in infantile or childish ways. Families should be counseled to set realistic expectations for the child based on age and abilities. For example, in the home, such children should have the same age-appropriate responsibilities as their siblings. As they approach adolescence, they should be encouraged to participate in group activities with peers. If abilities and strengths rather than physical size are emphasized, such children are more likely to develop a positive self-image.

Professionals and families can find resources for research, education, support, and advocacy from the Human Growth Foundation.[a]

[a]997 Glen Cove Ave., Suite 5, Glen Head, NY 11545; 800-451-6434; email: hgf1@hgfound.org; http://www.hgfound.org.

Treatment is expensive, but the cost is often partially covered by insurance if the child has a documented deficiency.

PITUITARY HYPERFUNCTION

Excess GH before closure of the epiphyseal shafts results in proportional overgrowth of the long bones until the individual reaches a height of 2.4 m (8 feet) or more. Vertical growth is accompanied by rapid and increased development of muscles and viscera. Weight is increased but is usually in proportion to height. Proportional enlargement of head circumference also occurs and may result in delayed closure of the fontanels in young children. Children with a pituitary-secreting tumor may also demonstrate signs of increasing intracranial pressure, especially headache.

If oversecretion of GH continues after epiphyseal closure (growth plate), growth occurs in the transverse direction, producing a condition known as **acromegaly**. Typical facial features include overgrowth of the head, lips, nose, tongue, jaw, and paranasal and mastoid sinuses; separation and malocclusion of the teeth in the enlarged jaw; disproportion of the face to the cerebral division of the skull; increased facial hair; thickened, deeply creased skin; and an increased tendency toward hyperglycemia and diabetes mellitus (DM). Acromegaly can develop slowly, leading to delays in diagnosis and treatment. Patients with acromegaly have a higher mortality rate due to an increased risk of cardiovascular, metabolic, skeletal, and pulmonary complications (Pivonello, Auriemma, Grasso, et al., 2017).

Diagnostic Evaluation

Excessive secretion of GH by a pituitary adenoma causes most cases of acromegaly (Colao, Grasso, Giustina, et al., 2019). Diagnosis is based on a history of excessive growth during childhood and evidence of increased levels of GH and IGF-1 (Colao et al., 2019). MRI may reveal a tumor or an enlarged sella turcica, normal bone age, enlargement of bones (e.g., the paranasal sinuses), and evidence of joint changes. Endocrine studies to confirm excess of other hormones, specifically thyroid, cortisol, and sex hormones, should also be included in the differential diagnosis.

Therapeutic Management

If a pituitary lesion is present, surgery may be performed to remove the tumor. Other therapies aimed at destroying pituitary tissue include external irradiation and radioactive implants. Pharmacologic agents, including somatostatin receptor ligands, dopamine agonists, or GH receptor antagonists, have been used individually or in combination with other treatment modalities to treat acromegaly (Colalo et al., 2019).

Nursing Care Management

Nurses can actively assist in the identification of children with excessive growth rates. Although medical management is unable to reduce a patient's height, further growth can be prevented. If treatment for acromegaly is initiated early, it improves a patient's chance of maintaining normal adult height. Nurses should also observe for signs of a tumor, especially headache, and evidence of concurrent hormonal excesses, particularly the gonadotropins, which cause sexual precocity. Children with excessive growth rates require as much emotional support as those with short stature.

PRECOCIOUS PUBERTY

It is now accepted that puberty is occurring earlier than in previous generations likely due to changes in hormonal, genetic, environmental, and nutritional factors over time (Alotaibi, 2019). Traditionally,

BOX 28.4 Causes of Precocious Puberty

Central Precocious Puberty
Idiopathic, with or without hypothalamic hamartoma
Secondary
- Congenital anomalies
- Postinflammatory: Encephalitis, meningitis, abscess, granulomatous disease
- Radiotherapy
- Trauma
- Neoplasms

After effective treatment of long-standing pseudosexual precocity

Peripheral Precocious Puberty
Familial male-limited precocious puberty
Albright syndrome
Gonadal or extragonadal tumors
Adrenal
- Congenital adrenal hyperplasia (CAH)
- Adenoma, carcinoma
- Glucocorticoid resistance

Exogenous sex hormones
Primary hypothyroidism

Incomplete Precocious Puberty
Premature thelarche
Premature menarche
Premature pubarche or adrenarche

Modified from Root, A. W. (2000). Precocious puberty. *Pediatrics in Review, 21*(1), 10–19.

sexual development before 9 years old in boys and 8 years old in girls is considered precocious, warranting further evaluation (Brito, Spinola-Castro, Kochi et al., 2016). New guidelines define puberty as precocious if it occurs in Caucasian girls younger than 7 years old and African-American girls younger than 6 years old (Brito, Spinola-Castro, Kochi, et al., 2016). Although previous data suggest that boys may be beginning maturation earlier as well (Herman-Giddens, 2006; Slyper, 2006), no changes have been made to the guidelines for evaluation of precocious puberty in boys (Brito et al., 2016).

Normally, the hypothalamic-releasing factors stimulate secretion of the gonadotropic hormones from the anterior pituitary at the time of puberty. In boys, interstitial cell–stimulating hormone stimulates Leydig cells of the testes to secrete testosterone; in girls, FSH and LH stimulate the ovarian follicles to secrete estrogens (Nebesio & Eugster, 2007). This sequence of events is known as the **hypothalamic-pituitary-gonadal axis.** If for some reason the cycle undergoes premature activation, the child will display evidence of advanced or precocious puberty. Causes of precocious puberty are found in Box 28.4.

Most children with precocious puberty have **central precocious puberty (CPP)**, in which pubertal development is stimulated by hypothalamic gonadotropin-releasing hormone (GnRH), following the same pattern as in normal puberty (Aguirre & Eugster, 2018). This produces early maturation and development of the gonads with secretion of sex hormones, development of secondary sex characteristics, and sometimes production of mature sperm and ova (Garibaldi & Chemaitilly, 2020). CPP may be the result of congenital anomalies; infectious, neoplastic, or traumatic insults to the central nervous system (CNS); or treatment of long-standing sex hormone exposure (Trivin, Couto-Silva, Sainte-Rose, et al, 2006). CPP occurs more frequently in girls and is usually idiopathic, with 90% to 95% demonstrating no causative factor (Aguirre & Eugster, 2018; Greiner & Kerrigan, 2006; Li, Li, & Yang, 2014; Nebesio & Eugster, 2007).

Peripheral precocious puberty (PPP) includes early puberty resulting from hormone stimulation other than the hypothalamic GnRH–stimulated pituitary gonadotropin release. Isolated manifestations that are usually associated with puberty may be seen as variations in normal sexual development (Brito et al., 2016). They appear without other signs of pubescence and are caused by excess secretion of sex hormones through the gonads or adrenal glands and may be isosexual or contrasexual. Included are premature thelarche (development of breasts in prepubertal girls), premature pubarche (premature adrenarche, early development of sexual hair), and premature menarche (isolated menses without other evidence of sexual development).

Therapeutic Management

Identification of precocious puberty warrants a referral to an endocrinologist for evaluation. Early exposure of growth plates to sex hormones can cause premature closure of the epiphyses, resulting in short stature. The goal of treatment is to prevent exposure and allow a child to achieve adult height (Chen & Eugster, 2015). Treatment of precocious puberty is directed toward the specific cause when known. In 50% of cases, precocious pubertal development regresses or stops advancing without any treatment (Carel & Léger, 2008). CPP usually is managed with monthly injections of a synthetic analog of **luteinizing hormone–releasing hormone (Lupron Depot)** in the United States (Chen & Eugster, 2015). The available preparation, leuprolide acetate (Lupron Depot), is given once every 4 to 12 weeks depending on the preparation. An alternative treatment is the GnRH analog (GnRHa) histrelin implant, which is placed subcutaneously in the upper arm and suppresses LH and testosterone levels for 1 to 2 years (Chen & Eugster, 2015; Garibaldi & Chemaitilly, 2020). Studies suggest that not all patients attain adult target heights with these treatments. The use of GH to improve adult height is being investigated in children with precocious puberty and advanced bone age (Garibaldi & Chemaitilly, 2020). Treatment for precocious puberty is discontinued at a chronologically appropriate time, allowing pubertal changes to resume.

Nursing Care Management

Both parents and the affected child should be taught to perform injections using return demonstration if possible. Psychological support and guidance of the child and family are the most important aspects of management. Parents need anticipatory guidance, support, information resources, and reassurance. GnRH agonists are associated with side effects such as headache, emotional lability, and vasodilation causing hot flashes (Harrington & Palmert, 2016). Nurses are essential in providing medical education to the patient and family. Dress and activities for the physically precocious child should be appropriate to the chronologic age. Sexual interest is not usually advanced beyond the child's chronologic age, and parents need to understand that the child's mental age is congruent with the chronologic age.

DIABETES INSIPIDUS

The principal disorder of posterior pituitary hypofunction is diabetes insipidus (DI), also known as **neurogenic DI** or **central DI**, which results from undersecretion of **antidiuretic hormone (ADH)**, or **vasopressin** (Pitressin), producing a state of uncontrolled diuresis (polyuria) and excessive thirst and water intake (polydipsia) (Levy, Prentice, & Wass, 2019). This disorder is not to be confused with nephrogenic DI, a rare hereditary disorder affecting primarily males and caused by unresponsiveness of the renal tubules to vasopressin. Nephrogenic DI can also be cause by electrolyte disturbance, renal disease, or medications such as lithium (Levy et al., 2019).

Central DI may result from a number of different causes. Primary causes are familial or idiopathic; of the total cases, approximately 20% to 50% are idiopathic (Di Iorgi, Allegri, Napoli, et al., 2014). Secondary causes include trauma (accidental or surgical), tumors, granulomatous disease, infections (meningitis or encephalitis), and vascular anomalies (aneurysm). Certain drugs, such as alcohol and phenytoin (diphenylhydantoin), can cause a transient polyuria. DI may be an early sign of an evolving cerebral process (Di Iorgri, Napoli, Allegri, et al., 2012).

The cardinal signs of DI are polyuria and polydipsia. In older children, signs such as excessive urination accompanied by a compensatory insatiable thirst may be so intense that the child does little more than go to the toilet and drink fluids. Frequently, the first sign is enuresis. In infants, the initial symptom is irritability that is relieved with feedings of water but not milk. These infants are also prone to dehydration, electrolyte imbalance, hyperthermia, azotemia, and potential circulatory collapse.

Dehydration is usually not a serious problem in older children, who are able to drink larger quantities of water. However, any period of unconsciousness (such as after trauma or anesthesia) may be life threatening because the voluntary demand for fluid is absent. During such instances, careful monitoring of urine volumes, blood concentration, and IV fluid replacement is essential to prevent dehydration.

! NURSING ALERT

Children with diabetes insipidus (DI) complicated by congenital absence of the thirst center must be encouraged to drink sufficient quantities of liquid to prevent electrolyte imbalance.

Diagnostic Evaluation

The simplest test used to diagnose this condition is restriction of oral fluids using the water deprivation test and observation of consequent changes in urine volume and concentration. Normally, reducing fluid intake results in concentrated urine and diminished volume. In DI, fluid restriction has little or no effect on urine formation and urine osmolality (Levy et al., 2019). If urine output decreases and urine osmolality increases during the water deprivation test, DI may be excluded (Levy et al., 2019). Accurate results from this procedure require strict monitoring of fluid intake and urinary output, measurement of urine concentration (specific gravity or osmolality), and frequent weight checks. A weight loss between 3% and 5% indicates significant dehydration and requires termination of the fluid restriction. An MRI should be performed to look for secondary causes of central DI, such as a tumor or central brain anomaly (Di Iorgi et al., 2012).

! NURSING ALERT

Small children require close observation during fluid deprivation to prevent them from drinking, even from toilet bowls, flower vases, and other unlikely sources of fluid.

If a water deprivation test is positive, the child should be given a test dose of desmopressin (DDAVP), which should alleviate the polyuria and polydipsia. Unresponsiveness to exogenous vasopressin usually indicates nephrogenic DI. An important diagnostic consideration is to differentiate DI from other causes of polyuria and polydipsia, especially DM.

Therapeutic Management

The usual treatment for DI is hormone replacement using DDAVP, which is a synthetic analog of the endogenous hormone arginine vasopressin (AVP). DDAVP can be administered orally, intranasally, or parenterally. The intranasal and oral forms of DDAVP are most commonly used in children. Oral DDAVP has few complications and is easier to give, which likely increases compliance (Di Iorgi et al., 2012).

NURSING TIP: To be effective, injectable desmopressin must be thoroughly resuspended before administration. If this is not done, the oil may be injected minus the antidiuretic hormone (ADH). Small brown particles, which indicate drug dispersion, must be seen in the suspension.

Nursing Care Management

An early sign of DI may be sudden enuresis in a child who is toilet trained. Excessive thirst with concurrent bedwetting indicates further investigation. Another clue is persistent irritability and crying in an infant that is relieved only by bottle feedings of water. After head trauma or certain neurosurgical procedures, the development of DI can be anticipated; therefore these patients must be closely monitored.

Nursing assessment includes frequent measurements of a patient's weight, serum electrolytes, blood urea nitrogen (BUN), hematocrit, and urine specific gravity. Fluid intake and output should be measured frequently and recorded. Alert patients are able to adjust fluid intake, but unconscious or very young patients require closer fluid observation. In children who are not toilet trained, collection of urine specimens may require application of a urine-collecting device.

After confirmation of DI, parents need comprehensive teaching. Specific clarification that DI is a different condition from DM should be reinforced. Parents and children must realize that treatment is lifelong. Caregivers should be taught the correct procedure for preparation and administration of vasopressin. When children are old enough, they should be encouraged to assume full responsibility for their care.

For emergency purposes, children with DI should wear medical alert identification. Older children should carry the nasal spray with them for temporary relief of symptoms. School personnel need to be aware of a child's diagnosis so that they can grant children unrestricted use of the lavatory. When admitted to the hospital, close attention should be paid to the scheduled doses of vasopressin. Missed doses or dosing errors could cause severe electrolyte abnormalities, causing significant harm or even death (Levy et al., 2019).

SYNDROME OF INAPPROPRIATE ANTIDIURETIC HORMONE SECRETION

The disorder that results from hypersecretion of ADH from the posterior pituitary hormone is known as syndrome of inappropriate antidiuretic hormone secretion (SIADH). It is observed with increased frequency in a variety of conditions, including infections, tumors, CNS disease, trauma, or medication use, and it is one of the most common causes of hyponatremia in hospitalized children (Moritz, 2019).

The manifestations are directly related to fluid retention and hyponatremia. Excess ADH causes most of the filtered water to be reabsorbed from the kidneys back into central circulation. Serum osmolality is low, and urine osmolality is inappropriately elevated. When serum sodium levels are diminished to 120 mEq/L, affected children may display anorexia, nausea, vomiting, stomach cramps, irritability, weakness, confusion, and personality changes. With progressive reduction in sodium, other neurologic signs, including stupor and seizure, may occur. When hyponatremia occurs acutely, swelling of the brain may occur. This is a medical emergency and can cause irreversible brain damage or even death (Giuliani & Peri, 2014). Children are at increased risk for developing hyponatremic encephalopathy when compared to adults (Moritz, 2019).

Fluid restriction is the first management of SIADH. Subsequent management depends on the cause and severity. Fluids continue to be restricted to one-fourth to one-half maintenance. When there are no fluid abnormalities but SIADH can be anticipated, fluids are often restricted expectantly at two-thirds to three-fourths maintenance.

! NURSING ALERT

Early symptoms of SIADH can be easily attributed to other causes: headache, nausea, vomiting, weakness, and general malaise (Moritz, 2019). These symptoms may precede the onset of more severe stages, such as disorientation, confusion, coma, and seizures (Gardner & Shoback, 2011).

Nursing Care Management

The first goal of nursing management is recognizing the presence of SIADH from symptoms described in patients at risk.

Accurately measuring intake and output, noting daily weight, and observing for signs of fluid overload are primary nursing functions and are essential when children are receiving IV fluids. Seizure precautions and neurologic checks may be implemented when a hospitalized child has SIADH. Hyponatremic encephalopathy is a medical emergency requiring hypertonic sodium chloride (3%) administration (Moritz, 2019). Patients and families need education on the rationale for fluid restrictions. The rare child with chronic SIADH will be placed on long-term ADH-antagonizing medication, and the child and family will require instructions for administration.

DISORDERS OF THYROID FUNCTION

The thyroid gland secretes two types of hormones: **thyroid hormone (TH)**, which consists of the hormones **thyroxine (T_4) and triiodothyronine (T_3)**, and **calcitonin**. The secretion of THs is controlled by TSH from the anterior pituitary, which in turn is regulated by thyrotropin-releasing factor (TRF) from the hypothalamus as a negative feedback response. Consequently, hypothyroidism or hyperthyroidism may result from a defect in the target gland or from a disturbance in the secretion of TSH or TRF. Because the functions of T_3 and T_4 are qualitatively the same, the term *thyroid hormone* is used throughout the discussion.

The synthesis of TH depends on available sources of dietary iodine and tyrosine. The thyroid is the only endocrine gland capable of storing excess amounts of hormones for release as needed. During circulation in the bloodstream, T_4 and T_3 are bound to carrier proteins (T_4-binding globulin). They must be unbound before they are able to exert their metabolic effect.

The main physiologic action of TH is to regulate the basal metabolic rate and thereby control the processes of growth and tissue differentiation. Unlike GH, TH is involved in many more diverse activities that influence the growth and development of body tissues. Therefore a deficiency of TH exerts a more profound effect on growth than that seen in GH deficiency.

Calcitonin helps maintain blood calcium levels by decreasing the calcium concentration. Its effect is the opposite of parathyroid hormone (PTH) in that it inhibits skeletal demineralization and promotes calcium deposition in the bone.

JUVENILE HYPOTHYROIDISM

Hypothyroidism is one of the most common endocrine problems of childhood. It may be either congenital (see Chapter 8) or acquired and represents a deficiency in secretion of TH (Patterson & Felner, 2020).

Beyond infancy, primary hypothyroidism may be caused by a number of defects. For example, a congenital hypoplastic thyroid gland may provide sufficient amounts of TH during the first year or two but be inadequate when rapid body growth increases demands on the gland. A partial or complete thyroidectomy for cancer or thyrotoxicosis can leave insufficient thyroid tissue to furnish hormones for body requirements. Radiotherapy for Hodgkin disease or other malignancies may lead to hypothyroidism (Metzger, Krasin, Choi, et al., 2016). Infectious processes may cause hypothyroidism. It can also occur when dietary iodine is deficient, although it is now rare in the United States because iodized salt is a readily available source of the nutrient.

Clinical manifestations depend on the extent of dysfunction and the child's age at onset. Primary congenital hypothyroidism is characterized by low levels of circulating THs and raised levels of TSH at birth (Kaplowitz, 2019). If left untreated, congenital hypothyroidism causes severe neurocognitive dysfunction (Wassner, 2018). Improvements in newborn screening have led to earlier detection and prevention of complications (American Academy of Pediatrics, Rose, Section on Endocrinology and Committee on Genetics of the American Thyroid Association, et al, 2006; Wassner, 2018). Children with acquired hypothyroidism, which occurs after the newborn period, may have decelerated growth from chronic deprivation of TH, or thyromegaly (enlargement of the thyroid) (Leung & Leung, 2019). Impaired growth and development are less severe when hypothyroidism is acquired at a later age, and because brain growth is nearly complete by 2 to 3 years old, intellectual disability and neurologic sequelae are not associated with juvenile hypothyroidism. Other manifestations are myxedematous skin changes (dry skin, puffiness around the eyes, sparse hair), constipation, lethargy, and mental decline (Box 28.5).

Therapy is TH replacement, the same as for hypothyroidism in infants, although the prompt treatment needed in infants is not required in children. Levothyroxine is administered over a period of 4 to 8 weeks to avoid symptoms of hyperthyroidism.

Nursing Care Management

The importance of early recognition in the infant is discussed in Chapter 8. Growth cessation or retardation in a child whose growth has previously been normal should alert the observer to the possibility of hypothyroidism. Treatment is daily oral TH replacement. The

BOX 28.5 Clinical Manifestations of Juvenile Hypothyroidism

Decelerated growth
- Less when acquired at later age

Myxedematous skin changes
- Dry skin
- Puffiness around eyes
- Sparse hair
- Constipation
- Sleepiness
- Mental decline

importance of daily compliance and the need for periodic monitoring of serum thyroid levels should be stressed to patients and their families.

GOITER

A goiter is an enlargement or hypertrophy of the thyroid gland. It may occur with deficient (hypothyroid), excessive (hyperthyroid), or normal (euthyroid) TH secretion. It can be congenital or acquired. Congenital disease occurs as a result of maternal administration of antithyroid drugs or iodides during pregnancy or as an inborn error of TH production (Leung & Leung, 2019). Acquired disease can result from increased secretion of pituitary TSH in response to decreased circulating levels of TH or from infiltrative neoplastic or inflammatory processes. In areas where dietary iodine (essential for TH production) is deficient, goiter can be endemic.

Enlargement of the thyroid gland may be mild and noticeable only when there is an increased demand for TH (e.g., during periods of rapid growth). Enlargement of the thyroid at birth can be sufficient to cause severe respiratory distress. Sporadic goiter is usually caused by lymphocytic thyroiditis or chronic autoimmune thyroiditis, otherwise known as Hashimoto thyroiditis (Leung & Leung, 2019). TH replacement is necessary to treat resulting hypothyroidism and reverse the TSH effect on the gland.

Nursing Care Management

Large goiters are identified by their obvious appearance. Smaller nodules may be evident only on palpation. Benign enlargement of the thyroid gland may occur during adolescence and should not be confused with pathologic states. Nodules rarely are caused by a cancerous tumor but always require evaluation. Nurses should be aware of the possibility of goiters and report findings. Questions regarding radiation exposure should be included in patient assessments.

> **! NURSING ALERT**
>
> If an infant is born with a goiter, immediate precautions are instituted for emergency ventilation, such as supplemental oxygen and a tracheostomy set nearby. Hyperextension of the neck often facilitates breathing.

Immediate surgery to remove part of the gland may be life-saving in infants born with a goiter. When thyroid replacement is necessary, parents have the same needs regarding its administration as discussed for the parents of children who have hypothyroidism.

LYMPHOCYTIC THYROIDITIS

Lymphocytic thyroiditis (**Hashimoto disease**, **chronic autoimmune thyroiditis**) is the most common cause of thyroid disease and goiter in children and adolescents and accounts for the largest percentage of juvenile hypothyroidism in iodine-sufficient parts of the world (Leung & Leung, 2019). Although lymphocytic thyroiditis can occur during the first 3 years of life, it occurs more frequently after 6 years old, with peak incidence occurring during adolescence. Some children may have subclinical hypothyroidism, but the presence of a goiter and elevated thyroglobulin antibody, with progressive increase in both thyroid peroxidase antibody and TSH, are predictive factors for future development of hypothyroidism (Hanley, Lord, & Bauer, 2016).

An enlarged thyroid gland is often detected during routine examination. Parents may notice it when a child swallows. In most children, the entire gland is enlarged symmetrically (although it may be asymmetric) and is firm, freely movable, and nontender. There may be manifestations of moderate tracheal compression (sense of fullness, hoarseness, and dysphagia). Many patients are euthyroid and asymptomatic (Leung & Leung, 2019). It is extremely rare for a nontoxic, diffuse goiter to cause airway obstruction. Other signs suggestive of thyroiditis are found in Box 28.6.

> **BOX 28.6 Clinical Manifestations of Lymphocytic Thyroiditis**
>
> **Enlarged Thyroid Gland**
> Usually symmetric
> Firm
> Freely movable
> Nontender
>
> **Tracheal Compression**
> Sense of fullness
> Hoarseness
> Dysphagia
>
> **Hyperthyroidism (Possible)**
> Nervousness
> Irritability
> Increased sweating
> Hyperactivity

Diagnostic Evaluation

Thyroid function test results are usually normal, although TSH levels may be slightly or moderately elevated. With progressive thyroiditis, the T_4 decreases, followed by a decrease in T_3 levels and an increase in TSH. Many children have antithyroid antibody titers (Caturegli, De Remiqis, & Rose, 2014). However, levels in children are lower than in adults; therefore repeated measurements may be needed in doubtful cases. The identification of genes involved in this disease has led to improved diagnostic testing and may lead to new treatments in the future (Tomer, 2014).

Therapeutic Management

In many cases, the goiter is transient and asymptomatic and regresses spontaneously within a year or two. Therapy of a nontoxic diffuse goiter is usually simple, uncomplicated, and effective. Oral administration of TH provides the feedback needed to suppress TSH stimulation and decrease the size of the thyroid gland. TSH levels should be monitored, with the goal of restoring normal growth and development. Surgery is contraindicated in this disorder. Untreated patients should be evaluated periodically.

Nursing Care Management

Nurses help identify children with thyroid enlargement and provide reassurance and education regarding therapy and positive outcome.

HYPERTHYROIDISM

Graves disease (GD) is the most common cause of hyperthyroidism in children (Leger & Carel, 2018). This disease often runs in families. GD-associated hyperthyroidism is caused by autoantibodies to the TSH receptor causing excess secretion of TH. Most cases of GD in children occur in adolescence, with a peak incidence between 12 and 14 years old. Transient GD may be present at birth in children of thyrotoxic mothers. The incidence is higher in girls than boys (Léger & Carel, 2013). There is no cure for GD, and treatment options

BOX 28.7 Clinical Manifestations of Hyperthyroidism (Graves Disease)

Cardinal Signs
Emotional lability
Physical restlessness, characteristically at rest
Decelerated school performance
Voracious appetite with weight loss in 50% of cases
Fatigue

Physical Signs
Tachycardia
Widened pulse pressure
Dyspnea on exertion
Exophthalmos (protruding eyeballs)
Wide-eyed, staring expression with eyelid lag
Tremor
Goiter (hypertrophy and hyperplasia)
Warm, moist skin
Accelerated linear growth
Heat intolerance (may be severe)
Hair fine and unable to hold a curl
Systolic murmurs

Thyroid Storm
Acute onset:
- Severe irritability and restlessness
- Vomiting
- Diarrhea
- Hyperthermia
- Hypertension
- Severe tachycardia
- Prostration

May progress rapidly to:
- Delirium
- Coma
- Death

continue to be debated among pediatric endocrinologists (Leger & Carel, 2018).

Signs and symptoms of GD develop gradually, with an interval between onset and diagnosis of approximately 6 to 12 months. Clinical features include irritability, hyperactivity, short attention span, tremors, insomnia, emotional lability, poor concentration, nervousness, and palpitations or tremor (Leger & Carel, 2018). Because of the variety of symptoms, some children may see many different subspecialists before consulting an endocrinologist (Leger & Carel, 2018). Clinical manifestations are presented in Box 28.7.

Exophthalmos (protruding eyeballs), which is observed in many children, is accompanied by a wide-eyed staring expression, increased blinking, eyelid lag, lack of convergence, and absence of wrinkling of the forehead when looking upward. As exophthalmos progresses, the eyelid may not fully cover the cornea. Visual disturbances may include blurred vision and loss of visual acuity. Eye disease associated with hyperthyroidism can develop before or after the clinical diagnosis.

Diagnostic Evaluation

Graves disease is established based on increased levels of T_4 and T_3. TSH is suppressed to unmeasurable levels (Leger & Carel, 2018).

Therapeutic Management

Therapy for hyperthyroidism is controversial, but the end goal is the same—decrease the circulating TH. The three acceptable modes available are antithyroid drugs, subtotal thyroidectomy, and ablation with radioiodine (^{131}I iodide) (Lee & Hwang, 2014; Leger & Carel, 2018). Each therapy has advantages and disadvantages.

When affected children exhibit signs and symptoms of hyperthyroidism (e.g., increased weight loss, pulse, pulse pressure, and blood pressure), their activity should be limited to classwork only. Vigorous exercise is restricted until thyroid levels are decreased to normal or near-normal values.

Thyrotoxicosis (thyroid "crisis" or thyroid "storm") may occur from sudden release of TH. Although thyrotoxicosis is unusual in children, it can be life threatening. Clinical signs of thyroid storm are acute onset of severe irritability and restlessness, vomiting, diarrhea, hyperthermia, hypertension, severe tachycardia, and prostration. There may be rapid progression to delirium, coma, and even death. A crisis may be precipitated by acute infection, surgical emergencies, or discontinuation of antithyroid therapy. In addition to antithyroid drugs, beta-blockers are used to control symptoms until normal thyroid function is achieved (Leger & Carel, 2018). Therapy is usually required for 2 to 3 weeks.

The American Thyroid Association[b] has an extensive website with information related to prevention, treatment, and cure of thyroid disease.

Nursing Care Management

Because the clinical manifestations often appear gradually, the goiter and ophthalmic changes may not be noticed, and the excessive activity may be attributed to behavioral problems. Nurses in ambulatory settings, particularly schools, need to be alert to signs that suggest this disorder. Weight loss despite an excellent appetite, academic difficulties resulting from a short attention span, inability to sit still, unexplained fatigue and sleeplessness, and difficulty with fine motor skills such as writing can all be signs of this disease. Exophthalmos may develop long before the onset of the signs and symptoms and may be the only presenting sign.

Nursing care focuses on treating physical symptoms before a response to drug therapy is achieved. Children with hyperthyroidism need a quiet, unstimulating environment that is conducive to rest. Increased metabolic rate may cause heat intolerance and increased food intake in these patients. Mood swings and irritability can disrupt relationships, creating difficulties within and outside the home. Nurses can help parents understand the medical reason for behavior changes and offer ways to minimize them. A school consultation is important to provide education and suggest ways to assist a child after diagnosis.

Nurses should know the side effects of antithyroid drug therapy, including urticarial rash, fever, arthralgias, vasculitis, liver dysfunction, and agranulocytosis. Lymphadenopathy, edema, and diminished taste can also occur. Parents must understand the signs of hypothyroidism, which can occur from overdose.

! NURSING ALERT

Children being treated with propylthiouracil or methimazole must be carefully monitored for side effects of the drug. Because sore throat and fever accompany the grave complication of leukopenia, these children should be seen by a practitioner if such symptoms occur. Parents and children should be taught to recognize and report symptoms immediately.

! NURSING ALERT

The earliest indication of hypoparathyroidism may be anxiety and mental depression followed by paresthesia and evidence of heightened neuromuscular excitability, such as:

Chvostek sign: Facial muscle spasm elicited by tapping the facial nerve in the region of the parotid gland

Trousseau sign: Carpal spasm elicited by pressure applied to nerves of the upper arm

Tetany: Carpopedal spasm (sharp flexion of wrist and ankle joints), muscle twitching, cramps, seizures, and stridor

[b]6066 Leesburg Pike, Suite 550, Falls Church, VA 22041; 800-THY-ROID; email: thyroid@thyroid.org; http://www.thyroid.org.

DISORDERS OF PARATHYROID FUNCTION

The parathyroid glands secrete **parathyroid hormone (PTH)**. Along with vitamin D and calcitonin, PTH regulates the homeostasis of serum calcium concentrations (Lal & Clark, 2011). The effect of PTH on calcium is opposite that of calcitonin. PTH and vitamin D work together to maintain serum calcium levels within a narrow normal range. They are required for bone mineralization. Secretion of PTH is controlled by a negative feedback system involving the serum calcium ion concentration. Low ionized calcium levels stimulate PTH secretion, causing absorption of calcium by the target tissues; high ionized calcium concentrations suppress PTH.

HYPOPARATHYROIDISM

Hypoparathyroidism can be inherited or acquired and is rare in children (Al-Azem & Khan, 2012; Cusano, Rubin, & Bilezikian, 2015). Impaired secretion of PTH results in hypocalcemia and hyperphosphatemia (Snyder, 2015). **Congenital hypoparathyroidism** may be caused by genetic defects in the synthesis or cellular processing of PTH or by aplasia or hypoplasia of the gland (Al-Azem & Khan, 2012; Lal & Clark, 2011). Hypoparathyroidism may occur secondary to other causes, including infection, radiation, low levels of magnesium, and autoimmune syndromes (Al-Azem & Khan, 2012; Snyder, 2015). Postoperative hypoparathyroidism may be a result of thyroid surgery and be due to damage or removal of the parathyroid glands or disruption of their blood supply (Monis & Monnstadt, 2015). Two forms of transient hypoparathyroidism may be present in newborns, both of which are the result of PTH deficiency. One type is caused by maternal hyperparathyroidism. A more common form appears almost exclusively in infants fed a milk formula with a high phosphate-to-calcium ratio.

Pseudohypoparathyroidism occurs when there is a genetic defect in the cellular receptors to PTH and a resistance to the hormone (Al-Azem & Khan, 2012; Linglart, Levine, & Juppner, 2018). The result is normal parathyroid gland and normal PTH levels (Linglart et al., 2018). Calcium and phosphorus levels are not affected by administration of PTH. These children typically have a short, stocky build; a round face; and abnormally shaped hands and fingers. Other endocrine dysfunction may be found concurrently (Shoback, 2008).

Clinical signs of hypoparathyroidism are found in Box 28.8. Muscle cramps are an early symptom, progressing to numbness, stiffness, and tingling in the hands and feet. A positive Chvostek or Trousseau sign or laryngeal spasms may be present. Convulsions with loss of consciousness may occur. These episodes may be preceded by abdominal discomfort, tonic rigidity, head retraction, and cyanosis. Headaches and vomiting with increased intracranial pressure and papilledema may occur and may suggest a brain tumor (Doyle, 2020a). Hypoparathyroidism is associated with poor growth in children (Waller, 2011).

Diagnostic Evaluation

The diagnosis of hypoparathyroidism is made based on clinical manifestations associated with **decreased serum calcium** and **increased serum phosphorus**. Levels of plasma PTH are low in hypoparathyroidism but high in pseudohypoparathyroidism. End-organ responsiveness is tested by the administration of PTH with measurement of urinary cyclic adenosine monophosphate (cAMP). Kidney function tests are included in the differential diagnosis to rule out renal insufficiency. Magnesium levels should also be tested. Although bone radiograph findings are usually normal, they may demonstrate increased bone density and suppressed growth.

BOX 28.8 Clinical Manifestations of Hypoparathyroidism

Pseudohypoparathyroidism

Short stature
Round face
Short, thick neck
Short, stubby fingers and toes
Dimpling of skin over knuckles
Subcutaneous soft tissue calcifications
Intellectual disability a prominent feature

Idiopathic Hypoparathyroidism

None of the above physical characteristics observed
May include papilledema
May have intellectual disability

Both Types

Dry, scaly, coarse skin with eruptions
Hair often brittle
Nails thin and brittle with characteristic transverse grooves
Dental and enamel hypoplasia
Muscle contractions:
- Tetany
- Carpopedal spasm
- Laryngospasm (laryngeal stridor)
- Muscle cramps and twitching
- Positive Chvostek or Trousseau sign
- Paresthesias, tingling

Neurologic:
- Headache
- Seizures (generalized, absence, or focal)
- Swings of emotion
- Loss of memory
- Depression
- Confusion possible

Gastrointestinal:
- Muscle cramps
- Diarrhea
- Vomiting
- Retarded skeletal growth

Therapeutic Management

The objective of treatment is to maintain normal serum calcium and phosphate levels with minimum complications. Acute or severe tetany is corrected immediately by IV and oral administration of calcium and follow-up daily doses to achieve normal levels. Twice-daily serum calcium measurements are taken to monitor the efficacy of therapy and prevent hypercalcemia. When diagnosis is confirmed, **vitamin D therapy** is begun (Snyder, 2015). Vitamin D therapy is somewhat difficult to regulate because the drug has a prolonged onset and a long half-life. Some advocate beginning with a lower dose with stepwise increases and careful monitoring of serum calcium until stable levels are achieved. Others prefer rapid induction with higher doses and rapid reduction to lower maintenance levels (Doyle, 2020a).

Long-term management usually consists of vitamin D and oral calcium supplementation. Blood calcium and phosphorus are monitored frequently until the levels have stabilized. Renal function, blood pressure, and serum vitamin D levels are measured every 6 months. Serum magnesium levels are measured to permit detection of hypomagnesemia, which may raise the requirement for vitamin D. The US Food

BOX 28.9 Clinical Manifestations of Hyperparathyroidism

Gastrointestinal
Nausea
Vomiting
Abdominal discomfort
Constipation

Central Nervous System
Delusions
Confusion
Hallucinations
Impaired memory
Lack of interest and initiative
Depression
Varying levels of consciousness

Neuromuscular
Weakness
Easy fatigability
Muscle atrophy (especially proximal muscles of lower limbs)
Tongue twitching
Paresthesias in extremities

Skeletal
Vague bone pain
Subperiosteal resorption of phalanges
Spontaneous fractures
Absence of lamina dura around teeth

Renal
Polyuria
Polydipsia
Renal colic
Hypertension

and Drug Administration has approved a daily subcutaneous injection of recombinant human PTH for use in adults, and clinical trials are studying its use in children (Snyder, 2015).

Nursing Care Management

Unexplained convulsions, irritability (especially to external stimuli), gastrointestinal symptoms (diarrhea, vomiting, cramping), and positive signs of tetany are signs of hypocalcemia related to hypoparathyroidism. Nursing care includes institution of seizure and safety precautions; reduction of environmental stimuli; and observation for signs of laryngospasm, such as stridor, hoarseness, and a feeling of tightness in the throat. A tracheostomy set and injectable calcium gluconate should be available for emergency use. The administration of calcium gluconate requires precautions against extravasation of the drug and tissue destruction.

The nurse educates the family about continuous daily calcium and vitamin D. Because vitamin D toxicity can be a serious consequence of therapy, parents are advised to watch for signs that include weakness, fatigue, lassitude, headache, nausea, vomiting, and diarrhea. Polyuria, polydipsia, and nocturia are signs of early renal impairment.

HYPERPARATHYROIDISM

Hyperparathyroidism is rare in childhood but can be primary or secondary. The most common cause of primary hyperparathyroidism is adenoma of the gland (Doyle, 2020b). The most common causes of secondary hyperparathyroidism are chronic renal disease, renal osteodystrophy, and congenital anomalies of the urinary tract. The most common symptom is hypercalcemia. The clinical signs of hyperparathyroidism are listed in Box 28.9.

Diagnostic Evaluation

Blood studies to identify elevated calcium and decreased phosphorus levels are routinely performed. Measurement of PTH and tests to isolate the cause of the hypercalcemia, such as renal function studies, should be included. If a parathyroid adenoma is suspected, imaging using ultrasound and a sestamibi nuclear subtraction study are recommended (Pashtan, Grogan, Kaplan, et al., 2013). Other procedures used to substantiate the physiologic consequences of the disorder include electrocardiography and radiographic bone surveys.

Therapeutic Management

Treatment depends on the cause of hyperparathyroidism. The treatment of primary hyperparathyroidism is medication, but if this fails, surgical removal of the tumor or radioactive iodine is used (Doyle, 2020b). Treatment of secondary hyperparathyroidism is directed at the underlying contributing cause, which subsequently restores the serum calcium balance. However, in some instances (such as in chronic renal failure), the underlying disorder is irreversible. In this case, treatment is aimed at raising serum calcium levels to inhibit the stimulatory effect of low levels on the parathyroids. This includes oral administration of calcium salts, high doses of vitamin D to enhance calcium absorption, a low-phosphorus diet, and administration of a phosphorus-mobilizing aluminum hydroxide to reduce phosphate absorption.

Nursing Care Management

The initial nursing objective is recognition of the disorder. Because secondary hyperparathyroidism is a consequence of chronic renal failure, the nurse is always alert to signs that suggest this complication, especially bone pain and fractures. Because urinary symptoms are the earliest indication, assessment of other body systems for evidence of high calcium levels is indicated when polyuria and polydipsia coexist. Clues to the possibility of hyperparathyroidism include change in behavior, especially inactivity; unexplained gastrointestinal symptoms; and cardiac irregularities.

DISORDERS OF ADRENAL FUNCTION

The **adrenal cortex** secretes three main groups of hormones collectively called **steroids** and classified according to their biologic activity: (1) **glucocorticoids** (cortisol, corticosterone), (2) **mineralocorticoids** (aldosterone), and (3) **sex steroids** (androgens, estrogens, and progestins). The glucocorticoids and mineralocorticoids affect metabolism and stress. The sex steroids influence sexual development but are not essential because the gonads secrete the major supply of these hormones.

The **adrenal medulla** secretes the **catecholamines epinephrine** and **norepinephrine**. Both hormones have the same effects on various organs as those caused by direct sympathetic stimulation, except that the hormonal effects last several times longer. Catecholamine-secreting tumors are the primary cause of adrenal medullary hyperfunction. Primary adrenal insufficiency (PAI) is a group of disorders of the adrenal cortex that impair secretion of glucocorticoids and may be accompanied by mineralocorticoid and androgen deficiency or overproduction (Kirkgoz & Guran, 2018). This condition is usually inherited in children (Kirkgoz & Guran, 2018). Central adrenal insufficiency (CAI) is life threatening, involves impaired communication of hormone secretion from the pituitary or hypothalamus in the brain, and can be seen in children with genetic or malformative syndromes (Patti, Guzzeti, Di Iorgi, et al., 2018). In each case, the adrenal cortex will not secrete appropriate steroids in response to stress

ACUTE ADRENOCORTICAL INSUFFICIENCY

The acute form of adrenocortical insufficiency (**adrenal crisis**) may have a number of causes during childhood. Acute causes of adrenal insufficiency in children include hemorrhage into the adrenal gland from trauma or childbirth; infections, such as meningococcemia; abrupt withdrawal of exogenous sources of cortisone; failure to increase exogenous steroids during stress; or congenital adrenogenital hyperplasia of the salt-losing type.

Early symptoms of acute adrenocortical insufficiency may include increased irritability, poor feeding, headache, abdominal pain,

BOX 28.10 Clinical Manifestations of Acute Adrenocortical Insufficiency

Early Symptoms
Increased irritability
Headache
Diffuse abdominal pain
Weakness
Nausea and vomiting
Diarrhea

Generalized Hemorrhagic Manifestations (Waterhouse-Friderichsen Syndrome)
Fever (increases as condition worsens)
Central nervous system (CNS) signs:
- Nuchal rigidity
- Seizures
- Stupor
- Coma

Shocklike State
Weak, rapid pulse
Decreased blood pressure
Shallow respirations
Cold, clammy skin
Cyanosis
Circulatory collapse (terminal event)

Newborn
Hyperpyrexia
Tachypnea
Cyanosis
Seizures
Gland evident as palpable retroperitoneal mass (hemorrhagic)

weakness, nausea, vomiting, and diarrhea. Other clinical signs are found in Box 28.10. In newborns, adrenal crisis may be accompanied by high fever, tachypnea, cyanosis, and seizures. Usually there is no evidence of infection or clinical signs of bleeding. However, hemorrhage into the adrenal gland may be evident as a palpable retroperitoneal mass.

Diagnostic Evaluation

There is no rapid, definitive test to confirm acute adrenocortical insufficiency. Diagnosis is often made based on clinical presentation, especially when a fulminating sepsis is accompanied by hemorrhagic manifestations and signs of circulatory collapse despite adequate antibiotic therapy. Because there is no real danger in administering a cortisol preparation for a short period, treatment is instituted immediately. Improvement with cortisol therapy confirms the diagnosis.

Therapeutic Management

Acutely, treatment involves replacement of cortisol, replacement of body fluids to combat dehydration and hypovolemia, administration of glucose solutions to correct hypoglycemia, and specific antibiotic therapy in the presence of infection. Initially, IV hydrocortisone (Solu-Cortef) is administered. Normal saline containing 5% glucose is given parenterally to replace lost fluid, electrolytes, and glucose. If hemorrhage has been severe, whole blood may be replaced. In the event that these measures do not reverse the circulatory collapse, vasopressors are used for immediate vasoconstriction and elevation of blood pressure.

After the child's condition has been stabilized, oral doses of cortisone, fluids, and salt are given, similar to the regimen used for chronic adrenal insufficiency. To maintain sodium retention, aldosterone is replaced by synthetic salt-retaining steroid. Once a patient is stable, if central adrenal insufficiency is suspected, morning serum cortisol levels should be measured, and a stimulation test to measure cortisol release may be warranted (Patti et al., 2018).

Nursing Care Management

Because of the abrupt onset and potentially fatal outcome of this condition, prompt recognition is essential. Vital signs and blood pressure are taken every 15 minutes. Seizure precautions are instituted. The nurse should monitor the child's response to fluid and cortisol replacement. Rapid administration of fluids can precipitate cardiac failure, and overdosage with cortisol may cause hypotension and a sudden fall in temperature.

When the acute phase is over and the hypovolemia has been corrected, the child is given oral fluids in small quantities. Rapid ingestion of oral fluids may induce vomiting, which increases dehydration. Therefore the nurse should plan a gradual schedule for reintroducing liquids.

! NURSING ALERT

Monitor serum electrolyte levels and observe for signs of hypokalemia or hyperkalemia (e.g., weakness, poor muscle control, paralysis, cardiac dysrhythmias, apnea). The condition is rapidly corrected with intravenous (IV) or oral potassium replacement.

NURSING TIP: When an oral potassium preparation is given, it should be mixed with a small amount of strongly flavored fruit juice to disguise its bitter taste.

The sudden, severe nature of this disorder necessitates a great deal of emotional support for the child and family. The child may be placed in an intensive care unit where the surroundings are strange and frightening. Despite the need for emergency intervention, the nurse must be sensitive to the family's psychologic needs and prepare them for each procedure even if this is a brief statement, such as "The IV infusion is necessary to replace fluid that the child is losing." Because recovery within 24 hours is often dramatic, the nurse should keep the parents apprised of the child's condition, emphasizing signs of improvement, such as a lowered temperature and elevated blood pressure.

PRIMARY ADRENAL INSUFFICIENCY (ADDISON DISEASE)

Chronic primary adrenal insufficiency is rare in children and is usually caused by a genetic disorder causing one of the following: abnormal development of the adrenal gland, dysfunctional synthesis of adrenal hormones, resistance to ACTH, or damage to the adrenal cortex (Kirkgoz & Guran, 2018). Other causes include infection, a destructive lesion of the adrenal gland, or an autoimmune process. Because 90% of adrenal tissue must be nonfunctional before signs of insufficiency are manifested, onset of symptoms is often gradual. However, during periods of stress, when demands for additional cortisol are increased, symptoms of acute adrenal insufficiency may appear in a previously well child (Box 28.11).

Definitive diagnosis is based on measurements of functional cortisol reserve. The fasting serum cortisol and urinary 17-hydroxycorticosteroid levels are low and fail to rise, and plasma **adrenocorticotropic**

BOX 28.11 Clinical Manifestations of Chronic Adrenocortical Insufficiency

Neurologic Symptoms
Muscular weakness
Mental fatigue
Irritability, apathy, and negativism
Increased sleeping, listlessness

Pigmentary Changes
Previous scars
Palmar creases
Mucous membranes
Hair
Hyperpigmentation over pressure points (elbows, knees, or waist)
Less frequently, vitiligo (loss of pigmentation)

Gastrointestinal Symptoms
Dehydration
Anorexia
Weight loss

Circulatory Symptoms
Hypotension
Small heart size
Dizziness
Syncopal (fainting) attacks

Hypoglycemia
Headache
Hunger
Weakness
Trembling
Sweating

Other Signs (Seen in Some Children)
Recurrent, unexplained seizures
Intense craving for salt
Acute abdominal pain
Electrolyte imbalances

hormone (ACTH) levels are elevated with corticotropin (ACTH) stimulation, the definitive test for the disease.

Therapeutic Management

Treatment involves replacement of glucocorticoids (cortisol) and mineralocorticoids (aldosterone). Some children are able to be maintained solely on oral supplements of cortisol (cortisone or hydrocortisone preparations) with a liberal intake of salt. During stressful situations (such as fever, infection, emotional upset, or surgery), the dosage must be tripled to accommodate the body's increased need for glucocorticoids. Failure to meet this requirement will precipitate an acute crisis. Overdosage produces appearance of cushingoid signs.

Children with more severe states of chronic adrenal insufficiency require mineralocorticoid replacement to maintain fluid and electrolyte balance. Other forms of therapy include monthly injections of desoxycorticosterone acetate or implantation of desoxycorticosterone acetate pellets subcutaneously every 9 to 12 months. Continuous subcutaneous hydrocortisone infusions via a pump have also been used, but are associated with higher costs and potential risk of complications (Kirkgoz & Guran, 2018).

Nursing Care Management

After the disorder is diagnosed, parents need guidance concerning drug therapy. They must be aware of the continuous need for cortisol replacement. Sudden termination of the drug because of inadequate supplies or inability to ingest the oral form because of vomiting places the child in danger of an acute adrenal crisis. Parents should always have a spare supply of medication. Ideally, families will have a prefilled syringe of hydrocortisone and have training to administer this drug during a crisis. Unnecessary administration of cortisone will not harm the child, but if it is needed, it may be life-saving. Any evidence of acute insufficiency should be reported to the practitioner immediately.

Undesirable side effects of cortisone include gastric irritation, which is minimized by ingestion with food or the use of an antacid; increased excitability and sleeplessness; weight gain, which may require dietary management to prevent obesity; and occasionally behavioral changes, including depression or euphoria. Parents should be aware of signs of overdose and report these to the practitioner. In addition, the drug has a bitter taste, which creates a challenge.

Because the body cannot supply endogenous sources of cortical hormones during times of stress, the home environment should be stable and relatively unstressful. Parents need to be aware that during periods of emotional or physical crisis, the child requires additional hormone replacement. The child should wear a medical identification bracelet, to notify medical personnel during emergency care.

BOX 28.12 Etiology of Cushing Syndrome

Pituitary: Cushing syndrome with adrenal hyperplasia, usually attributed to an excess of ACTH
Adrenal: Cushing syndrome with hypersecretion of glucocorticoids, generally a result of adrenocortical neoplasms
Ectopic: Cushing syndrome with autonomous secretion of ACTH, most often caused by extrapituitary neoplasms
Iatrogenic: Cushing syndrome, frequently a result of administration of large amounts of exogenous corticosteroids
Food dependent: Inappropriate sensitivity of adrenal glands to normal postprandial increases in secretion of gastric inhibitory polypeptide

Adapted from Magiakou, M. A., Mastorakos, G., Oldfield, E. H., et al. (1994). Cushing's syndrome in children and adolescents: Presentation, diagnosis, and therapy. *New England Journal of Medicine, 331*(10), 629–636.
ACTH, Adrenocorticotropic hormone.

CUSHING SYNDROME

Cushing syndrome (CS) is a characteristic group of conditions caused by excessive circulating free cortisol. This can result from a variety of causes, which generally fall into one of five categories (Box 28.12).

Cushing syndrome is uncommon in children. When seen, it is often caused by excessive or prolonged steroid therapy that produces a cushingoid appearance (Fig. 28.2). When caused by excess exogenous steroid therapy, CS is reversible after the steroids are gradually discontinued (Stratakis, 2016). Abrupt withdrawal will precipitate acute adrenal insufficiency. Gradual withdrawal of exogenous supplies is necessary to allow the anterior pituitary an opportunity to secrete increasing amounts of ACTH to stimulate the adrenals to produce cortisol.

Clinical Manifestations

Because the actions of cortisol are widespread, clinical manifestations are equally profound and diverse. The symptoms that produce changes in physical appearance occur early in the disorder and are of considerable concern to school-age and older children. The physiologic disturbances, such as hyperglycemia, susceptibility to infection, hypertension, and hypokalemia, may have life-threatening consequences unless they are recognized early and treated successfully. Children with short stature may be responding to increased cortisol levels, resulting in Cushing syndrome. Cortisol inhibits the action of GH.

Diagnostic Evaluation

Several tests are helpful in confirming Cushing syndrome. Serum cortisol levels should be measured at midnight and in the morning along with corticotropin hormone, urinary free cortisol, fasting blood glucose levels for hyperglycemia, serum electrolyte levels for hypokalemia and alkalosis, and 24-hour urinary levels of elevated 17-hydroxycorticoids and 17-ketosteroids (Lowitz & Keil, 2015). Imaging of the pituitary and

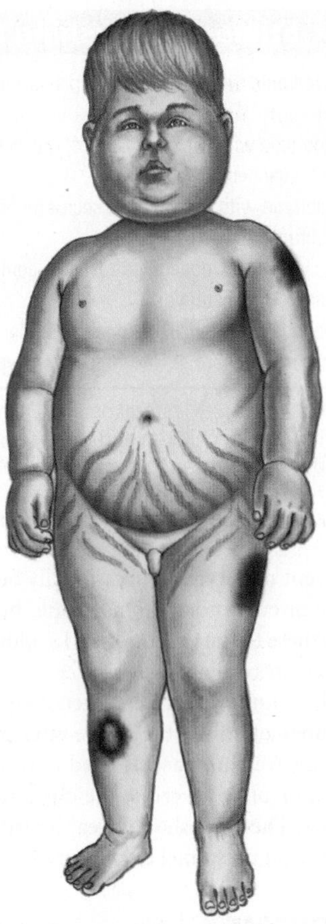

Fig. 28.2 Characteristics of Cushing syndrome.

adrenal glands to assess for tumors, bone density studies for evidence of osteoporosis, and skull radiographs to determine enlargement of the sella turcica may also aid in the diagnosis. Another procedure used to establish a more definitive diagnosis is the dexamethasone (cortisone) suppression test (Ceccato & Boscaro, 2016). Administration of an exogenous supply of cortisone normally suppresses ACTH production. However, in individuals with Cushing syndrome, cortisol levels remain elevated. This test is helpful in differentiating between children who are obese and those who appear to have cushingoid features.

Therapeutic Management

Treatment depends on the cause. If the cause is an adrenal tumor, surgery involves bilateral adrenalectomy and postoperative replacement of the cortical hormones (as outlined for primary adrenocortical insufficiency). If a pituitary tumor is found, surgical extirpation or irradiation may be chosen. In either of these instances, treatment of panhypopituitarism with replacement of GH, TH, ADH, gonadotropins, and steroids may be necessary for an indefinite period (Lau, Rutledge, & Aghi, 2015).

Nursing Care Management

Nursing care also depends on the cause. When cushingoid features are caused by steroid therapy, the effects may be lessened with administration of the drug early in the morning and on an alternate-day basis. Giving the drug early in the day maintains the normal diurnal pattern of cortisol secretion. If given during the evening, it is more likely to produce symptoms because endogenous cortisol levels are already low, and the additional supply exerts more pronounced effects. An alternate-day schedule allows the anterior pituitary an opportunity to maintain more normal hypothalamic-pituitary-adrenal control mechanisms.

If an organic cause is found, nursing care is related to the treatment regimen. Although a bilateral adrenalectomy permanently solves one condition, it reciprocally produces another syndrome. Before surgery, parents need to be adequately informed of the operative benefits and disadvantages. Postoperative teaching on drug replacement is the same as discussed in the previous section.

> **! NURSING ALERT**
>
> Postoperative complications of adrenalectomy are related to the sudden withdrawal of cortisol. Observe for shocklike symptoms (e.g., hypotension, hyperpyrexia).

Anorexia and nausea and vomiting are common and may be improved with the use of nasogastric decompression. Muscle and joint pain may be severe, requiring use of analgesics. The psychologic depression can be profound and may not improve for months. Parents should be aware of the physiologic reasons behind these symptoms in order to be supportive of the child.

CONGENITAL ADRENAL HYPERPLASIA

Congenital adrenal hyperplasia (CAH) is a family of inherited disorders caused by decreased enzyme activity required for cortisol production in the adrenal cortex and is the most common cause of primary adrenal insufficiency in children (Kirkgoz & Guran, 2018). The adrenal gland produces excessive amounts of cortisol precursors and androgens to compensate. The most common defect is **21-hydroxylase deficiency**, which constitutes more than 90% of all cases of CAH (El-Maouche, Arlt, & Merke, 2017). This deficiency is an autosomal recessive disorder that results in improper steroid hormone synthesis (Mendes, Vaz Matos, Ribeiro, et al., 2015).

Excessive androgens cause masculinization of the urogenital system at approximately the tenth week of fetal development. The most pronounced abnormalities occur in girls, who are born with varying degrees of ambiguous genitalia. Masculinization of external genitalia causes the clitoris to enlarge so that it appears as a small phallus. Fusion of the labia produces a saclike structure resembling the scrotum without testes. However, no abnormal changes occur in the internal sexual organs, although the vaginal orifice is usually closed by the fused labia. The label *ambiguous genitalia* should be applied to any infant with hypospadias or micropenis and no palpable gonads, and a diagnostic evaluation for CAH should be contemplated (Witchel, 2017).

Increased pigmentation of skin creases and genitalia caused by increased ACTH may be a subtle sign of adrenal insufficiency. A salt-wasting crisis frequently occurs, usually within the first few weeks of life, and is often the first presentation in boys, who have normal genital development (White, 2020a; Witchel, 2017). Infants fail to gain weight, and hyponatremia and hyperkalemia may be significant. Cardiac arrest can occur.

Untreated CAH results in early sexual maturation, with enlargement of the external sexual organs; development of axillary, pubic, and facial hair; deepening of the voice; acne; and a marked increase in musculature with changes toward an adult male physique. However, in contrast to precocious puberty, breasts do not develop in girls, and they remain amenorrheic and infertile. In boys, the testes remain small, and spermatogenesis does not occur. In both sexes, linear growth is accelerated, and epiphyseal closure is premature, resulting in short stature by the end of puberty.

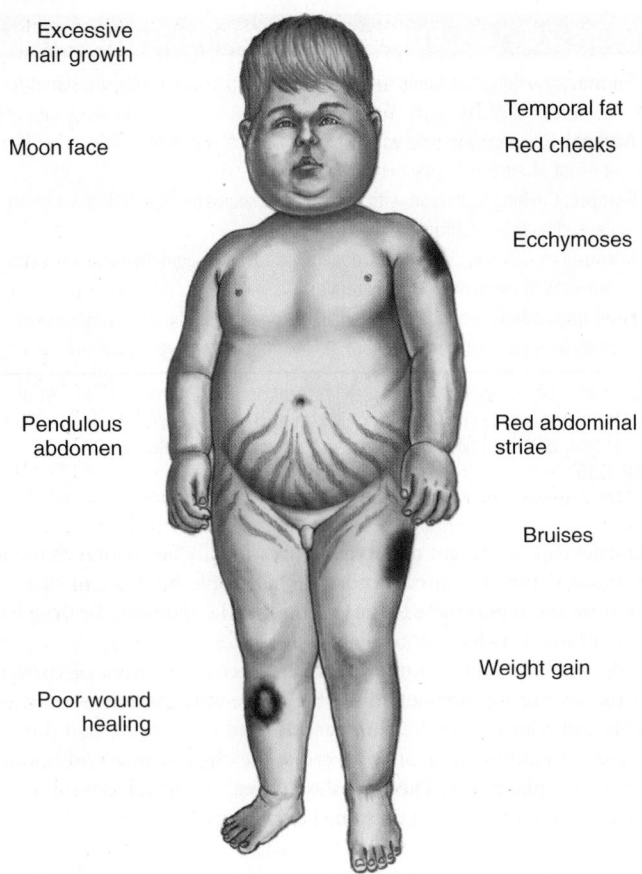

Diagnostic Evaluation

Clinical diagnosis is initially based on congenital abnormalities that lead to difficulty in assigning sex to the newborn and on signs and symptoms of adrenal insufficiency. Newborn screening is currently done in all 50 states by measurement of the cortisol precursor 17-hydroxyprogesterone. Definitive diagnosis is confirmed by evidence of increased 17-ketosteroid levels in most types of CAH (Kaye, Committee on Genetics, Accurso, et al., 2006). In complete 21-hydroxylase deficiency, blood electrolytes demonstrate loss of sodium and chloride and elevation of potassium. In older children, bone age is advanced, and linear growth is increased. Deoxyribonucleic acid (DNA) analysis for positive sex determination and to rule out any other genetic abnormality (e.g., Turner syndrome) is always done in any case of ambiguous genitalia.

Another test that can be used to visualize the presence of pelvic structures is ultrasonography, a noninvasive, painless imaging technique that does not require anesthesia or sedation. It is especially useful in CAH because it readily identifies the absence or presence of female reproductive organs or male testes in a newborn or child with ambiguous genitalia. Because ultrasonography yields immediate results, it has the advantage of determining the child's gender long before the more complex laboratory results for chromosome analysis or steroid levels are available.

Therapeutic Management

After diagnosis is confirmed, medical management includes administration of glucocorticoids to suppress the abnormally high secretions of ACTH and adrenal androgens. The goal of therapy is to achieve and maintain the timing of normal pubertal development and achieve adult height (Bomberg, Addo, Kyllo, et al., 2015; Witchel, 2017). If cortisone is begun early enough, it is very effective. Cortisone depresses the secretion of ACTH by the anterior pituitary, which in turn inhibits the secretion of adrenocorticosteroids, which stems the progressive virilization. The signs and symptoms of masculinization in girls gradually disappear, and excessive early linear growth is slowed. Puberty occurs normally at the appropriate age.

The recommended oral dosage is divided to simulate the normal diurnal pattern of ACTH secretion. Because these children are unable to produce cortisol in response to stress, it is necessary to increase the dosage during episodes of infection, fever, surgery, or other stresses. Acute emergencies require immediate IV or intramuscular administration. Children with the salt-losing type of CAH require aldosterone replacement, as outlined under chronic adrenal insufficiency, and supplementary dietary salt. Frequent laboratory tests are conducted to assess the effects on electrolytes, hormonal profiles, and renin levels. The frequency of testing is individualized to the child.

Gender assignment and surgical intervention in the newborn with ambiguous genitalia is complex and controversial. It is a significant stress for families, who need support from a multidisciplinary team of experienced specialists. Factors that influence gender assignment include genetic diagnosis, genital appearance, surgical options, fertility, and family and cultural preferences. Generally, genetically female (46XX) infants should be raised as girls. Early reconstructive surgery should be considered only in the case of severe virilization (El-Maouche et al., 2017). Emphasis is on functional rather than cosmetic outcomes, and surgery often can be delayed. Reports of sexual satisfaction after partial clitoridectomy indicate that the capacity for orgasm and sexual gratification is not necessarily impaired. Male infants may require phallic reconstruction by an experienced surgeon.

Unfortunately, not all children with CAH are diagnosed at birth and raised in accordance with their genetic sex. Particularly in the case of affected females, masculinization of the external genitalia may have led to sex assignment as a male. In males, diagnosis is usually delayed until early childhood, when signs of virilism appear. In these situations, it is advisable to continue rearing the child as a male in accordance with assigned sex and phenotype. Hormone replacement may be required to permit linear growth and to initiate male pubertal changes. Surgery is usually indicated to remove the female organs and reconstruct the phallus for satisfactory sexual relations. These individuals are not fertile.

Nursing Care Management

Of major importance is recognition of ambiguous genitalia and diagnostic confirmation in newborns. Parents need assistance in understanding and accepting the condition and time to grieve for the loss of perfection in their newborn child. As soon as the sex is determined, parents should be informed of the findings and encouraged to choose an appropriate name, and the child should be identified as a male or female with no reference to ambiguous sex.

In general, rearing a genetically female child as a girl is preferred because of the success of surgical intervention and the satisfactory results with hormones in reversing virilism and providing a prospect of normal puberty and the ability to conceive. This is in contrast to the choice of rearing the child as a boy, in which case the child is sterile and may never be able to function satisfactorily in heterosexual relationships. If the parents persist in their decision to assign a male sex to a genetically female child, a psychologic consultation should be requested to explore their motivations and ensure their understanding of the future consequences for the child.

Nursing care management regarding cortisol and aldosterone replacement is the same as discussed for chronic adrenocortical insufficiency. Because infants are especially prone to dehydration and salt-losing crises, parents need to be aware of signs of dehydration and the urgency of immediate medical intervention to stabilize the child's condition. Parents should have injectable hydrocortisone available and know how to prepare and administer the intramuscular injection (see Chapter 20).

In the unfortunate situation in which the sex is erroneously assigned and the correct sex is determined later, parents need a great deal of help in understanding the reason for the incorrect sex identification and the options for sex reassignment or medical-surgical intervention.

Parents should be referred for genetic counseling before they conceive another child because CAH is an autosomal recessive disorder. Prenatal diagnosis and treatment are available.

> **! NURSING ALERT**
>
> The parents should be advised that there is no physical harm in treating for suspected adrenal insufficiency that is not present, but the consequence of not treating acute adrenal insufficiency can be fatal.

PHEOCHROMOCYTOMA

Pheochromocytoma is a rare tumor characterized by secretion of catecholamines. The tumor most commonly arises from the chromaffin cells of the adrenal medulla but may occur wherever these cells are found, such as along the paraganglia of the aorta or thoracolumbar sympathetic chain. In children, they are frequently bilateral or multiple and are generally benign. Often there is a familial transmission of the condition as an autosomal dominant trait (White, 2020b).

The clinical manifestations of pheochromocytoma are caused by an increased production of catecholamines, producing hypertension, tachycardia, headache, decreased gastrointestinal activity and resulting constipation, increased metabolism with anorexia, weight loss, hyperglycemia, polyuria, polydipsia, hyperventilation, nervousness, heat intolerance, and diaphoresis. In severe cases, signs of congestive heart failure are evident. A child with sustained hypertension, family history of endocrine tumors, or syndromic features associated with endocrine tumor development should be screened (Jain, Baracco, & Kapur, 2019).

Diagnostic Evaluation

The clinical manifestations mimic those of other disorders, such as hyperthyroidism or DM. Usually the tumor is identified by computed tomography (CT) scan or MRI. Diagnostic tests include a 24-hour measurement of urinary levels of the catecholamine metabolites and plasma metanephrine measurement (Jain et al., 2019).

Therapeutic Management

Definitive treatment consists of surgical removal of the tumor. In children, the tumors may be bilateral, requiring a bilateral adrenalectomy and lifelong glucocorticoid and mineralocorticoid therapy. The major complications that can occur during surgery are severe hypertension, tachyarrhythmias, and hypotension. The first two are caused by excessive release of catecholamines during manipulation of the tumor, and the latter results from catecholamine withdrawal and hypovolemic shock. Treatment with alpha-adrenergic receptor blockers 7 to 14 days prior to surgery, volume expansion preoperatively, followed by beta-blockade, is necessary to reduce the incidence of complications (Jain et al., 2019). Success of therapy is judged by lowering of blood pressure to normal, absence of hypertensive attacks (flushing or blanching, fainting, headache, palpitations, tachycardia, nausea and vomiting, profuse sweating), heat tolerance, a decrease in perspiration, and disappearance of hyperglycemia.

Nursing Care Management

Children with hypertension and hypertensive attacks should be assessed for pheochromocytoma. Because of behavioral changes (nervousness, excitability, overactivity, and even psychosis), increased cardiac and respiratory activity may appear to be related to an acute anxiety attack. Therefore a careful history of the onset of symptoms and association with stressful events is helpful in distinguishing between an organic and a psychologic cause for the symptoms.

Preoperative nursing care involves frequent monitoring of vital signs and observation for evidence of hypertensive attacks and congestive heart failure. Therapeutic effects are evidenced by normal vital signs and absence of glycosuria. Daily blood glucose levels, urine acetone, and any signs of hyperglycemia are noted and reported immediately.

> **! NURSING ALERT**
>
> Do not palpate the mass. Preoperative palpation of the mass releases catecholamines, which can stimulate severe hypertension and tachyarrhythmias.

The environment is made conducive to rest and free of emotional stress. This requires adequate preparation during hospital admission and before surgery. Parents are encouraged to room-in with their child and to participate in care. Play activities need to be tailored to the child's energy level without being overly strenuous or challenging, because these activities can increase metabolic rate and promote frustration and anxiety.

After surgery, the child is observed for signs of shock from removal of excess catecholamines. If a bilateral adrenalectomy was performed, the nursing interventions are those discussed for chronic adrenocortical insufficiency.

DISORDERS OF PANCREATIC HORMONE SECRETION

DIABETES MELLITUS

DM is a chronic disorder of metabolism characterized by hyperglycemia and insulin resistance. It is the most common metabolic disease, resulting in metabolic adjustment or physiologic change in almost all areas of the body. The most recent statistics indicate that in the United States, approximately 208,000 children younger than 20 years old have either type 1 or type 2 diabetes (National Institutes of Health 2017). Type 1 diabetes has the highest number of new cases in non-Hispanic white children at a 4.2% annual increase.

Traditionally, DM was classified according to the type of treatment needed. The old categories were insulin-dependent diabetes mellitus (IDDM), or type I, and non–insulin-dependent diabetes mellitus (NIDDM), or type II. In 1997 these terms were eliminated because treatment can vary (some people with NIDDM require insulin) and because the terms do not indicate the underlying problem. The new terms are *type 1* and *type 2,* using Arabic symbols to avoid confusion (e.g., type II could be read as type eleven) (American Diabetes Association, 2001). The characteristics of type 1 DM and type 2 DM are outlined in Table 28.2.

TABLE 28.2 Characteristics of Type 1 and Type 2 Diabetes Mellitus

Characteristic	Type 1	Type 2
Age at onset	<20 years	Increasingly occurring in younger children
Type of onset	Abrupt	Gradual
Sex ratio	Affects males slightly more than females	Females outnumber males
Percentage of diabetic population	5%-8%	85%-90%
Heredity:		
Family history	Sometimes	Frequently
Human leukocyte antigen	Associations	No association
Twin concordance	25%-50%	90%-100%
Ethnic distribution	Primarily whites	Increased incidence in American Indians, Hispanics, African Americans
Presenting symptoms	Three Ps common—polyuria, polydipsia, polyphagia	May be related to long-term complications
Nutritional status	Underweight	Overweight
Insulin (natural):		
Pancreatic content	Usually none	>50% normal
Serum insulin	Low to absent	High or low
Primary resistance	Minimum	Marked
Islet cell antibodies	80%-85%	<5%
Therapy:		
Insulin	Always	20%-30% of patients
Oral agents	Ineffective	Often effective
Diet only	Ineffective	Often effective
Chronic complications	>80%	Variable
Ketoacidosis	Common	Infrequent

Type 1 diabetes most commonly presents between 4 and 6 years of age and then at 10 to 14 years of age; about 45% of children diagnosed will present before their tenth birthday. In 2003 type 2 diabetes represented 20% of pediatric diabetes cases, and half of those cases were adolescents between 15 and 19 years old (Levitsky & Misra, 2019a).

Type 1 diabetes is characterized by destruction of the pancreatic beta cells, which produce insulin; this usually leads to absolute insulin deficiency. Type 1 diabetes has two forms. Immune-mediated DM results from an autoimmune destruction of the beta cells; it typically starts in children or young adults who are slim, but it can arise in adults of any age. **Idiopathic type 1** refers to rare forms of the disease that have no known cause.

Type 2 diabetes usually arises because of insulin resistance in which the body fails to use insulin properly combined with relative (rather than absolute) insulin deficiency. People with type 2 DM can range from predominantly insulin resistant with relative insulin deficiency to predominantly deficient in insulin secretion with some insulin resistance. It typically occurs in those who are older than 45 years of age, are overweight and sedentary, and have a family history of diabetes.

The symptomatology of diabetes is more readily recognizable in children than in adults, so it is surprising that the diagnosis may sometimes be missed or delayed. Diabetes is a great imitator; influenza, gastroenteritis, and appendicitis are the conditions most often diagnosed when it turns out that the disease is really diabetes (Box 28.13).

Pathophysiology

Insulin is needed to support the metabolism of carbohydrates, fats, and proteins, primarily by facilitating the entry of these substances into the cells. Insulin is needed for the entry of glucose into the muscle and fat cells, prevention of mobilization of fats from fat cells, and storage of glucose as glycogen in the cells of liver and muscle. Insulin is not needed for the entry of glucose into nerve cells or vascular tissue. The chemical composition and molecular structure of insulin are such that it fits into receptor sites on the cell membrane. Here it initiates a sequence of poorly defined chemical reactions that alter the cell membrane to facilitate the entry of glucose into the cell and stimulate enzymatic systems outside the cell that metabolize the glucose for energy production.

With a deficiency of insulin, glucose is unable to enter the cells, and its concentration in the bloodstream increases. The increased concentration of glucose (**hyperglycemia**) produces an osmotic gradient that causes the movement of body fluid from the intracellular space to the interstitial space and then to the extracellular space and into the glomerular filtrate to "dilute" the hyperosmolar filtrate. Normally, the renal tubular capacity to transport glucose is adequate to reabsorb all the glucose in the glomerular filtrate. When the glucose concentration in the glomerular filtrate exceeds the renal threshold (180 mg/dl), glucose spills into the urine (**glycosuria**) along with an osmotic diversion of water (**polyuria**), a cardinal sign of diabetes. The urinary fluid losses cause the excessive thirst (**polydipsia**) observed in diabetes. This water "washout" results in a depletion of other essential chemicals, especially potassium.

Protein is also wasted during insulin deficiency. Because glucose is unable to enter the cells, protein is broken down and converted to glucose by the liver (**glucogenesis**); this glucose then contributes to the hyperglycemia. These mechanisms are similar to those seen in starvation when substrate (glucose) is absent. The body is actually in a state of starvation during insulin deficiency. Without the use of carbohydrates for energy, fat and protein stores are depleted as the body attempts to meet its energy needs. The hunger mechanism is triggered, but increased food intake (polyphagia) enhances the problem by further elevating blood glucose.

Ketoacidosis

When insulin is absent or insulin sensitivity is altered, glucose is unavailable for cellular metabolism, and the body chooses alternate sources of energy, principally fat. Consequently, fats break down into fatty acids, and glycerol in the fat cells is converted by the liver to ketone bodies (β-hydroxybutyric acid, acetoacetic acid, acetone). Any excess is eliminated in the urine (**ketonuria**) or the lungs (**acetone breath**). The ketone bodies in the blood (ketonemia) are strong acids that lower serum pH, producing **ketoacidosis**.

Ketones are organic acids that readily produce excessive quantities of free hydrogen ions, causing a fall in plasma pH. Then chemical buffers in the plasma, principally bicarbonate, combine with the hydrogen ions to form carbonic acid, which readily dissociates into water and carbon dioxide. The respiratory system attempts to eliminate the excess carbon dioxide by increased depth and rate (Kussmaul respirations, or the hyperventilation characteristic of metabolic acidosis). The ketones are buffered by sodium and potassium in the plasma. The kidneys attempt to compensate for the increased pH by increasing tubular secretion of hydrogen and ammonium ions in exchange for fixed base, thus depleting the base buffer concentration.

With cellular death, potassium is released from the cells (intracellular fluid) into the bloodstream (extracellular fluid) and excreted by the kidneys, where the loss is accelerated by osmotic diuresis. The total body potassium is then decreased even though the serum potassium level may be elevated as a result of the decreased fluid volume in which it circulates. Alteration in serum and tissue potassium can lead to cardiac arrest.

If these conditions are not reversed by insulin therapy in combination with correction of the fluid deficiency and electrolyte imbalance, progressive deterioration occurs, with dehydration, electrolyte imbalance, acidosis, coma, and death. **Diabetic ketoacidosis (DKA)** should be diagnosed promptly in a seriously ill patient and therapy instituted in an intensive care unit.

Long-Term Complications

Long-term complications of diabetes involve both the microvasculature and the macrovasculature. The principal microvascular complications are **nephropathy**, **retinopathy**, and **neuropathy**. Microvascular disease develops during the first 30 years of diabetes, beginning in the first 10 to 15 years after puberty, with renal involvement evidenced by proteinuria and clinically apparent retinopathy. Macrovascular disease

BOX 28.13 Clinical Manifestations of Type 1 Diabetes Mellitus

- Polyphagia
- Polyuria
- Polydipsia
- Weight loss
- Enuresis or nocturia
- Irritability; "not himself" or "not herself"
- Shortened attention span
- Lowered frustration tolerance
- Dry skin
- Blurred vision
- Poor wound healing
- Fatigue
- Flushed skin
- Headache
- Frequent infections
- Hyperglycemia
  - Elevated blood glucose levels
  - Glucosuria
- Diabetic ketosis
  - Ketones and glucose in urine
  - Dehydration in some cases
- Diabetic ketoacidosis (DKA)
  - Dehydration
  - Electrolyte imbalance
  - Acidosis
  - Deep, rapid breathing (Kussmaul respirations)

develops after 25 years of diabetes and creates the predominant problems in patients with type 2 DM. The process appears to be one of glycosylation, wherein proteins from the blood become deposited in the walls of small vessels (e.g., glomeruli), where they become trapped by "sticky" glucose compounds (glycosyl radicals). The buildup of these substances over time causes narrowing of the vessels, with subsequent interference with microcirculation to the affected areas (Rosenson & Herman, 2008).

With poor diabetic control, vascular changes can appear as early as 2½ to 3 years after diagnosis; however, with good to excellent control, changes can be postponed for 20 or more years. Intensive insulin therapy appears to delay the onset and slow the progression of retinopathy, nephropathy, and neuropathy. Hypertension and atherosclerotic cardiovascular disease are also major causes of morbidity and mortality in patients with DM (Karnik, Fields, & Shannon, 2007).

Other complications have been observed in children with type 1 DM. Hyperglycemia appears to influence thyroid function, and altered function is frequently observed at the time of diagnosis and in poorly controlled diabetes. Limited mobility of small joints of the hand occurs in 30% of 7- to 18-year-old children with type 1 DM and appears to be related to changes in the skin and soft tissues surrounding the joint as a result of glycosylation.

! NURSING ALERT

Recurrent vaginal and urinary tract infections, especially with *Candida albicans*, are often an early sign of type 2 diabetes mellitus, especially in adolescents.

Diagnostic Evaluation

Three groups of children who should be considered candidates for diabetes are (1) those who have glycosuria, polyuria, and a history of weight loss or failure to gain despite a voracious appetite; (2) those with transient or persistent glycosuria; and (3) those who display manifestations of metabolic acidosis, with or without stupor or coma. In every case, diabetes must be considered if there is glycosuria, with or without ketonuria, and unexplained hyperglycemia.

Glycosuria by itself is not diagnostic of diabetes. Other sugars, such as galactose, can produce a positive result with certain test strips, and a mild degree of glycosuria can be caused by other conditions, such as infection, trauma, emotional or physical stress, hyperalimentation, and some renal or endocrine diseases.

DM is diagnosed based on any of the following four abnormal glucose metabolites: (1) 8-hour fasting blood glucose level of 126 mg/dl or more, (2) a random blood glucose value of 200 mg/dl or more accompanied by classic signs of hyperglycemia, (3) an oral glucose tolerance test (OGTT) finding of 200 mg/dl or more in the 2-hour sample, and (4) hemoglobin A1c of 6.5% or more (Laffel & Svoren, 2018). Postprandial blood glucose determinations and the traditional OGTTs have yielded low detection rates in children and are not usually necessary for establishing a diagnosis. Serum insulin levels may be normal or moderately elevated at the onset of diabetes; delayed insulin response to glucose indicates impaired glucose tolerance.

Ketoacidosis must be differentiated from other causes of acidosis or coma, including hypoglycemia, uremia, gastroenteritis with metabolic acidosis, salicylate intoxication encephalitis, and other intracranial lesions. DKA is a state of relative insulin insufficiency and may include the presence of hyperglycemia (blood glucose level ≥200 mg/dl), ketonemia (strongly positive), acidosis (pH <7.30 and bicarbonate <15 mmol/L), glycosuria, and ketonuria (Wolsdorf, Craig, Daneman, et al., 2009). Tests used to determine glycosuria and ketonuria are the glucose oxidase tapes (Keto-Diastix).

Therapeutic Management

The management of the child with type 1 DM consists of a multidisciplinary approach involving the family; the child (when appropriate); and professionals, including a pediatric endocrinologist, diabetes nurse educator, nutritionist, and exercise physiologist. Often psychologic support from a mental health professional is also needed. Communication among the team members is essential and extends to other individuals in the child's life, such as teachers, school nurse, school guidance counselor, and coach.

The definitive treatment is replacement of insulin that the child is unable to produce. However, insulin needs are also affected by emotions, nutritional intake, activity, and other life events, such as illnesses and puberty. The complexity of the disease and its management requires that the child and family incorporate diabetes needs into their lifestyle. Medical and nutritional guidance are primary, but management also includes continuing diabetes education, family guidance, and emotional support.

Insulin Therapy

Insulin replacement is the cornerstone of management of type 1 DM. Insulin dosage is tailored to each child based on home blood glucose monitoring. The goal of insulin therapy is maintaining near-normal blood glucose values while avoiding too frequent episodes of hypoglycemia. Insulin is administered as two or more injections per day or as continuous subcutaneous infusion using a portable insulin pump.

Healthy pancreatic cells secrete insulin at a low but steady basal rate with superimposed bursts of increased secretion that coincide with intake of nutrients. Consequently, insulin levels in the blood increase and decrease coincidentally, with the rise and fall in blood glucose levels. In addition, insulin is secreted directly into the portal circulation; therefore the liver, which is the major site of glucose disposal, receives the largest concentration of insulin. No matter which method of insulin replacement is used, this normal pattern cannot be duplicated. Subcutaneous injection results in absorption of the drug into the general circulation, thus reducing the concentrations of insulin to which the liver is exposed.

Insulin Preparations

Insulin is available in highly purified pork preparations and in human insulin biosynthesized by and extracted from bacterial or yeast cultures. Most clinicians suggest human insulin as the treatment of choice. Insulin is available in rapid-, intermediate-, and long-acting preparations; and all are packaged in the strength of 100 units/ml. Some insulins are available as premixed insulins, such as 70/30 and 50/50 ratios, the first number indicating the percentage of intermediate-acting insulin and the second number the percentage of rapid-acting insulin. The different types of insulin are outlined in Box 28.14.

! NURSING ALERT

The human insulins from various manufacturers may be interchangeable, but human insulin and pork insulin or pure pork insulin should never be substituted for one another.

Dosage. Conventional management is a twice-daily insulin regimen of a combination of **rapid-acting** and **intermediate-acting** insulin drawn up into the same syringe and injected before breakfast and before the evening meal. The amount of morning regular insulin is determined by patterns in the late morning and lunchtime blood glucose values. The morning intermediate-acting dosage is determined by patterns in the late afternoon and supper blood glucose values.

Fasting blood glucose patterns at breakfast help determine the evening dose of intermediate insulin, and the blood glucose patterns at bedtime help determine the evening dose of rapid-acting (regular) insulin. For some children, better morning glucose control is achieved by a later (bedtime) injection of intermediate-acting insulin.

Regular insulin is best administered at least 30 minutes before meals. This allows sufficient time for absorption and results in a significantly greater reduction in the postprandial rise in blood glucose than if the meal were eaten immediately after the insulin injection. Intensive therapy consists of multiple injections throughout the day with a once- or twice-daily dose of long-acting (Ultralente) insulin to simulate the basal insulin secretion and injections of rapid-acting insulin before each meal. A multiple daily injection program reduces microvascular complications of diabetes in young, healthy patients who have type 1 DM.

The precise dose of insulin needed cannot be predicted. Therefore the total dosage and percentage of regular- to intermediate-acting insulin should be determined empirically for each child. Usually 60% to 75% of the total daily dose is given before breakfast, and the remainder is given before the evening meal. Furthermore, insulin requirements do not remain constant but change continuously during growth and development; the need varies according to the child's activity level and pubertal status. For example, less insulin is required during spring and summer months when children are more active. Illness also alters insulin requirements. Some children require more frequent insulin administration. This includes children with difficult-to-control diabetes and children during the adolescent growth spurt.

BOX 28.14 Types of Insulin

There are four types of insulin, based on the following criteria:

- How soon the insulin starts working (onset)
- When the insulin works the hardest (peak time)
- How long the insulin lasts in the body (duration)

However, each person responds to insulin in his or her own way. That is why onset, peak time, and duration are given as ranges.

Rapid-acting insulin (e.g., NovoLog) reaches the blood within 15 minutes after injection. The insulin peaks 30 to 90 minutes later and may last as long as 5 hours.

Short-acting (regular) insulin (e.g., Novolin R) usually reaches the blood within 30 minutes after injection. The insulin peaks 2 to 4 hours later and stays in the blood for about 4 to 8 hours.

Intermediate-acting insulins (e.g., Novolin N) reach the blood 2 to 6 hours after injection. The insulins peak 4 to 14 hours later and stay in the blood for about 14 to 20 hours.

Long-acting insulin (e.g., Lantus) takes 6 to 14 hours to start working. It has no peak or a very small peak 10 to 16 hours after injection. The insulin stays in the blood between 20 and 24 hours.

Some insulins come mixed together (e.g., Novolin 70/30). For example, you can buy regular insulin and NPH insulins already mixed in one bottle, which makes it easier to inject two kinds of insulin at the same time. However, you cannot adjust the amount of one insulin without also changing how much you get of the other insulin.

NPH, Neutral protamine Hagedorn.

Methods of administration. Daily insulin is administered subcutaneously by twice-daily injections, by multiple-dose injections, or by means of an insulin infusion pump. Insulin pumps are small computerized devices that deliver insulin in two ways: in a steady measured and continuous dose (the "basal" insulin) or as a surge ("bolus") dose, at your direction, around mealtime.

Doses are delivered through a flexible plastic tube called a catheter. With the aid of a small needle, the catheter is inserted through the skin into the fatty tissue and is taped in place. Pumps can be programmed to release small doses of insulin continuously (basal) or a bolus dose close to mealtime to control the rise in blood glucose after a meal. This delivery system most closely mimics the body's normal release of insulin (Insulin Pumps, 2018).

The system consists of a syringe to hold the insulin, a plunger, and a computerized mechanism to drive the plunger. The insulin flows from the syringe through a catheter to a needle inserted into subcutaneous tissue (the abdomen or thigh), and the lightweight device is worn on a belt or a shoulder holster. The needle and catheter are changed every 48 to 72 hours by the child or parent using aseptic technique and then taped in place.

Although the pump provides more consistent insulin delivery, it has certain disadvantages. Pump therapy is expensive and requires commitment from the parent and child. A certain level of math skills is required to calculate infusion rates. It should also not be removed for more than 1 hour at a time, which may limit some activities. Skin infections are common, and as with any other mechanical device, it is subject to malfunction. However, the pumps are equipped with alarms that signal problems, such as a depleted battery, an occluded needle or tubing, or a microprocessor malfunction.

Monitoring

Daily monitoring of blood glucose levels is an essential aspect of appropriate DM management. Plasma blood glucose and hemoglobin A1c goal ranges are found in Table 28.3.

Blood glucose. Self-monitoring of blood glucose (SMBG) has improved diabetes management and is used successfully by children from the onset of their diabetes. By testing their own blood, children are able to change their insulin regimen to maintain their glucose level in the euglycemic (normal) range of 80 to 120 mg/dl. Diabetes

TABLE 28.3 Plasma Blood Glucose and Hemoglobin A1c Goals for Type 1 Diabetes Mellitus by Age-Group

Age	Value[a] Before Meals (mg/dl)	Value[a] at Bedtime/ Overnight (mg/dl)	Hemoglobin A1c (%)	Implications
Toddlers and preschoolers (<6 years)	100-180	110-200	≤8.5% (but ≥7.5%)	High risk and vulnerability to hypoglycemia
School age (6-12 years)	90-180	100-180	<8%	Risks of hypoglycemia and relatively low risk of complications before puberty
Adolescents (>12 years) and young adults	90-130	90-150	<7.5%	Risk of hypoglycemia Developmental and psychologic issues

[a]Plasma blood glucose goal range.

Modified from American Diabetes Association. (2005). Standards of medical care in diabetes. *Diabetes Care, 28*(Suppl), S4–S36.

management depends to a great extent on SMBG. In general, children tolerate the testing well.

Glycosylated hemoglobin. The measurement of glycosylated hemoglobin (hemoglobin A1c) levels is a satisfactory method for assessing control of the diabetes. As red blood cells circulate in the bloodstream, glucose molecules gradually attach to the hemoglobin A molecules and remain there for the lifetime of the red blood cell, approximately 120 days. The attachment is not reversible; therefore this glycosylated hemoglobin reflects the average blood glucose levels over the previous 2 to 3 months. The test is a satisfactory method for assessing control, detecting incorrect testing, monitoring the effectiveness of changes in treatment, defining patients' goals, and detecting nonadherence. Nondiabetic hemoglobin A1c values are generally between 4% and 6% but can vary by laboratory. Well-controlled diabetes has a hemoglobin A1c goal of less than 7.5% for most children and adolescents (Levitsky & Misra, 2018; Silverstein, Klingensmith, Copeland, et al., 2005).

Urine. Urine testing for glucose is no longer used for diabetes management; there is poor correlation between simultaneous glycosuria and blood glucose concentrations. However, urine testing can be carried out to detect evidence of ketonuria.

! NURSING ALERT

It is recommended that urine be tested for ketones every 3 hours during an illness or whenever the blood glucose level is greater than 240 mg/dl when illness is not present.

Nutrition

Essentially, the nutritional needs of children with diabetes are no different from those of healthy children. Children with diabetes need no special foods or supplements. They need sufficient calories to balance daily expenditure for energy and to satisfy the requirement for growth and development. Unlike children without diabetes, whose insulin is secreted in response to food intake, insulin injected subcutaneously has a relatively predictable time of onset, peak effect, duration of action, and absorption rate depending on the type of insulin used. Consequently, the timing of food consumption must be regulated to correspond to the timing and action of the insulin prescribed.

Meals and snacks must be eaten according to peak insulin action, and the total number of calories and proportions of basic nutrients must be consistent from day to day. The constant release of insulin into the circulation makes the child prone to hypoglycemia between the three daily meals unless a snack is provided between meals and at bedtime. The distribution of calories should be calculated to fit the activity pattern of each child. For example, a child who is more active in the afternoon will need a larger snack at that time. This larger snack might also be split to allow some food at school and some food after school. Food intake should be altered to balance food, insulin, and exercise. Extra food is needed for increased activity.

Concentrated sweets are discouraged, and because of the increased risk of atherosclerosis in persons with DM, fat is reduced to 30% or less of the total caloric requirement. Dietary fiber has become increasingly important in dietary planning because of its influence on digestion, absorption, and metabolism of many nutrients. It has been found to diminish the rise in blood glucose after meals.

For growing children, food restriction should never be used for diabetes control, although caloric restrictions may be imposed for weight control if the child is overweight. In general, the child's appetite should be the guide for the amount of calories needed, with the total caloric intake adjusted to appetite and activity.

Exercise

Exercise is encouraged and never restricted unless indicated by other health conditions. Exercise lowers blood glucose levels, depending on the intensity and duration of the activity. Consequently, exercise should be included as part of diabetes management, and the type and amount of exercise should be planned around the child's interests and capabilities. However, in most instances, children's activities are unplanned, and the resulting decrease in blood glucose can be compensated for by providing extra snacks before (and if the exercise is prolonged, during) the activity. In addition to a feeling of well-being, regular exercise aids in use of food and often results in a reduction in insulin requirements.

! NURSING ALERT

Hypoglycemic episodes most commonly occur before meals or when the insulin effect is peaking.

Hypoglycemia

Occasional episodes of hypoglycemia are an integral part of insulin therapy, and an objective of diabetes management is to achieve the best possible glycemic control while minimizing the frequency and severity of hypoglycemia. Even with good control, a child may frequently experience mild symptoms of hypoglycemia. If the signs and symptoms are recognized early and promptly relieved by appropriate therapy, the child's activity should be interrupted for no more than a few minutes.

The signs and symptoms of hypoglycemia are caused by both increased adrenergic activity and impaired brain function. The increased adrenergic nervous system activity plus increased secretion of catecholamines produces tremor, pallor, rapid heart rate, palpitations, and diaphoresis (Levitsky & Misra, 2019b). Weakness, dizziness, headache, drowsiness, irritability, loss of coordination, seizures, and coma are more severe responses and reflect CNS glucose deprivation and the body's attempts to elevate the serum glucose levels.

It is often difficult to distinguish between hyperglycemia and a hypoglycemic reaction (Table 28.4). Because the symptoms are similar and usually begin with changes in behavior, the simplest way to differentiate between the two is to test the blood glucose level. The blood glucose level is low in hypoglycemia, but in hyperglycemia, the glucose level is significantly elevated. Urinary ketones may be present after hypoglycemia as a result of starvation ketone production. In doubtful situations, it is safer to give the child some simple carbohydrate. This will help alleviate the symptoms in the case of hypoglycemia but will do little harm if the child is hyperglycemic.

Children are usually able to detect the onset of hypoglycemia, but some are too young to implement treatment. Parents should become adept at recognizing the onset of symptoms—for example, a change in a child's behavior, such as tearfulness or euphoria. In the majority of cases, 10 to 15 g of simple carbohydrate, such as 1 Tbsp of table sugar, will elevate the blood glucose level and alleviate the symptoms. The simpler the carbohydrate, the more rapidly it will be absorbed (8 oz of milk equals 15 g of carbohydrate). The rapidly releasing sugar is followed by a complex carbohydrate (such as a slice of bread or a cracker) and by a protein (such as peanut butter or milk).

For a mild reaction, milk or fruit juice is a good food to use in children. Milk supplies them with lactose or milk sugar, as well as a more prolonged action from the protein and fat (aids in decreased absorption). Other glucose sources include Insta-Glucose (cherry-flavored glucose), carbonated drinks (not sugarless), sherbet, gelatin, or cake icing. All children with diabetes should carry with them glucose tabs, Insta-Glucose, sugar cubes, or sugar-containing candy, such as

TABLE 28.4 Comparison of Manifestations of Hypoglycemia and Hyperglycemia

Variable	Hypoglycemia	Hyperglycemia
Onset	Rapid (minutes)	Gradual (days)
Mood	Labile, irritable, nervous, weepy	Lethargic
Mental status	Difficulty concentrating, speaking, focusing, coordinating Nightmares	Dulled sensorium Confusion
Inward feeling	Shaky feeling	Thirst
	Hunger	Weakness
	Headache	Nausea and vomiting
	Dizziness	Abdominal pain
Skin	Pallor Sweating	Flushed Signs of dehydration
Mucous membranes	Normal	Dry, crusty
Respirations	Shallow, normal	Deep, rapid (Kussmaul)
Pulse	Tachycardia, palpitations	Less rapid, weak
Breath odor	Normal	Fruity, acetone
Neurologic	Tremors	Diminished reflexes Paresthesia
Ominous signs	Late: Hyperreflexia, dilated pupils, seizure Shock, coma	Acidosis, coma
Blood:		
Glucose	Low: <60 mg/dl	High: ≥200 mg/dl
Ketones	Negative	High, large
Osmolarity	Normal	High
pH	Normal	Low (≤7.25)
Hematocrit	Normal	High
Bicarbonate	Normal	<20 mEq/L
Urine:		
Output	Normal	Polyuria (early) to oliguria (late)
Glucose	Negative	Enuresis, nocturia
Ketones	Negative or trace	High
Visual	Diplopia	Blurred vision

LifeSavers or Charms. A difficulty with candies or icing is that the child may learn to fake a reaction to get the sweets; therefore commercial treatment products such as Insta-Glucose or glucose tabs may be preferred.

Glucagon is sometimes prescribed for home treatment of hypoglycemia. It is available as an emergency kit that must be mixed at the time of use and is administered intramuscularly or subcutaneously. Glucagon functions by releasing stored glycogen from the liver and requires about 15 to 20 minutes to elevate the blood glucose level.

! NURSING ALERT

Vomiting may occur after administration of glucagon; therefore precautions against aspiration must be taken (e.g., placing the child on the side) because the child often becomes unconscious.

Morning hyperglycemia. The management of elevated morning blood glucose levels depends on whether the increase is a true dawn phenomenon, **insulin waning**, or a rebound hyperglycemia (the **Somogyi effect**). Insulin waning is a progressive rise in blood glucose levels from bedtime to morning. It is treated by increasing the nocturnal insulin dose. The true dawn phenomenon shows relatively normal blood glucose level until about 3 AM, when the level begins to rise. The Somogyi effect may occur at any time but often entails an elevated blood glucose level at bedtime and a drop at 2 AM, with a rebound rise following. The treatment for this phenomenon is decreasing the nocturnal insulin dose to prevent the 2 AM hypoglycemia. The rebound rise in the blood glucose level is a result of counterregulatory hormones (epinephrine, GH, and corticosteroids), which are stimulated by hypoglycemia. More frequent blood monitoring (especially at times of anticipated peak insulin action) will usually identify these conditions. Trace amounts of urinary ketones aid in identifying undetected hypoglycemia.

Illness Management

Illness alters diabetes management, and maintaining control is usually related to the seriousness of the illness. In a well-controlled child, an illness will run its course as it does in unaffected children. The goals during an illness are to restore euglycemia, treat urinary ketones, and maintain hydration. Blood glucose levels and urinary ketones should be monitored every 3 hours. Some hyperglycemia and ketonuria are expected in most illnesses, even with diminished food intake, and are an indication for increased insulin. Insulin should never be omitted during an illness, although dosage requirements may increase, decrease, or remain unchanged, depending on the severity of the illness and the child's appetite. Often the child will need supplemental insulin between usual dose times. If the child vomits more than once, if blood glucose levels remain above 240 mg/dl, or if urinary ketones remain high, the health care practitioner should be notified. Simple carbohydrates may be substituted for carbohydrate-containing exchanges in the meal plan. Although insulin and diet are important tools in sick-day care, fluids are the most important intervention. Fluids must be encouraged to prevent dehydration and to flush out ketones.

Therapeutic Management of Diabetic Ketoacidosis

DKA, the most complete state of insulin deficiency, is a life-threatening situation. Management consists of rapid assessment, adequate insulin to reduce the elevated blood glucose level, fluids to overcome dehydration, and electrolyte replacement (especially potassium).

DKA constitutes an emergency situation, thus a child should be admitted to an intensive care facility for management. The priority is to obtain a venous access for administration of fluids, electrolytes, and insulin. The child should be weighed, measured, and placed on a cardiac monitor. Blood glucose and ketone levels are determined at the bedside, and samples are obtained for laboratory measurement of glucose, electrolytes, BUN, arterial pH, PaO_2, $PaCO_2$, hemoglobin, hematocrit, white blood cell count and differential, calcium, and phosphorus.

Oxygen may be administered to patients who are cyanotic and in whom arterial oxygen is less than 80%. Gastric suction is applied to unconscious children to avoid the possibility of pulmonary aspiration. Antibiotics may be administered to febrile children after appropriate specimens are obtained for culture. A Foley catheter may or may not be inserted for urine samples and measurement. Unless the child is unconscious, a collection bag is usually sufficient for accurate assessments.

Fluid and Electrolyte Therapy

All patients with DKA experience dehydration (10% of total body weight in severe ketoacidosis) because of the osmotic diuresis, accompanied by depletion of electrolytes, sodium, potassium, chloride, phosphate, and magnesium. Serum pH and bicarbonate reflect the degree of acidosis. Prompt and adequate fluid therapy restores tissue perfusion and suppresses the elevated levels of stress hormones.

The initial rehydration attempts should be 10 to 20 ml/kg of isotonic saline (normal saline or lactated Ringer solution given as an IV bolus). Repeat this bolus until fluid status is stable. Once stable, replace the remaining fluid deficit over the next 24 to 48 hours (Glaser, 2019).

! NURSING ALERT

Potassium must never be given until the serum potassium level is known to be normal or low and urinary voiding is observed. All maintenance intravenous (IV) fluids should include 30 to 40 mEq/L of potassium. Never give potassium as a rapid IV bolus, or cardiac arrest may result.

Serum potassium levels may be normal on admission, but after fluid and insulin administration, the rapid return of potassium to the cells can seriously deplete serum levels, with the attendant risk of cardiac arrhythmias. As soon as the child has established renal function (i.e., is voiding at least 25 ml/h) and insulin has been given, vigorous potassium replacement is implemented. The cardiac monitor is used as a guide to therapy, and configuration of T waves should be observed every 30 to 60 minutes to determine changes that might indicate alterations in potassium concentration (widening of the QT interval and the appearance of a U wave following a flattened T wave indicate hypokalemia; an elevated and spreading T wave and shortening of the QT interval indicate hyperkalemia).

Insulin should not be given until urinary ketones and a blood glucose level have been obtained. Continuous IV regular insulin is given at a dosage of 0.1 units/kg/h. Insulin therapy should be started after the initial rehydration bolus because serum glucose levels fall rapidly after volume expansion. Blood glucose levels should decrease by 50 to 100 mg/dl/h. When blood glucose levels fall to 250 to 300 mg/dl, dextrose is added to the IV solution. The goal is to maintain blood glucose levels between 120 and 240 mg/dl by adding 5% to 10% dextrose. Sodium bicarbonate is used conservatively; it is used for pH less than 7.0, severe hyperkalemia, or cardiac instability. Because sodium bicarbonate has been associated with an increased risk for cerebral edema, children receiving this substance must be carefully monitored for changes in level of consciousness.

When the critical period is over, the task of regulating the insulin dosage in relation to diet and activity is started. Children should be actively involved in their own care and are given responsibility according to their ability and the guidance of the nurse.

! NURSING ALERT

Because insulin can chemically bind to plastic tubing and in-line filters, thereby reducing the amount of medication reaching the systemic circulation, an insulin mixture is run through the tubing to saturate the insulin-binding sites before the infusion is started.

Nursing Care Management

Children with DM may be admitted to the hospital at the time of their initial diagnosis; during illness or surgery; or for episodes of ketoacidosis, which may be precipitated by any of a variety of factors (see Translating Evidence Into Practice box, which evaluates hospitalization compared with outpatient care for children newly diagnosed with type 1 DM). Many children are able to keep the disease under control with periodic assessment and adjustment of insulin, diet, and activity as needed under the supervision of a practitioner. Under most circumstances, these children can be managed well at home and require hospitalization only for serious illnesses or upsets.

However, a small number of children with diabetes exhibit a degree of metabolic lability and have repeated episodes of DKA that require hospitalization, which interferes with their education and social development. These children appear to display a characteristic personality structure. They tend to be unusually passive and nonassertive and to come from families that are inclined to smooth over conflicts without resolution. Children in this type of setting experience emotional arousal with little, if any, opportunity or ability to resolve it. Other children from psychosocially dysfunctional families display behavioral and personality problems. This emotional stress causes an increased production of endogenous catecholamines, which stimulate fat breakdown, leading to ketonemia and ketonuria.

TRANSLATING EVIDENCE INTO PRACTICE

Outpatient Treatment of Type I Diabetes

A *Cochrane Systematic Review* of seven studies evaluating whether children newly diagnosed with type 1 diabetes should be admitted to a hospital or treated in the outpatient setting found no disadvantages to allowing the child to remain an outpatient. Studies evaluated metabolic control, acute diabetic complications and hospitalizations, psychosocial variables and behavior, and total care costs (Clar, Waugh, & Thomas, 2007).

Hospital Management

Children with DKA require intensive nursing care. Vital signs should be observed and recorded frequently. Hypotension caused by the contracted blood volume of the dehydrated state may cause decreased peripheral blood flow, which can be particularly hazardous to the heart, lungs, and kidneys. An elevated temperature may indicate infection and should be reported so that treatment can be implemented immediately.

Careful and accurate records should be maintained, including vital signs (pulse, respiration, temperature, and blood pressure), weight, IV fluids, electrolytes, insulin, blood glucose level, and intake and output. A urine collection device or retention catheter is used to obtain the urine measurements, which include volume, specific gravity, and glucose and ketone values. The volume relative to the glucose content is important because 5% glucose in a 300-ml sample is a significantly greater amount than a similar reading from a 75-ml sample. A diabetic flowsheet maintained at the bedside provides an ongoing record of the vital signs, urine and blood tests, amount of insulin given, and intake and output. The level of consciousness is assessed and recorded at frequent intervals. The comatose child generally regains consciousness fairly soon after initiation of therapy but is managed like any unconscious child until then.

When the critical period is over, the task of regulating insulin dosage to diet and activity begins. The same meticulous records of intake and output, urine glucose and acetone levels, and insulin administration are maintained. Capable children should be actively involved in their own care and are given responsibility for keeping the intake and output record; testing the blood and urine; and, when appropriate, administering their own insulin—all under the supervision and guidance of the nurse (see the Next-Generation NCLEX® Examination-Style Unfolding Case Study box).

NEXT-GENERATION NCLEX® EXAMINATION-STYLE UNFOLDING CASE STUDY

The Child With Diabetes Mellitus

Day 1, 1:00 pm

1. An 8-year-old who has been healthy has lost weight in the past 2 weeks. His mother noticed that he is getting up several times during the night to go to the bathroom. He was drinking a great deal more in the past week, and she thought that was the reason for needing to use the bathroom. However, today he has a headache and is too tired to go to school. She also notices that he has wet the bed during the night. She becomes alarmed and calls the pediatrician for an appointment the next day. She has a brother with diabetes and thinks that the symptoms are similar to her brother's problems when he was first diagnosed as a child. The next day at the pediatrician's office the nurse performs a history and assessment. Which findings in the child's history and assessment findings would require the nurse to **immediately** investigate further? **Select all that apply.**
   A. Tiredness
   B. Headache
   C. Increased thirst
   D. Increased urination
   E. Wetting the bed at night
   F. Oral temperature 98.8 F
   G. Pulse 60 beats per minute
   H. Blood pressure= 94/60 mmHg
   I. Respirations 20 breaths per minute

Day 1, 2:30 pm

2. At the pediatrician's office, several tests are completed, and results are listed below.
   - random blood glucose = 230 mg/dl
   - hemoglobin (Hgb) A1c level = 10.5%.
   - hematocrit = 35%
   - platelets= 250,000/mm^3
   - white blood cells= 8,000/mm^3
   - urine dip test is positive for glucose and ketones

   He is admitted to the hospital for further evaluation to establish a diagnosis. **Choose the most likely options for the information missing from the statements below by selecting from the lists of options provided.**

   Based on the child's history and physical assessment, along with laboratory findings, the nurse suspects a diagnosis of ____1____ because his ____2____ and ____2____ are high. His symptoms may be caused by an increased concentration of ____3____ in the bloodstream.

Options for 1	Options for 2	Options for 3
Diabetes mellitus	platelets	Insulin
Addison disease	hematocrit	Glucose
Cushing syndrome	blood glucose	Potassium
Hyperparathyroidism	A1c level	Calcium
Pituitary hyperfunction	white blood cells	Sodium

Day 2, 12:00 noon

3. An 8-year-old who has been healthy has lost weight in the past 2 weeks. His mother noticed that he is getting up several times during the night to go to the bathroom. He was drinking a great deal more in the past week, and she thought that was the reason for needing to use the bathroom. However, today he has a headache and is too tired to go to school. She also notices that he has wet the bed during the night. She becomes alarmed and calls the pediatrician for an appointment the next day. She has a brother with diabetes and thinks that the symptoms are similar to her brother's problems when he was first diagnosed as a child.

   He was admitted yesterday for further evaluation. To obtain a fasting blood glucose he was given nothing to eat or drink but water for 8 hours before the test this morning. Laboratory results from this AM include the following:
   - 8 hour fasting glucose level =145 mg/dl
   - Oral Glucose tolerance test (OGTT)= 240 mg/dl in 2 hr sample
   - urine dip test is positive for glucose and ketones
   - Hgb A1C level= 10.5%

   He has met the criteria for the diagnosis of Type 1 Diabetes Mellitus. He will start with a twice-daily insulin regimen combining a rapid-acting (regular) insulin with an intermediate-acting (neutral protamine Hagedorn [NPH]/Lente) insulin. The nurse meets with the mother and patient to begin insulin therapy teaching. The mother asks why two types of insulin are needed. What are the **most appropriate** responses for the nurse to provide to help the mother and child understand about types of insulin? **Select all that apply.**
   A. "Rapid-acting insulin peaks in about 30-90 minutes and may last about 5 hours."
   B. "Short-acting insulin reaches the blood in about 5 minutes and peaks in about an hour."
   C. "Extended insulin takes 4 hours to start working and can stay in the blood for up to 14 hours."
   D. "Intermediate-acting insulin peaks in about 4-14 hours and can stay in the blood for 14-20 hours."
   E. "Long-acting insulin takes 6-14 hours to start working and can stay in the blood for up to 24 hours."
   F. "The types of insulin are based on how soon they start working, when the insulin works the hardest and how long it lasts."

NEXT-GENERATION NCLEX® EXAMINATION-STYLE UNFOLDING CASE STUDY—cont'd

The Child With Diabetes Mellitus

Day 2, 4:30 pm

4. The insulin injections are ordered to be given at least 30 minutes before breakfast. The second one will be given 30 minutes before dinner. Even though the patient will start off receiving insulin twice daily, he will still need to check his blood glucose before meals and at bedtime. Based on his age, his glucose goal range before meals should be 90 to 180 mg/dl and at bedtime should be 100 to 180 mg/dl. The nurse is planning the teaching session and is preparing to give an injection of insulin before dinner after checking his blood glucose level. She will demonstrate to the child and parents how to administer the medication with this injection and discuss important aspects of insulin administration at home.
Indicate which nursing action listed in the far-left column is appropriate for each potential complication listed in the middle column. Indicate the nursing action number in the far-right column.
Note that ONLY one nursing action can be used for each potential complication and that NOT all nursing actions will be used.

Nursing Action	Potential Complication	Nursing Action for Complication
1. Obtain blood glucose level before meals and at bedtime.	normal blood glucose level is not maintained	
2. Administer insulin as prescribed.	appropriate dose of insulin is not administered	
3. Monitor urine glucose before each meal.	appropriate type of insulin is not administered	
4. Use aseptic techniques when preparing and administering insulin.	infection occurs	
5. Store insulin in the freezer to preserve the medication.	absorption of insulin is impaired	
6. Understand the action of insulin: differences in composition, time of onset, and duration of action for the various preparations.		
7. Rotate insulin injection sites.		
8. Give less insulin before physical activity		

Day 3, 8:00 am

5. Before breakfast, the blood glucose was checked by the mother with guidance from the nurse. The mother administers the insulin into his left thigh; the patient wanted to have his mother give the insulin the first few times so that he can observe. An hour later the nurse is called to the bed site because he feels funny and his head hurts. He is dizzy when he stands, and his hands are shaking. The parents tell the nurse he did not eat breakfast because he is hoping to be discharged and wanted to eat on the way home.
For each nursing action, use an X to indicate whether it was Effective (helped to meet expected quality patient outcomes), Ineffective (did not help to meet expected quality patient outcomes), or Unrelated (not related to the quality patient outcomes).

Nursing Action	Effective	Ineffective	Unrelated
Immediately administer cup of fruit juice or a glass of nonfat or 1% milk.			
Check blood glucose after 15 minutes.			
Give a starch-protein snack.			
Start intravenous fluids with glucose.			
Provide information for the teacher on the child's diagnosis.			
Give parents instructions regarding signs and symptoms of hypoglycemia versus hyperglycemia.			
Teach parents how to administer intramuscular glucagon if unresponsive, unconscious, or seizing.			
Place the child on a portable insulin infusion pump.			

Day 3, 3:00 pm

6. The patient experienced hypoglycemia this morning after receiving the morning insulin injection. He did not eat breakfast after the injection. The nurse will use this experience to continue teaching the parents and child about how to monitor and manage his diabetes. What are the **most important** teaching topics for the nurse to include at this time? **Select all that apply.**
   A. "Signs of hyperglycemia or high blood sugar include fever, headache, seizures, and cough."
   B. " The blood sugar should be maintained within a target range of 90 to 180 mg/dl during the day."
   C. "Signs of hypoglycemia or low blood sugar include headache, dizziness, shaking, sweating and the pulse is fast."
   D. "Your child should no longer participate in any sports of physical activity that would cause his blood glucose to fall."
   E. "Learning how to plan meals, understanding specific good groups and making good food choices will be an important part of managing his diabetes."
   F. "The health care provider should be contacted when your child has fever for 2 days, vomiting and diarrhea, is unable to keep fluids down, and his glucose levels are above the target range."

Child and Family Education

Several organizations are prepared to assist with education and dissemination of knowledge about diabetes. The American Diabetes Association,[c] Canadian Diabetes Association,[d] Juvenile Diabetes Research Foundation International,[e] and American Association of Diabetes Educators[f] are valuable resources for a wide variety of educational materials. The National Institute of Diabetes and Digestive and Kidney Diseases[g] publishes a number of comprehensive annotated bibliographies, including "Educational Materials for and About Young People With Diabetes," a compilation of resource materials for children, siblings, parents, teachers, and health professionals, and "Sports and Exercise for People With Diabetes."

Medical Identification

One of the first things the nurse should call to the parents' attention is the need for the child to wear some means of medical identification. Usually recommended is the MedicAlert identification, a stainless steel or silver- or gold-plated identification bracelet that is visible and immediately recognizable. It contains a collect telephone number that medical personnel can call around the clock for medical records and personal information.

Nature of Diabetes

The better the parents understand the pathophysiology of diabetes and the function and action of insulin and glucagon in relation to caloric intake and exercise, the better they will understand the disease and its effects on the child. Parents need answers to a number of questions (voiced or unvoiced) to increase their confidence in coping with the disease. For example, they may want to know about the various procedures performed on their child and treatment rationale, such as what is being put in the IV bottle and the expected effect.

Meal Planning

Normal nutrition is a major aspect of the family education program. Diet instruction is usually conducted by the nutritionist, with reinforcement and guidance from the nurse. The emphasis is on adequate intake for age, consistent menus, complex carbohydrates, and consistent eating times. The family is taught how the meal plan relates to the requirements of growth and development, the disease process, and the insulin regimen. Meals and snacks are modified based on the child's preferences and current menu, preserving cultural patterns and preferences as much as possible. Extensive exchange lists that include foods compatible with most lifestyles are available.

Learning about foods within specific food groups helps in making choices. Weights and measures of foods are used as eye-training devices for defining serving sizes and should be practiced for about 3 months, with gradual progression to estimation of food portions. Even when the child and family become competent in estimating portion sizes, reassessment should take place weekly or monthly and when there is any change of brands.

Family members should also be guided in reading labels for the nutritional value of foods and food content. They need to become familiar with the carbohydrate content of food groups. Substitution with foods of equal carbohydrate content is the skill needed for successful carbohydrate counting. Substitution might be necessary if a food is not available in sufficient quantity or for the teenager who wishes to eat fast food with peers. The use of a multiple daily injection program lends flexibility to the timing of meals.

Lists of popular fast-food items and items served at the major fast-food chains can be obtained from the restaurants to help guide food selections. It is important that the child know the nutritional value of these items (the major chains are remarkably uniform), but the child should be cautioned to avoid high-fat and high-sugar/high-carbohydrate items; for example, the child could choose a plain hamburger instead of a double cheeseburger.

Children should use sugar substitutes in moderation in items such as soft drinks. Artificial sweeteners have been shown to be safe, but if there is any question about amounts, the physician, dietitian, or nurse specialist can provide guidelines based on body weight. Sugar-free chewing gum and candies made with sorbitol may be used in moderation by children with DM. Although sorbitol is less cariogenic than other varieties of sugar substitutes, it is an alcohol sugar that is metabolized to fructose and then to glucose. Furthermore, large amounts can cause osmotic diarrhea. Most dietetic foods contain sorbitol. They are more expensive than regular foods. Also, although a product may be sugar free, it is not necessarily carbohydrate free.

Traveling

Traveling requires planning, especially when a trip involves crossing time zones. A number of tips are included in pamphlets available free of charge. Suggestions for traveling encompass what will be needed from the practitioner before leaving, what and how much to take along, needs in transit, what to consider at the destination, and planning for when the child returns home. Planning is needed no matter what type of travel is considered—automobile, plane, bus, or train.

Insulin

Families need to understand the treatment method and the insulin prescribed, including the effective duration, onset, and peak action. They also need to know the characteristics of the various types of insulins, the proper mixing and dilution of insulins, and how to substitute another type when their usual brand is not available (insulin is a nonprescription drug). Insulin need not be refrigerated but should be maintained at a temperature between 15°C and 29.4°C (59°F and 85°F). Freezing renders insulin inactive.

Insulin bottles that have been "opened" (i.e., the stopper has been punctured) should be stored at room temperature or refrigerated for up to 28 to 30 days. After 1 month, these vials should be discarded. Unopened vials should be refrigerated and are good until the expiration date on the label. Diabetic supplies should not be left in a hot environment.

Injection Procedure

Learning to give insulin injections is a source of anxiety for both parents and children. It is helpful for the learner to know that this important aspect of care will become as routine as brushing the teeth. First, the basic injection technique is taught using an orange or similar item and sterile normal saline for practice. To gain children's confidence, the nurse can demonstrate the technique by giving a skillful injection to the parent and then having the parent return the demonstration by giving the nurse an injection. With practice and confidence, the parents will soon be able to give the insulin injection to their children, and their children will trust them. Another effective strategy is to instruct the children and then have them teach the technique to the parents while the nurse observes. Both parents should participate, and as little time as possible should elapse between instruction and the actual injection, especially with parents and teenage learners.

---

[c] 2451 Crystal Dr., Arlington, VA 22202; 800-342-2383; http://www.diabetes.org.

[d] 1300–522 University Ave., Toronto, ON M5G 2R5; 800-226-8464; http://www.diabetes.ca.

[e] 26 Broadway, 14th Floor, New York, NY 10004; 800-533-CURE; http://www.jdrf.org.

[f] 200 W. Madison St., Suite 800, Chicago, IL 60606; 800-338-3633; email: education@aadenet.org; http://www.diabeteseducator.org.

[g] Office of Communications and Public Liaison, NIDDK, NIH, Building 31, Room 9A06, 31 Center Drive, MSC 2560, Bethesda, MD 20892-2560; 301-496-3583; http://www.niddk.nih.gov.

Insulin can be injected into any area in which there is adipose (fat) tissue over muscle; the drug is injected at a 90-degree angle. Newly diagnosed children may have lost adipose tissue, and care should be exerted not to inject intramuscularly. The pinch technique is the most effective method for tenting the skin to allow easy entrance of the needle to subcutaneous tissues in children. The site selected will sometimes depend on whether children or parents administer the insulin. The arms, thighs, hips, and abdomen are usual injection sites for insulin. The children can reach the thighs, abdomen, and part of the hip and arm easily but may require help to inject other sites. For example, a parent can pinch a loose fold of skin of the arm while the child injects the insulin.

The parents and child are helped to work out a rotation pattern to various areas of the body to enhance absorption because insulin absorption is slowed by fat pads that develop in overused injection areas. The most efficient rotation plan involves giving about four to six injections in one area (each injection about 2.5 cm [1 inch] apart, or the diameter of the insulin vial from the previous injection) and then moving to another area.

Remember that the absorption rate varies in different parts of the body (Table 28.5). The methodical use of one anatomic area and then movement to another (as described in the previous paragraph) minimizes variations in absorption rates. However, absorption is also altered by vigorous exercise, which enhances absorption from exercised muscles; therefore it is recommended that a site be chosen other than the exercising extremity (e.g., avoiding legs and arms when playing in a tennis tournament).

Injection sites for an entire month can be determined in advance on a simple chart. For example, a "paper doll" (body outline) can be constructed and insulin sites marked by the child. After injection, the child places the date on the appropriate site. To keep in practice, it is a good idea for the parent to give two or three injections a week in areas that are difficult for the child to reach. The same basic methodology is used when teaching children to give their own insulin injections (Fig. 28.3). They should practice first on an orange or a doll, building courage gradually. Other devices are available for insulin injection, and these may offer advantages to some children. Children who do not wish to give themselves injections can be taught to use a syringe-loaded injector (Inject-Ease). With the device, puncture is always automatic. Adolescents respond well to a self-contained and compact device resembling a fountain pen (NovoPen), which eliminates conventional vials and syringes.

Continuous subcutaneous insulin infusion. Some children are considered candidates for use of a portable insulin pump, and even some young children with unsatisfactory metabolic control can benefit from its use. The child and the parents are taught to operate the device, including the mechanics of the pump, battery changes, and alarm systems. A number of devices that vary in the basal rates they are able to deliver and in the cost of the equipment are on the market. Families can investigate the various devices and select the model that best suits their needs. Product information is available from pump manufacturers and distributors.[h]

Parents and children learn (1) the technical aspects of the pump and SMBG; (2) prevention and treatment for hyperglycemia, sick-day management, and meal planning; (3) the effects of exercise, stress, and diet on blood glucose levels; and (4) decision-making strategies to evaluate blood glucose patterns and make adjustments in all aspects of the regimen.

Numerous blood glucose measurements (at least four times per day) are an essential part of infusion pump use. Intensive education and supervision are critical to obtaining maximum efficiency and control. This is particularly important if the family has been accustomed to a conventional insulin regimen. They must realize that simply wearing the pump will not normalize blood glucose. The pump is merely an insulin delivery device, and frequent, routine blood glucose determinations are necessary to adjust the insulin delivery rate.

The major problems with use of the insulin pump are inflammation from irritation and infection at the insertion site. The site should be cleaned thoroughly before the needle is inserted and then covered with a transparent dressing. The site is changed and rotated every 48 to 72 hours (this may vary) or at the first sign of inflammation. Nurses working where pumps are part of the therapeutic regimen should become familiar with the operation of the specific device being used and the protocol of disease management. Others should be aware of this management technique and be prepared to assist patients using the pump.

Monitoring

Nurses should also be prepared to teach and supervise blood glucose monitoring. SMBG is associated with few complications, and although it does not necessarily lead to improved metabolic control, it provides a more accurate assessment of blood glucose levels than can be obtained with the historical urine testing. Blood glucose monitoring has the added advantage that it can be performed anywhere (see Atraumatic Care box).

ATRAUMATIC CARE

Minimizing Pain of Blood Glucose Monitoring

- To enhance blood flow to the finger, hold it under warm water for a few seconds before the puncture.
- When obtaining blood samples, use the ring finger or thumb (blood flows more easily to these areas) and puncture the finger just to the side of the finger pad (more blood vessels and fewer nerve endings).
- To prevent a deep puncture, press the platform of the lancet device lightly against the skin and avoid steadying the finger against a hard surface.
- Use lancet devices with adjustable-depth tips. Begin with the shallowest setting.
- Use glucose monitors that require small blood samples (e.g., Ascensia Elite) to avoid repeated punctures.

[h]Medtronic MiniMed, http://www.medtronicdiabetes.com/home; Animas, http://www.animas.com.

TABLE 28.5 Onset and Duration of Action Related to Injection Site

	SITE OF INJECTION			
	Abdomen	**Arm**	**Leg**	**Buttock**
Rate	Very fast	Fast	Slow	Very slow
Duration	Very short	Short	Long	Very long

From Albisser, A. M., & Sperlich, M. (1992). Adjusting insulins. *Diabetes Educator, 18*(3), 211–218.

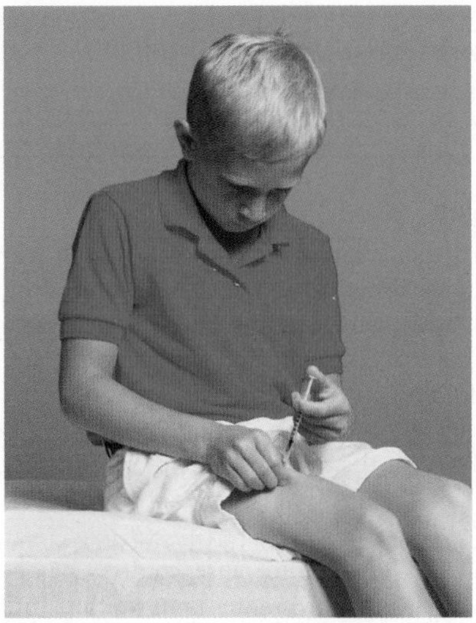

Fig. 28.3 School-age children can administer their own insulin.

Blood for testing can be obtained by two different methods: manually or with a mechanical bloodletting device. A mechanical device is recommended for children, although the child and family should learn to use both methods in the event of mechanical failure. Several lancet devices are available, and each provides a means for obtaining a large drop of blood for testing (Fig. 28.4).

> **! NURSING ALERT**
>
> Caution children not to allow anyone else to use their lancet because of the risk of contracting hepatitis B virus or human immunodeficiency virus infection.

The blood sample may be obtained from fingertips or alternate sites, such as the forearm. Alternate site testing requires a meter that can test a small volume of blood. Not all meters are capable of this.

Signs of redness and soreness at the site of finger puncture should be examined by the practitioner. It may be evidence of poor technique, poor hygiene, or poor skin healing relative to poor control. Many types of blood-testing meters are available for home use. Newer technology has brought about improvements in meter size and ease of use. The family should be shown features of several meters, including advantages and disadvantages, and allowed to choose equipment that best meets their needs.

The least expensive testing method uses a reagent strip to which blood is applied (Fig. 28.5). After blotting, the color change is compared against a color scale for an estimation of the blood glucose level. The strips can be cut in half (although not all professionals recommend this) to obtain two readings per strip. This method is not accepted practice but may be necessary for some families or situations.

Urine testing. Testing for urinary ketones is recommended during times of illness and when blood glucose values are elevated. Information on a specific ketone-testing product should include correct procedure, storage, and product expiration. Families need a clear understanding of home management of ketones (fluids and additional insulin as directed by the health care team).

Signs of Hyperglycemia

Severe hyperglycemia is most often caused by illness, growth, emotional upset, or missed insulin doses. Emotional stress from school finals or examinations or physical response to immunizations are examples of causes of hyperglycemia. With careful glucose monitoring, any elevation can be managed by adjustment of insulin or food intake. Parents should

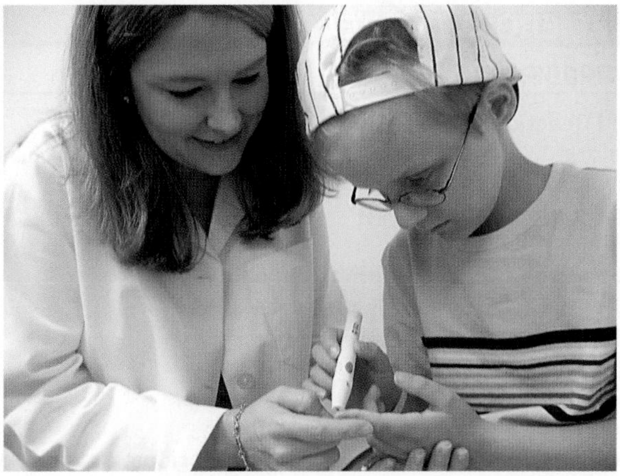

Fig. 28.4 Child using a finger-stick device to obtain a blood sample.

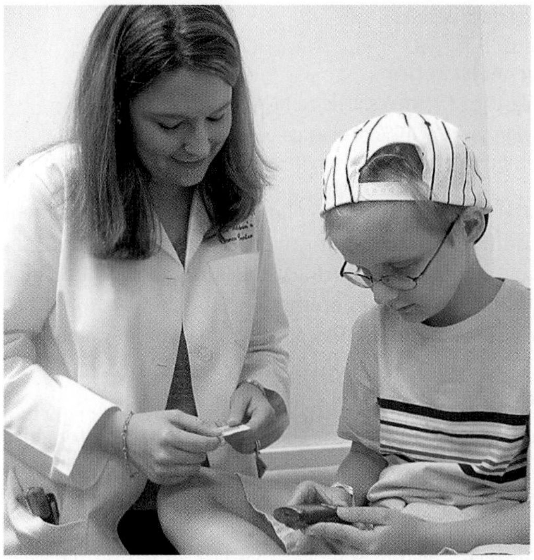

Fig. 28.5 Child using a blood glucose monitor and reagent strips to test his blood for glucose.

understand how to adjust food, activity, and insulin at the time of illness or when the child is treated for an illness with a medication known to raise the blood glucose level (e.g., steroids). The hyperglycemia is managed by increasing insulin soon after the increased glucose level is noted. Health care professionals should be aware that adolescent girls often become hyperglycemic around the time of their menses and should be advised to increase insulin dosages if necessary.

Signs of Hypoglycemia

Hypoglycemia is caused by imbalances of food intake, insulin, and activity. Ideally, hypoglycemia should be prevented, and parents need to be prepared to prevent, recognize, and treat the problem. They should be familiar with the signs of hypoglycemia and instructed in treatment, including care of the child with seizures. Early signs are adrenergic, including sweating and trembling, which help raise the blood glucose level, similar to the reaction when an individual is startled or anxious. The second set of symptoms that follow an untreated adrenergic reaction is neuroglycopenic (also called *brain hypoglycemia*). These symptoms typically include difficulty with balance, memory, attention, or concentration; dizziness or lightheadedness; and slurred speech. Severe and prolonged hypoglycemia leads to seizures, coma, and possible death (Levitsky & Misra, 2019b). Hypoglycemia can be managed effectively as outlined in the Emergency Treatment box.

EMERGENCY TREATMENT

Hypoglycemia

Mild Reaction: Adrenergic Symptoms

Give child 10 to 15 g of a simple, high-carbohydrate substance (preferably liquid; e.g., 3 to 6 oz of orange juice).

Follow with starch-protein snack.

Moderate Reaction: Neuroglycopenic Symptoms

Give child 10 to 15 g of a simple carbohydrate as above.

Repeat in 10 to 15 minutes if symptoms persist.

Follow with larger snack.

Watch child closely.

Severe Reaction: Unresponsive, Unconscious, or Seizures

Administer glucagon as prescribed.

Follow with planned meal or snack when child is able to eat or add a snack of 10% of daily calories.

Nocturnal Reaction

Give child 10 to 15 g of a simple carbohydrate.

Follow with snack of 10% of daily calories.

It is advisable for parents to plan for anticipated excitement or exercise. In addition, gastroenteritis may decrease insulin needs slightly as a result of poor appetite, vomiting, or diarrhea. If the blood glucose level is low but urinary ketones are present, the family should be aware of the increased need for simple carbohydrates and liquids.

Hygiene

All aspects of personal hygiene should be emphasized for children with diabetes. Children should be cautioned against wearing shoes without socks, wearing sandals, and walking barefoot. Correct nail and extremity care tailored to the individual child (with the guidance of a podiatrist) can begin health practices that last a lifetime. These children's eyes should be checked once a year unless the child wears glasses and then as directed by the ophthalmologist. Regular dental care is emphasized, and cuts and scratches should be treated with plain soap and water unless otherwise indicated. Diaper rash in infants and *Candida* infections in teens may indicate poor diabetes control.

Exercise

Exercise is an important component of the treatment plan. If the child is more active at one time of the day than at another time, food or insulin can be altered to meet that activity pattern. Food should be increased in the summer, when children tend to be more active. Decreased activity on return to school may require a decrease in food intake or increase in insulin dosage. Children who are active in team sports will need a snack about a half-hour before the anticipated activity. Races or other competitions may call for a slightly higher food intake than at practice times.

Food intake will usually need to be repeated for prolonged activity periods, often as frequently as every 45 minutes to 1 hour. Families should be informed that if increased food is not tolerated, decreased insulin is the next course of action. If the timing of the exercise is changed so that the supper meal is delayed, the insulin in the second or third dose of the day may be moved back to precede the mealtime. Sugar may sometimes be needed during exercise periods for quick response. Elevated blood glucose levels after extreme activity may represent the body's adrenergic response to exercise. If the blood glucose level is elevated (>240 mg/dl) before planned exercise, urinary ketones should be checked, and the activity may need to be postponed until the blood glucose is controlled.

NURSING ALERT

Ketonuria in the presence of hyperglycemia is an early sign of ketoacidosis and a contraindication to exercise.

Record Keeping

Home records are an invaluable aid to diabetes self-management. The nurse and family devise a method to chart insulin administered, blood glucose values, urine ketone results, and other factors and events that affect diabetes control. The child and family are encouraged to observe for patterns of blood glucose responses to events such as exercise. If lapses in management occur (e.g., eating a candy bar), the child should be encouraged to note this and not be criticized for the transgression.

Self-Management

Self-management is the key to close control. Being able to make changes when they are needed rather than waiting until the next contact with health care professionals is important for self-management and gives the individual and family the feeling that they have control over the disease. Psychologically, this helps family members believe they are useful and participating members of the team. Allowing the child to learn to look at records objectively promotes independence in self-management support. As children grow and assume more responsibility for self-management, they develop confidence in their ability to manage their disease and confidence in themselves as persons. They learn to respond to the disease and to make more accurate interpretations and changes in treatment when they become adults.

Puberty is associated with decreased sensitivity to insulin that normally would be compensated for by an increased insulin secretion. Health care professionals should anticipate that pubertal patients will have more difficulty maintaining glycemic control. Higher doses of insulin are often needed in pubertal children (Levitsky & Misra, 2019b). Patients should be taught to give themselves additional doses of rapid-acting insulin (5% to 10% of their daily dose) when their blood glucose levels are increased. The use of supplemental rapid-acting insulin is preferred to withholding food in adolescents.

Child or Adolescent and Family Support

Just as the physiologic responses affect the child, the parents and other family members of the child with newly diagnosed DM experience various emotional responses to the crisis. Care in the acute setting is short but may create fears and frustrations. The prospect of a chronic illness in their child engenders all of the feelings and concerns that are faced by parents of children with other chronic illnesses (see Chapter 17). The threat of complications and death is always present, as is the continuing drain on emotional and financial resources.

Certain fears may develop as a result of past experiences with the disease. A severe insulin reaction with seizures can contribute to fear of repetition. If parents observe a seizure or the adolescent has one in a public place, the desire to maintain better control is reinforced. They must understand how to prevent problems and how to handle problems calmly and coolly if they occur, and they must understand the complexities of the body, the disease, and its complications. Young children usually adjust well to problems related to the disease. With toddlers and preschoolers, insulin injections and glucose testing may be difficult at first. However, they usually accept the procedures when the parents use a matter-of-fact approach, without calling attention to a "hurt," and treat the procedure like any other routine part of the child's life. After the injection, time with some special and positive attention, such as reading or talking, or another pleasant activity, is one way to convert children who initially refuse injections to those who accept them.

In the years before adolescence, children probably accept their condition most easily. They are able to understand the basic concepts related to their disease and its treatment. They are able to test blood glucose and urine, recognize food groups, give injections, keep records, and distinguish fear or excitement from hypoglycemia. They understand how to recognize, prevent, and treat hypoglycemia. However, they still need considerable parental involvement.

NURSING TIP: Ongoing motivation to adhere to a regimen is difficult. An older child and parent (or another caregiver) may enjoy negotiating a day off when the responsibility for testing and recording blood glucose is delegated from the child to the caregiver (or vice versa).

Adolescents appear to have the most difficulty adjusting. Adolescence is a time of stress in trying to be perfect and similar to one's peers, and no matter what others say, having diabetes is being different. Some adolescents are more upset about not being able to have a candy bar than about injections, diet, and other aspects of management. If children can accept the difference as a part of life—in other words, that each person is different in some way—then, with adequate parental support, they should be able to adjust well (see Critical Thinking Case Study box).

Camping and other special group activities are useful. At diabetes camp, children learn that they are not alone. As a result, they become more independent and resourceful in other settings. Useful information about such camps and organizations can be obtained from the American Diabetes Association. A list of accredited camps specifically for children and teenagers with diabetes is also available from the American Camping Association.[i]

[i]5000 State Road 67 N., Martinsville, IN 46151; 765-342-8456; http://www.acacamps.org.

CRITICAL THINKING CASE STUDY

Type 1 Diabetes Mellitus

Shelly, a 14-year-old adolescent with a 3-year history of type 1 diabetes mellitus (DM), has been admitted to the pediatric intensive care unit for treatment of diabetic ketoacidosis (DKA). This is her fifth hospital admission for DKA in the past year. Shelly's parents are divorced, and she has four younger siblings, none of whom has diabetes. Shelly's mother has maintained two jobs for the past 5 years and frequently leaves Shelly in charge of the household. In anticipation of her discharge, you are planning a patient education program for Shelly and her mother. What important issues regarding Shelly's unstable diabetes management must you consider to plan the education program?

Initial Assessment. What are the concerns related to Shelly's recurrent DKA episodes and family stressors?

Expected Nursing Action. What education is necessary for Shelly and her parents to decrease the frequent hospitalizations?

Teaching Points

- Adolescence is a time of increasing independence, so while encouraging adolescents to take control of their diabetes management, minimal or no adult involvement results in poor glycemic control (Levitsky & Misra, 2019b).
- Adolescents with diabetes have a threefold increased risk of depression and eating disorders (Levitsky & Misra, 2019b).
- Socioeconomic factors such as single-parent homes, poor socioeconomic status, and physical or mental health problems with one parent are associated with poorer diabetes control and increased hospitalizations (Levitsky & Misra, 2019a).

Critical Thinking Answers

Initial Assessment. An adolescent with diabetes living in a single-parent home with a poor socioeconomic status is at an increased risk of poor glycemic control and increased hospitalizations.

Expected Nursing Action. Work with the family to develop a family-focused teamwork approach to Shelly's care. Parental involvement along with increased responsibility for the management of her diabetes will promote Shelly to have better glycemic control.

CLINICAL JUDGMENT AND NEXT-GENERATION NCLEX® EXAMINATION-STYLE QUESTIONS

1. An 8-year-old boy is diagnosed with diabetes insipidus (DI) and is being discharged on hormone replacement using DDAVP. The nurse will be completing discharge teaching with the parents and patient. What are the **most important** teaching topics for the nurse to include at this time? **Select all that apply.**
   - **A.** Education and support regarding the rationale for fluid restrictions.
   - **B.** Understanding that treatment will be needed only until the child reaches puberty.
   - **C.** Knowing that school-age children may assume full responsibility for their care.
   - **D.** Information for school personnel regarding the diagnosis so that they can grant children unrestricted use of the lavatory.
   - **E.** A thorough explanation regarding the condition, with specific clarification that DI is a different condition from diabetes mellitus (DM).
   - **F.** For emergency purposes, the child should wear a medical alert identification.
2. You are working with a nurse who is new to your endocrine unit and has never worked with an infant born with congenital adrenal hyperplasia (CAH). You want to make sure that the nurse has a full understanding of this diagnosis before she takes care of a new patient. What health teaching would the nurse include when teaching the parents about the infant's diagnosis? **Select all that apply.**
   - **A.** "Insulin is used to suppress high secretions of the hormones and can be very effective."
   - **B.** "A definitive diagnosis is confirmed by evidence of increased 17-ketosteroid levels in most types of CAH."
   - **C.** "Blood studies to identify elevated calcium and decreased phosphorus levels are routinely performed."
   - **D.** "Another test that can be used to visualize the presence of pelvic structures, such as female reproductive organs, is ultrasonography."
   - **E.** "This deficiency is an autosomal recessive disorder that results in improper steroid hormone synthesis."
   - **F.** "Genetic counseling is recommended before they conceive another child because CAH is a genetic disorder.

3. A nurse working in a pediatric clinic is completing an assessment of a 7-year-old girl who has breast development and pubertal hair. Her mother is concerned and scheduled the visit. The nurse performs a physical assessment and findings include:
   - Oral temperature = 98.4F
   - Pulse = 62 beats/min
   - Respiration = 18 breaths/min
   - Blood pressure = 102/60 mm Hg
   - Breast enlargement, Tanner Stage 3
   - Hair over entire pubis, Tanner Stage 3

   Choose the most likely options for the information missing from the statements below by selecting from the lists of options provided.
   As a result of the physical findings, the nurse is aware that these are signs of ____1____. This is treated with a ____2____that is administered once every ____3____depending on the medication preparation.

Options for 1	Options for 2	Options for 3
aplastic crisis	preparation of insulin	4-12 days
diabetes insipidus	luteinizing hormone-releasing hormone	2-3 weeks
diabetes mellitus	vasopressin injection	10-14 days
precocious puberty	vitamin-D injection	3-5 weeks
Cushing syndrome	corticosteroid agent	4-12 weeks

4. A 13-year-old girl is newly diagnosed with Graves disease based on her symptoms that gradually increased over the past 7 months. Her grades at school dropped and she was not able to concentrate. She was always restless and tired. Her appetite increased but she lost 20 lbs over the last several months. The diagnostic work up confirmed increased blood levels of T4 and T3 and the TCH level was low. The nurse will provide education to the child and parents before discharge. **Use an X to indicate whether the nursing education below is Indicated (appropriate or necessary), Contraindicated (could be harmful), or Non-Essential (makes no difference or not necessary).**

Nursing Action-Education	Indicated	Contraindicated	Non-Essential
When starting drug therapy encourage staying in a quiet, unstimulating environment that promotes rest.			
Heat tolerance is a common symptom experienced by individuals with Graves disease.			
Weight gain is a common symptom experienced by individuals with Graves disease.			
Mood swings and irritability are common symptoms experienced by individuals with Graves disease.			
Eating fruit and vegetables as part of a healthy diet is recommended for teenagers.			

REFERENCES

Aguirre, R. S., & Eugster, E. A. (2018). Central precocious puberty: From genetics to treatment. *Best Practice and Research Clinical Endocrinology and Metabolism*, *32*, 343–354.

Al-Azem, H., & Khan, A. A. (2012). Hypoparathyroidism. *Best Practice and Research Clinical Endocrinology and Metabolism*, *26*, 517–522.

Alotaibi, M. (2019). Physiology of puberty in boys and girls and pathological disorders affecting its onset. *Journal of Adolescence*, *71*, 63–71.

American Academy of Pediatrics, Rose, S. R., Section on Endocrinology and Committee on Genetics of the American Thyroid Association, et al. (2006). Update of newborn screening and therapy for congenital hypothyroidism. *Pediatrics*, *7*(6), 2290–2303.

American Diabetes Association. (2001). Report of the expert committee on the diagnosis and classification of diabetes mellitus. *Diabetes Care*, *24*(Suppl. 1), S5–S20.

Amin, N., Mushtaq, T., & Alvi, S. (2015). Fifteen-minute consultation: The child with short stature. *Archives of disease in childhood. Education and practice edition*, *100*(4), 180–184.

Bomberg, E. M., Addo, O. Y., Kyllo, J., et al. (2015). The relation of peripubertal and pubertal growth to final adult height in children with classic congenital adrenal hyperplasia. *The Journal of Pediatrics*, *166*(3), 743–750.

Brito, V. N., Spinola-Castro, A. M., Kochi, C., et al. (2016). Central precocious puberty: Revisiting the diagnosis and therapeutic management. *The Archives of Endocrinology and Metabolism*, *60*(2), 163–172.

Bryant, J., Baxter, L., Cave, C. B., et al. (2007). Recombinant growth hormone for idiopathic short stature in children and adolescents. *The Cochrane Database of Systematic Reviews*, (3), CD004440.

Carel, J. C., & Léger, J. (2008). Clinical practice: Precocious puberty. *The New England Journal of Medicine*, *358*(22), 2366–2377.

Caturegli, P., De Remiqis, A., & Rose, N. R. (2014). Hashimoto thyroiditis: Clinical and diagnostic criteria. *Autoimmunity Reviews*, *13*(4-5), 391–397.

Ceccato, F., & Boscaro, M. (2016). Cushing's syndrome: Screening and diagnosis. *High Blood Pressure & Cardiovascular Prevention*, *23*(3), 209–2015.

Cerbone, M., & Dattani, M. T. (2017). Progression from isolated growth hormone deficiency to combined pituitary hormone deficiency. *Growth Hormone and IGF Research*, *37*, 19–25.

Chen, M., & Eugster, E. A. (2015). Central precocious puberty: Updated on diagnosis and treatment. *Paediatric Drugs*, *17*(4), 273–281.

Clar, C., Waugh, N., & Thomas, S. (2007). Routine hospital admission versus out-patient or home care in children at diagnosis of type 1 diabetes mellitus. *The Cochrane Database of Systematic Reviews*, (2), CD004099.

Colao, A., Grasso, L. F. S., Giustina, A., et al. (2019). Acromegaly. *Primer*, *5*(20), 1–17.

Cusano, N. E., Rubin, M. R., & Bilezikian, J. P. (2015). Parathyroid hormone therapy for hypoparathyroidism. *Best Practice & Research: Clinical Endocrinology & Metabolism*, *29*(1), 47–55.

Deodati, A., & Cianfarani, S. (2011). Impact of growth hormone therapy on adult height of children with idiopathic short stature: Systematic review. *The BMJ*, *342*, c7157.

Di Iorgi, N., Allegri, A. E., Napoli, F., et al. (2014). Central diabetes insipidus in children and young adults: Etiological diagnosis and long-term outcome of idiopathic cases. *The Journal of Clinical Endocrinology & Metabolism*, *99*(4), 1264–1272.

Di Iorgi, N., Napoli, F., Allegri, A. E., et al. (2012). Diabetes insipidus-diagnosis and management. *Hormone Research in Paediatrics*, *77*, 69–84.

Doyle, D. A. (2020a). Hypoparathyroidism. In R. M. Kliegman, J. W. St Geme, N. L Blum, et al. (Eds.), *In Nelson textbook of pediatrics* (21th ed.). Philadelphia, PA: Elsevier.

Doyle, D. A. (2020b). Hyperthyroidism. In R. M. Kliegman, B. Stanton, J. W. St Geme, et al. (Eds.), *Nelson textbook of pediatrics* (20th ed.). Philadelphia: Saunders.

El-Maouche, D., Arlt, W., & Merke, D. P. (2017). Congenital adrenal hyperplasia. *Lancet*, *390*(10108), 2194–2210.

Gangat, M., & Radovick, S. (2017). Pituitary hypoplasia. *Endocrinology and Metabolism Clinics of North America*, *46*, 247–257.

Gardner, D., & Shoback, D. (2011). *Greenspan's basic and clinical endocrinology* (9th ed.). New York: Lange Medical Books/McGraw-Hill.

Garibaldi, L. R., & Chemaitilly, W. (2020). Disorders of pubertal development. In R. M. Kliegman, J. W. St Geme, N. L. Blum, et al. (Eds.), *In Nelson textbook of pediatrics* (21th ed.). Philadelphia, PA: Elsevier.

Giuliani, C., & Peri, A. (2014). Effects of hyponatremia on the brain. *Journal of Clinical Medicine*, *3*(4), 1163–1677.

Glaser, N. (2019). Treatment and complications of diabetic ketoacidosis in children and adolescents. In A. G. Hoppin (Ed.), *UpToDate*. Retrieved from https://www.uptodate.com/contents/treatment-and-complications-of-diabetic-ketoacidosis-in-children-and-adolescents?source=history.

Greiner, M. V., & Kerrigan, J. R. (2006). Puberty: Timing is everything. *Pediatric Annals*, *35*(12), 916–922.

Grimberg, A., Divall, S. A., Polychronakos, C., et al. (2016). Guidelines for growth hormone deficiency and insulin-like growth factor-1 treatment in children and adolescents: Growth hormone deficiency, idiopathic short stature, and primary insulin-like growth factor-1 deficiency. *Hormone Research in Paediatrics*, *86*(6), 361.

Hanley, P., Lord, K., & Bauer, A. J. (2016). Thyroid disorders in children and adolescents: A review. *JAMA Pediatrics*, *170*(10), 1008–1019.

Harrington, J, & Palmert, M .R. (2016) .Treatment of precocious puberty. In T. W. Post (Ed.), *UpToDate*, Waltham MA.

Herman-Giddens, M. E. (2006). Recent data on pubertal milestones in United States children: The secular trend toward earlier development. *International Journal of Andrology*, *29*(1), 241–246.

Hokken-Koelega, A. C. (2011). Diagnostic workup of the short child. *Hormone Research in Paediatrics*, *76*(Suppl. 3), 6–9.

Insulin Pumps. (2018). In www.diabetes.org. Retrieved from http://www.diabetes.org/living- with-diabetes/treatment-and-care/medication/insulin/insulin-pumps.html.

Jain, A., Baracco, R., & Kapur, G. (2019). Pheochromocytoma and paraganglioma-an update on diagnosis, evaluation, and management. *Pediatric Nephrology*, Advance online publication.

Kaplowitz, P. B. (2019). Neonatal thyroid disease. *Pediatric Clinics of North America*, *66*, 343–352.

Karnik, A. A., Fields, A. V., & Shannon, R. P. (2007). Diabetic cardiomyopathy. *Current Hypertension Reports*, *9*(6), 467–473.

Kaye, C. I., Committee on Genetics, Accurso, F., et al. (2006). Introduction to the newborn screening fact sheets. *Pediatrics*, *118*(3), 1304–1312.

Kirkgoz, T., & Guran, T. (2018). Primary adrenal insufficiency in children: Diagnosis and management. *Best Practice and Research Clinical Endocrinology and Metabolism*, *32*, 397–424.

Laffel, L. & Svoren, B. (2018). Epidemiology, presentation, and diagnosis of type 2 diabetes mellitus in children and adolescents. In A. G. Hoppin (Ed.), *UpToDate*. Retrieved from https://www.uptodate.com/contents/epidemiology-presentation-and-diagnosis-of-type-2-diabetes-mellitus-in-children-and-adolescents?source=bookmarks.

Lal, G., & Clark, O. H. (2011). Endocrine surgery. In D. G. Gardner, & D. Shoback (Eds.), *Basic and clinical endocrinology* (9th ed.). New York: Lang Medical Books/McGraw-Hill.

Lau, D., Rutledge, C., & Aghi, M. K. (2015). Cushing's disease: Current medical therapies and molecular insights guiding future therapies. *Neurosurgical Focus*, *38*(2), E11.

Lee, H. S., & Hwang, J. S. (2014). The treatment of Graves' disease in children and adolescents. *Annals of Pediatric Endocrinology & Metabolism*, *19*(3), 122–126.

Léger, J., & Carel, J. C. (2013). Hyperthyroidism in childhood: Causes, when and how to treat. *Journal of Clinical Research In Pediatric Endocrinology*, *5*(Suppl. 1), 50–56.

Leger, J., & Carel, J. C. (2018). Diagnosis and management of hyperthyroidism from prenatal life to adolescence. *Best Practice and Research clinical Endocrinology and Metabolism*, *32*, 373–386.

Leung, A. K. C., & Leung, A. A. C. (2019). *Evaluation and management of the child with hypothyroidism*. Springer: World Journal of Pediatrics.

Levitsky, L. L. & Misra, M. (2018). Management of type 1 diabetes mellitus in children and adolescents. In A. G. Hoppin (Ed.). *UpToDate*. Retrieved from https://www.uptodate.com/contents/management-of-type-1-diabetes-mellitus-in-children-and-adolescents?source=history.

Levitsky, L.L. & Misra, M. (2019a). Epidemiology, presentation, and diagnosis of type 1 diabetes mellitus in children and adolescents. In A. G. Hoppin (Ed.), *UpToDate*. Retrieved from https://www.uptodate.com/contents/epidemiology-presentation-and-diagnosis-of-type-1-diabetes-mellitus-in-children-and-adolescents?source=history.

Levitsky, L. L. & Misra, M. (2019b). Hypoglycemia in children and adolescents with type 1 diabetes mellitus. In A. G. Hoppin (Ed.). *UpToDate*. Retrieved from https://www.uptodate.com/contents/hypoglycemia-in-children-and-adolescents-with-type-1-diabetes-mellitus?source=history.

Levy, M., Prentice, M., & Wass, J. (2019). Diabetes insipidus. *The British Medical Journal*, *364*(l321), 1–5.

Li, P., Li, Y., & Yang, C. L. (2014). Gonadotropin releasing hormone agonist treatment to increase final status in children with precocious puberty: A meta-analysis. *Medicine*, *93*(27), e260.

Linglart, A., Levine, M. A., & Juppner, H. (2018). Pseudohypoparathyroidsm. *Endocrinology and Metabolism Clinics of North America*, *47*, 865–888.

Lowitz, & Keil, M. F. (2015). Cushing syndrome: Establishing timely diagnosis. *Journal of Pediatric Nursing*, *30*(3), 528–530.

Mendes, C., Vaz Matos, I., Ribeiro, L., et al. (2015). Congenital adrenal hyperplasia due to 21- hydroxylase deficiency: Genotype-phenotype correlation. *Acta Médica Portuguesa*, *28*(1), 56–62.

Metzger, M. L., Krasin, M. J., Choi, J. K., et al. (2016). Hodgkin lymphoma. In P. A. Pizzo, & D. G. Poplack (Eds.), *Principles and theories of pediatric oncology* (7th ed.). Philadelphia: Lippincott Williams and Wilkins.

Monis, E. L., & Mannstadt, M. (2015). Hypoparathyroidsm- disease update and emerging treatments. *Annales D Endocrinologie*, *76*(2), 84–88.

Moritz, M. L. (2019). Syndrome of inappropriate antidiuresis. *Pediatric Clinics of North America*, *66*, 209–226.

Murray, P. G., Dattani, M. T., & Clayton, P. E. (2016). Controversies in the diagnosis and management of growth hormone deficiency in childhood and adolescence. *Archives of Disease in Childhood*, *101*(1), 96–100.

National Institutes of Health. (2017). *Rates of new diagnosed cases of type 1 and type 2 diabetes on the raise among children, teens*. https://www.nih.gov/news-events/news-releases/rates-new-diagnosed-cases-type-1-type-2-diabetes-rise-among-children-teens.

Nebesio, T. D., & Eugster, E. A. (2007). Current concepts in normal and abnormal puberty. *Current Problems in Pediatric and Adolescent Health Care*, *37*(2), 50–72.

Pashtan, I., Grogan, R. H., Kaplan, S. P., et al. (2013). Primary hyperparathyroidism in adolescents: The same but different. *Pediatric Surgery International*, *29*(3), 275–279.

Patti, G., Guzzeti, C., Di Iorgi, N., et al. (2018). Central adrenal insufficiency in children and adolescents. *Best Practice and Research Clinical Endocrinology and Metabolism*, *32*, 425–444.

Patterson, B. C., & Felner, E. I. (2020). Hypopituitarism. In R. M. Kliegman, J. W. St Geme, N. L. Blum, et al. (Eds.), *In Nelson textbook of pediatrics* (21th ed.). Philadelphia, PA: Elsevier.

Pine-Twaddell, E., Romero, C., & Radovick, S. (2013). Vertical transmission of hypopituitarism: Critical importance of appropriate interpretation of thyroid function tests and levothyroxine therapy during pregnancy. *Thyroid*, *23*(7), 892–897.

Pivonello, R., Auriemma, R. S., Grasso, L. F., et al. (2017). Complications of acromegaly: Cardiovascular, respiratory, and metabolic comorbidities. *Pituitary*, *20*(1), 42–62.

Rosenson, R. S., & Herman, W. H. (2008). Glycated proteins and cardiovascular disease in glucose intolerance and type 11 diabetes. *Current Cardiovascular Risk Reports*, *2*(1), 43–46.

Schoenmaker, N., Alatzoglou, K. S., Chatterjee, V. K., et al. (2015). Recent advances in central congenital hypothyroidism. *The Journal of Endocrinology*, *227*(3), R51–R71.

Shoback, D. (2008). Clinical practice: Hypoparathyroidism. *The New England Journal of Medicine*, *359*(4), 391–403.

Silverstein, J., Klingensmith, G., Copeland, K., et al. (2005). Care of children and adolescents with type 1 diabetes: A statement of the American Diabetes Association. *Diabetes Care*, *28*(1), 186–212.

Slyper, A. H. (2006). The pubertal timing controversy in the USA, and a review of possible causative factors for the advance in timing of onset of puberty. *Clinical endocrinology*, *65*(1), 1–8.

Snyder, C. K. (2015). Hypoparathyroidism in children. In J. M. Foote (Ed.), *The Pediatric Endocrinology Nursing Society Department* (pp. 939–941). Elsevier.

Stanley, T. (2012). Diagnosis of growth hormone deficiency in childhood. *Current Opinion in Endocrinology, Diabetes and Obesity*, *19*(1), 47–52.

Stratakis, C. (2016). Diagnosis and clinical genetics of cushing syndrome in pediatrics. *Endocrinology and Metabolism Clinics of North America*, *45*, 311–328.

Tomer, Y. (2014). Mechanisms of autoimmune thyroid diseases: From genetics to epigenetics. *The Annual Review of Pathology*, *9*, 147–156.

Toogood, A. A., & Stewart, P. M. (2008). Hypopituitarism: Clinical features, diagnosis, and management. *Endocrinology and Metabolism Clinics of North America*, *37*, 235–261.

Trivin, C., Couto-Silva, A. C., Sainte-Rose, C., et al. (2006). Presentation and evolution of organic central precocious puberty according to the type of CNS lesion. *Clinical endocrinology*, *65*(2), 239–245.

Waller, S. (2011). Parathyroid hormone and growth in chronic kidney disease. *Pediatric Nephrology*, *26*(2), 195–204.

Wassner, A. J. (2018). Congenital hypothyroidism. *Clinics in Perinatology*, *45*, 1–18.

White, P. C. (2020a). Congenital adrenal hyperplasia and related disorders. In R. M. Kliegman, J. W. St Geme, N. L. Blum, et al. (Eds.), *In Nelson textbook of pediatrics* (21th ed.). Philadelphia, PA: Elsevier.

White, P. C. (2020b). Pheochromocytoma. In R. M. Kliegman, J. W. St Geme, N. L. Blum, et al. (Eds.), *In Nelson textbook of pediatrics* (21th ed.). Philadelphia, PA: Elsevier.

Witchel, S. F. (2017). Congenital adrenal hyperplasia. *North American Society for Pediatric and Adolescent Gynecology*, *30*, 520–534.

Wolsdorf, J., Craig, M. E., Daneman, D., et al. (2009). Diabetic ketoacidosis in children and adolescents with diabetes. *Pediatric Diabetes*, *10*(Suppl. 12), 118–133.

UNIT 12 The Child With a Problem That Interferes With Physical Mobility

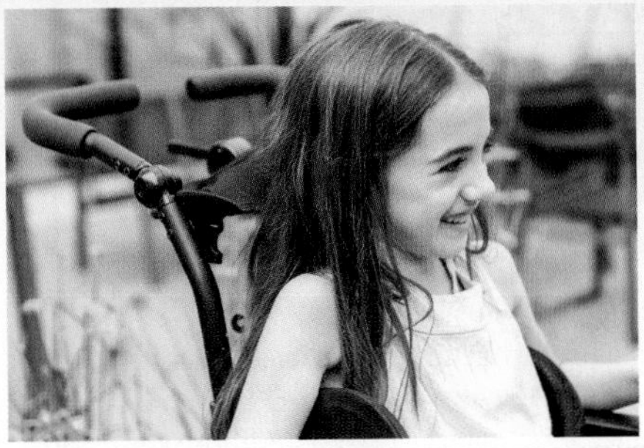

29

The Child With Musculoskeletal or Articular Dysfunction

Laura Tillman

http://evolve.elsevier.com/wong/essentials

CONCEPTS

- Infection
- Immunity
- Integrity
- Mobility

THE IMMOBILIZED CHILD

IMMOBILIZATION

One of the most difficult aspects of illness in children is the immobility it often imposes on a child. Children's natural tendency to be active influences all aspects of their growth and development. Impaired mobility presents a challenge to children, their families, and their caregivers.

Physiologic Effects of Immobilization

Many clinical studies, including space program research, have documented predictable consequences that occur after immobilization and the absence of gravitational force. Functional and metabolic responses to restricted movement can be noted in most of the body systems. Each has a direct influence on the child's growth and development because of homeostatic mechanisms that thrive on normal use and feedback to maintain dynamic equilibrium. Inactivity leads to a decrease in the functional capabilities of the whole body as dramatically as the lack of physical exercise leads to muscle weakness.

Disuse from illness, injury, or a sedentary lifestyle can limit function and potentially delay age-appropriate milestones. Most of the pathologic changes that occur during immobilization arise from decreased muscle strength and mass, decreased metabolism, and bone demineralization, which are closely interrelated, with one change leading to or affecting the others.

The major effects of immobilization are outlined briefly in Table 29.1 and are related directly or indirectly to decreased muscle activity, which produces numerous primary changes in the musculoskeletal system with secondary alterations in the cardiovascular, respiratory, skeletal, metabolic, and renal systems. The musculoskeletal changes that occur during disuse are a result of alterations in the effect of gravity and stress on the muscles, joints, and bones. Muscle disuse leads to tissue breakdown and loss of muscle mass (**atrophy**). Muscle atrophy causes decreased strength and endurance, which may take weeks or months to restore.

The daily stresses on bone created by motion and weight bearing maintain the balance between bone formation (osteoblastic activity) and bone resorption (osteoclastic activity). During immobilization, increased calcium leaves the bone, causing osteopenia (demineralization of the bones), which may predispose bone to pathologic fractures. A **joint contracture** begins when the arrangement of collagen, the main structural protein of connective tissues, is altered, resulting in a denser tissue that does not glide as easily. Eventually, muscles, tendons, and ligaments can shorten and reduce joint movement, ultimately producing contractures that restrict function. The major musculoskeletal consequences of immobilization are:

- Significant decrease in muscle size, strength, and endurance
- Bone demineralization leading to osteoporosis
- Contractures and decreased joint mobility

Circulatory stasis combined with hypercoagulability of the blood, which results from factors such as damage to the endothelium of blood vessels (Virchow's triad), can lead to thrombus and embolus formation. **Deep vein thrombosis (DVT)** involves the formation of a thrombus in a deep vein, such as the iliac and femoral veins, and can cause significant morbidity if it remains undetected and untreated. The larger the portion of the body immobilized and the longer the immobilization, the greater the risks of immobility.

Psychologic Effects of Immobilization

For children, one of the most difficult aspects of illness is immobilization. Throughout childhood, physical activity is an integral part of daily life and is essential for physical growth and development. It also serves children as an instrument for communication and expression and as a means for learning about and understanding their world. Activity helps them deal with a variety of feelings and impulses and

TABLE 29.1 Summary of Physical Effects of Immobilization With Nursing Interventions[a]

Primary Effects	Secondary Effects	Nursing Considerations
Muscular System		
Decreased muscle strength, tone, and endurance	Decreased venous return and cardiac output Decreased metabolism and need for oxygen	Use antiembolism stockings or intermittent compression devices to promote venous return (monitor circulatory and neurovascular status of extremities when such devices are used).
	Decreased exercise tolerance	Plan play activities to use uninvolved extremities.
	Bone demineralization	Place in upright posture when possible.
Disuse atrophy and loss of muscle mass	Catabolism Loss of strength	Have patient perform range-of-motion, active, passive, and stretching exercises.
Loss of joint mobility	Contractures, ankylosis of joints	Maintain correct body alignment. Use joint splints as indicated to prevent further deformity. Maintain range of motion.
Weak back muscles	Secondary spinal deformities	Maintain body alignment.
Weak abdominal muscles	Impaired respiration	See nursing considerations for respiratory system.
Skeletal System		
Bone demineralization—osteoporosis, hypercalcemia	Negative bone calcium uptake Pathologic fractures Calcium deposits Extraosseous bone formation, especially at hip, knee, elbow, and shoulder Renal calculi	With paralysis, use upright posture on tilt table. Handle extremities carefully when turning and positioning. Administer calcium-mobilizing drugs (diphosphonates) and normal saline infusions if ordered. Ensure adequate intake of fluid; monitor output. Acidify urine. Promptly treat urinary tract infections.
Negative bone calcium uptake	Life-threatening electrolyte imbalance	Monitor serum calcium levels. Provide electrolyte replacement as indicated.
Metabolism		
Decreased metabolic rate	Slowing of all systems Decreased food intake	Mobilize as soon as possible. Have patient perform active and passive resistance exercises and deep-breathing exercises. Ensure adequate food intake. Provide a high-protein, high-fiber diet.
Negative nitrogen balance	Decline in nutritional state Impaired healing	Encourage small, frequent feedings with protein and preferred foods. Prevent pressure areas.
Hypercalcemia	Electrolyte imbalance	See nursing consideration for skeletal system.
Decreased production of stress hormones	Decreased physical and emotional coping capacity	Identify causes of stress. Implement appropriate interventions to lower physical and psychosocial stresses.
Cardiovascular System		
Decreased efficiency of orthostatic neurovascular reflexes	Inability to adapt readily to upright position (orthostatic intolerance) Pooling of blood in extremities in upright posture	Monitor peripheral pulses and skin temperature changes. Use antiembolism stockings or intermittent compression devices to decrease pooling when upright.
Diminished vasopressor mechanism	Orthostatic intolerance with syncope, hypertension, deceased cerebral blood flow, tachycardia	Provide abdominal support. In severe cases, use antigravitational pants. Position horizontally.
Altered distribution of blood volume	Increased cardiac workload Decreased exercise tolerance	Monitor hydration, blood pressure, and urinary output.
Venous stasis	Pulmonary emboli or thrombi	Encourage and assist with frequent position changes. Elevate extremities without knee flexion. Ensure adequate fluid intake. Have patient perform active or passive exercises or movement as needed. Prescribe routine wearing of antiembolism stockings or intermittent compression devices. Monitor for signs of pulmonary embolism—sudden dyspnea, chest pain, respiratory arrest.

TABLE 29.1 Summary of Physical Effects of Immobilization With Nursing Interventions[a]—cont'd

Primary Effects	Secondary Effects	Nursing Considerations
		Promptly intervene to maintain adequate oxygenation if signs and symptoms of pulmonary emboli are noted. Measure circumference of extremities periodically. Give anticoagulant drugs as prescribed.
Dependent edema	Tissue breakdown and susceptibility to infection	Administer skin care. Turn every 2-4 h. Monitor skin color, temperature, and integrity. Use pressure-reduction surface as necessary to prevent skin breakdown (see Chapter 20).
Respiratory System		
Decreased need for oxygen	Altered oxygen/carbon dioxide exchange and metabolism	Promote exercise as tolerated. Encourage deep-breathing exercises.
Decreased chest expansion and diminished vital capacity	Diminished oxygen intake Dyspnea and inadequate arterial oxygen saturation; acidosis	Position for optimum chest expansion. Semi-Fowler position may assist in lung expansion if patient can tolerate. Use prone positioning without pressure on abdomen to allow gravity to aid in diaphragmatic excursion. Ensure that patient maintains proper alignment when sitting to prevent pressure on respiratory mechanism.
Poor abdominal tone and distention	Interference with diaphragmatic excursion	Avoid restriction of chest and abdominal musculature. Supply torso support to promote chest expansion.
Mechanical or biochemical secretion retention	Hypostatic pneumonia Bacterial and viral pneumonia Atelectasis	Change position frequently. Carry out chest percussion, vibration, and drainage (or suctioning) as necessary. Use incentive spirometer. Monitor breath sounds.
Loss of respiratory muscle strength	Poor cough	Encourage coughing and deep breathing. Support chest wall by splinting with pillow when patient coughs. Use incentive spirometer. Observe for signs of respiratory distress with pulse oximetry or blood gas measurement as necessary.
	Upper respiratory tract infection	Prevent contact with infected persons. Provide adequate hydration. Administer immunizations as necessary (pneumococcal, meningococcal).
Gastrointestinal System		
Distention caused by poor abdominal muscle tone	Interference with respiratory movements Difficulty in feeding in prone position	Monitor bowel sounds. Encourage small, frequent feedings.
No specific primary effect	Possible constipation caused by gravitational effect on feces through ascending colon or weakened smooth muscle tone	Have patient sit in upright position in bedside chair if possible. Carry out bowel training program with hydration, stool softeners, increased fiber intake, and mild laxatives if necessary.
	Anorexia	Stimulate appetite with favored foods.
Urinary System		
Alteration of gravitational force	Difficulty in voiding in prone position	Position as upright as possible to void.
Impaired ureteral peristalsis	Urinary retention in calyces and bladder Infection Renal calculi	Hydrate to ensure adequate urinary output for age. Stimulate bladder emptying with warm running water, as necessary. Catheterize only for severe urinary retention. Administer antibiotics as indicated.
Integumentary System		
Altered tissue integrity	Decreased circulation and pressure leading to tissue injury	Turn and reposition at least every 2-4 h. Frequently inspect total skin surface. Eliminate mechanical factors causing pressure, friction, moisture, or irritation. Place on pressure-reduction mattress.
	Difficulty with personal hygiene	Assess ability to perform self-care and assist with bathing, grooming, and toileting as needed. Encourage self-care to potential ability. Ensure adequate intake of protein, vitamins, and minerals.

[a]Individualize care according to child's needs; interventions may vary in different institutions.

provides a mechanism by which they can exert control over inner tensions. Children respond to anxiety with increased activity. Removal of this power deprives them of necessary input and a natural outlet for their feelings and fantasies. Through movement, children also gain sensory input, which provides an essential element for developing and maintaining body image.

When children are immobilized by disease or as part of a treatment regimen, they experience diminished environmental stimuli with a loss of tactile input and an altered perception of themselves and their environment. Sudden or gradual immobilization narrows the amount and variety of environmental stimuli children receive by means of all their senses: touch, sight, hearing, taste, smell, and proprioception (a feeling of where they are in their environment). This sensory deprivation frequently leads to feelings of isolation and boredom and of being forgotten, especially by peers.

The quest for mastery at every stage of development is related to mobility. Even speech and language skills require sensorimotor activity and experience. For toddlers, exploration and imitative behaviors are essential to developing a sense of autonomy. Preschoolers' expression of initiative is evidenced by the need for vigorous physical activity. School-age children's development is strongly influenced by physical achievement and competition. Adolescents rely on mobility to achieve independence.

Children may react to immobility by active protest, anger, and aggressive behavior, or they may become quiet, passive, and submissive. They may believe that the immobilization is a justified punishment for misbehavior. Children should be allowed to display their anger, but it should be within the limits of safety to their self-esteem and not damaging to the integrity of others (see Chapter 19, Providing Opportunities for Play and Expressive Activities). When children are unable to express anger, aggression is often displayed inappropriately through regressive behavior and outbursts of crying or temper tantrums.

Effect on Families

Even brief periods of immobilization may disrupt family function, and catastrophic illness or disability may severely tax a family's resources and coping abilities. The family's needs often must be met by the services of a multidisciplinary team, and nurses play a key role in anticipating the services that they will need and in coordinating conferences to plan care. Home management, including special considerations for addressing cultural, economic, physical, and psychologic needs, is frequently planned prior to discharge. A child with a severe disability is very dependent, and caregivers need respite to revitalize themselves. Individual and group counseling is beneficial for solving problems in advance and provides an emotional support system. Parent groups are also helpful and often allow nonthreatening social contact. The families of children with permanent disabilities need long-term resources because some of the most difficult problems arise as they try to sustain high-quality care for many years (see Chapter 17).

Nursing Care Management

Physical assessment of the child who is immobilized for any number of reasons (e.g., injury, illness) includes a focus not only on the injured part (e.g., fracture) but also on the functioning of other systems that may be affected secondarily—the circulatory, renal, respiratory, muscular, and gastrointestinal systems. With long-term immobilization, there may also be neurologic impairment and changes in electrolytes (especially calcium), nitrogen balance, and the general metabolic rate. The psychologic impact of immobilization should also be assessed.

Children who require prolonged total immobility and are unable to move themselves in bed should be placed on a pressure-reduction mattress to prevent skin breakdown. Frequent position changes also help prevent dependent edema and stimulate circulation, respiratory function, gastrointestinal motility, and neurologic sensation. Children at greater risk for skin breakdown include those with prolonged immobilization; mechanical ventilation; casts; and assistive devices including orthotics, prosthetics, and wheelchairs. Additional risk factors include poor nutrition, friction (from bed linens with traction), and moist skin (from urine or perspiration). Nursing care of children at risk includes strategies for preventing skin breakdown when such conditions are present. The Braden QD Scale is a reliable, objective tool that may be used in the assessment for pressure ulcer development in children who are acutely ill or who are at risk for skin breakdown from neurologic conditions and immobilization (Curley, Hasbani, Quigley, et al., 2018).

The use of antiembolism stockings or intermittent compression devices prevents circulatory stasis and dependent edema in the lower extremities and reduces the likelihood of developing a DVT. Anticoagulant therapy may also be implemented with low-molecular-weight heparin, unfractionated heparin, or vitamin K antagonists. The child should be allowed as much activity as possible within the limitations of the illness or treatment. Any functional mobility, however minimal, is preferred to total immobility.

High-protein, high-calorie foods are encouraged to prevent negative nitrogen balance, which may be difficult to correct by diet, especially if there is anorexia as a result of immobility and decreased gastrointestinal function (decreased motility and possibly constipation). Stimulating the appetite with small servings of attractively arranged, preferred foods may be sufficient. At times, supplementary nasogastric or gastrostomy feedings or intravenous (IV) nutrition or fluids may be needed, but these are reserved for serious disability in which oral intake is impossible. Adequate hydration and, when possible, an upright position and remobilization promote bowel and kidney function and help prevent complications in these systems.

Children are encouraged to be as active as their condition and restrictive devices allow. This poses few problems for children, whose innate ingenuity and natural inclination toward mobility provide them with the impetus for physical activity. They need the opportunity, the materials and objects to stimulate activity, and the encouragement and participation of others. Those who are unable to move may benefit from passive exercise and movement in consultation with a physical therapist.

Using dolls, stuffed animals, or puppets to illustrate and explain the immobilization method (e.g., traction, cast) is a valuable tool for small children. Placing a cast, tubing, or other restraining equipment on the doll offers the child a nonthreatening opportunity to express, through the doll, feelings about the restrictions and feelings toward the nurse and other health care providers. The doll or puppet may also be used for teaching the child and family procedures, such as IV therapy, procedural sedation, and general anesthesia.

Whenever possible, transporting the child outside the confines of the room increases environmental stimuli and allows social contact with others. Specially designed wheelchairs or carts for increased mobility and independence are available. While hospitalized, children benefit from visitors, computers, books, interactive video games, and other items brought from their own room at home. An activity center or slanting tray can be helpful for the child with limited mobility to use for drawing, coloring, writing, and playing with small toys, such as trucks and cars. Accessibility to clocks, calendars, and a program of diversional therapy are also beneficial. All of these interventions help children function in a more typical way while hospitalized. Children are able to express frustration, displeasure, and anger through play activities (see Chapter 19), which is helpful in their recovery. A child life specialist should be consulted for recreational planning.

All efforts should be made to minimize family disruption resulting from the hospitalization. Children should be allowed to wear their own clothes (street clothes, especially for preadolescent and adolescent girls) and resume school and preinjury activities if able. A parent or siblings should be allowed to stay overnight and room-in with the hospitalized child to prevent the effects of family disruption. Visits from significant persons, such as family members and friends, offer occasions for emotional support and provide opportunities for learning how to care for the child. Privacy is necessary, especially for adolescents.

One of the most useful interventions to help children cope with immobility is participation in their own care. Self-care to the maximum extent is usually well received by children. They can help plan their daily routine; select their diet; and choose "street clothes," including innovative adornment, such as a baseball cap or brightly colored stockings to express their autonomy and individuality. They are encouraged to do as much for themselves as they are able to keep their muscles active and their interest alive.

Although most of the suggestions discussed relate to hospital care, the same consultations (physical therapist, occupational therapist, child life specialist, speech therapist) and environment may be considered in the home to help the child and family achieve independence and normalization (see Chapter 18). For a child with greatly restricted movement (e.g., child with a bilateral hip spica cast or confined to bed rest), care is often a challenge. These situations require long-term management either in the hospital or at home. Wherever the care occurs, consistent planning and coordination of activities with other health care workers and caregivers are vital nursing functions.

Family Support and Home Care

The needs of a child with severe disabilities can be complex, and family members require time to assimilate the teachings and demonstrations needed to understand the child's situation and care. Even a child who is confined on a short-term basis can be a challenge for the family, which is usually unprepared for the problems imposed by the child's special needs. Home modification is usually needed for facilitating care, especially when it involves traction, a large cast, or extended confinement. Suitable child care may be needed for times when all family members work.

Just as in the hospital, the child at home is encouraged to be as independent as possible and to follow a schedule that approximates his or her normal lifestyle as nearly as possible, such as continuing school lessons, regular bedtime, and suitable recreational activities.

TRAUMATIC INJURY

SOFT-TISSUE INJURY

Injuries to the muscles, ligaments, and tendons are common in children (Fig. 29.1). In young children, soft-tissue injury usually results from mishaps during play. In older children and adolescents, participation in sports is a common cause of such injuries.

Contusions

A contusion (bruise) is damage to the soft tissue, subcutaneous structures, and muscle. The tearing of these tissues and small blood vessels and the inflammatory response lead to hemorrhage, edema, and associated pain when the child attempts to move the injured part. The escape of blood into the tissues is observed as **ecchymosis**, a black-and-blue discoloration.

Large contusions cause gross swelling, pain, and disability, and usually receive immediate attention from health personnel. Smaller injuries may go unnoticed, allowing continued participation. However,

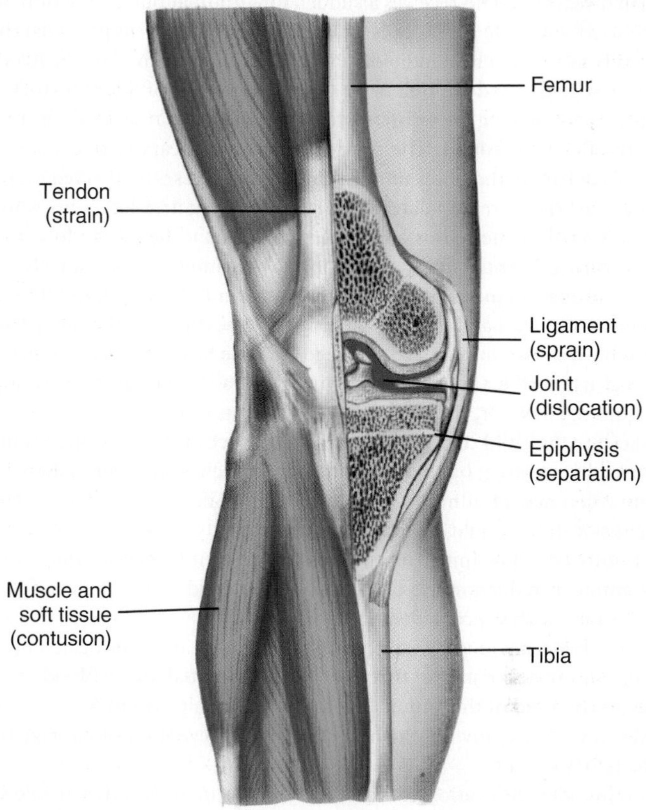

Fig. 29.1 Sites of injuries to bones, joints, and soft tissues.

they can become disabling after rest because of pain and muscle spasm. Immediate treatment consists of cold application, as in the treatment of sprains described later. Return to participation is allowed when the strength and range of motion of the affected extremity are equal to those of the opposite extremity or are demonstrated under conditions, such as sport-specific tests. **Myositis ossificans** may occur from deep contusions to the biceps or quadriceps muscles; this condition may result in a restriction of flexibility of the affected limb.

Crush injuries occur when children's extremities or digits are crushed (e.g., fingers slammed in doors, folding chairs, or equipment) or hit (as when hammering a nail). A severe crush injury involves the bone, with swelling and bleeding beneath the nail (subungual) and sometimes laceration of the pulp of the nail. The **subungual hematoma** can be released by creating a hole at the proximal end of the nail with a special cautery device or a heated sterile 18-gauge needle.

Dislocations

Long bones are held in approximation to one another at the joint by ligaments. A dislocation occurs when the force of stress on the ligament is so great as to displace the normal position of the opposing bone ends or the bone end to its socket. The predominant symptom is pain that increases with attempted passive or active movement of the extremity. In dislocations, there may be an obvious deformity and inability to move the joint. Children with naturally lax joints are more prone to dislocation of joints. Dislocation of the phalanges is the most common type seen in children, followed by elbow dislocation. In the adolescent population, shoulder dislocations are more common and dislocation unaccompanied by fracture is rare.

A common injury in young children is subluxation, or partial dislocation, of the radial head, also called *pulled elbow* or **nursemaid's elbow**. In the majority of cases, the injury occurs in a child younger than 5 years old who receives a sudden longitudinal pull or traction at the wrist while the arm is fully extended and the forearm pronated. It usually occurs when an individual who is holding the child by the hand or wrist gives a sudden pull or jerk to prevent a fall or attempts to lift the child by pulling the wrist or when the child pulls away by dropping to the floor or ground. The child often cries, appears anxious, complains of pain in the elbow or wrist, and refuses to use the affected limb. The practitioner manipulates the arm by applying firm finger pressure to the head of the radius and then supinates and flexes the forearm to return the bone structure to normal alignment. Alternatively, a hyperpronation method where the practitioner holds the child's flexed elbow with one hand while pronating the forearm with the other has also been shown to be effective. A click may be heard or felt, and functional use of the arm returns within minutes. Immobilization is not required. However, the longer the subluxation is present, the longer it takes for the child to recover mobility after treatment. No anesthetic is usually required, but a mild pain reliever such as acetaminophen or ibuprofen may be administered. In an older child, severe elbow injury or dislocation should be evaluated immediately by a practitioner. If a traumatic elbow injury in a younger child is not a subluxation or if attempts at reduction are unsuccessful, the child should be carefully evaluated, with the consideration of radiographs.

In children younger than 5 years old, the hip can be dislocated by a fall. The greatest risk after this injury is the potential loss of blood supply to the head of the femur. Relocation of the hip within 60 minutes after the injury provides the best chance for prevention of damage to the femoral head.

Shoulder dislocations and separations occur most often in older adolescents and are often sports related. Temporary restriction of the joint, with a sling or bandage that secures the arm to the chest in a shoulder dislocation, can provide sufficient comfort and immobilization until medical attention is received.

Simple dislocations should be reduced as soon as possible with the child under procedural sedation combined with local anesthesia. An unreduced dislocation may be complicated by increased swelling, making reduction difficult and increasing the risk of neurovascular problems. Treatment is determined by the severity of the injury.

Sprains

A sprain occurs when trauma to a joint is so severe that a ligament is partially or completely torn or stretched by the force created as a joint is twisted or wrenched, often accompanied by damage to associated blood vessels, muscles, tendons, and nerves. Common sprain sites include ankles and knees.

The presence of joint laxity is the most valid indicator of the severity of a sprain. In a severe injury, the child complains of the joint "feeling loose" or as if "something is coming apart" and may describe hearing a "snap," "pop," or "tearing." Pain may or may not be the principal subjective symptom, and in some children, it may prevent optimal examination of ligamentous instability. There is a rapid onset of swelling, often diffuse, accompanied by immediate disability and appreciable reluctance to use the injured joint.

Strains

A strain is a microscopic tear to the musculotendinous unit and has features in common with sprains. The area is painful to touch and swollen. Most strains are incurred over time rather than suddenly, and the rapidity of the appearance provides clues regarding severity. In general, the more rapidly the strain occurs, the more severe the injury. When the strain involves the muscular portion, there is more bleeding, often palpable soon after injury and before edema obscures the hematoma.

Therapeutic Management

The first 12 to 24 hours are the most critical period for virtually all soft-tissue injuries. Basic principles of managing sprains and other soft-tissue injuries are summarized in the acronyms RICE and ICES.

RICE	ICES
Rest	**I**ce
Ice	**C**ompression
Compression	**E**levation
Elevation	**S**upport

Soft-tissue injuries should be iced immediately. This is best accomplished with crushed ice wrapped in a towel, a screw-top ice bag, or a resealable plastic storage bag. Chemical-activated ice packs are also effective for immediate treatment but are not reusable and must be closely monitored for leakage. A wet elastic wrap, which transfers cold better than dry wrap, is applied to provide compression and to keep the ice pack in place. A cloth barrier should be used between the ice container and the skin to prevent trauma to the tissues. Ice has a rapid cooling effect on tissues that reduces edema and pain. Ice should never be applied for more than 30 minutes at a time.

> **NURSING TIP:** A plastic bag of frozen vegetables, such as peas, serves as a convenient ice pack for soft-tissue injuries. It is clean, watertight, and easily molded to the injured part. When available, snow placed in a plastic bag may also serve as an ice bag.

Elevating the extremity uses gravity to facilitate venous return and reduce edema formation in the damaged area. The point of injury should be kept several inches above the level of the heart for therapy to be effective. Several pillows can be used for elevation. Allowing the extremity to be dependent causes excessive fluid accumulation in the area of injury, delaying healing and causing painful swelling.

Torn ligaments, especially those in the knee, are usually treated by immobilization with a knee immobilizer or a knee brace that allows flexion and extension until the child is able to walk without a limp. Crutches are used for mobility to rest the affected extremity. Passive leg exercises, gradually increased to active ones, are begun as soon as sufficient healing has taken place. Parents and children are cautioned against using any form of liniment or other heat-producing preparation before examination. If the injury requires casting or splinting, the heat generated in the enclosed space can cause extreme discomfort and even tissue damage. In some cases, torn knee ligaments are managed with arthroscopy and ligament repair or reconstruction as necessary depending on the extent of the tear, the ligaments involved, and the child's age. Surgical reconstruction of the anterior cruciate ligament may be performed in young athletes who wish to continue in active sports.

FRACTURES

Bone fractures occur when the resistance of bone against the stress being exerted yields to the stress force. Fractures are a common injury at any age but are more likely to occur in children and older adults. Because childhood is a time of rapid bone growth, the pattern of fractures, problems of diagnosis, and methods of treatment differ in children compared with adults. In children, fractures heal much faster than in adults. Consequently, children may not require as long a period of immobilization of the affected extremity as an adult with a fracture.

Fracture injuries in children are most often a result of traumatic incidents at home, at school, in a motor vehicle, or in association with recreational activities. Children's everyday activities include vigorous play that predisposes them to injury, including climbing, falling down, running into immovable objects, skateboarding, trampolines, skiing, playground activities, and receiving blows to any part of their bodies by a solid, immovable object.

Aside from automobile accidents or falls from heights, true injuries that cause fractures rarely occur in infancy. Up to 25% of fractures in children younger than 12 months old have been attributed to nonaccidental trauma (child abuse) (Flaherty, Perez-Rossello, Levine, et al., 2014). Therefore bone injury in children of this age-group warrants further investigation. In any small child, radiographic evidence of fractures at various stages of healing is, with few exceptions, a result of nonaccidental trauma. Any investigation of fractures in infants, particularly multiple fractures, should include consideration of osteogenesis imperfecta (OI) after nonaccidental trauma has been ruled out.

Fractures in school-age children are often a result of playground falls or bicycle/automobile or skateboard injuries. Adolescents are vulnerable to multiple and severe trauma because they are mobile on bicycles, all-terrain vehicles, skateboards, skis, snowboards, trampolines, and motorcycles and are active in sports.

A distal forearm (radius, ulna, or both) fracture is the most common fracture in children. The clavicle is also a common fracture sustained in childhood, with approximately half of clavicle fractures occurring in children younger than 10 years old. Common mechanisms of injury include a fall with an outstretched hand or direct trauma to the bone. In neonates, a fractured clavicle may occur with a large newborn and a small maternal pelvis. This may be noted in the first few days after birth by a unilateral Moro reflex or at the 2-week well-child check, when a fracture callus is palpated on the infant's healing clavicle.

Types of Fractures

A fractured bone consists of fragments—the fragment closer to the midline, or the proximal fragment, and the fragment farther from the midline, or the distal fragment. When fracture fragments are separated, the fracture is complete; when fragments remain attached, the fracture is incomplete. The fracture line can be any of the following:

Transverse: Crosswise at right angles to the long axis of the bone

Oblique: Slanting but straight between a horizontal and a perpendicular direction

Spiral: Slanting and circular, twisting around the bone shaft

The twisting of an extremity while the bone is breaking results in a spiral break. If the fracture does not produce a break in the skin, it is a simple, or closed, fracture. Open, or compound, fractures are those with an open wound through which the bone protrudes. If the bone fragments cause damage to other organs or tissues (e.g., lung, liver), the injury is said to be a complicated fracture. When small fragments of bone are broken from the fractured shaft and lie in the surrounding tissue, the injury is a comminuted fracture. This type of fracture is rare in children. The types of fractures that are seen most often in children are described in Box 29.1 and Fig. 29.2.

Growth Plate (Physeal) Injuries

The weakest point of long bones is the cartilage growth plate, or the physis. Consequently, this is a frequent site of damage in childhood trauma. Growth plate fractures are classified with the Salter-Harris classification system (Fig. 29.3). Detection of physeal injuries is sometimes difficult but critical. Close monitoring and early treatment, if indicated, is essential to prevent longitudinal or angular growth deformities (or both). Treatment of these fractures may include surgical open reduction and internal fixation to prevent or reduce growth disturbances.

Immediately after a fracture occurs, the muscles contract and physiologically splint the injured area. This phenomenon accounts for the muscle tightness observed over a fracture site and the deformity that is produced as the muscles pull the bone ends out of alignment. This muscle response must be overcome by traction or complete muscle relaxation (e.g., anesthesia) to realign the distal bone fragment to the proximal bone fragment.

BOX 29.1 Types of Fractures in Children

Plastic deformation: Occurs when the bone is bent but not broken. A child's flexible bone can be bent 45 degrees or more before breaking. However, if bent, the bone will straighten slowly but not completely, producing some deformity but without the angulation seen when the bone breaks. Bends occur most commonly in the ulna and fibula, often in association with fractures of the radius and tibia.

Buckle, or torus, fracture: Produced by compression of the porous bone; appears as a raised or bulging projection at the fracture site. These fractures occur in the most porous portion of the bone near the metaphysis (the portion of the bone shaft adjacent to the epiphysis) and are more common in young children.

Greenstick fracture: Occurs when a bone is angulated beyond the limits of bending. The compressed side bends, and the tension side fails, causing an incomplete fracture similar to the break observed when a green stick is broken.

Complete fracture: Divides the bone fragments. These fragments often remain attached by a periosteal hinge, which can aid or hinder reduction.

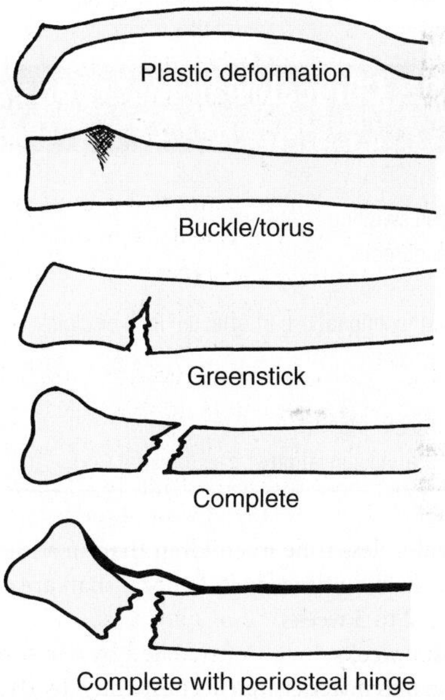

Fig. 29.2 Types of fractures in children.

Bone Healing and Remodeling

Bone healing is rapid in growing children because of the thickened periosteum and generous blood supply. When there is a break in the continuity of bone, the osteoblasts are stimulated to maximal activity. New bone cells are formed in immense numbers almost immediately after the injury and, in time, are evidenced by a bulging growth of new bone tissue between the fractured bone fragments. This is followed by deposition of calcium salts to form a callus. Remodeling is a process that occurs in the healing of long bone fractures in growing children. The irregularities produced by the fracture become indistinct as the angles and bone overgrowth are smoothed out, giving the bone a straighter appearance.

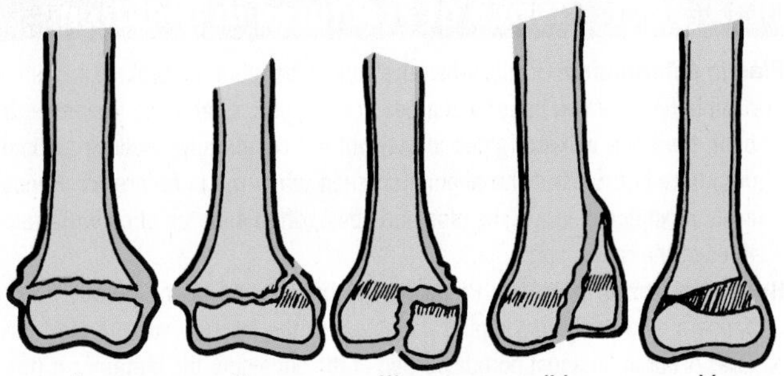

Fig. 29.3 Salter-Harris fracture classification. Types of epiphyseal injury in order of increasing risk for growth abnormalities. The injuries are classified as follows: *Type I,* separation or slip of growth plate without fracture of the bone; *type II,* separation of growth plate and breaking off of section of metaphysis; *type III,* fracture of epiphysis extending through joint surface; *type IV,* fracture of growth plate, epiphysis, and metaphysis; and *type V,* crushing injury of epiphysis (can be diagnosed only in retrospect). This classification of epiphyseal injuries was developed by orthopedists R. B. Salter and W. R. Harris. (First published in Salter, R. B., & Harris, W. R. [1963]. Injuries involving the physeal plate. *Journal of Bone and Joint Surgery, 45*[3], 587–622.)

BOX 29.2 Clinical Manifestations of a Fracture

Signs of injury:
- Generalized swelling
- Pain or tenderness
- Deformity
- Diminished functional use of affected limb or digit

May also demonstrate:
- Bruising
- Severe muscular rigidity
- Crepitus (grating sensation at fracture site)

Fractures heal in less time in children than in adults. For example, the approximate healing times for a femoral shaft are as follows:
Neonatal period: 2 to 3 weeks
Early childhood: 4 weeks
Later childhood: 6 to 8 weeks
Adolescence: 8 to 12 weeks

Diagnostic Evaluation

A history of the injury may be lacking in childhood injuries. Infants and toddlers are unable to communicate, and older children may not volunteer information (even under direct questioning) when the injury occurred during questionable activities. Whenever possible, it is helpful to obtain information from someone who witnessed the injury. In cases of nonaccidental trauma, providers may give false information to protect themselves or family members.

The child may exhibit the same manifestations seen in adults, which may include swelling, bruising, pain or tenderness, deformity, and diminished function (Box 29.2). However, often a fracture is remarkably stable because of intact periosteum. The child may even be able to use an affected arm or walk on a fractured leg. Because bones are highly vascular, a soft, pliable hematoma may be felt around the fracture site.

! NURSING ALERT

A fracture should be strongly suspected in a small child who refuses to walk or crawl.

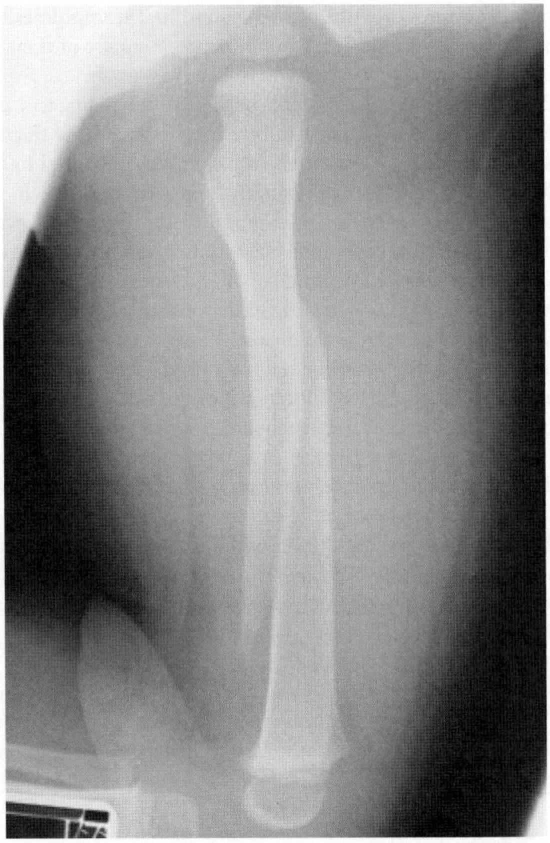

Fig. 29.4 Fractured femur. Most fractured femurs in childhood are of the spiral type shown here. (From Mark, J. A., Hockberger, R. S., & Walls, R. M. [2013]. *Rosen's emergency medicine: Concepts and clinical practice* [8th ed.]. St. Louis, MO: Elsevier.)

Radiographic examination is the most useful diagnostic tool for assessing skeletal trauma. The calcium deposits in bone make the entire structure radiopaque. Radiographic films are taken after fracture reduction and in some cases may be taken during the healing process to determine satisfactory progress.

Therapeutic Management

The goals of fracture management are:
- To regain alignment and length of the bony fragments (reduction)
- To retain alignment and length (immobilization)
- To restore function to the injured parts
- To prevent further injury and deformity

The majority of children's fractures heal well, and nonunion is rare. Fractures are splinted or casted to immobilize and protect the injured extremity. Children with displaced fractures may have immediate surgical reduction and fixation (internal or external) rather than being immobilized by traction (Fig. 29.4). This practice is more common and holds true for all types of fractures, including femur fractures, although there is variation based on provider preference and institutional practice. Some conditions require immediate medical attention, including open fractures, compartment syndrome, fractures associated with vascular or nerve injury, and joint dislocations that are unresponsive to reduction maneuvers.

In children, immobilization is used until adequate callus is formed. The position of the bone fragments in relation to one another influences the rapidity of healing and residual deformity. Weight bearing and active movement for the purpose of regaining function may begin after the fracture site is determined to be stable by the medical provider. The child's natural tendency to be active is usually sufficient to restore normal mobility, and physical or occupational therapy is rarely indicated.

Children are most frequently hospitalized for fractures of the femur and supracondylar area of the distal humerus. If simple reduction cannot be achieved or a neurovascular problem is detected after the injury, observation in a hospital setting may be indicated. The trend is to avoid hospitalization. The major methods for immobilizing a fracture, casting and traction, are described later.

Nursing Care Management

Nurses are frequently the persons who make the initial assessment of a child with a suspected fracture (see Emergency Treatment box). The child and parents may be frightened and upset, and the child is often in pain. Therefore if the child is alert and there is no evidence of hemorrhage, the initial nursing interventions are directed toward calming and reassuring the child and parents so that a more extensive assessment can be more easily accomplished.

EMERGENCY TREATMENT

Fracture

Determine the mechanism of injury.
Assess the 6 Ps (see Box 29.3).
Move the injured part as little as possible.
Cover open wounds with a sterile or clean dressing.
Immobilize the limb, including joints above and below the fracture site; do not attempt to reduce the fracture or push protruding bone under the skin.
Use a soft splint (pillow or folded towel) or rigid splint (rolled newspaper or magazine).
Uninjured leg can serve as a splint for a leg fracture if no splint is available.
Reassess neurovascular status.
Apply traction if circulatory compromise is present.
Elevate the injured limb if possible.
Apply cold to the injured area.
Call emergency medical services or transport to medical facility.

While remaining calm and speaking in a quiet voice, the nurse can ask the parents and older child to describe what happened. The child may arrive with the limb supported in some manner; if not, careful support or immobilization may be provided to the affected site. In the event that the limb is supported or immobilized, it may be best not to touch the child but to ask him or her to point to the painful area and to wiggle the fingers or toes. By this time the child may feel relatively safe and will allow someone to gently touch the area just enough to feel the pulses and test for sensation. A child's anxiety is greatly influenced by previous experiences with injury and with health personnel. However, he or she needs to be told what will happen and what to do to help. The affected limb need not be palpated, and it should not be moved unless properly splinted. If the child is at home or if the practitioner is not present to examine the child, some type of splint is applied carefully for transport to the medical facility. Parental anxiety may be heightened by the child's pain reaction and fear and possibly by other events surrounding the accident. It is important to communicate to the parent that the child will receive the necessary care, including pain management.

THE CHILD IN A CAST

The completeness of the fracture, the type of bone involved, and the amount of weight bearing influence how much of the extremity must be included in the cast to immobilize the fracture site completely. In most cases, the joints above and below the fracture are immobilized to eliminate the possibility of movement that might cause displacement at the fracture site. Four major categories of casts are used for fractures: **upper extremity** to immobilize the wrist or elbow, **lower extremity** to immobilize the ankle or knee, spinal and cervical to immobilize the spine, and spica casts to immobilize the hip and knee (Fig. 29.5).

! NURSING ALERT

Compartment syndrome is a serious complication that results from compression of nerves, blood vessels, and muscle inside a closed space. This injury may be devastating, resulting in tissue death, and thus requires emergency treatment (fasciotomy). The six Ps of ischemia from a vascular, soft-tissue, nerve, or bone injury should be included in an assessment of any injury:

1. Pain
2. Pulselessness
3. Pallor
4. Paresthesia
5. Paralysis
6. Pressure (Box 29.3)

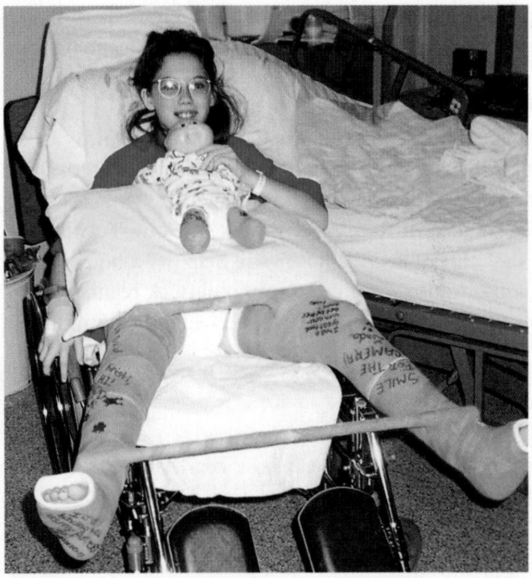

Fig. 29.5 Spica cast with hip abductor. Note casts on doll as well.

The Cast

Casts are constructed from gauze strips and bandages impregnated with plaster of Paris or, more commonly, from synthetic lighter weight and water-resistant materials (e.g., waterproof liners, fiberglass and polyurethane resin).

Both types of casting produce heat from chemical reaction activated by water immediately after application. Plaster casts are able to be molded closely to the body part, take 10 to 72 hours to dry, have a smooth exterior, and are inexpensive. The newer synthetic casting material is lightweight, dries in 5 to 20 minutes, permits earlier weight bearing, and is water resistant when applied with a waterproof liner. It is always desirable to give children choices, and synthetic casting materials come in a variety of colors. The disadvantages of synthetic casting are its inability to mold closely to body parts and its rough exterior, which may scratch surfaces. Synthetic casts are also difficult to write on; a waterproof marker or color markers may be used.

Cast Application

The child's developmental age should be considered before the cast is applied. For preschoolers who fear bodily harm and fantasize about the loss of an extremity, it may be helpful to use a plastic doll or stuffed animal to explain the procedure beforehand. Toddlers and preschoolers do not have easily defined body boundaries; if an extremity is wrapped in a bandage, cast, or splint, to the young child the extremity ceases to function or exist. It is also helpful to explain that some synthetic cast material will become warm during application but will not burn. During the application of the cast, various distraction methods can be used, including discussing favorite pets or activities at school, blowing bubbles, and so forth. In this age-group, explanations, such as "This will help your arm get better," are futile because the child has no concept of causality.

Before the cast is applied, the extremities are checked for any abrasions, cuts, or other alterations in the skin surface and for the presence of rings or other items that might cause constriction from swelling; such objects are removed. A tube of cloth stockinette or Gore-Tex liner is stretched over the area to be casted, and bony prominences are padded with soft cotton sheeting. Dry rolls of casting material are immersed in a pail of water. The wet rolls are put on in a bandage fashion and molded to the extremity. During application of the cast, the underlying stockinette is pulled over the rough edges of the cast and secured with casting material to form a padded edge to protect the skin.

Nursing Care Management

The complete evaporation of the water from a hip spica cast can take 24 to 48 hours when older types of plaster materials are used. Drying occurs within minutes with fiberglass cast material. The cast must remain uncovered to allow it to dry from the inside out. Turning the child in a plaster cast at least every 2 hours will help dry a body cast evenly and prevent complications related to immobility. A regular fan or cool-air hair dryer to circulate air may be helpful when the humidity is high.

! NURSING ALERT

Heated fans or dryers are not used because they cause the cast to dry on the outside and remain wet beneath or cause burns from heat conduction by way of the cast to the underlying tissue.

A wet plaster cast should be supported by a pillow that is covered with plastic and handled by the palms of the hands to prevent indenting the cast, which can create pressure areas. A dry plaster-of-Paris cast produces a hollow sound when it is tapped with the finger. After it has dried, "hot spots" felt on the cast surface or a foul-smelling odor may indicate an infection. This should be reported for further evaluation, and if concern continues, an opening, or a "window," may be exposed over the area of concern to evaluate the site.

During the first few hours after a cast is applied, the chief concern is that the extremity may continue to swell to the extent that the cast becomes a tourniquet, shutting off circulation and producing neurovascular complications (**compartment syndrome**) (see Box 29.3). To reduce the likelihood of this potential problem, the body part can be elevated, thereby increasing venous return. If edema is excessive, casts are bivalved (i.e., cut to make anterior and posterior halves that are held together with an elastic bandage). The cast and the involved extremity are observed frequently for neurovascular integrity and any signs of compromise. Permanent muscle and tissue damage can occur within a few hours.

BOX 29.3 Compartment Syndrome Evaluation

Assess the extent of injury—"the 6 Ps":

1. **Pain:** Severe pain that is not relieved by analgesics or elevation of the limb, movement that increases pain
2. **Pulselessness:** Inability to palpate a pulse distal to the fracture or compartment
3. **Pallor:** Pale-appearing skin, poor perfusion, capillary refill greater than 3 seconds
4. **Paresthesia:** Tingling or burning sensations
5. **Paralysis:** Inability to move extremity or digits
6. **Pressure:** Involved limb or digits may feel tense and warm; skin is tight, shiny; pressure within the compartment is elevated

! NURSING ALERT

Observations such as pain (unrelieved by pain medication 1 hour after administration, especially with passive range of motion), swelling, discoloration (pallor or cyanosis) of the exposed portions, decreased pulses, decreased temperature, paresthesia, or the inability to move the distal exposed part(s) should be reported immediately. Pallor, paralysis, and pulselessness are late signs (see Box 29.3).

When an extremity that has sustained an open fracture is casted, a window is often left over the wound area to allow for observation and dressing of the wound. For the first few hours after surgery, substantial bleeding may soak through the cast. Periodically, the circumscribed bloodstained area should be outlined with a waterproof marker and the time indicated to provide a guide for assessing the amount of bleeding.

Appropriate cast care guidelines for the child's caregiver are necessary before discharge. Instructions are also given for checking for signs and symptoms that indicate that the cast is too tight (see Family-Centered Care box). Parents should also be told to take the child to the health professional for attention if the cast becomes too loose because a loose cast no longer serves its purpose and can cause skin irritation or pressure sores.

FAMILY-CENTERED CARE

Cast Care

Keep the casted extremity elevated on pillows or similar support for the first day or as directed by the health professional.

Avoid denting the plaster cast with fingertips (use palms of hand to handle) while it is still wet to avoid creating pressure points.

Expose the plaster cast to air until dry.

Observe the extremities (fingers or toes) for any evidence of swelling or discoloration (darker or lighter than a comparable extremity) and contact the health professional if noted.

Check movement and sensation of the visible extremities frequently.

Follow health professional's orders regarding any restriction of activities.

Restrict strenuous activities for the first few days:

- Engage in quiet activities but encourage use of muscles.
- Move the joints above and below the cast on the affected extremity.

Encourage frequent rest for a few days, keeping the injured extremity elevated while resting.

Avoid allowing the affected limb to hang in a dependent position for any length of time:

- Keep an injured upper extremity elevated (e.g., in a sling) while upright.
- Elevate a lower limb when sitting and avoid standing for too long.

Do not allow the child to put anything inside the cast. Keep small items that might be placed inside the cast away from small children.

Keep a clear path for ambulation. Remove toys, hazardous floor rugs, pets, and other items over which the child might stumble.

Use crutches appropriately if lower limb fracture requires non–weight bearing on affected extremity.

The crutches should fit properly, have a soft rubber tip to prevent slipping, and be well padded at the axilla.

With crutch walking, the child's body weight is supported on the hand grips, not the axilla.

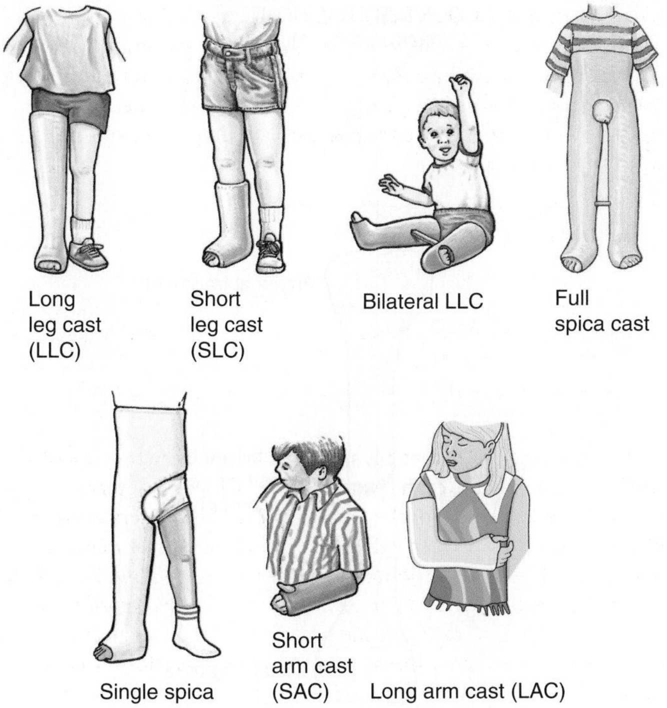

Fig. 29.6 Types of casts.

Nurses can help families adapt the child's home environment to meet the temporary encumbrance of a large cast or one that restricts the child's mobility (e.g., a long leg or spica cast [Fig. 29.6]). Commonplace situations become problematic (e.g., transporting a child safely and comfortably in a car). Standard seat belts and car seats may not be readily adapted for use by children in certain casts. Specially designed car seats and restraints that meet safety requirements are available.[a] Alterations to standard car seats to accommodate the cast are not recommended because the structure may be adversely altered and fail to properly restrain the child. A bedside commode or rental wheelchair maybe be necessary equipment for a child who is nonambulatory.

Parents are taught the proper care of the cast or brace, and are helped to devise means for maintaining cleanliness. A superabsorbent disposable diaper is tucked beneath the entire perineal opening of the cast. A larger diaper can be applied and fastened over the small diaper and cast to hold the smaller diaper in place. In the event that the larger diaper becomes wet or soiled, it is likely the cast is as well.

For tightly fitting casts, transparent film dressings can be cut into strips for petaling, with one edge applied to the cast edge and the other directly to the perineum; this forms a continuous, waterproof bridge between the perineum and the cast to prevent leakage. An additional advantage to the use of this transparent dressing is that it keeps both the skin and the cast dry while allowing for observation of skin beneath the dressing.

[a]For information on specially adapted molded-plastic chairs for children who have spica casts, contact R82 Inc. at 844-876-6245; http://www.r82.com. The E-Z-On vest is a special safety harness for larger children with poor trunk control. Additional safety restraints and a list of distributors are available from SafetyBeltSafe U.S.A., http://www.carseat.org. Another resource is the National Center for the Safe Transportation of Children with Special Health Care Needs; 800-543-6227; http://www.preventinjury.org/Special-Needs-Transportation/Child-Seats-for-Children-with-Special-Needs.

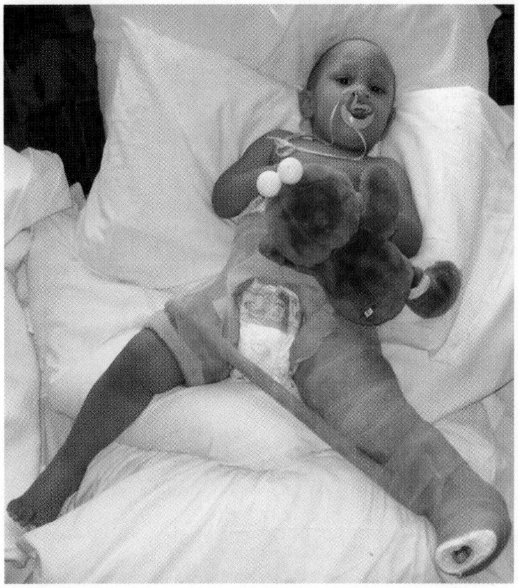

Fig. 29.7 Single spica cast. Note diaper to maintain dryness. (Courtesy Texas Children's Hospital, Houston, TX.)

Older infants and small children may stuff bits of food, small toys, or other items under the cast; parents should be alerted to this possibility so that they can initiate suitable preventive measures.

Feeding an infant in a hip spica cast offers problems in positioning. Very young infants can be fed in the supine position with the head elevated. With the infant's hips and legs supported on a pillow at the side, the parent can cuddle the infant in his or her arms during feeding. A somewhat similar position can be used for breastfeeding (i.e., with the infant supported on pillows or held in a "football" hold facing the mother with the legs behind her). An alternate position is to hold the infant upright on the caregiver's lap with the legs of the infant astride the adult's leg.

Children in spica casts usually find the prone position easier for self-feeding from a small table placed next to the dining table; alternatively, they may manage a semisitting position in bed or in a wheelchair (Fig. 29.7). The use of a conventional toilet is almost impossible. A bedside toilet can be adapted for use. Small bedpans or other containers offer alternatives for elimination. The nurse may suggest waterproofing methods by devising plastic wraps for elimination and showers. Baths are possible only if the plaster cast is kept out of the water and covered to prevent it from becoming wet.

Cast Removal

Cutting the cast to remove it or to relieve tightness is frequently a frightening experience for children. They fear the sound of the cast cutter and are terrified that their flesh, as well as the cast, will be cut. The oscillating blade vibrates rapidly back and forth and will not cut when placed *lightly* on the skin. Children have described it as producing a "tickly" sensation. The vibration also generates heat that may be felt by the child. Both of these feelings should be explained.

Preparation for the procedure will help reduce anxiety, especially if a trusting relationship has been established between the child and the nurse. Many young children come to regard the cast as part of themselves, which intensifies their fear of removal (Fig. 29.8). They need continual reassurance that all is going well and that their behavior is accepted. After the cast is removed, the parents and child should be given the option of keeping the cast. If the cast has been in place for a lengthy period, decreased muscle mass will be noted. The child should be reassured that resuming exercise and routine activities will return function and appearance (provided that there was no significant trauma beforehand).

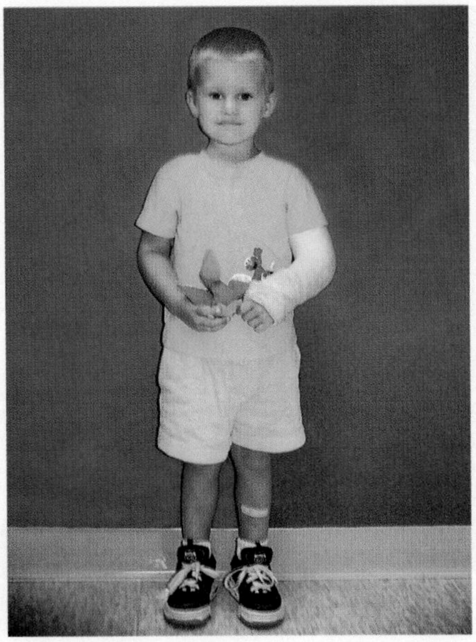

Fig. 29.8 Young children come to regard a cast as part of their body.

After the cast is removed, the skin surface will be caked with desquamated skin and sebaceous secretions. Application of mineral oil (e.g., baby oil) or lotion may remove the particles as well as provide comfort. Soaking the extremity in a bathtub is usually sufficient for their removal, but it may take several days to eliminate the accumulation completely. The parents and child should be instructed not to pull or forcibly remove this material with vigorous scrubbing because it may cause excoriation and bleeding.

THE CHILD IN TRACTION

The ever-changing health care arena has witnessed the demise of many long-term treatments involving lengthy hospitalization; one such change is in the area of traction. Most balanced skeletal traction is applied in children after a severe or complex injury to allow physiologic stability, align bone fragments, and permit closer evaluation of the injured site. Newer technology has produced orthopedic fixation devices that allow partial or full mobility, thus preventing long-term immobilization and its consequences. In many situations, surgical intervention may be carried out within a matter of days; therefore skeletal traction devices described herein may be used infrequently in pediatrics.

Purposes of Traction

The six primary purposes of traction are:

1. To fatigue the involved muscles and reduce muscle spasm so that bones can be realigned
2. To position the distal and proximal bone ends in desired realignment to promote satisfactory bone healing
3. To immobilize the fracture site until realignment has been achieved and sufficient healing has taken place to permit casting or splinting
4. To help prevent or improve contracture deformity
5. To provide immobilization of specific areas of the body
6. To reduce muscle spasms (rare in children)

The three essential components of traction management are traction, countertraction, and friction (Fig. 29.9). To reduce or realign a fracture site, **traction** (forward force) is produced by attaching weight to the distal bone fragment. Body weight provides **countertraction** (backward force), and the patient's contact with the bed constitutes the **frictional** force. These forces are used to align the distal and proximal

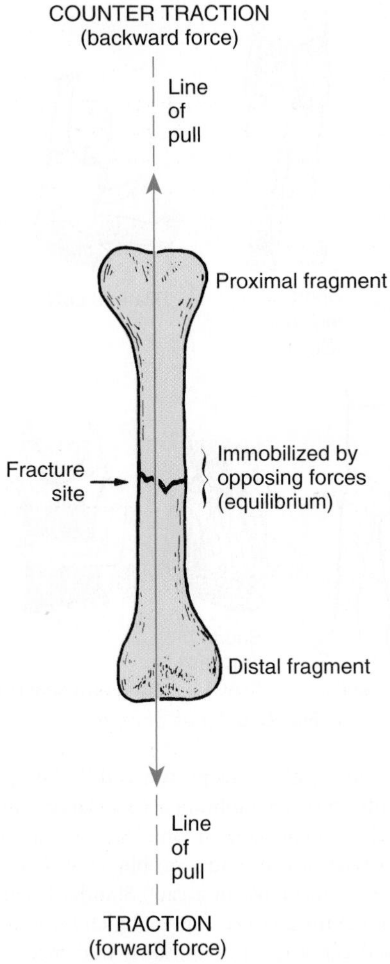

Fig. 29.9 Application of traction for maintaining equilibrium.

bone fragments by adjusting the line of pull upward or downward and adducting or abducting the extremity.

To attain equilibrium, the amount of forward force is adjusted by adding weight to or subtracting weight from the traction, or countertraction can be increased by elevating the foot of the bed to create a greater gravitational pull to the backward force.

The **all-or-none law**, characteristic of muscle contractibility, influences the complete relaxation. When muscles are stretched, muscle spasm ceases, which permits the realignment of the bone ends. The continuous maintenance of traction is important during this phase because releasing the traction allows the muscle's normal contracting ability to again cause a malpositioning of the bone ends.

The realignment of the fragments is a gradual process that is achieved more rapidly in infants, who have limited muscle tone, than in muscular teenagers. The desired vector force and callus formation are checked periodically by radiographic examination. The traction pull to some degree immobilizes the fracture site; however, adjunctive immobilizing devices such as splints or casts are sometimes used with skeletal traction. Immobilization with traction is maintained until the bone ends are in satisfactory realignment, after which a less confining type of immobilization—a cast, pins, or external stabilization device—is applied.

Types of Traction

The pull needed for traction can be applied to the distal bone fragment in several ways (Box 29.4). The type of traction applied is determined primarily by the child's age, the condition of the soft tissues, and the

BOX 29.4 Types of Traction

Manual traction: Applied to the body part by the hand placed distal to the fracture site. Manual traction may be provided during application of a cast but more commonly when a closed reduction is performed.

Skin traction: Applied directly to the skin surface and indirectly to the skeletal structures. The pulling mechanism is attached to the skin with adhesive material or an elastic bandage. Both types are applied over soft, foam-backed traction straps to distribute the traction pull.

Skeletal traction: Applied directly to the skeletal structure by a pin, wire, or tongs inserted into or through the diameter of the bone distal to the fracture.

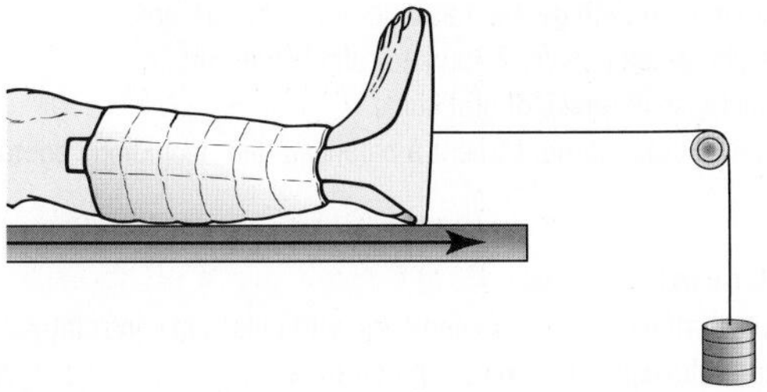

Fig. 29.10 Buck extension traction.

type and degree of displacement of the fracture. Fractures most commonly treated by application of traction are those involving the femur and vertebrae. The major types of traction for specific fractures are briefly discussed in the following paragraphs.

The use of upper extremity traction in children is uncommon. Newer surgical techniques allow for early mobilization and optimal results without traction. Nursing care of the child with upper extremity traction is the same as that for lower extremity traction, which is discussed later.

The frequent site for a femoral fracture is in the middle third of the shaft. With this fracture, there may be significant overriding but minimal displacement. In a fracture in the lower third of the shaft, the pull of the gastrocnemius muscle causes the distal fragment to become downwardly displaced.

Fractures of the femur can often be reduced with immediate application of a hip spica cast in young children. When traction is required, several types may be used based on the initial assessment.

Bryant traction is a type of running traction in which the pull is in only one direction. Skin traction is applied to the legs, which are flexed at a 90-degree angle at the hips. The child's trunk (with the buttocks raised slightly off the bed) provides countertraction.

Buck extension traction (Fig. 29.10) is a type of traction with the legs in an extended position. Except for fracture cases, turning from side to side with care is permitted to maintain the involved leg in alignment. Buck extension traction is used primarily for short-term immobilization, such as preoperative management of a child with a dislocated hip, or for correction of contractures or bone deformities, such as in Legg-Calvé-Perthes disease. Buck extension traction may be accomplished with either skin straps or a special foam boot designed for traction.

Russell traction uses skin traction on the lower leg and a padded sling under the knee. Two lines of pull, one along the longitudinal line of the lower leg and one perpendicular to the leg, are produced. This combination of pulls allows realignment of the lower extremity and immobilizes the hip and knee in a flexed position. The hip flexion must be kept at the prescribed angle to prevent fracture malalignment because there is no direct support under the fracture and the skin traction may slip. Special nursing measures include carefully checking the position of the traction so that the amount of desired hip flexion is maintained and damage to the common peroneal nerve under the knee does not produce foot drop.

A common skeletal traction is **90-degree–90-degree traction** (90-90 traction). The lower leg is supported by a boot cast or a calf sling, and a skeletal Steinmann pin or Kirschner wire is placed in the distal fragment of the femur, resulting in a 90-degree angle at both the hip and the knee. From a nursing standpoint, this traction facilitates position changes, toileting, and prevention of complications related to traction.

Balanced suspension traction may be used with or without skin or skeletal traction. Unless used with another traction, the balanced suspension merely suspends the leg in a desired flexed position to relax the hip and hamstring muscles and does not exert any traction directly on a body part. A **Thomas splint** extends from the groin to midair above the foot, and a **Pearson attachment** supports the lower leg. Towels or pieces of felt covered with stockinette are clipped or pinned to the splints for leg support. When the child is lifted off the bed, the traction lifts with the child without loss of alignment. This traction requires careful checking of splints and ropes to make certain that no slippage or fraying has occurred. The traction is of great value in an older and heavier child when it is essential to lift the patient for care.

The cervical area is a vulnerable site for flexion or extension injuries to muscle, vertebrae, or the spinal cord. Cervical muscle trauma without other complications is treated with a cervical hard collar to relieve the weight of the head from the fracture site. When a child displaces or fractures a cervical vertebra, it may be necessary to reduce and immobilize the site with cervical skeletal traction. The spinal cord runs through the intravertebral canal, and dislocation or fracture of the vertebrae can also cause spinal cord injury. Nursing assessment of neurologic function is essential to prevent further injury during the application and use of cervical skeletal traction.

Most cervical traction is accomplished with the use of a **halo brace** or **halo vest** (Fig. 29.11A). This device consists of a steel halo attached to the head by four screws inserted into the outer skull; several rigid bars connect the halo to a vest that is worn around the chest, thus providing greater mobility of the rest of the body while avoiding cervical spinal motion altogether. If the injury has been limited to a vertebral fracture without neurologic deficit, a halo brace can be applied to permit earlier ambulation. Gardner-Wells tongs may be used with cervical traction to immobilize the cervical spine (see Fig. 29.11B). Gardner-Wells tongs are spring loaded, so making burr holes and shaving hair are not required; a local anesthetic may be used during application. As the neck muscles fatigue with constant traction pull, the vertebral bodies gradually separate so that the cord is no longer pinched between the vertebrae. Immobilization until fracture healing or surgical fixation can occur is an essential goal of cervical traction. If immobilization is required in an infant or young child, a special cervical spine cast (Minerva cast) is applied.

Nursing Care Management

To assess the child in traction, it is essential to know the purpose for which the traction is applied and to understand the basic principles of traction. Regular assessment of both the child and the traction apparatus is required (see Nursing Care Guidelines box). Many of the nursing problems associated with a child in traction are related to immobility. Modifying the child's diet, encouraging fluids, increasing fiber, and offering a mild stool softener may be necessary to prevent constipation.

NURSING CARE GUIDELINES

Traction Care

Understand Therapy

Understand purpose of traction.

Understand function of traction in each specific situation.

Maintain Traction

Check desired line of pull and relationship of distal fragment to proximal fragment. Check whether fragment is being directed upward, adducted, or abducted.

Check function of each component:

- Position of bandages, frames, splints, specialized boot
- Ropes: In center track of pulley, taut, no fraying, knots tied securely
- Pulleys: In original position on attachment bar; have not slid from original site; wheels freely movable
- Weights: Correct amount of weight, hanging freely, in safe location

Check bed position: Head or foot elevated as directed for desired amount of pull and countertraction.

Do not remove skeletal traction or adhesive traction straps on skin traction.

Maintain Alignment

Observe for correct body alignment with emphasis on alignment of shoulder, hip, and leg.

Check after child has moved.

Maintain correct angles at joints.

Skin Traction

Replace nonadhesive straps or elastic bandage on skin traction *when permitted* or absolutely necessary, but make certain that traction on limb is maintained by someone during procedure.

Assess straps or bandages to ascertain if they are correctly applied (diagonal or spiral) and not too loose or too tight, which could cause slippage and malalignment of traction.

Assess traction boot to ensure that it has not slipped and is not causing compression of the foot, thus impairing the circulation.

Skeletal Traction

Check pin sites frequently for signs of bleeding, inflammation, or infection.

Cleanse and dress pin sites per institution protocol or as ordered.

Apply topical antiseptic or antibiotic to pin sites daily as ordered.

Cover ends of pins with protective rubber or padding to prevent child being scratched by pin.

Note pull of traction on pin; pull should be even.

Check pin screws to be certain that screws are tight in metal clamp that attaches traction apparatus to pin.

Prevent Skin Breakdown

Provide alternating-pressure mattress underneath hips and back.

Make total-body skin checks for redness or breakdown, especially over areas that receive greatest pressure.

Wash and dry skin at least daily.

Inspect pressure points daily or more often if risk for breakdown is observed.

Use a skin breakdown assessment scale, such as Braden Q.

Stimulate circulation with gentle massage over pressure areas.

Change position at least every 2 hours to relieve pressure.

Encourage increase in intake of oral fluids.

Provide and encourage patient to eat a balanced diet, including vegetables and fruits.

Prevent Complications

Check pulses in affected area and compare with pulses in contralateral site.

Assess circular dressings for excessive tightness.

Assess restrictive bandages or devices used to maintain traction on affected limb:

1. Make certain that they are not too loose or too tight.
2. Remove periodically and check for skin breakdown or pressure areas.

Encourage deep breathing or use of incentive spirometry:

- Monitor the 6 Ps (see Box 29.3).

Take immediate action to correct problem or report to practitioner if neurovascular changes are present.

Record findings of neurovascular changes.

Carry out passive, active, or active-with-resistance exercises of uninvolved joints.

Note if any tightness, weakness, edema, or contractures are developing in uninvolved joints and muscles.

Take measures to correct or prevent further development of weakness, such as applying footboard or foot orthoses to prevent foot drop.

When indicated by the attending practitioner, the nurse may remove nonadhesive skin traction. In these cases, intermittent traction is periodically released and reapplied as ordered. A child may have several types of traction at one time, and each one must be assessed separately to avoid problems.

! NURSING ALERT

Skeletal traction is never released by the nurse (except under direct supervision by the practitioner). This precaution includes not lifting the weights that are applying traction (e.g., for moving the child in bed, for repositioning).

In addition to routine skin observation and care, the child in skeletal traction will need special skin care at the pin sites according to hospital policy or practitioner preference. Pin sites should be frequently assessed and cleaned to prevent infection; after the first 48 to 72 hours, pin site care may be performed once daily or weekly for mechanically stable pins (Holmes, Brown, & Pin Site Care Expert Panel, 2005). Use of a 2-mg/ml chlorhexidine solution has been proposed as best practice care for skeletal pin sites by the National Association of Orthopaedic Nurses (Smith, Dahlen, Bruemmer, et al., 2013). A pressure-reduction device, such as a pressure-reduction mattress, decreases the chance of skin breakdown.

NURSING TIP: A small hand mirror facilitates visualization of inaccessible skin areas.

When the child is first placed in traction, increased discomfort is common as a result of the traction pull fatiguing the muscle. It has been determined that orthopedic conditions are associated with a higher-than-average number of painful events and a higher percentage of bodily symptoms than other common conditions. Analgesics, including IV opioids, and muscle relaxants help during this phase of care and should be administered liberally.

! NURSING ALERT

For skeletal traction to be effective, ensure that the weights are hanging freely at all times.

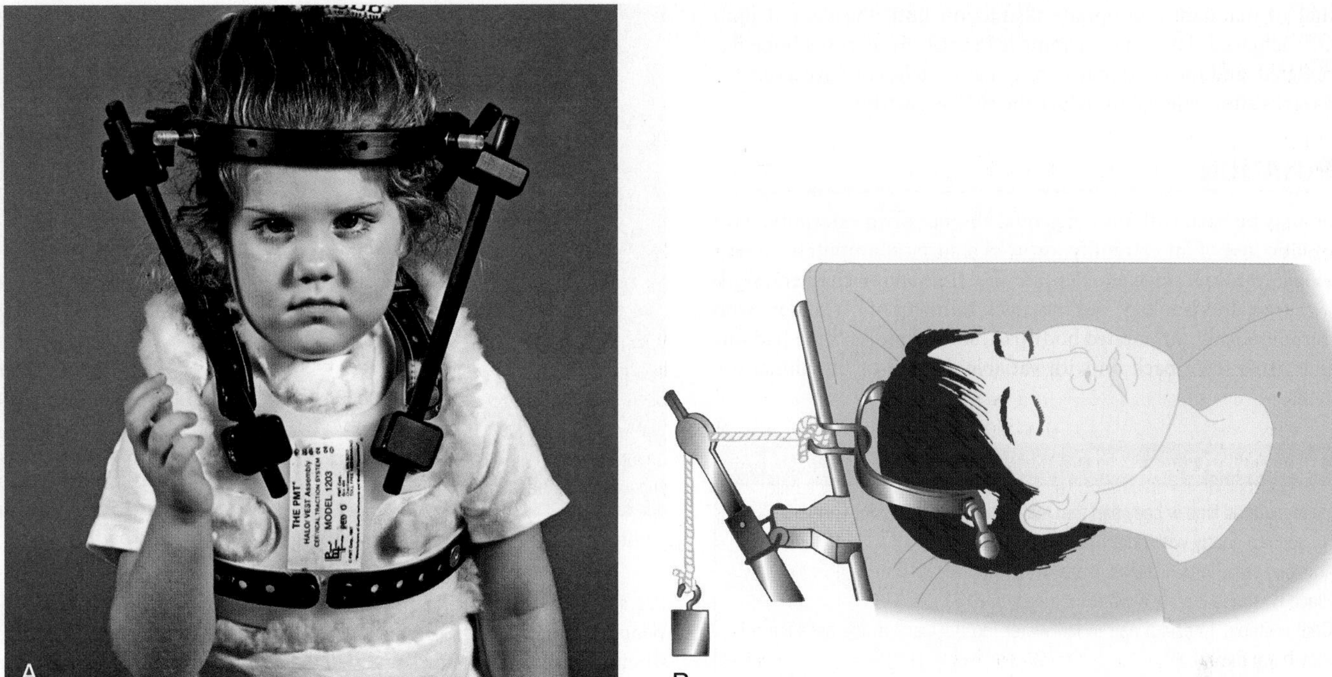
A
B
Fig. 29.11 A, Halo vest. B, Cervical traction with Gardner-Wells tong.

The specific nursing responsibilities for the patient in traction are outlined in the Nursing Care Guidelines box earlier.

DISTRACTION

Unlike traction, which helps bones realign and fuse properly, distraction is the process of separating opposing bone to encourage regeneration of new bone in the created space. Distraction can also be used when limbs are of unequal lengths and new bone is needed to elongate the shorter limb.

External Fixation

Monolateral, Taylor Spatial Frame, and Ilizarov external fixators (IEFs) are common external fixation devices. The IEF uses a system of wires, rings, and telescoping rods that permits limb lengthening to occur by manual distraction (Fig. 29.12). In addition to lengthening bones, the device can be used to correct angular or rotational defects or to immobilize fractures. The device is attached surgically by securing a series of external full or half rings to the bone with wires. External telescoping rods connect the rings to each other. Manual distraction is accomplished by manipulating the rods to increase the distance between the rings. A percutaneous osteotomy is performed when the device is applied to create a "false" growth plate. A special osteotomy or corticotomy involves cutting only the cortex of the bone while preserving its blood supply, bone marrow, endosteum, and periosteum. Capillary blood flow to the transected area is essential for proper bone growth. Cut bone ends typically grow at a rate of 1 cm (0.4 inch) per month. The IEF can result in up to a 15-cm (6-inch) gain in length.

Nursing Care Management

Success of the fixation devices depends on the child's and family's cooperation; therefore, before surgery, they must be fully informed of the appearance of the device, how it accomplishes bone growth and limits bone mobility, alterations in activities, and home and follow-up care. Children are involved in learning to adjust the device to

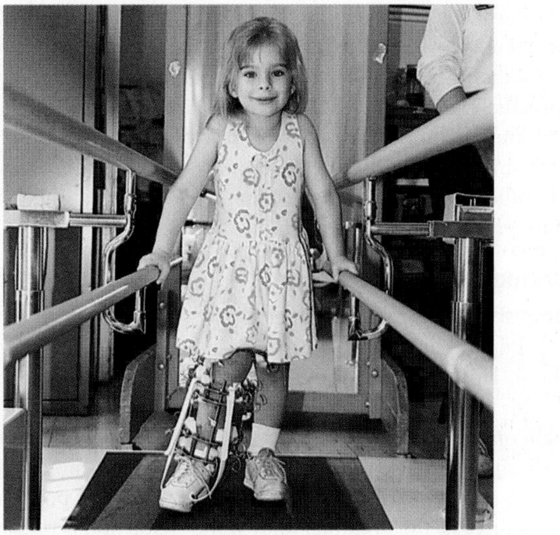
Fig. 29.12 Child with Ilizarov external fixator (IEF; on right leg) during physical therapy on parallel bars.

accomplish distraction. Children and parents should be instructed in pin care, including observation for infection and loosening of the pins. Cleaning routines for the pin sites vary among practitioners but should not traumatize the skin.

Children who participate actively in their care report less discomfort. Because the device is external, the child and family need to be prepared for the reactions of others and assisted in camouflaging the device with appropriate apparel, such as wide-legged pants that close with self-adhering fasteners around the device. A loose sock or stockinette may also be used over the device to decrease public awareness. Partial weight bearing is allowed, and the child learns to walk with crutches. Alterations in activity include modifications at school and in physical education (PE). Full weight bearing is not allowed until the distraction is completed and bone consolidation has occurred. Follow-up care is essential to maintain appropriate distraction until the desired limb length is achieved. The device is removed surgically after the bone has consolidated, and the child may need to use crutches or have a cast for 4 to 6 weeks after removal to reduce the risk of fracture.

AMPUTATION

A child may be born with the congenital absence of an extremity, have a traumatic loss of an extremity, or need a surgical amputation for a pathologic condition such as **osteosarcoma** (see later in chapter). With today's surgical technology and the quick thinking of bystanders who save a traumatically amputated body part, some children have had fingers and arms sewn back on with variable degrees of functional use regained.

! NURSING ALERT

For an amputated limb or body part that may be reattached, do the following:

1. Rinse limb gently with normal saline.
2. Loosely wrap limb in sterile gauze.
3. Place wrapped limb in a watertight bag.
4. Cool (without freezing) bag in ice water (do not pack in ice because this may harm tissue).
5. Label with child's name, date, and time, and transport with the child to the hospital.

Surgical amputation or the surgical repair of a permanently severed limb focuses on constructing an adequately nourished residual limb. A smooth, healthy, padded stump, free of nerve endings, is important in prosthesis fitting and subsequent ambulation. In some situations in which there is no vascular or neurologic deficit, a cast is applied to the stump immediately after the procedure, and a pylon, metal extension, and artificial foot are attached so that the patient can walk on the temporary prosthesis within a few hours.

Nursing Care Management

Stump shaping is done postoperatively with special elastic bandaging using a figure-eight bandage, which applies pressure in a cone-shaped fashion. This technique decreases stump edema, controls hemorrhage, and aids in developing desired contours so that the child will bear weight on the posterior aspect of the skin flap rather than on the end of the stump. Stump elevation may be used during the first 24 hours, but after this time the extremity should not be left in this position because contractures in the proximal joint will develop and seriously hamper ambulation. Monitoring proper body alignment will further decrease the risk of flexion contractures.

For older children and adolescents, arm exercises, bed pushups, and prosthesis-training programs using parallel bars help build up the arm muscles necessary for walking with crutches. Full range-of-motion exercises of joints above the amputation must be performed several times daily using active and isotonic exercises. Young children are often spontaneously active and require little encouragement.

Depending on the child's age, children or their parents will need to learn hygiene, including carefully washing with soap and water every day and checking for skin irritation, breakdown, and infection. A tube of stockinette or powder is used to slide the prosthesis on more easily. Skin must be checked carefully every time the prosthesis is removed, and prosthesis tolerance time must be adjusted to prevent skin breakdown.

For children who have had an amputation, **phantom limb sensation** is an expected experience because the nerve-brain connections are still present. Gradually, these sensations fade, although in many people who have had amputations, they persist for years. Preoperative discussion of this phenomenon will aid a child in understanding these "unusual feelings" and not hiding the experiences from others. Limb pain, especially pain that increases with ambulation, should be evaluated for the possibility of a **neuroma** at the free nerve endings in the stump or other problems such as a poorly fitting prosthesis or joint instability.

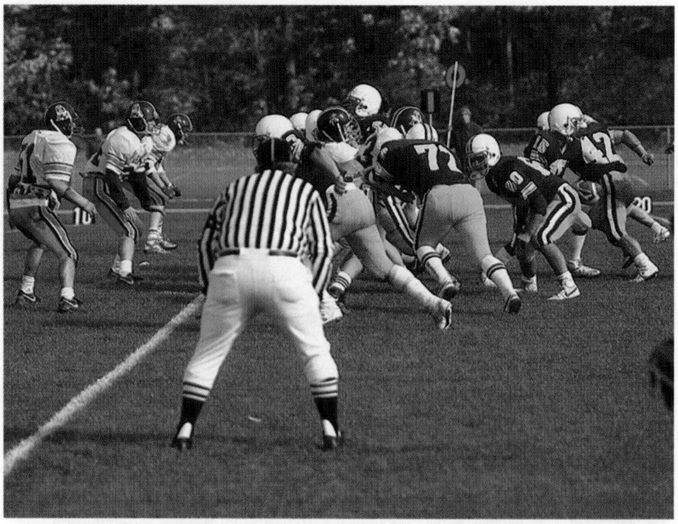

Fig. 29.13 A number of injuries may occur with sports participation.

SPORTS PARTICIPATION AND INJURY

Every sport has the potential for injury to participants—whether an adolescent engages in serious competition or participates for enjoyment. Serious injury occurs most often during rough contact sports or to persons who are not physically prepared for the activity. Injuries also occur when the children's or adolescents' bodies are not suited to the sport, when their muscles and body systems (respiratory and cardiovascular) are not conditioned to endure physical stress, or when they lack the insight and judgment to recognize that an activity exceeds their physical abilities. Rapidly growing bones, muscles, joints, and tendons are especially vulnerable to unusual strain. In general, more injuries occur during recreational sports participation than during organized athletic competition.

The environment and the sports or recreational equipment can also present risks (Fig. 29.13). Children and adolescents who participate in physical activity or sports do so in many different environments, including indoors and outdoors, on floors, on the ground and snow, on or beneath water surfaces, and sometimes in free air space. Most of these activities also involve equipment, which children and adolescents may not be physically mature enough to manage safely. A common example is skateboarding when the child or adolescent does not take safety precautions and perceives increased risk taking as a part of the sport.

Acute overload injuries are those that occur suddenly during an activity and produce immediate symptoms. A blow or overstretching, twisting, or sudden stress to tissues can cause these injuries. For descriptions and management of traumatic injuries, see earlier in the chapter.

OVERUSE SYNDROMES

To excel in sports, young athletes are forced to train longer, harder, and earlier in life than previously. The rewards are an increased level of fitness, better performance, faster times, and the satisfaction of attaining a personal goal. However, risks are associated when young people overtrain; these risks include recurrent upper respiratory infections, sleep and mood disturbances, loss of appetite, decreased interest in training and competition, and inability to concentrate (Winsley & Matos, 2011). Annually, 3.5 million children are injured participating in sports and athletic activities (Mickalide & Hansen, 2012). Growing numbers of young people participate in organized sports, resulting in an increase in overuse injuries. Nearly half of all injuries evaluated in pediatric sports medicine are overuse injuries (Biber & Gregory, 2010).

The risk of overuse injury is always present and can be related to several factors, including training errors, muscle or tendon imbalance, anatomic malalignment (e.g., femoral anteversion, excessive lumbar lordosis, tibial torsion), incorrect footwear or playing surface, an associated disease state, and growth (growth cartilage is less resistant to microtrauma). Chronic pain in athletes is often associated with overuse injury, which can occur at any level of athletic participation. The common feature in overuse injuries is the **repetitive microtrauma** that occurs to a particular anatomic structure. Performing the same movements repeatedly can cause several types of injury:

1. **Frictional,** or rubbing of one structure against another
2. **Tractional,** or repeated pull on a ligament or tendon
3. **Cyclic,** or repetitive loading of impact forces (stress fractures)

The end result is inflammation of the involved structure with complaints of pain, tenderness, swelling, and disability.

Stress Fractures

Stress fractures are a consequence of repetitive, excessive stress on the bone that causes microfractures within the bone. Continued stress to the bone can lead to spread of the microfracture and eventual macrofracture. The pathogenesis of stress injury to the bone is multifactorial and includes everything from the footwear to the fitness level of the athlete. Stress fractures occur most commonly in the lower extremities, particularly the tibia. High school athletes at high risk for stress fractures are those who participate in cross country running and gymnastics (Changstrom, Brou, Khodaee, et al., 2015).

The most common symptom of stress fracture is a sharp, persistent, progressive pain or a deep, persistent dull ache located over the bone. Sometimes there is pain on impact (heel strike), but the most important clinical sign is pain over the involved bony surface. Diagnosis is based on clinical observation and history. Plain radiographs are rarely diagnostic of stress fractures during the initial few weeks because callus formation is not yet evident. Magnetic resonance imaging (MRI) is used when other causes of pain must be ruled out.

Therapeutic Management

Development of inflammation is common to all overuse syndromes; therefore management involves rest or alteration of activities, physical therapy, and medication. Rest is the primary therapy, usually interpreted as reduced activity and the use of alternative exercise—not bed rest or immobilization with an orthosis. The main purpose is to alleviate the repetitive stress that initiated the symptoms. It is important to keep the adolescent mobile, and training can be continued. Alternative exercise that maintains conditioning without aggravating the injury is selected. For example, pool running (treading water in the deep end of a pool) can use the same movements as running but without the weight bearing; bicycling, swimming, and rowing are viable alternatives.

Other modalities include cryotherapy and cold whirlpool baths. Sometimes taping, bracing, splinting, and other orthoses are used, depending on the injury. **Nonsteroidal antiinflammatory drugs (NSAIDs)** are often prescribed to reduce inflammation and pain. Topical medications are of questionable value.

NURSE'S ROLE IN SPORTS FOR CHILDREN AND ADOLESCENTS

Nurses are often involved in sports activities in the areas of preparation and evaluation for activities, prevention of injury, treatment of injuries, and rehabilitation after injury. Selecting an appropriate sport for both recreation and competition is a joint effort of the adolescent, parents, and health professionals. The best approach to counseling children, adolescents, and parents regarding sports participation is to encourage activities that are most likely to provide pleasure and physical benefits throughout childhood and into adulthood. Exposure to a variety of activities is better for young children than limiting them to one sport. Parents should be cautioned against overcommitting children to sports activities so that they have time for other activities.

When children sustain athletic injuries, nurses are often responsible for instructions regarding care. Instructions (e.g., schedule for appointments, application of ice, any restrictions in activity) should be clear and accompanied by written directions. The importance of taking medications as prescribed is emphasized, especially if medications are needed for an extended period and if adherence is an issue. Antiinflammatory medications given an hour before practice or competition may help children continue their activities.

Prevention of sports injuries is the most important aspect of athletic programs. Children should be suited to the activity, and the environment and the equipment must be safe. Children should be prepared for the sport, especially if it requires strenuous or continuous physical exertion. Nurses, coaches, and athletic trainers must collaborate to ensure that safety measures are implemented. Stretching exercises, warm-up and cool-down activities, and appropriate training are requirements for safe participation. Protective measures such as pads, taping, and wrapping are also important to prevent injury. Finally, nurses must be aware of environmental safety risks (see Chapter 27, Head Injury).

BIRTH AND DEVELOPMENTAL DEFECTS

Some skeletal defects may be diagnosed at birth or within days, weeks, or months after birth. In other cases, the deviation may be difficult to detect without careful inspection. Therefore it is imperative that nurses become acquainted with signs of these defects and understand the principles of therapy in order to direct families in the care and management of these children.

DEVELOPMENTAL DYSPLASIA OF THE HIP

The broad term **developmental dysplasia of the hip (DDH)** describes a spectrum of disorders related to abnormal development of the hip that may occur at any time during fetal life, infancy, or childhood. A change in terminology from *congenital hip dysplasia* and *congenital dislocation of the hip* to DDH more properly reflects a variety of hip abnormalities in which there is a shallow acetabulum, subluxation, or dislocation.

The incidence of hip dysplasia varies depending on ethnicity or race but is approximately 1 to 2 infants per 1000 live births in the United States. Girls are affected more commonly than boys, and a positive family history increases a child's risk of having DDH. Approximately 7% to 40% of infants with DDH have a breech intrauterine position (Loder & Skopelja, 2011a).

Pathophysiology

The cause of DDH is unclear but is likely multifactorial. Certain factors such as gender, birth order, family history, intrauterine position, joint laxity, and postnatal positioning are believed to affect the risk of DDH.

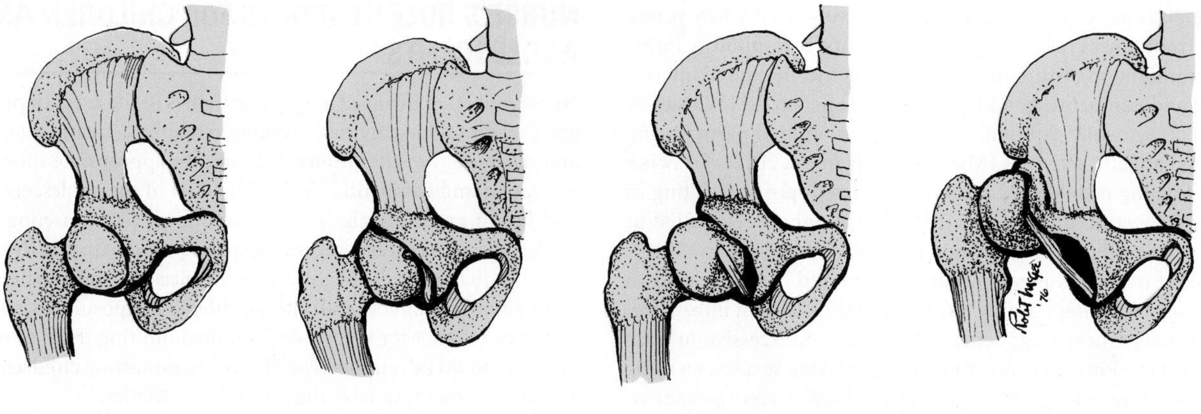

Fig. 29.14 Configuration and relationship of structures in developmental dysplasia of the hip (DDH).

Predisposing factors associated with DDH may be divided into three broad categories: (1) physiologic factors, which include maternal hormone secretion and intrauterine positioning; (2) mechanical factors, which involve breech presentation, multiple fetus, oligohydramnios, and large infant size as well as swaddling where the hips are maintained in adduction and extension, which in time may cause a dislocation; and (3) genetic factors, which entail a higher incidence of DDH in siblings of affected infants and an even greater incidence of recurrence if a sibling and one parent were affected.

Some experts categorize DDH into two major groups: (1) **idiopathic**, in which the infant is neurologically intact, and (2) **teratologic**, which involves a neuromuscular defect, such as arthrogryposis or myelodysplasia. The teratologic forms usually occur in utero and are much less common.

Three degrees of DDH are illustrated in Fig. 29.14.

1. **Acetabular dysplasia:** This is the mildest form of DDH, in which there is a delay in acetabular development evidenced by osseous hypoplasia of the acetabular roof that is oblique and shallow, although the cartilaginous roof is comparatively intact. The femoral head remains in the acetabulum.
2. **Subluxation:** The largest percentage of DDH, subluxation, implies incomplete dislocation of the hip. The femoral head remains in contact with the acetabulum, but a stretched capsule and ligamentum teres cause the head of the femur to be partially displaced. Pressure on the cartilaginous roof inhibits ossification and produces a flattening of the socket.
3. **Dislocation:** The femoral head loses contact with the acetabulum and is displaced posteriorly and superiorly over the fibrocartilaginous rim. The ligamentum teres is elongated and taut.

Factors related to infant handling are indicated in the Cultural Considerations box.

CULTURAL CONSIDERATIONS

Developmental Dysplasia of the Hip

A striking relationship exists between the development of hip dislocation and methods of swaddling the hips. Among the cultures with the highest incidence of dislocation (Navajo Indians and Canadian Natives), newly born infants are tightly wrapped with the hips adducted and extended in blankets or other swaddling material or are strapped to cradle boards. In cultures such as those in Central and South America, Asia, and Africa, where mothers traditionally carry infants on their backs with the infants' hips in the abducted and flexed position, hip dysplasia is much less common.

Recently, several prominent orthopedic specialty organizations recommended that infants' hips be placed in slight flexion and abduction during swaddling. It was further recommended that infants' knees be maintained in slight flexion and that forced or sustained passive hip extension in the first few months should be avoided (Price & Schwend, 2011). These recommendations were supported by evidence that demonstrated a significant relationship between tight swaddling and hip dysplasia, and are aimed at decreasing the incidence of hip dysplasia in infants.

Diagnostic Evaluation

DDH is often not detected at the initial examination after birth; thus all infants should be carefully monitored for hip dysplasia at follow-up visits throughout the first year of life at routine well-child checks. In the newborn period, hip dysplasia usually appears as hip joint laxity rather than as outright dislocation. Subluxation and the tendency to dislocate can be demonstrated by the Ortolani or Barlow maneuvers (Fig. 29.15D). The Ortolani and Barlow tests are most reliable from birth to 4 weeks of age. With the Barlow test, the thigh is adducted and light pressure is applied to see if the femoral head can be felt to slip posteriorly out of the acetabulum. The Ortolani test involves abducting the thighs and placing anterior pressure at the hip to see if the femoral head slips forward into the acetabulum. Other signs of DDH are shortening of the limb on the affected side (see Fig. 29.15C), asymmetric thigh and gluteal folds (see Fig. 29.15A), and decreased hip abduction on the affected side (see Fig. 29.15B). See Box 29.5.

! NURSING ALERT

These tests must be performed by an experienced clinician to prevent an injury to the infant's hip.

Radiographic examination in early infancy is not reliable because ossification of the femoral head does not normally take place until the fourth to sixth month of life. However, the cartilaginous head can be visualized directly by ultrasonography. Universal newborn screening with ultrasonography has been proposed; however, numerous studies reveal that this approach has a high rate of false-positive results and subsequent overtreatment. Therefore ultrasonography is recommended as an adjunct to the physical examination (Shaw & Segal, 2016).

In infants older than 6 months of age and in children, radiographic examination is useful in confirming the diagnosis. An upward slope in the roof of the acetabulum (acetabular angle) greater than 30 degrees with upward and outward displacement of the femoral head is seen in an infant with hip dysplasia, and the acetabular angle should continue to decrease with age.

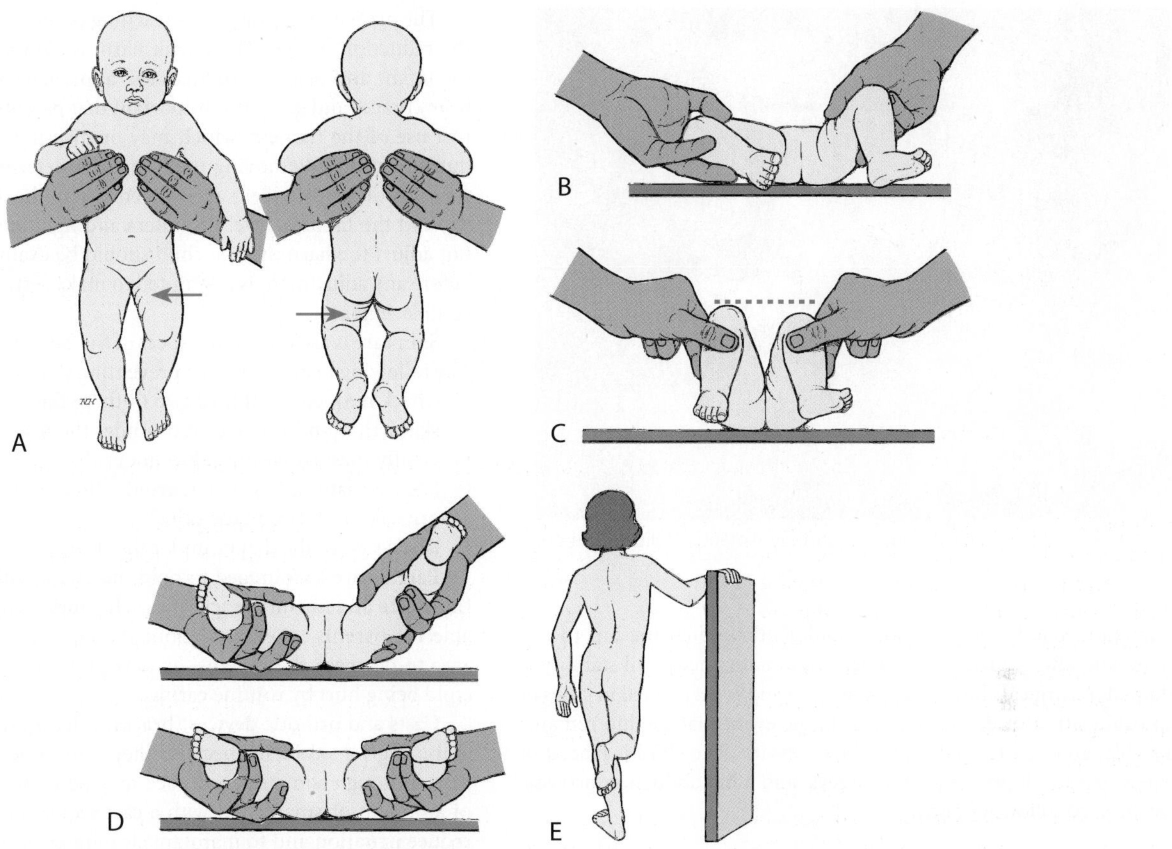

Fig. 29.15 Signs of developmental dysplasia of the hip (DDH). A, Asymmetry of gluteal and thigh folds. B, Limited hip abduction, as seen in flexion. C, Apparent shortening of the femur, as indicated by the level of the knees in flexion (Galeazzi sign). D, Ortolani maneuver with clunk elicited. E, Positive Trendelenburg sign (if child is weight bearing).

BOX 29.5 Clinical Manifestations of Developmental Dysplasia of the Hip

Infants

Shortening of limb on affected side (Galeazzi sign)
Restricted abduction of hip on affected side
Unequal gluteal folds (best visualized with infant prone)
Positive Ortolani test (hip is reduced by abduction)
Positive Barlow test (hip is dislocated by adduction)

Older Infants and Children

Affected leg appears shorter than the other
Telescoping or piston mobility of joint: Head of femur felt to move up and down in buttock when extended thigh is pushed first toward child's head and then pulled distally
Trendelenburg sign: When child stands first on one foot and then on the other (holding onto a chair, rail, or someone's hands) bearing weight on affected hip, pelvis tilts downward on normal side instead of upward, as it would with normal stability
Greater trochanter prominent and appearing above a line from anterosuperior iliac spine to tuberosity of ischium
Marked lordosis and waddling gait (bilateral hip dislocation)

Therapeutic Management

Treatment is begun as soon as the condition is recognized because early intervention is more favorable to the restoration of normal bony architecture and function. The longer treatment is delayed, the more severe the deformity, the more difficult the treatment, and the less favorable the prognosis. The treatment varies with the child's age and the extent of the dysplasia. The goal of treatment is to obtain and maintain a safe, congruent position of the hip joint to promote normal hip joint development.

Newborns to Age 6 Months

The hip joint is maintained, by dynamic splinting, in a safe position with the proximal femur centered in the acetabulum in a degree of flexion. Of the numerous devices available, the **Pavlik harness** is the most widely used, and with time, motion, and gravity, the hip works into a more abducted, reduced position (Fig. 29.16). The harness is worn continuously, 22 to 24 hours per day depending on the severity of dysplasia, until the hip is proved stable on both clinical and ultrasound examination, usually within 6 to 12 weeks.

When there is difficulty in maintaining stable reduction of the femoral head, a surgical closed reduction of the hip and application of a hip spica cast is performed. The cast is changed periodically to accommodate the child's growth. Once sufficient stability is acquired, after approximately 3 months, the child is transitioned to a removable hip abduction orthosis. The duration of treatment in the orthosis depends on development of the acetabulum.

Ages 6 to 24 Months

In this age-group, the dislocation is often not recognized until the child begins to stand and walk, when shortening of the limb and contractures of hip adductor and flexor muscles become apparent. In less severe DDH or acetabular dysplasia, use of a hip abduction orthosis may be initiated. Duration of treatment depends on development of the acetabulum. When adduction contracture is present, devices such

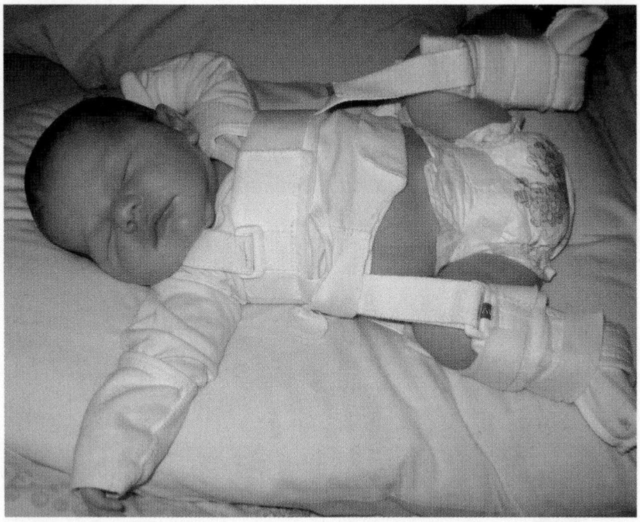

Fig. 29.16 Child in Pavlik harness. (Courtesy Amanda Politte, St. Louis, MO.)

as traction may be used to slowly and gently stretch the hip to full abduction, after which wide abduction is maintained until stability is attained. A surgical closed reduction of the hip is performed in cases of hip subluxation or dislocation, and in the event that the hip remains unstable, an open reduction may be necessary. The child is placed in a spica cast for approximately 12 weeks, and a hip abduction orthosis may be used following casting.

Older Children

Correction of the hip deformity in older children is inherently more difficult than in the preceding age-groups because secondary adaptive changes and other etiologic factors (such as juvenile arthritis and cerebral palsy) complicate the condition. Operative reduction, which may involve preoperative traction, lengthening of contracted muscles, and pelvic osteotomy procedures designed to construct an acetabular roof, often combined with proximal femoral osteotomy, are usually required. After cast removal, range-of-motion exercises help restore movement. Other rehabilitation measures may include muscle strengthening, a period of crutch or walker use, and gait training.

Nursing Care Management

Nurses are in a unique position to detect DDH in early infancy. During the infant assessment process and routine nursing activities, the hips and extremities are inspected for any deviations from normal. Any observations or concerns are reported to the attending provider. An ambulatory child who displays a limp or an unusual gait should be referred for evaluation. This may indicate an orthopedic or neurologic problem. Nonambulatory children with cerebral palsy should also be assessed for evidence of hip problems throughout their growing years.

The major nursing problems in the care of an infant or child in a cast or other device are related to maintenance of the device and adaptation of nurturing activities to meet the patient's needs. Generally, treatment and follow-up care of these children are carried out in an outpatient setting.

! NURSING ALERT

The former practice of double or triple diapering for developmental dysplasia of the hip (DDH) is not recommended because there is no evidence to support its efficacy.

The primary nursing goal is teaching parents to apply and maintain the reduction device. The Pavlik harness allows for easy handling of the infant and usually produces less apprehension in the parent than heavy braces and casts. It is important that parents understand the correct use of the harness, which may or may not allow for its removal during bathing. Removing the harness is determined individually on the basis of the provider's recommendation, the degree of hip instability, and the family's level of understanding. Parents are instructed to not adjust the harness. The child should be examined by the provider before any adjustment is attempted to make certain the hips are in correct placement.

Skin care is an important aspect of the care of an infant in a harness. The following instructions for preventing skin breakdown are stressed:

- Check frequently (at least two or three times a day) for red areas or skin irritation in skin folds or under the straps.
- Gently massage healthy skin under the straps once a day to stimulate circulation. In general, avoid lotions and powders because they can cake and irritate the skin.
- Always place the diaper under the straps.

Parents are encouraged to hold the infant with a harness and continue care and nurturing activities. The nurse can assist by being available for parents' questions about the necessary adaptations to daily care to decrease the parents' anxiety and possible feelings about the child being hurt by routine caring.

Casts and orthotic devices (braces) offer more challenging nursing and caregiver problems because they cannot be removed for routine care, although sometimes a brace may be removed for bathing. Care of an infant or small child with a cast requires nursing innovation to reduce irritation and to maintain cleanliness of both the child and the cast, particularly in the diaper area (see earlier in the chapter for care of the child in a cast).

It is important for nurses, parents, and other caregivers to understand that children in corrective devices need to be involved in all typical age-appropriate activities. Confinement in a cast or appliance should not exclude children from family (or unit) activities. They can be held astride the lap for comfort and transported to areas of activity. An adapted wheelchair, stroller, or wagon can offer mobility to an older infant or child.

CLUBFOOT

Clubfoot or talipes equinovarus (TEV) is a complex deformity of the ankle and foot that includes forefoot adduction, midfoot supination, hindfoot varus, and ankle equinus. The foot is pointed downward (plantarflexed) and inward in varying degrees of severity (Fig. 29.17). Clubfoot may occur as an isolated deformity or in association with other disorders or syndromes, such as chromosomal abnormalities, arthrogryposis, or spina bifida.

The incidence of clubfoot in the general population is approximately 1 per 1000 live births, with boys affected twice as often as girls. Bilateral clubfeet occur in 50% of the cases (Winell & Davidson, 2020). The precise cause of clubfoot is unknown. However, there is a strong familial tendency, with a 1 in 10 chance that a parent with clubfoot will have an affected offspring. Other possible theories as to the cause of clubfoot include arrested or abnormal fetal development or abnormal positioning and restricted movement in utero, although the evidence is not conclusive. Whereas arrested development during this early stage tends to result in a rigid deformity, mechanical pressures from intrauterine positioning are likely causes of more flexible deformities (Shyy, Wang, Sheffield, et al., 2010).

Clubfoot may be further divided into three categories: (1) positional clubfoot (also called *transitional, mild,* or *postural clubfoot*), which is

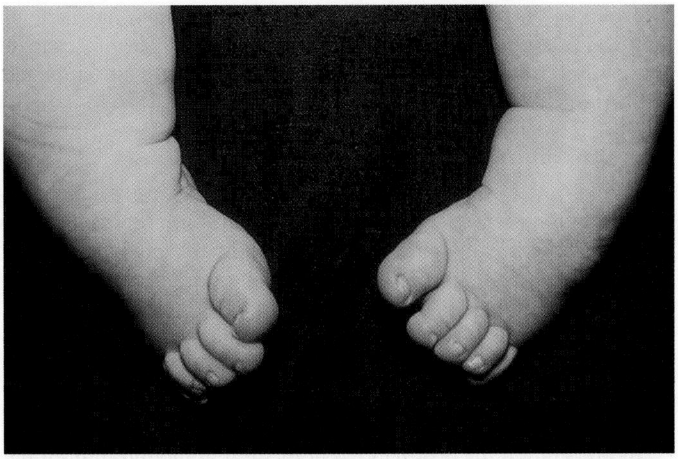

Fig. 29.17 Bilateral congenital talipes equinovarus (TEV; clubfoot) in a 2-month-old infant. (From Zitelli, B. J., McIntire, S. C., & Nowalk, A. J. [2012]. *Zitelli and Davis' atlas of pediatric physical diagnosis* [6th ed]. St. Louis, MO: Saunders/Elsevier.)

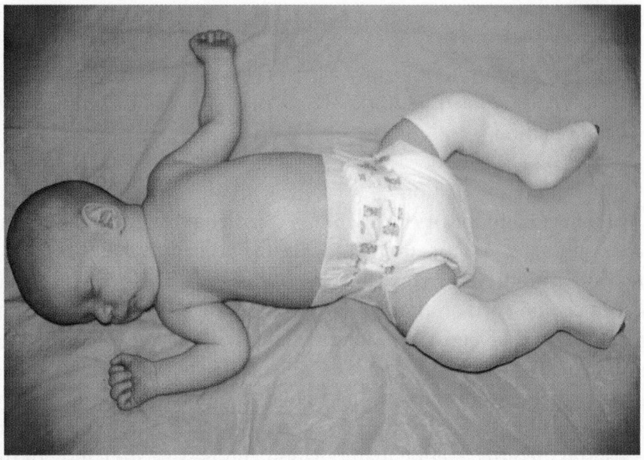

Fig. 29.18 Feet casted for correction of bilateral talipes equinovarus (TEV).

believed to occur primarily from intrauterine crowding and responds to simple stretching and casting; (2) congenital clubfoot, also referred to as *idiopathic*, which may occur in an otherwise normal child and has a wide range of rigidity and prognosis; and (3) syndromic (or teratologic) clubfoot, which is associated with other congenital anomalies (such as myelomeningocele or arthrogryposis) and is a more severe form of clubfoot that is often resistant to typical treatment.

Classification

The positional clubfoot may correct spontaneously or may require passive exercise or serial casting. There is no bony abnormality, but there may be tightness and shortening of the soft tissues medially and posteriorly. The teratologic clubfoot usually requires surgical correction and has a high incidence of recurrence. The congenital idiopathic clubfoot, or "true clubfoot," almost always requires casting coupled with surgical intervention, usually a heel-cord tenotomy.

Diagnostic Evaluation

The deformity is readily apparent at birth if it has not been detected prenatally through ultrasonography. However, it must be differentiated from some positional deformities that can be passively corrected. Once it is detected, a careful yet comprehensive physical assessment of the affected foot (or feet) should be completed to allow for appropriate decision making regarding treatment plans and prognosis. The affected foot (or feet) is usually smaller and shorter with an empty heel pad and midfoot medial crease. When the deformity is unilateral, the affected limb may be shorter and calf atrophy is present. Radiographs of the feet are generally not necessary. A thorough hip examination should be performed for all infants with clubfoot; an increased risk of hip dysplasia is associated with clubfoot deformities.

Therapeutic Management

The goal of treatment for clubfoot is to achieve a painless, plantigrade, and functional foot. Treatment of clubfoot involves three stages: (1) correction of the deformity, (2) maintenance of the correction until normal muscle balance is regained, and (3) follow-up observation to avert possible recurrence of the deformity. Some feet respond to treatment readily; some respond only to prolonged, vigorous, and sustained efforts; and the improvement in others remains disappointing even with maximal effort.

Recommended treatment of clubfoot is with the use of the Ponseti method. Serial casting is begun shortly after birth. Weekly gentle manipulation and stretching of the foot along with placement of serial long leg casts allow for gradual improvement in the alignment of the foot (Fig. 29.18). The extremity or extremities are casted until maximum correction is achieved, usually within 6 to 10 weeks. The majority of the time, a percutaneous heel-cord tenotomy is performed at the end of casting to correct the equinus deformity. After the tenotomy, a long leg cast is applied and left in place for 3 weeks. After casting is completed, children are transitioned to using Ponseti sandals with a bar set in abduction to help maintain the correction and prevent a recurrence of the foot deformity. Inability to achieve normal foot alignment after casting and tenotomy indicates the need for surgical intervention (Ponseti, 1996).

Nursing Care Management

Nursing care of the child with clubfoot is the same as for any child who has a cast (see earlier in the chapter). Because the child will spend considerable time in a corrective device, nursing care plans include both long- and short-term goals. Careful observation of the skin and circulation is particularly important in young infants because of their rapid growth rate.

Because treatment and follow-up care are handled in the orthopedic clinic or outpatient department, parent education and support are important in nursing care of these children. It is important for parents to understand the diagnosis, the overall treatment program, the importance of regular cast changes, and the role they play in the long-term effectiveness of the therapy. Reinforcing and clarifying the orthopedic provider's explanations and instructions, teaching parents about care of the cast or bracing (including vigilant observation for potential problems), and encouraging parents to facilitate normal development within the limitations imposed by the treatment are all part of nursing responsibilities.

METATARSUS ADDUCTUS (VARUS)

Metatarsus adductus, or metatarsus varus, is probably the most common congenital foot deformity. In most instances, it is a result of abnormal intrauterine positioning, particularly in a firstborn child, and is usually detected at birth. The deformity is characterized by medial adduction of the toes and forefoot, frequently in association with inversion and convexity of the lateral border of the foot (kidney shaped). Metatarsus adductus may be divided into three categories:

- Type I: The forefoot is flexible and corrects easily with manipulation
- Type II: The forefoot is only partial flexible and corrects passively past neutral position but only to neutral position with active manipulation
- Type III: The forefoot is rigid and will not stretch to neutral position with manipulation

Unlike a clubfoot, with which it is often confused, the angulation occurs at the tarsometatarsal joint while the heel and ankle remain in a neutral position. Ankle range of motion is normal. This deformity may cause a pigeon-toed or intoeing gait in the child. A thorough hip examination should be performed for all infants with metatarsus adductus, as an increased risk of hip dysplasia is associated with foot deformities.

Management depends on the rigidity and type of the deformity. Most cases of metatarsus adductus are types I and II and generally correct spontaneously. Gentle manipulation and passive stretching of the foot, which the parent is taught to perform, can be added and may help in this correcting more quickly. With type III, the child usually requires serial manipulation and casting to correct the deformity, after which a corrective shoe or orthosis may be used. Surgical correction is rarely required for the condition but may be performed in children older than 4 to 6 years of age who have considerable pain on ambulation or functional difficulties as a result of the deformity (Winell & Davidson, 2020).

Nursing Care Management

The nursing role primarily involves identifying the defect so that early therapy and instruction of the parents can be initiated. The nurse teaches the parents how to hold the heel firmly and to stretch only the forefoot; otherwise, undue force on the heel may produce a valgus deformity. If casting or an orthosis is required, the nurse instructs the parents in cast care and use of the brace.

SKELETAL LIMB DEFICIENCY

Congenital limb deficiencies, or reduction malformations, are manifested by a variety of degrees of loss of functional capacity. They are characterized by underdevelopment of skeletal elements of the extremities. The range of malformation can extend from minor defects of the digits to serious abnormalities, such as **amelia**, absence of an entire extremity, or **meromelia**, partial absence of an extremity, which includes **phocomelia** (seal limbs), an interposed deficiency of long bones with relatively good development of hands and feet attached at or near the shoulder or the hips. Most reduction defects are primary defects of development of the limb, but prenatal destruction of the limb can occur, such as full or partial amputation of a limb in utero from constriction of an amniotic band (**amniotic band syndrome**). Neonates with congenital limb deficiencies often have associated malformations and should be thoroughly assessed for cardiovascular, central nervous system (CNS), renal, and digestive abnormalities (Stoll, Alembik, Dott, et al., 2010).

Pathophysiology

Limb deficiencies can be attributed to both heredity and environment and can originate at any stage of limb development. Formation of limbs may be suppressed at the time of limb bud formation, or there may be interference in later stages of differentiation and growth. Heredity appears to play a prominent role, and prenatal environmental insults have been implicated in a number of cases, such as the well-publicized **thalidomide** tragedy of the 1950s and early 1960s, which demonstrated a clear relationship between the time of exposure of the pregnant woman to the antiemetic drug and the presence and type of limb deformity in the newborn. There are still drugs that may have similar **teratogenic** effects in the first trimester of pregnancy. Therefore medication administration during this period should be carefully evaluated by the provider.

Therapeutic Management

The child with a limb deficiency should be fitted with prosthetic devices, and the devices should be applied at the earliest possible stage of development in an attempt to match the infant's motor readiness. This favors natural progression of prosthetic use. For example, an infant with an upper extremity deficiency is fitted with a simple passive device between 3 to 6 months old to encourage limb exploration, sitting (with the extremities needed for support), and bilateral hand activities. Lower limb prostheses are applied when the infant is ready to pull to a standing position.

In preparation for prosthetic devices, surgical modification of the residual limb may be necessary to ensure the most effective use of the device or prosthetic. Phocomelic digits are preserved for controlling switches of externally powered appliances in the upper extremities. Digits (in both the upper and the lower extremities) provide the child with surfaces for tactile exploration and stimulation. Prostheses are replaced to accommodate the child's growth and increasing capabilities.

Nursing Care Management

Prosthetic application, training, and use are most successfully carried out in a center that specializes in meeting the special needs of these children, especially very young children and those with multiple amputations or missing limbs. Management involves a **prosthetist**, who specializes in the development, fitting, and maintenance of prosthetic limbs, and other health care providers, such as physical and occupational therapists. Parents need support and are encouraged to assist the child in making age-appropriate adjustments to the environment. Although these children need assistance, overprotection may produce overdependence, with later maladjustment to school and other situations.

OSTEOGENESIS IMPERFECTA

Osteogenesis imperfecta (OI) is a rare genetic disorder characterized by bones that fracture easily. Although inheritance follows an autosomal dominant pattern in most cases, rare autosomal recessive inheritance exists. Most types of OI have defects in the *COL1A1* or *COL1A2* genes, which code for polypeptide chains in type 1 procollagen, a precursor of type 1 collagen, which is a major structural component of bone. The error results in faulty bone mineralization, abnormal bone architecture, and increased susceptibility to fracture. There are at least 12 described types of OI, which accounts for significant disease variability. Clinical features may include varying degrees of bone fragility and deformity, short stature, blue sclerae, hearing loss, and dentinogenesis imperfecta (hypoplastic discolored teeth) (Marini & Blissett, 2013).

Classification is based on clinical features and patterns of inheritance (Box 29.6). Clinically, type I is the most common and mildest form, with most fractures occurring before puberty. Stature is near normal and bone deformity is minimal or absent. Type II is the most severe and is considered lethal in infancy. Type III OI is characterized by multiple fractures often present at birth, short stature, severe bone deformity, and disability with a shortened life expectancy. Type IV is similar to type I although slightly more severe, with short stature and mild to moderate bone deformities. Types V and VI do not have a type 1 collagen defect and are clinically similar to type IV. Both types demonstrate a unique pattern to their bone. Individuals affected have hypertrophic callus formation at fracture sites, a radiodense metaphyseal band, and calcification of the interosseous membrane of the forearm. In type VI, bone has

BOX 29.6 Classification of Osteogenesis Imperfecta[a]

Type I[a,b]
- **A:** Mild bone fragility; blue sclerae; normal teeth; hearing loss (occurs between 20 and 30 years old); autosomal dominant inheritance
- **B:** Same as A except dentinogenesis imperfecta instead of normal teeth
- **C:** Same as B but no bone fragility

Type II: Lethal; stillborn or die in early infancy; severe bone fragility, multiple fractures at birth; 10% of cases of OI; autosomal recessive inheritance

Type III: Severe bone fragility leading to severe progressive deformities; normal sclerae; marked growth failure; most autosomal recessive inheritance; few autosomal dominant inheritance

Type IV
- **A:** Mild to moderate bone fragility; normal sclerae; normal teeth; short stature; variable deformity; autosomal dominant inheritance
- **B:** Same as A except dentinogenesis imperfecta instead of normal teeth; approximately 6% of cases of OI

Type V: Clinically similar to type IV; hyperplastic callus; collagen mutation negative

Type VI: Sclerae and dentition normal; moderate to severe bone fragility; diagnosis by bone biopsy because of similarities to other types

Types VII and VIII (recessive form): Clinically overlap types II and III but have white sclerae, rhizomelia, and small to normal head circumference; severe osteochondroplastica and short stature in survivors. Type VII is associated with *CRTAP* gene, and type VIII is associated with the *LEPRE1* genetic mutation.

[a]Two-thirds of cases are type I.
[b]This classification is based on that proposed by Sillence, D. O., Senn, A., & Danks, D. M. (1979). Genetic heterogeneity in osteogenesis imperfecta. *Journal of Medical Genetics, 16*(2), 101–116, which originally included OI types I to IV. Additional types have been described but are not included herein.
OI, Osteogenesis imperfecta.

a characteristic mineralization defect or microscopic "fish scale" appearance with elevated alkaline phosphatase activity. Types VII through XII are rare, recessive forms of OI with different genetic defects being found. Clinical severity is variable and overlaps types II and III in relation to clinical features. Those who survive have white sclerae, short stature, and rhizomelia (Marini & Blissett, 2013).

Therapeutic Management

The treatment for OI has historically been primarily supportive, although patients and families are optimistic about new research advances. The use of bisphosphonate therapy with IV pamidronate to promote increased bone density and prevent fractures has become standard therapy for many children with OI. However, bisphosphonate therapy is reportedly more beneficial for increasing vertebral bone density and less effective for long bones (Marini, 2020).

The goals of a rehabilitative approach to management are directed toward preventing (1) positional contractures and deformities, (2) muscle weakness and osteoporosis, and (3) malalignment of lower extremity joints prohibiting weight bearing. Lightweight braces and splints help support limbs, prevent fractures, and aid in ambulation. Physical therapy helps prevent disuse osteoporosis and strengthens muscles, which in turn improves bone density. Surgery is sometimes used to help treat the manifestations of the disease. Surgical techniques are used to prevent or correct deformities that interfere with bracing, standing, or walking. The placement of intramedullary rods into the long bones can provide stability to bone, as well as prevent or correct deformities.

Nursing Care Management

Infants and children with this disorder require careful handling to prevent fractures. They must be supported when they are being turned, positioned, moved, and held. Even changing a diaper may cause a fracture in severely affected infants. These children should never be held by the ankles when being diapered but should be gently lifted by the buttocks or supported with pillows. However, nurses should not be afraid to touch or handle the infant or child with OI. Such children need compassionate handling and care as much as any other patient.

Both parents and the affected child need education on the child's limitations and guidelines in planning suitable activities that promote optimal development and protect the child from harm. Realistic occupational planning and genetic counseling are part of the long-term goals of care. Educational materials and information can be obtained from the Osteogenesis Imperfecta Foundation,[b] which also has a network that places families in contact with other families with a similar condition.

Children with current fractures or healing fractures should be screened for OI; the assumption that abuse or neglect is the cause of fractures in children must be carefully evaluated by a multidisciplinary team. A detailed history, no evidence of associated soft-tissue injury, and the presence of other symptoms related to OI help determine the diagnosis.

ACQUIRED DEFECTS

LEGG-CALVÉ-PERTHES DISEASE

Legg-Calvé-Perthes disease is a self-limiting disorder in which there is avascular necrosis of the femoral head. The disease affects children 2 to 12 years old, but most cases occur as an isolated event in boys between 4 and 8 years old, with a male-to-female ratio of 4:1. In approximately 10% of cases, the involvement is bilateral; most of the affected children have a skeletal age significantly below their chronologic age. Caucasian children are affected 10 times more frequently than African American children (Loder & Skopelja, 2011b).

Pathophysiology

The cause of the disease is unknown, but a temporary disturbance of circulation or vascular supply to the femoral capital epiphysis produces an ischemic avascular necrosis of the femoral head. During middle childhood, circulation to the femoral epiphysis is more tenuous than at other ages and can become obstructed by trauma, inflammation, coagulation defects, and a variety of other causes. The pathologic events seem to take place in four stages (Box 29.7). The entire disease process may encompass as little as 18 months or continue for several years. The reformed femoral head may be severely altered or minimally affected.

Clinical Manifestations and Diagnostic Evaluation

The onset of Legg-Calvé-Perthes disease is usually insidious, and the history may reveal only intermittent appearance of a limp on the affected side or a symptom complex, including hip soreness, ache, or stiffness, which can be constant or intermittent. The parents may report seeing the child limping, and the limp becomes more pronounced with increased activity. The pain may be experienced in the hip, along the entire thigh, or in the vicinity of the knee joint. The pain and limp are usually most evident on arising and at the end of a long day of activities. The pain is usually accompanied by joint dysfunction and limited range of motion at the hip. There may be a vague history of trauma but not necessarily. The diagnosis is established by characteristic radiographic findings, including medial joint space widening,

[b]804 W. Diamond Ave., Suite 210, Gaithersburg, MD 20878; 844-889-7579; http://www.oif.org.

BOX 29.7 Radiographic Stages of Legg-Calvé-Perthes Disease

Stage I: Initial, or **avascular, stage:** Avascular necrosis or infarction of the proximal femoral epiphysis with degenerative changes producing flattening of the upper surface of the femoral head or a decrease in femoral head height
Stage II: Fragmentation, or **resorptive, stage:** Femoral head resorption and revascularization produces collapse of the femoral head and fragmentation that gives a mottled appearance on radiographs
Stage III: Reossification stage: New bone formation, which is represented on radiographs as calcification and ossification or increased density in the areas of radiolucency; this filling-in process appears to begin in the periphery of the femoral head and progress centrally
Stage IV: Healing, or **remodeling, stage:** Gradual reformation of the head of the femur without radiolucency; this occurs until skeletal maturity

flattening of the femoral head with irregular ossification, and possible subchondral fracture. A perfusion MRI of the hip may be obtained to assess the blood flow to the femoral head.

Therapeutic Management

Because deformity occurs early in the disease process, the aims of treatment are to restore and maintain adequate hip range of motion; prevent femoral head collapse, extrusion, or subluxation; and preserve as well-rounded a femoral head as possible at the time of healing. Treatment varies according to the child's age at the time of diagnosis and the appearance of the femoral head and position within the acetabulum. Activity causes microfractures of the soft ischemic epiphysis, which tend to induce synovitis, stiffness, and adductor contracture.

The initial therapy is rest or activity restrictions and limited weight bearing, which helps reduce inflammation and irritability of the hip. The use of NSAIDs can provide relief of pain or discomfort; physical therapy or range-of-motion exercises help restore hip motion. In rare cases, traction is applied to stretch tight adductor muscles and improve containment of the femoral head. Abduction braces or casting may also be used for containment of the femoral head. If nonsurgical or conservative management is unsuccessful, surgical reconstruction or containment procedures such as a pelvic or proximal femoral osteotomy may be necessary.

The disease is self-limiting, but the ultimate outcome of therapy depends on early and efficient treatment. Children 5 years old and younger, whose epiphyses are more cartilaginous, tend to have the best prognosis or outcome. Children older than 8 years of age have a significant risk for degenerative arthritis, especially if they have femoral head deformity at the time of diagnosis. The later the diagnosis is made, the more femoral damage will have occurred before treatment is implemented (Herring, 2011).

Nursing Care Management

Because these children are largely cared for on an outpatient basis, the major emphasis of nursing care is teaching the family the required care and management. The family needs to comprehend the diagnosis and understand the purpose and function of activity restrictions and limitations in achieving the desired outcome. The child and family may rely on the nurse to help them understand and adjust to therapeutic measures.

One of the most difficult aspects associated with the disorder is the need to cope with a normally active child who feels well but must remain relatively inactive. It is important to emphasize that children should continue to attend school and engage in activities that can be adapted to the prescribed regimen. Suitable activities must be devised to meet the needs of a child in the process of developing a sense of initiative or industry. Activities that fulfill creative urges are well received.

BOX 29.8 Clinical Manifestations of Slipped Capital Femoral Epiphysis

Very often obese (body mass index >95%)
Limp on affected side
Possible inability to bear weight because of severe pain
Pain in groin, thigh, or knee
- May be acute, chronic, or acute-on-chronic
- Continuous or intermittent

Affected leg is externally rotated
Loss of hip flexion, abduction, and internal rotation as severity increases
Affected leg may appear shorter

SLIPPED CAPITAL FEMORAL EPIPHYSIS

Slipped capital femoral epiphysis (SCFE) refers to the spontaneous displacement of the proximal femoral epiphysis in a posterior and inferior direction. It develops most frequently shortly before or during accelerated growth and the onset of puberty (children between 8 and 15 years old; median age of 12 years old for boys and 11 years old for girls) and is seen more often in boys and obese children. The incidence is 0.3 to 24 cases per 100,000 children. Bilateral involvement occurs in up to 50% of cases (Loder & Skopelja, 2011c).

Pathophysiology

In a hip with SCFE, the capital femoral epiphysis remains in the acetabulum, but the femoral neck slips, deforming the femoral head and stretching blood vessels to the epiphysis. Most cases of SCFE are idiopathic, although it can be associated with endocrine disorders, such as hypothyroidism, low growth hormone levels, pituitary tumors, and renal osteodystrophy. The cause of idiopathic SCFE is multifactorial and includes obesity, physeal architecture and orientation, and pubertal hormone changes that affect physeal strength. Although obesity stresses the physeal plate, SCFE can also occur in children who are not obese.

Diagnostic Evaluation

SCFE is suspected when an adolescent or preadolescent displays clinical signs of a limp or complains of hip, groin, thigh, or knee pain. See Box 29.8 for additional clinical manifestations. The diagnosis is confirmed by anteroposterior and frog-leg hip radiographs that reflect a change in position of the proximal femoral epiphysis. Radiographs show medial displacement of the epiphysis and uncovered upper portion of the femoral neck adjacent to the physis. There is a widened growth plate and irregular metaphysis.

Therapeutic Management

The treatment goals of SCFE are to prevent further slipping of the femoral epiphysis until physeal closure, avoid further complication such as avascular necrosis, and maintain adequate hip function (Peck & Herrara-Soto, 2014). If the diagnosis is suspected or has been established, the child should be non–weight bearing to prevent further slippage. Surgical intervention is necessary and most often occurs within 24 hours to avoid further slippage and potential complications such as avascular necrosis.

Currently, in situ pinning using a single screw or alternatively multiple screws through the femoral neck into the proximal femoral epiphysis is the treatment of choice. For moderate to severe SCFE, an experienced surgeon may choose to perform a surgical hip dislocation to improve the anatomy at the site of the deformity (Tibor & Sink, 2013). Postsurgical care includes non–weight bearing or limited weight bearing with use of crutches for ambulation for weeks to months. Children may be restricted from certain sports or activities until fusion or closure of the proximal femoral physis has occurred in order to prevent further slippage.

Nursing Care Management

Nursing care involves preparing the child and family for the surgical procedure and recovery. Postoperative care involves hemodynamic stabilization, pain management, and assessment for complications. The adolescent is taught the proper use of crutches and the importance of avoiding weight bearing on the affected hip. Self-care and performance of activities of daily living to capability are encouraged to promote confidence and decrease a sense of helplessness.

> **! NURSING ALERT**
>
> Children with hip issues, such as Legg-Calvé-Perthes or slipped capital femoral epiphysis (SCFE), often present with groin, thigh, or knee pain. This is often because of referred pain and is anatomically related to the obturator nerve. Any time a child presents with groin, thigh, or knee pain, a complete hip examination is paramount to rule out underlying hip pathology.

KYPHOSIS AND LORDOSIS

The spine, which consists of numerous segments, can acquire deformity curves of three types: kyphosis, lordosis, and scoliosis (Fig. 29.19). **Kyphosis** is the lateral convex angulation in the curvature of the thoracic spine (see Fig. 29.19B). If it is increased (>45 degrees), it may occur secondary to disease processes, such as tuberculosis (TB), chronic arthritis, osteodystrophy, or compression fractures of the thoracic spine. The most common form of hyperkyphosis is posture related. Children, especially during the time when skeletal growth outpaces growth of muscle, are prone to exaggeration of a normal kyphosis. This is particularly common in self-conscious adolescent girls who assume a round-shouldered slouching posture in an attempt to hide their developing breasts and increasing height. **Scheuermann kyphosis** is a thoracic curve greater than 45 degrees with wedging of more than 5 degrees of at least three adjacent vertebral bodies and vertebral irregularity.

Postural (flexible) hyperkyphosis is almost always accompanied by a compensatory postural lordosis, an abnormally exaggerated concave lumbar curvature. Treatment of kyphosis consists of exercises to strengthen shoulder and abdominal muscles and bracing for more marked deformity. With adolescents who are significantly self-conscious about their appearance, the best approach is to emphasize the cosmetic value of corrective therapy and to place the responsibility on the adolescent for carrying out an exercise program at home with regular visits to and assessments by a physical therapist. Treatment with a brace may be indicated until skeletal maturity, and surgical fusion may be considered for severe, painful, or progressive thoracic curves, such as Scheuermann kyphosis.

Lordosis is the lateral inward curve of the cervical or lumbar curvature (see Fig. 29.19C). Hyperlordosis may be a secondary complication of a disease process, a result of trauma, or idiopathic. Hyperlordosis is a normal observation in toddlers and, in older children, is often seen in association with flexion contractures of the hip, obesity, DDH, and SCFE. During the pubertal growth spurt, lordosis of varying degrees is observed in teenagers, especially girls. In obese children, the weight of the abdominal fat alters the center of gravity, causing a compensatory lordosis. Unlike kyphosis, severe lordosis is usually accompanied by pain.

Treatment involves management of the predisposing cause when possible, such as weight loss and correction of deformities. Postural exercises or support garments are helpful in relieving symptoms in some cases; however, these do not usually provide a permanent cure.

IDIOPATHIC SCOLIOSIS

Scoliosis is a complex spinal deformity in three planes, usually involving lateral curvature, spinal rotation causing rib asymmetry, and when in the thoracic spine, often thoracic hypokyphosis (see Fig. 29.19E to G). It is the most common spinal deformity and is classified according to age of onset: *congenital* occurs in fetal development; *infantile* occurs at birth up to 3 years old; *juvenile* occurs in children ages 3 to 10 years old; and *adolescent* occurs at 10 years old or older.

Scoliosis can be caused by a number of conditions and may occur alone or in association with other diseases, particularly neuromuscular conditions (neuromuscular scoliosis). In most cases, however, there is no apparent cause, hence the name *idiopathic scoliosis.* There appears to be a genetic component to the etiology of idiopathic scoliosis; however, the exact relationship has yet to be established. The following section is limited to a discussion of adolescent idiopathic scoliosis.

Clinical Manifestations

Idiopathic scoliosis is most commonly identified during the preadolescent growth spurt. Parents frequently bring a child for follow-up on an abnormal school scoliosis screening or because of ill-fitting clothes, such as poorly fitting jeans. School screening is controversial because there are no controlled studies to demonstrate improved outcomes and a reported number of false-positive results lead to referrals. A recent US Preventive Services Task Force found insufficient evidence to determine whether screening for scoliosis in adolescents was of benefit (US Preventive Services Task Force, 2018). Nevertheless, a number of specialty organizations, including the American Academy of Orthopaedic Surgeons, Scoliosis Research Society, Pediatric Orthopaedic Society of North America, and American Academy of Pediatrics, advocate for routine screening of scoliosis in adolescents (Hresko, Talwakar, & Schwend, 2015). According to a joint statement released by the organizations, a medical professional educated in the detection of spinal deformity should screen girls at 10 and 12 years old and boys once at either 13 or 14 years old (Hresko et al., 2015).

Diagnostic Evaluation

Observation is performed behind a standing child wearing only shorts or undergarments. The child with scoliosis may exhibit asymmetry of shoulder height, scapular or flank shape, and hip height or pelvic obliquity. When the child bends forward at the waist so that the trunk is parallel with the floor and the arms hang free (the Adams forward bend test), asymmetry of the ribs and flanks may be appreciated (see Fig. 29.19G). A scoliometer is used in the initial screening to measure truncal rotation. Often a primary curve and a compensatory curve will place the head in alignment with the gluteal cleft. However, with an uncompensated curve, the head and hips are not aligned (see Fig. 29.19E and F).

Definitive diagnosis is made by radiographs of the child in the standing position and use of the Cobb technique, a standard measurement of angle curvature. The Risser scale is used to evaluate skeletal maturity on the radiograph. This scale assists in making a determination of the likely progression of the spinal curvature based on growth potential. The sexual maturity rating is also used to evaluate the risk of curve progression in adolescents. Not all spinal curvatures are scoliosis. A curve of less than 10 degrees is considered a postural variation. Curves measured between 10 and 25 degrees are mild and, if nonprogressive, do not require treatment (Hresko, 2013).

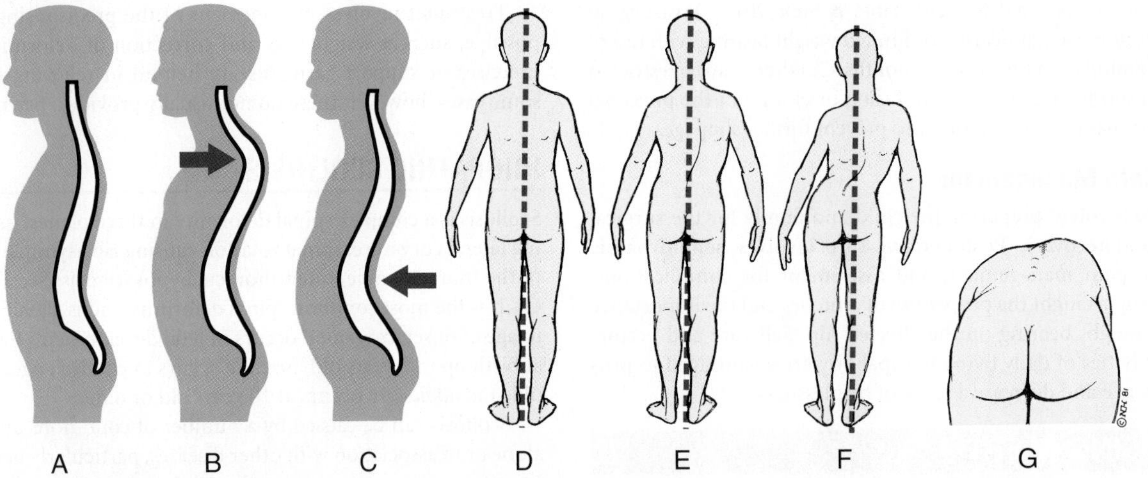

Fig. 29.19 Defects of spinal column. A, Normal spine. B, Kyphosis. C, Lordosis. D, Normal spine in balance. E, Mild scoliosis in balance. F, Severe scoliosis not in balance. G, Rib hump and flank asymmetry seen in flexion caused by rotary component. (Redrawn from Hilt, N. E., & Schmitt, E. W. [1975]. *Pediatric orthopedic nursing.* St. Louis, MO: Mosby.)

Intraspinal conditions or other disease processes that can cause scoliosis must be ruled out. The presence of pain, sacral dimpling or hairy patches, cutaneous vascular changes, absent or abnormal reflexes, bowel or bladder incontinence, or a left thoracic curve may indicate an intraspinal abnormality, such as syringomyelia, diastematomyelia, or tethered cord syndrome. An MRI scan of the spine is usually obtained for evaluation.

Therapeutic Management

Current management options include observation with regular clinical and radiographic evaluation, orthotic intervention (bracing), and surgical spinal fusion. Treatment decisions are based on the magnitude, location, and type of curve; the age and skeletal maturity of the child or adolescent; and any underlying or contributing disease process.

Bracing and Exercise

For moderate curves (25 to 45 degrees) in the growing child and adolescent, bracing may be the treatment of choice. Historically, bracing has not been shown to be curative; the goal is to slow the progression of the curvature to allow skeletal growth and maturity. The two most common types of bracing are the Boston and Wilmington braces, which are underarm orthoses customized from prefabricated plastic shells, with corrective forces using lateral pads and decreasing lumbar lordosis, and a thoracolumbosacral orthosis (TLSO), which is an underarm orthosis made of plastic that is custom molded to the body and then shaped to correct or hold the deformity (Fig. 29.20). The Milwaukee brace, which is an individually adapted brace that includes a neck ring, is rarely used in scoliosis but is sometimes used in the treatment of kyphosis. The Charleston nighttime bending brace is worn only when the child is in bed, as it prevents walking because of the severity of the trunk bend. Brace wear can be challenging due to the child's age and preoccupation with body image and appearance. Although bracing is not curative, using a rigid TLSO has been shown to be effective in reducing the likelihood of a curve progressing to a surgical magnitude while an individual finishes his or her growth. Bracing is discontinued once growth is complete and risk for further progression is negligible. One study found that of those with idiopathic progressive scoliosis, only 28% who used a TLSO progressed to needing surgery, whereas 52% who did not use a brace required surgery; in addition, the success rate of TLSO management increased with the more hours a brace was worn (Weinstein, Dolan, Wright, et al., 2013). There is very limited evidence regarding the effect of exercises and chiropractic treatment in the prevention of curve progression in scoliosis. Transcutaneous electrical nerve stimulation has proved to be an ineffective treatment. Exercises are of benefit when used in conjunction with bracing to maintain and increase the strength and range of motion of the spine.

Operative Management

Surgical intervention may be required for treatment of severe curves, which are typically greater than 45 to 50 degrees, as these curves generally continue to progress over time even after skeletal maturity is reached (Mistovich & Spiegel, 2020). The child's age, location of the curvature, and curve magnitude influence the decision for surgery. Any progressive or severe curve that does not respond to conservative orthotic measures (such as bracing) requires surgical correction. Bracing and exercise have been found to be ineffective in managing curves greater than 45 degrees. Neuromuscular, dysplastic, and congenital curves, which eventually progress, are best treated with surgical stabilization. Difficulties with balance or seating, respiratory compromise, or pain are also considered.

There are a number of surgical techniques for severe scoliosis. A spinal fusion consists of realignment and straightening of the spine with internal fixation and instrumentation combined with bony fusion (arthrodesis). Posterior and/or anterior surgical approaches may be implemented. The goals of surgical intervention are to improve the curvatures in the sagittal and coronal planes and to provide a solid, pain-free fusion in a well-balanced torso, with maximum mobility of the remaining spinal segments.

Advances in surgical technology currently being evaluated include thoracoscopic spinal fusion and placement of implants; metallic staples may also be placed into the vertebral bodies to achieve spinal fusion and to correct the deformity (Mistovich & Spiegel, 2020). The use of minimally invasive surgical techniques has gained acceptance for their small incisions, decreased blood loss, decreased recovery time, earlier mobilization, and decreased pain and need for pain medications (Sarwahi, Wollowick, Sugarman, et al., 2011).

Nursing Care Management

Treatment for scoliosis extends over a significant portion of the affected child's period of growth. In adolescents, this period is the one in which their identity, both physical and psychologic, is formed. The

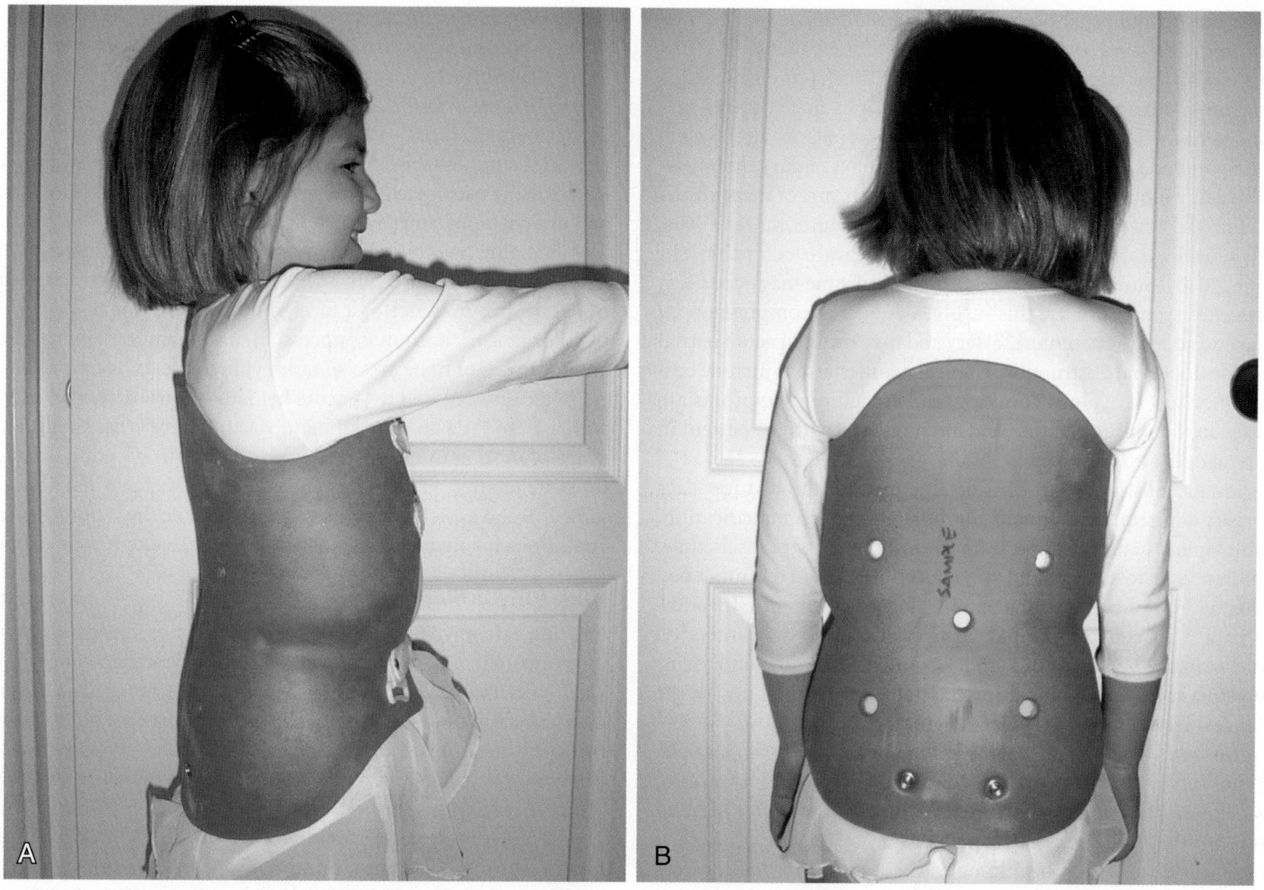

Fig. 29.20 A, Standard thoracolumbosacral orthotic (TLSO) brace for idiopathic scoliosis. The brace may be decorated to make it more acceptable to adolescents. B, Posterior view of the same brace.

identification of scoliosis as a "deformity," in combination with unattractive braces and a significant surgical procedure, can have a negative effect on the already fragile adolescent body image. The adolescent and family require excellent nursing care to meet not only physical needs but also psychologic needs associated with the diagnosis, surgery, postoperative recovery, and eventual rehabilitation.

Although adolescents with scoliosis are encouraged to participate in most peer activities, necessary therapeutic modifications are likely to make them feel different and isolated. Nursing care of the adolescent who is facing scoliosis surgery, potential social isolation, pain, and uncertainty, not to mention misunderstood emotions and body image issues, must be evaluated from the adolescent's perspective to be successful in meeting the individual's needs.

When a child or adolescent first faces the prospect of a prolonged period in a brace or other device, the therapy program and the nature of the device must be explained thoroughly to both the child and the parents so that they will understand the anticipated results, how the appliance corrects the defect, the freedoms and constraints imposed by the device, and what they can do to help achieve the desired goal. Management involves the skills and services of a team of specialists, including the orthopedist, physical therapist, orthotist (a specialist in fitting orthopedic braces), nurse, social worker, and sometimes a thoracic or pulmonary specialist.

Preoperative Care

The preoperative workup usually involves a radiographic series, including bending or traction spine films, pulmonary function studies, and serologic laboratory studies (including prothrombin, partial thromboplastin, and platelet function test; blood count; electrolyte levels; urinalysis and urine culture; and blood levels of any medications). Spinal surgery typically results in considerable blood loss, so several options are considered preoperatively to maintain or replace blood volume. These options include autologous blood donations obtained from the patient before the surgery; intraoperative blood salvage; intraoperative hemodilution; erythropoietin administration; and controlled induced hypotension, which must be carefully monitored at all times to prevent physiologic instability.

Surgery for spinal fusion is complex, and often adolescents who require the procedure due to idiopathic scoliosis are not familiar with medical terms or procedures. Preoperative teaching is critical for the adolescent to be able to cooperate and participate in his or her treatment and recovery. Because the surgery is extensive, the patient is taught how to manage his or her own patient-controlled analgesia (PCA) pump; how to log roll; and the use and function of other equipment, such as a chest tube (for anterior repair) and Foley urinary catheter. It is recommended that the child or adolescent bring a favorite toy (age dependent) or personal items such as a favorite stuffed animal, laptop computer, cell phone, MP3 player, or movie player for postoperative use. Meeting with a peer who has undergone a similar surgery may also be valuable.

Postoperative Care

Following surgery, patients are monitored in an acute care setting and log rolled when changing position to prevent damage to the fusion and instrumentation. In some cases, an immobilization brace or cast is used postoperatively depending on the type of surgical intervention and underlying diagnosis. Skin care is important, and pressure-relieving mattresses or beds may be needed to prevent pressure wounds (see Chapter 20, Maintaining Healthy Skin).

In addition to the usual postoperative assessments of wound, circulation, and vital signs, the neurologic status of the patient's extremities requires special attention. Prompt recognition of any neurologic impairment is imperative because delayed paralysis that requires surgical intervention may develop. Postoperative problems after spinal fusion may include neurologic injury or spinal cord injury, hypotension from acute blood loss, wound infection, syndrome of inappropriate antidiuretic hormone secretion, atelectasis, pneumothorax, ileus, delayed neurologic injury, and implanted hardware complications (Freeman, 2013). Superior mesenteric artery syndrome may occur several days after spinal surgery; this involves duodenal compression by the aorta and superior mesenteric artery and may result in acute partial or complete duodenal obstruction. Clinical manifestations include epigastric pain, nausea, copious vomiting, and eructation; symptoms are aggravated in the supine position and often relieved with the patient in a left lateral decubitus or prone position.

The adolescent usually has considerable pain for the first few days after surgery and requires frequent administration of pain medication, preferably opioids administered intravenously on a regular schedule. For children able to understand the concept, PCA is recommended (see Chapter 5, Pain Assessment and Pain Management). In addition to pain management, the patient is evaluated for skin integrity, adequate urinary output, fluid and electrolyte balance, and ileus. Discharge planning should include a timetable for follow-up with the provider and resumption of regular activities.

In most cases, the patient begins ambulation as soon as possible. Depending on the instrumentation used and the surgical approach, most patients are walking by the second or third postoperative day and discharged within 5 to 7 days. The patient may start physical therapy as soon as he or she is able, beginning with range-of-motion exercises on the first postoperative day and many of the activities of daily living in the following days. Self-care, such as washing and eating, is always encouraged. Throughout the hospitalization, age-appropriate activities and contact with family and friends are important parts of nursing care and planning (see Immobilization earlier in the chapter). The family is encouraged to become involved in the patient's care to facilitate the transition from hospital to home management. An organization that provides education and services to both families and professionals is the National Scoliosis Foundation.[c]

INFECTIONS OF BONES AND JOINTS

OSTEOMYELITIS

Osteomyelitis, an infectious process in the bone, can occur at any age but most frequently is seen in children 10 years old or younger. Boys are more commonly affected than girls, and the median age of diagnosis is 5 to 6 years old. The limbs most commonly affected include the foot, femur, tibia, and pelvis. *Staphylococcus aureus* is the most common causative organism. Neonates are also likely to have osteomyelitis caused by group B streptococci. Children with sickle cell disease may develop osteomyelitis from *Salmonella* organisms as well as *S. aureus*. *Neisseria gonorrhoeae* is a potential causative organism in sexually active adolescents. *Kingella kingae* has been reported as one of the most causative organisms in children younger than 5 years old (Robinette & Shah, 2020a).

Acute hematogenous osteomyelitis results when a bloodborne bacterium causes an infection in the bone. Common foci include infected lesions, upper respiratory tract infections, otitis media, tonsillitis, abscessed teeth, pyelonephritis, and infected burns. **Exogenous osteomyelitis** is acquired from direct inoculation of the bone from a puncture wound, open fracture, surgical contamination, or adjacent tissue infection. **Subacute osteomyelitis** has a longer course and may be caused by less virulent microbes with a walled-off abscess or **Brodie abscess**, typically in the proximal or distal tibia. **Chronic osteomyelitis** is a progression of acute osteomyelitis and is characterized by dead bone, bone loss, and drainage and sinus tracts.

Generally, healthy bone is not likely to become infected. Factors that contribute to infection include inoculation with a large number of organisms, presence of a foreign body, bone injury, high virulence of an organism, immunosuppression, and malnutrition; certain types and locations of bone are also more vulnerable to infection.

Typically, children with acute hematogenous osteomyelitis are seen with a 2- to 7-day history of pain, warmth, tenderness, and decreased range of motion in the affected limb along with systemic symptoms of fever, irritability, and lethargy (Box 29.9). Infants may have an adjacent joint effusion as well. Symptoms often resemble those observed in other conditions involving bones, such as arthritis, leukemia, or sarcoma.

Pathophysiology

In acute osteomyelitis, bacteria adhere to bone, causing a suppurative infection with inflammatory cells, edema, vascular congestion, and small-vessel thrombosis; the result is bone destruction, abscess formation, and dead bone (sequestra). Infection within the bone can rupture through the cortex into the subperiosteal space, stripping loose periosteum and forming an abscess. As dead bone is resorbed, new bone is formed along the live bone and infection borders. This surrounding sheath of live bone is called an **involucrum**. Sinus tracts from perforations in the involucrum may drain pus through soft tissue to the skin.

The pathology of osteomyelitis is different in infants, children older than 1 year old, and adults. In infants, blood vessels cross the growth plate into the epiphysis and joint space, which allows infection to spread into the joint. In children, the infection is contained by the growth plate, and joint infection is less likely (unless the infection is intracapsular). In older adolescents (with a closed growth plate), the

BOX 29.9 Causative Microorganisms of Osteomyelitis According to Age

Newborns
Staphylococcus aureus
Group B streptococcus
Gram-negative enteric rods

Infants
S. aureus (methicillin-sensitive *S. aureus*, methicillin-resistant *S. aureus* [MRSA])
Haemophilus influenzae

Older Children
S. aureus
Pseudomonas organisms
Salmonella organisms
Neisseria gonorrhoeae

Adolescents and Adults
Pseudomonas organisms
Mycobacterium tuberculosis

From McCance, K. L., & Huether, S. E. (2010). *Pathophysiology: The biological basis for disease in adults and children* (6th ed.). St. Louis, MO: Mosby/Elsevier.

[c] 5 Cabot Place, Stoughton, MA 02072; 800-673-6922; http://www.scoliosis.org.

infection is poorly contained and the joint is compromised. Adult periosteum is attached to bone; consequently, rupture through the periosteum and sinus drainage is more common in adults.

Diagnostic Evaluation

Organism identification and antibiotic susceptibility testing are essential for effective therapy. Cultures of aspirated purulent drainage along with cultures of blood, joint fluid, and infected skin samples should be obtained. Bone biopsy is indicated if blood culture results and radiographic findings are not consistent with osteomyelitis. Supporting evidence for osteomyelitis includes leukocytosis and elevated erythrocyte sedimentation rate (ESR) and C-reactive protein (CRP). Radiographic signs, except for soft-tissue swelling, are evident only after 2 to 3 weeks. A three-phase technetium bone scan can show areas of increased blood flow, such as occurs in early stages in infected bone, and is useful in locating multiple sites; however, it is not a diagnostic test. Computed tomography (CT) scan can detect bone destruction, and MRI provides anatomic details useful in delineating the area of involvement, especially if surgical intervention is planned. MRI is reported to be the most sensitive diagnostic radiologic tool for diagnosing osteomyelitis (Robinette & Shah, 2020a). Sometimes the osteomyelitis may be unrecognized if it occurs as a complication of a severe toxic and debilitating disease. Neonates may not present with clinical manifestations other than limited mobility of the affected extremity; fever may or may not be present, and the neonate may not appear to be sick (Robinette & Shah, 2020a).

Therapeutic Management

After culture specimens are obtained, empiric therapy is started with IV antibiotics covering the mostly likely organisms. For *S. aureus*, nafcillin or clindamycin is generally used. Consideration should be given to the increased rates of community-acquired methicillin-resistant *S. aureus* (MRSA) in the selection of first-line antibiotic therapy; MRSA may require vancomycin, or in some cases, clindamycin may be appropriate. When the infectious agent is identified, administration of the appropriate antibiotic is initiated and continued for at least 3 to 4 weeks, but the length of therapy is determined by the duration of the symptoms, the response to treatment, and the sensitivity of the organism; 6 weeks to 4 months may be required in some cases (Robinette & Shah, 2020a). In selected cases, oral antibiotic therapy may follow the IV treatment. Because of the prolonged duration of high-dose antibiotic therapy, it is important to monitor for hematologic, renal, hepatic, ototoxic, and other potential side effects. To prevent antibiotic-associated diarrhea in some children, administration of a probiotic may be considered.

Surgery may be indicated if there is no response to specific antibiotic therapy, a penetrating injury exists, persistent soft-tissue abscess is seen, or the infection spreads to the joint. Opinions differ regarding surgical intervention, but many advocate sequestrectomy and surgical drainage to decompress the metaphyseal space before purulent fluid erupts and spreads to the subperiosteal space, forming abscesses that strip the periosteum from bone or form draining sinuses. When these complications occur, a chronic infection usually persists, which may require antibiotic therapy for several months.

Nursing Care Management

During the acute phase of illness, movement of the affected limb will cause discomfort; therefore the child is positioned comfortably with the affected limb supported. A temporary splint or cast may be applied. Weight bearing is avoided in the acute phase, and moving and turning are carried out carefully to minimize pain. The child may require long-term pain medication to deal with the bone pain. Postoperatively, pain medication should be considered as with any other surgical procedure.

Antibiotic therapy requires careful observation and monitoring of the IV equipment and site. A peripherally inserted central catheter (PICC) may be inserted for long-term antibiotic therapy. Antibiotic therapy is often continued at home or through an outpatient infusion clinic.

Standard Precautions are implemented for all children with osteomyelitis. If there is an open wound, it is managed according to standard wound care precautions. If a PICC line or central venous catheter (CVC) is inserted, meticulous care should be taken to prevent catheter-related infection.

As the infection subsides, physical therapy is instituted to ensure restoration of optimum function. The child may eventually be transitioned to a regimen of oral antibiotics, and progress is followed closely for some time.

SEPTIC ARTHRITIS

Septic arthritis is a bacterial infection in the joint. It usually results from hematogenous spread or from direct extension of an adjacent cellulitis or osteomyelitis. Direct inoculation from trauma accounts for 15% to 20% of septic arthritis cases. The most common causative organism is *S. aureus.* Community-acquired MRSA is commonly a cause of septic arthritis. In addition to *S. aureus,* pathogens seen in neonates include group B streptococci, *Escherichia coli,* and *Candida albicans.* In children 2 months to 5 years old, *S. aureus, Streptococcus pyogenes, Streptococcus pneumoniae,* and *K. kingae* are the primary organisms causing infection. Children older than 5 years of age are more likely to be infected by *S. aureus* and *S. pyogenes,* and sexually active adolescents may be infected by *N. gonorrhoeae* (Gutierrez, 2005; Robinette & Shah, 2020a).

The knees, hips, ankles, and elbows are the most common joints affected. Clinical manifestations include severe joint pain, swelling, warmth of overlying tissue, and occasionally erythema. An infection involving the hip, however, is considered a surgical emergency to prevent compromised blood supply to the head of the femur (Robinette & Shah, 2020b).

The child is resistant to any joint movement. Features of systemic illness such as fever, malaise, headache, nausea, vomiting, and irritability may also be present.

Therapeutic Management and Nursing Care Management

The affected joint is aspirated and the specimen evaluated by Gram stain, cultures (including separate cultures for *H. influenzae* and *N. gonorrhoeae*), and determination of leukocyte count. In addition, perform blood cultures and obtain complete blood count with differential and ESR or CRP level. Early radiographic findings are limited to soft-tissue swelling but may reveal a foreign body, and such films always provide a baseline for comparison. Technetium scans reveal areas of increased blood flow but will not differentiate between sites. MRI and CT scans provide more detailed images of cartilage loss, joint narrowing, erosions, and ankylosis of progressive disease. Ultrasonography is helpful in the detection of joint effusions and fluid in the soft tissue and subperiosteum (Robinette & Shah, 2020b).

Treatment is IV antibiotic therapy based on Gram stain results and the clinical presentation. The benefits of serial aspirations to demonstrate sterility of synovium fluid and reduce pressure or pain are controversial. Pain management is an important aspect of nursing care, particularly with involvement of a large joint such as the hip. Surgical intervention may also be required if there was a penetrating wound or a foreign object was possibly involved. Physical therapy may be initiated for the child who is immobilized to prevent flexion contractures. Additional nursing care is the same as for osteomyelitis.

SKELETAL TUBERCULOSIS

In children, tubercular infection of the bones and joints is acquired by lymphohematogenous spread at the time of primary infection. Occasionally it is from chronic pulmonary TB. Skeletal tubercular infection is not common in the United States but should be considered in communities with high TB case rates. The condition is a late manifestation of TB and is most likely to involve the vertebrae, causing tubercular spondylitis. If the infection is progressive, it causes **Pott disease** with destruction of the vertebral bodies and results in kyphosis and spinal malalignment (Pigrau-Serrallach & Rodríguez-Pardo, 2013). Symptoms are insidious. The child may report persistent or intermittent pain. Other findings include joint swelling and stiffness; fever and weight loss are not common. Tubercular arthritis can also affect single joints (such as a knee or hip) and tends to cause severe destruction of adjacent bone. Infection in the fingers causes spina ventosa, a tuberculous dactylitis.

As with pulmonary TB, the index case should be located. A family and environmental history needs to be obtained and tuberculin skin tests (TSTs) performed. Results of TSTs are positive for most children with tuberculous arthritis; however, the results are not diagnostic, and the clinical and laboratory features do not differentiate tubercular arthritis from a nontubercular septic arthritis. Diagnosis requires isolation of *Mycobacterium tuberculosis* from the site. Patients with the susceptible organism start treatment with combined antituberculosis chemotherapy (isoniazid, rifampin, and pyrazinamide); directly observed therapy (DOT) is preferred.

Nursing Care Management

Nursing care depends on the site and extent of infection. Tuberculous spondylitis and hip infection may require immobilization, casting, and surgical fusion. Nursing care is individualized but is generally the same as for osteomyelitis and septic arthritis.

DISORDERS OF JOINTS

JUVENILE IDIOPATHIC ARTHRITIS

Juvenile idiopathic arthritis (JIA) refers to chronic childhood arthritis. A group of heterogeneous autoimmune diseases, JIA causes inflammation in the joint synovium and surrounding tissue. The cause of JIA is unknown. JIA starts before 16 years old with a peak onset between 1 and 3 years old. Twice as many girls as boys are affected. The reported incidence of chronic childhood arthritis varies from 1 to 20 cases per 100,000 children with a prevalence of 10 to 400 per 100,000 (Cassidy & Petty, 2011). Genetic factors and environmental triggers (e.g., rubella, Epstein-Barr virus, parvovirus B19) have been associated with the onset of JIA, but the etiology remains unclear.

Pathophysiology

The disease process is characterized by chronic inflammation of the synovium with joint effusion and eventual erosion, destruction, and fibrosis of the articular cartilage. Adhesions between joint surfaces and ankylosis of joints may occur if the inflammatory process persists.

Clinical Manifestations

Whether single or multiple joints are involved, swelling and loss of motion develop in the affected joint. The swollen joint may be slightly warm and mildly tender to touch, but it is not uncommon for pain not to be reported despite a large joint effusion. Loss of motion in the joint from joint inflammation and muscle spasm may be exacerbated by inactivity. Morning stiffness of the joint(s) is characteristic of JIA and may be present on arising or inactivity. Functional change may be an obvious limp or subtle limitations in joint motion, such as fisting to avoid wrist extension with pressure. Growth disturbances (either overgrowth or undergrowth) may occur, such as bony enlargement of the adjacent femoral or tibial condyles with a knee effusion or a receding chin from temporomandibular arthritis.

Classification of Juvenile Idiopathic Arthritis

JIA is not a single disease but a heterogeneous group of diseases. The universal Durban classification of JIA, developed in 1997 and revised in 1998 and 2001, lists several disease categories, each with its own set of criteria and exclusions, which continue to be revised (Petty, Southwood, Manners, et al., 2004).

- Systemic arthritis is arthritis in one or more joints associated with at least 2 weeks of quotidian fever and daily for at least 3 days and one or more of the following: rash, lymphadenopathy, hepatosplenomegaly, and serositis. **Exclusions: a, b, c, d*
- Oligoarthritis is arthritis in one to four joints for the first 6 months of disease. It is subdivided to persistent oligoarthritis if it remains in four joints or fewer, or becomes extended oligoarthritis if it involves more than four joints after 6 months. **Exclusions: a, b, c, d, e*
- Polyarthritis rheumatoid factor (RF) negative affects five or more joints in the first 6 months with a negative RF. **Exclusions: a, b, c, e*
- Polyarthritis RF positive also affects five or more joints in the first 6 months, but these children have a positive RF. **Exclusions: a, b, c, e*
- Psoriatic arthritis is arthritis with psoriasis or an associated dactylitis, nail pitting, or onycholysis or psoriasis in a first-degree relative. **Exclusions: b, c, d, e*
- Enthesitis-related arthritis is arthritis or enthesitis associated with at least two of the following: sacroiliac or lumbosacral pain, human leukocyte antigen B27 (HLA-B27) antigen, arthritis in a boy older than 6 years old, acute anterior uveitis, inflammatory bowel disease, Reiter syndrome, or acute anterior uveitis in a first-degree relative. [d]*Eclusions: a, d, e*
- Undifferentiated arthritis fits no other category above or fits more than one category.

Diagnostic Evaluation

JIA is a diagnosis of exclusion; there are no definitive tests. Classifications are based on the clinical criteria of age of onset before 16 years old, arthritis in one or more joints for 6 weeks or longer, and exclusion of other causes. Laboratory tests may provide supporting evidence of disease. The ESR/CRP may or may not be elevated. Leukocytosis is frequently present during exacerbations of systemic JIA. Antinuclear antibodies are common in JIA but are not specific for arthritis; however, they help identify children who are at greater risk for uveitis. Plain radiographs are the best initial imaging studies and may show soft-tissue swelling and joint space widening from increased synovial fluid in the joint. Later films can reveal osteoporosis, narrow joint space, erosions, subluxation, and ankylosis. A slit lamp eye examination is necessary to diagnose uveitis, inflammation in the anterior chamber of the eye, which is most common in antinuclear antibody–positive

[d]Exclusions: (a) Psoriasis or history of psoriasis in the patient or first-degree relative; (b) arthritis in an HLA-B27–positive male beginning after the sixth birthday; (c) ankylosing spondylitis, enthesitis-related arthritis, sacroiliitis with inflammatory bowel disease, Reiter syndrome, or symptomatic anterior uveitis, or a history of one of these disorders in a first-degree relative; (d) the presence of immunoglobulin M rheumatoid factor (RF) on at least two occasions at least 3 months apart; (e) the presence of systemic JIA in the patient.

young girls with oligoarthritis. Routine examinations are necessary for early diagnosis and treatment to avoid or minimize sight-threatening disease (Qian & Acharya, 2010).

Therapeutic Management

There is no cure for JIA. The major goals of therapy are to control pain, preserve joint range of motion and function, minimize effects of inflammation such as joint deformity, and promote normal growth and development. Outpatient care is the mainstay of therapy; lengthy hospitalizations are infrequent in this era of managed care. The treatment plan can be exhaustive and intrusive for the child and family, including medications, physical and occupational therapy, ophthalmologic slit lamp examinations, splints, comfort measures, dietary management, school modifications, and psychosocial support.

Medications

In 2011 the American College of Rheumatology published recommendations for the treatment of JIA intended to lend guidance to the provider. Additional recommendations were added in 2013 to further address treatment of systemic JIA as well as routine screening tests for those with JIA (Ringold, Weiss, Beukelman, et al., 2013). The guidelines are divided into four groups: children with (1) four or fewer affected joints, (2) five or more affected joints, (3) systemic arthritis and active systemic features, and (4) systemic arthritis with active arthritis. Each path provides recommendations for a stepwise escalation of the medication and therapy (Beukelman, Patkar, Saag, et al., 2011). All tracks consider poor prognostic indicators, such as erosions on radiograph; arthritis of the hip, cervical spine, ankle, or wrist; and a positive RF. In addition, each track takes into account disease activity levels that include elevated acute phase reactants and global assessments of both the provider and the patient and parents.

Medications included in the guidelines include those described in the following sections.

Nonsteroidal antiinflammatory drugs. NSAIDs (e.g., naproxen, ibuprofen) are used alone or in combination with other drugs depending on the amount of disease activity and poor prognostic features. NSAIDs offer an analgesic effect but may require higher dosing for an antiinflammatory effect. Patient and parent education is important and should include potential side effects of gastrointestinal, renal, hepatic, and prolonged coagulation.

Disease-modifying antirheumatic drugs. Disease-modifying antirheumatic drugs (DMARDs) include the nonbiologic drugs methotrexate and sulfasalazine. The decision to use a DMARD at initiation of therapy or later in the escalation of therapy is guided by the amount of disease activity and poor prognostic features. Effective against arthritis and uveitis, antirheumatic low-dose methotrexate has a time-proven safety profile, but parents may be overwhelmed by the potential adverse effects of liver disease, infections, bone marrow suppression, gastrointestinal disturbance, teratogenic effects, and alarming but unconfirmed risk of cancer. Patient and parent education includes frank discussion of sexual activity and birth defects. Sexually active teenagers need effective birth control. As a precaution, pregnant caregivers or those trying to conceive need to avoid contact with methotrexate. Instructions about avoiding live immunizations and alcohol are essential during patient education. Sulfasalazine may be used in children with axial arthritis, a positive test result for HLA-B27, or symptoms of inflammatory bowel disease, given this drug's success in these select groups of patients.

Biologic disease-modifying antirheumatic drugs. Biologic DMARDs are initiated when there is significant disease activity and/or poor prognostic indicators after unsuccessful treatment with methotrexate. Tumor necrosis factor–alpha (TNF-α) inhibitors are the most frequently used biologic DMARDs and include etanercept, infliximab, and adalimumab. All three reduce the proinflammatory response that promotes arthritis. Anakinra (interleukin-1 receptor antagonist), tocilizumab (interleukin-6 receptor antagonist), and abatacept (selective T-cell costimulation blocker) are also biologics that may be selected for use in systemic JIA (tocilizumab and off-label anakinra) or in children with JIA and limited response to other biologics (tocilizumab and abatacept). Patient education focuses on the increased risk for infection, holding the scheduled dose if the child has fever or symptoms of infection, and seeking medical attention at early onset of illness. All patients starting biologic DMARDs need a negative TST prior to starting. Although biologic DMARDs have been found to be safe and effective, the potential for malignancy needs to be addressed, and patients need routine safety monitoring (Ruperto & Martini, 2011; Tarkiainen, Tynjälä, Vähäsalo, et al., 2015).

Glucocorticoids. Glucocorticoids are potent antiinflammatory agents; however, the significant adverse effects of long-term systemic steroids are undesirable, so they are used in conjunction with other medications to provide prompt antiinflammatory response with acute arthritis, then tapered and discontinued. High-dose IV steroids may be used with acutely active arthritis or systemic features (fevers, rash, and pericarditis). Intra-articular long-acting steroid injections are effective in treating individual joint effusions with minimal adverse effects and frequently provide sustained control. Glucocorticoid education is extensive and includes discussion of potential risks of infection, adrenal insufficiency, Cushingoid features, weight gain, mood or sleep changes, hypertension, diabetes, and osteoporosis and avascular necrosis. Simultaneous dietary changes (low calorie and low salt) and, if possible, an active exercise program should be considered when steroids are initiated.

Physical and Occupational Therapy

Physical therapy programs are individualized for each child and designed to reach the ultimate goal—preserving function or preventing deformity. Physical therapy is directed toward specific joints, focusing on strengthening muscles, mobilizing restricted joint motion, and preventing or correcting deformities. Occupational therapists are responsible for evaluating and improving performance of activities of daily living.

Treatment or maintenance programs vary; a child may be seen a couple of times a week or monthly, but the mainstay of any program is the child doing the daily home exercise program, which is demonstrated and revised at each therapy session.

Exercising in a pool is excellent therapy because it allows an almost weightless freedom of movement against the gentle resistance of water. If there is pain on motion, a hot pack or warm bath before therapy may help.

Providers may recommend nighttime splinting to help minimize pain and reduce flexion deformity. Joints most frequently splinted are the knees, wrists, and hands. Loss of extension in the knee, hip, and wrist causes special problems and requires vigilance to detect the earliest signs of involvement and vigorous attention to prevent deformity with specialized passive stretching, positioning, and resting splints.

Nursing Care Management

Nursing the child with JIA involves assessment of the child's general health, the status of involved joints, and the child's emotional response to all ramifications of the disease—discomfort, physical restrictions, therapies, and self-concept.

The effects of JIA are manifest in every aspect of the child's life, including physical activities, social experiences, and personality development. Nursing interventions to support the parents may foster successful adaptation for the entire family. Parental concerns about the disease prognosis, financial and insurance issues, spouse and sibling relationships, and job and schedule conflicts must all be addressed. Referral to social workers, counselors, or support groups may be needed.

Relieve Pain

The pain of JIA is related to several aspects of the disease, including disease severity, functional status, individual pain threshold, family variables, and psychologic adjustment. The aim is to provide as much relief as possible with medication and other therapies to help children tolerate the pain and cope as effectively as possible. Nonpharmacologic modalities, such as behavioral therapy and relaxation techniques, have proved effective in modifying pain perception (see Chapter 5, Pain Management) and activities that aggravate pain. Opioid analgesics are typically avoided in juvenile arthritis; however, for children immobilized with refractory pain, short-term opioid analgesics can be part of a comprehensive plan that uses multiple pain-relief techniques (Connelly & Schanberg, 2006).

Promote General Health

The child's general health must be considered. A well-balanced diet with sufficient calories to maintain growth is essential. If the child is relatively inactive, caloric intake needs to match energy needs to avoid excessive weight gain, which places additional stress on affected joints. Sleep and rest are essential for children with JIA. Some children require rest during the day; however, daytime napping that interferes with nighttime sleepiness should be avoided. A bedtime routine that involves comfort measures can help induce sleep. A firm mattress, electric blanket, or sleeping bag helps provide warmth, comfort, and rest. Nighttime splints needed to maintain range of motion might initially be a source of bedtime conflict. The family needs to be instructed on how to use the splint appropriately; the splint should not be painful or impede sleep. Behavior modification programs that reward splint and exercise compliance may be helpful in reducing adherence barriers. Well-child care to assess growth, development, and immunization requirements needs to be coordinated between the primary care provider and the rheumatologist. Common childhood illnesses, such as upper respiratory tract infections, may cause arthritis to worsen; consequently, medical attention must be sought quickly for relatively minor illness to prevent arthritis flares. Effective communication among the family, the primary care provider, and the rheumatology team is essential for care coordination.

Children are encouraged to attend school even on days when they have some pain or discomfort. The school nurse's assistance is enlisted so that a child is permitted to take the prescribed medication at school and to arrange for rest in the nurse's office during the day. Split days or half days may help a child remain involved in school. Permitting the child to come to school late allows time to gain joint movement and reduces the time at school to avoid exhaustion. It is important that the child attend school to learn skills and engage in social interaction, especially if the JIA continues to limit physical skills. Arranging for two sets of textbooks—one for home and one for school—eliminates heavy backpacks, or rolling backpacks may be used. In addition, extra time to take tests, allowing the child to stand and stretch, participating in PE as tolerated or in a modified PE program, an elevator pass, and extra time to change classes can all reduce barriers and maximize the student's attendance and participation in school. A formal school hearing may be necessary to obtain an individualized educational program (IEP), ensured by public law, which includes intensive school modifications.

Facilitate Adherence

The child and family need to be actively involved in the treatment plan to commit to it. They need to know the purpose and correct use of any splints, exercise programs, and medications prescribed. Pill boxes can help foster adherence, although parents should continue to monitor adherence of the older child who is able to safely take medications independently. Nurses can facilitate adherence by demonstrating and providing written instructions on proper techniques for pill crushing or pill swallowing skills. Teaching parents and patients how to give subcutaneous injections lays the groundwork for future adherence by identifying and addressing potential barriers. Shots are never a pleasant activity; if available, enlist a child life specialist as a resource in providing the child with skills to cope and better understand and accept unpleasant but necessary medical treatments.

Comfort Measures and Exercise

Heat has been shown to be beneficial to children with arthritis. Moist heat is best for relieving pain and stiffness, and the most efficient and practical method is in the bathtub with warm water. In some cases, a daily whirlpool bath, paraffin bath, or hot packs may be used as needed for temporary relief of acute swelling and pain. Hot packs are easily applied using a damp hand towel wrung out after being immersed in hot water or heated in a microwave oven; after testing for heat, hot packs are applied to the area and covered with plastic to retain heat. Commercial pads that warm in only a few seconds in the microwave are also available. Painful hands or feet can be immersed in a pan of warm water or a paraffin unit.

Pool therapy is the easiest method for exercising a large number of joints. Swimming activities strengthen muscles and maintain mobility in larger joints. Very small children who are frightened of the water can carry out their exercises in the bathtub. Small children love to splash, kick, and throw things in the water. Remember, adult supervision is necessary for all water activities.

Activities of daily living provide satisfactory exercise for older children to maintain maximal mobility with minimal pain. These children are encouraged in their efforts to be independent and patiently allowed to dress and groom themselves, to assume daily tasks, and to care for their belongings. It is often difficult for children to manipulate buttons, comb or brush their hair, and turn faucets, but unless there is an acute flare with significant loss of motion and pain, parents and other caregivers should offer not assistance but extra time and encouragement to proceed independently. In turn, children should learn and understand why others do not help them. Many helpful devices, such as self-adhering fasteners, tongs for manipulating difficult items, and grab bars installed in bathrooms for safety, can be used to facilitate tasks. A raised (higher) toilet seat often makes the difference between dependent and independent toileting because weak quadriceps muscles and sore knees inhibit the ability to raise the body from a low sitting position.

A child's natural affinity for play offers many opportunities for incorporating therapeutic exercises. Throwing or kicking a ball and riding a tricycle (with the seat raised to achieve maximum leg extension) are excellent moving and stretching exercises for a young child whose activities of daily living are physically limited.

An effective approach to beginning the day's activities is to awaken children early to give them their medication and then to allow them to sleep for an hour. On arising, children take a hot bath (or shower) and perform a simple ritual of limbering-up exercises, after which they commence the activities of the day, such as going to school. Exercise, heat, and rest are spaced throughout the remainder of the day according to the child's individual needs and schedules. Parents are instructed in exercises that meet the child's needs.

The Arthritis Foundation and the American Juvenile Arthritis Alliance (an organization within the Arthritis Foundation) provide information and services for both parents and professionals, and nurses can refer families to these agencies as an added resource.

Support Child and Family

JIA affects every aspect of life for the child and family. Physical limitations may interfere with self-care, school participation, and recreational activities. The intensive treatment plan, including multiple medications, physical therapy, comfort measures, and medical appointments, is intrusive and disruptive to the parents' work schedule and the family routine. To prevent isolation and foster independence, the family is encouraged to pursue their normal activities. Unfortunately, the adaptations necessary to make that occur take resourcefulness and commitment from all family members. At diagnosis and throughout the span of JIA, it is essential to recognize signs of stress and counterproductive coping and provide the necessary support to maximize adaptation. The problems and needs of these families are discussed in Chapter 17, and readers are directed to that chapter for guidance in planning care.

SYSTEMIC LUPUS ERYTHEMATOSUS

Systemic lupus erythematosus (SLE) is a severe chronic autoimmune disease that results in inflammation and multiorgan system damage. Other forms of lupus include discoid lupus, which is limited to the skin, and neonatal lupus, which occurs when maternal autoantibodies cause a transient lupus-like syndrome in a newborn with the potential serious complication of heart block. The remaining discussion focuses on SLE.

The Lupus Foundation of America (2019) and National Kidney Foundation (2017) estimate that 5 million individuals worldwide have lupus, and 10% to 20% of these adults were diagnosed with SLE as children or adolescents. SLE in children tends to be more severe at onset and has a more aggressive clinical course than adult-onset SLE (Mina & Brunner, 2013).

SLE is more common in girls, with an approximate 4:3 female-to-male predominance before 10 years old and 4:1 in the second decade, indicating a potential hormonal trigger with maturation. There is a familial tendency, although many newly diagnosed patients are unaware of other affected family members. SLE has been reported in all cultures, but within the United States there has been a disproportionately higher incidence in African American, Asian, and Hispanic children.

The cause of SLE is not known. It appears to result from a complex interaction of genetics with an unidentified trigger that activates the disease. Suspected triggers include exposure to ultraviolet (UV) light, estrogen, pregnancy, infections, and drugs. Genetic predisposition to SLE is evidenced in an increased concordance rate in twins (tenfold), increased incidence within family members (10% to 16%), and increased frequency of certain gene alleles in population-based studies.

Clinical Manifestations and Diagnostic Evaluation

The child with SLE may have any of the clinical manifestations with mild to life-threatening severity (Box 29.10). The diagnosis is established when 4 of the 11 diagnostic criteria are met (Box 29.11). Kidney involvement heralds progressive disease and the need for rigorous therapeutic management.

Therapeutic Management

The goal of treatment is to ensure the child's health by balancing the medications necessary to avoid exacerbation and complications while preventing or minimizing treatment-associated morbidity. Therapy involves the use of specific medications and general supportive care. The drugs used to control inflammation are corticosteroids administered in doses sufficient to control inflammation and then tapered to the lowest suppressive dose or given intravenously during acute flares. Hydroxychloroquine, an antimalarial, is a useful medication for inflammatory control, rash, and arthritis. NSAIDs relieve muscle and joint inflammation, and immunosuppressive agents, such as cyclophosphamide, are administered for renal and CNS disease. Mycophenolate, azathioprine, and methotrexate are effective immunosuppressive drugs that may be used to control SLE and allow steroids to be reduced. Rituximab is a monoclonal antibody that results in decreased antibody formation and has been used off-label in pediatric patients with lupus who have not responded to standard therapy (Nwobi, Abitbol, Chandar, et al., 2008). Antihypertensives, low-dose aspirin (as a blood thinner), and calcium and vitamin D supplements are just a few of the additional remedies that may be necessary to treat or avoid complications.

General supportive care includes sufficient nutrition, sleep and rest, and exercise. Exposure to the sun and ultraviolet B (UVB) light is limited because of its association with SLE exacerbation.

BOX 29.10 Manifestations of Systemic Lupus Erythematosus

Constitutional: Fever, fatigue, weight loss, anorexia
Cutaneous: Erythematosus butterfly rash over bridge of nose and across cheeks, discoid rash, photosensitivity, mucocutaneous ulceration, alopecia, periungual telangiectasias
Musculoskeletal: Arthritis, arthralgia, myositis, myalgia, tenosynovitis
Neurologic: Headache, seizure, forgetfulness, behavior change, change in school performance, psychosis, chorea, stroke, cranial and peripheral neuropathy, pseudotumor cerebri
Pulmonary and cardiac: Pleuritis, basilar pneumonitis, atelectasis, pericarditis, myocarditis, and endocarditis
Renal: Glomerulonephritis, nephrotic syndrome, hypertension
Gastrointestinal: Abdominal pain, nausea, vomiting, blood in stool, abdominal crisis, esophageal dysfunction, colitis
Hepatic, splenic, and nodal: Hepatomegaly, splenomegaly, lymphadenopathy
Hematologic: Anemia, cytopenia
Ophthalmologic: Cotton wool spots, papilledema, retinopathy
Vascular: Raynaud phenomenon, thrombophlebitis, livedo reticularis

BOX 29.11 Classification Criteria for Systemic Lupus Erythematosus[a]

Malar rash: Fixed malar erythema
Discoid rash: Patchy erythematous lesions
Photosensitivity: Rash with sunlight exposure
Oronasal ulcers: Painless ulcers in mouth and nose
Arthritis: Swelling, tenderness, or effusion in two or more peripheral joints (nonerosive)
Serositis: Pleuritis, pericarditis
Renal disorder: Proteinuria, casts in urine
Neurologic disorder: Psychosis, seizures
Hematologic disorder: Hemolytic anemia, thrombocytopenia, leukopenia, lymphopenia
Immunologic disorder: Anti–double-stranded deoxyribonucleic acid, anti-Sm, antiphospholipid antibodies; lupus anticoagulant; false-positive result on syphilis test (rapid plasma reagin)
Antinuclear antibodies: Presence of antinuclear antibody by immunofluorescence or an equivalent assay

[a]The presence of four criteria is required for classification as systemic lupus erythematosus (SLE).

Nursing Care Management

The principal nursing goal is to help the child and family positively adjust to the disease and therapy. The child and family must learn to recognize subtle signs of disease exacerbation and potential complications of medication therapy and to communicate these concerns to their care provider. Consequently, patient and family education is an ongoing process initiated at diagnosis and tailored to the patient's individual needs. Referral to a social worker, psychologist, or support group may help the child and family make a successful adjustment. Support groups are associated with the Lupus Foundation of America and the Arthritis Foundation.

Key issues include therapy compliance; body image problems associated with rash, hair loss, and steroid therapy; school attendance; vocational activities; social relationships; sexual activity; and pregnancy (see Chapter 17 for a discussion on adjusting to a chronic illness). Specific instructions for avoiding exposure to the sun and UVB light, such as using sunscreens, wearing sun-resistant clothing, and altering outdoor activities, must be provided with great sensitivity to ensure compliance while minimizing the associated feeling of being different from peers. Patients need to be instructed to maintain regular medical supervision and seek attention quickly during illness or before elective surgical procedures, such as dental extraction, because of potential needs for increased steroids or prophylactic antibiotics. People with SLE should carry medical identification for their disease and steroid dependence.

CLINICAL JUDGMENT AND NEXT-GENERATION NCLEX® EXAMINATION-STYLE QUESTIONS

1. A 6-year-old boy has experienced significant trauma in a motor vehicle crash 4 days ago. He has been in the intensive care unit and is now stabilized and being transferred to the pediatric orthopedic unit to continue recovery. He is immobilized with a fractured femur and humerus, and multiple lacerations. **Use an X for the nursing action below that is Indicated (appropriate or necessary), Contraindicated (could be harmful), or Non-Essential (makes no difference or not necessary).**

Nursing Action	Indicated	Contraindicated	Non-Essential
Monitor peripheral pulses and skin temperature changes			
Use compression stockings or intermittent compression devices to decrease pooling			
Reposition every 8 hours			
Monitor intake and output closely			
Place on a hard mattress to prevent movement			
Encourage cough and deep breathing			
Complete a dietary assessment			
Monitor vital signs			

2. A 12-year-old who was in an all-terrain vehicle (ATV) accident has a long leg fiberglass cast on his left leg for a tibia-fibula fracture. He requests pain medication at 2:00 AM for pain he rates as 10/10 on the numeric scale. The nurse brings the pain medication and notes that he has removed the pillows that kept his leg elevated. He complains of pain in the left foot, and she notes that there is 3+ edema in the exposed leg and foot and she has difficulty slipping a finger under the cast; no pulse is found, and the capillary refill is difficult to visualize. **Choose the most likely options for the information missing from the statements below by selecting from the lists of options provided.** The nurse notes that these may be signs of a _____1_____. The nurse would immediately call the physician since permanent damage can occur within_____2_____. The nurse would _____3_____ and continue to assess for a pulse _____4_____the fracture.

Options for 1	Options for 2	Options for 3	Options for 4
bone fracture	days	keep limb at heart level	proximal to
severed nerve	hours	lower the limb	adjacent to
compartment syndrome	minutes	remove the cast	aligned with
bone contusion	seconds	turn patient on his side	alongside
bone rotation	weeks	provide pressure	distal to

3. The nurse is completing an assessment of a 2-month-old girl during a well-child visit. The infant was born breech and weighed 9 lbs. 2 oz. She is growing well and is being breast fed. She is to receive her 2-month vaccinations today. The nurse completes the assessment and finds the following on examination. Which findings would be **immediate** concern that **require follow-up? Select all that apply.**
   A. Back is rounded
   B. Limb may turn outward
   C. Limb may appear shorter
   D. Gluteal folds are unequal
   E. Posterior fontanel is closed
   F. Both limbs are of equal length
   G. Restricted abduction of the hip on one side

4. A 6-year-old girl is newly diagnosed with juvenile idiopathic arthritis after a 3-month history of swollen joints that are warm and painful to touch. Her symptoms also included morning stiffness. When she presented to the Emergency Department, she has bony enlargement of her left knee with an effusion. She is to be discharged today and the nurse is meeting with the parents to discuss the care she will need at home.
   Use an X for the health teaching evaluation below that is Indicated (appropriate or necessary), Contraindicated (could be harmful), or Non-Essential (makes no difference or not necessary).

Health Teaching	Indicated	Contraindicated	Non-Essential
"Opioid medications should be given to your child whenever she complains of pain."			
"Relaxation techniques can be effective in decreasing her pain."			
"Make sure your child takes the prescribed medications on time."			
"Keeping your child in bed when she has extremity pain will prevent swelling."			
"Swimming can help strengthen your child's muscles and maintain mobility."			
"Your child can sleep in her sister's bedroom at night if she wishes."			

REFERENCES

Beukelman, T., Patkar, N. M., Saag, K. G., Tolleson Rinehart, S., Cron, R. Q., DeWitt, E. M., et al. (2011). 2011 American College of Rheumatology recommendations for the treatment of juvenile idiopathic arthritis: Initiation and safety monitoring of therapeutic agents for the treatment of arthritis and systemic features. *Arthritis Care & Research, 63*(4), 465–482.

Biber, R., & Gregory, A. (2010). Overuse injuries in youth sports: Is there such a thing as too much sports? *Pediatric Annals, 39*(5), 286–292.

Cassidy, J. T., & Petty, R. E. (2011). Chronic arthritis in childhood. In J. T. Cassidy, R. E. Petty, R. M. Laxer, et al. (Eds.), *Textbook of pediatric rheumatology* (6th ed). Philadelphia, PA: Elsevier/Saunders.

Changstrom, B. G., Brou, L., Khodaee, M., Braund, C., & Comstock, R. D. (2015). Epidemiology of stress fracture injuries among US high school athletes, 2005-2006 through 2012-2013. *The American Journal of Sports Medicine, 43*(1), 26–33.

Connelly, M., & Schanberg, L. (2006). Opioid therapy for the treatment of refractory pain in children with juvenile rheumatoid arthritis. *Nature Reviews Rheumatology, 2*(12), 636.

Curley, M. A., Hasbani, N. R., Quigley, S. M., Stellar, J. J., Pasek, T. A., Shelley, S. S., et al. (2018). Predicting pressure injury risk in pediatric patients: The Braden QD Scale. *The Journal of Pediatrics, 192*, 189–195.

Flaherty, E. G., Perez-Rossello, J. M., Levine, M. A., Hennrikus, W. L., & American Academy of Pediatrics Committee on Child Abuse and Neglect. (2014). Evaluating children with fractures for child physical abuse. *Pediatrics, 133*(2), e477–e489.

Freeman, B. L., III. (2013). Scoliosis and kyphosis. In S. T. Canale, & J. H. Beaty (Eds.), *Campbell's operative orthopaedics* (12th ed.). Philadelphia, PA: Mosby.

Gutierrez, K. (2005). Bone and joint infections in children. *Pediatric Clinics, 52*(3), 779–794.

Herring, J. (2011). Legg-Calvé-Perthes disease at 100: A review of evidence-based treatment. *Journal of Pediatric Orthopedics, 31*(2 Suppl), S137–S140.

Holmes, S., Brown, S., & Panel, P. S. C. E. (2005). Skeletal pin site care: National Association of Orthopaedic Nurses guidelines for orthopaedic nursing. *Orthopaedic Nursing, 24*(2), 99–107.

Hresko, M. T. (2013). Idiopathic scoliosis in adolescents. *New England Journal of Medicine, 368*(9), 834–841.

Hresko, M. T., Talwakar, V. R., & Schwend, R. M. (2015). *SRS/POSNA/AAOS/AAP position statement: Screening for the early detection for idiopathic scoliosis in adolescents.* 2015. Accessed January 18th, 2019. https://www.srs.org/about-srs/news-and-announcements/position-statement---screening-for-the-early-detection-for-idiopathic-scoliosis-in-adolescents.

Robinette, E., & Shah, S. S. (2020a). Osteomyeltitis. In R. M. Kliegman, J. W. St Geme, N. L. Blum, et al. (Eds.), *Nelson textbook of pediatrics* (21th ed.). Philadelphia, PA: Elsevier.

Robinette, E., & Shah, S. S. (2020b). Septic arthrisits. In R. M. Kliegman, J. W. St Geme, N. L. Blum, et al. (Eds.), *Nelson textbook of pediatrics* (21th ed.). Philadelphia, PA: Elsevier.

Loder, R. T., & Skopelja, E. N. (2011a). The epidemiology and demographics of hip dysplasia. *ISRN Orthopedics.*

Loder, R. T., & Skopelja, E. N. (2011b). The epidemiology and demographics of Legg-Calvé-Perthes disease. *ISRN Orthopedics.*

Loder, R. T., & Skopelja, E. N. (2011c). The epidemiology and demographics of slipped capital femoral epiphysis. *ISRN Orthopedics.*

Lupus Foundation of America. (2019). Understanding lupus: what is lupus?. Retrieved from https://www.lupus.org/resources/what-is-lupus.

Marini, J. C. (2020). Osteogenesis imperfecta. In R. M. Kliegman, J. W. St Geme, N. L. Blum, et al. (Eds.), *Nelson textbook of pediatrics* (21th ed.). Philadelphia, PA: Elsevier.

Marini, J. C., & Blissett, A. R. (2013). New genes in bone development: What's new in osteogenesis imperfecta. *The Journal of Clinical Endocrinology & Metabolism, 98*(8).

Mickalide, A. D., & Hansen, L. M. (2012). *Coaching our kids to fewer injuries: A report on youth sports safety*. Washington, DC: Safe Kids Worldwide.

Mina, R., & Brunner, H. I. (2013). Update on differences between childhood-onset and adult-onset systemic lupus erythematosus. *Arthritis Research & Therapy, 15*(4), 218.

Mistovich, R. J., & Spiegel, D. A. (2020). Idiopathic scoliosis. In R. M. Kliegman, J. W. St Geme, N. L. Blum, et al. (Eds.), *Nelson textbook of pediatrics* (21th ed.). Philadelphia, PA: Elsevier.

National Kidney Foundation. (2017). *Lupus and kidney disease (lupus nephritis)*. Retrieved from https://www.kidney.org/atoz/content/lupus.

Nwobi, O., Abitbol, C. L., Chandar, J., Seeherunvong, W., & Zilleruelo, G. (2008). Rituximab therapy for juvenile-onset systemic lupus erythematosus. *Pediatric Nephrology, 23*(3), 413–419.

Peck, K., & Herrera-Soto, J. (2014). Slipped capital femoral epiphysis: What's new? *Orthopedic Clinics, 45*(1), 77–86.

Petty, R. E., Southwood, T. R., Manners, P., Baum, J., Glass, D. N., Goldenberg, J., et al. (2004). International league of associations for rheumatology classification of juvenile idiopathic arthritis: Second revision, Edmonton, 2001. *The Journal of Rheumatology, 31*(2), 390.

Pigrau-Serrallach, C., & Rodríguez-Pardo, D. (2013). Bone and joint tuberculosis. *European Spine Journal, 22*(4), 556–566.

Ponseti, I. V. (1996). Congenital clubfoot. *Fundamentals of treatment*, 37–48.

Price, C. T., & Schwend, R. M. (2011). Improper swaddling a risk factor for developmental dysplasia of hip. *American Academy of Pediatrics News, 32*(11).

Qian, Y., & Acharya, N. R. (2010). Juvenile idiopathic arthritis associated uveitis. *Current Opinion in Ophthalmology, 21*(6), 468.

Ringold, S., Weiss, P. F., Beukelman, T., DeWitt, E. M., Ilowite, N. T., Kimura, Y., et al. (2013). 2013 update of the 2011 American College of Rheumatology recommendations for the treatment of juvenile idiopathic arthritis: Recommendations for the medical therapy of children with systemic juvenile idiopathic arthritis and tuberculosis screening among children receiving biologic medications. *Arthritis & Rheumatism, 65*(10), 2499–2512.

Ruperto, N., & Martini, A. (2011). Pediatric rheumatology: JIA, treatment and possible risk of malignancies. *Nature Reviews Rheumatology, 7*(1), 6.

Sarwahi, V., Wollowick, A. L., Sugarman, E. P., Horn, J. J., Gambassi, M., & Amaral, T. D. (2011). Minimally invasive scoliosis surgery: An innovative technique in patients with adolescent idiopathic scoliosis. *Scoliosis, 6*(1), 16.

Shaw, B. A., & Segal, L. S. (2016). Evaluation and referral for developmental dysplasia of the hip in infants. *Pediatrics, 138*(6).

Shyy, W., Wang, K., Sheffield, V. C., & Morcuende, J. A. (2010). Evaluation of embryonic and perinatal myosin gene mutations and the etiology of congenital idiopathic clubfoot. *Journal of Pediatric Orthopedics, 30*(3).

Smith, M. A., Dahlen, N. R., Bruemmer, A., Davis, S., & Heishman, C. (2013). Clinical practice guideline surgical site infection prevention. *Orthopaedic Nursing, 32*(5), 242–248.

Stoll, C., Alembik, Y., Dott, B., & Roth, M. P. (2010). Associated malformations in patients with limb reduction deficiencies. *European Journal of Medical Genetics, 53*(5), 286–290.

Tarkiainen, M., Tynjälä, P., Vähäsalo, P., & Lahdenne, P. (2015). Occurrence of adverse events in patients with JIA receiving biologic agents: Long-term follow-up in a real-life setting. *Rheumatology, 54*(7), 1170–1176.

Tibor, L. M., & Sink, E. L. (2013). Risks and benefits of the modified Dunn approach for treatment of moderate or severe slipped capital femoral epiphysis. *Journal of Pediatric Orthopaedics, 33*, S99–S102.

US Preventive Services Task Force. (2018). Screening for adolescent idiopathic scoliosis: US Preventive Services Task Force Recommendation Statement. *The Journal of the American Medical Association, 319*(2), 165–172.

Weinstein, S. L., Dolan, L. A., Wright, J. G., & Dobbs, M. B. (2013). Effects of bracing in adolescents with idiopathic scoliosis. *New England Journal of Medicine, 369*(16), 1512–1521.

Winell, J. J., & Davidson, R. S. (2020). Talipes equinovarus (clubfoot). In R. M. Kliegman, J. W. St Geme, N. L. Blum, et al. (Eds.), *Nelson textbook of pediatrics* (21th ed.). Philadelphia, PA: Elsevier.

Winsley, R., & Matos, N. (2011). Overtraining and elite young athletes. In *The elite young athlete* (Vol.56) (pp. 97–105). Karger Publishers.

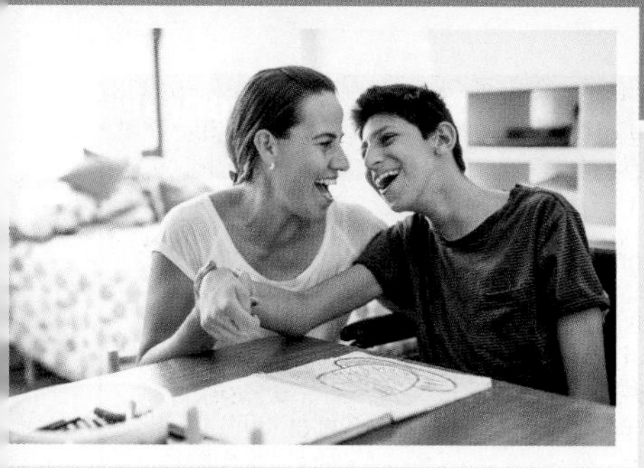

30

The Child With Neuromuscular or Muscular Dysfunction

Marilyn J. Hockenberry

http://evolve.elsevier.com/wong/essentials

CONCEPTS

- Mobility
- Sensory Perception

CONGENITAL NEUROMUSCULAR OR MUSCULAR DISORDERS

CEREBRAL PALSY

Cerebral palsy (CP) has been defined as a disorder of posture and movement from static brain injury perinatally or postnatally, which limits activity (Glader & Barkoudah, 2019; Nordqvist & Christian, 2017). In addition to motor disorders, the condition often involves disturbances of sensation, perception, communication, cognition, and behavior; secondary musculoskeletal problems; and epilepsy (Glader & Barkoudah, 2019; Nordqvist & Christian, 2017). The etiology, clinical features, and course vary and are characterized by abnormal muscle tone and coordination as the primary disturbances. CP is the most common permanent physical disability of childhood, and the incidence is reported to range from 1.5 to more than 4 per 1000 live births in various studies in the United States, affecting about 367,000 Americans (Centers for Disease Control and Prevention, 2019; Nordqvist & Christian, 2017). One systematic review and meta-analysis indicated a prevalence of 2.11 per 1000 live births, with the highest prevalence among infants weighing 1000 to 1499 g at birth; the prevalence of CP was higher among infants born before completion of 28 weeks of gestation (Oskoui, Coutinho, Dykeman, et al., 2013). Van Naarden Braun and colleagues (2016) studied spastic CP prevalence over 17 years, from 1985 to 2002, in Atlanta, Georgia, and found no significant trends by gestational age or birth weight; ethnic or racial disparities remained and warrant further investigation. In the 1960s the prevalence of CP rose approximately 20%, which most likely reflected the improved survival of extremely low birth weight (ELBW) and very low birth weight (VLBW) infants. However, in the past 2 decades there has been a decrease in the incidence of CP among ELBW and VLBW infants (Van Naarden Braun et al., 2016). The incidence is higher in males than females and more likely to occur in African Americans than in white or Hispanic children (Centers for Disease Control and Prevention, 2019).

Etiology

A variety of prenatal, perinatal, and postnatal factors contribute to the development of CP, singly or multifactorially. The human brain undergoes development during the prenatal period and up to 2 years of age. A brain insult or injury occurring during this period may result in CP.

Although the prevalent traditional hypothesis has been that CP results from perinatal problems, especially birth asphyxia, it is now believed that CP results more often from existing prenatal brain abnormalities. However, the exact cause of these abnormalities remains elusive. It has been estimated that as many as 70% to 80% of CP cases are caused by unknown prenatal factors (MacLennan, Thompson, & Gecz, 2015).

In general, infants exposed to maternal and perinatal infections are at increased risk for the development of CP as a result of the effects on the developing brain. Although CP occurs in term births, preterm birth of ELBW and VLBW infants continues to be the single most important risk factor for CP. Still, in some cases no identifiable cause is determined. Periventricular leukomalacia and intracerebral hemorrhage in low-birth-weight infants are significant risk factors in the development of CP. Perinatal ischemic stroke is also associated with a later diagnosis of CP (Golomb, Saha, Garg, et al., 2007). One study found a higher risk for CP occurring among infants born at 42 weeks of gestation or later than among those born at 37 or 38 weeks of gestation (Moster, Wilcox, Vollset, et al., 2010). Additional factors that may contribute to the development of CP postnatally include bacterial meningitis, multiple births, viral encephalitis, motor vehicle accidents, and child abuse (shaken baby syndrome [traumatic brain injury]). About 10% of children with CP acquired the condition after birth from causes such as falls, motor vehicle crashes (MVCs), and infections such as meningitis (Cerebral Palsy Guide, 2017). A significant number (4 in 10) of children with CP also have epilepsy (Centers for Disease Control and Prevention, 2019). In summary, as many as 80% of the total cases of CP may be linked to a perinatal or neonatal brain lesion or brain maldevelopment, regardless of the cause (Krageloh-Mann & Cans, 2009). A number of biochemical disorders may cause motor abnormalities often seen in CP and may be initially misdiagnosed as CP (Nehring, 2010).

Pathophysiology

It is difficult to establish a precise location of neurologic lesions on the basis of etiology or clinical signs because there is no characteristic pathologic picture. In some cases, there are gross malformations of the brain. In others, there may be evidence of vascular occlusion, atrophy, loss of neurons, and laminar degeneration that produce narrower gyri, wider sulci, and low brain weight. Anoxia appears to play the most significant role in the pathologic state of brain damage, which is often secondary to other causative mechanisms.

There are a few exceptions. In some cases, the manifestations or etiology is related to anatomic areas. For example, CP associated with preterm birth is usually spastic diplegia caused by hypoxic infarction or hemorrhage with periventricular leukomalacia in the area adjacent to the lateral ventricles. The athetoid (extrapyramidal) type of CP is most likely to be associated with birth asphyxia but can also be caused by kernicterus and metabolic genetic disorders such as mitochondrial disorders and glutaric aciduria (Johnston, 2020). Hemiplegic (hemiparetic) CP is often associated with a focal cerebral infarction (stroke) secondary to an intrauterine or perinatal thromboembolism, usually a result of maternal thrombosis or hereditary clotting disorder (Johnston, 2020). Cerebellar hypoplasia and sometimes severe neonatal hypoglycemia are related to ataxic CP. Generalized cortical and cerebral atrophy often cause severe quadriparesis with cognitive impairment and microcephaly.

Clinical Classification

A revision of the Winter classification was proposed in 2005 to reflect the child's actual clinical problems and their severity, an assessment of the child's physical and quality-of-life status across time, and long-term support needs (Nehring, 2010; Romeo, Ricci, Brogna, et al., 2016).

The proposed new definition has four major dimensions of classification (Bax, Goldstein, Rosenbaum, et al., 2005):

Motor abnormalities—Nature and typology of the motor disorder; functional motor abilities

Associated impairments—Seizures; hearing or vision impairment; attentional, behavioral, communicative, and/or cognitive deficits; oral motor and speech function

Anatomic and radiologic findings—Anatomic distribution or parts of the body affected by motor impairments or limitations; radiologic findings sometimes including white matter lesions or brain anomaly noted on computed tomography (CT) or magnetic resonance imaging (MRI)

Causation and timing—Identification of a clearly identified cause such as a postnatal event (e.g., meningitis, traumatic brain injury)

The International Classification of Functioning, Disability and Health (ICF) emphasizes participation and function, whereas the Gross Motor Function Classification System (GMFCS), Functional Mobility Scale (FMS) (Sehrawat, Marwaha, Bansal, et al., 2014), Manual Ability Classification System (MACS), and Communication Function Classification Scale (CFCS) have been widely used to assess fine motor, gross motor, and communication ability (Sun, Wang, Hou, et al., 2018). Several studies used the Hammersmith Infant Neurological Examination (HINE) as an examination tool in diagnosing CP.

CP has four primary types of movement disorders: spastic, dyskinetic, ataxic, and mixed (Box 30.1) (Nehring, 2010). The most common clinical type, spastic CP (75% to 85% reported by the Centers for Disease Control and Prevention [2019]), represents an upper motor neuron muscular weakness. The reflex arc is intact, and the characteristic physical signs are increased stretch reflexes, increased muscle tone, and (often) weakness. Early neurologic manifestations are usually generalized hypotonia or decreased tone that lasts for a few weeks or may extend for months or even as long as a year.

BOX 30.1 Clinical Classification of Cerebral Palsy

Spastic (Pyramidal)

- Characterized by persistent primitive reflexes, positive Babinski reflex, ankle clonus, exaggerated stretch reflexes, eventual development of contractures
- 70% to 80% of all cases of cerebral palsy (CP)
- **Diplegia**—All extremities affected; lower more than upper (30% to 40% of spastic CP)
- **Tetraplegia**—All four extremities involved: legs and trunk, mouth, pharynx, and tongue (10% to 15% of spastic CP)
- **Triplegia**—Three limbs involved
- **Monoplegia**—Only one limb involved
- **Hemiplegia**—Motor dysfunction on one side of the body; upper extremity more affected than lower (20% to 30% of spastic CP)
- Hypertonicity with poor control of posture, balance, and coordinated motion
- Impairment of fine and gross motor skills

Dyskinetic (Nonspastic, Extrapyramidal)

- **Athetoid**—Chorea (involuntary, irregular, jerking movements); characterized by slow, wormlike, writhing movements that usually involve the extremities, trunk, neck, facial muscles, and tongue
- **Dystonic**—Slow, twisting movements of the trunk or extremities; abnormal posture
- Involvement of the pharyngeal, laryngeal, and oral muscles causing drooling and dysarthria (imperfect speech articulation)

Ataxic (Nonspastic, Extrapyramidal)

- Wide-based gait
- Rapid, repetitive movements performed poorly
- Disintegration of movements of the upper extremities when the child reaches for objects

Mixed Type

- Combination of spastic CP and dyskinetic CP
- May be labeled *mixed* when no specific motor pattern is dominant; however, this term is losing favor to more precise descriptions of motor function and affected area of brain involved (Rosenbaum, Paneth, Leviton, et al., 2007)

Data from Nehring, W. (2010). Cerebral palsy. In P. J. Allen, J. A. Vessey, & N. A. Schapiro (Eds.), *Primary care of the child with a chronic condition* (5th ed.). St. Louis, MO: Mosby; Jones, M. W., Morgan, E., Shelton, J. E., et al. (2007). Cerebral palsy: Introduction and diagnosis, part 1. *Journal of Pediatric Health Care, 21*(3), 146–152; and National Institute of Neurologic Disorders and Stroke. (2006). Cerebral palsy: Hope through research. Retrieved from https://www.ninds.nih.gov/Disorders/Patient-Caregiver-Education/Hope-Through-Research/Cerebral-Palsy-Hope-Through-Research

Clinical Manifestations

The alert observer may suspect CP when a child demonstrates some of the groups of manifestations in Box 30.2.

Delayed Gross Motor Development

Delayed gross motor development is a universal manifestation of CP. The child shows a delay in all motor accomplishments, and the discrepancy between motor ability and expected achievement tends to increase with successive developmental milestones as growth advances. It is especially significant if other developmental behaviors, such as language and personal-social achievement, are normal. Delayed development of the ability to balance may also slow the progression of milestones.

Abnormal Motor Performance

Neuromotor dysfunction is particularly evident in motor performance. An early sign is preferential unilateral hand use that may be apparent at approximately 6 months of age. Hand dominance does not normally develop until the preschool years. Abnormal crawling

BOX 30.2 Clinical Manifestations of Cerebral Palsy (at Time of Diagnosis)

Delayed Gross Motor Development
- A universal manifestation
- Delay in all motor accomplishments
- Increases as growth advances
- Delays more obvious as growth advances

Abnormal Motor Performance
- Very early preferential unilateral hand preference
- Abnormal and asymmetric crawl
- Standing or walking on toes
- Uncoordinated or involuntary movements
- Poor sucking
- Feeding difficulties
- Persistent tongue thrust

Alterations of Muscle Tone
- Increased or decreased resistance to passive movements
- Opisthotonic posturing (arching of back)
- Feels stiff on handling or dressing
- Difficulty in diapering
- Rigid and unbending at the hip and knee joints when pulled to sitting position (early sign)

Abnormal Postures
- Maintains hips higher than trunk in prone position with legs and arms flexed or drawn under the body
- Scissoring and extension of legs with feet plantar flexed in supine position
- Persistent infantile resting and sleeping position
- Arms abducted at shoulders
- Elbows flexed
- Hands fisted

Reflex Abnormalities
- Persistence of primitive infantile reflexes
- Obligatory tonic neck reflex at any age
- Nonpersistence beyond 6 months of age
- Persistence or hyperactivity of the Moro, plantar, and palmar grasp reflexes
- Hyperreflexia, ankle clonus, and stretch reflexes elicited in many muscle groups on fast, passive movements

Associated Disabilities
- Altered learning and reasoning
- Seizures
- Impaired behavioral and interpersonal relationships
- Sensory impairment (vision, hearing)

From Nehring, W. M. (2010). Cerebral palsy. In P. J. Allen, J. A. Vessey, & N. A. Schapiro (Eds.), *Primary care of the child with a chronic condition* (5th ed.). St. Louis, MO: Mosby. Adapted from Jones, M. W., Morgan, E., & Shelton, J. E. (2007). Primary care of the child with cerebral palsy: A review of systems (part II). *Journal of Pediatric Health Care, 21*(4), 226–237.

with propulsion by hand movements only and with lower extremities and hips hiked along, much like a "bunny hop," occurs in diplegia. Children with hemiplegia have an asymmetric crawl, using the unaffected arm and leg to propel themselves on either the buttocks or the abdomen. Spasticity may cause the child to stand or walk on the toes. Uncoordinated or involuntary movements are characteristic of dyskinetic CP, and facial grimacing and writhing movements of the tongue, fingers, and toes are signs of athetosis. Other significant signs of motor dysfunction are poor sucking and feeding difficulties, with persistent tongue thrust. Head staggering, tremor on reaching, and truncal ataxia are also common. Hand preference in the first 2 years of life is reported to be a sign of hemiplegic CP (Berker & Yalçin, 2008).

Alterations of Muscle Tone

Increased or decreased resistance to passive movements is a sign of abnormal muscle tone. The child may exhibit opisthotonic postures (exaggerated arching of the back) and may feel stiff on handling or dressing. Also, there is difficulty in diapering because of spasticity of the hip adductor muscles and lower extremities. When pulled to a sitting position, the child may extend the entire body and be rigid and unbending at the hip and knee joints. This is an early sign of spasticity.

Abnormal Posture

Children with spastic CP assume abnormal postures at rest or when their position is changed. From an early age, a child lying in a prone position will maintain the hips higher than the trunk with the legs and arms flexed or drawn under the body. In the supine position spasticity is evident by scissoring (legs in crossed position; knees, hips, and ankles stiff) and extension of the legs, with the feet plantar flexed. This posture is exaggerated when the child is suspended vertically or when others try to make the child bear weight. Depending on the degree of impairment, spasticity may be mild or severe. A persistent infantile resting and sleeping posture (i.e., arms abducted at shoulders, elbows flexed, and hands fisted) is a sign of spasticity when it remains constant after 4 to 5 months of age. The hemiparetic child may rest with the affected arm adducted and held against the torso, with the elbow pronated and slightly flexed and the hand closed.

Reflex Abnormalities

Persistence of primitive reflexes is one of the earliest clues to CP (e.g., obligatory tonic neck reflex at any age or nonobligatory persistence beyond 6 months of age, and the persistence or even hyperactivity of the Moro, plantar, and palmar grasp reflexes). Hyperreflexia, ankle clonus, and stretch reflexes can be elicited from many muscle groups on fast passive movements (e.g., resistance to passive abduction when the hips are suddenly separated [adductor catch]).

Associated Disabilities and Problems

Some of the disabilities associated with CP are visual impairment, hearing impairment, behavioral problems, communication and speech difficulties, seizures, and intellectual impairment. Additional sensory deficits such as hypersensitivity, hyposensitivity, and balance difficulties may occur in children with CP (Nehring, 2010). According to the Centers for Disease Control and Prevention (2019), about 1 in 10 children with CP are also diagnosed with autism spectrum disorder.

Intellectual impairment is a concern, although children with CP have a wide range of intelligence, and 50% to 60% are within normal limits. Speech difficulties are often interpreted as a sign of cognitive impairment. Assessing the intelligence of a child with CP is often difficult because of the motor and sensory deficits. Tests carried out periodically over time should determine the degree of intelligence. Many persons with CP who have severely limiting physical involvement actually have the least intellectual impairment. As a group, children with athetosis and ataxia are intellectually superior to those with other types of CP. The incidence of severe or profound impairment is highest in rigid and atonic CP. Improved communication devices (e.g., communication jacket, computerized communication) have revealed that some people with quadriplegic spastic CP have normal intelligence. Rick Hoyt, for example, who has quadriplegic spastic CP, communicates with his eyes and slight head movement and a computer to spell what he wants to communicate; he graduated from University of Boston and serves as consultant for technology devices.

The manifestations of attention-deficit/hyperactivity disorder may occur in children with CP. The primary presenting symptoms are poor attention span, marked distractibility, hyperactive behavior, and defects of integration (see Chapter 16). Seizures are more likely to accompany postnatally acquired hemiplegia. They are an unusual finding in ataxia and diplegia. The most common types of seizures are generalized tonic-clonic seizures and minor motor types (Nehring, 2010). Epilepsy is reported to occur in 41% of children with CP; epilepsy was especially common in nonambulatory children (Christensen, Van Naarden Braun, Doernberg, et al., 2014).

Poor control of oral musculature may contribute to a number of problems. Abnormal posture and motor performance and alterations in muscle tone affect chewing, swallowing, and talking. Occupational and speech-language therapy interventions may be necessary to assist some children with feeding and speech. Coughing and choking, especially while eating, may predispose the child with CP to aspiration, which may not be readily apparent. Respiratory problems may result from and coexist with feeding difficulties in children with CP; respiratory symptoms observed during feedings include apnea, dyspnea, tachypnea, coughing and choking, and hypoxemia (Nehring, 2010). Many children with CP may also have gastroesophageal reflux.

Motor impairment associated with CP contributes to other problems. Children with CP who are nonambulatory have an increased risk of developing orthopedic complications such as unilateral or bilateral hip dislocations, scoliosis, and joint contractures resulting from unbalanced muscle tone. One study examined the Cobb angle for use in predicting the course of scoliosis in adolescents with CP (Oda, Takigawa, Sugimoto, et al., 2017).

A variety of factors, including decreased mobility, decreased fluid intake, a fear of toileting, poor positioning on the toilet, and lack of fiber intake, may be responsible for constipation (Nehring, 2010). Stool softeners, laxatives, and a bowel management program may be required to prevent chronic constipation.

Increased incidence of dental caries results from improper dental hygiene, congenital enamel defects (hypoplasia of primary teeth), high carbohydrate intake and retention, dietary imbalance with poor nutritional intake, inadequate fluoride, and difficulty in mouth closure and drooling. Spastic or clonic movements can cause gagging or biting down on the toothbrush, thus interfering with cleaning techniques. Oral hypersensitivity is also common, which causes the child to resist dental hygiene. Malocclusion can occur in as many as 90% of these children. Gingivitis is secondary to inadequate dental hygiene and may be further complicated by the use of antiepileptic drugs (AEDs) such as phenytoin (Nehring, 2010). Sehrawat and colleagues (2014) presented an eloquent coverage of the complexities and importance of dental care in children with CP. The CP multidisciplinary clinic within the University of Kansas Medical Center included a dental assistant at each clinic as part of the Kansas state initiative to improve oral health. The nurse may check with the state to see if it could provide this for special needs children. It was most helpful for families to receive teaching on oral health.

Skin breakdown may occur with prolonged positioning, especially with underweight children with bony prominences and those who are unable to reposition themselves or who may have insensate areas of skin.

Nystagmus and amblyopia are common and may require surgery, corrective lenses, or both. Hearing impairment is also common in children with CP. Some loss is caused by sensorineural involvement. Affected infants may spend increased amounts of time lying flat. This predisposes them to otitis media, which may result in conductive hearing loss.

Diagnostic Evaluation

Infants at risk according to known etiologic factors associated with CP warrant careful assessment during early infancy to identify the signs of muscular dysfunction as early as possible. Recent clinical practice guidelines recommend that a diagnosis of CP or of high risk of CP, can be made within the first 6 months postterm age (Spittle, Morgan, Olsen, et al., 2018). The neurologic examination and history are the primary modalities for diagnosis. Neuroimaging of the child with suspected brain abnormality and CP, is now recommended for diagnostic assessment, with MRI being a strong predictor of CP when performed at term (corrected age); general movements assessment also had a strong predictive value in children older than 2 years of age and younger than 5 years of age (Bosanquet, Copeland, Ware, et al., 2013). MRI has the capability of early identification of infants at risk for CP (George, Fiori, Fripp, et al., 2017). MRI was useful in predicting language development in people with certain brain lesions (Choi, Choi, & Park, 2017). Metabolic and genetic testing is recommended if no structural abnormality is identified by neuroimaging; laboratory tests are no longer recommended in the diagnostic process for CP.

Early recognition is made more difficult by the lack of reliable neonatal neurologic signs. However, the nurse should monitor infants with known etiologic risk factors and evaluate them closely in the first 2 years of life. Because cortical control of movement does not occur until later in infancy, motor impairment associated with voluntary control is usually not apparent until after 2 to 4 months of age at the earliest. More often the diagnosis cannot be confirmed until the age of 1 or 2 years because motor tone abnormalities may be indicative of another neuromuscular condition. In addition, some children who show signs consistent with CP before 2 years do not demonstrate such signs after 2 years (Nehring, 2010). However, there is no consensus regarding an age cutoff for the onset of symptoms.

Establishing a diagnosis may be easier with the persistence of primitive reflexes: either the asymmetric tonic neck reflex or the persistent Moro reflex (beyond 4 months of age), and the crossed extensor reflex. The tonic neck reflex normally disappears between 4 and 6 months of age. An obligatory response is considered abnormal. This is elicited by turning the infant's head to one side and holding it there for 20 seconds. When a crying infant is unable to move from the asymmetric posturing of the tonic neck reflex, it is considered obligatory and an abnormal response. The crossed extensor reflex, which normally disappears by 4 months, is elicited by applying a noxious stimulus to the sole of one foot with the knee extended. Normally the contralateral foot responds with extensor, abduction, and then adduction movements. The possibility of CP is suggested if these reflexes occur after 4 months.

A number of assessment instruments are available to evaluate muscle spasticity (Modified Ashworth Scale); functional independence in self-care, mobility, and cognition (Functional Independence Measure and WeeFIM [specific to children]); self-initiated movements over time (Gross Motor Function Measure); and capability and performance of functional activities in self-care, mobility, and social function (Pediatric Evaluation of Disability Inventory) (Krigger, 2006). Elastography is a new way to measure the flexibility of muscles, tendons, and nerves. A new technique, myotonometry, allows objective assessment of muscle spasticity by quantifying tissue displacement response to a standard measuring compression force, and it is suggested to be a sensitive method that can be used in daily clinical practice (Balci, 2018).

BOX 30.3 Therapeutic Interventions for Cerebral Palsy

Interdisciplinary developmental and physical assessment with recommendations may include the following:

Physical Therapy

Orthotic Devices
- Braces
- Splints
- Casting
- Molded orthoses

Adaptive Equipment
- Scooters, bicycles, and tricycles
- Wheelchairs
- Boards
- Standing devices

Functional (Neuromuscular) Electrical Stimulation (in Combination With Dynamic Splinting)

Occupational Therapy

Adaptive Equipment
- Utensils for functional use (e.g., eating, writing)
- Switches
- Computers

Speech-Language Therapy
- Oral-motor skills
- Adaptive communication techniques

Special Education
- Early intervention programs
- Specialized learning programs and support services in school
- Socialization to promote self-concept development

Surgical Intervention
- Orthopedic (e.g., tendon transfers, muscle lengthening, spinal deformities)
- Neurologic (e.g., neurectomies)
- Selective dorsal rhizotomy
- Feeding (e.g., gastrostomy)
- Dental

Medication Therapy
- Medications to treat the following:
  - Spasticity
  - Pain
  - Secondary conditions (e.g., seizure disorder, chronic constipation, urinary tract infections, gastroesophageal reflux)
- Primary care for health supervision and acute childhood illnesses

Behavioral Therapy

Care Coordination
- Care coordination of specialized services and community resources in collaboration with the child's family

Modified from Nehring, W. M. (2010). Cerebral palsy. In P. J. Allen, J. A. Vessey, & N. A. Schapiro (Eds.), *Primary care of the child with a chronic condition* (5th ed.). St. Louis, MO: Mosby.

A thorough knowledge of normal variations of motor development is required for detecting abnormal progress, and a careful history is necessary to detect possible etiologic factors. Observe the child's spontaneous movements and behavior, including posture; attitude; and muscle size, function, and tone. Because children with CP often have sensory deficits, it is appropriate to evaluate the child for hearing and vision deficits.

Therapeutic Management: General Concepts

The goals of therapy for children with CP are early recognition and promotion of an optimum developmental course to enable affected children to attain their potential within the limits of their dysfunction. The disorder is permanent, and therapy is chiefly symptomatic and preventive.

The beneficial influences of a habilitation program on both child and family are based on recognizing the disability as early as possible and implementing treatment. Parents are essential to a treatment program. Consider their goals and desires, their cooperation, and their confidence in all aspects of management. With early diagnosis parents can begin to provide the sensorimotor experiences essential to cognitive development because central nervous system (CNS) structures depend on stimulation and use to attain and maintain their functional integrity.

The broad aims of therapy are to (1) establish locomotion, communication, and self-help skills; (2) gain optimum appearance and integration of motor functions; (3) correct associated defects as early and effectively as possible; (4) provide educational opportunities adapted to the individual child's needs and capabilities; and (5) promote socialization experiences with other affected and unaffected children. Each child is evaluated and managed on an individual basis. The plan of therapy may involve a variety of settings, facilities, and specially trained persons. The scope of the child's needs requires multidisciplinary planning and care coordination among professionals and the child's family (Box 30.3). The outcome for the child and family with CP is normalization and promotion of self-care activities that empower the child and family to achieve maximum potential.

Mobilizing Devices

Many children with CP wear ankle–foot orthoses (AFOs) (braces) and a variety of orthotics. Orthotics are molded to fit the feet and are worn inside the shoes. Devices are often used to help prevent or reduce deformity, increase the energy efficiency of gait, and control alignment. Some of the more commonly used mobility devices include wheeled scooter boards that allow children to propel themselves while the abdomen or total body is supported and the legs are positioned with wedges to prevent scissoring. Wheeled go-carts provide good sitting balance and serve as an early "wheelchair" experience for young children. Strollers can be equipped with custom seats for dependent mobilization. Special devices for independent mobilization that may or may not allow the upper extremities to remain free are particularly valuable for children with lower extremity involvement (Fig. 30.1). A number of wheelchairs can be customized to meet the needs and preferences of older children (Fig. 30.2).

Surgery

Surgical intervention is usually reserved for the child who does not respond to more conservative measures such as orthotics, but it is also indicated for the child whose spasticity causes progressive deformities. Orthopedic surgery may be required to correct contracture or spastic deformities, to provide stability for an uncontrollable joint, to address bone malalignment (e.g., lever arm dysfunction), and to provide balanced muscle power. This includes tendon-lengthening procedures

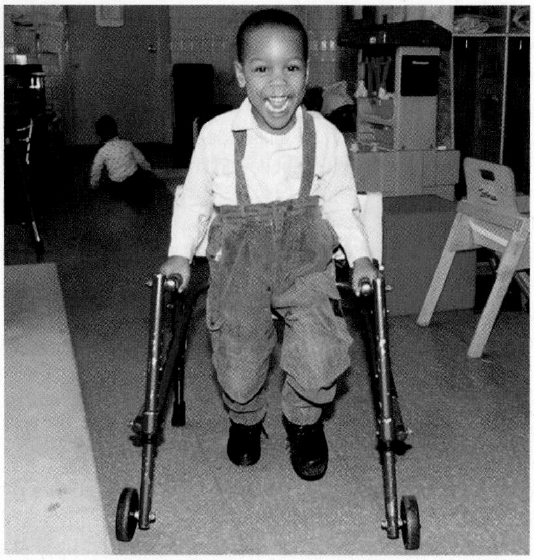

Fig. 30.1 Child ambulating with use of assistive device.

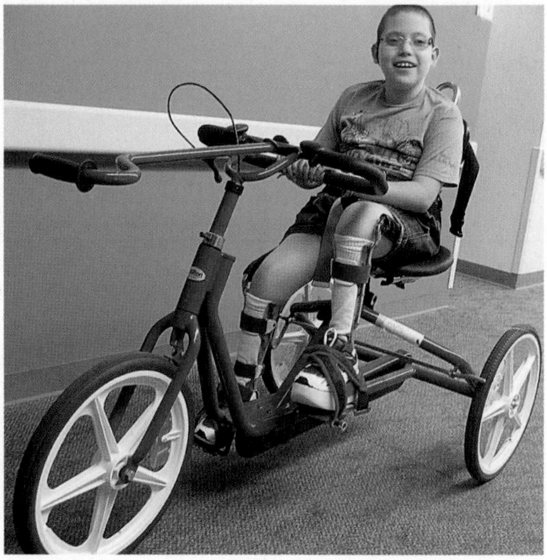

Fig. 30.2 Bike walker used to provide mobility and to enhance leg muscle strength.

(especially heel-cord lengthening), release of spastic wrist flexor muscles, and correction of hip and adductor muscle spasticity or contracture to improve locomotion. Orthopedic specialists with special interest in CP will implement hip observation protocols for children considered at risk for hip abnormalities. Hip surveillance and surgical salvage choices are individual for each person with CP. There is not one procedure that fits all. Orthopedic surgery is generally not performed until after the child is 6 years old (Nehring, 2010). Surgery is used primarily to improve function rather than for cosmetic purposes and is followed by physical therapy. Surgery may also be performed to improve caloric intake, correct gastroesophageal reflux disease, prevent aspiration, and correct associated dental problems (Nehring, 2010).

Neurosurgical procedures are used only in selected cases. Selective dorsal rhizotomy has provided marked improvement in some children with CP (Park, Dobbs, & Cho, 2018). After selective dorsal rhizotomy, gait was improved in children with CP (Rumberg, Bakir, Taylor, et al., 2016). However, achieving the benefits from the surgery requires intensive physical therapy and family commitment. Because the procedure results in flaccid muscles, the child must relearn to sit, stand, and walk.

Medication

Intense pain may occur with muscle spasms in patients with CP. Children with CP may also experience pain as a result of painful procedures such as injection with botulinum toxin type A (Botox), surgical procedures intended to reduce contracture deformities, abdominal pain related to position and gastroesophageal reflux, and pain associated with physical therapy. Therefore pain management is an important aspect of the care of the child with CP.

Pharmacologic agents given orally (dantrolene sodium [Dantrium], baclofen [Lioresal], and diazepam [Valium]) have had little effectiveness in improving muscle coordination in children with CP. However, they are effective in decreasing overall spasticity. The most common side effects of these agents include hepatotoxicity (dantrolene), drowsiness, fatigue, and muscle weakness. Less commonly, diaphoresis and constipation may occur with oral baclofen; other possible complications include hallucinations, mood changes, seizures, nausea, and urinary incontinence. Diazepam is used frequently but should be restricted to older children and adolescents.

Botulinum toxin A is also used to reduce spasticity in targeted muscles of the upper and lower extremities (Yana, Tutuola, Westwater-Wood, et al., 2019). Botulinum toxin A is injected into a selected muscle (commonly the quadriceps, gastrocnemius, or medial hamstrings), where it acts to inhibit the release of acetylcholine into a specific muscle group, thereby preventing muscle movement. When it is administered early in the course of the illness, this may prevent affected muscle contractures, particularly in lower extremities, thus avoiding surgical procedures with possible adverse effects. The goal is to allow stretching of the muscle; as it relaxes, it permits ambulation with an AFO. The major reported adverse effects of botulinum toxin A injection include pain at the injection site and a temporary weakness (Yana et al., 2019). Prime candidates for botulinum toxin A injections are children with spasticity confined to the lower extremities. The onset of action occurs within 24 to 72 hours, with a peak effect observed at 2 weeks and a duration of action of 3 to 6 months. Decreasing spasticity with botulinum toxin A may also result in less pain from spasms (Yana et al., 2019). One case study showed improvement with spinal balance after one botulinum toxin A injection (Chaléat-Valayer, Bernard, Deceuninck, et al., 2016).

The neurosurgical and pharmacologic approach to managing the spasticity associated with CP involves the implantation of a pump to infuse baclofen directly into the intrathecal space surrounding the spinal cord to provide relief of spasticity. High doses of oral baclofen are associated with significant side effects, including drowsiness and confusion, yet are often unable to provide adequate relief of spasticity. Direct infusion of baclofen into the intrathecal space is especially helpful in improving comfort without as many side effects (Eek, Olsson, Lindh, et al., 2018).

One study combined baclofen and antibiotic in the pump to prevent infection and maintain lasting stability and benefit of the pump (Aristedis, Dimitrios, Nikolaos, et al., 2017). Patients may be screened before pump placement by the infusion of a "test dose" of intrathecal baclofen delivered via a lumbar puncture. Close monitoring for side effects (e.g., hypotonia, somnolence, seizures, nausea, vomiting, headache, catheter- or pump-related problems) and relief of spasticity occurs for several hours after the infusion. If a positive effect occurs, the patient is considered a candidate for pump placement.

The pump is placed in the subcutaneous space of the midabdomen; it is about the size of a hockey puck. An intrathecal catheter is tunneled from the lumbar area to the abdomen and connected to the pump. The pump is filled with baclofen and programmed to provide a set dose using a telemetry wand and a computer. The patient remains hospitalized for several days to adjust the dosage and ensure proper healing. Outpatient visits to refill the pump and make dosage adjustments occur about every 4 to 6 weeks, depending on the patient's response to the treatment. Benefits of intrathecal baclofen include fewer systemic side effects, dosage titration for maximizing effects, and reversibility of therapy with removal of the pump if so desired. Abrupt withdrawal of intrathecal baclofen, especially at high doses, may result in adverse effects such as rebound spasticity, pruritus, hyperthermia, rhabdomyolysis, disseminated intravascular coagulation, multiorgan failure, and death; in some cases intrathecal baclofen withdrawal may mimic sepsis. Treatment of withdrawal centers on reestablishing the medication dosage, with improvements observed within 1 to 2 hours. Hospitalization and surgery may be required for withdrawal as a result of pump or catheter failure.

AEDs such as carbamazepine (Tegretol), divalproex (valproate sodium and valproic acid [Depakote]), oxcarbazepine (Trileptal), and lamotrigine (Lamictal) are prescribed routinely for children who have seizures. Gabapentin (Neurontin) has been used in adults with spinal cord injury (SCI) to decrease spasticity with success. Yuan-Kim Liow and colleagues (2016) found that gabapentin improved quality of life, pain, and dystonia in children with CP. The α_2-adrenergic agonists clonidine (Catapres) and tizanidine (Zanaflex) have been used to decrease spasticity in adults with SCI and multiple sclerosis; however, their use in children does not appear to have gained widespread acceptance in the United States. Oral tizanidine given in conjunction with botulinum type A has been reported to be more effective than oral baclofen and botulinum type A in one study of children with CP (Dai, Wasay, & Awan, 2008). Monitor all medications for maintenance of therapeutic levels and avoidance of subtherapeutic or toxic levels (see Quality Patient Outcomes box).

QUALITY PATIENT OUTCOMES: Seizures
- No physical injury as a result of seizure activity
- Prevention of seizure activity

Children with CP have been treated with a number of complementary and alternative medicine strategies, including Chinese herbs, acupuncture, growth hormone therapy, aquatic exercise, equine-assisted therapy, and hyperbaric oxygen (Nehring, 2010). Gasalberti (2006) reported some alternative therapies being used in children with disabilities that the practitioner may overlook during a health history but that may be beneficial to such children. These include pet therapy, massage, hippotherapy (horse riding), music, and color-light therapy. Other alternative therapies that may be used by families with children with disabilities include vitamins, prayer, meditation, hypnosis, and guided imagery.

Technical Aids

A wide variety of technical aids are available to improve the functioning of children with CP. These include electromechanical toys that use the concept of biofeedback and operate from a head unit. The toy is manipulated only when the head and trunk are in correct alignment. Computerized toys and games can also enhance eye-hand coordination.

Microcomputers combined with voice synthesizers help children with speech difficulties to "speak." Smart phones and tablets with speech applications are appropriate for some children. These and other devices print messages onto screen monitors and paper. These devices have made it apparent that some children have been erroneously considered to be cognitively impaired. Microcomputers have also increased the possibilities for increased mobility via wheelchairs and specially designed mobilization devices.

Many other electronic devices allow independent functioning. Computerized games have been studied to help with fine motor skills in school-age children (Kanitkar, Szturm, Parmar, et al., 2017). Robots were studied to help improve movement in children with CP; there is a need for more cost-effective robots to further evaluate effectiveness (Michmizos & Krebs, 2017). Combined brain stimulation and robotics improved upper limb functioning in adults with CP; more study is needed with children (Friel, Lee, Soles, et al., 2017).

Sensors can be activated and deactivated using a head-stick, a voluntary muscle such as the tongue, or any other voluntary muscle movement over which the child has control. The application of this technology makes it possible for older persons with CP to eventually function in their own apartments and can be extended into the workplace.

Associated Problems

Children with CP often have sensory deficits, which require the attention of appropriate specialists. Speech-language therapy involves the services of a speech-language pathologist (SLP) who may also assist with feeding problems (see Chapter 20). Dental care is especially important for children with CP and often is overlooked. Regular visits to the dentist and dental prophylaxis, including brushing, fluoride, and flossing (after several teeth are present), should begin as soon as the teeth erupt. This is especially important for children given phenytoin, who often develop gum hyperplasia. Additional problems common among children with CP include constipation caused by neurologic deficits and lack of exercise; poor bladder control and urinary retention; chronic respiratory tract infections and aspiration pneumonia, which occur as a result of gastroesophageal reflux, abnormal muscle tone, immobility, and altered positioning; and skin problems as a result of altered positioning, poor nutrition, and immobility. Hip dislocation occurs often in children with CP. Latex allergy has also been reported in children with CP (Nehring, 2010).

Therapeutic Management: Therapies, Education, Recreation

Physical Therapy

Physical therapy is one of the most commonly used treatment modalities in children with CP. In general, physical therapy is directed toward good skeletal alignment for the child with spasticity; training in purposeful acts, even in the face of involuntary motion, for the child with athetosis; and gait training and maximum development of proprioceptive sense for the child with ataxia.

An active therapy program involves the family, the physical therapist (PT), the occupational therapist (OT), and other members of the health care team. Developing a treatment program that can be carried out at home is of utmost importance. The major approach uses traditional types of therapeutic exercises that consist of stretching; passive, active, and resistive movements applied to specific muscle groups or joints to maintain or increase range of motion; strength; or endurance. Neuromuscular electrical stimulation combined with dynamic splinting may benefit some children (Wright, Durham, Ewins, et al., 2012). No therapeutic approach is able to achieve spectacular changes in the ultimate outcome of motor disability. Early efforts focus on alleviating abnormal postures by positioning and range-of-motion exercises. Passive range-of-motion exercises, stretching, and elongation exercises are valuable at any age, even when the child is too young to cooperate. Some active extension can be performed when the child is old enough to cooperate, with passive motion applied to complete joint extension. Prevention of contracture deformity is a prime function of physical therapy. Seating, mobility, strength, and endurance are other key goals.

Functional and Adaptive Training (Occupational Therapy)

Training in manual skills and activities of daily living (ADLs) proceeds along developmental lines and according to the child's functional level. Sitting, balancing, crawling, and walking are encouraged at appropriate ages and are accompanied by stimulation of protective extension and equilibrium reactions. Hand activities are begun early to improve motor function and provide the child with sensory experiences and information about the environment. As the child progresses from simple feeding and self-care activities, training is extended to include other tasks (e.g., cooking or use of keyboard or computer mouse) that are within the child's developmental and functional capabilities.

Incorporating play into the therapeutic program often requires great ingenuity and inventiveness from those involved in the child's care. Objects and toys are chosen to provide needed sensory input using a variety of shapes, forms, and textures. Nurses can help parents integrate therapy into play activities in natural ways.

Children with CP may need considerable help (and patience) in learning to feed and dress themselves and care for personal hygiene needs. A feeding program may be developed by an OT in conjunction with an SLP. Children should be fed in the normal eating position. When they have difficulty sucking and swallowing, it is tempting to hold them in a semireclining posture to make use of gravity flow. However, this method does not promote active swallowing, and the neck hyperextension may even interfere with swallowing. A more flexed sitting position, with the arms brought forward to decrease the tendency toward back and neck extension, is more natural during bottle- or spoon-feeding and encourages active swallowing.

Because jaw control is compromised, more normal control can be achieved if the feeder provides stability for the oral mechanism from the side or front of the face. When directed from the front, the middle finger of the nonfeeding hand is placed posterior to the bony portion of the chin, the thumb is placed below the bottom lip, and the index finger is placed parallel to the child's mandible (Fig. 30.3). Manual jaw control from the side assists with head control, correction of neck and trunk hyperextension, and jaw stabilization. The middle finger of the nonfeeding hand is placed posterior to the bony portion of the chin, the index finger is placed on the chin below the lower lip, and the thumb is placed obliquely across the cheek to provide lateral jaw stability (Fig. 30.4).

In all ADLs it is important to capitalize on the child's assets and compensate for liabilities. The level of expected independence is related to both gross and fine motor manipulation. Even when complete independence in a specific activity is not realistic, the child should learn any part of the task that he or she can master. However, motor function is not the sole purpose of learning to be as independent as possible. Any accomplishment promotes self-reliance and self-esteem for healthier personality development.

Speech Therapy

Speech training under the supervision of an SLP begins early, before the child learns poor habits of communication. Parents and others can help by following the directions of the speech therapist and by talking to the child slowly while using pictures or handling objects about which the adult is speaking. Feeding techniques such as forcing the child to use the lips and tongue in eating facilitate speech. An example of this technique is placing food at the side of the tongue, first one side

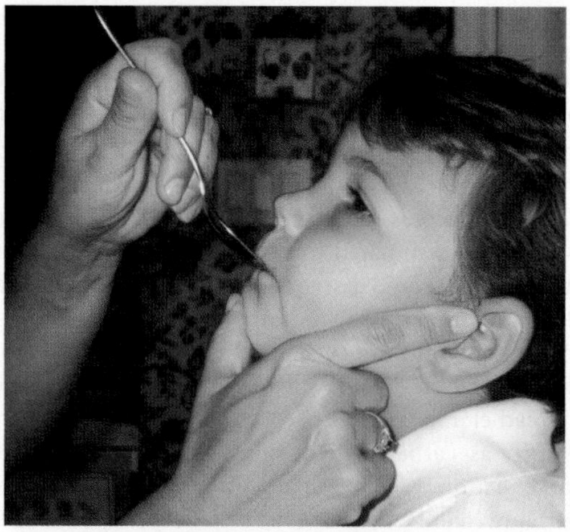

Fig. 30.3 Manual jaw control provided anteriorly.

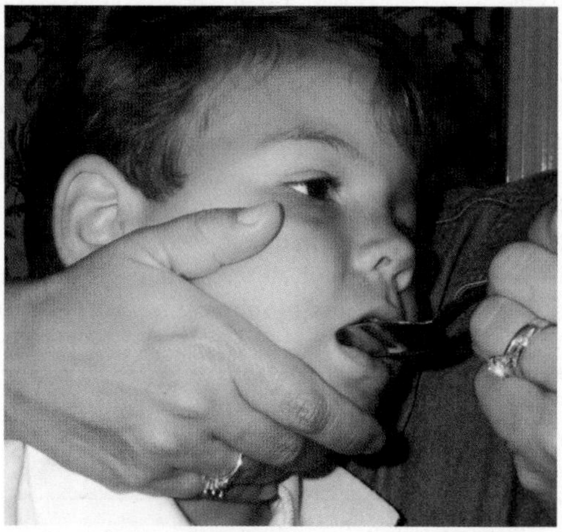

Fig. 30.4 Manual jaw control provided from the side.

and then the other, and making the child use the lips to take food from a spoon rather than placing it directly on the tongue. If severe dysarthria prevents articulate speech and the child has reasonable intelligence, the child learns nonverbal communication (e.g., sign language) (see Chapter 18).

Education

As in all aspects of care, educational requirements are determined by the child's needs and potential. This includes the severity of the child's disease and the presence and degree of associated conditions that affect learning and participation, such as learning impairment, abnormal actions or behaviors, impaired vision or hearing, and seizures. Children with mild to moderate cognitive involvement are generally able to participate, for varying amounts of time, in regular classes. Resource rooms are available in most schools to provide more individualized attention to a child's particular needs. Integration of these children into regular classrooms should be the initial goal. Teachers' assistants often work one-on-one with children in both settings. A training program may be appropriate for those children who are unable to benefit from formal education. Prevocational and vocational counseling and guidance are arranged at adolescence. Education is geared toward the child's assets at any phase or in any setting. Nurses should be aware of early intervention programs and provisions for special education and related services for children and should support parents in their efforts to obtain appropriate educational services for the child. Bourke-Taylor and colleagues (2017) emphasized the importance of collaboration among team members of school-age children with CP in schools, in the community, in health care, and across the life span for best outcomes.

Recreation

Recreational activities are also a necessary part of growing up. Recreational outlets and after-school activities should be an option for the child who is unable to participate in regular athletic and other peer activities. Some can compete in athletic and artistic endeavors, and many games and pastimes are suited to their capabilities. Sports, physical fitness, and recreation programs are encouraged for children with CP, and young children should be exposed to all physical activities available to children without disabilities. Individual sports such as the martial arts (e.g., Tae Kwon Do) in which groups are small and the emphasis is on discipline and balance are also enjoyable to many children with CP. Many states mandate adaptive physical education classes.

Numerous developmental centers have facilities for indoor and outdoor activities designed to appeal to children of all ages. If these are not available, they should be developed. However, such programs require adequate supervision to avoid any harmful effects. Recreational activities serve to stimulate children's interest and curiosity, help them adjust to their disability, improve their functional abilities, and build self-esteem. Competitive sports are also becoming increasingly available to children with disabilities and offer an added dimension to physical activities. For more information, access the United Cerebral Palsy website (http://www.ucp.org) and go to the Sports and Leisure link. Any accomplishment that helps children approach a normal way of life enhances their self-concept.

Prognosis

The prognosis for the child with CP depends largely on the type and severity of the condition. Children with mild to moderate involvement (85%) have the capability of achieving ambulation between the ages of 2 and 7 years (Berker & Yalçin, 2008). If the child does not achieve independent ambulation by this time, chances are poor for ambulation and independence. Approximately 30% to 50% of individuals with CP have significant cognitive impairments, and an even higher percentage have mild cognitive and learning deficits (National Institute of Neurological Disorders and Stroke, 2013). Children with profound cognitive impairment have a higher mortality rate, and less than one-half of those children reach adulthood (O'Shea, 2008). However, many children with severe spastic tetraplegic CP have normal intelligence. Growth is affected in children with spastic tetraplegia, and many children remain below the 5th percentile for age and sex.

As children with CP become adults, about 30% remain in the home and are cared for by a parent or caregiver; 50% of individuals with spastic tetraplegia live in independent settings and function at appropriate social levels considering their disability (Green & Hurvitz, 2007). Vocational rehabilitation and higher education are possible for adults with CP. Children with severe CP mobility impairment and feeding problems often succumb to respiratory tract infection in childhood. The few survival rate studies on children or adults with CP show that survival is influenced by existing comorbidities (Nehring, 2010). In general, the more medically fragile children are least likely to survive to adulthood (Westbom, Bergstrand, Wagner, et al., 2011) (see Quality Patient Outcomes box).

QUALITY PATIENT OUTCOMES: Pain

- Acceptable pain threshold experienced as defined by patient or caregiver, or a pain score of 4 or less on Wong-Baker FACES Pain Rating Scale.
- The occurrence of pain in people with cerebral palsy (CP) was measured and found to be similar to previous reports. More attention to the report and treatment of pain needs to be given (Westbom, Rimstedt, & Nordmark, 2017).
- Early detection, prevention, and treatment of pain in children with CP have been studied by several (Adolfsson, Johnson, & Nilsson, 2017).

Nursing Care Management

Assessment

Nursing assessment includes risk identification of infants with etiologic factors that are associated with CP. Ongoing assessment of infants for abnormal muscle tone, inability to achieve developmental milestones, and persistence of neonatal reflexes alert the nurse to investigate further.

Reinforce Therapeutic Plan and Assist in Normalization

Because children are being treated at an earlier age, parents are participating at an earlier stage in treatment programs for their disabled child. They learn the proper handling and home care of young children with CP and need carefully programmed steps so that their expanded parental role can be melded into the established relationship. Close work with other multidisciplinary team members is essential. Nurses reinforce the therapeutic plan and assist the family in devising and modifying equipment and activities to continue the therapy program in the home (see also Chapter 17).

Some children have difficulty keeping their head upright. Because of this, they can neither explore much of their environment nor process the information. Parents need to be complimented on their efforts to provide a stimulating environment for these children. These infants are at risk for delayed development in holding up their heads, righting their shoulders and trunks for stable posture, sitting, pulling, standing, and crawling. Most parents of children with impaired movements benefit from support and practical suggestions for feeding, moving, holding, and encouraging the infant to explore hands and feet and to play. Helping parents incorporate therapeutic suggestions into typical daily activities is an important normalizing strategy.

Although practical advice is important, the nurse, OT, or PT should offer suggestions at a pace that can be absorbed by the parents. Encourage the parents to define their concerns, acknowledge the concerns as genuine, and ask the parents what approaches they have tried and for how long. In this way the nurse is able to find out what works, what does not work, and what the parents would like to try next. Give the parents positive feedback for their observations of the infant, the progress they note, and how they differentiate the child's needs.

Address Health Maintenance Needs

Because children with CP expend so much energy in their efforts to accomplish ADLs, more frequent rest periods should be arranged to avoid the fatigue that may aggravate their limited capabilities. Meeting the child's nutritional needs may be a challenge because of gastroesophageal reflux, feeding and swallowing difficulties, chronic constipation and subsequent anorexia, and absence or diminished ability to independently feed himself or herself (Trivic & Hojsak, 2019). As a result of being ELBW or VLBW in combination with these feeding problems, children with CP are at risk for failure to thrive, and the nurse must ensure an adequate caloric intake. Children with spasticity expend more energy and often require more energy intake than same-age counterparts to maintain adequate growth. Nutritional supplements such as high-calorie milk products (e.g., Pediasure) may be necessary to provide adequate caloric intake after the child has reached 1 year of age. Additional nutritional concerns include providing adequate intake of fruits and fiber to enhance gastrointestinal (GI) motility, routinely monitoring the child's growth on a standardized growth chart, and avoiding overfeeding and obesity (Trivic & Hojsak, 2019).

Routine assessment of skin status is imperative in children with CP who are limited in movement or who must remain in assistive devices such as a wheelchair for a prolonged period. The overall nutritional status may also be a risk factor for skin breakdown. Care must be taken to ensure that adequate objective skin assessments are routinely performed. If skin breakdown does occur, consult a skin and wound specialist for treatment and further prevention.

Gastrostomy feedings may be necessary to supplement regular feedings and ensure adequate weight gain, particularly in children at risk for growth failure and chronic malnutrition, those with severe CP and subsequent oral feeding difficulties, and children whose well-being is affected by illness and decreased fluid or medication intake (Trivic & Hojsak, 2019). Oral feedings may be continued to maintain oral motor skills. Weight gain is perceived as an important measure of adequate oral feeding efficiency along with follow-up and body composition assessments (Trivic & Hojsak, 2019).

Parents may need assistance and advice with medication administration through a gastrostomy tube to prevent clogging. Pills may be crushed and mixed with small amounts of water but not with other liquids, such as formula or elixir medications, because these may act together to form a sludge that can interfere with gastrostomy tube function. When crushed pills or tablets are administered, flush the feeding tube with more water after instilling the dissolved pill in water. The pharmacist can provide information on crushed pills and tablets and elixirs, which should not be mixed together when administered via gastrostomy or nasogastric tube. A skin-level gastrostomy is particularly suited for the child with CP (see also Chapter 20, Gastrostomy Feeding).

Safety precautions are implemented, such as having children wear protective helmets if they are subject to falls or capable of injuring their heads on hard objects. Because the child with CP is at risk for altered proprioception and subsequent falls, parents should adapt the home and play environment to the child's particular needs to prevent bodily harm. Transportation of the child with motor problems and restricted mobility may be especially challenging for the family and child. Attention must be given to the child's safety when riding in a motor vehicle; a federally approved safety restraint should be used at all times. Lovette (2008) recommends that children with CP ride in a rear-facing position for as long as possible because of their poor head, neck, and trunk control. This author also provides a list of options for special car restraint systems for children with CP, including several restraints that are suitable for children with a hip spica cast.

Appropriate immunizations should be administered to prevent childhood illnesses and protect against respiratory tract infections such as influenza. Depending on the level of involvement, dental problems may be more common in children with CP, which creates a need for meticulous attention to all aspects of dental care.

Support the Family

The nursing interventions that are probably most valuable to the family are support and help in coping with the emotional aspects of the chronic disorder, many of which are discussed in Chapter 19. Initially the parents need information and support in understanding the implications of the diagnosis and all the feelings it engenders. Later they need clarification regarding what they can expect from the child and from health care professionals. Educating families in the principles of family-centered care and parent-professional collaboration is essential. The family also may require help to modify the home environment for care of the child. Transportation to the practitioner's office and other health care agencies often requires special considerations.

Care management for the child and family with CP is an important nursing role. In many cases the family assumes complete care of the child and becomes quite adept at caring for her or his individual needs. The home health nurse or case manager has an important role in the support and encouragement of families who assume the primary care of a child with CP. Having a child with CP implies numerous problems of daily management, with changes in family life, and the nurse needs to stress principles of normalization (see Chapter 17, Normalization and Transition).

Parents can also find help and support from parent groups, where they can share experiences, accomplishments, problems, and concerns while deriving comfort and practical information. For example, parents can understand from others what it is like to have a child with CP. United Cerebral Palsy has branches in most communities and provides a variety of services for children and families. A number of excellent books are available to guide parents and nurses who work with children with CP. Many of the books are written by people with CP who have triumphed (e.g., *My Left Foot,* a movie and book).

Care of the Hospitalized Child

CP is not a condition that requires hospitalization; therefore when children with CP are hospitalized, they are usually admitted for an associated illness or for corrective surgery. To facilitate the care and management of hospitalized children with CP, the therapy program should be continued (insofar as their condition allows) while they are hospitalized. This should be incorporated into the multidisciplinary care plan, with every effort expended to make certain the ground that has been so laboriously gained is not lost. Encouraging the parent to room-in and actively participate in the child's care facilitates a continuation of the home therapy program and helps the child adjust to an unfamiliar environment. However, it is equally important to remember that a hospitalization may be the first time a parent can defer care to a nurse and not be the primary caregiver. This respite may be crucial to the parent's well-being. Respect the parent's preference in this regard.

DEFECTS OF NEURAL TUBE CLOSURE

Abnormalities that derive from the embryonic neural tube (**neural tube defects [NTDs]**) constitute the largest group of congenital anomalies with multifactorial inheritance. Normally the spinal cord and cauda equina are encased in a protective sheath of bone and meninges (Fig. 30.5A). Failure of neural tube closure produces defects of varying degrees (Box 30.4). They may involve the entire length of the neural tube or may be restricted to a small area.

ETIOLOGY

Two of the defects, anencephaly and spina bifida (SB), occur in association with each other more often than would be expected by chance, suggesting a common origin. The CNS defects may alternate in siblings, which also tends to support the theory of a common origin. In the United States, approximately 1645 infants with spina bifida are born each year (Centers for Disease Control and Prevention: National Center on Birth Defects and Developmental Disabilities, 2019). The incidence of SB is higher in girls than in boys, and it is more likely to occur in Hispanic (3.8 per 10,000 births) women than in Caucasian

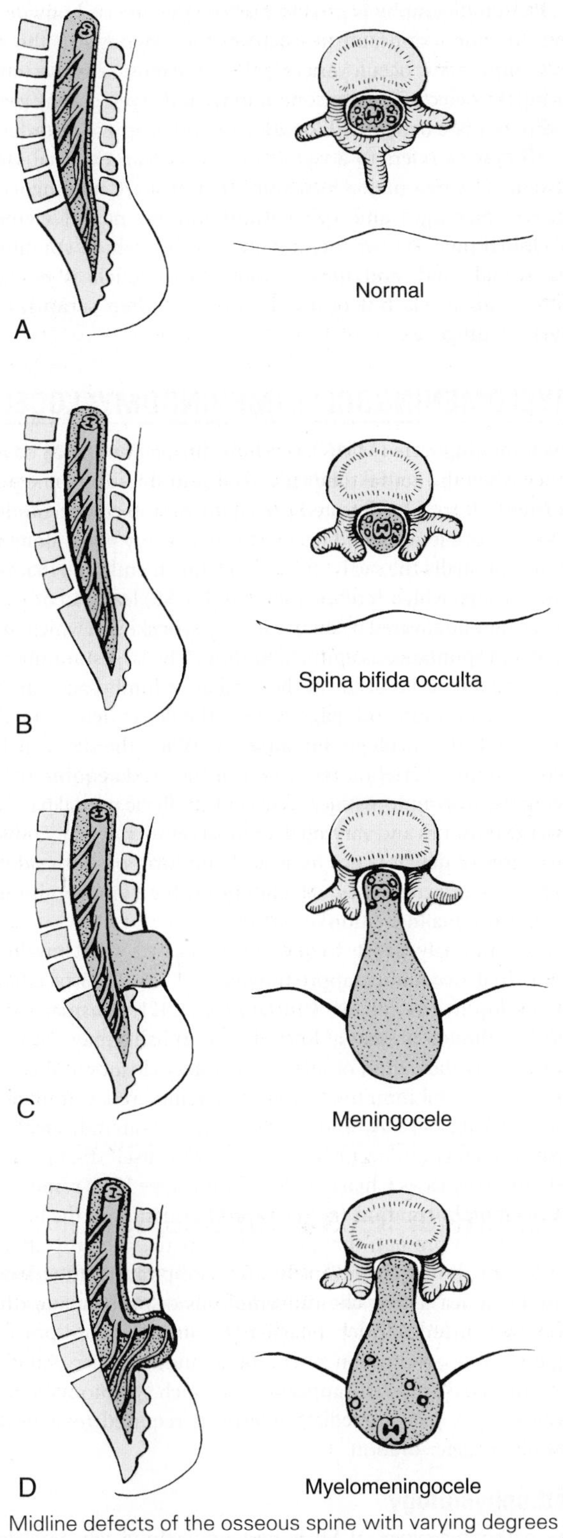

Fig. 30.5 Midline defects of the osseous spine with varying degrees or neural herniations. **A,** Normal. **B,** Spina bifida occulta. **C,** Meningocele. **D,** Myelomeningocele.

(3.09 per 10,000) or African American (2.73 per 10,000) women (Centers for Disease Control and Prevention: National Center on Birth Defects and Developmental Disabilities, 2019).

In the United States, rates of NTDs declined by as much as 23% between 1995 and 2000. NTD rates decreased an additional 6.9% between 2000 and 2005, primarily among African American mothers.

BOX 30.4 Neural Tube Defects

Cranioschisis—A skull defect through which various tissues protrude

Exencephaly—Brain totally exposed or extruded through an associated skull defect; fetus usually aborted

Anencephaly—Congenital malformation in which both cerebral hemispheres are absent

Encephalocele—Herniation of brain and meninges through a defect in the skull producing a fluid-filled sac

Rachischisis or spina bifida—Fissure in the spinal column that leaves the meninges and spinal cord exposed

Meningocele—Hernial protrusion of a saclike cyst of meninges filled with spinal fluid (see Fig. 30.5C)

Myelomeningocele (meningomyelocele)—Hernial protrusion of a saclike cyst containing meninges, spinal fluid, and a portion of the spinal cord with its nerves (see Fig. 30.5D)

One concern is that NTD rates have not decreased significantly among Hispanic and non-Hispanic Caucasian mothers since 1999 (Centers for Disease Control and Prevention, 2009). The decline in NTDs in the late 1990s has been attributed in large part to the addition of folic acid to cereal grain products (Williams, Mai, Mulinare, et al., 2015). Population-based studies have also witnessed a substantial decrease in NTDs since food fortification with folic acid and folic acid supplementation recommendations were made (Williams et al., 2015). Increased use of prenatal diagnostic techniques and termination of pregnancies have also affected the overall incidence of NTDs.

The National Spina Bifida Patient Registry is a data collection program funded by the Centers for Disease Control and Prevention. It was started in 2008 to provide a framework to standardize and improve treatment of children, adolescents, and adults older than 21 years of age. Detailed questionnaires from the participating 10 specialized, multidisciplinary spina bifida clinics provide data, which are sent to a Centers for Disease Control and Prevention database for analysis. This process helps identify the most beneficial care for patients.

Most authorities believe that the primary defect in NTDs is a failure of neural tube closure during the embryo's early development (between the third and fourth week). However, evidence also implicates a multifactorial origin, including drugs, radiation, maternal malnutrition, chemicals, and possibly a genetic mutation in folate pathways in some cases, which may result in abnormal development (Kinsman & Johnston, 2020).

Additional factors predisposing the infant to NTDs include maternal obesity, previous NTD pregnancy, Hispanic ancestry, low folic acid intake, gestational diabetes, hot tub or sauna use, low maternal vitamin B_{12} status, and the use of antiepileptic drugs (e.g., valproic acid) in pregnancy (Agopian, Tinker, Lupo, et al., 2013). The degree of neurologic dysfunction depends on where the sac protrudes through the vertebrae, the anatomic level of the defect, and the amount of nerve tissue involved (see Fig. 30.5). Most myelomeningoceles involve the lumbar or lumbosacral area.

The American Academy of Pediatrics, Committee on Genetics (2007) recommends daily intake of folic acid for all women of childbearing age. The recommended 0.4-mg daily dose is supplied safely in many multivitamin preparations. Because the greatest risk factor is a previous pregnancy affected by NTDs, women in this category should increase their daily folic acid dose to 4 mg, under a practitioner's supervision, beginning at least 1 month before they plan a pregnancy and through the first trimester because the neural tube closes about 1 month after conception. In 2009 the US Preventive Services Task Force published a statement indicating that there is ample evidence to support the recommendations for folic acid supplementation to decrease the incidence of NTDs (Williams et al., 2015). In 1998 the US Food and Drug Administration authorized the fortification of cereal grains (including cornmeal, grits, and wheat flour) with folic acid. It remains important for all women of childbearing age to take a multivitamin with 0.4 mg folic acid daily (American Academy of Pediatrics, Committee on Genetics, 2007). Sexually active females should be counseled on the risks of inadequate folate intake (Burke, Liptak, & Council on Children with Disabilities, 2011).

The following discussion of NTDs is limited to the two most common types: anencephaly, a defect incompatible with life, and SB, in particular myelomeningocele, an abnormality that causes significant disability.

ANENCEPHALY

Anencephaly, the most serious NTD, is a congenital malformation in which both cerebral hemispheres are absent. If the child with exencephaly (where brain protrudes from the skull), survives, degeneration of the brain to a spongiform mass occurs, with no bony covering. The condition is incompatible with life, and many affected infants are stillborn. For those who survive, no specific treatment is available. The infants have a portion of the brainstem and are able to maintain vital functions (such as temperature regulation and cardiac and respiratory function) for a few hours to several weeks but eventually die of respiratory failure.

Traditionally these infants have been provided comfort measures, but with no effort at resuscitation. Ethical and moral questions arise regarding treatment and withdrawal of support systems (e.g., feedings) if the newborn survives the first few days of life, as well as regarding use of the organs for donor transplants. During this time the family requires emotional support and counseling to cope with the birth of an infant with a fatal defect. Referral to neonatal palliative care or hospice should be made as soon as possible.

SPINA BIFIDA AND MYELODYSPLASIA

Myelodysplasia refers broadly to any malformation of the spinal canal and cord. Midline defects involving failure of the osseous (bony) spine to close are called **spina bifida**, the most common defect of the CNS. SB is categorized into two types: SB occulta and SB cystica.

SB occulta refers to a defect that is not visible externally. It occurs most commonly in the lumbosacral area (L5 and S1) (see Fig. 30.5B). Routine radiographic examinations indicate that the disorder may occur in as many as 10% to 30% of the general population. However, it may not be apparent unless there are associated cutaneous manifestations or neuromuscular disturbances. Superficial cutaneous indications include a skin depression or dimple (which may also mark the outlet of a dermal sinus tract that extends to the subarachnoid space); port-wine angiomatous nevi; dark tufts of hair; and soft, subcutaneous lipomas. These signs may be absent, appear singly, or be present in combination.

If associated neurologic involvement is present, the defect is known as occult spinal dysraphism. Fibrous bands and adhesions, an intraspinal **lipoma** (fatty tumor) or subcutaneous lipoma (lipomyelomeningocele), a dermoid or epidermoid cyst, diastematomyelia (spinal cord split in two), or a tethered cord can distort the spinal cord or roots. The usual cause is abnormal adhesion, or tethering, to a bony or fixed structure, resulting in traction on the spinal cord and cauda equina.

Neuromuscular disturbances usually consist of progressive or static changes in gait with foot weakness, foot deformity, or bowel and bladder sphincter disturbances. Some manifestations may not be evident until the child walks or is toilet trained.

Plain radiography is used to disclose the precise bony defect in the symptomatic lesion and to establish the diagnosis in the suspected, nonsymptomatic occult variety. MRI is the most sensitive tool for evaluating the defect. CT, ultrasonography, and myelography are also used to differentiate between SB occulta and other spinal disorders.

SB cystica refers to a visible defect with an external saclike protrusion. The two major forms of SB cystica are meningocele, which encases meninges and spinal fluid but no neural elements, and myelomeningocele (or meningomyelocele), which contains meninges, spinal fluid, and nerves. Neurologic deficit is not associated with meningocele but occurs in varying, often serious, degrees in myelomeningocele.

MYELOMENINGOCELE (MENINGOMYELOCELE)

Myelomeningocele (MMC) develops during the first 28 days of pregnancy when the neural tube fails to close and fuse at some point along its length. It may be detected prenatally or at birth, accounts for 90% of spinal cord lesions, and may be located at any point along the spinal column. Usually the sac is encased in a fine membrane that is prone to tears through which cerebrospinal fluid (CSF) leaks. In other instances the sac may be covered by dura, meninges, or skin, in which case there is rapid and spontaneous epithelialization. The largest number (75%) of myelomeningoceles occur in the lumbar or lumbosacral area (see Fig. 30.5). The location and magnitude of the defect determine the nature and extent of neurologic impairment. When the defect is below the second lumbar vertebra, the nerves of the cauda equina are involved, giving rise to symptoms such as flaccid, areflexic partial paralysis of the lower extremities and varying degrees of sensory deficit. Unlike an SCI, the degree of deficit is not necessarily uniform on both sides but may vary between extremities, depending on the compromise to specific nerves from malformation or tethering.

The anomaly most frequently associated with myelomeningocele is **hydrocephalus**; approximately 80% to 85% of children with SB develop hydrocephalus (Burke et al., 2011; Kinsman & Johnston, 2020). Although present at birth, hydrocephalus may not be apparent until shortly thereafter, or after the primary closure of the opening on the back. Careful monitoring of head circumference, fontanel tension, and ventricular size by head ultrasonography can indicate its presence. Hydrocephalus can occur because the NTD itself disrupts the flow of CSF. In many cases Chiari malformation (type II) is responsible. Type II **Chiari malformation** (a downward herniation of the brain into the brainstem) is present, though asymptomatic, in many children with SB. It can, however, adversely affect respiratory function, causing episodic apnea. Other clinical symptoms of problematic Chiari malformation include stridor, hoarse cry from vocal cord paralysis, feeding difficulties, aspiration pneumonia, and, in older children, upper extremity spasticity. The appearance of such symptoms should not be taken for granted; immediate referral is required to prevent further neurologic deterioration.

Pathophysiology

The pathophysiology of SB is best understood when related to the normal formative stages of the nervous system. At approximately 20 days of gestation, a decided depression, the neural groove, appears in the dorsal ectoderm of the embryo. During the fourth week of gestation, the groove deepens rapidly, and its elevated margins develop laterally and fuse dorsally to form the neural tube. Neural tube formation begins in the cervical region near the center of the embryo and advances in both directions—caudally and cephalically—until by the end of the fourth week of gestation, the ends of the neural tube, the anterior and posterior neuropores, close.

Most experts believe that the primary defect in neural tube malformations is a failure of neural tube closure. However, some evidence indicates that the defects are a result of splitting of the already closed neural tube as a result of an abnormal increase in CSF pressure during the first trimester.

There is evidence of a multifactorial etiology, including drugs, radiation, maternal malnutrition, chemicals, and possibly a genetic mutation in folate pathways in some cases, which may result in abnormal development. There is also evidence of a genetic component in the development of SB; myelomeningocele may occur in association with syndromes such as trisomy 18, PHAVER (limb **p**terygia, congenital **h**eart **a**nomalies, **v**ertebral defects, **e**ar anomalies, and **r**adial defects) syndrome, and Meckel-Gruber syndrome (Shaer, Chescheir, & Schulkin, 2007). The genetic predisposition is supported by evidence of the risk for recurrence after one affected child (3% to 4%) and a 10% risk for recurrence with two previously affected children (Kinsman & Johnston, 2020).

The degree of neurologic dysfunction depends on where the sac protrudes through the vertebrae, the anatomic level of the defect, and the amount of nerve tissue involved. One classification designates the level of functional mobility in relationship to the anatomic level of the defect. For example, children with a high lumbar-thoracic defect may be able to walk short distances using long leg braces and by early adolescence must use a wheelchair for mobility; children with a low lumbar defect can walk with short leg braces and forearm crutches (Liptak & Dosa, 2010). This classification system, however, does not describe genitourinary and bowel function. About 80% of patients with myelomeningocele develop a type II Chiari malformation (Kinsman & Johnston, 2020). There is some evidence that prolonged exposure of the MMC sac to amniotic fluid predisposes to the development of hindbrain herniation and Chiari II malformation (Adzick, 2013).

Clinical Manifestations

The manifestations of SB vary widely according to the degree of the spinal defect. The defect is readily apparent on inspection. The degree of neurologic dysfunction is directly related to the anatomic level of the defect and thus the nerves involved. Sensory disturbances usually parallel motor dysfunction. The upper level of sensory and motor impairment can be determined by observation of the infant's response to a pinprick over the legs and trunk. The infant responds to the sensory stimulus with limb movement, arousal, and crying. When withdrawal activity is used to determine the lowest level of spinal cord function, the response to pinprick should begin above the lesion.

Defective nerve supply to the bladder affects both sphincter and detrusor tone, which often causes constant dribbling of urine or produces overflow incontinence. This can often be mistaken for normal voiding patterns in the newborn. Some infants with SB, however, are able to void in a stream and achieve complete bladder emptying with each void.

Frequently the infant has poor anal sphincter tone and poor anal skin reflex, which result in lack of bowel control and sometimes rectal prolapse. Avoid taking rectal temperatures in affected infants. Because bowel sphincter function is frequently affected, the thermometer can cause irritation and rectal prolapse. If the defect is below the third sacral vertebra, the infant has no motor impairment but may have saddle anesthesia with bladder and anal sphincter paralysis.

Sometimes the denervation to the muscles of the lower extremities produces joint deformities in utero. These are primarily flexion or extension contractures, talipes valgus or varus contractures, kyphosis, lumbosacral scoliosis, and hip dislocations. The extent and severity of these associated orthopedic deformities again depend on the degree of nerve involvement. Most flexion deformities result from the pull of stronger, fully innervated muscles acting without the counterpull of their nonfunctioning paralyzed antagonists. Box 30.5 provides a summary of clinical manifestations of SB cystica and occulta.

BOX 30.5 Clinical Manifestations of Spina Bifida

Spina Bifida Cystica

- Sensory disturbances usually parallel to motor dysfunction
- Below second lumbar vertebra:
  - Flaccid, partial paralysis of lower extremities
  - Varying degrees of sensory deficit
  - Overflow incontinence with constant dribbling of urine
  - Lack of bowel control
  - Rectal prolapse (sometimes)
- Below third sacral vertebra:
  - No motor impairment
  - Bladder and anal sphincter paralysis
- Joint deformities (sometimes produced in utero):
  - Talipes valgus or varus (foot) contractures
  - Kyphosis
  - Lumbosacral scoliosis
  - Hip dislocation

Spina Bifida Occulta

- Frequently no observable manifestations
- May be associated with one or more cutaneous manifestations:
  - Skin depression or dimple
  - Port-wine angiomatous nevi
  - Dark tufts of hair
  - Soft, subcutaneous lipomas
- May be neuromuscular disturbances:
  - Progressive disturbance of gait with foot weakness
  - Bowel and bladder sphincter disturbances

Diagnostic Evaluation

The diagnosis of SB is made on the basis of clinical manifestations (see Box 30.5) and examination of the meningeal sac (Fig. 30.6A). Diagnostic measures used to evaluate the brain and spinal cord include MRI, ultrasonography, and CT. A neurologic evaluation will determine the extent of involvement of bowel and bladder function, as well as lower extremity neuromuscular involvement. Flaccid paralysis of the lower extremities is a common finding with absent deep tendon reflexes.

Prenatal Detection

It is possible to determine the presence of some major open NTDs prenatally. Ultrasonographic scanning of the uterus and elevated maternal concentrations of alpha-fetoprotein (AFP, or MS-AFP), a fetal-specific gamma-1-globulin, in amniotic fluid may indicate anencephaly or myelomeningocele. The optimum time for performing these diagnostic tests is between 16 and 18 weeks of gestation before AFP concentrations normally diminish and in sufficient time to permit a therapeutic abortion. It is recommended that such diagnostic procedures and genetic counseling be considered for all mothers who have borne an affected child, and testing is offered to all pregnant women (American College of Obstetrics and Gynecology, 2016). Chorionic villus sampling is also a method for prenatal diagnosis of NTDs; however, it carries certain risks (skeletal limb depletion) and is not recommended before 10 weeks of gestation (Simpson, Richards, & Otaño, 2012).

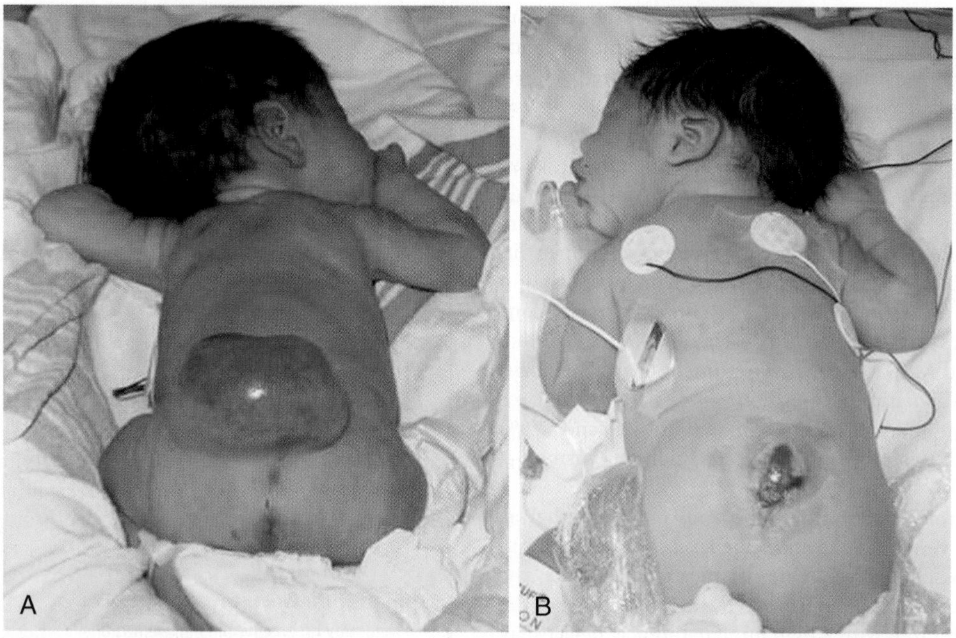

Fig. 30.6 **A,** Myelomeningocele with intact sac. **B,** Myelomeningocele with ruptured sac. (Courtesy Dr. Robert C. Dauser, Neurosurgery, Baylor College of Medicine, Houston, TX.)

Therapeutic Management

Management of the child who has a myelomeningocele requires a multidisciplinary team approach involving the specialties of neurology, neurosurgery, pediatrics, urology, orthopedics, rehabilitation, physical therapy, occupational therapy, and social services, as well as intensive nursing care in a variety of specialty areas. The collaborative efforts of these specialists focus on the following:

- The myelomeningocele and the problems associated with the defect—hydrocephalus, paralysis, orthopedic deformities (e.g., developmental dysplasia of the hip, clubfoot), and genitourinary abnormalities
- Possible acquired problems that may or may not be associated, such as Chiari II malformation, meningitis, seizures, hypoxia, tethered cord, and hemorrhage
- Other abnormalities, such as cardiac or GI malformations

Many hospitals have specialty clinics staffed by multidisciplinary teams to provide the complex follow-up care needed for children and families with myelodysplasia.

In 2008 the Centers for Disease Control and Prevention started a National Spina Bifida Patient Registry, based on results from a survey from spina bifida clinics across the United States. The Registry was initiated to provide a more organized approach to the care of all individuals with spina bifida. It seeks to improve and align the quality of care received at spina bifida clinics nationwide. The registry works to develop standards and best practices for patients with spina bifida. The data collected from the Registry clinics is sent to the Centers for Disease Control and Prevention to be analyzed so that it can be disseminated to other physicians and clinics. The Registry also hopes to gain insight into some of the secondary conditions of spina bifida, such as paralysis, neurogenic bladder and bowel, and hydrocephalus (Moldenhauer & Adzick, 2017).

Many authorities believe that early closure, within the first 24 to 72 hours, offers the most favorable outcome. Surgical closure within the first 24 hours is recommended if the sac is leaking CSF (Kinsman & Johnston, 2020). Surgical closure within 24 hours also results in improved bladder capacities and lower detrusor leak point pressures. Increased incidence of febrile urinary tract infections (UTIs), vesicoureteral reflux, and hydronephrosis have been shown when closure is delayed past 72 hours (Tarcan, Onol, Ilker, et al., 2006).

A variety of neurosurgical and plastic surgical procedures are used for skin closure without disturbing the neural elements or removing any portion of the sac. The objective is satisfactory skin coverage of the lesion and meticulous closure. Wide excision of the large membranous covering may damage functioning neural tissue.

Prenatal surgical closure of the myelomeningocele sac through fetal surgery has been evaluated in relation to prevention of injury to the exposed spinal cord tissue and the improvement of neurologic and urologic outcomes in the affected child. The Management of Myelomeningocele Study (MOMS), a clinical trial supported by the National Institutes of Health, found that prenatal surgery for myelomeningocele reduced the need for shunting (for hydrocephalus), evaluated at 12 months, and decreased the incidence of hindbrain herniation. In addition, there was an improvement in mental and motor function scores at 30 months in the children who had prenatal surgery (compared with children who had postnatal surgery) (Lapa, 2019). However, the surgery is not without risks to the fetus and mother, and premature delivery is common. Outcome data for urologic and bowel function, motor function, cognition, and spina bifida–associated outcomes are being gathered in the MOMS2 study, which ended in 2013 (Moldenhauer, Soni, Rintoul, et al., 2015).

Initial Care

Care of the newborn involves preventing infection; performing a neurologic assessment, including observation for associated anomalies; and dealing with the impact of the anomaly on the family. Although meningoceles are repaired early, especially if the sac is in danger of rupturing, the philosophy regarding skin closure of myelomeningocele varies. Most authorities believe that early closure, within the first 24 to 72 hours, offers the most favorable outcome. Surgical closure within the first 24 hours is recommended if the sac is leaking CSF (Kinsman & Johnston, 2020). Early closure, preferably in the first 12 to 18 hours, not only prevents local infection and trauma to the exposed tissues but also avoids stretching other nerve roots (which may occur as the meningeal sac expands during the first hours after birth), thus preventing further motor impairment. Broad-spectrum antibiotics are initiated, and neurotoxic substances such as povidone-iodine are avoided at the malformation.

Associated problems are assessed and managed by appropriate surgical and supportive measures. Shunt procedures provide relief from imminent or progressive hydrocephalus (see Chapter 27). When diagnosed, ventriculitis, meningitis, and UTI are treated with vigorous antibiotic therapy and supportive measures. Surgical intervention for Chiari II malformation is indicated only when the child is symptomatic (i.e., high-pitched crowing cry, stridor, respiratory difficulties, apnea, failure to thrive, gastroesophageal reflux, oral-motor difficulties, upper extremity spasticity).

Improved surgical techniques do not alter the major physical disability and deformity or chronic UTIs that affect the quality of life for these children. Superimposed on these physical problems are the disorder's effects on family life and finances and on school and hospital services.

Musculoskeletal Considerations

According to most orthopedists, musculoskeletal problems that will affect later locomotion should be evaluated early and treatment, where indicated, instituted without delay. Neurologic assessment determines the neurosegmental level of the lesion, spasticity and progressive paralysis, potential for deformity, and functional expectations. Orthopedic and musculoskeletal management includes preventing joint contractures, correcting the existing deformity, preventing or minimizing effects of motor and sensory deficits, preventing skin breakdown, and obtaining the best possible function of affected lower extremities. Common musculoskeletal problems requiring attention in SB include deformities of the knees, hips, feet, and spine; fractures and insensate skin further complicate orthopedic care. Other problems that may occur later include kyphosis and scoliosis (Lazzaretti & Pearson, 2010; Liptak & Dosa, 2010). An overwhelming majority of infants born with myelomeningocele will have clubfoot (Moldenhauer & Adzick, 2017). Because children with MMC often have decreased sensitivity in lower extremities, preventive skin care is important. A high percentage (60%) of children seen in a wound clinic for skin breakdown had myelomeningocele at birth (Samaniego, 2003). The most common wound sites were the foot and ankle, with the buttocks being the second most common site. Pressure wounds are more common in patients who use wheelchairs for mobility (Ottolini, Harris, Amling, et al., 2013).

The status of the neurologic deficit remains the most important factor in determining the child's ultimate functional abilities; however, many children with lumbar and sacral myelomeningocele are able to achieve functional ambulation (Kinsman & Johnston, 2020). With technologic advances, a variety of lightweight orthoses, including braces, special "walking" devices, and custom-built wheelchairs, are available to provide mobility to children with spinal cord lesions. Early in infancy, intervention with passive range-of-motion exercises, positioning, and stretching exercises may help decrease the incidence of muscle contractures. Corrective surgical procedures, when indicated, are best initiated at an early age so that the child will not lag significantly behind age-mates in developmental progress. The degree of lower extremity function guides decisions about whether orthopedic surgery will be needed.

Physical therapy and musculoskeletal management of children with myelomeningocele are continual processes to achieve optimum function and ambulation when possible. Problems such as type II Chiari malformation, hydrocephalus, and a tethered spinal cord can complicate expectations. A common complication is tethered cord syndrome in which there is a presumed traction injury to the distal spinal cord with subtle and progressive loss of neural function; this may occur any time but is more common during periods of rapid growth and can be precipitated by ventricular shunt failure (Burke et al., 2011).

Management of Genitourinary Function

Myelomeningocele is one of the most common causes of neuropathic (neurogenic) bladder dysfunction among children. Neurologic deficits can affect the innervation of the bladder, impairing the ability to store and empty urine. As many as 90% of children with SB will experience some form of voiding dysfunction. A child with a neuropathic bladder will require care across the life span. The goals of urologic treatment should be individualized to the child's developmental stage. In infants the goal of treatment is to preserve renal function. In older children the goal is to preserve renal function and achieve optimum urinary continence. Urinary incontinence is a chronic, often debilitating problem for the child. In addition, the neuropathic bladder may produce **urinary system distress**, characterized by symptomatic urinary tract infections, ureterohydronephrosis, vesicoureteral reflux, or renal insufficiency. The characteristics of bladder dysfunction in children vary according to the level of the neurologic lesion and the influence of bony growth and development of the spine. In addition, the presence of type II Chiari malformation and subsequent hydrocephalus has the potential to affect bladder function, although spinal influences predominate.

During infancy, urinary incontinence is normally physiologic, but urinary system distress may occur. Ongoing urologic monitoring is essential. Evidence is growing that early intervention, based on evaluation during the neonatal period and before complications occur, improves bladder function, reduces the subsequent risk of urinary system distress, and reduces the need for reconstructive surgery of the lower urinary tract. Ultrasonography of the bladder and ureters and routine urinalysis (and urine cultures when indicated) are used to detect urinary system distress before renal function is compromised. In addition, urodynamic testing is used to identify bladder dysfunction that predisposes the child to urinary system distress (Gray & Moore, 2009; Snodgrass & Gargollo, 2010). These conditions include high-pressure detrusor hyperreflexia (reflex contractions of the detrusor muscle) with vesicosphincter dyssynergia (incoordination of detrusor and sphincter muscles), low bladder wall compliance (poor distensibility of the bladder wall causing increased intravesical pressures during urine filling and storage), or detrusor areflexia (absence of detrusor contractions caused by the spinal defect).

Infants may have one of several predominant neuropathic bladder disorders. Detrusor contractions associated with vesicosphincter dyssynergia are particularly common. Some infants are able to empty the bladder efficiently despite incoordination between the sphincter mechanism and detrusor, but the majority experience chronic residual urine, UTIs, or more serious types of urinary system distress. A minority of infants have poor detrusor contraction strength or detrusor areflexia. This condition is particularly damaging to the urinary system when it coexists with low bladder wall compliance and an elevated detrusor leak point pressure. Low bladder wall compliance occurs when collagen or fibrosis causes stiffening of the bladder wall. This stiffened bladder wall raises intravesical pressures, obstructing the bladder, ureters, and, ultimately, the nephron. The impact of low bladder wall compliance is directly related to the influence of the bladder outlet. Among children with myelodysplasia, the urethral muscles are typically weakened, and collagen replaces much of the muscle tissue. As a result, the sphincter is fixed, so it neither closes efficiently to prevent urinary leakage nor opens well to allow urinary flow with a detrusor contraction. When the magnitude of the pressure required to drive urine across the abnormal sphincter is greater than 40 cm H_2O (the detrusor leak point pressure) and the compliance of the bladder wall is low (<10 cm H_2O), the risk of urinary system distress is high.

In contrast, a small number of infants experience effective detrusor contractions without vesicosphincter dyssynergia. Effective bladder evacuation is likely among this group, and the incidence of urinary system distress during the first year of life is low.

As the child grows, detrusor hyperreflexia is often replaced by deficient detrusor contraction strength and **stress urinary incontinence (SUI)** (leakage produced by physical exertion). The bladder wall is often poorly compliant (producing chronically elevated intravesical pressures), and the bladder outlet, while incompetent, obstructs the outflow of urine. When the detrusor leak point pressure exceeds 40 cm H_2O, the child is predisposed to chronic urinary leakage and urinary distress symptoms, including recurrent UTIs and reflux. When the detrusor leak point pressure is lower than 40 cm H_2O, urinary leakage is more severe, although the risk of urinary system distress is lessened. Thus the child with more severe urinary incontinence is less predisposed than the "drier" child to serious UTIs.

Infants with myelomeningocele and a neurogenic bladder who are not at risk for urinary system distress are managed by diaper containment and watchful waiting. The infant empties the bladder into a diaper, the urine is routinely monitored for infection, and the upper urinary tracts are monitored for evidence of urinary system distress (dilation of the ureters, renal pelves, or collecting systems) via serial ultrasonography.

In contrast, children with evidence of urinary system distress, or those considered at risk based on early urodynamic testing, undergo **clean intermittent catheterization (CIC)**, typically in combination with an antispasmodic medication such as oxybutynin or propantheline (Elzeneini, Waly, Marshall, et al., 2019; Gray & Moore, 2009). Anticholinergic medications are prescribed because they reduce detrusor muscle tone and reduce bladder pressures both during urine filling and storage and during micturition. CIC is not intended to prevent spontaneous voiding. Instead, it ensures routine, regular bladder evacuation, further preventing deleterious elevation of intravesical pressures. Usually the parents learn to catheterize the infant every 4 hours during the day and once each night. Follow-up evaluation, consisting of serial ultrasonography and urinalysis, is completed every 3 to 6 months as indicated.

Infants with significant urinary system distress and neuropathic bladder dysfunction at birth sometimes require temporary urinary diversion to ensure adequate urine outflow and prevent further damage to the upper urinary tracts. A vesicostomy is a relatively simple procedure wherein the anterior bladder wall is brought to the abdominal wall, creating a small stoma for urinary drainage. Urine is contained via a diaper, but double diapering or use of a larger diaper that can be placed higher on the abdomen is necessary for adequate urine containment. Meticulous skin care is necessary because the perineal skin is exposed to continuous urinary leakage.

Among older children the quest for continence typically begins with a CIC program. The parents learn the procedure and teach the child to self-catheterize as soon as possible, usually by 6 years of age (Gray & Moore, 2009). The child with detrusor hyperreflexia and dyssynergia often responds well to antispasmodic medications and CIC. In contrast, the child with poor bladder wall compliance and SUI often requires a combination of antispasmodic medications to reduce intravesical filling pressures and a sympathetic agonist (such as imipramine, pseudoephedrine, or phenylpropanolamine) to enhance sphincter competence. Unfortunately, the combination of medications and CIC is typically only partially effective, and more aggressive interventions are often required to render the neuropathic bladder both continent and free from its predisposition toward producing urinary system distress. It is important that a careful history is taken by the provider to identify other problems that may be contributing to persistent incontinence. Factors that can affect bladder continence include caffeinated drinks, constipation, or lack of access to bathrooms (Metcalfe, 2017).

When the child cannot attain continence by conservative measures, surgery is considered. Augmentation enterocystoplasty (or gastrocystoplasty) is a surgical procedure that increases bladder capacity, reverses or halts the negative effects of the poorly compliant bladder wall, and reduces harmfully high bladder pressures caused by detrusor hyperreflexia with vesicosphincter dyssynergia. A detubularized segment of large or small bowel or a wedge of the fundus of the stomach has been used to successfully augment bladder capacity. The choice of segment varies according to the surgeon's preference and the status of the patient's urinary and GI systems. Large and small bowel segments produce significant volumes of mucus that may clog catheters used for CIC. Augmentation with the stomach produces less mucus, and its acidic secretions may reduce the urinary system's predisposition to infection. The bladder must be irrigated to decrease mucus within the bladder; this also decreases the possible complications of infection, stones, and bladder perforation.

Even though augmentation of the bladder may improve or resolve urinary leakage related to detrusor hyperreflexia or urinary system distress caused by low bladder wall compliance, the SUI produced by the abnormal sphincter mechanism typically persists. Several surgical procedures help correct this intrinsic sphincter deficiency. The Mitrofanoff procedure uses the appendix to provide an alternative route for intermittent catheterization. The appendix is removed from the colon and used to create a continent conduit between the abdominal wall and the bladder. The resulting stoma is relatively small and produces minimum mucus. The ureter may be used as an alternative to the appendix for some children. If the appendix is insufficient, a segment of tapered intestine, ileum, or colon may be used to create a conduit (Monti tube) (Gray & Moore, 2009). CIC through the easily accessible abdominal route fosters greater independence in children, especially in those unable to transfer from wheelchair to toilet to perform CIC.

When intrinsic sphincter deficiency produces only mild stress urinary leakage, the construction of a Mitrofanoff route alone may be sufficient to achieve continence between catheterization episodes. However, when SUI is more severe, a suburethral sling or suburethral collagen injection is used to alleviate intrinsic sphincter deficiency.

The suburethral sling is a slip of fascia or synthetic material that is placed below the proximal third of the urethra. The sling may be placed in a fashion that uses only slight tension to obstruct the urethra and prevent SUI. The sling may be used for both boys and girls, and the procedure can be completed at the same time as the augmentation enterocystoplasty is constructed. After augmentation enterocystoplasty and placement of a suburethral sling, the patient can expect to evacuate the bladder by CIC of the appendiceal Mitrofanoff route (appendicovesicostomy) or the urethra if a Mitrofanoff route has not been constructed.

Suburethral injection of glutaraldehyde cross-linked (GAX) collagen also may be used to alleviate or prevent SUI caused by intrinsic sphincter deficiency. Collagen is used to bulk or expand the urethral tissue, promoting coaptation (approximation) of the mucosa. The collagen implant complements the urethra's ability to form a watertight seal, rather than obstructing the urethral lumen. Collagen may be injected using different approaches. Transurethral collagen is injected through the working channel of a cystoscope. Transperineal collagen is directed underneath the urethra using a needle inserted through the perineal skin. In this case the location of the urethra is confirmed by simultaneous cystoscopic visualization of the urethra. The antegrade approach requires creation of a suprapubic cystostomy tract. A flexible cystoscope is then inserted through the cystostomy tract, and collagen is injected into the proximal urethra. Multiple injections may be required to achieve optimum continence. Subsequent injections may be required when the collagen is dissipated or resorbed by the body over a period of years. Botulinum toxin (Botox) can also be injected into the detrusor muscle to increase bladder capacity and decrease intravesicular pressures, but this measure is only temporary (Ingham, Angotti, Lewis, et al., 2019).

The artificial urinary sphincter provides another alternative for the management of intrinsic sphincter deficiency in the child with myelomeningocele. The device consists of a urethral cuff, abdominal reservoir, and control pump. In the activated position, the cuff is filled, and the pressure of this cuff closes the urethral lumen. During micturition, the control pump is used to baffle fluid from the urethral cuff to the abdominal reservoir, opening the urethra for micturition or catheterization. However, because of the significant risk for infection, need for revision with growth, and mechanical failure, the popularity of the artificial urinary sphincter has declined.

Because of advances in neurogenic bladder management, adolescents and young adults with myelomeningocele and neurogenic bladder have been followed for up to 30 years without evidence of deterioration in renal function. Nevertheless, urinary and fecal incontinence are common, and these conditions lead to significant and sometimes devastating problems with growth and developmental tasks, including establishing independence and social and intimate relationships. This observation underscores the need to aggressively manage both continence and the threat of urinary system distress from an early age and to establish an expectation of social continence critical to providing these patients with the skills they need to thrive as adolescents and adults. Newborns with SB and normal urodynamics require close follow-up care during the first several years of life to prevent deterioration in urodynamic status as a result of neurologic deterioration.

Bowel Control

Some degree of fecal continence can be achieved in most children with myelomeningocele with diet modification, regular toilet habits, and prevention of constipation and impaction. It is frequently a lengthy process. Dietary fiber supplements (recommended: age of child in years + 5 g/day), laxatives, suppositories, or enemas aid in producing regular evacuation. Older children and adolescents seeking more independence may attain bowel continence and higher quality of life after undergoing an **antegrade continence enema** (ACE) procedure (Ayub, Zeidan, Larson, et al., 2019). In a procedure similar to the Mitrofanoff, the appendix or ileum is used to create a catheterizable channel with attachment of the proximal end to the colon. The distal end of the channel exits through a small abdominal stoma. Every 1 or 2 days, a catheter is passed through the stoma, allowing enema solution to be instilled directly into the colon. After administration of the enema solution, the child sits on the toilet for 30 to 60 minutes as stool is flushed out through the rectum. The frequency of enemas and volume of solution used to completely evacuate the bowel vary among individuals.

Prognosis

The early prognosis for the child with myelomeningocele depends on the neurologic deficit present at birth, including motor ability, bladder innervation, and associated neurologic anomalies. Early surgical repair of the spinal defect, antibiotic therapy to reduce the incidence of meningitis and ventriculitis, prevention of urinary system dysfunction, and early detection and correction of hydrocephalus have significantly increased the survival rate and quality of life in such children. Mortality rates are reported to be 10% to 15%, with many deaths occurring before the age of 4 years (Kinsman & Johnston, 2020). Many young adults with SB achieve partial independent living and gainful employment. Reports of survival rates vary, and many include adults who were born before medical advances and surgical techniques seen in the past 25 years. Coordinated care for adults with SB is essential; however, multidisciplinary adult care is often inadequate (Lazzaretti & Pearson, 2010). One of the factors associated with early death among adults with MMC is hydrocephalus and shunt failure (Mourtzinos & Stoffel, 2010). This chronic condition has an array of associated complications, including hydrocephalus and shunt malfunctions, tethered cord syndrome, scoliosis, Chiari II development, bowel and bladder management issues, latex allergy, and epilepsy. However, based on current medical knowledge and ethical considerations, aggressive, early management is favored for the child with myelomeningocele.

Prevention

The Centers for Disease Control and Prevention (2009) continues to affirm that 50% to 70% of NTDs can be prevented by daily consumption of 0.4 mg of folic acid by women of childbearing age. The data indicate that serum folate concentrations among women of childbearing age decreased 16% from 2003 to 2004 in all ethnic groups studied. Lowest serum folate levels were seen in non-Hispanic whites in 2003 to 2004; however, overall serum folate levels remained below recommended levels in non-Hispanic African Americans during all three periods studied (Centers for Disease Control and Prevention, 2007). These results indicate that nurses and other health care workers have an important task in disseminating information that may decrease the incidence of birth defects in children by promoting maternal consumption of folic acid.

To ensure adequate daily intake of the recommended amount of folic acid, women must take a folic acid supplement, eat a fortified breakfast cereal containing 100% of the recommended dietary allowance of folic acid (e.g., Kellogg's Product 19, General Mills Total, Multigrain Cheerios Plus), or increase their consumption of fortified foods (e.g., cereal, bread, rice, grits, pasta) and foods naturally rich in folate (e.g., green leafy vegetables, citrus fruits). For women who have had a previous pregnancy affected by NTDs, folic acid intake is increased to 4 mg/day under the supervision of a health care practitioner beginning 1 month before a planned pregnancy and continuing through the first trimester. Supplementation of 4 mg of folate should not be given solely in multivitamin preparations because of the risk for overdose of other vitamins. Drugs that affect folic acid metabolism and increase the risk for myelomeningocele should be avoided before pregnancy (if plans are to become pregnant in the near future) and during pregnancy; these include trimethoprim and the AEDs carbamazepine, phenytoin, phenobarbital, valproic acid, and primidone (Kinsman & Johnston, 2020).

Nursing Care Management

The basic needs of the infant with a myelomeningocele are essentially the same as for any newborn infant (see Chapter 8). Special needs related to the defect and potential complications are discussed in the following section. As the child matures, the problems increase and involve all aspects of daily living; therefore care is directly related to the child's habilitation at each stage of development.

Assessment

At the time of delivery an examination is performed to assess the intactness of the membranous cyst. During transport to the nursery, make every effort to prevent trauma to this protective covering. In addition to the routine assessment of the newborn (see Chapter 7), assess the infant for the level of neurologic involvement. Note movement of extremities or skin response, especially an anal reflex that might provide clues to the degree of motor or sensory impairment.

Care of the Myelomeningocele Sac

The infant is usually placed in an incubator or radiant warmer so that temperature can be maintained without clothing or covers that might irritate the CNS lesion. When an overhead warmer is used, the dressings over the defect require more frequent moistening because of the dehydrating effect of the radiant heat. Before surgical closure, the myelomeningocele is kept from drying by the application of a sterile, moist, nonadherent dressing. The moistening solution is usually sterile normal saline. Dressings are changed frequently (every 2 to 4 hours), and the sac is closely inspected for leaks, abrasions, irritation, and signs of infection. The sac must be carefully cleansed if it becomes soiled or contaminated. Sometimes the sac ruptures during delivery or transport, and any opening in the sac greatly increases the risk of infection to the CNS (see Fig. 30.6B).

Positioning

One of the most important and challenging aspects of early care of the infant with myelomeningocele is positioning. Before surgery the infant remains in the prone position to minimize tension on the sac and the risk of trauma. The prone position allows for optimum positioning of the legs, especially in cases of associated hip dysplasia. Various aids, including diaper rolls, foam pads, and specially designed frames and appliances, are available to maintain the desired position.

The prone position affects other aspects of the infant's care. For example, in this position the infant is more difficult to keep clean, pressure areas are a constant threat, and feeding becomes a problem. The infant's head is turned to one side for feeding. Fortunately, most defects are repaired early, and the infant can be held for feeding and routine care soon after surgery. Physical therapy consultation may be necessary for difficult positioning problems. Speech-language pathologist consultation may be needed for difficulty with oral-motor skills that may indicate complications caused by a Chiari malformation.

General Care

Diapering the infant may be contraindicated until the defect has been repaired and healing is well advanced or epithelialization has taken place. The padding beneath the diaper area is changed as needed to keep the skin dry and free of irritation. When the nurse detects urinary retention (the bladder is still an abdominal organ in early infancy), CIC is used. Because the bowel sphincter is frequently affected, there may be continual passage of stool, often misinterpreted as diarrhea, which is a constant irritant to the skin and a source of infection to the spinal lesion.

Areas of sensory and motor impairment are subject to skin breakdown and therefore require meticulous care. The infant may be placed on a pressure-reducing mattress or a mattress to prevent pressure on the knees and ankles (see Chapter 20, Skin Care and General Hygiene).

Gentle range-of-motion exercises are carried out to prevent contractures, and stretching of contractures is performed when indicated. However, these exercises may be restricted to the foot, ankle, and knee joint. When the hip joints are unstable, stretching against tight hip flexors or adductor muscles, which act much like bowstrings, may aggravate a tendency toward subluxation. A physical therapy consultation is often necessary to develop a multidisciplinary plan to prevent long-term complications.

Some infants with unrepaired myelomeningocele are unable to be held in the arms and cuddled as unaffected infants are, so their need for tactile stimulation is met by caressing, stroking, and other comfort measures. To facilitate handling and reduce parental anxiety, the infant can recline on a pillow placed in the parent's lap.

Ophthalmic complications may occur in children with SB and hydrocephalus. The appearance of a squint, other ocular motility, or papilledema usually denotes hydrocephalus and is reported. Ophthalmologic follow-up care, particularly in children with shunts, is generally included in the multidisciplinary care plan.

Postoperative Care

Postoperative care for the infant with myelomeningocele involves the same basic care as for any postsurgical infant: monitoring vital signs, weight, and intake and output; maintaining body temperature; assessing and relieving pain; providing nourishment; and observing for signs of infection. The wound is managed according to the surgeon's directions, and general care is continued as preoperatively.

The prone position is maintained after operative closure, although many neurosurgeons allow a side-lying or partial side-lying position unless it aggravates a coexisting hip dysplasia or permits undesirable hip flexion. This offers an opportunity for position changes, which reduces the risk of pressure sores and facilitates feeding. Once the effects of anesthesia have subsided and the infant is alert, feedings may resume unless there are other anomalies or associated complications.

Nursing assessments are carried out for implementation of comfort measures in the postoperative period. The infant can be held upright against the body, taking care to avoid pressure on the operative site. In the case of an unusually large defect, skin grafting may be required for wound closure; the infant must then be kept prone postoperatively with as little movement as possible to prevent tension on the skin graft.

The nurse can assist in determining the extent of neuromuscular involvement. Note movement of the extremities or skin response, especially an anal reflex, that might provide clues to the degree of motor or sensory status. Measure head circumference daily (see Chapter 4) and examine the fontanels for signs of tension or bulging. The nurse is also alert to early signs of infection, such as elevated or decreased temperature (axillary), irritability, and lethargy, and to signs of increased intracranial pressure. Urinary catheterization may be needed for urine retention. Although it may not have been a problem preoperatively, swelling around the operative site may cause transient urine retention, which resolves in 2 to 5 days.

Family Support and Home Care

As soon as the parents are able to cope with the infant's condition, encourage them to become involved in care. They need to learn how to continue at home the care that has been initiated in the hospital: positioning, feeding, skin care, and range-of-motion exercises when appropriate. Parents also need to learn CIC technique when prescribed. The family needs to know the signs of complications and how to reach assistance when needed.

As the child grows and develops, parents need guidance to encourage and stimulate the infant to accomplish age-appropriate developmental tasks within the limits imposed by the disabilities. Upper limb movement can be stimulated early by placing the infant on the floor in a prone position with toys within reach. Activities that encourage body consciousness, such as rolling over and pulling to a sitting position, are encouraged at the appropriate times. Creeping and crawling help the child explore the environment. The parents may need help to modify appliances and activities normally expected of a growing child. A standing table, frame, or parapodium is helpful for a variety of activities, and it is best for the child to begin supported weight bearing and standing as close as possible to the expected time for standing to occur.

It is important for the family to understand the nature of sensory deficit in a child with a spinal defect. The child will be insensitive to pressure or other sources of tissue injury. Therefore the family must be alert to hot or cold items that could cause thermal injury to tissues and remember to inspect the skin regularly for signs of pressure, especially over bony prominences. Because of sensory impairment, the child is unaware of bladder discomfort, and signs of UTIs may go unnoticed. Urinary tract infection is often considered when the child becomes ill.

The long-range planning with and support of the parents and newborn begin in the hospital and extend throughout childhood and even into young adulthood. The life expectancy of children with SB extends well into adulthood; therefore planning should involve long-term goals and plans for optimum function as an adult. Long-range planning goals should include a discussion of achievement of functional mobility, urinary continence, and as much bowel continence as physically possible. Discussion about aspects of adulthood such as having a mate, sexual relationships, and bearing and rearing children is important and should not be overlooked (Rowe & Jadhav, 2008). The unique service needs of adolescents with SB as they attempt to gain independence from family and establish a life of their own have not been adequately addressed in the literature (Sawyer & Macnee, 2010). Betz and colleagues (2010) interviewed young people with SB making the transition to adulthood. Some common themes that emerged among these young people were challenges in preparation for self-management, limited social relationships, awareness of their cognitive challenges, and the cost of independence. Advances in neurology, orthopedics, and urology have enabled adolescents to progress into adulthood with fewer deficits than observed in previous decades; one key factor is the recognition of subtle signs of neurologic deterioration and rapid intervention (Rowe & Jadhav, 2008).

Changes in functional ability, particularly in the lower extremities, bowel, or bladder, may indicate the presence of a tethered cord, one that is bound low or restricted in an abnormal position by scar tissue. These symptoms usually occur after a growth spurt and can best be detected with MRI. Tethering can be repaired surgically but, unfortunately, may recur.

Habilitation involves solving not only problems of self-help and locomotion but also the most distressing problem of incontinence, which threatens the child's social acceptability. Assistance in preparing the child and the school regarding the special needs of children with disabilities helps the parents provide a better initial adjustment to broader social experiences. A Life Course Model has been developed for patients, families, caregivers, teachers, and clinicians to facilitate, through a developmental approach, the care of the child and young person with SB; this program has been made into a web-based tool that can be used to assist in the transition to adulthood (Dicianno, Fairman, Juengst, et al., 2010). Additional information on this program is available through the Spina Bifida Association's website (https://www.spinabifidaassociation.org/).

Latex Allergy

Latex allergy, or latex hypersensitivity, was identified as a serious health hazard when a report linked intraoperative anaphylaxis with latex in children with SB. Latex, a natural product derived from the rubber tree, is used in combination with other chemicals to give elasticity, strength, and durability to many products. Children with SB are at high risk for developing latex allergy because of repeated exposure to latex products during surgery and procedures. Therefore such children should not be exposed to latex products from birth onward to minimize the occurrence of latex hypersensitivity. Allergic reactions range from urticaria, wheezing, watery eyes, and rashes to anaphylactic shock. More severe reactions tend to occur when latex comes in contact with mucous membranes, wet skin, the bloodstream, or an airway. There also can be cross-reactions to a number of foods (e.g., banana, avocado, kiwi, chestnut).

Allergic reactions to latex protein can also occur when the substance is transferred to food by food handlers wearing latex gloves, prompting several states to pass legislation that prohibits the use of latex gloves in food service. In addition to patients with SB, high-risk populations include patients with urogenital anomalies or multiple surgeries, as well as health care workers.

The most important goals are prevention of latex sensitivity and identification of children with a known hypersensitivity (see Nursing Care Guidelines box). High-risk and latex-allergic individuals must be managed in a **latex-free environment**. Take care that they do not come in direct or secondary contact with products or equipment containing latex at *any time* during medical treatment. Allergy testing can identify latex sensitivity with varying success. Skin prick testing and provocation testing carry the risk for allergic reaction or anaphylaxis. Several commercially available assays can be useful in confirming latex sensitivity. To date, none of these tests demonstrates complete diagnostic reliability, and they should not be the sole determinant of the presence or absence of an allergic response to latex.

NURSING CARE GUIDELINES

Identifying Latex Allergy

- Does your child have any symptoms, such as sneezing, coughing, rashes, or wheezing, when handling rubber products (e.g., balloons, tennis or Koosh balls, adhesive bandage strips) or when in contact with rubber hospital products, such as gloves or catheters?
- Has your child ever had an allergic reaction during surgery?
- Does your child have a history of rashes, asthma, or allergic reactions to medication or foods, especially milk, kiwi, bananas, or chestnuts?
- How would you identify or recognize an allergic reaction in your child?
- What would you do if an allergic reaction occurred?
- Has anyone ever discussed latex or rubber allergy or sensitivity with you?
- Has the child had any allergy testing?
- When did the child last come in contact with any type of rubber product? Were you present?

Because children who have SB are prone to develop sensitivity to latex, reducing exposure from birth on may decrease the chance of allergy development. Nonlatex products lists are available to parents and health care workers; these products may be substituted for those containing latex. In the health care arena, it is important to use products with the lowest potential risk for sensitizing patients and staff members.

The identification of those sensitive to latex is best accomplished through careful screening of all patients. During the health interview with the parent or child, ask *all* patients, not only those at risk, about sensitivity to latex. Be certain that this is a routine part of all preoperative and preprocedural histories. Stress the importance of the allergy history to all personnel (e.g., phlebotomists, respiratory therapists) (see Nursing Care Guidelines box for questions related to latex allergy). Children with latex hypersensitivity should carry some form of allergy identification, such as a MedicAlert bracelet. Education programs on latex hypersensitivity are aimed at those who care for high-risk groups, such as children with SB, and may include relatives, school nurses, teachers, child care workers, and babysitters. In addition to educating caregivers about the child's exposure to medical products that contain latex, nurses need to inform them of common nonmedical latex objects such as water toys, pacifiers, and plastic storage bags. Items brought to the hospital, such as floral bouquets, should also be screened for latex toys and balloons. Parents should also receive literature explaining signs and symptoms of latex hypersensitivity and appropriate emergency treatment (see Chapter 23, Anaphylaxis).

SPINAL MUSCULAR ATROPHY TYPE 1 (WERDNIG-HOFFMANN DISEASE)

Spinal muscular atrophy (SMA) type 1 (Werdnig-Hoffmann disease) is a disorder characterized by progressive weakness and wasting of skeletal muscles caused by degeneration of anterior horn cells. It is inherited as an autosomal recessive trait and is the most common paralytic form of the **floppy infant syndrome (congenital hypotonia)**. The sites of the pathologic condition are the anterior horn cells of the spinal cord and the motor nuclei of the brainstem, but the primary effect is atrophy of skeletal muscles.

Clinical Manifestations

The age of onset is variable, but the earlier the onset, the more disseminated and severe the motor weakness. The disorder may be manifested early—often at birth—and almost always before 2 years of age; death may occur as a result of respiratory failure by age 2 years (Arnold, Kassar, & Kissel, 2019).

The manifestations (Box 30.6) and prognosis are categorized according to the age of onset, severity of weakness, and clinical course; some children may fluctuate between exhibiting symptoms of types 1 and 2 or types 2 and 3 in regard to clinical function (Haliloglu, 2020). Some experts also categorize SMA according to the highest level of motor function; type 1 includes "nonsitters," type 2 includes "sitters," and type 3 includes "walkers" (Arnold et al., 2019). A severe rare fetal form of SMA, classified as type 0, is reported to be quite lethal in the perinatal period; motor neuron degeneration may be noted as early as midgestation in type 0 (Haliloglu, 2020). Type 4 may present between 20 and 30 years of age and may be referred to as proximal adult-type SMA (Arnold et al., 2019).

Diagnostic Evaluation

The diagnosis is based on the molecular genetic marker for the *SMN* (survival motor neuron) gene, which is located on chromosome *5q13*. Prenatal diagnosis may be made by genetic analysis of circulating fetal cells in maternal blood or circulating fetal cells in amniotic fluid. The risk for subsequent affected offspring in carriers of the mutant gene or in families with known cases of SMA may also be evaluated genetically. Further diagnostic studies include muscle electromyography (EMG), which demonstrates a denervation pattern, and muscle biopsy; however, the genetic analysis has become the gold standard for diagnosis of the condition (Haliloglu, 2020).

Therapeutic Management

There is no cure for the disease, and treatment is symptomatic and supportive, primarily preventing joint contractures and treating orthopedic problems, the most serious of which is scoliosis. Hip subluxation and dislocation may also occur. Many children benefit from powered wheelchairs, lifts, special pressure-adjustable mattresses, and accessible environmental controls. Muscle and joint contractures require careful attention and care to prevent further complications. Nutritional growth failure may occur in infants and toddlers as a result of poor feeding; supplemental gastrostomy feedings may be required to maintain adequate nutritional status and maintain weight gain. The use of lower extremity orthoses may assist with ambulation, but eventually the child may be confined to a wheelchair as muscle atrophy progresses. Restrictive lung disease is the most serious complication of SMA (Arnold et al., 2019). Upper respiratory tract infections often

BOX 30.6 Clinical Manifestations of Spinal Muscular Atrophy

Type 1 (Werdnig-Hoffmann Disease)

- Clinical manifestations within first few weeks or months of life
- Onset within 6 months of life
- Inactivity the most prominent feature
- Infant lying in a frog-leg position with legs externally rotated, abducted, and flexed at knees
- Generalized weakness
- Absent deep tendon reflexes
- Limited movements of shoulder and arm muscles
- Active movement usually limited to fingers and toes
- Diaphragmatic breathing with sternal retractions (diaphragmatic paralysis may occur)
- Abnormal tongue movements (at rest)
- Weak cry and cough
- Poor suck reflex
- Fatigues quickly during feedings (if breastfed, may lose weight before noticeable)
- Failure to thrive (nutritional)
- Alert facies
- Normal sensation and intellect
- Affected infants not able to sit alone, roll over, or walk
- Early death possible from respiratory failure or infection

Type 2 (Intermediate Spinal Muscular Atrophy)

- Onset before age 18 months
  - **Early**—Weakness confined to arms and legs
  - **Later**—Becomes generalized
- Legs usually involved to greater extent than arms
- Prominent pectus excavatum
- Movements absent during complete relaxation or sleep
- Some infants able to sit if placed in position, but few can ambulate
- For most, life span varies from 7 months to 7 years, although many have normal life expectancy

Type 3 (Kugelberg-Welander Syndrome; Mild Spinal Muscular Atrophy)

- Onset of symptoms after 18 months of age
- Normal head control and ability to sit unassisted by 6 to 8 months of age
- Thigh and hip muscles weak
- Scoliosis common
- Failure to walk a common presentation
- In those who manage to walk:
  - Waddling gait
  - Genu recurvatum
  - Protuberant abdomen
  - Ambulation becoming increasingly difficult
  - Confined to a wheelchair by second decade
- Deep tendon reflexes may be present early but disappear

Type IV (Adult Spinal Muscular Atrophy)

- Rare, adult-onset spinal muscular atrophy usually in second or third decade of life; muscle weakness is first symptom

Note: These classifications are general, but some research suggests that there may be variations in life span and other characteristics (Iannaccone & Burghes, 2002; Lunn & Wang, 2008; Russman, 1996; Russman, Iannaccone, Buncher, et al., 1992).

occur and are treated with antibiotic therapy; they are the cause of death in many children. Rapid eye movement (REM)–related sleep-disordered breathing is common in children with SMA type 1; this progresses to sleep-disordered breathing during REM and non-REM sleep followed by respiratory failure, which often requires nocturnal noninvasive mechanical ventilation (Arnold et al., 2019). Noninvasive ventilation methods such as bilevel positive airway pressure (BiPAP) have decreased the morbidity and increased the survival rate of children with SMA types 1 and 2. Children with SMA type 1 who undergo tracheotomy and invasive ventilation often remain ventilator dependent for the rest of their lives; some families choose to withdraw support when invasive ventilation becomes necessary (Mercuri, Bertini, & Iannaccone, 2012). Palliative care is an important aspect of care for families of children with SMA type 1. A decreased ability to cough and clear secretions may be managed with airway clearance therapies such as the cough-assist machine and manual cough assistance. Guidelines for the standardization of respiratory care for patients with SMA have been published elsewhere (Schroth, 2009).

In addition to noninvasive respiratory support, some infants and children may benefit from tracheostomy and mechanical ventilation. If untreated, some infants may die of respiratory complications in infancy.

Associated medical conditions in survivors include gastroesophageal reflux, scoliosis, early-onset puberty, hip dysplasia, and recurrent oral candidiasis (Bach, 2007). A referral to pediatric palliative care may help the families of children with SMA make decisions about the benefits and burdens of treatment options.

A new therapy to treat SMA has recently been approved by the US Food and Drug Administration. Spinraza (nusinersen) is an antisense oligonucleotide (ASO) that consists of small strings of synthetic nucleotides that selectively bind ribonucleic acid (RNA). It was designed to treat infants with SMA. In recent studies, treated infants experienced a statistically significant improvement in motor milestones compared with those not treated. The medication is given by intrathecal injection. This allows it to be delivered directly to the CSF around the spinal cord, where motor neurons degenerate in SMA patients due to insufficient levels of survival motor neuron (SMN) protein. Spinraza is designed to alter the splicing of *SMN2* to increase the production of full-length SMN protein. Although not a cure, it is showing promise of improving motor skills in infants with SMA (Meylemans & De Bleecker, 2019).

Nursing Care Management

An infant or a small child with progressive muscle weakness requires nursing care similar to that of an immobilized patient. However, the underlying goal of treatment should be to assist the child and family in dealing with the illness while progressing toward a life of normalization within the child's capabilities. Special attention should be directed to preventing muscle and joint contractures, promoting independence in performance of ADLs, and becoming incorporated into the mainstream of school when possible. In addition, parents need support and resources to be able to provide for the child and remain an intact family. Because children with neuromuscular disease have abnormal breathing patterns that often contribute to early death, it is important to assess adequate oxygenation, especially during the sleep phase when shallow breathing occurs and hypoxemia may develop. Home pulse oximetry may be used to assess the child during sleep and provide noninvasive mechanical ventilation as necessary (Young, Lowe, & Fitzgerald, 2007) (see Duchenne Muscular Dystrophy, later in the chapter, for respiratory management). Supportive care also includes management of orthoses and other orthopedic equipment as required. Because children with SMA are intellectually normal, verbal, tactile, and auditory stimulation are important aspects of developmental care. Supporting them so that they can see the activities around them and transporting them in appropriate equipment (e.g., wagon, power wheelchair) for a change of environment provide stimulation and a broader scope of contacts.

Children who are able to sit require proper support and attention to alignment to prevent deformities and other complications. Children who survive beyond infancy need attention to educational needs and opportunities for social interaction with other children. The parents of a child who is chronically ill require much support and encouragement (see Chapter 19). Parents who have not sought genetic counseling should be encouraged to do so to evaluate further risk potential.

JUVENILE SPINAL MUSCULAR ATROPHY (KUGELBERG-WELANDER DISEASE)

Spinal muscular atrophy type 3 (Kugelberg-Welander disease) is a result of anterior horn cell and motor nerve degeneration. The disease is characterized by a pattern of muscular weakness similar to that of infantile SMA (see Box 30.6). Several modes of inheritance have been reported for the disease: autosomal recessive, autosomal dominant, and X-linked recessive.

The onset occurs from younger than 1 year of age into adulthood, with symptoms resembling group 3 infantile SMA. Proximal muscle weakness (especially of the lower limbs) and muscular atrophy are the predominant features. The disease runs a slowly progressive course. Some children lose the ability to walk 8 to 9 years after the onset of symptoms, but many can still walk after 30 years or more. One source notes that approximately one-half of all children with SMA type 3 lose ambulation by age 14 years and may require a wheelchair when falls are more frequent (Mercuri et al., 2012). Many affected persons have a normal life expectancy.

Therapeutic and Nursing Care Management

Promising results from ongoing clinical trials suggest that treatments that increase SMN protein might provide clinical benefit to patients with spinal muscular atrophy (Sumner & Crawford, 2018). However, the management is primarily symptomatic and supportive and is related to maintaining mobility for as long as possible, preventing complications such as skin breakdown, optimizing and maintaining respiratory function, and providing support to the child and family. The discussion of family support in the section on Duchenne muscular dystrophy (later in the chapter) is also applicable to families of children with SMA.

GUILLAIN-BARRÉ SYNDROME

Guillain-Barré syndrome (GBS), also known as *infectious polyneuritis,* is an uncommon acute demyelinating polyneuropathy with a progressive, usually ascending flaccid paralysis. The hallmark of GBS is acute peripheral motor weakness. The paralysis usually occurs approximately 10 days after a nonspecific viral infection; GBS has also been reported after administration of certain vaccines (e.g., rabies, influenza, polio, meningococcal) (Haliloglu, 2020). Several subtypes of GBS include acute inflammatory demyelinating neuropathy, acute motor axonal neuropathy, acute motor sensory axonal neuropathy, and Miller Fisher syndrome. Children are less often affected than adults; among children, those between ages 4 and 10 years have higher susceptibility. The male-to-female ratio is reported to be 1.5 to 1. Two peak periods with an increased incidence of GBS have been identified: late adolescence and young adulthood.

Chronic inflammatory demyelinating polyradiculoneuropathies (CIDPs) are chronic types of GBS that recur intermittently or do not improve over a period of months to years (Ryan, 2020). The following discussion focuses on GBS.

Congenital GBS is rare, yet may occur in the neonatal period, and consists of hypotonia, weakness, and decreased or absent reflexes.

Maternal neuromuscular disease may or may not be present. Diagnosis is established by the same criteria as in older children, but the symptoms gradually subside over the first few months of life and disappear by 12 months (Ryan, 2020).

Pathophysiology

Guillain-Barré syndrome is an immune-mediated disease often associated with a number of viral or bacterial infections or the administration of certain vaccines. It has been associated with infectious mononucleosis, measles, mumps, *Campylobacter jejuni* (gastroenteritis), cytomegalovirus, *Borrelia burgdorferi* (Lyme disease), Epstein-Barr virus, *Helicobacter pylori,* and *Mycoplasma* and *Pneumocystis* infections. Onset of GBS symptoms usually occurs within 10 days of the primary infection. Pathologic changes in spinal and cranial nerves consist of inflammation and edema with rapid, segmented demyelination and compression of nerve roots within the dural sheath. Nerve conduction is impaired, producing ascending partial or complete paralysis of muscles innervated by the involved nerves. GBS has three phases:

1. Acute—Phase starts when symptoms begin and continues until new symptoms stop appearing or deterioration ceases; it may last as long as 4 weeks.
2. Plateau—Symptoms remain constant without further deterioration; it may last from days to weeks.
3. Recovery—Patient begins to improve and progress to optimal recovery; it usually lasts a few weeks to months, depending on the deficits incurred by the illness.

Clinical Manifestations

A mild influenza-like illness or sore throat usually precedes the paralytic manifestations of GBS. The onset can be rapid, reaching peak activity within 24 hours, or there may be a gradual progression of symptoms over days or weeks. Neurologic symptoms initially involve muscle tenderness that sometimes is accompanied by paresthesia and cramps. Proximal muscle weakness progressing to paralysis usually occurs before distal weakness, and there is a tendency toward symmetric involvement. In most patients paralysis ascends from the lower extremities, often involving the muscles of the trunk and upper extremities and those supplied by cranial nerves. The seventh cranial (facial) nerve is often affected.

Tendon reflexes are depressed or absent, and paralysis is flaccid. Paralysis may involve facial, extraocular, labial, lingual, pharyngeal, and laryngeal muscles. Evidence of intercostal and phrenic nerve involvement includes breathlessness in vocalizations and shallow, irregular respirations. There may be variable degrees of sensory impairment. Most patients complain of muscle tenderness or sensitivity to slight pressure. Lower limb pain and back pain are common in children with GBS. Urinary incontinence or retention and constipation are often present. Abdominal pain and fatigue have also been reported in children with GBS (Lyons, 2008).

Autonomic nervous system disturbances may occur in children and adolescents with severe muscle involvement and respiratory muscle paralysis. These include orthostatic hypotension; hypertension; and vagal responses such as bradycardia, asystole, and heart block (Piccione, Salame, & Katirji, 2014).

Diagnostic Evaluation

Diagnosis is based on the paralytic manifestations, CSF analysis, and EMG. Motor nerve conduction velocities are greatly reduced. Sensory nerve conduction time is often slowed. CSF analysis reveals an elevated protein concentration, fewer than 10 WBCs/mm^3, and normal glucose level (Ryan, 2020). Other laboratory studies are usually noncontributory. The symmetric nature of the paralysis helps differentiate this disorder from spinal paralytic poliomyelitis, which usually affects sporadic muscles.

Therapeutic Management

Treatment of GBS is primarily supportive. In the acute phase, patients are hospitalized because respiratory and pharyngeal involvement may require assisted ventilation, sometimes with a temporary tracheostomy. Treatment modalities include aggressive ventilatory support in the event of respiratory compromise, intravenous (IV) administration of immunoglobulin (IVIG), and sometimes steroids; plasmapheresis and immunosuppressive drugs may also be used. Plasmapheresis has been shown to decrease the length of recovery in patients with severe GBS; however, it is expensive, and side effects include hypotension, fever, bleeding disorders, chills, urticaria, and bradycardia. Further evidence reports equal benefits to treatment of GBS with IVIG administration or plasmapheresis; both sped up recovery time in studies reviewed (Liu, Dong, & Ubogu, 2018). However, there is evidence of significant improvement in children with high-dose IVIG therapy (vs. supportive treatment alone) (Liu et al., 2018). IVIG is now recommended as the primary treatment of GBS when administered within 2 weeks of disease onset (Piccione et al., 2014). Corticosteroids alone do not decrease the symptoms or shorten the duration of the disease.

Additional medications that may be administered during the acute phase include a low-molecular-weight heparin to prevent deep vein thrombosis (DVT), a mild laxative or stool softener to prevent constipation, pain medication such as acetaminophen, and a histamine-antagonist to prevent stress ulcer formation. Chronic neuropathic pain after GBS may be treated with gabapentin, which is reported to be more effective than carbamazepine (Ryan, 2020).

Rehabilitation after the acute phase may involve physical therapy, occupational therapy, and speech therapy. Additional consideration should be given to problems of general weakness and retraining for toileting and feeding (Lyons, 2008).

Prognosis

Better outcomes are associated with younger age, no requirement for mechanical respiratory assistance, slower progression of disease, normal peripheral nerve function on EMG, and treatment with either IVIG or plasmapheresis. Recovery usually begins within 2 to 3 weeks, and most patients regain full muscle strength. The recovery of muscle strength progresses in the reverse order of onset of paralysis, with lower extremity strength being the last to recover. Poor prognosis with subsequent residual effects in children is reportedly associated with cranial nerve involvement, extensive disability at time of presentation, and intubation.

Most deaths associated with GBS are caused by respiratory failure; therefore early diagnosis and access to respiratory support are especially important. The rate of recovery is usually related to the degree of involvement and may extend from a few weeks to months. The greater the degree of paralysis, the longer the recovery phase.

Nursing Care Management

Nursing care is primarily supportive and is the same as that required for children with immobilization and respiratory compromise. The emphasis of care is on close observation to assess the extent of paralysis and on prevention of complications, including aspiration, ventilator-associated pneumonia (VAP), atelectasis, DVT, pressure ulcer, fear and anxiety, autonomic dysfunction, and pain.

During the acute phase of the disease, the nurse should carefully observe the child's condition for possible difficulty in swallowing and respiratory involvement. The child's respiratory function is closely monitored, and oxygen source, appropriate-size insufflation bag and mask, endotracheal intubation and suctioning equipment, tracheotomy tray, and vasopressor drugs are kept available. Vital signs are monitored frequently, as are neurologic signs and level of consciousness. For children who develop respiratory impairment, the care is the same as that for any child with respiratory distress requiring mechanical ventilation.

Respiratory care, if intubation is required, requires close monitoring of oxygenation status (usually by pulse oximetry and sometimes arterial blood gases), maintenance of an open airway with suctioning, and postural changes to prevent pneumonia. Consideration should be given to preventing opportunistic infections such as VAP; meticulous oral care and hypopharynx suctioning, elevating the head of the bed 30 degrees, and strict asepsis with suctioning equipment (including catheters, a Yankauer device, or both) should be implemented to prevent VAP. Children with oral and pharyngeal involvement may be fed via a nasogastric or gastrostomy tube to ensure adequate feeding. It is also important to consider the possibility of stress ulcers in such patients and to administer a proton pump inhibitor. Immobilization, which occurs with GBS, decreases GI function; therefore problems such as decreased gastric emptying, constipation, and feeding residuals require nursing assessment and appropriate collaborative interventions. Temporary urinary catheterization may be required; urinary retention is common, and appropriate assessment of urinary output is vital. Sensory impairment and paralysis in the lower extremities make the child susceptible to skin breakdown, and attention should be given to meticulous skin care. Passive range-of-motion exercises and application of orthoses to prevent muscle contracture are important when paralysis is present. Prevention of DVT is accomplished with pneumatic compression (antiembolism) devices, administration of a low-molecular-weight heparin, and early mobilization and ambulation. Autonomic dysfunction may be life threatening; thus close monitoring of vital signs in the acute phase is essential.

A key to recovery in the child with GBS is the prevention of muscle and joint contractures, so passive range-of-motion exercises must be carried out routinely to maintain vital function. Although the child may have a generalized paralysis, cognitive function remains intact; therefore it is important for nursing care to involve communication with the child or adolescent regarding procedures and treatments that may be frightening, especially if mechanical ventilation is required. Encourage parents to talk to the child and make eye and physical contact and to reassure the child during this phase of the illness.

Pain management is crucial in the care of children with GBS. Although neuromuscular impairment may make pain perception more difficult to evaluate accurately, objective pain scales should be used. Gabapentin and carbamazepine may be used to manage neuropathic pain in patients with GBS.

Physical therapy may be limited to passive range-of-motion exercises during the evolving phase of the disease. Later, as the disease stabilizes and recovery begins, an active physical therapy program is implemented to prevent contracture deformities and facilitate muscle recovery. This may include active exercise, gait training, and bracing.

Throughout the course of the illness, child and parent support are paramount. The usual rapidity of the paralysis and the long recovery period greatly tax the emotional reserves of all family members. The parents and child benefit from repeated reassurance that recovery is occurring and from realistic information on the possibility of permanent disability. In the event of a residual disability, the family needs assistance in accepting and adjusting to the loss of function (see Chapter 17). The GBS/CIDP Foundation International is a nonprofit organization devoted to support, education, and research. It provides families with support from recovered persons, publishes informational literature and a newsletter, and maintains a list of health care practitioners experienced with the disease.

TETANUS

Tetanus, or lockjaw, is an acute, preventable, and sometimes fatal disease caused by an exotoxin produced by the anaerobic, spore-forming, gram-positive bacillus *Clostridium tetani.* It is characterized by painful muscular rigidity primarily involving the masseter and neck muscles. The development of tetanus has four requirements: (1) presence of tetanus spores or vegetative forms of the bacillus, (2) injury to the tissues, (3) wound conditions that encourage multiplication of the organism, and (4) a susceptible host.

Tetanus spores are found in soil, dust, and the intestinal tracts of humans and animals, especially herbivorous animals. The organisms are more prevalent in rural areas but are readily carried to urban areas by wind. They enter the body by way of wounds, particularly a puncture wound, burn, or crushed area. In the newborn, infection may occur through the umbilical cord, usually in situations in which infants are delivered in contaminated surroundings and the mother has not been properly immunized against tetanus. The disease has the greatest incidence during months in which persons are more involved in outdoor activities.

Prevention

Primary prevention is key and occurs through immunization and boosters and good wound care. Once an injury has occurred, further preventive measures are based on the child's immune status and the nature of the injury. Specific prophylactic therapy after trauma is administration of either tetanus toxoid or tetanus antitoxin. A dose of tetanus toxoid is not necessary for clean, minor wounds in children who have completed the immunization series (see Chapter 10) or who have received a booster within the previous 10 years. Protective levels of antibody are maintained for at least 10 years. Therefore antitoxin is not indicated for the fully immunized child. Children with more serious wounds (e.g., contaminated, puncture, crush, or burn wounds) are given a tetanus toxoid booster prophylactically as soon as possible after injury.

The unprotected or inadequately immunized child who sustains a "tetanus-prone" wound (including wounds contaminated with dirt, feces, soil, and saliva; puncture wounds; avulsions; and wounds resulting from missiles, crushing, burns, and frostbite) should receive tetanus immunoglobulin (TIG). Concurrent administration of both TIG and tetanus toxoid at separate sites is recommended both to provide protection and to initiate the active immune process (Kimberlin, Brady, Jackson, et al., 2018). Completion of active immunization is carried out according to the usual pattern. Proper surgical cleansing and debridement of contaminated wounds reduce the chance of infection.

Pathophysiology

When prevention efforts are not effective and conditions are favorable, the organisms multiply and form two exotoxins: (1) tetanospasmin, a potent toxin that affects the CNS to produce the clinical manifestations of the disease, and (2) tetanolysin, which appears to have no significance. The ideal conditions for growth of the organisms are devitalized tissues without access to air (e.g., puncture wounds); wounds that have not been washed or kept clean; and those that have crusted over, trapping pus beneath. The exotoxin appears to reach the CNS by way of either the neuron axons or the vascular system. The toxin becomes fixed on nerve cells of the brainstem and the anterior horn of the spinal cord. The toxin acts at the neuromuscular junction to produce muscular stiffness and to lower the threshold for reflex excitability.

The incubation period is 3 days to 3 weeks and averages 8 days. Most cases occur within 14 days; in neonates it is usually 5 to 14 days.

Shorter incubation periods have been associated with more heavily contaminated wounds, more severe disease, and a worse prognosis (Kimberlin et al., 2018).

Clinical Manifestations

There are several forms of the disease. Local tetanus is a less common but severe form characterized by persistent rigidity of muscles near the inoculation site, which may persist for weeks or months. Some cases resolve without sequelae. Neonatal tetanus results from contamination of the umbilical cord, which is rare in the United States but is common and often fatal in developing countries. The first symptom is difficulty in sucking, progressing to total inability to suck, excessive crying, irritability, and nuchal rigidity.

Generalized tetanus is the most common and dangerous form of the disease. The manner of onset varies, but the initial symptoms are usually a progressive stiffness and tenderness of the muscles in the neck and jaw. The characteristic difficulty in opening the mouth (**trismus**), which is caused by sustained contraction of the jaw-closing muscles, is evident early and gives the disease its common name, lockjaw. Spasm of facial muscles produces the so-called sardonic smile (**risus sardonicus**). Progressive involvement of the trunk muscles causes **opisthotonos** and a boardlike rigidity of abdominal and limb muscles. The patient has difficulty swallowing and is highly sensitive to external stimuli. The slightest noise, a gentle touch, or bright light triggers convulsive muscular contractions that last seconds to minutes. The paroxysmal contractions recur with increased frequency until they become almost continuous.

Mentation is unaffected; the patient remains alert, and pain and distress are reflected in a rapid pulse, sweating, and an anxious expression. Laryngospasm and tetany of respiratory muscles and accumulated secretions predispose the child to respiratory arrest, atelectasis, and pneumonia. Fever is usually absent or mild and generally indicates a poor prognosis. As the child recovers from the disease, the paroxysms become less frequent and gradually subside. Survival beyond 4 days usually indicates recovery, but complete recovery may take weeks.

Therapeutic Management

The unprotected or inadequately immunized child who sustains a "tetanus-prone" wound (as described earlier) should receive TIG. Concurrent administration of both TIG and tetanus toxoid at separate sites is recommended both to provide protection and to initiate the active immune process (Kimberlin et al., 2018). After the individual has received primary tetanus immunization, antitoxin is believed to provide protection for at least 10 years and for a longer period after booster immunization (Kimberlin et al., 2018) (see also Chapter 6, Immunizations).

Antibiotic treatment with penicillin G (or erythromycin or tetracycline in older children with allergy to penicillin) is important in the management of tetanus as an adjunct against clostridia; metronidazole is a viable alternative (Schleiss, 2020).

Aggressive supportive care is necessary to treat tetanus in the acute phase. The acutely ill child is best treated in an intensive care facility, where close and constant observation and equipment for monitoring and respiratory support are readily available.

General supportive care is indicated, including maintaining adequate airway and fluid and electrolyte balance, providing pain management, and ensuring adequate caloric intake. Indwelling oral or nasogastric feedings may be required to maintain adequate fluid and caloric intake; continued laryngospasm may necessitate total parenteral nutrition or gastrostomy feeding. Severe or recurrent laryngospasm or excessive secretions may require advanced airway management such as endotracheal intubation; in some cases a tracheotomy may be performed to provide an adequate airway.

TIG therapy to neutralize toxins is the most specific therapy for tetanus. In countries where TIG is not available, equine tetanus antitoxin (not available in the United States) should be administered. Antibiotics are administered to control the proliferation of the vegetative forms of the organism at the site of infection. When the child recovers, active immunization should take place because contraction of the disease does not confer a permanent immunity. Standard Precautions for the child with tetanus are recommended; isolation is not recommended.

Local care of the wound by surgical debridement and cleansing with an antiseptic solution helps reduce the number of proliferating organisms at the site of injury. The cleansing should be repeated several times during the first 48 hours. Deep, infected lacerations are usually exposed and debrided. Infiltration of the wound with TIG is no longer considered necessary (Kimberlin et al., 2018).

Diazepam is the drug of choice for seizure control and muscle relaxation (Schleiss, 2020), but lorazepam (Ativan) may be used in some cases. Other AEDs may be administered as well. Intrathecal baclofen, magnesium sulfate, dantrolene sodium, and midazolam may also be used in the management of tetanus; intrathecal baclofen may cause apnea and should be used only in the intensive care setting (Schleiss, 2020). Patients with severe tetanus and those who do not respond to other muscle relaxants may require the administration of a neuromuscular blocking agent, such as rocuronium or vecuronium. Because of their paralytic effect on respiratory muscles, use of these drugs requires mechanical ventilation with endotracheal intubation or tracheotomy and constant cardiopulmonary monitoring. Endotracheal tube insertion or tracheotomy is often indicated and should be performed before severe respiratory distress develops. Despite the absence of pain manifestation with these drugs, it is important to administer adequate analgesia. The administration of corticosteroids has met with success in some cases.

Nursing Care Management

The care of the child with tetanus requires supportive management with particular attention to airway and breathing. Respiratory status is carefully evaluated for any signs of distress, and appropriate emergency equipment is kept available at all times. The location, extent, and severity of muscle spasms are important nursing observations. Muscle relaxants, opioids, and sedatives that may be prescribed can also cause respiratory depression; therefore the child should be assessed for excessive CNS depression. Attention to hydration and nutrition involves monitoring an IV infusion, monitoring nasogastric or gastrostomy feedings, and suctioning oropharyngeal secretions when indicated.

In caring for a child with tetanus during the acute phase, every effort should be made to control or eliminate stimulation from sound, light, and touch. Although a darkened room is ideal, sufficient light is essential so that the child can be carefully observed; light appears to be less irritating than vibratory or auditory stimuli. The infant or child is handled as little as possible, and extra effort is expended to avoid any sudden or loud noise to prevent seizures.

If a potent muscle relaxant such as vecuronium is used, the total paralysis makes oral communication impossible. The drug is not a sedative, however, and anxiety should be considered in children who are intubated. Therefore all of the child's needs must be anticipated and procedures carefully explained beforehand. Additional care is focused on preventing the complications associated with prolonged immobility, including decreased bowel and bladder tone and subsequent constipation, anorexia, DVT, pneumonia, and skin breakdown.

BOTULISM

Botulism is serious food poisoning that results from ingestion of the preformed toxin produced by the anaerobic bacillus *Clostridium botulinum*. Botulism toxin exerts its effect by inhibiting the release of acetylcholine at the neuromuscular junction, thereby impairing motor activity of the muscles innervated by the affected nerves. The disease has a wide variation in severity, from constipation to progressive sequential loss of neurologic function and respiratory failure. Human botulism is caused by neurotoxins A, B, E, and rarely F (Kimberlin et al., 2018). Types A and B are the most common causes of infant botulism.

Several forms of botulism are recognized: foodborne, infant, wound, human made (for bioterrorism), and botulism from undetermined causes. This chapter covers only the first three forms.

Foodborne Botulism

This classic form of the disease usually occurs in adults but may occur in children and adolescents. The most common source of the toxin is improperly sterilized home-canned foods. CNS symptoms appear abruptly approximately 12 to 36 hours after ingestion of contaminated food and may or may not be preceded by acute digestive disturbance. Early symptoms include blurred vision, diplopia, weakness, dizziness, difficulty talking and speaking, vomiting, and dysphagia. These are followed by descending paralysis and dyspnea. Progressive respiratory paralysis is life threatening.

Infant Botulism

Infant botulism, unlike the disease in older persons, is caused by ingestion of spores or vegetative cells of *C. botulinum* and the subsequent release of the toxin from organisms colonizing the GI tract. *C. botulinum* types A and B are the most common causative strains of infant botulism. This form of botulism has become more prevalent than any other form. Many cases of infant botulism occur in breastfed infants who are being introduced to nonhuman milk substances (Kimberlin et al., 2018). Cases of infant botulism are still being reported in Europe, where honey is commonly given to infants. There appears to be no common food or drug source of the organisms; however, the *C. botulinum* organisms have been found in honey. Botulism may occur in infants from 1 week to 12 months of age, with peak incidence between 2 and 4 months of age.

The severity of the disease varies widely, from mild constipation to progressive sequential loss of neurologic function and respiratory failure. The affected infant is usually well before the onset of symptoms. Constipation is a common presenting symptom, and almost all infants exhibit generalized weakness and a decrease in spontaneous movements. Deep tendon reflexes are usually diminished or absent. Cranial nerve deficits are common, as evidenced by loss of head control, difficulty in feeding, weak cry, and reduced gag reflex. SMA type 1 and metabolic disorders are often mistaken for infant botulism in the initial diagnostic phase because of the similarities in clinical manifestations of hypotonia, lethargy, and poor feeding (Norton & Schleiss, 2020). Presenting clinical signs also often mimic those of sepsis in young infants. Botulism toxin exerts its effect by inhibiting the release of acetylcholine at the myoneural junction, thereby impairing motor activity of muscles innervated by affected nerves.

Diagnosis and Therapeutic Management

The diagnosis is made on the basis of the clinical history, physical examination, and laboratory detection of the organism in the patient's stool and, less commonly, blood. However, isolation of the organism may take several days; therefore suspicion of botulism by clinical presentation should require emergency treatment (Norton & Schleiss, 2020). EMG may be helpful in establishing the diagnosis; however, results may be normal early in the course of the illness.

Treatment consists of immediate administration of botulism immune globulin intravenously (BIG-IV) (Norton & Schleiss, 2020) without delaying for laboratory diagnosis. Early administration of BIG-IV neutralizes the toxin and stops the progression of the disease. The human-derived botulism antitoxin (BIG-IV) has been evaluated and is now available nationwide for use only in infant botulism. Infants treated with BIG-IV usually have a shortened hospital stay from approximately 6 days to 2 weeks, reportedly as a result of decreased requirements for mechanical ventilation and intensive care (Norton & Schleiss, 2020). Approximately 50% of affected infants require intubation and mechanical ventilation; therefore respiratory support is crucial, as is nutritional support because these infants are unable to feed. Trivalent equine botulinum antitoxin and bivalent antitoxin, used in adults and older children, are not administered to infants. Antibiotic therapy is not part of the management because the botulinum toxin is an intracellular molecule and antibiotics would not be effective; aminoglycosides in particular should not be administered because they may potentiate the blocking effects of the neurotoxin (Norton & Schleiss, 2020).

The prognosis is generally good if the patient is adequately treated, although recovery may be slow, requiring a few weeks after severe illness. Untreated patients may require a longer hospitalization.

! NURSING ALERT

Although the precise source of *Clostridium botulinum* spores has not been identified as originating from honey in many cases of infant botulism in the United States, it is still recommended that honey not be given to infants younger than 12 months because the spores have been found in honey.

Nursing Care Management

Nursing responsibilities include observing, recognizing, and reporting signs of poor feeding, constipation, and muscle impairment in the infant with botulism and providing intensive nursing care when an infant is hospitalized (see Nursing Care Management for the infant with SMA, earlier in the chapter, and Chapter 8, Care of High-Risk Newborns). Parental support and reassurance are important. Most infants recover when the disorder is recognized and BIG-IV therapy is implemented. Nursing care of the infant on mechanical ventilation requires observation of oxygenation status and vigilance for any complications (see Chapter 26). Parents should be aware that, during recovery, infants fatigue easily when muscular action is sustained. This has important implications for timing the resumption of feedings because of the risk of aspiration. They should also be advised that normal bowel activity may not return for several weeks. Therefore a stool softener can be beneficial.

One cultural consideration that requires further parent education and anticipatory guidance is the use of honey pacifiers among mothers with small infants; there is evidence that honey pacifiers are still commonly used among many mothers to soothe their infants (Benjamins, Gourishankar, Yataco-Marquez, et al., 2013).

SPINAL CORD INJURIES

SCIs with major neurologic involvement are not a common cause of physical disability in children. Pediatric SCI incidence is estimated at 14 per million, with the adolescent age-group predominating (Piatt & Imperato, 2018). However, many children with these injuries are admitted to major medical centers, and because of the increased survival rate resulting from improved management, nurses have an important role in the care of children with SCI.

The principles of management and nursing care of the child with a spinal cord lesion apply regardless of cause. In addition to care related to the immobilized child, as discussed in Chapter 17, children with damage to the spinal cord present additional problems—specifically, complications related to the neuropathology of the central and autonomic nervous systems. The extent of paralysis is determined by both neurologic and clinical assessment. Although most children with SCI are paraplegic, some are tetraplegic (quadriplegic). Some children with tetraplegia are able to move only their face and neck muscles, whereas others are able to lift and bend their arms but are unable to perform fine hand movements. Almost every physiologic system is disrupted in a child with high-level tetraplegia. Not only are the central and peripheral nerves impaired, but there is also autonomic nervous system dysfunction. Vital structures such as blood vessels, lungs, bladder, and bowel are affected. Therefore an understanding of neuromuscular physiology is essential to effectively care for the child with damage or injury to the spinal cord.

Essential Neuromuscular Physiology

The spinal cord extends from the medulla oblongata to the lower border of the first lumbar vertebra and contains millions of nerve fibers. However, because of its protected location, a considerable amount of direct trauma is required to cause injury. Posteriorly the cord is protected by the spinous processes, which are stabilized by related ligaments and muscles. It is further protected by the spinal fluid, which surrounds it and absorbs some of the shock.

Spinal Nerves

The 31 nerves of the spinal cord are divided into five segments. The cervical cord segments lie within the first seven vertebrae. The remaining cord segments—thoracic (12), lumbar (5), sacral (5), and coccygeal (1)—extend from the first thoracic vertebra to the lower level of the first lumbar vertebra. Therefore the cord constituents do not anatomically match by number the 33 associated vertebrae. However, nerves that arise from the spinal cord exit from the spinal column at the numerically corresponding vertebrae. In describing injuries to the spinal cord, the highest point at which there is normal function is referred to in relation to the vertebra; for example, an intact cord at the sixth cervical vertebra is designated a C6 injury.

Certain areas of the curved vertebral column are less stable and more prone to damage from severe flexion and twisting. These sites are the cervical area and the junction of the thoracic and lumbar regions. The cervical vertebrae are fractured most often, and this high level of injury causes extensive paralysis and many associated neurologic problems. Also, traumatic tearing or embolic occlusion of the arteries supplying these areas can markedly jeopardize the cord tissue. Impaired blood supply often produces severe neurologic deficit, which can extend to complete loss of cord function at the level of injury.

Cell bodies of interneurons and motor neurons within the spinal cord are identified as H-shaped gray matter surrounded by columns of white myelinated nerve fibers. Each column serves as a route for a specific type of impulse, such as touch, vibration, pain, and temperature. Nerve pathways in the spinal cord transmit sensory and motor impulses between peripheral receptors and the brain, conduct impulses through the reflex arc, and convey sympathetic and parasympathetic nerve impulses from the brain to peripheral structures.

Sensory transmission begins when peripheral receptors pick up a wide variety of stimuli and transfer the impulses, by means of peripheral nerves, to the spinal nerves, where they make ganglionic connections and enter the cord posteriorly. At this point the impulses travel in two directions: across the interneuron connection and then to the motor neurons (reflex arc) or up the spinal cord to predetermined areas of the brain. Motor impulses are transmitted from the cerebral cortex to the medulla (where nerve tracts cross) and proceed down descending motor pathways to the desired level within the spinal cord. Here they connect with the anterior horn cells and are transmitted to the muscle fibers by means of the lower motor neurons to complete a meaningful movement.

A network of nerves that serves the major muscle groups constitutes a plexus. Total involvement of any one of these plexuses seriously impairs function to the areas it innervates.

Upper Versus Lower Motor Neurons

Upper motor neurons extend from cerebral centers to cells in the spinal column; lower motor neurons consist of anterior horn cells and spinal and peripheral nerves. Motor fibers of the reflex arc are lower motor neurons. This is an important point because relative dominance of the CNS over reflex arcs suppresses some reflex responses. When the higher centers no longer exert an influence in SCI, spastic responses are observed in muscles innervated by the intact lower motor neurons. Most SCIs involve upper motor neurons; children born with spinal cord defects have primarily lower motor neuron deficits.

Effect on Sensory and Motor Tracts

Voluntary muscle control is lost after complete transection of the cord. In partial transection, function is altered to varying degrees depending on the areas innervated by involved nerves. The crossing of motor tracts at various levels makes it possible for an injured person to have motor paralysis in one leg but retain pain and temperature sensation in that leg, while the opposite leg retains its motor function but loses pain and temperature sensation.

Although a transected cord injury leads to sensory loss, it is not uncommon for the injured person to experience pain. For example, smooth or skeletal muscle spasms, destruction of the myelin sheath (impulses cross to adjacent nerves), and scar formation or irritation of nerve endings may cause pain. Pain suffered by a person with tetraplegia or paraplegia is often intensified because of loss of sensation in other parts. Severe and prolonged pain should be medically evaluated for a treatable pathologic condition.

Effect on Autonomic System

Sympathetic and parasympathetic systems receive both excitatory and inhibitory stimuli from autonomic centers in the cerebral cortex, limbic system, and hypothalamus. The stimuli are transmitted by means of a feedback mechanism within the ascending fibers of the cord that normally controls descending input. Axons of the many CNS neurons synapse with autonomic preganglionic fibers and thus are able to alter their patterned responses.

Etiology

The most common cause of serious spinal cord damage in children is trauma involving MVCs (including automobile/bicycle, all-terrain vehicles, and snowmobiles), sports injuries (especially from diving, trampoline activities, gymnastics, and football), birth trauma, and nonaccidental trauma. MVCs accounted for 31.9% of SCIs in children and 50% in adolescents, and falls accounted for 18.3% in children and 10% in adolescents (Piatt & Imperato, 2018). In the United States football injuries accounted for a high percentage of sport-related injuries in adolescents, whereas in Canada such injuries were associated with ice hockey (Mathison, Kadom, & Krug, 2008).

The increased use of recreational activities involving motorized vehicles such as jet water skis, all-terrain vehicles, and motorcycles has also increased the incidence of SCIs in children. Congenital defects of the spine such as myelomeningocele also may in some cases produce the effects of SCI (see discussion earlier in the chapter).

Transverse myelitis (inflammation of the spinal cord) may be caused by illness and has also been reported to develop from inadvertent intra-arterial administration of long-acting penicillin injected into the buttocks. Damage can be extensive enough to result in paraplegia or even lower limb amputation.

In MVCs, most SCIs in children are a result of indirect trauma caused by sudden hyperflexion or hyperextension of the neck, often combined with a rotational force. Trauma to the spinal cord without evidence of vertebral fracture or dislocation (**SCI without radiographic abnormality**, or SCIWORA) is particularly likely to occur in an MVC when proper safety restraints are not used. An unrestrained child becomes a projectile during sudden deceleration and is subject to injury from contact with various objects inside and outside the vehicle. Individuals who use only a lap seat belt restraint are at greater risk for SCI than those who use a combination lap and shoulder restraint. High cervical spine injuries have been reported in children younger than 2 years who are improperly restrained in forward-facing car seats. Infants who are improperly restrained in an infant car seat may experience cervical trauma in a car crash. Small children may also be severely injured by deploying front seat air bags.

Falling from heights occurs less often in children than in adults, but vertebral compression from blows to the head or buttocks can occur in water sports (diving and surfing), falls from horses, or other athletic activities. Birth injuries may occur in breech births from traction force on the spinal cord during birth of the head and shoulders. When shaken, infants commonly sustain cervical cord damage, as well as subdural hematoma and retinal hemorrhage; cognitive impairment and death may occur subsequent to the traumatic event. Infants have weak neck muscles, and during vigorous shaking their large and heavy heads rapidly wobble back and forth. A significant number of adolescents receive SCIs secondary to gunshot wounds, stabbings, and other violent inflicted injuries.

Because of the marked mobility of the neck, fracture or **subluxation** (partial dislocation) is the most common immediate cause of SCI, particularly in the lower cervical region. Although unusual in adults, SCI without fracture is common in children, whose spines are suppler, weaker, and more mobile than those of adults. Therefore the force is more easily dissipated over a larger number of segments. In infants and small children younger than 5 years, upper cervical spine fractures and spinal compression are more common, but adolescents tend to have lower cervical and thoracolumbar fracture dislocations (Proctor, 2020). Children who suffer SCI before puberty are reported to experience a higher incidence of musculoskeletal complications such as scoliosis and hip dislocation (Vogel, Betz, & Mulcahey, 2012).

Pathophysiology

The severity of the force, the mechanisms of the injury, and the degree of the individual's muscular relaxation at the time of the injury greatly influence the extent of the trauma. SCIs are classified as either *complete* or *incomplete.* In a complete injury, there is no motor or sensory function more than three segments below the neurologic level of the injury (Alizadeh, Dyck, & Karimi-Abdolrezaee, 2019). Incomplete lesions have several typical characteristics (Mathison et al., 2008):

- Central cord syndrome—Central gray matter destruction and preservation of peripheral tracts; tetraplegia with sacral sparing common; some motor recovery gained
- Anterior cord syndrome—Complete motor and sensory loss with trunk and lower extremity proprioception and sensation of pressure
- Posterior cord syndrome—Loss of sensation, pain, and proprioception with normal cord function, including motor function; able to move extremities but have difficulty controlling such movements
- Brown-Séquard syndrome—Unilateral cord lesion with a motor deficit on the opposite side of the body from the primary insult; absence of pain and temperature sensation on the opposite side from the injury
- Spinal cord concussion—Transient loss of neural function below the level of the acute spinal cord lesion, resulting in flaccid paralysis and loss of tendon, autonomic, and cutaneous reflex activity; may last hours to weeks

The American Spinal Injury Association (Alizadeh et al., 2019) International Standards for Neurological Classification of Spinal Cord Injury worksheet was recently revised and published in the cited reference. The American Spinal Injury Association Impairment Scale combines motor and sensory function and is used to determine the severity of impairment from the injury (complete or incomplete). It may also be used to measure neurologic changes and functional goals for rehabilitation (Alizadeh et al., 2019).

The injury sustained can affect any of the spinal nerves, and the higher the injury, the more extensive the damage. The child can be left with complete or partial paralysis of the lower extremities (**paraplegia**) or with damage at a higher level and without functional use of any of the four extremities (**tetraplegia**). A high cervical cord injury that affects the phrenic nerve paralyzes the diaphragm and leaves the child dependent on mechanical ventilation.

A mild but equally frightening form of cord trauma is **spinal cord compression**, a temporary neural dysfunction without visible damage to the cord. Complete tetraplegia can result but initially may not be differentiated from serious cord injury.

Clinical Manifestations

It is often difficult to determine the extent and severity of damage at first. Immediate loss of function is caused by both anatomic and impaired physiologic function, and improved function may not be evident for weeks or even months. Manifestation of the initial response to acute SCI is flaccid paralysis below the level of the damage. This stage is often referred to as **spinal shock syndrome** and is caused by the sudden disruption of central and autonomic pathways. Local effects of cord edema and ischemia produce a physiologic transection with or without an anatomic severance. Most children with an SCI experience some spinal shock. Manifestations include the absence of reflexes at or below the cord lesion, with flaccidity or limpness of the involved muscles, loss of sensation and motor function, and autonomic dysfunction (i.e., symptoms of hypotension, low or high body temperature, loss of bladder and bowel control, and autonomic dysreflexia). It is estimated that 25% to 50% of children with SCI will have a delay in the onset of neurologic abnormalities ranging from 30 minutes to 4 days (Vogel et al., 2012).

Autonomic paralysis also affects thermoregulatory functions. Afferent impulses from temperature receptors in the skin are not integrated; therefore the patient is subject to temperature increases or decreases in response to alterations in environmental temperature. Hyperthermia can result from excessive ambient temperature, such as too many covers.

Except in the situations previously mentioned, flaccid paralysis is replaced by spinal reflex activity and increasing spasticity or, in incomplete lesions, greater or lesser degree of neurologic recovery.

The paralytic nature of autonomic function is replaced by autonomic dysreflexia, especially when the lesions are above the midthoracic level. This autonomic phenomenon is caused by visceral distention or irritation, particularly of the bowel or bladder. Sensory impulses are triggered and travel to the cord lesion, where they are blocked, which causes activation of sympathetic reflex action with disturbed central inhibitory control. Excessive sympathetic activity is manifested by a flushing face, sweating forehead, pupillary constriction, marked hypertension, headache, and bradycardia. The precipitating stimulus may be merely a full bladder or rectum, or other internal or external sensory input. It can be a catastrophic event unless the irritation is relieved.

Additional clinical findings of SCI may include numbness, tingling, or burning; priapism; weakness; and loss of bowel and bladder control (Hayes & Arriola, 2005).

Neurogenic shock occurs as a result of a disruption in the descending sympathetic pathways with loss of vasomotor tone and sympathetic innervations to the cardiovascular system (Hagen, 2015). Hypotension, bradycardia, and peripheral vasodilation occur as a result of neurogenic shock.

Children with suspected SCI may have suffered multiple injuries (e.g., MVC); therefore multiple clinical manifestations that may mask those of an SCI may occur.

In the final stage, neurologic signs are stabilized in terms of loss and recovery of function. The major emphasis is on rehabilitation. A problem unique to injury in childhood is progressive spinal deformity usually not seen in adults or in adolescents near the end of the growth period. Scoliosis develops in most children with high thoracic and cervical lesions and is almost certain to occur in children with tetraplegia whose injury occurred in infancy or early childhood.

Diagnostic Evaluation

A history of the injury provides valuable clues regarding the possible type of damage incurred and directions for further assessment without the risk of additional damage. A complete neurologic examination determines whether damage was incurred and, if so, the level and extent of any nerve impairment. A neurologic unit of the CNS is considered normal if reflex arcs are functioning, sensory tracts are intact when each dermatome is examined separately, and voluntary motor response demonstrates an ability to move a body part against gravity on command.

Testing a reflex arc is accomplished by stimulating the peripheral receptors at a specific site, such as eliciting the patellar reflex. Symmetric testing is performed to determine unilateral or bilateral neurologic deficit. A sufficient number of reflexes are examined to test motor function thoroughly. The blunt end of a safety pin is used to assess pressure sensitivity, and the sharp point is used to elicit pain. Hot and cold water, a tuning fork, and cotton may also be used to determine specific sensory loss (e.g., temperature, vibration, light touch).

The American Spinal Injury Association dermatome classification worksheet is used to determine the extent of neurologic damage. Body surface zones, or dermatomes, accurately correspond to the spinal cord segment receiving the sensory input from the peripheral nerves in that zone. Systematically pinpricking the body surface in each zone determines intactness of sensory pathways. The examiner tests for each specific sensory fiber in the dermatome areas in which neurologic deficit is suspected.

Matching cord level to vertebra is more difficult in infants and young children than it is in older children and adults because the sacral and several lower lumbar cord segments lie at a lower position, especially during the first 2 years of life. The spinal anatomy approaches adult configuration by the time the child reaches age 7 or 8 years; by late adolescence the conus medullaris has usually reached the level of L1.

Motor system evaluation includes observing gait if the child is able to walk; noting balance maintenance with the child's eyes open and closed; and noting the ability to lift, flex, and extend the arms and legs. Testing muscle strength with and without resistance and against gravity provides clues to the specific nature and degree of motor dysfunction. The number of muscles in any muscle group that remain completely intact in the upper extremities makes a marked difference in the individual's ability to provide self-care, especially at high injury levels. Hip movement is necessary for ambulation with braces and crutches.

The degree to which supportive aids are needed for ambulation is determined by the strength, stability, and movement of the pelvis, trunk, hip flexor muscles, and quadriceps muscles. A general guideline for determining the capacity for self-help is that a person with paraplegia who has function down to and including the quadriceps muscle or muscle function below the L3 level will have little difficulty in learning to walk with or without braces and crutches. It is especially vital that children with lumbar levels of injury be taught to walk functionally so that they are weight bearing at least part of the time; this minimizes the risk of osteoporosis and hypercalcemia.

If a CNS pathologic disorder is detected, a body system assessment is performed to determine the degree of autonomic impairment. Because the cord and CNS directly influence the function of the autonomic nerves, the specific sympathetically related organ systems are examined for skeletal muscle and vascular tone and body temperature regulation. For example, bladder and GI functions have sympathetic and parasympathetic innervation and local reflexes.

CT and MRI scans are important for localizing the lesion, but the nature of the spine in childhood often creates difficulty in interpretation. Guidelines for diagnostic imaging of children with suspected SCI have been published elsewhere (Rozelle, Arabi, Dhall, et al., 2013). Small children often have no radiographic evidence of vertebral or spinal injury despite significant injuries ranging from complete transection with major hemorrhage to minor hemorrhage, edema, or normal neural findings. This condition, SCIWORA, is reported to occur in 17% to 20% of cervical spine injuries in toddlers ages 0 to 3 years and accounts for only 5% of cervical spine injuries in teenagers (Farrell, Hannon, & Lee, 2017). The younger the child, the more likely it is for SCIWORA to occur; it is seen in up to 72% of children 5 years old and younger (Schottler, Vogel, & Sturm, 2012). SCIWORA is also a common finding in very young children who are victims of abuse (primarily shaken baby syndrome) because of the elasticity and incomplete ossification of the vertebrae. SCIWORA is more common in children under the age of 8 years, and injury to the cervical spine is common. Diagnostic scans must be taken carefully and with sufficient help to prevent further damage to the spine.

Therapeutic Management

Initial care begins at the scene of the accident with proper immobilization of the cervical, thoracic, and lumbar spine. Immobilization should take into account the age and size of the child; smaller children have a larger head, which may make effective immobilization on a rigid board difficult (Rozelle et al., 2013). Because of the complexity of these injuries, it is usually recommended that these persons be transported to a spinal injury center for care by specially trained health care personnel as soon as possible after the injury for appropriate diagnostic evaluation and intervention.

The initial management of the child with a suspected SCI should begin with an assessment of the ABCs: **a**irway, **b**reathing, and circulation. The airway should be opened using the jaw-thrust technique to minimize damage to the cervical spine. The child is monitored for cardiovascular instability, and measures are taken to support systemic blood pressure and maintain optimal cardiac output. Because MVCs and other trauma in children may involve internal organ damage and potential bleeding, abdominal distention and other signs are acted on immediately to prevent further systemic shock. After the child is stabilized and transported to a regional trauma center, a thorough evaluation of neurologic status and any other associated trauma is carried out by the multidisciplinary team. In the emergency department, spinal immobilization should be maintained until a thorough neurologic assessment is completed and SCI is ruled out; in children, this typically involves a CT scan and possibly an MRI. Additional interventions are discussed in the Nursing Care Management section. Assessment of neurologic status using the Glasgow Coma Scale (see Chapter 27) is important; a helpful assessment is represented in the mnemonic AVPU: ***a***lert; responds to ***v***erbal stimuli; responds to ***p***ainful stimuli; and ***u***nresponsive. A secondary assessment tool in the emergency department follows the mnemonic AMPLE: ***a***llergies, ***m***edications, ***p***ast medical history, ***l***ast meal or fluids, and ***e***nvironment and events leading to the incident (Avarello & Cantor, 2007).

The American Association of Neurological Surgeons and the Congress of Neurological Surgeons have published management guidelines and standards of care for adult and pediatric patients with SCIs. Recently, evidence-based guidelines for the management of SCI in children were published (Rozelle et al., 2013).

IV methylprednisone may be started within the first 12 hours after the injury to decrease inflammation and minimize further injury; however, its use in small children is controversial. Studies of methylprednisone administration in adults with SCI have shown mixed results, with experts recommending against its use in acute SCI (Hurlbert, Hadley, Walters, et al., 2013).

In children with upper motor neuron involvement, the spasticity that develops may require administration of an antispasmodic medication such as diazepam. Baclofen is considered the drug of choice for reducing muscle spasticity (Vogel et al., 2012). Gabapentin may be used to treat neuropathic pain (Hauer & Houtrow, 2017). Botulinum toxin type A and α_2-adrenergic agonists may be used in older children with SCI to decrease muscle spasticity.

A number of progressive rehabilitation modalities that have the potential for increasing the quality of life for children with SCI have been developed in recent years. One treatment is functional electrical stimulation (FES), also referred to as *functional neuromuscular stimulation* or *neuromuscular electrical stimulation.* With this treatment, an electrical stimulator is surgically implanted under the skin in the abdomen and electrode leads are tunneled to paralyzed leg muscles, enabling the child to sit, stand, and walk with the aid of crutches, a walker, or other orthoses. The stimulator can also be used to elicit a voluntary grasp and release with the hand. Before the latter can be accomplished, a number of surgical tendon transfers may be required for elbow extension, wrist extension, and finger and thumb flexion. In addition, FES has therapeutic benefits, which include increased muscle strength, improved gait function, and increased cardiovascular fitness (Ho, Triolo, Elias, et al., 2014). Tendon transfers have been shown to be successful in enhancing hand and arm function, increasing pinch force, and facilitating independence in ADLs (van Zyl, Hill, Cooper, et al., 2019). Restoration of hand and arm function enables children with SCI to perform self-catheterization and achieve greater independence in personal hygiene.

Exercise is considered an integral part of SCI rehabilitation; exercise may enhance neuroplasticity and decrease further muscle atrophy. Examples of exercise modalities in SCI patients include upper body strength training and hand cycling (Hosalkar, Pandya, Hsu, et al., 2009).

Administration of pharmacologic agents such as clonidine hydrochloride may improve ambulation in patients with partial SCIs, and exercise therapy through interactive locomotor training has helped some individuals with SCI regain ambulatory function.

A number of orthoses or ambulation aids such as crutches may still be necessary to achieve upright mobility, yet as robotic technology advances, so do the chances for improved mobilization in children with SCI. Mechanical or robotic orthoses may be used in conjunction with FES to enable ambulation in persons with SCI (To, Kirsch, Kobetic, et al., 2005). Gait training may be achieved with a number of different modalities, including a stationary cycle; however, no specific method has proved superior to the others. FES has also been effective in reducing complications from bladder and bowel incontinence and in assisting males in achieving penile erection. Ambulation is an important part of rehabilitation in SCI; retrospective studies found that ambulation was dependent on age at injury and extent of neurologic injury (as measured by American Spinal Injury Association motor scales). Age (younger) and lesser neurologic impairment are key predictors for ambulation (Vogel et al., 2012). A knee-ankle-foot orthosis and reciprocating-gait orthosis may also be used to assist with early rehabilitation and ambulation (Vogel et al., 2012). Additional detailed information on ambulation and orthotics for children have been published elsewhere (Calhoun, Schottler, & Vogel, 2013).

Surgical interventions for SCI include early cord decompression (decompression laminectomy) and cervical or thoracic fusion. Crutchfield, Vinke, or Gardner-Wells tongs and skeletal traction may be used for early cervical vertebral stabilization. A halo vest or Minerva jacket may be suited for ambulation after the acute phase. After cervical spinal fusion, a hard cervical collar or sterno-occipital-mandibular immobilizer brace may be worn until the fusion is solidified. When SCI occurs in young children and preteens, scoliosis develops over time and often requires surgical consideration (Parent, Mac-Thiong, Roy-Beaudry, et al., 2011).

Prognosis

The ultimate outlook for spinal cord function after injury depends on the completeness of the cord transection, site of injury, complicating damage to the neuronal tissue, and success of treatment regimens aimed at recovery of lost muscle movement and ability. Healing of the injury and the return of neurologic function are related to two factors:

1. Although individual nerve fibers do regenerate, they do not necessarily reconnect or make synaptic connections with the distal portion of the severed fibers; the chance of numerous fibers reconnecting is highly unlikely.
2. The damage resulting from cord ischemia produces necrosis in the gray and white matter of the cord tissue, which does not regenerate if the axon cylinder is not intact.

In children the prognosis for recovery is considered better than in adults because children have rapid healing of bone and ligaments and increased potential for nervous system regeneration. Paraplegia is more common in children under age 12 years, whereas older children and adolescents tend to have incomplete injuries (Mathison et al., 2008). Shavelle and colleagues (2007) reported an increased likelihood of mortality among children younger than 16 years of age who suffered an SCI in comparison to adults with similar injuries. Children with incomplete injuries (and who are not ventilator dependent) had a projected 83% chance of normal life expectancy, whereas those with high-level cervical injuries who are not ventilator dependent had a 50% chance of having a normal life expectancy. One study found that adults who had an SCI as children (younger than 18 years of age at time of incident) had comparable or greater degrees of education in comparison to the general population of the same age (Vogel, Chlan, Zebracki, et al., 2011). The same study found lower employment rates for adults with pediatric-onset SCI, lower rates of independent living and independent driving, and lower rates of marriage in this select population.

In general, recovery of motor function in children with thoracic lesions is variable. Cervical injuries are also variable in the extent of damage. Incomplete lesions produce hemiplegia, whereas complete transection implies some involvement of all extremities—from partial use of the upper extremities to complete paralysis, including the need for some type of assisted ventilation. Lumbar injury may involve partial or complete loss of function in the lower extremities and bladder. With rapidly advancing surgical technology, use of microcomputers in medicine, and newer treatment modalities such as FES, there are increasing hope and evidence that functional mobility and independence can be restored in children with SCI (see Quality Patient Outcomes box).

QUALITY PATIENT OUTCOMES: Neurologic Impairment

- Neurologic status maintained or improved
- No further injuries

Nursing Care Management

The nursing care of the child affected by SCI is complex and challenging. A multidisciplinary SCI team is equipped to manage the acute phase of the injury, and some members, including the nurse, may follow the patient to eventual recovery. Nursing management is concerned with ensuring adequate initial stabilization of the entire spinal column with a rigid cervical collar with supportive blocks on a rigid backboard. The traumatic event causing the injury may or may not be recalled if the child lost consciousness; such events are extremely frightening to the child. The young child may also be frightened by the immobilization process and the inability to move extremities; therefore it is important to reassure and comfort the child during this process.

During the acute phase of the injury it is imperative that airway patency be ensured, complications prevented, and function maintained. Evaluate the extent of the neurologic damage early to establish a baseline for neurologic function. Continual assessment of sensory and motor function should occur to prevent further deterioration of neurologic status as a result of spinal cord edema. The American Spinal Injury Association Impairment Scale can be used to assess neurologic function on a routine basis during the patient's recovery. Once the patient is admitted, further evaluation of his or her ability to perform ADLs and need for assistance during recovery can be made with the Functional Independence Measure scale.

Nursing care during the acute phase should also focus on frequent monitoring of neurologic signs to determine any changes in neurologic function that require further intervention (e.g., level of consciousness using the Glasgow Coma Scale). In addition to airway maintenance, the nurse monitors for changes in hemodynamic status that may require immediate medical attention. Neurogenic shock consists of hypotension, bradycardia, and vasodilation. Inotropic medications may be required to maintain adequate perfusion. Renal function is closely monitored by measuring urinary output and fluids administered. The child with a head injury may experience elevated intracranial pressure; therefore changes in neurologic status are reported to the practitioner. Fluid restriction may be required if intracranial pressure is elevated, so fluid intake should be closely monitored.

The nursing care of the child with an SCI is, in most respects, the same as that of any immobilized child (see Chapter 29, The Immobilized Child). Additional aspects of care that should be addressed on an individual basis include hypercalcemia in adolescent boys, DVT, latex sensitization, pain, hypothermia and hyperthermia, spasticity, autonomic dysreflexia, and sleep-disordered breathing (Vogel et al., 2012).

Respiratory Care

The child with a high-level cervical injury (C3 and above) requires continuous ventilatory assistance. In most instances a tracheostomy is the method of choice for greater ease in clearing secretions and for less trauma to tissues during long-term ventilatory dependence. Patient-triggered synchronous intermittent mandatory ventilation (SIMV–assist/control mode) may be required to maintain adequate oxygenation. In an acute care center, respiratory therapy personnel are often responsible for establishing and maintaining the equipment, but the nurse must understand how it works and recognize mechanical malfunction and deviations from the prescribed rate and volume. In case of malfunction, the nurse must be prepared to maintain respirations manually with a self-inflating bag-valve-mask device. In many home care situations the family is responsible for the care of ventilatory assistance devices; therefore adequate family training and availability of the nurse (or durable medical equipment representative) for questions related to the equipment and evaluation of the child's breathing are essential. For some children, breathing pacemaker devices (phrenic nerve stimulators) are implanted to stimulate the phrenic nerve and produce diaphragmatic contractions and lung expansion without assisted ventilation.

Children with lesions below the C4 level are seldom ventilator dependent, but pulmonary vital capacity is significantly reduced. Position them for optimum chest expansion, and use a variety of breathing exercises and assistive devices to stimulate deep breathing. Chest physiotherapy is performed as needed to mobilize secretions, and flow-by oxygen may be needed occasionally. Regular monitoring of breath sounds to assess for adequate ventilation in all lung fields is part of routine care.

The cough reflex may be markedly diminished, which, combined with weak intercostal muscles, may mean that the child has difficulty with secretions. Increasing the elastic qualities of the lung by breathing exercises, mechanical cough assist techniques, and incentive spirometry helps the child achieve a productive cough. (See the discussion of airway management and airway clearance devices under Duchenne Muscular Dystrophy: Therapeutic Management later in the chapter.)

Cardiovascular Care

Children with SCI may experience cardiovascular instability as a result of loss of vagal tone, vagal stimulation during procedures such as oral suctioning or insertion of a nasogastric tube, turning, and endotracheal suctioning. Close monitoring of heart rate and blood pressure is essential to detect any signs of decreased cardiac output. Pneumothorax may occur, resulting in a mediastinal shift and decreased cardiac output. Autonomic dysreflexia may occur and result in decreased cardiac output (see discussion later in the chapter).

The child with loss of muscle tone and prolonged immobility may be at high risk for the development of DVT. In addition, major reparative surgery for associated injuries and spinal decompression place the child at risk for thrombus formation. DVT is prevented with the use of pneumatic compression devices and low-molecular-weight heparin during the acute phase of care. Fluid and electrolyte balance may be impaired as a result of trauma and associated injuries or decreased fluid intake during the recovery period. Fluid intake should be closely monitored, especially with regard to the development of pulmonary edema and intracranial pressure. The child may require nasogastric tube feedings due to anorexia and immobility.

Temperature Regulation

Temperature is often poorly regulated in children with SCI; therefore body temperature must be monitored closely for fluctuations. In small children hypothermia may occur relative to large body surface and inability to mount an appropriate metabolic response to the initial injury, so close attention should be given to preserving body temperature. Response to environmental temperature changes may be slow or absent, and the ability to dissipate heat through the process of shivering may be compromised.

During the spinal shock stage, the dilated capillaries conducting body heat to the subcutaneous tissues cause heat loss. Without the capacity to sweat, the body retains heat in hot weather. An elevated temperature that cannot be corrected by environmental measures should be evaluated to rule out urinary or upper respiratory tract infection. However, excessive perspiration observed in sentient areas usually indicates an elevated ambient temperature.

Skin Care

Children with SCI have unique needs in relation to skin care. Because of decreased sensation and impaired mobility, they depend on others to assess and assist in the management of intact skin. Skin care practices are the same as those for any child who is immobilized. A skin score scale such as the Braden Q Scale can objectively evaluate risks for skin breakdown and skin conditions (Noonan, Quigley, & Curley, 2011). Keep an alternating-pressure mattress or other pressure relief or reduction device underneath the child, and inspect the skin thoroughly at least twice a day for signs of pressure, especially over bony prominences. Prevention of skin breakdown is much easier than treatment. A number of factors contribute to the risk of skin breakdown in these children: decreased sensation, inadequate nutrition, muscle spasticity, impaired peripheral circulation, diaphoresis, mechanical shearing from assistive devices, and improper positioning (see Chapter 20, Maintaining Healthy Skin).

The areas most likely to be affected are the sacrum, scapulae, heels, and occiput when the child is supine; the trochanters and the lateral aspect of the ankles, heels, and knees when the child is in a side-lying position; and the ischial tuberosities when the child is sitting. The pressure wound may begin in deeper tissues and be visible on the surface only at a later stage. Therefore areas that feel firm, irregular, or warm or that appear to be only slightly reddened require careful evaluation. Keeping the skin clean and dry is particularly important in these children, especially those who are incontinent of urine or stool or those who have significant diaphoresis. When there is any evidence of skin breakdown, treatment to prevent further breakdown is implemented promptly. When orthotic devices such as AFOs and braces are used, skin care and vigilance for pressure areas are also important in the prevention of pressure ulcers. Prolonged use of wheelchairs without special sacral protection may also lead to skin ulceration.

The child who is heavily sedated or who is being given muscle paralytics should receive appropriate eye care to prevent corneal damage (e.g., artificial tears, ointment, impermeable eye shield). Additional nursing care may involve the administration of histamine blockers and proton pump inhibitors to prevent stress ulcers by reducing the secretion of hydrochloric acid.

Physical Therapy

An important consideration for the child with SCI is achievement of mobility and ambulation. A developmental approach should be considered in the rehabilitation phase (Calhoun et al., 2013). Range-of-motion, passive, and active exercises are carried out under the guidance of a physical therapist.

Unless there are contraindications, exercises during the period of immobilization are aimed at maintaining and increasing the strength of the child's intact musculature. Upper extremity strengthening is especially important to the paraplegic child, who must rely on these muscle groups for turning, transferring, dressing, parallel bar walking, gait training, and other activities. Children are usually eager to use their muscles and respond to interesting and innovative activities.

Neurogenic Bladder

When the bladder is denervated, as in the acute stage of spinal shock syndrome or after lower motor neuron damage, the bladder wall is flaccid. Lack of muscle tone inhibits the bladder's ability to respond to changes in passive pressure, causing overdistention. Therefore it is important to prevent distention by periodic emptying, even though there may be dribbling between emptying.

In contrast, an upper motor neuron lesion causes increased bladder tone and contractions that often include the urinary sphincter. Thus although the bladder empties periodically by reflex action, complete emptying is prevented, resulting in urinary retention and ureteral reflux. Administration of an anticholinergic drug such as dicyclomine (Bentyl) relaxes bladder musculature and promotes increased bladder capacity and more adequate emptying. Intervals of urination depend on many factors, including patterns of fluid intake and perspiration.

In school-age children and adolescents, achieving bladder and bowel continence is a significant developmental issue related to self-esteem and perception of self in relation to peers. Therefore it is imperative to consider options that best meet the child's physiologic and emotional needs.

Surgical options for children with neurogenic bladder include the creation of a urinary stoma, made possible by removing the appendix and creating a urinary diversion from the bladder to the exterior, usually the umbilicus, thus making self-catheterization more private, especially with the recovery of hand and elbow movement (with tendon transfers). Other options include surgical bladder augmentation to increase capacity and FES to restore micturition on command without a urinary catheter (Merenda & Hickey, 2005). There are promising recent research efforts to augment the bladder using tissue engineering technology (Osorio, Reyes, & Massagli, 2014).

Emptying the bladder by CIC is also an option for children with SCI; older children who are functionally capable can learn to perform self-catheterization. Encourage the child to adhere to a schedule for CIC and to maintain a regular pattern of fluid intake throughout the day; they should avoid large intakes of fluid without considering the need for more frequent CIC. Caffeinated beverages and other caffeinated foods are used sparingly to avoid bladder overdistention with increased urine formation (Francis, 2007). Latex catheters should be avoided to prevent the development of latex allergy (if it is not already present). Bladder-training programs usually begin with intermittent bladder emptying at regular intervals that are gradually increased. The Credé method (applying suprapubic pressure) for emptying the bladder may be used by some individuals with SCI, but this may result in high intravesical pressures, causing further bladder complications (Francis, 2007).

Urinary tract infections are common due to urinary stasis. A regular schedule of CIC may help prevent such infections. Encourage the child to increase fluid intake by approximately 240 ml/day and use CIC every 3 to 4 hours.

Maintenance of bladder dynamics and control of UTIs are of utmost importance. Pyelonephritis and renal failure are the most significant causes of death in long-standing paraplegia.

Bowel Training

The loss of bowel function is considered to be one of the most stressful events when quality-of-life issues are considered in persons with SCI; however, successful bowel training is easier to institute than bladder management. The aim is to control defecation until an appropriate time and place are found. Merenda and Hickey (2005) propose four components in a successful bowel management program: desired stool consistency (i.e., a soft stool), a regular evacuation pattern, upright positioning for planned evacuation, and motivation and commitment from the child and family.

A diet with sufficient fiber (age in years plus 5 g is recommended) for adequate stool bulk and insertion of a glycerin or bisacodyl (Dulcolax) suppository at a convenient time, either morning or evening, are often all that is necessary to induce a bowel movement within a short time. The probability of an accident between times diminishes once the bowel is completely evacuated. The key to adequate bowel training is to maintain consistency in the time of day for evacuation. Stool softeners, such as docusate sodium (Colace) and senna (Senokot), may be prescribed, and manual anal stimulation may help initiate evacuation, especially in spastic paraplegia. Sometimes an oral laxative such as bisacodyl may be necessary. Once an appropriate regimen is established, little modification is required.

One surgical option is the antegrade continence enema, which involves the creation of a stoma whereby colonic washouts may be performed with the child sitting on the toilet. FES has also been used successfully in some children with SCI to achieve bowel training.

Autonomic Dysreflexia

Children with high-level lesions are susceptible to the development of autonomic dysreflexia, which requires prompt action to prevent encephalopathy and shock. Clinical manifestations of autonomic dysreflexia include an increase in systemic blood pressure, headache, bradycardia, profuse diaphoresis, cardiac arrhythmias, flushing, piloerection, blurred vision, nasal congestion, anxiety, spots on the visual field, or absent or minimum symptoms. A quick assessment may rule out other causes, such as orthostatic intolerance. After that, vital signs, including blood pressure, are taken while the bladder is checked for distention (the usual precipitating cause). The bladder is drained slowly; if this does not relieve symptoms, any tight clothing is loosened, and the bowel is checked for the presence of impacted feces.

Other potential causes of autonomic dysreflexia in children with an SCI include bowel impaction and abdominal distention, pressure ulcers, tight clothing, burns, DVT, menses, trauma, fractures, pregnancy, labor, surgery or invasive procedures, any painful stimulus, and hyperthermia (Vogel et al., 2012). If removal of the causative agent is unsuccessful in controlling the syndrome, IV administration of an antihypertensive drug is indicated, followed by oral maintenance doses. Antispasmodics may also be administered.

Remobilization

As soon as the condition warrants, the child is moved from a reclining to an upright position. Cardiovascular deconditioning and impaired autonomic responses below the level of injury will cause pooling of blood in the extremities (because of peripheral vasodilation); a drop in blood pressure; and a feeling of lightheadedness, dizziness, or fainting on sudden assumption of an upright posture, often referred to as **orthostatic intolerance**. Therefore an upright position must be accomplished gradually by first placing the child (who is secured by passive restraint) on a head-up tilt table. The table is slowly elevated from a horizontal to a 30-degree semireclining position. This is performed twice daily for 20 to 30 minutes, with the angle gradually increased until the vertical angle is reached.

During the procedure the vital signs are monitored, and the child's behavior is observed for subjective symptoms of syncope. The pooling of blood is reduced by using elastic antiembolism stockings and sequential pneumatic compression devices, which consist of inflatable sleeves that fit on the legs and compress the leg muscles for cyclic emptying and filling of leg veins. The process of achieving an upright posture may require several weeks. After tolerance is achieved, the child will be ready to begin using a wheelchair. Getting the child up should be accomplished slowly by gradually elevating the bed over 20 to 30 minutes before placing the child in the wheelchair and then gradually lowering the legs after the child has been in the chair for a short time.

All adaptive devices help children increase their mobility, function, and endurance. The child with some lower extremity function progresses to parallel bars and then to a walker. The child with tetraplegia learns to use a wheelchair—among the most valuable aids available to the child with an SCI. The wheelchair should be selected carefully in relation to where it will be used, the architectural barriers, and the child's functional capacity. For children with severe upper extremity paralysis, a variety of motorized wheelchairs are used; however, the more complex they are, the greater their cost, weight, and tendency to break down. Wheelchair tolerance is gained over time and is accompanied by measures to prevent orthostatic hypotension and pressure sores.

A variety of orthoses and other appliances can be adapted for use by many children. The primary purpose of lower extremity bracing in the child with an SCI is for ambulation, although correction of deformities may be attempted. However, the efficacy is limited because of the tendency to develop pressure lesions over insensate areas. The higher the lesion, the more support is required, with the accompanying difficulties of getting into the orthosis and the greater energy expended in using the appliance. The energy required in walking with crutches and braces is two to four times greater than that required for normal walking.

Children, with their natural and overwhelming desire for mobility, usually attain or even surpass the maximum expectation in ambulation. However, as they approach adulthood, the increasing weight and energy cost usually cause them to resort to predominant use of the wheelchair for mobility and the pursuit of more intellectual and vocational interests. Wheelchair mobility has the advantages of requiring no more energy than normal walking and allowing the person with paraplegia to maintain the speed of other pedestrians on level ground.

Physical Rehabilitation

The process of physical rehabilitation usually begins once the child is medically stable and associated problems have been managed. The major aims of physical rehabilitation are to prepare the child and family to achieve normalization and resume life at home and in the community. Additional goals of rehabilitation in children with SCI are to promote independence in mobility and self-care skills, academic achievement, independent living, and employment.

Members of the multidisciplinary rehabilitation team cooperate with one another and the family to identify the child's needs and to plan realistic interventions. Integration of activities is coordinated by one team member, most often a specialist in physical medicine and rehabilitation. Members of the team attempt to achieve their collaborative goals through mutual trust, good communication, professional respect, and sincere interest in the child and family. Training in the rehabilitation center promotes maximum achievement commensurate with each child's physical capacities. Instruction for home routine is stressed and includes all precautions and management implemented in the acute care center (e.g., skin care, nutrition, bladder and bowel training, gait training) and an exercise program.

Inpatient physical rehabilitation of children with tetraplegia takes approximately 2 to 4 months; children with paraplegia can achieve these goals in 1 to 3 months but require constant vigilance to avoid complications. Emotional adjustments take longer, especially in older children and adolescents. In most children the outlook is favorable unless the life-threatening consequences of urinary pathologic condition are severe or the emotional adjustment is poor.

Psychosocial Rehabilitation

Early-acquired or congenital disability is usually more readily accepted by children than paralysis that appears later in childhood. Rehabilitation efforts should include not only the child's emotional responses but also those of the persons closest to the child. Intensive education is important so that family members understand the nature of the disability, the therapeutic regimen, and complications and are able to provide the physical and emotional support the child needs.

As with any disability, treat children as normally as possible and encourage them in developmental tasks at the age at which they would typically be expected to acquire abilities and perform activities. However, the goals must be realistic, and children should not be forced beyond their capabilities. Vogel and colleagues (2012) emphasize the need for children and adolescents with SCI to assume responsibility for their own care. When this is not physically possible, they should direct others in their care. Encouraging self-care is important in the emotional and physical rehabilitation of the child or adolescent with SCI.

Severe depression can be emotionally and intellectually immobilizing, but it indicates that the child is no longer hiding behind denial. In rehabilitation it is desirable for the child to begin to express negative feelings toward the situation because these feelings, redirected by efforts of the rehabilitation team, are the ones that will motivate the child toward learning a new way of life. Anxiety and depression in young children and adolescents with SCI are associated with a poorer quality of life (Osorio et al., 2014).

The needs of young children and adolescents who are permanently disabled must be reevaluated periodically by the total rehabilitation team, including the children and their families. Vocational rehabilitation is important for helping these adolescents find meaningful work activities and enroll in formal educational programs as desired.

The outlook for children and adolescents with SCI is increasingly favorable for integration into society. Increased awareness of the needs of persons with disabilities has removed many structural and occupational barriers. The success of a rehabilitation program is judged not by how well children and adolescents manage within the rehabilitation setting but by how well they function on the outside. In addition to agencies that offer assistance to children with disabilities in general, some agencies provide specific assistance to paralyzed persons, including children.

Sexuality

Issues related to loss of sexual function also apply to adolescents with debilitating neuromuscular diseases such as Duchenne muscular dystrophy (DMD) and SMA. The problems of self-image are particularly significant when children with SCI reach puberty, especially if the disability was acquired during early adolescence. Sexual development and awareness and changing perceptions of body image are prominent aspects of adolescence; a loss that affects these areas is often devastating. Development of secondary sexual characteristics does not seem to be altered by SCIs, and it is now believed that with comprehensive rehabilitation, motivated young people can look forward to successful participation in marital and family activities.

In females, if the injury occurs after the onset of menstruation, there is usually a temporary cessation and irregularity in menstrual flow, but menstruation resumes in the majority of cases. Ovulation and conception are possible, but only about 50% of females experience vaginal or clitoral orgasms, although they can learn to use other erogenous zones for a sexual experience. This is important to emphasize in sex education because many females have the misconception that they are unable to conceive because they lack sensation. FES may help some women with SCI to achieve orgasm. Education is important because the pregnant paraplegic or tetraplegic patient may be unaware that she is in labor, and those with a high-level injury are subject to autonomic dysreflexia during labor.

More attention has been focused on rehabilitating male sexual function (erection and ejaculation) than female sexual function until the last 2 decades. A number of pharmacologic (prostaglandin E_1) and mechanical devices (e.g., penile implants, vacuum pump devices) now make it possible for males to participate in sexual intercourse and produce offspring, provided that fertility has not been affected by associated complications. Penile injections with vasoactive substances (prostaglandin E_1) are reported to be effective in 90% of men (DeForge, Blackmer, Garritty, et al., 2006). However, sildenafil (Viagra) is now considered the treatment of choice for the sexually active male. Adolescents with SCI should be counseled regarding condom use and the symptoms of latex allergy.

As soon as adolescent males become aware of their functional loss, they will be concerned about sexual capacities, regardless of the type of sexual activities experienced before the SCI. The health care professional should take the initiative in discussing sexuality with adolescents and their families. Parents of younger children may want to know about their children's sexual and reproductive potential. As their interest and understanding increase, adolescents need to know the specifics of physiology, the prognosis, and sexual techniques related to their particular problems. The practitioner should provide them with information about what can be expected regarding erection, ejaculation, and other sexual experiences.

A knowledgeable rehabilitation team is valuable to adolescents as they experience concerns regarding loss as a sexual being. This is especially true in paraplegia or tetraplegia. Most sexual counseling for adolescents with SCI focuses on developing the idea that sex means different things to different people. Most rehabilitation teams have an active counseling program to help adolescents learn intimacy and how to function sexually within their limitations. Through individual and group counseling they gain new attitudes concerning sexuality and experiences exclusive or inclusive of intercourse. Guidelines for sexual and reproductive health care of persons with SCI are published elsewhere (Consortium for Spinal Cord Medicine, 2010).

Transition to Adulthood

With the ultimate goal of making an effective transition to adulthood, adolescents with SCI often face challenges similar to others with chronic and debilitating conditions. Issues such as housing, education, personal assistance care, transportation, medical care, and specialized medical care must be addressed in a coordinated transition program (Vogel et al., 2012). The concepts of care coordination for children and adolescents requiring home care also apply to adolescents making the transition to adulthood because different health care services may be needed or requirements may change for benefits for those no longer dependent on parents.

MUSCULAR DYSFUNCTION

JUVENILE DERMATOMYOSITIS

Juvenile dermatomyositis (JDM) is a relatively rare systemic autoimmune vasculopathy that often occurs after a triggering event such as infection with group A beta-hemolytic streptococci, enterovirus (coxsackievirus B), or parvovirus B19. An environmental trigger such as excessive sun exposure has also been proposed in some children. In children, one of the human leukocyte antigens (DQA1*0501, B8, DRB*0301, or DQA1*0301) is present on chromosome 6 and may be associated with increased susceptibility to the disease (Feldman, Rider, Reed, et al., 2008; Robinson & Reed, 2020). White girls are twice as likely to be affected as boys. The peak age at onset is between 4 and 10 years of age. Children with onset before age 7 years may experience milder symptoms.

The diagnosis is often established through the following clinical presentations: bilateral symmetric proximal weakness; a characteristic heliotropic rash of the eyelids; Gottron papules on the knuckles, knees, and elbows; Gottron sign; elevated serum enzymes (aldolase, creatine kinase, aspartase aminotransferase, and lactate dehydrogenase); altered EMG; and abnormal muscle biopsy. An atraumatic alternative to muscle biopsy is an MRI. Nailfold capillaroscopy shows decreased capillary density and presence of disease activity and may be used to diagnose the condition (Wakiguchi, 2019).

For approximately half of affected children, the disease is acute and progresses rapidly. Children younger than 6 years of age often are seen initially with fever and signs of an upper respiratory tract illness. There is proximal limb and trunk muscle weakness and loss of reflexes. Consequently, the child may not be able to rise from the floor to a standing position without walking the hands up the legs (Gower sign). The disease often affects the neck muscles, and the child may have difficulty lifting the head or supporting it in an upright position. Muscles tend to be stiff and sore. A generalized vasculitis of small arteries and capillaries is one prominent feature of the disease. Masseter involvement with atrophy may occur, which makes it difficult to chew food during the active stage of the disease. Soft palate dysfunction may make speech difficult and interfere with breathing. Distal muscle strength and reflex responses remain unaffected. JDM is characterized by a red erythematous rash over the malar areas and nose and a violet discoloration of the eyelids. The skin over extensor muscle surfaces may be erythematous, scaly, and atopic. Calcium deposits (calcinosis) develop in muscle tissues as the disease progresses. Dystrophic calcifications may develop over areas exposed to pressure, including the elbows, knees, digits, and buttocks. These lesions may result in skin ulceration with subsequent infection, pain, and functional disability from joint contractures. The vasculitis may cause GI, renal, cardiac, and ophthalmologic symptoms as the disease progresses. A common problem in JDM is aspiration pneumonia, and measures should be taken to ensure that the child has an adequate airway at all times. Additional pulmonary involvement includes interstitial lung disease, so pulmonary function testing should be part of the medical management. There is evidence that adults with pediatric-onset JDM may develop cardiac problems such as heart failure. If the child has difficulty feeding, a gastrostomy may be used to supplement caloric intake until the drug regimen controls the symptoms.

JDM responds to high-dose oral corticosteroid therapy and methotrexate; in some children high-dose intermittent IV methylprednisone may be required. All children with JDM should use a sunscreen to protect against ultraviolet A and B rays. Vitamin D and adequate dietary intake of calcium are also recommended to increase and maintain bone density and minimize osteopenia (Feldman et al., 2008; Huber, 2012). IVIG has been effective in some children who were intolerant of high-dose corticosteroids. Other treatments that have been effective in adult myositis and in isolated cases of JDM include hydroxychloroquine, systemic tacrolimus, etanercept or infliximab, rituximab, and cyclosporin (Wakiguchi, 2019).

Physical therapy is essential to prevent contracture deformity and to rebuild muscle strength. Meticulous skin care is an important nursing consideration in the care of these patients.

Although the prognosis for survival has steadily improved, JDM remains a serious chronic illness. Death can occur in the acute phase as a result of myocarditis, progressive unresponsive myositis, perforation of the bowel, or, occasionally, lung involvement. The current mortality rate is approximately 1% (Robinson & Reed, 2020).

MUSCULAR DYSTROPHIES

The muscular dystrophies (MDs) constitute the largest and most important single group of muscle diseases of childhood. They have a genetic origin in which there is gradual, progressive degeneration of muscle fibers, and they are characterized by progressive weakness and wasting of symmetric groups of skeletal muscles, with increasing disability and deformity. In all forms of MD there is insidious loss of strength, but each differs in regard to the muscle groups affected, age of onset, rate of progression, and inheritance patterns (Fig. 30.7).

Treatment of the MDs consists mainly of providing supportive measures (including physical therapy; orthopedic procedures to minimize deformity; and ventilatory support, including airway clearance techniques) and assisting the affected child in meeting the demands of daily living.

Facioscapulohumeral (Landouzy-Dejerine) muscular dystrophy is inherited as an autosomal dominant disorder with onset in early adolescence. It is characterized by difficulty in raising the arms over the head, lack of facial mobility, and a forward slope of the shoulders. The progression is slow, and the life span is usually unaffected.

Limb-girdle muscular dystrophy (LGMD) is a heterogenous group of disorders with autosomal dominant and recessive inheritance whose clinical manifestations often appear in later childhood, adolescence, or early adulthood with variable but usually slow progression (Quan, 2011). All types of LGMD are characterized by weakness of proximal muscles of the pelvic and shoulder girdles. Other forms of MD include myotonic dystrophy, scapulohumeral MD (Emery-Dreifuss MD), facioscapulohumeral MD (Landouzy-Dejerine disease), and congenital MD; these forms consist of subtypes of MD and are discussed at length elsewhere (Bharucha-Goebel, 2020). Duchenne muscular dystrophy is discussed in the following section.

DUCHENNE MUSCULAR DYSTROPHY

DMD is the most severe and most common MD of childhood. It is inherited as an X-linked recessive trait, and the single-gene defect is located on the short arm of the X chromosome. DMD has a high mutation rate, with a negative family history in approximately 65% to 75% of all cases; therefore genetic counseling is an important aspect of the care of the family. Approximately 30% of DMD patients are new mutations and the mother is not the carrier (Bharucha-Goebel, 2020).

As in all X-linked disorders, males are affected almost exclusively. The female carrier may have an elevated serum creatine kinase, but muscle weakness is usually not a problem; however, about 10% of female carriers develop cardiomyopathy (Manzur, Kinali, & Muntoni, 2008). In rare instances a female may be identified with DMD disease yet with muscular weakness that is milder than in boys

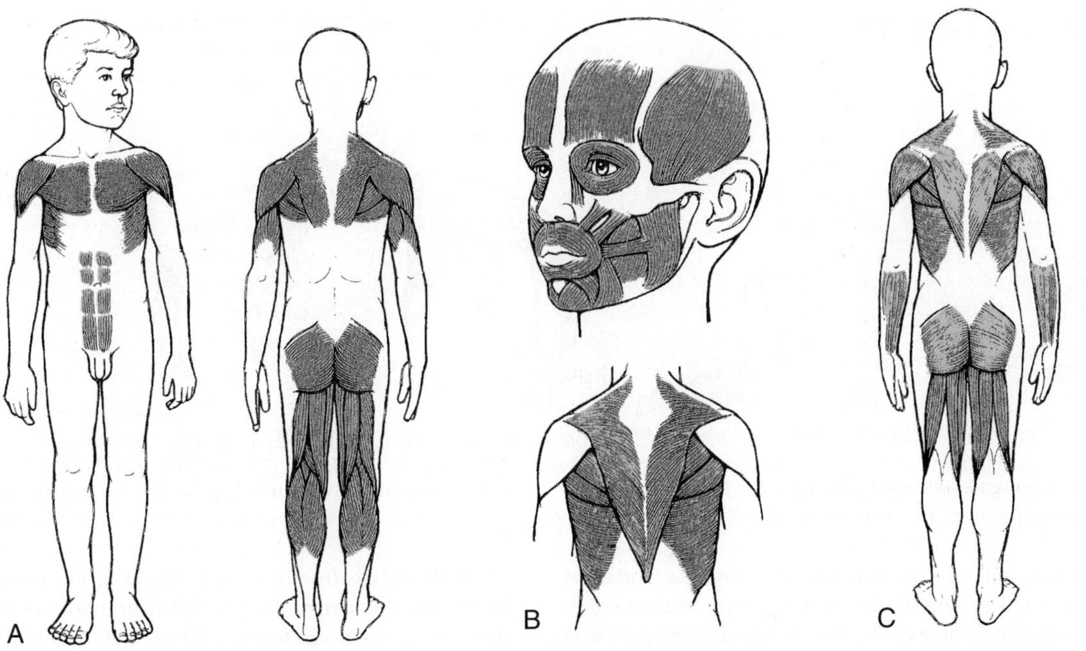

Fig. 30.7 Initial muscle groups involved in muscular dystrophies. **A,** Pseudohypertrophic (Duchenne). **B,** Facioscapulohumeral. **C,** Limb-girdle.

(Bharucha-Goebel, 2020). The incidence is approximately 1 in 3600 male births for the Duchenne form and approximately 1 in 30,000 live births for the Becker type, a milder variant (Bharucha-Goebel, 2020). Box 30.7 describes the characteristics of DMD.

At the genetic level, both DMD and Becker MD result from mutations of the gene that encodes dystrophin, a protein product in skeletal muscle. Dystrophin is absent from the muscle of children with DMD and is reduced or abnormal in children with Becker MD. The absence of dystrophin leads to a number of problems in muscle, including muscle fiber degeneration. A deficiency of dystrophin isoforms in brain tissue causes cognitive and intellectual impairment. Children with Becker MD have a later onset of symptoms, which are usually not as severe as those seen in DMD. There is a strong correlation between the clinical severity of these disorders and the type of genetic mutation and dystrophin protein alterations. Survival has increased with newer ventilation technologies, and median age is reported as high as 27 years in those being ventilated; types of ventilation used were not described in the report (Rall & Grimm, 2012).

Clinical Manifestations

Most children with DMD reach the appropriate developmental milestones early in life, although they may have mild, subtle delays. Evidence of muscle weakness usually appears during the third to seventh year, although there may have been a history of delay in motor development, particularly walking. Difficulties in running, riding a bicycle, and climbing stairs are usually the first symptoms noted. Later, abnormal gait on a level surface becomes apparent. In the early years, rapid developmental gains may mask the progression of the disease. Questioning the parents may reveal that the child has difficulty in rising from a sitting or supine position. Occasionally the parents notice enlarged calves.

Typically, affected boys have a waddling gait and lordosis, fall frequently, and develop a characteristic manner of rising from a squatting or sitting position on the floor (Gower sign) (Fig. 30.8). Lordosis occurs as a result of weakened pelvic muscles, and the waddling gait is a result of weakness in the gluteus medius and maximus muscles (Battista, 2010). Muscles, especially in the calves, thighs, and upper arms, become enlarged from fatty infiltration and feel unusually firm or woody on palpation. The term *pseudohypertrophy* is derived from this muscular enlargement. Profound muscular atrophy occurs in the later stages; contractures and deformities involving large and small joints are common complications as the disease progresses. Ambulation usually becomes impossible by 12 years of age. The loss of mobilization further increases the spectrum of complications, which may include osteoporosis, fractures, constipation, skin breakdown, and psychosocial and behavioral problems. Atrophy of facial, oropharyngeal, and respiratory muscles does not occur until the advanced stage of the disease. Ultimately the disease process involves the diaphragm and auxiliary muscles of respiration, and cardiomegaly is common.

BOX 30.7 Characteristics of Duchenne Muscular Dystrophy

- Early onset, usually between 3 and 5 years of age
- Progressive muscular weakness, wasting, and contractures
- Calf muscle hypertrophy in most patients
- Loss of independent ambulation by 9 to 12 years of age
- Slowly progressive generalized weakness during adolescence
- Relentless progression until death from respiratory or cardiac failure

Mild to moderate mental impairment is commonly associated with MD. The mean intelligence quotient (IQ) is approximately 20 points below normal, and frank mental deficit is present in 20% to 30% of these children. Verbal IQ is markedly low in males with DMD, and emotional disturbance is more common than in other children with disabilities; however, children with DMD should be involved in early learning programs and eventually moved into regular classrooms as much as possible.

Complications

The major complications of MD include contractures, scoliosis, disuse atrophy, infections, obesity, and respiratory and cardiopulmonary problems. Contracture deformities of the hips, knees, and ankles occur from early selective muscle involvement and often exaggerate

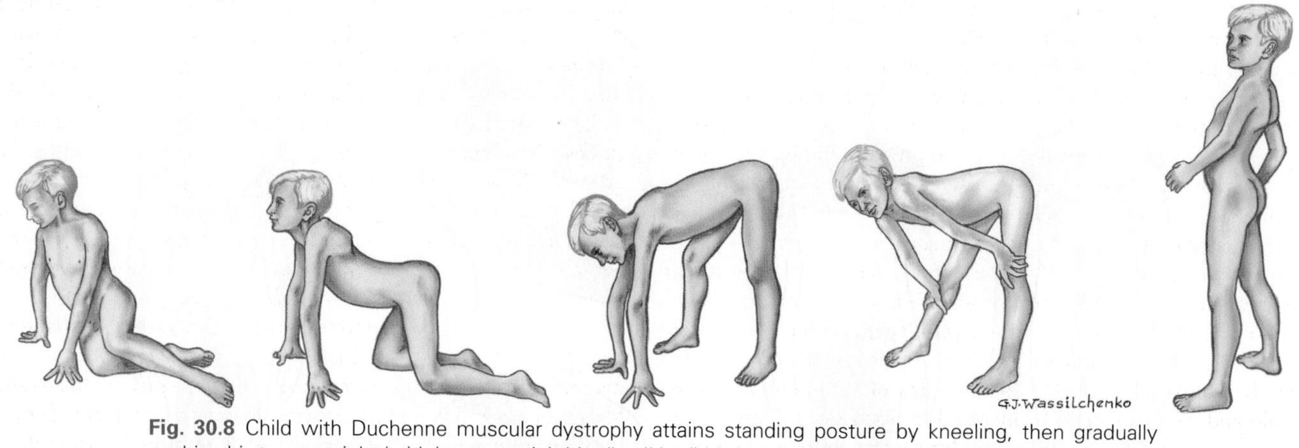

Fig. 30.8 Child with Duchenne muscular dystrophy attains standing posture by kneeling, then gradually pushing his torso upright (with knees straight) by "walking" his hands up his legs (Gower sign). Note marked lordosis in upright position.

the weakness. Passive range-of-motion exercises, stretching, and active exercises under the supervision of a PT are effective in treating reducible contractures. Nonreducible contractures require wedge casting or surgical reduction. Scoliosis caused by muscle imbalance is common in children who lose ambulatory capability and tends to progress even when the child becomes dependent on a wheelchair. Bracing with an orthosis may be required, but in many cases spinal fusion surgery is performed to prevent complications associated with cardiac and pulmonary restriction.

Atrophy of disuse from prolonged inactivity occurs readily when children are immobilized or confined to bed with illness, injury, or surgery. To minimize this complication, physical therapy should begin if bed rest extends beyond a few days. To maintain muscle strength, a daily goal for well children with moderate disability should be at least 3 hours of ambulation.

Pulmonary infections become increasingly frequent as the dystrophic process produces a progressive decrease in pulmonary vital capacity as a result of weakness of the primary, secondary, and associated muscles of respiration. Consequently, even minor upper respiratory tract infections may become serious in these children. The eventual cause of death is usually respiratory tract infection or cardiac failure; however, much progress has been made in providing ventilatory methods to prolong and maintain quality of life. Prompt and vigorous antibiotic therapy, supplemented by postural drainage and aggressive airway clearance methods, is effective. Because of the respiratory musculature weakness, these children are unable to cough effectively and secretions collect easily.

Obesity is a common complication that contributes to premature loss of ambulation. Children who have restricted opportunities for physical activity and who suffer from boredom easily consume calories in excess of their needs. This may be compounded by overfeeding by well-meaning family and friends. Proper dietary intake and a diversified recreational program help reduce the likelihood of obesity and enable children to maintain ambulation and functional independence for a longer time.

Cardiac manifestations are usually late events but may occur in ambulatory children. The most significant of these, cardiac failure, is difficult to correct in advanced cases, but treatment with digoxin and diuretics is often beneficial in the early stages of the disease.

Diagnostic Evaluation

DMD is suspected on the basis of clinical manifestations (see Box 30.7) and confirmed by molecular genetic detection of deficient dystrophin by DNA analysis from peripheral blood or in muscle tissue obtained by biopsy. The diagnosis of DMD is primarily established by blood polymerase chain reaction (PCR) for the dystrophin gene mutation (Bharucha-Goebel, 2020). Diagnostic techniques such as multiplex PCR have made it possible to diagnose 98% of the DMD mutations. Prenatal diagnosis is also possible as early as 12 weeks of gestation. However, ethical questions exist regarding diagnosing a condition in the fetus when no treatment exists.

Serum enzyme measurement, muscle biopsy, and EMG may also be used in establishing the diagnosis. Serum creatine kinase levels are extremely high in the first 2 years of life, before the onset of clinical weakness. If the child demonstrates the usual characteristics and has a positive family history for DMD and if the PCR is positive, the muscle biopsy may be deferred.

Muscle biopsy reveals degeneration of muscle fibers, with fibrosis and fatty tissue replacement. EMG readings show a decrease in amplitude and duration of motor unit potentials.

Therapeutic Management

Currently no curative treatment exists for childhood MD. Increased muscle bulk and muscle power have been reported after a course of corticosteroids. Several clinical trials demonstrated increased muscle strength and improved performance and pulmonary function, with significant decrease in the progression of weakness, when prednisone was administered for 6 months to 2 years (Manzur, Kuntzer, Pike, et al., 2008). Corticosteroid administration also prolonged ambulation, preserved respiratory function, and decreased the incidence of scoliosis and cardiomyopathy (Manzur, Kinali, & Muntoni, 2008). Major side effects in these studies included weight gain and a cushingoid facial appearance. The American Academy of Neurology has published a practice parameter for the administration of corticosteroids in the treatment of DMD (Moxley, Ashwal, Pandya, et al., 2005).

Maintaining optimum function in all muscles for as long as possible is the primary goal; secondary is the prevention of contractures. In general, children who remain as active as possible are able to avoid wheelchair confinement for a longer time. Maintenance of function often includes stretching exercises, strength and muscle training, breathing exercises and use of incentive spirometry to increase and maintain vital lung capacity, airway clearance, range-of-motion exercises, surgery to release contracture deformities, bracing, and performance of ADLs. Knee-ankle-foot orthoses have been shown to prolong ambulation for 18 to 24 months beyond the termination of independent ambulation. Serial casting of ankles has proven more effective than surgical release of Achilles tendons in many children with DMD to prevent contractures (Manzur, Kinali, & Muntoni, 2008).

Parents should always be involved in making decisions about the child's care, and teaching on home safety and prevention of falls is important as well. Also encourage parents to have the child keep follow-up appointments for medical care and physical and occupational therapy. Because respiratory tract infections are most troublesome in these children, encourage regular influenza and pneumococcal vaccines and avoidance of contact with persons with respiratory tract infections as much as possible. Baseline pulmonary function testing, electrocardiograms, and echocardiograms are also recommended.

Eventually, respiratory and cardiac problems become the central focus of the debilitating illness. Referral to palliative care may help the family evaluate the benefits and burdens of various treatments. The child and parents should be involved in discussion of long-term ventilation options. Cardiac and respiratory assessment during wake-sleep cycles is imperative. Children with neuromuscular disease eventually develop abnormal breathing patterns, particularly during REM sleep, and hypoxia occurs as a result of inadequate oxygenation. The sleep-disordered breathing of DMD results in symptoms such as frequent night awakenings, morning headache, and daytime sleepiness. Polysomnography should be performed once daytime symptoms of sleep-disordered breathing occur. Noninvasive positive-pressure ventilation should be considered in such children to prevent further hypoventilation and cardiorespiratory deterioration (Culebras, 2008). Respiratory care for children with neuromuscular conditions such as SMA and DMD may involve the use of noninvasive ventilation with BiPAP on a temporary or full-time basis, mechanically assisted coughing (MAC), or tracheostomy and relief of airway obstruction with coughing and suctioning devices; the tracheostomy, however, is associated with more complications (Simonds, 2006; Young et al., 2007). Home pulse oximetry may be used to monitor oxygenation during sleep or to aid in decision making regarding the use of MAC to clear the airways. A polysomnogram may be used to evaluate the effectiveness of supplemental oxygen and noninvasive ventilation devices.

Several devices are available for children with neuromuscular disease to assist in clearing the airway when the cough reflex is ineffective or diminished. The *mechanical in-exsufflator* (MIE) (also referred to as cough assist) has been found to be safe and effective in the daily management of respiratory function (Kravitz, 2009). The MIE delivers positive inspiratory pressures at a set rate, followed by negative pressure exsufflation coordinated with the patient's own breathing rhythm. The exsufflation is designed to mimic a cough reflex so that mucus can be cleared effectively. Airway suctioning after exsufflation is accomplished as necessary to clear the airways. In children, the MIE device may be connected directly to a tracheostomy or used with a mouthpiece or face mask. Boitano's (2009) article provides a variety of equipment options, including various masks that can be used to deliver noninvasive positive pressure.

Manual cough-assisting techniques include glossopharyngeal breathing or air stacking (frog breathing); the abdominal thrust, which is similar to the Heimlich maneuver (Kravitz, 2009); and manual hyperinflation with a self-inflating resuscitation bag (without oxygen) and a mouthpiece. Hyperinflation may be used in conjunction with abdominal thrusts to improve peak cough flows (Boitano, 2009).

The use of routine chest physiotherapy for DMD has not been adequately evaluated for its effectiveness in clearing the airway of mucus except when there is focal atelectasis and mucous plugging the airways (Kravitz, 2009).

Survival in individuals with DMD may be prolonged several years with the use of noninvasive ventilation and airway clearance devices such as cough assist as alternatives to tracheotomy and airway suctioning (Simonds, 2006). Care considerations for Duchenne muscular dystrophy, sponsored by the Centers for Disease Control and Prevention, were published in *Lancet Neurology* in 2010, and in 2018 these guidelines were updated (Birnkrant, Bushby, Bann, et al., 2018).

The American Academy of Pediatrics (2005) recommends an extensive cardiac evaluation of the child diagnosed with either DMD or Becker MD. Patients with neuromuscular conditions may not have the typical signs and symptoms of cardiac dysfunction. Therefore symptoms such as weight loss, nausea and vomiting, cough, increased fatigue on performance of ADLs, and orthopnea should be carefully evaluated to detect early signs of cardiomyopathy.

Research evaluating a number of treatments for DMD is in progress. These include clinical trials with glutamine and creatine monohydrate to preserve muscle strength; utrophin, a protein that is similar to dystrophin and that in large quantities may counteract the effects of the dystrophin deficiency (Chakkalakal, Thompson, Parks, et al., 2005; Miura & Jardin, 2006); and the enzyme CT GalNAc transferase, which blocks muscle wasting in mice. Deflazacort, a corticosteroid, was approved in 2017 by the US Food and Drug Administration for those age 5 years and older to work as an antiinflammatory and immunosuppressant. Oral albuterol administered daily for 12 weeks increased lean body mass and decreased fat mass in a group of 14 ambulatory boys with Becker MD and DMD; however, overall muscle strength improvement was not observed (Skura, Fowler, Wetzel, et al., 2008).

Guidelines for the standardization of diagnosis and therapeutic management of DMD have been published elsewhere (Bushby, Finkel, Birnkrant, et al., 2010).

Nursing Care Management

The care and management of a child with MD involve the combined efforts of a multidisciplinary health care team. Nurses can help clarify the roles of these health care professionals to family and others. The major emphasis of nursing care is to assist the child and family in coping with the progressive, incapacitating, and fatal nature of the disease; to help design a program that will afford a greater degree of independence and reduce the predictable and preventable disabilities associated with the disorder; and to help the child and family deal constructively with the limitations the disease imposes on their daily lives. Because of advances in technology, children with MD may live into early adulthood; therefore the goals of care should also involve decisions regarding quality of life, achievement of independence, and transition to adulthood.

Working closely with other team members, nurses assist the family in developing the child's self-help skills to give the child the satisfaction of being as independent as possible for as long as possible. It is tempting for parents to overprotect their affected children. Children derive pleasure and build self-esteem from performing actions that visibly please their parents. Therefore parents must be helped to develop a balance between limiting the child's activity because of muscular weakness and allowing the child to accomplish things alone. This requires continual evaluation of the child's capabilities, which are often difficult to assess. Most children with MD instinctively recognize the need to be as independent as possible and strive to do so.

Practical difficulties faced by families are the physical limitations of housing, transportation, and mobility. Housing accommodations must be made so that the wheelchair-bound child can be mobile in the home setting. Transportation in a car restraint seat adapted for the child with weakened neck and back musculature will be necessary, and eventually a wheelchair-accessible vehicle will be required. Discuss diet, nutritional needs, and nutrition modification according to the needs of the individual child and family. Nutritional needs decrease once the child becomes wheelchair bound, and dietary modifications should be made in conjunction with a pediatric dietitian to ensure that the child is receiving an adequate amount of the necessary nutrients to maintain bone health and prevent constipation.

Parents' social activities may be restricted, and the family's activities must be continually modified to meet the needs of the affected child. When the child becomes increasingly incapacitated, the family may consider home care to provide the care needed. The nurse as case manager can assist the family in making this difficult transition. Unless the child is severely incapacitated, he or she should also be involved in the decisions regarding such care. Nurses can assist with decision making by exploring all available options and resources and supporting the child and family in the decision.

Each child's therapy program is tailored to individual needs and capabilities, and family members should be active participants. Parents often need assistance with the physical therapy program and education on a home regimen of exercises and activity. Many parents erroneously believe that by exerting sufficient effort, the child can overcome the weakness and prevent progression of the disease process. They should also be advised to notify the nurse or other designated person when the child becomes even temporarily bedridden so that the exercise program can be modified and continued during this time.

Children with MD tend to become socially isolated as their physical condition deteriorates to the point that they can no longer keep up with friends and classmates. Their physical capabilities diminish, and their dependency increases at the age at which most children are expanding their range of interests and relationships. To gain peer associations, they often learn and use behaviors that bring them the rewards of other children's company. These friends are often children who have been rejected by more able-bodied classmates.

Older boys with MD may also need psychiatric or psychologic counseling to deal with issues such as depression, anger, and quality of life. Parents need encouragement to become involved in support groups because there is evidence that adequate social support from family, community, and other parents is crucial to appropriate coping in families with children with chronic illness.

Regardless of the success of the program and how well the family adapts to the disorder, superimposed on the physical and emotional problems associated with the child's long-term disability is the constant specter of the disease's ultimate outcome. These families encounter all the manifestations of the child with a chronic and fatal illness (see Chapter 17).

CLINICAL JUDGMENT AND NEXT-GENERATION NCLEX® EXAMINATION-STYLE QUESTIONS

1. A newborn is born with a myelomeningocele and a surgical repair is planned for the next day. What actions would the nurse take to care for the myelomonocyte sac before the surgical repair? **Select all that apply.**
   A. Apply a sterile, moist nonadherent dressing to the sac.
   B. Take a rectal temperature every 2 hours before surgery.
   C. Irrigate the sac and surrounding skin with chlorhexidine.
   D. Diaper the infant while making sure it does not touch the sac.
   E. Maintain the legs in abduction with a pad between the knees.
   F. Position the newborn in a prone position with hips slightly flexed.
   G. Place the newborn in an incubator or warmer without clothing or cover.

2. The nurse is completing an assessment on a 3-month-old male who is in the pediatrician's office because the infant had fever and diarrhea the past 2 days. The infant's history reveals he was exposed to maternal chorioamnionitis and born prematurely at 32 weeks' gestation. The nurse performs a history and assessment and finds the following. Which assessment **findings require follow-up** by the nurse? **Select all that apply.**
   A. head lag
   B. arms are stiff
   C. does not smile
   D. floppy posture
   E. unable to roll over
   F. feeding difficulties
   G. irritable and cries often
   H. unable to sit without support
   I. unable to pass object between hands

3. A 5-year-old boy with spina bifida has bladder dysfunction and is unable to empty his bladder without assistance. He also struggles with bowel control and is taking dietary fiber supplements, and suppositories to assist with regular bowel movements. He was born with a myelomeningocele and had surgical repair 48 hours after birth. **Choose the most likely options for the information missing from the statements below by selecting from the lists of options provided.** Based on the child's diagnosis and history, the nurse understands that a ____1____ may produce urinary system ____2____ The nurse would teach the parents and child a method to empty the bladder such as ____3____.

Options for 1	Options for 2	Options for 3
renal cyst	infection	foley catheter placement
kidney stone	failure	clean intermittent catheterization
neuropathic bladder	strictures	sterile intermittent catheterization
rectal fissure	distress	suprapubic aspiration

4. A 6-year-old boy is admitted with increasing symptoms of muscle weakness including difficulties running, riding his bike and climbing stairs. In the hospital he undergoes numerous lab tests, muscle biopsy and EMG. He is diagnosed with Duchene Muscular Dystrophy (DMD). The nurse plans to provide discharge teaching and answer questions the parents and patient ask. **Use an X for the health teaching statement below that is Indicated (appropriate or necessary), Contraindicated (could be harmful), or Non-Essential (makes no difference or not necessary).**

Health Teaching	Indicated	Contraindicated	Non-Essential
"DMD is inherited as an X-linked recessive trait and affects boys."			
"Your child may need to have casts on his legs to help him walk."			
"You will learn stretching exercises and strength and muscle training to help your child."			
"You should call your health care provider if any respiratory symptoms occur."			
"Your child should be hospitalized when ambulation becomes impossible."			
"It is important for your child to remain as independent as possible."			
"Breathing exercises will help maintain his vital lung capacity."			

REFERENCES

Adolfsson, M., Johnson, E., & Nilsson, S. (2017). Pain management for children with cerebral palsy in school settings in two cultures: Action and reaction approaches. *Disability and Rehabilitation*, 1–11.

Adzick, N. S. (2013). Fetal surgery for spina bifida: Past, present, future. *Seminars in Pediatric Surgery*, *22*(1), 10–17.

Agopian, A. J., Tinker, S. C., Lupo, P. J., et al. (2013). Proportion of neural tube defects attributable to known risk factors. Birth defects research. Part A. *Clinical and Molecular Teratology*, *97*(1), 42–46.

Alizadeh, A., Dyck, S. M., & Karimi-Abdolrezaee, S. (2019). Traumatic spinal cord injury: An overview of pathophysiology, models and acute injury mechanisms. *Frontiers in Neurology*, *10*, 282.

American Academy of Pediatrics, Committee on Genetics. (2007). Folic acid for the prevention of neural tube defects. *Pediatrics*, *119*(5), 1031.

American Academy of Pediatrics. (2005). Cardiovascular health supervision for individuals affected by Duchenne or Becker muscular dystrophy. *Pediatrics*, *116*(6), 1569–1573.

American College of Obstetrics and Gynecology. (2016). ACOG practice bulletin No. 163: Screening for fetal aneuploidy. *Obstetrics and Gynecology*, *127*(5), e124.

Aristedis, R., Dimitrios, P., Nikolaos, P., et al. (2017). Intrathecal baclofen pump infection treated by adjunct intrareservoir teicoplanin instillation. *Surgical Neurology International*, *8*, 38.

Arnold, W. D., Kassar, D., & Kissel, J. T. (2019). Spinal muscular atrophy: Diagnosis and management in a new therapeutic era. *Muscle Nerve*, *51*(2), 157–167.

Avarello, J. T., & Cantor, R. M. (2007). Pediatric major trauma: An approach to evaluation and management. *Emergency Medicine Clinics of North America*, *25*(3), 803–836.

Ayub, S. S., Zeidan, M., Larson, S. D., et al. (2019). Long-term outcomes of antegrade continence enema in children with chronic encopresis and incontinence: What is the optimal flush to use? *Pediatr Surg Int*, *35*(4), 431–438.

Bach, J. R. (2007). Medical considerations of long-term survival of Werdnig-Hoffmann disease. *American Journal of Physical Medicine and Rehabilitation*, *86*(5), 349–355.

Balci, B. P. (2018). Spasticity measurement. *Noro Psikiyatri Arsivi*, *55*(Suppl. 1), S49–S53.

Battista, V. (2010). Muscular dystrophy, Duchenne. In P. L. Jackson, J. A. Vessey, & N. A. Schapiro (Eds.), *Primary care of the child with a chronic illness* (5th ed.). St. Louis: Mosby.

Bax, M., Goldstein, M., Rosenbaum, P., et al. (2005). Proposed definition and classification of cerebral palsy. *Developmental Medicine and Child Neurology*, *47*(8), 571–576.

Benjamins, L. J., Gourishankar, A., Yataco-Marquez, V., et al. (2013). Honey pacifier use among an indigent pediatric population. *Pediatrics*, *131*(6), e1838–e1841.

Berker, A. N., & Yalçin, M. S. (2008). Cerebral palsy: Orthopedic aspects and rehabilitation. *Pediatric Clinics of North America*, *55*(5), 1209–1225.

Betz, C., Linroth, R., Butler, C., et al. (2010). Spina bifida: What we learned from consumers. *Pediatric Clinics of North America*, *57*(4), 935–944.

Bharucha-Goebel, D. X. (2020). Muscular dystrophies. In R. M. Kliegman, B. F. St. Geme, N. J. Blum, et al. (Eds.), *Nelson textbook of pediatrics* (21st ed.). Philadelphia: Elsevier.

Birnkrant, D. J., Bushby, K., Bann, C. M., et al. (2018). Diagnosis and management of Duchenne muscular dystrophy, part 2: Respiratory, cardiac, bone health, and orthopaedic management. *Lancet Neurol, 17*(4), 347–361.

Boitano, L. J. (2009). Equipment options for cough augmentation, ventilation, and noninvasive interfaces in neuromuscular respiratory management. *Pediatrics, 123*(Suppl. 4), S226–S230.

Bosanquet, M., Copeland, L., Ware, R., et al. (2013). A systematic review of tests to predict cerebral palsy in young children. *Developmental Medicine and Child Neurology, 55*(5), 418–426.

Bourke-Taylor, H. M., Cotter, C., Lalor, A., et al. (2017). School success and participation for students with cerebral palsy: A qualitative study exploring multiple perspectives. *Disability and Rehabilitation*, 1–9.

Burke, R., Liptak, G. S., & Council on Children with Disabilities. (2011). Providing a primary care medical home for children and youth with spina bifida. *Pediatrics, 128*(6), e1645–e1658.

Bushby, K., Finkel, R., Birnkrant, D. J., et al. (2010). Diagnosis and management of Duchenne muscular dystrophy, part 1: Diagnosis, and pharmacologicical and psychosocial management. *The Lancet. Neurology, 9*(1), 77–93. Retrieved from http://www.treat-nmd.eu/downloads/file/standardsofcare/dmd/lancet/the_diagnosis_and_management_of_dmd_lancet_complete_with_erratum.pdf.

Calhoun, C. L., Schottler, J., & Vogel, L. C. (2013). Recommendations for mobility in children with spinal cord injury. *Topics in Spinal Cord Injury Rehabilitation, 19*(2), 142–151.

Centers for Disease Control and Prevention. (2007). Folate status in women of childbearing age, by race/ethnicity—United States, 1999-2000, 2001-2002, and 2003-2004. *MMWR. Morbidity and Mortality Weekly Report, 55*(51), 1377–1380.

Centers for Disease Control and Prevention. (2009). Racial/ethnic differences in the birth prevalence of spina bifida—United States, 1995-2005. *MMWR. Morbidity and Mortality Weekly Report, 57*(53), 1409–1413.

Centers for Disease Control and Prevention. (2019). *11 Things to know about cerebral palsy*. Retrieved from https://www.cdc.gov/features/cerebral-palsy-11-things/index.html. [Accessed 19 June 2019].

Centers for Disease Control and Prevention: National center on birth defects and developmental disabilities United States, page last reviewed:August 19, 2019. Retrieved from http://www.cdc.gov/ncbddd/spinabifida/data.html.

Cerebral Palsy Guide. (2017). *Causes of cerebral palsy*. Retrieved from https://www.cerebralpalsyguide.com/cerebral-palsy/causes/. [Accessed 19 June 2019].

Chakkalakal, J. V., Thompson, J., Parks, R. J., et al. (2005). Molecular, cellular, and pharmacological therapies for Duchenne/Becker muscular dystrophies. *FASEB Journal: Official Publication of the Federation of American Societies for Experimental Biology, 19*(8), 880–891.

Chaléat-Valayer, E., Bernard, J. C., Deceuninck, J., et al. (2016). Pelvic-spinal analysis and the impact of onabotulinum toxin a injections on spinal balance in one child with cerebral palsy. *Journal of Child Neurology Open*, 3 2016.

Choi, J. Y., Choi, Y. S., & Park, E. S. (2017). Language development and brain magnetic resonance imaging characteristics in preschool children with cerebral palsy. *Journal of Speech, Language, and Hearing Research: JSLHR, 60*(5), 1330–1338.

Christensen, D., Van Naarden Braun, K., Doernberg, N. S., et al. (2014). Prevalence of cerebral palsy, co-occurring autism spectrum disorders, and motor functioning – autism and developmental disabilities monitoring network, USA, 2008. *Dev Med Child Neurol, 56*(1), 59–65.

Consortium for Spinal Cord Medicine. (2010). Sexuality and reproductive health in adults with spinal cord injury: A clinical practice guideline for health-care professionals. *The Journal of Spinal Cord Medicine, 33*(3), 281–336.

Culebras, A. (2008). Sleep-disordered breathing in neuromuscular disease. *Sleep Medicine Clinics, 3*(3), 377–386.

Dai, A. I., Wasay, M., & Awan, S. (2008). Botulinum toxin type A with oral baclofen versus oral tizanidine: A randomized pilot comparison in patients with cerebral palsy and equines foot deformity. *Journal of Child Neurology, 23*(12), 1464–1466.

DeForge, D., Blackmer, J., Garritty, C., et al. (2006). Male erectile dysfunction following spinal cord injury: A systematic review. *Spinal Cord, 44*(8), 465–473.

Dicianno, B. E., Fairman, A. D., Juengst, S. B., et al. (2010). Using the spina bifida life course model in clinical practice: An interdisciplinary approach. *Pediatric Clinics of North America, 57*(4), 945–957.

Eek, M. N., Olsson, K., Lindh, K., Askljung, B., et al. (2018). Intrathecal baclofen in dyskinetic cerebral palsy: Effects on function and activity. *Developmental Medicine & Child Neurology, 60*(1), 94–99.

Elzeneini, W., Waly, R., Marshall, D., & Bailie, A. (2019). Early start of clean intermittent catheterization versus expectant management in children with spina bifida. *Journal of Pediatric Surgery, 54*(2), 322–325.

Farrell, C. A., Hannon, M., & Lee, L. K. (2017). Pediatric spinal cord injury without radiographic abnormality in the era of advanced imaging. *Current Opinion in Pediatrics, 29*(3), 286–290.

Feldman, B. M., Rider, L. G., Reed, A. M., et al. (2008). Juvenile dermatomyositis and other idiopathic inflammatory myopathies of childhood. *Lancet, 371*(9631), 2201–2212.

Francis, R. (2007). Physiology and management of bladder and bowel continence following spinal cord injury. *Ostomy/Wound Management, 53*(12), 18–27.

Friel, K. M., Lee, P., Soles, L. V., et al. (2017). Combined transcranial direct current stimulation and robotic upper limb therapy improves upper limb function in an adult with cerebral palsy. *Neurorehabilitation.*

Gasalberti, D. (2006). Alternative therapies for children and youth with special health care needs. *Journal of Pediatric Health Care, 20*(2), 133–136.

George, J. M., Fiori, S., Fripp, J., et al. (2017). Validation of an MRI brain injury and growth scoring system in very preterm infants scanned at 29- to 35-week postmenstrual age. *American Journal of Neuroradiology (AJNR).*

Glader, L., & Barkoudah, E. (2019). *Cerebral palsy: Clinical features and classification.* In M. C. Patterson, & C. Brigemohan (Eds.), UpToDate, Retrieved June 21, 2019 https://www.uptodate.com/contents/cerebral-palsy-clinical-features-and-classification.

Golomb, M. R., Saha, C., Garg, B. P., et al. (2007). Association of cerebral palsy with other disabilities in children with perinatal arterial ischemic stroke. *Pediatric Neurology, 37*(4), 245–249.

Gray, M., & Moore, K. N. (2009). *Urologic disorders: Adult and pediatric care.* St. Louis: Mosby.

Green, L. B., & Hurvitz, E. A. (2007). Cerebral palsy. *Phys Med Rehabil Clin N Am, 18*(4), 859–882.

Hagen, E. M. (2015). Acute complications of spinal cord injuries. *World Journal of Orthopedics, 6*(1), 17–23.

Haliloglu, G. (2020). Spinal muscular atrophies. In R. M. Kliegman, B. F. St. Geme, N. J. Blum, et al. (Eds.), *Nelson textbook of pediatrics* (21st ed.). Philadelphia: Elsevier.

Hauer, J., & Houtrow, A. J. (2017). Pain assessment and treatment in children with significant impairment of the central nervous system. *Pediatrics, 139*(6), e20171002.

Hayes, J. S., & Arriola, T. (2005). Pediatric spinal injuries. *Pediatric Nursing, 31*(6), 464–467.

Ho, C. H., Triolo, R. J., Elias, A. L., et al. (2014). Functional electrical stimulation and spinal cord injury. *Physical Medicine and Rehabilitation Clinics of North America, 25*(3), 631–654.

Hosalkar, H., Pandya, N. K., Hsu, J., et al. (2009). Specialty update: What's new in orthopaedic rehabilitation. *The Journal of Bone and Joint Surgery. American, 91*(9), 2296–2310.

Huber, A. M. (2012). Idiopathic inflammatory myopathies in childhood: Current concepts. *Pediatric Clinics of North America, 59*(2), 365–380.

Hurlbert, R. J., Hadley, M. N., Walters, B. C., et al. (2013). Pharmacological therapy for acute spinal cord injury. *Neurosurgery, 72*(Suppl. 3), 93–105.

Iannaccone, S. T., & Burghes, A. (2002). Spinal muscular atrophies. *Advances in Neurology, 88*, 83–98.

Ingham, J., Angotti, R., Lewis, M., et al. (2019). Onabotulinum toxin A in children with refractory idiopathic overactive bladder: Medium-term outcomes. *Journal of Pediatric Urology, 15*(1), 32.e1–32.e5.

Johnston, M. V. (2020). Cerebral palsy. In R. M. Kliegman, B. F. St. Geme, N. J. Blum, et al. (Eds.), *Nelson textbook of pediatrics* (21st ed.). Philadelphia: Elsevier.

Kanitkar, A., Szturm, T., Parmar, S., et al. (2017). The effectiveness of a computer game-based rehabilitation platform for children with cerebral palsy: Protocol for a randomized clinical trial. *JMIR Research Protocols, 6*(5), e93.

Kimberlin, D. W., Brady, M. D., Jackson, M. A., et al. (Eds.). (2018). *Red book: Report of the committee on infectious diseases.* Elk Grove Village, Ill: American Academy of Pediatrics, Committee on infectious diseases.

Kinsman, S., & Johnston, M. (2020). Myelomeningocele. In R. M. Kliegman, B. F. St. Geme, N. J. Blum, et al. (Eds.), *Nelson textbook of pediatrics* (21st ed.). Philadelphia: Elsevier.

Krageloh-Mann, I., & Cans, C. (2009). Cerebral palsy update. *Brain and Development, 31*(7), 537–544.

Kravitz, R. M. (2009). Airway clearance in Duchenne muscular dystrophy. *Pediatrics, 123*(Suppl. 4), S231–S235.

Krigger, K. W. (2006). Cerebral palsy: An overview. *American Family Physician, 73*(1), 91–100, 101–102.

Lapa, D. A. (2019). Endoscopic fetal surgery for neural tube defects. *Best Pract Res Clin Obstet Gynaecol, 58*, 133–141.

Lazzaretti, C. C., & Pearson, C. (2010). Myelodysplasia. In P. J. Allen, J. A. Vessey, & N. A. Schapiro (Eds.), *Primary care of the child with a chronic condition* (5th ed.). St. Louis: Mosby.

Liptak, G. S., & Dosa, N. P. (2010). Myelomeningocele. *Pediatrics in Review, 31*(11), 443–450.

Liu, S., Dong, C., & Ubogu, E. E. (2018). Immunotherapy of Guillain-Barré syndrome. *Human Vaccines & Immunotherapeutics, 14*(11), 2568–2579.

Lovette, B. (2008). Safe transportation for children with special needs. *Journal of Pediatric Health Care, 22*(5), 323–328.

Lunn, M. R., & Wang, C. H. (2008). Spinal muscular atrophy. *Lancet, 371*(9630), 2120–2133.

Lyons, R. (2008). Elusive belly pain and Guillain-Barré syndrome. *Journal of Pediatric Health Care, 22*(5), 310–314.

MacLennan, A. H., Thompson, S. C., & Gecz, J. (2015). Cerebral palsy: Causes, pathways, and the role of genetic variants. *American Journal of Obstetrics and Gynecology, 213*(6), 779–788. http://www.ajog.org/article/S0002-9378(15)00510-4/fulltext?cc=y=.

Manzur, A. Y., Kinali, M., & Muntoni, F. (2008). Update on the management of Duchenne muscular dystrophy. *Archives of Disease in Childhood, 93*(11), 986–990.

Manzur, A. Y., Kuntzer, T., Pike, M., et al. (2008). Glucocorticoid corticosteroids for Duchenne muscular dystrophy. *Cochrane Database of Systematic Review* (1), CD003725.

Mathison, D. J., Kadom, N., & Krug, S. E. (2008). Spinal cord injury in the pediatric patient. *Clinical Pediatric Emergency Medicine, 9*(2), 106–123.

Mercuri, E., Bertini, E., & Iannaconne, S. T. (2012). Childhood spinal muscular atrophy: Controversies and challenges. *The Lancet. Neurology, 11*(5), 443–452.

Merenda, L. A., & Hickey, K. (2005). Key elements of a bladder and bowel management for children with spinal cord injuries. *SCI Nursing: A Publication of the American Association of Spinal Cord Injury Nurses, 22*(1), 8–14.

Metcalfe, P. D. (2017). Neuropathic bladder: Investigation and treatment through their lifetime. *Canadian Urological Association Journal, 11*(1–2 Suppl. 1).

Meylemans, A., & De Bleeker, J. (2019). Current evidence for treatment with nusinersen for spinal muscular atrophy: A systematic review. *Acta Neurologica Belgicapresents* Epub ahead of print.

Michmizos, K. P., & Krebs, H. I. (2017). Pediatric robotic rehabilitation: Current knowledge and future trends in treating children with sensorimotor impairments. *Neurorehabilitation, 41*(1), 69–76.

Miura, P., & Jardin, B. J. (2006). Utrophin upregulation for treating Duchenne or Becker muscular dystrophy: How close are we? *Trends in Molecular Medicine, 12*(3), 122–129.

Moldenhauer, J. S., & Adzick, N. S. (2017). Fetal surgery for myelomeningocele: After the Management of Myelomeningocele Study (MOMS). *Semin Fetal Neonatal Med, 22*(6), 360–366.

Moldenhauer, J. S., Soni, S., Rintoul, N. E., et al. (2015). Fetal myelomeningocele repair: The post-MOMS experience at the Children's Hospital of Philadelphia. *Fetal Diagnosis and Therapy, 37*(3), 235–240.

Moster, D., Wilcox, A. J., Vollset, S. E., et al. (2010). Cerebral palsy among term and postterm births. *JAMA: The Journal of the American Medical Association, 304*(9), 976–982.

Mourtzinos, A., & Stoffel, J. T. (2010). Management of goals for the spina bifida neurogenic bladder: A review from infancy to adulthood. *The Urologic Clinics of North America, 37*(4), 527–535.

Moxley, R. T., Ashwal, S., Pandya, S., et al. (2005). Practice parameter: Corticosteroid treatment on Duchenne dystrophy. *Neurology, 64*(1), 13–20.

National Institute of Neurological Disorders and Stroke. (2013). *Cerebral palsy: Hope through research.* NIH Publication. No. 13-159 https://www.ninds.nih.gov/Disorders/Patient-Caregiver-Education/Hope-Through-Research/Cerebral-Palsy-Hope-Through-Research.

Nehring, W. M. (2010). Cerebral palsy. In P. L. Jackson, J. A. Vessey, & N. A. Schapiro (Eds.), *Primary care of the child with a chronic illness* (5th ed.). St. Louis: Mosby.

Noonan, C., Quigley, S., & Curley, M. (2011). Using the Braden Q scale to predict pressure ulcer risk in pediatric patients. *Journal of Pediatric Nursing, 26*(6), 566–575.

Nordqvist, Christian. (2017). *Cerebral palsy: Symptoms, causes, and treatments.* http://www.medicalnewstoday.com/articles/152712.php.

Oda, Y., Takigawa, T., Sugimoto, Y., et al. (2017). Scoliosis in patients with severe cerebral palsy: Three different courses in adolescents. *Acta Medica Okayama, 71*(2), 119–126.

O'Shea, T. M. (2008). Diagnosis, treatment, and prevention of cerebral palsy. *Clinical Obstetrics and Gynecology, 51*(4), 816–828.

Oskoui, M., Coutinho, F., Dykeman, J., et al. (2013). An update on the prevalence of cerebral palsy: A systematic review and meta-analysis. *Developmental Medicine and Child Neurology, 55*(6), 509–519.

Osorio, M., Reyes, M. R., & Massagli, T. L. (2014). Pediatric spinal cord injury. *Current Physical Medicine and Rehabilitation Reports, 2*, 158.

Ottolini, K., Harris, A. B., Amling, J. K., et al. (2013). Wound care challenges in children and adults with spina bifida: An open-cohort study. *Journal of Pediatric Rehabilitation Medicine, 6*(1), 1–10.

Parent, S., Mac-Thiong, J. M., Roy-Beaudry, M., et al. (2011). Spinal cord injury in the pediatric population: A systematic review of the literature. *Journal of Neurotrauma, 28*(8), 1515–1524.

Park, T. S., Dobbs, M. B., & Cho, J. (2018). Evidence supporting selective dorsal rhizotomy for treatment of spastic cerebral palsy. *Cureus, 10*(10), e3466.

Piccione, E. A., Salame, K., & Katirji, B. (2014). Guillain-Barré syndrome and related disorders. In B. Katirji, H. Kaminski, & R. Ruff (Eds.), *Neuromuscular disorders in clinical practice.* New York, NY: Springer.

Proctor, M. R. (2020). Spinal cord injuries in children. In R. M. Kliegman, B. F. St. Geme, N. J. Blum, et al. (Eds.), *Nelson textbook of pediatrics* (21st ed.). Philadelphia: Elsevier.

Quan, D. (2011). Muscular dystrophies and neurologic diseases that present as myopathy. *Rheumatic Diseases Clinics of North America, 37*(2), 233–244.

Rall, S., & Grimm, T. (2012). Survival in Duchenne muscular dystrophy. *Acta Myologica: Myopathies and Cardiomyopathies, 31*(2), 117–120.

Robinson, A. B., & Reed, A. M. (2020). Juvenile dermatomyositis. In R. M. Kliegman, B. F. St. Geme, N. J. Blum, et al. (Eds.), *Nelson textbook of pediatrics* (21st ed.). Philadelphia: Elsevier.

Romeo, D. M., Ricci, D., Brogna, C., et al. (2016). Use of the hammersmith infant neurological examination in infants with cerebral palsy: A critical review of the literature. *Developmental Medicine and Child Neurology, 58*(3), 240–245.

Rosenbaum, P., Paneth, N., Leviton, A., et al. (2007). A report: The definition and classification of cerebral palsy, April 2006. *Developmental Medicine and Child Neurology, 49*(S109), 1–44.

Rowe, D. E., & Jadhav, A. L. (2008). Care of the adolescent with spina bifida. *Pediatric Clinics of North America, 55*(6), 1359–1374.

Rozelle, C. J., Arabi, B., Dhall, S. S., et al. (2013). Management of pediatric cervical spine and spinal cord injuries. *Neurosurgery, 72*(Suppl. 3), 205–226.

Rumberg, F., Bakir, M. S., Taylor, W. R., et al. (2016). The effects of selective dorsal rhizotomy on balance and symmetry of gait in children with cerebral palsy. *PLoS ONE, 11*(4), e0152930.

Russman, B. S. (1996). Function changes in spinal muscular atrophy II and III: The DCN/SMA Group. *Neurology, 47*(4), 973–976.

Russman, B. S., Iannaccone, S. T., Buncher, C. R., et al. (1992). Spinal muscular atrophy: New thoughts on the pathogenesis and classification schema. *Journal of Child Neurology, 7*(4), 347–353.

Ryan, M. M. (2020). Guillain-Barre syndrome. In R. M. Kliegman, B. F. St. Geme, N. J. Blum, et al. (Eds.), *Nelson textbook of pediatrics* (21st ed.). Philadelphia: Elsevier.

Samaniego, I. A. (2003). A sore spot in pediatrics: Risk factors for pressure ulcers. *Pediatric Nursing, 29*(4), 278–282.

Sawyer, S., & Macnee, S. (2010). Transition to adult healthcare for adolescents with spina bifida: Research issues. *Developmental Disabilities Research Reviews, 16*(1), 60–65.

Schleiss, M. R. (2020). Tetanus (*Clostridium tetani*). In R. M. Kliegman, B. F. St. Geme, N. J. Blum, et al. (Eds.), *Nelson textbook of pediatrics* (21st ed.). Philadelphia: Elsevier.

Schottler, J., Vogel, L., & Sturm, P. (2012). Spinal cord injuries in young children: A review of children injured at 5 years of age and younger. *Developmental Medicine and Child Neurology, 54*, 1138–1143.

Schroth, M. K. (2009). Special considerations in the respiratory management of spinal muscular atrophy. *Pediatrics, 123*(Suppl. 4), S245–S249.

Sehrawat, N., Marwaha, M., Bansal, K., et al. (2014). Cerebral palsy: A dental update. *International Journal of Clinical Pediatric Dentistry, 7*(2), 109–118.

Shaer, C. M., Chescheir, N., & Schulkin, J. (2007). Myelomeningocele: A review of the epidemiology, genetics, risk factors for conception, prenatal diagnosis, and prognosis for affected individuals. *Obstetrical and Gynecological Survey, 62*(7), 471–479.

Shavelle, R. M., DeVivo, M. J., Paculdo, D. R., et al. (2007). Long-term survival after childhood spinal cord injury. *The Journal of Spinal Cord Medicine, 30*(Suppl. 1), S48–S54.

Simonds, A. K. (2006). Recent advances in respiratory care for neuromuscular disease. *Chest, 130*(6), 1879–1886.

Simpson, J. L., Richards, D. S., & Otaño, L. (2012). Prenatal genetic diagnosis. In S. G. Gabbe, J. R. Niebyl, J. L. Simpson, et al. (Eds.), *Obstetrics: Normal and problem pregnancies* (6th ed.). Philadelphia: Saunders.

Skura, C. L., Fowler, E. G., Wetzel, G. T., et al. (2008). Albuterol increases lean body mass in ambulatory boys with duchenne or becker muscular dystrophy. *Neurology, 70*(2), 137–143.

Snodgrass, W., & Gargollo, P. (2010). Urologic care of the neurogenic bladder in children. *The Urologic Clinics of North America, 37*(2), 207–214.

Spittle, A. J., Morgan, C., Olsen, J. E., Novak, I., & Cheong, J. L. Y. (2018). Early diagnosis and treatment of cerebral palsy in children with a history of preterm birth. *Perinatology Clinics, 45*(3), 409–420.

Strobl, W., Theologis, T., Brunner, R., et al. (2015). Best clinical practice in botulinum toxin treatment for children with cerebral palsy. *Toxins, 7*(5), 1629–1648.

Sumner, C. J., & Crawford, T. O. (2018). Two breakthrough gene-targeted treatments for spinal muscular atrophy: Challenges remain. *Journal of Clinical Investigation, 128*(8), 3219–3277.

Sun, D., Wang, Q., Hou, M., et al. (2018). Clinical characteristics and functional status of children with different subtypes of dyskinetic cerebral palsy. *Medicine, 97*(21) e10817.

Tarcan, T., Onol, F. F., Ilker, Y., et al. (2006). The timing of primary neurosurgical repair significantly affects neurogenic bladder prognosis in children with myelomeningocele. *Journal of Urology, 176*, 1161.

To, C. S., Kirsch, R. F., Kobetic, R., et al. (2005). Simulation of a functional neuromuscular stimulation powered mechanical gait orthosis with coordinated joint locking. *IEEE Transactions on Neural Systems and Rehabilitation Engineering: A Publication of the IEEE Engineering in Medicine and Biology Society, 13*(2), 227–235.

Trivic, I., & Hojsak, I. (2019). Evaluation and treatment of malnutrition and associated gastrointestinal complications in children with cerebral palsy. *Pediatric Gastroenterology Hepatology and Nutrition, 22*(2), 122–131.

Van Naarden Braun, K., Doernberg, N., Schieve, L., et al. (2016). Birth prevalence of cerebral palsy: A population-based study. *Pediatrics, 137*(1).

van Zyl, N., Hill, B., Cooper, C., et al. (2019). Expanding traditional tendon-based techniques with nerve transfers for the restoration of upper limb function in tetraplegia: A prospective case series. *Lancet, 394*(10198), 565–575.

Vogel, L. C., Betz, R. R., & Mulcahey, M. J. (2012). Spinal cord injuries in children and adolescents. In J. Verhaagen, & J. W. MacDonald (Eds.), *Handbook of clinical neurology* (109) (pp. 131–148) 3.

Vogel, L. C., Chlan, K. M., Zebracki, K., et al. (2011). Long-term outcomes of adults with pediatric-onset spinal cord injuries as a function of neurologic impairment. *The Journal of Spinal Cord Medicine, 34*(1), 60–66.

Wakiguchi, H. (2019). Multispecialty approach for improving outcomes in juvenile dermatomyositis. *The Journal of Multidisciplinary Healthcare (JMDH), 12*, 387–394.

Westbom, L., Bergstrand, L., Wagner, P., et al. (2011). Survival at 19 years of age in a total population of children and young people with cerebral palsy. *Developmental Medicine and Child Neurology, 53*, 806–814.

Westbom, L., Rimstedt, A., & Nordmark, E. (2017). Assessments of pain in children and adolescents with cerebral palsy: A retrospective population-based registry study. *Developmental Medicine and Child Neurology, 59*(8), 858–863.

Williams, J., Mai, C. T., Mulinare, J., et al. (2015). Updated estimates of neural tube defects prevented by mandatory folic acid fortification — united states, 1995–2011. *Morbidity and Mortality Weekly Report (MMWR), 64*(01), 1–5.

Wright, P., Durham, S., Ewins, D., et al. (2012). Neuromuscular electrical stimulation for children with cerebral palsy: A review. *Archives of Disease in Childhood, 97*(4), 364–371.

Yana, M., Tutuola, F., Westwater-Wood, S., & Kavlak, E. (2019). The efficacy of botulinum toxin a lower limb injections in addition to physiotherapy approaches in children with cerebral palsy: A systematic review. *NeuroRehabilitation, 44*(2), 175–189.

Young, H. K., Lowe, A., & Fitzgerald, D. A. (2007). Outcome of noninvasive ventilation in children with neuromuscular disease. *Neurology, 68*(3), 198–201.

Yuan-Kim Liow, N., Gimeno, H., Lumsden, D. E., et al. (2016). Gabapentin can significantly improve dystonia severity and quality of life in children. *European Journal of Paediatric Neurology, 20*(1), 100–107.

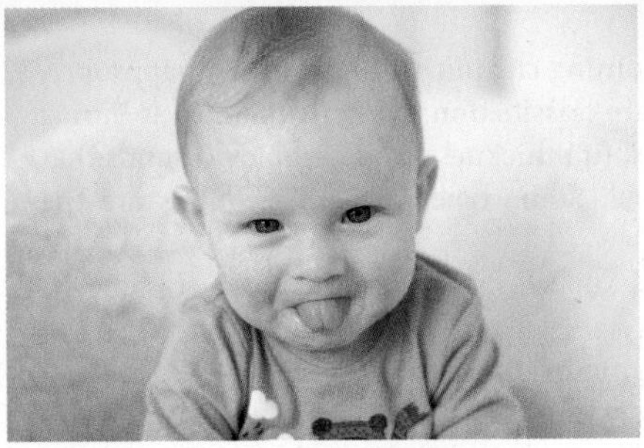

31

The Child With Integumentary Dysfunction

Rose Ann U. Baker, Mary Mondozzi, Marilyn J. Hockenberry

http://evolve.elsevier.com/wong/essentials

CONCEPTS

- Tissue Integrity
- Inflammation
- Infection

INTEGUMENTARY DYSFUNCTION

SKIN LESIONS

Lesions of the skin result from a variety of etiologic factors. Skin lesions originate from (1) contact with injurious agents, such as infective organisms, toxic chemicals, and physical trauma; (2) hereditary factors; (3) external factors, such as allergens; or (4) systemic diseases, such as varicella, lupus erythematosus, and nutritional deficiency diseases. Responses are highly individualized in children. An agent that is harmless to one individual may be damaging to another, and a single agent may produce varying degrees of responses in different individuals.

Another factor in the etiology of skin manifestations is the child's age. For example, infants and young children are subject to "birthmark" malformations and atopic dermatitis that appear early in life. The school-age child is susceptible to tinea (ringworm) of the scalp, and acne is a characteristic skin disorder of puberty. Children's typical social environments also make them susceptible to skin disorders; the most recent national survey notes that up to 20% of American children experience atopy. Exposure to smoke and children with food allergies, particularly peanut allergy, have also been associated with higher rates of atopic dermatitis and eczema. Contact dermatitis, such as poison ivy, is seen only when the noxious agent is found in the environment. Similarly, insect bites are associated with seasonal activities during the summer and fall months.

Skin of Younger Children

The major skin layers arise from different embryologic origins. Early in the embryonic period, a single layer of epithelium forms from the ectoderm while simultaneously the corium develops from the mesenchyme. In infants and small children, the epidermis is loosely bound to the dermis. This poor adherence causes the layers to separate easily during an inflammatory process to form blisters. This is especially true in preterm infants, who have a propensity to blister formation and separation of the skin with minor trauma such as the removal of adhesive tape. In contrast, the skin of older children is thinner, and the cells of all the strata are more compressed.

Pathophysiology of Dermatitis

More than half of the dermatologic problems in children are various forms of dermatitis. This implies a sequence of inflammatory changes in the skin that are grossly and microscopically similar but diverse in course and causation. Acute responses produce intercellular and intracellular edema, the formation of intradermal vesicles, and an initial infiltration of inflammatory cells into the epidermis. In the dermis, there is edema, vascular dilation, and early perivascular cellular infiltration. The location and manner of these reactions produce the lesions characteristic of each disorder. The changes are usually reversible, and the skin ordinarily recovers without blemish unless complicating factors such as ulceration from the primary irritant, scratching, and infection are introduced or underlying vascular disease develops. In chronic conditions, permanent effects are seen that vary according to the disorder, the general condition of the affected individual, and the available therapy.

Diagnostic Evaluation

Although the history and subjective symptoms of skin lesions are explored first, the obvious objective characteristics of the lesions are often noted simultaneously. Many skin lesions are diagnosed after careful inspection.

History and Symptoms

Many cutaneous lesions are associated with local symptoms. The most common local symptom is itching (**pruritus**), which varies in frequency and intensity. Pain or tenderness often accompanies some skin lesions. Other skin sensations such as burning, prickling, stinging, or crawling are also described. Alterations in local feeling include absence of sensation (**anesthesia**); excessive sensitivity (**hyperesthesia**); diminished sensation (**hypesthesia** or **hypoesthesia**); or abnormal sensation, such as burning or prickling (**paresthesia**). These symptoms may remain localized or migrate. They may also be constant or intermittent and may be aggravated by a specific activity, such as exposure to sunlight.

It is important to determine whether the child has an allergic condition such as asthma or history of a previous skin disease. Atopic dermatitis, often associated with allergies, frequently begins in infancy. Important questions for the parent include when the lesion or symptom first appeared; whether it occurred with ingestion of a food or other substance, including any medication; and whether the condition was related to activity such as contact with plants, insects, or chemicals. Finally, inquire if other children in the home or classroom have similar symptoms and if the child's parents or siblings have a history of atopy or allergic skin conditions.

Objective Findings

The skin lesions' distribution, size, location, and morphology provide significant information. Skin lesions assume distinct characteristics that are related to the pathologic process. Nurses should become familiar with the common terms that are applied to skin lesions because these terms are used in the processes of record keeping and communication. These terms include the following:

Erythema—A reddened area caused by increased amounts of oxygenated blood in the dermal vasculature

Ecchymoses (bruises)—Localized red or purple discolorations caused by extravasation of blood into dermis and subcutaneous tissues

Petechiae—Pinpoint, tiny, and sharp circumscribed spots in the superficial layers of the epidermis

Primary lesions—Skin changes produced by a causative factor; common primary lesions in pediatric skin disorders are macules, papules, and vesicles

Secondary lesions—Changes that result from alteration in the primary lesions, such as those caused by rubbing, scratching, medication, or involution and healing

Distribution pattern—The pattern in which lesions are distributed over the body, whether local or generalized, and the specific areas associated with the lesions

Configuration and arrangement—The size, shape, and arrangement of a lesion or groups of lesions (e.g., **discrete**, **clustered**, **diffuse**, or **confluent**)

Extrinsic causes usually result from physical, chemical, or allergic irritants or from an infectious agent such as bacteria, fungi, viruses, or animal parasites. Intrinsic causes such as a specific infection (e.g., measles, chickenpox), drug sensitization, or other allergic phenomena can produce skin manifestations.

Laboratory Studies

When it is suspected that a skin problem might be related to a systemic disease, such as one of the collagen diseases or an immunodeficiency disease, studies are needed to rule out these possibilities. Diagnostic techniques include microscopic examination, cultures, skin scrapings or biopsy, cytodiagnosis, patch testing, and Wood light examination. Allergic skin testing and other laboratory tests such as blood count and sedimentation rate are used when indicated.

WOUNDS

Wounds are structural or physiologic disruptions of the skin that activate normal or abnormal tissue repair responses. Wounds are classified as acute or chronic. **Acute wounds** are those that heal uneventfully within 2 to 3 weeks. **Chronic wounds** are those that do not heal in the expected time frame or are associated with complications. Cofactors that disrupt or delay wound healing include compromised perfusion, malnutrition, and infection. In children, most wounds are acute and can be prevented from becoming chronic wounds through appropriate nursing care. Wounds are classified in the same manner as burns: superficial, partial thickness, full thickness, and complex wounds that include muscle and/or bone. Some types of acute wounds are the following:

Abrasion—Removal of the superficial layers of skin by rubbing or scraping

Avulsion—Forcible pulling out or extraction of tissue

Laceration—Torn or jagged wound; accidental cut wound

Incision—Division of the skin made with a sharp object; cut

Penetrating wound—Disruption of the skin surface that extends into underlying tissue or into a body cavity

Puncture—Wound with a relatively small opening compared with the depth

Epidermal Injuries

Abrasions are the most common epidermal wounds in children, usually in the form of a skinned knee or elbow. In most injuries, the margins of the abraded area are superficial, involving only the outer layers of epidermis, although the central portion may extend into the dermis. Initially the defect is filled by a blood clot and necrotic debris, which subsequently dehydrate to form a scab. Epithelial tissue is composed of labile cells, which are constantly destroyed and replaced throughout the life span. Injury to these tissues results in **regeneration** (i.e., rapid replacement by similar cells).

Injury to Deeper Tissues

Tissues composed of **permanent cells** such as muscle and nerve cells are unable to regenerate. These tissues repair themselves by substituting fibrous connective tissue for the injured tissue. This fibrous tissue, or **scar**, serves as a patch to preserve or restore the continuity of the tissue. Wounds involving permanent cells include surgical incisions, lacerations, ulcers, evulsions, and full-thickness burns. Injured cells of glandular organs and bones, composed of stable cells, multiply less vigorously and heal more slowly. With some wounds an overgrowth of nerve endings may occur, resulting in **allodynia**, or the sensation of pain from normally nonpainful stimuli, such as light touch.

Process of Wound Healing

The nonspecific repair mechanism of wound healing with scar formation involves the processes of inflammation, fibroplasia, scar contraction, and scar maturation. The initial response at the site of injury is **inflammation**, a vascular and cellular response that prepares the tissues for the subsequent repair process. There is a transient constriction of transected blood vessels, lasting 5 to 10 minutes, followed by active vasodilation of all local small vessels and increased blood flow to the area. This is accompanied by increased permeability of small venules, which allows plasma to leak into surrounding tissues (edema). A blood clot is formed along wound edges, providing a framework for future growth of capillaries (**angiogenesis**) and epithelial cells.

At the same time, vessel walls become lined with leukocytes, primarily neutrophils, which pass through the walls and concentrate at the injured site, where they ingest bacteria and debris (**phagocytosis**). Neutrophils are superseded by macrophages, which continue phagocytosis, and by growth factors needed for skin repair and angiogenesis. Fibroblasts attracted to the area from blood vessels deposit fibrin throughout the clot. Adjacent capillaries begin to form buds that stretch across the supporting fibrin threads, and epithelial cells secrete a fibrolytic enzyme that allows their advancement across the wound. This initial phase of wound healing takes place during the first 3 to 5 days after injury. The wound is weakest at this time.

Fibroplasia (granulation or proliferation), the second phase of healing, continues for 5 days to 4 weeks. Fibroblasts, immature connective tissue cells, migrate to the healing site and begin to secrete collagen into the meshwork spaces. Granulation tissue is highly vascular, "beefy" red, shiny connective tissue that organizes and restructures, forming thicker, stronger fibers arranged in orderly layers. A thin layer of epithelial tissue is regenerated over the surface of the wound, and leukocytes gradually disappear from the area. The wound is fragile at this time, and granulation tissue bleeds profusely if disturbed.

During contraction and maturation, the third and fourth phases of wound healing, collagen continues to be deposited and organized into layers, compressing the new blood vessels and gradually stopping blood flow across the wound. Fibroblasts disappear as the wound becomes stronger. Fibroblast movement causes contraction of the healing area, which helps bring wound edges closer together. A mature scar is then formed. Initially the scar is pink or hypopigmented and elevated. With maturation, the scar becomes pale, does not tan when exposed to sunlight, will not sweat or produce hair, and may itch. The maturation process continues for years, the extent to which the scar remodels varies among individuals.

Types of Wound Healing

Children have a highly elastic skin quality. This quality, combined with the rapid healing process during the latency and puberty developmental growth periods, results in abundant scar tissue that pulls on wounds during the healing process. Healing of wounds takes place in one of three ways: by primary, secondary, or tertiary intention (Fig. 31.1). **Primary intention** healing takes place when all layers of the wound margins (skin, subcutaneous tissue, and muscle) are neatly approximated, as with a surgical incision. Unless infection interferes or the wound edges separate, these wounds heal with a minimum of scarring.

Repair by **secondary intention** takes place in wounds that occur from ulceration and lacerations in which the edges cannot be approximated, such as an avulsion or a third-degree burn. The inflammatory reaction may be greater, and the chance of infection is increased. Often debris, cells, and exudate must be cleaned away (debrided) before healing can take place. Healing takes place from the edges inward and from the bottom of the wound upward until the defect is filled. More granulation tissue and a larger scar are formed than in healing by primary intention.

Repair by **tertiary intention** takes place when suturing is delayed after injury or the wound later breaks down and is sutured or resutured when granulation is present. More granulation tissue is formed than in healing by primary intention, and there is a greater chance that microorganisms will invade the wound, resulting in a larger and deeper scar than healing by primary intention. Frequently, suturing of a contaminated wound is deliberately delayed to afford better removal of infection before closing.

Factors That Influence Healing

During the past decade, understanding of wound healing has revolutionized the interventions used to promote healing. Emphasis has shifted from interventions directed at maintaining a dry environment that promotes eschar formation to those that promote a moist, crust-free environment that enhances the migration of epithelial cells across the wound and facilitates resurfacing. An acute full-thickness wound kept in a moist environment usually reepithelializes in 12 to 15 days, whereas the same wound kept open to the air heals in approximately 25 to 30 days.

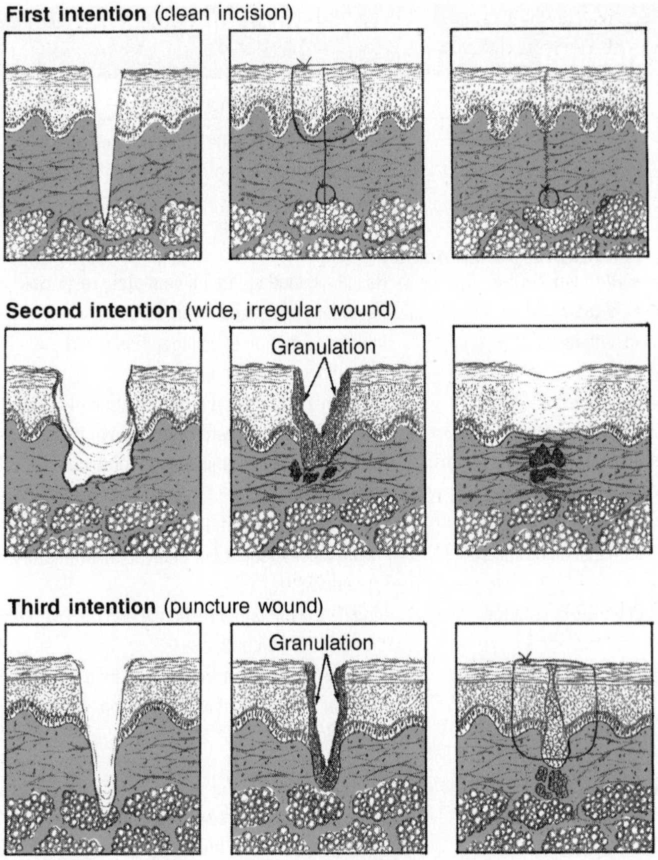

Fig. 31.1 Types of wound healing.

Eschar (thick, fibrin-containing necrotic tissue) also interferes with healing by preventing wound contraction. In most situations it is best to remove eschar and other dead tissue from the wound. Repeated application of occlusive dressings mobilizes the body's own enzymes to lyse the eschar, a process known as **autolysis**.

Adequate nutrition is essential for wound healing. In particular, sufficient protein, calories, vitamins C and D, and zinc are needed for healing of extensive wounds, such as burns. Supplemental nutrition is an integral aspect of treatment of severe wounds.

Numerous factors delay healing of the skin (Table 31.1). Some traditional practices are ineffective or even harmful; for example, antiseptics that were once used to help prevent infections (hydrogen peroxide and povidone-iodine [Betadine] solutions) are now known to have cytotoxic effects on healthy cells and minimal effect on controlling infections. Povidone-iodine may be absorbed through the skin in neonates and young children and must be used with caution in patients with thyroid or renal disease. Factors that delay wound healing, particularly in the home environment, include exposure to smoke or other allergens, dry or arid air, noncompliance or inconsistent adherence to the treatment regimen, and stress.

General Therapeutic Management

The human body intrinsically attempts to heal itself; therefore treatment is directed toward eliminating or ameliorating factors that interfere with normal healing processes. Some disorders may demand aggressive therapy, but by and large the major aim of any treatment is to prevent further damage, eliminate the cause, prevent complications, and provide relief from discomfort while tissues undergo healing. When possible, eliminate factors that contribute to the dermatitis and prolong the course of the disease. The most common offenders in

TABLE 31.1 Factors That Delay Wound Healing

Factor	Effect on Healing
Dry wound environment	Allows epithelial cells to dry out and die; impairs migration of epithelial cells across wound surface
Nutritional deficiencies	
• Vitamin A	Results in inadequate inflammatory response
• Vitamin B_1	Results in decreased collagen formation
• Vitamin C	Inhibits formation of collagen fibers and capillary development
• Vitamin D	Regulates growth and differentiation of cell types, inhibits hyperproliferation of cells
• Protein	Reduces supply of amino acids for tissue repair
• Zinc	Impairs epithelialization
Immunocompromised	Results in inadequate or delayed inflammatory response
Impaired circulation	Inhibits inflammatory response and removal of debris from wound area Reduces supply of nutrients to wound area
Stress (pain, poor sleep)	Releases catecholamines that cause vasoconstriction
Antiseptics	
• Hydrogen peroxide	Toxic to fibroblasts; can cause subcutaneous gas formation (mimics gas-forming infection)
• Povidone-iodine	Toxic to white and red blood cells and fibroblasts
• Chlorhexidine	Toxic to white blood cells
Medications	
• Corticosteroids	Impair phagocytosis Inhibit fibroblast proliferation Depress formation of granulation tissue Inhibit wound contraction
• Chemotherapy	Interrupts the cell cycle; damages DNA or prevents DNA repair
• Antiinflammatory drugs	Decrease the inflammatory phase
Foreign bodies	Increase inflammatory response Inhibit wound closure
Infection	Increases inflammatory response Increases tissue destruction
Mechanical friction	Damages or destroys granulation tissue
Fluid accumulation in area	Inhibits tissues from approximating
Radiation	Inhibits fibroblastic activity and capillary formation May cause tissue necrosis
Diseases	
• Diabetes mellitus	Inhibits collagen synthesis Impairs circulation and capillary growth Hyperglycemia impairs phagocytosis
• Anemia	Reduces oxygen supply to tissues
• Peripheral vascular disease	Reduces oxygen supply to wounds
• Uremia	Decreases collagen and granulation tissue

DNA, Deoxyribonucleic acid.

pediatrics are environmental factors, including soaps (bubble baths and shampoos) and lotions; garments that are made of synthetic materials, have a rough texture (wool), or are tight-fitting; prolonged exposure to damp undergarments or swimsuits; and natural elements (plants and insects, dirt, sand, heat, cold, moisture, and wind). Dermatitis can also be aggravated by home remedies, poor nutrition, exposure to smoke, scratching or physical irritation of the site, and medications.

Dressings

No one dressing meets the needs of all wounds. The traditional dry gauze dressing should not be used on open wounds because it allows the wound surface to dry, does little to prevent bacterial invasion, and adheres to the dried scab so that removal disturbs the newly regenerating epithelial cells. In most instances, traditional gauze dressings have been replaced by dressings that promote moist wound healing. Moist wound healing increases the rate of collagen synthesis and reepithelialization, and decreases pain and inflammation. It also creates an environment for autolytic debridement of necrotic tissue, which creates a clean wound bed and enhances granulation. However, a balance must be achieved between creating a moist wound bed and maintaining a dry periwound area that protects the skin and wound from maceration. The dressing type and frequency of dressing changes help achieve this balance. The frequency of dressing changes is based on the presence of infection, the type of dressing, the location of the wound, and the amount of drainage. Dressings should always be changed when they are loose or soiled. They should be changed more frequently in areas where contamination is likely (e.g., the sacral area, the buttocks, the tracheal area) or when wound infection is suspected or present.

Dressings serve the following functions: (1) provide a moist healing environment, (2) protect the wound from infection and trauma, (3) provide compression in the event of anticipated bleeding or swelling, (4) apply medication, (5) absorb drainage, (6) debride necrotic tissue, (7) reduce pain, and (8) control odor. To ensure a moist environment, cover wounds with an occlusive ointment or dressing (Table 31.2).

Occlusive dressings can be classified according to their degree of permeability. The term *occlusive* is synonymous with impermeable, *semiocclusive* is synonymous with semipermeable, and *nonocclusive* is synonymous with permeable. No one dressing meets the needs of all types of wounds. The traditional gauze dressing is a permeable dressing that reduces the moisture content in a wound by absorbing exudate and allowing it to evaporate. Dry gauze dressings have been replaced by new "active occlusive" dressings, which allow for moist wound healing rather than the traditional dry wound environment that created an increased risk for wound sepsis and trauma during removal. The use of silver-impregnated dressings for the treatment of wound care has reemerged. Although several studies suggest that silver decreases the bacteria and bioburden in the wound and improves short-term healing of wounds and ulcers, the long-term effects remain unclear. Due to the possibility of silver toxicity in children with silver-containing dressings, caution is strongly recommended when applying these dressings in the pediatric population (King, Stellar, Blevins, et al., 2014).

Topical Therapy

A variety of agents and methods are available for treatment of dermatologic problems. In selecting a therapeutic program, the practitioner considers (1) the active ingredient of the agent, (2) the vehicle or base, (3) the cosmetic effect, (4) the cost, (5) instructions for the agent's use, and (6) the family preference. Practitioners aim to avoid overtreatment, particularly in young children. For example, when the dermatitis is acute, short-term topical medications such as steroids are used to reduce irritation, inflammation, and spread of the disorder, then quickly tapered to mild

TABLE 31.2 Dressing Category Definitions and Examples of Products

Category	Description	Examples
Gauze or sponge for external use	Nonresorbable Sterile or nonsterile Strip, piece, or pad Woven or nonwoven mesh cotton cellulose Simple chemical derivatives of cellulose Intended for medical purposes	Pads Island dressings
Hydrophilic wound dressing	Sterile or nonsterile Nonresorbable Material with hydrophilic properties No added drugs or biologics Intended to cover wound and absorb exudate	Alginate dressings Foam dressings Hydropolymer dressings Sheet gel dressings Hydrocolloid dressings Composite dressings
Occlusive wound dressing	Sterile or nonsterile Nonresorbable Synthetic polymeric material with or without adhesive backing Intended to cover wound, provide or support moist wound environment, and allow exchange of gases	Transparent adhesive dressings Thin film dressings Foam dressings Hydrocolloid dressings Composite dressings Hydropolymer dressings
Hydrogel wound dressing	Sterile or nonsterile Nonresorbable Matrix of hydrophilic polymers or other material combined with at least 50% water Intended to cover wound; absorb wound exudates; control bleeding or fluid loss; and protect against abrasion, friction, desiccation, and contamination	Alginate dressings Hydropolymer dressings Hydrogel dressings Gauze dressing impregnated with hydrogel (without active ingredients)
Porcine wound dressing	Made from pigskin Temporary burn dressing	

or less frequent dosages to prevent side effects or long-term consequences. Chemicals that are nonirritating to intact skin (soaps and lotions) should be avoided because they can be quite irritating to inflamed or wounded skin, especially in children, whose skin is more absorbent.

Tepid or cool baths or the topical application of tepid or cool moist compresses may be used to treat the disorder, reduce the itching associated with many diseases, or decrease external stimuli. Baths are especially useful in the treatment of widespread dermatitis because they evenly distribute the soothing antipruritic and antiinflammatory solution, usually an oatmeal or mineral oil preparation. The temperature of the bathwater should be tepid, and the treatment usually lasts 15 to 30 minutes. Therapeutic baths are always more interesting for the child when toys are available in the tub for water play.

Topical agents are applied to skin lesions to ease discomfort, prevent further injury, and facilitate healing. The emollient action of ointments and allergen-free lotions provides a soothing film over the skin surface that reduces external stimuli. Most preparations are placed directly on the skin and left uncovered; some may be applied under an occlusive dressing. The occlusive dressing promotes moisture retention and decreases evaporation of the therapeutic preparation. A thin application of the ointment or cream is covered with plastic film and anchored with adhesive or covered with a commercial transparent dressing. Apply any topical applications in a systematic manner following the contour of the body surface (not simply up and down). Children love to be "painted," so lotion applications can be fun when an ordinary soft-bristle paintbrush is used. Regardless of the type of preparation used, parents need detailed information on the medication being applied, how to apply it, and how long the preparation should remain on the skin or under an occlusive dressing.

> **! NURSING ALERT**
>
> Application of heat tends to aggravate most conditions, and its use is generally reserved for reducing specific inflammatory processes, such as folliculitis and cellulitis.

Topical corticosteroid therapy. Glucocorticoids are the therapeutic agents used most frequently for skin disorders. Their local antiinflammatory effects are merely palliative, so the medication is applied until the condition undergoes a remission or the causative agent is eliminated. Corticosteroids are applied directly to the affected area, are essentially nonsensitizing, and have only minor side effects. As with the use of any steroids, their use in large amounts may mask signs of infection, and symptoms may be exacerbated after termination of the drug. Families are cautioned that the medication cannot be used for all skin disorders. The concentrations available without prescription are not adequate for stubborn skin conditions (e.g., psoriasis, eczema) and may further aggravate inflammation caused by fungus or bacteria. When appropriate, it is important to counsel parents to apply only a thin film and to massage it into the skin because most parents and children apply more topical hydrocortisone than necessary for effective treatment. Parents and children should also be advised to use the application for no more than 5 to 7 days because these agents may cause depigmentation and other changes in the skin with extended use.

Other topical therapies. Other topical treatments include chemical cautery (especially useful for warts), cryosurgery, electrodesiccation (chiefly used for warts, granulomas, and nevi), ultraviolet (UV) light therapy (primarily used in psoriasis and acne), laser therapy (especially for birthmarks), and special acne therapies such as dermabrasion and chemical peels. **Topical immunomodulators** are effective in reducing the itching of atopic dermatitis (eczema) and preventing flare-ups in children resistant to first-line treatment options. However, the US Food and Drug Administration issued a black box warning cautioning against the use of these topicals as first-line treatments in children younger than 2 years of age after chronic use of these medications was linked to possible skin cancer and lymphoma (Margolis, Abuabara, Hoffstad, et al., 2015). To date, no evidence has been published linking malignancy to the use of pimecrolimus cream (Elidel) in infants and children, but safety and efficacy are considered before using these medications in children (Margolis et al., 2015). Nonprescription and prescription topical antibiotics (lotions, gels, ointments, or creams) may also be used to treat minor wounds and acne. Again, families should be instructed to apply only a thin layer of medication at determined daily intervals for a limited number of days to the wound or affected area(s); each application of medication should be followed by careful hand washing.

! NURSING ALERT

Provide written instructions and demonstrate to parents the correct amount of topical medication to apply (e.g., size of a pea, thin film to cover). If more than one preparation is to be applied, mark the containers 1 and 2 to help parents remember the correct order for application to the skin. While educating children and their caregivers about medications, the nurse should emphasize that *more* medication or increased frequency of applications is *not better* when using topical medications and may carry the risk of being harmful, especially in the case of topical steroids.

Systemic Therapy

Systemic drugs may be used as an adjunct to topical therapy in some dermatologic disorders. The drugs most frequently used are corticosteroids, antibiotics, and antifungal agents. Corticosteroids are valuable in the treatment of severe skin disorders because of their capacity to inhibit inflammatory and allergic reactions. The dosage is carefully adjusted and gradually tapered to the minimum dosage that is effective and tolerated. Prolonged use of systematic corticosteroids may temporarily suppress the child's growth.

Antibiotics are used in cases of severe, chronic, or widespread skin infections. However, because these drugs tend to produce hypersensitivity in some patients, they are used with caution. Oral antifungal agents are the only effective means for treating systemic fungal infections and tinea capitus.

Nursing Care Management

To help establish a diagnosis, it is important for nurses to accurately describe any deviation in the character of the skin, using both inspection and palpation. Note the color, shape, size, character, and distribution of the lesions or wounds. Describe the individual lesions using the accepted terminology, understanding that there may be more than one type of wound, lesion, or rash. Assess wounds for depth of tissue damage, evidence of healing, and signs of infection (e.g., drainage, warmth, odor).

To confirm or amplify the assessment findings made by inspection, gently palpate the skin to detect characteristics such as temperature, moisture, texture, elasticity, and the presence of edema. Indicate whether the findings are restricted to the area of the lesion(s) or are generalized.

! NURSING ALERT

Signs of wound infection include the following:
- Increased erythema, especially beyond wound margin
- Edema
- Purulent exudate
- Odor
- Pain at the site or extending beyond the wound margin
- Increased temperature

A detailed history of the child's presenting illness, condition, or wound and the description (or appearance) of symptoms provide additional information. Older children may be able to tell you precipitating factors they may have been exposed to, timing of the disorder, and treatments they have already tried. They are also usually able to describe the condition as painful, itching, or tingling or use other descriptive terms and associated symptoms related to the condition. In younger children, the nurse can determine much by noting behavior during the intake interview and the caregivers' account of the symptoms or illness and the reaction to any home treatments. Besides asking about medical history and noting the allergy and medication list of the patient, a careful nursing history may provide clues that will assist in determining an uncertain diagnosis. During the interview process, the nurse should ask the following questions:

- How long has this been occurring?
- Is the child scratching the area?
- Is the child restless or irritable?
- Does the child favor or avoid using a certain body part?
- Has the child had a fever or other illnesses recently?
- Has the child been around chemicals, woodlands, gardens, or woodpiles?
- Has the child traveled recently or visited someone's home for the first time?
- Has the child recently eaten a new food?
- Do any classmates, playmates, or siblings have similar lesions or illnesses?
- What has been done to treat the symptoms so far? Have any medications or home remedies been used?

Therapeutic treatments of skin disorders are typically aimed at providing comfort measures: rest, protection from infection or spread of the condition, and relief of discomfort. Specific treatments, such as a definitive medication or physical treatment or technique, may be prescribed for chronic conditions or wounds. Only a few skin disorders are contagious, so it is usually not necessary to isolate the affected child unless there is a danger that the child may acquire a secondary infection (e.g., the child who is receiving large doses of corticosteroids or other immunosuppressant drugs or the child with an immunologic deficiency disorder). However, when the skin manifestation is a viral exanthem such as chickenpox or an easily spread vector such as lice, the recommendation is to prevent exposing other susceptible children until the disorder is almost healed or the treatment is complete.

Wound Care

Parents can generally manage small skin wounds at home. Instruct parents to wash their hands and then wash the wound gently with mild soap and water. Topical antibiotics and nonadherent dressings are usually applied to the wound while it is in the primary healing stage. Caution parents to avoid povidone-iodine, alcohol, and hydrogen peroxide because these products are toxic to wounds. Wounds covering a very large area (>15% of the body) need medical attention with the child undergoing conscious sedation and analgesia.

! NURSING ALERT

Do not put anything in a wound that you would not put in the eye. The safest solution is normal saline.

Open wounds are typically covered with a nonadherent dressing, such as a commercial adhesive bandage, although larger wounds may benefit from the use of occlusive dressings. If occlusive dressings are applied, instruct parents on their correct application and removal. For example, hydrocolloid dressings adhere best if a wide margin is left around the wound and the dressing is pressed against intact skin until it adheres. The edges of the dressing can be secured to the healthy skin margins with waterproof tape. The dressings are removed if leakage occurs or after specific time intervals, usually for a period of 7 days.

! NURSING ALERT

Advise parents that the yellow gel forming under hydrocolloid dressings may look like pus and has a distinct odor (somewhat fruity) but is normal leakage.

Dressings are removed carefully to protect intact skin and the epithelial surface of the wound. If the affected skin has significant hair growth, the nurse may consider removing a small patch or strip of hair surrounding the wound to improve dressing adherence and decrease discomfort for the child during dressing changes. When removing transparent or hydrocolloid dressings, the nurse or parent raises one edge of the dressing and pulls *parallel* to the skin to loosen the adhesive. The child may assist the nurse or caregiver in the dressing change procedure by firmly holding the skin taut as the adhesive dressing is removed. If a dressing sticks to the wound base when it is being removed, saturate the dressing with normal saline or clean water to loosen it and then proceed with care. Another useful technique for applying dressings to wounds is "picture-framing." The wound is "framed" on all sides with the application of a skin barrier dressing that stays in place around the wound (e.g., DuoDERM, Coloplast). This technique protects the healthy skin from injury during repeated dressing changes because the adhesive can be secured to the skin barrier surrounding the wound rather than directly to the skin. Lacerations present a special challenge with cleaning and dressing. The injured child and family are usually distressed by the bleeding associated with the wound and may be experiencing variable degrees of anxiety, fear, and shock. Because scalp and facial lacerations tend to bleed profusely, they are especially frightening. The initial nursing intervention is to calmly apply direct pressure to the area and to attempt to calm the child before further examination. Unless there is bleeding from a severed artery, the wound is cleansed with a forced stream of sterile tepid water or normal saline (via syringe). The wound is then examined for extent and depth of injury and presence of foreign material such as dirt, glass, or fabric fragments. Before suturing lacerations or wounds, a topical anesthetic or intradermal buffered lidocaine should be used to reduce discomfort and promote cooperation of the child during the procedure.

The location of the wound dictates careful physical assessment. For example, wounds over bony areas may contain bone chips, and clear fluid seeping from severe head wounds may indicate cerebrospinal fluid. For severe wounds that cannot be completely evaluated immediately and lacerations that require suturing, apply a clean pressure dressing over the affected area and transfer the child for emergency medical care. Puncture wounds should initially be irrigated with sterile saline and then soaked in a basin of warm soapy water for several minutes before applying a clean dressing. Causing the puncture wound to rebleed may be indicated to ensure that no foreign body is embedded in the wound. Puncture wounds of the head, chest, or abdomen, or those that could still contain a portion of the puncturing object must be evaluated further by a practitioner and may require an x-ray to confirm that all foreign material has been removed from the wound. Caution parents against opening ("popping") wounds, blisters, or vesicles, or kissing a wound "to make it better." The skin can easily become contaminated from germs in the human mouth. If scabs form, they are allowed to slough off without assistance; picking or early removal may cause scarring and secondary infection. Advise parents to seek medical help if there is evidence of infection.

Relief of Symptoms

Most of the therapeutic regimens are intended to promote wound healing, prevent infection, and provide relief of pruritus, the most common subjective complaint. Preventing scratching is of primary importance. Itching is believed to often result from stimulation of C fibers at the dermoepidermal junction and the release of histamine and endopeptidases. These fibers are similar to but distinct from pain fibers and may be stimulated with a single scratch. Cooling the affected area and increasing the skin pH with an alkaline-containing compress, such as a baking soda or Burow solution, or a tepid bath reduce the child's external stimuli and the urge to scratch. Older children usually can avoid self-contaminating the wound, though they may occasionally need to be reminded to stop scratching or rubbing. In younger and uncooperative children, techniques and devices such as mittens (especially during sleep) or special hand coverings are required. Keeping fingernails short and clean helps reduce scratching and the chance of secondary infection of the wound. Clothing and bed linens should be soft, smooth, lightweight, and made of natural fibers to decrease the irritation from friction and stimulation. Antipruritic medications such as diphenhydramine (Benadryl) or hydroxyzine (Atarax) may be prescribed for severe itching, especially if it disrupts the child's sleep.

Wet compresses or dressings cool the skin by evaporation, relieve itching and inflammation, and cleanse the area by loosening and removing crusts and debris. A variety of ingredients, such as plain water or Burow solution (available without a prescription), can be applied on Kerlix gauze; plain gauze; or (preferably) soft cotton cloths such as freshly laundered towels, bed sheets, or pillowcases.

Pain and discomfort are usually managed with nonpharmacologic measures such as positioning and rest, distraction techniques, and individual preferences of comfort. Occlusive dressings applied over wounds reduce pain similar to cool or tepid compresses. Doses of mild analgesics such as acetaminophen or ibuprofen, prescribed based on the patient's weight, may be recommended. Severe pain requires prescribed analgesic medication and careful nursing assessment for infection or an underlying cause of discomfort. For severe wounds and burns, prescribed analgesic medications should be administered before each dressing change, debridement procedure, or cleansing, allowing adequate time for the medicine to take therapeutic effect (see Chapter 5, Pain Management).

Wound healing may be facilitated by recombinant growth factor or a vacuum-assisted closure device. These therapies may be used when wounds are large and in a location that creates challenges for therapy (e.g., sacral or groin wound) or when the child has associated conditions such as malnutrition or a comprised immune system, putting "normal" wound healing at risk. Recombinant growth factors are human platelet–derived growth factors that are engineered outside the body. They foster the formation of new granulation tissue by stimulating the migration of fibroblasts, macrophages, smooth muscle cells, and capillary endothelial cells to the wound site.

The vacuum-assisted closure (VAC) device uses a technique that involves placing a foam dressing into the wound, covering it with an occlusive dressing, and applying gentle, continuous suction. The negative pressure of the suction is applied from the foam dressing to the wound surfaces. The mechanical force removes excess fluids from the wound, stimulates formation of granulation tissue, restores capillary flow, and fosters closure of the wound. VAC has been used to prepare wounds for a skin graft and to treat surgical wounds, burns, and pressure ulcers (Han & Ceilley, 2017). The safety and efficacy of the VAC technique for infants and children has been documented in recent studies (Koehler, Jinbo, Johnson, et al., 2014; Satteson, Crantford, Wood, et al., 2015; Takahara, Sai, Kagatani, et al., 2014).

Home Care and Family Support

Care of a child with a dermatologic condition always involves the family, but few situations require hospitalization, and most care is delivered at home. Because the family members must carry out the treatment plan, their cooperation is essential. Regimens that are routine for health care professionals to accomplish in the clinic, hospital, or primary care provider's office may be frustrating and baffling for caregivers in the home. The family may also need assistance in adapting equipment available for home therapy.

It is important that the child and family be given as detailed explanations as possible about both the expected and the unexpected results of treatment, including any side effects that might occur. If unexplained reactions develop, direct the family to discontinue treatment and report the reactions to the appropriate person. Discourage the use of over-the-counter medicines and homeopathic treatments unless the preparations have been discussed with the health care provider and have received approval.

Because the skin is the most visible portion of the body, defects in its surface alter its appearance and cause distress for the child. Skin problems may also result in rejection by others. Parents of other children may fear that their children will "catch" the disorder. Occasionally, the affected child's own family members reduce their interaction or physical contact with the child, especially close physical contact, or demonstrate distaste for the condition, which the child may interpret as rejection or punishment. This is seldom a concern for children with dermatitis of short duration, but chronic conditions can frequently create problems and affect the child's self-esteem.

INFECTIONS OF THE SKIN

BACTERIAL INFECTIONS

Normally, the skin harbors a variety of bacterial flora, including the major pathogenic varieties of staphylococci and streptococci. The degree of pathogenicity of the organism depends on its invasiveness and toxicity, the integrity of the skin (the host's barrier), and the host's immune and cellular defenses. Children with congenital or acquired immunodeficiency disorders (e.g., acquired immune deficiency syndrome [AIDS]), children receiving immunosuppressant therapy, and those with a malignancy such as leukemia or lymphoma are at risk for developing bacterial infections.

Because of the characteristic "walling-off" process of the inflammatory reaction (abscess formation), staphylococci are more difficult to treat, and the local infected area is associated with an increase in bacteria all over the skin surface that serves as a source of continuing infection. Since the early 2000s, the number of methicillin-resistant *Staphylococcus aureus* (MRSA) community-acquired infections rose dramatically until reaching a peak in 2007 and then steadily declined (Kaplan, 2016). These factors underline the importance of careful hand washing and cleanliness when caring for infected children and their lesions to prevent the spread of infection and as an essential prophylactic measure when caring for infants and small children. Common bacterial skin disorders are outlined in Table 31.3 (Figs. 31.2 and 31.3).

Nursing Care Management

The major nursing functions related to bacterial skin infections are to prevent the spread of infection and to prevent complications. Impetigo contagiosa and MRSA infection can easily spread by self-inoculation; therefore caution the child against touching the involved area. Hand washing is mandatory before and after contact with an affected child. Also emphasize hand washing to both the child and the family. Many children with atopic dermatitis are colonized with MRSA (Chaptini, Quinn, & Marshman, 2016). For many bacterial infections, and for MRSA infection in particular, the child should be provided with washcloths and towels separate from those of other family members. The child's clothes should be changed daily and washed in hot water. Razors used for shaving should be discarded after each use and not shared. To prevent recurrence, some infectious disease specialists recommend bathing in a chlorine bath daily for 5 to 14 days, although evidence of the effectiveness is inconclusive (Gupta, Lyons, & Rosen, 2015; Kaplan, Forbes, Hammerman, et al., 2014). For the chlorine bathing, 1 teaspoon of bleach is diluted in 13 gallons of water or ¼ cup of bleach is diluted in a standard 50-gallon tub one-fourth filled with water (Gupta et al., 2015). In addition, mupirocin can be applied to the nares of patients and families twice daily for 5 to 10 days to prevent reinfection (Gupta et al., 2015).

Children and parents are often tempted to squeeze follicular lesions. They must be warned that squeezing will not hasten the resolution of the infection and that there is a risk of making the lesion worse or spreading the infection. No attempt should be made to puncture the surface of the pustule with a needle or sharp instrument. A child with a sty may waken with the eyelids of the affected eye sealed shut with exudate. The child or the parents are instructed to gently wipe the eyelid from the inner to the outer edge with warm water and a clean washcloth until the exudate is removed.

The child with limited cellulitis of an extremity is usually managed at home on a regimen of oral antibiotics and warm compresses. The parents are taught the procedures and instructed in administration of the medication. Children with more extensive cellulitis, especially around a joint with lymphadenitis or on the face, are usually admitted to the hospital for parenteral antibiotics with continued treatment at home. Nurses are responsible for teaching the family to administer the medication and apply compresses.

VIRAL INFECTIONS

Viruses are intracellular parasites that produce their effect by using the intracellular substances of the host cells. Composed of only a deoxyribonucleic acid (DNA) or ribonucleic acid (RNA) core enclosed in an antigenic protein shell, viruses are unable to provide for their own metabolic needs or to reproduce themselves. After a virus penetrates a cell of the host organism, it sheds the outer shell and disappears within the cell, where the nucleic acid core stimulates the host cell to form more virus material from its intracellular substance. In a viral infection, the epidermal cells react with

TABLE 31.3 Bacterial Infections

Disorder and Organism	Manifestations	Management	Comments
Impetigo contagiosa—*Staphylococcus* (see Fig. 31.2)	Begins as a reddish macule Becomes vesicular Ruptures easily, leaving superficial, moist erosion Tends to spread peripherally in sharply marginated irregular outlines Exudate dries to form heavy, honey-colored crusts Pruritus common Systemic effects—Minimal or asymptomatic	Topical bactericidal ointment mupirocin or triple antibiotic ointment Oral or parenteral antibiotics (penicillin) in severe or extensive lesions Vancomycin for MRSA	Tends to heal without scarring unless secondary infection Autoinoculable and contagious Common in toddlers and preschoolers May be superimposed on eczema
Pyoderma—*Staphylococcus, Streptococcus*	Deeper extension of infection into dermis Tissue reaction more severe Systemic effects—Fever, lymphangitis, sepsis, liver disease, heart disease	Soap and water cleansing Topical antiseptic, such as chlorhexidine Mupirocin Antibiotics depending on causative organism: Cephalexin, nafcillin, intramuscular benzathine penicillin Bathing with antibacterial soap as prescribed Do not share washcloths or towels	Autoinoculable and contagious May heal with or without scarring
Folliculitis (pimple), furuncle (boil), carbuncle (multiple boils)—*Staphylococcus aureus*, MRSA	Folliculitis—Infection of hair follicle Furuncle—Larger lesion with more redness and swelling at a single follicle Carbuncle—More extensive lesion with widespread inflammation and "pointing" at several follicular orifices Systemic effects—Malaise if severe	Skin cleanliness Local warm, moist compresses Topical application of antibiotic agents Systemic antibiotics in severe cases Incision and drainage of severe lesions, followed by wound irrigations with antibiotics or suitable drain implantation MRSA infections: • 5-inch soak of ½ cup bleach diluted in a standard 50-gallon tub one-fourth filled with water once or twice weekly • No sharing of towels or washcloths, changing of clothes and underwear daily, and laundering in hot water • Disposal of razors after one use • Application of mupirocin to nares bid for 2-4 wk	Autoinoculable and contagious Furuncle and carbuncle tend to heal with scar formation Lesions should never be squeezed
Cellulitis—*Streptococcus, Staphylococcus, Haemophilus influenzae* (see Fig. 31.3)	Inflammation of skin and subcutaneous tissues with intense redness, swelling, and firm infiltration Lymphangitis "streaking" frequently seen Involvement of regional lymph nodes common May progress to abscess formation Systemic effects—Fever, malaise	Oral or parenteral antibiotics Rest and immobilization of both affected area and child	Hospitalization may be necessary for child with systemic symptoms Otitis media may be associated with facial cellulites
Staphylococcal scalded skin syndrome—*S. aureus*	Macular erythema with "sandpaper" texture of involved skin Epidermis becomes wrinkled (in days or less), and large bullae appear Localized bullous impetigo in older child	Systemic antibiotics Gentle cleansing with saline, Burow solution, or 0.25% silver nitrate compresses	Infants subject to fluid loss; impaired body temperature regulation; and secondary infection, such as pneumonia, cellulitis, and septicemia Heals without scarring

bid, Two times daily; *MRSA*, methicillin-resistant *Staphylococcus aureus*.

inflammation and vesiculation (as in herpes simplex) or by proliferating to form growths (warts).

Many of the communicable viral diseases of childhood are associated with rashes, and each rash is characteristic. The type of lesion and the configuration of rubeola, rubella, and chickenpox are described in Chapter 6, Table 6.3. Other common viral disorders of the skin are outlined in Table 31.4.

Dermatophytoses (Fungal Infections)

The dermatophytoses (ringworm) are infections caused by a group of closely related filamentous fungi that invade primarily the stratum corneum, hair, and nails. These are superficial infections by organisms that live on, not in, the skin. Dermatophytoses are designated by the Latin word *tinea*, with further designation relating to the area of the

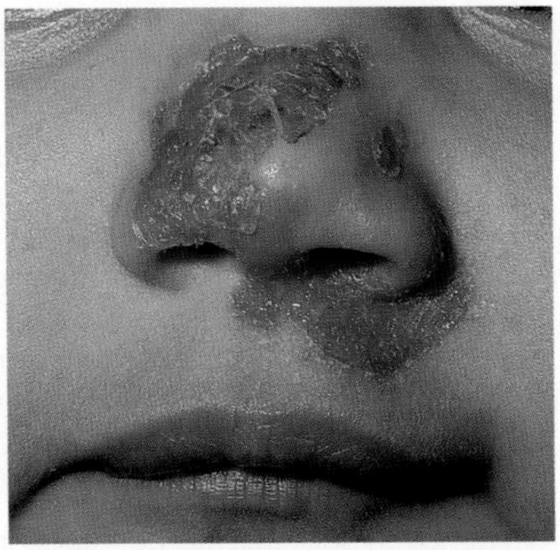

Fig. 31.2 Impetigo contagiosa. (From Weston, W. L., & Lane, A. T. [2007]. *Color textbook of pediatric dermatology* [4th ed.]. St. Louis, MO: Mosby.)

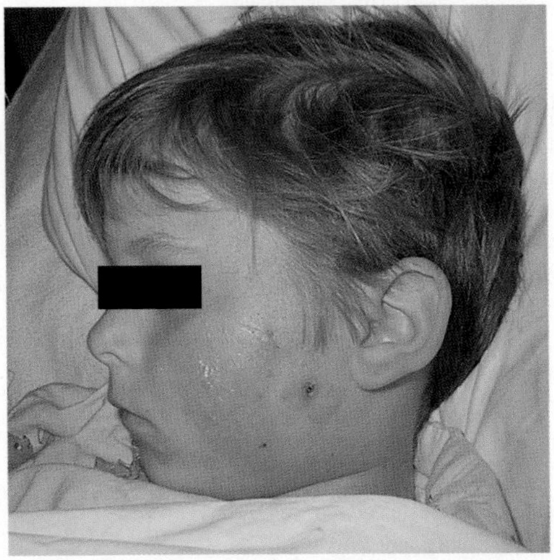

Fig. 31.3 Cellulitis of cheek from a puncture wound. (From Weston, W. L., & Lane, A. T. [2007]. *Color textbook of pediatric dermatology* [4th ed.]. St. Louis, MO: Mosby.)

body where they are found (e.g., tinea capitis [ringworm of the scalp]). Table 31.5 outlines common dermatophytoses (Fig. 31.4).

Dermatophyte infections are most often transmitted from one person to another or from infected animals to humans. Because the keratin is desquamated constantly, the fungus must multiply at a rate that equals the rate of keratin production to maintain itself; otherwise the infection would be shed with the discarded skin cells. Diagnosis is made from microscopic examination of scrapings taken from the advancing periphery of the lesion, which almost always produces a scale.

Nursing Care Management

When teaching families how to care for ringworm, the nurse should emphasize good health and hygiene. Because of the infectious nature of the disease, affected children should not exchange grooming items, headgear, scarves, or other articles of apparel that have been in proximity to the infected area with other children. Affected children are provided with their own towels and directed to wear a protective cap at night to avoid transmitting the fungus to bedding, especially if they sleep with another person. Because the infection can be acquired by animal-to-human transmission, all household pets should be examined for the disorder. Other sources of infection are seats in locker rooms, tanning beds, seats in public transportation vehicles, helmets, and gymnasium mats.

Both 2% ketoconazole and 1% selenium sulfide shampoos may reduce colony counts of dermatophytes. These shampoos can be used in combination with oral therapy to reduce the transmission of disease to others. The shampoo should be applied to the scalp for 5 to 10 minutes at least three times per week. The child may return to school after the therapy is initiated.

Alternatively, if the child is treated with the drug griseofulvin, the therapy frequently continues for weeks or months, and because subjective symptoms subside, children or parents may be tempted to decrease or discontinue the drug. The nurse should emphasize to family members the importance of maintaining the prescribed dosage schedule and of taking the medication with high-fat foods for best absorption. They are also instructed on possible drug side effects, such as headache, gastrointestinal upset, fatigue, insomnia, and photosensitivity. For children who take the drug over many months, periodic testing is required to monitor leukopenia and assess liver and renal function. Other antifungal medications such as terbinafine, itraconazole, and fluconazole can be used.

SYSTEMIC MYCOTIC (FUNGAL) INFECTIONS

Mycotic (systemic or deep fungal) infections have the capacity to invade the viscera, as well as the skin. The most common infections are the lung diseases, which are usually acquired by inhalation of fungal spores. These fungi produce a variable spectrum of disease, and some are common in certain geographic areas. They are not transmitted from person to person but appear to reside in the soil, from which their spores are airborne. The cutaneous lesions caused by deep fungal infections are granulomatous and appear as ulcers, plaques, nodules, fungating masses, and abscesses. The course of deep fungal diseases is chronic with slow progression that favors sensitization (Table 31.6).

SKIN DISORDERS RELATED TO CHEMICAL OR PHYSICAL CONTACTS

CONTACT DERMATITIS

Contact dermatitis is an inflammatory reaction of the skin to chemical substances, natural or synthetic, that evoke a hypersensitivity response or direct irritation. The initial reaction occurs in an exposed region, most commonly the face and neck, backs of the hands, forearms, male genitalia, and lower legs. There is characteristically a sharp demarcation between inflamed and normal skin that ranges from a faint, transient erythema to massive bullae on an erythematous swollen base. Itching is a constant symptom.

The cause may be a primary irritant or a sensitizing agent. A **primary irritant** is one that irritates any skin. A **sensitizing agent** produces an irritation on those individuals who have encountered the irritant or something chemically related to it, have undergone an immunologic change, and have become sensitized. Prior exposure is not necessarily a factor in the reaction. A sensitizer irritates in relatively low concentrations only persons who are allergic to it.

The major goal in treatment is to prevent further exposure of the skin to the offending substance. Provided there is no further irritation, the skin's normal recuperative powers will often produce healing without treatment. The most frequent offenders are plant (poison ivy, oak, or sumac), animal (wool, feathers, and furs), and metal irritants (nickel found in jewelry and the snaps on sleepers and denim). In infants, contact dermatitis occurs on the convex surfaces of the diaper area. Other agents that produce contact dermatitis include vegetable irritants (oleoresins, oils, and turpentine), synthetic fabrics (e.g., shoe components), dyes, cosmetics, perfumes, and soaps (including bubble baths).

TABLE 31.4 **Viral Infections**

Infection	Manifestations	Management	Comments
Verruca (warts) Cause—Human papillomavirus (various types)	Usually well-circumscribed, gray or brown, elevated, firm papules with a roughened, finely papillomatous texture Occur anywhere but usually appear on exposed areas such as fingers, hands, face, and soles May be single or multiple Asymptomatic	Not uniformly successful Local destructive therapy, individualized according to location, type, and number—surgical removal, electrocautery, curettage, cryotherapy (liquid nitrogen), caustic solutions (lactic acid and salicylic acid in flexible collodion, retinoic acid, salicylic acid plasters), laser ablation	Common in children Tend to disappear spontaneously Course unpredictable Most destructive techniques tend to leave scars Autoinoculable Repeated irritation will cause to enlarge
Verruca plantaris (plantar wart)	Located on plantar surface of feet and, because of pressure, are practically flat; may be surrounded by a collar of hyperkeratosis	Caustic chemical solution applied to wart and wear foam insole with hole cut to relieve pressure on wart; soak 20 min after 2-3 days; repeat until wart comes out	Destructive techniques tend to leave scars, which may cause problems with walking
Herpes simplex virus Type I (cold sore, fever blister) Type II (genital)	Grouped, burning, and itching vesicles on inflammatory base, usually on or near mucocutaneous junctions (lips, nose, genitalia, buttocks) Vesicles dry, forming a crust followed by exfoliation and spontaneous healing in 8-10 days May be accompanied by regional lymphadenopathy	Avoidance of secondary infection Burow solution compresses during weeping stages Oral antiviral (acyclovir [Zovirax]) for initial infection or to reduce severity in recurrence; may also be given prophylactically for recurrent Valacyclovir (Valtrex), an oral antiviral, used for episodic treatment of recurrent genital herpes; reduces pain, stops viral shedding, and has a more convenient administration schedule than acyclovir; primarily recommended for immunocompromised patients	Heal without scarring unless secondary infection Type I cold sores prevented by using sunscreens protecting against ultraviolet A and ultraviolet B light to prevent lip blisters Aggravated by corticosteroids Positive psychologic effect from treatment May be fatal in children with depressed immunity
Varicella-zoster virus (herpes zoster; shingles)	Caused by same virus that causes varicella (chickenpox) Virus has affinity for posterior root ganglia, posterior horn of spinal cord, and skin; crops of vesicles usually confined to dermatome following along course of affected nerve Usually preceded by neuralgic pain (rare in children), hyperesthesias, or itching May be accompanied by constitutional symptoms	Symptomatic Analgesics for pain Drying lotions sometimes helpful Ophthalmic variety: systemic corticotropin (adrenocorticotropic hormone) or corticosteroids Acyclovir or valacyclovir Preventive vaccine is available for persons >50 years old	Pain in children usually minimal Postherpetic pain does not occur in children Chickenpox may follow exposure; isolate affected child from other children in a hospital or school May occur in children with depressed immunity; can be fatal
Molluscum contagiosum Cause—Pox virus	Flesh-colored papules (1-20) with a central caseous plug (umbilicated) that occur on trunk, face and extremities; may be transmitted by sexual contact Usually asymptomatic	Cases in well children resolve spontaneously in about 18 months Treatment reserved for cosmetic purposes; alleviate discomfort; reduce autoinoculation; prevent secondary infection Numerous chemical removing agents, including tretinoin gel 0.01% or cantharidin (Cantharone) liquid; podophyllin; imiquimod cream These are painful treatments: Use local anesthesia Curettage, electrodessication, or cryotherapy	Common in school-age children Spread by skin-to-skin contact, including autoinoculation and fomite-to-skin contact Outbreaks in child care centers have been reported

Nursing Care Management

Nurses frequently detect evidence of contact dermatitis during routine physical assessments. Skin manifestations in specific areas suggest limited contact, such as around the eyes (mascara), areas of the body covered by clothing but not protected by undergarments (wool), or areas of the body not covered by clothing (UV injury). Generalized involvement is more likely to be caused by bubble bath, laundry soap, body soap, or lotion. Often nurses can determine the offending agent and counsel families on management. If the lesions persist, are extensive, or show evidence of infection, medical evaluation is indicated.

POISON IVY, OAK, AND SUMAC

Contact with the dry or succulent portions of any of three poisonous plants (ivy, oak, and sumac) produces localized, streaked or spotty, oozing, and painful impetiginous lesions that are often highly urticarial. The offending substance in these plants is an oil, **urushiol**, which is extremely potent. Sensitivity to urushiol is not inborn but is developed after one or two exposures and may change over a lifetime. All parts of the plants, including dried leaves and stems, contain the oil (Fig. 31.5A). Even smoke from burning brush piles can produce a reaction.

Animals do not seem to be affected by the oil; however, dogs or other animals that have run or played in the plants may carry the sap

TABLE 31.5 Dermatophytoses (Fungal Infections)

Disease and Organism	Manifestations	Management	Comments
Tinea capitis—*Trichophyton tonsurans, Microsporum audouinii, Microsporum canis* (see Fig. 31.4A)	Lesions in scalp but may extend to hairline or neck Characteristic configuration of scaly, circumscribed patches or patchy, scaling areas of alopecia Generally asymptomatic but severe, deep inflammatory reaction may occur that manifests as boggy, encrusted lesions (kerions) Pruritic Diagnosis: Microscopic examination of scales	Oral griseofulvin or terbinafine Oral ketoconazole for difficult cases Selenium sulfide shampoos, used twice a week, may decrease infection and fungal shedding (American Academy of Pediatrics, 2018) Kerion: Griseofulvin and possibly oral corticosteroids for 2 wk to achieve therapeutic effect (American Academy of Pediatrics, 2018)	Person-to-person transmission Animal-to-person transmission Rarely, permanent loss of hair *audouinii* transmitted from one human to another directly or from personal items; *M. canis* usually contracted from household pets, especially cats Atopic individuals more susceptible
Tinea corporis—*Trichophyton rubrum, Trichophyton mentagrophytes, M. canis, Epidermophyton* (see Fig. 31.4B)	Generally round or oval, erythematous scaling patch that spreads peripherally and clears centrally; may involve nails (tinea unguium) Diagnosis—Direct microscopic examination of scales Usually unilateral	Oral griseofulvin Local application of antifungal preparation such as tolnaftate, naftifine, miconazole, terbinafine, clotrimazole; applied 2.5 cm (1 inch) beyond periphery of lesion; application continued 1-2 wk after no sign of lesion Topical antifungals with high-potency steroids are not recommended as they may lead to further infection and have local and systemic side effects (American Academy of Pediatrics, 2018)	Usually of animal origin from infected pets but may occur from human transmission, soil, or fomites Majority of infections in children caused by *M. canis* and *M. audouinii* Tinea gladiatorum is commonly seen in wrestlers
Tinea cruris ("jock itch")—*Epidermophyton floccosum, T. rubrum, T. mentagrophytes*	Skin response similar to tinea corporis Localized to medial proximal aspect of thigh and crural fold; may involve scrotum in males Pruritic Diagnosis—Same as for tinea corporis	Local application of tolnaftate liquid, terbinafine, clotrimazole, ciclopirox twice daily for 2-4 wk	Rare in preadolescent children Health education on transmission via person-to-person (direct or indirect) Occurs in close association with tinea pedis and tinea unguium
Tinea pedis ("athlete's foot")—*T. rubrum, Trichophyton interdigitale, E. floccosum* Tinea unguium: Nail infection	On intertriginous areas between toes or on plantar surface of feet Lesions vary: Maceration and fissuring between toes Patches with pinhead-size vesicles on plantar surface Pruritic Diagnosis—Direct microscopic examination of scrapings	Local applications of terbinafine, ciclopirox or clotrimazole, or miconazole, or ketoconazole Oral itraconazole, terbinafine, or griseofulvin for severe infections or those that do not respond to topical acute infections—Compresses or soaks with Burow solution (1:80) (American Academy of Pediatrics, 2018) Elimination of conditions of heat and perspiration by use of clean, light socks and well-ventilated shoes; avoidance of occlusive shoes	Most frequent in adolescents and adults; rare in children, but occurrence increases with wearing of plastic shoes Common in locations such as showers, locker rooms, and swimming pools where fungi proliferate
Candidiasis (moniliasis)—*Candida albicans*	Grows in chronically moist areas Inflamed areas with white exudate, peeling, and easy bleeding Pruritic Diagnosis—Characteristic appearance; microscopic identification of scrapings; candidemia diagnosed from cultures (blood, cerebrospinal fluid, bone marrow); tissue biopsy Chronic or recurrent often seen with HIV infection and immunocompromised child	Neonatal thrush, oral nystatin Older children, clotrimazole troches applied to lesions (American Academy of Pediatrics, 2018) Fluconazole or itraconazole for immunocompromised Esophagitis: Treat with oral or IV fluconazole or itraconazole; IV amphotericin, voriconazole, micafungin Treat skin lesions with topical nystatin, miconazole, clotrimazole, ketoconazole, econazole, or ciclopirox (American Academy of Pediatrics, 2018) Vulvovaginal: Clotrimazole, miconazole, butoconazole, terconazole, and tioconazole used topically (American Academy of Pediatrics, 2018)	Common form of diaper dermatitis (see Fig. 31.10) Oral form common in infants (see Chapter 8) Vaginal form in females Disseminated disease in very low birth weight infants and immunosuppressed children

HIV, Human immunodeficiency virus; *IV*, intravenous.

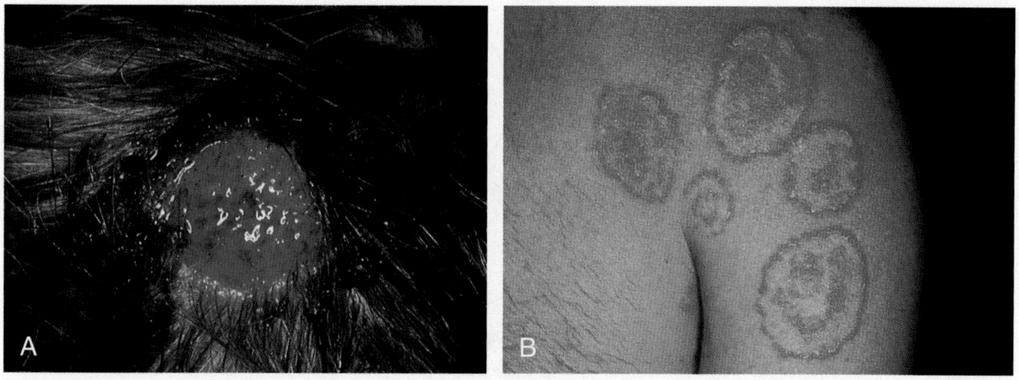

Fig. 31.4 **A,** Tinea capitis. **B,** Tinea corporis. Both infections are caused by *Microsporum canis,* the "kitten" or "puppy" fungus. (From Habif, T. P. [2004]. Clinical dermatology: *A color guide to diagnosis and therapy* [4th ed.]. St. Louis, MO: Mosby.)

TABLE 31.6 Systemic Mycoses

Disorder and Organism	Skin Manifestations	Systemic Manifestations	Management	Comments
North American blastomycosis—*Blastomyces dermatitidis*	Chronic granulomatous lesions and microabscesses in any part of body Initial lesion is a papule; undergoes ulceration and peripheral spread	Pulmonary symptoms, such as cough, fever, chest pain, weakness, and weight loss; rarely develop ARDS Possible skeletal involvement, with bone destruction and formation of cutaneous abscesses	IV amphotericin B Oral fluconazole or itraconazole for mild or moderate cases after amphotericin B (American Academy of Pediatrics, 2018)	Usual portal of entry is lungs Source of infection unknown Pulmonary infections may be mild and self-limiting and require no treatment Progressive disease often fatal
Cryptococcosis—*Cryptococcus neoformans* (*Torula histolytica*)	Usually on face; acneiform, firm, nodular, painless eruption	CNS manifestations—Headache, dizziness, stiff neck, and signs of increased intracranial pressure Low-grade fever, mild cough, lung infiltration	IV amphotericin B; may be administered intrathecal for CNS involvement Oral flucytosine then fluconazole for meningitis Excision and drainage of local lesions	Acquired by inhalation of contaminated soil (bird feces) Endemic in Mississippi and Ohio River valleys Increased incidence in persons with defects in T lymphocyte–mediated immunity (HIV, leukemia, systemic lupus, AIDS, or organ transplant) No person-to-person transmission
Histoplasmosis—*Histoplasma capsulatum*	Not distinctive or uniform but most appear as punched-out or granulomatous ulcers Erythema nodosum in adolescents	General systemic symptoms may include pallor, diarrhea, vomiting, irregular spiking temperature, hepatosplenomegaly, and pulmonary symptoms Any tissue of body may be involved with related symptoms	IV amphotericin B for severe cases Itraconazole for mild to moderate infections	Organism cultured from soil, especially where contaminated with fowl droppings Fungus enters through skin or mucous membranes of mouth and respiratory tract Endemic in Mississippi and Ohio River valleys Disseminated diseases most common in infants and children younger than 2 years
Coccidioidomycosis (valley fever)—*Coccidioides immitis* and *Coccidioides posadasii*	Erythema nodosum Erythema multiforme Erythematous maculopapular rash	Primary lung disease usually asymptomatic: 60% of children Symptoms: Cough, fever, malaise, myalgia, headache, chest pain May be sign of acute febrile illness Disseminated disease is very serious; occurs in infants (meningitis)	Fluconazole or itraconazole for 3-6 months IV amphotericin B if no response to above Surgical resection of persistent pulmonary cavities	Inhalation of aerospores from soil Endemic in southwestern United States (*C. immitis* occurs almost exclusively in California) Usually resolves spontaneously Increased incidence in dark-skinned races (Filipino, African American, Hispanic), pregnant women, diabetics, persons with cardiopulmonary disease, and infants <1 year old

AIDS, Acquired immune deficiency syndrome; *ARDS,* acute respiratory distress syndrome; *CNS,* central nervous system; *HIV,* human immunodeficiency virus; *IV,* intravenous.

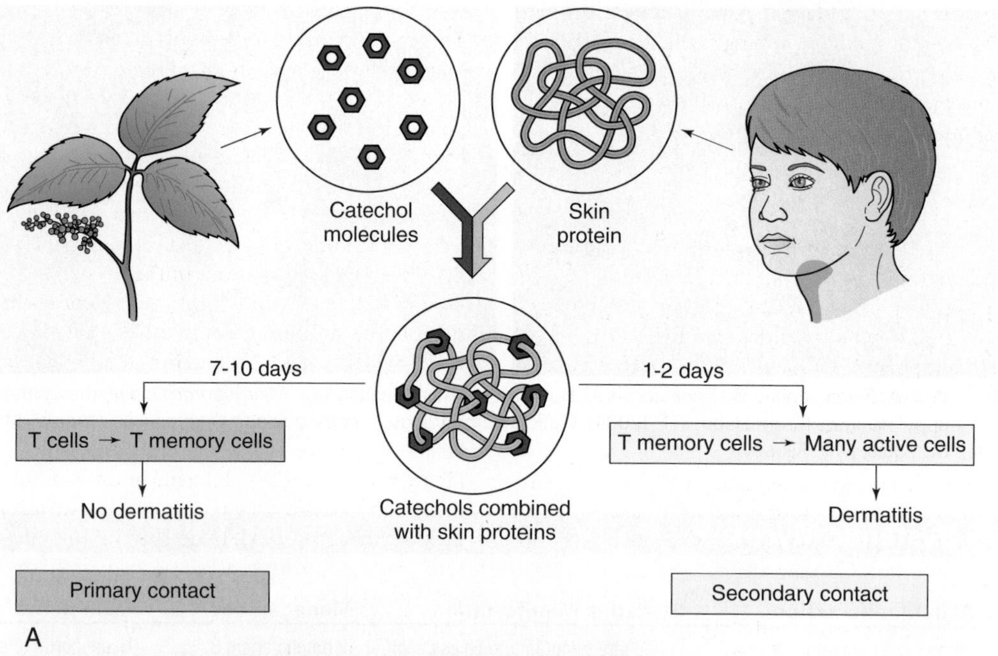

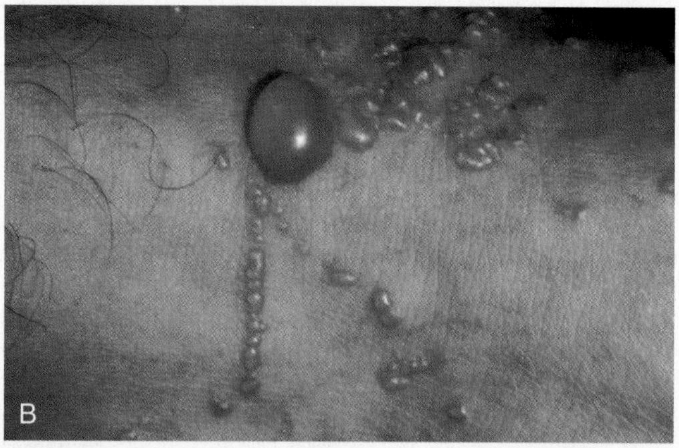

Fig. 31.5 **A,** Development of allergic contact dermatitis. **B,** Poison ivy lesions; note the "streaked" blisters surrounding one large blister. (**A,** From McCance, K., & Huether, S. [2010]. Pathophysiology: The biological basis for disease in adults and children [6th ed.]. St. Louis, MO: Mosby. **B,** From Habif, T. P. [2010]. Clinical dermatology: A color guide to diagnosis and therapy [5th ed.]. St. Louis, MO: Mosby.)

on their fur, and animals that eat the plants can transfer the oil in their saliva. Shoes, tools, and toys can transfer the oil. Golf balls that have been in the rough are another source of contact.

Urushiol takes effect as soon as it touches the skin. It penetrates through the epidermis as a mixture of compound molecules called *catechols.* These catechols bond skin proteins and initiate an immune response. The full-blown reaction is evident after about 2 days, with redness, swelling, and itching at the site of contact. Several days later, streaked or spotty blisters oozing serum from damaged cells produce the characteristic impetiginous lesions (see Fig. 31.5B). The lesions dry and heal spontaneously, and itching stops by 10 to 14 days.

Therapeutic Management

Treatment of the lesions includes application of calamine lotion, soothing Burow solution compresses, and/or Aveeno baths to relieve discomfort. Topical corticosteroid gel is effective for prevention or relief of inflammation, especially when applied before blisters form. Oral corticosteroids may be needed for severe reactions and those affecting the face, throat, or genital region. A sedative such as diphenhydramine may be ordered.

Nursing Care Management

The earlier the skin is cleansed, the greater the chance of removing the urushiol before it attaches to the skin. When it is known that the child has made contact with the plant, the area is immediately flushed (preferably within 15 minutes) with *cold* running water to neutralize the urushiol not yet bonded to the skin. Once the oil has been removed from the skin, the allergen has been neutralized. The rash that results from poison ivy cannot be spread to another child; only direct contact with the oil can cause the response. Harsh soap and scrubbing the exposed skin is contraindicated because it removes protective skin oils and dilutes the urushiol, allowing it to spread. All clothing that has come in contact with the plant is removed with care and thoroughly laundered in hot water and detergent. Every effort is made to prevent the child from scratching the lesions. Although the lesions do not spread by contact with the blister serum or from scratching, they can become secondarily infected.

Prevention

Prevention is best accomplished by avoiding contact and removing the plant from the environment. Teach all children, especially those known to be sensitive, to recognize the plant. Information regarding means for destroying plants can be obtained from the US Department of Agriculture or US Forestry Service. Home garden sprays that kill broad-leaf plants or all vegetation (e.g., Roundup, Spectracide) are ineffective. If poisonous plants are growing in public community area, the local authorities should be contacted to remove the plants.

DRUG REACTIONS

Although drugs can adversely affect any organ of the body, reactions to medications are seen more often in the skin than in any other organ. The reaction may be a result of toxicity related to drug concentration, individual intolerance to the therapeutic dosage of the drug, or an allergic or idiosyncratic response. The manifestations may be associated with side effects or secondary effects of a drug, either of which are unrelated to its primary pharmacologic actions.

Although any drug is capable of producing a reaction in the susceptible individual, some drugs have a tendency to produce a particular reaction consistently (e.g., hives after a dose of antibiotics in an individual with sensitivity), and others are more likely to produce an untoward effect (e.g., nausea, vomiting, diarrhea). Many are allergenic responses that occur after a previous administration of the drug, even a topical application. Other factors influence a drug response in a particular individual. For example, the incidence of adverse reaction increases with the dosage amount and number of drugs given simultaneously.

> **! NURSING ALERT**
>
> Intravenous drugs are more likely to cause a reaction than oral drugs. If a reaction occurs, stop the drug but maintain the infusion with normal saline.

Manifestations of drug reactions may be delayed or immediate. A period of 7 days is usually required for a child to develop sensitivity to a drug that has never been administered previously. With prior sensitivity, the manifestations appear almost immediately. Rashes that are exanthematous, urticarial, or eczematoid are the most common manifestation of adverse drug reactions in children. However, individual drug reactions may vary from a single lesion to extensive, generalized epidermal necrosis such as that seen in Stevens-Johnson syndrome. Cutaneous manifestations can resemble almost any skin disease and can be seen in almost any degree of severity. With few exceptions, the distribution of a drug eruption is widespread because it results from a circulating agent; appears as an inflammatory response with itching; is sudden in onset; and may be associated with constitutional symptoms such as fever, malaise, gastrointestinal upset, anemia, or liver and kidney damage.

Another common adverse medication response in children is a fixed eruption (i.e., a recurrent eruption at the same site with each administration of the offending drug). The lesion, a purplish red round or oval plaque with a sharp border seen most frequently on the extremities, disappears slowly, and the pigmentation deepens with each episode.

In most cases, treatment for simple cutaneous reactions consists of discontinuing the drug. Sometimes a decision is made to continue the drug (e.g., an antibiotic in a small child) until the cause of the rash is clearly indicated and the negative or mild effects of the rash outweigh the benefits of the antibiotic (or other medication) treatment. Once the medication reaction is identified, it is well documented in the patient's medical record and avoided in the future. The provider will either substitute the offending medication with treatment in a comparative class or simply discontinue treatment, depending on the patient scenario. Often antihistamines may be ordered to relieve urticaric rashes. A tapering course of corticosteroids may be used for widespread and severe rashes. Severe anaphylactic reactions are a medical emergency (see Chapter 23, Anaphylaxis).

Nursing Care Management

The most effective means of management is prevention, documentation, and assessment. Frequent offenders in drug reactions are penicillin and sulfonamides, and nurses must be alert to this possibility. However, even commonplace drugs such as aspirin and barbiturates, chemical agents in some foods, flavoring agents, and preservatives can produce an undesired response. Parents always remember details of their child's severe reaction. As the nurse takes a careful medical history, details of a previous drug reaction should include the name and dose of the drug, nature of the reaction, and how soon after administration the reaction occurred. This information should be carefully noted in the medical record (see Chapter 4, History Taking). A careful nursing assessment (observation, inspection, and palpation) of the skin is paramount for any child receiving medication, especially intravenously. Noting the child's behavior and frequency of scratching is also critical. Nurses who identify a new rash after medication is administered or suspect a medication sensitivity in a patient whose rash is enlarging, increasingly itchy, or widespread on the child's body should withhold any further dose and report the eruption to the practitioner. Persons who have severe reactions should wear a medical identification bracelet or necklace in case of emergency or inadvertent administration of the offending agent.

FOREIGN BODIES

Small wooden, glass, or metal splinters and thorns from plants can usually be safely removed with a pointed needle and tweezers that have been sterilized with either alcohol or a flame. The area around the sliver is washed thoroughly with soap and water before removal is attempted, and the child should be cooperative and calm before removal is attempted. The sliver is exposed with the needle and then grasped firmly by the tweezers and pulled out. Some foreign bodies, such as a fishhook, pieces of glass, a difficult-to-see object, or a deeply embedded object (e.g., a needle in a foot or near a joint), require medical evaluation.

Small cactus prickles or spines are troublesome to remove, and attempts may be distressing to the child and family. Large spines or clumps can be removed with tweezers. Small prickles or spines may be removed by the following methods:

- Apply a thin layer of water-soluble household glue and cover it with gauze; when the glue dries, peel off the gauze.
- Apply hair removal wax or body sugar, let it dry, and remove.
- Place cellophane tape, sticky side down, over the spines and lift it off.

SKIN DISORDERS RELATED TO ANIMAL CONTACTS

ARTHROPOD BITES AND STINGS

Arthropods include insects and arachnids, such as mites, ticks, spiders, and scorpions. Most arthropods in the United States, including tarantulas, are relatively harmless. Although all spiders produce venom that is injected via fangs, some are unable to pierce the skin, and others produce venom that is insufficiently toxic to be harmful. Only scorpions and two spiders—the brown recluse and the black widow—inject venom deadly enough to require immediate attention. Children bitten by these arachnids must receive medical attention as soon as possible. Major offending creatures, their manifestations, and management are outlined in Table 31.7. A brown recluse spider bite is shown in Fig. 31.6.

TABLE 31.7 Skin Lesions Caused by Arthropods

Mechanism and Characteristic	Manifestations	Management
Insect Bites—Flies, Gnats, Mosquitoes, Fleas		
Mechanism—Foreign protein in insects' saliva introduced when skin is penetrated for a blood meal Distribution: Almost everywhere—Fleas, mosquitoes, ants Suburbs and rural areas—Bees Urban areas—Hornets, wasps, yellow jackets	Hypersensitivity reaction Papular urticaria Firm papules; may be capped by vesicles or excoriated Little or no reaction in nonsensitized person	Treatment: Use antipruritic agents and baths Administer antihistamines Prevent secondary infection Prevention: Avoid contact Remove focus, such as untreated furniture, mattresses, carpets, and pets, where insects may live Apply insect repellent when exposure is anticipated
Chiggers—Harvest Mites		
Mechanism—Attach with claws and secrete a digestive substance that liquefies the host's epidermis	Erythematous papules Intense itching Favor warm areas of body, especially intertriginous areas and areas covered with clothing	Treatment: May require systemic steroids for extensive bites Prevention: Avoid contact, especially in areas of tall grass and underbrush Apply insect repellant when exposure is anticipated Spray insecticides such as diazinon in yards
Hymenopterans—Bees, Wasps, Hornets, Yellow Jackets, Fire Ants		
Mechanism: Injection of venom through stinging apparatus Venom contains histamine; allergenic proteins; and often a spreading factor, hyaluronidase Severe reactions caused by hypersensitivity or multiple stings	Local reaction—Small red area, wheal, itching, and heat Systemic reactions—May be mild to severe, including generalized edema, pain, nausea and vomiting, confusion, respiratory impairment, and shock	Treatment: Carefully scrape off stinger or pull out stinger as quickly as possible Cleanse with soap and water Apply cool compresses Apply common household product (e.g., lemon juice, paste made with aspirin or baking soda) Administer antihistamines Severe reactions—Administer epinephrine, corticosteroids; treat for shock Prevention: Teach child to wear shoes; to avoid wearing bright clothing, flowery prints, shiny jewelry, or perfumed grooming products (cologne, scented hairspray), which might attract the insect; and to avoid places where the insect may be contacted Hypersensitive children should wear medical identification to indicate allergy and therapy needed; family should keep emergency medication and be taught its administration
Black Widow Spider		
Mechanism—Venom injected through a clawlike appendage; has neurotoxic action Characteristics: Shiny black spider, with a body about 1.25 cm (0.5 inch) long and a red or orange hourglass-shaped marking on underside Avoids light and bites in self-defense	Mild sting at time of bite Area becomes swollen, painful, and erythematous Dizziness, weakness, and abdominal pain May produce delirium, paralysis, seizures, and (if large amount of venom absorbed) death	Treatment: Cleanse wound with antiseptic Apply cool compresses Administer antivenin Administer muscle relaxant, such as calcium gluconate; analgesics or sedatives; hydrocortisone or diazepam intravenously Prevention—Teach children to avoid places that harbor the spider (e.g., woodpiles)
Brown Recluse Spider		
Mechanism: Venom injected via fangs Venom contains powerful necrotoxin Characteristics: Slender spider, with long legs and body length of 1-2 cm; color is fawn to dark brown; recognized by fiddle-shaped mark on head Shy; bites only when annoyed or surprised Prefers dark areas where seldom disturbed	Mild sting at time of bite Transient erythema followed by bleb or blister; mild to severe pain in 2-8 h; purple, star-shaped area in 3-4 days; necrotic ulceration in 7-14 days (see Fig. 31.6) Systemic reactions may include fever, malaise, restlessness, nausea, vomiting, and joint pain Generalized petechial eruption Wounds heal with scar formation	Treatment: Apply cool compresses locally Administer antibiotics, corticosteroids Relieve pain Wound may require skin graft Prevention—Teach children to avoid possible nesting sites

TABLE 31.7 Skin Lesions Caused by Arthropods—cont'd

Mechanism and Characteristic	Manifestations	Management
Scorpions		
Mechanism: Sting by means of a hooked caudal stinger that discharges venom Venom of more venomous species contains hemolysins, endotheliolysins, and neurotoxins Characteristics—Usual habitat southwestern United States	Intense local pain, erythema, numbness, burning, restlessness, vomiting Ascending motor paralysis with seizures, weakness, rapid pulse, excessive salivation, thirst, dysuria, pulmonary edema, coma, and death Some species produce only local tissue reaction with swelling at puncture site (distinctive) Symptoms subside in a few hours Deaths occur among children <4 years of age, usually in first 24 h	Treatment: Delay absorption of venom by keeping child quiet; place involved area in dependent position Administer antivenin Relieve pain Admit to pediatric intensive care unit for surveillance Prevention—Teach children to avoid possible nesting sites
Ticks		
Mechanism—In process of sucking blood, head and mouth parts are buried in skin Characteristics: Feed on blood of mammals Significant in humans because of pathologic organism carried May be vectors of various infectious diseases, such as Rocky Mountain spotted fever, Q fever, tularemia, relapsing fever, Lyme disease, tick paralysis Must attach and feed for 1-2 h to transmit disease Usual habitat is wooded area	Tick usually attached to skin with head embedded Firm, discrete, intensely pruritic nodules at site of attachment May cause urticaria or persistent localized edema	Treatment: Grasp tick with tweezers (forceps) as close as possible to point of attachment Pull straight up with steady, even pressure; if using bare hands, use a tissue to touch tick during removal; wash hands thoroughly with soap and water Remove any remaining part (e.g., head) with sterile needle Cleanse wounds with soap and disinfectant Prevention—Teach children to avoid areas where prevalent Inspect skin (especially scalp) after being in wooded areas

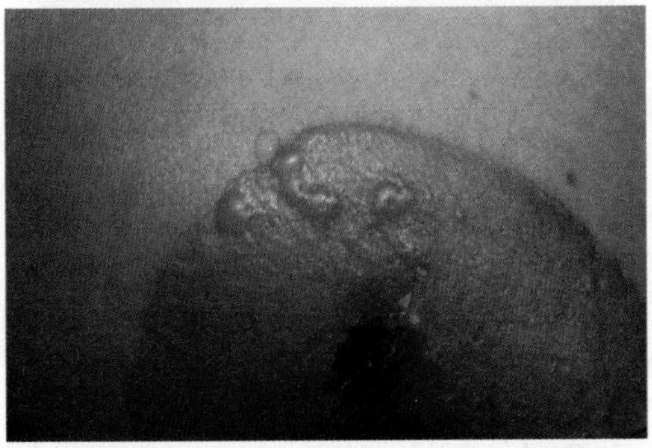

Fig. 31.6 Brown recluse spider bite. Note central necrosis surrounded by purplish area and blisters. (From Weston, W. L., & Lane, A. T. [2007]. *Color textbook of pediatric dermatology* [4th ed.]. St. Louis, MO: Mosby.)

When a hymenopteran (bees in particular) stings, its barbed stinger penetrates the skin. As long as the stinger remains in the skin, the muscles push the stinger deeper, and the venom is pumped into the wound. The best approach is to remove the stinger as quickly as possible and to get away from the vicinity of other insects to prevent further injury. Children who have become sensitized to hymenopteran bites may demonstrate a severe systemic response that can be life threatening. One sting can produce generalized urticaria, respiratory difficulty (from laryngeal edema), hypotension, and death. Intramuscular administration of epinephrine provides immediate relief and must be available for emergency use.

Hypersensitive children should wear a medical identification bracelet. They should also have a kit that contains epinephrine and a hypodermic syringe. Families are reminded to check the expiration date on the kit and to replace an outdated one. They should determine whether a nurse is available at the school and find out what the school policy is regarding administration of drugs. If a school nurse is not present, someone at the school should be designated to inject the epinephrine in case of an emergency.

SCABIES

Scabies is an endemic infestation caused by the scabies mite, *Sarcoptes scabiei*. Lesions are created as the impregnated female burrows into the stratum corneum of the epidermis (never into living tissue) to deposit her eggs and feces. The inflammatory response causes intense pruritus that leads to punctate discrete excoriations secondary to the itching (Box 31.1). Maculopapular lesions are characteristically distributed in intertriginous areas: interdigital surfaces, the axillary-cubital area, popliteal folds, and the inguinal region. The observer must look for discrete papules, burrows, or vesicles (Fig. 31.7). Scabies is transmitted primarily through prolonged close personal contact, and it affects persons regardless of age, sex, personal hygiene, or socioeconomic status.

Nursing Care Management

The treatment of scabies is the application of a scabicide. The drug of choice in children and infants older than 2 months of age is permethrin 5% cream (Elimite). Alternative drugs are 10% crotamiton (cream or lotion) or oral ivermectin. Lindane can be neurotoxic and is contraindicated by the American Academy of Pediatrics (2018).

BOX 31.1 Clinical Manifestations of Scabies

Lesion

Children—Minute grayish brown, threadlike (mite burrows), pruritic
- Black dot at end of burrow (mite)

Infants—Eczematous eruption, pruritic

Distribution

Generally in intertriginous areas—Interdigital, axillary-cubital, popliteal, inguinal
Children older than 2 years of age—Primarily hands and wrists
Children younger than 2 years—Primarily feet and ankles

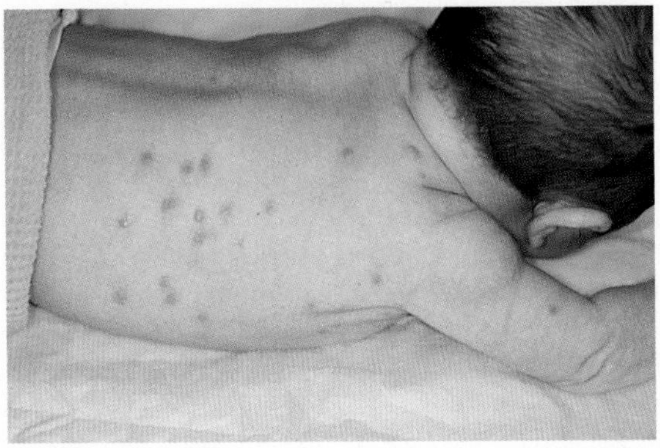

Fig. 31.7 Scabies. (From McCance, K., & Huether, S. [2010]. *Pathophysiology: The biological basis for disease in adults and children* [6th ed.]. St. Louis, MO: Mosby/Elsevier.)

Ivermectin, an oral medication, may be used to treat scabies in patients with secondary excoriations for whom topical scabicides are irritating and not well tolerated or whose infestation is refractory. However, the safety and efficacy of ivermectin for children weighing less than 15 kg (33 pounds) has not been established.

Because of the length of time between infestation and physical symptoms (30 to 60 days), all persons who were in close contact with the affected child need treatment. This may include boyfriends or girlfriends, babysitters, grandparents, and immediate family members. The objective is to treat as thoroughly as possible the first time. Enough medication for the entire family should be prescribed, with 2 oz allowed for each adult and 1 oz for each child.

PEDICULOSIS CAPITIS

Pediculosis capitis (head lice) is an infestation of the scalp by *Pediculus humanus capitis,* a common parasite in school-age children. These lice infestations create embarrassment and concern in the family and community. They can also cause a child to be ridiculed by other children. An important nursing role is education about pediculosis. Nurses should emphasize that anyone can get pediculosis; it has no respect for age, socioeconomic level, or cleanliness.

The adult louse lives only about 48 hours when away from a human host, and the life span of the average female is 1 month. The female lays her eggs at night at the junction of a hair shaft and close to the skin because the eggs need a warm environment. The **nits**, or eggs, hatch in approximately 7 to 10 days. Itching, caused by the crawling insect and saliva on the skin, is usually the only symptom. The louse is a blood-sucking organism that requires approximately five meals a day. Common areas involved are the occipital area, behind the ears, and the nape of the neck (Box 31.2).

BOX 31.2 Clinical Manifestations of Pediculosis

Pruritus (caused by crawling insects and insect saliva on skin)
Nits observable on hair shaft (see Fig. 31.8)

Distribution

Occipital area
Behind ears
Nape of neck
Eyebrows and eyelashes (occasionally) (caused by pubic lice)

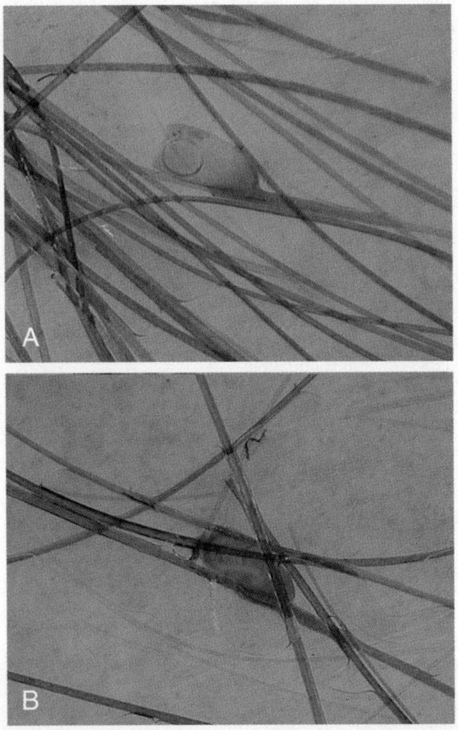

Fig. 31.8 **A,** Empty nit case. **B,** Viable nits. (From Stefani, A. D., Hofmann-Wellenhof, R., & Zalaudek, I. [2006]. Dermoscopy for diagnosis and treatment monitoring of pediculosis capitis. *Journal of the American Academy of Dermatology, 54*(5), 909–911.)

Diagnostic Evaluation

Diagnosis is made by observation of the white eggs (nits) firmly attached to the hair shafts (Fig. 31.8). Lice are small and grayish tan, have no wings, and are visible to the naked eye. Observation of the white eggs (nits) firmly attached to the hair shafts confirms the diagnosis. The nits, or eggs, appear as tiny whitish oval specks adhering to the hair shaft about 6 mm (0.25 inch) from the scalp. The adherent nature of the nits distinguishes them from dandruff, which falls off readily. Empty nit cases, indicating hatched lice, are translucent rather than white and are located more than 6 mm from the scalp. Because of their brief life span and mobility, adult lice are more difficult to locate. Nits must be differentiated from dandruff, lint, hair spray, and other items of similar size and shape. Scratch marks or inflammatory papules, caused by secondary infection, are also found on the scalp in the vulnerable areas.

Therapeutic Management

Treatment consists of the application of pediculicides and manual removal of nit cases. The drug of choice for infants and children is permethrin 1% cream rinse (Nix), which kills adult lice and nits. This product and preparations of pyrethrin with piperonyl butoxide (RID or A-200 Pyrinate) can be obtained without a prescription and are effective and safe. A second treatment at 7 to 10 days is advised to ensure a cure. If neither permethrin nor pyrethrin products are effective, the prescription drug 0.5% malathion, which has been approved for treatment of head lice, can be used. However, malathion is not recommended for children younger than 2 years of age.

Because of concerns that head lice may be developing resistance to chemical shampoos and that repeated exposure of children to strong chemicals on the scalp may be unwise, effective nonchemical control measures are essential. Removal of nits from the child's hair with a metal nit comb daily is a control measure following treatment with a pediculicide.

Nursing Care Management

An important nursing role is educating the parents about pediculosis. Nurses should emphasize that *anyone* can get pediculosis; it has no respect for age, gender, socioeconomic level, or cleanliness. Lice do not jump or fly, but they can be transmitted from one person to another on personal items. Children are cautioned against sharing combs, hair ornaments, hats, caps, scarves, coats, and other items used on or near the hair. Lice are not carried or transmitted by pets (Gunning, Kiraly, & Pippitt, 2019).

Nurses or parents should carefully inspect children who scratch their heads more than usual for bite marks, redness, and nits. The hair is systematically spread with two flat-sided sticks or tongue depressors, and the scalp is observed for any movement that indicates a louse. Nurses should wear gloves when examining the hair.

If evidence of infestation is found, it is important to treat the child according to the directions on the label of the pediculicide. Permethrin 1% lotion or shampoo (Nix) is recommended for first-line treatment. Alternative treatments should not be used unless permethrin fails after two treatments (Gunning et al., 2019). Parents are advised to read the directions carefully before beginning treatment. The child is made as comfortable as possible during the application process because the pediculicide must remain on the scalp and hair for several minutes. A useful strategy is playing "beauty parlor" while shampooing. The child lies supine with the head over a sink or basin and covers the eyes with a dry towel or washcloth. This prevents medication, which can cause chemical conjunctivitis, from splashing into the eyes. If eye irritation occurs, the eyes must be flushed well with tepid water. It is not necessary to remove the nits after treatment because only live lice cause infestation. However, because none of the pediculicides is 100% effective in killing all of the eggs, the makers of some pediculicides recommend manual removal of the nits after treatment. An extra-fine-tooth comb that is included in many commercial pediculicides or is available at community pharmacies facilitates manual removal. Live lice survive for up to 48 hours away from the host, but nits are shed into the environment and are capable of hatching in 7 to 10 days; retreatment is required. Therefore measures must be taken to prevent further infestation (see Community Focus box). Spraying with insecticide is not recommended because of the danger to children and animals. Families should also be advised that the pediculicide is relatively expensive, especially when several members of the household require treatment. Families may be inclined to try home remedies such as petroleum jelly, oils, vinegar, butter, alcohol, and mayonnaise to treat the lice; however, there is no evidence demonstrating the effectiveness of these remedies (Gunning et al., 2019).

COMMUNITY FOCUS

Focus Preventing the Spread and Recurrence of Pediculosis

- Machine wash all washable clothing, towels, and bed linens in water hotter than 130°F and dry them in a hot dryer for at least 20 minutes. Dry clean nonwashable items.
- Thoroughly vacuum carpets, car seats, pillows, stuffed animals, rugs, mattresses, and upholstered furniture.
- Seal nonwashable items in plastic bags for 14 days if unable to dry clean or vacuum.
- Soak combs, brushes, and hair accessories in lice-killing products for 1 hour or in boiling water for 10 minutes.
- In daycare centers, store children's clothing items such as hats and scarves and other headgear in separate cubicles.
- Discourage the sharing of items such as hats, scarves, hair accessories, combs, and brushes among children in group settings such as daycare centers and schools.
- Avoid physical contact with infected individuals and their belongings, especially clothing and bedding.
- Inspect children in a group setting regularly for head lice.
- Provide educational programs on the transmission of pediculosis, its detection, and treatment.

Modified from Chin, J. (Ed.). (2000). *Control of communicable diseases manual.* Washington, DC: American Public Health Association; and Gunning, K., Kiraly, B., & Pippitt, K. (2019). Lice and scabies: Treatment update. *American Family Physician, 99*(10), 635–642.

RICKETTSIAL DISEASES

The organisms responsible for a number of disorders are transmitted to human beings via arthropods (Table 31.8). Mammals become infected only through the bites of infected lice, fleas, ticks, and mites, all of which serve as both infectors and reservoirs. Rickettsiae are intracellular parasites, similar in size to bacteria that inhabit the alimentary tract of a wide range of natural hosts. Rickettsial diseases are more common in temperate and tropical climates where humans live in association with arthropods. Infection in humans is incidental (except epidemic typhus) and not necessary for the survival of the rickettsial species. However, after the organism invades a human, it causes a disease that varies in intensity from a benign, self-limiting illness to a disease that is fulminating and fatal.

LYME DISEASE

Lyme disease is the most common tickborne disorder in the United States. It is caused by the spirochete *Borrelia burgdorferi,* which enters the skin and bloodstream through the saliva and feces of ticks, especially the deer tick (Steere, Strle, Wormser, et al., 2016). Most cases of Lyme disease are reported in the Northeast from southern Maine to northern Virginia in the months of May through October and more commonly occur in children 5 to 15 years of age and adults 45 to 55 years of age (Steere et al., 2016).

Clinical Manifestations

The disease may be initially seen in any of three stages. The first stage, early localized disease, consists of the tick bite at the time of inoculation, followed in 3 to 30 days by the development of erythema migrans at the site of the bite. The lesion begins as a small erythematous papule that enlarges radially up to 30 cm (12 inches) over a period of days to weeks. It results in a large circumferential ring with a raised, edematous

TABLE 31.8 **Eruptions Caused by Rickettsiae**

Disorder, Organism, and Host	Manifestations	Management	Comments
Rocky Mountain spotted fever—*Rickettsia rickettsii* Arthropod—Tick Transmission—Tick Mammal source—Wild rodents, dogs	Gradual onset—Fever, malaise, anorexia, myalgia Abrupt onset—Rapid temperature elevation, chills, vomiting, myalgia, severe headache Maculopapular or petechial rash primarily on extremities (ankles and wrists) but may spread to other areas, characteristically on palms and soles	Control—Protection from tick bite by wearing proper apparel, tick repellent Tetracycline or chloramphenicol Vigorous supportive therapy	Usually self-limiting in children Onset in children may resemble any infectious disease Severe disease rare in children Inspect children and dogs regularly if they play in wooded areas See Table 31.7 for management of ticks
Epidemic typhus— *Rickettsia prowazekii* Arthropod—Body louse Transmission—Infected feces into broken skin Mammal source—Humans	Abrupt onset of chills, fever, diffuse myalgia, headache, malaise Maculopapular rash becoming petechial 4-7 days later, spreading from trunk outward	Control—Immediate destruction of vectors Tetracycline or chloramphenicol Supportive treatment	Isolate patient until deloused See discussion in this chapter for management of pediculosis Excreta from infected lice also in dust; patient's clothing, bedding, and possessions are disinfected and washed in hot water
Endemic typhus—*Rickettsia typhi* Arthropod—Rat fleas or lice Transmission—Flea bite; inhaling or ingesting flea excreta Mammal source—Rats	Headache, arthralgia, backache followed by fever; may last 9-14 days Maculopapular rash after 1-8 days of fever; begins in trunk and spreads to periphery; rarely involves face, palms, soles	Control—Eliminate rat reservoir, insect vectors, or both Tetracycline or chloramphenicol Supportive treatment	Fairly common in United States Shorter duration than epidemic typhus Mild, seldom fatal illness Difficult to distinguish from epidemic typhus
Rickettsialpox—*Rickettsia akari* Arthropod—Mouse mite Transmission—Mite Mammal source—House mouse	Maculopapular rash following primary lesion; eschar at site of bite; fever, chills, headache	Control—Eradication of rodent reservoir and mite vector Tetracycline or chloramphenicol Supportive treatment	Self-limiting nonfatal disease Initially endemic in New York City but now found in many cities in United States

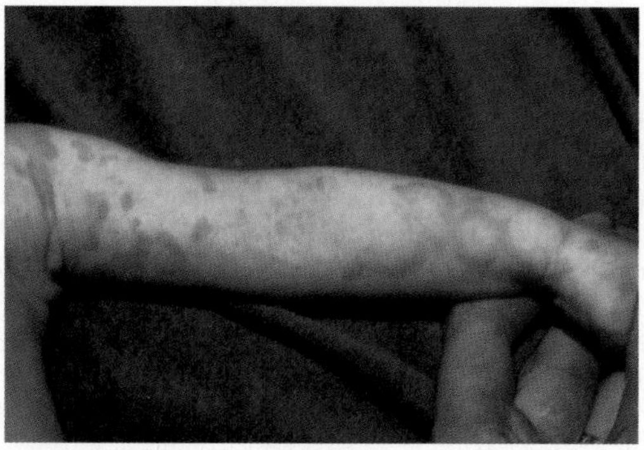

Fig. 31.9 Lyme disease. Note annular red rings in erythema chronicum migrans. (From Weston, W. L., & Lane, A. T. [2007]. *Color textbook of pediatric dermatology* [4th ed.]. St. Louis, MO: Mosby.)

doughnut-like border resulting in a bull's-eye appearance (Fig. 31.9). The thigh, groin, and axilla are common sites. The lesion is described as "burning," feels warm to the touch, and occasionally is pruritic. The single annular rash may be associated with fever, myalgia, headache, or malaise.

The second stage, early disseminated disease, occurs 3 to 10 weeks after inoculation. Many patients develop multiple smaller, secondary annular lesions without the indurated center. They may occur anywhere except on the palms and soles, and in untreated patients they disappear in 3 to 4 weeks. Constitutional symptoms, including fever, headache, malaise, fatigue, anorexia, stiff neck, generalized lymphadenopathy, splenomegaly, conjunctivitis, sore throat, abdominal pain, and cough, are often observed. A focal neurologic finding of cranial nerve palsy (seventh nerve palsy) occurs in 3% to 5% of cases. Additional manifestations include ophthalmic conditions such as optic neuritis, uveitis, conjunctivitis, and keratitis.

Finally, the third stage and the most serious stage of the disease is characterized by systemic involvement of neurologic, cardiac, and musculoskeletal systems that appears 2 to 12 months after inoculation. Lyme arthritis is the most common manifestation with pain, swelling, and effusion. In children the arthritis is characterized by intermittently painful swollen joints (primarily the knees), with spontaneous remissions and exacerbations. Rare neurologic features of pediatric Lyme disease may include meningitis, encephalitis, and polyneuritis (Koedel, Fingerle, & Pfister, 2015). Cardiac complications, which may appear in a small percentage of persons during the early phase of the infection, are commonly acute atrioventricular conduction abnormalities and less commonly pericarditis or mild left ventricular dysfunction (Steere et al., 2016).

Diagnostic Evaluation

Diagnosis is based primarily on the history, observation of the lesion, and clinical manifestations. Serologic testing for Lyme disease at the time of a recognized tick bite is not recommended because antibodies are not detectable in most persons (American Academy of Pediatrics, 2018). Laboratory diagnosis can be established in later stages with a two-step approach that includes the screening test enzyme immunoassay or immunofluorescent immunoassay and, if the results are equivocal or positive, with Western immunoblot testing, as outlined by the Centers for Disease Control and Prevention (2017) and adopted by the American Academy of Pediatrics (2018).

Therapeutic Management

Early and appropriate treatment is essential to prevent complications. Children older than 8 years of age are treated with oral doxycycline; amoxicillin is recommended for children younger than 8 years of age (American Academy of Pediatrics, 2018). For patients who are allergic to penicillin, alternative drugs include cefuroxime or erythromycin.

The length of treatment depends on the clinical response and other disease manifestations, but it usually lasts from 14 to 21 days (American Academy of Pediatrics, 2018). The treatment is effective in preventing second-stage manifestations in most cases. Persons who have removed ticks from themselves should be monitored closely for signs and symptoms of tickborne diseases for 30 days; in particular, they should be monitored for erythema migrans, a red expanding skin lesion at the site of the tick bite that may suggest Lyme disease. People who develop a skin lesion or viral infection–like illness within 1 month of an attached tick should seek prompt medical attention. Treatment of erythema migrans most often prevents development of later stages of Lyme disease.

Neurologic, cardiac, and arthritic manifestations are managed with oral or intravenous (IV) antibiotics, such as ceftriaxone, cefotaxime, or penicillin G. Follow-up care is important in ensuring that treatment is initiated or terminated as needed.

Nursing Care Management

The major emphasis of nursing care should be educating parents to protect their children from exposure to ticks. Children should avoid tick-infested areas or wear light-colored clothing so that ticks can be spotted easily, tuck pant legs into socks, and wear a long-sleeved shirt tucked into pants when in wooded areas. Parents and children need to perform regular tick checks when they are in infested areas (with special attention to the scalp, neck, armpits, and groin areas). Parents should also be alert for signs of the skin lesion, especially if their children have been in tick-infested areas. The American Academy of Pediatrics (2018) points out that the risk of infection after a deer tick bite, even in endemic regions of the United States, is 1% to 4%; children bitten by a deer tick in nonendemic regions should not receive antibiotic prophylaxis.

Parents should also be educated on tick removal in the event of a tick bite. The tick should be grasped firmly with tweezers and pulled straight out. The application of nail polish or petroleum jelly is not recommended and does not appear to affect tick withdrawal, as has been hypothesized. Concerns about tick engorgement or tick remains (such as the tick head) left in the person's body appear to be unfounded; there is no need for medical examination of the tick itself. After the tick is removed, wash the bite area with an iodine scrub, rubbing alcohol, or plain soap and water.

Insect repellents containing diethyltoluamide (DEET) and permethrin can protect against ticks, but parents should use these chemicals cautiously. Although there have been reports of serious neurologic complications in children resulting from frequent and excessive application of DEET repellants, the risk is low when they are used properly. Products with DEET should be applied sparingly according to label instructions and not applied to a child's face, hands, or any areas of irritated skin. Plant essential oils, such as juniper and Chinese weeping cedar essential oil, have been reported as being safe and effective as an insect repellent without the effects of chemicals (Eisen & Dolan, 2016). Permethrin-treated clothing has also been shown to be effective in repelling ticks (Eisen & Dolan, 2016). After the child returns indoors, treated skin should be washed with soap and water. Information about Lyme disease can be obtained from the American Lyme Disease Foundation, Inc.,[a] or from the Centers for Disease Control and Prevention (https://www.cdc.gov/lyme/).

Pet Bites

Animal bites are common in childhood. Wild animal bites are discussed in relation to rabies in Chapter 30. The present discussion is directed primarily toward dog bites because most animal bites to children are caused by dogs. Cat bites are less frequent, although cat scratches are extremely common (see Cat Scratch Disease later in the chapter).

Most injuries caused by dogs or cats are to the upper extremities. Small children are likely to be bitten or scratched on the head, face, and neck because they tend to put their heads near the animal's head and flail their arms rather than protecting their heads. Most dogs involved are owned by the family of the victim or by a neighbor. Injuries vary in intensity from small puncture wounds to complete evulsion of tissue that is associated with significant crush injury. Animal bites are potentially serious because of the likelihood of significant infection.

Therapeutic Management

General wound care consists of rinsing the wound with copious amounts of saline or lactated Ringer solution under pressure via a large syringe and of washing the surrounding skin with mild soap. A clean pressure dressing is applied, and the extremity is elevated if the wound is bleeding. Medical evaluation is advised because of the danger of tetanus and rabies, although dogs in most urban areas are required to be immunized against rabies. Bites from wild animals, such as squirrels, bats, raccoons, foxes, and skunks, are potentially dangerous.

Prophylactic antibiotics are indicated for puncture wounds and wounds in areas that may prove to be cosmetically or functionally impaired if infected. Extensive lacerations are debrided and loosely sutured to allow drainage in the event of infection. Tetanus toxoid is administered according to standard guidelines (see Chapter 6, Immunizations), and rabies protocol is followed (see Chapter 30, Rabies). Injuries to poorly vascularized areas, such as the hands, are more likely to become infected than those in more vascularized areas, such as the face; puncture wounds are more likely to become infected than lacerations.

Nursing Care Management

The most important aspect related to animal bites is prevention. Children should understand animal behavior and develop respect for animals (see Community Focus box). Parents should monitor their children's behavior with dogs and instruct them not to tease or surprise dogs, invade their territory, interfere with their feeding or sleeping, take their toys, or interact with sick or injured dogs or dogs with pups. Parents who are considering getting a pet, especially a dog, for themselves or their children, should select a dog that has a high level of sociability with, and is unlikely to be a danger to, children.

HUMAN BITES

Children often acquire lacerations from the teeth of other humans in rough play, during fights, or as victims of child abuse. Some young children bite others out of frustration or anger. Because human dental plaque and gingiva harbor pathogenic organisms, all human bites

[a]PO Box 466, Lyme, CT 06371; http://www.aldf.com.

COMMUNITY FOCUS

Animal Safety

To avoid bites and scratches

- Never bother a pet when it's eating or pull its food or water away.
- Don't tease a dog or cat or pull its tail or ears.
- Never bother a pet when it's sleeping.
- Don't take a toy or bone away from a cat or dog or hold it out of reach of the animal.
- Never try to get near a pet with its babies (like a cat with kittens or a dog with puppies). Animal mothers are very protective and will bite to keep you away.
- When lifting a rabbit, hamster, guinea pig, or gerbil from its cage, do it slowly. Be sure to hold the animal underneath its belly.
- Never pick up or hold a rabbit by its ears.
- When pulling an iguana, lizard, snake, or other reptile from its tank, do it slowly and carefully. Then wash your hands right away because reptiles can carry bacteria like Salmonella on their skin.
- Never stick your bare hand into a fish tank — most fish can't hurt you. But a few types of fish can and do sting if they get upset. The water also contains germs that could cause a skin infection.
- If a pet looks sick or is injured, stay far away. An animal that normally loves to be petted and played with may get very upset and even bite when it is feeling ill. Tell an adult so he or she can get help for the animal.

To keep your cool around dogs

- Never pet or touch a strange dog, even if it runs up to you and seems like it might be friendly.
- If a dog starts running toward you, don't run. Running away can make the dog want to chase after you — even if it doesn't want to hurt you, its instincts will tell it to chase.
- If a strange dog approaches you, try to stand very still. This may be scary for a minute or two, but often the dog will become bored and walk away. If the dog tries to sniff you, let it sniff — this is its way of checking you out.
- Walk away from a strange dog very slowly. Don't wave your arms around or make a lot of noise because these actions will only excite the dog. Look straight ahead and not into the dog's eyes.
- If you are very afraid of a strange dog or a strange dog tries to bite or attack you, tell an adult as soon as possible. He or she can find the dog's owner.

KidsHealth®
from Nemours

From KidsHealth (2019). Staying Safe Around Animals, https://kidshealth.org/en/kids/animals.html.

should receive attention. Delayed treatment increases the risk of infection.

The wound is washed vigorously with soap and water, and a pressure dressing is applied to stop bleeding. Ice applications minimize discomfort and swelling. Increased pain or redness at the wound site is an indication that the child should receive medical attention for antibiotic therapy. Tetanus toxoid is needed if the child is insufficiently immunized. Wounds larger than 6 mm should receive medical attention.

CAT SCRATCH DISEASE

Cat scratch disease is the most common cause of regional lymphadenitis in children and adolescents. It usually follows the scratch or bite of an animal (a cat or kitten in 99% of cases) and is caused by *Bartonella henselae*, a gram-negative bacterium. The disease is usually a benign, self-limiting illness that resolves spontaneously in about 4 to 6 weeks (American Academy of Pediatrics, 2018).

The usual manifestations are a painless, nonpruritic erythematous papule at the site of inoculation, followed by regional lymphadenitis. The lymph nodes most commonly involved are axillary epitrochlear, cervical, submandibular, inguinal, and preauricular. The disease may persist for several months before gradual resolution. In some children, especially those who are immunocompromised, the adenitis may progress to suppuration. Some children may develop serious complications that include encephalitis, hepatitis, and Parinaud oculoglandular syndrome. This syndrome is characterized by granulomatous lesions on the palpebral conjunctiva associated with swelling of the ipsilateral preauricular nodes.

Diagnosis is made on the basis of (1) history of contact with a cat or kitten, (2) the presence of regional lymphadenopathy for several days, and (3) serologic identification of the causative organism by indirect fluorescent antibody assay or polymerase chain reaction test (American Academy of Pediatrics, 2018).

Treatment is primarily supportive. Some experts recommend a 5-day course of oral azithromycin to hasten recovery (American Academy of Pediatrics, 2018). Antibiotics do not shorten the duration or prevent progression to suppuration but may be helpful in severe forms of the disease. Trimethoprim-sulfamethoxazole, ciprofloxacin, gentamicin, and rifampin have shown some benefit in uncontrolled clinical studies. Enlarged painful nodes may be treated by needle aspiration.

Children should be cautioned about playing with aggressive kittens that bite or scratch. Wounds should be washed with soap and water. Analgesics may be given for discomfort. Most children can continue normal activities during the disease. The animals are not ill during the time they transmit the disease, and most authorities do not recommend disposal of a cherished pet.

MISCELLANEOUS SKIN DISORDERS

A number of miscellaneous skin lesions occur in children. Some occur as a result of congenital disorders and are inherited as an autosomal dominant trait (Table 31.9). **Ichthyoses** are a heterogeneous group of disorders characterized by scaling that create challenging problems in treatment. These disorders are not discussed in detail here because of their wide variability.

SKIN DISORDERS ASSOCIATED WITH SPECIFIC AGE-GROUPS

Several common dermatologic conditions are confined to children in specific age-groups. These conditions include diaper, atopic, and seborrheic dermatitis, which occurs predominantly in infants, and acne, which is most common in adolescence.

DIAPER DERMATITIS

Diaper dermatitis is common in infants and one of several acute inflammatory skin disorders caused either directly or indirectly by wearing diapers. The peak age of occurrence is 9 to 12 months of age, and the incidence is greater in bottle-fed infants than in breastfed infants.

Pathophysiology and Clinical Manifestations

Diaper dermatitis is caused by prolonged and repetitive contact with an irritant (e.g., urine, feces, soaps, detergents, ointments, friction). Although the irritant in most cases is urine and feces, a combination of factors contributes to irritation.

Prolonged contact of the skin with diaper wetness produces higher friction, greater abrasion damage, increased transepidermal

TABLE 31.9 Miscellaneous Skin Disorders

Disease and Causative Agent	Local Manifestations	Management	Comments
Urticaria—Usually allergic response to drugs or infection	Development of wheals Vary in size and configuration and tend to appear quickly, spread irregularly, and fade within a few hours May be constant or intermittent, sparse or profuse, small or large, discrete or confluent May be acute, chronic, or recurrent in acute attacks	Topical soothing and antipruritic applications Antihistamines Cortisone in severe cases Severe involvement may require epinephrine	Known etiologic agents should be avoided May be accompanied by malaise, fever, lymphadenopathy Severe cases may involve mucous membranes, internal organs, and joints Obstruction to air passages constitutes medical emergency
Intertrigo—Mechanical trauma and aggravating factors of excessive heat, moisture, and sweat retention	Red, inflamed, moist, partially denuded, marginated areas, the shape of which is determined by location Appears where opposing skin surfaces rub together, such as intergluteal folds, groin, neck, and axilla Excessive moisture and obesity are often factors	Maintenance of cleanliness and dryness of affected areas Skinfolds kept separated with a generous supply of nonmedicated powder Expose to air and light Remove excess clothing	A form of diaper irritation Prevent recurrence by keeping susceptible areas clean and dry Frequently associated with overheating from too much clothing Common in tracheostomy patients with short necks and copious secretions
Psoriasis—Cause unknown; hereditary predisposition; may be triggered by stress	Round, thick, dry, reddish patches covered with coarse, silvery scales over trunk and extremities; first lesions commonly appear in scalp; facial lesions more common in children than in adults Affected cells proliferate at a much more rapid rate than normal cells	Tar preparations in combination with ultraviolet B light or natural sunlight Topical corticosteroids Topical vitamin D analog calcipotriene Phenol and saline solutions followed by a tar shampoo to remove scales Keratolytic agents (salicylic acid) Acitretin Emollients may provide relief	Uncommon in children younger than 6 years Affected patients are otherwise healthy Coal tar acts synergistically with ultraviolet light Keratolytic agents enhance absorption of corticosteroids Humidifiers may help in winter
Alopecia[a]			
Alopecia areata	Sudden onset of asymptomatic, noninflammatory, round, bald patches in hairy parts of body	Psychologic support Minoxidil (peripheral vasodilator)	Family history in 10%-26% of cases Some concern regarding drug therapy safety Refer to support groups[a]
Traumatic alopecia	Traction alopecia around scalp margins from tight hair styles (e.g., braids, ponytails, cornrows)	Counseling on hair styling, use of hair cosmetics, hot combs, rollers	More prevalent in African American children and adolescents Prolonged traction can produce fibrosis of hair root and permanent loss
Trichotillomania	Compulsive hair pulling	Determine and treat cause	Chronic hair pulling may require psychologic therapy
Tinea capitis	See Table 31.5	See Table 31.5	See Table 31.5
Erythema multiforme (Stevens-Johnson syndrome)—Cause unknown; associated with ingestion of some drugs; often follows upper respiratory tract infection	Erythematous papular rash Lesions enlarge by peripheral expansion, develop central vesicle Involves most skin surfaces except scalp May extend to mucous membranes, especially oral, ocular, and urethral	Symptomatic and supportive Maintenance of adequate intake of fluids (oral or intravenous), calories, and protein Moist wound care, hydrogels such as CarraGauze, Vaseline, or Aquaphor Appropriate treatment of complications Diligent monitoring of urine volume and specific gravity, hemoglobin and hematocrit, serum electrolyte levels, total body weight	Rash often preceded by fever and malaise Complications include renal failure and severe eye disease Respiratory involvement in a number of cases Self-limiting, but recovery may extend for weeks; skin lesions may subside without scarring; mucous membrane lesions may persist for months Recurrence rate, 20%; mortality rate as high as 10% High mutation rate
Neurofibromatosis—Inherited disorder; autosomal dominant inheritance pattern	Café-au-lait spots, pigmented nevi, axillary freckling Slow-growing cutaneous and subcutaneous neurofibromas	Symptomatic treatment of associated manifestations (e.g., speech defects, seizures, skeletal defects [scoliosis, kyphosis], learning disabilities) Surgical removal of troublesome tumors	Refer to support groups[b] Family needs to know about genetic implications

[a]National Alopecia Areata Foundation, 65 Mitchell Blvd., Suite 200-B, San Rafael, CA 94903; 415-472-3780; email: info@naaf.org; http://www.naaf.org.
[b]Children's Tumor Foundation, 120 Wall St., 16th Floor, New York, NY 10005-3904; 800-323-7938; email: info@ctf.org; http://www.ctf.org.

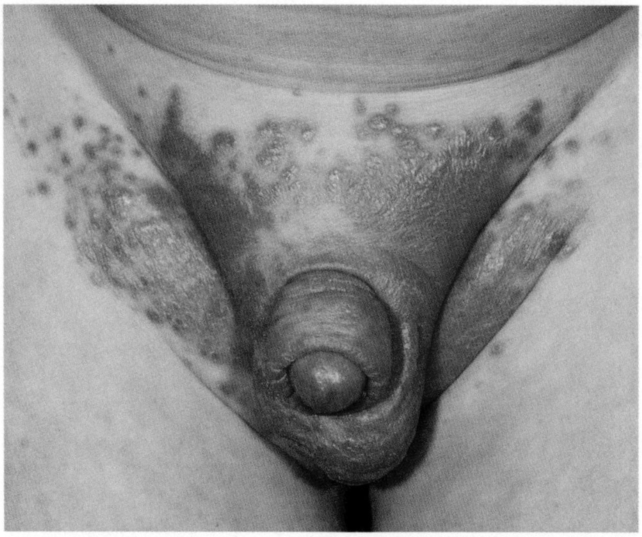

Fig. 31.10 Irritant diaper dermatitis. Note the sharply demarcated edges. (From Habif, T. P. [2010]. *Clinical dermatology: A color guide to diagnosis and therapy* [5th ed.]. St. Louis, MO: Mosby.)

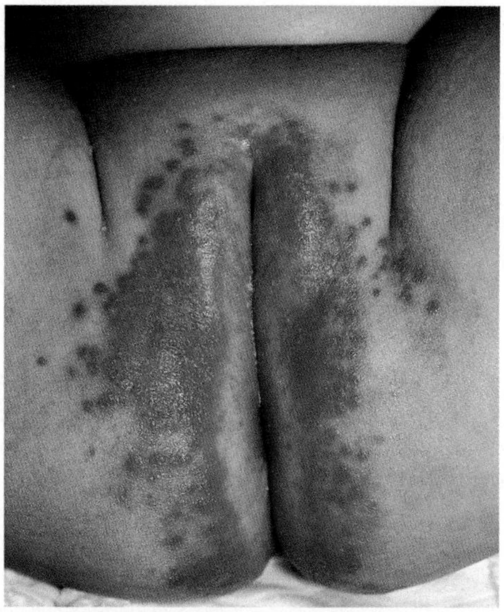

Fig. 31.11 Candidiasis of diaper area. Note the beefy red central erythema with satellite pustules. (From Paller, A. S., & Mancini, A. J. [2011]. *Hurwitz clinical pediatric dermatology* [4th ed.]. St. Louis, MO: Saunders Elsevier.)

permeability, and increased microbial counts. Healthy skin is less resistant to potential irritants.

Although ammonia was once thought to cause diaper rash because of the association between the strong odor on diapers and dermatitis, ammonia alone is not sufficient. The irritant quality of urine is related to an increase in pH from the breakdown of urea in the presence of fecal urease. The increased pH promotes the activity of fecal enzymes, principally the proteases and lipases, which act as irritants. Fecal enzymes also increase the permeability of skin to bile salts, another potential irritant in feces.

The eruption of diaper dermatitis is manifested primarily on convex surfaces or in folds. The lesions represent a variety of types and configurations. Eruptions involving the skin in most intimate contact with the diaper (e.g., the convex surfaces of buttocks, inner thighs, mons pubis, scrotum) but sparing the folds are likely to be caused by chemical irritants, especially from urine and feces (Fig. 31.10). Other causes are detergents or soaps from inadequately rinsed cloth diapers or the chemicals in disposable wipes. Perianal involvement is usually the result of chemical irritation from feces, especially diarrheal stools. *Candida albicans* infection produces perianal inflammation and a maculopapular rash with satellite lesions that may cross the inguinal fold (Fig. 31.11). It is seen in up to 90% of infants with chronic diaper dermatitis and should be considered in diaper rashes that are recalcitrant to treatment.

Nursing Care Management

Nursing interventions are aimed at altering the three factors that produce dermatitis: wetness, pH, and fecal irritants. The most significant factor amenable to intervention is the moist environment created in the diaper area. Changing the diaper as soon as it becomes wet eliminates a large part of the problem and removing the diaper to expose healthy skin to air facilitates drying. The use of a hair dryer or heat lamp is not recommended because these devices can cause burns.

Diaper construction has a significant impact on the incidence and severity of diaper dermatitis. Superabsorbent disposable paper diapers reduce diaper dermatitis. They contain an absorbent gelling material that binds water tightly to decrease skin wetness, maintains pH control by providing a buffering capacity, and decreases skin irritation by preventing mixing of urine and feces in the diaper. Guidelines for controlling diaper rash are presented in the Family-Centered Care box. A common misconception about using cornstarch on skin is that it promotes the growth of *C. albicans*. Neither cornstarch nor talcum powder promotes the growth of fungi under conditions normally found in the diaper area. Based on safety in terms of inhalation injury, cornstarch is the preferred product. Talcum powder should not be used.

FAMILY-CENTERED CARE

Controlling Diaper Rash

Keep skin dry.[a]
- Use superabsorbent disposable diapers to reduce skin wetness.
- Change diapers as soon as soiled—especially with stool—whenever possible, preferably once during the night.
- Expose healthy or only slightly irritated skin to air, not heat, to dry completely.

Apply ointment, such as zinc oxide or petrolatum, to protect skin, especially if skin is very red or has moist, open areas.
- Avoid removing skin barrier cream with each diaper change; remove waste material and reapply skin barrier cream.
- To completely remove ointment, especially zinc oxide, use mineral oil; do not wash vigorously.

Avoid overwashing the skin, especially with perfumed soaps or commercial wipes, which may be irritating.
- May use a moisturizer or nonsoap cleanser, such as cold cream or Cetaphil, to wipe urine from skin.
- Gently wipe stool from skin using a soft cloth and warm water.
- Use disposable diaper wipes that are detergent and alcohol-free.

[a]Powder helps keep the skin dry, but talcum powder is dangerous if breathed into the lungs. Plain cornstarch or cornstarch-based powder is safer. When using any powder product, first shake it into your hand and then apply it to the diaper area. Store the container away from the infant's reach; keep the container closed when not in use.

ATOPIC DERMATITIS (ECZEMA)

Atopic dermatitis (AD), also referred to as eczema, refers to a descriptive category of dermatologic diseases and not to a specific etiology. AD is a chronic relapsing inflammatory skin disorder that results in itching

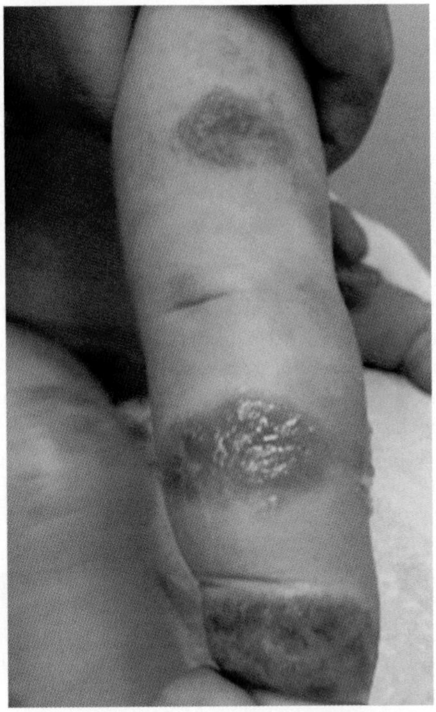

Fig. 31.12 Atopic dermatitis. (From Gupta, D. [2015]. Atopic dermatitis. *Medical Clinics of North America, 99*(6), 1269–1285.)

and lesions (Fig. 31.12; Grey & Maquiness, 2016). It occurs in 20% of children (Page, Weston, & Loh, 2016). AD manifests in three forms based on the child's age and the distribution of lesions:

1. **Infantile** (infantile eczema)—Usually begins at 2 to 6 months of age; generally undergoes spontaneous remission by 3 years of age
2. **Childhood**—May follow the infantile form; occurs at 2 to 3 years of age; 90% of children have manifestations by age 5 years
3. **Preadolescent and adolescent**—Begins at about 12 years of age; may continue into the early adult years or indefinitely

The diagnosis of AD is based on a combination of history and morphologic findings (Box 31.3). Although symptoms can vary among individuals, one common symptom is pruritus. Itching can be mild, moderate, or severe, and can intensify the inflammation and erythema associated with the lesions; itching can become so severe that the lesions bleed. Lesions gradually disappear when the scratching is stopped.

Although the cause is not fully understood, AD is believed to have genetic and environmental factors (Nguyen, Leonard, & Eichenfield, 2015). Most children with infantile AD have a family history of eczema, asthma, food allergies, or allergic rhinitis, which strongly supports a genetic predisposition. The cause is unknown but appears to be related to abnormal function of the skin, including alterations in perspiration, peripheral vascular function, and heat tolerance. Manifestations of the chronic disease improve in humid climates and get worse in the fall and winter, when homes are heated and environmental humidity is lower. The disorder can be controlled but not cured. A recent study of 250 patients with AD showed that the severity of AD significantly affected their quality of life, with more severe disease resulting in a lower quality of life (Holm, Agner, Causen, et al., 2016). Furthermore, the study reported a lower quality of life among females and among patients with eczema on their face (Holm et al., 2016).

Therapeutic Management

The major goals of management are to (1) hydrate the skin, (2) relieve pruritus, (3) reduce flare-ups or inflammation, and (4) prevent and control secondary infection. The general measures for

BOX 31.3 Clinical Manifestations of Atopic Dermatitis

Distribution of Lesions

Infantile form—Generalized, especially face, scalp, neck, and extensor surfaces of extremities

Childhood form—Flexural areas (antecubital and popliteal fossae, neck), wrists, ankles, and feet

Preadolescent and adolescent form—Face, sides of neck, hands, feet, face, and antecubital and popliteal fossae (to a lesser extent)

Appearance of Lesions

Infantile Form

Erythema
Vesicles
Papules
Weeping
Oozing
Crusting
Scaling
Often symmetric

Childhood Form

Symmetric involvement
Clusters of small erythematous or flesh-colored papules or minimally scaling patches
Dry and may be hyperpigmented
Lichenification (thickened skin with accentuation of creases)
Keratosis pilaris (follicular hyperkeratosis) common

Adolescent or Adult Form

Same as childhood manifestations
Dry, thick lesions (lichenified plaques) common
Confluent papules

Other Physical Manifestations

Intense itching
Unaffected skin dry and rough
African American children likely to exhibit more papular or follicular lesions than white children
May exhibit one or more of the following:

- Lymphadenopathy, especially near affected sites
- Increased palmar creases (many cases)
- Atopic pleats (extra line or groove of lower eyelid)
- Prone to cold hands
- Pityriasis alba (small, poorly defined areas of hypopigmentation)
- Facial pallor (especially around nose, mouth, and ears)
- Bluish discoloration beneath eyes ("allergic shiners")
- Increased susceptibility to unusual cutaneous infections (especially viral)

managing AD focus on reducing pruritus and other aspects of the disease. Management strategies include avoiding exposure to skin irritants or allergens; avoiding overheating; and administering medications such as antihistamines, topical immunomodulators, topical steroids, and (sometimes) mild sedatives as indicated.

Enhancing skin hydration and preventing dry, flaky skin are accomplished in a number of ways, depending on the child's skin characteristics and individual needs. A tepid bath with a mild soap (Dove or Neutrogena), no soap, or an emulsifying oil followed immediately by application of an emollient (within 3 minutes) assists in trapping moisture and preventing its loss. Bubble baths and harsh soaps should be avoided. The bath may need to be repeated once or twice daily, depending on the child's status; excessive bathing without emollient application only dries out the skin. Some lotions are not effective, and emollients should be chosen carefully to prevent excessive skin drying. Aquaphor, Cetaphil, and Eucerin are acceptable lotions for skin hydration. A nighttime bath followed by emollient application and dressing in soft cotton pajamas may help alleviate most nighttime pruritus.

Sometimes colloid baths, such as the addition of 2 cups of cornstarch to a tub of warm water, provide temporary relief of itching and may help the child sleep if given before bedtime. Cool wet compresses are soothing to the skin and provide antiseptic protection.

Oral antihistamine drugs (such as hydroxyzine or diphenhydramine) usually relieve moderate or severe pruritus. Nonsedating antihistamines such as loratadine (Claritin) or fexofenadine (Allegra) may be preferred for daytime pruritus relief. Because pruritus increases at night, a mildly sedating antihistamine may be needed.

Occasional flare-ups require the use of topical steroids to diminish inflammation. Low-, moderate-, or high-potency topical corticosteroids are prescribed, depending on the degree of involvement, the area of the body to be treated, the child's age, the potential for local side effects (striae, skin atrophy, and pigment changes), and the type of vehicle to be used (e.g., cream, lotion, ointment). Patients receiving topical corticosteroid therapy for chronic conditions should be evaluated for risk factors for suboptimal linear growth and reduced bone density. Topical immunomodulators, a nonsteroidal treatment for AD, are best used at the beginning of a "flare-up" just as the skin becomes red and itches. Second-line management for children with AD includes immunomodulator medications such as tacrolimus and pimecrolimus (Grey & Maquiness, 2016). These medications are approved for use in children 2 years of age and older (Grey & Maquiness, 2016). Both drugs can be used freely on the face without worrying about steroid side effects.

If secondary skin infections occur in children with AD, these infections are managed with appropriate systemic antibiotics. Obtaining cultures from affected areas and the child's nares is helpful to ensure appropriate therapy (Page et al., 2016).

Nursing Care Management

Assessment of the child with AD includes a family history for evidence of atopy, a history of previous involvement, and any environmental or dietary factors associated with the present and previous exacerbations. The skin lesions are examined for type, distribution, and evidence of secondary infection. Parents are interviewed regarding the child's behavior, especially in relation to scratching, irritability, and sleeping patterns. Exploration of the family's feelings and methods of coping is also important.

The nursing care of the child with AD is challenging. Controlling the intense pruritus is imperative if the disorder is to be successfully managed because scratching leads to new lesions and may cause secondary infection. In addition to the medical regimen, other measures can be taken to prevent or minimize the scratching. Fingernails and toenails are cut short, kept clean, and filed frequently to prevent sharp edges. Gloves or cotton stockings can be placed over the hands and pinned to shirtsleeves. One-piece outfits with long sleeves and long pants also decrease direct contact with the skin. If gloves or socks are used, the child needs time to be free from such restrictions. An excellent time to remove gloves, socks, or other protective devices is during the bath or after receiving sedative or antipruritic medication.

Conditions that increase itching are eliminated when possible. Woolen clothes or blankets, rough fabrics, and furry stuffed animals are removed from the child's environment. Because heat and humidity cause perspiration (which intensifies itching), proper dress for climatic conditions is essential. Pruritus is often precipitated by exposure to the irritant effects of certain components of common products such as soaps, detergents, fabric softeners, perfumes, and powders. During cold months, synthetic fabrics (not wool) should be used for overcoats, hats, gloves, and snowsuits. Exposure to latex products, such as gloves and balloons, should also be avoided.

Clothes and sheets are laundered in a mild detergent and rinsed thoroughly in clear water (without fabric softeners or antistatic chemicals). Putting the clothes through a second complete wash cycle without using detergent reduces the amount of residue remaining in the fabric.

Preventing infection is usually accomplished by preventing scratching. Baths are given as prescribed; the water is kept tepid; and soaps (except as indicated), bubble baths, oils, and powders are avoided. Skin folds and diaper areas need frequent cleansing with plain water. A room humidifier or vaporizer may benefit children with extremely dry skin. Skin lesions are examined for signs of infection—usually honey-colored crusts or pustules with surrounding erythema. Any signs of infection are reported to the practitioner.

> **! NURSING ALERT**
>
> If the child is being treated with baths, it is imperative that an emollient preparation be applied immediately after bathing (while the skin is still slightly moist) to prevent drying.

Wet soaks and compresses are applied and medications for pruritus or infection are administered as directed. The family is given explicit instructions on the preparation and use of soaks, special baths, and topical medications, including the order of application if more than one is prescribed. It is important to emphasize that one thick application of topical medication is *not* equivalent to several thin applications and that excessive use of an agent (particularly steroids) can be hazardous. If children have difficulty remaining still for a 10- or 15-minute soak, bath, or dressing application, these can be carried out at naptime or when the child is engrossed in watching television, listening to a story, or playing with tub toys.

Diet modification may prevent skin exacerbations. When a hypoallergenic diet is prescribed, parents need help to understand the reason for the diet and the guidelines for avoiding hyperallergenic foods. Because hypoallergenic diets take time before visible effects are apparent, parents need reassurance that results may not be seen immediately. If airborne allergens make eczema worse, the family is counseled about "allergy proofing" the home (see Chapter 21, Asthma).

Family Support

Parents are assured that the lesions will not produce scarring (unless secondarily infected) and that the disease is not contagious. However, the child may have repeated exacerbations and remissions. Spontaneous and permanent remission takes place at approximately 2 to 3 years of age in most children with the infantile disorder.

During acute phases, emotional stress can become intense for the family. They need time to discuss negative feelings and to be reassured that these feelings are normal. Stress tends to aggravate the severity of the condition. Therefore efforts to relieve as much anxiety as possible in both the parents and the child have a beneficial emotional and physical effect.

SEBORRHEIC DERMATITIS

Seborrheic dermatitis is a chronic, recurrent, inflammatory reaction of the skin. It occurs most commonly on the scalp (cradle cap) but may involve the eyelids (blepharitis), external ear canal (otitis externa), nasolabial folds, and inguinal region. The cause is unknown, although it is more common in early infancy, when sebum production is increased. The lesions are characteristically thick, adherent, yellowish, scaly, oily patches that may or may not be mildly pruritic. Unlike AD, seborrheic dermatitis is not associated with a positive family history for allergy and is common in infants shortly after birth and in adolescents after puberty. Diagnosis is made primarily based on the appearance and the location of the crusts or scales.

Nursing Care Management

Cradle cap may be prevented with adequate scalp hygiene. Frequently, parents omit shampooing the infant's hair for fear of damaging the "soft spots," or fontanels. The nurse should discuss how to shampoo the infant's hair and emphasize that the fontanel is similar to skin anywhere else on the body—it does not puncture or tear with mild pressure.

When seborrheic lesions are present, direct the treatment at removing the scales or crusts. Parents are taught the appropriate procedure to clean the scalp. Education may need to include a demonstration. Shampooing should be done daily with a mild soap or commercial baby shampoo; medicated shampoos are not necessary, but an antiseborrheic shampoo containing sulfur and salicylic acid may be used. Shampoo is applied to the scalp and allowed to remain on the scalp until the crusts soften. Then the scalp is thoroughly rinsed. A fine-tooth comb or a soft facial brush helps remove the loosened crusts from the strands of hair after shampooing.

ACNE

Acne vulgaris is the most common skin problem treated by physicians during adolescence. Acne is caused by testosterone, a hormone present in boys and girls that increases during puberty. It stimulates the sebaceous glands of the skin to enlarge, or produce oil, and plug the pores. Comedogenesis (formation of comedones) results in a noninflammatory lesion that may be either an open comedone ("blackhead") or a closed comedone ("whitehead").

More than half of the adolescent population experiences acne by the end of the teenage years. Although the disorder can appear before the age of 10 years, the peak incidence occurs in middle to late adolescence (ages 16 to 17 years in girls and 17 to 18 years in boys). It is more common in boys than in girls. After this age period, the disease usually decreases in severity, but it may persist into adulthood. The degree to which an individual is affected may range from nothing more than a few isolated comedones to a severe inflammatory reaction. Although the disease is self-limiting and not life threatening, it has great significance to adolescents. Health professionals should not underestimate the impact that acne has on teens.

Numerous factors affect the development and course of acne. Its distribution in families and a high degree of concordance in identical twins suggest hereditary factors. Premenstrual flare-ups of acne occur in nearly 70% of adolescent girls, suggesting a hormonal cause. Studies do not indicate a clear association between stress and acne, but adolescents commonly cite stress as a cause for acne outbreaks. Cosmetics containing lanolin, petrolatum, vegetable oils, lauryl alcohol, butyl stearate, and oleic acid can increase comedone production. Exposure to oils in cooking grease can be a precursor in adolescents who work over fast-food restaurant hot oils. There may be an association with the intake of dairy products and high glycemic index foods that may potentiate hormonal and inflammatory factors that contribute to acne severity (Fiedler, Stangl, Fiedler, et al., 2017).

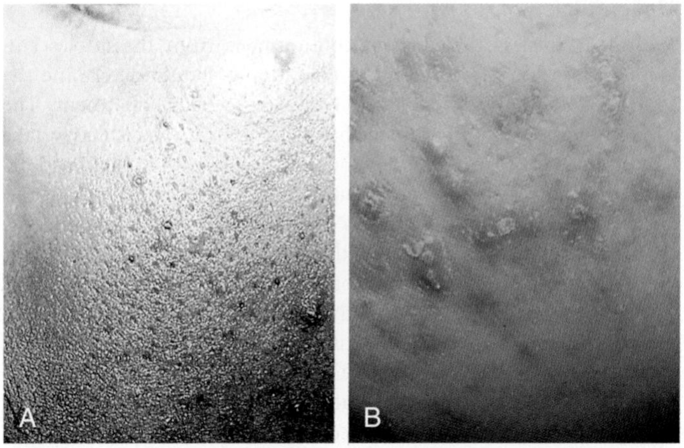

Fig. 31.13 Acne vulgaris. **A,** Acne vulgaris. **B,** Comedones with a few inflammatory pustules. (From Zitelli, B. J., McIntire, S. C., & Nowalk, A. J. [2012]. *Zitelli and Davis' atlas of pediatric physical diagnosis* [6th ed.]. St. Louis, MO: Saunders.)

Pathophysiology

Four pathophysiologic factors have the greatest influence on acne development: (1) excessive sebum production; (2) alterations in follicular growth; (3) differentiation with colonization of *Propionibacterium acnes;* and (4) an accompanying immune response and inflammation (Bhat, Latief, & Hassan, 2017). Acne severity is proportional to the sebum secretion rate, which is genetically determined and increases at the time of adrenocortical maturation. Inflammation occurs with the proliferation of *P. acnes,* which draws in neutrophils, causing inflammatory papules, pustules, nodules, and cysts (Fig. 31.13). Acne can be categorized as comedonal, inflammatory, or both and can be classified as mild, moderate, or severe based on the number and type of comedones and the extent of affected skin (Eichenfield, Krakowski, Piggott, et al., 2013).

Therapeutic Management

Successful management of acne depends on a cooperative effort among the health care provider, adolescent, and parents. Unlike many other dermatologic conditions, acne lesions resolve slowly, and improvement may not be apparent for at least 6 weeks. Individual comedones can take several weeks to months to resolve, and papules and pustules usually resolve in about 1 week. The multifactorial causes of acne necessitate a combined approach for successful treatment. Treatment consists of general measures of care and specific treatments determined by the type of lesions involved.

General Measures

The practitioner provides the adolescent with an overall explanation of the disease process, emphasizing the patient's involvement. Improvement of the adolescent's overall health status is part of the general management. Adequate rest, moderate exercise, a well-balanced diet, reduction of emotional stress, and elimination of any foci of infection are all part of general health promotion.

Cleansing

Dirt or oil on the surface of the skin does not cause acne. Gentle cleansing with a mild cleanser once or twice daily is usually sufficient. Antibacterial soaps are ineffective and may be drying when used in combination with topical acne medications. For some adolescents, hygiene of the hair and scalp appears to be related to the clinical activity of the acne. Acne on the forehead may improve with brushing the hair away from the forehead and more frequent shampooing.

Medications

Treatment success depends on commitment from the adolescent. Before prescribing treatment, the practitioner should determine the adolescent's level of comfort and readiness to begin treatment. The adolescent should be reminded that clinical improvement may take weeks to months. Early intervention, most often with topical medications, may prevent the development of more severe acne.

Tretinoin (Retin-A) is the only drug that effectively interrupts the abnormal follicular keratinization that produces microcomedones, the invisible precursors of the visible comedones. Tretinoin alone is usually sufficient for management of mild comedonal acne (Que, Whitaker-Worth, & Chang, 2016). Tretinoin is available as a cream, gel, or liquid. This drug can be extremely irritating to the skin and requires careful patient education for optimal usage. The patient should be instructed to begin with a pea-size dot of medication, which is divided into the three main areas of the face and then gently rubbed into each area. The medication should not be applied for at least 20 to 30 minutes after washing to decrease the burning sensation. The avoidance of the sun and the daily use of sunscreen must be emphasized because sun exposure can result in severe sunburn. Adolescents should be advised to apply the medication at night and to use a sunscreen with a sun protection factor (SPF) of at least 15 in the daytime.

Topical benzoyl peroxide is an antibacterial agent that inhibits the growth of *P. acnes* organisms. It is effective against both inflammatory and noninflammatory acne and is an effective first-line agent. This medication is available as a cream, lotion, gel, or wash. Benzoyl peroxide and salicylic acid are the most effective acne treatment kits available over the counter. The patient should be informed that the medication may have a bleaching effect on sheets, bedclothes, and towels. The adolescent can be reassured that skin bleaching will not occur. Accommodation to the medication can be gained with a gradual increase in the strength and frequency of application.

When inflammatory lesions accompany the comedones, a topical antibacterial agent may be prescribed. These agents are used to prevent new lesions and to treat preexisting acne. Clindamycin, erythromycin, metronidazole, and azelaic acid are currently available topical antibacterial therapy. A 5% dapsone gel has recently been approved for the treatment of inflammatory acne lesions and is reported to be effective when used in combination with a topical retinoid (Que et al., 2016). Retinoid in combination with antimicrobials also improves the penetration of these topical agents and is the only means to address three of the pathogenic causes of acne: keratinization, *P. acnes,* and inflammation. Side effects of the topical medications include erythema, dryness, and burning; using the medications every other day will decrease the adverse effects. Topical antimicrobials combined with benzoyl peroxide are more effective than either product alone; however, a yellowish discoloration of the skin occurs when topical dapsone is used in combination with benzoyl peroxide (Que et al., 2016).

Systemic antibiotic therapy is initiated when moderate to severe acne does not respond to topical treatments. The foundation for using systemic antibiotics in acne treatment has been the elimination of the inflammatory effects of *P. acnes* by suppressing the bacteria. Tetracycline, minocycline, and doxycycline are systematic antibiotics used to treat acne (Que et al., 2016). They are relatively free of side effects, with the exception of occasional gastrointestinal upset, photosensitivity, or vaginal candidiasis. Adolescent girls with mild to moderate acne may respond well to topical treatment and the addition of an oral contraceptive pill (OCP). OCPs reduce the endogenous androgen production and decrease the bioavailability of the woman's circulating androgens. Both of these actions result in decreased acne.

Isotretinoin, 13-cis-retinoic acid (Accutane), is a potent and effective oral agent that is reserved for severe cystic acne that has not responded to other treatments. Isotretinoin is the only agent available that affects factors involved in the development of acne. However, treatment with isotretinoin should be managed *only* by a dermatologist. Adolescents with multiple, active, deep dermal or subcutaneous cystic and nodular acne lesions are treated for 20 weeks. Multiple side effects can occur, including dry skin and mucous membranes, nasal irritation, dry eyes, decreased night vision, photosensitivity, arthralgia, headaches, mood changes, aggressive or violent behaviors, depression, and suicidal ideation. Adolescents taking this drug should be monitored for depression, depressive symptoms, and suicidal ideation (Oliveira, Sobreira, Velosa, et al., 2017). The drug should be given only at the recommended doses for no longer than the recommended duration. The most significant side effects of this drug are the teratogenic effects. Isotretinoin is absolutely contraindicated in pregnant women. Sexually active young women must use an effective contraceptive method during treatment and for 1 month after treatment. Patients receiving isotretinoin should also be monitored for elevated cholesterol and triglyceride levels. Significant elevation may require discontinuation of the medication.

Nursing Care Management

Because acne is so common and its appearance may seem so mild, the health care provider may underestimate the relative importance of the disease to the adolescent. The nurse should assess the individual adolescent's level of distress, current management, and perceived success of any regimen before initiating a referral. If adolescents do not perceive the acne to be a problem, they may lack motivation to follow the treatment plan.

The nurse can provide ongoing support for the adolescent when a treatment plan is initiated. Discuss the use of medications and basic skin care information in detail with the adolescent. Written instructions should accompany the verbal discussion. Information to dispel myths regarding the use of abrasive cleansing products can prevent unnecessary costs and trauma to the skin. Adolescents need education about the factors that aggravate and damage the skin, such as too vigorous scrubbing. In addition, picking, squeezing, and manual expression with fingernails break down the ductal walls of lesions and cause the acne to worsen. Mechanical irritation, such as vinyl helmet straps that rub areas predisposed to acne, can also cause the development of lesions.

BURNS

Burn injuries are usually attributed to extreme heat sources but may also result from exposure to cold, chemicals, electricity, or radiation. Most burns are relatively minor and can be treated in an outpatient setting. However, burns involving a large body surface area, critical body parts, or the geriatric or pediatric population often benefit from treatment in specialized burn centers. The American Burn Association has established criteria to guide decisions on the severity of injury and the need for transfer for specialized care.

The extent of tissue destruction is determined by the intensity of the heat source, the duration of contact or exposure, the conductivity of the tissue involved, and the rate at which the heat energy is dissipated by the skin. A brief exposure to high-intensity heat from a flame can produce burn injuries similar to those induced by long exposure to less intense heat in hot water.

When burns are categorized according to the patient's age and type of injury, the following patterns become apparent: (1) hot-water scalds are most frequent in toddlers; (2) flame-related burns are more common in older children; (3) when structural fires occur from children playing with matches or lighters, the majority are started by males, with 43% of those started by children under age 6 years (National Fire Protection Association, 2014); and (4) nonaccidental burns indicate maltreatment.

Etiology of the Injury

Most burns result from contact with thermal agents such as a flame, hot surfaces, or hot liquids. The death rate from fire and burn injury has declined by 53% from 1999 to 2013 (Safe Kids Worldwide, 2015). The leading cause of death from unintentional injury in the United States differs according to age-group, but fire and burns ranks third in children 5 to 9 years old. Approximately 237 children 14 years old and younger died from fire or burn injuries in 2016 (Centers for Disease Control and Prevention, 2018). Electrical injuries caused by household current have the greatest incidence in young children, who insert conductive objects into electrical outlets and bite or suck on connected electrical cords. These burns occur most commonly during the spring and summer months and are also associated with risk-taking behaviors in boys. Direct contact with high- or low-voltage current, as well as lightning strikes, is the most frequent mechanism of injury. Trauma results from resistance of the tissue and path of electric current through tissue, muscle compartments, nerves, and vital organs. Criteria for admission, as derived from evidence-based practice for electrical burn injuries, includes a history of loss of consciousness, electrocardiographic (ECG) changes, 10% total body surface area (TBSA) affected, or the need for monitoring an affected extremity. Cardiac monitoring is therefore included in standard burn care when ECG changes are identified on admission (McLeod, Maringo, Doyle, et al., 2018).

Chemical burns are seen in the pediatric population and can cause extensive injury since noxious agents exist in many cleaning products commonly found in the home. The severity of injury is related to the chemical agent (acid, alkali, or organic compound) and the duration of contact. The mechanism of injury differs from other burns in that there is a chemical disruption and alteration of the physical properties of the exposed body area. In addition to concern for localized damage, the potential for systemic toxicity must be addressed, including exposure of the eyes to chemical agents, the ingestion of caustic substances, and inhalation of toxic gases produced from chemicals.

Nonaccidental trauma due to maltreatment most commonly occurs in children 3 years old and younger. Children younger than 3 years old suffering a burn injury are at risk for future maltreatment of any type before the age of 6 years (Pawlik, Kemp, Maguire, et al., 2016). With nonaccidental burn trauma, scald burns from hot water are the most common injury followed by contact burns. Nonaccidental burn trauma should be suspected if the burn distribution on the body is inconsistent with the reported incident or with the child's developmental level and there was a delay in seeking treatment

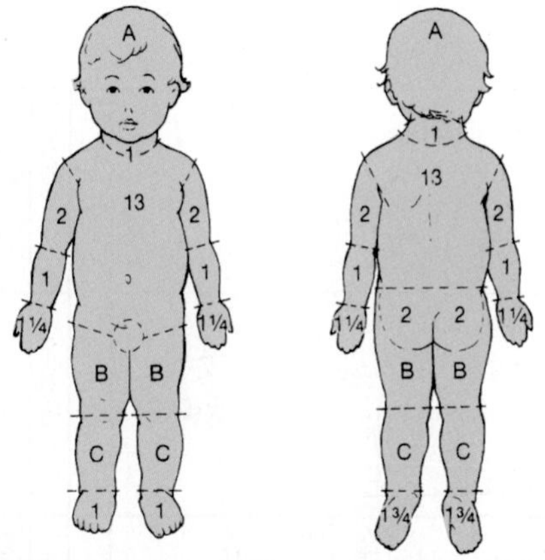

RELATIVE PERCENTAGES OF AREAS AFFECTED BY GROWTH

A

AREA	BIRTH	AGE 1 YR	AGE 5 YR
A = ½ of head	9½	8½	6½
B = ½ of one thigh	2¾	3¼	4
C = ½ of one leg	2½	2½	2¾

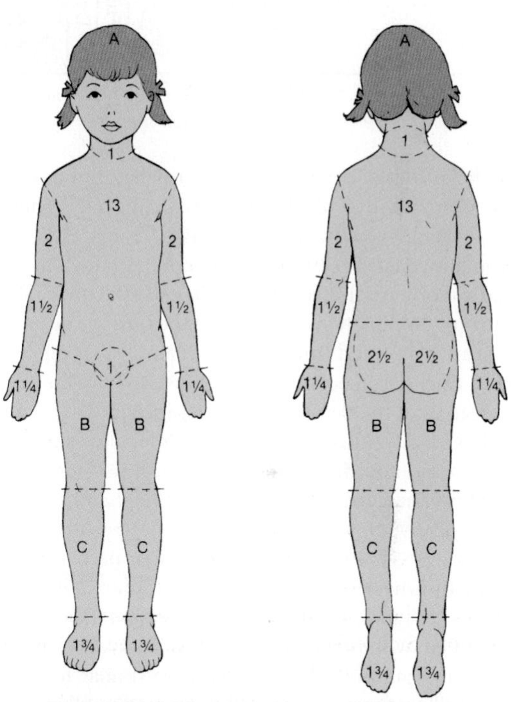

RELATIVE PERCENTAGES OF AREAS AFFECTED BY GROWTH

B

AREA	AGE 10 YR	AGE 15 YR	ADULT
A = ½ of head	5½	4½	3½
B = ½ of one thigh	4½	4½	4¾
C = ½ of one leg	3	3¼	3½

Fig. 31.14 Estimation of distribution of burns in children. **A,** Children from birth to age 5 years. **B,** Older children.

Characteristics of Burn Injury

The physiologic responses, treatment modalities, prognosis, and disposition of the injured child are all directly related to the *amount of tissue destroyed.* The severity of the burn injury is assessed based on the percentage of **total body surface area (TBSA)** burned and depth of the burn. Among children in the school-age group or younger age-groups, a burn that is 10% TBSA can be life threatening if not treated correctly. Other important factors in determining the seriousness of the injury are the child's age and general health, the causative agent, the location of the wounds, the presence of respiratory involvement, and any associated injury or condition.

Extent of Injury

The extent of a burn is expressed as a percentage of the TBSA. This is most accurately estimated by using specially designed age-related charts (Fig. 31.14). It is more efficient to use a chart designed to assign body proportions to children of different ages.

Depth of Injury

A burn is a three-dimensional wound that is also assessed in relation to depth of injury. Traditionally, the terms *first, second,* and *third degree* have been used to describe the depth of tissue injury. However, with the current emphasis on wound healing, these have been replaced by more descriptive terms based on the extent of destruction to the epithelializing elements of the skin (Fig. 31.15).

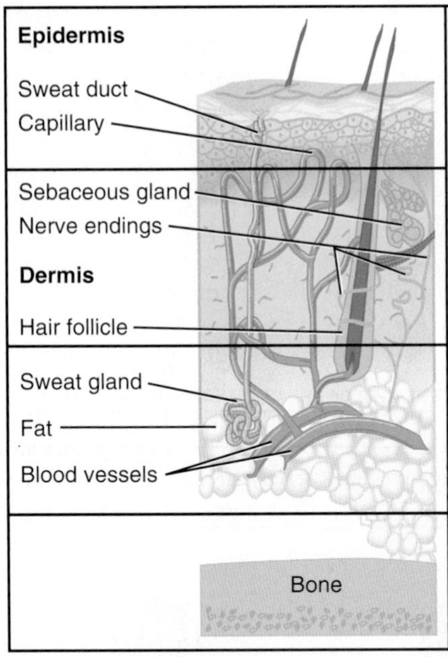

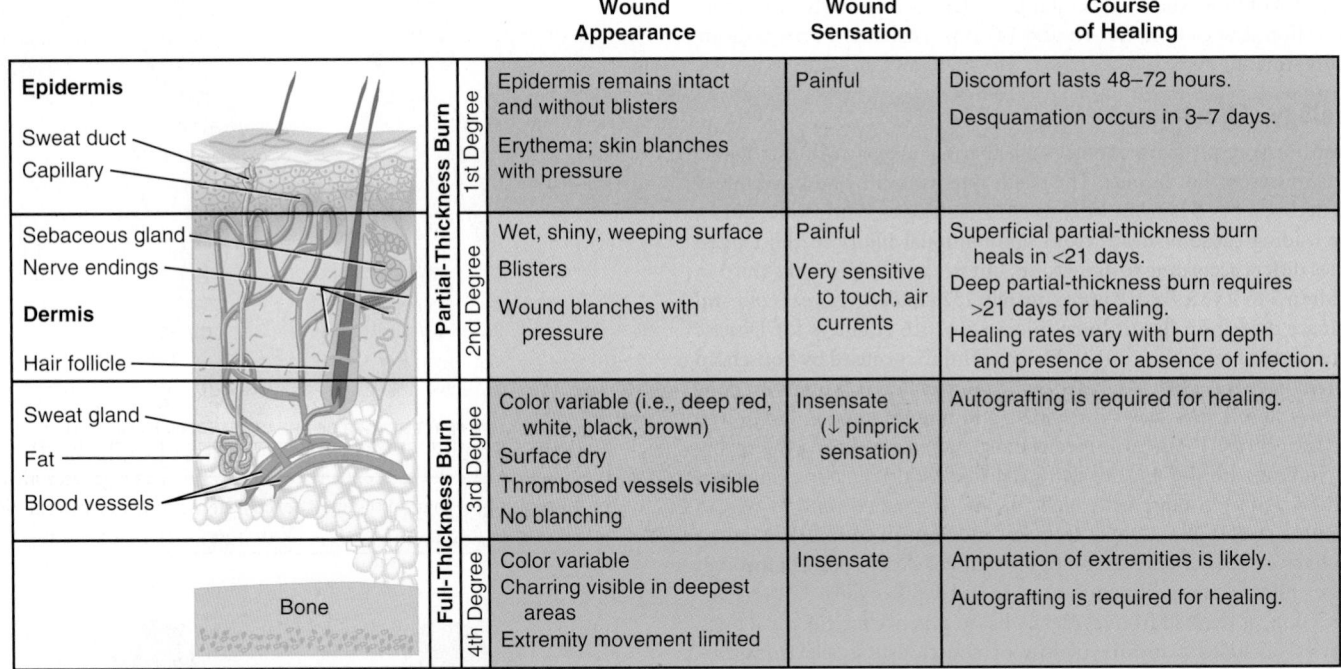

		Wound Appearance	Wound Sensation	Course of Healing
Partial-Thickness Burn	1st Degree	Epidermis remains intact and without blisters Erythema; skin blanches with pressure	Painful	Discomfort lasts 48–72 hours. Desquamation occurs in 3–7 days.
Partial-Thickness Burn	2nd Degree	Wet, shiny, weeping surface Blisters Wound blanches with pressure	Painful Very sensitive to touch, air currents	Superficial partial-thickness burn heals in <21 days. Deep partial-thickness burn requires >21 days for healing. Healing rates vary with burn depth and presence or absence of infection.
Full-Thickness Burn	3rd Degree	Color variable (i.e., deep red, white, black, brown) Surface dry Thrombosed vessels visible No blanching	Insensate (↓ pinprick sensation)	Autografting is required for healing.
Full-Thickness Burn	4th Degree	Color variable Charring visible in deepest areas Extremity movement limited	Insensate	Amputation of extremities is likely. Autografting is required for healing.

Fig. 31.15 Classification of burn depth according to depth of injury. (From Black, J. M. [2008]. *Medical-surgical nursing: Clinical management for positive outcomes* [8th ed.]. Philadelphia, PA: Saunders.)

Superficial (first-degree) burns are usually of minor significance. This type of injury involves the epidermal layer only. There is often a latent period followed by erythema. Tissue damage is minimal, and there is no blistering. The protective functions of the skin (such as bacterial and vapor barriers) remain intact, and systemic effects are rare. Pain is the predominant symptom, and the burn heals in 5 to 10 days without scarring. A mild sunburn is an example of a superficial burn.

Partial-thickness (second-degree) burns involve the epidermis and varying degrees of the dermal layer. These wounds are painful, moist, red, and blistered. With superficial partial-thickness burns, dermal elements are intact, and the wound should heal in approximately 14 to 21 days with variable amounts of scarring (Fig. 31.16). The wound is extremely sensitive to temperature changes, exposure to air, and light touch. Although classified as second-degree or partial-thickness burn, deep dermal burns resemble full-thickness injuries in many respects except that sweat glands and hair follicles remain intact. The burn may appear mottled, with pink, red, or waxy white areas exhibiting blisters and edema formation. Systemic effects are similar to those encountered with full-thickness burns. Although many of these wounds heal spontaneously, healing time may be extended beyond 21 days. These burn wounds often heal with extensive scarring.

Full-thickness (third-degree) burns are serious injuries that involve the entire epidermis and dermis and extend into subcutaneous tissue (see Fig. 31.15). Nerve endings, sweat glands, and hair follicles are destroyed. The burn varies in color from red to tan, waxy white, brown, or black. It is distinguished by a dry, leathery appearance and texture since the elasticity of the dermis is compromised (Fig. 31.17). Normally, full-thickness burns lack sensation in the area of injury because of the destruction of nerve endings. However, most full-thickness burns have superficial and partial-thickness burned areas at the periphery of the burn where nerve endings are intact and exposed. As the peripheral fibers regenerate, severe painful sensations return. Full-thickness wounds are not capable of reepithelialization and require surgical excision and grafting to close the wound.

Fourth-degree burns are full-thickness burns that involve underlying structures such as muscle, fascia, and bone. The wound appears dull and dry, and ligaments, tendons, and bone may be exposed (Fig. 31.18).

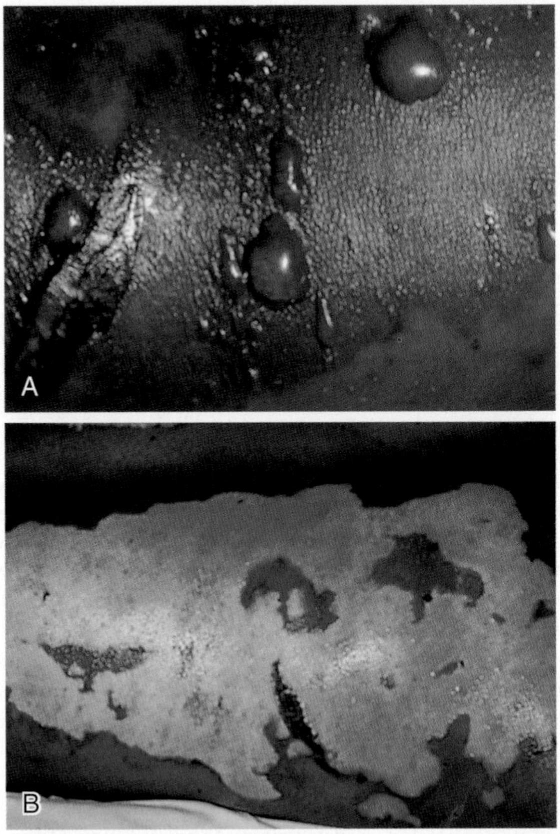

Fig. 31.16 Superficial partial-thickness burns on an African American child. **A,** Blisters intact. **B,** Blisters removed. (Courtesy Hillcrest Medical Center, Tulsa, OK.)

Severity of Injury

Burns are classified as minor, moderate, or major, which is useful in determining the disposition of the patient for treatment, which is guided by criteria developed by the American Burn Association (Table 31.10).

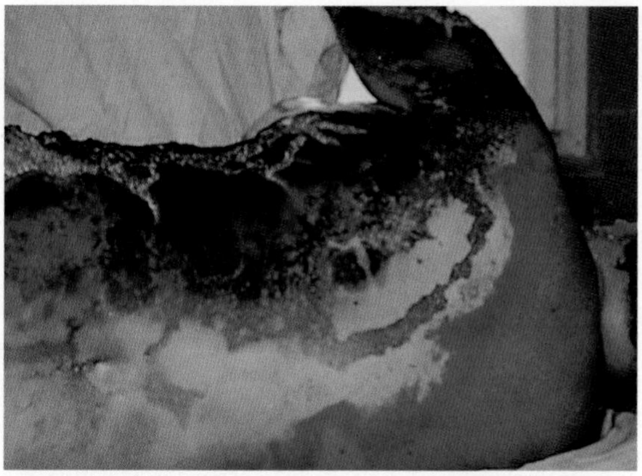

Fig. 31.17 *Bottom* to *top:* Deep partial-thickness burn (*red area*), full-thickness burn (*white area*), and full-thickness burn with eschar (*brown area*). (Courtesy Hillcrest Medical Center, Tulsa, OK.)

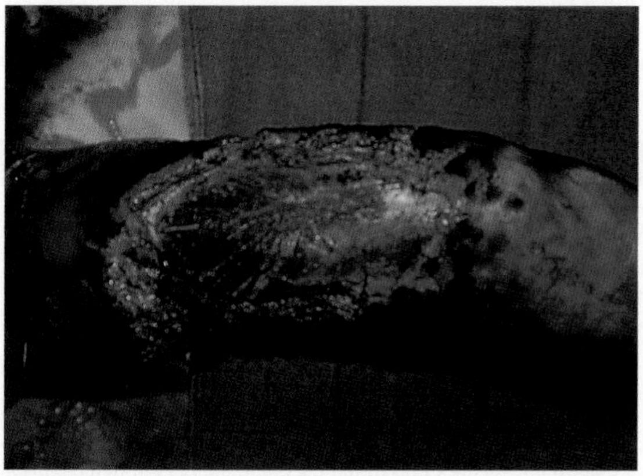

Fig. 31.18 Full-thickness burn with muscle and fascia involved. (Courtesy Hillcrest Medical Center, Tulsa, OK.)

Because the skin of infants is so thin, they are likely to sustain deeper injuries compared with older children. Children younger than 2 years old, especially those 6 months old or younger, have a significantly higher mortality rate than older children with burns of similar magnitude. Acute or chronic illnesses or superimposed injuries also complicate burn care and response to treatment.

Pathophysiology

Burn injuries produce both local and systemic effects that are related to the extent of tissue destruction. In superficial burns, the tissue damage is minimal. In partial-thickness burns, there is considerable edema and more severe capillary damage. With a major burn greater than 30% TBSA, there is a systemic response involving an increase in capillary permeability, allowing plasma proteins, fluids, and electrolytes to be lost. Maximum edema formation in a small burn occurs about 8 to 12 hours after injury (Rowan, Cancio, Elster, et al., 2015). After a larger burn, hypovolemia, associated with this phenomenon, will slow the rate of edema formation, with maximum effects at 18 to 24 hours.

Another systemic response is anemia, caused by direct heat destruction of red blood cells (RBCs), hemolysis of injured RBCs, and trapping of RBCs in the microvascular thrombi of damaged cells. A long-term decrease in the number of RBCs may occur as a result of increased RBC fragility. Initially, there is increased blood flow to the heart, brain, and kidneys, with decreased blood flow to the gastrointestinal tract. There is an increase in metabolism to maintain body heat, providing for the increased energy needs of the body.

Inhalation Injury

Trauma to the tracheobronchial tree often follows inhalation of heated gases and toxic chemicals produced during combustion. Although direct thermal injury to the upper airway may occur, heat damage below the vocal cords is rare. Inspired heated air is cooled in the upper airway before reaching the trachea. Reflex closure of the cords and laryngospasm also prevent full inhalation. However, evidence of direct thermal injury to the upper airway includes burns of the face and lips, singed nasal hairs, and laryngeal edema. Clinical manifestations may be delayed for as long as 24 to 48 hours (American Burn Association, 2016). Wheezing, increasing secretions, hoarseness, wet rales, and carbonaceous secretions are signs of respiratory tract involvement. Upper airway obstruction is often associated with burn shock and fluid resuscitation. In such situations, endotracheal intubation may also be necessary to preserve a patent airway.

Inhalation of carbon monoxide is suspected when the injury has occurred in an enclosed space. Carbon monoxide has a greater affinity for hemoglobin than oxygen, thereby depriving peripheral tissues and oxygen-dependent organs (e.g., heart, brain) of the oxygen needed for survival. Treatment is 100% oxygen, which reverses the situation rapidly. Mucosal erythema and edema followed by sloughing of the mucosa are manifestations of respiratory tract injury. A mucopurulent membrane replaces the mucosal lining and seriously compromises respiration and ventilation and possibly progresses to pneumonia. A significant increase in mortality has been observed with inhalation injury.

Complications

Burn-injured children are subject to a number of serious complications resulting from both the burn and systemic alterations. The immediate threat to life is related to airway compromise and profound burn shock. Burn shock occurs in the immediate postburn period and is marked by dramatic alterations in circulation. With fluid loss through the primary skin barrier, capillary permeability increases and vessels become dilated. Circulating blood volume decreases rapidly, and cardiac output is reduced. During healing, infection—both local and systemic sepsis—is the primary complication. Mortality associated with burns in children increases with the severity of the injury.

Pulmonary

Pulmonary problems are a major cause of fatality in children with direct burns or result in complications in the respiratory tract. Early in the postburn period, most pulmonary infections result from nosocomial exposure, immobility, and abdominal distention. The hematogenous variety occurs later and is related to the septic burn wound or other foci, such as phlebitis at the site of an invasive IV line. Respiratory problems include inhalation injuries, aspiration in unconscious patients, bacterial pneumonia, pulmonary edema, pulmonary embolus, posttraumatic pulmonary insufficiency, and atelectasis. The most common cause of respiratory failure in the pediatric age-group is bacterial pneumonia, which requires prolonged intubation and sometimes a tracheostomy. Tracheostomies increase the incidence of serious complications and are performed only in extreme cases.

A less common complication is pulmonary edema resulting from fluid overload or acute respiratory distress syndrome (ARDS) in association with gram-negative sepsis. ARDS results from pulmonary capillary damage and leakage of fluid into the interstitial spaces of the lung. A loss of compliance and interference with oxygenation are the consequences of pulmonary insufficiency in conjunction with systemic sepsis.

TABLE 31.10 Classification of Burn Severity Adapted From the American Burn Association's Criteria for Referral

	Minor[a]	Moderate	Major
% TBSA	<5% TBSA burn in young children <10% TBSA partial-thickness in children >10 years old	5-10% TBSA burn in young children	>10% TBSA burn in young children
Full-thickness burns	<2% full-thickness burn	2-5% full-thickness burn	>5% full-thickness burn
Other criteria		Suspected inhalation injury Circumferential burn Concomitant medical problem predisposing the patient to infection (e.g., diabetes, sickle cell disease)	Known inhalation injury Any significant burn to face, eyes, ears, genitalia, or joints Significant associated injuries (e.g., fracture, other major trauma)
Disposition	Usually outpatient	Admission to hospital, preferably one with expertise in burn care	Admission to a burn center

[a]Minor burns exclude any burn involving the face, hands, feet, perineum, or crossing joints; inhalation injury; circumferential burns; electrical injury; any injury with contaminant trauma; and children with psychosocial factors affecting the injury.
TBSA, Total body surface area.
Adapted from Committee on Trauma, American College of Surgeons. (2006). American Burn Association criteria for referral. In *Resources for optimal care of the injured patient.* Chicago, IL: American College of Surgeons.

Excessive Fluid Volume

Burns to the chest or abdomen decrease compliance and can contribute to a serious complication (increased intra-abdominal pressure) in burned individuals who receive larger than calculated amounts of fluids in the resuscitative period. Although children with increased intra-abdominal pressure readings tended to be younger, larger TBSA injuries and full-thickness components were significantly associated with elevated pressures and can result in tissue ischemia (Strang, Van Lieshout, Breederveld, et al., 2014). Increased intra-abdominal pressure has the potential to impair hemodynamics, pulmonary dysfunction, renal function, and hepatic malperfusion. Despite maintaining cardiac output with fluid replacement, renal function remains impaired in the presence of increased intra-abdominal pressure. To restore perfusion in children who have developed increased abdominal pressure, a decompressive laparotomy is necessary.

Wound Sepsis

Sepsis is a critical problem in the treatment of burns and an ever-present threat after the burn shock phase. Decreased level of consciousness and lethargy are early signs of sepsis. Initially, burn wounds are relatively pathogen free unless they are contaminated with potentially infectious material, such as dirt or polluted water. However, dead tissue and exudate provide a fertile field for bacterial growth. Early colonization of the wound surface by a preponderance of gram-positive organisms (primarily staphylococci) remains the chief cause of wound infection. Gram-negative organisms, particularly *Pseudomonas aeruginosa,* are ubiquitous and may cause invasive burn wound infections (Norbury, Herndon, Tanksley, et al., 2016). Early surgical excision of eschar together with placement of autograft reduces the incidence of sepsis.

Therapeutic Management

Emergency Care

The initial management of the burn patient begins at the scene of injury. The priority is to stop the burning process (see Emergency Treatment box). The child should then be transported immediately to the nearest medical facility for treatment and evaluation. The child and the family are usually extremely frightened and anxious; sensitivity to their emotional state and reassurance should be provided during the transport process.

EMERGENCY TREATMENT

Burns

Minor Burns

Stop the burning process:

- Remove burned clothing and jewelry.
- Apply cool water to the burn or hold the burned area under cool running water.
- Do not use ice.

Do not disturb any blisters that form unless the injury is from a chemical substance.

Do not apply anything to the burn.

Cover with a clean cloth if risk of damage or contamination.

Major Burns

Stop the burning process:

- Flame burns—smother the fire.
- Place victim in the horizontal position.
- Roll victim in a blanket or similar object; avoid covering the head.
- Remove burned clothing and jewelry.

Assess for an adequate airway and breathing.

If a child is not breathing, begin mouth-to-mouth resuscitation.

Cover the burn with a clean cloth.

Keep victim warm.

Begin intravenous fluids and oxygen therapy as prescribed.

Transport to medical aid.

Stop the burning process. The chief aim of rescue in flame burns is to smother the fire, not fan it. Children tend to panic and run, which spreads the flames and makes assistance more difficult. The burned child should be placed in a horizontal position and rolled in a blanket, rug, or similar article, with care taken not to cover the head and face because of the danger of inhalation of toxic fumes. If nothing is available, the victim should lie down and roll over slowly to extinguish the flames. Remaining in the vertical position may cause the hair to ignite or inhalation of flames, heat, or smoke.

Major burns should not be cooled for long periods of time. Heat is rapidly lost from burned areas, and additional cooling leads to a drop in core body temperature and potential circulatory collapse. Wet dressings also promote vasoconstriction because of cooling, resulting in impaired circulation to the burned area and increased tissue damage. Chemical burns require continuous flushing with large amounts of water before transport to a medical facility. The use of neutralizing agents on the skin is contraindicated because heat from a chemical reaction is initiated and further injury may result. If the chemical is in a powder form, adding water may spread the caustic agent. The powder should be brushed off, if possible, before flushing the area.

Burned clothing is removed to prevent further damage from smoldering fabric and hot beads of melted synthetic materials. Jewelry is removed to eliminate the transfer of heat from the metal and constriction resulting from edema formation. This also provides access to the burn and prevents painful removal later.

Assess the victim's condition. As soon as the flames are extinguished, the child is assessed. Airway, breathing, and circulation are the primary concerns. Cardiopulmonary complications may result from inhalation of toxic fumes and smoke, exposure to electric current, hypovolemia, and shock. Emergency measures are instituted as appropriate.

Cover the burn. The burn should be covered with a clean dry cloth to prevent hypothermia, decrease pain by eliminating air contact, and prevent contamination. No attempt should be made to treat the burn. Application of topical ointments, oils, or other home remedies is contraindicated.

Transport the child to medical aid. The child with an extensive burn is not given anything by mouth to avoid aspiration in the presence of upper airway edema. The child is transported to the nearest medical facility. If this cannot be accomplished within a relatively short period, IV access should be established, if possible, with a large-bore catheter. Oxygen is administered, if available, at 100%. A report of the initial assessment, suspected inhalation injury, associated trauma, and any interventions implemented is given to the medical facility assuming care of the child.

Provide reassurance. Providing reassurance and psychologic support to both the family and the child helps immeasurably during the period of postburn crisis. Reducing anxiety conserves energy that the family and child will need to cope with the physiologic and emotional stress of a burn.

Minor Burns

Treatment of burns classified as minor usually can be managed adequately on an outpatient basis when it is determined that the parent can be relied on to carry out instructions for care and observation. Patients with less than optimum circumstances may require close follow-up to ensure adherence with treatment.

Cleanse the burn with a mild soap and tepid water. Debridement of the burn includes removal of any embedded debris, chemicals, and devitalized tissue. Removal of intact blisters remains controversial (Smith, 2000). Some authorities argue that blisters provide a barrier against infection; others maintain that blister fluid is an effective medium for the growth of microorganisms. However, blisters should be broken if the burn is due to a chemical agent to control absorption or if the blisters are large enough that the buildup of fluid will cause pressure resulting in increased pain.

Most practitioners favor covering the burn with an antimicrobial ointment to reduce the risk of infection and to provide some form of pain relief. The dressing consists of nonadherent fine-mesh gauze placed over the ointment and a light wrap of gauze dressing that avoids interference with movement. This helps keep the burn clean and protects it from trauma. The caregiver is instructed to wash the burn, reapply the dressing, and return the child to the office or clinic as directed for burn wound observation. The frequency of dressing changes may vary from once a day to every other day or longer depending on the burn wound classification and dressing used. If there is a high probability of infection or other complications or if there is doubt about the ability to carry out instructions, the caregiver may be directed to bring the patient in more often for dressing changes and inspection. Another option is to have a nurse make a home visit to inspect the burn and perform the dressing change. Frequent removal of the dressing is an effective mode of debridement. Soaking the dressing in tepid water or normal saline before removal helps loosen the dressing and debris as well as reduces discomfort. Burns of the face are usually treated by an open method. Wash and debride the burn in the same manner and apply a thin film of antimicrobial ointment without a dressing. This is repeated at least twice a day.

Obtain a tetanus history on admission. Administer tetanus prophylaxis if there is no history of immunization or if more than 5 years have passed since the last immunization. A mild analgesic (such as acetaminophen) is usually sufficient to relieve discomfort; the antipyretic effect of the drug also alleviates the sensation of heat.

Most minor burns heal without difficulty. Hospitalization may be indicated if the burn margin becomes erythematous or grossly purulent or if the child develops evidence of a systemic reaction, such as fever or tachycardia. Evaluate the child for functional impairment. Instruct the caregiver in the exercise and ambulation program. After healing, an evaluation of scar maturation and range of motion will indicate any need for further therapy.

Major Burns

When a child with extensive burns is admitted to the hospital for treatment, various assessments are conducted and therapies initiated. Of these, the priority concerns include the establishment and maintenance of an adequate airway, initiation of fluid administration, and evaluation and treatment of the burn. Although the order of implementation may vary from institution to institution and the condition of the child, a number of procedures and activities are generally initiated on admission. Some are carried out simultaneously (Box 31.4).

QUALITY PATIENT OUTCOMES: Acute Management of Burns

- Stable body temperature
- Adequate fluid replacement and urinary output
- Adequate nutrition and reduction of metabolic losses
- No evidence of acute complications
- Pain controlled
- Evidence of wound healing
- No evidence of contractures
- Adequate emotional support

Establishment of adequate airway. The priority is airway maintenance. The inhalation of noxious agents or respiratory burns is suggested when there is a history of injury in an enclosed space; edema of the oral and nasal membranes; burn injury to the face, nares, and upper torso; hyperemia; and blisters or evidence of trauma to the upper respiratory passages. When respiratory involvement is suspected or evident, 100% oxygen is administered and blood gas values, including carbon monoxide levels, are determined.

If the child exhibits changes in sensorium, air hunger, or other signs of respiratory distress, an endotracheal tube is inserted to maintain the airway. When severe edema of the face and neck is anticipated, intubation is performed before swelling makes intubation difficult or impossible. Controlled intubation is preferred to an emergency intubation. Intubation allows for the delivery of humidified oxygen, the removal of secretions from respiratory passages, and the provision of ventilatory support. When full-thickness burns encircle the chest, constricting

BOX 31.4 Major Burn Management

- Ascertain the adequacy of the airway and provide oxygen, intubation, and ventilatory support as indicated.
- Assess breathing rate and depth. Note any use of accessary muscles, nasal flaring, or grunting, which may indicate respiratory compromise.
- Insert a large-bore intravenous (IV) line, preferably through unburned skin, to deliver fluids at a sufficiently rapid rate to effect resuscitation.
- Remove clothing and jewelry and examine for secondary trauma.
- Evaluate the burn wound and determine the extent and depth of injury.
- Obtain an admission weight.
- Calculate fluid requirements and establish the appropriate regimen.
- Obtain baseline laboratory studies.
- Provide IV medication for control of pain and anxiety only after adequate oxygenation is ensured and fluid resuscitation is initiated.
- Insert a nasogastric tube to empty stomach contents and maintain gastric decompression.
- Insert an indwelling Foley catheter to obtain specimens and monitor hourly output.
- Perform escharotomy or fasciotomy to the chest and extremities for constricting circumferential eschar, elevated compartment pressures, or impaired circulation.
- Apply topical antimicrobials and dressings to the burn wounds.
- Obtain a history regarding the injury and other pertinent data.
- Administer appropriate tetanus prophylaxis.
- Prophylactic antibiotic administration is not recommended.

eschar (dead tissue) may limit chest wall excursion, and ventilation of the child becomes more difficult. Young children are particularly at risk because of the pliability of the skeletal structure. Escharotomy of the chest, where the eschar is incised through to the fatty tissue, relieves this constriction and improves ventilation.

Fluid replacement therapy. The objectives of fluid therapy are to (1) compensate for water and sodium lost to traumatized areas and interstitial spaces; (2) reestablish sodium balance; (3) restore circulating volume; (4) provide adequate perfusion; (5) correct acidosis; and (6) improve renal function.

Fluid replacement is required during the first 24 hours because of fluid shifts that occur after the burn. Various formulas are used to calculate fluid needs, and the one adopted depends on practitioner preference. Crystalloid solutions are used during this initial phase of therapy. Parameters (such as urinary output volume, vital signs [especially heart rate], adequacy of capillary filling, and state of sensorium) determine adequacy of fluid resuscitation.

After the initial 24-hour period, theoretically there is a capillary seal, and capillary permeability is restored. Colloid solutions (such as albumin or fresh-frozen plasma) are useful in maintaining plasma volume. However, children with burns usually require fluids in excess of their calculated maintenance and replacement volume. Reasons for this may include underestimation of burn size (particularly in pediatric patients), delay in the initiation of fluid resuscitation, pulmonary injury that sequesters resuscitation fluid in the lung, and electrical injury with greater tissue destruction than that which is visible. Irreversible burn shock that persists despite aggressive fluid resuscitation remains a significant cause of death in the immediate postburn period. Fluid balance may continue to be a problem throughout the course of treatment, especially during periods in which there may be considerable evaporative loss from the burn.

Nutrition. The enhanced metabolic requirements and catabolism in severe burns make nutritional needs of paramount importance and often difficult to satisfy. To avoid protein breakdown, the diet must provide sufficient calories to meet the increased metabolic needs and enough protein. Hypoglycemia can result from the stress of the burn because the liver glycogen stores are rapidly depleted.

A high-protein, high-calorie diet is encouraged. Many children have poor appetites and are unable to meet energy requirements solely by oral feeding. Oral feedings are encouraged unless the child is intubated or paralytic ileus develops. Most children with burns in excess of 25% TBSA require supplementation with enteral feedings. Early and continued nutritional support is an important part of therapy for seriously burned patients. Children who require enteral supplementation must be monitored for adequacy of feeds, feeding intolerance, and tube malposition. The nurse should also monitor and report any abdominal distention, diarrhea, or electrolyte and metabolic deviations. If nutritional requirements cannot be met entirely by the enteral route, parenteral hyperalimentation is used to supplement intake. However, enteral feedings increase blood flow in the intestinal tract, preserve gastrointestinal function, and minimize bacterial translocation by decreasing mucosal atrophy of the intestines. These factors make enteral feeding the preferred route of nutritional support (Clark, Imran, Madni, et al., 2017).

To facilitate growth and proliferation of epithelial cells, administration of vitamins A and C is begun early in the post-burn period. Zinc is also supplemented because of its important role in burn healing and epithelialization.

Medication. Antibiotics are usually not administered prophylactically. The administration of systemic antibiotics to control wound colonization is not indicated because decreased circulation to the burned area prevents delivery of the medication to areas of deepest burn injury. The most reliable indicator of developing wound infection is changes in the appearance of the wound (Greenhalgh, 2017). Appropriate antibiotics are instituted to treat the specific identified organism. Remember, otitis media can also be a source of fever in the pediatric patient.

Some form of sedation and analgesia is required in the care of the burned child. There is no consensus for practice guidelines for procedural sedation and analgesia for pediatric patients across burn centers. Choice of the agent should depend on efficacy and safety of the agent as well as consideration of the age of the child, burn depth, extent and location, and length of the procedure (Fagin & Palmieri, 2017). The unstable circulatory status and edema formation preclude intramuscular or subcutaneous administration of these medications for effectiveness. Opioids, such as fentanyl (Sublimaze) and morphine, midazolam (Versed), propofol, ketamine, and dexmedetomidine, are the most commonly used agents. Dosage monitoring is important because tolerance to opioids may develop.

The use of short-acting anesthetic agents, such as propofol (Diprivan) and nitrous oxide, has proven beneficial in eliminating procedural pain. Pharyngeal reflexes remain intact, thus ensuring a patent airway. Propofol is an IV sedative hypnotic agent that produces sedation in less than 1 minute and lasts only a few minutes. For any conscious or unconscious sedation, the child must be monitored continuously during the procedure (see Chapter 20, Preoperative Care, and Chapter 5).

Management of the burn wound. After the initial period of burn shock and the restoration of fluid balance, the primary concern is the burn itself. The objectives of burn management include prevention of infection, removal of devitalized tissue, and closure of the burn. The application of dressings and topical antimicrobial therapy reduce pain by minimizing the exposure to air.

Primary excision. In children with large, full-thickness burns, excision is performed as soon as the patient is hemodynamically stable after initial resuscitation. Because the burn wound precipitates an exaggerated physiologic response, many complications do not resolve until the eschar is excised and the wound is closed. Early excision of the burn is an effective therapy to reduce the incidence of infection and the threat of sepsis, thus decreasing mortality (Rowan et al., 2015).

Debridement. Partial-thickness burns require debridement of devitalized tissue to promote healing. Debridement is painful and requires analgesia and a sedative before the procedure. IV analgesics are most effective when they are administered just before the onset of procedural pain. Early usage of appropriate sedation for burn wound care allows for early aggressive wound debridement (Fagin & Palmieri, 2017). Medications given for pain need to be readily available during this procedure and may need to be titrated up during the procedure.

Hydrotherapy is used to cleanse the burn and involves either showering (spraying off the burn) or immersion (soaking in a tub) at least once a day. Immersion hydrotherapy is becoming less common and is being replaced by shower hydrotherapy. The water acts to loosen and remove sloughing tissue, exudate, and topical medications. Any loose tissue is carefully trimmed away before the burn is redressed. Hydrotherapy helps cleanse not only the burn, but also the entire body and aids in maintenance of range of motion.

Topical agents. Methods used for managing the burn include:

- **Open**—involves applying the topical antibacterial cream or ointment directly to the wound without use of gauze or any type of covering. This process may be repeated throughout the day, two to three times, as ordered. Burns of the face and ears are often treated by an open method type of wound care.
- **Semiocclusive/occlusive (closed)**—the wound care agent is prepared on some type of sterile gauze or comes prepackaged. When this method is used, during application all edges of the wound should be covered completely. Once this is completed the area is usually covered with an overwrapped layer of gauze (secondary dressing) and then held in place or secured. Some prepackaged long-acting prepared dressings are not changed daily.

These methods of care provide burn wound coverage and use some type of topical agent. Topical agents do not eliminate organisms from the burn but can effectively inhibit bacterial growth. To be effective, a topical application must be nontoxic, capable of diffusing through eschar, harmless to viable tissue, inexpensive, and easy to apply. A variety of specific agents are available; examples include bacitracin, silver sulfadiazine (Silvadene), and mafenide acetate (Sulfamylon). Some topical agents are packaged and prepared on fine-mesh gauze that allows ease of application. The gauze provides necessary protection for the burn, is nonadherent, maximizes patient comfort, increases rate of healing, decreases the need for frequent dressing changes, and is cost effective. Examples include a flexible low-adherent polyester layer coated with silver (Acticoat Flex 3 or Flex 7), a silicone foam dressing with silver (Mepilex Ag), and a wound contact layer consisting of a polyamide net coated with soft silicone (Mepitel). Assessment of the dressing, drainage (if any), and other complications is still completed daily.

Temporary skin substitutes. Permanent coverage of extensive burns is a prolonged process that requires repeated operative procedures using general anesthesia for atraumatic care in debridement and grafting. Early closure shortens the period of metabolic stress and decreases the likelihood of burn wound sepsis. In the acute phase, temporary skin substitutes cover and protect the burn from contamination, reduce fluid and protein loss, increase the rate of epithelialization, reduce pain, and facilitate movement of joints to retain range of motion.

Allograft (homograft) skin is obtained from human cadavers that are screened for communicable diseases. Allograft is particularly useful as a temporary skin covering of surgically excised deep partial- and full-thickness burns and extensive burns when available donor sites are limited. Severe immunosuppression occurs in massively burned children, and the allograft becomes adherent. The allograft can remain in place until suitable donor sites become available. Typically, rejection is seen approximately 14 to 21 days after application (Rezaei, Beiraghi-Toosi, Ahmadabadi, et al., 2017). The availability of tissue banks and a supply of suitable donors limit the use of allografts.

Xenograft from a variety of species, most notably pigs, is commercially available. Porcine xenograft will adhere to a clean superficial burn and provide excellent pain control while the burn heals (Vloemans, Hermans, van der Wal, et al., 2014). Porcine xenograft dressings are replaced daily or every 2 to 3 days. They are particularly effective in children with partial-thickness scald burns of the hands and face because they allow relatively pain-free movement, which can reduce contracture formation.

When applied early to superficial partial-thickness burns, skin substitutes stimulate epithelial growth and faster wound healing. However, they must be applied to clean burns. If the dressing covers areas of heavy microbial contamination, infection occurs beneath the dressing. In the case of partial-thickness burns, such infection may convert the burn to a full-thickness injury.

Synthetic skin coverings are available for the management of partial-thickness burns and donor sites. Ideally, the dressing should provide the properties of human skin, including adherence, elasticity, durability, and hemostasis. Synthetic skin coverings are readily available and are composed of a variety of materials that are usually permeable to air, vapor, and fluids.

Since these dressings do not contain antimicrobial properties, it is important that the burn is free of debris before the dressing is applied. Body temperature elevation or evidence of purulence, erythema, or cellulitis around the wound edges may indicate that the burn has become infected beneath the dressing. If this occurs, prompt discontinuation of the synthetic dressing is indicated. Examples include a pertrolatum dressing (Xeroform), a hydrocolloid dressing (DuoDERM), and transparent adhesive films (OpSite and Tegaderm). All synthetic dressings are reputed to hasten burn wound healing and reduce discomfort.

Permanent skin coverings. Permanent coverage of deep partial- and full-thickness burns is usually accomplished with a split-thickness skin graft (autograft). The graft consists of the epidermis and a portion of the dermis removed from the donor site of an intact area of skin by a special instrument called a dermatome (Fig. 31.19). With extensive burns, it is often difficult to find enough viable skin to cover the burns;

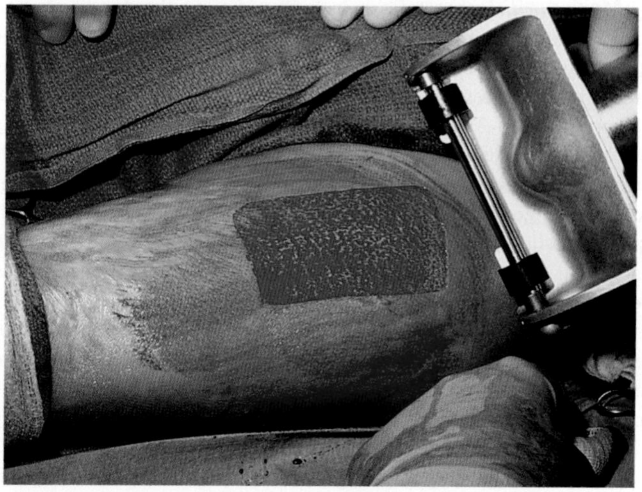

Fig. 31.19 Removal of split-thickness skin graft with a dermatome.

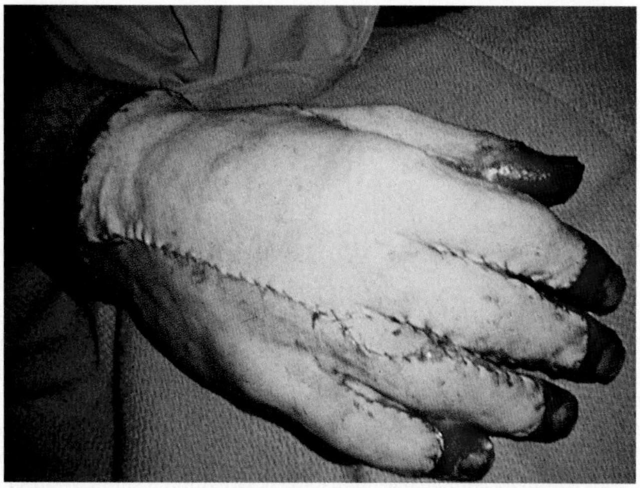

Fig. 31.20 Sheet graft.

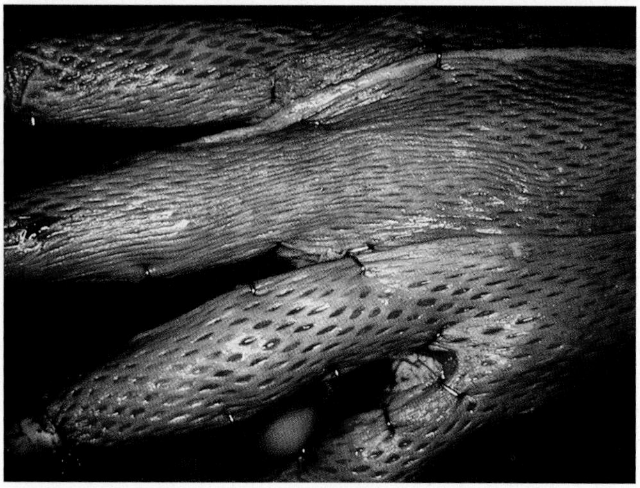

Fig. 31.21 Mesh graft.

therefore available donor sites and special techniques are used. Split-thickness skin grafts may be sheet graft or mesh graft.

Sheet graft. A sheet of skin removed from the donor site is placed intact over the recipient site and sutured in place; this is used in areas where cosmetic results are most visible—for example, the face (Fig. 31.20).

Mesh graft. A sheet of skin is removed from the donor site and passed through a mesher, which produces tiny slits in the skin before application that allow the skin to cover 1.5 to 9 times the area of the sheet graft; this results in a less desirable cosmetic, but functional outcome (Fig. 31.21).

The donor site is dressed with synthetic wound coverings until the dressing separates at 10 to 14 days when the wound is healed. Dressings are not changed on donor sites to avoid damage to newly healed, delicate epithelium. Healed donor sites are available for reharvesting in patients with extensive burns and limited undamaged skin, but the quality of skin is decreased when multiple grafts are taken.

Dermal replacements. The development of products that replace or allow the dermis to regenerate has produced significant improvement in burn wound healing and decreased scar formation. Integra (artificial skin) is a two-layer membrane made of collagen (a fibrous protein from animal tendons and cartilage) and silicone. Applied over the burn following excision, the outer silicone layer is later peeled off after the dermis is formed. The application of artificial skin does not replace the grafting procedure but prepares the burn wound to accept an ultrathin autograft.

AlloDerm is another product that is used similarly to artificial skin. It is made from human cadaveric tissue that is processed to remove cells that can lead to tissue rejection. The resulting acellular tissue contains epithelial elements that provide a foundation for new tissue regeneration. With dermal replacements, advantages include faster healing of the burn wound when integrity of the dermis is restored, faster healing of donor sites with the use of ultrathin grafts, and restoration of sweat glands and hair follicles. A disadvantage is its high cost.

Cultured epithelium. When burns are extensive and donor sites for split-thickness skin grafting are limited, it is possible to culture cells from a full-thickness skin biopsy and produce coherent sheets that can be applied to clean, excised full-thickness burns. Epithelial cell culture grafts offer the possibility of an unlimited source of autografts in patients with extensive burns. Cultured epithelial autografts (CEAs) are effective in early wound closure. The child's own skin is fractionated and cultured in a porcine media to form a thin epithelial layer that is applied to the burn. This technique offers an improved rate of survival in patients with extensive burns and limited donor sites.

Application of skin cells. New technologies are emerging for skin repair of the burn patient. ReCell is one such device that processes a solution of the patient's harvested skin cells using minimal donor site skin. The device produces an autologous skin cell suspension that the burn surgeon then sprays onto the open wound in surgery to repair skin texture and color (Holmes, Molnar, Carter, et al., 2018).

Nursing Care Management

Because the care of burned children encompasses a broad range of skills, nursing care has been divided into segments that correspond with the major phases of burn treatment. The **acute phase**, also referred to as the *emergent* or *resuscitative phase,* involves the first 24 to 48 hours. The **management phase** extends from the completion of adequate resuscitation through burn coverage. The **rehabilitative phase** begins when the majority of the burns have healed and rehabilitation has become the predominant focus of the care plan. This phase continues until all reconstructive procedures and corrective measures are accomplished (often a period of months or years).

Acute Phase

The primary emphasis during the emergent phase is the treatment of burn shock and the management of pulmonary status. Monitoring vital signs, urine output, fluid infusion, and respiratory parameters are ongoing activities in the hours immediately after injury. IV infusion is begun immediately and is regulated to maintain an hourly urinary output of at least 0.5 to 1 ml/kg in children weighing less than 30 kg (66 pounds) or 30 ml/h in children weighing more than 30 kg (American Burn Association, 2016). Urinary output, vital signs, laboratory data, and objective signs of adequate hydration guide the rate of fluid administration.

Children who are hospitalized with burns require constant observation and assessment for complications. Alterations in electrolyte balance produce clinical symptoms of confusion, weakness, cardiac irregularities, and seizures. Changes in respiratory function and gas exchange are reflected clinically by restlessness, irritability, increased work of breathing, and alterations in blood gas values. The loss of protective function of the skin exposes burned children to increased risk of hypothermia. Edema formation and circulatory impairment result in the loss of sensation and deep, throbbing pain.

Burn centers maintain a pictorial record of the burns to record progress and for legal purposes (if nonaccidental trauma is suspected). Burn wounds are treated according to the protocol of the specific burn

> **! NURSING ALERT**
>
> Evaluate the burned extremity and check the pulse every hour. If unable to palpate, use a Doppler (an ultrasonic pulse probe that can detect blood flow) to ascertain loss of circulation and pulse. If the pulse is lost, escharotomy may be necessary to relieve the edema causing pressure on blood vessels to restore adequate circulation.

center. The burn team monitors infection control procedures and ensures that staff and visitors comply with established protocols to prevent cross-contamination in the burn unit.

Throughout the acute phase of care, the psychosocial needs of the child and his or her family are carefully considered. The child is frightened, uncomfortable, and often confused. The child may be isolated from familiar persons and surroundings; the overwhelming physical needs at this time are the primary focus of the staff and parents.

Management and Rehabilitative Phases

After the patient's condition is stabilized, the management phase begins. The interprofessional team concentrates on preventing burn wound infections, closing the burn as quickly as possible, and managing the numerous complications. Although the rehabilitative phase begins when permanent burn wound closure has been achieved, rehabilitation issues are identified on admission and are included in the care plan throughout the hospital course.

> **! NURSING ALERT**
>
> In a pediatric burn patient, a decreased level of consciousness, increased restlessness, and lethargy are some of the first signs of overwhelming sepsis and may indicate inadequate hydration. A decrease in blood pressure is considered a late sign in a pediatric patient with sepsis. Assessment of capillary refill and pulses are another important indicator of the adequacy of hydration. With inadequate hydration, a spiking fever and diminished bowel sounds accompanied by paralytic ileus are noted and progressively increase over 48 to 72 hours, after which the temperature falls to subnormal limits. At this time the wound deteriorates, the white blood cell count is depressed, and septic shock becomes manifest.

Comfort Management

The severe pain of the burn and resultant therapies, the anxiety generated by these experiences, sleep deprivation, itching related to burn wound healing, and the conscious and unconscious interpretations of traumatic events contribute to the psychologic behaviors commonly observed in children with burns. It is always difficult to deal with a child in pain, and inflicting pain on a helpless child is contrary to the empathic nature of nursing. Interventions to promote comfort may include medications (as previously mentioned), relaxation techniques, distraction therapy, behavioral techniques, operant conditioning (e.g., tokens, star chart), and family participation (Fagin & Palmieri, 2017).

Children need age-appropriate explanations before all procedures. When children appear to accept pain with little or no response, psychologic consultation may be needed. Consistency in caregivers is important. If this is not possible, a carefully developed, interprofessional care plan is necessary to provide consistency.

Care of the Burn Wound

The nurse has a major responsibility for cleansing, debriding, and applying topical agents and dressings to the burn. Pain medication should be administered so that the peak effect of the drug coincides with the procedure. Children who understand the procedure to be performed and have some perceived control demonstrate less maladaptive behavior. Children also respond well to participating in decisions (see Atraumatic Care box).

> **ATRAUMATIC CARE**
>
> ***Reducing the Stress of Burn Care Procedures***
>
> - Have all materials ready before beginning the procedure.
> - Administer appropriate analgesics and sedatives.
> - Remind the child of the impending procedure to allow sufficient time to prepare.
> - Allow the child to test and approve the temperature of the water.
> - Allow the child to select the area of the body on which to begin.
> - Allow the child to request a short rest period during the procedure.
> - Allow the child to remove the dressings if desired.
> - Provide something constructive for the child to do during the procedure (e.g., holding a package of dressings or a roll of gauze).
> - Inform the child when the procedure is near completion.
> - Praise the child for cooperation.

Outer dressings are removed first. Any dressings that have adhered to the burn can be easily removed by applying tepid water or normal saline. Loose or easily detached tissue is debrided during the cleansing process. In dressing the burn, it is important that all areas be clean, that medication is amply applied, and that no two burned surfaces touch each other (e.g., fingers or toes, ears touching the side of the head). If they are touching, the burned surfaces will heal together, causing deformity or dysfunction.

Topical agents may be applied directly to the burn with a tongue blade or gloved hand as well as using impregnated fine-mesh gauze or prepackaged products. All dressings applied circumferentially should be wrapped in a distal-to-proximal manner. The dressing is applied with sufficient tension to remain in place but not so tightly as to impair circulation or limit motion. Elastic net is then applied to secure the dressing in place. A stable dressing is especially important when the child is ambulatory.

Standard Precautions, including the use of personal protective equipment as indicated, should be followed when caring for patients with burns. Frequent hand and forearm washing is the single most important element of the infection control program. Strict policies for cleaning the environment and patient care equipment should be implemented to minimize the risk of cross-contamination. All visitors and members of other departments should be oriented to the infection control policies, including the importance of hand and forearm washing and use of protective garb. Visitors should be screened for infection and contagious diseases before patient contact.

Prevention of Complications

Acute care. The maintenance of body temperature is important to children with burns. Core body temperature is supported when energy is conserved with an environmental temperature of 28°C to 33°C (82.4°F to 91.4°F). Large areas of the body should not be exposed simultaneously during dressing changes. Warmed solutions, linens, occlusive dressings, heat shields, radiant warmers, and warming blankets assist in preventing hypothermia.

The chief danger during acute care is infection: wound infection, generalized sepsis, or bacterial pneumonia. Accurate and ongoing assessments of all parameters that provide clues to the early diagnosis and treatment of infection are essential. Symptoms of sepsis include a decreased level of consciousness, a rising or falling white blood cell count, hyperthermia progressing to hypothermia, increasing fluid

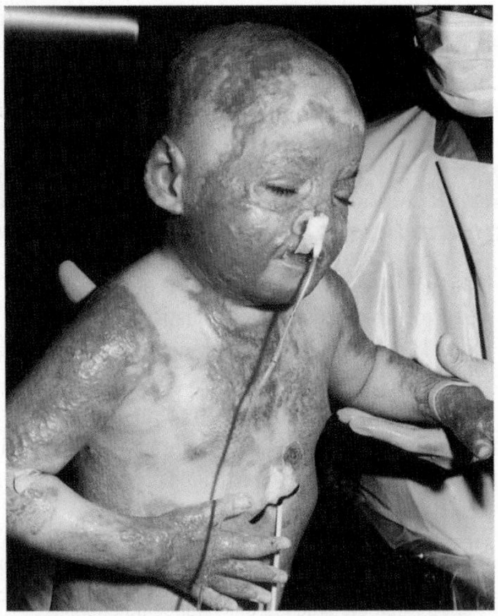

Fig. 31.22 Extensive scars from a flame burn. (Courtesy The Paul and Carol David Foundation Burn Institute, Akron, OH.)

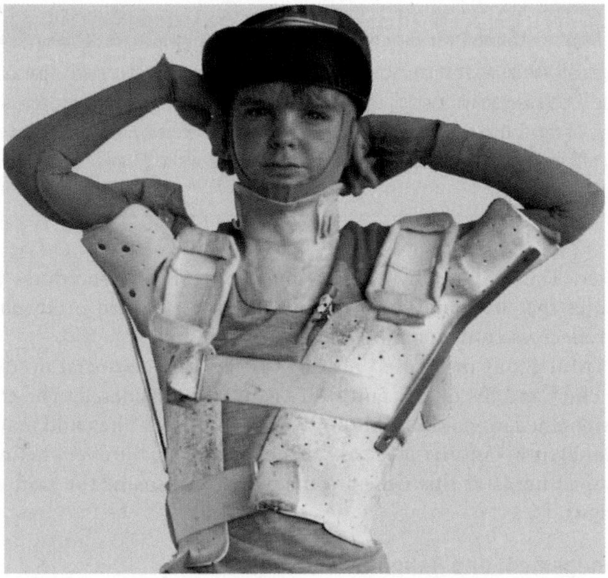

Fig. 31.23 Child in an elasticized (Jobst) garment and "airplane" splints.

requirements, hypoactive or absent bowel sounds, a rising or falling blood glucose level, tachycardia, tachypnea, and thrombocytopenia. Infection delays the progress of burn wound healing.

Children are reluctant to move if movement causes pain, and they are likely to assume a position of comfort. Unfortunately, the most comfortable position often encourages the formation of contractures and loss of function. Ongoing efforts to prevent contractures include maintaining proper body alignment, positioning and splinting the involved extremities in extension, providing active and passive physical therapy, and encouraging spontaneous movement when feasible. Frequent position changes are important to promote adequate bronchopulmonary hygiene and capillary perfusion to common pressure areas. Low–air loss beds are beneficial for morbidly obese children or children with posterior grafts. Special attention should be given to areas at risk for increased pressure, such as the posterior scalp, heels, sacrum, and areas exposed to mechanical irritation from splints and dressings.

Long-term care. When the burn heals, the rehabilitative phase of care begins. Scar formation becomes a major problem as the burn heals (Fig. 31.22). Contractile properties of the scar tissue can result in disabling contractures, deformity, and disfigurement.

Uniform pressure applied to the scar decreases the blood supply. When pressure is removed, blood supply to the scar is immediately increased; therefore periods without pressure should be brief to avoid nourishment of the hypertrophic tissue. Continuous pressure to areas of scarring can be achieved by elastic tubular bandages or commercially available pressure garments. Because these custom-made garments are often worn for months, revisions may be required as the child grows. It is much easier to prevent scarring and contracture of the burn than to resolve an existing problem. Splints and appliances may also be needed until wound maturation is achieved (Fig. 31.23).

Scar tissue has certain significant properties, particularly for growing children. Intense itching may occur in healing burn wounds and scar tissue until the scar is no longer active. Itching is usually treated with a variety of medications; hydroxyzine and diphenhydramine are examples of two such medications.

Frequently apply a moisturizer such as Aveeno Baby, Alpha Keri, Vaseline Intensive Care, or cocoa butter. Other brands with the word "ultra-healing" in their title that are fragrance-free and do not contain alcohol can be used. Massage therapy during the application of moisturizers is also beneficial to stretch scar tissue and aid in contracture prevention. Scar tissue has no sweat glands, and children with extensive scarring may experience difficulty during hot weather. Caregivers should be alerted to this possibility and be prepared to institute alternate methods of cooling when necessary.

Scar tissue does not grow and expand as does normal tissue, which may create difficulties, especially in functional areas such as on the hands and over joints. Additional surgery is sometimes required to allow independent functioning in daily activities, to improve cosmetic appearance, or to restore anatomic integrity.

The nursing activities in the rehabilitative phase of treatment focus on the child's and family's adaptation to the burn and their ability to reintegrate into the community. The psychologic pain and sequelae of severe burn injury are as intense as the physical trauma. The impact of severe burns taxes the coping mechanisms at all ages. Very young children, who suffer acutely from separation anxiety, and adolescents, who are developing an identity, are probably the most affected psychologically. Toddlers cannot understand why the parents they love and who protect them can leave them in such a frightening and unfamiliar place. Adolescents, in the process of achieving independence from the family, find themselves in a dependent role with a damaged body. Being different from others, especially at a time when conformity with peers is so important may be difficult to accept.

Anticipation of the return to school can be overwhelming and frightening. It is essential that health care professionals recognize the importance of preparing teachers and classmates for the child's return. Teachers need to be provided with information to assist the child and family and to promote the child's optimal adjustment. Hospital-sponsored school reentry programs use a variety of methods to provide education and information about the implications of the injury, the garments and appliances, and the need for support and acceptance. Telephone calls, videotapes, information packets, and visits by members of the health care team offer opportunities to help with reintegration into the school environment—a focal point of the child's life.

Psychosocial Support of the Child

Children should begin early to do as much for themselves as possible and to be active participants in their care. Loss of control and perceived helplessness may result in acting-out behaviors. During illness, children can regress to a previous developmental level that allows them to deal with stress. As children begin to participate in their care, they gain confidence and self-esteem. Fears and anxieties diminish with accomplishment and self-confidence. If the child demonstrates nonadherence in the rehabilitative phase, a behavior modification program can be initiated to promote or reward the child's accomplishments in care.

Play is a normal part of a young child's life. This normalcy becomes disrupted and compromised when a burn injury occurs and various treatments and therapies are necessary. In the hospital, a child life specialist can be of assistance in decreasing distress, fear, and sometimes pain during procedures or care. Having a child life specialist assess the child and introduce distraction techniques and play therapy can be instrumental throughout hospitalization (Fagin & Palmieri, 2017).

Children need to know that their injury and the treatments are not punishment for real or imagined transgressions and that the nurse understands their fear, anger, and discomfort. They also need human touch. This is often difficult to arrange for the child with massive burns. Stroking areas of unburned skin is comforting. Even older children enjoy sitting on the parent's or caregiver's lap and being cuddled and hugged. This can be a reward or a comfort in times of stress, but most of all it should be kept in mind that it is a natural part of childhood.

Psychosocial Support of the Family

Recognizing and respecting each family's strengths, differences, and methods of coping allow the nurse to respond to their unique needs by implementing a family-centered approach to care. In the acute phase, most of the attention is focused on the child, and the parents or caregivers may feel powerless and ineffectual. Parents or caregivers may feel overwhelming guilt, whether or not this guilt is justified. They feel responsible for the injury. These feelings may impede the child's rehabilitation. Parents or caregivers may indulge the child and allow nonadherent behaviors that affect physical and emotional recovery. They need to be informed of the child's progress and helped to cope with their feelings while providing support to their child. The nurse can help them understand that it is not selfish to look after themselves and their own needs in order to meet their child's needs. It is important to recognize the parents' or caregivers' need to grieve the change in their child's normal appearance as part of the grieving process. Definitive professional help may be needed for those whose response to the injury is severe or whose response to stress is manifested in destructive behavior.

The parents or caregivers are members of the interprofessional team and participate in the development of the care plan. It is important to facilitate their input; to consider all aspects of the physical, emotional, social, and cultural factors affecting the child and family; and to establish a realistic home therapy program. The family's willingness to assume responsibility for care and their ability to implement the therapeutic regimen are assessed. Home, school, and other environmental factors are explored; financial concerns and available community resources are discussed; and a specific care plan for the child, with an anticipated follow-up program, is developed.

Prevention of Burn Injury

The best intervention is to prevent burns from occurring. Hot liquids in the kitchen and bathroom most commonly injure infants and toddlers. Hot liquids should be kept out of reach; tablecloths and dangling appliance cords are often pulled by toddlers, who spill hot grease and liquids on themselves. Electrical cords and outlets represent a potential risk to small children, who may chew on accessible cords and insert objects into outlets.

The Consumer Product Safety Commission recommends a reduction of water heater thermostats to a maximum of 48.9° C (120° F). The "dial-down" recommendation has been suggested by utility companies, burn treatment centers, medical personnel, and others interested in public safety. However, many water heaters continue to remain set at levels well above the safe level. Small children are especially at risk for scald injuries from hot tap water because of their decreased reaction time and agility, their curiosity, and the thermal sensitivity of their skin. Third degree burns can develop within 5 seconds at a temperature of 140° F and within 2 seconds at 148° F. When bathing a child the caregiver should never leave the child unattended. Always test the water before placing the child into the tub or shower.

BOX 31.5 Microwave Safety

- Do not let small children operate the microwave.
- Place microwave ovens at a safe height (but higher than children's faces) and within easy reach to avoid spills.
- Never leave a young child alone while food is heating in the microwave.
- For food heated in containers, puncture plastic wrap, use vented lids, or wait 1 minute before removing a sealed covering; then lift the covering from the corner farthest away from face or arm.
- Never heat baby formula or milk in a plastic bottle liner because it may burst.
- Before adding a cold liquid to a liquid that has been heated in the microwave, insert a spoon to prevent bubbling over of the hot liquid.
- Stir food well or let it stand for 1 minute before tasting it so the heat can distribute evenly.

The increased use of microwave ovens has resulted in burn injuries from the extremely hot internal temperatures generated in heated items. Baby formula, jelly-filled pastries, noodles, and hot liquids or dishes may result in cutaneous scalds or the ingestion of overheated liquids. Caregivers should use caution when removing items from the microwave oven and should always mix and test the food before giving it to children (Box 31.5).

As children mature, risk-taking behaviors increase. Matches and lighters are dangerous in the hands of children. Adults must remember to keep potentially hazardous items out of the reach of children; a lighter, like a match, is a tool for adult use.

Education related to fire safety and survival should begin with very young children. They can practice "stop, drop, and roll" to extinguish a fire. The fire escape route, including a safe meeting place away from the home in case of fire, also should be practiced. A working smoke alarm greatly reduces the chance of dying in a home fire. Additional information on burn care and prevention can be obtained from the American Burn Association[b] and the National Safety Council.[c]

Community activities are also helpful in supporting burn survivors and preventing burns. Aluminum Cans for Burned Children is an exemplary effort based at The Paul and Carol David Foundation Burn Institute in Akron, Ohio.[d] Activities funded by Aluminum Cans for Burned Children include a burn survivors support group, Burn Camp, and meetings of Juvenile Firestoppers (for children with fire-setting behavior). Adult weekend retreats and school and family education sessions are a part of this program. The burn center and fire department provide the personnel to present programs.

[b]311 S. Wacker Dr., Suite 4150, Chicago, IL 60606; 312-642-9260, email: info@ameriburn.org; http://ameriburn.org/prevention/prevention-resources/.

[c]1121 Spring Lake Drive, Itasca, IL 60143; 800-621-7619, email: customerservice@nsc.org; http://www.nsc.org.

[d]Akron Children's Hospital, One Perkins Square, Akron, OH 44308-1062; 330-543-1000; fax: 330-543-9998; http://www.akronchildrens.org.

SUNBURN

Sunburn is a common skin injury caused by overexposure to UV light waves—either sunlight or artificial light in the UV range. The sun emits a continuous spectrum of visible and nonvisible light rays that range in length from very short to very long. The shorter, higher frequency waves are more damaging than longer wavelengths, but much of the light is filtered out as it travels through the atmosphere. Of the light that does filter through, **ultraviolet A (UVA) waves** are the longest and cause only minimum burning, but they play a significant role in photosensitive and photoallergic reactions. They are also responsible for premature aging of the skin and potentiate the effects of **ultraviolet B (UVB) waves**, which are shorter and responsible for tanning, burning, and most of the harmful effects attributed to sunlight, especially skin cancer.

Numerous factors influence the amount of UVB exposure. Maximum exposure occurs at midday (10 AM to 3 PM), when the distance from the sun to a given spot on the Earth is shortest. Solar intensity varies with the seasons, time zones, and altitude. Exposure is greater at higher altitudes and near the equator and less when the sky is hazy (although the effect is easily underestimated). Window glass effectively screens out UVB but not UVA rays. Fresh snow, water, and sand reflect UV rays, especially when the sun is directly overhead.

Excessive or long-term exposure to the sun and UV rays permanently damages the skin. Ninety percent of skin cancers occur in areas of the skin that are exposed to UV rays, and rates of skin cancers are higher in parts of the world where sunlight is more intense.

Nursing Care Management

Treatment involves stopping the burning process, decreasing the inflammatory response, and rehydrating the skin. Local application of cool tap water soaks or immersion in a tepid-water bath (temperature slightly below 36.7°C [98°F]) for 20 minutes or until the skin is cool limits tissue destruction and relieves the discomfort. After the cool applications, aloe gel or a bland oil-in-water moisturizing lotion can be applied. Partial-thickness burns are treated in the same way as those from any heat source (see earlier discussion on burns).

Protection from sunburn is the major goal of management, and the harmful effects of the sun on the delicate skin of infants and children are currently receiving increased attention. To protect skin exposed to the sun for extended periods, skin should be covered with clothing, and sun protection agents approved by the US Food and Drug Administration should be applied. Two types of products are available for sun protection: (1) **topical sunscreens**, which partially absorb UV light; and (2) **sun blockers**, which block out UV rays by reflecting sunlight. The most frequently recommended sun blockers are zinc oxide and titanium dioxide ointments.

Sunscreens are products containing a **sun protection factor (SPF)** based on evaluation of effectiveness against UV rays. Most sunscreens have an SPF ranging from 2 to more than 30; the higher the number, the greater the protection. For example, if an individual normally burns in 10 minutes without a sunscreen, use of a sunscreen with SPF 15 allows them to remain in the sun 15 times 10, or 150 minutes (2½ hours) before acquiring the same degree of burns. The most effective sunscreens against UVB are ***p-aminobenzoic acid (PABA)*** and **PABA-esters**. However, many individuals are allergic to PABA, and sunscreens without PABA are encouraged to prevent these reactions in children.

Sunscreens are applied evenly to all exposed areas, with special attention to skin folds and areas that might become exposed as clothing shifts. Avoid eye contact. Parents are directed to read labels of sunscreen products carefully for the SPF and follow manufacturer's directions for application.

> **! NURSING ALERT**
>
> Sunscreens are not recommended for infants younger than 6 months old. However, infants younger than 6 months old may have sunscreen applied over small areas of skin (such as the back of hands) that may not be adequately covered by clothing when they are in the sun. Infants should be kept out of the sun or physically shaded from it. Fabric with a tight weave, such as cotton, offers good protection.
>
> Individuals who work in the community, such as teachers, daycare workers, coaches, and youth group leaders, and relatives should all be made aware of sun safety for children. Sunscreens must be applied *liberally to exposed skin and reapplied often.*

COLD INJURY

In cold injuries the nature of the heat-regulating mechanisms of the body is such that the inner portion of the body, or core, produces heat, and the periphery, or outer area, conserves or dissipates heat. When the body attempts to conserve heat, the outer tissues are subjected to low temperatures, and local trauma may result.

Chilblain, redness and swelling of the skin, occurs when extremities, usually the hands, are exposed intermittently to temperatures of 1.1°C to 15.5°C (30°F to 60° F). The response may vary but is characterized by intense vasodilation that increases the temperature of involved tissues above that of unaffected tissue and produces edematous, reddish blue patches that itch and burn. As warming takes place, the sensations become more intense, but ordinarily they subside in a few days.

Frostbite is the term used to describe tissue damage caused when excessive heat loss to local tissues allows ice crystals to form in tissues. The frostbitten part appears white or blanched, feels solid, and is without sensation. Rapid rewarming is associated with less tissue necrosis than slow thawing. It restores blood flow and shortens the period of cellular damage. Rewarming produces a flush (sometimes deep purple) and a return of sensation, which is extremely painful. Large blisters may appear in 24 to 48 hours after rewarming and begin to reabsorb within 5 to 10 days, followed by the formation of a hard black eschar.

Nursing Care Management

Treatment involves rapid rewarming of the affected areas. Rewarming is accomplished by immersing the part in well-agitated water at 37.8°C to 42.2°C (100°F to 108°F). Discomfort is managed with analgesics and sedatives. Care of blistered skin is similar to that described for burns. Superficial injury often heals without incident. It is seldom possible to estimate the extent of tissue loss until new skin layers are revealed after the eschar layer separates. Treatment of the wound is comparable to burn wound care. In extreme cases amputation may be necessary.

CLINICAL JUDGMENT AND NEXT-GENERATION NCLEX® EXAMINATION-STYLE QUESTIONS

1. A 16-year-old male is admitted with burns on both arms and face after trying to light a gas grill. He had put gasoline on it because it would not light. The nurse notes that the patient has superficial partial thickness burns on both lower front arms and the top of the hands. He has superficial burns on both sides of his face, specifically on the cheeks. **Choose the most likely options for the information missing from the statements below by selecting from the lists of options provided.**
Using the Rule of Nines, the nurse calculates the patient has burns on approximately _____1_____ of his total body surface area. The nurse is aware that with superficial partial thickness burns, _____2_____ are intact and the wound should heal in approximately _____3_____ with possible scarring.

Options for 1	Options for 2	Options for 3
3%	bony structures	3-4 days
5 ½ %	muscle structures	5-7 days
10 ½ %	dermal elements	7-14 days
22%	fascia elements	14-21 days
6 ½%	nerve structures	30 days

2. A 9-month-old girl is in the pediatrician office because of a diaper rash that is getting worse. The child has no fever, is bottle fed and is in the 50% for weight and height for age. On examination the nurse notes a soiled diaper with a strong ammonia odor. The skin is beefy red with numerous maculopapular lesions across the front. The lesions extend into the skin folds and across the upper thighs. The child's axillary temperature is 98.9° F, pulse = 80 beats/min, respirations = 28/min. Which of the following would the nurse discuss with the mother? **For each nursing action, use an X to indicate whether it was Effective (helped to meet expected quality patient outcomes), Ineffective (did not help to meet expected quality patient outcomes), or Unrelated (not related to the quality patient outcomes).**

Nursing Action	Effective	Ineffective	Unrelated
"Change the diaper as soon as it becomes wet or soiled."			
"Use a hair dryer or heat lamp to dry the area."			
"Use a superabsorbent disposable diaper if you can."			
"Keep the skin dry."			
"Wash the area often as possible using a wipe."			
"Diapers that are unscented can be purchased."			
"Apply ointment such as zinc oxide or petrolatum to the skin."			
"Avoid removing the skin barrier cream with each diaper change."			

3. A school nurse is seeing several children who have evidence of pediculosis capitis. Most of these children are coming from one first grade class. Children have been evaluated by carefully assessing the scalp by spreading the hair to look for lice and observing for nits or eggs that adhere to the hair shafts close to the scalp. These children were treated with a lice treatment and recommended to treat the scalp again in 10 days. The nurse is working with the teacher to educate parents on how to prevent pediculosis. What are the **most appropriate** responses for the nurse to provide to help prevent another outbreak? **Select all that apply.**
   - **A.** Inspect the child for head lice on a regular basis once an outbreak occurs.
   - **B.** Seal non-washable items in plastic bags for 2 months before using again.
   - **C.** Keep clothing items such as hats and scarves in separate cubicles at school.
   - **D.** Treat infected children monthly with a lice treatment during the school year.
   - **E.** Teach children not to share hats, scarves, hair accessories, combs or brushes.
   - **F.** Machine wash all washable clothing, towels and linens in water hotter than 130° F.

4. A 9-year-old boy in the emergency department for a "skin rash." His boy scout troop was camping three weeks ago. The mother noted a large red raised lesion on his ankle when he returned from camp, but the child did not complain about it. The nurse completes a history and physical assessment and notes the following. Which assessment findings **require follow-up** by the nurse? **Select all that apply.**
   - **A.** Fatigue
   - **B.** Headache
   - **C.** Temperature 100.4° F
   - **D.** Cough for past week
   - **E.** Pulse = 88 beats/minute
   - **F.** Respirations = 20/minute
   - **G.** Blood pressure = 100/66 mmHg
   - **H.** Spleen 1 cm below left costal margin
   - **I.** Small, red, annular lesions on the lower legs and arms
   - **J.** Inguinal and axillar lymph nodes 1 cm in circumference

REFERENCES

American Academy of Pediatrics, & Committee on Infectious Diseases. (2018). In D. W Kimberline (Ed.), *2018 Red book: Report of the committee on infectious diseases* (31th ed.). Elk Grove Village, IL: The Academy.

American Burn Association (ABA). (2016). *Advanced burn life support provider manual 2016 update*. Chicago, IL.

Bhat, Y. J., Latief, I., & Hassan, I. (2017). Update on etiopathogenesis and treatment of acne. *Indian Journal of Dermatology Venereology and Leprology, 83*(3), 298–306.

Centers for Disease Control and Prevention. (2017). *Lyme disease (Borrelia burgdorferi)*. Retrieved from https://www.cdc.gov/nndss/conditions/lyme-disease/case-definition/2017/.

Centers for Disease Control and Prevention (CDC). (2018). *Ten leading causes of death by age groups highlighting unintentional injury deaths*. Atlanta, GA: United States-2016. Retrieved from https://www.cdc.gov/injury/wisqars/pdf/leading_causes_of_injury_deaths_highlighting_unintentional_injury_2016-508.pdf.

Chaptini, C., Quinn, S., & Marshman, G. (2016). Methicillin-resistant staphylococcus aureus in children with atopic dermatitis from 1999 to 2014: A longitudinal study. *The Australasian Journal of Dermatology, 57*(2), 122–127.

Clark, A., Imran, J., Madni, T., et al. (2017). Nutrition and metabolism in burn patients. *Burns & Trauma, 5*, 11.

Eichenfield, L. F., Krakowski, A. C., Piggott, C., et al. (2013). Evidence-based recommendations for the diagnosis and treatment of pediatric acne. *Pediatrics, 131*(Suppl. 3), S163–S183.

Eisen, L., & Dolan, M. C. (2016). Evidence for personal protective measures to reduce human contact with blacklegged ticks and for environmentally based control methods to suppress host-seeking blacklegged ticks and reduce infection with lyme disease spirochetes in tick vectors and rodent reservoirs. *Journal of Medical Entomology, 53*, 1063–1092.

Fagin, A., & Palmieri, T. L. (2017). Considerations for pediatric burn sedation and analgesia. *Burns & Trauma, 5*, 28.

Fiedler, F., Stangl, G. I., Fiedler, E., et al. (2017). Acne and nutrition: A systematic review. *Acta Dermato-Venereologica, 97*(1), 7–9.

Greenhalgh, D. G. (2017). Sepsis in the burn patient: A different problem than sepsis in the general population. *Burns & Trauma, 5*, 23.

Grey, K., & Maquiness, S. (2016). Atopic dermatitis: Update for pediatricians. *Pediatric Annals, 45*(8), e280–e286.

Gupta, A. K., Lyons, D. C., & Rosen, T. (2015). New and emerging concepts in managing and preventing community-associated methicillin-resistant staphylococcus aureus infections. *International Journal of Dermatology, 54*(11), 1226–1232.

Gunning, K., Kiraly, B., & Pippitt, K. (2019). Lice and scabies: Treatment update. *American Family Physician, 99*(10), 635–642.

Han, G., & Ceilley, R. (2017). Chronic wound healing: A review of current management and treatments. *Advances in Therapy, 34*, 599–610.

Holm, J. G., Agner, T., Clausen, M. L., et al. (2016). Quality of life and disease severity in patients with atopic dermatitis. *Journal of the European Academy of Dermatology and Venereology, 30*(1), 1760–1767.

Holmes, J. H., Molnar, J. A., Carter, J. E., et al. (2018). A comparison study of the ReCell® device and autologous split-thickness meshed skin graft in the treatment of acute burn injuries. *Journal of Burn Care & Research, 39*(5), 694–701.

Kaplan, S. L. (2016). Staphylococcus aureus infections in children: The implications of changing trends. *Pediatrics, 137*(4), e20160101.

Kaplan, S. L., Forbes, A., Hammerman, W. A., et al. (2014). Randomized trial of "bleach baths" plus routine hygienic measures vs routine hygienic measures alone for prevention of recurrent infections. *Clinical Infectious Diseases, 58*(5), 679–682.

King, A., Stellar, J. J., Blevins, A., et al. (2014). Dressing and products in pediatric wound care. *Advances in Wound Care, 3*(4), 324–334.

Koedel, U., Fingerle, V., & Pfister, H. (2015). Lyme neuroborreliosis – epidemiology, diagnosis and management. *Nature Reviews. Neurology, 11*, 446–456.

Koehler, S., Jinbo, A., Johnson, S., et al. (2014). Negative pressure dressing assisted healing in pediatric burn patients. *Journal of Pediatric Surgery, 49*(7), 1142–1145.

Margolis, D. J., Abuabara, K., Hoffstad, O. J., et al. (2015). Association between malignancy and topical use of pimecrolimus. *Journal of the American Medical Association Dermatology, 151*(6), 594–599.

McLeod, J. S., Maringo, A. E., Doyle, P. J., et al. (2018). Analysis of electrocardiograms associated with pediatric electrical burns. *Journal of Burn Care & Research, 39*(1), 65–72.

National Fire Protection Association (NFPA). (2014). *Playing with fire*. Retrieved from http:www.nfpa.org/News-and-Research/Data-research-and-tools/US-Fire-Problem/Children-playing-with-fire.

Nguyen, T. A., Leonard, S. A., & Eichenfield, L. F. (2015). An update on pediatric atopic dermatitis and food allergies. *The Journal of Pediatrics, 167*(3), 752–756.

Norbury, W., Herndon, D. N., Tanksley, J., et al. (2016). Infections in burns. *Surgical Infections, 7*(2), 250–255.

Oliveira, J. M., Sobreira, G., Velosa, J., et al. (2017). Association of isotretinoin with depression and suicide: A review of current literature. *Journal of Cutaneous Medicine and Surgery*.

Page, S. S., Weston, S., & Loh, R. (2016). Atopic dermatitis in children. *Australian Family Physician, 45*(5), 293–296.

Pawlik, M. C., Kemp, A., Maguire, S., et al. (2016). Children with burns referred for child abuse evaluation: Burn characteristics and co-existing injuries. *Child Abuse & Neglect, 55*, 52–56. https://doi.org/10.1016/j.chiabu.2016.03.006. Epub 2016 Apr 16.

Que, S. K. T., Whitaker-Worth, D. L., & Chang, M. W. (2016). Acne: Kids are not just little people. *Clinics in Dermatology, 34*, 710–716.

Rezaei, E., Beiraghi-Toosi, A., Ahmadabadi, A., et al. (2017). Can skin allograft occasionally act as a permanent coverage in deep burns? A pilot study. *World Journal of Plastic Surgery, 6*(1), 94–99.

Rowan, M. P., Cancio, L. C., Elster, E. A., et al. (2015). Burn wound healing and treatment: Review and advancements. *Critical Care, 19*, 243. https://doi.org/10.1186/s13054-015-0961-2.

Safe Kids Worldwide (SKW). (2015). *Burn and scald safety*. Washington, DC. Retrieved from https://www.safekids.org/sites/default/files/documents/skw_burns_fact_sheet_feb_2015.pdf.

Satteson, E. S., Crantford, J. C., Wood, J., et al. (2015). Outcomes of vacuum-assisted therapy in the treatment of head and neck wounds. *The Journal of Craniofacial Surgery, 26*(7), e599–e602.

Smith, M. L. (2000). Pediatric burns: Management of thermal, electrical, and chemical burns and burn-like dermatologic conditions. *Pediatric Annals, 29*(6), 367–378.

Steere, A. C., Strle, F., Wormser, G. P., et al. (2016). Lyme borreliosis. *Nature Reviews, 2*, 1–18.

Strang, S. G., Van Lieshout, E. M. M., Breederveld, R. S., et al. (2014). A systematic review on intra-abdominal pressure in severely burned patients. *Burns, 40*, 9–16.

Takahara, S., Sai, S., Kagatani, T., et al. (2014). Efficacy and haemodynamic effects of vacuum-assisted closure for post-sternotomy mediastinitis in children. *Interactive Cardiovascular and Thoracic Surgery, 19*(4), 627–631.

Vloemans, A. F., Hermans, M. H., van der Wal, M. B., et al. (2014). Optimal treatment of partial thickness burns in children: A systematic review. *Burns, 40*, 177–190.

Clinical Judgment and Next-Generation NCLEX® Examination-Style Questions Answer Key

CHAPTER 1 PERSPECTIVES OF PEDIATRIC NURSING

1. C, D
2. A, C, E, G
3.

CJMM Skill	Nursing Process	Match the Nursing Process Skill With CJMM Skill
1. Recognize Cues	Analysis	**2 or 3**
2. Analyze Cues	Planning	**4**
3. Prioritize Hypotheses	Implementation	**5**
4. Generate Solutions	Evaluation	**6**
5. Take Action	Assessment	**1**
6. Evaluate Outcomes		

4.

Nursing Action	Indicated	Contrain-dicated	Non-Essential
Eating preferences and attitudes related to food are established by family influences and culture.	X		
Breastfeeding provides micronutrients and immunologic properties.	X		
Most children establish lifelong eating habits by 18 months of age.		X	
Because of the stress of returning to work, most mothers use this as a time to stop breastfeeding.		X	
During adolescence, parental influence diminishes, and adolescents make food choices related to peer acceptability and sociability.			X
Chronic illness can cause a young child to not want to eat.		X	

CHAPTER 2 SOCIAL, CULTURAL, RELIGIOUS, AND FAMILY INFLUENCES ON CHILD HEALTH PROMOTION

1.

Options for 1	Options for 2	Options for 3 and 4
Stage I	**Autonomy**	**Marital**
Stage II	Trust	Sibling
Stage III	Identity	**Career**
Stage IV	Fear	Home
Stage V	Growth	Retirement
Stage VI	Height	Insurance

2.

Nursing Action: Quality Patient Outcomes	Indicated	Contrain-dicated	Non-Essential
Realize that parenting roles are learned behaviors and the mother is not prepared to take the child home.			X
The family strengths and unique functional style can be a resource for the nurse.	X		
Parenting styles are all the same, and the mother should be forced to listen to the discharge plan.		X	
Despite difficulty trying to meet with the mother, a sense of purpose to care for this child at home can promote a successful discharge.	X		
This must be a single family, and counseling should be contacted to work with the mother.		X	

3. A, B, C, D, E
4. A, C, E

CHAPTER 3 DEVELOPMENTAL AND GENETIC INFLUENCES ON CHILD HEALTH PROMOTION

1. C, E
2. B, C, D
3.

History and Assessment	Indicated	Contraindicated	Non-Essential
Family history should include information going back at least three generations.	X		
Family history should include environmental assessment, including neighbors and friends.		X	
Assessment should focus only on the infant's ability to move the arms and legs.		X	
Assessment should evaluate for Turner syndrome since girls have a prepubertal growth spurt and then mostly stop growing.			X
Awareness of parents' feelings of guilt about causing the disorder is important for the nurse to consider.	X		

4.

Options for 1	Options for 2	Options for 3
Chromosome analysis	**risk factors**	etiology
Family health history	medical records	**inheritance patterns**
Ultrasound	severity	rate of occurrence
Metabolic screening	birth defects	
Anorexia	platelets	
Fever	weight	

CHAPTER 4 COMMUNICATION AND PHYSICAL ASSESSMENT OF THE CHILD AND FAMILY

1. A, B, D
2.

Options for 1	Options for 2
20%	radial arterial
30%	radial venous
40%	dorsal arterial
50%	popliteal venous
60%	**brachial arterial**

3.

Nursing Action: Approach to Physical Examination	Effective	Ineffective	Unrelated
With toddlers, restraints help keep the child still, and requesting a parent's assistance is inappropriate.		X	
An infant's physical examination is always done head to toe, similar to that for an adult.		X	
When examining a preschooler, giving a choice of which body parts to examine first may be helpful in gaining the child's cooperation.	X		
Giving explanations about body systems can make adolescents nervous due to their egocentricities.			X
With an adolescent, it is best to have a parent present during the examination.		X	
The parent's knowledge of stethoscopes can help with cooperation during the examination			X

4.

Nursing Action	Indicated	Contraindicated	Non-Essential
Understand the difference in measurement for children who can stand alone and for those who must lie recumbent.	X		
Use a stadiometer to measure infant length.		X	
Two measurers are required for a recumbent child.			X
Reposition the child and repeat the procedure. Measure at least twice (ideally three times). Average the measurements for the final value.	X		
Demonstrate competency when measuring the growth of infants, children, and adolescents. Refresher sessions should be taken when a lack of standardization occurs.	X		
Understand the difference in body mass index (BMI) in children versus adults.			X

CHAPTER 5 PAIN ASSESSMENT AND MANAGEMENT IN CHILDREN

1.

Nursing Action	Indicated	Contrain-dicated	Non-Essential
"Infants don't feel pain as adults do because their pain receptors are not fully developed yet."		X	
"Although we try to give the baby medicine before pain is felt, we watch very closely and use different techniques to help relieve the pain."	X		
"The nurse gives pain medication to all hospitalized patients before the infant really feels the pain."			X
"We assess pain using a pain assessment tool for children of all ages and give the medicine as needed."		X	
"We wait until the infant cries or is fussy, and then we know that pain is being experienced."		X	

2. A, G, I, J
3.

Pain Assessment Scale	Patient and Type of Pain Experienced	Correct Pain Scale
1. CRIES: **C**rying, **R**equiring increased oxygen, **I**nability to console, **E**xpression, and **S**leeplessness	2-year-old with Down syndrome in recovery from morning surgery	**2**
2. FLACC Pain Assessment Tool: **F**acial expression, **L**eg movement, **A**ctivity, **C**ry, and **C**onsolability	Newborn in intensive care for low birth weight and born to an addicted mother	**1**
3. Non-Communicating Children's Pain Checklist (NCCPC): Parent and health care giver questionnaire assessing acute and chronic pain	17-year-old admitted for sickle cell crisis	**7**
4. Neonatal Pain, Agitation, and Sedation Scale (NPASS): For infants from 3 to 6 months old	5-year-old with leukemia undergoing a lumbar puncture	**5**
5. Wong-Baker FACES Pain Rating Scale		
6. Premature Infant Pain Profile (PIPP)		
7. Visual Analogue Scale		

4.

Options for 1	Options for 2	Options for 3
intermittent	**bolus**	increasing
continuous	triple	changing
as needed	half	stopping
prn	full	**tapering**
one-time	continuous	adjusting
daily	daily	holding

CHAPTER 6 CHILDHOOD COMMUNICABLE AND INFECTIOUS DISEASES

1.

Standard Precautions	History and Assessment Findings	Type of Precaution to Implement
1. Transfusion-Based Precautions	15-year-old returning from summer in India who presents with symptoms of tuberculosis	**2**
2. Airborne Precautions	3-year-old who has a respiratory illness with cough	**5**
3. Standard Precautions	5-year-old admitted with fever and productive cough; bacterial pneumonia confirmed by lab and x-ray	**4**
4. Droplet Precautions	7-year-old admitted for tonsillectomy	**3**
5. Respiratory Hygiene / Cough Etiquette		
6. No precautions needed		

2.

Options for 1	Options for 2	Options for 3
A Virus	subcutaneously	dorsogluteal
B Virus	intravenously	**vastus lateralis**
Tetanus	**intramuscularly**	pectoral
Infection	intrathecally	subclavicular

3. A, D, E, G, H, I
4. A, C, E

CHAPTER 7 HEALTH PROMOTION OF THE NEWBORN AND FAMILY

1. A, B, D, E, F
2.

Nursing Action: Early Discharge Newborn Care	Topic	Appropriate Nursing Education Action
1. The newborn should be fed every 1.5-3 hours.	Wet Diapers	**8**
2. This could occur within 24 hours of birth and hemolysis or ABO/Rh problem suspected.	Position of Sleep	**6**
3. The newborn should be fed 1-2 oz every 4-6 hours.	Umbilical Cord	**5**
4. Wash with warm water and check for bleeding.	Stools	**9**
5. Keep it above the diaper line, allow to dry, and check for drainage.	Breastfeeding	**1**
6. Place the newborn on his back.	Pathologic Jaundice	**2**
7. The newborn should have 4-5 wakeful periods a day.		
8. The newborn should have 6-10 wakeful periods a day after 14 days of age.		
9. The newborn should have 2-3 stools a day if breastfeeding.		

3. A, C, E
4.

Health Teaching	Indicated	Contraindicated	Non-Essential
Human immunodeficiency virus (HIV) is rarely transmitted to the newborn through maternal milk.		X	
In such infants, antiretroviral medication will be started within 12 hours of birth.			X
Breastfeeding will be avoided completely in mothers with high-risk behaviors.		X	
Breastfeeding will be withheld until HIV status (maternal) is determined.	X		

CHAPTER 8 HEALTH PROBLEMS OF NEWBORNS

1.

Options for 1	Options for 2
oral	mouth
rectal	ear
axillary	**rectum**
temporal	nose

2.

Nursing Action	Indicated	Contraindicated	Non-Essential
Review the medical history to assess what laboratory studies were performed after birth.	X		
Encourage frequent breastfeeding.	X		
Switch to formula feeding for 72 hours.		X	
Teach mother how to swaddle the newborn.			X
Administer intravenous (IV) immunoglobulin.		X	

3. B, C, D, E
4. B, C, E, F, G

CHAPTER 9 HEALTH PROMOTION OF THE INFANT AND FAMILY

1. B, D, E
2.

Health Teaching	Indicated	Contraindicated	Non-Essential
The infant will be taking a vitamin D supplement daily.	X		
The infant will be receiving a fluoride supplement.		X	
The infant will be receiving an iron supplement.		X	
The infant's head will be covered when breastfeeding.			X
Breast milk can be stored in the refrigerator for up to 5 days.	X		

3.

Options for 1	Options for 2	Options for 3
obesity	1-2 days	**food allergies**
iron-deficiency anemia	10-12 days	infection
rickets	**4-7 days**	growth delay
infant botulism	14 days	urinary tract infection

4.

Nursing Education	Potential Injury	Appropriate Nursing Action to Promote Safety
1. Keep buttons, beads, or other small objects out of infant's reach.	Falls	**2**
2. Restrain in a highchair.	Aspiration	**1**
3. Know the local poison control number.	Suffocation	**5**
4. Keep out of reach of water faucets.	Poisoning	**3**
5. Keep latex balloons out of reach.	Burns	**4**
6. Keep bathroom doors closed.		
7. Keep large objects that could be overturned off furniture.		

CHAPTER 10 HEALTH PROBLEMS OF INFANTS

1. A, B, D, E
2.

Options for 1	Options for 2
diarrhea	goat's milk
eczema	**soy milk or a hydrolyzed formula**
sneezing	whole milk
urticaria	evaporated milk
fever	milk
swelling	eggs

3. B, C, D, F
4.

Nursing Action: Health Teaching	Indicated	Contrain-dicated	Non-Essential
Reassure the mother that she is correct in keeping the infant on his side.		X	
Discuss with the mother that keeping the infant in bed with her can actually increase the risk of sudden infant death syndrome (SIDS).	X		
Advise the mother that the waterbed is a type of "soft bedding" and the infant should not sleep on the waterbed.	X		
Discuss with the mother that a warm bath before bedtime can help minimize risk.			X
Advise the mother to keep stuffed animals and toys in the crib to provide comfort.		X	

CHAPTER 11 HEALTH PROMOTION OF THE TODDLER AND FAMILY

1. A, B, D, E
2. A, C, D
3.

Health Teaching	Indicated	Contrain-dicated	Non-Essential
Avoid placing large food portions on the toddler's plate.	X		
Allow the child to graze on snacks during the day.		X	
Insist that the child sit at the table until all persons have completed their meals.		X	
Allow the child to make certain food choices (within reasonable limits).	X		
Provide meals at the same time of day as much as possible so that the toddler has a sense of consistency.	X		
Offer the child oranges or apples each day.			X
Make the child eat all of the food provided and use disciplinary actions if the plate is not cleaned.		X	

4.

Options for 1	Options for 2
rear-facing	until the child is 2 years of age
front seat	**for as long as possible**
forward-facing	until the child can sit in the front seat
booster that is front facing	until the child weighs 50 pounds

CHAPTER 12 HEALTH PROMOTION OF THE PRESCHOOLER AND FAMILY

1. A, B, E
2.

Health Teaching	Indicated	Contrain-dicated	Non-Essential
Most preschoolers weigh between 10 and 12 kilograms.		X	
The legs of a preschooler, rather than the trunk, increase in length, which may make him look thinner.	X		
Preschoolers usually keep that pot-bellied appearance until about 6 years old.		X	
Most preschoolers gain ½ to 1 pound per year.		X	
Most preschoolers do not like to get their weight and height checked.			X

3.

Options for 1	Options for 2	Options for 3
understand	**prejudice**	**perspective**
wonder	change	likeness
question	colors	family
fear	hardship	status
realize	temperature	parents

4. C, D, E

CHAPTER 13 HEALTH PROBLEMS OF TODDLERS AND PRESCHOOLERS

1. A, D, E
2. A, C, E, F
3.

Options for 1	Options for 2
surveillance	**1 month**
treatment	1 week
chelation	6 months
nutrition	6 weeks
iron supplements	1 year

4. A, C, E

CHAPTER 14 FAMILY-CENTERED CARE OF THE SCHOOL-AGE CHILD AND ADOLESCENT

1.

Health Teaching	Indicated	Contrain-dicated	Non-Essential
"Children this age are able to see things from another's point of view, and it is important to keep communication open with your son."	X		
"He may be having difficulty making judgments about his surroundings and may need further evaluation."		X	
"It would be helpful to sit beside him and watch a favorite movie to show support."			X
"School-age children often use their past experiences to evaluate their present situation, and moving to a new school is a tough adjustment for him."	X		

2. B, D, F
3.

Sex Education Nursing Action	Effective	Inef-fective	Unrelated
Separate the boys and girls into same-sex groups with a leader of the same sex.	X		
Answer questions in a matter-of-fact way that is honest and appropriate to the children's level of understanding.	X		
Use vernacular or slang terms to describe human physiologic functions.		X	
Avoid discussing sexually transmitted infections in this age-group.		X	
Discuss what it is like to have your first boyfriend or girlfriend.			X
Discuss common myths and misconceptions associated with sex and the reproductive process.	X		

4.

Options for 1	Options for 2
peer pressure	bullying
physical awkwardness	clumsiness
parents' lack of supervision	feeling small
wanting to impress the opposite sex	**risk-taking behaviors**
hormones	feeling invincible
underdeveloped skeletal muscles	showing off

CHAPTER 15 HEALTH PROMOTION OF THE ADOLESCENT AND FAMILY

1.

Options for 1	Options for 2
facial hair	muscle
height	**breast**
testicular enlargement	penile
ejaculation	testicular
axillary hair	larynx
voice changes	neck

2. B, C, D, F
3. A, B, C
4. B, D, F

CHAPTER 16 HEALTH PROBLEMS OF SCHOOL-AGE CHILDREN AND ADOLESCENTS

1. dry eyes, decreased night vision, headaches, depression, mood swings
2. A, D, E, F
3.

Option 1	Option 2	Option 3	Option 4
Abstinence	>99% effective	Irregular menstrual bleeding	Not recommended for women >90 kg
Calendar methods	Regulates menses	Latex sensitivity may occur	Risk of perforation
Oral contraceptives	Prevents ovarian cancers	**High failure rate unless combined with condom**	May cause headaches
Progestin	**Easy to use, minimal side effects**	May cause nausea	May cause dysmenorrhea
Cervical cap	Prevents endometriosis	May cause vaginitis	**Requires fitting by medical personnel, minimal sexually transmitted infection (STI) protection**

4.

Option 1	Option 2	Option 3
Neisseria gonorrhoeae	*Neisseria gonorrhoeae*	**Neisseria gonorrhoeae**
Chlamydia trachomatis	*Chlamydia trachomatis*	*Chlamydia trachomatis*
Treponema pallidum	*Treponema pallidum*	*Treponema pallidum*
Human papillomavirus (HPV)	**Human papillomavirus (HPV)**	Human papillomavirus (HPV)
Trichomonas vaginalis	*Trichomonas vaginalis*	*Trichomonas vaginalis*

CHAPTER 17 FAMILY-CENTERED CARE OF THE CHILD WITH SPECIAL NEEDS

1.

Health Teaching	Indicated	Contrain-dicated	Non-Essential
"'Giving in' is not a detriment to your child when he or she has a disability and limitations."		X	
"When parents establish reasonable limits, children are likely to develop independence that is appropriate for their age and achievement equal to their limitations."	X		
"It is best to wait to explain any procedure to the child until they are at the health care setting or just before the procedure to avoid unduly upsetting your child."		X	
"I recommend talking to other mothers in your neighborhood about how they parent their children."			X
"It is important to realize that it would be unfair to the siblings to expect similar rules to apply to all children in the family."		X	

2. A, C, F
3. A, B, E, F

4.

Nursing Action	Potential Communication Problems	Appropriate Nursing Action for Potential Communication Problem
1. Listen to the mother's perception of the seriousness or severity of the illness.	Lack of support from family and friends	**7**
2. Provide an opportunity for the mother to discuss her concerns and worries.	Nurse unaware of the mother's understanding of the child	**1**
3. Acknowledge that language constraints may make it necessary for the health care team to make some decisions.	Lack of support from health care providers	**2**
4. Ask the mother how her extended family feels about the child's illness.		
5. Tell the mother not to talk to anyone else about her concerns.		
6. Explore alternative medicines and therapies.		
7. Explore the mother's support network to find others that can help.		

CHAPTER 18 IMPACT OF COGNITIVE OR SENSORY IMPAIRMENT ON THE CHILD AND FAMILY

1. A, C, F, G, H
2. A, B, C, D
3.

Health Teaching	Indicated	Contra-indicated	Non-Essential
"It is unfortunate that you waited so long to have children; most children with Down syndrome are born to older women."		X	
"When feeding your infant, use a small, straight-handled spoon to push food to the side and back of the mouth."	X		
"Parents like you believe that the experience of having this special child makes them stronger and more accepting of others."			X
"As your child gets older, it has been found that school is detrimental to the child with Down syndrome due to lack of one-on-one teaching."		X	
"I am going to listen closely to your child's heart because congenital heart problems can occur in a child with Down syndrome."	X		

4.

Options for 1	Options for 2
antibiotics	**thimerosal**
vitamins	arsenic
vaccines	penicillin
milk	hormones
fruit juices	amoxicillin

CHAPTER 19 THE CHILD WHO IS HOSPITALIZED

1.

Health Teaching	Indicated	Contrain-dicated	Non-Essential
"Separation anxiety may be seen in your child by refusing to eat, having trouble sleeping, crying quietly for you when gone, or withdrawing from others."	X		
"Separation anxiety comes in stages: denial, despair, and detachment."		X	
"Loss of peer group contact may pose a severe emotional threat because of loss of group status and loss of group acceptance."		X	
"Your child may need and desire parental guidance or support from other adult figures as she returns to school."			X
"Young children can react 'negatively' to their parents during hospitalization; they may cling to you to ensure your continued presence."	X		

2. B, C, D, G
3. A, B, C, E, G, H
4. A, B, D, E

CHAPTER 20 PEDIATRIC NURSING INTERVENTIONS AND SKILLS

1. A, B, C, E, F
2.

Options for 1	Options for 2
5 ml	deltoid
2 ml	**dorsogluteal**
1 ml	ventrogluteal
8 ml	vastus lateralis

3. A, C, E, F
4.

Nursing Action	Indicated	Contrain-dicated	Non-Essential
An 18-gauge catheter needs to be inserted.		X	
A blunt plastic cannula needs to be used because it prevents the need for steel needles.	X		
An injection port site is used to deliver medications.	X		
An opaque covering of the intravenous (IV) site needs to be used.		X	
Music should be played in the background when performing the insertion.			X
A padded board should be placed below the hand where the catheter is inserted.		X	
Fingers are left unoccluded by tape or dressing to assess circulation.	X		

CHAPTER 21 THE CHILD WITH RESPIRATORY DYSFUNCTION

1. A, B, C, D, F
2. A, B, D, E
3.

Options for 1	Options for 2	Options for 3
Acute laryngotracheobronchitis	fungal	flashlight
Acute tracheitis	protozoic	**tongue depressor**
Acute epiglottitis	**bacterial**	microscope
Acute spasmodic laryngitis	idiopathic	otoscope light

4. A, B, D, E

CHAPTER 22 THE CHILD WITH GASTROINTESTINAL DYSFUNCTION

1.

Home Care Instruction	Indicated	Contrain-dicated	Non-Essential
Keep on clear liquids and toast for 24 hours.		X	
Offer a regular diet as child's appetite warrants.	X		
Sterilize the infant's eating utensils before each meal.			X
Give a BRAT diet (bananas, rice, applesauce, and toast) for 24 hours, then a soft diet as tolerated.		X	
Find out what the infant's favorite food is.			X
Give chicken or beef broth for 24 hours, then resume a soft diet.		X	

2.

Options for 1	Options for 2	Options for 3
Sugar	Yogurt	**Iron-deficiency anemia**
Meat	Corn on the cob	Bleeding
Gluten	Lettuce and tomato salad	Asthma
Salt	**Toast**	Hepatitis
Milk	Baked chicken	Pyloric stenosis
Eggs	Carrot sticks	Hoarseness and difficulty swallowing

3. A, E, F, G
4.

Options for 1	Options for 2	Options for 3	Options for 4
Hepatitis A	parenteral	**hepatitis A virus (HAV)**	Four
Hepatitis C	**fecal-oral**	hepatitis C virus (HCV)	**Two**
Hepatitis B	contaminated water	polio vaccine	Three
Hepatitis D	perinatal	hepatitis B virus (HBV)	One

CHAPTER 23 THE CHILD WITH CARDIOVASCULAR DYSFUNCTION

1. A, D
2.

1	2	3 and 4
Atrial septal defect (ASD)	Decreased pulmonary blood flow	**Abnormal opening between right and left ventricles = 3**
Coarctation of the aorta	**Resistance of blood flow in the left ventricle, causing decreased cardiac output**	Four defects of the heart disrupt blood flow
Heart failure	Increased pressure proximal to the defect and decreased pressure distal to the obstruction	**Valve fails to develop, leaving no communication from the right atrium to the right ventricle = 4**
Hypoplastic left heart syndrome	Blood flows from the left to right atrium, causing increased flow of blood to the right side of the heart	Local narrowing near the insertion of the ductus arteriosus

3. C, E
4. A, D, E, F, H, I

CHAPTER 24 THE CHILD WITH HEMATOLOGIC OR IMMUNOLOGIC DYSFUNCTION

1. A, B, C, E, H, I, J
2.

Health Teaching	Indicated	Contraindi-cated	Non-Essential
"We need to check your iron level to make sure you are not anemic."		X	
"I believe your disease is most common in those of Hispanic descent, although you are Mediterranean."		X	
"I would like to talk to you about the diagnosis and provide you with some information about beta thalassemia."	X		
"You look much younger than I would expect. I guess you are a late bloomer."			X
"I think a transfusion will be ordered because your hemoglobin level is 9.5."		X	

3. A, D, F, G
4.

Health Teaching	Indicated	Contraindicated	Non-Essential
"Your child should remain active to decrease joint problems, and most children with hemophilia can participate in the same activities as their peers."		X	
"Care should be taken to avoid bleeding of gums; softening the toothbrush in warm water before brushing or using a sponge-tipped disposable toothbrush may be helpful."	X		
"Signs of internal bleeding should be recognized, such as headache, slurred speech, loss of consciousness (from cerebral bleeding), and black, tarry stools (from gastrointestinal bleeding)."	X		
"If there is bleeding in a joint, elevation, ice, and rest should prevent the need for factor VIII replacement."		X	
"All of your son's teachers need to be aware of what to do if he gets a bloody nose."	X		
"Your child should drink a lot of fluids to decrease the possibility of dehydration."			X

CHAPTER 25 THE CHILD WITH CANCER

1. A, B, C, D, F
2.

Nursing Action	Indicated	Contraindicated	Non-Essential
Viscous lidocaine should be used to swish the mouth three times per day.		X	
Perform mouth care routinely before and after feeding.	X		
Lemon glycerin swabs are helpful because they remind children of lemon drops.		X	
Allowing the child to sleep 8 hours will help recovery.			X
Using a soft sponge–type toothbrush will decrease the tendency of gums to bleed.	X		
Sodium bicarbonate and salt water rinses can be used.	X		

3.

Options for 1	Options for 2	Options for 3
absolute red blood	subtracting	platelets
absolute platelet	**multiplying**	monocytes
absolute neutrophil	dividing	**neutrophils**
absolute white blood	adding	eosinophils

4. A, B, C, E

CHAPTER 26 THE CHILD WITH GENITOURINARY DYSFUNCTION

1. A, E
2.

Options for 1	Options for 2	Options for 3
post staphylococcal	**Group A beta-hemolytic streptococci**	Blood
post meningitis	Group B beta-hemolytic streptococci	**Urine**
post streptococcal	Group A beta-hemolytic staphylococcus	Radiographic
post pneumococcal	Group B beta-hemolytic staphylococcus	Ultrasound

3. B, C, D, F, G
4. B, C

CHAPTER 27 THE CHILD WITH CEREBRAL DYSFUNCTION

1. A, B, E, F, G
2.

Options for 1	Options for 2	Options for 3
Aplastic crisis	intubation	meningococcal
Bacterial meningitis	suctioning	**pneumococcal**
Acute chest syndrome	**isolation**	polio
Reye syndrome	vaccination	tetanus
COVID-19	blood transfusion	pertussis

3. A, E, F
4. A, B, E, F

CHAPTER 28 THE CHILD WITH ENDOCRINE DYSFUNCTION

1. C, D, E, F
2. B, D, E, F
3.

Options for 1	Options for 2	Options for 3
aplastic crisis	preparation of insulin	4-12 days
diabetes insipidus	**luteinizing hormone-releasing hormone**	2-3 weeks
diabetes mellitus	vasopressin injection	10-14 days
precocious puberty	vitamin D injection	3-5 weeks
Cushing syndrome	corticosteroid agent	**4-12 weeks**

4.

Nursing Action: Education	Indicated	Contrain-dicated	Non-Essential
When starting drug therapy, encourage staying in a quiet, unstimulating environment that promotes rest.	X		
Heat tolerance is a common symptom experienced by individuals with Graves' disease.	X		
Weight gain is a common symptom experienced by individuals with Graves' disease.		X	
Mood swings and irritability are common symptoms experienced by individuals with Graves' disease.	X		
Eating fruit and vegetables as part of a healthy diet is recommended for teenagers.			X

CHAPTER 29 THE CHILD WITH MUSCULOSKELETAL OR ARTICULAR DYSFUNCTION

1.

Nursing Action	Indicated	Contrain-dicated	Non-Essential
Monitor peripheral pulses and skin temperature changes.	X		
Use compression stockings or intermittent compression devices to decrease pooling.	X		
Reposition every 8 hours.		X	
Monitor intake and output closely.	X		
Place on a hard mattress to prevent movement.		X	
Encourage cough and deep breathing.	X		
Complete a dietary assessment.			X
Monitor vital signs.	X		

2.

Options for 1	Options for 2	Options for 3	Options for 4
bone fracture	days	**keep limb at heart level**	proximal to
severed nerve	**hours**	lower the limb	adjacent to
compartment syndrome	minutes	remove the cast	aligned with
bone contusion	seconds	turn patient on his side	alongside
bone rotation	weeks	provide pressure	**distal to**

3. B, C, D, G
4.

Health Teaching	Indicated	Contraindi-cated	Non-Essential
"Opioid medications should be given to your child whenever she complains of pain."		X	
"Relaxation techniques can be effective in decreasing her pain."	X		
"Make sure your child takes the prescribed medications on time."	X		
"Keeping your child in bed when she has extremity pain will prevent swelling."		X	
"Swimming can help strengthen your child's muscles and maintain mobility."	X		
"Your child can sleep in her sister's bedroom at night if she wishes."			X

CHAPTER 30 THE CHILD WITH NEUROMUSCULAR OR MUSCULAR DYSFUNCTION

1. A, E, F, G
2. A, B, C, D, F, G
3.

Options for 1	Options for 2	Options for 3
renal cyst	infection	Foley catheter placement
kidney stone	failure	**clean intermittent catheterization**
neuropathic bladder	strictures	sterile intermittent catheterization
rectal fissure	**distress**	suprapubic aspiration

4.

Health Teaching	Indicated	Contraindicated	Non-Essential
"DMD is inherited as an X-linked recessive trait and affects boys."			X
"Your child may need to have casts on his legs to help him walk."		X	
"You will learn stretching exercises and strength and muscle training to help your child."	X		
"You should call your health care provider if any respiratory symptoms occur."	X		
"Your child should be hospitalized when ambulation becomes impossible."		X	
"It is important for your child to remain as independent as possible."	X		
"Breathing exercises will help maintain his vital lung capacity."	X		

CHAPTER 31 THE CHILD WITH INTEGUMENTARY DYSFUNCTION

1.

Options for 1	Options for 2	Options for 3
3%	bony structures	3-4 days
5.5%	muscle structures	5-7 days
10.5%	**dermal elements**	7-14 days
22%	fascia elements	**14-21 days**
6.5%	nerve structures	30 days

2.

Nursing Action	Effective	Ineffective	Unrelated
"Change the diaper as soon as it becomes wet or soiled."	X		
"Use a hair dryer or heat lamp to dry the area."		X	
"Use a superabsorbent disposable diaper if you can."	X		
"Keep the skin dry."	X		
"Wash the area as often as possible using a wipe."		X	
"Diapers that are unscented can be purchased."			X
"Apply ointment such as zinc oxide or petrolatum to the skin."	X		
"Avoid removing the skin barrier cream with each diaper change."	X		

3. A, C, E, F
4. A, B, C, D, H, I, J

Next-Generation NCLEX® Examination-Style Unfolding Case Study Answer Key

CHAPTER 17 FAMILY-CENTERED CARE OF THE CHILD WITH SPECIAL NEEDS

Unfolding Case Study: Care at the End of Life

1. C, E, F, G, H, I
2.

Option 1	Option 2
1.0-2.0 mg/kg	**4 hours**
0.1-0.2 mg/kg	15 min
0.5-1.0 mg/kg	2 hours
0.1-1.0 mg/kg	6 hours
1.0-2.0 mg/kg	10 min

3. A, B, C, E, G
4.

Nursing Action	Potential Complication	Nursing Action for Complication
1. Administer morphine safely. Observe the patient for excessive sedation and respiratory depression.	To reduce unfounded fears.	3
2. Monitor for side effects of morphine: decreased respiratory rate, urinary retention, constipation, and pruritus.	To prevent unwanted side effects that may cause additional discomfort.	2
3. Educate parents on the safety and effectiveness of the pain-relieving medications.	To ensure optimal pain relief.	4
4. Reassess the pain level after administering pain medication. Assess within 1 hour of oral morphine and 30 minutes after intravenous (IV) administration.	To prevent adverse effects and overdose.	1
5. Recognize when pain is not well controlled on morphine.	To ensure satisfactory pain relief.	5
6. Provide appropriate bowel regimen and monitor urine output.		
7. Provide distraction and counseling to assure parents that everything possible is being done.		

5.

Nursing Action	Effective	Ineffective	Unrelated
Assure parents that the intravenous (IV) morphine dose can be the same dose they administer at home.		X	
Instruct parents to continue around-the-clock medications at home.	X		
Encourage parents to communicate any signs of pain; observe patient for nonverbal signs of pain.	X		
A home bowel regimen should be included in the discharge teaching.	X		
Instruct parents to talk to other family members about their feelings toward pain management.			X
Stress with the parents that escalating doses will not be needed and that tolerance to pain medications never occurs in children.		X	
Discuss appropriate nonpharmacologic options that can relieve pain.	X		

6. B, C, E, G

CHAPTER 21 THE CHILD WITH RESPIRATORY DYSFUNCTION

Unfolding Case Study: The Child With Acute Respiratory Tract Illness

1. A, B, C, D, E, F, G, H, J, K
2.

Options for 1	Options for 2	Options for 3
pneumonia	**Persistent dry, hacking cough worse at night, more productive in 2-3 days**	Inhaled corticosteroids, antibiotics
bronchiolitis	Retractions, labored respirations	Allergen and "triggers control"
emphysema	Poor feeding, inability to sleep, gastrointestinal symptoms	**Supplemental oxygen, fluid intake, suctioning as needed**
wheezing	Seizures, altered consciousness, inability to focus	Long-term antiinflammatory medications

3.

Options for 1	Options for 2	Options for 3
upper	skin	1-2
middle	**epithelial**	2-3
lower	blood	**5-8**
extreme	muscle	10-14
left	nasal	14-18
right	bone	21-24

4.

Nursing Action	Potential Complication	Nursing Action for Complication
1. Position infant for maximum ventilation and airway patency.	Inability to identify alterations in temperature, respiratory status, or circulation and need for additional interventions is missed	**2**
2. Monitor vital signs, including temperature and respiratory, cardiac, and oxygen status.	Nasal mucosal membrane drying	**3**
3. Provide humidified oxygen as indicated.	Fever	**6**
4. Suction airway (nares, mouth, nasopharynx) as indicated.	Bronchial constriction and decreased ventilation	**7**
5. Provide gentle chest percussion and chest physical therapy (CPT) as indicated.	Secretions causing lack of airway patency	**4**
6. Administer antipyretics as indicated.	Infection	**8**
7. Administer bronchodilators as indicated.	Spread of infection	**10**
8. Administer antibiotics if indicated.	Dehydration or fluid overload	**11**
9. Obtain specimens (e.g., secretions, blood) as indicated.		
10. Maintain appropriate precautions such as Standard Precautions, droplet isolation, and frequent hand washing.		
11. Monitor hydration status through strict intake and output and daily weights.		
12. Implement comfort measures such as allowing parent presence, parent holding infant, and comfort item such as favorite blanket or stuffed animal.		

5. A, C, E, F

6.

Health Teaching Evaluation	Indicated	Contrain-dicated	Non-Essential
Parents able to verbalize definition and characteristics of acute respiratory tract infection.	X		
Parents able to verbalize treatment, including medication and interventions that promote ventilation and airway clearance.	X		
Parents can identify discharge medications, including antipyretics, bronchodilators, and antibiotics as prescribed.	X		
Parents want to purchase a pulse oximeter before taking the infant home so they can constantly monitor the oxygen level.		X	
Parents feel that keeping the infant supine will assist with any nasal secretions the infant may have.		X	
Parents want to purchase another bed for the infant to keep her close to them at night.			X

Unfolding Case Study: The Child With Acute Asthma Exacerbation

7. B, C, D, F, G, H
8. A, C, E, G, H, I
9.

Nursing Action	Emergent	Not Emergent
Administer humidified oxygen to keep the oxygen saturation (SpO_2) above 90%.	X	
Administer methylprednisolone per the physician order.	X	
Administer albuterol per hospital protocol.	X	
Place the patient in a comfortable standing, sitting upright, or learning forward position.	X	
Discuss possible allergens in the home that might have triggered the attack.		X
Review how to use the metered-dose inhaler.		X

10.

Nursing Action	Potential Complication	Nursing Action to Prevent Complication
1. Allow patient to assume position of comfort.	To minimize drying of nasal mucous membranes.	**3**
2. Administer rescue medications (as prescribed) that can include inhalers, nebulization, and/or oral or intravenous (IV) steroids.	To prevent airway obstruction.	**1**
3. Administer humidified oxygen to maintain oxygen saturation (SaO_2) above 90%.	Decreased patient's awareness of factors that exacerbate asthma.	**5**
4. Assess patient's response to rescue medications.	To prevent constricted airways and decreased air exchange.	**2**
5. Assist patient in recognizing factors that trigger asthma symptoms.	Lack of awareness of need for more aggressive interventions.	**4**
6. Assure respirations will be easy and nonlabored at a rate within normal limits for age.		
7. Teach the patient how to use the peak expiratory flow meter (PEFM).		
8. Evaluate the use of the PEFM.		

11. A, D, E, F, H
12.

Options for 1	Options for 2	Options for 3	Options for 4
flow of air	5 seconds	**80%-100%**	4-5 weeks
flow of oxygen	10 seconds	50%-70%	**2-3 weeks**
flow of water	**1 second**	60%-80%	1-2 days

CHAPTER 22 THE CHILD WITH GASTROINTESTINAL DYSFUNCTION

Unfolding Case Study: The Child With Appendicitis

1. D, E, F, H, I
2.

Options for 1	Options for 2	Options for 3
Anemia	Blood pressure of 108/74	Ruptured kidney
Pain	Pulse of 80	**Acute abdomen**
Bleeding	**C-reactive protein (CRP)**	Influenza
Infection	Hemoglobin	Urinary tract infection
Heart failure	Platelets	Vomiting
Cancer	Serum sodium	Anxiety

3. A, C, D, F, H, I
4.

Nursing Action	Potential Postoperative Complication	Nursing Action for Postoperative Complication
1. Administer pain medications.	Inflammation at the wound site	**10**
2. Initiate intravenous (IV) fluids and assess intake and output (I&O).	Electrolyte imbalance	**6**
3. Assess temperature and report elevation.	Fluid deficit	**2**
4. Administer antiemetics.	Pain	**1**
5. Administer IV sodium heparin.	Nausea and vomiting	**4**
6. Draw blood as scheduled and evaluate results.	Infection	**8**
7. Report changes in vital signs, behavior, and level of consciousness.	Fever	**3**
8. Administer IV antibiotics.		
9. Administer a blood transfusion.		
10. Observe wound site.		

5.

Nursing Action	Effective	Ineffective	Unrelated
Exhibits no signs of infection.	**X**		
Pain is controlled.	**X**		
Referral is made to a physical therapist.			**X**
No complaints of nausea or vomiting and a regular diet is tolerated.	**X**		
No complaints of headaches.			**X**
Temperature remains in the normal range.	**X**		
Child spending all of the time in bed.		**X**	

6.

Health Teaching	Indicated	Contraindicated	Non-Essential
"Take your child's temperature if she feels warm and call the surgeon if she has a fever over 101°F."	**X**		
"Give ibuprofen every 6 hours for the next 5 days."		**X**	
"Sit beside her all day and watch her favorite movies."			**X**
"Inspect the surgical incision every day for increased redness, heat, or drainage; if present, call the surgeon immediately."	**X**		
Ask the parents, "What are your concerns regarding your daughter's care at home?"	**X**		
"Apply a topical antibiotic to the surgical wound for the next week."		**X**	

CHAPTER 23 THE CHILD WITH CARDIOVASCULAR DYSFUNCTION

Unfolding Case Study: The Child With Coarctation of the Aorta

1. A, B, D, E, G, I, J
2.

Options for 1	Options for 2	Options for 3 and 4
widening	increased	**bounding = 3**
absence	**decreased**	widening
narrowing	lack of	**weak or absent = 4**
crossing	absent	narrowing
absence	complex	unstable

3.

Nursing Action	Emergent	Not Emergent
Frequently assess and record heart rate, respiratory rate, blood pressure (BP), and any signs or symptoms of decreased cardiac output.	X	
Administer cardiac drugs on schedule. Assess and record any side effects or any signs and symptoms of toxicity. Follow hospital protocol for administration.	X	
Administer cool humidified oxygen to increase available oxygen during inspiration.	X	
Change the infant's position every 2 hours to prevent skin breakdown.		X
Keep accurate record of intake and output.	X	
Weigh infant on same scale at same time of day.		X
Maintain a 3-hour feeding schedule.		X
Restrict fluids if the intake and output is unbalanced.		X

4.

Nursing Action	Potential Complication	Nursing Action to Prevent Complication
1. Assess and record heart rate, respiratory rate, blood pressure (BP), and any signs or symptoms of altered cardiac output every 2 to 4 hours.	Decreased urinary output is a symptom of heart failure and could go unnoticed.	3
2. Administer cardiac drugs on schedule. Assess and record any side effects or any signs and symptoms of toxicity. Follow hospital protocol for administration.	Undetected changes in vital signs and infant's physical status that reflect altered cardiac output and high BP.	1
3. Keep accurate record of intake and output.	Excess water and salt because fluid retention commonly occurs with heart failure.	5
4. Weigh infant on same scale at same time of day as previously. Document results and compare to previous weight.	Dangers inherent in failure to administer cardiac drugs as prescribed and to perform careful assessment before administration.	2
5. Administer diuretics on schedule. Assess and record effectiveness and any side effects noted.		
6. Offer small, frequent feedings to infant's tolerance.		
7. Organize nursing care to allow infant uninterrupted rest.		

5. A, B, C, D, E, H, I

6.

Health Teaching	Indicated	Contraindicated	Non-Essential
Discuss the characteristics of coarctation of the aorta (COA) and the surgery done to repair the obstructive defect.	X		
Review the infant's daily care, including medication administration.	X		
Review signs and symptoms that could be of concern (fever, blue skin color, poor eating).	X		
Inform parents to purchase a pulse oximeter before taking the infant home so they can constantly monitor the oxygen level.		X	
Keep the infant supine at all times to assist with blood flow.		X	
Parents want to purchase another bed for the infant to keep her close to them at night.			X
Give parents the opportunity to express their fears and concerns.	X		

CHAPTER 24 THE CHILD WITH HEMATOLOGIC OR IMMUNOLOGIC DYSFUNCTION

Unfolding Case Study: The Child With Sickle Cell Anemia

1. C, E, F, G, J

2.

Options for 1	Options for 2
Aplastic crisis	High blood pressure
Sequestration crisis	**Ischemia**
Acute chest syndrome	Bleeding
Vasoocclusive crisis	Infection
Hyperhemolytic crisis	Diminished red blood cell production
Cerebral vascular accident	Decreased serum sodium

3. A, D, E

4.

Nursing Action	Potential Complication	Nursing Action for Complication
1. Discuss schedule of medication around the clock with parents.	Uncontrolled pain	**1**
2. Encourage high level of fluid intake.	Breakthrough pain	**3**
3. Recognize that various analgesics, including opioids, and medication schedules may need to be tried.	To avoid needless suffering because of unfounded fears	**4**
4. Reassure child and family that analgesics, including opioids, are medically indicated; that high doses may be needed; and that children rarely become addicted.	To prevent vasoconstriction that may enhance sickling with cold applications	**5**
5. Apply heat application or massage to affected area. Avoid applying cold compresses.	Dehydration	**2**
6. Provide protein shake with each meal.		
7. Weigh the child each morning with the same scale.		

5.

Options for 1	Options for 2	Options for 3	Options for 4
6	**0.4**	2.2	5 min
4	0.2	1.8	6 min
8	0.8	**1.4**	8 min
2	0.9	1.2	**10 min**

6.

Nursing Action	Effective	Ineffective	Unrelated
Administer morphine and ketorolac safely.	X		
Monitor for side effects of morphine; assess respiratory status closely and prevent constipation.	X		
Monitor for side effects of ketorolac; assess for bleeding (gastrointestinal [GI] or renal) closely.	X		
Educate parents on the safety and effectiveness of intravenous (IV) morphine and ketorolac when using them at home.		X	
Reassess the child's pain level once a shift after administering morphine and ketorolac.		X	
Read a children's book to the child while he is asleep.			X
Recognize that various analgesics and doses may need to be tried.	X		

CHAPTER 25 THE CHILD WITH CANCER

Unfolding Case Study: The Child With Acute Lymphoblastic Leukemia

1. A, C, D, E, H, I, J
2.

Option 1	Option 2	Option 3
Seizure	**Decreased production of red blood cells (RBCs)**	Lack of appetite and weight loss
Blindness	Increased production of plasma cells	Headache and seizure
Hemorrhage	Decreased production of central nervous system (CNS) fluid	Enlarged spleen
Hearing loss	Increased production of bilirubin	**Fever and infection**

3.

Options for 1	Options for 2	Options for 3
cardiac	**rapid**	production
cellular	slow	growth
metabolic	intermittent	**lysis**
neurologic	prolonged	mitosis

4.

Nursing Action	Effective	Ineffective	Unrelated
Explain the procedure to the patient and family and obtain informed consent.	X		
Monitor vital signs during the procedure (pulse rate, oxygen saturation, respirations, blood pressure).	X		
Administer a bolus of intravenous (IV) fluids before the procedure begins.		X	
Administer sedation during the procedure to provide optimal comfort and minimize pain.	X		
Provide comfort and reassure the patient and family throughout the procedure.	X		
Allow the child to watch a favorite show before the procedure.			X
Watch for signs of bleeding from the puncture site.	X		

5. B, C, D, E, F, H

6.

Nursing Action	Potential Complication	Nursing Action to Prevent Complication
1. Explain the disease course of treatment and adverse effects to the family.	Skin as an entry point for infection	**4**
2. Teach the patient and family ways to prevent infection through hand washing, bathing frequently, and not using cups and utensils used by another person.	Lack of recognition of infection	**3**
3. Teach the family how to recognize symptoms of infection such as fever, chills, cough, and sore throat and report these to the health care worker immediately.	Lack of understanding of leukemia treatment	**1**
4. Provide skin care to patient by keeping the skin and perianal area clean and apply mild lotion.	Mouth ulceration	**8**
5. Provide a high-protein and high-calorie diet.	Lack of knowledge on how to prevent infection in the home	**2**
6. Provide adequate hydration and encourage a high-fiber diet and stool softeners.	Bleeding	**7**
7. Educate family and patient on how to recognize and report abnormal bleeding through bruising and petechiae.		
8. Provide frequent mouth care and saline rinses and check for ulcers in the mouth and gum swelling.		
9. Instruct patient and family to avoid contact sports.		

CHAPTER 26 THE CHILD WITH GENITOURINARY DYSFUNCTION

Unfolding Case Study: The Child With Chronic Kidney Disease

1. A, B, C, D, E, G, I, M
2.

Nursing Action	Potential Complication	Nursing Action to Prevent Complication
1. Close monitoring of the patient's status. Follow clinical and laboratory findings. Blood studies include complete blood count (CBC), electrolytes, and kidney status.	Waste products accumulate	**2**
2. Observe for evidence of accumulated waste products.	Increased excretory kidney demands	**3**
3. Provide dietary instructions for foods that reduce excretory demands on kidneys and provide sufficient calories and protein for growth.	Changes in kidney status go unrecognized	**1**
4. Limit phosphorus, salt, and potassium as prescribed.	Growth failure unrecognized	**5**
5. Monitor growth closely since short stature is a significant side effect.	Accumulation of minerals	**4**
6. Monitor cardiovascular status, including blood pressure measurement.	Renal bone disease	**7**
7. Minimize renal bone disease by maintaining optimal calcium, phosphorus, and intact parathyroid hormone levels, and acid-base balance.		
8. Monitor for anemia. Child may require school accommodations and rest periods due to fatigue.		
9. Identify patient and family stressors that may accompany a diagnosis of chronic kidney disease (CKD).		

3. A, B, C, F, G, H
4. A, B, G, I, J, K
5. A, D, G
6. B, C, D, E, F

CHAPTER 27 THE CHILD WITH CEREBRAL DYSFUNCTION

Unfolding Case Study: The Child With Seizures

1. A, B, C, D, E, G, H
2.

Nursing Action	Potential Complication	Nursing Action to Prevent Complication
1. Monitor time (onset and duration), movements, and level of consciousness (LOC) during seizure.	Child experiences anxiety and fear.	**4**
2. If child is at risk of falling, ease child to floor. Prevent child from hitting head on objects. Do not attempt to restrain child or use force.	An accurate description of the seizure is not obtained.	**1**
3. During seizure, place child in a side-lying position on a flat surface such as floor. Do not put anything in child's mouth.	Parents unable to cope with the diagnosis and management of their son.	**5**
4. Stay with the child and reassure the child when awakening from seizure.	Physical harm occurs.	**2**
5. Involve child and parents in discussion of fears, anxieties, and resources and support options available to patient and family.	Aspiration can occur.	**3**
	Lack of description of the postictal state.	
	Further seizures occur.	

3. A, B, C, D, E
4.

Options for 1	Options for 2	Options for 3
simple partial seizure	blood pressure	intrathecal
complex partial seizure	seizure activity	intravenous
status epilepticus	**circulation, airway, and breathing (CAB)**	rectal
absence seizure	blood levels	**buccal**

5.

Nursing Action	Effective	Ineffective	Unrelated
Monitor circulation, airway, and breathing closely.	**X**		
Ensure antiepileptic drugs are being administered as directed.	**X**		
Monitor and record characteristics, onset, and duration of any new seizures, including motor effects, alterations in consciousness, and postictal state.	**X**		
Attempt to stop the seizure if one occurs again; keep the child upright.		**X**	
Do not place anything in child's mouth during the seizure.	**X**		
Place child in a side-lying position; suction the oral cavity and posterior oropharynx as needed.	**X**		
Closely monitor hemoglobin and platelet count.			**X**
Observe for hyperthermia, hypertension, and respiratory depression.	**X**		

6. B, D, E, F, G, H, I, J

CHAPTER 28 THE CHILD WITH ENDOCRINE DYSFUNCTION

Unfolding Case Study: The Child With Diabetes Mellitus

1. A, B, C, D, E
2.

Options for 1	Options for 2	Options for 3
Diabetes mellitus	platelets	insulin
Addison disease	hematocrit	**glucose**
Cushing syndrome	**blood glucose**	potassium
Hyperparathyroidism	**A1c level**	calcium
Pituitary hyperfunction	white blood cells	sodium

3. A, D, E, F

4.

Nursing Action	Potential Complication	Nursing Action for Complication
1. Obtain blood glucose level before meals and at bedtime.	Normal blood glucose level is not maintained.	**2**
2. Administer insulin as prescribed.	Appropriate dose of insulin is not administered.	**1**
3. Monitor urine glucose before each meal.	Appropriate type of insulin is not administered.	**6**
4. Use aseptic techniques when preparing and administering insulin.	Infection occurs.	**4**
5. Store insulin in the freezer to preserve the medication.	Absorption of insulin is impaired.	**7**
6. Understand the action of insulin: differences in composition, time of onset, and duration of action for the various preparations.		
7. Rotate insulin injection sites.		
8. Give less insulin before physical activity.		

5.

Nursing Action	Effective	Ineffective	Unrelated
Immediately administer cup of fruit juice or glass of nonfat or 1% milk.	**X**		
Check blood glucose after 15 minutes.	**X**		
Give a starch-protein snack.	**X**		
Start intravenous fluids with glucose.		**X**	
Provide information for the teacher on the child's diagnosis.			**X**
Give parents instructions on signs and symptoms of hypoglycemia versus hyperglycemia.	**X**		
Teach parents how to administer intramuscular glucagon if unresponsive, unconscious, or seizing.	**X**		
Place the child on a portable insulin infusion pump.		**X**	

6. B, C, E, F

INDEX

Note: Page numbers followed by "f" refer to illustrations; page numbers followed by "t" refer to tables; page numbers followed by "b" refer to boxes.

B

D

E

F